Hagan and Bruner's Microbiology and Infectious Diseases of Domestic Animals

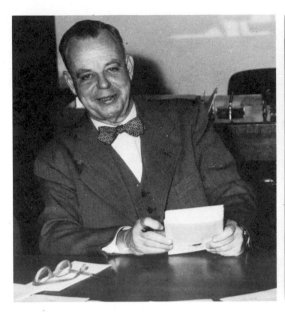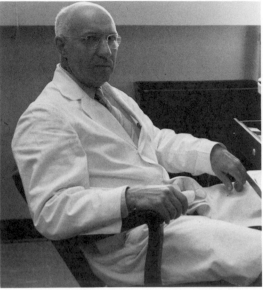

(*Left*) William A. Hagan (1893–1963), M.S., D.V.M., Honorary Doctor of Veterinary Science (Kansas State University, 1938), and Honorary Doctor of Letters (University of Toronto, 1962), was Professor of Veterinary Bacteriology and Dean of the College and Chairman, Department of Pathology and Bacteriology, New York State College of Veterinary Medicine at Cornell University. An excellent teacher, he taught courses in pathogenic microbiology and in infectious diseases of domestic animals to veterinary students for many years. This textbook was an outgrowth of his courses, and he served as senior author of the first four editions. He was also an eminent bacteriologist, whose research contributed fundamental knowledge about tuberculosis of animals and humans, Johne's disease of cattle, and other mycobacterial diseases of animals.

Dr. Hagan excelled as a teacher, scholar, scientist, administrator, and academician. He received many awards and honors for his distinguished contributions to the veterinary profession and society, including in 1960 the International Veterinary Congress Award of the American Veterinary Medical Association.

(*Right*) Dorsey W. Bruner (1906–   ), B.S., D.V.M., Ph.D., is Emeritus Professor of Veterinary Micro-biology and former Chairman, Department of Veterinary Microbiology, New York State College of Veterinary Medicine at Cornell University. A student of Dr. Hagan, he joined him as a colleague in 1949 after conducting research at the University of Kentucky and serving in the United States Army during World War II. At Cornell Dr. Bruner assumed responsibility for the course in pathogenic microbiology. He was co-author of the second, third, and fourth editions of this textbook and became senior author of the next two editions. He was also editor of and reviewer for the *Cornell Veterinarian* for twenty years.

A world-renowned expert on the enteric bacteria of animals and humans, particularly the salmonellae, Dr. Bruner has been awarded many honors, including the prestigious International Veterinary Congress Award in 1972. He will long be known as an outstanding teacher, research scientist, editor, scholar, administrator, and humanitarian.

Hagan and Bruner's Microbiology and Infectious Diseases of Domestic Animals

WITH REFERENCE TO ETIOLOGY, EPIZOOTIOLOGY, PATHOGENESIS, IMMUNITY, DIAGNOSIS, AND ANTIMICROBIAL SUSCEPTIBILITY

John F. Timoney, B.S., M.V.B., M.S., PH.D., D.SC.

Professor of Veterinary Bacteriology
New York State College of Veterinary Medicine
Cornell University

James H. Gillespie, V.M.D.

Professor Emeritus of Veterinary Microbiology
New York State College of Veterinary Medicine
Cornell University

Fredric W. Scott, D.V.M., PH.D.

Professor of Virology
New York State College of Veterinary Medicine
Cornell University

Jeffrey E. Barlough, D.V.M., PH.D.

Lecturer in Veterinary Microbiology
New York State College of Veterinary Medicine
Cornell University

EIGHTH EDITION

Comstock Publishing Associates

A division of Cornell University Press
Ithaca and London

Library of Congress Cataloging-in-Publication Data

Hagan, William Arthur, 1893–1963.
  Hagan and Bruner's microbiology and infectious
diseases of domestic animals.

    Rev. ed. of: Hagan and Bruner's infectious diseases
of domestic animals. 7th ed. 1981.
    Includes bibliographies and index.
    1. Communicable diseases in animals.   I. Bruner,
Dorsey William, 1906–   .   II. Timoney, John Francis.
III. Hagan,William Arthur, 1893–1963.   Infectious
diseases of domestic animals.   IV. Title.   V. Title:
Microbiology and infectious diseases of domestic
animals.   [DNLM: 1. Animals, Domestic.   2. Communicable
Diseases—veterinary.   3. Microbiology.   SF 781 H141i]
SF781.H3   1988   636.089′69   87-47848
ISBN 0-8014-1896-8 (alk. paper)

**For Bea C. Bruner, Virginia A. Gillespie,
Lois Scott, and M. Enid Timoney**

First edition, 1943, titled THE INFECTIOUS DISEASES OF DOMESTIC ANIMALS, by W. A. Hagan. Second edition, 1951, by W. A. Hagan and D. W. Bruner. Third edition, 1957. Fourth edition, 1961.

Fifth edition, 1966, titled HAGAN'S INFECTIOUS DISEASES OF DOMESTIC ANIMALS, by D. W. Bruner and J. H. Gillespie. Sixth edition, 1973.

Seventh edition, 1981, titled HAGAN AND BRUNER'S INFECTIOUS DISEASES OF DOMESTIC ANIMALS, by J. H. Gillespie and J. F. Timoney.

Eighth edition, 1988, published by Cornell University Press.

Printed in the United States of America

The paper in this book is acid-free and meets the guidelines for permanence and durability of the Committee on Production Guidelines for Book Longevity of the Council on Library Resources.

Contents

Part I   The Pathogenic Bacteria

Part III   The Virales

Preface to the Eighth Edition

Our primary goal in preparing this revision remains the same as that for previous editions: to produce an up-to-date resource for veterinary students enrolled in courses in infectious diseases, bacteriology, mycology, virology, pathogenic microbiology, clinical microbiology, and preventive medicine. The detailed treatment of topics and the extensive reference lists should also make the book uniquely valuable to clinicians, research scientists, laboratory diagnosticians, public health officials, and all who seek information on the microbiology and infectious diseases of domestic animals.

The 1980s have signaled what promises to be the most exciting and productive era in the history of infectious disease microbiology since the late 1800s, when Louis Pasteur, Robert Koch, and the other great microbiologists of the time conducted their pioneering research. Powerful new techniques have at last provided the means to define microbial virulence in molecular terms, resulting in an understanding of infectious diseases never before possible. As we prepared this edition, we were excited and inspired by the reports of the first applications of these new methodologies to the study of infectious diseases in animals. Clearly, individuals trained in the biology of both host and pathogen have almost boundless opportunities for fruitful application of these approaches, and we sincerely hope that some of the students who read this text will choose careers in which they can share in the opportunities of this unique time.

Almost all the chapters on the pathogenic bacteria have been completely reorganized and updated to reflect current thinking on taxonomy; for example, three species long thought to belong to the genus *Corynebacterium* are described in this edition under the new names *Rhodococcus equi, Actinomyces pyogenes,* and *Eubacterium suis.* For taxa whose revision has not yet been firmly established, the species are discussed under their familiar designations, with a statement that reclassification is imminent. Many of the virology chapters have also been extensively rewritten and reorganized to conform with the latest taxonomic thinking. Throughout, recently recognized infectious agents are described and many new illustrations appear. These additions have inevitably increased the length of the book, a consequence that we hope will not be too discouraging for the already burdened student.

Work on this edition was begun in 1985, and its completion nearly three years later has required the competent and generous efforts of many fine people. Joanne Lee, Mina Lee, Mary Neilans, Kim Newberry, Jennifer Schroeder, Raymond Scott, and Cynthia Wojcicki all helped with literature searches. Kathryn Freese, Doris June, Gwendolyn Frost, and Daisy Wallace were responsible for reducing many thousands of pages of rough manuscript to more than 3,000 pages of typed, legible text.

Colleagues at Cornell University and elsewhere reviewed most of the chapters and made valuable and much-appreciated suggestions for improvement. Dr. George Baer critiqued the chapter on the Rhabdoviridae, Dr. Howard Bachrach assisted James Gillespie in writing the section on foot-and-mouth disease, and Dr. Natasha Neef proofread many of the bacteriology and mycology chapters. We thank the many colleagues who generously provided photographs that have greatly improved the value and readability of the book, and we also gratefully acknowledge the assistance provided to John Timoney by Dr. Dwight Hirsh of the University of California, Davis, and to James Gillespie by Dr. Emerson Colby of Dartmouth Medical School during the sabbatic leaves spent writing portions of this edition.

Editing and final preparation of the text were ably guided by Helene Maddux of Cornell University Press, who tactfully and effectively prodded dilatory authors, who spotted a myriad of tiny (and not so tiny) blemishes in style, organization, and references, and who has, we believe, given the eighth edition a standard of editorial excellence never before achieved.

After contributing to four editions of this book, James Gillespie has decided that this edition will be his last. For the past thirty-nine years, he and Dorsey Bruner have provided the thrust for the continuation of the book. The addition of Fredric Scott and Jeffrey Barlough as authors of several of the virology chapters (Chapters 41–45, 48, 52–54, 57, and 58) will, we hope, ensure that the burden ably carried by Dr. Gillespie for so long will be in safe hands for the future; however, the exponential growth of information on infectious diseases, and the effort, expertise, and time required to survey and distill the scientific literature, will inevitably lead to the addition of more authors for future editions.

Finally, we acknowledge those individuals whose support or inspiration has significantly influenced our lives and careers. Dr. John F. Timoney, Sr., was the example that guided the senior author toward a career in infectious diseases of animals. Without the encouragement and sacrifice of his parents, sister, and brother, James Gillespie would never have had the opportunity to obtain his professional degree during the Great Depression. Clifton and Mildred Scott provided the critical encouragement that enabled their son to enter the veterinary profession and eventually to specialize in viral diseases of animals. We humbly pay tribute to these wonderful people.

JOHN F. TIMONEY
JAMES H. GILLESPIE
FREDRIC W. SCOTT
JEFFREY E. BARLOUGH

Ithaca, New York

Preface to the First Edition

This book is an outgrowth of a lecture course on pathogenic bacteriology and immunology which the author has given during the last twenty years to students of veterinary medicine. The work is less than a textbook of bacteriology in that a knowledge of the general principles of the subject is taken for granted and this part of the usual text is omitted. It is somewhat more, on the other hand, in that the fungi, protozoa, and viruses that are pathogenic for the domestic animals are included in addition to the bacteria. Also, somewhat greater consideration is given to the nature of the diseases produced by the various agents and to the biological products which are available for their diagnosis, prevention, and cure than is found in most texts of this type.

Since students of animal diseases are interested in microorganisms more because of what they do than for what they are, the work is not a systematic discussion of disease-producing organisms but rather a discussion of the infectious diseases of animals with special reference to their etiological factors.

With regard to the difficult matter of nomenclature of bacteria, *Bergey's Manual* has been followed in general except in the case of the Gram-negative enteric organisms, for which the old name *Bacterium* is retained. This is done because it is felt that the numerous divisions which have been made in this group on the basis of cultural features are highly artificial. The newer methods of antigenic analysis do not support these divisions but rather suggest that we have a large group in which there are minor gradations from the colon bacillus at one end to the dysentery organisms at the other without sharp divisions

anywhere. Until lines can be drawn more sharply it is felt that there is no justification for the creation of numerous genera within this group.

In instances in which the animal pathogens are transmissible to man, this fact is pointed out and brief discussions of the nature of the human diseases are given, together with what is known of the manner in which the transmission to man occurs. It is felt that veterinarians should be informed on these matters both for their own protection and for the assistance which they often can give to physicians in such cases.

The text will be used by the author in connection with his course in infectious diseases of animals. It is hoped that it will prove suitable for such courses in other schools. In addition it is hoped also that the compilation of brief accounts of the biological characteristics of the etiological agents of all of the more important infectious diseases of animals in a single volume will make it useful to veterinary practitioners, laboratory workers who are called upon to make diagnoses of these conditions, and research workers who utilize animals in their daily work. Because of the wide scope of the field covered and the necessary limitations in a book designed for student use, the discussions are not exhaustive. Diseases which are known to occur in North America are treated more exhaustively than those which do not occur here. Since experience shows, however, that diseases which are thought to occur only in remote parts of the world often exist here in an unrecognized form, and that it is always possible that remote diseases may be imported, an effort has been made to include brief descriptions of all of the more important of such diseases and their causative agents. A few references are given at the end of each subject so those who wish to read more exhaustively may find the more important papers in the literature. Since most students and practitioners do not have a working knowledge of foreign languages, the greater part of the references are to papers published in English. By consulting the bibliographies given in most of these papers one can obtain leads which will open the entire literature to him.

The author is indebted to many friends for various kinds of assistance. The illustrations, in particular, have been borrowed from many sources, acknowledgment being made in each case. The author is especially grateful to Dr. William H. Feldman, of the Mayo Foundation, for reading and making numerous criticisms of the copy, criticisms which undoubtedly have contributed to greater clarity and greater accuracy in the volume. To all of those who have helped he wishes to extend his hearty thanks.

In a first edition of this kind many errors undoubtedly have been included. The author will appreciate having these called to his attention in order that they may be eliminated from future editions if the reception of the work warrants future revisions. In many instances it is realized that subjects are still in the stage of controversy. An attempt has been made not to be too didactic in the treating of such matters; however, in the interest of good pedagogical practice some sort of a stand usually is taken in such matters after it has been indicated that uncertainty exists.

W. A. HAGAN

New York State Veterinary College
Cornell University, Ithaca, New York
June 1942

Part I The Pathogenic Bacteria

1 The Mechanisms and Consequences of Infection

Disease is an alteration of the state of a body or of some of its organs that interrupts or disturbs proper performance of bodily functions. Such functional disturbance is manifested by physical signs that the patient detects by his or her sensations and that usually can be detected by others. The causes of disease can be external or internal. The intrinsic causes of disease include metabolic and endocrine abnormalities, degeneration of organs from age, some neoplasms, genetic defects, and autoimmunity. The external causes of disease include living agents such as bacteria, protozoa, or viruses, or nonliving agents such as trauma, heat, cold, irradiation, chemical poisons, or deficiencies of vitamins or trace elements.

When living agents enter an animal's body and set up a disturbance of function in any part, *infection* is said to have occurred. The word *infection* is derived from the Latin word *inficere,* meaning "to put into." An *infectious disease* is one caused by the presence of a foreign living organism in or on an animal's body that creates a disturbance leading to the development of signs of illness.

Most infections are caused by living organisms that have escaped from another individual of the same species, but they sometimes come from another species. This occurs when a human develops rabies from a dog bite or when a lap dog contracts tuberculosis from its consumptive owner. The infection sometimes is obtained indirectly, as when a cow contracts leptospirosis from contaminated drinking water or when a horse in midwinter contracts anthrax from eating hay that was grown the previous summer on anthrax-infected soil.

Some infections originate from organisms that normally live a free existence in nature, as, for example, *Clostridium tetani.* Presumably, at some remote period in evolutionary history, all disease-producing organisms lived a free existence, becoming parasitic and pathogenic either through gradual adaptation or by the sudden acquisition of plasmid- or bacteriophage-encoded virulence traits.

The Fates of Infecting Organisms

Several possible fates await organisms that cause infections. The actual fate is a matter of considerable practical interest because transmission of a disease to other individuals by vertical or horizontal means implies survival and multiplication in the primary host.

1. Some organisms are destroyed by the host tissue. The host-parasite relationship is not a natural one; therefore, infections are not accomplished without resistance on the part of the host. The capacity of the host to destroy invading agents is such that most microorganisms that reach living tissues and fluids of the body are rapidly and completely destroyed. This is a continual process. In some instances resistance is unable to prevent initial growth and multiplication in the tissues, but the infection does not become extensive, and after a brief time the invading organisms are destroyed. Sometimes the agent persists, in which case the infection is called *chronic.* In a few infections, such as anthrax in herbivorous animals, the resistance of the host is overwhelmed so quickly that

the organism multiplies in all parts and the death of the host rapidly ensues. These infections are known as *acute* or *peracute* infections.

2. Some organisms usually are eliminated in the secretions or excretions of the host. Except in peracute infections when possibly no infecting organisms escape from the host, the diseased animal usually eliminates, in a manner that varies with the disease, the causative organism. In chronic infections the host usually eliminates large numbers of the infecting agent. Sometimes the agent is shed through pus, as when an abscess bursts or is lanced; sometimes it is shed through droplets that are discharged when the individual is suffering from a respiratory infection, such as canine distemper, enzootic pneumonia in swine, bovine tuberculosis, or avian coryza; sometimes it is shed in the feces, as in the case of salmonellosis or paratuberculosis; sometimes it is shed in the urine, as in leptospirosis in dogs and *Corynebacterium renale* infection in cows. Some infectious agents are shed in discharges from the reproductive tract or in milk, for example, *Brucella abortus,* and *Listeria monocytogenes.* In some diseases that become extensive and even fatal, the causative organisms can be eliminated in small numbers or not at all, as in some cases of tuberculosis. In systemic fungal infections such as histoplasmosis and blastomycosis, the tissue form of the infectious agent is shed in respiratory or other discharges but is not infectious for a new host in that form.

3. If the disease proves fatal to the host, many of the infecting organisms are destroyed with the carcass. Death of the host from infection always traps in the carcass a large number of the involved organisms. If the carcass is disposed of properly by incineration or deep burial, these organisms perish. Improper disposal of the dead bodies of animals can result in serious outbreaks of disease.

4. In some instances the organism and host reach an impasse. The organism is unable to cause serious damage to the host and yet the host is unable to eliminate the organism. This situation may continue throughout the animal's life or it may be terminated either by the final elimination of the infection or by a change in which the infection becomes more active and signs of disease are manifested by the host. In tuberculosis, the tubercle bacilli may become walled off by dense tissue in some organs; the case then is said to be *arrested.* Such cases are not entirely cured because living tubercle organisms can continue to exist in the tissues, and they sometimes break forth and cause a flare-up of the disease. In cattle, recovery from *Salmonella dublin* infection sometimes results in a situation in which the individual animal sheds organisms in its milk and feces for an indefinite period. Individuals that discharge virulent organisms with their excretions, al-

though apparently normal otherwise, are said to be *carriers.* An animal that has had a recognized disease and that has not rid itself of the infecting agent is said to be a *convalescent carrier.* Individual animals sometimes eliminate virulent infection although they have not had the disease themselves. These individuals are resistant but are a source of great danger to others who lack the same amount of resistance. They are known as immune carriers or sometimes as *asymptomatic carriers.* Sometimes an animal harbors and eliminates a dangerous organism that it has picked up from close contact with another individual. Such animals are known as *contact carriers.* Another important example of the carrier state is latent *B. abortus* infection in prepubescent heifers from infected dams. These animals harbor an infection without shedding it until they calve. A *passive carrier* is an animal that acquires an organism from its environment and passes it through its intestine.

The carrier is one of the great problems in the control of many infectious diseases. Animals that are obviously diseased are readily recognized, but the carrier animal may be difficult to recognize.

Sources of Infection

The routes by which infections reach new hosts often are indirect and complicated. Some of the more common ways in which infections are contracted by new hosts are as follows:

1. Direct or immediate contact with a diseased individual. This involves actual contact, such as when a cow licks the genitals of another animal and thereby picks up *B. abortus,* the organism of Bang's disease, or when ringworm is contracted by an animal's rubbing against the affected skin of another, or when venereal infections are transferred through sexual contact, or when an infection is transmitted by an animal's bite.

2. Contact through fomites. *Fomites* (fomes) are inanimate objects that serve to carry infections from one animal to another, such as a feed sack that conveys the dried discharge of an aborting cow to another cow, perhaps in a different herd, or a truck that has not been properly cleaned and disinfected after carrying diseased stock. Pails for drinking water or feed are frequently the means by which *Streptococcus equi* is transmitted from one horse to another. Similarly, riding tack can serve to carry arthroconidia or hyphal fragments of *Microsporum* or *Trichophyton* species between horses. Surgical instruments are also potentially significant as fomites.

3. Contact with disease carriers. Carrier animals are potentially more serious sources of infection for disease-

free populations than are diseased individuals because they cannot be recognized as easily and because they can shed infecting organisms for considerable periods. *Salmonella dublin* and *Mycoplasma hyopneumoniae* can be introduced onto disease-free premises in this way.

4. Infection from the environment. Spore-forming organisms such as *Clostridium perfringens* or *Bacillus anthracis* found in soil or pasture can enter wounds or the intestine and produce disease. *Coccidioides immitis, Microsporum gypseum,* and *Sporothrix schenckii* are examples of fungi that have their normal habitat in the soil and vegetation but that can cause disease in individuals given the appropriate circumstances.

5. Infections from food and water. Streams, rivers, and water holes are well known as means by which organisms such as salmonellas and leptospiras can be spread from one farm or herd to another. *B. anthracis* is sometimes conveyed to animals through hay and straw raised on lowlands contaminated with spores. *Listeria monocytogenes* infections are frequently associated with the consumption of contaminated silage of high pH. Similarly, offals and other feeds that carry *Clostridium botulinum* may be a source of botulinum toxin for animals such as mink or cattle.

6. Air-borne infections. Disease resulting from the spread of microorganisms over long distances in the air is highly unlikely because of dilution effects. Air-borne transmission, however, is very important in the spread of bacterial and viral respiratory diseases in animals kept close together and especially when housed indoors under intensive conditions. Kennel cough of dogs, enzootic pneumonia of swine, and bovine tuberculosis are examples of diseases transmitted by the airborne route. Dust particles can be important in the transmission of such diseases as coccidioidomycosis, histoplasmosis, and bronchopneumonia in foals caused by *Rhodococcus equi.*

7. Infections from bloodsucking arthropods. Some diseases of animals are normally transmitted through the bites of living vectors such as flies, fleas, lice, or ticks. Rickettsial disease such as anaplasmosis, eperythrozoonosis, and ehrlichiosis are examples of diseases transmitted in this manner. In some cases the infectious agent may replicate in cells of the vector. In other instances such as anthrax, horseflies carry the organism mechanically.

8. Iatrogenic infections. Medical or surgical interferences such as intramammary infusion of an antibiotic, passing of a stomach tube or urinary catheter, and debeaking or dehorning may inadvertently result in introduction of disease-producing organisms into a hitherto uninfected host.

9. Nosocomial infections. Infections acquired during an animal's hospitalization are known as nosocomial in-

fections. Salmonellosis is commonly acquired in this way. So too are *Pseudomonas, Klebsiella,* and *Staphylococcus* infections. The majority of nosocomial infections are caused by antibiotic-resistant organisms that survive in hospital environments and that often have enhanced communicability, survivability, or virulence encoded by plasmid-based genes. Important host factors in the epizootiology of nosocomial infections are diminished resistance to infection because of disease or surgery and administration of antibiotic that lowers colonization resistance of the gastrointestinal tract.

10. Endogenous infections from organisms normally present. *Pasteurella,* organisms mycoplasmas, streptococci that are ordinarily nonpathogenic, *Escherichia coli, Actinomyces bovis,* and other members of the normal flora of the nasopharynx, intestine, and skin can be invasive and can cause disease given the appropriate circumstances. Trauma, stress, viral infection, and immunosupressive therapy are examples. Endogenous infections are often termed *opportunistic* because the appropriate circumstances provide normally nonpathogenic organisms with the opportunity to cause disease.

Infection and Contagion

A contagious disease is one that can be transmitted from one individual to another by direct or indirect contact. All contagious diseases are also infectious, but infectious diseases are not necessarily contagious. Tetanus and gas gangrene infections, which are caused by organisms that live in the soil, are infectious but not contagious because they are not transmitted from one animal to another. The contagiousness of infectious diseases depends on the way the parasites are eliminated from the body of the diseased animal and the opportunity they have of reaching others. Some infectious diseases are highly contagious, some are slightly contagious, and a few are not contagious at all.

Superinfection, Mixed Infection, and Synergistic Relationships

Superinfection refers to a fresh invasion or reinfection by a pathogen in an animal that already has an existing infection. Treating respiratory disease with oral antibiotics, for example, can sometimes result in enteric disease owing to overgrowth of a resistant *Salmonella, Staphylococcus,* or *Pseudomonas* species in the intestine. Similarly, *Candida* species may overgrow and cause lesions in the oropharynx, stomach, and intestine of individual animals in which colonization resistance is diminished by antimicrobial administration.

A *mixed infection* is one in which more than one species of organism is present. This phenomenon is sometimes referred to as a *secondary infection* when it is established that the primary infection presents conditions favorable for invasion by another organism. Mixed infections are often present in the respiratory tract and in lesions of the nasopharynx, digestive tract, and feet. Shipping fever and the respiratory disease complex of cattle are good examples of mixed infections that usually involve viruses and secondary invasions by *Pasteurella* species, *Actinomyces (Cornyebacterium) pyogenes,* and *Haemophilus somnus.* Infections of the intestine and feet of the animal are usually populated by a mixture of microorganisms that reflects the local flora of the intestine and feces.

Mixed infections are usually synergistic in that lesion development depends on the cooperative interaction of two or more bacteria. Suppurative lesions of the liver fall into this category. *Fusobacterium necrophorum* and *A. pyogenes* are frequently found in combination, the latter being established in the reducing conditions of the necrosed liver tissue. Swine dysentery is caused by a synergy among *Treponema hyodysenteriae, Bacteroides* organisms, and *Campylobacter* species or intestinal spirochetes. Footrot in sheep is caused by *Bacteroides nodosus,* *F. necrophorum,* and *A. pyogenes.* Each of the participants is dependent on factors or conditions supplied by the other for its own growth.

Properties of Pathogenic Organisms

Virulence is an attribute of all pathogenic or disease-producing organisms and usually involves a set of morphologic, biochemical, and functional traits that must be present together for successful infection and disease production. The term refers to the disease-producing power or malignancy of an organism. A highly virulent organism has great malignancy, a slightly virulent one has little, and a nonvirulent one has none. The property of virulence varies greatly, both among different species of pathogenic bacteria and among different strains of the same species. Some strains of *Chlamydia,* for instance, cause disease after entry of only a few organisms into a susceptible host. In contrast, some salmonella serotypes do not produce enteric disease unless present in numbers greater than 5×10^5.

Virulence factors are specific attributes of a bacterium or fungus that are essential to its ability to cause disease. They include adhesins, toxins, antiphagocytic factors, IgA proteases, resistance to the bactericidal effect of complement, an ability to sequester iron, an ability to penetrate epithelium, and an ability to survive and multiply in phagocytes. Loss of a virulence factor usually results in loss of virulence. Mutations in characteristics not primarily involved with virulence, however, such as metabolic capabilities or cell wall synthesis, can also result in loss of virulence. Mutants of virulent organisms that have specific growth factor requirements may be unable to replicate in the body because the required growth factor is not available in tissue or blood. Mutants of this kind can be useful vaccine strains because they retain virulence antigens that can stimulate appropriate protective or neutralizing antibodies.

Many virulence characteristics are plasmid encoded or controlled. Loss of the plasmid therefore results in loss of virulence.

The virulence of some disease-producing bacteria can be readily altered in the laboratory. The process of diminishing the virulence of an organism is known as *attenuation* and is commonly used in the production of vaccines. Some of the methods used for attenuating virulent bacteria are as follows:

1. Cultivating the organism at an unfavorable temperature. Pasteur found that anthrax bacilli quickly lost virulence when incubated at 42° to 43°C, a temperature about 5 degrees above their optimum. This effect has recently been shown to be due to loss of a heat-sensitive plasmid that encodes the protective antigen.

2. Heating cultures or infective material for a short time to a temperature a little below the thermal death point of the organism.

3. Plating the organism on a suitable medium and selecting a rough, or granular, colony. Rough (R-type) colonies are usually defective in cell wall synthesis and have enhanced susceptibility to complement-mediated lysis.

4. Injecting the organism into a naturally resistant host and recovering it later. Passage of the organism by a series of transfers through a naturally resistant host can result in adaptation to that host and loss of virulence for the original host.

5. Applying a variety of mutagenesis techniques. Mutagens commonly used include ultraviolet, gamma, or x irradiation and chemical agents such as nitrosoguanidine, methane sulfonate, nitrous acid, acridine half-mustards, and base analogues (e.g., 5-bromouracil). Transposon mutagenesis is also a very powerful and commonly used genetic tool for obtaining avirulent mutants of a virulent organism.

Many diseases become less destructive with time, a phenomenon related to changes in both host and parasite. The development of herd immunity and the selection of genetically more resistant hosts are important factors, as are changes in the parasite that result in its better adaptation to its host.

In 1913 Theobald Smith suggested that infectious diseases could be expected to evolve into more chronic, less virulent forms with time, even if host resistance did not change. He reasoned that in acute disease the parasite quickly destroys its host and thus ends its own chances of escaping to new hosts, whereas in chronic disease the opportunity for escape is much better because of the prolonged course of the disease. Under such conditions, Smith concluded, the chronic form had a better chance of propagating itself and would, in time, become the predominant form.

Under conditions of intensive animal raising, however, pathogens can rapidly acquire enhanced virulence when the opportunity exists for dissemination of infection among large numbers of highly susceptible hosts. Moreover, the selective effect of feed-additive and parenterally administered antibiotics under conditions of intensive animal raising for the transfer of R factors and plasmid-encoded virulence genes is a very powerful force in the maintenance of virulence and the emergence of new combinations of virulence traits in enteric pathogens. Thus *E. coli* with genes for enterotoxins, antibiotic resistance, and hemolysin and adhesin production can rapidly become predominant in weanling swine raised intensively and exposed to antibiotic selection pressure.

Organ Colonization

Depending on the organ system or body location involved, pathogenic bacteria and fungi have a great variety of properties that allow them to colonize mucosal surfaces, penetrate epithelium, and evade destruction by the host defenses. Colonization often requires firm attachment of the microorganism to receptors on host cells by means of specific adhesin molecules present on its surface. Examples of these phenomena include adherence of K88 and K99 positive *E. coli* to mucosal cells of the small intestine of swine, attachment of *Bordetella bronchiseptica* to cilia of the trachea and larger bronchi of dogs, attachment of *Mycoplasma gallisepticum* to bronchial epithelium of chickens, adherence of *Streptococcus equi* to pharyngeal epithelium of horses, and of *Staphylococcus aureus* to epithelial cells of the mammary ducts of cows. Attached organisms resist being swept away by the natural cleansing forces of peristalsis, ciliary action, and fluid flow, and the like, and can therefore quickly attain large populations at specific target sites where other virulence factors such as toxins and enzymes can be released. Colonization may also be necessary for subsequent entry of the organism through the epithelium because it is the basis for production of microbial numbers great enough to overwhelm natural defenses at that site.

A characteristic feature of colonizing factors is their specificity—only specific organ sites in a specific host or genetic strain of a host have the appropriate surface receptors to mediate adhesion. This phenomenon is an important component of host adaptation or host specificity. Colonization can also involve the ability to penetrate and move in the mucus layer that coats the intestine. This is probably a very important virulence attribute of *Campylobacter jejuni* (Lee et al. 1986) and possibly of *Treponema hyodysenteriae*.

Epithelial Invasion

The molecular basis of epithelial penetration by virulent bacteria is still poorly understood. Outer membrane proteins that are often plasmid encoded are believed to be important in invasion of intestinal epithelium by *Salmonella typhimurium*, *S. dublin*, and *Yersinia enterocolitica*. These proteins likely bind to receptors on the host cell surface and then induce endocytosis of the bacterium.

Rickettsias also enter host cells by attaching to them, thereby inducing phagocytosis. After entry, the organism escapes from the phagolysosome by releasing a phospholipase A. It then multiplies and lives either in the cytoplasm of the host cell or in invaginations of the erythrocyte membrane.

Survival and Multiplication in Tissue and Blood

Bacteria and fungi utilize an impressive array of morphologic and functional components to evade or disarm host defenses (Joiner et al. 1984, Ogata 1983). Examples of these are listed on Table 1.1 and include mechanisms that affect phagocytosis, intracellular killing, serum bactericidal reaction, and the ability to scavenge iron. Some bacteria also have inhibitory or depressive effects on cell mediated and other immune functions in the animal. *Ehrlichia* species are believed to increase host susceptibility to opportunistic bacterial infections because of leukocyte function impaired by the presence of intracellular *Ehrlichia*. Secondary infections are therefore important contributors to mortality in cases of canine and equine ehrlichosis. The capsular galactan of *Mycoplasma mycoides* subsp. *mycoides* has potent immunosuppressive effects that results in depressed phagocytosis and persisting bacteremia. Similarly, the capsular polysaccharide of

Table 1.1. Morphologic and functional bacterial components involved in evasion and circumvention of host defenses

Component	Organism	Effect
Capsule	*Bacillus anthracis, Klebsiella pneumoniae, Streptococcus equi, Pseudomonas aeruginosa*	Antiphagocytic
M protein	*S. equi*	Antiphagocytic
Adenylate cyclase toxin	*Bordetella pertussis*	Inhibition of chemotaxis, phagocytosis, and immune effector cell function
Cytotoxin	*Pasteurella hemolytica*	Damage to alveolar macrophages and to polymorphonuclear leukocytes
Leucocidin	*Staphylococcus aureus*	Damage to leukocytes
O polysaccharide structure	*Salmonella* spp.	Diminished activation of complement
Serum (complement) resistance	*Escherichia coli*	Diminished complement mediated killing
Iron capture	*E. coli*	Enhanced growth rate
Cell wall sulfolipids	*Mycobacterium* spp.	Inhibition of phagolysosomal fusion
Phospholipase	*Rickettsia* spp.	Lysis of phagolysosomal membrane
IgA protease	*Haemophilis* spp. *Neisseria* spp.	Proteolysis of IgA

Cryptococcus neoformans inhibits leukocyte migration and depresses antibody synthesis (Murphy and Cozad 1972). The immunological paralysis produced is not specific to cryptococcal antigen and involves responsiveness to both T and B cell antigens.

Resistance to intracellular killing is characteristic of the facultative intracellular pathogens such as the brucellas, *Erysipelothrix rhusiopathiae,* salmonellas, *Listeria monocytogenes,* mycobacteria, and *Francisella tularensis.* In general, this phenomenon has its basis in resistance of the organism to oxygen-dependent killing systems in the phagocyte or to the antimicrobial effects of cationic proteins and to lysozyme and lactoferrin. Some organisms such as mycobacteria and rickettsias have cell wall constituents that inhibit fusion of phagosomal-lysosomal membranes and thus are able to escape the lethal consequences of exposure to lysosomal enzymes.

Injury to Tissue

The ability of bacteria and more especially of fungi to invade living tissue varies greatly. Some organisms that produce malignant diseases have little invasive ability and do most of their damage while growing in restricted parts of the body, where they produce potent toxins that then circulate throughout the body. *Clostridium tetani,* for example, is usually found in a small puncture wound in a superficial location, from where its potent neurotoxin tetanospasmin is carried in the blood or by neuronal retrograde transport to the nervous system; there it blocks the inhibitory nerve networks of the spinal cord and brain. Similarly, the phospholipases and neurotoxins of *Clostridium perfringens* type D, although produced in the intestine, can be carried in the blood to target sites remote from the site of production.

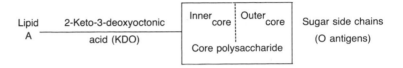

Figure 1.1. Schematic structure of bacterial lipo-polysaccharide. Endotoxin activity is associated with the lipid A component.

Other organisms produce severe tissue damage at or near the site of entry. Examples of such infections include clostridial myositis resulting from accidental entry of *Clostridium* organisms into wounds or injection sites; *Staphylococcus aureus* abscessation of the mammary gland or skin; otitis externa caused by *Pseudomonas aeruginosa;* pyelonephritis caused by *Corynebacterium renale;* foot-rot of cattle and sheep caused by *Fusobacterium necrophorum, Bacteroides nodosus,* and *Actinomyces pyogenes;* pinkeye of cattle caused by *Moraxella bovis;* and dermatitis caused by *Dermatophilus congolensis.* In each of these examples, toxins, enzymes, and other microbial constituents are important in local lesion development and tissue injury.

More invasive bacteria with properties that confer resistance to complement and phagocytes typically survive well in the bloodstream and lymphatics and are carried therein throughout the body. Their presence in the blood constitutes the condition known as *bacteremia* and is evidence that the bacterial clearance mechanisms of the blood and reticuloendothelial system have been circumvented or overloaded. A more extreme and life-threatening form of bacteremia is the condition known as *septicemia,* in which large numbers of organisms and their toxins and other constituents are present in the blood and tissues and cause degenerative effects on tissues and physiological processes. Examples of bacterial bacteremias or septicemias include anthrax, systemic salmonellosis, pasteurellosis, listeriosis, canine brucellosis, leptospirosis, and erysipelas. Newborn animals deprived of colostrum almost always succumb to septicemia caused by opportunistic bacteria that normally would be controlled by antibody and serum complement.

Pathogenic bacteria that have become established in tissue can elaborate and release toxins and enzymes that damage contiguous tissue. Examples include the collagenases, proteases, and phospholipases of *Clostridium perfringens, C. septicum, C. chauvoei,* and *C. novyi,* which damage cell membranes and other body components that contain complexes of lecithin and other phospholipids; streptococcal and staphylococcal hemolysins; and staphylococcal coagulase, *Pasteurella multocida* dermonecrotoxin, *A. pyogenes* protease and hemolysin, and the edema factor of *Bacillus anthracis.*

Much of the local and systemic damage associated with bacterial infection, however, can be attributed to interactions of bacterial components with host target cells and plasma components. The two most important of these are cell wall lipopolysaccharide (endotoxin) and peptidoglycan.

Endotoxin. Endotoxin activity is found in the lipopolysaccharide of the cell wall of Gram-negative bacteria. The structure of a typical endotoxin molecule is shown on Figure 1.1.

The biological activity of endotoxin resides in the lipid A component. This component is composed of long-chain fatty acids (lauric, palmitic, or myristoxymystic), D-glucosamine 4-phosphate, and ethanolamine. Lipid A is therefore a phospholipid that uses D-glucosamine instead of glycerol as a skeleton. The core polysaccharide is linked via 2-keto-3-deoxyoctonic acid (KDO) to lipid A and contains three hexoses in the outer core and heptose, ethanolamine, and phosphate in the inner core. Endotoxin is resistant to boiling and proteolytic enzymes and is usually considerably less toxic than proteinaceous bacterial toxins. Antiserum does not appreciably reduce its toxicity unless prepared against the core polysaccharide. Antibody to core polysaccharide is neutralizing because of steric inhibition of the adjacent lipid A component. The more important biological effects of endotoxin as mediated by lipid A are listed in Table 1.2. They include fever, shock, neutropenia, petechial and ecchymotic hemorrhages, pulmonary edema and congestion, hemorrhagic gastritis, and sometimes adrenal cortical necrosis. The often fatal circulatory collapse observed in Gram-negative septicemias is in part due to the release of vasamines such as scrotonin and histamine by marginated neutrophils and platelets (Hinshaw 1971). For further information on the biological effects of endotoxin and the pathophysiology of endotoxemia in horses, see the excellent review by Burrows (1981).

Peptidoglycan. Peptidoglycan is the cell wall component of both Gram-negative and Gram-positive bacteria that confers skeletal rigidity, structural integrity, and shape to the organism. It consists of linear polymers of N-acetylglucosamine and N-acetylmuramic acid and short side chains of four amino acids (tetrapeptides) attached to N-acetylmuramic acid (Figure 1.2). The tetrapeptides on adjoining chains are linked by short peptides.

Gram-positive bacteria have a thick layer of pep-

Table 1.2. Biological activity of endotoxin

Effect	Mechanism
Fever	Release of endogenous pyrogen from neutrophils and monocytes
Hypotension; pooling of blood in splanchnic vasculature	Fall in cardiac output owing to constriction of pulmonary, hepatic, and mesenteric veins
Intravascular coagulation	Production of fibrin polymers that stick to endothelial cells injured by endotoxin
Hemorrhages	Anticoagulant activity of fibrin degradation products via inhibition of fibrinogen proteolysis and platelet aggregation
Neutropenia and thrombocytopenia	Margination of neutrophils and platelets in capillaries
Hyperglycemia	Decline in hepatic glycogen owing to inhibition of gluconeogenesis
Complement depletion	Activation of complement by the alternative and classic pathways
Adjuvant effect	T lymphocyte-independent stimulation of immunoglobulin synthesis by B lymphocytes

tidoglycan in contrast to the thin layer present in Gram-negative organisms.

The biological effects of peptidoglycan resemble in part those of endotoxin. It is pyrogenic, lytic for platelets, and a potent activator of complement by both pathways. It induces inflammatory skin lesions and its persistence in tissues can result in host granulomatous responses such as botryomycosis in horses or chronic mastitis in cows. Activation of complement and release of C5a results in a potent chemotactic effect on neutrophils, which are drawn to the site of infection and contribute to lesion development. A good example of this phenomenon is lymphatic abscess development in *Streptococcus equi* infection in

horses. The role of peptidoglycan in lesion development is discussed more fully by Verhoef and Verbrugh (1981).

Contribution of the Host Immune Response to Lesion Development and Maintenance

The direct and indirect effects of bacterial toxins, enzymes, and cell wall constituents on tissues and physiological processes are clearly of great importance in the pathogenesis of bacterial disease. However, subsequent specific immune responses to persisting microorganisms or their constituents can also be of great importance in disease production and maintenance.

Examples of this phenomenon include chronic erysipelas or mycoplasma arthritis in swine, tuberculosis, *Brucella canis* infection of the canine testes, chronic leptospira nephritis, feline hemobartonellosis, purpura hemorrhagica and periodic ophthalmia in horses, and fungal granulomas. A variety of immune phenomena are involved in these disease processes, including humoral and cell-mediated responses to entrapped and nondegradable antigens and formation of antibody to ordinarily sequestered host antigens in the eye, erythrocyte stroma, or testes. Formation of immune complexes that attach to blood vessels, activate complement, and attract neutrophils is yet another way in which the host's immune response can contribute to lesion development. So too is the cytotoxic effect of killer T lymphocytes for host cells that contain facultative intracellular bacteria or fungi such as *Brucella abortus* or *Sporothrix schenckii*. These and other examples will be discussed in more detail in the chapters that follow.

REFERENCES

Burrows, G.E. 1981. Endotoxemia in the horse. Eq. Vet. J. 13:89–94.

Hinshaw, L.B. 1971. Release of vasoactive agents and the vascular

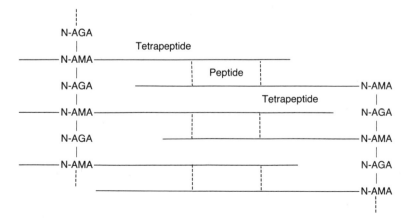

Figure 1.2. Schematic structure of peptidoglycan. N-acetylglucosamine (N-AGA) and N-acetylmuramic acid (N-AMA) form linear polymers linked by cross bridges of tetrapeptides, which are linked to each other by other peptides.

effects of endotoxin. In S. Kadis, G. Weinbaum, and S.J. Aji, eds., Microbial Toxins, vol. 5. Academic Press, New York, Pp. 209–260.

Joiner, K.A., Brown, E.J., and Frank, M.M. 1984. Complement and bacteria: Chemistry and biology in host defense. Ann. Rev. Immunol. 2:461–491.

Lee, A., O'Rourke, J.L., Barrington, P.J., and Trust, T.J. 1986. Mucus colonization as a determinant of pathogenicity in intestinal infection by *Campylobacter jejuni:* A mouse cecal model. Infect. Immun. 51:536–546.

Murphy, J.W., and Cozad, G.C. 1972. Immunological unresponsiveness induced by cryptococcal capsular polysaccharide assayed by the hemolytic plaque technique. Infect. Immun. 5:896–899.

Ogata, R.T. 1983. Factors determining bacterial pathogenicity. Clin. Physiol. Biochem. 1:145–159.

Verhoef, J., and Vergrugh, H.A. 1981. Host determinants in staphylococcal disease. Ann. Rev. Med. 32:107–122.

2 The Host's Response to Infection

After microorganisms penetrate into or through the primary epithelial barriers, they are usually quickly recognized as foreign by the host, which then mounts a sequence of responses; these responses can be local, systemic, or both. The nature and extent of these responses vary according to the site of invasion, the pathogenicity of the invading microorganisms, and the immunological status and genetic constitution of the host. In the case of microorganisms such as *Bordetella bronchiseptica,* mycoplasmas, or enterotoxigenic *Escherichia coli,* there may be no actual penetration of the epithelium by the organism itself; rather, the organism's toxins or metabolites are absorbed and cause various ill effects. Some infections may be superficial and clinically inapparent, as in the case with colonization of the tonsils of pigs by *Erysipelothrix rhusiopathiae* or *Mycoplasma hyosynoviae.* Although the infection may be clinically inapparent, the host animal often detects its presence and produces antibody.

In this chapter we describe the salient features of the host's response to infection beginning with inflammation and fever and progressing to the humoral and cellular phases of the immune response as they relate to infection by bacteria and fungi at both the systemic and local levels. As much as possible, infections in domestic animals are used to illustrate the immunological phenomena involved. A knowledge of the general principles of pathology and immunology is assumed; excellent sources on these subjects are Tizard (1987), Slauson and Cooper (1982), and Roitt (1981). The host response to viral infection is described in Chapter 38.

Inflammation and Microbial Clearance

After penetrating the epithelial barrier, microorganisms are physically hindered from spreading more deeply by the interlacing meshwork of connective tissue fibers in the subepithelial or submucosal tissues. Within a few minutes, the invader's presence is detected and results in rapid changes in the caliber and flow of the local vasculature. Vasodilation, plasma leakage, and movement of cells from the bloodstream through the walls of the blood vessels into the extravascular tissue then ensue. Initially the blood cells are predominantly neutrophils, which, before moving through the walls of the blood vessels, become adherent to the vascular endothelium.

The directed migration (chemotaxis) of neutrophils to the invasion site is mediated by bacterial products, especially N-formylated peptides, by complement component C5a, by lymphokines, and by chemoattractants released from leukocytes already recruited to the area. Complement component C5a is produced following complement activation by both the classical and alternate pathways (Figure 2.1). Reaction of preexisting antibody with microbial antigen results in binding and activation of complement by the classical pathway. Complement can also be activated (alternate pathway), however, directly by interaction of the properdin system of complement components with bacterial lipopolysaccharide and with peptidoglycan and lipoteichoic acids of Gram-positive organisms such as *Streptococcus equi.* The lipopolysaccharide of Gram-negative organisms such as *E.coli* can activate complement by both the classical and alternate pathways. The migrating neutrophils soon make contact with the invading microorganisms and, in many cases, adhere to them. Activation of C5 is associated with an increase in stickiness of the surface of neutrophils. These "sticky" neutrophils adhere more readily to each other and to the lining of blood vessels.

Recognition of the microorganisms by neutrophils is based on attachment of the cell receptor for C3b or the Fc region of IgG. Both C3b and IgG therefore can serve in recognition and attachment and are termed *opsonins.* The presence of a capsule may prevent binding of antibody or complement factors and so encapsulated organisms may escape the attention of neutrophils. The M protein on the surface of groups A, C, and G streptococci is believed to frustrate access of the neutrophil (C3b) receptor to complement bound on the surface of the bacterial cell wall.

The presence of specific antibody greatly enhances phagocytosis because it coats or opsonizes the microorganism, thus facilitating adhesion to the phagocytic cells and thereby stimulating phagocytosis. Complement in the extravascular transudate also is bound and activated by

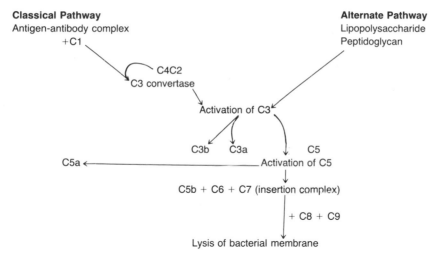

Figure 2.1. Activation of complement by the classical and alternate pathways.

the reaction of antibody with its antigen on the microbial surface. Complement activation enhances immune adherence in addition to promoting lysis of Gram-negative bacterial cells by damaging the membrane surface and allowing lysozyme to hydrolyze the peptidoglycan layer beneath. In addition, activation of complement results in formation of (1) anaphylatoxin (C3a, C5a), which triggers release of histamine from mast cells and results in a further increase in vascular permeability at the invasion site, and (2) chemotactic factors (C5a, C5b67), which attract even more neutrophils to the area. Following adherence, the neutrophil engulfs the microorganism within newly formed projections of its cytoplasm. These projections wrap around the organism and form a phagosome. The phagosome subsequently fuses with a lysosomal granule to form a phagolysosome, which has a high concentration of lytic enzymes that are lethal to many microorganisms. In the case of capsulated bacteria and fungi such as *Klebsiella pneumoniae, Bacillus anthracis,* and *Cryptococcus neoformans,* phagocytosis is greatly hindered. *B. anthracis, Pasteurella haemolytica* and some other bacteria also produce substances that are lethal to neutrophils and other phagocytic cells either before or after ingestion.

Some bacteria, such as *Brucella abortus, Listeria monocytogenes,* and *Erysipelothrix rhusiopathiae,* exhibit a high rate of survival in the phagolysosome and are known as *facultative intracellular parasites.* Infections caused by these organisms tend to be persistent, and their eventual control or elimination requires the production of cell-mediated immunity in the host animal.

In the case of rickettsias, the organisms escape from the phagosome into the cytoplasm and multiply. *Chlamydia psittaci* blocks phagolysosomal fusion and thus thwarts the capacity of phagocytes to destroy it.

In the peritoneum, neutrophils suspended in a transudate of plasma are the dominant cells for the first day of the infection. They are then replaced by eosinophils and mononuclear cells. The mononuclear response is much greater in immune animals than in nonimmune animals. The mononuclear cells include many macrophages, which, after they ingest bacteria or other foreign material, tend to clump together by intertwining their cytoplasmic processes (Spiers and Spiers 1974). These clumps also include lymphocytes and neutrophils and in a few days attach to the omentum where they become vascularized and organize into granulomas. Fibroblasts then appear and synthesize collagenic fibers. Histologically, the granuloma consists of a central area composed of necrotic cells, bacteria, or other foreign material, and scattered macrophages and neutrophils. The outer layer consists of macrophages, plasma cells, lymphocytes, eosinophils, fibroblasts, epithelioid cells, and giant cells. The latter two cell types are derivatives of macrophages and are actively pinocytotic rather than phagocytic. Giant cells are formed when epithelioid cells fuse together. Bacteria and fungi such as *Mycobacterium bovis* or *Histoplasma capsulatum* can survive indefinitely in macrophages in chronic granulomata.

Microorganisms that enter the blood stream are filtered out by fixed macrophages in the blood sinusoids of the liver, lymph nodes, bone marrow, and spleen. In bacteremic or septicemic infections these organs remove great numbers of bacteria. Virulent bacteria such as *B. anthracis, Salmonella typhimurium, E. rhusiopathiae* and virulent pneumococci eventually overcome the ability

Table 2.1. Numbers of pneumococci in the peripheral blood of normal rabbits after single intravenous doses

Time after injection	Avirulent	Slightly virulent	Highly virulent
Immediately	8,900,000	1,030,000	1,070,000
2 hours	206	20,800	137,000
5 hours	2	340	25,000
24 hours	0	1,300	1,510,000
48 hours	—	134	Animal dead
96 hours	—	0	—

From Wright, 1927, courtesy of *Journal of Pathology and Bacteriology*.

of the reticuloendothelial system to remove them, and their numbers then increase progressively in the blood (Table 2.1). Immune animals, particularly those that have developed a cell-mediated response, exhibit very rapid and permanent clearance.

Fever

Elevation of body temperature is usually the earliest and most readily recognized host response to infection, since most infectious processes follow a febrile course of varying degree and duration. A variety of microbial components including endotoxin of Gram-negative organisms, peptidoglycan of Gram-positive organisms, and staphylococcal enterotoxin have the ability to directly cause fever. Fever-causing substances derived from outside the animal are often termed *exogenous pyrogens*. Endogenous pyrogen (EP) is the lymphokine interleukin 1 (IL-1), a protein with a molecular weight of about 15,000 and produced by macrophages and monocytes following exposure to exogenous pyrogen or immune complexes or following recognition of antigens presented to T cells by macrophages (Atkins 1985, Dinarello 1983).

Endogenous pyrogen circulates in the blood stream following its release from monocytes and macrophages and impinges on the thermosensitive neurons in the anterior hypothalamus. These neurons in turn inhibit the "thermal blind" or thermoresistant neurons of the posterior hypothalamus. When the latter are no longer inhibited, peripheral vasoconstriction occurs and heat loss is reduced. Production of EP by monocytes and macrophages is later followed by synthesis of proteins known as shock proteins, which in turn inhibit further synthesis and secretion of EP.

The effect of fever on the host defense mechanism is not completely understood. Interleukin 1 (EP) stimulates expansion and maturation of T cells and so has a potent influence on the response of the immune system to specific immunogenic determinants of the invading infectious agent.

Another significant effect of fever in relation to microbial multiplication is depression of free iron in plasma. Organisms such as salmonellae, listerias, or clostridia that require iron for multiplication or toxin synthesis are therefore less virulent. Simultaneously, the elevated temperature causes a decrease in the production of iron-binding protein (siderophore) by the invading bacterium and so reduces its ability to capture the diminished supply of free iron in the plasma.

Fever also stimulates synthesis of complement components by the liver as well as mobilization of immature neutrophils from the bone marrow. Both of these phenomena clearly could benefit the host defense mechanism.

The Immune Response to Infection

Exposure to an infectious microorganism or its products usually results in stimulation of an immune response by the host animal. This response becomes evident between 1 and 2 weeks after exposure and is first characterized by formation of antibodies specific for the microbial invader. In the case of some microbial infections, there is onset of enhanced cell-mediated immunity.

Microbial protein antigens such as toxins can be directly recognized by B lymphocytes that carry the corresponding immunoglobulin receptor. These B lymphocytes then multiply following cooperative interactions with macrophages and T helper lymphocytes and differentiate into antibody-producing plasma cells. More commonly, the bacterial antigen requires processing by macrophages, which then interact with T helper lymphocytes that carry the specific antigen receptor. These T helper lymphocytes interact only if they have the correct receptor for the major histocompatibility glycoprotein antigen (class 2) carried on the macrophage. The genetic background of the host thus is an important factor in its responsiveness to microbial infections. The activated T helper lymphocytes in turn stimulate formation of antibody-producing plasma cells. Later populations of suppressor T lymphocytes arise and serve to limit secretion of immunoglobulin by these plasma cells.

The immunoglobulin marker on the surface of B lymphocytes can be IgG, IgM, or IgD and reflects the synthetic capacity of the cells. B lymphocytes also carry receptors for antigen-antibody complexes (Fc receptor) and for antigen-antibody-complement complexes (C3 receptor).

Table 2.2. Properties and defensive functions of the immunoglobulins

Immunoglobulin class	Molecular weight	Sedimentation constant	Serum concentration	Complement fixing	Defensive function
IgA	160,000 (serum) 350,000 (colostrum and secretions)	7S 11S	1.0–4.0 mg/ml	No	Protects mucosal surfaces by blocking microbial adherence, inhibiting bacterial growth, immobilizing motile bacteria, neutralizing viruses and toxins, and limiting entry of nonviable antigens
IgG	150,000	7S	8.0–16.0 mg/ml	Some isotypes (IgG1 only in cattle)	Combats microbial infections in blood, tissues, and extravascular spaces by neutralizing bacterial toxins, neutralizing viruses and toxins, opsonizing bacteria, lysing bacteria (bacteriolysis) in presence of complement, and inhibiting bacterial metabolism and multiplication
IgM	900,000	19S	0.5–2.0 mg/ml	Yes	Combats microbial infections in their early stages by opsonizing bacteria and lysing bacteria in presence of complement
IgD	185,000	7S	3.4 µg/ml	—	Antigen receptor?
IgE	190,000	8S	0–1.0 µg/ml	—	Functions in defense against parasites

The Humoral (Immunoglobulin) Response

Antibody activity has long been known to be associated with the gamma globulin fraction of serum. This fraction contains five major structural classes that have been designated immunoglobulins G, M, A, D, and E (IgG, IgM, IgA, IgD, and IgE). Their main properties and functions in defense against infection are summarized in Table 2.2.

Following its first exposure to a particular infectious agent, the infected animal produces a primary antibody response, which is slow to develop and of low intensity. It is characterized by a relatively high proportion of IgM-type antibodies.

If the infection persists or if there is a second exposure to the infectious agent or its antigen, the host produces antibodies principally of the IgG class at a more rapid rate and at a higher level. This is known as the anamnestic or secondary response. The immunological memory for the anamnestic response is stored in T and B lymphocytes.

IgA. IgA is present in serum mainly as a 7S monomer but occurs as a dimer in secretions. The latter is composed of two 7S molecules joined by a polypeptide chain (J chain) and also containing a secretory component. The dimer with secretory component is more resistant to digestive enzymes. Two subclasses, IgA1 and IgA2, have been described. IgA2 is resistant to bacterial IgA proteases.

Assembly of secretory IgA occurs in two phases. The dimer is formed by attachment of the J chain within plasma cells of the submucosa. The dimeric IgA is then secreted into the fluid surrounding the cell. Most of it becomes associated with serous epithelial cells of the nearby mucosa and is bound to secretory component (SC) polypeptide on the surfaces of these cells. The dimeric IgA thus bound is endocytosed and transported through the cell to the mucosal surface. During the time it is inside the cell, assembly of the SC polypeptide and the IgA dimer is completed.

IgA antibodies are the dominant defensive antibodies on mucosal surfaces of the eye, the nasopharynx, and the lower respiratory, intestinal, and reproductive tracts. Their importance in local protection is demonstrated by a concentration in swine intestinal juice that is 13 times higher than that of IgG (Bourne 1976). In sow's milk the level of IgA is twice that of IgG, whereas levels of the latter are 10 times higher in serum. IgA antibodies have been shown to block adherence of *E. coli* that have the K88 adhesive antigen (Miler et al. 1975). There is also evidence that they inhibit or otherwise modify bacterial growth (Brandtzaeg et al. 1968). IgA antibodies in the vaginas of cows have been shown to immobilize *Campylobacter fetus* (Corbeil et al. 1975). In the tracheas and bronchi of dogs they may prevent adhesion of *Bordetella bronchiseptica* to cilia of the tracheobronchial epithelium. It is known that in the lamina propria of the respiratory mucosa, plasma cells producing IgA are much more numerous than cells producing IgG or IgM (Breeze et al. 1976).

IgA secreted in colostrum has been shown to be rapidly absorbed into the blood streams of foals and then exported onto the nasopharyngeal mucosa (Galan and Timoney 1986), where it provides protection against respiratory pathogens such as *Streptococcus equi*.

An important function of secretory IgA in serum is removal of antigens from the bloodstream. Blood-borne complexes of antigen and polymeric IgA are carried to the liver, where the SC polypeptide binds to a receptor on Kuppfer's cells. The complexes are endocytosed and transported across hepatic cells to the biliary drainage system, where they are removed in the bile (Rifai and Mannik 1984).

IgA can fix complement by the alternate pathway, can participate in antibody-dependent, cell-mediated cytotoxic reactions, and can attach to some phagocytic cells by means of Fc receptors (Fanger et al. 1980, Pfaffenbach et al. 1982).

IgA is the immunoglobulin found in circulating immune complexes in the purpura that follows strangles in horses. It is complexed to the M protein of *S. equi* and its level in the serums of affected animals is about four times that found in normal horses (Galan et al. 1985a). The vasculitis characteristic of purpura is explained by degranulation of polymorphs following their attachment to IgA-M protein aggregates entrapped in the smaller blood vessels.

Levels of specific IgA on mucosal surfaces tend to wane a few weeks to months after induction, and maintenance of protective levels requires periodic restimulation. IgA memory is established so that responses to subsequent exposures to the pathogen are more rapid (Keren et al. 1982).

Mucosal IgA responses can be independent of the systemic responses (Galan and Timoney 1985b). Systemic priming, however, can result in mucosal synthesis of specific IgA. Migration of lymphoblasts primed in one location produces the potential for specific IgA synthesis at a mucosal site remote from that location. Replicating anti-gens are more effective than inert antigens at stimulating mucosal IgA responses, probably because of their ability to persist on or in the mucosa and stimulate the local immune system.

IgG. Antibodies of the IgG immunoglobulin class are important in the neutralization of bacterial toxins and viruses, in opsonization and complement-mediated lysis of Gram-negative bacteria, and in inhibition of bacterial growth. IgG immunoglobulins are further divided into subclasses, IgG1, IgG2, and so forth depending on host species.

In cattle, IgG2, unlike IgG1, does not bind complement. IgG1 is the predominant IgG subclass in animals infected by *Brucella abortus*. It is also the major immunoglobulin in bovine uterine fluids and ruminant colostrum and milk, and is produced locally in the mammary gland (Chang et al. 1980).

Other IgG subclasses are present in serum in much lower concentrations than IgG1 or IgG2. The biological role of each IgG subclass in immune defense has not yet been defined.

IgM. IgM antibodies are circular pentameric molecules that have 10 combining sites, of which 5 may not be expressed. They are therefore much more efficient than dimeric IgG molecules in agglutinating particulate antigens, in opsonization (by means of complement fixation), and in binding complement because only one molecule of IgM is required to initiate complement fixation, whereas two closely spaced IgG molecules are needed to initiate it. IgM antibodies appear earliest in the immune response and are therefore associated with the acute phase of infectious disease. They are primarily synthesized in the spleen.

There is evidence that IgM antibodies have a much more potent antibacterial action than do IgG antibodies (Chidlow and Porter 1978), especially in newborn piglets, calves, and the neonates of other species in which prevention of Gram-negative bacteremia is critical. They also neutralize some of the effects of endotoxin (Kim and Watson 1965). Another important characteristic of colostral IgM antibodies in newborns is that they do not suppress the individual animal's own active immune responses when infectious agents are encountered against which the individual already has IgM antibodies.

The microscopic agglutination test for leptospiral antibody is a test based on IgM antibody (Hanson 1974). In leptospirosis, however, these antibodies are not important in protection.

IgD. The IgD immunoglobulin class is present in only trace amounts in serum. It is found on the surface of large numbers of lymphocytes and is apparently an immunoglobulin receptor for antigen.

IgE. IgE, which, like IgD, is also a minor immunoglobulin with respect to concentration in serum, is the immunoglobulin class that contains the reaginic antibodies. These are antibodies produced by the host against allergens and are responsible for immediate hypersensitivity or allergy. The role of IgE in the host's response to an infectious agent is poorly understood. It may function indirectly by means of the inflammation it induces. The resulting transudation of fluid into the area may bring with it high concentrations of protective antibody. This fluid may also have a flushing effect on the mucosa.

Cell-Mediated Immunity

The host's immune response to facultative or obligate intracellular parasites includes not only an antibody response, but also, and of much greater importance in protection, a cell-mediated immune response characterized by delayed-type hypersensitivity (DTH), a heightened microbicidal activity of macrophages (Figure 2.2) and other effects.

Cell-mediated immunity is critical in acquired host resistance to many bacterial and fungal diseases including actinomycosis, brucellosis, listeriosis, tuberculosis, swine erysipelas, salmonellosis, candidiasis, histoplasmosis, and coccidioidomycosis. These infections are usually characterized by the accumulation of large numbers of macrophages, lymphocytes, and neutrophils at sites of microbial invasion or proliferation. These cellular accumulations are known as granulomatous responses. Chronic granulomas usually contain large numbers of macrophages with enhanced microbicidal activity for the pathogen. These macrophages are described as activated or angry macrophages and have enhanced motility and phagocytic ability. Their metabolic rates and lysosomal enzyme content are also increased.

Induction of DTH responses involves stimulation of specific T cell (T_D) clones by antigen presented on the macrophage surface in association with class 2 major histocompatibility antigen. T_D cells with the appropriate antigen receptors engage the macrophage-associated antigen in combination with the major histocompatibility antigen. The committed T_D lymphocyte is then signaled by means of interleukin 1, which is released by the macrophage, to express interleukin 2 receptors on its surface. Interleukin 2 production by the T_D lymphocytes then occurs following mitosis and blast transformation. Interleukin 2 is a helper lymphokine with a molecular weight of about 30,000. Its role is to enhance cellular immunity nonspecifically by stimulating expansion of the antigen-specific T_D cell, by promoting and maintaining long-term T_D cell growth, and by augmenting cytotoxic T_C cell responses (Klesius 1982).

Cytotoxic T lymphocytes (T_C) are derived from precursor T_C cells following their interaction with antigen presenting macrophages and T helper lymphocytes and interleukin 2.

T lymphocytes sensitized to antigens of the infectious agent begin to appear about 6 to 10 days after a primary infection begins. Their induction is highly specific—animals previously sensitized to mycobacterial antigens have an immunological memory of the sensitization that can be recalled only by the same antigen. The enhanced microbicidal activity of macrophages produced as a result of the sensitization is not specific, however, and can be expressed against unrelated bacteria. The activated state lasts only a few weeks but can be rapidly regained following another encounter of sensitized long-lived T lymphocytes with antigens of the infectious agent. These lymphocytes release lymphokines that are chemotactic for and activate macrophages. Many other lymphokines participate in the induction and expression of cellular immunity, including macrophage inhibition factor (MIF), a variety of chemotactic factors, immune interferon, and transfer factor.

Cell-mediated responses involving activated macrophages have been described in infections caused by *Brucella abortus*, *Mycobacterium tuberculosis*, *Listeria monocytogenes*, *Salmonella enteritidis*, *Francisella tula-*

Figure 2.2. Curves showing the intracellular inactivation of *Erysipelothrix rhusiopathiae* in macrophages from normal mice and from immune mice infected with *E. rhusiopathiae*. (From Timoney, 1969, courtesy of *Research in Veterinary Science*.)

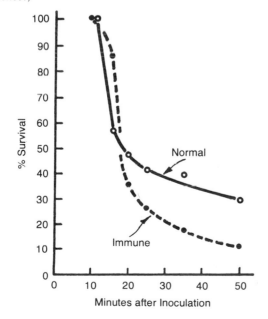

rensis, and *Erysipelothrix rhusiopathiae* (Blanden et al. 1966, Collins and Campbell 1982, Timoney 1969). They are also produced in response to living vaccines of these organisms, and activation persists as long as the vaccine strain survives in the tissues (Kuramasu et al. 1963).

The DTH reaction is characterized by swelling of the skin of a sensitized individual about 24 to 48 hours after the intradermal inoculation of the antigen (bacterial, fungal) to which it is hypersensitive. The area is edematous and contains infiltrates of lymphocytes and macrophages. The DTH reaction is of great diagnostic importance in veterinary medicine. It is used in the detection of infection by *Mycobacterium bovis, M. avium, M. paratuberculosis,* and *M. tuberculosis; Histoplasma capsulatum;* and *Coccidioides immitis.* Its protective value in the host response, however, is not always clear. It may actually be harmful because it can cause quiescent lesions to become hyperactive, resulting in necrosis, liquefaction, and release of bacteria from their intracellular nidi. Vascularization of the area may lead to possible systemic dissemination of the bacteria via the bloodstream following their entry into blood vessels close to the lesion. In contagious bovine pleuropneumonia caused by *Mycoplasma mycoides* subsp. *mycoides,* there is evidence that the DTH reaction contributes to the severe pathological conditions observed in this disease, whereas in enzootic pneumonia of swine caused by *M. hyopneumoniae* cell-mediated immunity to the organism is suppressed. Bacterial infections therefore can have a variety of different effects on cell-mediated immune responses. The mechanisms by which these divergent effects are produced are unknown.

The cytotoxic manifestation of cell-mediated immunity is a direct effect of mediators released by immune T_C lymphocytes on other attached cells that contain antigen to which the lymphocytes are sensitized. Interaction of T_C lymphocytes with target cells requires simultaneous recognition of foreign and self (major histocompatibility) antigens. The resulting intimate contact of plasma membranes triggers release of factors that destroy the target cell. This arm of the cell-mediated response is important in viral or mycoplasma infections in which a microbial antigen is associated with or inserted in a cell membrane.

Cytotoxic effects as mediated by T_C cells can also be important in acquired resistance to ringworm in which infections of *Microsporum* and *Trichophyton* species affect the nonliving stratum corneum and are remote from the direct effect of macrophages and other phagocytic cells. The cell-mediated response in this situation has to be mediated by means of soluble factors that diffuse outward from lymphocytes in the dermis to the stratum corneum.

In some infectious diseases, cell-mediated immune re-sponses tend to be inversely related to antibody response. Individuals with progressive fungal infections, for instance, often have high antibody titers but a diminished cell-mediated response. Similarly, in Johne's disease in cattle, animals with the highest titers of antibody are more severely affected, shed greater numbers of *Mycobacterium paratuberculosis,* and have a poor prognosis (de Lisle 1979). This phenomenon has been aptly termed the "immunoprotective niche."

Local Immune Responses

Respiratory Tract. Evidence for a local immune response in the nasal cavity was first obtained by Walsh and Cannon in the 1930s (1938). It was later shown that antibody to influenza virus in mice is stimulated most effectively when the antigen is applied intranasally and that the resulting antibody is produced locally (Fazekas de St. Groth and Donnelley 1950).

The tonsils are an important site of local antibody production for the nasopharynx, as first shown in studies of immunity to poliomyelitis virus in children. Children whose tonsils had been removed had much lower titers of antibody to the virus in their nasopharyngeal secretions (Tomasi 1976). Furthermore, paralytic polio has long been known to be less common in children who have not undergone tonsillectomy. Both secretory dimeric IgA and IgG are produced in pharyngeal and palatine tonsils, and the oral tonsils contain more cells that produce IgG than IgA (Ishikawa et al. 1972, Matthews and Basu 1982). In calves, IgA is quantitatively the most important immunoglobulin in nasal secretions, whereas, in secretions of the lower respiratory tract both IgA and IgG are important. Species differences play a role in the relative amounts of each immunoglobulin in the respiratory secretions. In horses, nasopharyngeal mucus from animals that have recently recovered from strangles caused by *Streptococcus equi* had higher IgG-associated antibody activity against M protein than IgA (Figure 2.3) (Galan and Timoney 1985b).

In the lower respiratory tract, the lamina propria of the trachea and bronchi contains many macrophages, neutrophils, lymphocytes, eosinophils, and plasma cells. The subepithelial tissues of the lung airways of healthy calves have a preponderance of IgA-producing cells in contrast to the situation in pneumonic calves and older cattle, in which cells that produce IgG1 are most numerous (Allan et al. 1979). Some plasma cells producing IgE are also present.

IgA acquired in colostrum can be transferred into respiratory secretions of sheep, cattle, pigs, and foals (Morgan et al. 1977, Galan et al. 1986, Smith et al. 1976); how-

vagina and cervix produce IgA antibodies that
mobilizing effect on the flagella of the organ-
ereby inhibit its spread in the tract. In the
bodies are predominantly of the IgG1 isotype
ry effective in clearing the infection by func-
opsonins for neutrophils and macrophages.
n in the cervicovaginal area tends to be per-
vever. This is probably in part due to the organ-
y to change its surface antigens, which allows
survive that have antigenic configurations that
t with the IgA antibody being synthesized at the
eil et al. 1975).
ies of IgG1 and IgG2 isotypes can be detected
and vaginal fluids following systemic vaccina-
acterin. These antibodies are protective, as are
timulated antibodies in bulls. There also is evi-
ocal antibody synthesis in the reproductive tract
fected with *Mycoplasma bovigenitalium* (Win-
Systemic vaccination is effective in curing bulls
tanding campylobacteriosis, suggesting that
can diffuse from the plasma to the preputial
n.

Tract. Infection of the urinary tract by *Cor-
ium renale* in cows causes a purulent urethritis
is that later may extend via the ureter to the
nd cause pyelonephritis. At this stage of the
gglutinating antibodies appear in the serum and
coated bacteria appear in the urine (Nicolet and
). These antibodies are mostly IgG, but some
odies also are present. The IgA antibodies are
of local origin; the IgG antibodies are derived
sudates of plasma that have leaked out of the
tory focus in the kidney.
dneys of dogs with acute interstitial nephritis
Leptospira canicola* have extensive accumula-
plasma cells (Morrison and Wright 1975). The
s produced by these cells appear to be ineffective
g renal infection because infected dogs continue
he organism. There is evidence, however, that
s are selective for leptospira clones of reduced
(Hirschberg and Vaughn 1973).
st immune response in the urinary tract is gener-
bited by the high urea content, poor phagocytic
of neutrophils, and diminished effect of com-

Plasma cells containing IgA are numerous in the
al region of lacrimal glands, and IgA is the only
globulin found in human tears (Tomasi 1976). It
he predominant immunoglobulin in bovine tears
et al. 1972). In cattle, a local resistance has been
d following infection of the eye by *Moraxella*
d by *Mycoplasma bovoculi*. This resistance corre-

wer respiratory tract,
3.0 μm (Kaltreider et
immune response ap-
ipate in a wider traffic
a number of mucosal

n shown to be impor-
ons in swine, in *Bor-*
dogs and pigs, and in
calves (Taylor and
sult in specific anti-
ce of the pathogen to
a.
sponses also play a
act against microbial
y necessary for a lo-
and systemic immu-
egard. The effector
s are found through-
.

l component of the
icroorganisms that
nd destroyed. Vir-
ttle, however, can
hese macrophages,
ptible to secondary
ord 1978, Lopez et
re immunized with
the virus-induced
ges was less effec-
ion to the cellular
crophages, locally
monstrated in the
lenney 1971). IgG
c lungs and there-
lular killing. Pha-
owever, if the in-
otoxin-producing
lytica. The mac-
are quickly killed
ly therefore must

ction in the intes-
antibody synthe-
ria. IgM and IgG
derived from the
n the intestinal
eric IgA and is
digestion.
bsorbed through
own as M cells
vidence that the

plasma cells in the lamina propria that produce IgA originate as lymphoid precursor cells in Peyer's patches or other lymphoid areas on the intestinal mucosa. Plasma cells are originally transformed by exposure to locally available antigen and then migrate through the mesenteric and ileocccal lymph nodes, thoracic duct, and bloodstream. Some of these cells travel back, or home, through the bloodstream to the lamina propria of the intestine. Others home to the mammary glands, respiratory mucosa, and the spleen. In neonates these plasma cells synthesize IgM immunoglobulin for the first week after birth; they then mature and make IgA.

Locally synthesized IgA prevents microbial adhesion, inhibits bacterial growth, and blocks attachment of *E. coli* enterotoxins to receptor sites on intestinal epithelium. It also binds to and prevents absorption of other potentially harmful molecules in the luminal fluid.

IgA has been shown to be bactericidal when acting in concert with monocytes (Befus and Bienenstock 1982). This effect may help protect the intestinal epithelium against bacterial invaders.

Intestinal IgA responses can be stimulated by intraperitoneal inoculation of antigen followed by an oral booster. Oral immunization by itself can also be successful provided the antigen can be protected against gastric acidity and digestive and microbial enzymes and can bind to a receptor on the intestinal mucosa. The intestinal IgA system has a memory mediated by long-lived T lymphocytes in the lamina propria, which can home to other locations such as the mammary gland (Pierce and Cray 1982).

Local cell-mediated immune responses in the intestine that are independent of systemic responses have been described (Frederick and Bohl 1976). Moreover, substantial macrophage and neutrophil populations occur in the lamina propria, and great numbers of neutrophils may pass through the mucosa in diseases such as enteric salmonellosis and can be found in the stool.

The local intestinal immune response also undoubtedly plays an important role in control of regional colonization of the intestine by the normal flora, but the manner by which this control is achieved is not yet understood.

Reproductive Tract.   The local immune response of cows to infection by *Brucella abortus, Campylobacter fetus venerealis*, and the protozoon parasite *Trichomonas fetus* has been recognized for many years and has often been used in the diagnosis of infection by these organisms.

The local immune response to *C. fetus venerealis* has been studied extensively (Winter 1982). Neutrophils are present in the early stages and are later replaced by foci of mononuclear cells including plasma cells. The plasma

cells in the
have an im
ism and t
uterus, an
and are ve
tioning as
Infectio
sistent, ho
ism's abil
variants tc
do not reac
time (Cor
Antibo
in uterine
tion with
similarly
dence for
of bulls ir
ter 1982).
of long-s
antibodie
epitheliur
Urinar
ynebacter
and cysti
kidneys
disease,
antibody
Fey 197
IgA anti
probably
from tra
inflamm
The k
caused b
tions of
antibodi
in cleari
to shed
antibodi
virulenc
The h
ally inh
activity
plement
Eye.
interstit
immun
is also
(Dunca
observe
bovis a

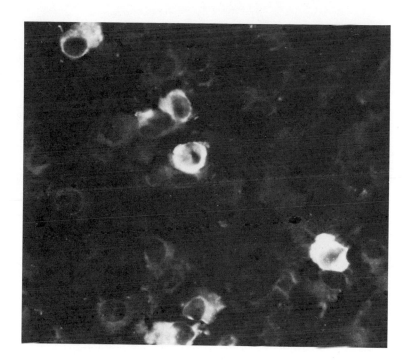

Figure 2.4. Plasma cells containing antibody to *Erysipelothrix rhusiopathiae* (ER) in the synovial tissue of a pig affected with arthritis caused by ER. The tissue section was treated with a soluble extract of ER followed by a fluorescent antiserum to ER.

lates with the presence of specific precipitins in the lacrimal secretions (Nayar and Saunders 1975).

Local immune mechanisms appear to be more important than systemic responses in protection against infection by *M. bovis* (Weech and Renshaw 1983). Systemic immunization, however, does increase resistance to challenge by homologous strains, suggesting that both phases of the immune response contribute to protection.

Oral immunization has also been shown to be effective in eliciting IgA antibodies in tears, a finding that supports the conclusion that the eye is a component of a common mucosal immune system (Montgomery et al. 1983).

During acute inflammation, bovine IgG1 is selectively transferred from the blood to the tears (Pedersen 1973), and may be responsible for the precipitin activity present. This is suggested because the highest and most persistent antibody titers in cattle are associated with IgG1 and not IgA (Killinger et al. 1978). IgG2 and IgM also pass from the plasma into the bovine lacrimal secretion.

Joints. Synovial tissue has the capacity to develop immunocompetence and mount a local immune response. Infection of the joints of pigs by *Erysipelothrix rhusiopathiae* (Timoney and Berman 1970) and by *Mycoplasma hyorhinis* (Ross 1973) results in accumulations of plasma cells. In the case of *E. rhusiopathiae* arthritis, these plasma cells contain antibodies to the causative bacterium and these antibodies are predominantly of the IgG class (Timoney and Yarkoni 1976) (Figure 2.4).

The type A synoviocytes of the synovial lining are phagocytic but, being fixed, are unable to escape from the joint with their burden of ingested microorganisms. Antigens of infectious agents therefore tend to be held in the synovial tissue and in cartilage and so are a continuing local source of immune stimulus. This may explain the chronicity of some forms of infectious arthritis in animals and humans.

Mammary Gland. Neutrophils are probably the most important component of the host defense mechanism in bovine mammary glands. They rapidly reproduce in the milk following bacterial invasion of the quarter and phagocytose and kill large numbers of bacteria. Endotoxin from Gram-negative bacteria and peptidoglycan from Gram-positive bacteria are very effective chemotactic stimuli for neutrophils within the udder. Endotoxin can be used in the treatment of persisting infections when the response of the udder by itself appears to be insufficient.

The immunoglobulin content of colostrum is much higher than that of milk (Table 2.3). The milk of pigs, horses, and dogs has a higher concentration of IgA than IgG, whereas in ruminants IgG levels are higher. Selective transfer of immunoglobulins from the bloodstream to lacteal secretions occurs and is supplemented by local synthesis of IgA, IgM, and small amounts of IgG (see review by Norcross 1982).

The mammary immune response in some species (but not in sheep or cattle) is linked to the mucosal immune

Table 2.3. Immunoglobulin concentrations (mg/ml) in colostrum and milk of domestic animals

Species	Colostrum			Milk		
	IgA	IgG	IgM	IgA	IgG	IgM
Horse	1.5	7.9–13.5	1.0–1.5	0.80	0.7	0.10
Cattle	1.5	37.5	3.9	0.06	0.3	0.06
Sheep	2.0	60.0	4.1	0.06	0.3	0.03
Pig	9.7	61.8	3.2	3.00	1.4	0.90
Dog	3.3	14.6	2.2	0.79	0.3	0.10

system so that lymphoblasts primed in the intestinal lymphoid aggregates (Peyer's patches) home to the mammary gland through the mesenteric lymph nodes, thoracic duct, and bloodstream. In this way immunocytes with the ability to synthesize specific IgA antibodies against enteric pathogens colonize the mammary gland and produce antibodies protective for the neonate when the latter ingests colostrum. In pigs and horses, secretion of these antibodies in milk continues for some weeks after parturition.

Protection of the bovine mammary gland against infection by Gram-positive cocci is mediated mainly by opsonizing and antitoxic antibodies that belong to the IgG isotype (Norcross 1977). Local antibody synthesis occurs in the supramammary lymph node and in plasma cells scattered through the secretory parenchyma (Willoughby 1966). IgA antibody against antigens of *Streptococcus agalactiae* can be stimulated by intramammary vaccination and may serve to block adhesion of the organism to ductular epithelium. IgM antibodies also play a role in protection of the gland against invasion by *S. agalactiae*.

IgA and IgG1 antibodies enhance the bacteriostatic effect of the iron-binding milk protein lactoferrin for organisms that require iron such as *E. coli*.

Both IgG1 and IgG2 are cytophilic for bovine mammary macrophages and probably function to enhance phagocytosis.

Attempts to vaccinate cattle against mastitis by immunization with bacterins or toxoids have not been very successful (Nickerson 1985). Although antibody responses can be detected in the milk (Opdebeeck 1982), the great dilution of antibody by the milk flow and the relative absence of complement components are factors that greatly reduce their contribution to protection. Cell-mediated responses including DTH play a role in protection and in the pathogenesis of chronic forms of mastitis caused by organisms such as *Staphylococcus aureus* or *Nocardia asteroides*. There is some evidence that T lymphocytes in milk are a selected population of cells with antigenic experiences different from those found at other body sites. These lymphocytes are less responsive than those from

blood and this may be a factor in the greater susceptibility of mammary parenchyma to bacterial invasion as compared with other tissues (see review by Opdebeeck 1982).

Response of the Fetus and Newborn Animal to Infectious Agents

The immune system of the fetus develops some time before birth (Figure 2.5) and is independent of antigenic stimulation. A calf is capable of responding to infectious agents about halfway through gestation (Schultz 1973, Schultz et al. 1971) whereas piglets develop immunocompetence about 3 months after conception. Puppies, perhaps because of their relatively short gestation period, do not develop humoral immune responsiveness to bacterial antigens until a week or two after birth.

Of all domestic animals, fetal ruminants are most prone to invasion by infectious agents. Examples of these agents are *Brucella abortus*, *Leptospira pomona*, *Campylobacter fetus*, *Aspergillus fumigatus*, and a number of pathogenic viruses. Infection before immunocompetence can result in postnatal tolerance to antigens of the infectious agent. This phenomenon may play a role in the latent

Figure 2.5. The development of the immune system in the fetal calf. (From Schultz, 1973, courtesy of *Cornell Veterinarian*.)

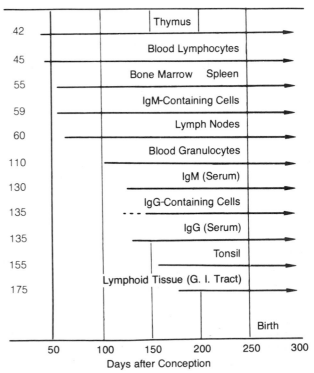

carrier state sometimes observed later in life in ruminants infected with *B. abortus* or *Leptospira* species. Most bacterial infections result in fetal death irrespective of the stage of fetal development.

Because plasma concentrations of complement components are much lower in the fetus than in the older animal, the fetus has a reduced or nonexistent neutrophil response (Osburn et al. 1982). Fetal neutrophils have good phagocytic and bactericidal ability, however.

The immune response of the fetus to infection is characterized by lymphoreticular hyperplasia and production of significant levels of immunoglobulins in the serum. Normally, only trace amounts of immunoglobulins are present at this time. IgM levels are raised in most species. In a calf infected in utero, IgG1 as well as IgG2 is present in amounts in excess of 300 µg/ml of serum. IgG2 is normally absent from calf serum at birth and so its presence in serum at birth is good evidence for fetal infection in utero.

Bovine fetuses develop the ability to mount cell-mediated responses to *Mycobacterium bovis* and *B. abortus* after 175 days of gestation (Osburn et al. 1982). However, calves infected in utero with *Mycobacterium bovis*, although sensitized to tuberculin, may be unable to mount a delayed hypersensitivity response because of fetal glucocorticoid synthesis just before parturition.

A newborn animal faces challenge by a variety of infectious agents as soon as it passes out of the sterile environment of the uterus. Its immune defenses are greatly reinforced by the ingestion of colostrum with its rich supply of immunoglobulins and complement factors. During the first weeks and months of life its ability to synthesize complement components and specific antibody gradually develops. The rate of this development varies with the species of host animal and with the microbial antigens encountered. For instance, calves develop antibodies earlier in life to salmonella flagellar protein than to salmonella lipopolysaccharide. Antibody responses of a newborn calf to *B. abortus* are slow and of low magnitude and no memory is established (Husband and Lascelles 1975).

Local intestinal immune responses develop during the first weeks of life. IgM antibodies appear first and are later replaced by IgA. Newborn calves and pigs can mount specific local antibody responses within 10 days of antigen exposure but do not have the ability to retain a memory of the exposure.

The immunological unresponsiveness of newborn animals is due in part to suppression of immunoglobulin synthesis by maternal immunoglobulin, by high levels of glucocorticoids, and by the activity of suppressor T lymphocytes (Banks 1982). Maternal immunoglobulin has a half-life of between 6 and 20 days for IgG, 4 to 5 days for IgM, and 2 to 3 days for IgA (Banks 1982). The hormonal

immunosuppressive effect persists for about 10 to 14 days in ruminants and for up to 60 days in pigs.

REFERENCES

Allan, E.M., Pirre, H.M., and Selman, I.E. 1979. Immunoglobulin containing cells in the bronchopulmonary system of non-pneumonic and pneumonic calves. Res. Vet. Sci. 26:349–355.

Atkins, E. 1985. Fever: The old and the new. J. Infect. Dis. 151:570.

Banks, K.L. 1982. Host defense in the newborn animal. J. Am. Vet. Med. Assoc. 181:1053–1056.

Befus, A.D., and Bienenstock, J. 1982. Factors involved in symbiosis and host resistance at the mucosa-parasite interface. Prog. Allerg. 31:76–177.

Bienenstock, J., and Befus, A.D. 1980. Mucosal immunology. Immunology 41:249–270.

Blanden, R.V., Mackaness, G.B., and Collins, F.M. 1966. Mechanisms of acquired resistance in mouse typhoid. J. Exp. Med. 124:585–599.

Bourne, F.J. 1976. Humoral immunity in the pig. Vet. Rec. 98:499–501.

Brandtzaeg, P., Fjellanger, I., Gjeruldsen, S.T. 1968. Immunoglobulin M: Local synthesis and selective secretion in patients with immunoglobulin A deficiency. Science 160:789–791.

Breeze, R.G., Wheeldon, E.B., and Pirie, H.M. 1976. Cell structure and function in the mammalian lung: The trachea, bronch and bronchioles. Vet. Bull. 46:319–337.

Chang, C.C., Winter, A.J., and Norcross, N.L. 1980. Antibody-producing cells in bovine lacteal secretions after local immunization. Am. J. Vet. Res. 41:1416–1418.

Charley, B., and Corthier, G. 1977. Local immunity in the pig respiratory tract. II. Relationship of serum and local antibodies. Ann. Microbiol. (Paris) 128:109–119.

Chidlow, J.W., and Porter, P. 1977. Uptake of maternal antibody by the neonatal pig following intramuscular and intramammary vaccination of the preparturient sow. Res. Vet. Sci. 23:185–190.

Collins, F.M., and Campbell, S.G. 1982. Immunity to intracellular bacteria. Vet. Immunol. Immunopathol. 3:5–66.

Corbeil, L.B., Schurig, G.G.D., Bier, P.J., and Winter, A.J. 1975. Bovine venereal vibriosis: Antigenic variation of the bacterium during infection. Infect. Immunol. 11:240–244.

de Lisle, G. 1979. Johne's disease: A study of the immunological responses of cattle infected with *Mycobacterium paratuberculosis*. Ph.D. dissertation, Cornell University, Ithaca, N.Y.

Dinarello, C.A. 1983. Molecular mechanisms in endotoxin fever. Agents Actions 13:470–486.

Duncan, J.R., Wilkie, B.N., Winter, A.J., and Hiestand, F. 1972. The serum and secretory immunoglobulins of cattle: Characterization and quantitation. J. Immunol. 108:965–976.

Fanger, M.W., Shen, L., Pugh, J., and Bernier, G.M. 1980. Subpopulations of human peripheral granulocytes and monocytes express receptors for IgA. Proc. Natl. Acad. Sci. USA 77:3640–3644.

Fazekas de St. Groth, S., and Donnelley, S. 1950. Studies in experimental immunology of influenza. III. The antibody response. Aust. J. Exp. Biol. Med. Sci. 28:61–75.

Frederick, G.T., and Bohl, E.H. 1976. Local and systemic cell-mediated immunity against transmissible gastroenteritis, an intestinal viral infection of swine. J. Immunol. 116:1000–1004.

Galan, J.E., and Timoney, J.F. 1985a. Immune complexes in purpura hemorrhagica of the horse contain IgA and M antigen of *Streptococcus equi*. J. Immunol. 135:3134–3137.

Galan, J.E., and Timoney, J.F. 1985b. Mucosal nasopharyngeal immune responses of horses to protein antigens of *Streptococcus equi*. Infect. Immun. 47:623–628.

Galan, J.E., Timoney, J.F., and Lengemann, F.W. 1986. Passive transfer of mucosal antibody to *Streptococcus equi* in the foal. Infect. Immun. 54:202–206.

Hanson, L.E. 1974. Bovine leptospirosis. J. Dairy Sci. 59:1166–1170.

Hirschberg, N., and Vaughn, J. 1973. Antibodies in bovine urine in leptospirosis. Vet. Med./Small Anim. Clin. 68:67.

Husband, A.J., and Lascelles, A.K. 1975. Antibody responses to neonatal immunization in calves. Res. Vet. Sci. 18:201–207.

Ishikawa, T., Wicher, K., and Arbesman, C.E. 1972. Distribution of immunoglobulins in palatine and pharyngeal tonsils. Int. Arch. Allergy Appl. Immunol. 43:801–812.

Jakab, G.J., and Green, G.M. 1973. Immune enhancement of pulmonary bactericidal activity in murine virus pneumonia. J. Clin. Invest. 52:2878–2884.

Jericho, K.W.F., and Langford, E.V. 1978. Pneumonia in calves produced with aerosols of bovine herpesvirus 1 and *Pasteurella haemolytica*. Can. J. Comp. Med. 42:269–277.

Kaltreider, H.G., Caldwell, J.C., and Adam, E. 1977. The fate and consequence of an organic particulate antigen instilled into bronchoalveolar spaces of normal canine lungs. Am. Rev. Respir. Dis. 116:267–280.

Keren, D.F., Kern, S.E., and Bauer, D.H. 1982. Direct demonstration in intestinal secretions of an IgA memory response to orally administered *Shigella flexneri* antigens. J. Immunol. 128:475–479.

Killinger, A.H., Weisiger, R.M., Helper, L.C., and Mansfield, M.E. 1978. Detection of *Moraxella bovis* antibodies in the SIgA, IgG and IgM classes of immunoglobulin in bovine lacrimal secretions by an indirect fluorescent antibody test. Am. J. Vet. Res. 39:931–934.

Kim, Y.B., and Watson, D.W. 1965. Modification of host responses to bacterial endotoxins. J. Exp. Med. 121:751–759.

Klesius, P.H. 1982. Intercellular communication: Role of soluble factors in cellular immune responses. J. Am. Vet. Med. Assoc. 181:1015–1021.

Kuramasu, S., Imamura, Y., Sameshima, T., and Tajima, Y. 1963. Studies on erysipelosis. II. Changes in the characters of bacteria and in the responses of mice after inoculation with the acriflavin-attenuated strain chiran. Zentralbl. Veterinärmed. [B] 9:362–379.

Lopez, A., Thompson, R.G., and Savan, M. 1976. The pulmonary clearance of *Pasteurella haemolytica* in calves infected with bovine parainfluenza-3 virus. Can. J. Comp. Med. 40:385–391.

Matthews, J.B., and Basu, K.M. 1982. Oral tonsils: An immunoperoxidase study. Int. Arch. Allergy Appl. Immunol. 69:21–25.

Miler, I., Cerna, J., Travnicek, J., and Rejnek, J. 1975. The protective effect of antibodies to *Escherichia coli* in newborn germfree piglets. Folia Microbiol. (Praha) 20:83.

Montgomery, P.C., Ayyildiz, A. Lemiatre-Coelho, I.M., Vaerman, J.P., and Rockey, J.H. 1983. Induction and expression of antibodies in secretions: The ocular immune system. Ann. N.Y. Acad. Sci. 409:428–440.

Morgan, K., Bradley, P., and Bourne, F.J. 1977. The immune system of the bovine respiratory tract. Commission of the European Community Seminar on Respiratory Diseases of Cattle. Edinburgh, Scotland.

Morgan, K.L., and Bourne, F.J. 1980. Immunoglobulin levels in porcine nasal and tracheal secretions—The influence of the method of collection. J. Immunol. Methods 37:165–173.

Morrison, W.I., and Wright, N.G. 1975. Canine leptospirosis: An immunopathological study of interstitial nephritis due to *Leptospira canicola*. J. Pathol. 120:83–89.

Nayar, P.S.G., and Saunders, J.R. 1975. Infectious bovine keratoconjunctivitis I. Experimental production. Can. J. Comp. Med. 39:22–31.

Nickerson, S.C. 1985. Immune mechanisms of the bovine udder: An overview. J. Am. Vet. Med. Assoc. 187:41–45.

Nicolet, J., and Fey, H. 1979. Antibody coated bacteria in urine sediment from cattle infected with *Corynebacterium renale*. Vet. Rec. 105:301–303.

Norcross, N.L. 1977. Immune response of the mammary gland and role of immunization in mastitis control. J. Am. Vet. Med. Assoc. 170:1228–1231.

Norcross, N.L. 1982. Secretion and composition of colostrum and milk. J. Am. Vet. Med. Assoc. 181:1057–1060.

Opdebeeck, J.P. 1982. Mammary gland immunity. J. Am. Vet. Med. Assoc. 181:1061–1065.

Osburn, B.I., Maclachlan, N.J., and Terrell, T.G. 1982. Ontogeny of the immune system. J. Am. Vet. Med. Assoc. 181:1049–1052.

Owen, R.L., and P. Nemanic. 1978. Antigenic processing structures of the mammalian intestinal tract: An SEM study of lymphoepithelial organs. In: Becker, R.P., Johari, O. eds. Scanning Electron Microscopy. II AMF, O'Hare, Ill. pp. 367–378.

Pedersen, K.B. 1973. The origin of immunoglobulin-G in bovine tears. Acta Pathol. Microbiol. Scand. [B] 81:245–252.

Pfaffenbach, G., Lamm, M.E., and Gigli, I. 1982. Activation of guinea pig alternative complement pathway by mouse IgA immune complexes. J. Exp. Med. 155:231–247.

Pierce, N.F., and Cray, W.C., Jr. 1982. Determinants of the localization, magnitude and duration of specific mucosal IgA plasma cell response in enterically immunized rats. J. Immunol. 128:1311–1315.

Rifai, A., and Mannik, M. 1984. Clearance of circulating IgA immune complexes is mediated by specific receptor on kupffer cells in mice. J. Exp. Med. 160:125–130.

Roitt, I. 1981. Essential Immunology. Blackwell Scientific Publications, Oxford, England.

Ross, R.F. 1973. Pathogenicity of swine mycoplasmas. Ann. N.Y. Acad. Sci. 225:347–368.

Schultz, R.D. 1973. Developmental aspects of the fetal bovine immune response: A review. Cornell Vet. 63:507–535.

Schultz, R.D., Wang, J.T., and Dunne, H.W. 1971. Development of the humoral immune response of the pig. Am. J. Vet. Res. 32:1331–1336.

Slauson, D.O., and Cooper, B.J. Mechanisms of Diseases: A Textbook of Comparative General Pathology, 1st ed. Williams & Wilkins, Baltimore.

Smith, W.D., Dawson, A., and Wells, P.W. 1976. Immunoglobulins in the serum and nasal secretions of lambs following vaccination and aerosol challenge with parainfluenza 3 virus. Res. Vet. Sci. 21:341–348.

Spiers, L., and Spiers, I. 1974. Quantitative studies of inflammation and granuloma formation. In G. Van Arman, ed., White Cells in Inflammation. Charles C Thomas, Springfield, Ill. Pp 54–92.

Taylor, G., and Howard, C.J. 1981. Importance of local antibody in resistance to mycoplasma infections of the respiratory tract. In F. Bourne, ed., The Mucosal Immune System. Martinus Nijhoff, The Netherlands. Pp. 330–333.

Timoney, J.F. 1969. Inactivation of *Erysipelothrix rhusiopathiae* in macrophages from normal and immune mice. Res. Vet. Sci. 10:301–302.

Timoney, J.F., and Berman, D.T. 1970. Erysipelothrix arthritis in swine: Serum–synovial fluid gradients for antibody and serum proteins in normal and arthritic joints. Am. J. Vet. Res. 31:1405–1409.

Timoney, J.F., and Galan, J.E. 1985. The protective response of the horse to an avirulent strain of *Streptococcus equi*. In Y. Kimura, S. Kotami, and Y. Shikokawa, eds., Recent Advances in Streptococci and Streptococcal Diseases. Reedbooks, Surrey, England.

Timoney, J.F., and Yarkoni, U. 1976. Immunoglobulins IgG and IgM in synovial fluids of swine with erysipelothrix polyarthritis. Vet. Microbiol. 1:467–474.

Tizard, I.R. 1982. An Introduction to Veterinary Immunology. W.B. Saunders, Philadelphia.

Tomasi, T.B. 1976. Mucosal immune system. A general review. Ann. Otol. Rhinol. Laryngol. 85(2 Suppl. 25, Pt. 2):87–89.

Waldman, R.H., and Henney, C.S. 1971. Cell-mediated immunity and antibody responses in the respiratory tract after local and systemic immunization. J. Exp. Med. 134:482–494.

Walsh, T.E., and Cannon, P.R. 1938. Immunization of the respiratory tract. A comparative study of the antibody content of the respiratory and other tissues following active, passive and regional immunization. J. Immunol. 35:31–45.

Weech, G.M., and Renshaw, H.W. 1983. Infectious bovine keratoconjunctivitis: Bacteriologic, immunologic and clinical responses to experimental exposure with *Moraxella bovis*. Comp. Immunol. Microbiol. Infect. Dis. 6:81–94.

Wilkie, B.N. 1982. Respiratory tract immune response to microbial pathogens. J. Am. Vet. Med. Assoc. 181:1074–1079.

Wilkie, B.N., and Markham, R.J.F. 1979. Sequential titration of bovine lung and serum antibodies after parenteral or pulmonary inoculation with *Pasteurella haemolytica*. Am. J. Vet. Res. 40:1690–1693.

Wilkie, B.N., Markham, R.J.F., and Shewen, P.E. 1980. Response of calves to lung challenge exposure with *Pasteurella haemolytica* after parenteral or pulmonary immunization. Am. J. Vet. Res. 41:1773–1778.

Willoughby, R.A. 1966. Bovine staphylococcic mastitis: An immunohistochemical study of the cellular sites of antibody formation. Am. J. Vet. Res. 27:522–532.

Winter, A.J. 1982. Microbial immunity in the reproductive tract. J. Am. Vet. Med. Assoc. 181:1069–1073.

Wright, N.D. 1927. Experimental pneumococcal septicemia and antipneumococcal immunity. J. Pathol. Bacteriol. 30:189–252.

3 The Genetics of Virulence and Antibiotic Resistance

Since the late 1970s the companion sciences of bacterial genetics and molecular biology have had a tremendous impact on the knowledge and understanding of cellular functions and the properties of bacteria that contribute to virulence and to their ability to survive in the presence of antibiotics and other antimicrobials used in disease prevention and control. In this chapter we will briefly describe and discuss some important genetic and biochemical features of virulence and antibiotic resistance of the pathogenic bacteria found in the infectious diseases of animals described in later chapters. A working knowledge of bacterial physiology and nucleic acid and protein biochemistry is assumed; for further information on these topics, see other more detailed sources (Birge 1981, Kopecko and Baron 1985, Lin et al. 1984).

The Bacterial Chromosome

The complement of genes representing the genetic potential of the bacterial cell is referred to as its genotype, whereas bacterial traits that can be observed constitute the phenotype. Genetic information in bacteria is mainly encoded in the deoxyribonucleic acid (DNA) of the single chromosome, and to a lesser extent, in plasmids and bacteriophages. The DNA is composed of two complementary polynucleotide strands arranged in a double helix (Figure 3.1). Each strand is composed of nucleotide units made up of combinations of the bases adenine, thymine, guanine, and cytosine. Junctions between nucleotides on opposite strands involve hydrogen bonding between the complementary bases adenine and thymine (two bonds) and between guanine and cytosine (three bonds). Linkages within each strand are formed by deoxyribose phosphate covalent bands. Each successive three-base sequence is the code for one amino acid in a protein. A protein of 300 amino acids therefore requires a coding sequence of about 900 nucleotides on the DNA strand. The term *gene* is applied to a DNA segment encoding a specific protein, ribososomal or transfer ribonucleic acid, or a regulatory function.

The DNA of the bacterial chromosome genome forms a closed circle and varies in coding capacity depending on the structural and organizational sophistication of the source organism. A typical *Escherichia coli* has a genome with a molecular mass of about 2.5×10^3 megadaltons (MDa), that is, it contains about 3.8×10^6 nucleotides or bases and can theoretically code for several thousand proteins. Mycoplasmas have much smaller genomes (500 MDa), which reflect their simpler structures and reliance on the host for many metabolites. *Chlamydia* and *Rickettsia* organisms also have smaller genomes (660 MDa and 1,000 MDa, respectively) than other bacteria because their intracellular habitat allows them to take advantage of the hosts' cell supply of ATP and other compounds necessary for maintenance and synthesis of new cell mass.

Plasmids

Plasmids are covalently closed circular molecules of DNA that are stably inherited and replicate somewhat independently of the bacterial chromosome. They range in size from less than 1 MDa to several hundred and are usually isolated by detergent lysis followed by selective precipitation of membrane-associated chromosomal DNA. They can then be separated and their sizes estimated by electrophoresis in agarose gels (Figure 3.2). Purified plasmid DNA can be photographed in the electron microscope and the contour length of the molecule measured to estimate its molecular mass (Figure 3.3).

Another method of plasmid purification is dye-bouyant density centrifugation in cesium chloride. In this procedure, the dye, ethidium bromide, is bound to a much greater extent by linear fragments of DNA than by the closed circular, supercoiled plasmid molecules and bands at a different level in a cesium chloride gradient during ultracentrifugation.

Genes carried on plasmids can mediate a wide variety of important functions, including antibiotic and heavy metal resistance, toxin production, cell penetration, iron chelation, complement resistance, and metabolic characteristics such as sucrose and lactose fermentation. In the

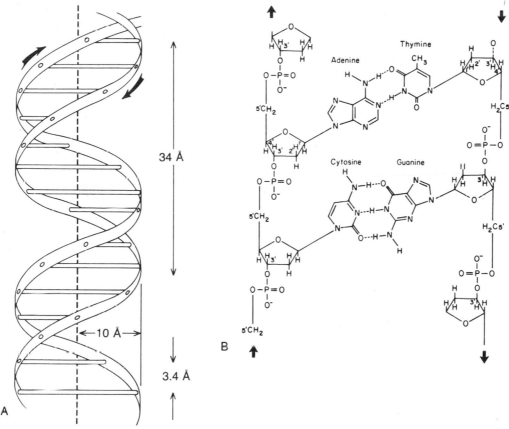

Figure 3.1. The stereochemical structure of bacterial DNA. (*A*) Diagram of the DNA double helix. Bacterial DNA is composed of two polynucleotide chains organized in a regular, right-handed double helix, with a diameter of 20 Å. Each turn of the helix contains 10 base pairs and is 34 Å long. (*B*) A segment of a DNA duplex showing the antiparallel nature of the complementary chains. The stereochemical consequence of hydrogen bond base pairing between adenine and thymine or between guanine and cytosine is that the two chains must run in opposite directions with respect to the 3′, 5′ sugar-phosphate linkages within each chain. (From Kopecko and Baron, 1985, courtesy of W. B. Saunders Co.)

case of *E. coli,* heat-stable and heat-labile enterotoxin production, adhesion and colonization factors, edema disease toxin, colicin and hemolysin production, and other factors involved in lethality can be plasmid mediated.

Mutations

A mutation is an alteration in nucleotide sequence and may be recognized by changes in the phenotype of cells such as loss of a biochemical function, change in morphology, or the appearance of colonial roughness. They can occur spontaneously, usually at a frequency of less than 10^{-6} but often much less frequently. Mutations that affect the organism's ability to absorb or synthesize an essential growth factor may render a virulent organism avirulent even though the mutation itself did not involve a primary virulence trait such as toxin or capsule produc-

tion. In fact, mutations of this kind are desirable in vaccine strains because they do not affect important protective antigenic determinants, which are usually on toxins or on the surface of the organism. An example of such a vaccine is a mutant strain of *Salmonella typhimurium* that is unable to synthesize galactose epimerase and that therefore undergoes growth inhibition and cell lysis in the body of the host animal following uncontrolled uptake of galactose. These events occur before the organism can cause damage to the host but not before the protective antigens are taken up by the immune system.

Following infection of the animal, there is often a selection for mutants or variants of the infectious bacterium that have increased virulence. This selection is the basis of passaging used experimentally to enhance the virulence of an organism. Conversely, passaging can be used to reduce virulence by repeated sequential inoculation and reisolation from a naturally resistant host. In this situation, there

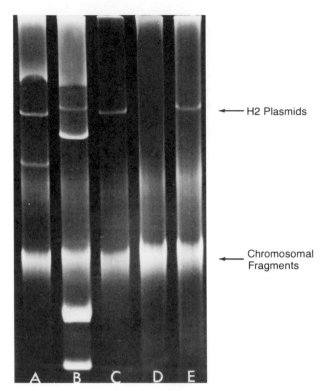

Figure 3.2. Agarose gel electrophoresis of plasmid DNAs from a series of *Salmonella typhimurium* strains with multiple antibiotic resistance and from an antibiotic-sensitive strain (track D). The narrow bands at the top of the picture are H2 incompatibility group plasmids of molecular mass greater than 140 MDa. The wide bands at the same level on all the tracks in the lower half of the picture are produced by chromosomal fragments (10 MDa). The two bands toward the lower end of track B are small plasmids of less than 6 MDa. The logarithm$_{10}$ of the distance of plasmid migration is inversely proportional to the logarithm$_{10}$ of its molecular mass.

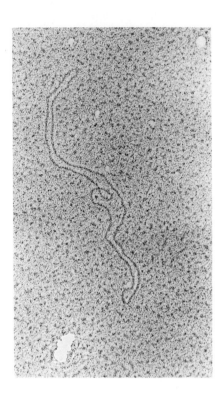

Figure 3.3. Electron micrograph of a small plasmid (6.1 MDa). $\times$ 60,000.

is a selection effect for mutants or variants that lack virulence factors. Because synthesis of these factors is a metabolic burden to the pathogen, mutants that have lost the trait (which is useless in the naturally resistant host) tend to be selected and become dominant. Similarly, pathogenic bacteria often lose virulence traits when plated on artificial media because virulence traits are usually of no survival value for the organism on culture media.

Mutational resistance to penicillin, the tetracyclines, kanamycin, and some other antibiotics arises in a stepwise fashion: mutants with low-level resistance appear first, and then mutants with a higher level of resistance are selected from among these clones. Resistance to streptomycin, however, can be found at a high level in the first generation of mutants, and these are described as "one-step" mutants. Mutational resistance to antibiotics is more common among Gram-positive pathogenic bacteria

than among Gram-negative ones because resistance in the latter group is usually due to genes acquired on plasmids, as is described later in this chapter.

Many antibiotic resistance genes as well as genes for other characteristics are carried on DNA segments that can move (transpose) from one location on the chromosome to another. They can also pass back and forth between plasmid locations and between plasmid locations and the chromosome. These transposable sequences are known as transposons (Tn) and have also been called "jumping genes." All carry a genetic marker as well as genes that encode transposition functions. Most transposons are flanked at each end by inverted repeat sequences that can be inserted within complementary sequences in the chromosome known as insertion sequences (IS). Thus sites on the chromosome or on a plasmid that contains IS elements are prone to acquisition, loss, or inversion of transposons. The IS sites can constitute up to 5 percent of the chromosomal DNA in the Enterobacteriaceae.

Transposons have played an important role in the acquisition of virulence traits and antibiotic resistance by pathogenic bacteria. Their ability to pass from chromosomal to plasmid DNA has facilitated their transfer from one bacterial genus or species to another during conjugation. Antibiotic selection pressure for prophylaxis and therapy is a potent force both for transfer and recombinational events thereby resulting in emergence of new, more complex resistance phenotypes in pathogenic bacteria. An example of this phenomenon has been the emergence of chloramphenicol- and trimethoprim-resistant *S. typhimurium* strains in cattle populations in Britain (Threlfall et al. 1978, 1980). Resistance to beta-lactam antibiotics and to streptomycin, erythromycin-lincomycin, gentamicin-tobramycin, sulfonamide, tetracycline, and fosfononomycin in Gram-negative organisms are encoded on transposons (Davis 1981).

Insertion of a transposon can inactivate a gene and affect the function of nearby genes. Insertional mutation by means of transposons with genes for ampicillin or tetracycline resistance, for example, has become a widely used and effective tool for the study of the contribution of specific genes and their products to virulence of an organism as it allows experimentation with isogenic pairs of strains that differ only in one characteristic.

Gene Transfer Mechanisms in Pathogenic Bacteria

Conjugation

Conjugation is the physical association of two bacteria during which DNA is passed directly from one cell to the other. The transfer can involve chromosomal genes, plasmid genes, or both. Conjugation has been described in several genera of Gram-positive bacteria and in the genera *Salmonella, Shigella, Klebsiella, Vibrio, Escherichia, Pseudomonas, Clostridium,* and *Bacillus.* Conjugation due to the presence of the F, or sex, plasmid in *E. coli* has been thoroughly studied (Falkow 1975). Donor *E. coli* cells (F+) containing the sex plasmid produce a hollow sex pilus, which serves to attach the donor and recipient cells so that the cell surfaces are brought together. It is not known whether the DNA passes through the hollow pilus or directly through the cell walls of the conjugating pair of bacteria. The F factor and part of all of the chromosomal DNA pass across into the recipient cell. In some cells the F factor may integrate into the host chromosome and cause the new host bacterium to exhibit a high frequency of recombination (Hfr). This means that Hfr donors rarely transfer the F factor to recipients but instead transfer their own chromosomal genes at a high frequency.

Many other plasmids can be transferred between bacteria via a conjugative mechanism similar to that of the F factor. The synthesis and transfer functions can be carried on the plasmid, which is then described as conjugative. However, many nonconjugative plasmids exist that lack genes for transfer. Nonconjugative plasmids that lack transfer functions are often mobilized by other coexisting conjugative plasmids; they apparently slip across behind the conjugative plasmid. Because intergeneric and interspecific conjugation is common among the Enterobacteriaceae, genes encoding a variety of traits can be freely exchanged within the intestine and in the environment among members of this family. In this way genes encoding chloramphenicol resistance can quickly pass from a harmless *E. coli* to a virulent *S. typhimurium* when a sick calf, for example, receives chloramphenicol as therapy for salmonellosis. Although such transfer events may be of low frequency, the presence of high concentrations of the antibiotic in the calf's intestine exerts a strong selection pressure for salmonella transconjugants that have received the resistance gene.

Phage Transduction and Conversion

Phage transduction is the process by which bacterial viruses or bacteriophages transfer bacterial genes from one cell to another. The process is called *generalized transduction* when the bacteriophage accidentally incorporates and transfers any bacterial gene. *Restricted,* or *specialized, transduction* is the term used when the phage transfers only the bacterial genes adjoining the prophage position on the bacterial chromosome. Thus, specialized transduction is seen only in the case of bacteriophage that cause temperate infection characterized by survival of some of the infected bacterial cells and incorporation of the phage genome either into the host chromosome or as a plasmidlike molecule in the bacterial cytoplasm.

The plasmid containing the gene for beta lactamase (penicillinase) in *Staphylococcus aureus* can be transferred in this way, and this transfer can occur within the body of the animal. Production of botulinum toxin by *Clostridium botulinum* types C and D and of alpha toxin by *C. novyi* type B is also phage transduced, although the exact mechanism has not yet been determined. Other examples of the involvement of genes carried by bacteriophage in the production or expression of bacterial constituents are the synthesis of O antigens 15 and 36 in *Salmonella* species, the synthesis of hyaluronidase by *Streptococcus equi,* and the production of alpha hemolysin and enterotoxin by *Staphylococcus aureus.*

Transformation

When free DNA released by one bacterium is taken in through the cell wall of another, and the new gene or genes are expressed in the host bacterium, the latter is described as having undergone transformation. Transformation is important in conversion of rough, avirulent pneumococci to the smooth, virulent form. It is also involved in genetic changes in species of *Haemophilus*, *Moraxella*, *Streptococcus*, and *Bacillus*. Its full significance in veterinary bacteriology has still to be discovered.

Antibiotic Resistance

The availability of antibiotics for clinical use in the 1940s was soon followed by the appearance of resistant strains of bacteria. By 1980 world production of antibiotics had reached a level in excess of 25,000 tons, of which a substantial proportion was added to animal feed. The National Academy of Sciences (1980) calculated that in 1978 about 1,600 tons of tetracycline were added to the feed of the 88 million hogs marketed in the United States that year. Another 2,100 tons of antibiotics were added to the diet of other U.S. food-producing species in the same year. The bacterial flora of livestock therefore has been and continues to be exposed to a continuous and relentless selection pressure from the use of antibiotics in feed for growth promotion and prevention as well as for therapy. The effect of this selection pressure has been the appearance of numerous resistant strains of *Escherichia coli*, *Salmonella* species, *Staphylococcus aureus*, *Pasteurella haemolytica*, *P. multocida*, *Streptococcus agalactiae*, *Pseudomonas aeruginosa*, *Klebsiella pneumoniae*, *Haemophilus pleuropneumoniae*, *Clostridium perfringens*, *Treponema hyodysenteriae*, *Bacteroides* species, and many other bacterial species (Table 3.1).

Most of the resistance in these strains has been shown to be mediated by plasmid-encoded genes. Plasmids of this kind are usually described as resistance (R) plasmids, or R factors. R factors were first found in members of the genus *Shigella* in 1959 in Japan and since then have been found in all the other genera of the Enterobacteri-

aceae and in the genera *Pasteurella*, *Vibrio*, *Campylobacter*, *Haemophilus*, *Bacteroides*, *Neisseria*, *Staphylococcus*, *Streptococcus*, *Clostridium*, and *Pseudomonas*. Resistance to a number of different antibiotics can be mediated by the same R factor and is known as multiple antibiotic resistance. This is an important characteristic of R factors and contrasts with mutational type resistance encoded by chromosomal genes in which resistance is against a single antibiotic.

Many of the genes for antibiotic resistance are carried on transposons that can insert on the R factor plasmid at special insertion sites in a region known as the r-determinant. Transposons carrying antibiotic resistance genes can move freely from one plasmid to another and back and forth from similar insertion sites on the chromosome. It is therefore possible for plasmids in virulent bacteria to rapidly acquire new resistance genes from other resistant commensal bacteria in the face of changing antibiotic therapy.

Another important characteristic of many R plasmids of Gram-negative bacteria is that they are conjugative and can mediate their own transfer from organism to organism. This function is carried on a part of the plasmid termed the *resistance transfer factor* (RTF). Conjugative R factor plasmids can also mobilize transfer of other nonconjugative plasmids, which are usually smaller because they lack the DNA necessary for encoding the RTF. Some types of R factor plasmids, such as Inc H, found commonly in *S. typhimurium*, are thermosensitive for transfer and do not transfer at antibody temperature. They appear to be acquired and transferred in the animal's environment (Timoney and Linton 1982).

Classification of R factor plasmids is based mainly on incompatibility (Inc) grouping, DNA homology, and endonuclease digest pattern (Figure 3.3) studies, but other characteristics can be helpful in classification, such as thermosensitivity of transfer, phage restriction, fertility

Table 3.1. Frequency of antibiotic resistance in some important bacterial pathogens of animals

Antibiotic	*E. coli*[*]	*P. multocida*[†]	*P. haemolytica*[‡]	*Salmonella* spp.[§]	*S. aureus*[‖]	*S. aureus*[¶]	*H. pleuropneumoniae*[#]
Ampicillin	35	22	41	31	60	64	6
Kanamycin	22	—	—	40	3	10	8
Streptomycin	60	58	90	66	55	—	83
Sulfonamides	—	88	24	57	—	78	42
Tetracycline	44	23	90	46	33	50	32

[*]Jackson 1981. Cattle.
[†]Fales et al. 1982. Cattle.
[‡]Amstutz et al. 1982. Cattle.
[§]Blackburn et al. 1984. All domestic food animal species.
[‖]Biberstein et al. 1974. All domestic species.
[¶]Prescott et al. 1984. Cattle, horses, dogs, cats.
[#]Libel 1982. Swine.

Table 3.2. The occurrence of H incompatibility group plasmids in multiresistant *Salmonella typhimurium* and enteropathogenic *Escherichia coli* from calves in New York State (1974–1978)

Host organism	Percentages of strains with			
	H only	H and non H*	Non H* only	No transfer
S. typhimurium (134)†	37	37	16	10
E. coli (115)†	1	0	69	30

*Plasmids of incompatibility groups other than H.
†The numbers in parentheses are the number of strains studied.

inhibition, the level of resistance mediated, the resistance determinants carried, and the type of pilus produced (Anderson et al. 1975, Datta 1974). Incompatibility grouping is based on the fact that similar plasmids cannot coexist in the same cell: one will be segregated from daughter cells during cell division. Unrelated plasmids, however, are compatible. Inc groups are designated by letters, for example, FI, FII, H1, H2, I, N, and so forth.

Restriction endonuclease fingerprinting of plasmids in strains of *Salmonella, Klebsiella,* and other potentially pathogenic organisms has proved to be a valuable epidemiological tool in source tracing and in the study of the evolution of resistance plasmids during an epidemic (Holmberg, Osterholm, et al. 1984; Holmberg, Wells, and Cohen 1984; O'Brien et al. 1982). Identical plasmids generate similar-sized fragments when digested by the same restriction endonuclease.

Inc H2 plasmids are of special interest because of the thermosensitivity of their transfer function and because they are associated with epidemics of salmonellosis in humans or animals in which the strain of salmonella hosting the Inc H2 plasmid dominates the salmonella population in a particular geographic area for an extended period. A good example of this phenomenon was observed in calves in New York during the late 1970s (Table 3.2) (Timoney 1978, 1981). The probable basis for this dominance is that the Inc H2 plasmid carries genes that enhance the host organism's ability to persist in the intestine and so enhance the degree and duration of shedding of the organism in the feces (Timoney and Linton 1982).

Inc H plasmids can also acquire genes for metabolic traits such as lactose fermentation. *S. typhimurium* strains carrying such traits are highly virulent in calves receiving a diet containing lactose (Timoney et al. 1980). Laboratory diagnosis is greatly complicated because lactose-positive salmonellas cannot be distinguished from *E. coli* on most differential enteric media.

Many R factors in Gram-positive organisms are non-

conjugative, although conjugative plasmids have been found in *Bacillus, Streptococcus,* and *Clostridium.* Transfer of nonconjugative plasmids must rely on such mechanisms as bacteriophage transduction or on transformation of plasmid DNA, but the involvement of these mechanisms in transfer among Gram-positive organisms in the body is not well understood. Conjugative transposons that can transfer independently of plasmids between Gram-positive species have been described and could be a means by which resistance genes can pass from one Gram-positive strain to another under conditions of antibiotic selection pressure (Clewell 1981).

Mechanisms of Resistance

R factors encode at least four basically different biochemical mechanisms. These involve either enzymic degradation or alteration of the antibiotic, altered uptake or retention of the antibiotic by the cell, alteration of the target site of the antibiotic, and, finally, synthesis of a resistant form of an essential metabolic enzyme that is normally sensitive to the antimicrobial. Some examples of mechanisms of R factor resistance against commonly used antibiotics are shown on Table 3.3 and are discussed in more detail by Davies (1981) and by Hardy (1986). The only chromosomally mediated resistances of importance in clinical situations appear to be those that involve mutational resistance to nitrofurans, nalidixic acid, rifampin, and streptomycin.

The Public Health Significance of Antibiotic Resistance in Animals

The feeding of low levels of antibiotics such as tetracycline and penicillin to poultry, swine, and calves in order to promote growth has resulted in a great increase in the reservoir of resistant bacteria. This increase has been such that resistant bacteria from animals may be contrib-

Table 3.3. Mechanisms of R factor resistance to some commonly used antibiotics and other antimicrobials

Antibiotic or antimicrobial	Resistance mechanism
Ampicillin, penicillin, carbenicillin, cephalosporins	Beta-lactamases cause hydrolysis of lactam ring
Chloramphenicol	Transacetylation resulting in an inactive form of the antibiotic
Erythromycin	Methylation of 23S ribosomal RNA
Amikacin, gentamicin, streptomycin, kanamycin	Acetyl- or phosphotransferase modification of antibiotic that prevents its transport into the cell
Sulfonamides	Formation of a dihydropteroate synthetase resistant to sulfonamide. This enzyme is needed for synthesis of dihydrofolate
Tetracyclines	Reduced uptake and retention
Trimethoprim	Formation of a dihydrofolate reductase resistant to trimethoprim

uting to the reservoir of antibiotic resistance in the bacterial flora of humans, and this may be compromising the efficacy of antimicrobial therapy in humans. Although there is considerable evidence that some antibiotic-resistant *E. coli* can colonize the intestine of humans long enough for transfer of antibiotic resistance to occur (Wells and James 1973), there is as yet no general consensus on whether resistant *E.coli* or other bacteria selected in animals by the feeding of subtherapeutic level of antibiotics contribute substantially to the pool of resistance genes in human pathogens. In fact, it has been determined that it is scientifically impractical to obtain even a crude measure of such a transfer (National Academy of Sciences 1980). The problem is compounded by the fact that R factors from human and animal sources are similar (Anderson and Threlfall 1974). Moreover, the same resistance genes occur in a wide range of pathogenic bacteria, a distribution that transcends distinctions based on genus and family and is related to the transposability of most of the genes involved. However, there have been many well-authenticated outbreaks of transmission of resistant salmonellas from animal sources to humans (Anderson 1968; Holmberg, Osterholm, et al. 1984; Holmberg, Wells, and Cohen 1984; O'Brien et al. 1982; Threlfall et al. 1978).

In some of these reports, the use of antibiotics as feed additives was incriminated as the selection pressure involved in emergence of the resistant *Salmonella* strain. This conclusion is generally incorrect because clinical salmonellosis in animals is usually a serious illness with a high morbidity and mortality and is therefore routinely and aggressively treated by the parenteral administration of antibiotics at therapeutic levels. Thus, the antibiotic selection pressure on virulent *Salmonella* strains in animals is predominantly therapeutic and is, to a great degree, unavoidable.

Human salmonellosis arising from ingestion of meat from salmonella-infected livestock can best be prevented by antemortem and postmortem inspection of the animals at the slaughterhouse by well-trained veterinarians along with routine bacteriological surveillance of packing plants and their end-products.

The effect of subtherapeutic levels of antibiotics on the salmonella flora of carrier animals such as swine and poultry has not been intensively studied, although there are indications that the practice does eventually result in emergence of resistant strains. Moreover, the salmonellas in carrier swine and poultry usually are the less virulent so-called exotic serotypes and not the more virulent multiresistant *S. typhimurium*, *S. dublin*, *S. thompson*, and *S. newport* strains seen in epidemics of human salmonellosis traceable to cattle.

Genetics of Virulence in Bacteria Pathogenic for Animals

Many important virulence properties of bacteria are plasmid encoded and include characteristics of the organism involved in colonization, invasion of intestinal epithelium, toxin production, complement resistance, hemolysis, iron scavenging, lethality, and persistence in the intestine (Table 3.4).

Colonizing Antigens. A number of fimbrial and capsule-associated antigens are known to be important in colonization of the small intestine of pigs, calves, lambs, and humans by enteropathogenic *E. coli* (Figure 3.4). These include the K88 (F4) and K99 (F5), F41, F165, and P987 fimbrial antigens. The K88 gene is flanked by an IS1 insertion sequence and is therefore readily transposable from one plasmid site to another. K88 genes thus have been found on different sized plasmids. Of some interest is the fact that the genes for LT or ST enterotoxins are rarely found on the same plasmid as the K88 gene, although both toxin and colonizing ability are required for production of disease in piglets (Smith and Huggins 1978). The presence of colonizing antigens such as the K88 and K99 antigen allows *E. coli* to attach to the appro-

Table 3.4. Plasmid-encoded virulence characteristics of bacterial pathogens of animals

Virulence trait	Occurrence	Host affected
K88 (F4) colonizing antigen	*Escherichia coli* O groups 8, 45, 138, 141, 147, 149	Piglet
K99 (F5) colonizing antigen	*E. coli* O groups 8, 9, 20, 64, 101	Calf, lamb, piglet
Heat-labile (LT) enterotoxin Heat-stable (ST) enterotoxins	*E. coli*	Calf, lamb, piglet
Hemolysin	*E. coli*	Pig?
Resistance to serum-mediated killing	*E. coli* O groups 78, 8, 1, 2, 36	Calf, piglet, chicken
Iron scavenging	*E. coli* O groups 78, 8, 1, 2, 36	Calf, piglet, chicken
Toxin receptor Capsule	*Bacillus anthracis*	Herbivores and other noncarnivorous species
Tetanus neurotoxin	*Clostridium tetani*	Most domestic species
Penetration of intestinal epithelium	*Salmonella* spp.	All domestic species
Resistance to serum-mediated killing; invasiveness	*Yersinia* spp.	Guinea pig, humans

priate ganglioside on the microvilli of the small intestine and so establish itself in large numbers despite the effect of peristalsis (Figure 3.5). It is only at this site that enterotoxin (ST or LT) can take effect.

The K99 (F5) fimbrial antigen is encoded on a conjugative plasmid of about 52 MDa (Van Embden et al. 1980). The genetic basis of other colonizing antigens such as F41 and P987 has not been as well studied as that of K88 or K99. F41 fimbriae are often found on *E. coli* of O groups 101 and 9 in association with K99 fimbriae (de Graaf and Roords 1982).

Enterotoxins (*E. coli*). Both heat-stable ST and heat-labile LT enterotoxin production is plasmid encoded, the genetic determinants for which can occur together on the same or on separate plasmids (Gyles et al. 1974). Plasmids carrying genes for each of the toxins usually lie in the size range 55 to 60 MDa, whereas genes for ST enterotoxin are found on plasmids whose size is much more variable. The transposability of the ST gene, which is bounded by inverted repeat sequences of IS1, probably accounts for its occurrence on plasmids of varying size.

Genes for enterotoxin production do not usually occur on the same plasmid as are carrying genes for K88 or K99 antigens but can be found in association with genes for antibiotic resistance. Antibiotic selection pressure therefore is a means by which the pool of enterotoxin genes can be increased. The gene for LT toxin has also been found on *E. coli* bacteriophage.

Edema Disease Toxin (*E. coli*). The gene or genes controlling the production of edema disease toxin, although normally chromosomally encoded, are sometimes carried on plasmids that vary between 42 and 55 MDa (Timoney 1986).

Resistance to Complement-Mediated Killing. *E. coli* isolated from invasive septicemic infections in animals have been shown to frequently carry plasmids that encode production of a surface protein that blocks action of the membrane attack complex of complement factors (Timmis et al. 1981).

Plasmid-Mediated Uptake of Iron. Many of the *E. coli* Col V plasmids that have been studied carry genes not only for synthesis of colicin V but also for iron-chelating

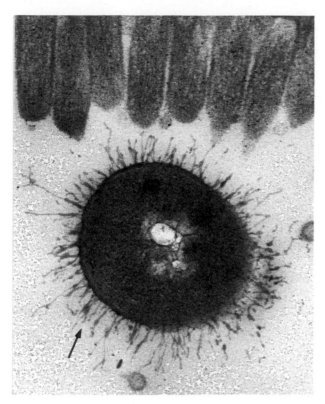

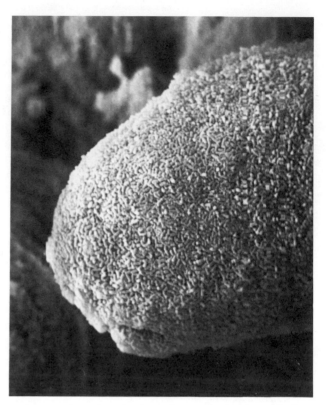

Figure 3.4. Transmission electron micrograph showing K99 (F5) fimbrial antigen on an *Escherichia coli* strain from a calf (*arrow*). These fimbriae are plasmid encoded and mediate adhesion to the microvilli of the anterior small intestine. (Courtesy Harley Moon.)

Figure 3.5. Scanning electron micrograph showing colonization of an intestinal villus of the small intestine of a calf by a K99-positive *Escherichia coli*. (Courtesy Harley Moon.)

hydroxamates that capture iron in the tissues and bloodstream. Because iron is an essential growth factor for *E. coli,* the ability to scavenge iron in competition with host iron-binding proteins is an important virulence trait for invasive strains of the organism.

Hemolysin.   Enteropathogenic *E. coli* in swine are usually hemolytic, a property related to production of a plasmid-encoded hemolysin with a molecular weight of about 107,000 (Bhakdi et al. 1986). The hemolysin gene occurs on conjugative plasmids of varying size and is usually independent of and carried on different plasmids than those carrying genes for enterotoxins or colonizing factors. The role of hemolysin in virulence of *E. coli* in the intestine is not understood. Populations of beta-hemolytic *E. coli* greatly increase in the intestine of pigs immediately after weaning when the animals are introduced to solid feed. It is possible that some other characteristic of value to *E. coli* in the changing milieu of the pigs' intestine at weaning is encoded on the same plasmid as the hemolysin gene and that selection for the latter is therefore "accidental."

Anthrax Capsule and Toxin.   Production of the polyglutamic acid capsule of *Bacillus anthracis* is a necessary

requirement for virulence, and strains that are nonencapsulated, although capable of lethal toxin synthesis, are avirulent. Such strains have been widely used as vaccines. The genes that control encapsulation have been shown to be carried on a 60-MDa plasmid, loss of which results in failure of the organism to produce capsule (Uchida et al. 1985). Similarly, the gene or genes for the protective antigen, the receptor-binding molecule of the anthrax holotoxin, are carried on a 110-MDa plasmid (Mikesell et al. 1983, Vodkin and Leppla 1983). This plasmid is thermosensitive and readily lost at 42.5°C. The loss of virulence at 42.5°C originally observed by Louis Pasteur in 1881 during preparation of the first anthrax vaccine was therefore the result of curing of a theromosensitive plasmid encoding an essential part of the toxin molecule.

Tetanus Neurotoxin.   The thermolabile neurotoxin, tetanospasmin, that is responsible for the clinical signs of tetanus, has been shown to be encoded by a large plasmid of about 50 MDa (Finn et al. 1984). Loss of the plasmid results in loss of toxigenicity by the organism.

Virulence of *Salmonella typhimurium, S. dublin,* and *S. enteritidis*.   Plasmid encoded genes have been shown to contribute to the enteroinvasiveness and virulence of

Salmonella typhimurium (Jones et al. 1982), *S. dublin* (Terakado et al. 1983), and *S. enteriditis* (Nakamura et al. 1985). Homologous DNA regions in plasmids of *S. typhimurium* and *S. dublin* involved in virulence suggest that the plasmid-encoded virulence function is the same in these serotypes. There is some preliminary evidence that it operates during the initial invasion phase of the intestinal epithelium.

Virulence of *Yersinia* species. Although *Yersinia pestis* and *Y. enterocolitica* are not serious pathogens of domestic animals, wild and domestic animal species can be important in the epidemiology of human infection by these bacteria. In laboratory rodents these two *Yersinia* species and *Y. pseudotuberculosis* harbor a related plasmid associated with virulence and Ca^{++}-dependent growth at 37°C. Genes on this plasmid encode a series of outer membrane proteins that are believed to increase resistance of the host cell to the bactericidal activity of normal human serum as well as the ability to penetrate epithelial cells.

REFERENCES

Amstutz, H.E., Morter, R.C., and Armstrong, C.H. 1982. Antimicrobial resistance of strains of *Pasteurella haemolytica* from feedlot cattle. Bovine Pract. 17:52–55.

Anderson, E.S. 1968. The ecology of transferable drug resistance in the enterobacteria. Ann. Rev. Microbiol. 22:131–180.

Anderson, E.S., and Threlfall, E.J. 1974. The characterization of plasmids in the enterobacteria. J. Hyg. 72:471–487.

Anderson, E.S., Humphreys, G.O. and Willshaw, G.A. 1975. The molecular relatedness of R factors in enterobacteria of human and animal origin. J. Gen. Microbiol. 91:376–382.

Bhakdi, S., Mackman, N., Nicaud, J., and Holland, I.B. 1986. *Escherichia coli* may damage target cell membranes by generating transmembrane pores. Infect. Immun. 52:63–69.

Biberstein, E.L., Franti, C.E., Jang, S.S., and Ruby, A. 1974. Antimicrobial sensitivity patterns in *Staphylococcus aureus* from animals. J. Am. Vet. Med. Assoc. 164:1183–1186.

Birge, E.A. 1981. Bacterial and Bacteriophage Genetics. Springer-Verlag, New York.

Blackburn, B.O., Schlater, L.K., and Swanson, M.R. 1984. Antibiotic resistance of the genus *Salmonella* isolated from chickens, turkeys, cattle and swine in the U.S. during October 1981 through September 1982. Am. J. Vet. Res. 45:1247–1249.

Clewell, D.B. 1981. Conjugation and resistance transfer in streptococci and other Gram-positive species: Plasmids, sex pheromones, and "conjugative transposons" (a review). In S.B. Levy, R.C. Clowes, and E.L. Koenig, eds., Molecular Biology, Pathogenicity, and Ecology of Bacterial Plasmids. Plenum Press, New York. Pp. 191–205.

Datta, N. 1974. Epidemiology and classification of plasmids. In D. Schlessinger, ed., Microbiology—1974. American Society of Microbiology, Washington, D.C. Pp. 9–15.

Davis, J.E. 1981. Antibiotic resistance—a survey. In S.B. Levy, R.C. Clowes, and E.L. Koenig, ed., Molecular Biology, Pathogenicity, and Ecology of Bacterial Plasmids. Plenum Press, New York. Pp. 145–156.

de Graaf, F.K., and Roords, I. 1982. Production, purification and characterization of the fimbrial adhesive antigen F41 isolated from calf enteropathogenic *Escherichia coli* strain B41 M. Infect. Immun. 36:751–758.

Dorn, C.R., Tsutakawa, R.K., Fein, D., Burton, G.C., and Blenden, D.C. 1975. Antibiotic resistance patterns of *Escherichia coli* isolated from farm families consuming home-raised meat. Am. J. Epidemiol. 102:319–326.

Fales, W.H., Selby, L.A., and Webber, J.J. 1982. Antimicrobial resistance among *Pasteurella* spp. recovered from Missouri and Iowa cattle with bovine respiratory disease complex. J. Am. Vet. Med. Assoc. 181:477–479.

Falkow, S. 1975. Infectious Multiple Drug Resistance. Pion, London.

Finn, C.W., Silver, R.P., Habig, W.H., Herdegree, M.C., and Garon, C.F. 1984. The structural gene for tetanus neurotoxin is on a plasmid. Science 224:881–884.

Gyles, C., So, M. and Falkow, S. 1974. The enterotoxin plasmid of *Escherichia coli*. J. Infect. Dis. 130:40–49.

Hardy, K. 1986. Bacterial Plasmids, 2d ed. American Society for Microbiology, Washington, D.C.

Holmberg, S.D., Osterholm, M.T., Senger, K.A., and Cohen, M.L. 1984. Drug-resistant *Salmonella* from animals fed antimicrobials. N. Engl. J. Med. 311:617–622.

Holmberg, S.D., Wells, J.G., and Cohen, M.L. 1984. Animal-to-man transmission of antimicrobial-resistant *Salmonella*: Investigations of U.S. outbreaks, 1971–1983. Science 224:833–835.

Jackson, G. 1981. A survey of antibiotic resistance of *Escherichia coli* isolated from farm animals in Great Britain from 1971–1977. Vet. Rec. 108:325–328.

Jones, G.W., Robert, D.K., Svinarich, D.M., and Whitefield, M.J. 1982. Association of adhesive, invasive, and virulent phenotypes of *Salmonella typhimurium* with autonomous 60 megadalton plasmids. Infect. Immun. 38:476–487.

Kopecko, D.J., and Baron, L.S. 1985. Gene expression and evolution in bacteria: Genetic and molecular bases. In B.A. Freeman, ed., Burrows Textbook of Microbiology, 22d ed. W.B. Saunders, Philadelphia. Pp. 161–227.

Libel, M.C., and Gates, C.E. 1982. Antimicrobial sensitivity patterns of *Haemophilus pleuropneumoniae* isolates from pigs with pneumonia. J. Am. Vet. Med. Assoc. 180:399–403.

Lin, E.C.C., Goldstein, R., and Syvanen, M. 1984. Bacteria, Plasmids, and Phages. An Introduction to Molecular Biology. Harvard University Press, Cambridge, Mass.

Mikesell, P.L., Ivins, B.E., Ristroph, J.D., and Dreier, T.M. 1983. Evidence for plasmid-mediated toxin production in *Bacillus anthracis*. Infect. Immun. 39:371–376.

Nakamura, M., Sato, S., Ohya, T., Suzuki, S., and Ikeda, S. 1985. Possible relationship of a 36-megadalton *Salmonella enteritidis* plasmid to virulence in mice. Infect. Immun. 47:831–833.

National Academy of Sciences. 1980. The Effects on Human Health of Subtherapeutic Use of Antimicrobials in Animal Foods. Report. NAS, Washington, D.C. P. 333.

O'Brien, T.F., Hopkins, J.D., Gilleece, E.S., Medeiros, A.A., and Kent, R.L. 1982. Molecular epidemiology of antibiotic resistance in salmonella from animals and human beings in the United States. N. Engl. J. Med. 307:1–6.

Prescott, J.F., Gannon, V.P., Kittler, G., and Hlywka, G. 1984. Antimicrobial drug susceptibility of bacteria isolated from disease processes in cattle, horses, dogs, and cats. Can. Vet. J. 25:289–292.

Smith, H.W., and Huggins, M.B. 1978. The influence of plasmid and other characteristics of enteropathogenic *E. coli* on their ability to proliferate on the alimentary tracts of piglets, calves and lambs. J. Med. Microbiol. 11:471–477.

Terakado, N., Sekizaki, T., Hashimoto, K., and Naitoh, S. 1983. Correlation between the presence of a fifty-megadalton plasmid in *Salmonella dublin* and virulence for mice. Infect. Immun. 41:443–444.

Threlfall, E.J., Ward, L.R., Ashley, A.S., and Rowe, B. 1980. Plasmid encoded trimethoprim resistance in multiresistant epidemic *Salmonella typhimurium* phage types 204 and 193 in Britain. Br. Med. J. 1:1210–1213.

Threlfall, E.J., Ward, L.R., and Rowe, B. 1978. Spread of multiresistant strains of *S. typhimurium* phage types 204 and 193 in Britain. Br. Med. J. 2:997.

Timmis, K.E., Manning, P.A., Echarti, C., Timmis, F.K., and Moll, A. 1981. Serum resistance in *E. coli*. In S.B. Levy, R.C. Clowes, and

E.L. Koenig, eds., Molecular Biology, Pathogenicity, and Ecology of Bacterial Plasmids. Plenum Press, New York. Pp. 133–144.

Timoney, J.F. 1978. The epidemiology and genetics of antibiotic resistance of *Salmonella typhimurium* isolated from diseased animals in New York. J. Infect. Dis. 137:67–73.

Timoney, J.F. 1981. R plasmids in pathogenic Enterobacteriaceae from calves. In S.B. Levy, R.C. Clowes, and E.L. Koenig, eds., Molecular Biology, Pathogenicity, and Ecology of Bacterial Plasmids. Plenum Press, New York. Pp. 547–555.

Timoney, J.F. 1986. Genetic and characterization studies on edema disease toxin. Proceedings of the 9th International Pig Veterinary Society Congress, Barcelona, Spain. P. 199.

Timoney, J.F., and Linton, A.H. 1982. Experimental ecological studies on H2 plasmids in the intestine and faeces of the calf. J. Appl. Bacteriol. 52:417–424.

Timoney, J.F., Taylor, D.E., Shin, S., and McDonough, P. 1980. pJT2: Unusual H1 plasmid in a highly virulent lactose-positive and chloramphenicol-resistant *Salmonella typhimurium* strain from calves. Antimicrob. Agents Chemother. 18:480–482.

Uchida, I., Sekizaki, T., Hashimoto, K., and Terakado, N. 1985. Association of the encapsulation of *Bacillus anthracis* with a 60 megadalton plasmid. J. Gen. Microbiol. 131:363–367.

Van Embden, J.D.A., de Graaf, F.K., Schouls, C.M., and Teppema, J.S. 1980. Cloning and expression of a deoxyribonucleic acid fragment that encodes for the adhesive antigen K99. Infect. Immun. 29:1125–1133.

Vodkin, M.H., and Leppla, S.H. 1983. Cloning of the protective antigen gene of *Bacillus anthracis*. Cell 34:693–697.

Wells, D.M., and James, O.B. 1973. Transmission of infectious drug resistance from animals to man. J. Hyg. 71:209–215.

4 The Genus *Pseudomonas*

Members of the genus *Pseudomonas* are commonly found in aquatic habitats and in soil. One species, *P. mallei,* is a specialized mammalian parasite. Two others, *P. pseudomallei* and *P. aeruginosa,* are occasional parasites of animals. All except *P. mallei* are motile by means of polar flagella and are rod-shaped and oxidase-positive. The mol% G + C of the DNA ranges from 58 to 71.

Pseudomonas aeruginosa

SYNONYMS: Bacillus of green pus,
Pseudomonas pyocyaneus

P. aeruginosa is an organism of comparatively low virulence that is frequently the cause of suppurative infections in domestic animals. Many infections are opportunistic and are commonly associated with wounds, immunosuppressive therapy, prolonged administration of broad-spectrum antibiotics, burns, or debilitating surgery. *P. aeruginosa* can cause severe epizootics of respiratory disease in mink and chinchillas. The organism is especially common in the intestinal contents of chickens and can result in early spoilage of chicken meat. It causes "green wool" in sheep—a condition associated with wetting of the fleece.

Morphology and Staining Reactions. *P. aeruginosa* is a straight, slender rod that measures 2.5 by 0.4 μm. Organisms in young cultures are rapidly motile by means of one to three polar flagella. Spores are not formed and a capsule is sometimes present. The organism is Gram-negative and stains readily with the ordinary dyes.

Cultural and Biochemical Features. *P. aeruginosa* is readily recognized by its bright green pigment and the characteristic grapclike odor (aminoacetophenone) it produces. The pigment consists of fluorescein (a pyoverdin), which is yellowish green and becomes oxidized to yellow, and pyocyanin, a bluish green pigment that oxidizes to brown. Both fluorescein and pyocyanin are water soluble, but only pyocyanin is soluble in chloroform. Some strains lose their ability to produce pigment upon prolonged culture. Apyocyanogenic strains are fairly common and must be identified by their mucoid growth on potassium gluconate medium.

P. aeruginosa is an obligate aerobe that uses oxygen as a terminal electron receptor. It can be cultivated on the simplest of media (Figure 4.1). Most strains produce smooth, shiny, moist, fimbriate, and spreading colonies. Colonies have thin, irregular margins, and the translucent centers are cream-colored, although this color often is disguised by the green pigment that stains the surroundings. An opalescent sheen characteristically appears on the surface of growths on solid media. The organism grows well at a range of incubation temperatures (4° to 42°C).

The organism does not ferment carbohydrates, but some strains have been shown to produce acid from D-arabinose, L-arabinose, D-glucose, D-mannose, and D-xylose. It is indole-, methyl red–, and Voges-Proskauer-negative and is catalase- and oxidase-positive. Most strains from disease lesions liquefy gelatin and are urease-positive and hemolytic. The mol% G + C of the DNA is 67.2.

Antigens and Toxins. There are 17 somatic O antigens

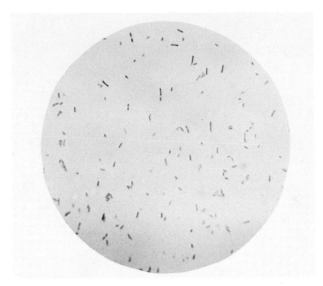

Figure 4.1. *Pseudomonas aeruginosa* from a culture on a slant agar incubated for 18 hours at 37°C. × 1,150.

(Bergan 1975, Pitt and Erdman 1977) and 6 H, or flagellar, antigens (Pitt 1981).

P. aeruginosa produces several toxic products, including toxin A, alkaline proteases, and elastase. Elastase, which destroys elastin in lung parenchyma, has been shown to be an important virulence factor in the pathogenesis of experimentally induced pneumonia (Blackwood et al. 1983). Toxin A, an inhibitor of protein synthesis, contributes significantly to lesion development in burn infections.

Bacteriocin Typing.   Strains of *P. aeruginosa* produce bacteriocins, substances that kill other strains of the same species. The particular bacteriocins produced by *P. aeruginosa* are proteins known as pyocins. Pyocin typing can be performed either by testing an extract of an unknown organism against a collection of indicator strains or by testing the sensitivity of the unknown strain to known pyocins. The technique has been reviewed by Brokopp and Farmer (1979). In North America, strains from animals seem to produce mainly pyocin types 1 and 3 (Lusis and Soltys 1971). Strains that produce type 1 also dominate among strains from cases of mastitis in Israel (Murkin and Ziv 1972).

Phage Typing.   The technique of phage typing is used to distinguish between *P. aeruginosa* strains of the same O group. It is useful epidemiologically only in conjunction with other typing procedures. Its lack of reproducibility is such that at least three differences in reaction must be obtained for the strains to be considered different phage types. The procedure involves spotting known phage suspensions on an overlay of the test strain

and noting the lysis pattern after incubation (Bergan 1978).

Epizootiology and Pathogenesis.   *P. aeruginosa* is often a component of the normal flora of the skin, mucous membranes, and intestine of healthy animals. Its presence in these locations reflects the animal's exposure to environmental sources such as water and soil. It is an opportunistic pathogen, and disease in animals is usually associated with such predisposing circumstances as wounds, corneal injury, parasitic or fungal infections of the skin, pneumovagina, otitis externa, excessive wetting of the fleece, exposure to contaminated disinfectants or therapeutics, heavy and prolonged exposure to antimicrobials, or poor sanitation.

Toxin A and proteases appear to be important in the production of the edema, induration, hemorrhage, and necrosis that is observed in skin lesions. Focal necrosis and hemorrhages are also a feature of pseudomonas pneumonia in mink (Long et al. 1980).

Toxin production in vivo is apparently enhanced by the ready availability of the amino acids aspartic acid, glutamic acid, and alpha-alanine in animal tissue. The extracellular slime produced by the organism is antiphagocytic and facilitates the organism's penetration of tissue. Protease production is greater in tissue with an elevated lactic acid concentration; thus the organism has greater penetration ability in injured tissue. Strains from lesions are more virulent than environmental strains and often produce hemolysis, a trait that is rare in the latter.

P. aeruginosa is often found in necrotic pneumonias, enteritis, and rhinitis of swine and in lesions associated with traumatic reticulopericarditis in cattle. The organism is a frequent cause of bovine mastitis, and outbreaks involving all four quarters simultaneously have been traced to contaminated intramammary infusions (Nicholls et al. 1980, Tucker 1950). The affected cows exhibited signs of endotoxemia and some died. Malmo et al. (1972) reported that water used for washing udders, or rinsing milking machines was also a source of pseudomonas infection for bovine mammary glands. In this outbreak, carrier cows were later responsible for secondary cases. In England, the incidence of pseudomonas mastitis appears to increase in August, September, and October (Anon. 1977); the reason for this is unclear. The disease may be characterized by chronic inflammation with periodic flare-ups, and the organism may be difficult to culture from affected animals. Infusion of endotoxin sometimes cures the infection because of the leukocytosis it induces.

P. aeruginosa has been implicated as a cause of bovine infertility (Corradini and Binato 1961). Heifers inseminated with semen containing this pathogen develop varying degrees of uteritis, cervicitis, and vaginitis. It has also been reported as the cause of sporadic abortions in cattle. The organism has been shown to be spermicidal (Schwerdtner 1961) and has caused balanoposthitis in bulls (Corrias and Molliniar 1958). It is also transmitted by stallions and can cause metritis and infertility in mares (Atherton and Pitt 1982; Gorg et al. 1983; Hughes, Asbury, et al. 1966; Hughes, Loy, et al. 1966). Type O3, H3 accounted for 50 percent of isolates from the United Kingdom and Ireland in the study by Atherton and Pitt. Other O serotypes were O2a, O4, O6, O9, and O10. After a difficult parturition, mares appear to be at greater risk of developing metritis after insemination by an infected stallion. Abortion caused by *P. aeruginosa* has also been described in mares.

In dogs the organism causes a suppurative otitis externa as a complication of injury, mange, or other bacterial and fungal infections. Postoperative septicemia caused by *P. aeruginosa* has been described in dogs that have undergone experimental cardiovascular surgery (Cross et al. 1975).

P. aeruginosa infection is perhaps most devastating in mink (Farrell et al. 1958) and chinchillas, in which it causes hemorrhagic pneumonia (Figure 4.2). The disease occurs throughout the world and has a mortality of up to 50 percent. It is common in the fall when kits are growing most rapidly. The organism apparently enters when the animal sniffs its food. The clinical course is short. Affected mink may be depressed and show tachypnea. A frothy, red fluid is characteristically expressed from the nares. The lungs are hemorrhagic with areas of necrosis, and the organism is present as microscopic colonies in these areas and free in the airways and parenchyma. In North America most epizootics of pseudomonas pneumonia in mink are caused by strains of serotype O1 (group G) (Long and Gorham 1981).

"Green wool," or fleece-rot, in sheep results from the growth of *Pseudomonas* species in fleeces subjected to prolonged wetting (Merritt and Watts 1978). Multiplication of the organism is favored by the presence of protein that leaks out of the macerated skin. A dermatitis results, and the wool fibers separate. The protein in the accumulated exudate degrades, resulting in an odor that stimulates oviposition by flies. Sheep affected with fleece-rot are thereby predisposed to the development of strike.

P. aeruginosa is also an opportunistic invader of the traumatized cornea. The corneas of racing horses are sometimes damaged by sand grains. The injured cornea is then invaded by *P. aeruginosa*, and the subsequent opacification and ulcer formation is difficult to treat (Ueda, Sanai, and Homma 1982). The lesions result from the activity of the toxin A, proteases, and elastase produced by the organism.

Immunity. Protective antibodies against *P. aeruginosa* may be opsonizing and directed against either the cell wall lipopolysaccharide, which is strain specific, or the endotoxin-associated protein (OEP), which is not

Figure 4.2. A colony of *Pseudomonas aeruginosa* in a section of lung from a mink with hemorrhagic pneumonia. × 700. (From Farrell et al., 1958, courtesy of *Cornell Veterinarian*.)

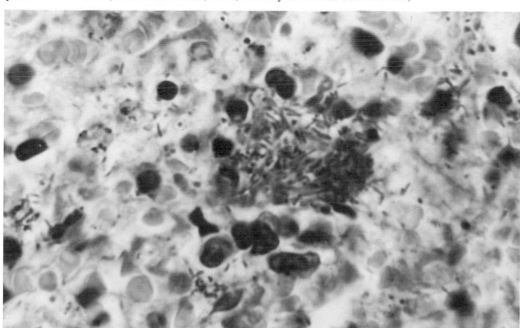

(Abe et al. 1977). Antibodies against toxin A, proteases, and elastase are also protective (Homma et al. 1978) and, as with OEP, are not strain or O type specific.

Vaccination of mink with bacterins and toxoids has been practiced widely and successfully for many years. Recent work by Homma and his colleagues (1978, 1980) has shown that a combination of OEP, protease, and elastase toxoids is much superior to formalinized cells in stimulating a protective response in mink. Furthermore, the response is not strain specific. This type of vaccine has also been used in the treatment of horses with corneal ulceration caused by *P. aeruginosa* (Ueda, Homma, and Abe 1982). Lesions in immunized horses are much less severe and heal more rapidly than those in nonimmunized control animals. Intracorneal injection of immunoglobulins from immunized horses has also proved to be effective therapy for corneal ulcers in experimentally infected horses (Ueda, Sanai, and Homma 1982). The antibody treatment neutralizes the proteases released by *P. aeruginosa*.

Antimicrobial Susceptibility.   Most strains of *P. aeruginosa* found in animal lesions have multiple resistance patterns that are commonly mediated by R factors. Antimicrobials that are likely to be effective against the different strains include gentamicin, tobramycin, carbenicillin (Hirsh et al. 1979), polymyxin B, amikacin, and colistin (Cox and Luther 1980). Silver sulfadiazine (1 percent) has been shown to be very active against multiresistant strains recovered from dogs with otitis externa (van den Bogaard et al. 1982).

REFERENCES

Abe, C., Tanamoto, K. and Homma, J.Y. 1977. Infection protective property of the common antigen (OEP) of *Pseudomonas aeruginosa* and its chemical composition. Jpn. J. Exp. Med. 47:393–402.

Anonymous. 1977. Coliform and psuedomonad mastitis: Epidemiology and control. Vet. Rec. 100:441–442.

Atherton, J.G., and Pitt, T.L. 1982. Types of *Pseudomonas aeruginosa* isolated from horses. Equine Vet. J. 14:329–332.

Bergan, T. 1975. Epidemiologic typing of *Pseudomonas aeruginosa*. In M.R.W. Brown, ed., Resistance of *Pseudomonas aeruginosa*. John Wiley & Sons, London. Pp. 189–235.

Bergan, T. 1978. Phage typing of *Pseudomonas aeruginosa*. In T. Bergan and J.R. Norris, eds., Methods in Microbiology, vol. 10. Academic Press, London. Pp. 169–199.

Blackwood, L.L., Stone, R.M., Iglewski, B.H., and Pennington, J.E. 1983. Evaluation of *Pseudomonas aeruginosa* exotoxin A and elastase as virulence factors in acute lung infection. Infect. Immun. 39:198–201.

Brokopp, C.D., and Farmer, J.J. 1979. Typing methods for *Pseudomonas aeruginosa*. In R.G. Doggett ed., *Pseudomonas aeruginosa*. Clinical Manifestations of Infection and Current Therapy. Academic Press, New York. Pp. 89–133.

Corc, H.U., and Luther, D.G. 1980. Determination of antimicrobial susceptibility of *Pseudomonas aeruginosa* by disk diffusion and microdilution methods. Am. J. Vet. Res. 41:906–909.

Corradini, L., and Binato, L. 1961. Su un caso di aborto da *Pseudomoinas* nel bovino. Vet. Ital. 12:320–322.

Corrias, A., and Molinari, G. 1958. Grave infezione da *Pseudomonasaeruginosa* in un gruppo di tori adibiti alla fecondazione artificiale. Atti Soc. Ital. Sci. Vet. 123:243–248.

Cross, M.R., Cooper, J.E., and Needham, J.R. 1975. Observations on a post-operative septicaemia in experimental dogs with particular reference to *Pseudomonas aeruginosa*. J. Comp. Pathol. 85:445–451.

Farrell, R.K., Leader, R.W., and Gorham, J.R. 1958. An outbreak of hemorrhagic pneumonia in mink. A case report. Cornell Vet. 48:378–383.

Gorg, D.N., Manchanda, V.P., and Chandiramons, N.K. 1983. *Pseudomonas aeruginosa* associated equine abortion, mare infertility and foal mortality. Indian J. Anim. Sci. 53:36–40.

Hirsh, D.C., Wiger, N., and Knox, S.J. 1979. Susceptibility of clinical isolates of *Pseudomonas aeruginosa* to antimicrobial agents. J. Vet. Pharmacol. Ther. 2:275–278.

Homma, J.Y. 1980. Roles of exoenzymes and exotoxin in the pathogenicity of *Pseudomonas aeruginosa* and the development of a new vaccine. Jpn. J. Exp. Med. 47:393–402.

Homma, J.Y., Abe, C., and Tanamoto, K. 1978. Effectiveness of immunization with single and multicomponent vaccines prepared from a common antigen (OEP) and protease and elastase toxoids of *Pseudomonas aeruginosa* on protection against hemorrhagic pneumonia in mink due to *P. aeruginosa*. Jpn. J. Exp. Med. 48:111–113.

Hughes, J.P., Asbury, A.C., Loy, R.G., and Burd, H.E. 1966. The occurrence of *Pseudomonas* in the genital tract of stallions and its effect on fertility. Cornell Vet. 57:53–69.

Hughes, J.P., Loy, R.G., Asbury, A.C., and Burd, H.E. 1966. The occurrence of *Pseudomonas* in the reproductive tract of mares and its effect on fertility. Cornell Vet. 56:595.

Long, G.G., and Gorham, J.R. 1981. Field studies: Pseudomonas pneumonia of mink. Am. J. Vet. Res. 42:2129–2133.

Long, G.G., Gallina, A.M., and Gorham, J.R. 1980. Pseudomonas pneumonia of mink. Pathogenesis, vaccination and serologic studies. Am. J. Vet. Res. 41:1720–1725.

Lusis, P.I., and Soltys, M.A. 1971. *Pseudomonas aeruginosa*. Vet. Bull. 41:169–172.

Malmo, J., Robinson, B., and Morris, R.S. 1972. An outbreak of mastitis due to *Pseudomonas aeruginosa* in a dairy herd. Aust. Vet. J. 48:137–139.

Merritt, G.C., and Watts, J.E. 1978. The changes in protein concentration and bacteria of fleece and skin during the development of fleece-rot and body strike in sheep. Aust. Vet. J. 54:517–520.

Murkin, R., and Ziv, G. 1973. An epidemiological study of *Pseudomonas aeruginosa* in cattle and other animals by pyocine typing. J. Hyg. 71:113–122.

Nicholls, T.J., Barton, M.G., and Anderson, B.P. 1980. An outbreak of mastitis in a dairy herd due to *Pseudomonas aeruginosa* contamination of dry-cow therapy at manufacture. Vet. Rec. 108:93–96.

Pitt, T.L. 1981. Preparation of agglutination antisera specific for the flagellar antigens of *Pseudomonas aeruginosa*. J. Med. Microbiol. 14:254–260.

Pitt, T.L., and Erdman, Y.J. 1977. The specificity of agglutination reactions of *Pseudomonas aeruginosa* with O antisera. J. Med. Microbiol. 11:15–23.

Schwerdtner, H. Von. 1961. Über das Vorkommen und die Bedeutung von *Pseudomonas aeruginosa* bei Besamungsbullen. Zuchthyg. Forpl. Stor. Besam. Haustiere 5:260–264.

Tucker, E.W. 1950. Pseudomonas infection of bovine udder apparently contracted from contaminated treatment equipment and material. Cornell Vet. 40:95–96.

Ueda, Y., Homma, J.Y., and Abe, C. 1982. Effects of immunization of horses with common antigen (OEP) protease toxoid, and elastase toxoid on corneal ulceration due to *P. aeruginosa* infection. Jpn. J. Vet. Sci. 44:289–300.

Ueda, Y., Sanai, Y., and Homma, J.Y. 1982. Therapeutic effect of intracorneal injection of immunoglobulins on corneal ulcers in horses experimentally infected with *Pseudomonas aeruginosa*. Jpn. J. Vet. Sci. 44:301–308.

van den Bogaard, A.E.J.M., Maes, J.H.J., and Simons, H.P. 1982. Silver sulfadiazine cream in the treatment of chronic pseudomonas infection of the external auditory canal in 15 dogs. Tijdschr. Diergeneesk. 107:224–228.

Pseudomonas pseudomallei

SYNONYMS: Bacillus of Whitmore, *Malleomyces pseudomallei, Malleomyces whitmori*

P. pseudomallei causes melioidosis, a glanderslike disease first described by Whitmore and Krishnaswami (1912) in Rangoon. The organism is widely distributed in tropical regions in Southeast Asia but has also been observed in wild and domestic animals in France, Australia, and the Caribbean. In endemic areas it is widespread in soil and water.

Morphology and Staining Reactions. *P. pseudomallei* is a Gram-negative bacillus (1.5 by 0.8 μm) with polar flagella. The organism closely resembles *P. aeruginosa*. It may show bipolar staining.

Cultural and Biochemical Features. Colonies are readily formed on simple media. They range from rough to mucoid and from cream-colored to orange. Strains of *P. pseudomallei* usually produce acid from glucose, maltose, sucrose, and mannitol. They liquefy gelatin and produce oxidase, although not pyoverdin. They usually reduce nitrate, producing gas as well. Some strains are hemolytic. Growth occurs at 42°C. The mol% G + C of the DNA is 69.5.

Epizootiology and Pathogenesis. The organism is widely distributed in the soil and water of endemic areas. In Australia it has been known to survive for up to 30 months in moist soil (Thomas et al. 1981). The organism can also occur in feces and therefore may be disseminated by manure spreading. Animals become infected either by inhaling the organism or by its entry through a wound. Although humans and most animals are susceptible to infection, the naturally occurring infection appears to involve rodents primarily. Transmission to these animals can occur through insect bites (Mirick et al. 1946). Direct transmission of infection between animals or from animals to humans is rare. Melioidosis has been observed in cats, dogs, pigs, goats, sheep, horses, and dolphins.

The characteristic lesion is a small caseous nodule. These nodules can coalesce to form large areas of caseation, or they can break down into abscesses. The nodules can be found in the lymph nodes, spleen, lungs, liver, joints, nasal cavity, tonsils, and other organs (Omar 1963). Most infections, however, are clinically inapparent.

Guinea pigs and rabbits are highly susceptible to infection, and inoculated male guinea pigs may develop the Straus reaction, a purulent orchitis. *P. pseudomallei* has been isolated from an aborted goat fetus (Retnasabapathy 1966). It has been reported as the cause of vertebral abscesses on the spinal cord of lambs, which leads to posterior flaccid paralysis (Ketterer and Bamford 1967). Cattle with an acute fatal infection show pneumonia, placentitis, and endometritis; those with a chronic infection have encapsulated caseous lesions in the lungs and arthritis (Ketterer et al. 1975). Infection was common in military dogs used in the Vietnam War. The affected animals exhibited fever, myalgia, dermal abscesses, and epididymitis (Moe et al. 1972).

Diagnosis. Diagnosis of melioidosis depends on isolation and identification of the organism rather than on clinical findings or serologic tests. Moe et al. (1972) diagnosed canine melioidosis by culturing blood and lesions and by using a hemagglutination test on serum. Fluorescent antiserum is available for laboratory identification of *P. pseudomallei*. Complement-fixation tests and agglutination tests can provide additional laboratory confirmation of infection (Nigg and Johnston 1961, Omar 1962). A complement-fixing antibody titer of 1:20 indicates active or recent infection.

Antimicrobial Susceptibility. *P. pseudomallei* is sensitive to a combination of trimethoprim and sulfamethoxazole (Bassett 1971) and to a combination of novobiocin and tetracycline (Calabi 1973). Strains from the environment and various animal species have shown resistance to a variety of antimicrobials, including cloxacillin, colistin, gentamicin, and polymyxin B (Thomas and Forbes-Faulkner 1981).

REFERENCES

Bassett, D.C.J. 1971. The sensitivity of *Pseudomonas pseudomallei* to trimethoprim and sulphamethoxazole in vitro. J. Clin. Pathol. 24:798–800.

Calabi, O. 1973. Bactericidal synergism of novobiocin and tetracycline against *Pseudomonas pseudomallei*. J. Med. Microbiol. 6:293–305.

Ketterer, P.J., and Bamford, V.W. 1967. A case of melioidosis in lambs in South Western Australia. Aust. Vet. J. 43:79–80.

Ketterer, P.J., Donald, B., Rogers, R.J. 1975. Bovine melioidosis in South-Eastern Queensland. Aust. Vet. J. 51:395–398.

Mirick, G.S., Zimmerman, H.M., Maner, G.D., and Humphrey, A.A. 1946. Melioidosis in Guam. J.A.M.A. 130:1063–1067.

Moe, J.B., Stedham, M.A., Jennings, P.B. 1972. Canine melioidosis. Am. J. Trop. Med. Hyg. 21:351–355.

Nigg, C., and Johnston, M.M. 1961. Complement fixation test in experimental, clinical and subclinical melioidosis. J. Bacteriol. 82:159–168.

Omar, A.R. 1962. Observations on porcine melioidosis in Malaya. Br. Vet. J. 118:421–429.

Omar, A.R. 1963. Pathology of melioidosis in pigs, goats, and a horse. J. Comp. Path. Ther. 73:357–372.

Retnasabapathy, A. 1966. Isolation of *Pseudomonas pseudomallei* from an aborted goat fetus. Vet. Rec. 79:166.

Thomas, A.D., and Forbes-Faulkner, J.C. 1981. Persistence of *Pseudomonas pseudomallei* in soil. Aust. Vet. J. 57:535–536.

Thomas, A.D., Forbes-Faulkner, J.C., and Duffield, B.J. 1981. Susceptibility of *Pseudomonas pseudomallei* isolates of non-human origin to chemotherapeutic agents by the single disc sensitivity method. Vet. Microbiol. 6:367–374.

Whitmore, A., and Krishnaswami, C.S. 1912. A glanders-like disease occurring in Rangoon. Indian Med. Gaz. 47:262.

Pseudomonas mallei

SYNONYMS: *Actinobacillus mallei, Bacillus mallei, Bacterium mallei, Corynebacterium mallei, Loefferella mallei, Malleomyces mallei, Mycobacterium mallei, Pfeifferella mallei*

P. mallei is the cause of glanders, a disease primarily of solipeds (members of the horse family). Humans and dogs are susceptible to the disease, as are lions that have eaten infected horse meat. The disease is one of the oldest known and was described by the ancient Greeks and Romans. It was recognized as contagious as early as the seventeenth century, but it was not until 1882 that Loeffler and Schultz isolated *P. mallei* and showed it to be the etiologic agent.

Morphology and Staining Reactions. In young cultures the organisms are long, slender rods. Older cultures often are quite pleomorphic, with the bacilli varying from coccoid elements to long, slender filaments. The longer rods usually are distinctively beaded with accumulated granules of poly-β-hydroxybutyrate. Shorter rods can appear bipolar because of granules that lie at each end of the cell. The width of the organism is 0.3 to 0.5 μm and the length is 0.7 to 5.0 μm. The organisms are always Gram-negative. Spores are not formed. There are no capsules or flagella. The organism stains poorly with the weaker dyes.

Cultural and Biochemical Features. *P. mallei* grows well but slowly on ordinary laboratory media. A selective medium for isolating the organism has been developed by Xie et al. (1980). It contains polymyxin B (10 IU/ml), bacitracin (12.5 IU/ml), and actidione (2.5 μm/ml). Growth is enhanced by the addition of glycerol. Colonies are small, round, convex, translucent, and yellowish. As they age, they become brownish. In the presence of glycerol, the growth can become honeylike and confluent. The organism usually does not liquefy gelatin. Carbohydrates, with the exception of glucose, are not fermented or are only weakly fermented. *P. mallei* is not hemolytic, does not reduce nitrates, and does not grow at 42°C. The mol% G + C of the DNA is 69.

Epizootiology and Pathogenesis. *P. mallei* is an obligate parasite of horses, mules, and donkeys. Humans, dogs, members of the family Felidae (e.g., lions), and other carnivorous animals have been infected accidentally either by contact with diseased horses or after consumption of meat from diseased animals. A number of serious outbreaks of glanders have occurred in zoological parks from the practice of feeding horse meat to tigers, lions, and other felids (Galati et al. 1974). Horses are infected either from ingestion of food and water contaminated with infected discharges or from inhalation of infectious droplets. Since *P. mallei* is easily destroyed by heat, sunlight, and drying, the disease in endemic areas is most frequent in the rainy season in animals penned without shelter. Such animals are simultaneously stressed by the lack of shelter and exposed to large numbers of viable *P. mallei* organisms on the ground and pasture (Verma 1981).

Glanders historically has been a scourge of army horses. Wars have always been accompanied by epizootics of the disease. The disease is still a problem among army mules and horses in endemic zones in India and other parts of Asia (Verma 1981). When introduced into dense concentrations of recently grouped susceptible animals, animals with open clinical cases of the disease rapidly spread the infection through their nasal discharge.

Acute glanders is more common in mules than in horses. In horses the disease is usually chronic. After infection, the organism penetrates the nasopharyngeal and intestinal mucosa and enters the regional lymphatics, through which it spreads to various sites in the animal. Nodules may form in the lymph channels; these then become thickened. Breakdown of the nodules results in the formation of craterlike ulcers that discharge a sticky, honeylike exudate containing *P. mallei*. This form of glanders is known as *farcy* (Figure 4.3). After dissemination in the lymphatics, the organism enters the bloodstream and lodges in the lungs.

The lung lesions take the form of either nodules or a diffuse pneumonic process (Figure 4.4). The nodules have a characteristic histological structure not unlike that of a tubercle (Duval and White 1907, McFadyean 1904). Other characteristic lesions frequently develop in the upper air passages when the lung nodules rupture into the bronchi and the infective material is carried upward. These lesions apparently can also occur in animals by direct infection through the nose, since well-defined lesions are sometimes found in the upper air passages when few or none exist in the lungs. The lesions in the nasal passages begin as submucosal nodules, which quickly rupture and form shallow, craterlike ulcers that exude a thick, sticky, purulent material (Figure 4.5). This is discharged from the nostrils, constituting a highly infectious exudate. Glanders nodules can also occur in the liver and spleen.

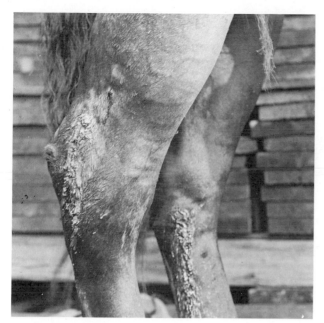

Figure 4.3. Skin glanders (farcy) on the legs of a horse.

Immunity. Horses that recover from glanders can become resistant to reinfection, indicating that a protective immune response is stimulated by infection (Liang et al. 1980). Chronic infection often persists, however, with periodic recrudescence of active lesions and shedding of the organism.

A humoral and cell-mediated immune response is elicited by the infection. A variety of antibodies are produced, which can be detected in complement-fixation, indirect hemagglutination, agglutination, and counter immunoelectrophoresis assays. These tests can also detect antibodies that cross-react with *P. pseudomallei* and so can give false-positive reactions in regions where melioidosis is endemic.

Diagnosis. *P. mallei* can be easily cultured on agar enriched with glycerol or on selective medium (Xie et al. 1980). Specimens taken from sick animals can also be inoculated into guinea pigs. Male guinea pigs inoculated intraperitoneally with material containing *P. mallei* develop a localized peritonitis involving the scrotal sac, which becomes enlarged, painful, and filled with caseous pus. In a few days the lesion discharges to the surface, and *P. mallei* can be recognized in pure culture. This is known

Figure 4.4. Lesions of glanders in the lung of a horse. The lung is extensively involved: not only are there nodules, but the hemorrhages indicate that there is a diffuse glanderous pneumonia.

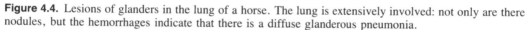

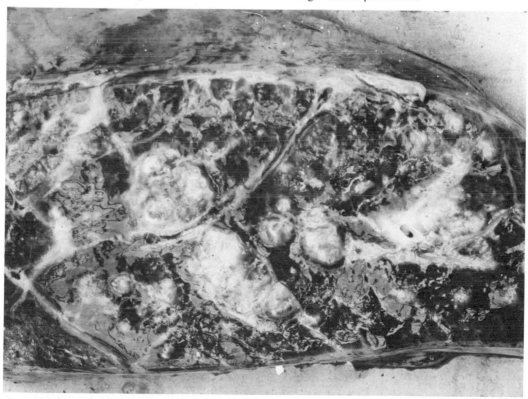

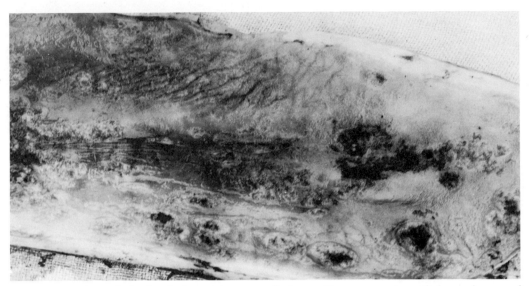

Figure 4.5. Lesions of glanders in the nasal septum of a horse. Shown are ecchymotic hemorrhages and superficial ulcers from which a sticky discharge exudes.

as the Straus reaction (Frothingham 1901). Serologic tests and mallein tests can also be used in the diagnosis of glanders.

Serologic tests.   The following four serologic tests have proved to be useful.

1. Complement-fixation. The complement-fixation test is the most accurate of the serologic methods of diagnosing glanders. It was first applied to the disease in Germany about 1909 and soon afterward was introduced to the United States as a diagnostic procedure.

2. Agglutination. The agglutination test is not as accurate as the complement-fixation test. Failures occur in chronic cases. Normal agglutinins exist in a concentration as high as 1:500 in many horses, whereas infected animals usually react in dilutions of 1:1,000 or higher (Moore and Taylor 1907).

3. Hemagglutination. Gangulee et al. (1966) proposed that the indirect hemagglutination test be used for the diagnosis of glanders, claiming that it is more sensitive than mallein test. A hemagglutinin titer above 1:640 is considered to be diagnostic for the disease.

4. Counter immunelectrophoresis (CIE). Counter immunoelectrophoresis is the most rapid, simple, and economical method for testing large numbers of serums (Jana et al. 1982). The antigen is a filtrate of a sonicate of a suspension of *P. mallei*. Its accuracy is equivalent to that of the complement-fixation or indirect hemagglutination tests.

Mallein tests.   Mallein is a glycoprotein somewhat analogous to tuberculin produced by *P. mallei* in glycerol broth. It can be extracted by alcohol precipitation. Mallein is nontoxic for healthy animals; however, animals infected with *P. mallei* are allergic to mallein and exhibit local and systemic hypersensitivity after its inoculation.

Mallein is used in three ways: (1) subcutaneous test, (2) ophthalmic test, (3) intrapalpebral test. When injected subcutaneously, it causes fever, which appears and subsides within 24 hours after the injection. There is usually a marked swelling at the point of injection. Normal horses can also show some swelling at this point, but the temperature curve is absent. The ophthalmic test consists of instilling some concentrated mallein into the eye (conjunctival sac). When the animal is glanderous, a pus-forming inflammation of the eye occurs within a few hours. The intrapalpebral test consists of injecting a small amount of concentrated mallein into the skin of the lower eyelid (Figure 4.6). A local swelling and a pus-forming inflammation of the eye occur in glanderous animals. The intrapalpebral test is more accurate than the ophthalmic test and accordingly is used more often.

Shumilov (1974) has reported that the subcutaneous and ophthalmic mallein tests are more reliable when double rather than single inoculations are used. A double subcutaneous mallein test detected twice as many infected horses in Mongolia as a double ophthalmic test. The inoculations of mallein did not induce complement-fixing antibody.

A useful diagnostic feature of mallein tests is that partially healed lesions of the nasal mucosa are activated and become easy to see some 12 to 36 hours after inoculation.

Control.   Since spontaneous recovery from chronic infections is rare in this disease and since no efficacious vaccines have been developed, control of the disease has been accomplished wholly by clinical examinations at

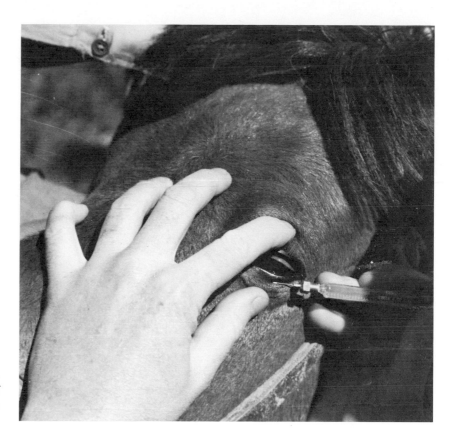

Figure 4.6. Injection of mallein in the intrapalpebral test for the detection of glanders. (Courtesy Col. W. E. Jennings, Veterinary Corps, U.S. Army.)

frequent intervals, the use of the mallein tests and the serologic tests, and the destruction of animals that show evidence of infection by any of these tests. These methods have proved adequate and have eliminated the disease from many parts of the world. Eradication of *P. mallei* is possible because the organism is an obligate parasite with a restricted host range.

Antimicrobial Susceptibility. *P. mallei* is sensitive to sulfonamides and tetracyclines (Ipatenko 1972).

The Disease in Humans.   Humans are not highly susceptible to glanders, yet numerous infections have occurred in persons caring for glanderous animals, especially stablehands and veterinarians (Coleman and Ewing 1903). The disease is characterized by swelling and pain at the point of infection (usually the hand, lip, or eye), which develops in 3 to 5 days, swelling of the neighboring lymph glands, development of nasal and mouth ulcers in about half the patients, development of abscesses and pustules in the skin, joint inflammations, and malaise accompanied by fever. The cases usually end fatally in 2 to 4 weeks. Chronic glanders in humans has been vividly described by Gaiger (1913, 1916), a British veterinarian who contracted the disease in India.

REFERENCES

Coleman, W., and Ewing, J. 1903. A case of septicemic glanders in the human subject. J. Med. Res. 4:223–240.

Duval, C.W., and White, P.G. 1907. The histological lesions of experimental glanders. J. Exp. Med. 9:352–380.

Frothingham, L. 1901. The diagnosis of glanders by the Straus method. J. Med. Res. 1:331–340.

Gaiger, S.H. 1913. Glanders in man. J. Comp. Pathol. Ther. 26:223–236.

Gaiger, S.H. 1916. Glanders in man. J. Comp. Pathol. Ther. 29:26–46.

Galati, P., Puccini V., and Contento, F. 1974. An outbreak of glanders in lions. Histopathologic findings. Vet. Pathol. 11:445.

Gangulee, P.C., Sen, G.P., and Sharma, G.L. 1966. Serological diagnosis of glanders by haemagglutination test. Indian Vet. J. 43:386–391.

Ipatenko, N.G. 1972. Bacteriostatic and bactericidal effects of some antibiotics on the glanders bacillus, *Bacillus (Actinobacillus) mallei*. Tr. Moscow Vet. Akad. 61:142–148.

Jana, A.M., Gupta, A.K., Pandya, G., Verma, R.D., and Rao, K.M. 1982. Rapid diagnosis of glanders in equines by counter-immunoelectrophoresis. Indian Vet. J. 59:5–9.

Liang, S.Y., Wei, J.S., Mei, W.H., Xie, X., Duan, X.W., and Gong, R.X. 1980. Post-infection immunity of horses after recovery from glanders. Collected Papers of Veterinary Research. Control Institute of Veterinary Bioproducts, Ministry of Agriculture, Peking, China, vol. 6. Pp. 77–82.

McFadyean, J. 1904. Glanders. J. Comp. Pathol. Ther. 17:295–317.

Moore, V.A., and Taylor, W.J. 1907. The agglutination method of diagnosis in the control of glanders. J. Infect. Dis. (Suppl.) 3:85–94.

Shumilov, K.V. 1974. Comparative study of methods of diagnosing glanders in horses (in Mongolia). Tr. Vsesoyuz Inst. Eksper. Vet. 42:274–278.

Verma, R.D. 1981. Glanders in India with special reference to incidence and epidemiology. Indian Vet. J. 58:177–183.

Xie, X., Xu, H.F., Xu, B.J., Duan, X.W., and Gong, R.X. 1980. A new selective medium for isolation of glanders bacilli. Collected Papers of Veterinary Research. Control Institute of Veterinary Bioproducts, Ministry of Agriculture, Peking, China, vol. 6. Pp. 83–90.

5 The Spirochetes

The spirochetes are slender, flexuous, helically coiled unicellular bacteria that range from 3 to 250 μm in length. The cell is enclosed in an outer sheath, which in turn encloses the helical protoplasmic cylinder. A variable number of flagella, which arise near each end of the protoplasmic cylinder, are wrapped around the cylinder and overlap at its center. These flagella have also been called axial filaments and differ from those of other bacteria in that they are enclosed by the outer sheath. They are responsible for forward movement, flexion, and rotation of the spirochete. The spirals can be tightly coiled or open and far apart.

The spirochetes are either anaerobic or facultatively anaerobic, and the parasitic members generally require elaborate media for growth. The organisms are Gram-negative and stain well with Giemsa stain. They also stain well with silver stains such as used in Levaditi's method. Live organisms can be visualized under a microscope by dark-field illumination or with the aid of a contrast medium such as India ink.

The family Spirochaetaceae contains three genera with species that cause diseases in domestic animals. These genera are *Borrelia*, *Leptospira*, and *Treponema*.

The Genus *Borrelia*

Borreliae are highly adapted arthropod-borne parasites of the blood of humans, other mammalian species, and birds. The *Borrelia* species that cause disease in domestic animals are *B. theileri*, *B. anserina*, and *B. burgdorferi*.

B. burgdorferi causes Lyme disease in humans and animals, and it may also be the agent of epizootic abortion in cattle in the western United States. The other *Borrelia* species cause relapsing fevers of humans. The species that cause relapsing fevers vary with the locality. Transmission occurs either from an animal reservoir through tick feeding (*Ornithodoros* spp.) or indirectly from other persons through infected body lice *(Pediculus humanus corporis)*. The organisms are carried in the hemolymph of infected lice, which, when squashed by human fingers, release borreliae onto the skin and into scratches and bite wounds.

Tick-borne relapsing fever is found in California, Arizona, Oregon, Washington, Colorado, New Mexico, Idaho, and Texas (Burgdorfer 1985) and appears to be closely associated with the distribution of *Ornithodoros hermsi* or *O. turicata* (Texas). The infection can survive in ticks for as long as 6½ years and can be transmitted through a number of generations (Francis 1938).

Borrelia theileri

SYNONYMS: *Spirocheta theileri, Treponema theileri*

B. theileri was first observed by Theiler (1904) in the blood of South African cattle and has since also been found in Australia. It is a large, loosely twisted spiral, measuring 20 to 30 μm in length. The organism can be easily demonstrated in the blood during the febrile state of the infection, but it disappears later. It is actively motile by means of 15 to 20 periplasmic flagella. Artificial culture of this organism has not been reported.

The disease is fairly benign. The symptoms resemble those of anaplasmosis but are less severe. There is weight loss, weakness, and anemia. One or more febrile attacks are followed by recovery. The ticks *Margaropus decoloratus* and *Rhipicephalus evertsi* transmit the disease. *Boophilus annulatus* also can be an efficient vector for *B. theileri*.

An organism similar to *B. theileri* has been associated with febrile attacks of minor clinical significance in sheep and horses.

REFERENCES

Burgdorfer, W. 1985. Borrelia. In E.M. Lennetti, A. Balows, W.J. Hausler, and M.J. Shadomy, eds., Manual of Clinical Microbiology, 4th ed. American Society for Microbiology, Washington, D.C. Pp. 479–484.

Francis, E. 1938. Longevity of the tick *Ornithodoros turicata* and of *Spirochaeta recurrentis* within this tick. Public Health Rpt. 53:2220–2241.

Theiler, A. 1904. Spirillosis of cattle. J. Comp. Pathol. Ther. 17:47–55.

Borrelia anserina

SYNONYMS: *Borrelia gallinarum*,
Spirochaeta anserina, *Spirochaeta*
gallinarum, *Spironema gallinarum*

B. anserina was first described in 1891 by Sakharoff in Russia as the cause of "goose septicemia." It has since been found to be a cause of borreliosis in geese, chickens, ducks, and turkeys throughout the world. In some regions the organism is the source of great economic losses for poultry raisers.

Morphology and Staining Reactions. *B. anserina* is about 8 to 20 μm long and 0.3 μm wide and has about 5 to 8 coils (Figure 5.1). It stains well with Giemsa stain.

Cultural and Biochemical Features. In vitro culture of *B. anserina* has not been confirmed. It grows well in chick embryos and can be maintained by passage (intraperitoneal inoculation) in day-old chicks. It can also be maintained in citrated blood and plasma with 15 percent

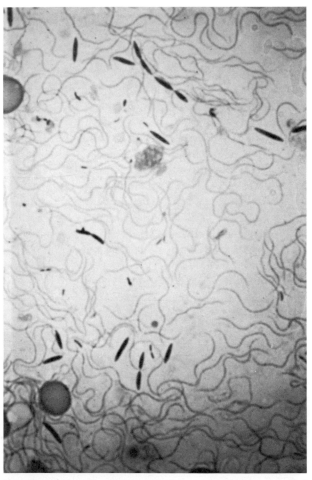

Figure 5.1. *Borrelia anserina* in plasma of a chicken that died of borreliosis. Giemsa stain.

glycerol at 4°C for 4 to 5 weeks and at −70°C for 8 weeks (Ginawi and Shammein 1980).

Antigens. *Borrelia* species are known to contain muramic acid and ornithine in their cell walls. The chemistry of the outer sheath in unknown but is of potential interest because of the great antigenic variability exhibited by the organism. Strain variations are known to occur that affect the efficacy of the protective immune response (Soni and Joski 1980).

Soluble borrelia antigen is present in the plasma of infected chickens 4 to 10 days after infection, but this antigen has not been characterized (Lad and Soni 1983).

Epizootiology and Pathogenesis. Avian borreliosis is transmitted by argasid ticks, in which transovarial transmission has been demonstrated. The chicken mite, *Dermanyssus gallinae,* has also been suspected as a transmitting agent, as have mosquitoes that have fed recently on infected birds. Infected droppings have been incriminated in the transmission of avian borreliosis in some California outbreaks (Loomis 1953, Mathey and Siddle 1955). In argasid ticks the spiral forms of *B. anserina* disappear in 3 to 4 months but the ticks remain infected. The infective form of *B. anserina* in this situation is probably the so-called granular form, which can be detected by fluorescent antibody methods in ticks known to be capable of transmitting infection. Ticks obtained from backyard flocks produce higher infection rates than those from commercial flocks and male ticks are more infective than female ticks (Buriro 1979).

Avian borreliosis is easily transmitted to a variety of birds, such as sparrows, canaries, and guinea fowl. Pigeons are relatively resistant. Ten or fewer spirochetes constitute an infective dose for susceptible chickens. After a bird has been infected the organisms are first found in the spleen, then within a few days they appear in the blood and other organs. Anemia resulting from a severely reduced erythrocyte count appears at the same time as bacteremia becomes evident.

Affected birds develop fever, become depressed, develop a profuse diarrhea, and die within a day or two. Infections by virulent stains are characterized by a very high mortality. At necropsy birds that have died of *B. anserina* infection have splenomegaly, liver enlargement, and a serofibrinous exudate in the pericardial sac. They also exhibit an intense erythrophagocytosis.

The basis for the anemia is not understood. Suspensions of ultrasonically disintegrated *Borrelia* organisms have a thromboplastinlike action and lyse thrombocytes (Dzhankov et al. 1982). Cold agglutinins appear in the plasma 5 to 7 days after infection and these can stimulate erythrophagocytosis. Soluble borrelia antigen complexed to antibody can also stimulate erythrophagocytosis after attachment of complexes to erythrocytes.

Immunity. Birds that survive the acute phase of the disease develop an immunity that persists for at least 6 months. Serum obtained from convalescent birds contains lytic antibodies that are protective in passively immunized birds. There is some evidence of strain specificity (Soni and Joski 1980).

Marchoux and Salimbeni (1903) prepared an effective vaccine by heating the fresh blood of affected birds to 55°C for 5 minutes. They also found that the organism loses its virulence when stored in blood for 48 hours and that such blood can be used as a vaccine. Embryonated egg vaccines that confer durable immunity in vaccinated birds are now commonly used in the field. A hemotissue vaccine derived from cocks infected with local strains can also be used in the field.

Antibodies have been demonstrated in the eggs of vaccinated hens 8 weeks after vaccination, and these antibodies protected chicks for the first 2 weeks of life (Dutta et al. 1977). Chicks do not develop effective protective immune responses when vaccinated at less than 6 weeks of age.

Diagnosis. The organism is easily detected in Giemsa-stained smears of blood from birds in the acute phase of the disease. Antigen can be detected by immunodiffusion in liver extracts of birds that are no longer bacteremic. A fluorescent antibody technique can also be used to detect borrelia antigen in the livers of birds recovering from the disease (Wadalker and Soni 1982).

Antimicrobial Susceptibility. *B. anserina* is sensitive to penicillin, tetracyclines, tylosin, erythromycin, and spectinomycin (Bok et al. 1975).

Benzathine chlortetracycline given subcutaneously or procaine penicillin (4,000 IU/lb) given intramuscularly are effective during the peak of the bacteremia.

REFERENCES

Bok, R., Samberg, Y., Rubina, M., and Hadoni, A. 1975. Studies on fowl spirochaetosis-survival of *Borrelia anserina* at various temperatures and its sensitivity to antibiotics. Refuah Vet. 32:147–153.

Buriro, S.N. 1979. Role of *Argas (Persiargas) persicus* in transmission of spirochaetosis. Pakistan J. Zool. 11:221–224.

Dutta, G.N., Mehta, M.L., and Muley, A.R. 1977. Studies on immunity in fowl spirochaetosis. Indian J. Anim. Sci. 47:554–558.

Dzhankov, I., Nikolov, N., and Kirev, T. 1982. Recent findings in the pathogenesis of avian spirochaetosis (*Borrelia anserina* infection).Vet. Med. Nauki 19:14–21.

Ginawi, M.A., and Shammein, A.M. 1980. Preservation of *Borrelia anserina* at different temperatures. Bull. Anim. Health Prod. Afr. 28:221–223.

Lad, P.L., and Soni, J.L. 1983. Soluble spirochaete antigen-antibody immune complex in plasma of *Borrelia anserina* –infected chickens. Indian J. Anim. Sci. 53:538–541.

Loomis, E.C. 1953. Avian spirochetosis in California turkeys. Am. J. Vet. Res. 14:612–615.

Marchoux, E., and Salimbeni, A. 1903. La spirillose des poules. Ann. Inst. Pasteur 17:569–580.

Mathey, W.J., and Siddle, P.J. 1955. Spirochetosis in pheasants. J. Am. Vet. Med. Assoc. 126:123–126.

Soni, J.L., and Joski, A.G. 1980. A note on strain variation in Akola and Jabalpur strains of *Borrelia anserina*. Zentralbl. Veterinärmed. [B] 27:70–72.

Wadalker, B.G., and Soni, J.L. 1980. Immunological basis of localization of spirochaeta antigen in prepeak and post spirochaetemic phases. Indian Vet. J. 57:93–98.

Borrelia burgdorferi

B. burgdorferi was first observed in hard ticks *(Ixodes dammini)* from Shelter Island, New York, which is part of an area in which an epidemic inflammatory disorder of humans known as Lyme disease was prevalent (Burgdorfer et al. 1982). *B. burgdorferi* has since been confirmed as the causative agent of Lyme disease, a disorder common during the tick season in the northeastern United States. A similar disease occurs in other parts of the United States and in Europe (Burgdorfer 1985). *B. burgdorferi* may also be the cause of epizootic abortion in cattle in the western United States (Lane et al. 1985).

Antigens. A number of antigens have been identified, including two abundant cellular proteins with molecular weights of 31,000 and 34,000. These proteins occur on the organism's outer membrane (Barbour et al. 1984).

Epizootiology and Pathogenesis. Although ixodid ticks of the *Ixodes ricinus* complex are of proven importance in transmission, it is probable that other bloodsucking arthropods are also involved. In the northeastern United States, white-footed mice and white-tailed deer are important vertebrate reservoirs. Because *B. burgdorferi* is found only in the midgut of infected ticks, it has been postulated that transmission is through fecal droplets or regurgitation of midgut contents during feeding (Burgdorfer 1985). Unlike other *Borrelia* species, *B. burgdorferi* appears to be antigenically stable.

The first report of Lyme disease in a domestic animal was that of a case in a 3-year-old Doberman pinscher with signs of polyarthritis (Lissman et al. 1984). Other cases have since been described (Kornblatt et al. 1985, Magnarelli et al. 1985). A typical history includes exposure to ticks followed by a sudden onset of lameness involving one or more joints. The affected joints are swollen and painful, and the arthritis typically is migratory, involving one joint for a few days and then another (Figure 5.2). Large numbers of polymorphonuclear leukocytes are present in the synovial fluid, in which spirochetes can be seen under dark-field microscopy or by fluorescent antibody techniques. Lymphadenopathy and

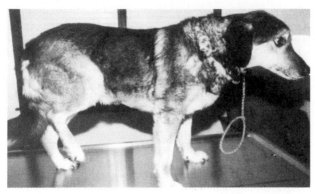

Figure 5.2. Dog with typical appearance of arthritis caused by *Borrelia burgdorferi*. Examination of 1.5 ml of fluid from the tarsal joint revealed a leukocyte count of 2,400/mm³. (From Kornblatt et al., 1985, courtesy of *Journal of the American Veterinary Medical Association*.)

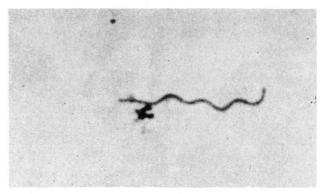

Figure 5.3. *Borrelia burgdorferi* in joint fluid from a dog. The length of the organism ranges from 10 to 30 μm. Giemsa stain. × 2,340. (From Kornblatt et al., 1985, courtesy of *Journal of the American Veterinary Medical Association*.)

fever have been observed in some sick animals and may be a common feature of the disease but one that escapes detection by the owner of the animal.

Encephalitis, arthritis, and panuveitis have been described in a horse (Burgess and Mattison 1987) and a pony (Burgess et al. 1986) in an endemic area in Wisconsin. Arthritis accompanied by mycocarditis, nephritis, and pneumonitis have also been observed in a cow in the same area (Burgess et al. 1987).

Immunity. Dogs with arthritis generally do not have antibodies of the IgM isotype, suggesting that the arthritis does not appear for some time after infection. Antibody levels are measured by indirect immunofluorescence (Steere et al. 1983). Protective antibodies have been stimulated in hamsters by subcutaneous immunization with whole cells (Johnson et al. 1986).

Diagnosis. *B. burgdorferi* can be detected by fluorescent antibody or immunoperoxidase-labeled monoclonal antibody in biopsy specimens (Figure 5.3). Citrated blood (0.1 ml) or synovial fluid should be inoculated into modified Kelley's medium, and the cultures examined weekly by dark-field microscopy for spirochete growth (Barbour et al. 1983).

REFERENCES

Barbour, A.G., Burgdorfer, W., Hayes, S.F., Peter, O., and Aeschlimann, T. 1983. Isolation of a cultivable spirochete from *Ixcodes ricinus* ticks of Switzerland. Curr. Microbiol. 8:123–126.

Barbour, A.G., Tessier, S.L., and Hayes, S.F. 1984. Variation in a major surface protein of Lyme disease spirochetes. Infect. Immun. 45:94–100.

Burgdorfer, W. 1985. Borrelia. In E.H. Lennette, A. Balows, W.J. Hausler, and H.J. Shadomy, eds., Manual of Clinical Microbiology, 6th ed. American Society for Microbiology, Washington, D.C. Pp. 479–484.

Burgdorfer, W., Barbour, A.G., Hayes, S.F., Benach, J.L., Grun-
waldt, E., and Davis, J.P. 1982. Lyme disease—A tickborne spirochetosis? Science 216:1317–1319.

Burgess, E.C., and Mattison, M. 1987. Encephalitis associated with *Borrelia burgdorferi* infection in a horse. J. Am. Vet. Med. Assoc. 191:1457–1458.

Burgess, E.C., Gendron-Fitzpatrick, A., and Wright, W.O. 1987. Arthritis and systemic disease caused by *Borrelia burgdorferi* infection in a cow. J. Am. Vet. Med. Assoc. 191:1468–1469.

Burgess, E.C., Gillette, D., and Pickett, J.P. 1986. Arthritis and panuveitis as manifestations of *Borrelia burgdorferi* infection in a Wisconsin pony. J. Am. Vet. Med. Assoc. 189:1340–1342.

Johnson, R.C., Kodner, C., and Russell, M. 1986. Active immunization of hamsters against experimental infection with *Borrelia burgdorferi*. Infect. Immun. 54:897–898.

Kornblatt, A.N., Urband, P.H., and Steere, A.S. 1985. Arthritis caused by *Borrelia burgdorferi* in dogs. J. Am. Vet. Med. Assoc. 186:960–964.

Lane, R.S., Burgdorfer, W., Hayes, S.F., and Barbour, A.G. 1985. Isolation of a spirochete from the soft tick, *Ornithodoros coriaceus:* A possible agent of epizootic bovine abortion. Science. 230:85–86.

Lissman, B.A., Bosler, E.M., Camay, H., Ormiston, B.G., and Benach, J.L. 1984. Spirochete-associated arthritis (Lyme disease) in a dog. J. Am. Vet. Med. Assoc. 185:219–220.

Magnarelli, L.A., Anderson, A.F., Kaufmann, A.F., Lieberman, C.C., and Whitney, G.D. 1985. Borreliosis in dogs from southern Connecticut. J. Am. Vet. Med. Assoc. 186:955–958.

Steere, A.C., Grodzicki, R.L., and Kornblatt, A.N. 1983. The spirochetal etiology of Lyme disease. N. Engl. J. Med. 308:733–740.

The Genus *Leptospira*

Leptospirae are chiefly saprophytic aquatic spirochetes found in a variety of moist habitats. There are two species: *Leptospira interrogans* and *L. biflexa*. The pathogenic leptospirae belong to the species *L. interrogans,* which is subdivided on the basis of surface agglutinins into at least 200 different serovars. The serovar is the basic taxon; serovars cannot be distinguished by morphologic, physiological, or biochemical criteria. Clinical signs of infec-

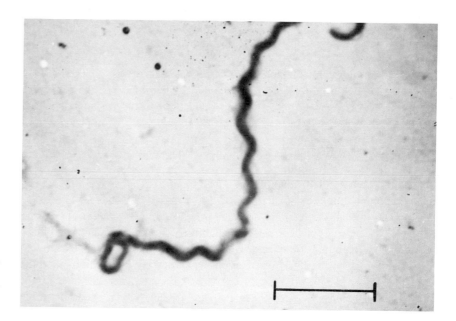

Figure 5.4. Electron micrograph of a *Leptospira* organism from a cow. Scale = 1 μm. × 20,100, approximately. (Courtesy J. A. Baker.)

tion include abortion, milk drop, hemoglobinuria, fever, jaundice, and death, although the great majority of leptospiral infections in animals are subclinical.

Morphology and Staining Reactions. Leptospirae are helical, flexible bacteria, the ends of which are typically hooked (Figure 5.4). The cells have a diameter of about 0.1 μm and their length lies in the range 6 to 30 μm. They are motile by means of two periplasmic flagella that arise subterminally and extend toward the middle of the cell but do not overlap. An external sheath encloses the helical body and flagella. Their motion consists of a writhing and flexing movement and a rapid rotation around the long axis. They stain only faintly with aniline dyes but are readily visualized under dark-field microscopy and by silver impregnation stains. They are readily filterable through bacteriological filters with pore sizes of 0.22 to 0.45 μm.

Cultural and Biochemical Features. Media for the culture of leptospirae usually contain either rabbit serum (Fletcher medium, Stuart broth) or bovine serum albumin (Ellinghausen medium) plus long-chain fatty acids and vitamins B_1 (thiamine) and B_{12} (cyanocobalamin). Protein-free media have also been devised (Bey and Johnson 1978). The optimum pH is 7.2. Leptospirae require long-chain fatty acids as energy sources and for cellular synthesis. These fatty acids are provided in a form bound to albumin or in an esterified detoxified form such as is found in polysorbates (Tween 80 and 40). Leptospirae cannot use carbohydrates as sources of energy and can use ammonium salts but not amino acids as sources of nitrogen. Pyruvate enhances the growth of primary cultures. The cell wall pepidoglycan contains alpha,epsilon-di-

aminopimelic acid. The leptospirae are catalase- and peroxidase-positive.

Leptospira organisms are obligate aerobes and are oxidase positive because of the presence of cytochromes a, b, and c, which serve as terminal electron receptors. The optimum growth temperature is 30°C, and cultures should be incubated in the dark. Although liquid or semisolid media are most commonly used for culture of *Leptospira*, colonies are formed by some serovars on or in solid media (1 or 2 percent agar). The mol% G + C of the DNA is 35 to 41 (Tm).

Antigens. Although the leptospiral antigens responsible for serologic reactions and protective immune responses have been studied by numerous investigators, many of these antigens have not yet been well defined (Stalheim 1984). The extremely small quantities and the chemical associations of these antigens with each other have made their definition and characterization very difficult. The type-specific (TM) antigen is similar to the endotoxin of Gram-negative organisms and contains carbohydrates, lipids, proteins, and phosphorous. A number of different epitopes exist on the molecule, some of which are common to other serovars. One of these, an oligosaccharide rich in rhamnose and arabinose, has been characterized in *L. interrogans* serovar *canicola* (Ono et al. 1984).

The outer sheath of leptospirae appears to carry most of the protective antigenic activity (Auran et al. 1972). It consists of a complex of proteins, carbohydrates, and lipids arranged in layers. Both serovar-specific and genus-broad antigens are present. Removal of the sheath greatly reduces the agglutinability of the leptospirae in immune serum. The sheath material is protective when administered as a vaccine (Takashima and Yanagawa 1975).

The immunologically reactive proteins on the sheath of serovar *hardjo* exhibit a range of molecular weights from about 21,000 to 50,000 (Nunes-Edwards et al. 1985). The major proteins are shared by serovars *pomona* and *balcanica*.

The axial filament (flagella) bears antigens that stimulate antibodies that agglutinate whole leptospirae. These agglutinins are distinct from those produced against outer sheath antigens.

Serovars that are antigenically related are placed in a serogroup. There are 26 of these, including Australis, Autumnalis, Ballum, Bataviae, Butembo, Canicola, Celledoni, Cynopteri, Djasiman, Grippotyphosa, Hebdomadis, Icterohaemorrhagiae, Javanica, Panama, Pomona, Pyrogenes, Sejroe, Shermani, and Tarassovi.

Serovars are distinguished from one another by agglutinin absorption tests with representative strains of serovars.

Epizootiology and Pathogenesis. Survival of pathogenic leptospirae in the environment is usually brief and requires suitable conditions of moisture, pH, and temperature. Slightly alkaline conditions favor survival (Twigg et al. 1972). Serovar *pomona* has been shown to survive for at least 30 days at 15°C in the kidneys of infected pigs (Ho and Blackmore 1979). The natural reservoir of pathogenic leptospirae is the lumen of nephritic tubules, from which the organism is shed in the urine and spread to other hosts. Shedding in the urine takes place during the later clinical phase and during the convalescent and recovery phases and persists for variable periods. Shedding is usually heavy for the first few months after infection in dogs, cattle, and swine and then becomes lighter or may cease altogether. Rodents are often persistently heavy shedders. Although urine is the most important vehicle of infection, milk, placental material, and aborted fetuses have also been sources of the organism for spread to other animals. The lability of pathogenic leptospirae to environmental influences reflects the high level of their adaptation to certain hosts and their reliance on these hosts for their survival. These hosts are maintenance hosts for the serovar that is adapted to them. Thus populations of serovar *hardjo* are maintained in cattle. This serovar is poorly adapted to pigs and infections in this species are often a result of accidental direct or indirect exposures to cattle (Hathaway et al. 1983).

Many serovars are maintained in wild animals and such animals can serve as sources of accidental infections in domestic animals or humans. For instance, Norway rats serve as maintenance hosts of serovar *icterohaemor-*

rhagiae, which is shed in great numbers in the urine throughout life of the animal. Dogs or humans exposed to this urine can become accidentally infected. The same animal species can be a maintenance host for more than one serovar and itself can be accidentally infected by a nonadapted serovar. Furthermore, a maintenance host in one region for a particular serovar may not function as such in a different region. Serovar *pomona,* for example, is maintained in cattle in the United States but not in New Zealand. The epizootiology of leptospiral infection thus can be quite complex.

Maintenance hosts are characterized by a high susceptibility to infection, long-term kidney infection with urinary shedding, and very efficient transmission within the host species. In contrast, accidental hosts usually have a low susceptibility to infection, but severe disease often results if infection occurs. Kidney infection is usually of short duration, and intraspecies transmission is inefficient and sporadic (Hathaway 1981). Leptospirae enter a new host through mucuous membranes or damaged skin. They quickly reach the bloodstream, where they multiply. Within a few days large numbers of organisms are present in the blood, spleen, liver, and brain and damage blood vessels and liver cells. Many are destroyed by the serum leptospiricidal activity of beta-macroglobulin acting in concert with complement and lysozyme. Those that survive are carried in the bloodstream to the kidneys where they move through the vascular endothelium and eventually reach the lumina of the proximal convoluted tubules, where they multiply in close proximity to the microvilli. Penetration of the placenta can occur in pregnant animals, with multiplication in the mesenchyme or fetal cotyledonary tissue. The organism eventually, moves into the fetus and multiplies in its bloodstream. Fetal death and resorption can result, or the mother may abort or produce a dead or weakly offspring. Placental infection during the last third of pregnancy can stimulate specific antibody formation in the fetus, which is then able to overcome the invading leptospirae. Placental and fetal infections by leptospirae thus are not always lethal for the fetus. For instance serovar *hardjo* has been observed in normal bovine fetuses removed in an abattoir (Ellis et al. 1982).

Antibody production begins a few days after the onset of leptospiremia and rapidly stimulates clearance of the organism from the blood and tissues. Body sites that do not have much antibody activity can provide a niche for leptospirae to survive and persist. They thus are found and persist in the renal tubules, the eyes, the uterus, and fetuses. Urinary excretion of leptospirae can persist for years in hosts to which the serovar is adapted. Urease production may be a factor in the persistance of leptospirae in the kidneys (Kadis and Pugh 1974). A hemolytic substance produced by strains of the Autumnalis, Grippotyphosa, Icterohaemorrhagiae, and Pomona serogroups is probably responsible for the hemoglobinuria (redwater disease) observed in young calves infected with members of these serogroups. Cold agglutinins of the IgM immunoglobulin isotype, however, can also contribute to intravascular hemolysis by sensitizing erythrocytes.

The disease in cattle. The predominant serovar in cattle varies from one geographic region to another. In the United States, serovars *balcaani, canicola, grippotyphosa, hardjo, icterohaemorrhagiae, pomona,* and *szwajizak* have been isolated from outbreaks of leptospirosis. There are two genotypes of serovar *hardjo: L. hardjobovis* and *L. hardjoprajitno;* the latter appears to be more common in U.S. cattle. Serovars *hardjo* and *pomona* are adapted to and maintained in cattle populations in many areas, whereas the other serovars are the causes of accidental infections derived from rodents and other wild species. The incubation period varies from 4 to 10 days and is followed by a leptospiremia that lasts for 1 to 5 days. This phase is terminated by the appearance of antibody in the animal's blood, which promotes complement-lysozyme–mediated immune lysis. The organism then is rapidly cleared from the bloodstream but localizes and remains in the kidneys (Burnstein and Baker 1954). The organism multiplies in the lumen of the convoluted tubules and is shed in the urine. Leptospiruria lasts for 1 to 3 months, but the organism can persist in the kidneys for longer periods.

Animals with acute leptospirosis have a transient fever and loss of appetite. Lactating cows exhibit agalactia and a milk secretion that is yellow, clotted, and often blood-stained. The fall in milk production, in the absence of other severe clinical signs, has been termed the *milk-drop syndrome.* It can last for 2 to 10 days and is usually associated with infection by serovar *hardjo* (Ellis and Michna 1976). Severely affected animals develop anemia, jaundice, hemoglobinuria, and pneumonia. These effects can be fatal in calves. Some animals show signs of meningitis (Stoenner et al. 1963).

Abortion and neonatal mortality are important sequelae to the acute phase of bovine leptospirosis but may not be observed for 2 to 4 months after the acute phase. Accidental infection by nonadapted serovars usually causes abortion only in the last trimester of pregnancy, whereas serovar *hardjo* can adversely affect pregnancy at any stage (Ellis 1984b). However, the abortion rate associated with serovar *hardjo* is generally much lower.

Infertility as a result of early abortions or fetal resorption has been a common observation in herds infected with serovar *hardjo* (Hanson and Brodie 1967). It has also been suggested that the local immune response of the animal's endometrium plays a role in the infertility caused by serovar *hardjo* (Belloni and Ruggeri 1969).

The disease in swine. At least twelve different serovars are known to infect swine, the most important of which are *canicola, icterohaemorrhagiae, pomona,* and *tarassovi.* Swine, which are the maintenance host of serovar *pomona,* have been a source of infection for their caretakers—whose resultant disease has been appropriately named *swineherd's disease.*

Contaminated urine is the most important vehicle by which leptospirae are transferred between or to swine. It is also possible that piglets can be infected from the milk of leptospiremic sows. Infection with serovar *pomona* results primarily in interstitial nephritis. Many infections are subclinical and only recognizable by seroconversion, isolation of the organism from the kidneys at slaughter, or, indirectly, by the occurrence of cases of leptospirosis in swineherds or abattoir personnel. Other signs of infection include fever, focal nonsuppurative mastitis (Tripathy et al. 1981), and leptospiremia. Signs can be severe in young pigs infected by serovars *icterohaemorrhagiae* or *canicola* and include fever, anorexia, jaundice, hemoglobinuria, and a heavy mortality (Bezdenezhnuikh and Kashanova 1956, Nisbet 1951). Petechiae occur in the lungs, kidneys, and other abdominal viscera. Diarrhea, irritability, conjunctivitis, tremors of the legs, weakness of the hind limbs, stiffness of the neck, and encephalitic symptoms have also been described (Sippel 1953).

Infertility, abortions, and stillbirths associated with serovars *canicola,* and *icterohaemorrhagiae,* and *pomona* are also widely observed (Michna 1970). Aborted fetuses are jaundiced, and piglets borne alive are weak and die soon after birth. Infections by serovar *pomona* early in gestation result in fetal death and resorption and the sow appears to be infertile. Fetal infection at 2 to 3 months' gestation can result either in death and abortion or carriage to term of a dead or weakened piglet. Infection toward the end of pregnancy can result in birth of live, normal, but chronically infected piglets that controlled the infection by their own antibody responses.

Serovar *hardjo* can cause accidental infections of swine in regions where this serovar is enzootic in cattle (Hathaway et al. 1983).

The disease in dogs. Canines are the maintenance hosts of serovar *canicola,* and infections by this serovar and by accidentally acquired serovar *icterohaemorrhagiae* are very common in dogs throughout the world. Other serovars occasionally encountered in this host include *ballum, bratislava, grippotyphosa, hardjo, poi, pomona, sejroe,* and *tarassovi* (Hartman 1984, Mackintosh et al. 1980).

Infection is more common in males (Ryu 1975), which

perhaps is a consequence of the male dogs' propensity to sniff in places contaminated with urine. Serovar *canicola* is more common in urban than in rural or sporting dog populations, in which infection by serovar *icterohaemorrhagiae* is most common. However, dogs in some urban areas can be infected predominantly with serovar *icterohaemorrhagiae* (Thiermann 1980). Infections by this serovar are most common in young dogs during the summer and autumn. Serovar *canicola* infections tend to be more evenly distributed throughout the year (Hartman 1984). Three clinical forms of leptospirosis in dogs are recognized: (1) the acute hemorrhagic type, (2) the less acute icteric type, and (3) the uremic type, commonly known as *Stuttgart disease.*

Serovar *icterohaemorrhagiae* has been associated with the first two syndromes, whereas serovar *canicola* has been most often implicated in renal disease (Figures 5.5 and 5.6). There is evidence, however, that serovar *icterohaemorrhagiae* also causes a substantial proportion of renal lesions in dogs (Hartman 1984, Timoney et al. 1974). Meningeal involvement can also result from infection by either serotype.

The acute hemorrhagic disease is characterized by high fever, prostration, and early death. Hemorrhages occur throughout the organs, especially in the lungs and alimentary tract. The second type is less acute and is characterized by intense icterus, depression, fever, hemorrhages with blood-stained feces, and pigmented urine. The third type is characterized by uremia associated with extensive kidney damage; by a foul odor from the mouth as a result of ulcerative stomatitis; and by hemorrhagic enteritis, coma, and death in a high percentage of cases. The serum biochemical changes in dogs with serovar *icterohaemor-*

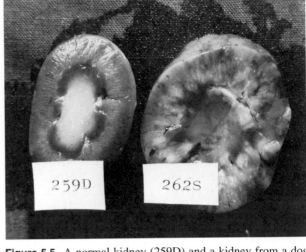

Figure 5.5. A normal kidney (259D) and a kidney from a dog with chronic interstitial nephritis caused by *Leptospira interrogans* serovar *icterohaemorrhagiae.*

rhagia infection include increased levels of aspartate aminotransferase and alanine aminotransferase (Navarro et al. 1981).

The kidneys of dogs with acute interstitial nephritis caused by serovar *canicola* exhibit extensive accumulations of plasma cells, which have been shown to contain IgG antibodies to leptospiral antigens (Morrison and Wright 1976). These antibodies appear to be ineffective in clearing renal infection, since many dogs continue to shed the organism in their urine. It is possible, however, that these organisms are less virulent than organisms shed during the early infection phase before antibody is produced,

Figure 5.6. *Leptospira interrogans* serovar *canicola* in the kidney of an artificially infected guinea pig. Warthin-Starry stain. × 2,300. (Courtesy J. T. Bryans and P. C. Kennedy.)

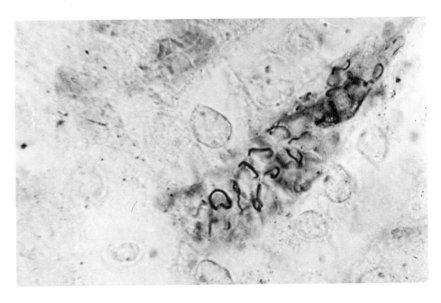

a phenomenon that has been well established in mice (Faine 1962, Hirshberg and Vaughn 1973).

Uremic leptospirosis is associated with renal failure resulting from extensive kidney damage. Most commonly this is a sequel to chronic leptospiral infection. The lesions are those of a chronic interstitial nephritis (CIN), which is progressive whether or not the inciting leptospirae remain in the kidneys. Immune complex deposition or autoantibodies, however, do not appear to be important in the pathogenesis of CIN (Spencer and Wright 1981).

Chronic active hepatitis associated with serologic evidence of infection by serovar *grippotyphosa* has been observed in a kennel of American foxhounds (Bishop et al. 1979). The organisms persisted within the hepatic cords causing focal necrosis and extensive fibrosis.

The disease in horses. Leptospirosis in general is a much less important disease in horses than in cattle, pigs, or dogs. Most infections in horses are accidental and are caused by serovars *hardjo, icterohaemorrhagiae,* and *pomona* (Ellis, O'Brien, et al. 1983; Hall and Bryans 1954; Jackson et al. 1957; Swart et al. 1982). In Ireland there is evidence that serovar *bratislava* may be adapted to and maintained by horses (Ellis, O'Brien, et al. 1983).

Leptospirae have been associated with equine abortion of fetuses from 6 months to term (Ellis, Bryson, et al. 1983; Jackson et al. 1957), with a condition known as periodic ophthalmia (recurrent iridocyclitis), and, rarely, with a typical acute leptospiral syndrome consisting of fever, anorexia, depression, and icterus (Hall and Bryans 1954, Roberts et al. 1952).

The association of leptospiral infection with periodic opthalmia is strongly circumstantial. Affected animals have high serum antibody titers and even higher titers in their aqueous humor (Heusser 1948), but leptospirae have not been found in the affected eyes. The disease occurs about 1 to 2 years after naturally occurring or experimentally induced infection (Morter et al. 1969, Yager et al. 1950). Injection of soluble leptospiral antigen into the corneas of dogs with high serum antibody titers to the same serovar has been shown to result in lesions resembling postleptospiral ophthalmia (Torten et al. 1967). An experimental basis for the involvement of an immune reaction in periodic ophthalmia thus has been laid. The disease is characterized by periodic recurrences of conjunctivitis, hypopyon, and iridocyclitis that can result in blindness.

The disease in sheep and goats. Serovar *pomona* is the most frequently incriminated serovar in outbreaks of leptospirosis in sheep, goats, and lambs (Davidson and Hirsh 1980, Hodges 1974). Serovar *hardjo* infection of sheep, which was apparently related to contact with infected cat-

tle, has been observed in England (Hathaway et al. 1984).

Acute leptospirosis in sheep is typical of that described in other hosts. There is depression, dyspnea, hemoglobinuria, jaundice, and anemia and a high mortality in lambs (Hartley 1952).

The disease in cats. Serum antibody surveys suggest that cats are infected with a variety of leptospiral serovars (Michna 1970). However, disease appears to be uncommon in this host (White et al. 1961).

Immunity. Antibodies of the IgM class are detectable a few days after the febrile and leptospiremic phases. These antibodies are agglutinins and are responsible for the initial clearance of the organism from the bloodstream. Antibodies of IgG class appear a few days after the IgM antibodies. These antibodies have neutralizing activity and are detectable by the hamster passive-protection test (Negi et al. 1971). They persist for several years.

Agglutinin titers peak after a month or two and persist at a high level for up to 2 years (Hanson 1974). Protective antibodies are not agglutinating and are serovar-specific, although there is some evidence for cross-immunity in animals that recover from infection but not in animals immunized with bacterin (Kemenes 1964).

Baby mice whose mothers do not have antibodies become chronic renal carriers if they are infected during the first day of life. They develop tolerance to the leptospiral antigens and do not form serum antibodies. The numbers of these seronegative renal carrier mice in an area is a critical factor in the epizootiology of accidental leptospirosis in livestock that share the same environment (Birnbaum et al. 1972). The frequency of occurrence of seronegative renal carriers among livestock appears to be much less, probably because late fetal or neonatal infections occur after the immune system has become competent. This fact notwithstanding, a poor correlation has been noted between the presence of serovar *hardjo* in bovine kidneys and the presence of serum antibody (Ellis 1984a).

Vaccination with killed bacterins protects against clinical leptospirosis for up to a year, but the bacterin must contain the antigens of the strain to which the cattle are subsequently exposed. Both IgM and IgG antibodies are produced. The IgM antibodies are present in low titer and fall below diagnostic levels in a few weeks (Tripathy et al. 1975). The protective antibodies, which are nonagglutinating and belong to the IgG class, persist for 6 months to a year. Most herds are vaccinated at intervals of 6 months to a year depending on the expected level of field exposure (Hanson et al. 1972).

Animals introduced into a herd should be vaccinated at or before the time of entry and, ideally, isolated for a short period until antibody titers have had a chance to develop.

Calves born of immunized dams are protected by colostral antibodies for the first few months of life. Passively immune calves should not be vaccinated before 3 months of age.

The use of vaccine in animals that have had a prior natural infection with the homologous serovar results in much higher antibody titers that persist for longer than does the use of the same vaccine in previously nonsensitized animals (Stringfellow et al. 1983). Vaccinal immunity, unlike that derived from natural infection, is short-lived. Furthermore, although greatly reducing the number of urinary shedders, infection by adapted serovars such as *hardjo* can continue in a vaccinated herd. Reduction in the number of naturally infected and immunized animals in such a herd could predispose the herd to a more severe clinical disease should vaccination not be continued or should it be applied haphazardly (Hathaway 1981).

Cattle vaccinated at 9 to 10 months of age are much less likely to become urinary shedders than animals vaccinated as adults (Hancock et al. 1984). Thus vaccination of younger stock, by reducing leptospiruria, should eventually lead to eradication of adapted serovars from populations of cattle isolated from exogenous sources of that serovar.

There is convincing evidence that leptospiral bacterin will protect swine against abortion and fetal mortality as well as reduce the urinary excretion of leptospirae (Bey and Johnson 1983, Caleffi 1966, Whyte et al. 1982). Gilts and sows should be vaccinated twice at an interval of 3 weeks at breeding age. Vaccination at 6 weeks of age has also been successfully used to eradicate serovar *pomona* in an intensive piggery (Gill and Williamson 1978).

Canine leptospiral vaccines also confer a high level of protection against clinical disease. They usually contain formalin-killed or phenol-killed suspensions of serovars *canicola* and *icterohaemorrhagiae*. Both IgM and IgG responses occur to primary vaccination. However, a booster vaccination is required to obtain an adequate IgG response, and annual revaccinations are needed to stimulate persistently high protective IgG antibody titers (Hartman et al. 1984). Some vaccines have been shown to protect against the renal carrier state (Kerr and Marshall 1974).

Hyperimmune serum has been used for passive protection and for treatment of early cases (Michna 1970). Horses have been protected against serovar *L. pomona* infection by vaccination with bacterin (Brown et al. 1956).

Diagnosis.   Diagnosis of leptospiral infections can be made by a variety of techniques.

Direct examination.   Direct dark-field microscopic ex-

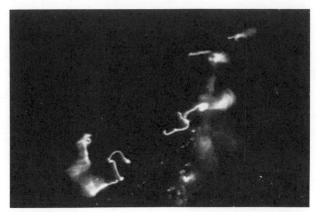

Figure 5.7. *Leptospira interrogans* serovar *hardjo* in a liver impression smear from an aborted bovine fetus. Fluorescent antibody stain.

amination of body or tissue fluids from acutely affected animals can be used to detect the organism. Blood (heparinized) should be centrifuged at low speed to deposit cellular elements and then the plasma should be examined. These techniques are of value only when large numbers of leptospirae are present.

The fluorescent antibody technique is more sensitive and is of particular value for examining urinary sediments or preparations of liver and kidney from aborted fetuses (Figure 5.7). It also can be used on tissue sections or impressions and to identify serotypes (Dacres 1961).

Silver impregnation or immunoperoxidase staining techniques (Terpstra et al. 1980) are also of value for the detection of leptospirae in clinical specimens. The immunoperoxidase staining technique has the advantage of rapidity.

Cultural examination.   During the acute phase of the disease, blood culture in Fletcher medium, Stuart broth, or Ellinghausen medium is the most reliable method of detecting the organism. In the later phases of the disease, when leptospiruria has commenced, urine samples collected aseptically can be inoculated into these media. Both undiluted and 10-fold dilutions of urine should be inoculated because the undiluted urine can contain growth-inhibitory substances. To inhibit other contaminating bacteria, one can also add 5-fluorouracil (200 μg/ml). Cultures should be examined at weekly intervals for 5 weeks before being discarded. Contaminated fluid specimens can be purified by filtration through bacteriological filters (0.22 to 0.45 μm).

Animal inoculation.   Inoculation of weanling hamsters or guinea pigs is the most sensitive method of detecting leptospirae. Material is inoculated intraperitoneally. If signs of disease appear, blood is collected and examined microscopically for the organism. If signs of disease do not appear, blood samples are collected at 4-day intervals and examined.

Detection of antibodies. Serologic examination is of immense value for retrospective diagnosis. Serum from acutely ill and convalescent animals should be examined. A positive diagnosis requires a four-fold or greater increase in titer. A high titer that remains stationary indicates past infection.

The tests for antibody that are commonly used are (1) the microscopic agglutination test using live or killed leptospirae, (2) the plate-and-tube agglutination test using formalin-treated leptospirae, (3) the hamster passive-protection test, (4) the growth-inhibition test, and (5) enzyme-linked immunosorbent assay (ELISA) (Thiermann and Garrett 1983).

The microscopic agglutination test is the most reliable and widely used of the serologic diagnostic methods. Titers can reach enormous levels in some animals, and a titer of 1:100 or greater is evidence of past exposure to *Leptospira* antigen. This test detects IgM agglutinins about 7 to 9 days after the onset of the clinical disease. The agglutination test with killed antigen is less reliable and is more difficult to read. The hamster passive-protection test and the growth-inhibition tests detect neutralizing antibodies and become positive about 2 to 3 weeks after signs of clinical disease. These antibodies are of the IgG isotype and persist much longer than IgM antibodies (Hanson 1974). The ELISA procedures allow separate measurements of antibody activity caused by IgG and IgM antibodies and thus are helpful in determining whether an infection is recent. Furthermore, they allow use of purified antigens such as the group-specific antigen when the infecting serovar is unknown.

Antimicrobial Susceptibility. Leptospirae are sensitive in vitro to penicillin G, ampicillin, ceftizoxime, erythromycin, kanamycin, streptomycin, and tetracyclines (Oie et al. 1983). Streptomycin is widely used to cure cattle, pigs and dogs that are renal carriers. Streptomycin therapy (25 mg/kg of body weight) in combination with vaccination is an effective method for controlling clinical leptospirosis in cattle herds (Ellis 1984b, South and Stoenner 1974). Abortions in swine (Wandurski 1982) have been controlled by routine streptomycin treatment. Brunner (1949) successfully used streptomycin to eliminate serovars *canicola* and *icterohaemorrhagiae* from the tissues and urine of heavily infected dogs. Tetracycline (1,000 g/ton of feed) has also been used to eliminate leptospiruria in swine (Baker et al. 1957).

The Disease in Humans. Leptospirosis in humans is predominantly an occupational disease. Thus serovar *icterohaemorrhagiae* infections (Weil's disease) are frequently observed in miners and in sewer and abattoir workers; serovar *canicola* infections (canicola fever) are found in veterinarians and in breeders and owners of dogs; serovar *grippotyphosa* attacks farmers and agricultural and flax workers; serovar *pomona* infection occurs in swineherds, creamery workers, abattoir workers, and cheesemakers; serovar *australis* infection is found in sugarcane plantation workers (canecutter's fever); serovar *bataviae* attacks rice-field workers (harvest fever); and serovar *hardjo* infects dairy farmers.

Infection of humans occurs either directly from urine, milk, or tissues from a diseased animal or indirectly through contact with water or soil contaminated by animals. In the United States, the animals most likely to be involved are dogs, rats, cattle, swine, and certain wild animals that contaminate streams. The portals of entry are the mucous membranes of the eyes, nose, and mouth or abraded skin.

Symptoms of leptospirosis in humans vary, and although they are frequently severe, mortality is low. The disease is manifested by fever, headache, conjunctivitis, muscle pains, and encephalitic symptoms. There can be muscular tenderness, pharyngeal inflammation, skin rash, and minor hemorrhagic episodes. In some patients meningitis is a conspicuous symptom. Orchitis has been reported. The urine frequently contains albumin, a few erythrocytes, and casts. Jaundice is not present in many patients. Agglutinins and lytic antibodies for leptospirae appear during the second week of the disease and reach maximum titers several weeks later. The specific organism has often been isolated from the blood during the febrile period and from the urine some days or weeks after this.

REFERENCES

Auran, N.E., Johnson, R.C., and Ritzi, D.M. 1972. Isolation of the outer sheath of *Leptospira* and its immunogenic properties in hamsters. Infect. Immun. 5:968–975.

Baker, C.E., Gallian, M.J., Price, K.E., and White, E.A. 1957. Leptospirosis. 1. Therapeutic studies on the eradication of renal carriers of porcine leptospirosis. Vet. Med. 52:103–107.

Belloni, L., and Ruggeri, L. 1968. Aborto enzootico e infecondita da leptospirosi bovina in val padana (Osservazioni e rilievi). Clin. Veterinaria 91:237–243.

Bey, R.F., and Johnson, R.C. 1983. Leptospiral vaccines: Immunogenicity of protein-free medium cultivated whole cell bacterins in swine. Am. J. Vet. Res. 44:2299–2301.

Bezdenezhnuikh, N.I., and Kashanova, N.I. 1956. Porcine leptospirosis (*L. canicola* infection) on Sakhalin Island. J. Microbiol. (Moscow) 27:101–104.

Birnbaum, S., Shenberg, E., and Torten, M. 1972. The influence of maternal antibodies on the epidemiology of leptospiral carrier state in mice. Am. J. Epidemiol. 96:313–317.

Bishop, L., Strandberg, J.D., Adams, R.J., Brownstein, D.G., and Patterson, R. 1979. Chronic active hepatitis in dogs associated with leptospires. Am. J. Vet. Res. 40:839–844.

Brown, A.L., Creamer, A.A., and Scheidy, S.F. 1956. Immunization of horses against leptospirosis by vaccination. Vet. Med. 51:556–558.

Brunner, T.K. 1949. Canine leptospirosis. North Am. Vet. 30:517–519.

Burnstein, T., and Baker, J.A. 1954. Leptospirosis in swine caused by *Leptospira pomona*. J. Infect. Dis. 94:53–64.

Caleffi, D.F. 1966. Sulla vaccinazione antileptospira dei suini (nota pratica). Clin. Vet. 89:215–218.

Dacres, W.G. 1961. Fluorescein-labeled antibody technique for identification of leptospiral serotypes. Am. J. Vet. Res. 22:570–572.

Davidson, J.N., and Hirsh, D.C. 1980. Leptospirosis in lambs. J. Am. Vet. Med. Assoc. 176:124–125.

Ellis, W.A. 1984a. A study of related aspects of leptospirosis in naturally infected cattle. Fellowship thesis, Royal College of Veterinary Surgeons, London.

Ellis, W.A. 1984b. Bovine leptospirosis in the tropics: Prevalence, pathogenesis and control. Prev. Vet. Med. 2:411–421.

Ellis, W.A., and Michna, S.W. 1976. Bovine leptospirosis: Infection by the *Hebdomadis* serogroup and abortion—A herd study. Vet. Rec. 99:409–412.

Ellis, W.A., Bryson, D.G., O'Brien, J.J., and Neill, S.D. 1983. Leptospiral infection in aborted equine fetuses. Equine Vet. J. 15:321–324.

Ellis, W.A., Neill, S.D., O'Brien, J.J., Cassells, J.A., and Hanna, J. 1982. Bovine leptospirosis: Microbiological and serological findings in normal fetuses removed from uteri after slaughter. Vet. Rec. 110:192–194.

Ellis, W.A., O'Brien, J.J., Cassells, J.A. and Montgomery, J. 1983. Leptospiral infection in horses in Northern Ireland: Serological and microbiological findings. Equine Vet. J. 15:317–320.

Faine, S. 1962. The growth of *Leptospira australis* B in the kidneys of mice in the incipient experimental carrier state. J. Hyg. 60:435–442.

Gill, I.J., and Williamson, P.L. 1978. Efficacy of vaccination in eradicating disease caused by *Leptospira interrogans* serotype *pomona* in an intensive piggery. Victorian Vet. Proc. 36:38–40.

Hall, C.E., and Bryans, J.T. 1954. A case of leptospirosis in a horse. Cornell Vet. 44:345–348.

Hancock, G.A., Wilks, C.R., Kotiw, M., and Allen, J.D. 1984. The long-term efficacy of a Hardjo-pomona vaccine in preventing leptospiruria in cattle exposed to natural challenge with *Leptospira interrogans* serovar *hardjo*. Aust. Vet. J. 61:54–56.

Hanson, L.E. 1974. Bovine leptospirosis. J. Dairy Sci. 59:1166–1170.

Hanson, L.E., and Brodie, B.O. 1967. *Leptospira hardjo* infections in cattle. In Proceedings of the 71st Annual Meeting of the U.S. Livestock and Sanitary Association, Arizona Pp. 210–215.

Hanson, L.E., Tripathy, D.N., and Killinger, A.H. 1972. Current status of leptospirosis immunization in swine and cattle. J. Am. Vet. Med. Assoc. 161:1235–1243.

Hartley, W.J. 1952. Ovine leptospirosis. Aust. Vet. J. 28:169–170.

Hartman, E.G. 1984. Epidemiologic aspects of canine leptospirosis in the Netherlands. Zentralbl. Bakteriol. Mickrobiol. Hyg. [A] 258:350–359.

Hartman, E.G., van Houten, M., Frik, J.F., and van der Donk, J.A. 1984. Humoral immune response of dogs after vaccination against leptospirosis measured by an IgM and IgG-specific ELISA. Vet. Immunol. Immunopathol. 7:245–254.

Hathaway, S.C. 1981. Leptospirosis in New Zealand: An ecological view. N.Z. Vet. J. 29:109–112.

Hathaway, S.C., Ellis, W.A., Little, T.W.A., Stevens, A.E., and Ferguson, M.W. 1983. *Leptospira interrogans* serovar *hardjo* in pigs: A new host-parasite relationship in the United Kingdom. Vet. Rec. 113:153–154.

Hathaway, S.C., Wilesmith, J.W., and Little, T.W. 1984. Some population parameters of *Leptospira interrogans* serovar *hardjo* infection in sheep. Vet. Rec. 114:428–429.

Heusser, H. 1948. Die periodische Augenentzündung, eine Leptospirose? Schweiz. Arch. Tierheilk. 90:287–312.

Hirshberg, N., and Vaughn, J. 1973. Antibodies in bovine urine in leptospirosis. Vet. Med./Small Anim. Clin. 68:67.

Ho, H.F., and Blackmore, D.K. 1979. Effect of chilling and freezing on survival of *Leptospira interrogans* serovar *pomona* in naturally infected pig kidneys. N.Z. Vet. J. 27:121–123.

Hodges, R.T. 1974. Some observations on experimental *Leptospira* serotype *pomona* infection in sheep. N.Z. Vet. J. 22:151–154.

Jackson, R.S., Jones, E.E., and Clark, D.S. 1957. Abortion in mares associated with leptospirosis. J. Am. Vet. Med. Assoc. 131:564–565.

Kadis, S., and Pugh, W.A. 1974. Urea utilization by leptospires. Infect. Immun. 10:793–801.

Kemenes, F. 1964. Cross-immunity studies on virulent strains of leptospirae belonging to different serotypes. Z. Immun. Allergieforschr. 127:209–229.

Kerr, D.D., and Marshall, V. 1974. Protection against the renal carrier state by a canine leptospirosis vaccine. Vet. Med./Small Anim. Clin. 69:1157–1160.

Mackintosh, C.G., Blackmore, D.K., and Marshall, R.B. 1980. Isolation of *Leptospira interrogans* serovars *tarassovi* and *pomona* from dogs. N.Z. Vet. J. 28:100.

Michna, S.W. 1970. Leptospirosis. Vet. Rec. 86:484–496.

Morrison, W.I., and Wright, N.G. 1976. Canine leptospirosis: An immunopathological study of interstitial nephritis due to *Leptospira canicola*. J. Pathol. 120:83–89.

Morter, R.L., Williams, R.D., Bolte, H., and Freeman, M.J. 1969. Equine leptospirosis. J. Am. Vet. Med. Assoc. 155:436–444.

Navarro, C.E.K., Kociba, G.J., and Kowalski, J.J. 1981. Serum biochemical changes in dogs with experimental *Leptospira interrogans* serovar *icterohaemorrhagiae*. Am. J. Vet. Res. 42:1125–1129.

Negi, S.K., Meyers, W.L., and Segre, D. 1971. Antibody response of cattle to *Leptospira pomona*: Response as measured by hemagglutination, microscopic agglutination, and hamster protection tests. Am. J. Vet. Res. 32:1915–1920.

Nisbet, D.I. 1951. *Leptospira icterohaemorrhagiae* infection in pigs. J. Comp. Pathol. Ther. 61:155–160.

Nunes-Edwards, P.L., Thiermann, A.B., Bassford, P.J., and Stamm, L.V. 1985. Identification and characterization of the protein antigens of *Leptospira interrogans* serovar *hardjo*. Infect. Immun. 48:492–497.

Oie, S., Hironaga, K., Konishi, H., and Yoshii, Z. 1983. In vitro susceptibilities of five leptospira strains to 16 antimicrobial agents. Antimicrob. Agents Chemother. 24:905–908.

Ono, E., Naiki, M., and Yanagawa, R. 1984. Isolation of an antigenic oligosaccharide fraction from *Leptospira interrogans* serovar *canicola* with a monoclonal antibody. J. Gen. Microbiol. 130:1429–1435.

Roberts, S.J., York, C.J., and Robinson, J.W. 1952. An outbreak of leptospirosis in horses on a small farm. J. Am. Vet. Med. Assoc. 121:237–242.

Ryu, E. 1975. An investigation of canine antileptospiral antibodies in Japan. Int. J. Zoonoses 2:16–34.

Sippel, W.L. 1953. Leptospirosis. North Am. Vet. 34:111–112.

South, P.J., and Stoenner, H.G. 1974. The control of outbreaks of leptospirosis in beef cattle by simultaneous vaccination and treatment with dihydrostreptomycin. Proc. U.S. Anim. Health Assoc. 78:126–130.

Spencer, A.J., and Wright, N.G. 1981. Chronic interstitial nephritis in the dog: An immunofluorescence and elution study. Res. Vet. Sci. 30:226–232.

Stalheim, O.M.V. 1985. Leptospira. In H. Blobel and T. Schliesser, eds., Handbuch der bakteriellen Infektionen bei Tieren, Band V. VEB Gustav Fischer Verlag, Jena. Pp. 90–154.

Stoenner, H.G., Hadlow, W.J., and Ward, J.K. 1963. Neurologic manifestations of leptospirosis in a dairy cow. J. Am. Vet. Med. Assoc. 142:491–493.

Stringfellow, D.A., Brown, R.R., Hanson, L., Schurrenberger, P.R., and Johnson, J. 1983. Can antibody responses in cattle vaccinated with a multivalent leptospiral bacterin interfere with serologic diagnosis of disease? J. Am. Vet. Med. Assoc. 182:165–167.

Swart, K.S., Calvert, K., and Meney, C. 1982. The prevalence of antibodies to serovars of *Leptospira interrogans* in horses. Aust. Vet. J. 59:25–27.

Takashima, I., Shinagawa, M., and Yanagowa, R. 1975. Serological studies of leptospiras by immunodiffusion. Zentralbl. Bakteriol. Mikrobiol. Hyg. [A] 228:369–377.

Terpstra, E.J., Ligthart, G.S., and Schoone, G.J. 1980. Serodiagnosis of human leptospirosis by enzyme-linked immunosorbent assay for the detection of antibodies to *Leptospira interrogans* serovars *hardjo* and *pomona* in cattle. Am. J. Vet. Res. 44:884–888.

Thiermann, A.B. 1980. Canine leptospirosis in Detroit. Am. J. Vet. Res. 41:1659–1661.

Thiermann, A.B., and Garrett, L.A. 1983. Enzyme linked immunosorbent assay for the detection of antibodies to *Leptospira interrogans* serovars *hardjo* and *pomona* in cattle. Am. J. Vet. Res. 44:884–887.

Timoney, J.F., Sheahan, B.J., and Timoney, P.J. 1974. Leptospira and infectious canine hepatitis (ICH) virus antibodies and nephritis in Dublin dogs. Vet. Rec. 94:316–319.

Torten, M., Ben-Efraim, S., Shenberg, E., Beemer, A.M., and van der Hoeden, J. 1967. Experimental induction of ocular reaction resembling post leptospiral ophthalmia and its relation to skin reactions and circulating antibodies. Clin. Exp. Immunol. 2:573–580.

Tripathy, D.N., Hanson, L.E., Mansfield, M., and Thilsted, J.P. 1981. Pathogenesis of *Leptospira pomona* in lactating sows and transmission to piglets. Proc. U.S. Anim. Health Assoc. 85:188–191.

Tripathy, D.N., Smith, A.R., and Hanson, L.E. 1975. Immunoglobulins in cattle vaccinated with leptospiral bacterins. Am. J. Vet. Res. 36:1735–1736.

Twigg, G.I., Hughes, D.M., and McDiarmid, A. 1972. Leptospiral antibodies in dairy cattle: Some ecological considerations. Vet. Rec. 90:598–602.

Wandurski, A. 1982. Effect of infection with various serotypes of *Leptospira interrogans* on the fertility of swine. Med. Weterynaryjna 38:218–220.

White, F.H., Stoliker, H.E., and Galton, M.M. 1961. Detection of *Leptospires* in naturally infected dogs, using fluorescein-labeled antibody. Am. J. Vet. Res. 22:650–654.

Whyte, P.B.D., Ratcliff, R.M., Cargill, C., and Dobson, K.J. 1982. Protection of pregnant swine by vaccination against leptospira infection. Aust. Vet. J. 59:41–45.

Yager, R.H., Gochenour, N.S., Jr., and Wetmore, P.W. 1950. Recurrent iridocyclitis (periodic ophthalmia) of horses. J. Am. Vet. Med. Assoc. 117:207–209.

The Genus *Treponema*

Members of the genus *Treponema* are found in the oral cavity, intestinal tract, and genital region of humans and animals. They are unicellular helical rods, 5 to 20 μm long, with tight regular or irregular spirals. The cells have one or more periplasmic flagella inserted at each end of the protoplasmic cylinder. Those that have been cultivated are anaerobic.

Only two species are of known significance in veterinary bacteriology: *T. hyodysenteriae* and *T. cuniculi*. These organisms cause dysentery and vent disease in swine and rabbits, respectively.

Treponema hyodysenteriae

Although *swine dysentery (bloody scours)* was first described by Whiting et al. in 1921, demonstration of *T. hyodysenteriae* as the primary infectious agent was not accomplished until the early 1970s (Harris et al. 1972, Taylor 1970). The delay in proving the cause was in great part because the disease process requires the interaction of other components of the normal colonic flora (Brandenburg et al. 1977, Harris et al. 1978, Meyer 1974). *Bacteroides vulgatus* and *Fusobacterium necrophorum* are two such organisms. Swine dysentery cannot be produced in gnotobiotic pigs unless *T. dysenteriae* and these organisms are administered together.

Morphology and Staining Reactions. *T. hyodysenteriae* is 6 to 9 μm in length and 0.4 μm in diameter (Figure 5.8). It is loosely coiled, tapered at the ends, and possesses 7 to 9 periplasmic flagella inserted at each end. These flagella overlap near the middle of the cell. *T. hyodysenteriae* can be stained with crystal violet or dilute carbol-fuchsin stain. The organism can be stained by the Goodpasture or Warthin-Starry procedures in sections of mucosa. It is Gram-negative.

Figure 5.8. Micrograph of *Treponema hyodysenteriae*, demonstrating the spiral shape of the organism. Carbol-fuchsin stain. × 1,400. (From Harris et al., 1972, courtesy of *Veterinary Medicine/Small Animal Clinicians*.)

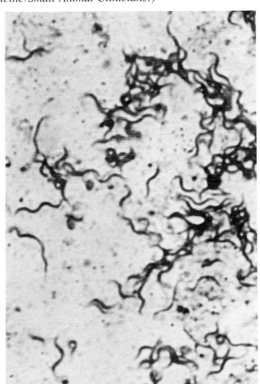

Cultural and Biochemical Features. Although *T. hyodysenteriae* is an anaerobe, it is tolerant of oxygen. It grows readily under anaerobic conditions on freshly poured trypticase-soy agar containing 5 percent bovine or equine blood. The plates should be examined for hemolysis every 2 days. The organism produces small, gray, hazy colonies within the hemolytic zones and can be transferred by taking a piece of agar from the edge of the zone and using it as inoculum for a new culture. Prereduced trypticase-soy broth containing 10 percent fetal calf serum can also be used for propagation. A selective medium containing spectinomycin (400 μm/ml) is commonly used to isolate *T. hyodysenteriae* from enteric specimens.

T. hyodysenteriae is readily separated from other intestinal bacteria by passing it through cellulose acetate filters with pore sizes of 0.8, 0.65, and 0.45 μm and culturing the filtrate on blood agar.

T. hyodysenteriae is oxidase- and catalase-negative and produces acid from glucose. It can be distinguished from the similar but nonpathogenic *T. innocens* by its production of a strong beta-hemolytic reaction and its failure to ferment fructose or esculin. *T. innocens* also produces an unusual galactolipid not found in *T. hyodysenteriae* (Matthews et al. 1980). The mol% G + C of the DNA is 26.0.

Antigens. At least four serovars have been proposed based on water-soluble antigens released after hot phenol water extraction (Baum and Joens 1979). Protective antigens occur among the outer envelope proteins (Peterson 1983).

Epizootiology and Pathogenesis. Survival of *T. hyodysenteriae* in soil or pig feces is brief (24 to 48 hours), and pigs exposed to soil that previously held infected animals are unlikely to become infected (Egan 1982). Depopulation is an effective measure to eliminate infection in a herd but it must be accompanied by sanitation measures and a rest period of 30 to 60 days. However, the organism can be maintained in the intestines of wild rats and mice for months, and it has been suggested that these animals are primary reservoir hosts (Blaha et al. 1984, Joens and Kinyon 1982). Experimental transmission from the feces of infected mice has been demonstrated (Joens 1980).

Within-group transmission occurs by means of the feces from clinically affected or carrier animals. Swine dysentery is most common in feeder swine that weigh between 30 and 140 pounds. After it enters into a susceptible pig, the organism invades goblet cells of the colonic mucosa and multiplies in the crypts of Lieberkühn (Figures 5.9 and 5.10). It is also found on the surface epithelium. The presence of the organism in goblet cells and in the adjoining mucosa induces mucus secretion and cell

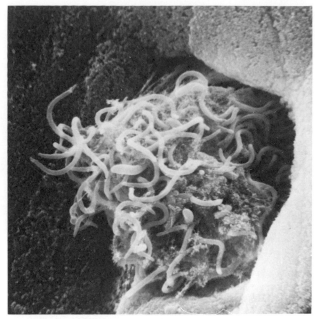

Figure 5.9. *Treponema hyodysenteriae* in a colonic crypt of a pig affected with swine dysentery. (From Kennedy and Strafuss, 1977, courtesy of Chicago Press Inc.)

Figure 5.10. Scanning electron micrograph of spirochetes and associated vibriolike organisms (*V*) in the colon of a pig affected with dysentery. × 9,300. (From Kennedy et al., 1973, courtesy of *Journal of American Veterinary Medical Association*.)

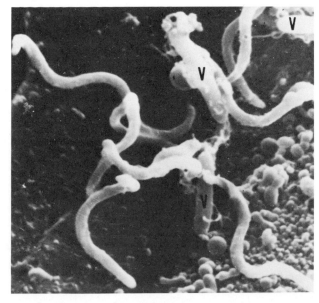

proliferation (Pohlenz et al. 1983). A mucohemorrhagic colitis results, and blood and mucus or mucus alone is passed in the feces, which is thin, dark, and watery. Some pigs have elevated temperatures. Fibronecrotic membranous material is formed on the colonic mucosa, and large numbers of *T. hyodysenteriae* and other vibriolike organisms are present in this material. The walls and mesentery of the large intestine are hyperemic and edematous, and the rugose texture of the mucosal surface is lost.

The lipopolysaccharide (LPS) of the organism is believed to play a role in the pathogenicity of *T. hyodysenteriae* (Nuessen et al. 1983). LPS-resistant mice are resistant to *T. hyodysenteriae* but LPS-sensitive, genetically related mice are not and develop severe colitis.

The pathophysiological transport alteration in swine dysentery is a colonic malabsorption characterized by a net decrease in lumen-to-blood flux of Na^+ and Cl^-. There is no evidence of a role for adenyl or guanyl cyclase activities in the pathogenesis of the diarrhea (Schmall et al. 1983).

Up to 50 percent of untreated swine die of the disease. Death is caused by dehydration and acidosis. Animals that recover can continue to shed the organism for 3 months or longer and can infect other animals with which they come in contact.

Immunity. Pigs that recover are resistant to challenge by homologous strains of *T. hyodysenteriae* but not by heterologous strains (Joens et al. 1983, Olson 1974), and antibodies have been found in the serums of convalescent animals. Intravenous hyperimmunization with formalin-killed antigen has been shown to increase serum antibody titers and to protect animals against challenge with a homologous strain (Glock et al. 1976). Formalinized vaccines in oil adjuvant have also been shown to reduce the incidence and severity of the disease in experimentally challenged animals (Fernie et al. 1983).

Passively immunized pigs are not protected against infection, but the onset of the disease is delayed (Schwartz and Glock 1976).

The fluorescent antibody test (Terpstra et al. 1968), passive hemolysis test (Jenkins et al. 1976), microtiter agglutination test (Joens et al. 1978), and ELISA (Joens et al. 1982) have been used to assay antibodies. ELISA appears to have the most potential for detection of asymptomatic carriers.

Diagnosis. Confirmation of clinical diagnosis must be made in the laboratory. The presence of numerous large, loosely coiled spirochetelike organisms in mucosal scrapings, as detected under phase or dark-field microscopy, by the fluorescent antibody test, or in stained preparations is tentative evidence for a diagnosis of swine dysentery. Attempts to culture the organism from filtrates of mucosal scrapings should also be made.

Campylobacter species and loosely coiled spirochetes can also be present in animals with swine dysentery and in other enteric conditions of swine and can complicate interpretation of microscopic preparations. Olson and Fales (1983) have concluded that diagnosis must be based on a combination of clinical signs and examination of stained smears and culturing.

Antimicrobial Susceptibility. *T. hyodysenteriae* is sensitive to penicillin, ampicillin, cephalothin, erythromycin, tylosin, tiamulin, polymyxin B, ronidazole, and furazolidone. Carbox and carbox plus sulfamethazine are effective feed additives for prophylaxis and control (Raynaud et al. 1981).

REFERENCES

Baum, D.H., and Joens, L.A. 1979. Serotypes of beta-hemolytic *Treponema hyodysenteriae*. Infect. Immun. 25:792–796.

Blaha, T., Gunther, H., Flossmann, K.D., and Erler, W. 1984. Epidemiological basis of swine dysentery. Zentralbl. Veterinärmed. [B] 31:451–465.

Brandenburg, A.C., Miniats, O.P., Geissenger, H.D., and Ewert, E. 1977. Swine dysentery: Inoculation of gnotobiotic pigs with *Treponema hyodysenteriae* and *Vibrio coli* and a peptostreptococcus. Can. J. Comp. Med. 41:294–301.

Egan, I.H.T. 1982. Epidemiology aspects of swine dysentery in the Midwestern United States. Dissertation Abstracts Int.[B] 42:4320.

Fernie, D.S., Ripley, P.H., and Walker, P.D. 1983. Swine dysentery: Protection against experimental challenge following single dose parenteral immunization with activated *Treponema hyodysenteriae*. Res. Vet. Sci. 35:217–221.

Glock, R.D., Schwartz, K.J., and Harris, D.L. 1976. Experimental immunization of pigs against *Treponema hyodysenteriae*. In Proceedings of the 4th International Pig Veterinary Society Congress, Ames, Iowa.

Harris, D.L., Alexander, T.J.L., Whipp, S.C., Robinson, I.M., Glock, R.D., and Matthews, P.J. 1978. Swine dysentery: Studies of gnotobiotic pigs inoculated with *Treponema hyodysenteriae*, *Bacteroides vulgatus*, and *Fusobacterium necrophorum*. J. Am. Vet. Med. Assoc. 172:468–471.

Harris, D.L., Glock, R.D., Christensen, C.R., and Kinyon, I.M. 1972. Swine dysentery. I. Inoculation of pigs with *Treponema hyodysenteriae* (new species) and reproduction of the disease. Vet. Med./Small Anim. Clin. 67:61–64.

Jenkins, E.M., Sinha, P.P., Vance, R.T., and Resse, G.L. 1976. Passive hemolysis test for antibody to *Treponema hyodysenteriae*. Infect. Immun.

Joens, L.A. 1980. Experimental transmission of *Treponema hyodysenteriae* from mice to pigs. Am. J. Vet. Res. 41:1225–1226.

Joens, L.A., and Kinyon, J.M. 1982. Isolation of *Treponema hyodysenteriae* from wild rodents. J. Clin. Microbiol. 15:994–997.

Joens, L.A., Harris, D.L., Kinyon, J.M., and Kaeberk, M.I. 1978. Microtitration agglutination for detection of *Treponema hyodysenteriae* antibody. J. Clin. Microbiol. 8:293–298.

Joens, L.A., Nord, N.A., Kinyon, J.M., and Egan, I.T. 1982. Enzyme-linked immuno-absorbent assay for detection of antibody to *T. hyodysenteriae* antigens. J. Clin. Microbiol. 15:249–252.

Joens, L.A., Whipp, S.C., Glock, R.D., and Neussen, M.E. 1983. Serotype-specific protection against *Treponema hyodysenteriae* infection in ligated colonic loops of pigs recovered from swine dysentery. Infect. Immun. 39:460–462.

Kennedy, G.A., and Strafuss, A.C. 1977. Scanning electron microscopy of the lesions of swine dysentery. In O. Johari and R. Becker, eds.,

Scanning Electron Microscopy, vol. 2. Chicago Press Inc., Chicago. Pp. 283–290.

Kennedy, G.A., Strafuss, A.C., and Schoneweis, D.A. 1973. Scanning electron microscope observations on swine dysentery. J. Am. Vet. Med. Assoc. 163:53–55.

Matthews, H.M., Yang, T.K., and Jenkin, H.M. 1980. *Treponema innocens* lipids and further description of an unusual galactolipid of *T. hyodysenteriae*. J. Bacteriol. 143:1151–1155.

Meyer, R.C., Simon, J., and Byerly, C.S. 1974. The etiology of swine dysentery. I. Oral inoculation of germ-free swine with *Treponema hyodysenteriae* and *Vibrio coli*. II. Effect of a known microbial flora, weaning and diet on disease production in gnotobiotic and conventional swine. Vet. Pathol. 11:515–526, 527–534.

Nuessen, M.E., Joens, L.A., and Glock, R.D. 1983. Involvement of lipopolysaccharide in the pathogenicity of *Treponema hyodysenteriae*. J. Immunol. 131:997–999.

Olson, L.D. 1974. Clinical and pathological observations on the experimental passage of swine dysentery. Can. J. Comp. Med. 38:7–13.

Olson, L.D., and Fales, W.H. 1983. Comparison of stained smears and culturing for identification of *Treponema hyodysenteriae*. J. Clin. Microbiol. 18:940–955.

Peterson, L.H. 1983. Immunologic response of swine to solubilized outer envelope components of *Treponema hyodysenteriae*. Diss. Abstr. Int. [B] 43:3500–3501.

Pohlenz, J.E.L., Whipp, S.C., and Robinson, I.M. 1983. Pathogenesis of swine dysentery caused by *Treponema hyodysenteriae*. D.T.W. 90:363–367.

Raynaud, J.P., Brunault, G., and Patterson, E.B. 1981. A swine dysentery model for evaluation of drug prophylaxis. I. Development of a model involving oral infection plus pen contamination. II. Efficacy of various drugs in the control of swine dysentery. Am. J. Vet. Res. 42:49–53.

Schmall, L.M., Argenzio, R.A., and Whipp, S.C. 1983. Pathophysiologic features of swine dysentery: Cyclic nucleotide-independent production of diarrhea. Am. J. Vet. Res. 44:1309–1316.

Schwartz, K., and Glock, R.D. 1976. Resistance to *Treponema hyodysenteriae* in passively immunized pigs. In Proceedings of the 4th International Pig Veterinary Society Congress, Ames, Iowa.

Taylor, D.J. 1970. An agent possibly associated with swine dysentery. Vet. Rec. 86:416.

Terpstra, J.I., Akkermans, J.P.W.M., and Ouwerkerk, H. 1968. Investigations into the etiology of vibrionic dysentery (Doyle) in pigs. Neth. J. Vet. Sci. 1:5–13.

Whiting, R.A., Doyle, L.P., and Spray, R.S. 1921. Swine dysentery. Indiana Agric. Exp. Sta. Bull. 257. Pp. 3–15.

Treponema cuniculi

SYNONYM: *Treponema paraluiscuniculi*

T. cuniculi is the cause of *rabbit syphilis (vent disease)* and is spread during sexual activity. The lesions are superficial ulcerated areas on the genital and perineal areas. The organism is very slender, is 6 to 14 μm long, and has not been cultured.

Organic arsenicals and penicillin are effective in therapy. Small and Newman (1972) give a good description of the disease.

REFERENCE

Small, J.D., and Newman, B. 1972. Venereal spirochetosis of rabbits (rabbit syphilis) due to *Treponema cuniculi*: A clinical, serological, and histopathological study. Lab. Anim. Sci. 22:77–89.

with genes that encode for lactose fermentation. The slow lactose fermentation of *Salmonella arizonae* is chromosomally encoded. The distinguishing characteristics of the genera of importance in veterinary bacteriology are shown in Table 6.1.

6 The Enterobacteriaceae— The Lactose Fermenters

Members of the family Enterobacteriaceae are facultatively anaerobic Gram-negative rods that can be motile or nonmotile; the motile strains have peritrichous flagella. All species grow well on artificial media and attack glucose, from which they form acid or acid and gas. They also produce catalase. With some exceptions in the genus *Erwinia*, members of Enterobacteriaceae reduce nitrates to nitrites. Their antigenic composition constitutes a mosaic of interlocking serologic relationships among the several genera. The family contains saprophytes and many animal and some plant parasites.

DNA homology studies have shown that the species within most genera of the Enterobacteriaceae are at least 20 percent related to one another and to the type species, *Escherichia coli*. Almost all species share a common enterobacterial antigen. Only a small number of genera have species that cause disease in animals. These are *Enterobacter, Escherichia, Klebsiella, Proteus, Salmonella, Serratia,* and *Yersinia*.

For convenience of presentation, the members of Enterobacteriaceae are divided into lactose-fermenting and non-lactose-fermenting groups. This chapter will deal with the lactose-fermenters; Chapter 8 will cover the genera that do not ferment lactose. Among the genera that ferment lactose are *Enterobacter, Escherichia,* and *Klebsiella*. Chromogenic *Serratia* organisms have been reported in bovine mastitis and in septicemias in humans and are assuming increasing importance as opportunistic pathogens. *Enterobacter* species occasionally cause mastitis and invade the urinary tract in dogs.

Isolates of *Salmonella* that ferment lactose are occasionally found. These strains generally carry plasmids

The Genus *Escherichia*

Escherichia coli

E. coli is a normal inhabitant of the lower intestine of all warm-blooded animals and is usually absent from the intestines of fish and other cold-blooded animals. Few or no *E. coli* organisms are found in the stomach and anterior portions of the bowel. Carnivores and omnivores usually harbor the organisms in greater abundance than herbivores. The feces of cows and horses usually contain only 10^3 to 10^4 *E. coli* per gram. *E. coli* is sought in bacteriological examination of water, and its presence is taken as evidence of fecal pollution.

Morphology and Staining Reactions. *E. coli* is a Gram-negative, rod-shaped organism 1.0 to 1.5 μm in width by 2.0 to 6.0 μm in length that varies widely in morphology under different conditions. Usually it is a short, plump rod; sometimes rather long filaments are seen. It can be motile by means of peritrichous flagella or it can be nonmotile. *E. coli* never forms spores, and capsular material is present on some strains. It stains readily and evenly with ordinary stains. Fimbriae are frequently present.

Cultural and Biochemical Features. *E. coli* grows readily on all ordinary media. The optimum temperature for growth is 37°C, but it will grow at a wide range of temperatures. It is aerobic and facultatively anaerobic. Colonies grown on agar media are raised, smooth, glistening, gray, and circular in outline. Heavily encapsulated strains appear mucoid. Rough colonial forms also occur. Some strains are beta-hemolytic on blood agar.

E. coli does not liquefy gelatin and does not use citrate. It ferments glucose and other carbohydrates by means of the conversion of pyruvate into lactic acid. Most strains ferment lactose.

E. coli forms indole usually in abundance; vigorously reduces nitrates; and reacts negatively to the Voges-Proskauer test. The Voges-Proskauer test is valuable in distinguishing *E. coli* from *Enterobacter aerogenes*, which reacts positively. The mol% G + C of the DNA is 48 to 52 (Tm).

Antigens. The surface structures of *E. coli* are expressed as O (somatic), K (capsular), H (flagellar), and F (fimbrial) antigens. At least 170 O, 80 K, and 56 H antigens are recognized. Each serotype is designated by the numbers of the antigens it carries, for example,

Table 6.1. Some differential characteristics of genera of the Enterobacteriaceae associated with animal disease

Enteric groups	Semisolid motility medium	Gelatinase	Hydrogen sulfide	Indole	Urease	Methyl red	Voges-Proskauer	Citrate	Glucose	Lactose	Sucrose	Salicin
Escherichia coli	v	−	−	+	−	+	−	−	ag	ag	v	v
Klebsiella	−	−	−	−	s	v	v	+	ag	ag	ag	ag
Enterobacter	+	−	−	−	v	v	+	+	ag	ag	ag	ag
Proteus	+	+	+	+	+	−	−	−	av	−	av	−
Salmonella	+	−	+	−	−	+	−	+	ag	−	−	−
Salmonella arizonae	+	s	+	−	−	+	−	+	ag	s	−	−
Serratia	+	+	−	−	v	v	+	+	av	(−)	+	+
Yersinia	−	−	−	v	+	+	−	−	av	−	+	v

v = variable; − = negative; (−) = usually negative, but important exceptions occur; + = positive; s = slow utilization; ag = acid and gas; av = acid with or without gas.

O139:K82:H2. The O antigen is determined by the sugar sidechains on the lipopolysaccharide molecule. Although K antigens are polysaccharides, some well-known proteinaceous fimbrial antigens such as F4 and F5 have been traditionally but incorrectly termed K antigens, for example, K88 and K99. The H antigens are proteinaceous and are found in the flagella.

There are a number of different fimbrial antigens (F1, F2, etc.), with the possibility of subtypes within a single antigen. Fimbrial antigens usually have important adhesive functions that allow an *E. coli* strain to colonize the intestine or other body sites (Figure 6.1). F1 fimbrial antigens exhibit an ability to hemagglutinate erythrocytes; this ability is blocked by mannose (mannose-sensitive).

The F1 fimbrial antigens mediate adhesion to mucus on mucosal surfaces. The F2, F3, F4, F5, F41, F165 fimbrial antigens are not mannose sensitive and mediate adhesion to specific ganglioside receptors on the intestinal mucosa. The best known fimbrial antigen, K88, is now termed F4 (Orskov and Orskov 1984).

F4 (K88) fimbriae are plasmid-encoded and composed of multimers of a protein subunit with a molecular weight of about 25,000 (Moon et al. 1979). *E. coli* strains carrying this antigen are common in swine. The intestinal receptor is inherited as a dominant characteristic in a simple Mendelian way (Sellwood 1979). Therefore, only homozygous dominants and heterozygotes carry the receptor and are susceptible to colonization by *E. coli* that

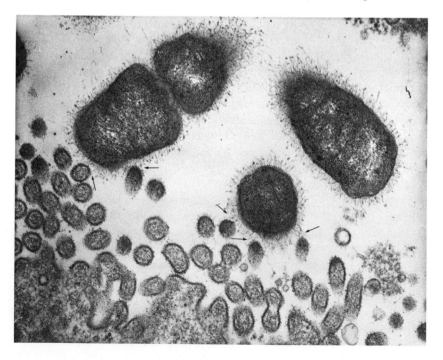

Figure 6.1. Transmission electron micrograph of K99 (F5)–positive *Escherichia coli* in the small intestine of a pig. The hairlike fimbriae (pili) on the surface of the *E. coli* are adherant to the host microvilli (*arrows*). (Courtesy Harley Moon.)

have F4 fimbriae. At least four variants of the F4 antigen—K88 ab 1, K88 ab 2, K88 ac, and K88 ad—that differ in amino acid composition of certain antigenic domains exist (Dykes et al. 1985).

The F5 fimbria or K99 antigen is also plasmid-encoded and is found on *E. coli* strains enterotoxigenic for calves, lambs, and piglets. It is composed of a single repeating protein subunit with a molecular mass of 18,500 (de Graaf et al. 1980). Its receptor is a complex glycolipid similar to GM_3 ganglioside (Smit et al. 1984).

Other fimbrial antigens important in colonization of the intestines of pigs, include F41, F165, and P987. Moreover, there is circumstantial evidence for the existence of other as yet uncharacterized fimbrial antigens (Moon et al. 1980).

Enterotoxins. Plasmid-encoded heat-labile (LT) and heat-stable (ST) enterotoxins can be produced singly or in combination by enterotoxic *E. coli* strains. They are always present in association with colonizing antigens such as F4 or F5 (K88 and K99) in isolates from animals with diarrhea. The heat-labile enterotoxin is plasmid-encoded and consists of two dissimilar polypeptide subunits A and B. There are five B and one A (molecular weight 27,500) subunits in each entire toxin molecule. The B subunits (molecular weight 11,500) have a receptor function and bind to ganglioside GM_1 on mucosal cells of the small intestine. After entry into the cell, the A subunit activates adenylate cyclase by NAD-dependent ADP ribosylation of its regulatory subunit (Gill and Richardson 1980). Levels of intracellular cyclic AMP increase and this in some way causes a net outflow of Na^+, Cl^-, and H_2O from the cell.

Heat-stable enterotoxin exists as STa and STb. Sta is found in enterotoxigenic *E. coli* from baby piglets and consists of a polypeptide with a molecular weight that varies from 1,500 to 2,000. It is soluble in methanol, has biological activity in suckling mice and activates guanylate cyclase in intestinal mucosal cells resulting in inhibition of Na^+ and Cl^- absorption by the brush-border membrane. Its intestinal receptor appears to be protein or glycoprotein with a molecular weight of about 100,000 (Dreyfus and Robertson 1984).

STb is found in enterotoxigenic *E. coli* from weanling swine, is insoluble in methanol, has no biological activity in suckling mice, and has no effect on cyclic GMP levels of intestinal mucosal cells (Kennedy et al. 1984). The mechanism of fluid efflux is unknown and is characterized by an early onset of action that is evident for as long as 18 hours in pig intestine (Kashiwazaki et al. 1981). Some important characteristics of the *E. coli* enterotoxins are summarized in Table 6.2.

Edema disease toxin. Edema disease toxin was the first of the *E. coli* toxins to be demonstrated and partially characterized (Timoney 1949, 1950, 1957). It is a thermolabile protein, insoluble at acid pH but soluble at alkaline pH, with a molecular weight of about 66,000 (Timoney 1986). It is related to the shigalike toxin 2 (SLT 2) of *E. coli* found in human cases of hemorrhagic colitis. The toxin produces paralysis and death in mice and toxic changes in Vero cells. Its mode of action may be to inhibit protein synthesis in endothelial cells of blood vessels. The end effect in the animal is hypertension with panarteritis (Kurtz and Quast 1976). It is antigenic, and antiserums are antitoxic (Timoney 1956). Antiserum to Shiga toxin does not neutralize the edema disease toxin.

Shigalike toxin (SLT). Most enteropathogenic *E. coli* from cases of enteritis in human infants produce proteinaceous toxins (SLT 1, 2, or both) that biologically and structurally resemble the cytotoxin of *Shigella dysenteriae* type 1 (Shiga). They contain A and B subunits, the B subunit having a toxin-binding function (O'Brien and Holmes 1987). The *E. coli* and Shiga cytotoxins are cell-associated, inhibit protein synthesis, are produced under conditions of iron deprivation, and are lethal for mice and enterotoxic for rabbits in microgram doses (O'Brien and LaVeck 1983). Infections by SLT-producing *E. coli* are associated with destruction of gut epithelial cell microvilli where there is dense adherence of *E. coli* (Figure 6.2). This effect is termed *effacement,* and *E. coli* that produce SLT are therefore known as effacing *E. coli*. Effacing *E. coli* belonging to O groups 26 and 111 have been isolated from cases of enteric colibacillosis in newborn pigs and calves.

Epizootiology and Pathogenesis. Pathogenic strains of *E. coli* are associated with disease of the intestine and with fulminating septicemias of newborn or young animals and with respiratory tract disease of poultry. Normally nonpathogenic strains also can cause opportunistic infections in the udder, uterus, and other body sites. *E. coli* strains that cause enteritis have been arbitrarily classified as enterotoxigenic (ETEC), enteropathogenic (EPEC), enteroinvasive (EIEC), and attaching and effacing (AEEC). ETEC strains produce enterotoxins; EPEC strains do not apparently produce enterotoxins or Shigalike toxin and cause enteritis by other unknown mechanisms; EIEC strains invade enterocytes and the deeper layers of the mucosa of the intestine; and AEEC strains colonize the small intestine, produce Shigalike toxins, and destroy the microvillus layer by unknown means. Most of these strains are host-specific, and a limited number of well-defined serotypes are closely associated with specific disease entities in each animal host. These diseases are characteristically found in newborn or young animals and a variety of epizootiological factors can be involved. Moreover, etiological agents other than

Table 6.2. Properties and effects of *E. coli* enterotoxins

Property	Heat-labile toxin (LT)	Heat-stable toxin (Sta)	Heat-stable toxin (Stb)
Molecular weight	85,000	1,500–2,000	4,000?
Antigenic	Yes	Only as a hapten	Only as a hapten
Occurrence	*E. coli* from diarrhea	*E. coli* from porcine and bovine neonatal diarrhea	*E. coli* from porcine weanling diarrhea
Mode of action	Stimulates adenyl activity of intestinal and capillary epithelium	Stimulates guanylate cyclase activity of ileal epithelial cells	Unknown
Onset and duration	Slow onset, prolonged action	Rapid onset, extended duration of action in baby pigs	Rapid onset, prolonged action
Effect	Cyclic AMP levels elevated with deregulation of ionic pump in intestinal epithelial cells. Efflux of Na^+, H_2O, and HCO_3^- and reduced absorption of Cl^-	Cyclic GMP levels elevated with deregulation of ionic pump in intestinal epithelial cells. Efflux of Na^+, H_2O, and HCO_3^- and reduced absorption of Cl^-	Efflux of Na^+, H_2O, and HCO_3^-

Figure 6.2. Electron micrographs showing attaching and effacing *Escherichia coli* (AEEC) in the colonic epithelium of a calf. In the photograph on the left, taken at low magnification, the intestinal microvilli have been effaced, and the *E. coli* are adhering to the host cell membrane. (Courtesy Harley Moon.) The photograph on the right shows the intimate association of bacterium and host cell in more detail. (From H. W. Moon, R. E. Isaacson, and J. Pohlenz, © *Am. J. Clin. Nutr.*, 32 (1979):119–127, courtesy of the American Society for Clinical Nutrition and Harley Moon.)

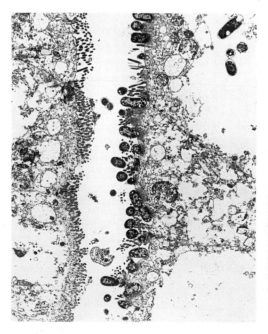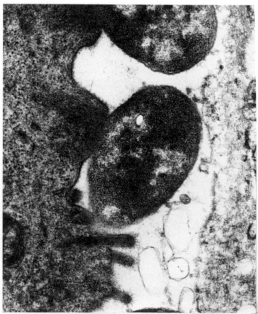

E. coli can be present at the same time. A critical factor is the immune status of the newborn animal. If the animal fails to absorb an adequate amount of colostral immunoglobulins with the appropriate antibody specificities it will have a much-enhanced susceptibility to *E. coli* enteritis or septicemia. Circumstances such as poor mothering, excessive cold, a weak constitution, or a dam that had no prior exposure to the pathogenic *E. coli* strain thus may indirectly predispose the newborn to colibacillosis. Intensive husbandry practices are important because they favor rapid passage of pathogenic clones. The primary source of pathogenic *E. coli* is feces, and factors and management practices that result in a build-up of fecal contamination favor feco-oral cycling with a high probability of exposure to large numbers of the pathogen. The degree and intensity of this exposure can be such as to overwhelm colostral immunity.

The disease in swine. There are three distinct manifestations of enteric colibacillosis in swine: (1) neonatal *E. coli* enteritis—enteritis of piglets 1 to 4 days old; (2) weanling enteritis—enteritis shortly after weaning; (3) edema disease—edema in various body tissues of pigs soon after weaning.

Neonatal *E. coli* enteritis occurs during the first 4 days of life in piglets raised under intensive conditions of husbandry. The serotypes involved mainly belong to groups O8, O9, O20, O101, O138, O139, O141, O147, O149, and O157. Closed herds are affected by only one or two serotypes, open herds by up to seven. After infection of the baby piglet, the *E. coli* strain colonizes the epithelium of the small intestine. This phase is favored by the possession of colonizing antigens such as the F4 (K88) pilus protein, which mediates adhesion to the microvilli of the epithelial cells of the anterior small intestine (Figure 6.3). Production and release of enterotoxin then follows. The majority of *E. coli* isolates from piglet enteritis are enterotoxigenic by the available assays. Both LT and STa forms can be found in the same strains. All strains produce STa and some also produce LT toxin (Smith and Gyles 1970). The piglets appear normal for the first 12 hours of life and then develop a profuse pale yellow watery diarrhea, which frequently leads to fatal dehydration within 18 hours. Most of the litter is usually affected, and mortality can be as high as 90 percent. At necropsy the small intestine is dilated, thin walled, and filled with a beige fluid. Predisposing factors include poor sanitation and ventilation, high humidity, and stress caused by cold. The disease is especially a problem in farrowing units in which a large proportion of young sows are farrowing for the first time. The litters of older sows are less likely to be severely affected.

Weanling enteritis (postweaning diarrhea) is caused by hemolytic *E. coli* of O groups 8, 9, 20, 138, 139, 141, and

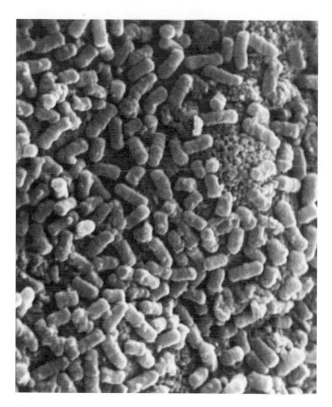

Figure 6.3. Scanning electron micrograph showing colonization by K88 (F4)–positive *Escherichia coli* of a villus on the small intestine of a pig. (Courtesy Harley Moon.)

149 in feeder pigs and is a very common complication of weaning. The disease is usually seen a short time after weaning in pigs that are thriving on a heavy grain diet. Change of diet leads to massive colonization of the anterior small intestine by an enteropathogenic clone carrying an adhesion antigen such as F4 (K88) or F5 (K99). Affected pigs develop diarrhea, depression, anorexia, and fever, which may persist for 2 to 3 days. Although large thriving pigs often collapse and die after a short period of diarrhea, the overall mortality from weanling diarrhea is much lower than that caused by neonatal *E. coli* diarrhea. The pathogenesis of the diseases is similar and involves adhesion to the brush border of the small intestine. Release of STb and LT enterotoxins results in a net efflux of Na^+, H_2O, HCO_3^-, and Cl^- into the bowel lumen. Shiga-toxin-producing strains (O26 and O111) can cause necrosis of the intestinal mucosa. At necropsy, the small intestine is dilated, thin-walled, and filled with watery, beige contents.

Edema disease (enterotoxemia, bowel edema) was first described in Ireland in 1938 and has since been reported from swine-raising areas throughout the world. It is associated with *E. coli* O groups 139 and 141.

Four fairly constant conditions are associated with the

occurrence of edema disease: (1) age—weanlings are most commonly involved but pigs of any age can be affected; (2) change of feed—frequently a change either in feed or methods of feeding has been made, a natural occurrence at weaning time; (3) rapid growth—the disease is seen most frequently in thriving animals; (4) diarrhea—mild diarrhea often occurs a day or two before the attack (Lamont 1950, Timoney 1950).

These factors in some unknown way predispose animals toward colonization of the small intestine by a toxin-producing serotype (most frequently 0139:K82) (Bertschinger and Pohlenz 1983). Edema disease (ED) toxin is released, absorbed, and carried in the bloodstream to various target sites in the animal. Its action is predominantly on the small arteries, which undergo mural edema, hyaline degeneration, and become permeable to fluid. The net outward movement of fluid accounts for the noninflammatory edema that is typical of the disease (Clugston et al. 1974).

The disease occurs suddenly, has a short course, and usually ends in the death of the pig. Affected animals exhibit a staggering gait, which may be slight at first but becomes more severe, and the animal is eventually unable to rise. Muscular tremors and spasms can also be present. The squeal is hoarse, and edema of the eyelids and face can be present. Body temperature is usually normal or subnormal, and the animal is often constipated. Some affected animals exhibit diarrhea, however, which may be a reflection of simultaneous enterotoxin production by the causative *E. coli* strain.

Edema is found in the eyelids, the facial area, the cardiac zone of the stomach between the mucosa and the muscle layers, the mesentery and the mesenteric lymph nodes, the gallbladder, the larynx, and other tissues (Figure 6.4). The extent of the edema is variable, and some animals may show very little.

Kurtz and Quast (1976) found areas of malacia in the brain stem that they felt were the result of ischemia. They characterized the lesions of edema disease as a vascular myolysis and panarteritis of the central nervous system.

Clugston and Nielsen (1974) have proposed that ED toxin be termed a vasotoxin because of its effect on arteries and its hypertensive effect. Onset of hypertension coincided with the development of the characteristic nervous signs of edema disease.

Invasive serotypes such as O8:K88 and O78:K80 sometimes cause infections in baby pigs that result in death within 48 hours of birth. Diarrhea can accompany or precede the onset of neonatal septicemia. Failure to ingest an adequate quantity of colostrum or ingestion of colostrum lacking in specific antibody are important predisposing factors.

Cerebrospinal angiopathy has been observed as a sequel to *E. coli* infection in weanling swine (Bertschinger and Pohlenz 1974). Affected swine exhibit a variety of neurological signs as a result of malacia, demyelination, and angiopathy of the nervous system and other organs. The disease may be a chronic form of edema disease. The prognosis is poor; affected animals waste and eventually die.

E. coli also has been shown to be a cause of acute meningitis and fibrinous polyserositis in piglets (Wilkie 1981). A rapidly progressing anorexia with weakness followed by death within 24 hours were the signs observed.

E. coli derived from the environment can be introduced into the sow's udder through wounds caused by the teeth of the piglets. The udder becomes swollen, edematous, and the sow has a high fever (Jones 1979).

The disease in cattle. Enteric disease (*white scour*) in calves caused by specific serotypes of *E. coli* is a very frequent and serious disorder during the first week of life. It occurs in all breeds of beef and dairy calves, and outbreaks of the disease occur constantly on premises where large numbers of calves are raised in confinement. In small herds the disease will be seen only sporadically during the calving season. Calves left with their dams on pasture rarely develop white scour.

The strains involved belong principally to O groups 8, 9, 20, and 101 (Orskov and Orskov 1979) and carry the F5 (K99) fimbrial or other colonizing antigen. STa entero-

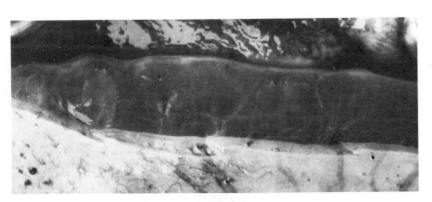

Figure 6.4. Edema disease of swine. Section of stomach wall showing thick layer of edema.

toxin is usually produced. Specific serotypes predominate on certain farms.

After infection by an enterotoxigenic strain, there is colonization and rapid multiplication of the middle and lower small intestine. The F5 (K99) adhesive antigen plays a critical role in this phase. Release of STa enterotoxin then results in deregulation of the ion pump mechanism by stimulation of cyclic guanylate cyclase in epithelial cells and net outward flux of Cl^-, Na^+, HCO_3, and water into the intestinal lumen. The animal develops a severe diarrhea, with feces full of gas bubbles, and may die in a few days from dehydration and acidosis.

Shiga-toxin-producing strains have been isolated from calves with enteric disease. These strains also have fimbrial antigens for attachment. The septicemic form of colibacillosis in calves is a common sequel to colostrum deprivation and is often preceded or accompanied by diarrhea (Sojka 1973).

An important distinction must be made between the serotypes found in enteritis and those found in cases of septicemia where the *E. coli* invades and multiplies in the bloodstream and tissues of the calf. Serotypes belonging to O groups 15, 26, 35, 78, 86, 115, 117, and 137 (Orskov and Orskov 1979) commonly are involved in the invasive form of colibacillosis in calves. Resistance to complement-mediated lysis and ability to scavenge iron can be important virulence attributes of the invasive strains. However, endotoxin from the cell wall of the organism is responsible for the events that culminate in shock and other clinical signs exhibited by the animal. Septicemic calves become weak and sleepy and soon die. Some animals survive longer but exhibit polyarthritis and meningitis, which is frequently fatal.

E. coli is by far the most important of the Gram-negative environmental organisms that cause mastitis in dairy cattle (Anonymous 1977). The incidence can be very high on certain farms and usually peaks during the winter months. The disease is more frequent in herds where dry cow therapy and teat dipping are practiced (Marr 1978) because these procedures reduce the population of commensal organisms such as *Corynebacterium bovis* and nonpathogenic staphylococci on and in the udder. Such commensal organisms normally promote a low-level cellular response in the secretion which helps protect against other infections.

There is also a positive correlation between contamination of the environment by *E. coli* and the occurrence of *E. coli* mastitis (Eberhart et al. 1979). The wide range of serotypes involved provides further circumstantial evidence that environmental rather than cow-to-cow transfer occurs.

Irregular vacuum fluctuations and inadequate milking machine sanitation contribute to the incidence of the disease (Bramley and Neave 1975). Entry of the organism occurs through the meatus. Adherence of some strains of fimbriate *E. coli* to epithelial cells in the mammary gland can be important in the pathogenesis of the disease (Anderson et al. 1977, Harper et al. 1978). In some cases colonization can be limited to the streak canal and the lower teat cistern. These organisms release endotoxin that incites an inflammatory response in more remote parts of the gland. In most cases of *E. coli* mastitis, however, there is true intramammary infection by the organism. Endotoxin released during bacteriolysis causes a great increase in mammary blood flow and diapedesis of blood neutrophils into the milk (Dhondt et al. 1977). There is marked swelling of the gland, and a serous fluid replaces the milk. Absorption of endotoxin into the animal's bloodstream leads to high fever, depression, a leukopenia followed by a leukocytosis, prolonged hypoglycemia, and, in severe cases, irreversible shock and death. Because recovery of damaged mammary tissue is slow, losses in milk production can be substantial. For a more extensive discussion of coliform mastitis, see the excellent review by Eberhart (1984).

The disease in lambs. Colibacillosis in lambs is basically similar in epizootiology and pathogenesis to that described in pigs and calves. Enteric and bacteremic forms of the disease occur. The enteric form occurs in lambs 2 to 8 days old and is caused by the proliferation of enteropathogenic, noninvasive strains in the upper small intestine.

The serotypes studied have been similar to those producing enterotoxemia in calves and often have F5 (K99) antigen and produce ST enterotoxin. However, Ansari et al. (1978) found that only a proportion of diarrhea-producing strains in lambs have produced enterotoxin in a ligated loop test in lambs, suggesting that another category of enteropathogenic *E. coli* exists in lambs.

Lambs with enteric colibacillosis exhibit diarrhea, depression, and some mortality. The bacteremic form often results in sudden death. Less severe manifestations include meningitis or arthritis or both. Ansari et al. (1978) found that in an intensive shed lambing operation, colibacillosis appeared sooner in lambs born during inclement weather than in those born during good weather.

Strains that produce bacteremia are different serotypically from the strains that produce enteric disease, the most prevalent serotype being O78:K88 (Terlecki and Sojka 1965).

The disease in horses. *E. coli* accounts for approximately 1 percent of the abortions observed in mares and for about 25 percent of the deaths of foals (Dimock et al. 1947). Foals that succumb to *E. coli* infection usually are congenitally abnormal and fail to suckle and to obtain an adequate quantity of colostrum (Gunning 1947, Platt 1973).

Signs include increased temperature and pulse, dullness, and weakness. Death frequently occurs within 24 hours after the onset of the disease. In foals examined before postmortem invasion occurs, *E. coli* can be isolated from the internal organs and from synovial fluids. *E. coli* is not an important cause of enteritis in foals, although the F4 (K88) antigen has been shown to bind strongly to horse brush-border membranes (Tzipori et al. 1984).

In mares *E. coli* (groups O2, O4, O6, O75) often is an invader of the genital tract after dystocia but usually is rapidly cleared from the tract. Occasionally, *E. coli* causes acute metritis.

The disease in dogs. In puppies bacteremias caused by *E. coli* (group O42) have been implicated in the "fading-puppy syndrome," in which affected puppies become weak and anorectic and die. Because this syndrome is also associated with herpesvirus infection, the etiology can be multifactorial.

E. coli is present in about 70 percent of cases of pyometra in bitches but is not believed to have primary etiological signnificance. Serotypes in O groups 4, 6, and 22 predominate (Chaffaux et al. 1978, Grindlay et al. 1973). *E. coli* is the most common opportunistic invader of the urinary tract of dogs and cats. Virulence factors for the urinary tract have not been well studied.

LT- and ST-producing strains of *E. coli* have been recovered from cascs of enteritis in young dogs (Olson et al. 1984, Richter 1984).

The disease in poultry. *E. coli* is rarely implicated in avian diarrheal disease; the diarrhea seen in avian colibacillosis is a result of urinary water loss and is not a sequel to enteritis. Typical colibacillosis in older chickens and turkeys involves primarily the respiratory tract as a result of inhalation of feces-contaminated dust. The organism then spreads into the bloodstream and causes acute colisepticemia with high mortality, fibrinopurulent serositis, or coligranuloma (Hjarre's disease). The virulence of invasive strains may be related to their adhesive and iron-uptake abilities (Dho and Lafont 1984). Hjarre's disease is usually chronic in course and is characterized by granulomatous lesions in the wall of the intestinal tract, the liver, and the lungs. Ammonia, dust, fluctuating air temperature, and concurrent viral infections are factors that increase the pathogenicity of *E. coli* in broilers (Pages and Costa 1985).

Colibacillosis in newly hatched chickens usually results from *E. coli* contamination of eggs, either from feces or from infection in the ovary of the hen. The chicks exhibit omphalitis and mushy chick disease. The serotypes involved in avian colibacillosis belong predominantly to groups O1, O2, O36, and O78 (Orskov and Orskov 1979).

The disease in rabbits. Outbreaks of *E. coli* enteritis in fattening rabbits have been recorded (Camguilhem 1985, Peeters et al. 1984). *E. coli* type O103 was isolated in one outbreak and shown in experiments to cause cecitis accompanied by dysentery and a high mortality.

Immunity. Antibodies to the F4 (K88), F5 (K99), F41, and 987P antigens are effective in reducing or preventing colonization of the intestine of piglets or calves by *E. coli* strains that carry these fimbrial antigens (Moon et al. 1979). The newborn animal is passively protected by colostrum that contains antibody stimulated in the dam by vaccination or natural infection. These antibodies are mostly of the IgA isotype (Kortbeek-Jacobs and van Houten 1982).

Vaccination of gilts and sows with vaccines prepared from the fimbrial K88 antigen or other pilus-associated antigens has been shown to reduce morbidity and mortality caused by *E. coli* neonatal enteritis (Brinton et al. 1983, Nagy and Walker 1983, Nagy et al. 1978, Rijke et al. 1983).

Heat-inactivated bacterins given in the feed to pregnant sows have also been shown to be effective in reducing losses caused by colibacillosis. The vaccine is given in the feed from 8 weeks after service until parturition and is supplemented by a booster intramuscular injection of the same antigen a few weeks before farrowing (Allen and Porter 1983). However, sows that are homozygous recessive for the F4 (K88) receptor do not develop immune responses to the corresponding antigen.

Piglets from nonimmune sows can be immunized by intramuscular inoculation shortly after birth and develop protection against weanling enteritis. Piglets that receive colostral antibody do not develop an active antibody response if vaccinated within 4 weeks of birth (Rijke et al. 1983). Young pigs have also been shown to be capable of responding to orally administered vaccine (Baljer 1979, Dziaba et al. 1983). Responses are rapid and unaffected by colostral antibody provided very large doses of antigen of the appropriate O group are given.

Although most of the commercially available vaccines are based on fimbrial antigens, local antibodies (IgA) to LT enterotoxin can be stimulated by feeding antigen (Pesti and Lukacs 1984a). Immunization of pregnant sows with heated, aggregated cholera toxin (procholerogenoid) stimulates formation of IgG antibodies to the immunologically similar *E. coli* LT enterotoxin. These antibodies will protect piglets after transfer in the colostrum (Furer et al. 1983).

ST enterotoxins, although poorly antigenic by themselves, are effective antigens when cross-linked to carrier proteins. STa enterotoxin linked in this way has been shown to be a good antigen in pigs (Pesti and Lukacs

1984b). Edema disease toxin is also a good antigen, and pigs can be passively protected with antiserum (Timoney 1956).

Passive protection of calves and goat kids against enteric colibacillosis can also be accomplished by vaccination of pregnant cows or does. An important protective antigen is the F5 (K99) antigen, and the highest K99 antibody titers are obtained with a vaccine that contains saponin and aluminum hydroxide as an adjuvant. Cows vaccinated at 8 and 4 weeks before calving secreted large quantities of antibody in the colostrum and in the milk for a week after calving (Bachmann et al. 1984). The importance of K99 antibodies in protection is supported by the high correlation between resistance of newborn calves to severe diarrhea and colostral titers of K99 antibody (Acres et al. 1982). Calves can also be protected against disease caused by enterotoxigenic *E. coli* that carries F5 (K99) fimbrial antigen by oral administration of K99-specific monoclonal antibody or by pooled colostrum from hyperimmunized cows (Chantal et al. 1984, Renault et al. 1984, Sherman et al. 1983).

Lambs and kid goats can be protected by vaccination of ewes or does before lambing (Contrepois and Guillimin 1984, Gregory et al. 1983).

Vaccination of chickens with inactivated *E. coli* O78:K80 strains has been shown to confer protection against coligranuloma (Cheville and Arp 1978). Similarly, an oil-emulsion preparation of *E. coli* (O1:K1) protected chicks against respiratory infection (Panigrahy et al. 1984). K88 and K99 antibody can be assayed by enzyme-linked immunosorbent assay (ELISA) (Nagy et al. 1984). Antibodies to LT enterotoxin have been assayed in a toxin neutralization test in adrenal cell cultures and in an ELISA (Dobrescu and Renault 1981).

Diagnosis. Enteric colibacillosis of newborn pigs, calves, and lambs is characteristically associated with abnormally large numbers of a single clone of *E. coli* (usually nonhemolytic and mucoid) in the anterior and distal segments of the small intestine. Postweaning colibacillosis in swine is usually caused by beta-hemolytic mucoid strains. Culture of fresh intestinal contents or of freshly voided stool will frequently yield almost pure cultures of *E. coli*.

The fluorescent antibody test using conjugates prepared against each of the common colonizing antigens F4 (K88), F5 (K99), 987P, and F41 is used in the diagnosis of enteric colibacillosis. In this procedure, sections of ileum from fresh carcasses are stained with conjugate. The test is rapid and allows early recognition of the colonizing antigen type involved.

ELISA methods are also available for the detection of K88 and K99 antigens in feces from cases of neonatal pig

or calf diarrhea (Holley et al. 1984, Mills et al. 1983, van Zijderveld and Overdijk 1983). The test is valid only in the first few days of life before the calf's own local antibody synthesis begins.

LT enterotoxin can be assayed in ligated intestinal loops, by a vascular permeability assay, by its effect on 3-ketosteroid production in adrenal cell monolayers, by its effect on Vero cells, by hemagglutination, by solid-phase radioimmunoassay, by ELISA, and by binding to polystyrene-absorbed GM_1 ganglioside (reviewed by Raskowa and Raska 1980). An ELISA based on monoclonal antibody is probably the most sensitive, specific, and reliable of the assays that have been developed for LT enterotoxin (Thompson et al. 1984).

STa enterotoxin can be assayed in suckling mice and in the ligated loop assay. An in vitro competitive ELISA is also available (Lockwood and Robertson 1984). STb enterotoxin is assayed in weaned pig and rabbit intestinal loops (Raskowa and Raska 1980).

Edema disease toxin can be detected in a Vero cell culture and in a mouse assay. Signs of posterior paralysis developing 24 to 72 hours after intraperitoneal or intravenous inoculation of polymyxin B extracts of suspect *E. coli* are evidence for the presence of the toxin.

Septicemic and avian colibacilloses are diagnosed by demonstrating pure cultures of *E. coli* in the blood, parenchymatous organs, and lesions. In cases of mastitis the organism can be difficult to culture; however, endotoxin can be detected by the limulus amebocyte lysate test.

Antimicrobial Susceptibility. *E. coli* strains that are susceptible to commonly used antimicrobials are somewhat rare in populations of animals raised in intensive management systems (Timoney 1980). *E. coli* strains from animals not exposed to antibiotic selection pressure are sensitive to amoxycillin, ampicillin, apramycin, chloramphenicol, furazolidone, kanamycin, spectinomycin, streptomycin, sulfonamides, tetracycline, and trimethoprim. The choice of antimicrobial must be based on sensitivity testing of representative isolates from an affected herd.

REFERENCES

Acres, S.D., Forman, A.J., and Kapitany, R.A. 1982. Antigen-extinction profile in pregnant cows, using a K99-containing whole-cell bacterin to induce passive protection against enterotoxigenic colibacillosis of calves. Am. J. Vet. Res. 43:569–575.
Allen, W.D., and Porter, P. 1983. Evaluation of "in feed" vaccination of piglets and sows against enteropathogenic *E. coli* using environmental production parameters. Dev. Biol. Stand. 53:147–153.
Anderson, J.C., Burrows, M.R., and Bramley, A.J. 1977. Bacterial adherence in mastitis caused by *Escherichia coli*. Vet. Pathol. 14:681–628.
Anonymous. 1977. Coliform and pseudomonad mastitis: Epidemiology and control. Vet. Rec. 100:441–442.

Ansari, M.M., Renshaw, H.W., and Gates, N.L. 1978. Colibacillosis in neonatal lambs: Onset of diarrheal disease and isolation and characterization of enterotoxigenic *Escherichia coli* from enteric and septicemic forms of the disease. Am. J. Vet. Res. 39:11–14.

Bachmann, P.A., Baljer, G., Gmelch, X., Eichhorn, W., Plank, P., and Mayr, A. 1984. Vaccination of cows with K99 and rotavirus antigen: Potency of K99 combined with different adjuvants in stimulating milk antibody secretion. Zentralbl. Veterinärmed. [B] 31:660–668.

Baljer, G. 1979. Possibilities and limitations of oral immunization against *Escherichia coli* in piglets and calves. In H. Willinger and A. Weber, eds., *Escherichia coli* Infections in Domestic Animals. Advances in Veterinary Medicine, Supplements to Zentralblatt für Veterinärimedizin, no. 29. Pp. 64–72.

Bertschinger, H.V., and Pohlenz. J. 1974. Cerebrospinal angiopathy in piglets with experimental *E. coli* enterotoxaemia. Schweiz. Arch. Tierheilkd. 116:543–554.

Bertschinger, H.V., and Pohlenz, J. 1983. Bacterial colonization and morphology of the intestine in porcine *Escherichia coli* enterotoxemia (edema disease). Vet. Pathol. 20:99–110.

Bramley, A.J., and Neave, F.K. 1975. Studies on the control of coliform mastitis in dairy cows. Br. Vet. J. 131:160–168.

Brinton, C.C. Jr., Rusco, P., Wood, S., Yappa, H.G., Goodnow, R.A., and Strayer, J.G. 1983. A complete vaccine for neonatal swine colibacillosis and the prevalence of *Escherichia coli* pili on swine isolates. Vet. Med./Small Anim. Clin. 78:962–966.

Camguilhem, R. 1985. Isolation of *Escherichia coli* serogroup O 103 causing enteritis in fattening rabbits; Demonstration of its pathogenicity. Rev. Méd. Vét. 136:61–68.

Chaffaux, S., Person, J.M., and L. Renault. 1978. Etude bactériologique de l'infection utérine des carnivores domestiques. Recl. Méd. Vét. 154:465–471.

Chantal, J., Lacheretz, A., Tulasne, J.J., Panier, C., Desmettre, P., Amine-Khodja, C.A., Picavet, D.P., and Stellmann, C. 1984. Activity of colostral whey in preventing enteritis in the newborn calf due to enterotoxinogenic *Escherichia coli* K99. Experimental model and results. Rev. Méd. Vét. 135:755–774.

Cheville, N.F., and Arp, L.H. 1978. Comparative pathological findings of *Escherichia coli* infection in birds. J. Am. Vet. Med. Assoc. 173:584–587.

Clugston, R.E., and Nielson, N.O. 1974. Experimental edema disease of swine (*E. coli* enterotoxemia). I. Detection and preparation of an active principle. Can. J. Comp. Med. 38:22–28.

Clugston, R.E., Nielson, N.O., and Smith, D.L.T. 1974. Experimental edema disease of swine (*E. coli* enterotoxemia). III. Pathology and pathogenesis. Can. J. Comp. Med. 38:34–43.

Contrepois, M., and Guillimin, P. 1984. Vaccination of goats against *Escherichia coli* K99. In Les maladies de la chèvre, colloque international, Niort (France), 9–11 octobre 1984. Paris, Institut National de la Recherche Agronomique. Pp. 473–476.

de Graaf, F.K., Klemm, P., and Gaastra, W. 1980. Purification, characterization and partial covalent structure of *Escherichia coli* adhesive antigen K99. Infect. Immun. 33:877–883.

Dho, M., and Lafont, J.P. 1984. Adhesive properties and iron uptake ability in *Escherichia coli* lethal and nonlethal for chicks. Avian Dis. 28:1016–1025.

Dhondt, G., Burvenich, C., and Peeters, G. 1977. Mammary blood flow during experimental *Escherichia coli* endotoxin-induced mastitis in goats and cows. J. Dairy Res. 44:433–440.

Dimock, W.W., Edwards, P.R., and Bruner, D.W. 1947. Infections observed in equine fetuses and foals. Cornell Vet. 37:89–99.

Dobrescu, L., and Renault, L. 1981. Detection of antibody to *E. coli* heat-labile enterotoxin in bovine sera samples from various regions of France. Zentralbl. Veterinärimed. [B] 28:341–343.

Dreyfus, L.A., and Robertson, D.C. 1984. Solubilization and partial characterization of the intestinal receptor for *Escherichia coli* heat-stable enterotoxin. Infect. Immun. 46:537–543.

Dykes, C.W., Halliday, I.J., Read, M.J., Hohden, A.N., and Harford, S. 1985. Nucleotide sequences of four variants of the K88 gene of porcine enterotoxigenic *Escherichia coli*. Infect. Immun. 50:279–283.

Dziaba, K., Kertrampf, B., and von Mickwitz, G. 1983. Oral active immunization of gnotobiotic piglets against *Escherichia coli* with formalin-inactivated *E. coli* whole antigen. Praktische Tierärzt. 64:300, 302–307.

Eberhart, R.J. 1984. Coliform mastitis. Vet. Clin. North Am. [Large Anim. Pract.] 6:287–300.

Eberhart, R.J., Natzke, R.P., and Newbould, F.H.S. 1979. Coliform mastitis—a review. J. Dairy Sci. 62:1–22.

Furer, E., Cryz, S.L. Jr., Domer, F., Nicolet, J., Wanner, M., and Germainier, R. 1982. Protection against colibacillosis in neonatal piglets by immunization of dams with procholerageroid. Infect. Immun. 35:887–894.

Gill, D.M., and Richardson, S.H. 1980. Adenosine diphosphate-ribosylation of adenylate cyclase catalyzed by heat labile enterotoxin *Escherichia coli:* Comparison with cholera toxin. J. Infect. Dis. 141:64–70.

Gregory, D.W., Cardella, M.A., and Myers, L.L. 1983. Lamb model in the study of immunity to enteropathogenic *Escherichia coli* infections. Am. J. Vet. Res. 44:2073–2077.

Grindlay, M., Renton, J.P., and Ramsay, D.H. 1973. O-groups of *Escherichia coli* associated with canine pyometra. Res. Vet. Sci. 14:75–77.

Gunning, O.V. 1947. Joint-ill in foals (pyosepticaemia), with special reference to the prophylactic treatment of the foal at birth. Vet. J. 103:47–67.

Harper, M., Turvey, A., and Bramley, A.J. 1978. Adhesion of fimbriate *Escherichia coli* to bovine mammary-gland epithelial cells in vitro. J. Med. Microbiol. 11:117–123.

Holley, D.L., Allen, S.D., and Barnett, B.B. 1984. Enzyme-linked immunosorbent assay, using monoclonal antibody, to detect *Escherichia coli* K99 antigen in feces of dairy calves. Am. J. Vet. Res. 45:2613–2616.

Jones, J.E.T. 1979. Coliform mastitis in the sow. Vet. Annual 19:97–101.

Kashiwazaki, M., Akaike, Y., Miyachi. T., Ogawa, T., Sugawara, M., and Isayema, Y. 1981. Production of heat-stable enterotoxin component by *Escherichia coli* strains enteropathogenic for swine. Natl. Inst. Anim. Health Q. 21:21–25.

Kennedy, D.J., Greenberg, R.N., Dunn, J.A., Abernathy, R., Ryers, J.S., and Guerrant, R.L. 1984. Effects of *Escherichia coli* heat-stable enterotoxin STb on intestines of mice, rats, rabbits and piglets. Infect. Immun. 46:639–643.

Kortbeek-Jacobs, N., and van Houten, M. 1982. Oral immunization of sows: Anti-K88 antibodies in serum and milk of the sow and in serum of the piglets. Vet. Q. 4:19–22.

Kurtz, H.J., and Quast, J.F. 1976. Encephalopathy in swine with edema disease. In Proceedings of the 4th International Pig Veterinary Society Congress, Ames, Iowa.

Lamont, H.G., Luke, D., and Gordon, W.A.M. 1950. Some pig diseases. Vet. Rec. 62:737–743.

Lockwood, D.E., and Robertson, D.C. 1984. Development of a competitive enzyme-linked immunosorbent assay (ELISA) for *Escherichia coli* heat-stable enterotoxin (ST). J. Immunol. Methods 75:295–307.

Marr, A. 1978. Bovine mastitis control: A need for appraisal? Vet. Rec. 102:132–134.

Mills, K.W., Tietze, K.L., and Phillips, R.M. 1983. Use of enzyme-linked immunosorbent assay for detection of K88 pili in fecal specimens from swine. Am. J. Vet. Res. 44:2188–2189.

Moon, H.W., Isaacson, R.E., and Pohlenz, J. 1979. Mechanism of association of enteropathogenic *Escherichia coli* with intestinal epithelium. Am. J. Clin. Nutr. 32:119–127.

Moon, H.W., Kohler, E.M., Schneider, R.A., and Whipp, S.C. 1980. Prevalence of pilus antigen enterotoxin types and enteropathogenicity among K88-negative enterotoxigenic *Escherichia coli* from neonatal pigs. Infect. Immun. 27:222–230.

Nagy, L.K., and Walker, P.D. 1983. Multi-adhesion vaccines for the protection of the neonatal pig against *E. coli* infections. Dev. Biol. Stand. 53:189–196.

Nagy, G., Barna, V.I., and Nagy, B. 1984. ELISA test to measure the antibody production elicited by K99 vaccine in cattle. Magy. Allatorv. Lapja 39:657–600.

Nagy, B., Moon, H.W., Isaacson, R.E., To, C.-C., and Brinton, C.C. 1978. Immunization of suckling pigs against enteric enterotoxigenic *Escherichia coli* infection by vaccinating dams with purified pili. Infect. Immun. 21:269–274.

O'Brien, A.D., and Holmes, R.K. 1987. Shiga and shiga-like toxins. Microbiol. Rev. 51:206–220.

O'Brien, A.D., and LaVeck, G.D. 1983. Purification and characterization of *Shigella dysenteriae* 1-like toxin produced by *Escherichia coli*. Infect. Immun. 40:675–683.

Olson, P., Hedhammar, A., and Wadstrom, T. 1984. Enterotoxigenic *Escherichia coli* infection in two dogs with acute diarrhea. J. Am. Vet. Med. Assoc. 184:952–983.

Orskov, F., and Orskov, I. 1979. Special *Escherichia coli* serotypes from enteropathies in domestic animals and man. In H. Willinger and A. Weber, eds., *Escherichia coli* Infections in Domestic Animals. Advances in Veterinary Medicine, Supplements to Zentralblatt für Veterinärimedizin, no. 29. Pp. 7–14.

Orskov, F., and Orskov, I. 1984. Serotyping of *Escherichia coli*. In T. Bergan and J.R. Norris, eds., Methods in Microbiology, vol. 14. Academic Press, New York.

Pages, A., and Costa, L. 1985. Factors potentiating the pathogenicity of *Escherichia coli* in broilers. Med. Vet. 2:23–40.

Panigrahy, B., Gyimah, J.E., Hall, C.F., and Williams, J.D. 1984. Immunogenic potency of an oil-emulsified *Escherichia coli* bacterin. Avian Dis. 28:475–481.

Peeters, J.E., Pohl, P., and Charlier, G. 1984. Infectious agents associated with diarrhea in commercial rabbits: A field study. Ann. Rech. Vet. 15:335–340.

Pesti, L., and Lukacs, K. 1984a. Local intestinal immune response to *Escherichia coli* heat-labile (LT) enterotoxin: LT antitoxin levels in healthy, diseased and antigen-fed pigs. Comp. Immunol. Microbiol. Infect. Dis. 7:149–155.

Pesti, L., and Lukacs, K. 1984b. Immunological properties of porcine enterotoxigenic *Escherichia coli* heat-stable (ST) enterotoxins. Comp. Immunol. Microbiol. Infect. Dis. 7:157–164.

Platt, H. 1973. Septicaemia in the foal: A review of 61 cases. Br. Vet. J. 129:221–229.

Raskowa, H., and Raska, K. 1980. Enterotoxins from Gram-negative bacteria relevant for veterinary medicine. Vet. Res. Commun. 41:195–224.

Renault, L., Espinasse, J., and Courtay, B. 1984. Prevention of *Escherichia coli* neonatal diarrhea in calves by administering immune colostral whey against K99 antigen. Bull. Mens. Soc. Vet. Prot. France 68:141–154.

Richter, T. 1984. Occurrence and properties of enterotoxin-forming strains of *Escherichia coli* from puppies with enteritis. Dtsch. Veterinärmed. Ges. Pp. 186–192.

Rijke, E.O., Webster, J., and Baars, J.C. 1983. Vaccination of piglets against post-weaning "*E. coli*" enterotoxicosis. Dev. Biol. Stand. 53:155–160.

Sellwood, R. 1979. *Escherichia coli* diarrhoea in pigs with or without the K88 receptor. Vet. Rec. 105:228–230.

Sherman, D.M., Acres, S.D., Saldowski, P.L., Springer, J.A., Bray, B., Raybould, T.J.G., and Muscoplat, C.C. 1983. Protection of calves against fatal enteric colibacillosis by orally administered *Escherichia coli* K99 specific monoclonal antibody. Infect. Immun. 42:653–658.

Smit, H., Gaastra, W., Kamerling, J.P., Vliegenthart, J.F.G., and de Graaf, F.K. 1984. Isolation and structural characterization of the equine erythrocyte receptor for enterotoxigenic *Escherichia coli* K99 fimbrial adhesion. Infect. Immun. 46:578–584.

Smith, H.W. 1974. A search for transmissible pathogenic characters in invasive strains of *Escherichia coli*: The discovery of plasmid-controlled toxin and plasmid-controlled lethal character closely associated or identical with colicin V. J. Gen. Microbiol. 83:95–111.

Smith, H.W., and Gyles, C.L. 1970. The relationship between two apparently different enterotoxins produced by enteropathogenic strains of *E. coli* of porcine origin. J. Med. Microbiol. 3:387–401.

Sojka, W.J. 1973. Enteropathogenic *Escherichia coli* in man and farm animals. Can. Inst. Food Sci. Technol. J. 6:52–63.

Terlecki, S., and Sojka, W.J. 1965. The pathogenicity for lambs of *Escherichia coli* of certain serotypes. Br. Vet. J. 121:462–470.

Thompson, M.R., Brandwein, H., LaBine-Racke, M., and Giannella, R.A. 1984. Simple and reliable enzyme-linked immunosorbent assay with monoclonal antibodies for detection of *Escherichia coli* heat-stable enterotoxins. J. Clin. Microbiol. 20:59–64.

Timoney, J.F. 1949. Experimental production of oedema disease of swine. Vet. Rec. 61:710.

Timoney, J.F. 1950. Oedema disease of swine. Vet. Rec. 62:748–756.

Timoney, J.F. 1956. Oedema disease of swine. Vet. Rec. 68:849–851.

Timoney, J.F. 1957. Oedema disease of swine. Vet. Rec. 69:1160–1175.

Timoney, J.F. 1986. Genetics and characterization of edema disease toxin. In Proceedings of the International Pig Veterinary Society's 9th Congress, Barcelona, Spain. P. 199.

Tzipori, S., Withers, M., Hayes, J., Robins-Browne, R., and Ward, K.L. 1984. Attachment of *E. coli* –bearing K88 antigen to equine brush-border membranes. Vet. Microbiol. 9:561–570.

van Zijderveld, F.G. and Overdijk, E. 1983. Experiences with the ELISA for detection of the *E. coli* K99 antigen in calf faeces. Ann. Rech. Vét. 14:395–399.

Wilkie, I.W. 1981. Polyserositis and meningitis associated with *Escherichia coli* infection of piglets. Can. Vet. J. 22:171–173.

The Genus *Klebsiella*

There are four species in the genus *Klebsiella*, of which only *K. pneumoniae* is a pathogen of animals. Although it is a member of the family Enterobacteriaceae and occurs as a minority commensal in the intestine, *K. pneumoniae* rarely causes disease in this location. Rather, it is an opportunistic invader of the reproductive tract of mares, the bovine mammary gland, and the urinary tract of bitches. Its ability to acquire multiple antibiotic resistance and to spread in hospital environments has earned it considerable respect as a nosocomial infection of human and animal hospital patients.

Klebsiella pneumoniae
SYNONYM: Friedlander's bacillus

Morphology and Staining Reactions. *K. pneumoniae* is a Gram-negative, non-spore-bearing, heavily encapsulated rod 0.3 to 1.0 μm in width by 0.6 to 6.0 μm long. There are no flagella.

Cultural and Biochemical Features. *K. pneumoniae* grows well on the commonly used laboratory media. The colonies are moist, spreading, glistening, and very viscid. Capsule production is enhanced in a carbohydrate-rich medium. *K. pneumoniae* is a facultative anaerobe, is oxidase-negative, and uses tartrate and malonate. It produces H_2S and urease, and produces negative results in the methyl red test and positive results in the Voges-Proskauer test. Lactose positivity is in part plasmid-encoded. Bacteriocins (klebicins) are produced and can be used in typing strains. The mol% G + C of the DNA is 56 to 58 (Tm).

Antigens. There are at least 82 capsular type (designated 1, 2, 3, etc.) and 11 different O type antigens. Only the capsular type is used in serologic typing. The capsular antigens are heat-stable polysaccharides and composed of one charged monosaccharide (usually glucuronic acid) and two or more sugars such as galactose, fucose, mannose, D-glucose, or L-rhamnose.

Epizootiology and Pathogenesis. *K. pneumoniae* is an intestinal commensal but also occurs in the environment. Heavy populations occur on wood shavings and other timber products and can be an important source of infection in outbreaks of *K. pneumoniae* mastitis in cattle (Newman and Kowalski 1973). *K. pneumoniae* populations in sawdust bedding increase with wetness (Thomas et al. 1983). However, a great diversity of serotypes and biotypes is found in cases of *K. pneumoniae* mastitis, a finding consistent with the opportunistic and contaminative nature of the infection (Braman et al. 1973, Nonnecke and Newbould 1984).

K. pneumoniae is a significant cause of nosocomial infection in small animal hospitals (Glickman 1981). Infections involve surgical wounds, the urinary tract, and the bloodstream. Use of antibiotics is an important predisposing factor—most isolates are multiresistant.

Invasive strains are resistant to serum bactericidal factors. Serum resistance is related to the presence of somatic antigens on the resistant strain (Ward and Sebunya 1981).

Mares have been shown to carry strains of *K. pneumoniae* in the vestibule, urethra, or clitoris as normal flora. These infections do not usually involve the cervix or uterus (Greenwood and Ellis 1976). In some mares opportunistic invasion of these sites does occur and results in vaginal discharge, metritis, infertility, and abortion. Strains isolated from mares with metritis predominantly belong to capsular types 1, 5, and 7 (Platt et al. 1976). A stallion can transmit infection from mare to mare but is usually not important as a reservoir of infection. Stallions clear infections within 10 to 12 days of ceasing service (Calazza and Sampieri 1973). However, an instance of prolonged symptomless carriage by a stallion has been recorded (Weiss et al. 1985). Contaminated instruments and hands can also serve to transmit the bacterium. A case of abortion with dissemination to the brain of the mare has been described (Timoney et al. 1983).

K. pneumoniae is an important component of the etiology of coliform mastitis in cattle. The disease frequently occurs within a few days of calving. Infection is derived from the animals' environment and causes an acute or peracute form of mastitis (Braman et al. 1973). There is hyperemia, edema, and swelling of the udder and milk secretion is reduced and altered to a serous fluid. The cow has a high fever initially, which may subside in a few hours if the animal develops often fatal endotoxic shock. A severe outbreak of hemorrhagic, necrotizing mastitis has been reported in a herd following intensive antibiotic treatment for streptococcal mastitis (Neumann and Wendy 1985).

K. pneumoniae mastitis has also been reported in sows (Done 1975, Ross et al. 1975), and an outbreak of pneumonia in goats has been reported (Kaushik and Kalra 1983).

Immunity. Little is known about protective immunity to *K. pneumoniae* infections in animals. Only strains resistant to serum bactericidal factor are invasive. A substantial number of persistent infections occur in mares, suggesting that local immune responses are not very effective in horses. Serum antibody as measured by the capsular swelling technique did not rise above 1:8 in infected mares (Brown et al. 1979).

Diagnosis. The heavily encapsulated appearance of *K. pneumoniae* in smears together with the very mucoid form of the colonies on agar constitute good presumptive evidence for its presence. Tampons left in place for 10 minutes are more effective in detecting uterine infections in mares than simple swabbing (Brown et al. 1979).

Antimicrobial Susceptibility. *K. pneumoniae* is usually resistant to ampicillin and carbenicillin, but may be sensitive to other antimicrobials effective against *E. coli*. However, because nosocomial infections are characteristically caused by multiresistant strains, sensitivity testing must routinely be performed on isolates of *K. pneumoniae*. Cephalexin is very effective in the treatment of canine urinary tract infections (Ling and Ruby 1983).

REFERENCES

Braman, S.K., Eberhart, R.J., Asbury, M.A., and Hermann, G.J. 1973. Capsular types of *Klebsiella pneumoniae* associated with bovine mastitis. J. Am. Vet. Med. Assoc. 162:109–111.

Brown, J.E., Corstvet, R.E., and Stranton, L.G. 1979. A study of *Klebsiella pneumoniae* infection in the uterus of the mare. Am. J. Vet. Res. 40:1523–1530.

Calazza, D., and Sampieri, G. 1973. Su akuni aspetti epizoologici delle affezioni genitali da *Klebsiella pneumoniae* negli equine. Folia Vet. Lat. 3:424–437.

Done, S.H. 1975. Observations on an outbreak of *Klebsiella* mastitis in sows. Acta Vet. Acad. Sci. Hung. 25:211–215.

Glickman, L.T. 1981. Veterinary nosocomial (hospital-acquired) *Klebsiella* infections. J. Am. Vet. Med. Assoc. 179:1389–1392.

Greenwood, R.E.S., and Ellis, D.R. 1976. *Klebsiella aerogenes* in mares. Vet. Rec. 99:439.

Kaushik, R.K., and Kalra, D.S. 1983. Investigations into outbreaks of caprine pneumoniae associated with *Klebsiella pneumoniae* "type 24." Indian J. Anim. Sci. 53:275–279.

Ling, G.V., and Ruby, A.L. 1983. Cephalexin for oral treatment of canine urinary tract infection caused by *Klebsiella pneumoniae*. J. Am. Vet. Med. Assoc. 182:1346–1347.

Neumann, P., and Wendt, K. 1985. Aetiopathogenesis of bovine mastitis due to *Klebsiella pneumoniae*. Monatsh. Veterinärmed. 40:120–123.

Newman, L.E., and Kowalski, J.J. 1973. Fresh sawdust bedding—A possible source of *Klebsiella* organisms. Am. J. Vet. Res. 7:979–980.

Nonnecke, B.J., and Newbould, F.H.S. 1984. Biochemical and serologic characterization of *Klebsiella* strains from bovine mastitis and the environment of the dairy cow. Am. J. Vet. Res. 45:2451–2454.

Platt, H., Atherton, J.G., and Orskov, I. 1976. *Klebsiella* and *Enterobacter* organisms isolated from horses. J. Hyg. 77:401–408.

Ross, R.F., Zimmerman, B.J., Wagner, W.C., and Cox, D.F. 1975. A field study of coliform mastitis in sows. J. Am. Vet. Med. Assoc. 167:231–235.

Thomas, C.B., Jasper, D.E., Rollins, M.H., Bushnell, R.B., and Carroll, E.J. 1983. Enterobacteriaceae bedding populations, rainfall and mastitis in a California dairy. Prevent. Vet. Med. 1:227–242.

Timoney, P.J., McArdle, J.F., and Bryne, M.J. 1983. Abortion and meningitis in a thoroughbred mare associated with *Klebsiella pneumoniae*, type 1. Equine Vet. J. 15:64–65.

Ward, G.E. and Sebunya, T.K. 1981. Somatic and capsular factors of coliforms which affect resistance to bovine serum bactericidal activity. Am. J. Vet. Res. 42:1937–1940.

Weiss, R., Tillmann, H., and Drager, K.G. 1985. Genital disease in horses due to *Klebsiella pneumoniae*, type 1. Praktische Tierarzt. 66:114–120.

7 The Enterobacteriaceae— The Non-Lactose-Fermenters

The non-lactose-fermenting genera of the Enterobacteriaceae that are of importance with respect to animal disease are *Salmonella*, *Proteus*, and *Yersinia*.

The Genus *Salmonella*

The genus *Salmonella* owes its name to D. E. Salmon, a veterinary bacteriologist who with Theobald Smith isolated and described the "hog cholera bacillus" for the first time (Salmon 1885). The organism was later named *Salmonella choleraesuis* and became the type species. More than 2,000 different serovars or serotypes of salmonellae producing many varied diseases have since been isolated from a great variety of hosts throughout the world.

DNA-DNA hybridization studies have shown that all salmonellae and the organisms formerly known as *S. arizonae* form a single genetic species (Crosa et al. 1973). This species consists of five subgroups (subgenera or subspecies) (Le Minor 1982):

I. Typical salmonellae, e.g., *S. choleraesuis*, *S. enteritidis*, *S. gallinarum*, *S. typhi*, *S. typhimurium*
II. Atypical salmonellae, e.g., *S. salamae*
III. *S. arizonae* and related organisms
IV. *S. houtenae* and related organisms
V. *S. bongor* and related organisms

The majority of salmonellae are in subgroup I. The significant animal pathogens mostly belong to this subgroup. A few belong to subgroup III.

Salmonellae have been named either for the disease they produce or for the animal or place in which they were first isolated, for example, *S. choleraesuis*, *S. dublin*. The use of specific epithets, although taxonomically incorrect, is so widespread in the medical and veterinary literature and so useful that it is certain to continue; however, the International Subcommittee on Enterobacteriaceae (Le Minor 1984) has recommended that new serovars of subgroups II, III, IV, and V be designated by their antigenic formulas.

Morphology and Staining Reactions. The cells are Gram-negative, noncapsulated, short rods (2 to 4 by 0.5 to 1.0 μm) that have peritrichous flagella and frequently also carry fimbriae (Figure 7.1). *S. gallinarum* and *S. pullorum* do not have flagella.

Cultural and Biochemical Features. Salmonellae are aerobic and facultatively anerobic and will grow on defined media without special growth factors. Many specially formulated differential and selective media for the isolation of salmonellae have been devised. The most useful of these in veterinary bacteriology are brilliant green, MacConkey, and bismuth sulfite agars. Colonies are usually 3 to 4 mm in diameter, but some serotypes produce small colonies (1 mm). The common biochemical characteristics are listed in Table 7.1. Salmonellae can selectively use tetrathionate or sodium selenite; thus, very small numbers can be detected in highly contaminated specimens when these substrates are used as enrichment media.

The optimum growth temperature is 37°C, but salmonellae also grow well at 43°C—a characteristic often used to reduce the growth of other bacteria in highly contaminated specimens.

Salmonellae usually produce gas from glucose and can use citrate as a carbon source. They reduce nitrates to nitrites but do not produce indole or urease. Lysine and ornithine decarboxylase reactions are usually positive. Hydrogen sulfide is produced by most serotypes. Lactose is not fermented unless the strain hosts a plasmid that encodes for this trait or the isolate is an *S. arizonae* strain. Some strains of *S. arizonae* ferment lactose slowly, others ferment it rapidly.

Biotypes. Biotypes are different fermentation phenotypes produced by strains of a single serotype. The characteristics used for biotyping are genetically stable and include in the case of *S. typhimurium*, fermentation of Bitter's rhamnose, *meso*-inositol, L-rhamnose, *d*-tartrate, and *meso*-tartrate (Duguid et al. 1975). The more ancient and widespread a serotype, the more likely it is to have a variety of biotypes. For instance, the lack of variant biotypes shown by *S. agona* compared with *S. typhimurium* has been taken as evidence that *S. typhimurium* is of more ancient origin (Barker et al. 1982).

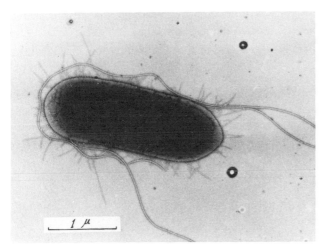

Figure 7.1. *Salmonella typhimurium* showing flagella and many short fimbriae. Negative stain. × 25,300. (From Tanaka and Katsube, 1978, courtesy of *Japanese Journal of Veterinary Science.*)

Biotyping in conjunction with phage typing has proved of great value in epidemiological studies of *S. typhimurium* in human and animal populations (Barker et al. 1980).

Phage Typing. Phage typing is based on the sensitivity of cultures to a series of bacteriophages at appropriate dilutions. The technique was first used on *S. typhi* and has since been applied to *S. typhimurium* and to other salmonellae (Anderson 1964). It is of great value for source tracing in epidemiological studies. The different phage typing schemes for salmonellae developed over the years have been reviewed by Guinee and van Leeuwen (1978). Phage typing of *S. typhimurium* has been widely practiced in Great Britain for many years. Recently a modification of the original method developed in England (Felix 1956) has become available, so that North American strains of this serotype can now be phage typed and compared with strains isolated elsewhere (Khakria and Lior 1980).

Plasmids can alter the phage type of a *Salmonella* strain by altering receptor sites on the cell surface or by encoding restriction endonucleases (Tschape et al. 1974).

Table 7.1. Antigenic formulas of some common *Salmonella* serotypes

Serotype	Antigenic formula
S. abortus ovis	4,12: c-1,6
S. choleraesuis	6,7: c-1,5 (diphasic)
S. dublin	9,12: g,p-(monophasic)
S. pullorum	9,12: -(nonmotile)
S. typhimurium	1,4,5,12: i-1,2 (diphasic)

Antigens. The three kinds of antigens used for the identification of salmonellae are the O (somatic), the H (flagellar), and the Vi (virulence) antigens. The specificity of the O antigen is determined by the structure and composition of the lipopolysaccharide of the cell wall, and the different O antigens are designated by Arabic figures, for example, 4, 12. The O antigens may change following lysogeny and this may result in change of serotype. In *S. pullorum*, the O12 antigen is present in three forms, 12, 12_2, and 12_3. Strains of *S. pullorum* rich in form 12_2 sometimes cause infections in poultry flocks and special antigen prepared from this variant therefore must be used to screen serums for antibody in these flocks (Edwards and Bruner 1946).

Another variation in the O antigen can result in a change in the colonial appearance of the strain from smooth (S) to rough (R). This change is accompanied by loss of the O antigen and sometimes of virulence. The H antigens, unlike the O antigens, are heat-labile and composed of protein. They can exist in either a single (monophasic) or in two separate forms (diphasic), only one of which is expressed at a given time. This phenomenon is known as the phase variation of Andrewes. Antigens of phase 1 are assigned lower case letters (e.g., *a* and *b*), and those of phase 2 are given Arabic numbers or lower case letters.

The antigens of phase 1 and phase 2 flagella are determined by two genes, H1 and H2, which code for the flagellar protein, flagellin. H2 flagellin synthesis is controlled by a recombinational event that inverts the section of the chromosome containing the H2 gene. When the H2 gene is activated, another gene close by is also active and synthesizes a repressor substance that inhibits expression of the H1 gene (Silverman et al. 1979).

The Vi antigen is found only on *S. typhi*, the cause of typhoid in humans.

The antigenic formulas (serotypes or serovars) of some common salmonellae are given in Table 7.1.

The cell wall protein antigens of salmonellae have not been as well studied as the somatic, flagellar, and virulence antigens. Outer membrane proteins ranging in molecular weight from 12,000 to 120,000 have been observed in *S. anatum*, *S. enteritidis*, *S. infantis*, and *S. typhimurium*. The protein profiles of each serotype varied greatly, although some proteins were common to all serotypes. These proteins when complexed to lipopolysaccharide were capable of eliciting specific immunoglobulin responses in mice (Kudrna et al. 1985). Porin proteins from *S. typhimurium* have also been shown to elicit antibodies that are protective for mice (Kuusi et al. 1979).

Epizootiology and Pathogenesis. Although the feco-

Table 7.2. Some host-adapted and non-host-adapted *Salmonella* serotypes

Host-adapted	Non-host-adapted
S. abortus equi	*S. anatum*
S. abortus ovis	*S. derby*
S. choleraesuis	*S. newport*
S. dublin	*S. tennessee*
S. gallinarum	*S. typhimurium*
S. paratyphi (A, C)	
S. pullorum	
S. typhi	

oral route is the most important mode of transmission of salmonellae in animals, the cycle of infection may be more complex in some animal populations; in poultry, for example, the primary source of infection may be contaminated feed, and subsequent spread may occur by means of the feco-oral route or from egg to chick in the hatchery. A variable percentage of animals, once infected, remain carriers and shed the organism intermittently in feces or sometimes in milk. The distribution of serotypes varies from one geographic region to another. *S. typhimurium,* however, is universally distributed.

The serotypes are classified as either host-adapted or non-host-adapted depending on their host range (Table 7.2). The host-adapted serotypes rarely cause disease in hosts other than the one to which they are adapted. *S. dublin* is traditionally host-adapted to cattle but in some areas has shown a tendency to spread to swine (McErlean 1968, Timoney 1970).

Young animals are more susceptible to salmonellosis than older ones. Poor sanitation, overcrowding, inclement weather, the stress of hospitalization and surgery, parturition, parasitism, transportation, overtraining, and concurrent viral infections are all factors that predispose animals to clinical salmonellosis. Many animals, particularly swine and poultry fed rations that contain salmonellae suffer inapparent infections during their lifetimes.

Animal feeds are often contaminated by a variety of serotypes (Pomeroy and Grady 1962), which usually enter the feed mixture in protein supplements such as meat and bone meal, fish meal, and soybean meal. The salmonellae enter these materials during or after processing. In the case of meat and bone meal, the percolator phase that removes fat after cooking is an important contaminative stage; the organisms are maintained and multiply in the material as it cools (Timoney 1968).

Wild birds and rodents such as rats and mice can also be a source of infection for livestock through feces contamination of feed or buildings.

Salmonellas, with the exception of some heat-resistant strains of *S. senftenberg,* are killed at 56°C in about 10 to 20 minutes. They survive for months or longer in manure, feces (Josland 1951), and the sediments of streams and ponds (Hendricks 1971).

Salmonellosis usually begins as an enteric infection that may subsequently generalize after entry of the organism into the bloodstream. The animal may develop septicemia, meningitis, arthritis, pneumonia, abortion, or a combination of these diseases.

The pathogenesis of salmonella enteritis follows three distinct phases: (1) colonization of the intestine, (2) invasion of the intestinal epithelium, and (3) stimulation of fluid exsorption.

Phase 1: Colonization of the intestine. Colonization of the distal small intestine and the colon is a necessary first step in the pathogenesis of enteric salmonellosis. Indigenous fusiform bacteria that lie in the mucous layer investing the epithelium of the large intestine normally inhibit growth of salmonellae by producing volatile organic acids (Hentges and Maier 1970). The normal flora also block access to attachment sites needed by the salmonellas. Factors that disrupt the normal colonic flora, such as antibiotic therapy, diet, and water deprivation, greatly increase the host's susceptibility to enteric and septicemic salmonellosis (Holmberg et al. 1984, Nelson 1971, Tannock and Smith 1972, Timoney et al. 1978). The importance of fimbriae in attachment and colonization of salmonellae during the initial phase of the pathogenesis of enteritis has been shown in mice by Tanaka (1982a, 1982b). Fimbriate salmonellae adhered better to ileal mucosa than nonfimbriate isogenic strains and were more infective.

Newly hatched chicks whose intestinal flora has not been established are much more prone to colonization by salmonellae than are chicks given cecal contents to establish a normal intestinal flora.

Reduced peristalsis also predisposes an animal to colonization by salmonellae because it allows temporary overgrowth to occur, especially in the small intestine. Peristalsis is stimulated by an active indigenous microflora, suppression of which increases the host's susceptibility to colonization.

Swine that are stressed by transport exhibit greatly increased rates of colonization by a variety of salmonellae (Williams and Newell 1968). The physiological basis of this phenomenon is poorly understood.

Phase 2: Invasion of the intestinal epithelium. The invasion phase involves the villous tips of the ileum and colon. The brush border is penetrated, and the salmonellae enter the cell (Figure 7.2), apparently without killing it, since there is no morphologic change until later

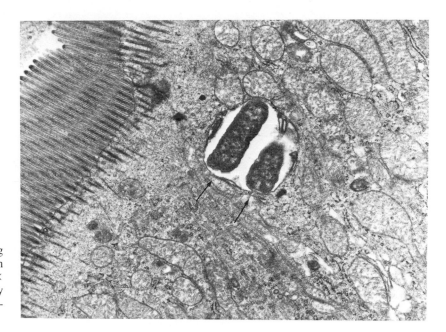

Figure 7.2. Electron micrograph showing cells of *Salmonella heidelberg* (*arrows*) in a villous absorptive cell of pig ileum. × 14,280. (From Reed et al., 1985, courtesy of *American Journal of Veterinary Research.*)

in the disease process. The organisms may multiply and infect other adjoining cells or pass into the lamina propria, where they continue to multiply and are phagocytosed and trapped in the regional lymph nodes. After invasion, the villous tips contract and are invaded by neutrophils.

The invasive abilities of some strains of *S. typhimurium* have been shown to be increased by genes encoded on a 60–70-megadalton plasmid (Jones et al. 1982). The biochemical basis of the enhanced virulence is unknown. Plasmid-encoded genes that enhance the virulence of *S. dublin* have also been observed (Terakado et al. 1983).

The invasiveness of salmonellae is also in part determined by the number and type of special monosaccharides in their O polysaccharide side chains. The rare 3,6-dideoxyhexoses are found only in virulent, invasive salmonellae such as *S. dublin, S. typhi,* and *S. typhimurium* (Ronatree 1967). It has been suggested that the 3,6-dideoxyhexoses in some way mask determinants on the bacterial cell surface that bind complement and activate it by means of the alternate pathway (Takasaki et al. 1983). Failure to activate complement would clearly have a survival advantage for the salmonellae since it would reduce the chances of phagocytosis.

Phase 3: Stimulation of fluid exsorption. The inflammatory response in the intestinal mucosa is an important factor in intestinal fluid exsorption. Prostaglandins, which are released as a result of this response, activate adenylate cyclase with resultant net secretion of water, bicarbonate, and chloride into the intestinal lumen (Giannella et al. 1975). The inflammatory response also triggers release of vasoactive substances that increase the permeability of the mucosal vasculature and so lead to fluid exsorption.

There is evidence that an enterotoxin similar to *E. coli* LT enterotoxin is produced by some *Salmonella* strains (Finkelstein et al. 1983). Both LT and ST enterotoxins have been observed in cell-free extracts of *S. enteritidis* (Ketyi et al. 1979). In *S. typhimurium* the amount of LT enterotoxin appears to be very low and requires induction by mitomycin C. The toxin gene itself is not phage-encoded (Houston et al. 1981). Other workers (Blaser et al. 1982) have failed to find enterotoxins in a variety of *Salmonella* serotypes from patients with enteric salmonellosis characterized by water diarrhea. It therefore appears that small amounts of cell-associated LT enterotoxin may be present in strains of *Salmonella* but probably are unimportant for the fluid exsorption seen in salmonella enteritis.

Fluid exsorption is accompanied by extensive neutrophil invasion of villous cores with acute ileitis and colitis. Neutrophils are also shed in the stool (Figure 7.3), and their presence has diagnostic value.

The pathogenesis of salmonella septicemia is closely related to the effects of endotoxin released from bacterial cell walls. Endotoxic activity is associated with the lipid A component of cell wall lipopolysaccharide (see Chapter 1). Many of the signs of salmonella septicemia are similar to those produced in experimental animals by the injection of purified endotoxin. These effects include fever, hemorrhages associated with consumption of coagulation factors, leukopenia followed by leukocytosis, hypotension and shock that is often fatal, and depletion of liver glycogen with resultant hypoglycemia.

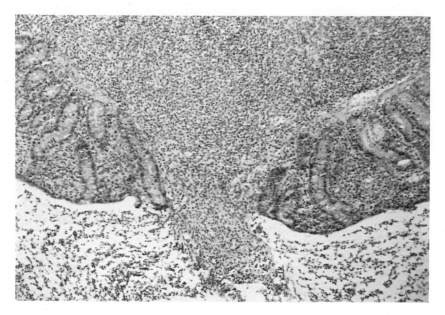

Figure 7.3. Section of ileum from a pig killed 48 hours after inoculation with *Salmonella heidelberg*. The villi have atrophied and the dome area has "exploded," resulting in exudation of inflammatory cells into the intestinal lumen. Hematoxylin and eosin stain. × 75. (From Reed et al., 1985, courtesy of *American Journal of Veterinary Research.*)

The disease in cattle. The two serotypes of greatest importance in bovine salmonellosis are *S. dublin* and *S. typhimurium.* Occasional outbreaks are caused by other, mostly feed-derived, serotypes. *S. dublin* is host-adapted to cattle and occurs in Europe, the western United States, and South Africa. *S. typhimurium* is found throughout the world and infects humans and a wide variety of wild and domestic animals.

Carrier animals are the main reservoir of *S. dublin.* Clinically normal adult cows serve as a source of infection for their calves. If the calf's passive immunity is poor, clinical disease may result. Adult carrier animals may excrete the organism for prolonged periods. Concurrent infection with *Fasciola hepatica* increases the susceptibility of cattle to *S. dublin* and increases the frequency of carrier animals (Aitken et al. 1982). Latent adult carriers of *S. dublin* are also common (Lawson et al. 1974). These animals may excrete the organism when stressed—for example, by parturition or concurrent disease.

Most *S. dublin* infections occur when animals are on pasture. Animals housed in stalls have a much lower likelihood of becoming infected than loose-housed animals. In the latter, infection is maintained and most animals eventually become either actively or passively infected (Williams 1980). Streams and rivers may become contaminated and serve to disseminate the organism to drinking places downstream. *S. dublin* can survive in feces for at least 4 months and elsewhere in the environment for more than a year (Gibson 1961).

Enteric disease caused by *S. dublin* is usually observed in calves between 3 and 6 weeks old. The disease in calves is characterized by foul-smelling diarrhea, depression, anorexia, fever, weakness, and death in a day or two. The stool may be bloodstained and contain mucus and shreds of mucosa. Postmortem examination reveals petechiae in the peritoneum and areas of hemorrhagic inflammation on the colon and distal small intestine. The mesenteric lymph nodes are also hemorrhagic and edematous. There may be areas of necrosis in the liver.

Calves that do not die in the acute phase of the disease may develop later signs of joint involvement and, rarely, ischemic necrosis of the tips of the ears, tail, and feet. Mortality may be as high as 75 percent, but losses are usually on the order of 5 to 10 percent. Losses are generally much higher among purchased than among home-bred calves (Hughes 1964).

The disease in adult cattle can be very severe, with a sudden onset of fever, depression, anorexia, or agalactia followed by severe diarrhea with blood and mucus in the feces. Death may occur in a substantial proportion of these animals if they are left untreated. Animals that survive usually take 2 to 3 months to return to their original condition. The acute form of the disease is seen in herds in which there has been no previous history of *S. dublin* infection and which therefore are fully susceptible. The subacute disease is seen in herds in which the infection is enzootic and is characterized by a much less severe clinical course of diarrhea, slight fever, and decreased milk production. Cows may have clinically inapparent infections of the mammary glands and shed the organism in the milk (Sharp et al. 1980).

Abortion is another common sequel to infection and may or may not be preceded by the other clinical signs of the disease. Fever may precede the occurrence of abortion but is rarely noticed. *S. dublin* abortions are more common from August to November in Europe (Frik 1969). The organism apparently enters the fetus from the maternal circulation via the placenta and causes septicemia and death of the fetus. There is no evidence of venereal transmission. The aborted fetus exhibits edema of the subcutis and serosanguineous fluid in the peritoneal cavity. Abortion occurs on average about 200 days after conception (Frik 1969).

Lesions in adult cattle with acute *S. dublin* infection usually include a mucoid-necrotic enteritis and petechiae on mucosal surfaces. Degenerative changes may be present in the liver and the wall of the gallbladder may be inflamed.

The epizootiology and pathogenesis of infection by *S. typhimurium* differs in several important respects from that just described for *S. dublin* infection. *S. typhimurium* is the most commonly isolated serotype from outbreaks and cases of salmonellosis in cattle. Although it is widely distributed in the environment and in a variety of wild animal hosts, the source of the majority of infections in cattle is other cattle (Hughes et al 1971). Specific clones of *S. typhimurium* recognizable by their phage type and plasmid complement dominate in cattle populations for extended periods and then are replaced by a new clone (Threlfall et al. 1978). This phenomenon is most apparent in calf populations and has been extensively documented in Britain and to a lesser extent in the northeastern United States (McDonough 1985, Timoney 1981). Calf marketing and distribution practices in which calves from widely separated sources are grouped and then redistributed over a wide geographic area ensure the distribution of specific clones. Subsequent antibiotic selection pressures imposed to minimize disease losses in these calves then ensure the maintenance and persistence of the enzootic clone of *S. typhimurium*. Furthermore, because the R factor plasmids in an enzootic clone may encode for traits such as enhanced persistence in the intestine, they contribute to epidemicity (Timoney and Linton 1982).

Cases of salmonellosis in intensively raised calves usually appear within a few days of entry of infected calves into the unit, and the number of cases peaks at about 3 weeks. The spread of infection is greater among calves penned loosely and able to contact one another than among calves that are isolated in individual pens (Linton et al. 1974); one reason for this is that calves with salmonellosis excrete the organism in the saliva and thus may pass the infection to others by licking or by contaminating buckets. However, feco-oral transfer among calves is the most important mode of transmission.

Since persistently shedding carrier animals are highly unusual, the disease in calves and adult cattle tends to be self-limiting. The infection therefore often dies out in a group or herd maintained under hygienic conditions and free of exposure to exogenous sources of infection.

Other possible sources of infection for cattle include contaminated feed, rodents and wild birds, sewage, poultry litter, and contaminated water courses (Wray and Callow 1985).

S. typhimurium causes enteritis and septicemia in susceptible calves. The morbidity may be high and mortalities of 50 percent or higher have sometimes been observed. Clones carrying plasmids with genes for lactose fermentation are highly virulent and cause a very high mortality (Timoney et al. 1980).

The lesions in calves and older cattle are similar to those described for *S. dublin*, although *S. typhimurium* does not cause gangrene of the extremities or meningitis and is rarely associated with abortion.

A variety of other *Salmonella* serotypes can also cause enteric or invasive salmonellosis in cattle. Many of these serotypes are derived from feed, droppings of wild birds or sewage contamination of pasture or water courses. Examples of serotypes other than *S. dublin* or *S. typhimurium* which cause bovine infections are *S. anatum* (Glickman et al. 1981), *S. montevideo* (Sharp et al. 1983), *S. newport* (Clegg et al. 1983), and *S. saint-paul* (Jones et al. 1983). The diseases and lesions produced by these serotypes generally resembled those described for *S. typhimurium*.

The disease in sheep and goats. Salmonellosis in sheep is associated with the host-adapted serotype *S. abortus ovis* and with *S. dublin*, *S. montevideo*, and *S. typhimurium*, and occasionally with other uncommon serotypes.

S. abortus ovis is found in Europe and the Middle East and is a cause of abortion in sheep during the last 2 months of pregnancy. It is usually introduced into a flock in an infected sheep (Jack 1968). Animals become infected by ingesting the organism, which then causes a bacteremia that may or may not be accompanied by a low fever. The organism invades the placenta and abortion results. The placenta and fetus show no visible evidence of the infection.

S. montevideo abortion is common in Scotland and is similar to that caused by *S. abortus ovis*. Ewes infected at 16 weeks or later in pregnancy are unaffected and produce normal lambs. Animals that are infected earlier abort a few weeks later. The placental membranes are heavily contaminated and are a source of infection for other animals (Sharp et al. 1983).

S. dublin and *S. typhimurium* cause enteritis, septicemia, and abortion that is similar in most respects to that described for cattle. Cattle are the usual source of *S. dublin* for sheep and goats, while *S. typhimurium* can be contracted from a variety of animal and environmental sources. Disease caused by *S. typhimurium* or *S. dublin* is usually seen in situations of defective flock or herd management (Findlay 1978).

Salmonellosis in goats has been reviewed by Bulgin and Anderson (1981).

The disease in horses.   It has been estimated that 5 to 10 percent of the horses in the United States become infected with salmonellae during their lifetimes (Morse et al. 1976).

S. typhimurium is by far the most common serotype isolated, but *S. enteritidis, S. heidelberg, S. newport,* and other exotic serotypes are also occasionally found. *S. abortus equi* is found in horses in Europe, South Africa, and South America but has apparently disappeared in the United States, where it was once a common cause of abortion.

A variety of stressful influences affect the susceptibility of horses to salmonellae. Latent infections are common (Biesinger 1983) and can be activated by transport, over-training, worming, early weaning, hot weather, hospitalization, and antibiotic administration (Morse et al. 1976).

Foals can become infected from their dams, from the droppings of infected wild birds, and from direct or indirect contact with other infected livestock. Acute salmonellosis in horses is characterized by fever, anorexia, depression, and diarrhea with signs of severe abdominal pain. The animal quickly becomes dehydrated, goes into shock, and dies within a few days. In foals, a peracute, septicemic, highly fatal infection is frequently observed. Endotoxin from the salmonella cell wall is responsible for the pyrexia, hypotension, and neutropenia that is observed.

Animals that survive the acute phase of the disease frequently progress to a chronic form characterized by intransigent diarrhea that persists for months. The feces may have a "cow pie" consistency (Morse et al. 1976). Foals that recover may have polyarthritis. Some horses with chronic enteric salmonellosis steadily loose condition and eventually are unable to rise.

S. abortus equi is spread mainly on the pasture. Infective discharges from aborting mares contaminate the grass, which then is eaten by others in the group. Just before abortion occurs, the mare usually has a fever and other signs of a systemic reaction that suggests the presence of a bacteremia. The fetal membranes are edematous and show hemorrhages and areas of necrosis.

The disease in swine.   The serotypes most frequently implicated in swine are *S. choleraesuis* and *S. ty-*

phimurium. A variety of other serotypes can be carried in the cecum and intestinal lymph nodes of many normal pigs and reflect the salmonella content of the animals' feed (Timoney 1970). Some of these serotypes, such as *S. anatum, S. derby, S. heidelberg, S. newport, S. panama,* and *S. saint-paul* can cause clinical salmonellosis in susceptible piglets or in older pigs stressed by other factors.

S. choleraesuis is maintained in the intestine and mesenteric lymphoid tissue of carrier swine. The organism is shed by most pigs for about 3 months following clinical recovery and indefinitely by a few pigs. It survives well in manure, and persistence for up to 20 weeks in slurry has been reported (Jones 1976). Contamination of housing is therefore important in the epizootiology of disease caused by this and by other serotypes. Feed is an important primary source of *S. typhimurium.*

The disease caused by *S. choleraesuis* is known as paratyphoid. Most cases in the United States and Europe are caused by the monophasic (6,7: −1,5) (Kunzendorf) variety. The other varieties, *S. typhisuis* and *S. choleraesuis* (diphasic), are rarely isolated. Paratyphoid occurs in pigs of all ages but is most common in fattening pigs after weaning. A variety of stresses can predispose the animal to infection. The organism was called the "hog cholera bacillus" by Salmon and Smith (1885) because infection by hog cholera (swine fever) virus was invariably followed by a secondary invasion of *S. choleraesuis.*

The acute disease is characterized by purplish areas on the ears, rump, and abdomen, high fever, conjunctivitis, anorexia, and death in 1 to 3 days. At postmortem examination, petechiation and other signs of septicemia are present. Pneumonia may also be observed. A less acute form is characterized by foul-smelling diarrhea, which can eventually result in death or extreme loss of condition. In animals with chronic cases, thickening of the intestine and mucosal necrosis are caused by secondary invasions of *Fusobacterium* and *Bacteroides* species.

Swine salmonellosis caused by *S. dublin* is characterized by enteritis and meningoencephalitis (McErlean 1968). Disease caused by *S. typhimurium* and other serotypes is usually enteric, septicemic, or both. *S. heidelberg* has been shown to produce a severe catarrhal enterocolitis followed by a persistent carrier state (Reed 1983).

The disease in dogs and cats.   Clinical salmonellosis is uncommon in dogs and cats, although a variety of serotypes may be carried (Borland 1975) by normal animals.

Timoney et al. (1978) described a nosocomial outbreak of *S. typhimurium* gastroenteritis and septicemia with a mortality of 61 percent in young cats in a veterinary hospital. Administration of ampicillin to affected cats in this

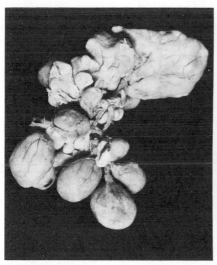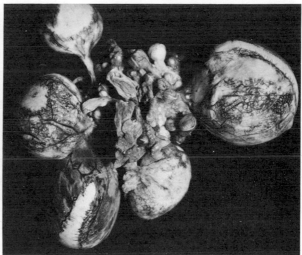

Figure 7.4. Pullorum disease in a chicken ovary. The diseased ovary is on the left. On the right is a normal ovary for comparison. The ova of a diseased bird are small, misshapen, discolored, and sometimes hemorrhagic.

outbreak apparently was a factor in the severity of the clinical signs. The causative *S. typhimurium* was resistant to ampicillin, and the antibiotic, by suppressing normal intestinal flora, allowed the resistant salmonella clone to attain overwhelming numbers in the intestine.

Salmonellosis is a complication of cancer chemotherapy in dogs. Dogs with lymphosarcoma developed enteric and septicemic salmonellosis within 3 days of the start of chemotherapy (Calvert and Leifer 1982).

Abortion, stillbirths, and neonatal deaths in breeding kennels have been caused by *S. panama* (Redwood and Bell 1983).

The disease in poultry. *S. pullorum* and *S. gallinarum* cause *bacillary white diarrhea* and *fowl typhoid,* respectively, in chickens. *S. typhimurium* and other non-host-adapted serotypes, most of which are feed-borne, also cause infections and disease in poultry. In broiler flocks, infections are very common but clinically inapparent and are of significance only from the standpoint of subsequent contamination of carcasses for human consumption.

S. pullorum has been isolated from turkeys, chickens, pheasants, canaries, parrots, calves, swine, dogs, foxes, mink, cats, chinchillas, and humans. It occurs most frequently in chickens raised in barnyard flocks and less often in turkeys. Eradication programs have been highly successful in the United States and Europe, and *S. pullorum* is now rarely isolated in these regions.

S. pullorum is highly fatal to young chicks during the first few days of life, and particularly if the chicks are stressed by chilling. Older chicks are more resistant.

The organism is maintained in the ovaries of adult birds (Figure 7.4), and infection is transmitted transovarily.

Some infected eggs may fail to hatch, others produce infected chicks, which, if stressed, become ill with diarrhea and septicemia. The feces contains large numbers of organisms that quickly serve to infect the remainder of the group of chicks in the incubator. Contaminated down is also an important source of infection for other chicks. Thus exposed to air-borne infection, these chicks contract the disease by inhaling the organism.

Affected chicks huddle near a source of heat, do not eat, appear sleepy, may have diarrhea, and usually die within a few hours. Meningoencephalitis may be seen in some affected chicks (Coelho et al. 1983). The lesions vary according to the method of infection. Chicks infected by inhaling the organism usually have caseous areas in the lungs. Similar caseous areas often are seen in the wall of the gizzard and in the heart muscle. The losses vary greatly depending on how the chicks are handled. Stresses such as chilling, handling, or transport may greatly increase losses.

Outbreaks in pheasants and Japanese quail (Krauss 1981) have also been described. *S. gallinarum* causes fowl typhoid in turkeys and chickens. Its distribution is limited almost entirely to these fowls, and its occurrence is considerably less than that of *S. agona, S. bareilly, S. hadar, S. oranienburg, S. pullorum, S. typhimurium,* and other feed-borne serotypes in regions where poultry is raised intensively. Because it is traditionally an infection of barnyard flocks, its incidence has been greatly reduced by changes in poultry husbandry, and also by the eradication of *S. pullorum,* which, because of common antigens (see Table 7.1), cross-reacts with *S. gallinarum* in the plate test.

The organism is maintained in the ovary of carrier birds and is transmitted vertically in the yolk. It is also transmitted horizontally through feces and broken eggs and by the tick *Argas persicus* (Gyurov 1983). Fowl typhoid typically affects adult birds. The symptoms are those of an acute septicemic disease with weakness, drowsiness, wing drooping, hyperexcitability, paresis, and diarrhea. There is rapidly developing anemia and a leukocytosis. In many cases, the birds are found dead under the roosts in the morning before any symptoms have been noticed. The lesions consists of hemorrhages in the subcutis and parenchymatous organs, multiple small necrotic areas in the liver and heart, and an enlarged spleen.

Carcasses of birds that died of fowl typhoid have yielded viable bacteria from the liver up to 11 days and from the bone marrow up to 25 days after death. The organisms have also been obtained from maggots feeding on the carcasses (Jordan 1954).

S. typhimurium is a common salmonella infection of poultry in regions where pullorum disease has been controlled and can cause severe losses in young birds. The disease is known as *paratyphoid* and is manifested by enteritis, diarrhea, and septicemia in severe cases. Arthritis in ducks has also been described (Bisgaard 1981). The organism can localize in the ovary and can be transmitted in the egg, although many infections are derived from feed.

In pigeon lofts, losses from *S. typhimurium* often are very great. Disease is typically seen in the squabs, which either die soon after hatching or develop swollen wing joints that render them unable to fly. Pigeon fanciers often call this disease *megrims*. Joint swelling is caused by infection and the formation of a gelatinous exudate in the joint capsule. Adult pigeons show no outward evidence of the disease ordinarily, but may have infection in the ovary. The organism can be found in many of the developing yolks and is vertically transmitted to the developing embryo.

Many other so-called exotic *Salmonella* serotypes that are derived from feed are frequently isolated from broiler flocks and from eggs, although salmonella contamination of eggs in New York State has greatly declined (Baker et al. 1980). Contamination of poultry meats by salmonellae that enter flocks in contaminated feed is of great public health significance because many cases of human salmonellosis are derived from this source in the United States and elsewhere each year.

The *S. arizonae* group contains two serotypes ($18:Z_4$, Z_{23} and $18:Z_4$, $Z_{32}-$) that cause enteritis or septicemia in turkeys. These serotypes are frequently designated *Arizona* 7:1,2,6 and 7:1,7,8, respectively. Members differ from other salmonellae mainly in being slow lactose fer-

menters. The disease they cause, which is of considerable economic importance and is known as arizonosis, resembles that caused by other salmonellae (Kowalski and Stephens 1968, West and Mohanty 1973). Because *S. arizonae* may localize in the ovary, it can be vertically transmitted. A chronic form of the disease is characterized by nervous signs and formation of cataracts.

Immunity. There is fairly general agreement that cell-mediated immunity is more important than humoral antibodies in resistance to systemic salmonellosis (Eisenstein and Sultzer 1983). Because salmonellae are facultative intracellular parasites, they have enhanced survival ability in the phagocyte. They are resistant to degradation by lysosomal enzymes and can survive and multiply in the acid environment of the phagolysosome. Cell-mediated immunity has its basis in increased bactericidal activity of the host's macrophages for the pathogen and is not serotype-specific (Mackaness et al. 1966).

Live salmonella vaccines are more effective than bacterins in stimulating cell-mediated immune responses. Live vaccines may persist in the tissues long after strong cell-mediated protective responses have been elicited (Nauciel et al. 1985). Thus, *Salmonella* serotypes such as *S. dublin* that are prone to establish carrier states at the same time are associated with a high level of protective immunity. This protective immunity may, however, be compromised if the animal is stressed or immunosuppressed.

Calves vaccinated with attenuated *S. typhimurium* vaccine develop cutaneous delayed hypersensitivity and a high degree of macrophage migration inhibition. Both of these correlates of cell-mediated immunity are associated with enhanced protection against experimental challenge (Chaturvedi and Sharma 1981, Habasha et al. 1985, Merritt et al. 1984).

Salmonella lipopolysaccharide has been shown to be capable of eliciting delayed-type hypersensitivity responses similar to those elicited by immunization with sublethal doses of live organisms (Desiderio and Campbell 1984). However, the antigen must be incorporated into liposomes for a delayed-type hypersensitivity effect to occur.

Studies on the major outer membrane protein of *S. typhimurium* have shown that it must be mixed with lipopolysaccharide to induce the synthesis of protective antibodies (Kuusi et al. 1981, Svenson et al. 1979).

Humoral antibodies are directed against the O antigen side chains of the lipopolysaccharide and against outer membrane proteins, O antibodies are agglutinating, and if they are of the IgM isotype, they can instigate complement-mediated bacteriolysis (Robbins et al. 1965). Antibodies to membrane proteins, although not serotype specific, can act as opsonins and can be protective (Johnson et al. 1985, Kuusi et al. 1979).

Antibodies to the common core glycolipid (2-keto, 3-deoxyoctonate-lipid A) of the lipopolysaccharide are effective in neutralizing the endotoxic effects of salmonella lipopolysaccharide. This effect can be expressed in all Gram-negative bacterial infections in which the same common core glycolipid is involved.

Local enteric mucosal immune responses to salmonella antigens have been observed (Mitze et al. 1981), but the nature and role of these responses in local protection of the mucosa require much further study. Antibodies have been detected in the jejunal secretions following oral administration of heat-inactivated S. typhimurium. Vaccinated calves shed fewer S. typhimurium following challenge than control animals (Hellmann 1983).

A variety of vaccines against S. abortus ovis have been described (Table 7.3). Inactivated vaccines appear to give only limited protection, doubtless because they fail to stimulate an adequate cell-mediated immune response. However, the intradermal route can be used to stimulate a protective cell-mediated response with a heat-killed bacterin (Aitken et al. 1982). In contrast, S. abortus equi bacterins have been very successfully used, with the result that the disease has disappeared from the United States and many other parts of the world.

A number of live S. choleraesuis vaccines have been used successfully in swine populations (Table 7.3) in which protective immunity appears about 2 weeks after vaccination. Because concurrent antibiotic administration may inactivate the vaccine, vaccinated animals may fail to mount a protective response.

Live S. gallinarum vaccines stimulate better protection than bacterins, and protection is not dependent on a humoral immune response (Padmanaban et al. 1981). Immunization of chickens with the attenuated 9 R strain did not protect against intestinal colonization by S. typhimurium or S. infantis (Silva et al. 1981).

Immunization of calves with rough S. dublin resulted in marked cellular immune but poor humoral responsiveness (Chaturvedi and Sharma 1981). Immunization of pregnant cows a few weeks before calving with formalinized S. dublin bacterin resulted in passive protection of calves in which an active immunity could later be stimulated (6 weeks later) by oral administration of a live streptomycin-dependent mutant of S. dublin (Hahn and Scholl 1984).

The rough S. dublin mutant widely used as a vaccine in Great Britain, (Smith 1965), also protects against disease caused by S. typhimurium. However, the level of protection against either serotype is modest and can be overcome when exposure to virulent strains is excessive.

S. typhimurium vaccines are even more varied and creative than those developed for other serotypes. Genetically modified strains include those lacking galactose epimerase that undergo growth inhibition and cell lysis following uptake of galactose. Aromatic-dependent mutants require para-amino benzoic benzoate and dihydroxybenzoate for folate and enterochelin synthesis, respectively. These metabolites are not available in the host tissues, so the vaccine strain eventually dies in the host. Streptomycin-dependent mutants survive only so long as the antibiotic is available. Because the most effective live vaccines are those that persist in the reticuloendothelial system, mutants such as those just described are unlikely to produce a long-lived cell-mediated protective response. S. typhimurium bacterins elicit only a low level protective response and cannot stimulate any response in neonatal calves.

Live vaccines are subject to inactivation by antibiotics given parenterally or in the animal's diet. Another disadvantage is that although live vaccines are avirulent for normal calves, they may be pathogenic in colostrum-deprived or immune-deficient animals.

Serology. Antibody responses to salmonella infection can be measured by the agglutination test, antiglobulin test, and enzyme-linked immunosorbent assay (ELISA). Antibody determinations in cattle are unreliable for the detection of individuals infected with S. dublin but are of great value in the detection of infected herds (Wray et al. 1977). Both O and H titers can be measured. Many infected animals do not have positive titers, however, because the serum was collected too early, the infection was not severe enough to stimulate an immune response, or the animal did not respond. It also is possible for animals to passively transfer the organism along their intestines without developing an immune response. The antigenic stimulus associated with clinical salmonellosis is usually effective in eliciting an antibody response (Richardson 1975), and recovered animals or cows that have aborted therefore usually have positive titers (Frik 1969).

Since calves are much more responsive to the H than the O antigens of salmonellae, H titers must be measured in these animals. Ideally, paired serum samples should be tested. O antibodies against S. typhimurium in intestinal fluids of calves have been measured with an ELISA (Schmidberger 1983). An ELISA has also been shown to be an effective method of measuring antibody to the O antigens of S. typhimurium in colostrum of cows vaccinated with bacterin and in the serums of their calves (Robertsson and Carlsson 1980).

Serums of horses infected with S. abortus equi usually agglutinate in dilutions from 1:500 to 1:5,000. Normal animals may have titers of 1:200 (Good and Corbett

Table 7.3. Examples of salmonella vaccines

Serotype	Designation	Type of vaccine	Route of administration	Reference
S. abortus ovis		Adjuvanated extract	Subcutaneous	Sidorchuk (1982)
	RG	Attenuated live	Subcutaneous	Pardon et al. (1980)
	Rv6	Streptomycin-independent reverse mutant, live	Subcutaneous	Lantier et al. (1983)
		Enzymic extract	Intramuscular	Arkangel'skii et al. (1979)
		Heat, formalin inactivated	Subcutaneous	Tadjbakhche and Nadalian (1980)
		Virulent, live	Oral	
S. abortus equi		Formalinized bacterin	Intramuscular, subcutaneous	Good and Dimock (1927)
		Thallium acetate attenuated live	Intramuscular	Fang et al. (1978b)
S. cholerae suis	C500	Thallium acetate attenuated live	Subcutaneous, intramuscular	Fang et al. (1978a)
	Suisaloral Dessau	Attenuated live (hypoxanthine auxotroph)	Subcutaneous, oral	Scholl et al. (1980)
	Suscovax	Rough mutant, live	Intramuscular, subcutaneous	Smith (1965)
S. dublin	Dessau	Avirulent, live	Oral	Steinbach et al. (1981)
		Formalinized bacterin	Intramuscular, subcutaneous	
		Streptomycin-dependent mutant, live	Oral	Hahn and Scholl (1984)
	51	Attenuated rough mutant, live	Subcutaneous	Smith (1965)
	SL 1438	Aromatic-dependent mutant, live	Intramuscular	Smith et al. (1984a, 1984b)
S. gallinarum		Attenuated live	Subcutaneous	Smith (1965)
	9R	Attenuated live	Subcutaneous	Silva et al. (1981)
	E20	Attenuated live		Cameron and Buys (1979)
	E37	Formalinized bacterin	Subcutaneous, intramuscular	Padmanaban et al. (1981)
S. typhimurium		Formalinized, adjuvanated bacterin	Subcutaneous, intramuscular	
	G30D	Galactose epimeraseless, live	Oral	Baljer et al. (1981), Suphabphant et al. (1983)
	SL 1479	Aromatic-dependent mutant, live	Intramuscular, oral	Smith et al. (1984b)

1913). H agglutinins are present before O agglutinins and are therefore indicative of recent infection.

Control of *S. pullorum* disease depends greatly on serologic detection and elimination of carrier breeder hens. Serum agglutinins are detected either by the tube, the serum-plate, or the whole-blood–plate method. A titer of 1:25 or greater in the tube test is evidence of infection. A positive plate test carries the same interpretation. The antigen in this test is a heavy suspension of stained *S. pullorum*. A microagglutination test is more effective in the detection of low levels of antibody (Thain and Blandford 1981). Antibody can also be detected in the egg yolk of infected birds.

S. gallinarum antibodies can be detected in the same way and with the same stained antigen as used in *S. pullorum* disease control. Other serologic tests for these antibodies include indirect hemagglutination, antiglobulin hemagglutination, and opsonophagocytic, cytophilic, and bactericidal antibodies (Padmanaban et al. 1981).

Agglutinin titers of 1:25 to the O and H antigens of *S. typhimurium* are suggestive of infection in turkeys

(Hinshaw and McNeil 1943), but many infected birds may be serologically negative. The test therefore is most useful when applied to a whole flock. An indirect hemagglutination test has also been described for the detection of infected birds (Sieburth 1957).

Serum agglutinins or complement-fixing antibodies to the O and H antigens of *S. abortus ovis* appear about a week after infection (Sanchis and Pardon 1984). Agglutinin titers peak 8 to 15 days after oral inoculation and persist for about 16 weeks. Serologic procedures are not routinely used for the detection of carrier ewes, and little information exists on their value for such determinations.

Antibody responses of swine to *S. choleraesuis* are not consistent or predictable enough to be useful in the diagnosis of carriers.

Diagnosis. Enteric salmonellosis can be diagnosed by direct plating of fecal specimens and intestinal scrapings on a selective and differential medium such as MacConkey, brilliant green, salmonella-shigella, xylose-lysine, deoxycholate, Hektoen enteric, and bismuth sulfite (Wilson and Blair) agars. The characteristics of salmonella colonies on these media are shown in Table 7.4. Lactose-fermenting salmonellae can best be recognized on bismuth sulfite agar. Some salmonellae, for example, *S. dublin* and *S. abortus ovis,* produce tiny colonies.

Samples (10 percent by volume) should also be inoculated into enrichment medium such as selenite or tetrathionate broth, incubated at 43°C, and then plated after 24 hours on a selective medium. *S. choleraesuis* cannot be isolated in a medium that contains selenite. Instead, a medium such as modified Rappaports' should be used for its isolation.

Giemsa-stained smears of feces from animals with salmonellosis usually contain large numbers of polymorphonuclear neutrophils and are therefore helpful in

diagnosis. Salmonella lipopolysaccharide (serogroup B or C2) can be detected by an ELISA in poultry feces, litter, or carcass washings (Rigby 1984).

In cases of abortion, the organisms can be observed in smears of the fetal stomach contents and placental tissue. A peroxidase-antiperoxidase immunoassay has been developed for the recognition of *S. choleraesuis, S. dublin,* and *S. typhimurium* in tissue (McRill et al. 1984).

Serologic methods of diagnosis are most valuable when applied to a whole herd or when paired acute and covalescent serum samples are available for comparison. Antibody responses are most consistently present in animals that have recently recovered from severe invasive infections.

Cattle that recovered from clinical *S. dublin* infection developed O titers in the range of 1:80 to 1:320 and H titers in the range of 1:640 to 1:5,120 about 3 to 4 weeks after the illness began (Clarenberg and Vink 1949, Williams 1980). Some latently infected cattle are serologically negative.

Antimicrobial Susceptibility. Salmonellae are sensitive to amikacin, ampicillin, apramycin, cephalothin, chloramphenicol, furazolidone, gentamicin, kanamycin, streptomycin, sulfamethoxazole-trimethoprim, and tetracycline. Although only ampicillin, choramphenicol, and sulfamethoxazole-trimethoprim have validated efficacy in the therapy of invasive salmonella infection, there is evidence that apramycin may be useful in therapy of systemic salmonellosis in calves (Theys et al. 1983).

S. typhimurium, and, to a lesser extent, other *Salmonella* strains from domesticated animals exhibit a high frequency of multiple antibiotic resistance (Blackburn et al. 1984, Timoney 1978, van Leeuwen et al. 1982, Wishart and Eddy 1985). The selection of an antimicrobial must therefore be based on sensitivity testing. Administration of an antibiotic to an animal infected with a salmonella resistant to that antibiotic is likely to increase the severity of the infection and convert a local enteric infection into a septicemia. In treated animals destruction of the protective colonic flora allows rapid overgrowth of the resistant organism. Furthermore, the number of animals that shed and the duration and volume of shedding can be greatly increased after antimicrobial therapy. The massive antimicrobial selection pressures applied in intensive calf-raising operations, for instance, have resulted in emergence of multiresistant *S. typhimurium* strains with plasmids that encode traits such as lactose fermentation or enhanced persistence in the intestine (Timoney and Linton 1982, Timoney et al. 1980). These traits clearly enhance epidemicity, increase pathogenic potential, and confuse the laboratory diagnostician.

Many clinicians favor use of antimicrobials only for the

Table 7.4. Characteristics of salmonella colonies on selective and differential media

Medium	Colonial characteristics
MacConkey agar	Colorless to grayish colonies
Brilliant green agar	Red colonies. Some strains of *Proteus, Pseudomonas,* and *Citrobacter* species also produce red colonies on this medium
Xylose-lysine agar Deoxycholate agar	Pink-red colonies with black centers
Hektoen enteric agar	Green colonies with black centers
Bismuth sulfite agar	Black colonies with a metallic sheen
Salmonella-shigella agar	Colorless colonies with black centers

parenteral treatment of systemic or invasive salmonellosis and avoid oral administration of antimicrobials.

The Disease in Humans.   Salmonellae cause a febrile gastroenteritis accompanied sometimes by bacteremia. The disease is self-limiting but may be severe in the young and the elderly. Many human infections in the developed countries of the world result from ingestion of animal products including eggs, poultry meat, pork, and beef.

REFERENCES

Aitken, M.M., Jones, P.W., and Brown, G.T.H. 1982. Protection of cattle against experimentally induced salmonellosis by intradermal injection of heat-killed *Salmonella dublin*. Res. Vet. Sci. 32:368–373.

Anderson, E.S. 1964. The phage typing of salmonellae other than *S.typhi*. In E. Van Oye, ed., The World Problem of Salmonellosis. Junk, The Hague. Pp. 89–110.

Arkhangel'skii, I.I., Sidorchuk, A.A., Karavaev, Yu. D, Kreinin, L.S., Kaverina, K.G., and Vasil'eva, I.N. 1979. Preparation and testing of a chemically treated vaccine against salmonellosis in sheep. Trud. Vsesoyuz. Inst. Eksp. Vet. 49:69–75.

Baker, R.C., Goff, J.P., and Timoney, J.F. 1980. Prevalence of salmonellae on eggs from poultry farms in New York State. Poult. Sci. 59:289–292.

Baljer, G., Hoerstke, M., Dirksen, G., Seitz, A., Sailer, J., and Mayr, A. 1981. Comparison of the efficacy of oral immunization with heat-inactivated and live, avirulent (gal E⁻) *S. typhimurium* against salmonellosis in calves. Zentralbl. Veterinärmed [B] 28:759–766.

Barker, R.M., and Old, D.C. 1980. Biotypes of strains of *Salmonella typhimurium* of phage types 49, 204 and 193. J. Med. Microbiol. 13:369–371.

Barker, R., Old, D.C., and Tyc, Z. 1982. Differential typing of *Salmonella agona:* Type divergence in a new serotype. J. Hyg. 88:413–423.

Biesinger, B. 1983. Occurrence of latent *Salmonella* infections in horses. Inaugural dissertation, Fachbereich Veterinärmedizin, Freie Universität, Berlin. Pp. 79.

Bisgaard, M. 1981. Arthritis in ducks. I. Aetiology and public health aspects. Avian Pathol. 10:11–21.

Blackburn, B.O., Schlater, L.K., and Swanson, M.R. 1984. Antibiotic resistance of members of the genus *Salmonella* isolated from chickens, turkeys, cattle, and swine in the United States during October 1981 through September 1982. Am. J. Vet. Res. 45:1245–1249.

Blaser, M.J., Hug, M.I., Glass, R.I., Zimicki. S., and Birkness, K.A. 1982. Salmonellosis at rural and urban clinics in Bangladesh. Epidemiological and clinical characteristics. Am. J. Epidemiol. 116:266–275.

Borland, E.D. 1975. *Salmonella* infection in dogs, cats, tortoises and terrapins. Vet. Rec. 96:401–402.

Bulgin, M.S., and Anderson, B.C. 1981. Salmonellosis in goats. J. Am. Vet. Med. Assoc. 178:720–723.

Calvert, C.A., and Leifer, C.E. 1982. Salmonellosis in dogs with lymphosarcoma. J. Am. Vet. Med. Assoc. 180:56–58.

Cameron, C.M., and Buys, S.B. 1979. Production and application of a live *Salmonella gallinarum* vaccine. Onderstepoort J. Vet. Res. 46:185–189.

Chaturvedi, G.C., and Sharma, V.K. 1981. Cell-mediated immunoprotection in calves immunized with rough *Salmonella dublin*. Br. Vet. J. 137:421–430.

Clarenburg, A.. and Vink, H.H. 1949. *Salmonella dublin* carriers in cattle. In Report of the 14th International Veterinary Congress, London, vol. 2. Pp. 262–266.

Clegg, F.G., Chiejina, S.N., Duncan, A.L., Kay, R.N., and Wray, C. 1983. Outbreaks of *Salmonella newport* infection in dairy herds and

their relationship to management and contamination of the environment. Vet. Rec. 112:580–584.

Coelho, H.E., Nogueira, R.H.G., de Silva, J.M.L., Girao, F.G.F., and do Nascimento, E.F. 1983. Purulent meninogencephalitis caused by *Salmonella pullorum* in chicks. Arq. Bras. Med. Vet. Zootec. 35:283–285.

Crosa, J.M., Brenner, D.J., Ewing, W.H., and Falkow, S. 1973. Molecular relationships among the Salmonelleae. J. Bacteriol. 115:307–315.

Desiderio, J.V., and Campbell, S.G. 1984. Vaccination against experimental murine salmonellosis with liposome-associated antigens. J. Leukocyte Biol. 36:399.

Duguid, J.P., Anderson, E.S., Alfredsson, G.A., Barker, R., and Ole, D.C. 1975. A new biotyping scheme for *Salmonella typhimurium* and its phylogenetic significance. J. Med. Microbiol. 8:149–166.

Edwards, P.R., and Bruner, D.W. 1946. Form variation in *Salmonella pullorum* and its relation to X strains. Cornell Vet. 38:318–325.

Eisenstein, T.K., and Sultzer, B.M. 1983. Immunity to salmonella infection. Adv. Exp. Med. Biol. 162:261–296.

Fang, H,-W., Li, Y.-L., Huang, C.-B., Zheng, M., Feng, W.-Ta., and Sun, W. 1978. Live vaccine against swine paratyphoid from the attenuated smooth strain C 500 of *Salmonella choleraesuis*. In Collected Papers of Veterinary Research, vol. 4. Control Institute of Veterinary-Bioproducts and Pharmaceuticals, Ministry of Agriculture and Forestry, Beijing, China. Pp. 1–13.

Fang, H.-W., Yan, T.-J., Chang, S.-Y., Chang, H.-C., Theng, M., Feng, W.-T., Wu, P.-G., and Cheng, S.-S. 1978. Studies on *Salmonella abortus equi* attenuated vaccine. In Collected Papers of Veterinary Research, vol. 5. Control Institute of Veterinary-Bioproducts and Pharmaceuticals, Ministry of Agriculture and Forestry, Beijing, China. Pp. 1–14.

Felix, A. 1956. Phage typing of *Salmonella typhimurium:* Its place in epidemiological and epizootiological investigations. J. Gen. Microbiol. 14:208–222.

Findlay, C.R. 1978. Epidemiological aspects of an outbreak of salmonellosis in sheep. Vet. Rec. 103:113–114.

Finkelstein, R.A., Marchlewicz, B.A., McDonald, R.J., and Boesman-Finkelstein, M. 1983. Isolation and characterization of a cholera-related enterotoxin from *Salmonella typhimurium*. FEMS Microbiol. Lett. 17:239–241.

Frik, J.F. 1969. *Salmonella dublin* infection in cattle in the Netherlands. Epidemiology, pathogenesis and relationship to fascioliasis. Proefschrift Facultat Diergeneesk. Rijksuniv. Utrecht.

Gianella, R.A., Gots, R.E., Charney, A.N., Greenough, W.B., and Formal, S.B. 1975. Pathogenesis of *Salmonella*-mediated intestinal fluid secretion: Activation of adenylate cyclase and inhibition by indomethacin. Gastroenterology 69:1238–1245.

Gibson, E.A. 1961. Symposium: Salmonellosis in man and animals. 1. Salmonellosis in calves. Vet. Rec. 73:1284–1295.

Glickman, L.T., McDonough, P.L., Shin, S.J., Fairbrother, J.M., LaDue, R.L., and King, S.E. 1981. Bovine salmonellosis attributed to *Salmonella anatum*– contaminated haylage and dietary stress. J. Am. Vet. Med. Assoc. 178:1268–1272.

Good, E.S., and Corbett, L.S. 1913. Investigation of the etiology of infectious abortion of mares and jennets in Kentucky. J. Infect. Dis. 13:53–68.

Good, E.S., and Dimock, W.W. 1927. Studies on abortion in mares. J. Am. Vet. Med. Assoc. 71:31–34.

Guinee, P.A.M., and van Leeuwen, W.J. 1978. Phage typing of *Salmonella*. In T. Bergan and J.R. Norris, eds., Methods in Microbiology, vol. 2. Academic Press, New York. Pp. 157–181.

Gyurov, B. 1983. Role of *Argas persicus* in the epidemiology of fowl typhoid. Vet. Sbirka 81:22–24.

Habasha, F.G., Smith, B.P., Schwartz, L., Ardans, A., and Reina-Guerra, M. 1985. Correlation of macrophage migration inhibition factor and protection from challenge exposure in calves vaccinated with *Salmonella typhimurium*. Am. J. Vet. Res. 46:1415–1421.

Hahn, I., and Scholl, W., 1984. Complete immunization program for control and eradication of *Salmonella dublin* in herds of cattle. Monatshft. Vet. 39:208–213.

Hellmann, E. 1983. Efficacy of oral vaccination against *Salmonella* infections: Results of different experimental approaches. Tierärztl. Umsch. 38:695–704.

Hendricks, C.W. 1971. Increased recovery rate of salmonellae from stream bottom sediments versus surface waters. Appl. Microbiol. 21:379–380.

Hentges, D.J., and Maier, B.R. 1970. Inhibition of *Shigella flexneri* by the normal intestinal flora. III. Interactions with *Bacteroides fragilis* strains in vitro. Infect. Immun. 2:364–370.

Hinshaw, W.R., and McNeil, E. 1943. The use of the agglutination test in detecting *Salmonella typhimurium* carriers in turkey flocks. Proc. Ann. Meet. U.S. Livestock Sanit. Assoc. 47:106–121.

Holmberg, S.D., Osterholm, M.T., Senger, K.A., and Cohen, M.L. 1984. Drug-resistant salmonella from animals fed subtherapeutic antimicrobials. N. Engl. J. Med. 311:617–622.

Houston, C.W., Koo, F.C.W., and Peterson, J.W. 1981. Characterization of *Salmonella* toxin released by mitomycin C-treated cells. Infect. Immun. 32:916–926.

Hughes, L.E. 1964. Infectious diseases of calves in Great Britain. Bull. Off. Int. Epizoot. 62:525–532.

Hughes, L.E., Gibson, E.A., Roberts, H.E., and Davis, E.T. 1971. Bovine salmonellosis in England and Wales. Br. Vet. J. 127:225–237.

Jack, E.J. 1968. *Salmonella abortus ovis:* An atypical *Salmonella*. Vet. Rec. 82:558–561.

Johnson, E.M., Hictala, S., and Smith, B.P. 1985. Chemiluminescence of bovine alveolar macrophages as an indicator of developing immunity in calves vaccinated with aromatic-dependent *Salmonella*. Vet. Microbiol. 10:451–464.

Jones, G.W., Robert, D.K., Svinarich, D.M., and Whitfield, M.J. 1982. Association of adhesive, invasive, and virulent phenotypes of *Salmonella typhimurium* with autonomous 60-megadalton plasmids. Infect. Immun. 38:476–486.

Jones, P.W. 1976. The effect of temperature, solids content and pH on the survival of salmonellas in cattle slurry. Br. Vet. J. 132:284–293.

Jones, P.W., Collins, P., Brown, G.T.H., and Aitken, M.N. 1983. *Salmonella saint-paul* infection in two dairy herds. J. Hyg. 91:243–257.

Jordan, F.T.W. 1954. The survival of *Salmonella gallinarum* in poultry carcasses. Br. Vet. J. 110:387–392.

Josland, S.W. 1951. Survival of *Salmonella typhimurium* on various substances under natural conditions. Aust. Vet. J. 27.264–266.

Ketyi, I., Pasca, S., Emody, A., Vertengi, A., Kocsis, B., and Kuch, B. 1979. *Shigella dysenteriae* I-like cytotoxic enterotoxins produced by *Salmonella* strains. Acta. Microbiol. Acad. Sci. Hung. 26:217–223.

Khakria, R., and Lior, H. 1980. Distribution of phagovars of *Salmonella typhimurium* in Canada (1969–1976). Zentralbl. Bacteriol Mikrobiol. Hyg. [A] 248:50–63.

Kowalski, L.M., and Stephens, J.F. 1968. *Arizona* 7:1, 7, 8 infection in young turkeys. Avian Dis. 12:317–326.

Krauss, H. 1981. Some epidemiological aspects of *Salmonella gallinarum* infection in Japanese quail. Zentralbl. Veterinärmed. 28:704–712.

Kudrna, D.A., Teresa, G.W., Arnzen, J.M., and Beard, K.S. 1985. Immunoglobulin M and immunoglobulin G responses in BALB/c mice to conjugated outer membrane extracts of four *Salmonella* serotypes. Infect. Immun. 49:598–608.

Kuusi, N., Nurminen, M., Saxen, H., and Makela, P.H. 1981. Immunization with major outer membrane protein (porin) preparations in experimental murine salmonellosis: Effect of lipopolysaccharide. Infect. Immun. 34:328–332.

Kuusi, N., Numinen, M., Saxen, H., Valtonen, M., and Makela, P.H. 1979. Immunization with major outer membrane proteins in experimental salmonellosis of mice. Infect. Immun. 25:857–862.

Lantier, F., Pardon, P., and Marly, J. 1983. Immunogenicity of a low-virulence vaccinal strain against *Salmonella abortus ovis* infection in mice. Infect. Immun. 40:601–607.

Lawson, G.H.K., McPherson, E.A., Laing, A.H., and Wooding, P. 1974. The epidemiology of *Salmonella dublin* infection in a dairy herd. J. Hyg. 72:311–328.

Le Minor, C.C. 1984. Salmonella. In N.R. Kreig and J. G. Holt, eds., Bergey's Manual of Systematic Bacteriology, vol. I. Williams & Wilkins, Baltimore. Pp. 446.

Le Minor, C.C., Veron, M., and Popoff, M. 1982. The taxonomy of *Salmonella*. Ann. Microbiol. (Paris) 133B:245–254.

Linton, A.H.K., Howe, K., Pethiyagoda, S., and Osborne, A.D. 1974. Epidemiology of *Salmonella* infection in calves: Its relation to their husbandry and management. Vet. Rec. 94:581–585.

McDonough, P.M. 1985. Ph.D. dissertation, Cornell University, Ithaca, N.Y.

McErlean, B.A. 1968. *Salmonella dublin* meningitis in piglets. Vet. Rec. 82:257–258.

Mackaness, G.B., Blanden, R.V., and Collins, F.M. 1966. Host-parasite relations in mouse typhoid. J. Exp. Med. 124:573–583.

McRill, C.M., Kramer, T.T., and Griffith, R.W. 1984. Application of the peroxidase-antiperoxidase immunoassay to the identification of salmonellae from pure culture and animal tissue. J. Clin. Microbiol. 20:281–284.

Merritt, F.F., Smith, B.P., Rcina-Guerra, M., Habasha, F., and Johnson, E. 1984. Relationship of cutaneous delayed hypersensitivity to protection from challenge exposure with *Salmonella typhimurium* in calves. Am. J. Vet. Res. 45:1081–1085.

Mitze, H., Hellmann, E., Staak, C., Pietzsch, O., and Bulling, E. 1981. Immune response and resistance to infection of calves after oral immunization against *S. typhimurium* with an inactivated vaccine. Zentralbl. Veterinärmed [B] 28:767–777.

Morse, E.V., Duncan, M.A., Page, E.A., and Fessler, J.F. 1976. Salmonellosis in Equidae: A study of 26 cases. Cornell Vet. 66:198–213.

Nauciel, C., Vilde, F., and Ronco, E. 1985. Host response to infection with a temperature-sensitive mutant of *Salmonella typhimurium* in a susceptible and a resistant strain of mice. Infect. Immun. 49:523–527.

Padmanaban, V.D., Mittall, K.R., and Gupta, B.R. 1981. Cross protection against fowl typhoid: Immunization trials and humoral tissue response. Dev. Comp. Immunol. 5:301–312.

Pardon, P., Lantier, F., Marly, J., and Sanchis, R. 1980. Preparation of a live vaccine against salmonellosis in sheep. Bull. Mens. Soc. Vet. Pract. France 64:449–452.

Pomeroy, B.S., and Grady, M.L. 1962. *Salmonella* organisms isolated from feed ingredients. Proc. Annu. Meet. U.S. Livestock Sanit. Assoc. 65:449–452.

Redwood, D.W., and Bell, D.A. 1983. *Salmonella panama:* Isolation from aborted and newborn canine fetuses. Vet. Rec. 112:362.

Reed, W.M. 1983. Studies on the pathogenesis of *Salmonella heidelberg, Salmonella typhimurium* and *Salmonella choleraesuis* var. *kunzendorf* infection in weanling pigs. Diss. Abstr. Int. B 43:3875–3876.

Reed, W.M., Olander, H.J., and Thacker, H.L. 1985. Studies on the pathogenesis of *Salmonella heidelberg* infection in weanling pigs. Am. J. Vet. Res. 46:2300–2310.

Richardson, A. 1975. Salmonellosis in cattle. Vet. Rec. 96:329–331.

Rigby, C.E. 1984. Enzyme-linked immunosorbent assay for detection of salmonella lipopolysaccharide in poultry specimens. Appl. Environ. Microbiol. 47:1327–1330.

Roantree, R.J. 1967. *Salmonella* O antigens and virulence. Ann. Rev. Microbiol. 21:443–466.

Robbins, J.B., Kenny, K., and Suter, E. 1965. The isolation and biological activities of rabbit M and G anti-*Salmonella typhimurium* antibodies. J. Exp. Med. 122:385–402.

Robertson, J.A., and Carlsson, H.E. 1980. ELISA for measurement of antibody response to a killed *Salmonella typhimurium* vaccine in cattle. Zentralbl. Veterinärmed. [B] 27:28–35.

Salmon, D.E. 1885. On swine plague. U.S. Bur. Anim. Indus. Annu. Rep. 2:184–246.

Sanchis, R., and Pardon, P. 1984. Experimental infection of ewes with *Salmonella abortus ovis:* Effect of stage of pregnancy. Ann. Rech. Vét. 15:97–103.

Schmidberger, K. 1983. Local immune processes in the small intestine of calves orally immunized against *Salmonella typhimurium.* Inaugural Dissertation, Tierärztliche Fakultät der Ludwig-Maximilians-Universität, München. 87 pp.

Scholl, W., and Grunert, G. 1980. "Suisaloral Dessau" a *Salmonella choleraesuis* live vaccine for oral, parenteral and combined use. Arch. Exp. Vet. 34:91–97.

Sharp, J.C.M., Paterson, G.M., and Forbes, G.I. 1980. Milk-borne salmonellosis in Scotland. J. Infect. 2:333–340.

Sharp, J.C.M., Reilly, W.J., Linklater, K.A., Inglis, D.M., Johnston, W.S., and Miller, J.K. 1983. *Salmonella montevideo* infection in sheep and cattle in Scotland, 1970–81. J. Hyg. 90:225–232.

Sidorchuk, A.A. 1982. Vaccinating sheep against salmonellosis (*Salmonella abortus ovis* infection). Vestn. Sel'skokhozaistvennoi Nauki 2:77–80.

Sieburth, J.M. 1957. Indirect hemagglutination studies on salmonellosis of chickens. J. Immun. 78:380–386.

Silva, E.N., Snoeyenbos, G.H., Weinock, O.M., and Smyser, C.F. 1981. Studies on the use of 9 R strain of *Salmonella gallinarum* as a vaccine in chickens. Avian Dis. 25:38–52.

Silverman, M., Zieg, J., and Simon, M. 1979. Flagellar-phase variation: Isolation of the rhl gene. J. Bacteriol. 137:517–522.

Smith, B.P., Reina-Guerra, M., Hoiseth, S.K., Stocker, B.A.D., Habasha, F., Johnson, E., and Merritt, F. 1984. Aromatic-dependent *Salmonella typhimurium* as modified live vaccines for calves. Am. J. Vet. Res. 45:59–66.

Smith, B.P., Reina-Guerra, M., Stocker, B.A.D., Hoiseth, S.K., and Johnson, E.H. 1984a. Vaccination of calves against *Salmonella dublin* with aromatic-dependent *Salmonella typhimurium.* Am. J. Vet. Res. 45:1858–1861.

Smith, B.P., Reina-Guerra, M., Stocker, B.A.D., Hoiseth, S.K., and Johnson, E.H. 1984b. Aromatic-dependent *Salmonella dublin* as a parenteral modified live vaccine for calves. Am. J. Vet. Res. 45:2231–2235.

Smith, H.W. 1965. The immunization of mice, calves and pigs against *Salmonella dublin* and *Salmonella cholerae-suis* infections. J. Hyg. 63:117–135.

Steinbach, G., Koch, H., Meyer, H., and Hartmann, H. 1981. Mode of action of an orally administered *Salmonella dublin* live vaccine. Arch. Vet. 15:103–111.

Suphabphant, W., York, M.D., and Pomeroy, B.S. 1983. Use of two vaccines (live G3OD or killed RW16) in the prevention of *Salmonella typhimurium* infections of chickens. Avian Dis. 27:602–216.

Svenson, S.B., Nurminen, M., and Lindberg, A.A. 1979. Artificial salmonella vaccines: O-antigenic oligosaccharide-protein conjugates induce protection against infection with *Salmonella typhimurium.* Infect. Immun. 25:863–872.

Tadjbakhche, H., and Nadalian, M. 1980. Immunity induced experimentally in ewes by *Salmonella abortusovis.* Rev. Méd. Vét. 131:247–250, 253–254.

Takasaki, C.J., Saxen, H., Makela, P.H., and Leive, L. 1983. Complement activation by polysaccharide of lipopolysaccharide: An important virulence determinant of salmonellae. Infect. Immun. 41:563–569.

Tanaka, Y. 1982a. Further studies on the infectivity to mice of *Salmonella typhimurium* strains with or without fimbriae. Jpn. J. Vet. Sci. 44:517–521.

Tanaka, Y. 1982b. Multiplication of the fimbriate and nonfimbriate *Salmonella typhimurium* organisms in the intestinal mucosa of mice treated with antibiotics. Jpn. J. Vet. Sci. 44:523–527.

Tanaka, Y., and Katsube, Y. 1978. Infectivity of *Salmonella typhimurium* for mice in relation to fimbriae. Jpn. J. Vet. Sci. 40:671–681.

Tannock, G.W., and Smith, J.M.B. 1972. The effect of food and water

deprivation (stress) on *Salmonella*-carrier mice. J. Med. Microbiol. 5:283–289.

Terakado, N., Sekizaki, T., Hashimoto, K., and Naitoh, S. 1983. Correlation between the presence of a fifty-megadalton plasmid in *Salmonella dublin* and virulence for mice. Infect. Immun. 41:443–444.

Thain, J.A., and Blandford, T.B. 1981. A long-term serological study of a flock of chickens naturally infected with *Salmonella pullorum.* Vet. Rec. 109:136–138.

Theys, H., Verhees, I., and Griman, A. 1983. Apramycin for salmonellosis and colibacillosis in veal calves. Vlaams Diergeneeskd. Tijdschr. 52:18–20.

Threlfall, E.J., Ward, L.R., and Rowe, B. 1978. Spread of multiresistant strains of *Salmonella typhimurium* phage types 204 and 193 in Britain. Br. Med. J. 2:997.

Timoney, J. 1968. The sources and extent of *Salmonella* contamination in rendering plants. Vet. Rec. 83:541–543.

Timoney, J. 1970. Salmonellae in Irish pigs at slaughter. Irish Vet. J. 24:141–145.

Timoney, J.F. 1978. The epidemiology and genetics of antibiotic resistance of *Salmonella typhimurium* isolated from diseased animals in New York. J. Infect. Dis. 137:67–73.

Timoney, J.F. 1981. R Plasmids in pathogenic enterobacteriaceae from calves. In S.B. Levy, R.C. Clowes, and E.L. Koenig, eds., Proceedings of the International Plasmid Conference, Santo Domingo. Plenum Press, New York. Pp. 547–556.

Timoney, J.F., and Linton, A.H. 1982. Experimental ecological studies on H2 plasmids in the intestine and feces of the calf. J. Appl. Bacteriol. 52:417–424.

Timoney, J.F., Neibert, H.C., and Scott, F.W. 1978. Feline salmonellosis. A nosocomial outbreak and experimental studies. Cornell Vet. 68:211–219.

Timoney, J.F., Taylor, D.E., Shin, S., and McDonough, P. 1980. PJT2: Unusual HI plasmid in a highly virulent lactose-positive and chloramphenicol-resistant *Salmonella typhimurium* strain from calves. Antimicrob. Agents Chemother. 18:680–682.

Tschape, H., Ana-Zlata D., Rische, H., and Kuhn, H. 1974. Conversion of phage types of *S. typhimurium* due to different R plasmids. Zentralbl. Bakteriol. Mikrobiol. Hyg. [A] 226:184–193.

van Leeuwen, W.J., Voogd, C.E., Guinee, P.A., and Manten, A., 1982. Incidence of resistance to ampicillin, chloramphenicol, kanamycin, tetracycline, and trimethoprim of salmonella strains isolated in the Netherlands during 1975–1980. Antonie Van Leeuwenhoek 48:85–96.

Williams, B.M. 1980. Bovine salmonellosis. Bovine Pract. 15:122–128.

Williams, L.P., Jr., and Newell, K.W. 1968. Sources of salmonellas in market swine. J. Hyg. 66:281–293.

Wishart, D.F., and Eddy, R.G. 1985. *Salmonella typhimurium* phage type 204c and antimicrobial resistance. Vet. Rec. 116:195.

West, J.L., and Mohanty, G.C. 1973. *Arizona hinshawii* infection in turkey poults: Pathological changes. Avian Dis. 17:314–324.

Wray, C., and Callow, R.J. 1985. A note on potential hazards to animals grazing on pasture improperly treated with sewage sludge. J. Appl. Bacteriol. 58:257–258.

Wray, C., Sojka, W.J., and Callow, R.J. 1977. The serological response in cattle to *Salmonella* infection. Br. Vet. J. 133:25–32.

The Genus *Proteus*

There are only four species of *Proteus,* and of these, *P. mirabilis* is of greatest significance as an opportunistic pathogen of animals.

Morphology and Staining Reactions. *Proteus* organisms are straight, Gram-negative rods, 0.5 μm in width by

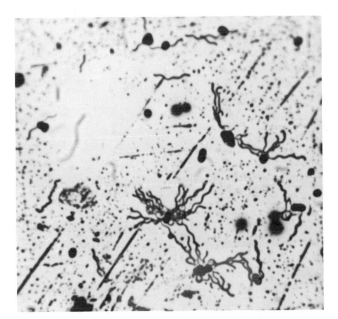

Figure 7.5. *Proteus mirabilis* showing peritrichous flagella. Leifson stain. × 1,400.

1.0 to 3.0 μm in length, with many peritrichous flagella (Figure 7.5).

Cultural and Biochemical Features. Most strains of *Proteus* produce a swarming growth on agar media which forms a uniform film over the surface. This layer is hardly distinguishable from the medium and makes the isolation of other enteric bacteria from a mixed culture very difficult. *Proteus* species produce urease, phenylalanine deaminase, and hydrogen sulfide. Only glucose and xylose are fermented. *P. vulgaris* produces indole, but *P. mirabilis* does not. The differentiation of *Proteus* species from other Enterobacteriaceae is shown in Table 6.1.

Swarming can be prevented by the addition of 8 mg/ml sulfadiazine to the medium or by the use of 6 percent agar.

Epizootiology and Pathogenesis. *Proteus* species are widely distributed in nature. Although easily demonstrable in the feces of animals, especially those of dogs and hogs, they rarely are found in large numbers except when the normal intestinal microflora is deranged. They have been associated with diarrhea in young animals, with otitis externa (*P. mirabilis*) in dogs, and with urinary tract infections in spayed bitches. Production of urease is an important virulence factor since the resultant ammonia is histotoxic.

Proteus species are also important in the spoilage of meat because they grow and spread readily on moist surfaces at low temperatures and produce a number of proteases.

Antimicrobial Susceptibility. *P. mirabilis* is generally sensitive to ampicillin, cephalosporins, chloramphenicol,

kanamycin, penicillins, and streptomycin. *P. vulgaris* is often resistant to penicillins and cephalosporins. Both species are naturally resistant to bacitracin, colistin, and polymyxin B. Since many strains carry plasmid-encoded resistance to tetracycline and other antibiotics, routine susceptibility testing is advisable.

The Genus *Yersinia*

The genus *Yersinia* was named after the French bacteriologist Yersin, who first isolated *Y. pestis*, the cause of plague, in 1894. There are seven species of *Yersinia*, of which only *Y. pseudotuberculosis* is important as a cause of disease in animals. *Y. enterocolitica* is frequently present in the alimentary tract of animals and can therefore serve as a source of infection for humans. *Y. pestis*, the cause of plague in humans, is primarily a disease of rodents, but carnivorous species such as dogs and cats may be naturally infected.

Yersinia pseudotuberculosis
SYNONYMS: *Bacterium pseudotuberculosis rodentium, Corynebacterium rodentium, Pasteurella pseudotuberculosis*

Y. pseudotuberculosis is the cause of a plaguelike disease of guinea pigs, sometimes of rats, and occasionally of other rodents. The organism has little importance for animals other than colonies of guinea pigs. Rare infections have been reported in cattle, sheep, goats, horses, pigs, foxes, mink, rabbits, chinchillas, birds, monkeys, and humans.

Morphology and Staining Reactions. *Y. pseudotuberculosis* is pleomorphic and varies from coccoid to bacillary forms 5 μm or more long. The cells may be single but also occur occasionally in chains. Bipolar staining is sometimes evident. *Y. pseudotuberculosis* is Gram-negative, non-acid-fast, and not encapsulated. Peritrichous flagella are present when the organism is cultured at 18° to 30°C but not when it is cultured at 37°C.

Cultural and Biochemical Features. The colonies are nonhemolytic, small (0.1 to 1.0 mm), translucent, and granular. The centers of old colonies are raised and more opaque than the periphery, which may have radial striations. The optimum growth temperature is 28°C. *Y. pseudotuberculosis* ferments glucose and some other carbohydrates but produces little or no gas. It does not ferment lactose, raffinose, dulcitol and sorbitol; it does produce urease. Some strains are citrate- and malonate-positive. The characteristics that differentiate *Y. pseudotuber-*

Table 7.5. Biochemical differentiation of *Y. pestis,*
Y. enterocolitica, and *Y. pseudotuberculosis*

	Y. pestis	*Y. entero-colitica*	*Y. pseudo-tuberculosis*
Urease	−	−	+
Motility (28°C)	−	+	+
Sorbitol fermentation	−	+	−
Rhamnose fermentation	−	−	+
Ornithine decarboxylase	−	+	−
H₂S production	+	−	−

culosis from *Y. pestis* and *Y. enterocolitica* are shown in Table 7.5.

The mol% G + C of the DNA is 46.5 (Tm).

Antigens. *P. pseudotuberculosis* expresses the enterobacterial common antigen as well as a number of other antigens that it shares with *Y. pestis* and *Y. enterocolitica.* An envelope antigen, F1, composed of protein and carbohydrate is also found on *Y. pestis* and is an important virulence factor (Quan et al. 1965). Plasmid-encoded V and W virulence antigens are also found on *Y. pseudotuberculosis* and *Y. pestis* (Gemski et al. 1980).

There are six serogroups based on the thermostable O antigens (I–VI) and five H or flagellar antigens (a–e) (Thal and Krapp 1971). Antigenic relationships exist between some O antigens of *Y. pseudotuberculosis* and salmonella O groups B and D and *E. coli* O groups 17, 55, and 77 (Mair and Fox 1973).

Epizootiology and Pathogenesis. *Y. pseudotuberculosis* occurs worldwide in wild rodents, birds, and soil. Animals become infected by ingestion of the organism, and most infections occur during cold weather. Outbreaks of pseudotuberculosis have been encountered in chinchilla colonies (Laughton et al. 1963) and mink colonies, and the organism has been isolated from a bovine (Mair and Harbourne 1963) and an ovine fetus (Watson and Hunter 1960). Infections in cattle have been associated with pneumonia as well as with abortion (Langford 1969), and in cats they have been characterized by abdominal and urinary disturbances (Mair et al. 1967). Pseudotuberculosis is a relatively common disease of captive birds and can cause outbreaks, although these are usually sporadic (Harcourt-Brown 1978).

The disease often occurs spontaneously in stocks of guinea pigs. The affected animals sicken, lose weight, develop diarrhea, and die in 3 to 4 weeks. The mesenteric lymph nodes are greatly swollen and caseous, and there may be nodular abscesses in the Peyer's patches. Similar nodules are usually numerous in the liver and spleen. Administration of tetracycline will induce disease in carrier animals.

The presence of the F1 and V and W antigens is necessary for virulence. Incubation of the organism at 37°C results in loss of the plasmid-encoded V and W antigens and loss of invasive ability.

Immunity. Intranasal instillation of live avirulent cultures are capable of producing a solid immunity in guinea pigs against virulent strains (Thal et al. 1964). The organism is a facultative intracellular parasite; cell-mediated immunity is therefore important in the protective immune response.

Diagnosis. Although *Y. pseudotuberculosis* resembles *Y. pestis* in cultural characteristics and in the disease it produces in guinea pigs, it can be differentiated from the latter by the urease test and by its ability to grow well on deoxycholate-citrate agar. *Y. pestis* does not attack urea and grows poorly in deoxycholate-citrate agar. Other tests of value in differentiation are shown in Table 7.5.

Antimicrobial Susceptibility. *Y. pseudotuberculosis* is sensitive to chloramphenicol, nalidixic acid, streptomycin, sulfonamides, and tetracyclines.

The Disease in Humans. Although the disease is rare in humans, *Y. pseudotuberculosis* can opportunistically produce severe, even fatal infections. The symptoms are those of mesenteric adenitis or septicemia.

REFERENCES

Gemski, P., Lazere, J.R., Casey, T., and Wohieter, I.A. 1980. Presence of a virulence-associated plasmid in *Yersinia pseudotuberculosis.* Infect. Immun. 28:1044–1047.

Harcourt-Brown, N.H. 1978. *Yersinia pseudotuberculosis* infection in birds. Vet. Rec. 102:315.

Langford, E.V. 1969. *Pasteurella pseudotuberculosis* associated with abortion and pneumonia in the bovine. Can. Vet. J. 10:208–211.

Laughton, N., Till, D.H., and Noble, D. 1963. An outbreak of acute pseudotuberculosis in a chinchilla colony. Vet. Rec. 75:835–838.

Mair, N.S., and Fox, E. 1973. An antigenic relationship between *Yersinia pseudotuberculosis* type G and *Escherichia coli* O-group 55. Contr. Microbiol. Immunol. 2:180–183.

Mair, N.S., and Harbourne, J.F. 1963. The isolation of *Pasteurella pseudotuberculosis* from a bovine foetus. Vet. Rec. 75:559–560.

Mair, N.S., Harbourne, J.F., Greenwood, M.T., and White, G. 1967. *Pasteurella pseudotuberculosis* infection in the cat; two cases. Vet. Rec. 81:461–462.

Thal, E., and Knapp, W. 1971. A revised antigenic scheme of *Yersinia pseudotuberculosis.* Progr. Immunobiol. Stand. 15:219–222.

Thal, E., Hanko, E., and Knapp, W. 1964. Intranasal vaccination of guinea-pigs with avirulent *Pasteurella pseudotuberculosis.* Acta Vet. Scand. 5:179–187.

Watson, W.A., and Hunter, D. 1960. The isolation of *Pasteurella pseudotuberculosis* from an ovine foetus. Vet. Rec. 72:770–772.

Yersinia enterocolitica

Y. enterocolitica is ubiquitous and since the mid-1970s has been isolated with increasing frequency from humans and chinchillas with alimentary tract disturbances, from healthy cattle and swine, and from meat, shellfish, and ice

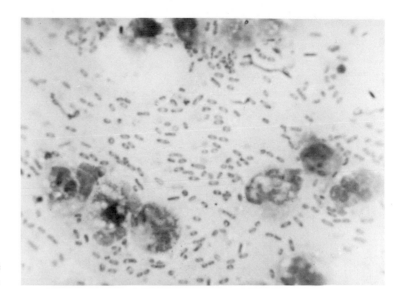

Figure 7.6. *Yersinia pestis* in a splenic smear. Note the bipolar-staining rods. Gram's stain. × 1,200.

cream. It resembles *Y. pseudotuberculosis* in colonial and microscopic morphology and can be differentiated from it and from *Y. pestis* by the characteristics in Table 7.5.

There are at least 34 O groups; O3 is found in pigs and O3, O8, and O9 in humans. A heat-stable enterotoxin is produced at 30°C, and the same plasmid-encoded virulence antigens (V,W\O) as found in *C. pseudotuberculosis* are present.

The disease in humans is a terminal ileitis with diarrhea, mesenteric adenitis, and symptoms that simulate appendicitis. Some human infections are derived from animal sources and from water contaminated with animal feces. However, most human cases appear to be associated with consumption of food contaminated by human carriers.

Yersinia pestis
SYNONYMS: *Pasteurella pestis*, plague bacillus

Y. pestis is the cause of bubonic plague, or the black death, in humans. In warm climates the disease usually assumes the *bubonic* form, so called from the swollen lymph nodes, known as *buboes,* which characterize it. In cold climates the disease occurs in the *pneumonic* form, which is highly fatal and contagious.

The organism resembles *Y. pseudotuberculosis* in microscopic and colonial morphology and in its antigenic make-up. It can be differentiated from *Y. enterocolitica* and *Y. pseudotuberculosis* by the characteristics shown in Table 7.5. In tissue it is a bipolar staining rod (0.5 by 1.5 μm) (Figure 7.6).

Bubonic plague is not a disease of domestic animals. It occurs naturally in rats, which become infected through the bite of infected rat fleas (*Xenopsylla cheopis*). The organism multiplies in the fleas. Once introduced into a rat population, the disease spreads rapidly. The disease also occurs naturally in marmots, ground squirrels, and many other rodents. Unlike rats, these creatures usually live in areas sparsely inhabited by humans. When plague spreads in such areas, it is known as the *sylvatic* form and has a much greater tendency to assume the more highly contagious pneumonic form.

In the United States, wild rodent populations constitute the natural reservoir of infection. The hosts involved include prairie dogs, ground squirrels, wood rats, and mice (Hubbert et al. 1966). New Mexico, Arizona, California, and Colorado report the highest incidence of human infections (Link 1955). These infections are contracted from the bites of ectoparasites that have inhabited wild rodents.

REFERENCES
Hubbert, W.T., Goldenberg, M.I., Kartman, L., and Prince, F.M. 1966. Public health potential of sylvatic plague. J. Am. Vet. Med. Assoc. 149:1651–1654.

Link, V.B. 1955. A History of Plague in the United States of America. U.S. Public Health Service Monograph no. 26.

8 The Genus *Haemophilus*

Organisms in the genus *Haemophilus* are minute to medium-sized, Gram-negative coccobacilli or bacilli that have a tendency to pleomorphism. They are strict parasites of respiratory or genital mucous membranes. Given the right conditions, pathogenic species can cause disease in a variety of organ systems.

The genus *Haemophilus* has traditionally included Gram-negative rods or coccobacilli that reduce nitrate and require hemin (X), niacinamide adenine nucleotide (V), and either or both of the growth factors. The validity of using these growth factor requirements as qualifications for inclusion in the genus is now in doubt because of the existence of organisms in unrelated genera that have similar requirements. It is therefore likely that the membership of *Haemophilus* will change as the DNA relationships of *Haemophilus*, *Pasteurella*, *Actinobacillus*, and other Gramnegative genera and species are more thoroughly investigated.

There are 16 *Haemophilus* species currently recognized in *Bergey's Manual of Systematic Bacteriology*, of which *H. pleuropneumoniae*, *H. parasuis*, and *H. paragallinarum* are important causes of disease in swine and chickens. *H. somnus* and *H. agni*, which cause septicemia and meningoencephalitis of cattle and sheep, respectively, are listed as *species incertae sedis*. *H. agni* and the organism known as *Histophilus ovis*, a common pathogen of sheep in Australia and New Zealand, are now widely regarded as variants of *H. somnus*.

H. hemoglobinophilus (canis) is found on the genitalia of dogs and has been associated with neonatal mortality in puppies (Maclachlan and Hopkins 1978). An unofficial

species, *H. ovis*, was isolated in 1925 from an outbreak of bronchopneumonia in sheep in Canada. A similar organism was later isolated from a ewe with mastitis (Roberts 1956). These organisms were subsequently lost. However, an organism resembling *H. ovis* has been isolated recently from the oropharynx of sheep (Little et al. 1980).

Haemophilus pleuropneumoniae
SYNONYMS: *Actinobacillus pleuropneumoniae*, *Haemophilus parahemolyticus*

H. pleuropneumoniae is the cause of contagious pleuropneumonia in swine, a disease of great economic importance in most swine-raising areas of the world. Although listed in 1984 as an official species of *Haemophilus*, transfer of *H. pleuropneumoniae* to the genus *Actinobacillus* has been proposed on the basis of DNA relatedness and phenotypic characteristics (Pohl et al. 1983).

Morphology and Staining Reactions. The organism forms short Gram-negative coccobacilli, rods, and tangled filaments. Capsules are present on organisms from virulent strains.

Cultural and Biochemical Features. *H. pleuropneumoniae* grows rapidly on blood agar and other enriched media. The colonies are mucoid and iridescent and about 1 to 2 mm in diameter. A zone of beta hemolysis on sheep- or calf-blood agar is produced and is enhanced by the beta-toxin of *Staphylococcus aureus*. The hemolysin is extracellular.

H. pleuropneumoniae is facultatively anaerobic and often requires an atmosphere with increased CO_2 for primary growth. It is V-factor dependent. It produces urease and ferments xylose, ribose, glucose, fructose, mannose, sucrose, and mannitol. It produces porphyrin from delta-aminolevulinic acid. The mol% G + C of the DNA is 42 (Tm).

Antigens. There are at least eight serotypes, numbered 1 through 8 (Nielsen and O'Connor 1984). Serotyping is based on surface antigens associated with capsular material. The thermolabile and thermostable type-specific antigens are routinely detected by agglutination, immunodiffusion, absorption, complement-fixation, and ring precipitation tests (Mittal et al. 1982, Sebunya and Saunders 1983).

The distribution of serotypes varies with geographic region: serotypes 1, 3, 4, and 5 are found in the United States, whereas only serotype 2 has been found in Denmark (reviewed by Sebunya and Saunders 1983). Serotype 5 is most common in Saskatchewan, whereas serotype 1 predominates in Quebec (Mittal et al. 1982).

Cross-protection experiments have shown that protection obtained through parenteral immunization is sero-type-specific. The protective antigen(s) have not been characterized.

Epizootiology and Pathogenesis. Transmission is apparently by means of the respiratory route and introduction or spread is usually associated with importation of infected animals. There is evidence, however, that serotype 2 can be carried in the nasal cavities of healthy pigs (Kume et al. 1984). Subclinical infections are common in many outbreaks and can develop into cases of acute disease as a result of stress associated with transport for slaughter (Greenaway 1981). Spread of infection is greatly enhanced under conditions of intensive husbandry. Inclement weather, poor ventilation, and intercurrent infection by other respiratory pathogens also can be important factors in the severity of outbreaks. The disease incidence peaks in late fall and winter. Pigs about 3 months old appear to be most susceptible.

The pathogenesis of porcine haemophilus pleuropneumonia has not been fully worked out. Endotoxin is believed to play an important role in the formation of thrombi and interlobular edema and in other changes resulting from damage to the vasculature. The lesions in the peracute form of the disease closely resemble those of endotoxic shock. The pathogenesis of the chronic lesions is not understood.

Clearance of the organism from the lungs is poor and in part may be the result of a heat-stable cytotoxin secreted by *H. pleuropneumoniae* which disarms lung macrophages (Bendixen et al. 1981). This cytotoxin is probably identical to the 7000-dalton, heat-stable hemolysin described by Kume et al. (1986). The hemolysin is carbohydrate in nature, antigenic, and readily neutralized by antibody. A cell-associated, heat-labile cytotoxic effect may also contribute to impairment of lung macrophage function (Bendixen et al. 1981). A glycoprotein produced by *H. pleuropneumoniae* may allow the organism to penetrate deeper into the lungs by reducing droplet size in the airways. It is likely that capsular material is of importance in survival and multiplication of *H. pleuropneumoniae* in the lungs because of its negative effects on phagocytosis.

In susceptible swine the disease may have an acute form characterized by trembling, anorexia, dyspnea, emesis, cyanosis, fever, and hemorrhaging from the nose and mouth (Schiefer et al. 1974). Death can occur within 24 hours of clinical onset. Animals that develop a less acute form of the disease usually recover within a few weeks, but residual lung or pleuritic lesions may be found at slaughter. These lesions adversely affect growth and food-conversion efficiency. As herd immunity develops, the severity of the disease decreases, and clinical signs are vague and lesions mild (Nielsen 1975).

The lesions consist of an exudative and proliferative desquamative bronchopneumonia with fibrinous pleuritis. In more chronic cases the lesions tend to become sequestrated. The lesions in the peracute form, and in the initial stages of less acute forms, include alveolar and interlobular edema with dilatation of lymph vessels, congestion, hemorrhage, and intravascular fibrinous thrombosis (Hani et al. 1973). These lesions appear to be a direct effect of the haemophilus endotoxin. A nodular form of chronic pneumonia caused by *H. pleuropneumoniae* has also been described (Chan et al. 1978).

Immunity. A protective immunity develops after an animal recovers from an experimental or naturally occurring infection. Levels of complement-fixing antibodies and protective immunity are closely correlated. Protective antibody is also passively transferred in colostrum to baby pigs. Animals with high titers of serum antibody are unlikely to harbor the organism with the possible exception of occasional tonsillar carriers or animals with sequestrated lung or pleuritic lesions (Nielsen and Mandrup 1977).

A variety of serologic tests are available for the detection and assay of antibody. These include complement fixation, agglutination, ring precipitation, and enzyme-linked immunosorbent assay (ELISA) (reviewed by Sebunya and Saunders et al. 1983). Because the complement-fixing antibody rises rapidly after subclinical infection, it is of value in the detection of current or recent infection (Lowbin et al. 1982). A 2-mercaptoethanol tube agglutination test has been shown to be more sensitive than the complement-fixation test, possibly because of the removal of the nonspecific blocking effects of IgM (Mittal et al. 1984).

Nielsen (1976) used the complement-fixation test in control of the disease in progeny testing stations. The test was of value provided it was carried out within a week of the pigs' arrival at the stations.

Vaccines prepared from 6-hour cultures have inferior protective properties (Nielsen 1976) that are apparently serotype-specific when administered parenterally (Nielsen 1984). However, pigs that recover from natural infection are immune to both homologous and heterologous serotypes (Nielsen 1979). Local nasopharyngeal immune responses are stimulated by natural infection and apparently are directed against antigenic sites on the organism that are not serotype-specific. A live intranasal vaccine therefore would not have to be multivalent to protect against heterologous challenge in the field. Bacterins have produced reasonably good results in the field (Kielstein et al. 1982, Nielsen 1976) by reducing mortality but do not eliminate infection from a herd and do not prevent lung and pleural lesions. Antibody to the core polysaccharide of *Escherichia coli* J5 endotoxin protects against the thrombogenic potential of rapidly multiplying *H. pleuropneumoniae* but does not prevent bacteremia or promote pulmonary clearance (Fenwick et al. 1986).

Diagnosis. *H. pleuropneumoniae* is readily isolated by culture of specimens on blood agar. Its requirement for V factor, its urease positivity, and the presence of beta-hemolysin are useful diagnostic characteristics. A coagglutination test for detection of serotype-specific antigen in the lungs of infected pigs has been described (Mittal et al. 1983).

Antimicrobial Susceptibility. *H. pleuropneumoniae* is sensitive to penicillin, ampicillin, streptomycin, chloramphenicol, tetracycline, sulfonamides, trimethoprim, furazolidone, polymyxin B, and gentamicin. Strains resistant to some of these antimicrobials have been isolated, however (Gilbride and Rosendal 1984).

REFERENCES

Bendixen, P.H., Shewen, P.E., Rosendal, S., and Wilkie, B.N. 1981. Toxicity of *Hemophilus pleuropneumoniae* for porcine lung macrophages, peripheral blood monocytes and testicular cells. Infect. Immun. 33:673–676.

Chan, C., Yamamoto, K., Konishi, S., and Ogata, M. 1978. Isolation and antigenic characterization of *Haemophilus parahemolyticus* from porcine pneumonia. Jpn. J. Vet. Sci. 40:103–107.

Fenwick, B.W., Cullor, J.S., Osburn, B.I., and Olander, H.J. 1986. Mechanisms involved in protection provided by immunization against core lipopolysaccharides of *Escherichia coli* J5 from lethal *Haemophilus pleuropneumoniae* infections in swine. Infect. Immun. 53:298–304.

Gilbride, K.A., and Rosendal, S. 1984. Antimicrobial susceptibility of 51 strains of *Haemophilus pleuropneumoniae*. Can. J. Comp. Med. 48:47–50.

Greenaway, J.A. 1981. *Haemophilus* pneumonia in B. C. swine. Can. Vet. J. 22:20–21.

Hani, H., Konig, H., Nicolet, J., and Scholl, E. 1973. Zur *Haemophiluspleuropneumoniae* beim Schwein. V. Pathomorphologie. Schweiz Arch. Tierheilkd. 115: 191–203.

Kielstein, P., School, W., Mirle, P., Michael, M., Boesler, M., Liesegang, M., and Grunert, G. 1982. Efficacy of an inactivated adsorbed vaccine against *Haemophilus pleuropneumoniae* in pig herds. Monatsh. Veterinärmed. 37:126–132.

Kume, K., Nakai, T., and Sawata, A. 1984. Isolation of *Haemophilus pleuropneumoniae* from the nasal cavities of healthy pigs. Jpn. J. Vet. Sci. 46:641–647.

Kume, K., Nakai, T., and Sawata, A. 1986. Interaction between heat-stable hemolytic substance from *Haemophilus pleuropneumoniae* and porcine pulmonary macrophages in vitro. Infect. Immun. 51:563–570.

Little, T.W.A., Pritchard, D.G., and Shreeve, J.E. 1980. Isolation of *Haemophilus* species from the oropharynx of British sheep. Res. Vet. Sci. 29:41–44.

Lowbin, L.H., Rosendal, S., and Mitchell, W.R. 1982. Evaluation of the complement fixation test for the diagnosis of pleuropneumonia of swine caused by *Hemophilus pleuropneumoniae*. Can. J. Comp. Med. 46:109–114.

Maclachlan, G.K., and Hopkins, G.F. 1978. Early death in pups due to *Haemophilus haemoglobinophilus* (*canis*) infection. Vet. Rec. 103:409–410.

Mittal, K.R., Higgins, R., and Lariviere, S. 1982. Evaluation of slide agglutination and ring precipitation tests for capsular serotyping of *Haemophilus pleuropneumoniae*. J. Clin. Microbiol. 15:1019–1023.

Mittal, K.R., Higgins, R., and Lariviere, S. 1983. Determination of antigenic specificity and relationship among *Haemophilus pleuropneumoniae* serotypes by an indirect hemagglutination test. J. Clin. Microbiol. 17:787–780.

Mittal, K.R., Higgins, R., Lariviere, S., and Leblanc, D. 1984. A 2-mercaptoethanol tube agglutination test for diagnosis of *Haemophilus pleuropneumoniae* infection in pigs. Am. J. Vet. Res. 45:715–719.

Nielsen, R. 1975. Colostral transfer of immunity to *Haemophilus parahemolyticus*. Nord. Vet. Med. 27:319–328.

Nielsen, R. 1976. Pleuropneumonia of swine caused by *Haemophilus parahemolyticus*. Nord. Vet. Med. 28:337–348.

Nielsen, R. 1979. *Haemophilus parahemolyticus* serotypes and serological response. Nord. Vet. Med. 31:401–413.

Nielsen, R. 1984. *Haemophilus pleuropneumoniae* serotypes—Cross protection experiments. Nord. Vet. Med. 36:221–234.

Nielsen, R., and Mandrup, M. 1977. Pleuropneumonia in swine caused by *Haemophilus parahemolyticus*. A study of the epidemiology of infection. Nord. Vet. Med. 29:465–473.

Nielsen, R., and O'Connor, P.J. 1984. Serological characterization of 8 *Haemophilus pleuropneumoniae* strains and proposal of a new serotype: Serotype 8. Acta Vet. Scand. 25:96–106.

Pohl, S., Bertschinger, H.U., Frederiksen, W., and Mannhein, W. 1983. Transfer of *Haemophilus pleuropneumoniae* and the *Pasteurella haemolytica*-like organism causing porcine necrotic pleuropneumonia to the genus *Actinobacillus* (*Actinobacillus pleuropneumoniae* comb. nov.) on the basis of phenotypic and deoxyribonucleic acid relatedness. Int. J. Syst. Bacteriol. 33:510–514.

Roberts, D.S. 1956. A new pathogen from a ewe with mastitis. Aust. Vet. J. 33:330–332.

Schiefer, B., Moffatt, R.E., Greenfield, J., Agar, J.L., and Majka, J.A. 1974. Porcine *Haemophilus parahemolyticus* pneumonia in Saskatchewan. I. Natural occurrence and findings. Can. J. Comp. Med. 38:99–104.

Sebunya, T.N.K., and Saunders, J.R. 1983. *Haemophilus pleuropneumoniae* infection in swine. J. Am. Vet. Med. Assoc. 182:1331–1337.

Haemophilus parasuis

SYNONYM: *Haemophilus suis*

The organism now known as *H. parasuis* was first described by Lewis and Shope (1931), who discovered it during studies of swine influenza virus. They named the organism *H. suis* and observed that it was relatively harmless by itself but highly pathogenic in the presence of influenza virus (Shope 1931). The isolate of Lewis and Shope required X and V factors. Many years later, Biberstein and White (1969) described an organism isolated from swine that was identical to *H. suis* in all respects except that it was not dependent on X factor and produced porphyrin from delta-aminolevulinic acid. This organism was named *H. parasuis* and now has precedence in *Bergey's Manual of Systematic Bacteriology* over *H. suis*. *H. parasuis* is a cause of respiratory tract disease and polyserositis (Glasser's disease) in swine.

Morphology and Staining Reactions. *H. parasuis* forms Gram-negative coccobacilli that have a tendency to develop filaments in old cultures.

Cultural and Biochemical Features. Growth of *H. parasuis* on chocolate agar is very slow and colonies are tiny unless a source of V factor is provided. Much larger colonies are produced, in the presence of a *Staphylococcus* species. This phenomenon is termed *satellitism*. The colonies are clear and smooth and about 0.5 mm in diameter. There is no hemolysis. *H. parasuis* produces acid from glucose, fructose, sucrose, ribose, and mannose in serum-enriched media but does not produce urease.

Antigens. Four serotypes (A, B, C, D) based on capsular polysaccharide have been described (Bakos et al. 1952).

Epizootiology and Pathogenesis. *H. parasuis* appears to be carried in the nasopharynx of many normal swine. Invasion by the swine influenza virus, which usually begins to circulate actively in susceptible pig populations in the autumn when temperatures fall suddenly, predisposes swine to invasion by *H. parasuis*. Influenzalike symptoms result, with coughing, fever, inappetence, and, in severe cases, lobular pneumonia and death of the animal. The disease is highly contagious and spreads rapidly.

H. parasuis has also been associated with a polyserositis syndrome in swine (*Glasser's disease*) in which there is fibrinous inflammation of the serous surfaces. Lesions are seen in the pericardium, pleura, peritoneum, joints, and, in animals with severe cases, the meninges. There is no viral involvement in Glasser's disease, but stresses such as weaning and transport are important predisposing factors. Affected pigs can have swollen joints, lameness, signs of bronchitis and pleuritis, fever, and, occasionally, meningitis. The disease is fatal in a small proportion of affected animals. Riley et al. (1977) described a fatal septicemia in swine that developed a few days after transport and was shown to be caused by *H. parasuis*.

Immunity. Nielsen and Danielsen (1975) protected swine against Glasser's disease with an autogenous bacterin prepared from a strain of *H. parasuis* isolated on the farm where the vaccine was used. Complement-fixing antibodies were formed in vaccinated pigs but not in unvaccinated litter mates. Baehler et al. (1974) also reported success with a *H. parasuis* bacterin.

Diagnosis. *H. parasuis* is usually isolated easily from lesions in acute cases by streaking material on chocolate agar and then inoculating a *Staphylococcus* species across the center of the plate as a source of V factor.

Antimicrobial Susceptibility. *H. parasuis* has a spectrum of sensitivity to antimicrobials similar to that of *H. pleuropneumoniae*.

REFERENCES

Baehler, J.F., Burgisser, H., De Meuron, P.A., and Nicolet, J. 1974. Infection à *Haemophilus parasuis* chez le porc. Schweiz. Arch. Tierheilkd. 116:183–188.

Bakos, K., Nilsson, A., and Thal, E. 1952. Untersuchungen über *Haemophilus suis*. Nord. Vet. Med. 4:241–255.

Biberstein, E.I., and White, D.C. 1969. A proposal for the establishment of two new *Haemophilus* species. J. Med. Microbiol. 2:75–78.

Lewis, P.A., and Shope, R.E. 1931. Swine influenza. II. A hemophilic bacillus from the respiratory tract of infected swine. J. Exp. Med. 54:361–371.

Nielsen, R., and Danielsen, V. 1975. An outbreak of Glasser's disease. Nord. Vet. Med. 27:20–25.

Riley, M.G.I., Russell, E.G., and Callinan, R.B. 1977. *Haemophilus parasuis* infection in swine. J. Am. Vet. Med. Assoc. 171:649–651.

Shope, R.E. 1931. Swine influenza. I. Experimental transmission and pathology. III. Filtration experiments and etiology. J. Exp. Med. 54:349–385.

Haemophilus paragallinarum

SYNONYMS: *Bacillus hemoglobinophilus coryzae gallinarum, Haemophilus gallinarum*

H. paragallinarum is the cause of a serious and widespread disease of chickens known as *fowl coryza*. The organism is much like the influenza bacilli of humans and swine in that it is frequently associated with viral infection. The species includes organisms previously labeled *H. gallinarum*.

Morphology and Staining Reactions. Colonies grown on chocolate agar are smooth, semiopaque, and iridescent, and attain a diameter of about 0.5 to 1 mm. The organism is a facultative anaerobe that grows best on primary isolation in an atmosphere of 10 percent CO_2. *H. paragallinarum* requires V factor but not X factor for growth. It is rather inactive biochemically and does not produce indole or hydrogen sulfide. It does not change litmus or methylene blue milk or liquefy gelatin. It regularly ferments glucose and variably ferments mannose, galactose, levulose, maltose, sucrose, and dextrin (Bornstein and Samberg 1954). One percent sodium chloride is required in medium for growth. It is catalase- and alpha-glucosidase-negative. The mol% G + C of the DNA is 42 (Tm).

Antigens. Heat-labile surface antigens have been used to establish three serotypes (A, B, C) (Page 1962). More recent studies in Japan based on hemagglutinating antigens from strains of *H. paragallinarum* have indicated that there are at least seven serotypes, designated HA1, HA2, HA3, etc. (Kume, Sawata, Nakai, and Matsumoto 1983). This typing system is known as the HA-L method. HA-L hemagglutinins are on the outer membrane of the bacterial cell, are heat-labile and trypsin-sensitive, and are the antigens responsible for protective immunity (Kume, Sawata, and Nakai 1983; Sawata et al. 1984). These antigens are found only on encapsulated organisms that produce iridescent colonies (Kume et al. 1980).

Epizootiology and Pathogenesis. The organism is

maintained in birds that recover from disease but continue to carry the organism. Transmission occurs by means of the respiratory route, but contaminated drinking water can also serve as a source of infection. Although it is a virulent primary pathogen, *H. paragallinarum* causes more severe disease in the presence of viral or mycoplasmal infections such as Newcastle disease, infectious bronchitis, infectious laryngotracheitis, and *Mycoplasma gallisepticum* infection. The signs produced in fowl by *H. paragallinarum* are acute inflammation of the turbinates and sinus epithelium, disruption of the trachea without cellular infiltration, and acute air sacculitis characterized by swelling and heterophilic response (Adler and Page 1962). The exudate in naturally occurring cases of fowl coryza is highly infectious when introduced into the palatine cleft of susceptible birds. The mortality can be high in the presence of other viral pathogens. Turkeys, pigeons, and many other species of birds are resistant to infection.

Immunity. Hemagglutination-inhibiting, agglutinating, and precipitating antibodies are formed in the serums of infected chickens, but the levels of these antibodies do not appear to affect the duration and severity of symptoms in experimentally infected chickens (Iritani et al. 1977). Vaccinal immunity is serotype-specific. However, birds that recover from infection by one immunotype are refractory to reinfection by another that is heterologous (Rimler et al. 1977). Colonization immunity as expressed in the respiratory tract may play an important role in protection. Bacterins appear to be rather ineffective in this regard, although they stimulate a useful level of resistance to systemic disease.

Diagnosis. The organism is easily cultured on chocolate agar in 10 percent CO_2. It can be distinguished from *H. avium*, a nonpathogenic commensal, by the absence of catalase and alpha-glucosidase and by its failure to produce acid from galactose and trehalose (Blackall and Reid 1982).

Antimicrobial Susceptibility. *H. paragallinarum* is sensitive to chloramphenicol, erythromycin, furazolidone, gentamicin, neomycin, spectinomycin, tetracycline, and sulfachlor-pyridazi-trimethoprim.

REFERENCES

Adler, H.E., and Page, L.A. 1962. Haemophilus infections in chickens. II. The pathology of the respiratory tract. Avian Dis. 6:1–6.
Blackall, P.J., and Reid, G.G. 1982. Further characterization of *Haemophilus paragallinarum* and *Haemophilus avium*. Vet. Microbiol. 7:359–367.
Bornstein, S., and Samberg, Y. 1954. The therapeutic effect of streptomycin on infectious coryza of chickens caused by *Haemophilus gallinarum*. II. Isolation and culture of *H. gallinarum*, and some of its biochemical reactions. Am. J. Vet. Res. 15:612–616.
Iritani, Y., Sugimori, G., and Katagiri, K. 1977. Serologic response to

Haemophilus gallinarum in artifically infected and vaccinated chickens. Avian Dis. 21:1–8.
Kume, K., Sawata, A., and Nakai, T. 1983. Serologic and immunologic studies on three types of hemagglutinin of *Haemophilus paragallinarum* serotype 1 organisms. Jpn. J. Vet. Sci. 45:783–792.
Kume, K., Sawata, A., Nakai, T., and Matsumoto, M. 1983. Serological classification of *Haemophilus paragallinarum* with a hemagglutinin system. J. Clin. Microbiol. 17:958–964.
Kume, K., Sawata, A., and Nakase, Y. 1980. Relationship between protective activity and antigen structure of *Haemophilus paragallinarum* serotypes 1 and 2. Am. J. Vet. Res. 41:97–100.
Page, L.A. 1962. Haemophilus in chickens. I. Characteristics of 12 *Haemophilus* isolates recovered from diseased chickens. Am. J. Vet. Res. 23:85–95.
Rimler, R.B., Davis, R.B., and Page, R.K. 1977. Infectious coryza: Cross protection studies, using seven strains of *Haemophilus gallinarum*. Am. J. Vet. Res. 38:1587–1589.
Sawata, A., Kume, K., and Nakai, T. 1984. Hemagglutinins of *Haemophilus paragallinarum* serotype 1 organisms. Jpn. J. Vet. Sci. 46:21–29.

Haemophilus somnus

H. somnus is the cause of infectious thromboembolic meningoencephalitis (TEME) in cattle, a disease that was first reported in Colorado (Griner et al. 1956) and has since been reported throughout the United States, Canada, and parts of Europe. A bacterium resembling *Haemophilus* organisms was isolated from sick cattle by Kennedy et al. (1960), and the species name was later proposed by Bailie (1969). Infections of the bovine genital tract and abortion have also been reported (Chladek 1975, van Dreumel and Kierstead 1975, Waldhalm et al. 1974).

H. somnus is not an official *Haemophilus* species. Similar organisms known in the clinical literature as *H. agni* and *Histophilus ovis* cause neonatal mortality and septicemia in lambs and epididymitis and mastitis in older sheep (reviewed by Humphrey and Stephens 1983).

Morphology and Staining Reactions. *H. somnus* is a very small, Gram-negative, nonmotile coccobacillus. It may stain in a bipolar fashion. Capsules, pili, or other surface appendages have not been seen.

Cultural and Biochemical Features. Colonies grown on blood or chocolate agar are circular, convex, shiny, butyrous, and about 1 to 2 mm in diameter in 48 hours. They may show be slightly yellowish. Older colonies may dehydrate, which gives them a granular appearance. Some strains are beta-hemolytic. The organism on primary isolation is CO_2-dependent, and although not responsive to X and V factors, it has a strict requirement for cocarboxylase and other unknown factors in blood and yeast. It also exhibits satellitism when grown near a suitable feeder bacterium.

H. somnus is oxidase-positive but does not hydrolyze gelatin. It produces H_2S by the filter strip method, and the

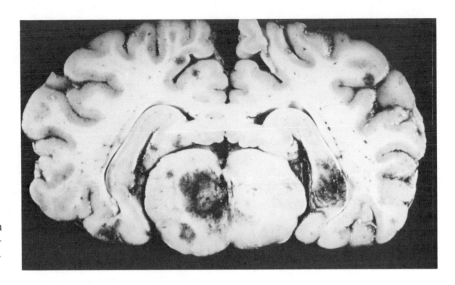

Figure 8.1. Hemorrhagic areas in the brain of a steer with infectious meningoencephalitis caused by *Haemophilus somnus*. (Courtesy Joseph Kowalski.)

majority of strains produce indole. It reduces nitrates and variably produces catalase. It does not produce urease. All strains ferment glucose, whereas most strains ferment fructose, maltose, xylose, trehalose, and sorbitol. The mol% G + C of the DNA is 37.3.

Antigens. At least three sets of antigens have been observed in U.S. and Swiss strains. These appear in various combinations that constitute four agglutination groups (Canto and Biberstein 1982). Variations in the molecular weights of proteins between 11,500 and 16,000 have been observed in mucoid and smooth variants of *H. somnus* (Corboz and Wild 1981). *H. somnus, H. agni, Histophilus ovis,* and *Actinobacillus seminis* share at least two common antigens, and the protein profiles of their cell envelopes are similar (Stephens et al. 1983).

Epizootiology and Pathogenesis. *H. somnus* colonizes the nasal cavities of normal healthy calves, the preputial cavity of male cattle, and the genital cavity of female cattle. Preputial isolates are relatively avirulent. Colonization of the nasal cavity can be mediated by specific adhesins on the bacterial surface. The organism is readily transmitted to other noninfected animals (Crandell 1977). Isolation rates from cattle remain relatively constant between seasons but increase in groups of animals where TEME is occurring (Corstvet et al. 1973).

The stresses of shipping, climatic change, and regrouping under crowded conditions predispose animals to TEME. The disease is therefore common in cattle some weeks after arrival in feedlots (Saunders et al. 1980). The mechanism by which endogenous inapparent infection is triggered to cause severe disease is unknown. Both bacterial and host factors are probably involved. The organism's ability to survive and multiply within bovine monocytes may be a factor in its survival in subacute and chronic lesions. Lateral spread of TEME is not a promi-

nent feature of the epizootiology, although the number of culturally positive animals increases during an outbreak.

Affected animals exhibit weakness, fever, staggering, stiffness, knuckling of the fetlocks, dyspnea, somnolence (hence the name *H. somnus*), erratic behavior, paralysis, and sudden death. The mortality among affected animals can be very high (Dirksen et al. 1978).

The lesions of *H. somnus* infection consist of a fibrinous meningitis with arterial thrombosis and necrosis. Hemorrhages on serous surfaces and in muscles are widespread. The lymph nodes are enlarged, dark, and edematous, and the brain contains hemorrhagic areas that can be several centimeters in diameter (Figure 8.1). A suppurative polyarthritis can also be present.

Fibrin thrombi can be found in the vessels of the brain and meninges, and there are multifocal areas of necrosis and infiltrations of polymorphonuclear cells (Smith and Biberstein 1977) (Figure 8.2). Momotani et al. (1985) found that the vasculature of the liver, spleen, kidney, lung, heart, and brain of animals with spontaneously occurring cases of TEME contained numerous fibrin thrombi distributed in a pattern consistent with disseminated intravascular coagulation.

H. somnus is also frequently associated with bovine respiratory disease, but the pathogenesis of this is not understood (Figure 8.3). The disease, a fibrinous pneumonia with pleuritis and arthritis, is most prevalent in spring and summer in nursing calves at pasture (Saunders and Janzen 1980). Other respiratory pathogens such as *Pasteurella* species, *Actinomyces pyogenes,* and *Mycoplasma* species may also be present. Strains of *H. somnus* from pneumonic lesions have been shown in experiments to be capable of causing TEME (Corboz and Pohlenz 1976).

H. somnus has been implicated as a cause of endo-

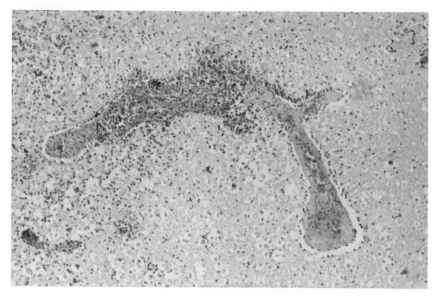

Figure 8.2. Vasculitis and thrombus formation in the brain of a steer with thromboembolic meningoencephalitis caused by *Haemophilus somnus*. Hematoxylin and eosin stain. (Courtesy John King.)

metritis, metritis, and late abortions in cattle (Chladek 1975). It has also been associated with mastitis and with acute granular vulvovaginitis (Rhunke et al. 1978). The organism has been isolated from a fatal case of septicemia in a ram (Groom et al. 1984). In New Zealand and Australia a variant of *H. somnus*, commonly known as *Histophilus ovis*, has been associated with mastitis, epididymitis, orchitis, synovitis, and bacteremia and

septicemia in lambs. The systemic disease is characterized by formation of emboli and thrombi in the smaller vessels (Rahaley 1978).

Immunity. Bactericidal antibody develops in animals after infection or immunization. The activity is complement-dependent (Simonson and Maheswaran 1982). A variety of serologic tests are available for assay of antibody to *H. somnus*. These include agglutination, comple-

Figure 8.3. Section of a bovine lung showing pneumonia caused by *Haemophilus somnus*. The circumscribed area of necrosis is the result of arterial blockage caused by fibrin thrombi.

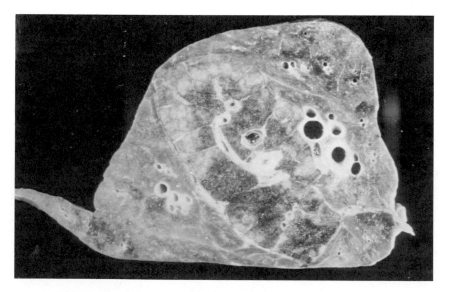

ment fixation, gel immunodiffusion, and ELISA (Humphrey and Stephens 1983). Many cattle have serum antibodies to *H. somnus*, a reflection in part of carrying the organism in the nasopharynx or reproductive tract. Since antibody titers rise in clinically normal animals in a herd where TEME is occurring, suggesting increased exposure to the organism, antibody titers are not of great value by themselves as diagnostic evidence. Susceptibility to experimental intravenous challenge is poorly correlated with titers of serum antibodies, indicating that the assays commonly used do not measure protective antibodies.

Protective antigens occur in protein extracts, sonicates, and saline extracts but not in polysaccharide fractions of the organism (Nayar et al. 1977). The protective antigen is an anionic component of the outer membrane complex (Stephens et al. 1984). Protective antiserums react strongly with 78- and 40-kilodalton proteins and with polysaccharide (Gogolewski et al. 1987).

Bacterins consisting of killed bacteria absorbed to aluminum hydroxide have been widely used and appear to be protective (Williams et al. 1978). However, TEME has been observed in vaccinated populations (Saunders and Janzen 1980).

Diagnosis. *H. somnus* can be cultured from the blood, brain, liver, and spleen of animals with TEME. Cultures must be grown on media enriched with yeast extract and in an atmosphere of 10 percent CO_2. Because the organism is difficult to isolate from sites heavily contaminated with other bacteria, such samples should either be diluted or plated on selective medium (Slee and Stephens 1985).

Antimicrobial Susceptibility. *H. somnus* is sensitive to penicillin G, ampicillin, colistin, novobiocin, chloramphenicol, erythromycin, tetracycline, and sulfachlorpyridazine trimethoprim. Susceptibility testing should be routinely performed on representative isolates because resistant strains have been detected.

REFERENCES

Bailie, W.E. 1969. Characterization of *Haemophilus somnus* (new species), a microorganism isolated from infectious thromboembolic meningoencephalomyelitis of cattle. Diss. Abstr. 30B:2482.

Canto, G.J., and Biberstein, E.L. 1982. Serological diversity in *Haemophilus somnus*. J. Clin. Microbiol. 15:1009–1015.

Chladek, D.W. 1975. Bovine abortion associated with *Haemophilus somnus*. Am. J. Vet. Res. 36:1041.

Corboz, L., and Pohlenz, T. 1976. Experimentelle Infektionen mit sogenanntem *Haemophilus somnus* beim Kalb: Vergleich von Stammen mit sinterscherdlicher Virulenz. Schweiz. Arch. Tierheilkd. 118.429–440.

Corboz, L., and Wild, P. 1981. Epidemiologie der *Haemophilus somnus*–Infektion beim Rind: Vergleich von Stammen in der Polyacrylomidgel–Elektrophorese (PAGE). Schweiz. Arch. Tierheilkd. 123:79–88.

Corstvet, R.E., Panciera, R.J., Rinker, H.B., Starks, B.L., and Howard, C. 1973. Survey of tracheas of feedlot cattle for *Haemophilus somnus* and other selected bacteria. J. Am. Vet. Med. Assoc. 163:870–873.

Crandell, R.A., Smith, A.R., and Kissil, M. 1977. Colonization and transmission of *Haemophilus somnus* in cattle. Am. J. Vet. Res. 38:1749–1751.

Dirksen, G., Kaiser, E., and Schels, H. 1978. Erstes Auftreten der infektiösen septikamisch-thrombosierenden Meningoenzephalitis (ISTME) bei Mastrindern in Suddeutschland. Praktische Tierärzt. 59:766–770.

Gogolewski, R.P., Kania, S.A., Ingzana, T.J., Widders, P.R., Liggitt, H.D., and Corbeil, L.B. 1987. Protective ability and specificity of convalescent serum from calves with *Haemophilus somnus* pneumonia. Infect. Immun. 55:1403–1411.

Griner, L.A., Jensen, R., and Brown, W.W. (1956). Infectious embolic meningoencephalitis in cattle. J. Am. Vet. Med. Assoc. 129:417–421.

Groom, S.G., Miller, R.B., and Hoover, D. 1984. Isolation of *Haemophilus somnus* from a ram with fatal septicemia. Can. Vet. J. 25:409–410.

Humphrey, J.D., and Stephens, L.R. 1983. *Haemophilus somnus*: A review. Vet. Bull. 53:987–1004.

Kennedy, P.C., Biberstein, E.L., Howarth, J.A., Frazier, L.M., and Dungworth, D.L. 1960. Infectious meningo-encephalitis in cattle, caused by *Haemophilus*-like organism. Am. J. Vet. Res. 21:403–409.

Momotani, E., Yabuki, Y., Miho, H., Ishikawa, Y., and Yoshino, T. 1985. Histopathological evaluation of disseminated intravascular coagulation in *Haemophilus somnus* infection in cattle. J. Comp. Pathol. 95:15–23.

Nayar, P.S.G., Ward, G.E., Saunders, J.R., and MacWilliams, P. 1977. Diagnostic procedures in experimental *Haemophilus somnus* infection in cattle. Can. Vet. J. 18:159–163.

Rahaley, R.S. 1978. Pathology of experimental *Histophilus ovis* infection in sheep. I. Lambs. Vet. Pathol. 15:631–637.

Rhunke, H.L., Doig, P.A., Mackay, A.L., Gagnov, A., and Kierstead, M. 1978. Isolation of ureaplasma from bovine granular vulvitis. Can. J. Comp. Med. 42:151–155.

Saunders, J.R., and Janzen, E.D. 1980. *Haemophilus somnus* infections. II. A Canadian field trial of a commercial bacterin: Clinical and serological results. Can. Vet. J. 21:219–224.

Saunders, J.R., Thiessen, W.A., and Janzen, E.D. 1980. *Haemophilus somnus* infections. I. A ten-year (1969–1978) retrospective study of losses in cattle herds in western Canada. Can. Vet. J. 21:119–123.

Simonson, R.R., and Maheswaran, S.K. 1982. Host humoral factors in natural resistance to *Haemophilus somnus*. Am. J. Vet. Res. 43:1160–1164.

Slee, K.J., and Stephens, L.R. 1985. Selective medium for isolation of *H. somnus* from cattle and sheep. Vet. Rec. 116:215–217.

Smith, B.P., and Biberstein, E.L. 1977. Septicemia and meningoencephalitis in pastured cattle caused by a hemophilus-like organism ("*Haemophilus somnus*"). Cornell Vet. 67:300–305.

Stephens, L.R., Humphrey, J.D., Little, P.B., and Barnum, D.A. 1983. Morphological, biochemical, antigenic, and cytochemical relationships among *Haemophilus somnus*, *Haemophilus agni*, *Haemophilus haemoglobinophilus*, *Histophilus ovis*, and *Actinobacillus seminis*. J. Clin. Microbiol. 17:728–737.

Stephens, L.R., Little, P.B., Wilkie, B.N., and Barnum, D.A. 1984. Isolation of *Haemophilus somnus* antigens and their use as vaccines for prevention of bovine thromboembolic meningoencephalitis. Am. J. Vet. Res. 45:234–239.

van Dreumel, A.A., and Kierstead, M. 1975. Abortion associated with *Haemophilus somnus* infection in a bovine fetus. Can. Vet. J. 16:367–370.

Waldhalm, D.G., Hall, R.F., Meinershagen, W.A., Card, C.S., and Frank, F.W. 1974. *Haemophilus somnus* infection in the cow as a possible contributing factor to weak calf syndrome: Isolation and animal inoculation studies. Am. J. Vet. Res. 35:1401–1403.

Williams, J.M., Smith, G.L., and Murdock, F.M. 1978. Immunogenicity of a *Haemophilus somnus* bacterin in cattle. Am. J. Vet. Res. 39:1756–1762.

9 The Genus *Taylorella*

The genus *Taylorella* was established to accommodate *Haemophilus equigenitalis* after evidence emerged that the organism was not a legitimate member of the genus *Haemophilus* (Sugimoto et al. 1984). The evidence resulted from studies of DNA base composition and DNA-DNA hybridization as well as numerical analysis of phenotypic characteristics. There is only species in the genus, *T. equigenitalis,* the cause of contagious equine metritis (CEM).

Taylorella equigenitalis

SYNONYM: *Haemophilus equigenitalis*

The microaerophilic organism *T. equigenitalis* was first described in 1977 by Platt et al. (1977), Ricketts et al. (1977), and Timoney et al. (1977) from outbreaks of a highly contagious venereal disease on stud farms in Britain and Ireland. Another report (O'Driscoll et al. 1977) published in the same year described a clinically similar disease that occurred in Ireland in 1976—an indication that the infection was present for some time before the causative agent was described. The disease was named *contagious equine metritis*. In addition to Britain and Ireland, CEM has been confirmed in Austria, Australia, Brazil, Belgium, Denmark, France, Germany, Italy, Japan, Norway, Sweden, the United States, and Yugoslavia.

Morphology and Staining Reactions. *T. equigenitalis* is a short, Gram-negative rod that is frequently described as a coccobacillus. In cultures from carrier mares it occasionally has filaments 5 to 6 μm long. It may stain in a bipolar fashion. There are no flagella or pili, although a thin threadlike capsule has been observed.

Cultural and Biochemical Features. It takes 2 to 5 days for *T. equigenitalis* colonies to grow on chocolate agar at 37°C. Incubation should be performed in 5 percent CO^2. Some strains grow to a limited extent aerobically following primary isolation. *T. equigenitalis* is a facultative anaerobe, and excellent growth occurs in an atmosphere of 90 percent H_2 and 10 percent CO_2. The colonies are raised, shining, smooth, butyrous, gray pinpoints (Figure 9.1). They are nonhemolytic. After prolonged incubation, they become larger and more opaque. *T. equigenitalis* grows well in brain-heart infusion, in thiol and cystine trypticase broths, and in Robertson's cooked-meat medium.

T. equigenitalis is oxidase-, catalase-, and phosphatase-positive but is otherwise unreactive biochemically. Neither X nor V factor is required, although some response to X factor occurs. The mol% G + C of the DNA is 36.1.

Antigens. There are at least 11 separate antigens, 2 of which are located on the cell surface. The surface antigens are composed of polysaccharide and lipopolysaccharide-protein (Brewer 1983). A surface protein binds equine IgG but is as yet uncharacterized (Widders et al. 1985).

Cattle and humans frequently have serum antibodies to *T. equigenitalis*. Their occurrence may reflect exposure to organisms with cross-reacting antigens, since *T. equigenitalis* has never been isolated from these hosts.

Epizootiology and Pathogenesis. In infected horses *T. equigenitalis* is carried as an obligate parasite in the urethral fossa and terminal urethra of stallions and in the clitoral sinuses and fossa of mares. It has also been found in the genitalia of colts and fillies that are not yet sexually mature (Timoney and Powell 1982).

Its origins are unknown. It may have arisen de novo in the early 1970s from an as yet unidentified progenitor organism. Its adaptation to the external genitalia of the male and female suggests that its ancestor may be a commensal of this region.

T. equigenitalis has been experimentally transmitted to donkey mares (Timoney, McArdle, et al. 1979) and to mice, rabbits, and guinea pigs (Timoney, Geraghty, et al. 1978). However, cattle, sheep, and pigs appear to be refractive to infection (Timoney, O'Reilly, et al. 1978).

The organism is transmitted naturally by the stallion during mating, but contaminated fomites can also serve to convey the organism to an uninfected female. The disease is therefore highly contagious. Infected mares can develop a profuse vulvar discharge with evidence of endometritis, cervicitis, or vaginitis 2 to 12 days after being bred to a carrier stallion and may return to estrus after a

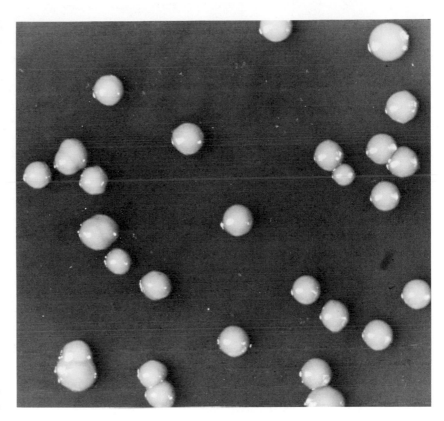

Figure 9.1. Colonies of *Taylorella equigenitalis* on Eugon blood agar at 72 hours.

shortened diestrous period. The discharge consists of a copious flow of thin grayish white exudate, which pours out of the vulva, soils the hindquarters, and matts the tail hairs. Since the causal organism causes no clinical signs and stimulates no local tissue response or any detectable serologic response in the stallion, it is regarded as a surface commensal in the male.

Cases of inapparent *T. equigenitalis* infection have been reported in both barren and in-foal mares. Infection does not preclude a normal pregnancy and the birth of a healthy foal. The organism has been recovered from the placental membranes from known infected mares.

The vulvar discharge from infected mares contains large numbers of neutrophils, some of which contain ingested organisms. Untreated mares can continue to discharge for 10 to 11 days. The organism can be shed either constantly or intermittently for long periods after the discharge ceases, and in many carrier mares it remains sequestered in the clitoral sinuses (Simpson and Eaton-Evans 1978). Shedding can be independent of the estrous cycle. Mares with acute CEM infection exhibit edema of the uterine mucosa (Figure 9.2), migration of neutrophils into the lumen, and infiltration of mononuclear cells into the lamina propria. Mild, multifocal salpingitis is a common finding. The endometritis and cervicitis become pre-

dominantly plasmacytic by 14 days (Acland and Kenney 1983

Immunity. Detectable antibody responses have been demonstrated only in mares and not in stallions. The resistance of recovered mares may be due to locally produced antibodies because systemic antibody responses are lower after the second than after the first infection.

Both local and systemic antibodies are produced after

Figure 9.2. Uterine mucosa of a mare 6 days after experimental infection with *Taylorella equigenitalis*. The mucosal edema is characteristic.

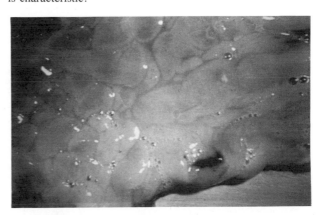

infection of mares, and these can be measured by enzyme-linked immunosorbent assay (ELISA) and by agglutination, antiglobulin, indirect fluorescent antibody, complement-fixation (CF), and passive hemagglutination (PHA) tests (Sahu et al. 1983). A combination of rapid plate agglutination, ELISA, and PHA tests has been recommended for serologic diagnosis in thoroughbreds (Sahu et al. 1983). These tests are unreliable for detecting disease in chronically infected mares, however, because many such animals do not have measurable antibody titers.

Although chronically infected mares tend to have CF test titers that persist much longer than agglutination or antiglobulin titers, the CF test is not reliable for identification of carrier animals (Bryans et al. 1979). CF test titers in animals with endometritis are detectable after 10 days, peak at 3 weeks, and decline within 8 to 10 weeks (Dawson et al. 1978). The anticomplementary activity of some horse serums after freezing must be neutralized before use in the CF test.

Bacterins have been shown to reduce the clinical severity of experimental infection. High titers of serum antibodies are stimulated, but these are relatively ineffective in local protection of the tract.

Diagnosis. Although the presence of large numbers of neutrophils in the characteristically profuse exudate together with the presence of Gram-negative coccobacilli both intra- and extracellulary is suggestive of CEM, isolation of *T. equigenitalis* is the only absolute means of confirming the disease in either a mare or stallion. Swabs from barren, maiden, or postparturient mares should preferably be taken during estrus and should include swabs from the uterus or cervix, the clitoral fossa and sinus, and any discharge present. The clitoral sinus is the recommended sampling site for pregnant mares. The swabbing sites in stallions are the urethral fossa, the terminal urethra, the prepuce, and preejaculatory fluid.

All swabs should be carried to the laboratory in Amie's or Stuart's transport media and should be shipped frozen or refrigerated. Specimens should be plated out promptly on chocolate agar or Eugonagar (Becton-Dickinson) in an atmosphere of 5 percent CO_2. Streptomycin (200–400 μg/ml) and amphotericin B (5 μg/ml) can be incorporated into the medium to suppress contaminants, but antibiotic-free medium should be inoculated at the same time because some strains of *T. equigenitalis* are streptomycin-sensitive. Because the organism is very slow growing, plates should be examined daily for 7 to 10 days. Colonies are frequently visible by the second or third day of incubation. A selective medium that contains trimethoprim, clindamycin, and amphotericin B is very effective in suppressing *Proteus* species (Timoney et al. 1982).

The serologic tests described above can also be helpful

adjuncts in diagnosis of acute infection but are of little value in the detection of carrier animals.

Antimicrobial Susceptibility. *T. equigenitalis* is sensitive to a wide range of antimicrobial agents including penicillin, ampicillin, neomycin, chloramphenicol, nitrofurazone, gentamicin, tetracycline, and chlorhexidine. Strains of the organism isolated so far are either resistant or sensitive to streptomycin. Cefotaxime has been shown to be very effective in the treatment and bacteriological cure of naturally occurring cases of CEM (Timoney et al. 1983).

Treated mares exhibit a rapid clinical response but can remain carriers of the organism. Local treatment of the external genitalia of carrier stallions has been very successful in clearing injection. The fertility of treated mares and stallions is not impaired after recovery from CEM.

Addition of antibiotics to semen inactivates the organism and is therefore potentially useful in the control of the disease (Timoney, O'Reilly, Harrington, et al. 1979). The most effective method of eliminating infection in carrier mares is surgical removal of the clitoral sinuses.

REFERENCES

Acland, H.M., and Kenney, R.M. 1983. Lesions of contagious equine metritis in mares. Vet. Pathol. 20:330–341.

Brewer, R.A. 1983. Contagious equine metritis: A review/summary. Vet. Bull. 53:881–891.

Bryans, J.T., Darlington, R.W., Smith, B., and Brooks, R.R. 1979. Development of a complement fixation test and its application to diagnosis of contagious equine metritis. J. Equine Med. Surg. 3:467–472.

Dawson, F.L.M., Benson, J.A., and Croxton-Smith, P. 1978. The course of serum antibody development in two ponies experimentally infected with contagious metritis. Equine Vet. J. 10:145–147.

O'Driscoll, J.G., Troy, P.T., and Geoghegan, F.J. 1977. An epidemic of venereal infection in thoroughbreds. Vet. Rec. 101:359–360.

Platt, H., Atherton, J.G., Simpson, D.J., Taylor, C.E.D., Rosenthal, R.O., Brown, D.F.J., and Wreghitt, T.G. 1977. Genital infection in mares. Vet. Rec. 101:20.

Ricketts, S.W., Rossdale, P.D., Wingfield-Digby, N.J., Falk, M.M., Hopes, R., Hunt, M.D.N., and Peace, C.K. 1977. Genital infection in mares. Vet. Rec. 101:65.

Sahu, S.P., Rommel, F.A., Fales, W.H., Hamdy, F.M., Swerczek, T.W., Youngquist, R.S., and Bryans, J.T. 1983. Evaluation of various serotests to detect antibodies in ponies and horses infected with contagious equine metritis bacteria. Am. J. Vet. Res. 44:1405–1409.

Simpson, D.J., and Eaton-Evans, W. 1978. Sites of CEM infection. Vet. Rec. 102:488.

Sugimoto, C., Isayama, Y., Sakazaki, R., and Kuramochi, S. 1984. Transfer of *Haemophilus equigenitalis* Taylor et al. 1978 to the genus *Taylorella* gen. nov. as *Talorella equigenitalis* comb. nov. Curr. Microbiol. 9:155–162.

Timoney, P.J., and Powell, D.G. 1982. Isolation of the contagious equine metritis organism from colts and fillies in the United Kingdom and Ireland. Vet. Rec. 111:478–482.

Timoney, P.J., Geraghty, V.P., Dillon, P.B., and McArdle, J.F. 1978. Susceptibility of laboratory animals to infection with *Haemophilus equigenitalis*. Vet. Rec. 103:563–564.

Timoney, P.J., McArdle, J.F., O'Reilly, P.J., Ward, J., and Harrington, A.M. 1979. Successful transmission of CEM to the donkey. Vet. Rec. 104:84.

Timoney, P.J., O'Reilly, P.J., Harrington, A.M., McCormack, R., and McArdle, J.F. 1979. Survival of *Haemophilus equigenitalis* in different antibiotic-containing semen extenders. J. Reprod. Fertil. (Suppl.) 27:377–381.

Timoney, P.J., O'Reilly, P.J., McArdle, J., and Ward, J. 1978. Attempted transmission of contagious equine metritis 1977 to other domestic animal species. Vet. Rec. 102:152.

Timoney, P.J., O'Reilly, P.J., McArdle, J.F., Ward, J., and Harrington, A.M. 1979. Responses of mares to rechallenge with the organism of contagious equine metritis. Vet. Rec. 104:264.

Timoney, P.J., Shin, S.J., Huntress, C., and Strickland, K.L. 1983. Activity of cefotazime, a β-lactam antibiotic, against the contagious equine metritis organism. Vet. Rec. 112:569–570.

Timoney, P.J., Shin, S.J., and Jacobson, R.H. 1982. Improved selective medium for isolation of the contagious equine metritis organism. Vet. Rec. 111:107–108.

Timoney, P.J., Ward, J., and Kelly, P. 1977. A contagious genital infection of mares. Vet. Rec. 101:103.

Widders, P.R., Stokes, C.R., Newby, T.J., and Bourne, F.J. 1985. Nonimmune binding of equine immunoglobulin by the causative organism of contagious equine metritis, *Taylorella equigenitalis*. Infect. Immun. 48:417–421.

10 The Genus *Pasteurella*

The genus *Pasteurella* belongs to the family Pasteurellaceae, a complex group of highly adapted parasitic organisms that includes the genera *Actinobacillus* and *Haemophilus*.

Pasteurella organisms occur most frequently as tiny, Gram-negative, pleomorphic coccobacilli that stain in a bipolar fashion in smears made from specimens taken from lesions. They are nonmotile, usually oxidase- and catalase-positive, and aerobic to microaerophilic or facultatively anaerobic.

P. multocida is the type species and embraces a variety of biotypes and serotypes. The other species currently recognized in *Bergey's Manual of Systematic Bacteriology* (1984) are *P. aerogenes*, *P. gallinarum*, *P. haemolytica*, *P. pneumotropica*, and *P. ureae*. *P. anatipestifer*, a cause of septicemia in ducks and other fowl, is listed as *species incertae sedis*. Although there is convincing evidence that it is not a *Pasteurella* species, its correct affiliation is as yet unknown. We will therefore describe it in this chapter with the other official species.

Shortly after the publication of *Bergey's Manual of Systematic Bacteriology* in 1984, Mutters et al. (1985) published a classification study of the genus *Pasteurella* based on DNA homology in which they concluded that the genus comprises at least 11 species. Although this reclassification has not yet affected the nomenclature in the veterinary literature, it clearly carries important etiological and epizootiological implications for an understanding of the diseases caused by members of the genus. The 11 species, their distinguishing characteristics, and their relationships to some of the species listed above are shown in Table 10.1.

Mutters et al. recommended that *P. ureae*, *P. haemolytica* biotypes A and T, and some biotypes of *P. pneumotropica* be removed from the genus *Pasteurella*, claiming that these organisms are more closely related to the *Actinobacillus* group and should probably be placed in this genus.

P. multocida and *P. haemolytica* are important pathogens of domestic and wild animals. *P. multocida* causes primary septicemias in cattle and in domestic and wild birds and is also an important opportunistic invader of the respiratory tract of a variety of species. *P. haemolytica* is important both as a primary and opportunistic respiratory pathogen of cattle and sheep and as a cause of septicemia and mastitis in sheep. *P. haemolytica* and, to a lesser extent, *P. multocida* are key constituents of the *shipping fever* complex in cattle. The other *Pasturella* species are relatively avirulent and are only occasionally found in secondary opportunistic invasions.

REFERENCE

Mutters, R., Ihm, P., Pohl, S., Frederiksen, W., and Mannheim, W. 1985. Reclassification of the genus *Pasteurella* Trevisan 1887 on the basis of deoxyribonucleic acid homology, with proposals for the new species *Pasteurella dagmatis*, *Pasteurella canis*, *Pasteurella stomatis*, *Pasteurella anatis*, and *Pasteurella langaa*. Int. J. Syst. Bacteriol. 35:309–322.

Pasteurella multocida

SYNONYM: *Pasteurella gallicida*

Morphology and Staining Reactions. *P. multocida* forms tiny ovoid rods about 0.3 μm wide by 0.4 to 0.8 μm long. When seen in carefully stained films obtained from tissue, the ends of the rod are more deeply stained than the central portion, giving it a distinct bipolar appearance. This characteristic is not so marked in bacilli obtained from cultures and can easily be obscured by overstaining. Wright's stain or Giemsa stain is recommended for demonstrating bipolar staining, although careful staining with methylene blue usually is satisfactory.

The pasteurellas are Gram-negative and non-spore-forming. Many strains form a capsular substance when freshly isolated, but usually this property is quickly lost. Pasteurellas have no flagella or pili.

Cultural and Biochemical Features. *P. multocida* grows very well on blood agar. It also grows on infusion agars; this growth can be enhanced by the addition of serum. Colonies on blood agar are smooth, buyrous, convex, and about 1 to 2 mm in diameter, with a characteristic odor.

Heavily encapsulated strains produce mucoid or watery colonies. Blood agar is not altered except for the presence of a slight greenish haze. Growth rarely occurs on Mac-

Table 10.1. Proposed classification and differentiation of the species of the genus *Pasteurella*

Species	Previous name	Source	NAD requirement	Ornithine	Indole	Urease	Trehalose	Maltose	D-Xylose	L-Arabinose	Mannitol	Sorbitol	Dulcitol
							Acid produced within 24 to 48 hours from						
Pasteurella species A	*Haemophilus avium*	Chicken	+	−	−	−	+	v	v	+	v	−	−
Pasteurella species B	None	Mouth of dogs and cats	−	+	+	−	+	+	+	−	−	−	+
P. anatis	None	Intestine of ducks	−	−	−	−	+	−	+	−	+	−	−
P. avium	NA	Chickens	v	−	−	−	+	−	v	−	−	−	−
P. canis	*P. multocida* biotype B	Mouth of dogs and calves; bite wounds	−	+	d	−	v	−	v	−	−	−	−
P. dagmatis	*P. pneumotropica*	Mouth of dogs and cats; bite wounds	−	−	+	+	+	+	−	−	−	−	−
P. gallinarum	*P. gallinarum*	Chickens; fowl cholera	−	−	−	−	+	+	−	−	−	−	−
P. langaa	NA	Respiratory tract of healthy chickens	−	−	−	−	−	−	−	−	+	−	−
P. multocida subsp. *multocida*	*P. multocida*	Mammals, birds; bite wounds	−	+	+	−	v	−	v	−	+	+	−
subsp. *septica*	*P. septica*	Mammals, birds; bite wounds	−	+	+	−	+	−	+	−	+		
subsp. *gallicida*	*P. gallicida*	Birds	−	+	+	−	−	−	+	v	+	+	+
P. stomatis	None	Respiratory tract of cats and dogs	−	−	+	−	+	−	−	−	−		
P. volantium	NA	Chickens	+	v	−	−	+	+	v	−	+	v	−

v = variable; d = delayed.
NA = not applicable, new species.
Modified from Mutters et al., 1985, courtesy of *International Journal of Systematic Bacteriology*.

Conkey agar. Growth in infusion (broth) with serum added is manifest by slight clouding and a viscid sediment. *P. multocida* does not liquefy gelatin, but does produce indole and reduce nitrates to nitrites. Most strains produce hydrogen sulfide, catalase, cytochrome c, and ornithine decarboxylase. The features that have commonly been used to distinguish *P. multocida* from the other species listed in *Bergey's Manual of Systematic Bacteriology* are shown in Table 10.2. The mol% G + C of the DNA is 40 to 45 (Tm).

Biotypes. Frederiksen (1971, 1973) has proposed seven biotypes or biovars of *P. multocida* based on fermentation of arabinose, xylose, maltose, trehalose, sorbitol, and mannitol. Strains from dogs constitute a biotype that is distinct from the other six and that is characterized by failure to attack sorbitol and mannitol. Other workers (Ghoniem et al. 1973) have found that strains from dogs usually ferment maltose but not mannitol, whereas porcine strains produce converse reactions.

Carter (1976) has developed another scheme of biotyping based on tests for hyaluronidase, decapsulation, acriflavine flocculation, colonial iridescence, carbohydrate fermentation, murine pathogenicity, and serum protection. Carter's biotypes are the following: 1, mucoid; 2, hemorrhagic septicemic; 3, porcine; 4, canine; and 5, feline.

Antigens and Serologic Classification. Colonies of *P. multocida* grown on agar have dissociation patterns show-

Table 10.2. Differentiation of *Pasteurella* species

Characteristic	*P. multocida*	*P. haemolytica*	*P. pneumotropica*	*P. gallinarum*	*P. aerogenes*	*P. ureae*	*P. anatipestifer*[†]
Hemolysis	−	+	−	−	−	−	−
Growth on MacConkey agar	−	+	−	−	+	−	−
Urease	−	−	+	−	+	+	−
Indole	+	−	+	−	+	+	−
Acid from mannitol	+[*]	+	−	−	−	+	−
Gas from glucose	−	−	−	−	+	−	−
Gelatin hydrolysis	−	−	−	−	−	−	+

[*]Strains from dogs may produce a negative result.
[†]Not a legitimate member of the genus; its correct affiliation is unknown.

Table 10.3. Common serotypes of *P. multocida* in animals

Host	Disease	Serotypes encountered
Cattle	Hemorrhagic septicemia	B2, E2
	Pneumonia	A2
Chickens	Fowl cholera	A1, A3, A5, A8
Turkeys	Cholera	A9
Pigs	Pneumonia	A3, D4, D10
	Atrophic rhinitis	A3, D3
Sheep	Pneumonia	D1, D4
Rabbits	Snuffles	A12

ing three principal colonial variants: (1) mucoid colonies that are large, flowing, moderately virulent for mice, and not typable by the usual serologic methods; (2) smooth or fluorescent colonies that are medium-sized, discrete, quite virulent for mice, and typable; and (3) rough or blue colonies that are small, discrete, low in virulence for mice, and autoagglutinable.

Mucoid and smooth colonial variants carry the specific soluble antigens associated with capsular acidic polysaccharide. These type-specific antigens are the basis of Roberts's (1947) and Carter's (1955) classifications. There are four Carter types: A, B, D, and E. These are usually determined by a hemagglutination test with known antiserums in which human erythrocytes are sensitized with extracts of the strain to be typed.

Type A is the most prevalent capsular type among *P. multocida* isolates from cattle, swine, poultry, and rabbits. *P. multocida* has also been shown to carry somatic and O antigens (Namioka and Murata 1961), of which there are at least 11. Arabic numbers are used to denote the different O antigens. The O antigens are recognized by using acid-treated cells in an agglutination test with typing antiserums. A gel diffusion test based on extracts obtained by boiling a suspension of cells is also used to determine the O antigen of strains from poultry (Heddleston et al. 1972). Isolates from outbreaks of disease in cattle are much more likely to be typable than isolates from the nasopharynx of healthy cattle and other animals.

Some common disease-producing serotypes of *P. multocida* are shown in Table 10.3.

Epizootiology and Pathogenesis. *P. multocida* is normally maintained as a commensal of the oropharynx of mammals. Unlike mammals, though, healthy birds do not carry the organism, and its presence in birds is almost invariably associated with acute or chronic disease.

The organism survives only briefly in the environment but can survive in the carcasses of animals for extended periods. Transmission between animals is usually by airborne droplets of by food or water contamination. These modes of spread are of great importance in the epizootiology of fowl cholera and hemorrhagic septicemia of cattle and buffaloes in the tropics.

Many outbreaks of respiratory disease in pigs and cattle caused by *P. multocida,* however, are apparently the result of invasions by endogenous infections of the nasopharynx. A variety of stressful situations such as shipment, viral infection, bad weather, poor nutrition, and overcrowding can impair the physical and immunological defenses of animals and allow *P. multocida* to multiply on the nasopharyngeal mucosa, with subsequent penetration of the lower respiratory tract.

Primary viral and mycoplasmal infections predispose animals to secondary invasions by *P. multocida* by impairing alveolar macrophage function and by damaging the mucociliary clearance mechanism in the trachea and bronchi. The local inflammatory effect they cause leads to increased fluidity of the mucus blanket, with consequent sneezing and coughing and, inevitably, formation of endogenous aerosols in the respiratory tree. During inspiration the aerosols can result in downward carriage of bacteria from the upper parts of the tract. These are just some of the possible conditions that predispose animals to pneumonic pasteurellosis. Much has yet to be learned about the factors that control initial multiplication of *P. multocida* in the nasopharynx and about the mechanism by which it subsequently invades the lower respiratory tract. The role of *P. multocida* in bovine respiratory disease and the possible influence of viral agents is discussed in greater detail by Yates (1982).

Stress or concurrent or antecedent viral infection is of less importance in the pathogenesis of hemorrhagic septicemia of cattle and sheep and of fowl cholera. The strains of *P. multocida* involved in these diseases are highly invasive by themselves and the organisms therefore behave as primary pathogens.

Hemorrhagic septicemia is a disease of cattle, buffalo, goats, and sheep that causes serious economic losses in tropical and subtropical zones of Asia and Africa. Serotype B2 is responsible for the disease found in Asia, and serotype E2 is the cause of the disease found in Africa (Carter 1984). The disease occurs during the rainy season. Outbreaks begin with the death of one or two animals, which during their illness shed huge numbers of *P. multocida*. These organisms are transmitted directly or indirectly to nearby animals. Very quickly an enzootic develops among exposed susceptible animals. Affected animals develop a high temperature (41° to 42°C), dysentery, edema, and, in advanced cases, cyanosis of the mucous membranes. Mortality is high.

The signs in hemorrhagic septicemia include hemorrhages on serous surfaces, blood-stained fluid in the thorax and abdomen, enteritis, and edema in the subcutaneous tissues. Edema is characteristic of the less acute forms of the disease. In subacute forms also, lesions can be confined to the pectoral region and include fluid in the pleural and pericardial sacs. Areas of pneumonia are present in the lungs together with greatly thickened septa. Large numbers of *P. multocida* are present in tissues and fluids. Some animals can be subclinically or chronically infected and therefore are of importance in maintaining the infection between enzootics. In carrier animals the organism is found in the tonsils and on the pharyngeal mucosa.

Fowl cholera, the pasteurellosis of birds, affects chickens principally, although ducks, geese, turkeys, swans, and other birds are susceptible. Wild birds frequently become infected and at times may be the source of infection for domestic flocks. *P. multocida* O antigen types 1, 3, and 4 and capsular type A are the most prevalent (Bhasin 1982). Carrier birds maintain the infection between enzootics. Transmission is by the oral and respiratory routes. Entry can occur through the eye and also through skin abrasions (Bierer and Derieux 1978). In many cases the disease is peracute and is manifested by an overwhelming bacteremia. Films prepared from blood or spleen pulp show large numbers of minute, bipolar-stained organisms. Outbreaks generally begin in a few birds in apparently healthy flocks. The daily mortality in a flock usually rises sharply, the peak normally being reached within a few days (Alberts and Graham 1948). The mortality varies from 10 to 75 percent.

The affected birds generally exhibit signs of depression, sleepiness, inappetence, and diarrhea. Death can occur within a few hours, or after 2 or 3 days. In some birds the course is much longer.

P. multocida is often associated with chronic infections of the air sacs, accompanied by accumulations of dry caseous material; with inflammatory processes in the wattles, especially of male birds, which frequently cause necrosis; and with infections of the mucous membranes of the head, a condition commonly called *colds.* The organism is frequently found in the peritoneal cavity of young laying birds mixed with yolk material from ruptured ova.

Fowl cholera causes serious economic losses on the duck farms of Long Island, New York, and on turkey farms in the western United States. Necropsy findings usually consist of a few petechiae of the heart, a slightly swollen spleen, and reddening of the mucosa of the anterior part of the intestine.

Rabbit septicemia can be very acute with hardly any premonitory signs. The causative organisms can easily be found in films prepared from blood or spleen pulp after death of the animal. A more common form of the disease is less acute. The affected animals are clearly ill for some days, during which they have fever, a seropurulent nasal discharge, inappetence, and, finally, difficult breathing. These animals suffer from fibrinous pneumonia, the greater part of the lungs often being hepatized and the pleura covered with fibrinous deposit. If such animals do not die within a few days, they become emaciated and usually are worthless afterward.

Snuffles is the common name applied to a milder respiratory infection caused by *P. multocida.* This disease initially involves only the upper respiratory tract. Affected animals exhibit mucopurulent exudate, which partially occludes the nares and frequently the conjunctiva. The animals have difficulty in breathing. The noises made by a colony of affected rabbits are characteristic and are responsible for the common name of the disease. In some cases the rabbits develop fibrinous pneumonia and die.

The lesions are minimal in rabbits with peracute cases of *P. multocida* septicemia and generally are limited to a few petechiae on the heart and some serous membranes. In rabbits with chronic cases the lesions as a rule are limited to the organs of the thorax.

P. multocida is also an important secondary invader of pneumonic lesions in cattle, sheep, swine, and goats, in which it is often a significant contributor to the morbidity and mortality associated with the syndrome commonly known as *shipping fever.* There is a marked tendency toward a seasonal incidence of shipping fever that corresponds with the activity of certain respiratory viral (parainfluenza 3, infectious bovine rhinotracheitis, bovine respiratory syncytial virus) and mycoplasmal infections. In the United States, this occurs in fall and early winter and is especially notable in large feedlot operations where young susceptible cattle are grouped together. In these populations respiratory viruses and mycoplasmas circulate rapidly and possibly pave the way for secondary invasions by pasteurellas.

Shipping fever characteristically begins a few days to a few weeks after transport. Affected animals cough, are febrile, and have a nasal discharge. The basic lesion is a bronchopneumonia with moderate amounts of fibrin on the lung surface. Other organisms are frequently present either concurrently (*P. haemolytica, Haemophilus somnus*) or later (*Actinomyces pyogenes*).

Factors other than transport are involved in outbreaks of *P. multocida* pneumonia of dairy cattle, in which *P. multocida* produces a high mortality in the northeastern United States (Rebhun and Fox 1981).

P. multocida has been associated with a fibrinous pneumonia in swine that in some animals is accompanied by

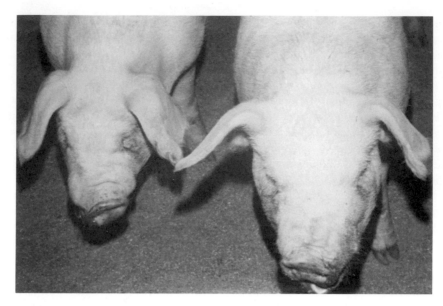

Figure 10.1. Atrophic rhinitis in swine. Note the lateral deviation of the snout. (Courtesy Barbara Straw.)

septicemia. Secondary opportunistic invasions also occur as complications of other viral or bacterial diseases such as enzootic pneumonia, contagious pleuropneumonia, influenza, and low-grade swine fever (hog cholera). The lungs have the same lesions as seen in cattle and rabbits. The anterior as well as the diaphragmatic lobes have a firm, liverlike texture. The surface is covered with a serofibrinous exudate, and a turbid fluid containing flakes of fibrin is found in the thoracic cavity. The cut surface of the involved lung is firm and mottled, some lobules being dark red and others grayish. The lobules often are widely separated by the interlobular connective tissue, which is distended by serofibrinous fluid. Other signs occasionally seen in swine include vegetative endocarditis, arthritis, and placentitis.

P. multocida capsular type D is involved with *Bordetella bronchiseptica* (see Chapter 11) in the pathogenesis of atrophic rhinitis (Figure 10.1). A proteinaceous dermonecrotoxin produced by type D and some type A strains of *P. multocida* can stimulate bone resorption in the area of the turbinates by suppressing osteoid synthesis (Pedersen and Elling 1984). The toxin alone has been shown to produce extensive degenerative lesions of the turbinates in 3-week-old gnotobiotic pigs (Rutter and Mackenzie 1984).

In addition to the diseases described above, *P. multocida* has been isolated from cases of mastitis in ewes and cows (Tucker 1953, Tunnicliff 1949), from outbreaks of keratoconjunctivitis in cattle (Garoiu et al. 1981), from a case of purulent leptomeningitis in a dog (Rogers and

Elder 1967), and from horses and a donkey with septicemia (Pavri and Apte 1967). The organism is a common contaminant of bite wounds inflicted by dogs and cats. Carter (1981) has provided an excellent review of the many recorded examples of sporadic *P. multocida* infections of humans and animals.

Immunity. Fowl cholera is notable as the first bacterial disease against which a successful vaccine was prepared (Pasteur 1880). Pasteur's vaccine was attenuated and consisted of living cultures of two grades of virulence administered a few days apart.

A protective antigen is found in the capsule of some *P. multocida* serotypes (Penn and Nagy 1974, 1976). The protective immunogen appears to be distinct from the typing antigens, and the protective immunologic relationship of strains cannot be predicted from their serologic characteristics (Cameron et al. 1980). Erler et al. (1983) found that protective antigen is present in saline extracts and stimulates both serum agglutinins and tracheal mucus IgA titers in calves immunized subcutaneously. Immunized calves were protected only against experimental challenge by the homologous serotype. A protective antigen for turkeys of type 1 and type 3 strains has been shown to be a protein of molecular weight 69,000 (Kajikawa and Matsumoto 1984). In type A organisms the protective immunogen may be a glycoprotein. In one study this antigen elicited an agglutinating and bactericidal antibody response in calves (Mukkur 1978).

Commercial *P. multocida* bacterins are most effective in stimulating protection against hemorrhagic septicemia and fowl cholera caused by homologous serotypes. Although widely used in cattle, they are relatively ineffective in stimulating local protection in the bovine respiratory tract. Vaccine failure may in part be due to the poor quality of available bacterins and to the fact that *P. multocida* is a much less frequent cause of bovine pneumonic pasteurellosis than is *P. haemolytica*. There are, however, reports of successful use of bacterins in the prevention of pneumonia in pigs (Bennewitz et al. 1983).

Vaccination programs based on bacterins that contain the essential protective surface antigens have been successfully used in the control of hemorrhagic septicemia in Africa and Asia (Carter 1967). The strain used for bacterin production must be the same as that causing the disease in the field. Preliminary field vaccination trials with a live streptomycin-dependent mutant of *P. multocida* type B have been encouraging (Alivis and Carter 1980). A similar vaccine has been shown to be protective for rabbits (Chengappa et al. 1980). A live *P. multocida* vaccine has also been shown to produce significant antibody and protective responses in beef calves and other animals (Kucera et al. 1981, Panciera et al. 1984).

Live avirulent vaccines administered in drinking water are widely used in the control of cholera in chickens, ducks, and turkeys (Bierer and Derieux 1972). A combination of oral and wing-web administration has also been used and appears to provide protection that is superior to that produced by oral administration alone (Ghazikhanian et al. 1983). Attenuated fowl cholera vaccine (strain CA) has been shown to be effective in the field in protecting swine against pasteurellosis caused by *P. multocida* types 5A and 8A (Chen et al. 1985).

P. multocida bacterins combined with *B. bronchiseptica* have been used in some areas to successfully reduce the prevalence and severity of clinical atrophic rhinitis in swine (Baars et al. 1986, De Jong et al. 1986). Vaccination of sows yields antibody to the dermonecrotoxin of *P. multocida* type D that is available to the sucking piglet in the colostrum and milk. Bording and Riising (1986) found, however, that a combination of vaccination of sows and immunization of 5- to 8-week-old piglets reduced the prevalence of atrophic rhinitis to a statistically greater extent than when only sows were vaccinated.

Diagnosis. *P. multocida* is readily seen in smears prepared from blood or spleen tissue of animals with septicemia or bacteremia. Smears prepared from material from pneumonic lesions can also reveal the organism, although it can be difficult to see because of its small size.

P. multocida grows well on blood but not on Mac-Conkey agar. Final identification is based on the criteria listed in Table 10.2. The results from commercially available identification systems may not be reliable and should be supplemented with tests based on media prepared in the laboratory. Counterimmunoelectrophoresis has been used to identify antigens of *P. multocida* types B and E in serum or tissues of animals with septicemia (Carter and Chengappa 1981).

Antimicrobial Susceptibility. *P. multocida* is sensitive to penicillin, ampicillin, cephalothin, chloramphenicol, gentamicin, tetracycline, nitrofurans, kanamycin, streptomycin, sulfonamides, trimethoprim, tylosin, spiramycin, and spectinomycin. Since strains from feedlot cattle and from poultry can be resistant to one or more of these antimicrobials for (Berman and Hirsh 1978, Fales et al. 1982), selection of antimicrobials treatment or prevention should be based on the results of susceptibility testing.

The Disease in Humans. Animals constitute the most important source of pasteurellosis for humans, although many of these infections cannot be proved to have resulted from animal contact (Biberstein 1979). The species of *Pasteurella* involved include *multocida, dagmatis,* and *canis* (Mutters et al. 1985). Resultant diseases include meningitis, abscesses, septicemia, and wound infections. Most wound infections result from animal bites. Infected bite wounds are slow to heal and exude a dirty, watery discharge.

REFERENCES

Alberts, J.D., and Graham, R. 1948. Fowl cholera in turkeys. North Am. Vet. 29:24–26.

Baars, J.C., Pennings, A., and Storm, P.K. 1986. Challenge and field experiments with an experimental atrophic rhinitis vaccine containing *Pasteurella multocida* DNT-toxoid and *Bordetella bronchiseptica*. In Proceedings of the 9th International Congress of the Pig Veterinary Society, Barcelona, Spain. P. 247.

Bennewitz, D., Achtzehn, W., and Kessel, H. 1983. Preventing pneumonia due to *Pasteurella multocida* in weaned piglets and fattening pigs by means of Dessau *Pasteurella* absorbed vaccine. Monatsh. Veterinärmed. 38:448–451.

Berman, S.M., and Hirsh, D.C. 1978. Partial characterization of R-plasmids from *Pasteurella multocida* isolated from turkeys. Antimicrob. Agents Chemother. 14:348–352.

Bhasin, J.L. 1982. Serological types of *Pasteurella multocida* isolated from turkeys and chickens in Canada. Can. J. Microbiol. 28:1078–1080.

Biberstein, E.L., 1979. The pasteurelloses. In J.H. Steele, ed, CRC Handbook Series in Zoonoses. Section A: Bacterial, Rickettsial and Mycotic Diseases. CRC Press, Boca Raton, Fla. Pp. 485–514.

Bierer, B.W., and Derieux, W.T. 1972. Immunologic response of turkeys to an avirulent *Pasteurella multocida* vaccine in the drinking water. Poult. Sci. 51:408–416.

Bierer, B.W., and Derieux, W.T. 1978. Exposing turkeys by various routes to an avirulent and virulent strains of *Pasteurella multocida*. Poult. Sci. 52:2290–2298.

Bording, A., and Riising, H.-J. 1986. Vaccination against atrophic rhinitis. A field study on Atrinord. In Proceedings of the 9th International Congress of the Pig Veterinary Society, Barcelona, Spain. P. 247.

Cameron, C.M., Piennaar, L., and Vermeulen, A.S. 1980. Lack of cross-immunity among *Pasteurella multocida* type A strains. Onderstepoort J. Vet. Res. 47:213–219.

Carter, G.R. 1955. Studies on *Pasteurella multocida* I. A hemagglutination test for the identification of serological types. Am. J. Vet. Res. 16:481–484.

Carter, G.R. 1967. Pasteurellosis: *Pasteurella multocida* and *Pasteurella haemolytica*. Adv. Vet. Sci. 11:321–379.

Carter, G.R. 1976. A proposal for five biotypes of *Pasteurella multocida*. In 19th Annual Proceedings of the American Association of Veterinary Laboratory Diagnosticians. AAVLD, Inc., Brookings, S. Dak. Pp. 189–196.

Carter, G.R. 1981. Pasteurelloses. In J. Balows and B. Hausler, eds., Diagnostic Procedures in Bacterial, Mycotic and Parasitic Infections, 6th ed. American Public Health Association, Washington, D.C. Pp. 551–563.

Carter, G.R. 1984. *Pasteurella*. In J.G. Holt and N.R. Kreig, eds., Bergey's Manual of Systematic Bacteriology, vol. 1. Williams & Wilkins, Baltimore. Pp. 552–557.

Carter, G.R., and Chengappa, M.M. 1986. Identification of types B and E *Pasteurella multocida* by counterimmunoelectrophoresis. Vet. Rec. 108:145–146.

Chen, T.J., Liang, J.H., Li, H.J., Zong, M.Z., and Wang, Z.M. 1985. Immunity conferred by attenuated fowl cholera vaccines to pasteurellosis (serotype A) in pigs. Guangdong Agric. Sc. 2:37–41.

Chengappa, M.M., Myers, R.C., and Carter, G.R. 1980. A streptomycin-dependent live *Pasteurella multocida* vaccine for the prevention of rabbit pasteurellosis. Lab. Anim. Sci. 30:515–518.

de Alivis, M.C.L., and Carter, G.R. 1980. Preliminary field trials with a streptomycin-dependent vaccine against haemorrhagic septicaemia. Vet. Rec. 106:435–437.

De Jong, M.F., Bouwkamp, F.T., and Oosterwoud, R.A. 1986. The results of a field evaluation with the Nobi-Vac AR vaccine after a period of three years. In Proceedings of the 9th International Congress of the Pig Veterinary Society, Barcelona, Spain. P. 243.

Erler, W., Schonherr, W., Heilmann, P., Kielstein, P., Muller, G., First, H., and Flossmann, K.D. 1983. Immunogenicity of *Pasteurella multocida* extracts in calves against pasteurellosis. Monatsh. Veterinärmed. 38:87–92.

Fales, W.H., Selby, L.A., Webber, J.J., Hoffman, L.J., Kintner, L.D., Nelson, S.C., Miller, R.B., Thorne, J.G., McGinity, J.T., and Smith, D.K. 1982. Antimicrobial resistance among *Pasteurella* spp. recovered from Missouri and Iowa cattle with bovine respiratory disease complex. J. Am. Vet. Med. Assoc. 181:477–479.

Frederiksen, W. 1971. A taxonomic study of *Pasteurella* and *Actinobacillus* strains. J. Gen. Microbiol. 69:viii.

Frederiksen, W. 1973. *Pasteurella* taxonomy and nomenclature. Contrib. Microbiol. Immunol. 2:170.

Garoiu, M., Levinschi, A., and Istrate, N. 1981. Isolation of *Pasteurella multocida* during an outbreak of infectious keratoconjunctivitis in cattle. Rev. Cresterea Anim. 31:55–58.

Ghazikhanian, G.Y., Duncan, W.M., and Kelly, B.J. 1983. Immunization of turkey breeder hens against fowl cholera by combined oral and wing-web administration of attenuated (CU) *Pasteurella multocida*. Avian Dis. 27:133–140.

Ghoniem, N., Amtsberg, G., and Bisping, W. 1973. Comparative studies of the biochemical reactions of *Pasteurella multocida* strains from dogs and pigs. Zentralbl. Veterinärmed. [B] 20:310–317.

Heddleston, K.L., Gallagher, J.E., and Rebers, P.A. 1972. Fowl cholera: Gel diffusion precipitin test for serotyping *Pasteurella multocida* from avian species. Avian Dis. 16:925–936.

Kajikawa, O., and Matsumoto, M., 1984. A protective antigen for turkeys purified from a type 1 strain of *Pasteurella multocida*. Vet. Microbiol. 10:43–55.

Kucera, C.J., Wong, J.C.S., and Eis, R.C. 1981. Development of a chemically altered *Pasteurella multocida* vaccinal strain. Am. J. Vet. Res. 42:1389–1394.

Mukkur, T.K.S. 1978. Immunologic and physiologic responses of calves inoculated with potassium thiocyanate extract of *Pasteurella multocida* type A. Am. J. Vet. Res. 39:1269–1273.

Namioka, S., and Murata, M. 1961. Serological studies on *Pasteurella multocida*. II. Characteristics of somatic (O) antigen of the organism. Cornell Vet. 51:507–521.

Panciera, R.J., Corstvet, R.E., Confer, A.W., and Greshen, C.N. 1984. Bovine pneumonic pasteurellosis: Effect of vaccination with live *Pasteurella* species. Am. J. Vet. Res. 45:2538–2542.

Pasteur, M. 1880. Mémoires et communications des membres et des correspondants de L'Académie. Sur le choléra des poules; études des conditions de la non-récidive de la maladie et de quelques autres de ses caractères. C. R. Acad. Sci. 90:239–257, 952–958, 1030–1033.

Pavri, K.M., and Apte, V.H. 1967. Isolation of *Pasteurella multocida* from a fatal disease of horses and donkeys in India. Vet. Rec. 80:437–439.

Pedersen, K.B., and Elling, F. 1984. The pathogenesis of atrophic rhinitis in pigs induced by toxigenic *Pasteurella multocida*. J. Comp. Pathol. 94:203–214.

Penn, C.W., and Nagy, L.K. 1974. Capsular and somatic antigens of *Pasteurella multocida* types B and E. Res. Vet. Sci. 16:251–259.

Penn, C.W., and Nagy, L.K. 1976. Isolation of a protective, non-toxic capsular antigen from *Pasteurella multocida* types B and E. Res. Vet. Sci. 20:90–96.

Rebhun, W.C., and Fox, F.H. 1981. *Pasteurella* bronchopneumonia in adult dairy cattle. Med. Vet. Proc. 62:763–765.

Roberts, R.S. 1947. An immunological study of *Pasteurella septica*. J. Comp. Pathol. 57:261–278.

Rogers, R.J., and Elder, J.K. 1967. Purulent leptomeningitis in a dog associated with an aerogenic *Pasteurella multocida*. Aust. Vet. J. 43:81–82.

Rutter, J.M., and Mackenzie, A. 1984. Pathogenesis of atrophic rhinitis in pigs: A new perspective. Vet. Rec. 114:89–90.

Tucker, E.W. 1953. A case of natural *Pasteurella multocida* mastitis. Cornell Vet. 43:378–380.

Tunnicliff, E.A. 1949. *Pasteurella* mastitis in ewes. Vet. Med. 44:498–502.

Yates, W.D.G. 1982. A review of infectious bovine rhinotracheitis, shipping fever pneumonia, and viral-bacterial synergism in respiratory disease of cattle. Can. J. Comp. Med. 46:225–263.

Pasteurella haemolytica

P. haemolytica was first recognized during studies of bovine hemorrhagic septicemia (Jones 1921). Because the hemolytic colonies were readily distinguishable from those of *P. multocida*, the new organism was named *P. haemolytica*. It has since been recognized as an important cause of pneumonia in domestic ruminants and of mastitis (bluebag) and septicemia in sheep, and as an essential component of the etiology of shipping fever in cattle. It has been isolated from poultry on a few occasions (Heddleston 1975).

Although two biotypes (A and T) of *P. haemolytica* have been recognized for many years, there is now compelling evidence that *P. haemolytica* biotype A should be transferred to the genus *Actinobacillus* (Mutters et al. 1985, Pohl 1981). Because this change has not yet appeared in the primary literature, the traditional nomenclature will be followed in this chapter.

Morphology and Staining Reactions. The cells of *P. haemolytica* are very similar in shape and staining reaction to those of *P. multocida*, although they may be larger.

Table 10.4. Host distribution and frequency of occurrence of biotypes and serotypes of *P. haemolytica*

Host	Biotype and serotype	Disease	Frequency
Cattle	A1	Bronchopneumonia (shipping fever, transit fever)	Most frequent
	A2	Bronchopneumonia	Frequent
	A6, T3, T4	Bronchopneumonia, mastitis	Sporadic
	A7, A9, A11	Septicemia, meningitis	
	Untypable	Bronchopneumonia	Sporadic
Sheep	A2	Bronchopneumonia, mastitis	Most frequent
	T3, T4, T10, T15	Septicemia, arthritis	Sporadic
	A1, A6	Bronchopneumonia, mastitis	Sporadic
	A5, A7, A9, A11, A13, A14	Bronchopneumonia	Infrequent
	Untypable	Bronchopneumonia	Infrequent

Capsules are present on new isolates but can be lost on subculture unless maintained on Sawata's medium.

Cultural and Biochemical Features. The colonies of biotype A are gray and surrounded by a zone of hemolysis. Colonies of biotype T are larger (2 mm) and have brownish centers. They are also hemolytic. Biotype A strains ferment arabinose within 7 days, and biotype T ferments trehalose within 2 days. Biotype A strains have a much greater sensitivity to penicillin. The mol% G + C of the DNA is 42.3 to 43.6 (Tm).

The differentiation of *P. haemolytica* from *P. multocida* and other *Pasteurella* species is shown in Table 10.2.

Antigens and Serologic Classification. There are at least 15 serotypes based on capsular antigens. Serotyping is performed by passive hemagglutination or by a rapid plate agglutination test and can be done only on strains that are encapsulated (Biberstein et al. 1960). Biotype A comprises serotypes 1, 2, 5, 6, 7, 8, 9, 11, 12, 13, and 14. Serotypes 3, 4, 10, and 15 are found only among biotype T strains.

Strains are usually designated by biotype and serotype—for example, A1. Table 10.4 shows the distribution of serotypes and biotypes by host species, disease produced, and frequency of occurrence of the serotypes and biotypes within a given host species. For further information, see the reviews by Gilmour (1980), Frank (1979), and Yates (1982).

Epizootiology and Pathogenesis. *P. haemolytica* is maintained as a commensal of the nasopharynx of cattle, sheep, and goats. Given the appropriate circumstances it is a devastating pathogen of great economic importance to the beef cattle and feeder lamb industries.

The disease in cattle. Naturally occurring outbreaks of disease in cattle caused by *P. haemolytica* are typically associated with the presence of predisposing factors. These include a variety of stresses such as transport, harsh climate, castration, and dipping. The disease usually appears within 2 weeks of arrival in the feedlot. *P. haemolytica* type A1 is the strain commonly found in epizootics of shipping fever, or transit fever, in cattle and in enzootic pneumonia of calves. Type A2 and other, untypable strains occasionally occur. Several studies have indicated that the number of *P. haemolytica* type A1 organisms increases greatly in the nasopharynx of cattle during and after shipment (Frank and Smith 1983, Hoerlein et al. 1961, Thomson et al. 1969); this type replaces type A2, the type most common in normal calves before shipment (Frank and Smith 1983). The proliferation of type A1 in the nasopharynx of calves that have been transported or otherwise stressed results in many more organisms entering the trachea, thereby increasing the probability of deposition of organisms in the lung parenchyma. Production and release of cytotoxin then compromises lung clearance, which is mediated by alveolar macrophages and other phagocytic cells.

All serotypes of *P. haemolytica* produce a chromosomally encoded proteinaceous cytotoxin consisting of two proteins of molecular weights 20,000 and 102,000. The toxin incapacitates alveolar macrophages and polymorphonuclear neutrophils (Berggren et al. 1981, Lo et al. 1987, Markham and Wilkie 1980). It can thus directly impair lung defenses as well as indirectly contribute to the inflammatory process by causing release of inflammatory mediators and enzymes from leukocytes. The toxin is related to the alpha toxin of *Escherichia coli* and is released in the early growth phase of the organism (Lo et al. 1987, Shewen and Wilkie 1985). Its mechanism of action is unknown but probably involves formation of pores in host cell membranes. A protease with specificity for sialoglycopeptides has been detected in the supernatant of cytotoxic cultures, but its relationship to cytotoxin has not been determined (Otulakowski et al. 1983).

The organism survives and multiplies, producing lesions of fibrinous pleuropenumonia in the anteroventral areas of the lungs. The distribution of the lesions is not as would be expected if microdroplets were the only means of transfer of the organism. Because inhaled microdroplets are distributed more evenly in the lung parenchyma, it has been suggested that the lesions are predominantly ventral owing to downward drainage of exudates initially produced in the posterodorsal regions of the lung (Lillie 1974).

Selective proliferation of type A1 in the nasopharynx of stressed cattle has not been explained. Nasopharyngeal mucus production is greatly increased in these animals, and the resulting larger volume of exudate clearly would favor formation of endogenous droplets that during inspiration could carry the proliferating *P. haemolytica* deeper into the respiratory tract. Perhaps more virulent clones emerge during the initial proliferation in the nasopharynx and are subsequently transmitted from calf to calf in aerosols, thereby helping to maintain and extend the epizootic after the effects of the initial shipment or other stress have passed. This might explain the observed transmission of the disease to unstressed animals that come in contact with infected animals (Gibbs et al. 1984, Lillie 1974).

Even though the above sequence of events is plausible for the pathogenesis of *P. haemolytica* pneumonia in cattle, it must be emphasized that the lower respiratory tract of healthy cattle is highly resistant to invasion by *P. haemolytica*; experimental production of lung lesions in such animals has required the administration of heroic numbers of the organism directly into the lung or lower trachea (Friend et al. 1977, Panciera and Corstvet 1984b, Wilkie et al. 1980). Only a very few of the many researchers of this disease have succeeded in producing pneumonia with a mode of exposure that closely mimics the one that probably occurs in the field (Gibbs et al. 1984). Why it is difficult to produce disease under experimental conditions is not yet known. Perhaps the challenge strain is changed during in vitro culture, or perhaps researchers have failed to duplicate the physiological and microbiological conditions that exist in the nasopharynx of a calf that is stressed by transport and is mixed with other animals of varied origin and microbiological status.

The role of antecedent or concurrent viral infection in the pathogenesis of *P. haemolytica* pneumonia of cattle has been studied and debated for many years (Yates 1982, 1984). A variety of microbial agents including parainfluenza 3 (PI-3) virus, bovine respiratory syncytial virus, bovine virus diarrhea virus, infectious bovine rhinotracheitis virus (herpes 1), *Mycoplasma* species, and *Ehrlichia phagocytophilia* can circulate rapidly in recently grouped populations of young cattle, participating in the pathogenesis of respiratory disease.

Experimental infections with PI-3 virus or infectious bovine rhinotracheitis virus have been shown to predispose calves to *P. haemolytica* pneumonia when the animals were exposed to the bacteria at least 4 days after exposure to the viral agents (Jericho and Langford 1978, Lopez et al. 1976). In the case of PI-3 virus infection the greatest effect on clearance of *P. haemolytica* was observed when the bacterial challenge was given 7 days after the virus challenge. Sheep exhibit a similar enhanced susceptibility when PI-3 virus is given 6 days before challenge with *P. haemolytica* (Davies et al. 1981). Viral infection impairs the bacterial-clearance abilities of alveolar macrophages, possibly increases the number of receptor sites for bacterial adhesion, damages the mucociliary clearance mechanism, and causes accumulation of exudate that can act as a substrate for bacterial growth.

The clinical signs of *P. haemolytica* pneumonia in cattle include severe dyspnea, fever, a soft cough, nasal discharge, and anorexia. The course of the disease is more acute than that caused by *P. multocida*, and animals may be found dead without premonitory signs. The lesions are those of fibrinous pleuropneumonia, predominantly affecting the anteroventral areas of the lungs.

The disease in sheep.   Two distinct syndromes, pneumonia and septicemia, are associated with *P. haemolytica* infection in sheep. Organisms of biotype A are involved in enzootic and sporadic pneumonias, whereas biotype T strains commonly cause an acute septicemic disease of lambs during fall and early winter. Biotype T strains have a special tropism for the tonsils of sheep and are rarely found elsewhere in healthy animals (Gilmore et al. 1974).

Young lambs quickly acquire biotype A strains from the ewe. These strains dominate in the tonsils for the first few weeks of life. As the animal gets older, the biotype A strains are gradually replaced by biotype T strains (Al-Sulton and Aitken 1985).

The enzootic and sporadic pneumonias resemble shipping fever in calves. However, transport is not as notable a component in the pathogenesis of the disease in sheep. Rather, other stresses such as bad weather, dipping, or castration as well as infections by other microbial agents are the important predisposing factors (Gilmour 1980).

In Europe, outbreaks of pneumonia are seen in late spring and early summer and can involve both lambs and ewes. In lambs raised intensively, outbreaks can occur immediately after grouping or subsequently.

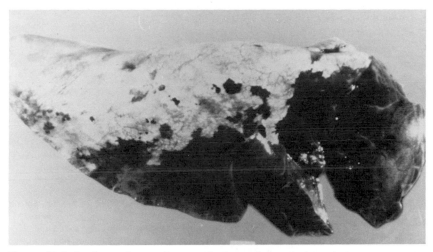

Figure 10.2. Lesions of acute *Pasteurella haemolytica* pneumonia in the lung of a sheep. (Courtesy Dept. of Pathology, Ontario Veterinary College.)

The onset of the disease is rapid and is usually characterized by the deaths of one or two lambs and respiratory illness of varying degrees of severity in the remainder of the group. Acutely affected animals are febrile, cough, and have ocular and nasal discharges and diarrhea. As much as 10 percent of the flock can be affected acutely. Chronically affected animals are unthrifty and usually have secondary lesions caused by *Actinomyces pyogenes.*

The lesions in acute enzootic pneumonia of sheep are hemorrhagic bronchopneumonia with effusive pleurisy and pericarditis. Lung lesions involve the anterior and ventral areas (Figure 10.2). Young lambs can develop an acutely swollen and edematous lung together with evidence of generalized septicemia (Gilmour 1980).

A form of mastitis known as *bluebag* is caused by *P. haemolytica* in ewes near the end of lactation. It is probable that the infection is derived from the noses or mouths of suckling lambs. The affected portion of the gland may slough.

Septicemic pasteurellosis associated with biotype T strains of *P. haemolytica* is usually seen in older sheep. The stress of dietary change is a well-established predisposing factor. Mucosal damage in the pharynx and intestine allows entry of organisms that are normally maintained as commensals in the tonsils. Simultaneously, the elevated hydrocortisone levels induced by the stress of dietary change result in immunosuppression, which allows multiplication of the invading *P. haemolytica* in the regional lymphatics. The organisms are then carried to the lungs, where they lodge, multiply, and release endotoxin

(Gilmour 1980, Suarez-Guemes 1985). The lesions consist of necrotic erosions of the posterior pharynx and abomasum, subcutaneous hemorrhages, and uniform distention of the lungs with fluid. Necrotic foci can also be present in the liver. Death is sudden. The sporadic occurrence of cases in a flock emphasizes the endogenous nature of the infection.

The disease in swine. *P. haemolytica* has been observed in localized lung lesions in pigs. No clinical abnormalities were associated with the lesions (Taylor 1983).

The disease in horses. Ulcerative lymphangitis caused by *P. haemolytica* has been reported in two horses on the same farm (Miller and Dresher 1981).

Immunity. *P. haemolytica* is very sensitive to antibody and complement-mediated killing in bovine serum (MacDonald et al. 1983). Clearance from the lung in calves is enhanced by previous exposure to the organism, and pulmonary lavage fluid shows antibody activity of both IgA and IgG isotypes (Walker et al. 1980). Prior natural exposure of calves to *P. haemolytica* confers a heightened resistance of lung tissue to experimental challenge (Confer et al. 1984). Pancicra et al. (1984) found that a similar level of protection was obtained by exposing calves to an aerosol of *P. haemolytica*, and levels of serum antibodies were correlated with resistance of the lungs to the development of lesions.

Protection is mediated by antibodies to cytotoxin (Cho et al. 1984) and to capsular antigen (Confer et al. 1987, Gonzalez-Rayos et al. 1986). Both of these protective antigens are present in culture supernatants of *P.*

haemolytica and were probably the basis of the success of the aggressin-type vaccines used years ago to reduce losses in U.S. stockyards (Buckley and Gochenour 1924, Miller 1927). Commercially available bacterins, however, have been found to be ineffective in the field and can actually potentiate rather than diminish the clinical signs and pathologic lesions (Confer et al. 1984, Martin 1983), although addition of Freund's complete or incomplete adjuvant to bacterins has been shown to improve their ability to stimulate resistance to experimental challenge (Confer et al. 1987). The failure of bacterins may in part be due to a lack of cytotoxin, because stationary phase cultures are commonly used for commercial bacterin production (Shewen and Wilkie 1985). Cytotoxin is associated mainly with logarithmic phase culture.

A live intradermal vaccine has been shown to be effective in reducing losses of beef and dairy calves due to pneumonia (Confer et al. 1985, Panciera et al. 1984, Smith et al. 1985). The success of this form of vaccine appears to be due to antigenic stimulation by cytotoxin released during replication of the live vaccine in the host. In lambs serum antibody protects against septicemic pasteurellosis (Cowen and McBeath 1982). Vaccines for control of ovine enzootic pneumonia have also been available for many years despite a lack of convincing proof of efficacy. Since protective immunity is serotype-specific, successful field vaccination programs require the use of multivalent vaccines (Gilmour 1980). Type A2, a common strain in the field, is poorly immunogenic, thus researchers have been unable to produce a vaccine against infection by this strain. Vaccines against septicemia caused by biotype T strains have not been widely used.

Diagnosis. The presence of *P. haemolytica* in nasal swabs is of little diagnostic value. Material from tracheal aspirates or from lung lesions at necropsy must be cultured on blood agar. Examination of sections of affected lung tissue will reveal the presence of "oat cells"—a pathognomic finding in enzootic pneumonia (Gilmour 1980). Antibody assays yield little useful information for diagnosis.

Antimicrobial Susceptibility. *P. haemolytica* is sensitive to the same wide range of antimicrobials as *P. multocida*. But because resistant strains are frequently encountered, susceptibility testing should be routinely practiced.

REFERENCES

Al-Sulton, I.I., and Aitken, I.D. 1985. The tonsillar carriage of *Pasteurella haemolytica* in lambs. J. Comp. Pathol. 95:193–210.

Berggren, K.A., Baluyut, C.S., Simonson, R.R., Bemrick, W.J., and

Maheswaranm, S.K. 1981. Cytotoxic effects of *Pasteurella haemolytica* on bovine neutrophils. Am. J. Vet. Res. 42:1383–1388.

Biberstein, E.L., Gills, M., and Knight, H. 1960. Serological types of *Pasteurella haemolytica*. Cornell Vet. 50:283–300.

Buckley, J.S., and Gochenour, W.S. 1924. Immunization against hemorrhagic septicemia. J. Am. Vet. Med. Assoc. 66:308–311.

Cho, H.J., Bohac, J.G., Yates, W.D.G., and Ohmann, H.B. 1984. Anticytotoxin-activity of bovine sera and body fluids against *Pasteurella haemolytica* A1 cytotoxin. Can. J. Comp. Med. 48:151–155.

Confer, A.W., Panciera, R.J., and Fulton, R.W. 1984. Effect of prior natural exposure to *Pasteurella haemolytica* on resistance to experimental bovine pneumonic pasteurellosis. Am. J. Vet. Res. 45:2622–2624.

Confer, A.W., Panciera, R.J., Fulton, R.W., Gentry, M.J., and Rummage, J.A. 1985. Effect of vaccination with live or killed *Pasteurella haemolytica* on resistance to experimental bovine pneumonic pasteurellosis. Am. J. Vet. Res. 46:342-346.

Confer, A.W., Panciera, R.J., Gentry, M.J., and Fulton, R.W. 1987. Immunologic response to *Pasteurella haemolytica* and resistance against experimental bovine pneumonic pasteurellosis, induced by bacterins in oil adjuvants. Am. J. Vet. Res. 48:163–168.

Cowan, S., and McBeath, D.G. 1982. Passive protection of lambs against septicaemic pasteurellosis. Vet. Rec. 111:185–186.

Davies, D.H., Herceg, M., Jones, B.A.H., and Thurley, D.C. 1981. The pathogenesis of sequential infection with parainfluenza virus type 3 and *Pasteurella haemolytica* in sheep. Vet. Microbiol. 6:173–182.

Frank, G.H. 1979. *Pasteurella haemolytica* and respiratory disease in cattle. Proc. U.S. Anim. Health. Assoc. 83:153–160.

Frank, G.H., and Smith, P.C. 1983. Prevalence of *Pasteurella haemolytica* in transported calves. Am. J. Vet. Res. 44:981–985.

Friend, S.C.E., Thomson, R.G., Wilkie, B.N., and Barnum, D.A. 1977. Bovine pneumonic pasteurellosis: Experimental induction in vaccinated and unvaccinated calves. Can. J. Comp. Med. 41:77–83.

Gibbs, H.A. 1983. Experimental bovine pneumonic pasteurellosis. (Correspondence.) Vet. Rec. 113:144.

Gibbs, H.A., Allan, E.M., Wiseman, A., and Selman, I.E. 1984. Experimental production of bovine pneumonic pasteurellosis. Res. Vet. Sci. 37:154–166.

Gibbs, H.A., Allen, M.J., Wiseman, A., and Selman, I.E. 1983. Pneumonic pasteurellosis in housed, weaned single suckled calves. Vet. Rec. 112:87.

Gilmour, N.J.L. 1980. *Pasteurella haemolytica* infections in sheep. Vet. Quart. 2:191–198.

Gilmour, N.J.L., Thompson, D.A., and Fraser, J. 1974. The recovery of *Pasteurella haemolytica* from the tonsils of adult sheep. Res. Vet. Sci. 17:413–414.

Gonzalez-Rayos, C., Lo, R.Y.C., Shewen, P.E., and Beneridge, T.J. 1986. Cloning of a serotype-specific antigen from *Pasteurella haemolytica* A1. Infect. Immun. 53:505–510.

Heddleston, K.L. 1975. Pasteurellosis. In S.B. Hitchner, C.H. Domermuth, H.G. Purchase, and J.E. Williams, eds., Isolation and Identification of Avian Pathogens. Arnold Printing Corp., Ithaca, N.Y. Pp. 38–50.

Hoerlein, A.B., Sazena, S.P., and Mansfield, M.E. 1961. Studies on shipping fever of cattle. II. Prevalence of *Pasteurella* species in nasal secretions from normal calves and calves with shipping fever. Am. J. Vet. Res. 22:470–472.

Jericho, K.W.F., and Langford, E.V. 1978. Pneumonia in calves produced with aerosols of bovine herpesvirus 1 and *Pasteurella haemolytica*. Can. J. Comp. Med. 42:269–277.

Jones, F.S. 1921. A study of *Bacillus bovisepticus*. J. Exp. Med. 34:561.

Lillie, L.E. 1974. The bovine respiratory disease complex. Can. Vet. J. 15:233–242.

Lo, R.Y., Strathdee, C.A., and Shewen, P.E. 1987. Nucleotide sequence of the leukotoxin genes of *Pasteurella haemolytica* A1. Infect. Immun. 55:1987–1996.

Lopez, A., Thomson, R.G., and Savan, M. 1976. The pulmonary clearance of *Pasteurella hemolytica* in calves infected with bovine parainfluenza-3 virus. Can. J. Comp. Med. 40:385–391.

MacDonald, J.T., Matheswaran, S.K., Opuda-Asibo, J., Townsend, E.L., and Thies, E.S. 1983. Susceptibility of *Pasteurella haemolytica* to the bactericidal effects of serum, nasal secretions and bronchoalveolar washings from cattle. Vet. Microbiol. 8:585–599.

Markham, R.J.F., and Wilkie, B.N. 1980. Interaction between *Pasteurella haemolytica* and bovine alveolar macrophages: Cytotoxic effect on macrophages and impaired phagocytosis. Am. J. Vet. Res. 41:18–22.

Martin, S.W. 1983. Vaccination: Is it effective in preventing respiratory disease or influencing weight gains in feedlot calves? Can. Vet. J. 24:10–19.

Miller, A.W. 1927. Report of committee on miscellaneous transmissible diseases: Hemorrhagic septicemia. J. Am. Vet. Med. Assoc. 70:952–955.

Miller, R.M., and Dresher, L.K. 1981. Equine ulcerative lymphangitis caused by *Pasteurella hemolytica* (2 case reports). Vet. Med./Small Anim. Clin. 76:1335–1338.

Mutters, R., Ihm, P., Pohl, S., Frederiksen, W., and Mannheim, W. 1985. Reclassification of the genus *Pasteurella* Trevisan 1887 on the basis of deoxyribonucleic acid homology, with proposals for the new species *Pasteurella dagmatis*, *Pasteurella canis*, *Pasteurella stomatis*, *Pasteurella anatis*, and *Pasteurella langaa*. Int. J. Syst. Bacteriol. 35:309–322.

Otulakowski, G.L., Shewen, P.E., Udoh, A.E., Mellors, A., and Wilkie, B.N. 1983. Proteolysis of sialoglycoprotein by *Pasteurella haemolytica* cytotoxic culture supernatant. Infect. Immun. 42:64–70.

Panciera, R.J., and Corstvet, R.E. 1984. Bovine pneumonic pasteurellosis: Model for *Pasteurella haemolytica* and *Pasteurella multocida*–induced pneumonia in cattle. Am. J. Vet. Res. 45:2532–2537.

Panciera, R.J., Corstvet, R.E., Confer, A.W., and Gresham, C.N. 1984. Bovine pneumonic pasteurellosis: Effect of vaccination with live *Pasteurella* species. Am. J. Vet. Res. 45:2538–2542.

Pohl, S. 1981. DNA relatedness among members of *Actinobacillus*, *Haemophilus* and *Pasteurella*. In M. Kilian, W. Frederiksen, and E.L. Biberstein, eds., *Haemophilus, Pasteurella and Actinobacillus*. Academic Press, London. Pp. 246–253.

Shewen, P.E., and Wilkie, B.N. 1985. Evidence for the *Pasteurella haemolytica* cytotoxin as a product of actively growing bacteria. Am. J. Vet. Res. 46:1212–1214.

Smith, C.K., Davidson, J.N., and Henry, C.W. 1985. Evaluating a live vaccine for *Pasteurella haemolytica* in dairy calves. Vet. Med. 80:78–80.

Suarez-Guemes, F., Collins, M.T., and Whiteman, C.E. 1985. Experimental reproduction of septicemic pasteurellosis in feedlot lambs: Bacteriologic and pathologic examinations. Am. J. Vet. Res. 46:193–201.

Taylor, D.J. 1983. Pig Diseases, 3d ed. Burlington Press, Cambridge, England. Pp. 111–114.

Thomson, G.S., Benson, M.L., and Savan, M. 1969. Pneumonic pasteurellosis of cattle: Microbiology and immunology. Can. J. Comp. Med. 33:194–206.

Walker, R.D., Corstvet, R.E., Lessley, B.A., and Panciera, R.J. 1980. Study of bovine pulmonary response to *Pasteurella haemolytica*: Specificity of immunoglobulins isolated from the bovine lung. Am. J. Vet. Res. 41:1015–1023.

Wilkie, B.N., Markham, R.J.F., and Shewen, P.E. 1980. Response of calves to lung challenge exposure with *Pasteurella haemolytica* after parenteral or pulmonary vaccination. Am. J. Vet. Res. 41:1773–1778.

Yates, W.D.G. 1982. A review of infectious bovine rhinotracheitis, shipping fever pneumonia, and viral-bacterial synergism in respiratory disease of cattle. Can. J. Comp. Med. 46:225–263.

Yates, W.D.G. 1984. Interaction between viruses and bacteria in bovine respiratory disease. Can. Vet. J. 25:37–41.

Pasteurella pneumotropica

P. pneumotropica is found in the nasopharynx of normal rodents, dogs, and cats. It has caused outbreaks of pneumonia in colonies of laboratory rodents and occasionally has been isolated from infected bite wounds of humans (Olson and Meadows 1969). Its distinguishing features are listed in Table 10.2.

REFERENCE

Olson, J.R., and Meadows, T.R. 1969. *Pasteurella pneumotropica* infection resulting from a cat bite. Am. J. Clin. Pathol. 51:709.

Pasteurella ureae

P. ureae is regarded as a commensal of pigs and has a very weak potential to cause disease and fetal death (Corkish and Naylor 1982, Suzuki 1980).

REFERENCES

Corkish, J.D., and Naylor, R.D. 1982. Abortion in sows and the isolation of *Pasteurella ureae*. Vet. Rec. 110:582.

Suzuki, T. 1980. Fetal death in swine with the isolation of *Pasteurella ureae*. J. Jpn. Vet. Med. Assoc. 33:219–222.

Pasteurella anatipestifer

SYNONYMS: *Moraxella anatipestifer, Pfeifferella anatipestifer*

P. anatipestifer is the cause of a septicemic disease of ducks known as *infectious serositis, new duck disease* (Dougherty 1953), or *antipestifer infection*. It has been described under the generic names of *Moraxella* and *Pfeifferella* but does not belong to either of these genera or to the genus *Pasteurella* (Bangun et al. 1981). In morphology the organism resembles *P. multocida*. In cultural features it differs in that it is able to liquefy gelatin as well as coagulated serum and egg. It does not ferment sugars. The best growth is obtained on primary isolation if the infected material is seeded on a medium that contains blood or serum and is incubated under 10 percent CO_2. *P. anatipestifer* is a strict aerobe and does not reduce nitrates. Its distinguishing characteristics are listed in Table 10.2.

Epizootiology and Pathogenesis. Young ducklings are most susceptible to infection, but because the organism has also been found in pheasants, turkeys, and a black swan, it may have a wide distribution among bird species (Bruner et al. 1970, Helfer and Helmboldt 1977, Munday et al. 1970). The organism enters through the respiratory tract. The clinical signs in ducklings include lethargy, diarrhea, incoordination, tremors, and other nervous abnormalities. Lesions include fibrinous epicarditis, airsacculitis, and perihepatitis.

Diagnosis. The organism can be identified in smears by the fluorescent antibody technique (Marshall et al. 1961) and can be distinguished from *P. multocida* by its proteolytic behavior and its strict requirement for oxygen.

Immunity. A formalinized vaccine has been shown to stimulate protective immunity (Harry and Deb 1979).

Antimicrobial Susceptibility. *P. anatipestifer* is sensitive to novobiocin, lincomycin, ampicillin, and sulfaquinoxaline. Novobiocin and lincomycin are the most effective for oral therapy, sulfaquinoxaline somewhat less so (Sandhu and Dean 1980). Drugs that are ineffective orally are chlortetracycline, tylosin-sulfamethazine, fosfomycin, furazolidone, penicillin, bacitracin, and erythromycin. Penicillin, penicillin-streptomycin, and oxytetracycline are effective, however, when administered subcutaneously early in the course of the infection.

REFERENCES

Bangun, A., Tripathy, D.N., and Hanson, L.E. 1981. Studies of *Pasteurella anatipestifer:* An approach to its classification. Avian Dis. 25:326–337.

Bruner, D.W., Angstrom, C.I., and Price, J.E. 1970. *Pasteurella anatipestifer* infection in pheasants. A case report. Cornell Vet. 50:491–494.

Dougherty, E. 1953. The efficacy of several immunizing agents for the control of fowl cholera in the White Pekin duck. Cornell Vet. 43:421–427.

Harry, E.G., and Deb, J.R. 1979. Laboratory and field trials on a formalin inactivated vaccine for the control of *Pasteurella anatipestifer* septicemia in ducks. Res. Vet. Sci. 27:329–333.

Helfer, D.H., and Helmboldt, C.F. 1977. *Pasteurella anatipestifer* infection in turkeys. Avian Dis. 21:712–715.

Marshall, J.D., Jr., Hansen, P.A., and Eveland, W.C. 1961. Histobacteriology of the genus *Pasteurella*. I. *Pasteurella anatipestifer*. Cornell Vet. 51:24–34.

Munday, B.L., Corbould, A., Heddleston, K.L., and Harry, E.G. 1970. Isolation of *Pasteurella anatipestifer* from black swan (*Cygnus atratus*). Aust. Vet. J. 46:322–325.

Sandhu, T.S., and Dean, W.F. 1980. Effect of chemotherapeutic agents on *Pasteurella anatipestifer* infection in White Pekin ducklings. Poult. Sci. 59:1027–1030.

11 The Genus *Bordetella*

There are four species in the genus *Bordetella: B. avium, B. bronchiseptica, B. parapertussis, B. pertussis.* All are related serologically, and all except *B. avium* produce a dermonecrotic toxin that is neutralized by *B. pertussis* antiserum. *B. bronchiseptica* is important as a cause of disease in the respiratory tract of dogs, pigs, laboratory rodents, and a variety of wild mammalian species. *B. avium* causes respiratory disease in turkeys and other birds.

Bordetella bronchiseptica

B. bronchiseptica was first described by Ferry (1910, 1911). It was isolated from the upper respiratory tract of a dog suffering from distemper and was erroneously believed to be the causative agent.

Morphology and Staining Reactions. *B. bronchiseptica* is a small (0.2 to 0.5 μm by 1.5 μm), Gram-negative, piliated coccobacillus (Figure 11.1) that can show bipolar staining. It is motile by means of peritrichous flagella.

Cultural and Biochemical Features. *B. bronchiseptica* is an obligate aerobe and grows rapidly on an ordinary laboratory media including MacConkey agar. On MacConkey agar supplemented with 1 percent glucose, it produces characteristic blue gray colonies. Colonies on blood agar are smooth, round, convex, shiny, and nearly transparent. Most strains are hemolytic; however, a variety of colonial phenotypes can be observed (Pepper and Schrumpf 1984). Large and small hemolytic and non-hemolytic dissociants can be present together. *B. bron-*

chiseptica does not ferment carbohydrates. It produces oxidase, catalase, lysine decarboxylase, and urease; reduces tetrazolium to red, insoluble formazan, and uses citrate. It also produces a strongly alkaline reaction in litmus milk and requires nicotinamide for growth. Most strains are sensitive to potassium tellurite (Bemis and Appel 1977), and most exhibit D -mannose-insensitive hemagglutination of sheep erythrocytes (Bemis et al. 1977a). There appears to be little variation between strains from different host species (Bemis et al. 1977a). The mol% G + C of its DNA is 67 to 69.

Antigens. *B. bronchiseptica* shares a genus-specific heat-stable somatic O antigen, a common host-labile agglutinogen, and a heat-labile dermonecrotic toxin with *B. pertussis* and *B. parapertussis.* It also carries a species-specific agglutinogen and shares 10 other agglutinogens with *B. pertussis* and *B. parapertussis* (see review by Goodnow 1980). Agglutinogens are found on the flagella (H) and the cell surface (K and O). The K and O antigens are heat-labile and heat-stable, respectively. Nakase (1957) extensively categorized the antigens of *B. bronchiseptica.*

The lipopolysaccharide for *B. bronchiseptica* has not been studied extensively but is probably similar to that of *B. pertussis*, which has been shown to be chemically different from enterobacterial lipopolysaccharide and to have a much lower pyrogenicity (Chaby et al. 1979).

The envelope proteins of bordetellas consist of a major protein of molecular weight 37,000 to 60,000 and at least six other minor proteins of lower molecular weight (Ezzell et al. 1981). An outer membrane protein with a molecular weight of 68,000 has been shown to stimulate protective antibodies in mice (Montaraz et al. 1985). Pilus protein is composed of as many as three different subunit variants with molecular weights of 21,000, 22,000, and 24,000. The subunit variants are serologically related, and all three can be present on a single strain (Lee et al. 1986).

The fimbrial antigen has been shown to be an important protective antigen for pigs (Hansen et al. 1983). The protein antigens that are expressed vary with colonial phenotype (Pepper and Schrumpf 1984), but the significance of this in the context of virulence is not yet known.

Epizootiology and Pathogenesis. *B. bronchiseptica* is an obligate parasite of the upper respiratory tract of dogs, pigs, and rodents. It is found mainly in young animals with or recovering from subclinical or clinical respiratory disease and is later cleared from the respiratory tract of the majority of these animals. The extent to which carrier animals occur is not known. Bemis et al. (1977b) feel that the organism cannot be regarded as normal flora in dogs.

The disease in dogs. *B. bronchiseptica* causes a highly

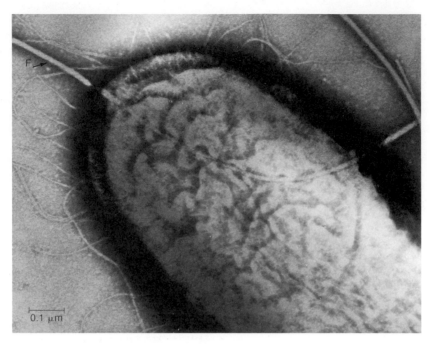

Figure 11.1. Electron micrograph of *Bordetella bronchiseptica*. Numerous pili (fimbriae) are visible on the surface. Portions of flagella (*F*) are also visible. Negative stain. (Courtesy David Bemis.)

infectious and contagious tracheobronchitis of young dogs (kennel cough), although older animals are susceptible if not previously exposed to the organism (Bemis et al. 1977b, Wright et al. 1973). The organism is also an important secondary invader following distemper viral infection and is mainly responsible for the bronchopneumonia that is often a fatal sequel to distemper.

Infection has been shown to be transmitted by aerosol, and colonization and persistence of the bacteria in the trachea involve adhesion to tracheal cilia by means of fibrillar material (Bemis et al. 1977b). After invasion and attachment, cilial movement is paralyzed and is followed by an inflammatory response characterized by neutrophilic invasion of the ciliated respiratory mucosa, which remains intact. The role of the dermonecrotic toxin (Morse 1976) in this effect is known; it causes dermonecrotic lesions in the skin of rabbits. The ciliostatic effect of *B. bronchiseptica* requires close association between metabolically active organisms and cilia (Bemis and Kennedy 1981). A heat-stable adenylate cyclase released by the organism inhibits chemotaxis, phagocytosis, and intracellular killing. Mucus accumulates in the trachea and causes the animal to cough continuously. The cough, which lasts for 1 to 3 weeks, is harsh, moist and hacking and is often followed by retching and vomiting. Puppies shed the organism for 2 to 3 months.

Clinical recovery coincides with the appearance of local immunity and is associated with a reduction in the number of organisms in the trachea. Immunity is probably mediated by blocking of adhesion. Total clearance of the organism does not occur until up to 3 months after infection. Dogs that have recovered maintain an immunity to reinfection for up to 14 months (Bemis et al. 1977b). Serum antibodies do not appear to be important in local clearance of infection.

The disease in pigs. B. bronchiseptica is a common inhabitant of the upper respiratory tract of swine, where it can be present in a carrier state or in association with disease of the upper respiratory tract characterized by sneezing, coughing, and, later, deformity of the bony structures of the nose known as *atrophic rhinitis* (see Figure 10.1). Atrophic rhinitis may result from infection by *B. bronchiseptica* alone (Kemeney 1972, Switzer 1956) or from a combined infection by *Pasteurella multocida* type D and *B. bronchiseptica* (Harris and Switzer 1968). Porcine cytomegalovirus has also been found in association with *B. bronchiseptica* in outbreaks of atrophic rhinitis but is not believed to be important in causing the lesions that result in atrophy of the turbinate bones (Edington et al. 1976, von Schoss 1977).

The organism adheres to epithelial cells on the turbinates. The cilia swell to a polyhedral shape, decrease in number, and become abnormally spaced (Duncan and Ramsey 1965). Osteoblasts and osteocytes in the underlying bone show swollen mitochondria, distention of the cisternae of the endoplasmic reticula, and cell lysis (Letter et al. 1975). Advanced turbinate atrophy has been seen as soon as 3 weeks after experimental inoculation (Tornoe and Nielsen 1976); however, turbinate atrophy induced in pigs a few weeks old may not persist until slaughter because turinate regeneration apparently can occur in swine infected early in life (Tornoe and Nielsen 1976). Turbinate atrophy may also develop in pigs infected at 11 to 13 weeks of age (Blackstrom and Bergstrom 1977), but the incidence of the disease is less than in pigs infected at an earlier age.

Pigs with severe atrophic rhinitis exhibit shortening of the upper jaw and twisting of the snout to one side; however, lesions in the turbinates may be detected radiographically before gross clinical changes are evident (Done 1976).

The disease in laboratory rodents and other hosts. B. bronchiseptica is a common cause of bronchopneumonia, other respiratory infections, and septicemia in laboratory rodents (see review by Goodnow 1980).

Bordetellosis has been reported as a cause of respiratory disease in cats (Fisk and Soave 1973, Snyder et al. 1973). Bronchopneumonia in hospitalized horses has also been described (Bayly et al. 1982). Predisposing factors may have included anesthesia stress and penicillin therapy.

Immunity. The localized nature of *B. bronchiseptica* infection in the respiratory tract of susceptible hosts strongly suggests that antibody at the mucosal surface is critical in protection. Bacterins have failed to protect dogs against experimental challenge (Bemis et al. 1977b), although immunized animals developed high titers of agglutinating antibodies and developed a less severe clinical disease than control dogs. Avirulent live vaccines administered intranasally, however, have been shown to be effective in stimulating high-level protective responses in dogs (Chladek et al. 1981, Shade and Goodnow 1979). Furthermore, a correlation between *B. bronchiseptica* – specific immunoglobulin A in the nasal secretions of intranasally vaccinated dogs and resistance to infection has been noted (Goodnow 1980). Pilus antigen is protective for mice (Lee et al. 1986).

Agglutinating antibodies appear in the serum of swine between 2 and 4 weeks after infection (Brassine et al. 1976, Kemeny 1973) and persist for at least 4 months. Kaong et al. (1971) found that in pig populations in which *B. bronchiseptica* infection was most frequent between 10 and 20 weeks of age, antibodies were not detectable until about 12 weeks of age. The frequency of positive titers

(greater than 1:10) in herds increases steadily with advancing age (Kemeney and Amtomer 1973).

Colostrum-deprived piglets develop turbinate atrophy more frequently than nondeprived animals, but colostral antibody may delay active antibody formation in passively immunized piglets (Kemeney 1973). Vaccination of sows has been shown to slightly reduce the incidence of the disease in herds with endemic infection (Pedersen and Barfod 1977).

The value of subsequent vaccination of young piglets has been questioned (see review by Giles and Smith 1983). Colostral antibody interferes with active immune responses to the vaccine (Kemeney 1973). Available nonliving vaccines also appear to be poorly immunogenic in pigs. A live attenuated intranasal vaccine has recently been developed, however, that provides a high level of protection against experimental challenge (Sakano et al. 1984). This type of vaccine may be a solution to the control of the disease in swine.

The serum agglutination test is widely used in the study of antibody responses both in serum and nasal secretions (see review by Giles and Smith 1983). This test is likely to be superseded by the much more sensitive enzyme-linked immunosorbent assay (ELISA) (Venier et al. 1984).

Diagnosis. Infected carrier swine can be detected by laboratory culture of nasal swabbings (Farrington and Switzer 1977), whereas bordetellosis in dogs is best determined by culture of transtracheal aspirates. A variety of media including blood agar, Bordet-Gengou agar, and selective media containing antimicrobials can be used for primary isolation. One such formulation that includes 5 percent sheep blood per milligram, clindamycin hydrochloride (5 mg/liter), gentamicin sulfate (0.75 mg/liter), potassium tellurite (2.5 mg/liter), amphotericin B (5 mg/liter), and bacitracin (15 mg/liter) has been shown to be useful for isolation of *B. bronchiseptica* from contaminated specimens from swine.

Antimicrobial Susceptibility. *B. bronchiseptica* is sensitive to carbenicillin, chloramphenicol, tetracycline, sulfamethazine, erythromycin, aminoglycosides, and polymyxin B. It is naturally resistant to penicillin. Bemis and Appel (1977) found that aerosols of kanamycin, gentamicin, or polymyxin B are effective in reducing populations of *B. bronchiseptica* in the airways of infected dogs and in producing clinical improvement. Parenterally administered antimicrobials are much less effective in the treatment of canines. In swine, sulfamethazine at a level of 100 g/ton of feed was effective in curing experimental infections (Switzer 1963). Because resistant strains are frequent in swine populations (Terakado et al. 1973), isolates from this host should be routinely checked in a susceptibility test.

REFERENCES

Backstrom, L., and Gergstrom, G. 1977. Atrophic rhinitis in swine fattener herds. A field study of the spread of the disease with infected pigs bought at market. Nord. Vet. Med. 29:539–542.

Bayly, W.M., Reed, S.M., Foreman, J.H., Traub, J.L., and McMurphy, R.M. 1982. Equine bronchopneumonia due to *Bordetella bronchiseptica*. Equine Pract. 4:25–27.

Bemis, D.A., and Appel, M.J.G. 1977. Aerosol, parenteral, and oral antibiotic treatment of *Bordetella bronchiseptica* infections in dogs. J. Am. Vet. Med. Assoc. 170:1082–1086.

Bemis, D.A., and Kennedy, J.R. 1981. An improved system for studying the effect of *Bordetella bronchiseptica* on the ciliary activity of canine tracheal epithelial cells. J. Infect. Dis. 44:349–357.

Bemis, D.A., Greisen, H.A., and Appel, M.J.G. 1977a. Bacteriological variation among *Bordetella bronchiseptica* isolates from dogs and other species. J. Clin. Microbiol. 5:471–480.

Bemis, D.A., Greisen, H.A., and Appel, M.J.G. 1977b. Pathogenesis of canine bordetellosis. J. Infect. Dis. 135:753–762.

Brassinne, M., Dewaele, A., and Gouffaux, M. 1976. Intranasal infection with *Bordetella bronchiseptica* in gnotobiotic piglets. Res. Vet. Sci. 20:162–166.

Chaby, R.G., Ayme, A., Caroff, M., Donikian, R., and Szabo, L. 1979. Structural features and separation of some of the biological activities of the *Bordetella pertussis* endotoxin by chemical fractionation. In I. Manclark and C.R. Hill II, eds., International Symposium on Pertussis. U.S. Government Printing Office, Washington, D.C. Pp. 185–190.

Chladek, S.W., Williams, J.M., Gerber, D.L., Harris, L.L., and Murdock, F.M. 1981. Canine parainfluenza—*Bordetella bronchiseptica* vaccine: Immunogenicity. Am. J. Vet. Res. 42:266–270.

Done, J.T. 1976. Porcine atrophic rhinitis: Snout radiography as an aid to diagnosis and detection of the disease. Vet. Rec. 98:23–28.

Duncan, J.R., and Ramsey, F.K. 1965. Fine structural changes in the porcine nasal ciliated epithelial cell produced by *Bordetella bronchiseptica* rhinitis. Am. J. Pathol. 47:601–612.

Edington, N., Smith, I.M., Plowright, W., and Watt, R.G. 1976. Relationship of porcine cytomegalovirus and *Bordetella bronchiseptica* to atrophic rhinitis in gnotobiotic piglets. Vet. Rec. 98:42–45.

Ezzell, J.W., Dobrogosy, W.J., Kloos, W.E., and Manclark, C.R. 1981. Phase-shift markers in *Bordetella*: Alterations in envelope proteins. J. Infect. Dis. 143:562–569.

Farrington, D.O., and Switzer, W.P. 1977. Evaluation of nasal culturing procedures for the control of atrophic rhinitis caused by *Bordetella bronchiseptica* in swine. J. Am. Vet. Med. Assoc. 170:34–36.

Ferry, N.S. 1910. A preliminary report of the bacterial findings in canine distemper. Am. Vet. Rev. 37:499–504.

Ferry, N.S. 1911. Etiology of canine distemper. J. Infect. Dis. 8:399–420.

Fisk, S.K., and Soave, O.A. 1973. *Bordetella bronchiseptica* in laboratory cats from central California. Lab. Anim. Sci. 23:33–35.

Giles, C.J., and Smith, I.M. 1983. Vaccination of pigs with *Bordetella bronchiseptica*. Vet. Bull. 53:327–338.

Goodnow, R.A. 1980. Biology of *Bordetella bronchiseptica*. Microbiol. Rev. 44:722–738.

Goodnow, R.A. 1984. Veterinary biologics: Something new—something old. Calif. Vet. 38:10–12.

Hansen, G.A., Pedersen, K.B., and Riising, H.-J. 1983. Protection against colonization of *Bordetella bronchiseptica* in the upper respiratory tract of the pig. In K.B. Pedersen and N.C. Nielsen, eds., Atrophic Rhinitis in Pigs. Commission of the European Communities, Luxembourg. Pp. 89–97.

Harris, D.L., and Switzer, W.P. 1968. Turbinate atrophy in young pigs exposed to *Bordetella bronchiseptica*, *Pasteurella multocida* and combined inoculum. Am. J. Vet. Res. 29:777–785.

Kang, B.K., Koshimuzu, K., and Ogata, M. 1971. Studies on the etiology of infectious atrophic rhinitis of swine. III. Field survey by agglutination test in relation to incidence of *B. bronchiseptica* and turbinate atrophy. Jpn. J. Vet. Sci. 33:17–23.

Kemeney, L.J. 1972. Experimental atrophic rhinitis produced by *Bordetella bronchiseptica* culture in young pigs. Cornell Vet. 62:477–485.

Kemeney, L.J. 1973. Agglutinin response of pigs to intranasal infection by *Bordetella bronchiseptica*. Cornell Vet. 63:130–137.

Kemeney, L.J., and Amtomer, W.C. 1973. *Bordetella* agglutinating antibody in swine—a herd survey. Can. J. Comp. Med. 37:409–412.

Lee, S.W., Way, A.W., and Ossen, E.G. 1986. Purification and subunit heterogeneity of pili of *Bordetella bronchiseptica*. Infect. Immun. 51:586–593.

Letter, A.W., Switzer, W.P., and Copen, C.C. 1975. Electron microscopic evaluation of bone cells in pigs with experimentally induced *Bordetella* rhinitis (turbine osteoporosis). Am. J. Vet. Res. 36:15–22.

Montaraz, J.A., Novotny, P., and Ivanyi, J. 1985. Identification of a 68-kilodalton protective protein antigen from *Bordetella bronchiseptica*. Infect. Immun. 47:744–751.

Morse, S.I. 1976. Biologically active components and properties of *Bordetella pertussis*. In D. Perlman, ed., Advances in Applied Microbiology, vol. 20. Academic Press, New York. Pp. 9–26.

Nakase, Y. 1957. Studies on *Haemophilus bronchisepticus*. I. The antigenic structures of *H. bronchisepticus* from guinea pigs. Kitasato Arch. Exp. Med. 30:57–72.

Pedersen, K.B., and Barfod, K. 1977. Effect of vaccination of sows with *Bordetella bronchiseptica* on the incidence of atrophic rhinitis in swine. Nord. Vet. Med. 29:369–375.

Peppers, M.S., and Schrumpf, M.E. 1984. Phenotypic variation and modulation in *Bordetella bronchiseptica*. Infect. Immun. 44:681–687.

Sakano, T., Sakurai, K.I., Furutani, T., and Shimuzu, T. 1984. Immunogenicity and safety of an attenuated *Bordetella bronchiseptica* vaccine in pigs. Am. J. Vet. Res. 45:1814–1817.

Shade, F.J., and Goodnow, R.A. 1979. Intranasal immunization of dogs against *Bordetella bronchiseptica*–induced tracheobronchitis (kennel cough) with modified live *Bordetella bronchiseptica* vaccine. Am. J. Vet. Res. 40:1241–1243.

Snyder, S.B., Fisk, S.K., Fox, J.G., and Soave, O.A. 1973. Respiratory tract disease associated with *Bordetella bronchiseptica* infection in cats. J. Am. Vet. Med. Assoc. 163:293–294.

Switzer, W.P. 1956. Studies on infectious atrophic rhinitis. V. Concept that several agents may cause turbinate atrophy. Am. J. Vet. Res. 17:478–484.

Switzer, W.P. 1963. Elimination of *Bordetella bronchiseptica* from the nasal cavity of swine by sulfonamide therapy. Vet. Med. 58:571–574.

Terakado, N., Azechi, H., Ninomiya, K., and Shimizu, T. 1973. Demonstration of R factors in *Bordetella bronchiseptica* isolated from pigs. Antimicrob. Agents Chemother. 3:555–558.

Tornoe, N., and Nielsen, N.C. 1976. Inoculation experiments with *Bordetella bronchiseptica* strains in SPF pigs. Nord. Vet. Med. 28:233–242.

Venier, L., Rothschild, M.F., and Warner, C.M. 1984. Measurement of serum antibody in swine vaccinated with *B. bronchiseptica*: Comparison of agglutination and enzyme-linked immunosorbent assay methods. Am. J. Vet. Res. 45:2634–2636.

Von Schoss, P. 1977. Sammelreferat. Einschluss korperchen—Rhinitis der Schweine und Rhinitis Atrophicans. D.T.W. 84:440–441.

Wright, N.G., Thompson, H., Taylor, D., and Cornwall, H.J.C. 1973. *Bordetella bronchiseptica*: A re-assessment of its role in canine respiratory diseases. Vet. Rec. 93:486–487.

Bordetella avium

SYNONYM: *Alcaligenes faecalis*

B. avium is the cause of *turkey coryza,* a highly contagious upper respiratory disease of turkeys. In the first description of the disease, Fillion et al. (1967) in Canada noted that the organism resembled *Bordetella* species. It was later erroneously identified as *Alcaligenes faecalis*. Subsequent studies of phenotypic and serologic characteristics as well as of DNA-hybridization led to the recommendation that the organism be named *B. avium* (Jackwood et al. 1985, Kersters et al. 1984).

Morphology and Staining Reactions. *B. avium* resembles *B. bronchiseptica* in morphology. It is a small (0.2 to 0.5 μm by 1.5 μm), Gram-negative, piliated coccobacillus that is motile by peritrichous flagella.

Cultural and Biochemical Features. *B. avium* is an obligate aerobe and grows well on ordinary laboratory media. The colonies are similar to those of *B. bronchiseptica* and exist as two types, 1 and 2. Type 1 colonies are round, raised, and colorless, with a well-defined border. Type 2 colonies are round and slightly raised, with an opaque mucoidlike surface. They are larger than type 1 colonies (Jackwood et al. 1985). Type 1, but not type 2, isolates agglutinate guinea pig erythrocytes. Only type 2 isolates grow on minimal essential medium and in 6.5 percent sodium chloride broth. Approximately one-third of all isolates of *B. avium* are hemolytic for cow erythrocytes. The oxidation fermentation test on glucose is negative. *B. avium* does not liquefy gelatin, does not produce indole, and does not reduce nitrate and nitrite. It does produce oxidase and catalase but not urease. The mol% G + C ranges from 61.6 to 62.6.

Antigens. Although antigens made of type 1 isolates react with type 2 antiserums, most type 2 antigens react only weakly with type 1 antiscrums (Jackwood et al. 1985). An O antigen is shared with *B. bronchiseptica*. At least three serotypes have been distinguished (Hertle and Hinz 1984).

Epizootiology and Pathogenesis. *B. avium* survives well in dust at low relative humidity, and dust is probably an important means of transmission. The organism is widely distributed in turkey populations and has also been found in a variety of other avian species (Hinz and Glunder 1985). Only type 2 isolates have been associated with disease.

The organism adheres to and colonizes the ciliated epithelial cells in the upper respiratory tract. Colonization results in loss of cilia and epithelium, accumulation of mucus, and tracheal collapse (Gary et al. 1983). Although the rate of tracheal mucus transport is reduced, clearance of particles is not depressed until late in the infection (Ficken et al. 1986).

The disease appears in 4- to 10-week-old turkey poults about 10 to 12 days following experimental exposure and is characterized by conjunctivitis, nasal discharge, coughing, moist rales, gaping, and reduced food intake. Turkey coryza is highly contagious, with a morbidity of up to 50 percent, and is exacerbated in birds stressed by concurrent infections with other pathogens or by vaccination. Mortality may reach 25 percent within 3 weeks after exposure. The signs are conjunctivitis and rhinotracheitis with epithelial hyperplasia and infiltration of the mucosa by lymphocytes and macrophages.

Immunity. Infection results in development of serum antibodies, which can be detected by the agglutination test. The immunological basis for protection probably involves production of local antibody. Garcia (1984) found that a live attenuated vaccine given into the conjunctiva and in the drinking water is protective. A bacterin in Freund's adjuvant given subcutaneously has also been shown to protect against disease but not against colonization (Glunder et al. 1980).

Diagnosis. *B. avium* is readily isolated on common laboratory media. Type 1 isolates are distinguished from *B. bronchiseptica* by their failure to grow on minimal essential medium or to produce urease. *B. avium* type 1 is differentiated from *A. faecalis* by its ability to agglutinate guinea pig erythrocytes. In addition, *A. faecalis*, unlike type 1 isolates, grows well on minimal essential medium and in 6.5 percent sodium chloride broth (Jackwood et al. 1985).

Antimicrobial Susceptibility. *B. avium* is sensitive to tetracycline, nitrofurantoin, and erythromycin but resistant to penicillin, streptomycin, and sulfonamides.

REFERENCES

Ficken, M.D., Edwards, J.F., and Lax, J.C. 1986. Clearance of bacteria in turkeys with *Bordetella avium*–induced tracheitis. Avian Dis. 30:352–357.

Filion, A.S., Cloutier, S., Vrancken, E.R., and Bernier, G. 1967. Respiratory infection in the turkey caused by a bacterium related to *Bordetella bronchiseptica*. Can. J. Comp. Med. 31:129–134.

Garcia, R. 1984. *Alcaligenes faecalis*— Laboratory and field studies evaluating the efficacy and safety of a live ART vaccine. In Proceedings of the 33d Western Poultry Disease Conference, Davis, California. Pp. 23–27.

Glunder, G., Hinz, K.H., Siegmann, O., and Stilurek, B. 1980. Immunization of turkey poults against bordetellosis with an adjuvant vaccine. Avian Pathol. 9:427–435.

Gray, J.G., Roberts, J.F., Dillman, R.C., and Simmons, D.G. 1983. Pathogenesis of change in the upper respiratory tracts of turkeys experimentally infected with an *Alcaligenes faecalis* isolate. Infect. Immun. 42:350–355.

Hertle, A., and Hinz, K.H. 1984. Serological studies on antigenic structure of *Bordetella avium* sp. nov. Berl. Münch. Tierärztl. Wochenschr. 97:58–60.

Hinz, K.H., and Glunder, G. 1985. Occurrence of *Bordetella avium* (new species) and *Bordetella bronchiseptica* in birds. Berl. Münch. Tierärztl. Wochenschr. 98:369–373.

Kersters, K., Hinz, K.H., Hertle, A., Segers, P., Lievens, A., Siegmann, O., and DeLey, J. 1984. *Bordetella avium* sp. nov. isolated from the respiratory tracts of turkeys and other birds. Int. J. Syst. Bacteriol. 34:56–70.

Jackwood, M.W., Saif, Y.M., Moorhead, P.D., and Dearth, R.N. 1985. Further characterization of the agent causing coryza in turkeys. Avian Dis. 29:690–705.

12 The Genus *Moraxella*

Members of the genus *Moraxella* are small, short, rod-shaped organisms that occur in pairs; they are therefore termed *diplobacilli*. *Bergey's Manual of Systematic Bacteriology* (1984) lists 10 species, of which only *M. bovis* is of veterinary importance. *M. ovis* is found in the conjunctival sac of sheep and appears to be a harmless commensal.

Moraxella bovis

SYNONYM: *Haemophilus bovis*

M. bovis causes *infectious keratoconjunctivitis,* or *pinkeye*, in cattle. Punch and Slatter (1984) have written an excellent review of this disease.

Morphology and Staining Reactions. *M. bovis* is a Gram-negative diplobacillus about 2 μm long and 1 μm wide. It is nonmotile and does not form spores. Rough forms of the organism are fimbriated (piliated). There are a number of pilus antigenic types (Gil-Turnes and Araujo 1982). *M. bovis* pilus protein shares extensive homology with pilus protein of *Bacteroides nodosus* (Marrs et al. 1985). It is very hydrophobic and exists in two forms: α (alpha) and β (beta).

Cultural and Biochemical Features. Colonies of *M. bovis* grown on cow-blood agar are smooth, circular, translucent, grayish, and beta-hemolytic; however, only the fimbriated (piliated) agar-eroding variants can colonize the conjunctiva (Pedersen et al. 1972). Because the pili are necessary for colonization, the loss of pili correlates with losses of virulence, ability to erode agar, and autoagglutinability (Pedersen et al. 1972, Sandhu et al.

1974). "Smooth" colony forms do not erode agar and are avirulent. The loss of hemolysin also correlates with a loss of virulence.

M. bovis needs serum or blood for good growth. The organism is proteolytic; it does not reduce nitrates and it does not ferment carbohydrates. It is aerobic, oxidase-positive, and catalase-variable. The mol% G + C of the DNA is 41.0 to 44.5.

Epizootiology and Pathogenesis. Pinkeye occurs throughout the cattle-raising areas of the world and is most prevalent in the warmer months. Factors that predispose cattle to develop pinkeye include prolonged exposure of the cornea to sunlight; the presence of many flies, such as face flies (*Musca autumnalis*); breed susceptibility; mechanical irritants, such as dust; and concurrent viral or mycoplasmal infections. Transmission can occur by direct contact between cattle (Hughes and Pugh 1970) or by mechanical transfer from the legs and mouthparts of flies (*M. autumnalis, M. domestica,* and *Stomoxys calcitrans*).

Carrier animals are a major source of infection for calves (Pugh, Kopecky, et al. 1982). Between outbreaks *M. bovis* resides in the conjunctiva and nares of carrier animals, where the organism may multiply and subsequently spread to uninfected cattle after the animals are exposed to sunlight or after they have been infected by other microbial or viral agents, such as infectious bovine rhinotracheitis virus (Pugh et al. 1968).

Pinkeye is highly contagious among cattle less than 2 years old, but may also spread rapidly among older susceptible animals. Clinically apparent disease is more common in younger cattle (Hughes and Pugh 1970). Breeds of *Bos indicus* are more resistant than breeds of *B. taurus*. The "hooded" structure of the eyelids of *B. indicus* may help protect the cornea from the effects of sunlight. Hereford cattle are the most severely affected.

Only strains of *M. bovis* that have pili can adhere to corneal epithelial cells (Chandler et al. 1983, Pedersen et al. 1983). The bacteria adhere to older, dark epithelial cells, and pitlike depressions form on the surface of the cells beneath the bacteria (Figure 12.1). Masses of *M. bovis* and neutrophils are visible in these shallow ulcers. The pili not only mediate adherence but also promote endocytosis and are cytotoxic. The surface epithelium becomes edematous and swollen, and there is some infiltration by lymphocytes. As the lesions become chronic, hyperplasia develops and the number of lymphocytes and plasma cells increases. Deeper layers are hyperemic and infiltrated by lymphocytes and polymorphonuclear leukocytes.

A dermonecrotic toxin in the cell wall of *M. bovis* produces the corneal lesions typical of pinkeye (Henson

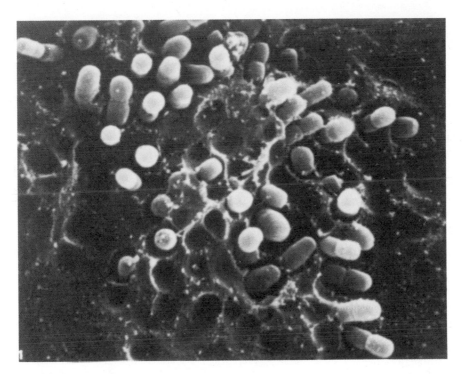

Figure 12.1. Scanning electron micrograph showing *Moraxella bovis* in pitlike depressions on the cornea of a cow. × 11,200. (From Chandler et al., 1985, courtesy of *Journal of Comparative Pathology.*)

and Grumbles 1960, 1961). The role of the hemolysin in lesion development has not been defined. Pugh et al. (1973), however, have shown that there is a specific oculopathic substance in the cell sap of *M. bovis* that induces ocular pruritis and lacrimation in cattle.

Animals with pinkeye exhibit photophobia, simple conjunctivitis, and a copious serous discharge. After several days the cornea shows a slight haziness and can then become edematous and opaque. The center of the edematous area can slough, leaving an ulcer. Sometimes a descemetocele forms; if so, the animal can lose the eye because of rupture of the anterior chamber.

Immunity. Animals that have recovered from pinkeye are relatively resistant to reinfection (Barner 1952), although this resistance is effective only against homologous strains of *M. bovis* carrying the same pilus protein antigen as the original infecting strain. Immunoglobulins IgA, IgM, and IgG have been detected in the lacrimal secretions of calves in a herd with enzootic pinkeye (Pugh et al. 1968), and the highest and most persistent titers to *M. bovis* were found to be caused by IgA antibodies. However, these antibodies did not prevent clinical disease (Killinger et al. 1978).

Bishop et al. (1982), using an enzyme-linked immunosorbent assay (ELISA), showed that IgA-type antibodies are predominant in lacrimal secretions, whereas the serum antibody response is mainly IgG. Some workers (Kopecky et al. 1983) have concluded that resistance to reinfection is the result of a generalized rather that a localized immune response. Others (Weech and Renshaw 1983) have provided evidence that local immunity is more important.

Several different experimental vaccines have been studied in attempts to stimulate a protective response. Baptista (1975) reported good protection against homologous strains from a live vaccine. Similarly, Pugh, McDonald, and Kopecky (1982) obtained some degree of protection with a nonhemolytic live vaccine. The bacterin must contain adequate amounts of pilus antigen in order to stimulate a protective response (Pugh et al. 1977). The immune response to pili is improved by using oil as an adjuvant. There is evidence (Pugh et al. 1976) that vaccines must be polyvalent to succeed in the field because of the strain specificity of the immune response.

Vaccinated calves are not protected until about 4 weeks after vaccination, during which time they are liable to contract infection from carrier dams and other cattle. Vaccination of pregnant cows with pilus vaccine is effective in raising antibody levels in the colostrum and thereby passively protecting calves (Pugh, Kopecky, et al. 1982).

Antimicrobial Susceptibility. *M. bovis* usually is sensitive to a wide variety of antibiotics and antimicrobials including penicillin, chloramphenicol, tetracycline, neomycin, erythromycin, ethidium bromide (a carcinogen), and furazolidone. However, because strains resistant to aminoglycosides, penicillin, cloxacillin, sulfonamides, and lincomycins have been reported (Pugh and McDonald 1977), susceptibility testing should be routinely practiced. Antibiotics can be administered topically, subconjunctivally, or parenterally.

REFERENCES

Baptista, P.J.H.P. 1975. Querato-conjunctivite infecciosa dos bovinos. I. Resistencia de bovinos vacinados com culturas vivas a agressao experimental com amostras homologa e heterologa de *Moraxella bovis*. II. Etiologia. III. Immunologia. Bol. Inst. Pesqui. Vet. Desiderio Finamor 3:5–16, 17–27, 29–35.

Barner, R.D. 1952. A study of *Moraxella bovis* and its relation to bovine keratitis. Am. J. Vet. Res. 13:132–144.

Bishop, B., Schurig, G.G., and Troutt, H.F. 1982. Enzyme-linked immunosorbent assay for measurement of anti–*Moraxella bovis* antibodies. Am. J. Vet. Res. 42:1443–1445.

Chandler, R.L., Bird, R.G., Smith, M.D., Anger, H.S., and Turfrey, B.A. 1983. Scanning electron microscope studies on preparations of bovine cornea exposed to *Moraxella bovis*. J. Comp. Pathol. 93:1–8.

Chandler, R.L., Smith, K., and Turfrey, B.A. 1985. Exposure of bovine cornea to different strains of *Moraxella bovis* and to other bacterial species in vitro. J. Comp. Pathol. 95:415–423.

Gil-Turnes, C., and de Araujo, F.O. 1982. Serological characterization of strains of *Moraxella bovis* using double immunodiffusion. Can. J. Comp. Med. 46:165–168.

Henson, J.B., and Grumbles, L.C. 1960. Infectious bovine keratoconjunctivitis. II. Susceptibility of laboratory animals to *Moraxella (Hemophilus) bovis*. Cornell Vet. 50:445–458.

Henson, J.B., and Grumbles, L.C. 1961. Infectious bovine keratoconjunctivitis. III. Demonstration of toxins in *Moraxella (Haemophilus) bovis* cultures. Cornell Vet. 51:267–284.

Hughes, D.E., and Pugh, G.W. 1970. A five-year study of infectious bovine keratoconjunctivitis in a beef herd. J. Am. Vet. Med. Assoc. 157:443–451.

Killinger, A.H., Weisiger, R.M., Helper, L.C., and Mansfield, M.E. 1978. Detection of *Moraxella bovis* antibodies in the SIgA, IgG and IgM classes of immunoglobulin in bovine lacrimal secretions by an indirect fluorescent antibody test. Am. J. Vet. Res. 39:931–934.

Kopecky, K.E., Pugh, G.W., and McDonald, T.J. 1983. Infectious bovine keratoconjunctivitis: Evidence for general immunity. Am. J. Vet. Res. 44:260–262.

Marrs, C.F., Schoolnik, G., Kooney, J.M., Hardy, J., Rothbard, J., and Falkow, S. 1985. Cloning and sequencing of a *Moraxella bovis* pilin gene. J. Bacteriol. 163:132–139.

Pedersen, K.B., Froholm, L.O., and Bovre, K. 1972. Fimbriation and colony type of *Moraxella bovis* in relation to conjunctival colonization and development of keratoconjunctivitis in cattle. Acta Pathol. Microbiol. Scand. [B] 80:911–918.

Pugh, G.W., and McDonald, T.J. 1977. Infectious bovine keratoconjunctivitis: Treatment of *Moraxella bovis* infections with antibiotics. Proc. Annu. Meet. U.S. Animal Health Assoc. 81:120–130.

Pugh, G.W., Hughes, D.E., and Booth, G.D. 1977. Experimentally induced infectious bovine keratoconjunctivitis: Effectiveness of a pilus vaccine against exposure to homologous strains of *Moraxella bovis*. Am. J. Vet. Res. 38:1519–1522.

Pugh, G.W., Hughes, D.E., and McDonald, T.J. 1968. Keratoconjunctivitis produced by *Moraxella bovis* in laboratory animals. Am. J. Vet. Res. 29:2057–2061.

Pugh, G.W., Hughes, D.E., and Schultz, V.D. 1973. The pathophysiological effects of *Moraxella bovis* toxins on cattle, mice and guinea pigs. Can. J. Comp. Med. 37:70–80.

Pugh, G.W., Hughes, D.E., Schultz, V.D., and Graham, C.K. 1976. Experimentally induced infectious bovine keratoconjunctivitis: Resistance of vaccinated cattle to homologous and heterologous strains of *Moraxella bovis*. Am. J. Vet. Res. 37:57–60.

Pugh, G.W., Kopecky, K.E., Kvasnicka, W.G., McDonald, T.J., and Booth, G.D. 1982. Infectious bovine keratoconjunctivitis in cattle vaccinated and medicated against *Moraxella bovis* before parturition. Am. J. Vet. Res. 43:320–325.

Pugh, G.W., McDonald, T.J., and Kopecky, K.E. 1982. Experimental infectious bovine keratoconjunctivitis: Efficacy of a vaccine prepared from non-hemolytic strains of *Moraxella bovis*. Am. J. Vet. Res. 43:1081–1084.

Punch, P.I., and Slatter, D.H. 1984. A review of infectious bovine keratoconjunctivitis. Vet. Bull. 54:193–207.

Sandhu, T.S., White, F.H., and Simpson, C.F. 1974. Association of pili with rough colony type of *Moraxella bovis*. Am. J. Vet. Res. 35:437–439.

Weech, G.M., and Renshaw, H.W. 1983. Infectious bovine keratoconjunctivitis: Bacteriologic, immunologic, and clinical responses to experimental exposure with *Moraxella bovis*. Comp. Immunol. Microbiol. Infect. Dis. 6:81–94.

13 The Genus *Actinobacillus*

The genus *Actinobacillus* consists of pleomorphic, Gram-negative, nonmotile organisms that are catalase- and oxidase-variable and ferment sugars without producing gas. Cultures are very sticky on primary isolation. All species of *Actinobacillus* grow on MacConkey agar, produce beta galactosidase but not indole, and reduce nitrates to nitrites. The mol% G + C of the DNA is 40 to 43 (Tm). Three species of importance as pathogens of domestic animals are described in *Bergey's Manual of Systematic Bacteriology* (1984). These are *A. lignieresii*, *A. equuli*, and *A. suis*. *A. seminis*, a cause of ovine epididymitis, and *A. salpingitidis*, a cause of salpingitis in laying hens, are not closely related to the actinobacilli but are described in this chapter because their correct affiliation has yet to be determined.

Recent DNA hybridization studies indicate that *Haemophilus pleuropneumoniae* (*parahemolyticus*) and *Pasteurella haemolytica* biovar A should be included in the genus *Actinobacillus* (Pohl et al. 1983). In this edition, however, these organisms will be described in chapters 9 and 10, on *Haemophilus* and *Pasteurella* respectively.

REFERENCE

Pohl, S., Bertschinger, H.U., Frederiksen, W., and Mannheim, W. 1983. Transfer of *Haemophilus pleuropneumoniae* and the *Pasteurella haemolytica*-like organism causing porcine necrotic pleuropneumonia to the genus *Actinobacillus* (*Actinobacillus pleuropneumoniae* comb. nov.) on the basis of phenotypic and deoxyribonucleic acid relatedness. Int. J. Syst. Bacteriol. 33:510–514.

Actinobacillus lignieresii

A. lignieresii was first described by Lignieres and Spitz (1902), who isolated it from Argentine cattle suffering from a disease that clinically resembled actinomycosis. Actinobacillosis later was recognized in Europe, the United States and South Africa.

Morphology and Staining Reactions. The rod-shaped cells of *A. lignieresii* are encased in small cheeselike granules in the pus of lesions. These are quite similar to the "sulfur granules" of actinomycosis but generally are much smaller, measuring less than 1 mm in diameter. If these granules are picked out of the pus and crushed between slides, moderate magnification will show clublike bodies radiating out from the centers of the masses (Figure 13.1). Stains made from the crushed granules show small Gram-negative bacilli.

In cultures *A. lignieresii* exhibits considerable variation in morphology depending on the medium used and on whether surface growth or deep growth on solid media is examined. Diplococci and slender rods are seen in fluid cultures. Long curved forms are often seen in colonies growing in the depths of solid media. The bacilli are about 0.4 μm wide and 1 to 15 μm long (Figure 13.2). They are nonmotile, are stained by the usual dyes, and are Gram-negative.

Cultural and Biochemical Features. *A. lignieresii* is quite serophilic, and little growth occurs in most media unless some serum or blood is present. It is rather strongly aerobic, to the extent that growth almost always fails under anaerobic conditions. On the other hand, primary cultures in fluid media or in stabs made in solid media are more apt to succeed than surface cultures. Primary cultures succeed best when they are incubated in an atmosphere consisting of 10 percent CO_2.

Delicate, naillike growths appear along the length of a stab made in serum agar. Surface colonies are bluish white and very delicate. They are smooth, glistening, convex, and 0.5 to 1 mm in diameter. *A. lignieresii* grows well in serum gelatin but does not liquefy the medium. In glucose serum broth *A. lignieresii* usually develops into small grayish granules that adhere to the sides of the tube but are easily broken loose by shaking. The remainder of the broth is clear. Litmus milk usually remains unchanged by *A. lignieresii*, but it sometimes develops slight acidity. Excellent growth occurs on coagulated blood serum. The medium is not softened or liquefied. *A. lignieresii* ferments glucose, lactose, sucrose, maltose, raffinose, and mannitol when these sugars are dissolved in serum broth. It ferments xylose irregularly, and it does not attack arabinose, dulcitol, salicin, or inulin. Indole is formed in

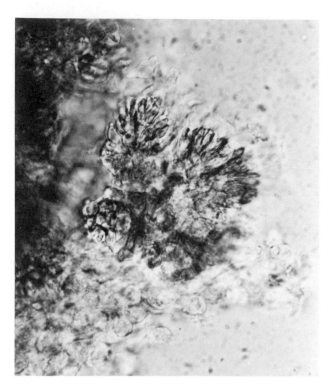

Figure 13.1. *Actinobacillus lignieresii,* with club-bearing rosettes, in pus from a lymph node lesion. Unstained. × 720. (From Campbell et al., 1975, courtesy of *Journal of the American Veterinary Medical Association.*)

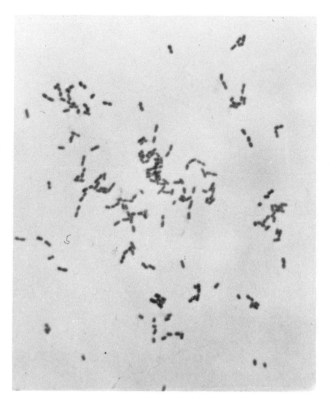

Figure 13.2. *Actinobacillus lignieresii* from a culture on serum agar incubated 24 hours at 37°C. × 1,400. (Courtesy L. R. Vawter.)

small amounts. Cultures must be transferred every 4 days or they will lose viability.

Antigens. Six antigenic types can be distinguished by differences in heat-stable antigens (Phillips 1967). Cattle strains are usually type 1 and sheep strains are usually types 3 and 4. Heat-labile antigens also occur and are common to the various heat-stable antigenic types.

Epizootiology and Pathogenesis. *A. lignieresii* is a normal commensal of the buccal mucous membrane of cattle and sheep, and it enters into the deeper tissues through penetration of wounds in the buccal epithelium caused by foreign material or some other type of trauma.

The natural disease in cattle is manifested most commonly by slowly developing tumors, which may occur in any part of the body but are seen most frequently in the region of the lower jaw and neck (Figure 13.3). These tumors are hard and often lobular. Sooner or later softened areas become evident; these fluctuate when palpated, indicating the presence of fluid, which in reality is a mucoid, nonodorous pus. This breaks through the skin, creating a deep ulcer that will not heal. In the meantime the tumorous mass usually continues to enlarge and additional ulcers may form. Lesions in the internal organs, particularly lymphoid structures, the lungs, and the walls

of the four compartments of the stomach, are not uncommon. A characteristic form of *A. lignieresii* infection is the so-called wooden-tongue of cattle. In this form of the disease a hard tumorous mass develops in the substance of the tongue, causing serious disability.

Hebeler et al. (1961) reported an outbreak in a dairy herd with about 7 percent morbidity and a high incidence of lesions of the skin and related lymph nodes rather than tongue or alimentary tract involvement. Campbell et al. (1975) described an outbreak in a group of 52 heifers where the morbidity was 73 percent. An important predisposing factor in that outbreak was dry, stemmy haylage, which when eaten abrased and penetrated the buccal mucosa. Some of this plant material was imbedded in the lesions (Figure 13.4). Although the lesions of *A. lignieresii* tend to localize, generalized actinobacillosis also occurs in cattle.

Actinobacillosis is often confused with actinomycosis. True actinomycosis, which is caused by the "ray fungus," *Actinomyces bovis*, is found mostly in the bone of the lower jaw and seldom occurs in the soft structures.

According to Taylor (1944), actinobacillosis is fairly common in sheep in Scotland. In one report (Johnston 1954) lesions of the disease were found in the head region

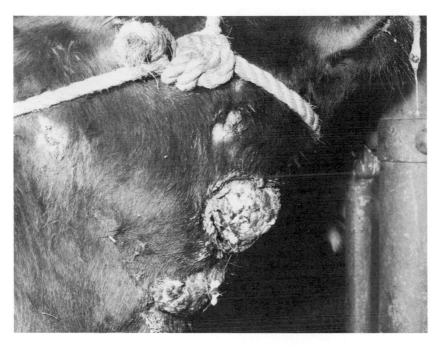

Figure 13.3. Actinobacillosis in a heifer. (From Campbell et al., 1975, courtesy of *Journal of the American Veterinary Medical Association.*)

Figure 13.4. Plant material in a granuloma from which *Actinobacillus lignieresii* was isolated. The granuloma is transected by plant fibers (*A, B*). A giant cell is also present (*C*), (From Campbell et al., 1975, courtesy of *Journal of the American Veterinary Medical Association.*)

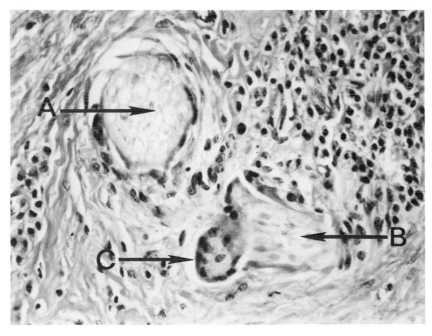

with involvement of the cheeks, nose, lips, and lymph glands. Abscesses were seen in the soft palate, pharynx, and lungs. Skin lesions have also been reported. The organism has been described as a cause of mastitis in ewes (Laws and Elder 1969).

Sautter et al. (1953) and Fletcher (1956) reported cases in dogs; however, their isolates did not have all the characteristics of *A. lignieresii*. In 1969 Carb and Liu (1969) found *A. lignieresii* to be the causative agent of a large, diffusely infiltrating granulomatous mass in the thigh of a 7½-year-old Boston Terrier.

Immunity. Many normal cattle have specific agglutinins in their serum (Fletcher et al. 1956), which is presumably a result of the presence of the organism as a commensal in the buccal cavity. There may be a significant rise in the titer in serum from affected cows (Davies and Torrence, 1930).

The granulomatous nature of the lesion suggests that cell-mediated immunity is important in the host response and possibly in resolution of the infection. A report (Hebeler et al. 1961) on the use of formalinized bacterin during an outbreak of actinobacillosis in a herd of 543 cattle concluded that the vaccine reduced the number of animals that relapsed and prevented the occurrence of new cases.

Diagnosis. Gram-stained smears of sulfur granules will reveal club-bearing rosettes that contain central masses of Gram-negative rods and cocci.

Antimicrobial Sensitivity. *A. lignieresii* is sensitive to streptomycin, sulfonamides, tetracyclines, and chloramphenicol (Sanders and Ristic 1956, Smith 1951). The infection is iodine-sensitive, and local lesions may be successfully treated by injecting them with an aqueous solution of iodine (Lugol's solution). Clinical experience has shown that sodium iodide administered intravenously or orally is highly successful in treating wooden tongue and other forms of actinobacillosis in which the lesions are inaccessible to local applications of iodine.

REFERENCES

Campbell, S.G., Whitlock, R.H., Timoney, J.F., and Underwood, A.M. 1975. An unusual epizootic of actinobacillosis in dairy heifers. J. Am. Vet. Med. Assoc. 166:604–606.
Carb, A.V., and Liu, S. 1969. *Actinobacillus lignieresii* infection in a dog. J. Am. Vet. Med. Assoc. 154:1062–1067.
Davies, G.O., and Torrence, H.L. 1930 Observations regarding the etiology of actinomycosis in cattle and swine. J. Comp. Pathol. Ther. 43:216–233.
Fletcher, R.B., Linton, A.H., and Osborne, A.D. 1956. Actinobacillosis of the tongue of a dog. Vet. Rec. 68:645–646.
Hebeler, H.F., Linton, A.H., and Osborne, A.D. 1961. Atypical actinobacillosis in a dairy herd. Vet. Rec. 73:517–521.
Johnston, K.G. 1954. Nasal actinobacillosis in sheep. Aust. Vet. J. 30:105–106.
Laws, L., and Elder, J.K. 1969. Mastitis in sheep caused by *Actinobacillus lignieresii*. Aust. Vet. J. 45:401–403.
Lignières, J., and Spitz, J. 1902. Actinobacillosis. Rev. Soc. Med. Argentina 11:169–230.
Phillips, J.E. 1967. Antigenic structure and serological typing of *Actinobacillus lignieresii*. J. Pathol. Bacteriol. 93:464–475.
Sanders, D.A., and Ristic, M. 1956. *Actinobacillus* of cattle. J. Am. Vet. Med. Assoc. 129:478–481.
Sautter, J.H., Rowsell, H.C., and Hohn, R.B. 1953. Actinomycosis and actinobacillosis in dogs. North Am. Vet. 34:341–346.
Smith. H.W. 1951. A laboratory consideration of the treatment of *Actinobacillus lignieresii* infection. Vet. Rec. 63:674–675.
Taylor, A.W. 1944. Actinobacillosis in sheep. J. Comp. Pathol. Ther. 54:228–237.

Actinobacillus equuli

SYNONYMS: *Bacterium pyosepticus equi, Bacillus nephritidis equi, Bacterium viscosum equi, Shigella equi, Shigella equirulis, Shigella viscosa*

A. equuli causes purulent infections of the joints and kidney abscesses in very young foals. It has also been found in adult horses. In foals the disease is often termed *sleepy foal disease*. *A. equuli* was first described by Meyer (1909), who found it in kidney abscesses in horses in South Africa and gave it the name *Bacillus nephritidis equi*.

Because this organism has been renamed each time a new classification has appeared and because the names that have been applied to the disease produced by the organism are no longer valid we propose that the infection be named *equulosis*, a designation based on the specific part of the binomial and thus more likely to remain unchanged.

Morphology and Staining Reactions. *A. equuli* is a small rod-shaped organism. Short chains and filaments are often seen. Capsules have been described, but generally *A. equuli* is believed to be noncapsulated. *A. equuli* is nonmotile, is easily stained with the ordinary stains, and is Gram-negative.

Cultural and Biochemical Features. *A. equuli* grows readily in ordinary media, producing rather abundant growth. Colonies on agar plates are smooth, rather dry in appearance, and tough. Dissociation readily occurs, especially when the medium is acidic and the incubation temperature high, the product being small, smooth, glistening colonies, some of which are dwarf types. On agar slants the growth is diffuse, grayish white, and highly mucoid. A ropy sediment forms in broth, and old cultures become very cloudy and mucoid. A grayish pellicle sometimes appears. Cultures grown in stabs made in gelatin show a filiform growth. There is no liquefaction. *A. equuli* slowly acidifies and sometimes coagulates litmus milk. The uncoagulated cultures generally are quite slimy. The organism does not form indole and reacts negatively to the

Voges-Proskauer test. It does not generate toxins. When grown with glucose, lactose, sucrose, galactose, maltose, raffinose, xylose, or mannitol, *A. equuli* forms acid but not gas. Freshly isolated cultures must be transferred at weekly intervals to maintain viability. *A. equuli* is usually nonhemolytic, but hemolytic variants have been described (Carter et al. 1971).

Epizootiology and Pathogenesis. *A. equuli* commonly occurs in the tonsils and intestines of normal horses and causes disease only in animals debilitated by overtraining, parasitism, or exposure to bad weather. Platt (1973) concluded from a review of 61 cases of septicemia caused by *A. equuli* that the organism was opportunistic and invaded foals that were congenitally defective in some way. Foals are infected either in utero or during or after birth. Dimock et al. (1947) noted that common verminous aneurysms of the mesenteric arteries are often infected with this organism, even when it cannot be demonstrated elsewhere. Apparently the larvae of *Strongylus vulgaris*, migrating from the intestinal lumen into the arteries, carry *A. equuli* with them and in this way set up infections in young susceptible animals. In prenatal infection it is possible that invasion of the fetal circulation by strongylid larvae from the dam may be a contributing factor. About one third of the foals that succumbed to equulosis died within the first 24 hours, and the majority succumbed before the fourth day of life. In foals that died within the first 24 hours, the only visible lesion consisted of a severe enteritis. Rarely was there any evidence of nephritis. In foals that died at 2 or 3 days of age, the lesions observed at postmortem examination were more marked. These foals often exhibited a purulent nephritis, small abscesses being scattered throughout the cortex of the kidney. Many times the joints of the legs were affected. The joint lesions ranged from a slight increase in synovial fluid and congestion of the joint capsule to a purulent arthritis involving the joint cavity and tendon sheaths, with accumulation of large amounts of fluid and extreme swelling. A few foals showed a severe purulent pleuropneumonia. The diagnosis was made by isolating the causative microorganism from the infected organs and joints of the diseased foal. Goy (1980) has described peritonitis in horses associated with *A. equuli*. In three animals there was an acute onset of intestinal and abdominal pain. Two animals showed a chronic syndrome with weight loss and a highly cellular peritoneal fluid. Pedersen (1977) described a series of cases of septicemia in piglets which were caused by a nonhemolytic strain of *A. equuli*.

Immunity. Antiserum has been used in the treatment of foals with equulosis but the results were disappointing. Maguire (1958) observed that vaccination of mares was an effective form of passive protection for foals.

Diagnosis. Blood, kidney lesions, synovial fluids, and cervical swabs from mares should be cultured on blood agar.

Antimicrobial Susceptibility. *A. equuli* is sensitive to streptomycin, chlortetracycline, and chloramphenicol. Streptomycin has been employed with very good results in the prevention and treatment of equulosis.

REFERENCES

Carter, P.L., Marshall, R.B., and Jolly, R.D. 1971. A haemolytic variant of *Actinobacillus equuli* causing an acute septicaemia in a foal. N.Z. Vet. J. 19:264–265.

Dimock, W.W., Edwards, P.R., and Bruner, D.W. 1947. Infections of fetuses and foal. Ky. Agric. Exp. Sta. Bull. 509.

Goy, C.L. 1980. Peritonitis in horses associated with *Actinobacillus equuli*. Aust. Vet. J. 56:296–300.

Maguire, L.C. 1958. The role of *Bacterium viscosum equi* in the causation of equine disease. Vet. Rec. 70:989–991.

Meyer, K.F. 1909. Notes on the pathological anatomy of pleuro-pneumonia. Transvaal Dept. of Agriculture, Report, Government Bacteriologist. Pp. 132–162.

Pedersen, K.B. 1977. *Actinobacillus* infection in swine. Nord. Vet. Med. 29:137–140.

Platt, H. 1973. Septicaemia in the foal: A review of 61 cases. Br. Vet. J. 129:221–229.

Actinobacillus suis

A. suis was first described by van Dorssen and Jaarsveld (1962). Their isolations were made from a variety of lesions and from septicemic disease in pigs.

Morphology and Staining Reactions. The cells are rod-shaped and 0.5 to 3 μm long and occur singly, in filaments, and in masses. They are nonmotile and Gram-negative.

Cultural and Biochemical Features. The colonies are moderately sticky and may adhere to the agar surface. *A. suis* produces a viscous growth in serum broth, and it will grow on MacConkey agar. It produces narrow, distinct zones of alpha hemolysis on horse-blood agar and a wide zone of beta (complete) hemolysis on sheep-blood agar. *A. suis* may produce hydrogen sulfide, but it does not produce indole or urease. When grown with glucose, lactose, arabinose, mannitol, or salicin, *A. suis* produces acid. It hydrolyzes esculin. The mol% G + C of the DNA is 40.5 (Tm).

Pathogenesis. *A. suis* has caused fatal acute septicemias in piglets aged 1 to 8 weeks (Liven et al. 1978, Moir et al. 1974, Zimmerman 1964). Affected pigs develop rapid respiration and cyanosis of the extremities. At necropsy there may be a mucopurulent coating of the nasal mucosa, pleural edema, an enlarged spleen, and focal hepatic necrosis (Liven et al. 1978). A verrucous endocarditis or a pericarditis may also be present. Petechiae can be found throughout the abdominal organs

(Moir et al. 1974). In older pigs *A. suis* has been associated with arthritis, pneumonia, and subcutaneous abscesses (Zimmerman 1964).

In New Zealand the organism has also been isolated from the nose of a healthy horse, aborted equine fetuses, foals dying within a week of birth, and from animals with respiratory or genital infections (Carman and Hodges 1982). However, the significance of this organism as a cause of disease in horses is as yet unclear. Kim et al. (1976) found that only 10 percent of isolates from horses were associated with pathological material; the remainder were obtained from the respiratory tracts of normal animals. It is probable that the organism is a normal commensal and opportunistically causes disease given the appropriate predisposing conditions.

Antimicrobial Susceptibility. *A. suis* is sensitive to ampicillin, chloramphenicol, streptomycin, gentamicin, and tetracyclines (Mair et al. 1974).

REFERENCES

Carman, M.G., and Hodges, R.T. 1982. *Actinobacillus suis* infection of horses. N.Z. Vet. J. 30:82–84.
Kim, B.H., Phillips, J.G., and Atherton, J.G. 1956. *Actinobacillus suis* in the horse. Vet. Rec. 98:239.
Liven, E., Larson, H., and Lium, B. 1978. Infection with *Actinobacillus suis* in pigs. Acta Vet. Scand. 19:313–315.
Mair, N.S., Randall, C.J., Thomas, G.W., Harbourne, J.F., McCrae, C.T., Cowl, K.P. 1974. *Actinobacillus suis* infection in pigs. A report of four outbreaks and two sporadic cases. J. Comp. Pathol. 84:113–119.
Van Dorssen, C.A., and Jaarsveld, F.H.J. 1962. *Actinobacillus suis* (novo species). A bacterium occurring in swine. Tidj. Diergeneeskd. 87:450–458.
Zimmerman, V.T. 1964. Untersuchungen über die Actinobazillosen des Schweines. D.T.W. 71:457–461.

Actinobacillus salpingitidis

Mraz et al. (1976) proposed that the organism resembling *Actinobacillus* which they isolated from 25 outbreaks of disease in chickens and from the cloacae of healthy pullets be named *A. salpingitidis*. Kohlert (1968) earlier had isolated a similar organism from an outbreak of salpingitis and peritonitis in laying hens and named his isolate *Pasteurella salpingitidis*.

The isolates of Mraz et al. (1976) were hemolytic on sheep-blood agar, showed the basic properties of the *Pasteurella-Actinobacillus* group, and grew on MacConkey agar containing crystal violet, a trait characteristic of *Actinobacillus*. Pohl (1981), however, demonstrated through DNA hybridization studies that *A. salpingitidis* is not closely related to the actinobacilli. Its true affiliation remains to be determined.

Other reports of organisms similar to *Actinobacillus*

species in cultures from waterfowl with salpingitis, airsacculitis, or bronchopneumonia have been made by Bisgaard (1975) and Hacking and Sileo (1977).

REFERENCES

Bisgaard, M. 1975. Characterization of atypical *Actinobacillus lignieresii* isolated from ducks with salpingitis and peritonitis. Nord. Vet. Med. 27:378–383.
Hacking, M.A., and Sileo, L. 1977. Isolation of a hemolytic *Actinobacillus* from waterfowl. J. Wildl. Dis. 13:68–73.
Kohlert, R. 1968. Aetiology of salpingitis in fowls. Vet. Med. 23:392–395.
Mraz, O., Vladik, P., and Bohacek, J. 1976. Actinobacilli in domestic fowl. Zentrabl. Bakteriol. [A]. 236:294–307.
Pohl, S. 1981. DNA relatedness among members of *Actinobacillus, Haemophilus,* and *Pasteurella.* In M. Kilian, W. Frederiksen, and E.L. Biberstein, eds., *Haemophilus, Pasteurella,* and *Actinobacillus.* Academic Press, New York. Pp. 246–253.

Actinobacillus seminis

First described in Australia by Baynes and Simmons (1960), *A. seminis* has since been shown to be widespread in sheep populations in Australia and South Africa. Although its classification is uncertain, it is included here in the genus *Actinobacillus* for convenience and because this is the classification used in the literature.

Morphology and Staining Reactions. The cells are pleomorphic, Gram-negative, nonmotile rods and coccobacilli (1 μm by 4 μm) that occur singly, in pairs, or short chains. The organism is nonencapsulated.

Cultural and Biochemical Features. Primary growth is best on media enriched with blood or serum and incubated in an atmosphere of 20 percent CO_2 (Van Tonder 1979). Colonies on 5 percent horse-blood tryptose agar are pinpoint to droplike at 24 hours and become enlarged (4 mm), and umbonate, with a transparent periphery and grayish center. *A. seminis* is nonhemolytic and does not grow on MacConkey agar. The organism does not ferment carbohydrates, does produce catalase, and usually does not reduce nitrates. It produces only slight amounts of H_2S if at all. *A. seminis* reacts negatively to the following tests or reactions: oxidase, methyl red, Voges-Proskauer, indole, phosphatase, gelatinase, and citrate utilization. The mol% G + C of the DNA is 43.7 (Tm).

Epizootiology and Pathogenesis. *A. seminis* is widely distributed in sheep populations in South Africa (Van Tonder 1979) and has also been isolated in different areas of Australia (Simmons et al. 1966, Walt et al. 1970). There is only one record of its occurrence in the United States (Livingston and Hardy 1964). The organism can enter the animal through the genitals but also by other routes. It localizes in the epididymus and the testis and is transmitted in the semen. In South Africa the incidence of clinical lesions in sheep is highest in the Dorper breed (5.7 percent) followed by the Karakal (3.0 percent) and Merino breeds (2.1 percent) (Van Tonder 1979). However, many rams can have clinically inapparent infections and spread the organism in their semen.

Watt et al. (1970) described the isolation of *A. seminis* from rams in western Australia with polyarthritis and posthitis. The organism has also been isolated from fetal and uterine samples obtained from ewes and goat does that aborted (Van Tonder 1973) and from uterine exudates of cows that delivered stillborn calves or had late abortions.

Immunity. Little is known about the immune response to *A. seminis*. A number of serologically different variants exist. Complement-fixing antibody is present in the serum of about 25 percent of rams with detectable lesions and in about 16 percent of animals culturally positive but without visible lesions (Van Tonder 1979). The test is therefore of little value for detection of infected individuals. When used as a flock test, complement fixation detects about 75 percent of infected flocks.

Diagnosis. The organism is difficult to identify because of its lack of biochemical activity. Differentiation from *B. ovis* is based on morphology and the modified Ziehl-Neelsen staining technique. *B. ovis* forms coccoid to short rods, whereas *A. seminis* is pleomorphic with rods as long as 5 μm. Unlike *B. ovis, A. seminis* is not stained red by modified Ziehl-Neelsen stain (Van Tonder 1979). An immunofluorescence technique for the diagnosis of *A. seminis* epididymitis has been described (Ajar 1980).

Antimicrobial Susceptibility. All strains of *A. seminis* are sensitive to penicillin, tetracycline, chloramphenicol, and novobiocin. They are resistant to streptomycin.

REFERENCES

Ajar, C.O. 1980. Diagnosing ovine epididymitis by immunofluorescence. Vet. Rec. 107:412–424.

Baynes, I.D. and G. C. Simmons. 1960. Ovine epididymitis caused by *Actinobacillus seminis* N.S.P. Aust. Vet. J. 36:454–459.

Livingston, C.W. and W.T. Hardy. 1964. Isolation of *Actinobacillus seminis* from ovine epidiymitis. Am. J. Vet. Res. 25:660–663.

Simmons, G.S., Baynes, I.D., and Ludford, C.G. 1966. Epidemiology of *Actinobacillus seminis* in a flock of border Leicester sheep. Aust. Vet. J. 42:183–187.

Van Tonder, E.M. 1973. Infection of rams with *Actinobacillus seminis*. J. S. Afr. Vet. Assoc. 44:235–240.

Van Tonder, E.M. 1979. *Actinobacillus seminis* infection in sheep in the Republic of South Africa. Onderstepoort J. Vet. Res. 46:129–148.

Watt, D.A., V. Bamford and M.E. Vlacin. 1970. *Actinobacillus seminis* as a cause of polyarthritis and posthitis in sheep. Aust. Vet. J. 46:515–520.

14 The Genus *Francisella*

Francisella tularensis

SYNONYMS: *Bacterium tularense, Brucella tularensis, Pasteurella tularensis*

F. tularensis is the cause of *tularemia*, also known as *deer-fly fever, rabbit fever,* and *Ohara's disease.* The disease affects various rodents, especially wild cottontail rabbits, water rats, and beavers, and occasionally certain birds and sheep. It has been reported in dogs and in coyotes. Humans become infected from these animals through the agency of ticks, lice (Price 1956), and blood-sucking flies.

Tularemia was first recognized in ground squirrels in California by McCoy in 1911. These animals became fatally infected with lesions resembling those of bubonic plague, with which tularemia was at first confused. Mc-Coy and Chapin (1912) isolated and described the causative organism. In 1914 Wherry and Lamb reported the first recognized case of tularemia in a human.

Some years later Francis (1922) identified the organism as the cause of a serious disease of humans in Utah. Francis named the disease *tularemia* after Tulare County, California, the location of McCoy's discovery of the disease in ground squirrels. For some years it was thought that the disease was confined to the United States, but it is now known to exist in the Scandinavian countries, the Soviet Union, and Japan. Its occurrence in humans has become quite important in these countries as well as in the United States.

An avirulent strain, *F. novicida*, has been described (Larson, et al. 1955) that is similar to *F. tularensis* but is avirulent for rabbits, white mice, and pigeons.

Morphology and Staining Reactions. *F. tularensis* is a particularly small (0.2 to 0.7 μm), nonmotile, poorly staining, bipolar rod. In older cultures bacillary forms as long as 2 and even 3 μm may be seen. Coccoid forms usually are mixed with the bacillary types. Polar granules can sometimes be seen, but these do not regularly occur. The organism is Gram-negative and can be stained with the usual stains. A relatively thick capsule can be present.

Cultural and Biochemical Features. Cysteine or cystine is required for growth of *F. tularensis* and or stimulates growth of *F. novicida*. Colonies of *F. tularensis* grown on glucose-cysteine-blood agar are smooth, gray, and surrounded by a green zone not associated with true hemolysis. It is a strict aerobe. It does not liquefy gelatin and grows poorly in milk. Suitable liquid media include peptone-cysteine broth, casein hydrolysate, and several chemically defined media. It produces acid from maltose, glycerol, and glucose. It is weakly catalase-positive and oxidase-negative. The mol% G + C of the DNA is 33 to 36.

Final characterization depends on growth requirements, solubility in sodium recinoleate, and reaction with specific antibody. The biovars *tularensis* and *palaearctica* are distinguished by the failure of palaearctica to hydrolyze glycerol or to produce citrulline ureidase.

Epizootiology and Pathogenesis. *F. tularensis* is found throughout the world with the exception of Australia and Antartica. Most human infections have occurred in the United States and the southern Soviet Union. Biovar *tularensis* occurs only in North America and is widespread in wildlife, whereas biovar *palaearctica* is found worldwide, is less virulent, and has as its reservoir hosts voles, water rats, muskrats, and beavers. The greatest reservoir of tularemia in the United States is the wild rabbit population, especially in the many midwestern states. Most of the human cases in this country originate from the handling of the carcasses of such rabbits. Of 266 authenticated cases of tularemia in California reported during 1927 to 1951, 81 percent were contracted from rabbits; jackrabbits were involved more frequently than cottontail rabbits. Cases are also contracted from the bites of bloodsucking insects that have fed on infected rabbits (Hillman and Morgan 1937). Washburn and Tuohy (1949) reported that tick-borne infection was almost twice as common in Arkansas as rabbit-borne infection. Later it was shown by Calhoun (1954) that the Lone Star tick (*Amblyomma americanum*) was the important carrier of *F. tularensis* in Arkansas and that the bacterium multiplied in this arthropod. Argasid ticks as well as members of the genus *Dermacentor* can also transmit tularemia. The bacterium sometimes becomes prevalent in water holes and small streams, being spread from the bodies of infected water animals such as water rats and beavers. Cases in humans have been reported from contact with such water. In general, strains of *F. tularensis* obtained from North American ticks, lagomorphs, and sheep are highly virulent and those obtained from beavers, rodents, and water are less so (Thorpe et al. 1965).

There is serologic evidence that the western elk may be a significant reservoir in the United States (Merrell and Wright 1978). More than 50 percent of these animals are serologically positive.

Parker and Dade (1929) have reported severe losses in lambs pastured on land in Montana that was heavily infested with wood ticks and have shown that this tick carried the infection. The ticks became infected by feeding on wild rodents in which the disease was enzootic. Tularemia in range sheep is associated with the stress of inclement weather, lambing, and ectoparasitism and causes unthriftiness and mortality (Bell et al. 1978). Affected sheep may show stiffness of gait, dorsiflexion of the head, diarrhea, weakness, and loss of fleece. Normal sheep are resistant to challenge from the virulent strains. The disease has been reported in epizootics in sheep in Idaho (Frank and Meinershagen 1961) and in Wyoming (Ryff et al. 1961), in pen-raised beavers in Oregon (Bell et al. 1962), and in rabbits in South Carolina (McCahan et al. 1962). It has occurred in cats, dogs, calves, and domestic chickens. *F. tularensis* can infect practically all rodents and has been isolated from beavers, foxes, skunks, coyotes, bobcats, deer, snakes, quail, prairie chickens, pheasants, shrikes, ducks, gulls, hawks, owls, muskrats, water rats, monkeys, and mink.

Because the guinea pig is easily infected with *F. tularensis,* it is frequently used in diagnostic work. A generalized, fatal disease develops in which the most striking lesions are multiple necrotic areas in the liver and spleen.

Immunity. *F. tularensis* is a facultative intracellular parasite, and effective immunity is cell-mediated (Koskela and Herva 1982). Although of diagnostic importance, humoral antibodies are not protective. A live, avirulent vaccine has been used to protect against laboratory-acquired tularemia (Burke 1977). Only one antigenic type of *F. tularensis* has been observed.

Agglutinins in convalescent serums react with *Brucella abortus,* which carries a cross-reacting antigen. Agglutination tests must therefore be performed with antigens of both organisms. The higher titer is usually produced by the homologous reaction.

Diagnosis. The procedures for collection, storage, and transport of clinical specimens is described by Eigelsbach (1974). After collection, specimens should be refrigerated. A portion should be stored at $-70°C$ as insurance against failure of attempts at direct culture. As much as possible, specimens should be cultured immediately on glucose-cysteine-blood agar. Normal contaminants can be controlled by the addition of penicillin (100,000 IU/ml), polymyxin B sulfate (100,000 IU/ml), and cycloheximide (0.1 mg/ml) to the medium.

If adequate containment is available, guinea pig inoculation is a very sensitive method of detecting *F. tularensis* in specimens. Death occurs in 5 to 10 days. At necropsy the guinea pigs have enlarged spleens, and the organism can be isolated from the blood, liver, and spleen (necrotic foci). The direct or indirect fluorescent antibody techniques are highly sensitive procedures for detecting *F. tularensis* in smears.

Antimicrobial Susceptibility. Streptomycin is bactericidal for *F. tularensis* and is the antibiotic of choice for treating tularemia (Howe et al. 1946). Other aminoglycosides such as gentamicin and kanamycin are also effective. The tetracyclines have been used successfully to treat sheep (Frank and Meinershagen 1961).

The Disease in Humans. Tularemia in humans is an acute, febrile, granulomatous disease. The organism is very invasive and can penetrate unbroken skin. A dose as low as 10^5 organisms can be infectious when inhaled. Many laboratory workers studying the disease have contracted it themselves. The incubation period is usually 3 to 4 days, and before the advent of antibiotics a mortality of 5 to 30 percent was observed. The disease can occur in either a glandular or an ulceroglandular form. A papule may appear at the site of entry and later ulcerate. In the typhoidal form there are no local lesions; instead, lesions occur in the respiratory tract.

REFERENCES

Bell, J.F., Owen C.R., Jellison W.L., Moore, G.J., and Buker, E.D. 1962. Epizootic tuleremia in pen-raised beavers, and field trials of vaccines. Am. J. Vet. Res. 23:884–888.

Bell, J.F., Wikel, S.K., Hawkins, W.W., and Owen, C.R. 1978. Enigmatic resistance of sheep (*Ovis aries*) to infection by virulent *Francisella tularensis*. Can. J. Comp. Med. 42:310–315.

Burke, D.G. 1977. Immunization against tularemia: Analysis of the effectiveness of live *Francisella tularensis* vaccine in prevention of laboratory-acquired tularemia. J. Infect. Dis. 135:55–60.

Calhoun, E.L. 1954. Natural occurrence of tularemia in the Lone Star tick, *Amblyomma americanum* (Linn.), and in dogs in Arkansas. Am. J. Trop. Med. Hyg. 3:360–366.

Eigelsbach, H.T. 1974. *Francisella tularensis*. In H. Lennette, E. H. Spaulding, and J.P. Truant, eds., Manual of Clinical Microbiology, 2d ed. American Society for Microbiology, Washington, D.C. Pp. 316–319.

Francis, E. 1922. Tularemia: A new disease of man. J.A.M.A. 78:1015–1018.

Frank, F.W., and Meinershagen, W.A. 1961. Tularemia epizootic in sheep: A review of the disease and controlled clinical study of treatment. Vet. Med. 56:374–378.

Hillman, C.C., and Morgan, M.T. 1937. Tularemia: Report of a fulminant epidemic transmitted by the deer fly. J.A.M.A. 108:538–540.

Howe, C., Coriell, L.L., Bookwalter, J.H.L., and Ellingson, H.V. 1946. Streptomycin treatment of tularemia. J.A.M.A. 132:195–200.

Koskela, P., and Herva, E. 1982. Cell-mediated and humoral immunity induced by a live *Francisella tularensis* vaccine. Infect. Immun. 36:983-989.

Larson, C.L., Wicht, W., and Jellison, W.C. 1955. A new organism resembling *F. tularensis* isolated from water. Pub. Health Rep. 70:253–258.

McCahan, G.R., M.D. Moody and F.A. Hayes. 1962. An epizootic of tularemia among rabbits in northwestern South Carolina. Am. J. Hyg. 75:335–338.

McCoy, G.W. 1911. A plague-like disease of rodents. U.S. Public Health Service Bulletin 43. Pp. 53–71.

McCoy, G.W., and Chapin, C.W. 1912. Further observations on a plague-like disease of rodents with a preliminary note on the causative agent, *Bacterium tularense*. J. Infect. Dis. 10:61–72.

Merrell, C.L., and Wright, D.N. 1978. A serologic survey of mule deer and elk in Utah. J. Wildlife. Dis. 14:471–478.

Parker, R.R., and H. Dade, 1929. Tularemia: Its transmission to sheep by the wood tick, *Dermacentor andersoni stiles*. J. Am. Vet. Med. Assoc. 75:173–191.

Price, R.D. 1956. The multiplication of *Pasterella tularensis* in human body lice. Am. J. Hyg. 63:186–197.

Ryff, J.F., Michael, H.A., and Norton, E.S. 1961. Tularemia in Wyoming sheep. J. Am. Vet. Med. Assoc. 138:309–310.

Thorpe, B.D., Sidwell, R.W., Johnson, D.E., Smart, K.L., and Parker, D.D. 1965. Tularemia in the wildlife and livestock of the Great Salt Lake Desert region, 1951 through 1964. Am. J. Trop. Med. and Hyg. 14:622–637.

Washburn, A.M., and Tuohy, J.H. 1949. The changing picture of tularemia transmission in Arkansas. South. Med. J. 42:60–62.

Wherry, W.B., and Lamb, B.H. 1914. Infection of man with *Bacterium tularense*. J. Infect. Dis. 15:331–340.

15 The Genus *Brucella*

The genus *Brucella* contains six species, *B. abortus*, *B. canis*, *B. melitensis*, *B. neotomae*, *B. ovis*, and *B. suis*, all of which, except *B. neotomae*, are important pathogens of domestic animals and humans (Table 15.1), causing the disease known as brucellosis. Infections typically are found in the reproductive organs and in the reticuloendothelial tissues. In cattle, sheep, and goats, lesions of the female reproductive tract and of the placenta and fetus can lead to abortion with consequent severe economic loss. Moreover, the ease with which some *Brucella* species can be transmitted directly or indirectly from infected animals to humans gives the genus considerable zoonotic importance and has been an additional stimulus for eradication programs in many of the developed countries.

The first member of the genus *Brucella* was isolated in 1887 by David Bruce from the spleens of patients who died of Mediterranean or Malta fever. The organism was appropriately named *Brucella melitensis*. Ten years later, a Danish veterinarian, Fredrick Bang, isolated and named *Brucella abortus* from an aborted bovine fetus. *B. suis* was isolated in 1914 by Jacob Traum from an aborted piglet, and *B. ovis* and *B. canis* were first described in 1956 and 1969, respectively. The latter two species are more highly host-adapted than *B. abortus*, *B. melitensis*, or *B. suis*.

Morphologic and cultural features are not sufficiently characteristic to differentiate the six species or their various biotypes. Nor can the host from which the organism is isolated be entirely relied on for identification, although each species does have a predilection for certain hosts, as shown in Table 15.1.

Isolation of a Gram-negative rod from a suspected case of brucellosis requires reliance on the results of the laboratory tests outlined in Table 15.2 before final identification of the species and biotype can be made.

Brucella abortus

SYNONYMS: *Bacillus abortus*, Bang's bacillus

B. abortus is found in cattle populations throughout the world, although it is rare or absent in some countries where eradication programs have been actively pursued.

Morphology and Staining Reactions. *B. abortus* is a short rod or a coccobacillus measuring 0.5 to 0.7 µm by 0.6 to 1.5 µm. The rods are frequently so short that they can be easily mistaken for cocci. They are usually arranged singly, although in cultures short chains may form. Because it is a facultative intracellular bacterium, *B. abortus* is frequently found in clumps and smears made from exudates. *B. abortus* is Gram-negative and stains with ordinary stains although with some difficulty. It is not acid-fast but can resist decolorization with some mild acids; this property provides the basis for some differential staining procedures, such as the Koster stain in which the organism stains deep red.

B. abortus is nonmotile, does not form spores, and does not have a well-developed capsule. Poorly developed capsules have been demonstrated on freshly isolated strains using special stains.

Cultural and Biochemical Features. Growth is aerobic, but many strains require increased tensions of CO_2 for growth, especially on primary isolation. *B. abortus* is catalase and oxidase positive and usually produces H_2S from protein or peptides rich in amino acids containing

Table 15.1. The species of *Brucella* and their principal hosts

Host	Principal pathogenic *Brucella* sp. isolated	Other pathogenic *Brucella* sp. isolated
Cattle	*B. abortus*	*B. melitensis* *B. suis*
Sheep	*B. melitensis* *B. ovis* (epididymitis)	*B. abortus*
Goats	*B. melitensis*	*B. abortus*
Horses	*B. abortus*	*B. suis*
Pigs	*B. suis*	*B. melitensis* *B. abortus*
Dogs	*B. canis*	*B. abortus* *B. melitensis* *B. suis*
Wood rats	*B. neotomae*	
Humans	*B. abortus* *B. melitensis* *B. suis*	*B. canis*

Table 15.2. Classification scheme for species and biotypes in the genus *Brucella*

Species	Biotype	CO$_2$ for growth	H$_2$S produced	Thionin 10*	20	50	Fuchsin 10	20	Tb	Wb	Bk$_2$	Fi	A	M	Anti-rough serums	L-Alanine	L-Asparagi
B. abortus	1	+,−	+	−	−	−	+	+	+	+	+	+	+	−	−	+	+
	2	+	+	−	−	−	−	−	+	+	+	+	+	−	−		
	3	+,−	+	+	+	−	+	+	+	+	+	+	+	−	−		
	4	+,−	+	−	−	−	+	+	+	+	+	+	−	+	−		
	5	−	−	+	+	−	+	+	+	+	+	+	−	+	−		
	6	−	−,+	+	+	−	+	+	+	+	+	+	+	−	−		
	7	−	−,+	+	+	−	+	+	+	+	+	+‡	+	+	−		
	9	−	+	+	+	−	+	+	+	+	+	+‡	−	+	−		
B. suis	1	−	+	+	+	+	−	−	−	+	+	+‡	+	−	−	+,−	−
	2	−	+,−	+	−	−	−	−	−	+	+	+‡	+	−	−	−	+,−
	3	−	−	+	+	+	+	+	−	+	+	+‡	+	−	−	+,−	−
	4	−	−	+	+	+	+	+	−	+	+	+‡	+	+	−	−	−
B. melitensis	1	−	−	+	+	−	+	+	−	−	+	−	−	+	−	+	+
	2	−	−	+	+	−	+	+	−	−	+	−	+	−	−		
	3	−	−	+	+	−	+	+	−	−	+	−	+	+	−		
B. neotomae		−	+	+	−	−	−	−	−	+	+	+	+	−	−	+,−	+
B. ovis		+	−	+	+	−	+	+	−	−	−	−	−	−	+	+,−	+
B. canis		−	−	+	+	+	+	−	−	−	−	−	−	−	+	+	−

*Micrograms of dye per milliliter of medium.
†+ = utilization rate above (QO$_2$N) rate of 50; − = no utilization; +,− = strain variability within species.
‡Partial lysis.
RTD = routine test dilution. Modified from Meyer (1974).

sulfur. It usually produces urease. Eight biotypes are currently recognized and are distinguished by dye sensitivity tests, CO$_2$ requirement, H$_2$S production, and the presence of A or M surface antigens (Table 15.2). *B. abortus* is not hemolytic, does not liquefy gelatin, and does not produce acid from glucose or other carbohydrates. It has a characteristic substrate oxidation pattern as shown in Table 15.2.

Growth of *B. abortus* is enhanced by serum or blood. Complex media such as serum dextrose agar or Albimi brucella agar or broth must be used for primary isolation and maintenance. A variety of antibiotics are sometimes added to these basal media to inhibit contaminants in specimens such as milk and vaginal discharges (Corbel and Hendry 1985).

On primary isolation, colonies of *B. abortus* are slow-growing and barely visible at 48 hours. They reach maximum size after 5 to 7 days at the optimum growth temperature (37°C). The isolates may be of the smooth type, characterized by round convex colonies with an entire edge, or they may dissociate to the rough type, characterized by large flat colonies with a dull granular appearance. Growth is sparse in fluid media and appears as a faint clouding.

The mol% G + C of the DNA is 57 (Tm). *B. abortus* shows 100 percent homology with the other *Brucella* species except *B. ovis*.

Bacteriophage Typing. Bacteriophages are often used for identifying and typing cultures of *Brucella* species spp. including *B. abortus*. The phages currently in routine use are the Tb, Wb, Fi, Bk$_2$, and R strains (Corbel and Hendry 1985). The dilution of the phage used is known as the routine test dilution (RTD) and usually is about 10^4 to 10^5 plaque-forming units per milliliter. The RTD is the minimum number of phages that will produce confluent lysis on a lawn of the propagating strain. The procedures for phage typing *Brucella* species are described in more detail by Corbel and Hendry (1985). Phage typing is a

			Substrate oxidation[†]						
L-Glutamate	DL-Ornithine	DL-Citrulline	DL-Citrulline	L-Lysine	L-Arabinose	D-Galactose	D-Ribose	D-Glucose	i-Erythritol
−	−	−	+	+	+	+	+	+	+
All *B. abortus* biotypes are identical									
−	+	+	+	+	+	+	+	+	+
+	+	+	+	+	+	+,−	+	+	+
+,−	+	+	+	+	−	−	+	+	+
+,−	+	+	+	+	−	−	+	+	+
+	−	−	−	−	−	−	−	l	−
+	−	−	−	+	+	+	+,−	+	+
+	−	−	−	−	−	−	−	−	−
−	+	+	+	+	+	+	+,−	+	+,−

rapid and very useful method of identifying *B. abortus* (Table 15.2).

Antigens. The cell wall of *B. abortus* consists of an outer layer of lipopolysaccharide protein on which the polysaccharide chains are exposed. The polysaccharide chains carry the major surface antigens (A and M) involved in the agglutination reaction. These antigens on smooth *B. abortus* are closely related to the surface antigens on *Yersinia enterocolitica* O9 and are a potential source of confusion in the interpretation of serologic tests for brucellosis (Mittal and Tizard 1981).

The cell wall proteins have been grouped into three categories according to molecular weight on SDS-PAGE gels (Verstreate and Winter 1984). The categories are proteins with molecular weights of 88,000 to 94,000, 35,000 to 40,000 (porins); and 25,000 to 30,000. One antigen is shared among the porin proteins of all *B. abortus* strains and three antigens are shared among the proteins of the lowest molecular weight category. It is gener-

ally accepted that the brucella antigen that stimulates delayed type hypersensitivity is a protein, probably porin (Winter et al. 1983). The antigen(s) involved in stimulating cell-mediated immune responses have not been identified.

Epizootiology and Pathogenesis. *B. abortus* is an obligate facultative intracellular parasite of cattle and some wild ruminants and is freely transmitted by ingestion of contaminated discharges or feed. Venereal transmission is possible but unusual. Intramammary and congenital transmission also occur. Horses, sheep, chickens, and dogs can also be infected, but transmission from these species to the primary host is highly unlikely. The organism is found in most cattle raising areas of the world except in countries where eradication programs have been successfully implemented.

B. abortus is not very resistant to sunlight and drying and therefore survives better in winter than summer. It survives well in milk but is destroyed by pasteurization.

Table 15.3. Survival times of *B. abortus* under various environmental conditions

Medium	Temperature or season	Environmental conditions	Survival time (days)	Reference
Uterine exudate	February	Placed on ground	10	Cotton (1919)
Placenta, fetal organs	Winter and spring	Covered with leaves in forest	135	Cotton (1919)
Milk	15°C	Milk samples from infected cows	38	Huddelson et al. (1927)
Butter			142	Carpenter and Boak (1928)
Cheese	4.4°C		180	Gilman et al. (1946)
Grass	10–70°F, February	0.6 in. rain	6	Ky. Agric. Exp. Sta. 43d Annu. Rep., 1931, p. 14.
	60–81°F, May	Sunny	<1	Ky. Agric. Exp. Sta. 43d Annu. Rep., 1931, p. 14.
	36–70°F, February		5	Ky. Agric. Exp. Sta. 43d Annu. Rep., 1931, p. 14.
Open plate cultures	October and November	Sunny	2–3	Ky. Agric. Exp. Sta. 43d Annu. Rep., 1931, p. 14.
Water	−40°C		800	Kuzdas and Morse (1954)
	37°C, 25°C, 8°C		57	
Infected guinea pig carcass	January (Wisconsin)	Placed on ground	44	Kuzdas and Morse (1954)
	June and August (Wisconsin)	Placed on ground	1	Kuzdas and Morse (1954)
	January (Wisconsin)	Buried	29	Kuzdas and Morse (1954)
Meat and salted meat	0–20°C		65	Prost (1957)
Manure pit	158°F	In tubes at bottom of pit	<4 hours	King (1957)
Manure pit		In tubes at top of pit	2	King (1957)
In manure	12°C		250	Plommet (1972)

Table 15.3 summarizes studies on the survival times of *B. abortus* under different conditions.

In the United States 85 percent of infections are caused by biotype 1, the remainder mostly by biotypes 2 and 4. Large dairy herds are more likely than smaller herds to be infected with a higher prevalence of infection within the herd. The greater level of intensivism and opportunity for transmission within large herds together with the greater likelihood of introduction of a latently infected animal are some of the factors that contribute to the higher risk of infection in larger herds (Nicoletti 1981). The use of community pastures can be a factor in transmission of *B. abortus* between herds, as can contamination of streams and the activities of carrion feeders.

Evidence of brucella infection is found in several species of free-living animals, for example, bison, moose, and elk, in North America. Comingling of these species with cattle enhances the possibility of cross-infection, but there is no evidence that this represents a substantial source of infection for domesticated animals. In Africa, however, Thimm and Nauwerck (1974) found large-scale involvement of game animals in the epizootiology of bovine brucellosis. Although prepubescent animals are generally resistant to infection by *B. abortus* and susceptibility increases with sexual development and pregnancy, heifer calves can be infected early in life either in utero from infected dams or by ingestion of contaminated milk. Calves exposed in this way develop latent infections that are not detectable by serologic tests. The frequency of such latent infections has been estimated at 2 to 3 percent of exposed calves (Wilesmith 1978). Latently infected animals can later have an infected calving and disseminate infection in a clean herd. Male cattle are resistant to infection but infection of the epididymus and testicle has been recorded. Such bulls can transmit the infection in their semen (Bendixen and Blom 1947).

The main portals of entry for *B. abortus* are the oral mucosa of calves that drink infected milk, the nasopharynx and conjunctivae of cattle exposed to the organism, and occasionally the genital tract in both bulls and cows. Under experimental conditions the organism has been shown to penetrate the unbroken skin of guinea pigs and cattle (Cotton and Buck 1932). After penetration of the host, *B. abortus* initially localizes in the regional lymph node and then enters the blood stream. The bacteremic phase results in dissemination of the organism to the udder, uterus, and associated nodes. *B. abortus* is a facultative intracellular bacterium and can survive and grow in host macrophages and epithelial cells. Survival of the organism in phagocytic cells is in part related to failure of the organism to stimulate an effective level of degranulation after ingestion. This effect is more apparent with smooth than with rough strains of *B. abortus* (Riley and Robertson 1984). *B. abortus* also has an unusually high resistance to intraleukocytic killing (Riley and Robertson 1984). The organism proliferates massively in cells with high levels of erythritol such as are found in the genital tracts of the male and pregnant female (Smith et al. 1962). *B. abortus* penetrates the epithelial cells of the chorion and proliferates, producing a placentitis. An endometritis is produced with ulceration of the epithelial lining of the uterus. Lesions of the fetus include edema and congestion of the lungs along with hemorrhages of the epicardium and splenic capsule. Fetal death follows, but it is unclear whether this is attributable to the endotoxin of *B. abortus* or to interference with placental function. The presence of the organism induces an inflammation of the membranes; this interference with the circulation of the fetus may explain why abortion occurs. The organism is also found in the stomach and lungs of aborted fetuses. Abortions occur late in pregnancy.

After calving or abortion, *B. abortus* is present in large numbers in uterine discharges for a few days but is then gradually cleared from the reproductive tract. The infection is, however, maintained in the reticuloendothelial tissue and the udder. Large numbers are shed in the milk, which is therefore a source of infection for calves and humans. Most infected animals remain carriers for life and shed the organism in uterine exudates and in milk after each calving. Abortions are usually seen only during the first pregnancy after infection and not subsequently, although the placenta is infected during each pregnancy.

B. abortus has occasionally been found in lymph nodes of the digestive tract and in the spleen of infected cattle. It has also been isolated from the blood and from hygromas of the knee. Hygroma of the knee shows a high correlation with brucella abortion in African cattle and it has been proposed as an easily discernible sign of the infection (Domenech et al. 1982). Large numbers of virulent organisms are present in the hygroma fluid.

B. abortus can infect horses but with much less frequency than cattle. In horses, it frequently localizes in bursae, joints, or tendon sheaths and has been found in poll evil and fistulous withers, supra-atlantal bursitis, and supraspinous bursitis (Roderick et al. 1948) as well as in lesions of the fetlock and sternum (Van der Hoeden 1930). It can also infect sheep (Luchsinger and Anderson 1967), goats (Doyle 1939), and pigs (McCullough et al. 1951) but much less frequently than other species of *Brucella*.

Immunity. *B. abortus* is a facultative intracellular parasite and so readily escapes the bactericidal effects of antibody and complement in plasma. Protective immunity depends mainly on cell-mediated responses in which the microbicidal activity of macrophages is enhanced following activation by lymphokines from sensitized T lymphocytes. Opsonic antibody does, however, enhance intracellular killing. The organism has been shown to multiply more slowly in the macrophages of vaccinated calves than in control animals (Fitzgeorge et al. 1967).

Humoral antibodies correlate poorly with protective immunity. Cattle vaccinated as calves with strain 19 vaccine have been shown to be resistant to challenge after antibody titers fall below detectable levels (Cunningham and O'Reilly 1968, McDiarmid 1957). However, large doses of hyperimmune serum can arrest the spread of *Brucella* organisms in infected animals.

Following infection, IgM agglutinins are the first antibodies to appear in the plasma and their levels reach a peak at about 2 weeks. IgG antibodies appear later but exceed IgM titers by 4 to 6 weeks and remain the dominant antibody thereafter. Infected cattle have high titers of nonagglutinating antibody of the IgG1 subclass. These nonagglutinating antibodies have been shown to have no opsonizing activity and to have no effect on clearance of the organism and so it has been suggested that they contribute to the chronicity of *B. abortus* infection (Parma et al. 1984). They also competitively block agglutinating IgM and IgG2 antibodies. Treatment with acid at pH 3.6 activates their agglutinating ability.

In calves vaccinated with strain 19, IgM antibody levels increase rapidly. IgG1 antibody levels rise more slowly, do not attain high levels, and do not persist (Beh 1974). Also, levels of nonagglutinating IgG1 antibodies are much lower than in naturally infected animals.

The protective immune responses of cows to *B. abortus* appear to be most effective when infection occurs before puberty. Only 2.6 percent of calves infected at birth or shortly thereafter remain infected as adults whereas the majority of infections in sexually mature animals persist for life although the immune response does reduce the severity of disease in the uterus and placenta so that such animals are more likely to carry to term in later pregnancies.

Vaccines. Two vaccines are important in the control of *B. abortus* infection: strain 19 vaccine and the McEwen killed 45/20 vaccine. The strain 19 vaccine consists of a viable culture of a strain that was discovered to have very little virulence for guinea pigs and cattle but to possess excellent immunizing properties. The strain has great stability; many deliberate attempts to change its virulence have failed, and it has not changed since 1930.

Strain 19 is a smooth strain of *B. abortus* that is mildly pathogenic for guinea pigs. Pregnant cattle can be made to abort by inoculating them with large doses of strain 19. In these cases the vaccine organism can usually be demonstrated without difficulty in the fetal membranes and the fetus itself. Susceptible cattle, associating with those that have aborted as a result of inoculation with the vaccine strain, do not become infected. Much experience has shown that strain 19 is unlikely to be transmitted from one animal to another; if any damage is done by the use of this vaccine, it is limited to the animal injected. Strain 19 is rarely shed in the milk of vaccinated animals. It can cause infection in humans (Spink and Thompson 1953), although it is usually mild with recovery in a much shorter time than with virulent strains. The vaccine, in view of its dangers for humans, should be handled with caution.

Calves are vaccinated at 2 to 10 months of age. Vaccination at this age is advocated to avoid persistent agglutinins that could create diagnostic problems later in the animal's life. Strain 19 protects about 65 to 70 percent of animals for 4 or 5 pregnancies and is most effective for protection of young breeding animals when applied on a herd basis. Animals vaccinated as adults are also protected but develop persisting agglutinins. There is evidence that a reduced dose of vaccine causes fewer persisting agglutinin responses (Alton et al. 1984, Nicoletti 1981). Latently infected animals or animals in the early stages of infection do not benefit from vaccination. Colostral antibodies may interfere with the response to strain 19 during the first 5 months of the calf's life (Cunningham 1977a).

Vaccination of cows in early pregnancy with large doses (6×10^9 organisms) of strain 19 produces a high probability of uterine infection. This risk is greatly diminished when the dose is reduced to 3×10^8 organisms.

Horses with fistulous withers caused by *B. abortus* are sometimes treated by vaccination with strain 19 or 45/20.

The McEwen killed 45/20 strain of *B. abortus* is a rough strain that is inactivated and adjuvanated for use as a vaccine or antigen in the anamnestic diagnostic test. It is administered in two doses 6 to 12 weeks apart. It stimulates complement fixing antibodies and agglutinins for rough *B. abortus* antigens of the IgG1 subclass. These antibodies do not react with the antigens used in the standard agglutination tube or plate tests. The 45/20 vaccine has been used widely in Ireland and other parts of Europe for the control of bovine brucellosis.

Diagnosis. *B. abortus* infection can be diagnosed bacteriologically or serologically.

Bacteriological diagnosis. Isolation and recognition of *B. abortus* are often accomplished by direct culture on a basal medium such as tryptose agar or Albimi agar to which serum and selected antibiotics are added. The cultures are incubated at 37°C in an atmosphere of 10 percent CO_2 tension and are examined in 2 to 3 days. Final identification is made on the basis of the characteristics listed in Table 15.2. Serologic typing of *Brucella* strains and phage typing with the Tbilisi (Tb) strain of bacteriophage are useful aids to definitive identification, but their use is restricted to specifically equipped reference laboratories.

Specimens should be examined from the following:

1. The aborted fetus. Direct cultures of specimens of the stomach contents, the intestinal contents, or the lung tissue will usually demonstrate *B. abortus*.

2. The placenta. Direct stained smears from the outer surface of the chorion, especially from the margins of the characteristic thickenings, will usually suffice to make a positive diagnosis without the need for cultural methods. The organism occurs free or enclosed in epithelial cells. It is these intracellular organisms that can be recognized with certainty, even though many other bacteria may have invaded the placenta. They are easily visualized using the modified Koster strain by which they appear red against a blue background (Christofferson and Ottosen 1961). New fetal membranes can be washed in water and rinsed in saline before attempts are made to culture the organism. After washing, obvious lesions are incised and the cut surface rubbed onto plates of selective media (Corbel and Hendry 1985).

3. The uterine exudate. After abortion or calving, when the placenta has been infected, *B. abortus* is present in the lochia and can be recognized by guinea pig inoculation. Within a few days, however, the organism seems to disappear and usually cannot be found in the uterus until

the animal is again pregnant and reinfection of the organ occurs.

4. Milk. When the udder is infected, *B. abortus* can be readily detected by the intraperitoneal injection of milk into guinea pigs or by direct cultural means. The cream layer and pellet formed after centrifugation should be cultured.

5. Abscesses. Direct culture of specimens from abscesses of the testicle and epididymis usually produce pure cultures of *B. abortus*, and isolations have been made from hygromas in cattle and from infected bursae in horses. Isolation of *B. abortus* from infected tissue is not always easy, therefore, it is advisable to preserve aliquots for later reculturing, guinea pig inoculation, or serologic examination.

Inoculation of guinea pigs is the most reliable method of detecting *B. abortus* in infected materials. Macerated tissue or fluid is inoculated into two guinea pigs, which are killed 3 and 6 weeks later. Their serums are examined for the presence of antibodies and specimens from the spleen, liver, regional lymph nodes, and testicles are cultured.

The direct examination of tissues with a fluorescent-antibody preparation can be an aid to diagnosis. This method is particularly useful for examining material that may be contaminated, such as placental membranes, cotyledons, or fetal or vaginal discharges.

Serologic diagnosis. There is, perhaps, no other infectious disease of animals for which there is a greater variety of serologic diagnostic tests than brucellosis. These tests are applied to serum, whole blood, vaginal mucus, seminal plasma, whey, or milk. The following descriptions deal only with those tests in routine use in eradication schemes. For additional information, consult the reviews by Nicoletti (1980), Stemshorn (1984), and Sutherland (1980).

The serum tube agglutination test (SAT) has been successfully used in eradication programs in many countries. The antigen and conditions of the test have been the subject of international standards. The test is performed in small test tubes on dilutions of serum (Figure 15.1). Complete agglutination at a serum dilution of 1:100 and higher is considered positive. In Great Britain a titer of at least 50 percent agglutination at 1:40 is considered positive. The test is subject to considerable error. False-positive reactions can be caused by reactions of antibodies to *Yersinia enterocolitica* 09 and other Gram-negative organisms. Antibodies stimulated by vaccination with strain 19 can also confuse interpretation of the test. False-negative reactions occur in a significant number of serum samples from latently or chronically infected animals. Animals in the early stages of infection similarly may fail to react. In

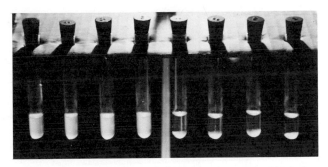

Figure 15.1. The tube agglutination test. Two tests are represented here. The four tubes on the left contain serum dilutions of 1:25, 1:50, 1:100, and 1:200. This serum is negative (devoid of agglutinins), as indicated by the fact that the bacteria remain in suspension. The tubes on the right contain the same dilutions of a strongly positive serum; the bacteria have flocculated and settled to the bottom, leaving the fluid perfectly clear.

some countries, buffered antigen plate agglutination tests have replaced the standard SAT because the use of buffered antigen reduces the frequency of false-positive reactions (Stemshorn 1984).

The antigen in the rose bengal plate test consists of *B. abortus* cells stained with rose bengal and suspended in acidic buffer to inhibit nonspecific agglutinins. The test can be used as a screen or definitive test. It detects IgM antibodies more efficiently than IgG1 or IgG2 and so readily picks up IgM antibodies stimulated by strain 19. The frequency of false-negative reactions is less than for the SAT.

In the card test the antigen is a buffered, stained, whole-cell suspension of *B. abortus* strain 1119-3. The antibody source is plasma separated from blood following clumping of erythrocytes by lectins. Only one antigen plasma or serum dilution is made. The test is useful for the detection of early infections where IgM is the dominant antibody. It is easily performed under range conditions.

The antigen in the plate agglutination, or rapid, test is a heavy suspension of strains of *B. abortus* stained with gentian violet and brilliant green to make the test easier to read. Because the antigen is standardized, it should give results comparable with those of the tube method. Serum, whole blood, or whey can may be used in this test. The test is done on a glass slide or plate and the reactions can be read in several minutes (Figure 15.2). A fair degree of accuracy can be obtained by using whole blood instead of serum. The whole-blood method is often used for testing range cattle when it is desirable to hold the animals in chutes until the results are known. A drop of blood is collected on a glass slide from an incision in the end of the tail. A drop of antigen is mixed with the blood and the results are obtained in a few minutes.

In the milk ring test the antigen is a hematoxylin-

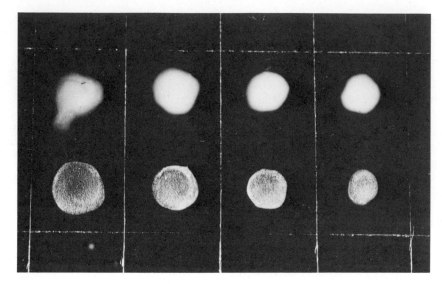

Figure 15.2. The plate agglutination, or rapid, test. Two tests are depicted, four dilutions of serum being tested in each case. These correspond to dilutions of 1:25, 1:50, 1:100, and 1:200, reading from left to right. The sample above is negative; the one below is positive in all dilutions.

stained suspension of killed *B. abortus*. It is mixed with fresh milk in a tube in the proportion of one drop per milliliter of milk. The mixture is then incubated in a water bath at 37°C for 1 hour.

Clumps of agglutinated organisms are carried to the surface by the rising fat globules. Thus, a positive test is indicated by a bluish violet cream layer and a decolorized milk column. Sources of error include mastitis or the presence of colostrum. The test is widely used for the examination of bulk milk samples and so allows herds in an area to be quickly and economically screened. Positive herds are then subjected to blood tests on individual animals.

The complement-fixation test is one of the most accurate tests in widespread use for the diagnosis of *B. abortus* infection. It detects IgM and IgG1 antibodies only. Fewer false-positive reactions due to strain 19 vaccination are seen in animals vaccinated as calves than as adults because complement-fixing antibodies do not persist as long as agglutinating antibodies in calf serum. However, the test does not differentiate infected animals from animals recently vaccinated with strain 19 or 45/20. Although it is subject to prozone effects owing to IgG2 antibodies competitively blocking access of IgG1 or IgM to antigen sites and does not detect latently infected animals, when used a week after the administration of 45/20 antigen in an anamnestic test, it can be very effective in detecting latently infected cattle (Cunningham and O'Connor 1971).

The test has been automated in many laboratories, resulting in greater precision. A complement-fixation test

designed to test antibody to the 45/20 vaccine is also available (Miller et al. 1976).

The antiglobulin (Coombs) test measures binding of nonagglutinating antibodies to *B. abortus* antigen. Its value is in defining the status of cattle for which the results in the complement-fixation test are inconclusive (Sutherland 1980).

The rivanol and mercaptoethanol tests are used to help distinguish between agglutinin titers caused by chronic infection and those caused by vaccination with strain 19. IgM antibodies are sensitive to mercaptoethanol and so a drop in titer following treatment with the reagent is indicative of a vaccine titer. Chronically infected animals have higher IgG1 antibody titers than IgM.

A variety of assays such as enzyme-linked immunosorbent assay (ELISA) (van Aert et al. 1984) have been developed in recent years that offer promise of greater sensitivity and specificity than the tests described above. Allergic skin tests based on purified antigens also promise to be a valuable addition to serology for detecting animals that have been infected by *B. abortus* (Stemshorn 1984).

Control. The economic losses from brucellosis together with the hazards posed to human health have prompted many countries to impose measures for the control and eradication of the disease. Many approaches have been followed for its control, but the following principles are usually incorporated, depending on local conditions of husbandry and the numbers of animals involved.

1. Affected animals are detected and eliminated from

the herd. Detection is usually by serologic methods, using the milk-ring test for rapid herd screening, followed by an agglutination test on each animal's serum. Slaughter of these serologically positive animals follows, with indemnity paid by a regulatory agency.

2. The resistance of the remaining animals or any replacements is increased by vaccination.

3. General principles of hygiene are imposed to prevent spread or reintroduction of infection.

In herds that are only lightly infected, blood testing and removal of reactors are begun immediately. If there is any danger of exposure, it is wise to conduct systematic calf vaccination as a protective measure. In heavily infected herds, in which many valuable animals would have to be removed, the so-called test-and-slaughter plan is not logical. In such herds systematic calfhood vaccination with strain 19 or 45/20 is practiced. If this is done for several years, clinical evidence of the disease generally disappears within 2 years, and at the end of 5 years natural attrition will have eliminated most of the chronically infected cows. Blood testing at this time usually will show few or no reactors, and these may then be eliminated. Calfhood vaccination is maintained in such a herd as long as there is a real danger of exposure to the disease from any source.

Surveillance of herds is maintained thereafter by means of periodic milk-ring tests on bulk milk samples and by random testing of serum samples of animals when they are sent for slaughter. Back-tagging of these animals allows any infection to be traced back to the herd of origin.

Antimicrobial Susceptibility. B. *abortus* is sensitive to gentamicin, kanamycin, tetracycline, and rifampicin. Tetracycline is often combined with streptomycin for treatment of human brucellosis (Young 1983). The combination of cotrimoxazole with rifampin or tetracycline and streptomycin with rifampin is also used.

The intracellular location of the organism requires that therapy be prolonged. Cattle are not usually given antimicrobials for prophylaxis or therapy of B. *abortus* infection.

REFERENCES

Alton, C.G., Corner, L.A., and Plackett, P. 1984. Vaccination against bovine brucellosis. Third International Symposium on Brucellosis, Algiers, Algeria, 1983. Dev. Biol. Stand. 56:643–647.

Beh, K.J. 1974. Quantitative distribution of brucella antibody amongst immunoglobulin classes in vaccinated and infected cattle. Res. Vet. Sci. 17:1–4.

Bendixen, H.C., and Blom, E. 1947. Investigations on brucellosis in the male with special regard to the spread of the disease by artificial insemination. Br. Vet. J. 103:337–345.

Carpenter, C.M., and Boak, R. 1928. *Brucella abortus* in milk and dairy products. Am. J. Public Health 18:743–751.

Christoffersen, F.A., and Ottosen, H.E. 1961. Recent staining methods. Skand. Vettidskr. 31:599–607.

Corbel, M.J. and Hendry, D. 1985. Brucellas. In C.H. Collins and I.M. Grange, eds., Isolation and Identification of Micro-Organisms of Medical and Veterinary Importance. Society for Applied Bacteriology Technical Series, no. 21. Academic Press, New York.

Cotton, W.E. 1919. Abortion disease of cattle. J. Am. Vet. Med. Assoc. 55:504–528.

Cotton, W.E., and Buck, J.M. 1932. Further researches on Bang's disease. J. Am. Vet. Med. Assoc. 80:342–352.

Cunningham, B. 1977a. Protective effects of colostral antibodies to *Brucella abortus* on strain 19 vaccination and field infection. Vet. Rec. 101:521–524.

Cunningham, B. 1977b. The transfer of *Brucella abortus* antibodies from dam to calf. Vet. Rec. 100:522–524.

Cunningham, B., and O'Connor, M. 1971. The use of killed 45/20 adjuvant vaccine as a diagnostic agent in the final stages of the eradication of brucellosis: The clearance of brucellosis from problem herds by interpretation of anamnestic serological responses. Vet. Rec. 89:680–686.

Cunningham, B., and O'Reilly, D.J. 1968. Agglutinin responses in blood serum and milk following vaccination of cattle of various ages with live S19 and killed 45/20 adjuvant *Brucella abortus* vaccines. Vet. Rec. 82:678–680.

Domenech, J., Lucet, P., and Coudert, M. 1982. Bovine brucellosis in central Africa. V. Description of a simplified survey technique. Rev. Elev. Méd. Vét. Pays Trop. 35:125–129.

Doyle, T.M. 1939. *Brucella abortus* infection of goats. J. Comp. Pathol. Ther. 52:89–115.

Fitzgeorge, R.B., Solotorovsky, M., and Smith, H. 1967. The behaviour of *Brucella abortus* within macrophages separated from the blood of normal and immune cattle by adherence to glass. Br. J. Exp. Pathol. 48:522–528.

Gilman, H.L., Dahlberg, A.C., and Marquardt, J.C. 1946. The occurrence and survival of *Brucella abortus* in cheddar and limburger cheese. J. Dairy Sci. 29:71–85.

Huddelson, I.F., Hasley, D.E., and Torrey, J.P. 1927. Further studies on the isolation and cultivation of *Bacterium abortus* (Bang). J. Infect. Dis. 40:352–368.

King, N.B. 1957. The survival of *Brucella abortus* (U.S.D.A. strain 2308) in manure. J. Am. Vet. Med. Assoc. 131:349–352.

Kuzdas, C.D., and Morse, E.V. 1954. The survival of *Brucella abortus* USDA strain 2308 under controlled conditions in nature. Cornell Vet. 44:216–221.

Luchsinger, D.W., and Anderson, R.K. 1967. Epizootiology of brucellosis in a flock of sheep. J. Am. Vet. Med. Assoc. 150:1017–1021.

McCullough, N.B., Eisele, C.W., and Pavelchek, E. 1951. Survey of brucellosis in slaughtered hogs. U.S. Public Health Rep. 66:205–208.

McDiarmid, A. 1957. The degree and duration of immunity in cattle resulting from vaccination with S19 B. *abortus* vaccine and its implications in the future control and eradication of brucellosis. Vet. Rec. 69:877–879.

Meyer, M.E. 1974. Advances in research on brucellosis, 1957–1972. Adv. Vet. Sci. 18:231–250.

Miller, J.K., Kelly, J.I., and Roerink, J.H.G. 1976. A complement fixation method for quantitative differentiation of reactions to 45/20 vaccine and brucella infection. Vet. Rec. 98:210–215.

Mittal, K.R., and Tizard, I. 1981. Serological cross-reactions between *Brucella abortus* and *Yersinia enterocolitica* serotype 09. Vet. Bull. 51:501–506.

Nicoletti, P. 1981. The epidemiology of bovine brucellosis. Adv. Vet. Sci. Comp. Med. 24:69–98.

Parma, A.E., Sahtisteban, G., and Margni, R.A. 1984. Analysis and in vivo assay of B. *abortus* agglutinating and non-agglutinating antibodies. Vet. Microbiol. 9:391–398.

Plommet, M. 1972. Survival of *Brucella abortus* in bovine manure. Ann. Rech. Vét. 3:621–632.

Prost. 1957. Ann. Univ. Marie Curie-Sklodowska. 12:163–173.

Riley, L.K., and Robertson, D.C. 1984. Ingestion and intracellular survival of *Brucella abortus* in human and bovine polymorphonuclear leukocytes. Infect. Immun. 46:224–230.

Roderick, L.M., Kimball, A., McLeod, W.M., and Frank, E.R. 1948. A study of equine fistulous withers and poll evil. A complex infection with *Actinomyces bovis* and *Brucella*. Am. J. Vet. Res. 9:5–10.

Smith, H., Williams, A.E., Pearce, J.H., Keppie, J., Harris-Smith, P.W., Fitzgeorge, R.B., and Witt, K. 1962. Foetal erythritol: A cause of the localization of *Brucella abortus* in bovine contagious abortion. Nature 193:47–49.

Spink, W.W., and Thompson, H. 1953. Human brucellosis caused by *Brucella abortus*, strain 19. J.A.M.A. 153:1162–1165.

Stemshorn, B.W. 1984. Recent progress in the diagnosis of brucellosis. Third International Symposium on Brucellosis, Algiers, Algeria, 1983. Dev. Biol. Stand. 56:325–340.

Sutherland, S.S. 1980. Immunology of bovine brucellosis. Vet. Bull. 50:359–368.

Thimm, B., and Nauwerck, G. 1974. Bovine brucellosis in Guinea and West Africa. Zentralbl. Veterinärmed. [B] 21:692–705.

van Aert, A., Brioen, P., Dekeyser, P., Uyt-Terhagegen, L., Sijens, R.J., and Boeye, A. 1984. A comparative study of ELISA and other methods for the detection of *Brucella* antibodies in bovine sera. Vet. Microbiol. 10:13–21.

Van der Hoeden, J. 1930. De abortusbacterie van het Rund (*Brucella* Bang) Ziekteverwekker Paard. Tijdschr. Diergeneeskd. 57:15–36.

Verstreate, D.R., and Winter. A.J. 1984. Comparison of sodium dodecyl sulfate-polyacrylamide gel electrophoresis profiles and antigenic relatedness among outer membrane proteins of 49 *Brucella abortus* strains. Infect. Immun. 46:192–187.

Wilesmith, J.W. 1978. The persistence of *Brucella abortus* infection in calves:A retrospective study of heavily infected herds. Vet. Rec. 103:149–153.

Winter, A.J., Verstreate, D.R., Hall, C.E., Jacobson, R.H., Castleman, W.L., Meredith, M.P., and McLaughlin, C.A. 1983. Immune response to porin in cattle immunized with whole cell, outer membrane, and outer membrane protein antigens of *Brucella abortus* combined with trehalose dimycolate and muramyl dipeptide adjuvants. Infect. Immun. 42:1159–1167.

Young, E.J., 1983. Human brucellosis. Rev. Infect. Dis. 5:821–842.

Brucella suis

SYNONYM: Porcine type of *Brucella*

B. suis causes brucellosis in swine. It has a wider range of host specificity than the other *Brucella* species and can infect humans, dogs, rodents, horses, reindeer, musk oxen, and wild carnivores. Five types are recognized. Biotypes 1, 2, and 3 have the pig as their natural host but can be transmitted to other hosts. Biotype 2 also occurs naturally in horses and is relatively avirulent for humans. Reindeer and rodents are the primary natural hosts of biotypes 4 and 5, respectively, but other host species can be infected.

Morphology and Staining Reactions. *B. suis* closely resembles *B. abortus* in morphology and staining reactions.

Cultural and Biochemical Features. *B. suis* does not require increased levels of CO_2 for growth. Large amounts of H_2S are produced by biotype 1 but more is produced by the other biotypes. Urea is rapidly hydrolyzed. The features by which *B. suis* is distinguished from the other *Brucella* species are shown in Table 15.2.

Antigens. The A surface antigen predominates on smooth cultures of all biotypes except biotypes 4 and 5. Biotype 4 has both A and M antigens in equal amounts, and biotype 5 has mostly M antigen on its surface. Many protein antigens are shared with the other *Brucella* species (Freeman et al. 1970).

Epizootiology and Pathogenesis. *B. suis* occurs in most swine raising areas of the world but has not been reported in Great Britain, Iceland, or Canada. Survival in the environment has not been well studied but probably is similar to that of *B. abortus*. The organism survives in feces and urine for at least 6 weeks.

About 0.1 percent of domesticated swine in the United States are infected compared with a prevalence rate of 6 percent in feral swine (Zygmont et al. 1982). *B. suis* biotype 1 has been isolated from tissues of wild swine in the southern United States.

In Germany wild hares and wild boars have been shown to be important reservoirs of *B. suis* biotype 2. Pastures contaminated from these hosts could be source of infection for domestic pigs (Dedek 1983). Feral pigs also have been shown to be a source of *B. suis* infection for cattle (Cook and Noble 1984).

Brucellosis is an important disease of reindeer (*Rangifer tarandus*) found in Russia as well as in Alaska and Canada. *B. suis* biotype 4 has been isolated from infected animals; it causes bursitis, spondylitis, arthritis, and orchitis (Huntley et al. 1963). The same biotype of *B. suis* has been isolated from the larvae of the reindeer warble fly, and there is some speculation that this insect may act as a vector of the disease. Biotype 4 has also been isolated from wolves in Siberia and from sled dogs in Alaska fed on infected reindeer meat. This form of brucellosis is of particular interest and significance to the Soviet Union because of the large number of free-living reindeer and because of the importance of domesticated reindeer in that country's northern regions. A domestic guard dog has been shown to be a carrier of *B. suis* biotype 2 and to have been a source of infection for a herd of domestic swine (Kormendy and Nagy 1982).

Although feral animals can be a source of *B. suis* infection for pigs, the organism is transmitted almost exclusively from pig to pig and is spread by coitus or by the ingestion of feed contaminated by urine or genital excretions from infected sows and boars. Because of the current intensive methods of pig husbandry, spread is rapid in a susceptible herd. An outbreak of the disease is often followed by intermittent cases as susceptible newcomers contact chronically infected pigs.

Upon initial infection *B. suis* is localized in the regional lymph nodes. There it proliferates and may cause an extended bacteremia with subsequent generalized infection of the spleen, lymph nodes, joints, udder, and genitalia.

As with *B. abortus*, *B. suis* is a facultative intracellular parasite and owes a great deal of its pathogenic properties to its ability to survive in the host's phagocytic cells. Erythritol has been shown to have a growth-stimulating effect upon *B. suis* and is found in the placenta of sows and the seminal vesicles of boars. Keppie et al. (1965) suggested that the stimulatory action of erythritol on *B. suis* and its presence in these tisues explains the production of lesions in the male and female genital tracts. The clinical signs and lesions produced vary considerably, depending on the animal's age, previous exposure, and the organ or organs involved. The disease may affect suckling and weanling piglets, but it is more common in adults, where it produces abortion, metritis, spondylitis, lameness, and paralysis. Infections that localize in the bodies of the vertebrae (spondylitis), especially of the lumbar and sacral regions, are not uncommon. These sometimes are unsuspected and are found only after slaughter. More often signs of posterior paralysis caused by pressure from the necrotic tissue on the spinal cord are seen. Nodular splenitis in swine can also be associated with brucellosis and in the absence of other lesions justifies a presumptive diagnosis of this disease (Anderson and Davis 1957). Many cases are clinically inapparent.

Immunity. Both field and experimental evidence indicate that swine immunity to brucellosis is very slight and that after a period of herd resistance, animals are again susceptible to the disease. Abortions do not usually occur after the first exposure, but most animals readily contract the disease when reexposed. Because *B. suis* is a facultative intracellular organism, cell-mediated immunity is likely to be important in protecting the host.

An effective vaccine has not been developed. Attempts to immunize boars and sows with a bacterin of *B. suis* biotype 2 resulted in only partial protection (Xie et al. 1981).

Diagnosis. Brucellosis in swine can be positively diagnosed by cultural methods and by the agglutination test. *B. suis* can be readily isolated from the blood, spleen, uterus, lymph nodes, and mammary glands of sows and the testes and semen of boars. The methods are the same as those used for *B. abortus* except that an increase of the CO_2 tension of the culture jar is unnecessary. The cultural characteristics of *B. suis* are given in Table 15.2.

The agglutination test is used as an aid to diagnosis, but it is not as reliable in swine as it is in cattle. Positive titers do not appear until 2 months after infection; many infected pigs have low titers, and nonspecific reactions occur, producing low titers. Incubation of the tubes (standard *B. abortus* antigen is used) at 56°C for 16 hours will eliminate the nonspecific but not the specific reactions.

The card test or rose bengal test is superior to most other serologic tests for detection of antibody in swine serum.

The agglutination test is valuable in determining whether infection exists in a herd. Hubbard and Hoerlein (1952) consider a herd free of brucellosis if, on two consecutive tests of the entire herd, there are no pigs with titers greater than 1:100. They also suggest that animals in an infected herd with titers of 1:25 or higher be considered infected. An ELISA has been developed that will probably replace tube agglutination tests (Thoen et al. 1980).

Control. The simplest way to eradicate the disease in commercial swine herds, is to sell all stock for slaughter once they reach market weight. The premises should then be thoroughly cleaned and disinfected. After it has been kept free of all swine for at least 2 months (longer in winter), it can then be restocked from sources known to be brucellosis-free.

For breeding herds in which blood lines must be preserved, Cameron (1946) suggested a system that was endorsed by Hutchings and Washko (1947) and Spink and Hutchings 1949. Pigs are raised from the infected unit. They are weaned when 8 weeks old and tested individually by the agglutination test. If negative, they are removed from the infected herd, placed on clean ground, and raised in isolation from the main herd. All pigs are tested periodically, and reactors are immediately removed. When of breeding age, serologically negative gilts are bred to noninfected boars. The original herd is disposed of as soon as the replacement unit has grown to sufficient size.

Antimicrobial Susceptibility. Although sensitive in vitro to aminoglycosides, rifampicin, and tetracyclines, the clinical efficacy of these antimicrobials in treatment of *B. suis* infection is very low.

REFERENCES

Anderson, W.A., and Davis, C.L. 1957. Nodular splenitis in swine associated with brucellosis. J. Am. Vet. Med. Assoc. 131:141–145.

Cameron, H.S. 1946. Brucellosis of swine. IV. The unit-segregation system of eradication. Am. J. Vet. Res. 7:21–26.

Cook, D.R., and Noble, J.W. 1984. Isolation of *Brucella suis* from cattle. Aust. Vet. J. 61:263–264.

Dedek, J. 1983. Epidemiology of brucellosis in swine, particularly reservoirs of *Brucella suis*. Monatsheft. Veterinärmed. 38:852–856.

Freeman, B.A., McGhee, J.R., and Baughn, R.E. 1970. Some physical, chemical and taxonomic features of the soluble antigens of the brucellae. J. Infect. Dis. 121:522–527.

Hubbard, E.D., and Hoerlein, A.B. 1952. Studies on swine brucellosis. II. Control in farm herds. J. Am. Vet. Med. Assoc. 120:138–143.

Huntley, B.E., Phillip, R.N., and Maynard, J.E. 1963. Survey of brucellosis in Alaska. J. Infect. Dis. 112:100–106.

Hutchings, L.M., and Wasko, F.V. 1947. Brucellosis in swine. VII. Field control experiments. J. Am. Vet. Med. Assoc. 110:171–174.

Keppie, J., Williams, A.E., Witt, K., and Smith, H. 1965. The role of erythritol in the tissue localization of the brucellae. Br. J. Exp. Pathol. 46:104–108.

Kormendy, B., and Nagy, G. 1982. *Brucella suis* infection in the dog and its probable epidemiological significance. Magy. Allatorv. Lapja 37:91–93.

Spink, W.W., and Hutchings, L.M. 1949. Control and eradication of brucellosis in animals. J.A.M.A. 141:326–329.

Thoen, C.P., Hopkins, M.D., Armbust, A.L., Angus, R.D., and Pietz, D.E. 1980. Development of an enzyme-linked immunosorbent assay for detecting antibodies in sera of *B. suis*-infected swine. Can. J. Comp. Med. 44:294–298.

Xie, X., Xihao, L., Xin, W., Zhiqu, T., and Cuiying, T. 1981. Immunization of sheep, goats, cattle and swine with *Brucella suis* strain 2 vaccine. III. Test on swine. Acta Vet. Zootech. Sin. 12:175–180.

Zygmont, S.M., Nettles, V.F., Shotts, E.B., Jr., Carmen, W.A., and Blackburn, B.O. 1982. Brucellosis in wild swine: A serologic and bacteriologic survey in the southeastern United States and Hawaii. J. Am. Vet. Med. Assoc. 181:1285–1287.

Brucella melitensis

SYNONYMS: *Bacterium melitensis,* caprine type of *Brucella, Micrococcus melitensis*

B. melitensis, the type species for the genus, was first isolated by Bruce in 1887 from the spleen of a resident of the Island of Malta who had died of a disease known as *Malta fever* or *Mediterranean fever*. Brucellosis of goats and sheep caused by *B. melitensis* is prevalent in southern Europe, Mexico, the southwestern United States, Africa, and Central America.

Morphology and Staining Reactions. *B. melitensis* forms small rods that are so short they may be mistaken for cocci. Its staining characteristics are similar to those described for *B. abortus.*

Cultural and Biochemical Features. *B. melitensis* does not require supplementary CO_2 for growth and either does not produce H_2S or does so only in trace amounts. The solid and fluid media used for *B. abortus* are suitable for *B. melitensis.*

The criteria by which it can be differentiated from the other *Brucella* species are shown in Table 15.2. There are three biotypes, 1, 2, and 3, of which biotype 1 is by far the most common (Feinhaken and Dafni 1980).

Antigens. Smooth cultures have the A or M antigens or both antigens together. Many protein antigens are shared with the other brucellas.

Epizootiology and Pathogenesis. The usual natural hosts for *B. melitensis* are goats and sheep, but pigs, cattle, camels, and humans are also easily infected. Infection has been found in many species of feral animals, including hares (Jacotot et al. 1951) and impala (Scheimann and Staak 1971).

Goats are more susceptible than sheep. Most infections are acquired by ingestion of feed or water contaminated by uterine and vaginal discharges from infected does. Milk from these animals also contains large numbers of *B. melitensis* organisms. The pathogenesis of *B. melitensis* infection in goats and sheep is similar to that of *B. abortus* in cows.

B. melitensis is a facultative intracellular parasite and survives and multiplies within phagocytic cells of the reticuloendothelial system (Maruashvili et al. 1980). Its growth is stimulated by erythritol, and extended bacteremia with fever of 5 to 10 weeks or longer is followed by abortion in late pregnancy (Shimi et al. 1981). An abortion storm may be observed in a highly susceptible goat herd or sheep flock. Infected does may show lameness, hygromas, and mastitis. Billy goats sometimes develop orchitis. As herd immunity develops, clinical signs of infection abate. Kid goats can remain latently infected until sexually mature (Alton 1966).

Immunity. Goats and sheep develop effective protective immune responses to *B. melitensis* that eventually clear the infection (Papadopoulos et al. 1981). Humoral antibody appears about 2 to 3 weeks after infection. Cell-mediated immune responses have not been well studied in goats or sheep, but most infected sheep develop delayed type hypersensitivity to antigens of *B. melitensis.*

Vaccines used to prevent and control *B. melitensis* infection in goats and sheep are the live avirulent Rev 1 and a bacterin prepared from strain 53H38. Rev 1 is more effective than 53H38 and protects goats against abortion as well as reducing shedding of the organism (Gaumont et al. 1984). 53H38 stimulates a more persistent antibody response than Rev 1. Animals immunized with Rev 1 usually become serologically negative 6 months later (Falade 1981). A disadvantage of Rev 1 is that it may localize in the placenta of pregnant does and cause abortion. Localization in the mammary gland and shedding in the milk also occurs.

Diagnosis. The bacteriological methods are the same as those used to detect brucellosis in other species. Isolates may be identified by phage sensitivity, by agglutination with monospecific antiserums and by the criteria shown in Table 15.2, or through guinea pig inoculation. Alternatively, serologic tests, including complement fixation, agar-gel immunodiffusion, and the rose bengal plate test, are now available and give results comparable with the classic agglutination test (Waghela 1978). Whey tests can also be performed, but milk ring tests are unreliable on sheep milk.

An intrapalpebral allergic test has been shown to be more sensitive, but slightly less specific than serologic assays for detection of infection in sheep flocks (Ebadi and Zowghi 1983).

Antimicrobial Susceptibility. *B. melitensis* is sensitive to aminoglycosides, rifampicin, and tetracyclines, but the efficacy of these antimicrobials in therapy or prophylaxis of sheep and goats has not been reported.

REFERENCES

Alton, G.G. 1966. Duration of the immunity produced in goats by the Rev. 1 *Brucella melitensis* vaccine. J. Comp. Pathol. 76:241–253.

Ebadi, A., and Zowghi, E. 1983. The use of allergic test in the diagnosis of *Brucella melitensis* infection in sheep. Br. Vet. J. 139:456–461.

Falade, S. 1981. Studies on *Brucella melitensis* Rev. 1 vaccine in goats. Zentralbl. Veterinärmed. [B] 28:749–758.

Feinhaker, D., and Dafni, I. 1980. Identification of *Brucella* isolates in Israel, 1970–1979. Refu. Vet. 37:117–123.

Gaumont, R., Trap, D., and Dhennin, L. 1984. Immunization of primiparous goats against experimental *Brucella melitensis* infection. Comparison of Rev 1 and 53H38 vaccines. In Les maladies de la chèvre, colloque international, Niort (France), 9–11 octobre 1984. Institut National de la Récherche Agronomique, Paris. Pp. 111–120.

Jacotot, H., Vallee, A., and Barriere, J. 1951. Brucellosis of the hare in France. Bull. Acad. Vet. France 24:283–285.

Maruashvili, G.M., Baramidze, I.V., Tsagareli, Z.G., and Vtyurin, B.V. 1980. Electron microscopical study of the morphology of *Brucella melitensis* and the mechanism of its phagocytosis by blood cells. Arch. Patol. 8:70–75.

Papadopoulos, O., Sarris, K., and Papanastasopoulou, M. 1981. Long term observations on sheep experimentally infected with *Brucella melitensis*. Delt. Hell. Kteniatr. Hetair. (Bulletin of the Hellenic Veterinary Medical Society) 32:283–289.

Schiemann, G., and Staak, C. 1971. *Brucella melitensis* in impala (*Aepyceras melampus*). Vet. Rec. 88:344.

Shimi, A., and Tabatabayi, A.H. 1981. Pathological bacteriological and serological responses of ewes experimentally infected with *Brucella melitensis*. Bull. Off. Int. Epizoot. 93:1411–1422.

Waghela, S. 1978. Serological response of adult goats infected with live *Brucella melitensis*. Br. Vet. J. 134:565–571.

Brucella neotomae

First isolated by Stoenner and Lockman (1957) from a desert wood rat, *Neotoma lepida*, trapped alive in the Great Salt Desert of Utah, *B. neotomae* has not been recovered from any other naturally infected host. It is well tolerated by wood rats, and upon experimental infection it persists for at least a year without producing significant lesions. The characteristics that differentiate it from other species are given in Table 15.2.

REFERENCE

Stoenner, H.B., and Lockman, D.B. 1957. A new species of *Brucella* isolated from the desert wood rat *Neotoma lepida* Thomas. Am. J. Vet. Res. 18:942–951.

Brucella ovis

B. ovis causes epididymitis in rams, and since its early isolation in New Zealand and Australia (Buddle and Boyes 1953) it has been described in many of the world's sheep-raising countries, including the United States, South America, South Africa, and the Soviet Union. In addition to epididymitis in rams, the organism produces late abortions in females (Simmons and Hall 1953) and lowers flock fertility.

Morphology and Staining Characteristics. *B. ovis* has a morphology typical of the genus. It is somewhat acid-fast under certain conditions of staining (Stamp et al. 1950). It stains blue, not red, by the Koster staining method.

Cultural and Biochemical Features. *B. ovis* requires supplementary CO_2 for growth. It does not produce H_2S, and most strains are urease negative. It does not metabolize erythritol or other carbohydrates. Although the colonies superficially appear smooth, they are always in the rough phase on primary isolation. The features by which *B. ovis* can be differentiated from other brucellas are shown on Table 15.2. There are no biotypes. *B. ovis* is the only species to show less than 100 percent DNA homology with other species in the genus.

Antigens. *B. ovis* has an R surface antigen that cross-reacts with rough strains of other *Brucella* species and does not react with A or M antigens. It shares a large number of protein antigens with other *Brucella* species.

Epizootiology and Pathogenesis. Sheep are the only natural hosts of *B. ovis*. The British breeds are more susceptible than Merinos, and rams are clinically affected much more frequently than ewes. Transmission appears to be venereal, and rams become infected by mating with ewes previously covered by other infected rams. Although the infection in the ewe is often rapidly cleared, some ewes may develop placental infections with subsequent abortion.

Because *B. ovis* can survive for a month or two on pasture, ingestion is another possible route of natural infection. It has been shown that rams can be experimentally infected by the oral route as can ewes in the early stages of pregnancy (Hall et al. 1955). The possibility of the oral route as a natural mode of infection is further supported by the observation that rams as young as 4 months old can become infected (Burgess et al. 1982).

Infection is followed by a transient, inapparent bacteremia with subsequent localization of the organism in the epididymis of the male. The tail of the epididymis is affected, often unilaterally. The ram may show no clinical signs at this time, but shed the organism in its semen for a prolonged period (Hall 1955). In the epididymis a permatocele forms and ruptures, and finally spermatic granulomas form with later testicular atrophy (Biberstein et al. 1964, Kennedy et al. 1956). Such rams have lowered fertility.

There is evidence that type 3 hypersensitivity responses play a role in the pathogenesis of the epididymitis because lesions in experimentally challenged rams are more severe in animals previously vaccinated than in nonvaccinated controls (Rahaley 1983).

Ewes are somewhat less susceptible to infection by *B.*

ovis (Hughes 1972), but lesions can occur. They vary from a superficial purulent exudate on an intact chorioallantoic membrane to advanced fibrosis and necrosis of this membrane (McGowan et al. 1961, Osborn and Kennedy 1966).

The organism is pathogenic for lambs in utero, but the fetus may survive in the presence of infection. The placentitis interferes with fetal nutrition, and Hughes (1972) suggests that this may account for low birth weights in lambs. Frank abortion has not been the cardinal sign of this disease, but it has been reported under experimental (Buddle 1955) as well as under natural conditions in New Zealand (Simmons and Hall 1953).

Immunity. The immunological basis of the protective immune response has not been defined but is probably cell-mediated. Many rams that become infected do not develop epididymitis. Humoral antibodies are detectable about 3 to 4 weeks after infection, and delayed cutaneous hypersensitivity to *B. ovis* antigens develops later.

Vaccines consist of saline in oil adjuvant bacterins of formalinized *B. ovis* or live *B. melitensis* Rev 1 (Buddle 1958, Van Heerden and Van Rensburg 1962). In the Soviet Union a live vaccine, *B. ovis* 7-26, was shown to be effective in 6- to 10-week-old ram lambs against experimental challenge and was not transmitted to unvaccinated sheep. Vaccination of ewes apparently does not influence spread of infection in a flock.

There is evidence that agglutinin titers persist for several years in vaccinated rams (Ris 1967).

Diagnosis. Diagnosis is accomplished by palpation of the testicles, culture of the semen, and demonstration of antibodies in the serum. Palpation is of limited value since many advanced cases show no palpable lesions of the testes. However, an enlarged epididymis with testicular atrophy is valuable in diagnosis. Culture of the semen is also an important adjunct to diagnosis and has been facilitated by the use of selective media modified for the growth of *B. ovis* (Brown et al. 1971, Jones et al. 1975).

Fluorescent antibody can be used to detect the organism in a semen smear, and the complement-fixation, ELISA, immunodiffusion, and hemagglutination tests are used for detection of antibody in serum. The ELISA has been shown to be at least as accurate and sensitive as the complement-fixation text and is easier to perform (Rahaley et al. 1983, Ris et al. 1984). In infected flocks rams are five times more likely than ewes to be positive in the complement-fixation test (Dolley et al. 1982).

Control. Control of *B. ovis* infection depends on preventing spread of infection between rams. Infected older rams must therefore be kept separate from young rams, and the latter are used only on ewes known to be free of infection. Vaccination of young rams is also helpful.

Eradication of the disease in some areas is based on testing and the slaughter of rams that react in the complement-fixation test or the ELISA.

REFERENCES

Biberstein, E.L., McGowan, B., Olander, H., and Kennedy, P.C. 1964. Epididymitis in rams: Studies on pathogenesis. Cornell Vet. 54:27–41.

Brown, G.M., Ranger, C.R., and Kelley, D.J. 1971. Selective media for the isolation of *Brucella ovis*. Cornell Vet. 61:265–280.

Buddle, M.B. 1955. Observations on the transmission of brucella infection in sheep. N.Z. Vet. J. 3:10–19.

Buddle, M.B. 1958. Vaccination in the control of *Brucella ovis* infection in sheep. N.Z. Vet. J. 6:41–46.

Buddle, M.B., and Boyes, B.W. 1953. A *Brucella* mutant causing genital disease of sheep in New Zealand. Aust. Vet. J. 29:145–153.

Burgess, G.W., McDonald, J.W., Norris, M.J. 1982. Epidemiological studies on ovine brucellosis in selected ram flocks. Aust. Vet. J. 59:45–47.

Dolley, P., Geral, M.F., Pellerin, J.L., Milon, A., and Lautie, R. 1982. Contagious epididymitis of the ram (*Brucella ovis* infection). I. Use of three serological methods for diagnosis. Rev. Méd. Vét. 133:187–195.

Hall, W.T.K. 1955. Epididymitis of rams—Studies on skin sensitivity and pathology. Aust. Vet. J. 31:7–9.

Hughes, K.L. 1972. Experimental *Brucella ovis* infection in ewes. I. Breeding performances of infected ewes. Aust. Vet. J. 48:12–17.

Jones, L.M., Dubray, G., and Marly, J. 1975. Comparison of methods of diagnosis of *Brucella ovis* infection of rams. Ann. Rech. Vét. 6:11–22.

Kennedy, P.C., Frazier, L.M., and McGowan, B. 1956. Epididymitis in rams: Pathology and bacteriology. Cornell Vet. 46:303–319.

McGowan, B., Biberstein, E.L., Harrold, D.R., and Robinson, E.A. 1961. Epididymitis in rams: The effect of the ram epididymitis organism (REO) on the pregnant ewe. Proc. U.S. Livestock Assoc. 65:291–296.

Osborn, B.I., and Kennedy, P.C. 1966. Pathologic and immunologic responses of the fetal lamb to *Brucella ovis*. Pathol. Vet. 3:110–136.

Rahaley, R.S. 1983. Studies on the development of brucellosis in rams. Diss. Abstr. Int. B 44:1373–1374.

Rahaley, R.S., Dennis, S.M., and Smeltzer, M.S. 1983. Comparison of the enzyme-linked immunosorbent assay and complement fixation for detecting *Brucella ovis* antibodies in sheep. Vet. Rec. 113:467–470.

Ris, D.R. 1967. The persistence of antibodies against *Brucella ovis* and *Brucella abortus* in rams following vaccination: A field study. N.Z. Vet. J. 15:94–98.

Ris, D.R., Hamel, K.L., Long, D.L. 1984. Comparison of an enzyme-linked immunospecific assay (ELISA) with the cold complement fixation test for the serodiagnosis of *Brucella ovis* infection. N.Z. Vet. J. 32:18–20.

Simmons, G.C., and Hall, W.T.K. 1953. Epididymitis of rams. Aust. Vet. J. 29:33–40.

Stamp, J.T., McEwen, A.D., Watt, A.A., and Nisbet, D. 1950. Enzootic abortion in ewes. I. Transmission of the disease. Vet. Rec. 62:251–255.

Van Heerden, K.M., and Van Rensburg, S.W.J. 1962. The immunization of rams against ovine brucellosis. J.S. Afr. Vet. Med. Assoc. 33:143–148.

Brucella canis

SYNONYM: canine type of *Brucella*

The first isolations of *B. canis* were made in 1966 from outbreaks of abortion and whelping failures among dogs in the United States and Great Britain. In 1968 the organism was characterized and named *Brucella canis* (Carmichael and Bruner 1968). It is highly adapted to domestic dogs and is not readily transmitted to other animals, although it will infect humans.

Morphology and Staining Reactions. The organism is a small rod-shaped coccobacillus similar to the other *Brucella* species in morphology and staining reactions.

Cultural and Biochemical Features. *B. canis* produces only rough or mucoid colonies and a smooth phase has not been observed. Unlike other brucellas, *B. canis* is inhibited by 10 percent CO_2. After several days of incubation, growth becomes quite mucoid and a ropy, viscous sediment is formed in broth. It does not utilize erythritol as a preferred nutrient. It produces large amounts of urease but does not form H_2S. The features by which *B. canis* can be distinguished from other brucellas are shown in Table 15.2.

Antigens. *B. canis* carries R but not A or M surface antigens. A species-specific antigen is associated with the mucoid antigen shed by the organism (Zoha and Carmichael 1981). A number of protein antigens are shared with the other *Brucella* species. Cross-reactivity with *Actinobacillus equuli, Pseudomonas aeruginosa,* and *P. multocida* also occurs. *B. canis* has been found in breeding kennels, pet and stray dogs, and in laboratory colonies of beagles in the United States, Europe, Japan, and Central and South America. Infection appears to be more prevalent in stray dogs than in pets (Ciuchini et al. 1982, Myers and Varela-Diaz 1980) and can vary from about 1 percent to as high as 30 percent. A study performed in Illinois revealed that dogs in the 2- to 3-year age group had a higher prevalence of seropositivity (33.3 percent) than did older dogs (Ghoneim and Woods 1984).

Transmission occurs principally at the time of abortion, when many bacteria are shed in the persistent vaginal discharge. Transmission by this route may continue for 4 to 6 weeks after an abortion (Carmichael 1976). Males harbor the organism in their genital tracts, from which it is shed intermittently, and it can be transmitted to the female by coitus.

Infection can occur through all mucosae and by many routes of inoculation. Bacteremia follows, and although it may be intermittent, it is prolonged and may persist for 2 years after the initial infection (Carmichael and Kenney 1968). Infected dogs do not have elevated temperatures, and most show no clinical signs. Those that do exhibit clinical signs have generalized lymphadenitis, splenitis, and embryonic deaths and abortions at approximately 50 days of gestation. Infected males have epididymitis, scrotal dermatitis, and testicular atrophy, which is often unilateral. George and Carmichael (1984) demonstrated sperm agglutination in the semen of infected dogs, phagocytosis of spermatozoa, and delayed skin hypersensitivity to testicular antigens and suggested that isoimmune responses to sperm antigens play a role in the pathogenesis of *B. canis* infections and in male fertility.

There is evidence that damage to epithelial cells of the testes, epididymis, and prostate caused by *B. canis* triggers production of sperm antibody (Serikawa et al. 1984).

Immunity. The protective immune response to *B. canis* is probably cell-mediated but has not been well studied. Humoral antibodies appear at between 2 to 7 weeks and are present in highest concentration in bacteremic animals (Larsson et al. 1984). Titers diminish with resolution of the bacteremia.

There is no successful vaccine against *B. canis* infection in dogs. Experiments have shown that a live *B. ovis* vaccine can stimulate some resistance to *B. canis,* but this resistance is much inferior to that observed in dogs following recovery from *B. canis* infection (George 1974).

Diagnosis. Diagnosis is easy in animals that show clinical signs of abortion and infertility (females) or epididymis (males). It is also easy in kennel outbreaks that involve a number of animals, but the individual animal that is infected yet appears normal presents a diagnostic problem. Clinical signs, direct culture of blood, lymph nodes, or bone marrow; and serologic tests are used in diagnosis. The latter include mercaptoethanol, tube agglutination (Carmichael 1968), complement fixation, counter immunoelectrophoresis, agar-gel immunodiffusion (Meyers et al. 1972), and a rapid slide agglutination test (George and Carmichael 1974). These tests are still not completely standardized and are subject to occasional but important "false-positives" and hard-to-interpret "low titers" and to the broad heterotypic reactivity shown by *B. canis* antigens.

An agar-gel immunodiffusion test that is based on internal antigens of *B. canis* is the most sensitive and accurate serologic means of detecting infection (Zoha and Carmichael 1981). However, isolation of *B. canis* from infected dogs is still the most certain diagnostic method.

Antimicrobial Susceptibility. Although *B. canis* is sensitive in vitro to aminoglycosides, rifampicin, and tetracycline, treatment of *B. canis* infection is unlikely to be successful. One study showed that aminocycline (25 mg/lb twice daily) in combination with streptomycin (25 mg/lb) given by intramuscular injection for 7 days was effective in curing only 3 out of 11 experimentally infected dogs (Flores-Castro and Carmichael 1981).

REFERENCES

Carmichael, L.E. 1968. Canine brucellosis: Isolation, diagnosis, transmission. Proc. U.S. Livestock Sanit. Assoc. 71:517–527.

Carmichael, L.E. 1976. Canine brucellosis: An annotated review with selected cautionary comments. Theriogenology 6:105–116.

Carmichael, L.E., and Bruner, D.W. 1968. Characteristics of a newly recognized species of *Brucella* responsible for infectious canine abortions. Cornell Vet. 58:579–592.

Carmichael, L.D., and Kenney, R.M. 1968. Canine abortion caused by *Brucella canis*. J. Am. Vet. Med. Assoc. 152:605–616.

Ciuchini, F., Pistoia, V., Piccininno, G., Pievaroli, A., and Fantini, C. 1982. Brucellosis caused by *Brucella canis*: Antibody levels in dogs from Rome and its suburbs. Clin. Vet. 105:138–144.

Flores-Castro, R., and Carmichael, L.E. 1981. *Brucella canis* infection in dogs: Treatment trials. Rev. Latinoam. Microbiol. 23:75–79.

George, L.W. 1974. Studies on the immune response in canine brucellosis. Ph.D. dissertation, Cornell University, Ithaca, N.Y.

George, L.W., and Carmichael, L.E. 1974. A plate agglutination test for the rapid diagnosis of canine brucellosis. Am. J. Vet. Res. 35:905–909.

George, L.W., and Carmichael, L.E. 1984. Antisperm responses in male dogs with chronic *Brucella canis* infection. Am. J. Vet. Res. 45:274–281.

Ghoneim, N.H., and Woods, G. 1984. Serological epidemiology of *Brucella canis* in a hospitalized and referral population of dogs and cats in Illinois. Canine Prac. 11:17–127.

Larsson, M.H.M.A., Larsson, C.E., da Costa, E.O., and Guerra, J.L. 1984. Experimental brucellosis in dogs: Bacteriological, serological and pathological studies. Arq. Bras. Med. Vet. Zootec. 36:141–156.

Myers, D.M., and Varela-Diaz, V.M. 1980. Serological and bacteriological detection of *Brucella canis* infection of stray dogs in Moreno, Argentina. Cornell Vet. 70:258–265.

Myers, D.M., Jones, L.M., and Varela-Diaz, V.M. 1972. Studies of antigens for complement fixation and gel diffusion tests in the diagnosis of infections caused by *Brucella ovis* and other *Brucella*. Appl. Microbiol. 23:894–902.

Serikawa, T., Takada, H., Kondo, Y., Muragachi, T., and Yamada, J. 1984. Multiplication of *Brucella canis* in male reproductive organs and detection of autoantibody to spermatozoa in canine brucellosis. Dev. Biol. Stand. 56:295–305.

Zoha, S.J., and Carmichael, L.E. 1981. Properties of *Brucella canis* (sic) surface antigens associated with colonial mucoidiness. Cornell Vet. 71:428–438.

Zoha, S.J., and Carmichael, L.E. 1982. Serological responses of dogs to cell wall and internal antigens of *Brucella canis* (*B. canis*). Vet. Microbiol. 7:35–50.

Brucellosis (Undulant Fever) of Humans

Brucellosis in humans can be caused by *B. abortus, B. canis, B. melitensis,* and *B. suis* (all biotypes). The species involved is in great part determined by opportunity for exposure. For instance, in the swine belt (north central states of the United States), *B. suis* infections are most common, whereas in the southeastern United States *B. abortus* is more often found. *B. melitensis* infections are most common in Mexico and in certain localized areas of the southwestern part of the United States. This species is also found with some frequency in the midwestern states, where it is contracted from swine. In Alaska clinical cases of brucellosis in humans have been derived from caribou (the North American reindeer *Rangifer tarandus*) infected with *B. suis* biotype 4.

In the decade after *B. canis* was first isolated, many people were found to be infected with this species (Mun-

ford et al. 1975). Half were laboratory personnel who were working with the organism, and most of the others were owners of infected pet dogs (Carmichael 1976).

Cases of *B. abortus,* or *B. suis* infection are usually seen in veterinarians, farmers, slaughterhouse personnel, and others who are exposed on the job to infected cattle or swine. Thus, although both males and females are about equally susceptible, at least two-thirds of the cases occurring in one study in Iowa were in men (Hardy et al. 1930). These were partly *B. abortus* and partly *B. suis* infections. Iowa is largely a rural state and most of the cases were in farm families where the men usually handled the livestock. Direct contact is apparently more hazardous than drinking infected milk, because infections in men are more common even in areas where the predominant type is *B. abortus*. Brucellosis, or undulant fever, can occur at any age, but the greatest number of clinically recognized cases occur in the age group between 20 and 45 years (Hardy et al. 1930). Infants, who consume a much larger volume of milk proportionally than adults, seldom become infected, although the disease has been diagnosed in children as young as 4 years old.

B. suis is more virulent for humans than *B. abortus* and is most often contracted by exposure to blood or tissue fluids from infected swine in the slaughterhouse.

Brucellosis as an Occupational Hazard for Veterinarians. Brucellosis poses a hazard to veterinarians in rural practice because they often come in contact with infected secretions. Blood-test surveys made before 1940 indicated that a comparatively large percentage of veterinarians reacted positively, although many had no clinical history of the disease. At the same time, infection in students in veterinary colleges was not uncommon. In a survey carried out in 1974 in New Zealand, Robinson and Metcalfe (1976) found antibody titers in 90 percent of the veterinarians sampled. The veterinarians who showed no evidence of antibodies to brucella infection were either recent graduates or involved in commerce, laboratory work, or teaching.

The practicing veterinarian is exposed to more viable *Brucella* organisms than are other people, even those in rural communities. During the common procedure of removing a retained placenta from a cow, the veterinarian comes in intimate contact with uterine discharges rich in organisms that can enter his or her body through the conjunctiva or the intact skin, or by inhalation. Wounds on the hands and arms are not uncommon during obstetrical procedures, and they make ideal sites of entry.

The other major source of infection for veterinarians is accidental inoculation with *B. abortus* strain 19 while vaccinating cattle. In the course of vaccinating frisky young calves, the veterinarian may jab the needle into his or her thigh or scratch a thumb. Kerr et al. (1966) reported that about one-third of the veterinarians surveyed had inoculated themselves at least once. Spink and Thompson (1953) described the course of the disease in two veterinarians accidently inoculated with strain 19. Strain 19 usually does not cause chronic infections in humans but can cause severe effects in those previously infected with *B. abortus*. The reactions are particularly severe when the vaccine is splashed into the eye of a sensitized person.

Diagnosis. The acute disease is frequently overlooked or misdiagnosed. Patients frequently decide they have influenza or chills and then recover. Even when a medical practitioner is consulted in the acute stage, the disease may be misdiagnosed because of its sporadic nature and its vague signs. Diagnosis is based on the patient's history, clinical signs, isolation of the organism, and serologic tests.

In the early, severe phase of the disease the individual is acutely ill, suffers from prostration and weakness, develops daily fever in the afternoon and evening, and suffers chills and night sweats during which the fever disappears only to have the cycle recur on following days. The intermittent fever is responsible for the name *undulant fever*. Such acute symptoms usually lessen after a few days, but, following an interval of varying length during which the patient feels better, another period of acute symptoms may appear. There may be several such remissions. The symptoms are the same, no matter which type of *Brucella* is the infecting agent. Infections with *B. melitensis* and *B. suis* are usually more severe than those with *B. abortus*, but this is not always the case. The mortality is low, but recovery from infections often is very slow. Many persons never fully recover from the effects of the disease.

The symptoms of chronic cases vary greatly, and this form of the disease is more difficult to diagnose. Usually the patient suffers from great debility, weakness, a low-grade remittent fever, and joint pains; there may be sweating, lassitude and malaise, gastritis, abdominal pain, skin rashes, headache, irritability, depression, insomnia, arthritis, and backache. Kerr et al. (1966) note that patients may be labeled neurotic because their complaints are hard to substantiate by laboratory tests.

An osteoarticular complication of brucellosis is the melitococcic spondylitis of humans reported in Italy. *B. suis* has also been reported in septic arthritis of the hip. *Brucella* organisms have been implicated in cases of osteomyelitis (Kelly et al. 1960) and in diseases of the nervous system (Fincham et al. 1963). Perry and Belter (1960) have published a review on fatal brucellosis and heart disease.

Blood cultures, when positive, are diagnostic, but the isolation of the organism from the blood is usually diffi-

cult and often impossible, particularly when the offending organism is *B. abortus*. Greater success is achieved in acute rather than in chronic cases, but repeated attempts often have to be made, even in the acute forms.

Three serologic tests have been used as an aid to diagnosis: the standard agglutination test, the antiglobulin test, and the complement-fixation test. The agglutination test has been used for years, but it must be interpreted with great caution because it may produce aberrant results, such as occasional prozones, and "nonagglutination" antibodies may be present, giving a negative test even in persons who have had the disease for a long time. Nevertheless, it is useful, particularly in recently acquired acute cases of brucellosis (Robinson and Metcalfe 1976). The antiglobulin test (Coomb's test) and the complement-fixation test (Kerr et al. 1968) are supplementary, and while they too are subject to some variability in results, they are of value in the diagnosis of long-standing brucellosis.

Treatment. Because the intracellular nature of brucellas makes them relatively inaccessible to chemotherapeutic agents, brucellosis, especially chronic brucellosis in humans, is often very refractory to treatment. In 1958 a joint FAO/WHO Expert Committee on Brucellosis recommended that tetracyclines be given for 21 days and that a combination of tetracycline and streptomycin be given for severe infections and for all *B. suis* infections (Joint FAO/WHO Committee 1958). The committee also suggested that chloramphenicol is of value but urged caution in its prolonged use. Although these antibiotics often produce a good initial clinical response, a large percentage of patients suffer recurrence of the disease.

REFERENCES

Carmichael, L.E. 1976. Canine brucellosis: An annotated review with selected cautionary comments. Theriogenology 6:105–116.

Fincham, R.W., Saks, A.L., and Joynt, R.J. 1963. Protean manifestations of nervous system brucellosis. J.A.M.A. 184:269–275.

Hardy, A.V., Jordan, C.F., Borts, I.M., and Hardy, A.V. 1930. Undulant fever with special reference to a study of *Brucella* infection. U.S. Nat. Inst. Health Bull. 158. Pp. 81–89.

Joint FAO/WHO Expert Committee on Brucellosis. 1958. Third Report. WHO Technical Report Series, no. 148. World Health Organization, Geneva.

Kelly, P.J., Martin, W.J., Shirger, A., and Weed, L.A. 1960. Brucellosis of the bones and joints. J.A.M.A. 174:347–353.

Kerr, W.R., Coghlan, J.D., Payne, D.J.H., and Robertson, L. 1966. Chronic brucellosis in the practicing veterinary surgeon. Vet. Rec. 79:602–606.

Kerr, W.R., McCaughey, W.J., Coghlan, J.D., Payne, D.J.H., Quaife, R.A., Robertson, L., and Farrell, I.D. 1968. Techniques and interpretations in the serological diagnosis of brucellosis in man. J. Med. Microbiol. 1:181–193.

Munford, R.S., Weaver, R.E., Patton, C., Feeley, J.C., and Feldman,

R.A. 1975. Human disease caused by *Brucella canis*. J.A.M.A. 231:1267–1269.

Perry, T.M., and Belter, C.F. 1960. Brucellosis and heart disease. Am. J. Pathol. 36:673–696.

Robinson, R.A., and Metcalfe, R.V. 1976. Zoonotic infections in veterinarians. N.Z. Vet. J. 24:201–210.

Spink, W.W., and Thompson, H. 1953. Human brucellosis caused by *Brucella abortus,* strain 19. J.A.M.A. 153:1162–1165.

16 The Genus *Campylobacter*

The genus *Campylobacter* is composed of organisms that are short, curved, rigid rods arranged singly or united into spiral forms. When they were first discovered organisms in the genus *Campylobacter* were classified as vibrios because of their curved shape and rapid corkscrew-type mobility. The name of the genus was *Vibrio* for many years until Sebald and Veron (1963) found that many of the member species were sufficiently different to merit classification under the separate generic name *Campylobacter*. The term *vibriosis* is still applied to the diseases caused by pathogenic species of this genus. Campylobacters are found in the reproductive and alimentary tracts of humans and animals.

Biochemically, species of *Campylobacter* are rather inactive, but all are oxidase-positive and most produce catalase. The pathogenic *Campylobacter* species have been classified by their ability to grow at temperatures between 25° and 45°C.

Table 16.1 lists the *Campylobacter* species and subspecies found in animals and humans together with their more important characteristics. The thermophilic species do not grow at 25°C but grow well at 42° to 45°C (Table 16.2). Since the 1970s they have been shown to be an important cause of acute enteritis in humans and dogs and therefore have considerable zoonotic importance. However, much work has yet to be done to classify and categorize strains from diarrheal disease in humans and animals.

Organisms that resemble the campylobacters and that tolerate exposure to atmospheric oxygen have been isolated from aborted bovine and porcine fetuses (Ellis et al.

1977, 1978) and mastitic bovine milk (Logan et al. 1982). The cells are very long, helical, and do not share known antigens with *C. fetus*. They have not yet been classified.

REFERENCES

Ellis, W.A., Neill, S.D., O'Brien, J.J., Ferguson, H.W., and Harma, J. 1977. Isolation of spirillum/vibrio-like organisms from bovine fetuses. Vet. Rec. 100:451–452.

Ellis, W.A., Neill, S.D., O'Brien, J.J., and Harma, J. 1978. Isolation of spirillum-like organisms from pig fetuses. Vet. Rec. 102:106–108.

Logan, E.F., Neill, S.D., Mackie, D.P. 1982. Mastitis in dairy cows associated with an aerotolerant campylobacter. Vet. Rec. 100:229–230.

Sebald, M., and Veron, M. 1963. Teneur en bases de l'ADN et classification des vibrions. Ann. Inst. Pasteur 105:897–910.

Campylobacter fetus

There are two subspecies of *C. fetus*: *C. fetus* subspecies *venerealis* and *C. fetus* subspecies *fetus*. *C. fetus* subsp. *venerealis* is highly adapted to the bovine reproductive tract; *C. fetus* subsp. *fetus* is found in the intestine and as a cause of abortion in sheep and cattle. The morphologic, cultural, and biochemical features of these subspecies will be described together. Their other features will be covered separately. For more detailed information, see the excellent review by Garcia et al. (1983).

Morphology and Staining Reactions. *C. fetus* subsp. *venerealis* and *C. fetus* subsp. *fetus* characteristically produce comma-shaped or S-shaped Gram-negative bodies (0.2 to 0.5 µm by 1.5 to 4.0 µm). The comma forms have a single polar flagellum while the S forms may have bipolar flagella. The catalase-positive species form spirals when a number of S forms remain joined together. Cells in old cultures form coccoid or spherical bodies. *C. fetus* subsp. *fetus* has a glycoproteinaceous microcapsule (McCoy et al. 1975).

Cultural and Biochemical Features. Growth is microaerophilic to anaerobic. The organisms require an atmosphere of 10 to 20 percent CO_2, and the oxygen concentration should be reduced to 5 percent or less. Optimal growth occurs at 37°C on serum, blood agar, thiol agar, cystine-heart agar, and brain-heart infusion agar. Antibiotics such as novobiocin and bacitracin can be added to inhibit the growth of contaminants (Plastridge et al. 1964).

Colonies usually are visible 2 days after inoculation. They are round, raised, and regular in shape and butyrous in consistency. They may be translucent at first but later become opaque. Colony diameter ranges from 1 to 3 mm. The subspecies of *C. fetus* do not ferment or oxidize carbohydrates and do not hydrolyze gelatin or urea. The mol% G + C of the DNA ranges from 33 to 36.

153

Table 16.1. Some characteristics of the species and subspecies of *Campylobacter* found in animals and humans

Species	Habitat	Disease	Catalase	Thermophilic (growth at 42°C)
C. fetus subsp. *venerealis*	Genital tract of cattle	Infertility and abortion	+	−
C. fetus subsp. *fetus*	Intestine of sheep, cattle, other mammals, birds	Abortion in sheep; occasional abortion in cattle	+	−
C. jejuni	Intestine of mammals, birds	Abortion in sheep and mink; fever, bacteremia and enteritis in humans, foals, and mink; hepatitis in birds; mortality in cattle	+	+
C. coli	Intestine of swine, poultry, and humans	Enteritis in piglets, foals, and humans	+	+
C. sputorum subsp. *mucosalis*	Mouth and intestine of swine	Intestinal adenomatosis and necrotic enteritis in swine	−	+
C. sputorum subsp. *bubulus*	Genital tract of cattle and sheep	None reported	−	−
C. fecalis	Sheep feces, semen and vagina of cattle	None reported	+	+
C. hyointestinalis	Intestine of swine	Proliferative ileitis	+	−

REFERENCES

Garcia, M.M., Eaglesome, M.D., and Rigley, C. 1983. Campylobacters important in veterinary medicine. Vet. Bull. 53:793–818.

McCoy, E.C., Doyle, D., Wiltberger, H., Burda, K., and Winter, A.J. 1975. Flagellar ultrastructure and flagella-associated antigens of *Campylobacter fetus*. J. Bacteriol. 122:307–315.

Plastridge, W.N., Stula, E.F., and Williams, L.F., 1964. *Vibrio fetus* infection and reinfection in heifers, as determined by cultural tests using blood agar plus antibiotics. Am. J. Vet. Res. 25:710–713.

Campylobacter fetus subspecies *venerealis*

Antigens. Both *C. fetus* subsp. *venerealis* and *C. fetus* subsp. *fetus* have heat-stable somatic (O) antigens, flagellar (H) antigens, and heat-labile superficial protein antigens that mask the underlying O antigen. The O antigens in *C. fetus* subsp. *venerealis* are A-1 and A-sub 1. At least

Table 16.2. Differentiation of *Campylobacter* species found in animals

Species/subspecies	Growth at 25°C	Growth at 43°C	Catalase	Glycine (1%)	H₂S production (TSI)	Hydrolysis of hippurate	Nalidixic acid susceptibility
C. fetus subsp. *venerealis*	+	−	+	−	−	−	−
C. fetus subsp. *fetus*	+	−	+	+	−*	−	−
C. jejuni	−	+	+	+	−	+	+
C. coli	−	+	+	+	−	−	+
C. sputorum subsp. *mucosalis*	+	−	−	−	+	−	−
C. sputorum subsp. *bubulus*	+	−	−	+	+	−	−
C. fecalis	variable	+	+	+	+	−	−
C. hyointestinalis	+	−	+	+	+	−	−

*Positive on lead acetate strip; the reaction of *C. fetus* subsp. *venerealis* on lead acetate strip is negative.

three antigens are associated with flagella (McCoy et al. 1975), but they are not used in routine serotyping. The superficial protein antigens exhibit variations during an infection (Corbeil et al. 1975), but the biochemical basis of this variation has not been studied.

Epizootiology and Pathogenesis. *C. fetus* subsp. *venerealis* is an obligate parasite of the bovine genitalia. In bulls infection is inapparent and involves the epithelium of the penis and the fornix of the prepuce. Transmission is by coitus or artificial insemination. In a susceptible herd introduction of the organism is followed by a period of infertility in all breeding females (120 days). In chronically infected herds only newly introduced susceptible animals show signs of infertility.

The organism localizes in the anterior vagina and cervix during the ovulatory phase but does not invade the uterus and oviducts until the progestational phase. A moderate endometritis and salpingitis then results and persists for several weeks to a few months (Vandeplassche et al. 1963). During this time the animal is infertile either because of failure of implantation or because of early abortion. On rare occasions the pregnancy may continue to a later stage (5 to 7 months) before placental damage becomes sufficient to cause fetal death and abortion.

The inflammatory reaction in the cervical and endometrial mucosa involves a neutrophil invasion in the earlier stages. The cells are eventually replaced by foci of mononuclear cells.

Animals usually regain fertility within 5 months as a result of elimination of the infection from the uterus and oviducts. In some animals infection can persist in the cervicovaginal area for many months in spite of the presence of local antibodies. During this time the organism can exhibit a series of antigenic changes that allow it to survive and avoid the effects of local antibody production (Corbeil et al. 1975).

Immunity. The antibodies in the vaginal secretions are predominantly of the IgA class (Corbeil et al. 1974), and their effect is to immobilize the organism so that it cannot penetrate higher into the tract. They can also inhibit bacterial adherence. Unlike antibodies of the IgM and IgG classes, which are present only for a short time, IgA antibodies can persist for many months. IgG antibodies, which have good opsonizing activity, dominate in the uterine fluid, and their effect is to clear the organism from the uterus during the early convalescent phase.

Systemic vaccination with bacterins has been shown to be effective in preventing infertility in cattle (Hoerlein and Kramer 1964) by stimulating serum antibodies of the IgG variety (Corbeil et al. 1974). When complete Freund's adjuvant is included with the bacterin, a heightened resistance is induced that will prevent not only infer-

tility but the carrier state as well (Wilkie and Winter 1971). Vaccination has been used to prevent and terminate natural infection in bulls (Bouters et al. 1973). It has been recommended that breeding herds be vaccinated twice before breeding so that adequate serum titers of protective antibody are present at the time of insemination.

C. fetus subsp. *venerealis* infection in cattle herds that breed naturally is self-limiting because of the normal immune response in infected animals. However, infection persists in some cows and bulls; thus clinical disease will continue to occur in susceptible virgin heifers and in newly introduced stock. Vaccination is important to protect these animals.

Diagnosis. If the fetal membranes are available, a direct microscopic examination is made of the cotyledons. The presence of distinctly spiral-shaped organisms is regarded as positive evidence of the infection. Transport enrichment medium (TEM) as described by Clark and Dufty (1978) will maintain the organism for at least 2 days at ambient temperature. Cultures are made in serial dilution on semisolid thiol medium from stomach fluids, lung tissue, heart blood, amniotic fluid, and suspensions of ground cotyledons. The tubes are incubated under CO_2 tension at 37°C for 3 to 9 days and then examined. Careful culturing of cervicovaginal mucus, preputial samples, or semen by the millipore filter technique (Plumer et al. 1962) will sometimes reveal the organism in infected animals. Vaginal mucus samples are best cultured around the time of estrus, especially the 2 days before and the 2 days after estrus (Clark et al. 1969). The use of the filter technique is less sensitive than direct culturing but has the advantage that it can be used with noninhibitory media. Media that contain antibiotics such as novobiocin and bacitracin are valuable for isolating the organism from contaminated materials such as preputial scrapings or washings (Plastridge et al. 1964). When contaminated materials are cultured, it is good practice to use both the filter technique and direct culture onto inhibitory medium.

Serologic diagnosis of infection by the agglutination reaction on serums is unreliable because many infected animals do not develop detectable titers. Also, O antibodies to *C. fetus* subsp. *venerealis* are normally present in the serums of mature cattle (Winter 1965).

The detection of agglutinating antibodies in cervical mucus is much more useful in diagnosis but should be combined with mucus culture and should be performed on a number of animals in a herd because a high rate of false-negative and false-positive results is inherent in the use of cervical mucus as a source of diagnostic antibodies. The availability of a more sensitive enzyme-linked immunosorbent assay (ELISA) (Hewson et al. 1985) combined with a purified antigen preparation should soon allow development of a more sensitive and reliable test.

A fluorescent antibody test is available for the detection of *C. fetus* specific antigen in smears or sections. The test, however, does not distinguish between the subspecies.

REFERENCES

Bouters, R., de Keyser, J., Vandeplassche, M., van Aert A., Brone, E., and Bonte, P. 1973. *Vibrio fetus* infection in bulls: Curative and preventative vaccination. Br. Vet. J. 129:52–57.

Clark, B.L., and Dufty, J.H. 1978. Isolation of *Campylobacter fetus* from bulls. Aust. Vet. J. 54:262–263.

Clark, B.L., Monsbourgh, M.J., and Dufty, J.H. 1969. Observations on the isolation of *Vibrio fetus* (*venerealis*) from the vaginal mucus of experimentally infected heifers. Aust. Vet. J. 45:209–211.

Corbeil, L.B., Schurig, G.D., Bier, P.J., and Winter, A.J. 1975. Bovine venereal vibriosis: Antigenic variation of the bacterium during infection. Infect. Immun. 11:240–244.

Corbeil, L.B., Schurig, G.D., Duncan, J.R., Corbeil, R.R., and Winter, A.J. 1974. Immunoglobulin classes and biological functions of *Campylobacter (Vibrio) fetus* antibodies in serum and cervicovaginal mucus. Infect. Immun. 10:422–429.

Hewson, P.I., Lander, K.P., and Gill, K.P.W. 1985. Enzyme-linked immunosorbent assay for antibodies to *C. fetus venerealis* in bovine genital mucus. Res. Vet. Sci. 38:41–45.

Hoerlein, A.B., and Kramer, T. 1964. Artificial stimulation of resistance to bovine vibriosis: Use of bacterins. Am. J. Vet. Res. 25:371–373.

McCoy, E.C., Doyle, D., Wiltberger, H., Burda, K., and Winter, A.J. 1975. Flagellar ultrastructure and flagella-associated antigens of *Campylobacter fetus*. J. Bacteriol. 122:307–315.

Plastridge, W.N., Stula, E.F., and Williams, L.F. 1964. *Vibrio fetus* infection and reinfection in heifers, as determined by cultural tests using blood agar plus antibiotics. Am. J. Vet. Res. 25:710–713.

Plumer, G.J., Duvall, W.C., and Shepler, V.M. 1962. A preliminary report on a new technique for isolation of *Vibrio fetus* from carrier bulls. Cornell Vet. 52:110–122.

Vandeplassche, M., Florent, A., Bouters, R., Huysmin, A., Brone, E., and Dekeyser, P. 1963. The pathogenesis, epidemiology, and treatment of *Vibrio fetus* infection in cattle. C. R. Recherches 29:1–90.

Wilkie, B.N., and Winter, A.J. 1971. Bovine vibriosis: The distribution and specificity of antibodies induced by vaccination and infection and the immunofluorescent localization of the organism in infected heifers. Can. J. Comp. Med. 35:301–312.

Winter, A.J. 1965. Characterization of the antibody for *Vibrio fetus* endotoxin in sera of normal and *V. fetus* infected cattle. J. Immunol. 95:1002–1012.

Campylobacter fetus subspecies *fetus*
SYNONYMS: *Campylobacter fetus intestinalis, Vibrio fetus intestinalis*

Antigens. There are two serovars of *C. fetus* subspecies *fetus*, A-2 and B, based on heat-resistant O antigens (Berg et al. 1971). Protein antigens found on the surface of the organism are the basis for at least five serotypes (1, 2, 3, 4, and 5), of which 1 and 5 are most common in the United States, Great Britain, and Australia (Clark and Monsbourgh 1974, Marsh and Firehammer

1953). The microcapsular glycoprotein antigen is antiphagocytic (Corbeil et al. 1975).

Epizootiology and Pathogenesis. *C. fetus* subsp. *fetus* is an occasional cause of abortion during the latter half of gestation in cattle. The pathogenesis of the infection is similar to that caused by *C. fetus* subsp. *venerealis*, but the organism probably enters the animal by ingestion of infectious material.

Ovine infection by *C. fetus* subsp. *fetus* is contracted by ingestion of the organism (Frank et al. 1957). There is evidence that magpies (Meinershagen et al. 1965), ravens (Dennis 1967), and other carriers (Firehammer et al. 1962) are involved in spreading the disease, and it is possible that some sheep are asymptomatic carriers (Smibert 1965). Venereal transmission does not occur. The organism localizes in the placentomes after a period of bacteremia (Miller et al. 1959), placentitis develops, and abortion occurs toward the end of the gestation period. Infection of ewes in the first half of the gestation period does not result in abortion. Only heavily gravid animals are susceptible to bacterial invasion of the placenta with subsequent abortion. The incubation period is from 7 to 25 days. Animals usually exhibit a vaginal discharge for several days before they abort.

In outbreaks of ovine vibriosis the percentage of ewes having abortions or immature lambs can be high. The pathological changes observed in naturally infected sheep are chiefly confined to the uterus, placenta, and fetus. The uterine wall as well as the fetal membranes are edematous. Necrotizing and fibrinoid changes in the walls of arteries are followed by thrombus formation. The subcutaneous tissues of the fetus are edematous, and the peritoneal, pleural, and pericardial cavities can contain blood-tinged fluid. The presence of necrotic spots in the liver has also been reported. Foci of mononuclear cells or reticuloendothelial hyperplasia are present in many tissues. As a rule ewes do not abort in the years after an outbreak and appear not to carry the infection, although Smibert (1965) was able to isolate *C. fetus* subsp. *fetus* from the fecal and intestinal contents of clinically normal sheep. Vibrionic abortion also occurs in goats, but its importance as a cause of abortion is unknown (Dobbs and McIntyre 1951).

Immunity. Vaccination has been shown to be effective in the prevention of *C. fetus* subsp. *fetus* abortion in sheep flocks (Storz et al. 1966). Vaccinal immunity is serotype-specific; thus polyvalent vaccines that contain at least serotypes 1 and 5 (the common serotypes associated with ovine abortion) should be used. Thompson and Gilmour (1978) showed that good antibody responses to these different serotypes in a single vaccine can be obtained simultaneously. They also showed that vaccination at the beginning of an outbreak can be valuable in preventing later abortions in other members of the flock (Gilmour et al. 1975).

Williams et al. (1976) developed an in vitro bactericidal test that can be used to evaluate the immune response to bacterins. A pregnant guinea pig model is also effective in demonstrating the efficacy of commercial vaccines against *C. fetus*.

Diagnosis. *C. fetus* subsp. *fetus* can readily be seen in impression smears of fresh cotyledons, fetal stomach contents, and lungs. Culture on cystine-heart sheep-blood agar plates with and without antibiotic selection (Plastridge et al. 1961) in 10 percent CO_2 and reduced oxygen concentration usually establishes the cause of the abortion. A fluorescent antibody technique is also widely used but may be subject to error if the specimen has been contaminated with feces (Andrews and Frank 1974).

REFERENCES

Andrews, J., and Frank, F.W. 1974. Comparison of four diagnostic tests for detection of bovine genital vibriosis. J. Am. Vet. Med. Assoc. 165:695–697.

Berg, R.L., Jutila, J.W., and Firehammer, B.D. 1971. A revised classification of *Vibrio fetus*. Am. J. Vet. Res. 32:11–22.

Clark, B.L., and Monsbourgh, M.J. 1974. Serological types of *Vibrio fetus* var. *intestinalis* causing ovine vibriosis in southern Australia. Aust. Vet. J. 50:16–18.

Corbeil, L.B., Schurig, G.D., Bier, P.J., and Winter, A.J. 1975. Bovine venereal vibriosis: Antigenic variation of the bacterium during infection. Infect. Immun. 11:240–244.

Dennis, S.M. 1967. The possible role of the raven in the transmission of ovine vibriosis. Aust. Vet. J. 43:45–48.

Dobbs, E.M., and McIntyre, R.W. 1951. A case report of vibrionic abortion in a goat herd. Calif. Vet. 4:19.

Firehammer, B.D., Lovelace, S.A., and Hawkins, W.W. 1962. The isolation of *Vibrio fetus* from the ovine gallbladder. Cornell Vet. 52:21–35.

Frank, F.W., Bailey, J.W., and Heithecker, D. 1957. Experimental oral transmission of vibrionic abortion of sheep. J. Am. Vet. Med. Assoc. 131:472–473.

Gilmour, N.J.L., Thompson, D.A., and Fraser, J. 1975. Vaccination against *Vibrio (Campylobacter) fetus* infection in sheep in late pregnancy. Vet. Rec. 96:129–131.

Marsh, H., and Firehammer, B.D. 1953. Serological relationships of twenty-three ovine and three bovine strains of *Vibrio fetus*. Am. J. Vet. Res. 14:396–398.

Meinershagen, W.A., Waldhalm, D.G., Frank, F.W., and Scrivner, L.H. 1965. Magpies as a reservoir of infection for ovine vibriosis. J. Am. Vet. Med. Assoc. 147:843–845.

Miller, V.A., Jensen, R., and Gilroy, J.J. 1959. Bacteremia in pregnant sheep following oral administration of *Vibrio fetus*. Am. J. Vet. Res. 20:677–679.

Plastridge, W.N., Koths, M.E., and Williams, L.F. 1961. Antibiotic mediums for the isolation of vibrios from bull semen. Am. J. Vet. Res. 22:867–870.

Smibert, R.M. 1965. *Vibrio fetus* var. *intestinalis* isolated from fecal and intestinal contents of clinically normal sheep: Biochemical and cultural characteristics of microaerophilic vibrios isolated from the intestinal contents of sheep. Am. J. Vet. Res. 26:320–327.

Storz, J., Miner, M.L., Olson, A.E., Marriott, M.E., and Elsner, Y.Y. 1966. Prevention of ovine vibriosis by vaccination: Effect of yearly vaccination of replacement ewes. Am. J. Vet. Res. 27:115–120.

Thompson, D.A., and Gilmour, N.J.L. 1978. The serological response of sheep to a trivalent *Campylobacter (Vibrio) fetus* var. *intestinalis* vaccine. Vet. Rec. 102:530.

Williams, C.E., Renshaw, H.W., Meinershagen, W.A., Everson, D.O., Chamberlain, R.K., Hall, R.F., and Waldhalm, D.G. 1976. Ovine campylobacterosis: Preliminary studies of the efficacy of the in vitro serum bactericidal test as an assay for the potency of *Campylobacter (Vibrio) fetus* subsp. *intestinalis* bacterins. Am. J. Vet. Res. 37:409–415.

Campylobacter sputorum

There are three subspecies of *C. sputorum*: *C. sputorum* subsp. *sputorum*, *C. sputorum* subsp. *mucosalis*, and *C. sputorum* subsp. *bubulus*. Only the latter two are found in animals.

Campylobacter sputorum subspecies *mucosalis*

C. sputorum subsp. *mucosalis* was first isolated from swine with lesions of a disease known as *porcine intestinal adenomatosis* (Lawson and Rowland 1974) and has since been observed in most parts of the world. It is also a cause of necrotic enteritis, regional ileitis, and proliferative hemorrhagic enteropathy in swine (Love et al. 1977, Roland and Lawson 1975).

Morphology and Staining Reactions. The cells are short and irregularly curved (0.3 μm by 1.0 to 3.0 μm). Filamentous forms can be present in old cultures. Spirals of attached cells are not seen.

Cultural and Biochemical Features. Colonies are circular, raised, and have a flat surface and a dirty yellowish color; swarming can occur on moist agar. Good growth on cystine-blood agar with horse blood (7 percent) occurs as long as the oxygen content is reduced to 3 percent and 10 percent CO_2 is provided. Thioglycollate-blood agar can also be used as a plating medium.

C. sputorum subsp. *mucosalis* grows in 3.5 percent sodium chloride. Hydrogen is required as an electron donor. The organism contains large amounts of cytochrome c. It converts fumarate to succinate, but has no urease, lipase, lecithinase, or gelatinase activities. The mol% G + C of the DNA is 34.

Antigens. Strains of *C. sputorum* subsp. *mucosalis* are closely related antigenically. Three serovars—A, B, and C—have been reported (Lawson et al. 1981).

Epizootiology and Pathogenesis. The organism is found in the oral cavity of piglets for about 2 weeks after weaning and then disappears (Roberts 1981). Later catalase-negative organisms similar to but antigenically different from *C. sputorum* subsp. *mucosalis* can be found (reviewed by Garcia et al. 1983). It is therefore possible that antigenic variants are selected by antibody selection pressures in the oral cavity.

Transmission experiments, although occasionally successful, have revealed a high level of resistance to infection in normal pigs. It thus is probable that another predisposing factor is required which damages intestinal cells and allows intracellular multiplication of the organism. Lesion development is definitely related to how many organisms are in the intestinal mucosa (Roberts et al. 1980). The disease is characterized by excessive proliferation of immature epithelial cells, which carry the organism within the apical cytoplasm. It is not yet clear whether the adenomatous change in the epithelium precedes or is a sequel to the bacterial invasion.

The disease has a high mortality in highly susceptible swine (Love et al. 1977). Some degree of herd immunity usually exists, however, which protects swine against the most severe form of the disease. In such herds newly introduced nonimmune pigs are liable to be more severely affected.

Affected pigs do not thrive and their appetites are capricious. The lesions are found in the lower ileum and cecum and consist of proliferating epithelial cells throughout the entire depth of the mucosa. There is loss of villi and development of polypoid masses. In the absence of secondary infection most animals recover in about 6 weeks and have normal intestines at slaughter.

Necrotic enteritis characterized by thickening and coagulative necrosis of the ileal mucosa has also been associated with the presence of large numbers of *C. sputorum* subsp. *mucosalis* (Rowland and Lawson 1975). Another condition of swine known as *regional ileitis,* in which the lumen is obstructed by tissue proliferation, has also been associated with large numbers of the organism in the affected area.

Immunity. The protective immune responses of swine to the organism have not been studied. Agglutinins are present in the serums of infected animals (Rowland and Lawson 1974).

Diagnosis. The gross and microscopic morphology of the lesions together with evidence of the organism in the lesions constitute a basis for diagnosis of porcine intestinal adenomatosis. The organism can be isolated on a selective medium composed of a nutrient base, horse blood (5 percent), brilliant green, and novobiocin (Lawson and Rowland 1974). A fluorescent antibody technique for detection of the organism is also available (Roland and Lawson 1974).

REFERENCES

Garcia, M.M., Eaglesome, M.D., and Rigley, C. 1983. Campylobacters important in veterinary medicine. Vet. Bull. 53:793–818.

Lawson, G.H.K., and Rowland, A.C. 1974. Intestinal adenomatosis in the pig: A bacteriological study. Res. Vet. Sci. 17:331–336.
Lawson, G.H.K., Leaver, J.L., Pettigrew, G.W., and Rowland, A.C. 1981. Some features of *Campylobacter sputorum* subsp. *mucosalis* and their taxonomic significance. Int. J. Syst. Bacteriol. 31:385–391.
Love, D.N., Love, R.J., and Bailey, M. 1977. Comparison of *Campylobacter sputorum* subsp. *mucosalis* strains in PIA and PHE. Vet. Rec. 101:407–409.
Roberts, L. 1981. Natural infection of the oral cavity of young piglets with *Campylobacter sputorum* subsp. *mucosalis*. Vet. Rec. 109:170–172.
Roberts, L., Lawson, G.H.K., and Rowland, A.C. 1980. The experimental infection of neonatal pigs with *Campylobacter sputorum* subsp.*mucosalis*. Res. Vet. Sci. 28:145–147.
Rowland, A.C., and Lawson, G.H.K. 1974. Intestinal adenomatosis in the pig: Immunofluorescent and electron microscopic studies. Res. Vet. Sci. 17:323–330.
Rowland, A.C., and Lawson, G.H.K. 1975. Porcine intestinal adenomatosis: A possible relationship with necrotic enteritis, regional ileitis, and proliferative haemorrhagic enteropathy. Vet. Rec. 97:178–181.

Campylobacter sputorum subspecies *bubulus*

C. sputorum subsp. *bubulus* is a common commensal of the preputial epithelium of bulls (Samuelson and Winter 1966). It can be distinguished from the pathogenic *C. fetus* subsp. *venerealis* by its failure to produce catalase. Colonies are characteristically greenish and surrounded by a zone of alpha hemolysis.

REFERENCE

Samuelson, J.D., and Winter, A.J. 1966. Bovine vibriosis: The nature of the carrier state in the bull. J. Infect. Dis. 116:581–592.

Campylobacter hyointestinalis

C. hyointestinalis has been isolated in the United States from pigs with proliferative ileitis (Gebhart et al. 1983).

Morphology and Staining Reactions. *C. hyointestinalis* forms curved rods (0.2 to 0.5 μm by 1.2 to 2.5 μm) that have a single polar flagellum at one or both ends. Long, loose spirals are formed on solid media.

Cultural and Biochemical Features. On Mueller-Hinton agar with 5 percent sheep blood the colonies are yellowish, slightly mucoid, round, convex,and about 2 mm in diameter. Swarming does not occur. The organism produces catalase, grows in 1 percent glycine, produces H_2S, reduces nitrates, and grows well at 25°C but not at 43°C. It does not grow in 1.75 percent sodium chloride, is resistant to nalidixic acid, and is sensitive to cephalothin (Table 16.2).

Epizootiology and Pathogenesis. *C. hyointestinalis* was isolated from 18 of 27 pigs with proliferative ileitis and from only 1 of 21 pigs with other enteric diseases

(Gebhart et al. 1983). The organism was detected in the apical cytoplasm of proliferative cryptal epithelium but not in normal epithelium (Chang et al. 1984).

Diagnosis. The organism is readily isolated from 0.8-μm or 0.65-μm filtrates of intestinal macerate on Mueller-Hinton agar with 5 percent sheep blood, trimethoprim (2.5 μg/ml), and sulfamethoxazole (47.5 μg/ml). A fluorescent antibody procedure can also be used to detect the organism in smears (Chang et al. 1984).

REFERENCES

Chang, K., Kurtz, H.J., Ward, G.E., and Gebhart, C.J. 1984. Immunofluorescent demonstration of *Campylobacter hyointestinalis* and *Campylobacter sputorum* subsp. *mucosalis* in swine intestines with lesions of proliferative enteritis. Am. J. Vet. Res. 45:703–710.

Gebhart, C.J., Ward, G.E., Chang, K., and Kurtz, H.J. 1983. *Campylobacter hyointestinalis* (new species) isolated from swine with lesions of proliferative ileitis. Am. J. Vet. Res. 44:361–367.

Campylobacter jejuni

SYNONYMS: *Campylobacter fetus* serotype C, *Campylobacter fetus* subspecies *jejuni*

C. jejuni is a thermophilic campylobacter (Table 16.2) that has emerged in the 1970s as an important zoonotic pathogen. Milk, minced meat, dogs, cats, and poultry have been shown to be important sources of infection for humans. It is a component of the normal flora of most domestic and wild animals and a common contaminant of streams and other bodies of fresh water.

Morphology and Staining Reactions. *C. jejuni* forms small, tightly coiled, Gram negative cells 0.2 to 0.3 μm in diameter and 1.5 to 5.0 μm long. Coccoid bodies are formed when the organism is exposed to air. A polar flagellum is present.

Cultural and Biochemical Features. Colonies can be either flat, grayish, translucent, and granular with an irregular edge that tends to spread along the line of inoculation or round, convex, and smooth with an entire edge and a brownish center. There is no hemolysis. The important distinguishing characteristics are listed in Table 16.2. The mol% G + C of the DNA is 31. An extended biotyping scheme for *C. jejuni* and *C. coli* has been devised (Roop et al. 1984).

Antigens. The heat-resistant somatic (O) antigen of *C. jejuni* is designated C. Soluble heat-stable antigens are the basis of a serotyping scheme that is commonly used in epidemiological studies (Penner and Hennessy 1980). Another serotyping scheme is based on heat-labile antigens (Lior et al. 1982) and is apparently as effective in epidemiological studies as that of Penner and Hennessy.

Epizootiology and Pathogenesis. *C. jejuni* is widely distributed in the intestine of domestic and wild animals but is rarely isolated from the feces of normal humans. The organism is quite pathogenic for humans, and as few as 500 organisms in milk have caused enteritis. It has been implicated in the etiology of winter dysentery or black scours of cattle, diarrhea in calves, dogs, cats, and foals, hepatitis in chickens, and abortion in sheep and mink.

Jones and co-workers (1931) were the first to propose *C. jejuni* as a causative agent of winter dysentery in calves and older cattle, but this has never been satisfactorily confirmed. The disease is seen most often in housed dairy cattle in the northeastern United States in the autumn and winter and frequently takes the form of an acute herd outbreak of diarrhea. The feces are greenish to black and thin but not foul-smelling. Most animals recover in 2 to 3 days. In the original description of *C. jejuni* infection the organism was most abundant in the jejunum; although some of the more recent studies have failed to demonstrate a microbial etiology of the disease (Scott and Kahrs 1973), *C. jejuni* has been shown to be capable of producing diarrhea and sporadic dysentery in experimentally infected calves (Al-Moshat and Taylor 1980, Firehammer and Myers 1981). Further studies clearly are needed to define the etiology of the naturally occurring disease.

Diarrhea caused by *C. jejuni* has been described in dogs (Slee 1979). Dullness, emesis, thirst, and bloody diarrhea were the signs observed, and the lesions at necropsy included a hemorrhagic enteritis, ascites, and congestion and mottling of the liver. Some workers (Hosie et al. 1979), however, have concluded that *Campylobacter* species are not a significant cause of diarrhea in dogs, while others (Fleming 1983, Seifert and Weber 1983) have observed much higher rates of isolation of *Campylobacter* species from diarrheic animals than from normal animals.

C. jejuni has also been isolated from foals less than 4 months old with signs of acute enteritis (Atherton and Ricketts 1980). In the United States *C. jejuni* is a common cause of contagious abortion in sheep (Williams et al. 1976). The disease is similar to that described above for *C. fetus* subsp. *fetus*. Ewes are resistant for some years after abortion.

Avian vibrionic hepatitis (Hofstad 1956), a disease of poultry characterized by listlessness, poor egg production, and degenerative changes in the liver and other organs, is also caused by *C. jejuni*. The organism is widespread in poultry populations and spread rapidly in young, noninfected populations.

The organism has recently been shown to cause bovine mastitis (Lander and Gill 1980, Morgan et al. 1985). The report of Morgan et al. (1985) showed that the organism could be shed for 12 weeks from a subclinically infected quarter and produced gastroenteritis in people who consumed unpasteurized milk from the cow.

Diagnosis. A variety of selective media have been described for the isolation of *C. jejuni* from feces. These include Skirrows', Butzlers', and Blasers' media and modifications thereof (reviewed by Bolton et al. 1983). These media contain a base, 5 percent lysed horse blood, and antimicrobials such as polymyxin B (2,500 or 5,000 IU/liter), rifampicin (10 μl/liter), trimethoprim (10 mg/liter), and cycloheximide (100 mg/liter) to suppress fecal contaminants. Incubation at 42°C further enhances the selective abilities of these media.

REFERENCES

Al-Moshat, R.R., and Taylor, D.J. 1980. Production of diarrhoea and dysentery in experimental calves by feeding pure cultures of *Campylobacter fetus* subsp. *jejuni.* Vet. Rec. 107:459–464.

Atherton, J.G., and Ricketts, S.W. 1980. Campylobacter infection from foals. Vet. Rec. 107:264–265.

Bolton, F.J., Coates, D., Hinchliffe, P.M., and Robertson, L. 1983. Comparison of selective media for isolation of *Campylobacter jejuni/coli.* J. Clin. Pathol. 36:78–83.

Firehammer, B.D., and Myers, C.C. 1981. *Campylobacter fetus* subsp. *jejuni:* Its possible significance in enteric disease of calves and lambs. Am. J. Vet. Res. 42:918–922.

Fleming, M.P. 1983. Association of *Campylobacter jejuni* with enteritis in dogs and cats. Vet. Rec. 13:372–374.

Hofstad, M.S. 1956. Hepatitis in chickens. A report of progress in veterinary medical research. Veterinary Medicine Research Institute of the State College, Ames, Iowa.

Hosie, B.D., Nicolson, T.B., and Henderson, D.B. 1979. Campylobacter infections in normal and diarrhoeic dogs. Vet. Rec. 105:80–81.

Jones, F.S., Orcutt, M., and Little, R.B. 1931. Vibrios (*Vibrio jejuni,* n. sp.) associated with intestinal disorders of cows and calves. J. Exp. Med. 53:853–864.

Lander, K.P., and Gill, K.P.W. 1980. Experimental infection of the bovine udder with *Campylobacter coli/jejuni.* J. Hyg. 84:421–428.

Lior, H., Woodward, D.C., Edgar, J.A., Laroche, L.J., and Gill, P. 1982. Serotyping of *Campylobacter jejuni* by slide agglutination based on heat-labile antigenic factors. J. Clin. Microbiol. 15:761–768.

Morgan, G., Chadwick, P., Lander, K.P., and Gill, P. 1985. *Campylobacter jejuni* mastitis in a cow: A zoonosis-related incident. Vet. Rec. 116:111–112.

Penner, J.L., and Hennessy, J.N. 1980. Passive hemagglutination technique for serotyping *Campylobacter fetus* subsp. *jejuni* on the basis of soluble heat-stable antigens. J. Clin. Microbiol. 12:732–737.

Roop, R.M., Swibert, R.M., and Krieg, N.R. 1984. Improved biotyping schemes for *Campylobacter jejuni* and *Campylobacter coli.* J. Clin. Microbiol. 20:990–992.

Scott, F.W., and Kahrs, R.F. 1973. Etiologic studies on bovine winter dysentery. Bovine Pract. 8:40–43.

Siefert, U., and Weber, A. 1983. Detection of *C. jejuni* in dogs and cats with and without enteritis. Kleintierpraxis 28:371–372.

Slee, A. 1979. Haemorrhagic gastroenteritis in a dog. Vet. Rec. 104:14–15.

Williams, C.E., Renshaw, H.W., Meinershagen, W.A., Everson, D.O., Chamberlain, R.K., Hall, R.F., and Waldheim, D.G. 1976. Ovine campylobacteriosis: Preliminary studies of the efficacy of the in vitro serum bactericidal test as an assay for the potency of *Campylobacter (Vibrio) fetus* subsp. *intestinalis* bacterins. Am. J. Vet. Res. 37:409–415.

Campylobacter coli

C. coli greatly resembles *C. jejuni* except that it is unable to hydrolyze hippurate. It is an inhabitant of the intestinal tract of swine, poultry, and humans. Although it has been implicated as a cause of enteritis in weaned piglets with clinical signs of mild swine dysentery (Taylor and Olubunmi 1981), it does not appear to be an important pathogen of domestic animals. The mol% G + C of its DNA is 31.

REFERENCE

Taylor, D.J., and Olubunmi, P.A. 1981. A re-examination of the role of *Campylobacter fetus* subsp. *coli* in enteric disease of the pig. Vet. Rec. 109:112–115.

Antimicrobial Susceptibility of *Campylobacter* Species

Campylobacter species in general are sensitive to chloramphenicol, tetracyclines, erythromycin, streptomycin, and gentamicin. Pig strains of *C. sputorum* subsp. *mucosalis* and *C. hyointestinalis* are also sensitive to carbadox, furazolidone, nitrofurantoin, and dimetridazole (Gebhart et al. 1985).

REFERENCE

Gebhart, C.J., Ward, G.E., and Kurtz, H.J. 1985. In vitro activities of 47 antimicrobial agents against three *Campylobacter* spp. from pigs. Antimicrob. Agents Chemother. 27:55–59.

17 The Genera *Fusobacterium* and *Bacteroides*

The Bacteroidaceae, a family of Gram-negative, non-sporulating, obligate anaerobes that inhabit the alimentary tract of humans and animals, comprises 13 genera, of which only the genera *Fusobacterium* and *Bacteroides* contain species that commonly cause disease. Members of the family are differentiated by gas chromatographic analysis of fatty acid formation from peptone or glucose. *Bacteroides* species produce varying amounts of succinic, acetic, formic, lactic, and propionic acids. The major fermentation product of *Fusobacterium* species is butyric acid.

The Genus *Fusobacterium*

Among the species of *Fusobacterium* only *F. necrophorum* regularly causes disease in domestic animals.

Fusobacterium necrophorum

SYNONYMS: *Actinomyces necrophorus,*
   Bacillus diphtheriae vitulorum,
   Bacterium necrophorum, calf diptheria
   bacillus, *Cladothrix cuniculi,*
   Corynebacterium necrophorum,
   Fusiformis necrophorus, necrosis
   bacillus, *Spheropherus necrophorus,*
   Streptothrix cuniculi

F. necrophorum is found in necrotic lesions in warm-blooded animals. It produces the diseases commonly known under the collective term *necrobacilloses*.

Morphology and Staining Reactions. In infected tissues *F. necrophorum* is ordinarily seen in the form of long filaments, but shorter elements and even coccoid forms occur. The rods are about 1 μm wide and can be more than 100 μm long. In some cultures swollen rods are seen which may be nearly twice as thick as the usual forms. Freshly isolated strains growing in cooked-meat medium usually show a predominance of long filaments. The sides of these filaments are parallel and regular and are either straight or in the form of sweeping curves. After prolonged artificial culture the predominant forms usually are short. Very young cultures stain uniformly, but the filaments in cultures older than 24 hours usually are vacuolated, that is, the stained portions are separated by sections that are free or almost free of stain. The irregular distribution of cytoplasm along the filaments can easily be seen in unstained preparations (Figure 17.1). Flagella have not been demonstrated and motility is absent. Young cultures are readily stained with the ordinary stains. The organism is always Gram-negative.

Cultural and Biochemical Features. *F. necrophorum* is very sensitive to oxygen and strict anaerobic conditions must be provided. The presence of 5 to 10 percent CO_2 enhances growth. A medium containing peptone (1 percent), yeast extract (1 percent), vitamin K, hemin, or blood and a reducing agent such as cysteine is necessary for good growth. Cultures die soon after initial growth. Thioglycollate medium, without enrichment, is a good maintenance medium but cultures must be passaged every week. Maintenance and storage media should not contain fermentable carbohydrate.

Under favorable conditions *F. necrophorum* forms acid and gas from glucose, lactose, sucrose, maltose, and salicin. The amount of acid formed is not great, and gas formation is limited. *F. necrophorum* regularly forms a large bubble of gas in cooked-meat medium covered with a vaspar seal (petrolatum and paraffin in equal parts). It hemolyzes horse blood, does not liquefy serum gelatin, does not digest coagulated serum, and does not produce lecithinase. In clear, solid medium colonies are fuzzy when the medium is fairly soft and dense when it is more solid. Colonies are round, convex, gray, and 1 to 3 mm in diameter, with scalloped to erose edges and often an uneven surface.

A selective medium consisting of an egg yolk–agar base containing 0.02 percent crystal violet, 0.01 percent brilliant green, and phenethyl alcohol (to suppress Gram-negative facultative anaerobes) has been described (Fales and Teresa 1972). When incubated in CO_2, colonies of *F. necrophorum* are blue and are surrounded by opaque and clear zones. Antibiotics such as kanamycin, erythromycin, vancomycin, and bacitracin have also been used in

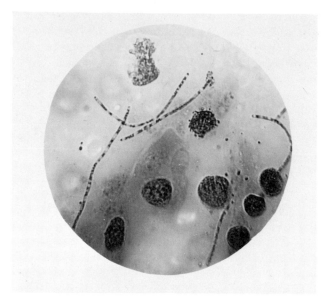

Figure 17.1. *Fusobacterium necrophorum* in a lung abscess in a calf. The long filaments with irregular distribution of chromatic material are characteristic. Gram's stain. × 1,040.

selective media (Balows et al. 1975). Cultures may be preserved by freezing them at −70°C in calf serum or by lyophilization in skim milk (Fales and Teresa 1972).

F. necrophorum can be differentiated from other species of *Fusobacterium* by its ability to produce indole and to form propionic acid from lactate. *Fusobacterium* species may be differentiated from *Bacteroides* species by the failure of *Fusobacterium* species to synthesize 3-hydroxy fatty acids (Fritsche and Boehmer 1974). The mol% G + C of the DNA is 31 to 34.

Antigens. *Fusobacterium* species do not cross-react serologically with *Bacteroides* (Werner and Sebald 1968) and fluorescent antiserums against *F. necrophorum* do not react with other *Fusobacterium* species. Both heat-labile and heat-stable antigens are present in *F. necrophorum*, and there is considerable antigenic heterogeneity among strains. Serotyping thus does not appear to have much potential in the study of the epizootiology of fusobacterial diseases unless these antigens can be shown to be important in protection. Feldman et al. (1936) described four distinct antigenic groups among 14 strains of *F. necrophorum* from bovine liver abscesses.

Biotypes. There are four biotypes of *F. necrophorum* designated A, B, AB, and C. They are distinguished by differences in cellular and colonial morphology and biological characteristics including mouse pathogenicity and hemolytic and hemagglutinating properties (Fievez 1963, Scanlan and Hathcock 1983). Biotype A strains are usually found in liver abscesses, are very pathogenic for

mice, and agglutinate chicken erythrocytes. Biotype B strains are less virulent for mice, are nonhemolytic, and usually are found in mixed cultures with biotype A strains or other bacteria in lesions and the contents of the rumen. Strains of biotype C are avirulent and have no hemolytic or hemagglutinating ability. Biotype AB strains represent a blend of the characteristics of A and B strains. They are less pathogenic than biotype A strains (Scanlan and Hathcock 1983).

Epizootiology and Pathogenesis. *F. necrophorum* is a commensal of the alimentary tract of many animal species and humans. Infections in animals generally occur when they are kept in filthy surroundings. especially when there are accumulations of manure underfoot. The organism remains viable in soil for short periods of time. Marsh and Tunnicliff (1934) were able to demonstrate the presence of the organism in a wet pasture 10 months after sheep affected with foot-rot had run on it, but they could not demonstrate its presence after a second 10-month period. The organism has little or no ability to invade normal epithelia but readily enters and multiplies in tissues damaged by trauma, viral or bacterial infection, or maceration.

In all species, the typical lesion is characterized by necrosis, abscess formation, and putrid odor. Bacteremia can occur in some instances, with dissemination to the liver and other organs. Strains of *F. necrophorum* contain a classical lipopolysaccharide endotoxin that is associated with the cell wall and in which lipid A is a major toxic component (Garcia, Alexander, and McKay 1975). Other components of the organism also have toxic activity. Garcia, Charlton, and McKay (1975) have described a cytoplasmic proteinaceous toxin that has hemolytic activity and is protectively immunogenic, and Roberts (1967a) described a leukocidin that is apparently distinct from this hemolysin. Leukotoxin-producing strains are more pathogenic for rat livers than strains that do not produce leukotoxin (Coyle-Dennis and Lauerman 1979). Biotype A strains produce more leukotoxin than biotype AB strains. Biotype B strains produce only trace amounts (Scanlan et al. 1982). The presence of leukotoxin thus correlates well with the known virulence of different biotypes. Experimental infections of mice indicate that the organism multiplies in the liver, causing focal necrosis and accumulation of mononuclear cells including macrophages (Garcia et al. 1977). The organism is found within the macrophages, which are eventually killed by the leukocidin. Fales et al. (1977) examined this toxic effect in isolated rabbit peritoneal macrophages and found that 90 percent of macrophages were killed within 6 hours. The cytotoxic effect of *F. necrophorum* for liver cells and other cells has not yet been fully defined but may

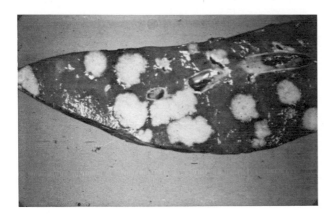

Figure 17.2. Lesions caused by *Fusobacterium necrophorum* in the liver of a cow.

be an effect of endotoxin because the latter produces necrosis when rabbits are inoculated intradermally.

Cattle. Infection of the mouth and pharynx of calves, known as *calf diphtheria,* is an especially malignant form of necrobacillosis. The disease usually occurs in young calves that are bucket-fed under unsanitary conditions, but it has also been observed in cattle up to 2 years old. The lesions may extend to the larynx, with subsequent aspiration of necrotic material into the lungs, resulting in fatal pneumonia.

Rumenitis and liver abscesses caused by *F. necrophorum* in cattle result in serious economic loss to the meat industry in many parts of the world. Lesions in the liver are light yellow, firm, dry, sharply circumscribed areas (Figure 17.2). Sometimes the lesions are well-encapsulated abscesses, in which case other bacteria such as *Actinomyces pyogenes* may also be present. Liver abscesses caused by *F. necrophorum* are especially common in feedlot cattle and are a part of a complex where ruminal lesions induced by acid from fermentable carbohydrate predisposes the animal toward invasion by *F. necrophorum.* Focal abscesses are formed in the rumen wall and serve as a source of infective emboli that are carried in the portal venous system to the liver (Smith 1944). Biotype B organisms dominate in ruminal lesions, whereas biotype A organisms dominate in liver abscesses (Berg and Scanlan 1982). It has been postulated that the possession of leukotoxin gives biotype A strains an advantage against host defenses, thus they are more invasive (Berg and Scanlan 1982).

Foot-rot, or foul in the foot, in cattle (Figure 17.3) has frequently been associated with *F. necrophorum,* but the role of the organism in the genesis of the lesions is uncertain. Berg and Loan (1975) isolated both *F. necrophorum* and *Bacteroides melaninogenicus* in large numbers from biopsy specimens of naturally occurring and experimen-

tally produced lesions in cattle in the United States. Thorley et al. (1977) reported the presence of *Bacteroides nodosus* in necrotic lesions of the interdigital skin in cattle in Britain.

Attempts to produce the disease experimentally with pure cultures of *F. necrophorum* have not been successful (Flint and Jensen 1951); however, typical foot-rot lesions were produced with a combination of fusiformlike organisms and staphylococci (Gupta et al. 1964). It is probable that concurrent infection by *F. necrophorum* plus any of several other bacteria can produce foot-rot in cattle. Trauma and maceration are well-known predisposing factors. The milder form of the disease involves only the interdigital space where a fissure lined by foul-smelling necrotic tissues develops. The bacteria found in more severe lesions involving the laminar structures, bacteria found include *F. necrophorum, B. nodosus,* and *A. pyogenes.*

Lesions associated with *F. necrophorum* have also been seen on the udders and teats of cattle. Uterine infections are not uncommon, and ulceration of the mucosa of the abomasum is often ascribed to this bacillus. The organism has been encountered in bovine mastitis and in rumenitis in calves reared on an early weaning feeding system.

The disease in sheep. F. necrophorum lesions in sheep are similar to those in cattle. The organism has been associated with the disease known as ovine interdigital dermatitis, lip and leg ulceration, foot-rot, and infective bulbar necrosis (boot abscess) of ewes lambing in wet conditions. The most important bacterium in foot-rot of sheep, however, is *B. nodosus. F. necrophorum* is of importance in creating invasion sites for *B. nodosus, A.*

Figure 17.3. Bovine foot-rot.

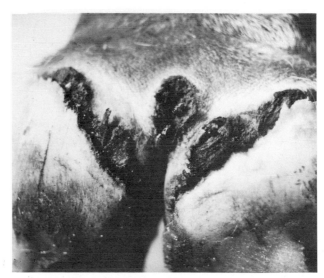

pyogenes, and *Spirochaeta penortha,* which are also commonly found in lesions as secondary invaders. Ovine interdigital dermatitis is a skin condition associated with an intense invasion by *F. necrophorum* of the posterior interdigital epidermis when subjected to continuous wet conditions, and foot-rot associated with *B. nodosus* may be a sequel to this disease. Ovine foot abscesses are caused by *F. necrophorum* and *A. pyogenes* in synergy (Roberts 1967a, 1967b). *F. necrophorum* facilitates the establishment and growth of *A. pyogenes* in the tissues through the leukocidal action of its exotoxin and prevention of phagocytosis, whereas *A. pyogenes* produces a macromolecular substance that stimulates the growth and invasiveness of *F. necrophorum. A. pyogenes* also contributes to the growth of *F. necrophorum* by removing oxygen and decreasing Eh.

The disease in swine. F. necrophorum in swine is associated with ulcerative stomatitis (sore mouth) and the condition known as bullnose, in which there is an infection of the subcutaneous tissues of the face frequently originating in the wound resulting from placing a ring in the nose. It is also associated with necrosis of the epithelium and deeper layers of the intestines, a condition known as necrotic enteritis. Necrobacillosis has also been described in rabbits, in which it involves the lips and mouth; in horses, in which the lower posterior aspects of the legs may be involved (scratches); and in chickens as a sequel to fowlpox virus infection (Emmel 1948).

Immunity. Attempts to vaccinate animals with formalinized cell preparations and with culture filtrates of *F. necrophorum* have not been successful. However, liver abscessation in cattle has been prevented by using a cytoplasmic fraction of sonically treated *F. necrophorum* (Garcia et al. 1974). During a 6-month trial precipitating antibodies were produced in almost all animals receiving the highest dose of vaccine, whereas only 35 percent of control cattle produced precipitins. Feldman et al. (1936) found that healthy adult animals exhibit a high rate of seropositivity in the agglutination reaction and that young animals such as calves show little or no seropositivity. It thus appears that most animals develop antibodies as they age and are exposed to the organism. Furthermore, these workers were able to relate the presence and severity of abscessation to the magnitude of agglutinin titers, an indication that these antibodies are not important in protection against the disease.

Diagnosis. Gram-stained smears obtained from the edges of lesions frequently reveal the organism. Cultures should be quickly made on suitable prereduced selective media, such as that of Fales and Teresa (1972), and placed under anaerobic conditions. Determination of genus is then made by gas liquid chromatography of the fatty acids

produced in peptone glucose broth. No serologic methods of diagnosis are available.

Antimicrobial Susceptibility. *F. necrophorum* is sensitive to tetracyclines, chloramphenicol, penicillin, clindamycin, cephalothin, erythromycin, tylosin, and sulfonamides; however, the amounts of erythromycin or tylosin needed to obtain therapeutically adequate serum levels after intramuscular administration are excessively high (Berg and Scanlan 1982).

Sulfapyridine or tetracyclines are effective in treatment of calf diphtheria. Sodium sulfadimidine or penicillin given parenterally in conjunction with local treatment is effective in treatment of foot-rot.

Feeding chlortetracycline (75 mg/day) or tylosin (70 mg/day) to feedlot cattle is effective in reducing the incidence of liver abscesses and in allowing normal weight gain. Spiramycin given at the rate of 10 mg/kg of body weight (20 percent solution intramuscularly) four times a year has been found to prevent foot-rot in cattle on premises where the disease was endemic (Chauvau and Royer 1977). Larger amounts given in two doses 48 hours apart are also effective in the treatment of acute foot-rot.

REFERENCES

Balows, A., DeHaan, R.M., Dowell, V.R., and Guze, L.B., eds. 1975. Anaerobic Bacteria: Role in Disease. American Lecture Series in Microbiology, no. 940. Charles C. Thomas, Springfield, Ill.

Berg, J.N., and Loan, R.W. 1975. *Fusobacterium necrophorum* and *Bacteroides melaninogenicus* as etiologic agents of foot rot in cattle. Am. J. Vet. Res. 36:1115–1122.

Berg, J.N., and Scanlan, C.M. 1982. Studies of *Fusobacterium necrophorum* from bovine hepatic abcesses, biotypes, quantitation, virulence and antibiotic susceptibility. Am. J. Vet. Res. 43:1580–1586.

Chauveau, J., and Royer, P. 1977. Interdigital foot rot in cattle. Treatment with spiramycin. Bull. Mens. Soc. Vét. Prat. France 61:255–266.

Coyle-Dennis, J.E., and Lauerman, L.H. 1979. Correlations between leukocidin production and virulence of two isolates of *Fusobacterium necrophorum.* Am. J. Vet. Res. 40:274–276.

Emmel, M.W. 1948. *Necrophorus* infection in chickens. J. Am. Vet. Med. Assoc. 113:169–171.

Fales, W.H., and Teresa, G.W. 1972. A selective medium for the isolation of *Sphaerophorus necrophorus.* Am. J. Vet. Res. 33:2317–2321.

Fales, W.H., Warner, J.F., and Teresa, G.W. 1977. Effects of *Fusobacterium necrophorum* leukotoxin on rabbit peritoneal macrophages in vitro. Am. J. Vet. Res. 38:491–495.

Feldman, W.H., Hester, H.R., and Wherry, R.P. 1936. the occurrence of *Bacillus necrophorus* agglutinins in different species of animals. J. Infect. Dis. 59:159–170.

Fievez, L. 1963. Etude comparée des souches de *Spaerophorus necrophorus* isolée chez l'homme et l'animal. Brussells, Presses Académiques Européenes.

Flint, J.C., and Jensen, R. 1951. Pathology of necrobacillosis of the bovine foot. Am. J. Vet. Res. 12:5–13.

Fritsche, D., and Boehmer, H. 1974. Die Zuordnung buttersäure-bildender Anaerobier zum Genus *Bacteroides* mit Hilfe ihres Lipoid-Stoffwechsels. Zentralbl. Bakteriol. Mikrobiol. Hyg. [A] 226:248–256.

Garcia, M.M., Alexander, D.C., and McKay, K.A. 1975. Biological characterization of *Fusobacterium necrophorum* cell fractions in preparation for toxin and immunization studies. Infect Immun. 11:609–616.

Garcia, M.M., Charlton, K.M., and McKay, K.A. 1975. Characterization of endotoxin from *Fusobacterium necrophorum*. Infect. Immun. 11:371–379.

Garcia, M.M., Charlton, K.M., and McKay, K.A. 1977. Hepatic lesions and bacterial changes in mice during infection of *Fusobacterium necrophorum*. Can. J. Microbiol. 23:1465–1477.

Garcia, M.M., Dorward, W.J., Alexander, D.C., Magwood, S.E., and McKay, K.A. 1974. Results of a preliminary trial with *Sphaerophorus necrophorus* toxoids to control liver abscesses in feedlot cattle. Can J. Comp. Med. 38:222–226.

Gupta, R.B., Fincher, M.G., and Bruner, D.W. 1964. A study of the etiology of foot-rot in cattle. Cornell Vet. 54:66–77.

Marsh, H., and Tunnicliff, E.A. 1934. Experimental studies of foot-rot in sheep. Mont. Agric. Exp. Sta. Bull. 285. Pp. 3–16.

Roberts, D.S. 1967a. The pathogenic synergy of *Fusiformis necrophorus* and *Corynebacterium pyogenes*. I. Influence of the leucocidal exotoxin of *F. necrophorus* to a filterable product of *F. necrophorus*. Br. J. Exp. Pathol. 48:665–673.

Roberts, D.S. 1967b. The pathogenic synergy of *Fusiformis necrophorus* and *Corynebacterium pyogenes*. II. The response of *F. necrophorus* to a filterable product of *C. pyogenes*. Br. J. Exp. Pathol. 48:674–679.

Scanlan, C.M., and Hathcock, T.C. 1983. Bovine rumenitis–liver abscess complex: A bacteriological review. Cornell Vet. 73:288–297.

Scanlan, C.M., Berg, J.N., and Fales, W. H. 1982. Comparative in vitro leukotoxin production of three bovine strains of *Fusobacterium necrophorum*. Am. J. Vet. Res. 43:1329–1333.

Smith, H.A. 1944. Ulcerative lesions of the bovine rumen and their possible relation to hepatic abscesses. Am. J. Vet. Res. 5:234–242.

Thorley, C.M., Calder, H.A.M., and Harrison, W.J. 1977. Recognition in Great Britain of *Bacteroides nodosus* in foot lesions of cattle. Vet. Rec. 100:387.

Werner, H., and Sebald, M. 1968. Etude sérologique dianaerobies gram-négatifs asporules, et particulièrement de *Bacteroides convexus* et *Bacteroides melaninogenicus*. Ann. Inst. Pasteur 115:350–366.

The Genus *Bacteroides*

Although *B. nodosus* is the only *Bacteroides* species of importance as a cause of a specific disease in domestic animals, a number of other opportunistic *Bacteroides* species have been isolated from suppurative and necrotic lesions in a variety of body sites. Examples of these infections together with the *Bacteroides* species isolated are shown in Table 17.1.

B. fragilis with enterotoxinlike activity has been isolated from outbreaks of acute diarrheal disease in 24- to 48-hour-old lambs in the northwestern United States. Isolates have been used to produce a similar disease in experimentally infected newborn lambs (Myers et al. 1984). The incidence of this disease in the United States and elsewhere remains to be determined.

REFERENCE

Myers, L.L., Firehammer, B.D., Shoop, D.S., and Border, M.M. 1984. *Bacteroides fragilis*: A possible cause of acute diarrheal disease in newborn lambs. Infect. Immun. 44:241–244.

Bacteroides nodosus

SYNONYMS: *Actinomyces nodosus,*
Fusiformis nodosus, Ristella nodosa

B. nodosus is an essential transmitting agent of foot-rot in sheep and was first described by Beveridge in Australia (1941).

Table 17.1. *Bacteroides* species (other than *B. nodosus*) isolated from suppurative lesions in domestic animals

Species	Lesion	Host	Reference
Bacteroides spp. (asaccharolytic pigmented spp. and saccharolytic spp.)	Soft tissue infection, pyothorax	Cat	Love et al. 1981, 1984
B. asaccharolyticus	Osteomyelitis	Dogs, cats, horses, cattle	Walker et al. 1983
B. fragilis	Diarrheal disease Mastitis Abscesses	Newborn lambs Cattle Swine	Myers et al. 1984 Preez et al. 1982 Benno et al. 1982
B. helcogenes *B. intermedius* *B. pyogenes* *B. suis*	Abscesses	Swine	Benno et al. 1982
B. melaninogenicus	Suppurative effusions of abdomen and thorax	Dogs, cats, cattle	Biberstein et al. 1968
	Bite wounds Foot-rot	Dogs, cats Cattle	Berg 1975

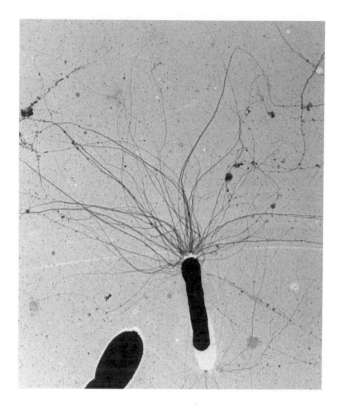

Figure 17.4. *Bacteroides nodosus* strain 80, a virulent cause of foot-rot, grown in liquid culture and negatively stained with uranyl acetate. Numerous pili emerge from one pole. (From Every and Skerman, 1980, courtesy of *Journal of Bacteriology* and T. M. Skerman.)

Morphology and Staining Reactions. The organism is a large, piliated, rod-shaped bacterium characterized by the presence of terminal enlargements, usually at both ends. These enlargements are more pronounced in the organisms seen in tissue smears than in those that have been developed in culture. The rods usually are straight but may be slightly curved. They are 0.6 to 0.8 μm in diameter and 3 to 10 μm in length, although few are more than 6 μm long. Numerous pili are attached to one pole (Figure 17.4). In cultures the organisms tend to be shorter, and in old cultures they may even be coccoid in form. They are nonmotile, do not form spores, and stain readily with all ordinary dyes. They are Gram-negative and non-acid-fast. Organisms stained with methylene blue often show one or several metachromatic granules, usually located at the ends of the rod.

Cultural and Biochemical Features. The organism is an obligate anaerobe. Growth is enhanced when 10 percent or more CO_2 is introduced into the anaerobic culture jar. Cultures grow best at 37°C in neutral or alkaline media that contain trypticase and arginine (0.05 M). Growth is also enhanced by the addition of 10 percent horse serum. Serums from other species are usually not satisfactory. Surface colonies on agar media containing peptic

digest of beef muscle and liver or horse serum are 0.5 to 2.0 mm in diameter, smooth, convex, and semiopaque or translucent. Virulent isolates from animals with foot-rot produce papillate or beaded colonies that etch the medium. Less virulent isolates produce mucoid colonies. Cultures grown in broth are slightly turbid and granular. A simple medium recommended for the isolation of *B. nodosus* consists of pulverized suspended sheep horn (4 percent) in an anaerobic medium with 10 percent CO_2 (Thomas 1958). A liquid medium used by Thomas (1963) contained hydrolyzed sheep hoof (2 percent) as a basic ingredient. Heavy inocula will often cause milk to curdle after several days' incubation without a change in reaction; later the curd is digested. The organisms in old cultures form tyrosine crystals. *B. nodosus* does not ferment any of the ordinary carbohydrates. It does not reduce nitrates, but it does form hydrogen sulfide and produces gelatinase and keratinase.

Antigens and Serotypes. Both K (specific) and O (group) antigens have been described. The K antigen, a protein, is associated with the fimbriae (pili) and is a protective antigen (Stewart 1978). Egerton (1973) examined the K antigens of different strains and found that each was serologically distinct. He designated the prevalent

Australian K antigens as A, B, and C, but all strains possessed the same heat-stable or O antigens. The O antigen lipopolysaccharide is biologically, chemically, and ultrastructurally similar to that of the Enterobacteriaceae and consists of a polysaccharide joined to lipid A through an acid-labile 2-keto-3-deoxyoctonic acid link (Stewart 1977).

The K or fimbrial antigens have been used to establish at least eight major serogroups and a number of subtypes. They consist of a single repeated polypeptide unit that varies in size from one serotype to another with a mean molecular weight of about 18,500. In serotype A1 the molecular weight is 17,500. A polypeptide with a molecular weight of about 80,000 appears to serve as a link between the fimbria and the surface of the cell (Mattick et al. 1984). The gene encoding the structural subunit of serogroup A fimbriae has been cloned and expressed in *E. coli* (Anderson et al. 1984).

Epizootiology and Pathogenesis. *B. nodosus* is an obligate parasite of the hooves of sheep, goats, and cattle. It survives for only a few days on pasture or in soil. The infection can be transmitted between cattle and sheep, but the disease is not transmitted to sheep from cattle under natural conditions (Laing and Egerton 1978). Strains that occur in the hooves of cattle are less virulent for sheep. Since the organism survives only in the hoof, carrier animals serve as sources for uninfected stock. The infection spreads rapidly when sheep are grazing on lush, damp pasture in rainy weather. Foot-rot is thus more common in late spring and early fall. Besides maceration of the feet, minor wounds, abrasions from stony surfaces, and damage caused by migrating *Strongyloides* larvae are other predisposing factors for the development of foot-rot in sheep.

Much of the recent definitive work on the pathogenesis of foot-rot in sheep has been done in Australia and New Zealand. Invasion of the interdigital epidermis by *B. nodosus* is preceded by colonization of the stratum corneum by *F. necrophorum*, which is apparently derived from feces. *F. necrophorum* damages the epidermis sufficiently to allow entry and multiplication of *B. nodosus*. *B. nodosus* has little inflammatory destructive action but produces a powerful protease that digests horn (Broad and Skerman 1976) and permits invasion of the epidermal matrix of the hoof. *B. nodosus* grows slowly when nutrients are scarce and thus can sustain itself between the brief waves of growth of *F. necrophorum* and so persist in the lesion. It also produces a heat-stable soluble factor that promotes the growth and invasiveness of *F. necrophorum*.

Although Beveridge (1941) has indicated that *Spirochaeta penortha* is the accessory factor in producing foot-rot in sheep, Roberts and Egerton (1969) have concluded that spirochetes and motile fusiforms are probably not essential to the pathogenesis of this disease but are derived from the environment. *Actinomyces pyogenes* and other aerobic diptheroids, which usually have a superficial location in the lesion, remove oxygen and reduce Eh, thus facilitating the growth of the anaerobes. The separation of horn in foot-rot is caused by lysis of the epidermal matrix as a result of the local inflammatory response to the infection and is not a result of direct bacterial attack (Egerton et al. 1969).

The role of *B. nodosus* in the pathogenesis of foot-rot in cattle is not as well defined as in foot-rot in sheep, but the organism has been recognized in bovine foot lesions in Australia (Egerton and Parsonson 1966), Holland, and Great Britain (Thorley et al. 1977). Typical lesions in cattle consisted of necrosis of the interdigital epidermis, which became eroded. The posterior skin area between the claws showed a swollen gray seborrheic area with a pronounced foul odor. Cracking of the skin at its junction with the horn in the interdigital space was a common sequel. Also, the horn in the heel area sometimes became separated. The isoenzyme patterns of the proteases from ovine virulent and benign isolates and bovine isolates are distinguishable from one another (Every 1982), suggesting that distinct groups of strains with varying virulence and host preference exist. The involvement of Bacteroidaceae in diseases of the foot in cattle and sheep is summarized in Table 17.2.

Immunity. *B. nodosus* is excluded from the dermis by the bactericidal effects of serum and by phagocytes. After infection IgG1 antibodies are produced against the fimbrial (K) antigen of the organism, and these antibodies are protective when present in high titers (Stewart 1978). Successful vaccines against ovine foot-rot must contain K antigen (Egerton and Roberts 1971). Furthermore, type-specific K antigen is required (Egerton 1973, Egerton et al. 1972).

Multivalent vaccines that contain all the K specificities of strains that occur in a flock thus are necessary for good protection against disease in that flock. Antigenic heterogeneity of *B. nodosus* has been an important source of failure of vaccination programs.

Immunity to foot-rot requires very high titers of antibody (Egerton and Roberts 1971), and protection has been correlated with the titer of serum antibodies to the fimbrial antigen (Lee et al. 1983). To be effective against *B. nodosus* in the epidermal layers, antibodies in adequate

Table 17.2. Involvement of Bacteroidaceae in diseases of the foot in cattle and sheep

Disease and host	Area affected	Bacteria and their role in pathogenesis	
1. Interdigital dermatitis (cattle, sheep)	Interdigital epidermis	*F. necrophorum*	Causes epidermal necrosis and secretes a leucocidal toxin that aids establishment of *A. pyogenes*
		A. pyogenes	Elaborates a substance that stimulates growth of *F. necrophorum*. It also lowers Eh
2. Scald (sheep)	Interdigital epidermis	*F. necrophorum, C. minutissime*	Causes epidermal necrosis and secretes a leukocidal toxin that may aid invasion by *C. minutissime*
3. Foot-rot (sheep)	Laminar structure of hoof	*F. necrophorum*	Causes epidermal necrosis and makes way for entry of *B. nodosus*
		B. nodosus	Secretes protease that digests epidermal matrix and facilitates entry of other bacteria. Secretes growth factor for *F. necrophorum*
		A. pyogenes	As in No. 1
		Spirochaeta penortha	Unknown, probably of minor significance
4. Foot-rot or foul in the foot (cattle), heel abscess, infective bulbar necrosis (sheep)	Deeper tissues of the foot	*F. necrophorum, A. pyogenes*	As in No. 1
5. Pododermatitis, stinky foot (cattle)	Interdigital epidermis (posterior region near bulbs of heel)	*F. necrophorum, B. nodosus*	As in No. 1

concentration must diffuse out of the capillary bed beneath the stratum germinativum and through the nonliving layers of the epidermis toward the skin surface.

Higher and more persistent titers are obtained with vaccines that incorporate an oil adjuvant than with alum-based vaccines (Egerton and Thorley 1981). However, vaccines containing oil are irritants and frequently cause persisting granulomas at the injection site.

Diagnosis. Smears prepared from the edge of lesions beneath the epidermal matrix and stained with Gram's stain may reveal the characteristically shaped *B. nodosus* (Figure 17.5). It may be necessary to examine a number of smears to confirm the presence of the organism. Culture of *B. nodosus* from foot smears can be attempted on selective medium containing Eugon agar, 0.2 percent yeast extract, 10 percent horse blood, and 1 μg lincomycin per milliliter (Gradin and Schmitz 1977).

Antimicrobial Susceptibility. *B. nodosus* is sensitive to penicillin, tetracycline, chloramphenicol, clindamycin, and cefamandole (Gradin and Schmitz 1983). Although *B. nodosus* does not respond to streptomycin, a combination of this antibiotic and penicillin is synergistic (Egerton et al. 1968). The organism is also sensitive to

copper sulfate, zinc sulfate (10 percent) and formalin (10 percent) and these compounds are commonly included in baths for foot disinfection after surgical debridement of affected areas. Lincomycin in combination with spectinomycin injected daily for 3 days has been reported to be therapeutically effective (Spais and Arguroudis 1982).

REFERENCES

Anderson, B.J., Bills, M.M., Egerton, J.R., and Mattick, J.S. 1984. Cloning and expression in *Escherichia coli* of the gene encoding the structural subunit of *Bacteroides nodosus* fimbriae. J. Bacteriol. 160:749–754.

Benno, Y., Mitsuoka, T., and Shirasaka, S. 1982. Anaerobic bacteria isolated from abscesses in pigs. Jpn. J. Vet. Sci. 44:309–315.

Berg, J. 1975. *Fusobacterium necrophorum* and *Bacteroides melaninogenicus* as etiologic agents of footrot in cattle. Am. J. Vet. Res. 36:1115–1122.

Beveridge, W.I.B. 1941. Foot-rot in sheep: A transmissible disease due to infection with *Fusoformis nodosus* (n. sp.). Aust. Counc. Sci. Indus. Res. Bull. 140.

Biberstein, E.L., Knight, H.D., and England, K. 1968. *Bacteroides melaninogenicus* in diseases of domestic animals. J. Am. Vet. Med. Assoc. 153:1045–1047.

Broad, T.E. and Skerman, T.M. 1976. Partial purification and properties of extracellular proteolytic activity of *Bacteroides nodosus*. N.Z. J. Agr. Res. 19:317–322.

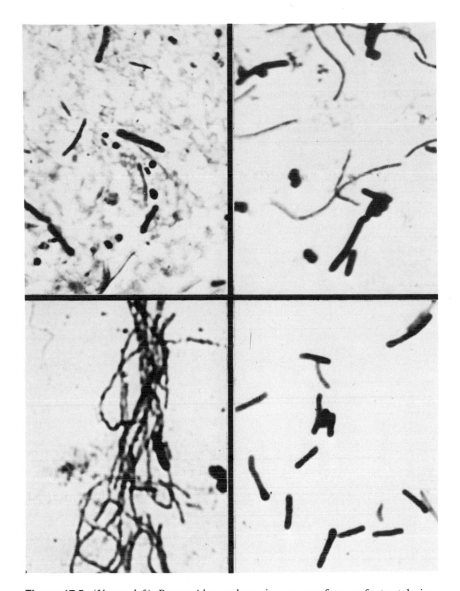

Figure 17.5. (*Upper left*) *Bacteroides nodosus* in a smear from a foot-rot lesion. Carbol-fuchsin stain. × 1,500 (*Upper right*) Spirochetelike organism in a smear from a foot-rot lesion. Krajian silver stain. × 1,450. (*Lower left*) Mass of spirochetelike organisms in a smear from a foot-rot lesion. Krajian silver stain. × 1,450. (*Lower right*) *Bacteroides nodosus* from a 3-day-old colony on agar. Carbol-fuchsin stain. × 1,450. (Courtesy of H. Marsh and K.D. Claus, *Cornell Veterinarian*.)

Egerton, J.R. 1973. Surface and somatic antigens of *Fusiformis nodosus*. J. Comp. Pathol. 83:151–159.

Egerton, J.R., and Parsonson, I.M. 1966. Isolation of *Fusiformis nodosus* from cattle. Aust. Vet. J. 42:425–429.

Egerton, J.R., and Roberts, D.S. 1971. Vaccination against ovine foot-rot. J. Comp. Pathol. 81:179–185.

Egerton, J.R., and Thorley, C.M. 1981. Effect of alum-precipitated or oil-adjuvant *Bacteroides nodosus* vaccines on the resistance of sheep to experimental foot rot. Res. Vet. Sci. 30:28–31.

Egerton, J.R., Morgan, I.R., and Burrell, D.H. 1972. Foot-rot in vaccinated and unvaccinated sheep. Vet. Rec. 91:447–452.

Egerton, J.R., Parsonson, I.M., and Graham, N.P.H. 1968. Parenteral chemotherapy of ovine foot rot. Aust. Vet. J. 44:275–283.

Egerton, J.R., Roberts, D.S., and Parsonson, I.M. 1969. The aetiology and pathogenesis of ovine foot-rot. I. A histological study of the bacterial invasion. J. Comp. Pathol. 79:207–215.

Every, D., and Skerman, T.M. 1980. Ultrastructure of the *Bacteroides nodosus* cell envelope layers and surface. J. Bacteriol. 141:845–857.

Every, E. 1982. Proteinase isoenzyme patterns of *Bacteroides nodosus*: Distinction between ovine virulent isolates, ovine benign isolates and bovine isolates. J. Gen. Microbiol. 128:809–812.

Gradin, J.L., and Schmitz, J.A. 1977. Selective medium for isolation of *Bacteroides nodosus*. J. Clin. Microbiol. 6:298–302.

Gradin, J.L., and Schmitz, J.A. 1983. Susceptibility of *Bacteroides nodosus* to various antimicrobial agents. J. Am. Vet. Med. Assoc. 183:434–437.

Laing, E.A., and Egerton, J.R. 1978. The occurrence, prevalence and transmission of *Bacteroides nodosus* infection in cattle. Res. Vet. Sci. 24:300–304.

Lee, S.W., Alexander, B., and McGowan, B. 1983. Characterization and serologic characteristics of *Bacteroides nodosus* pili and use of purified pili vaccine in sheep. Am. J. Vet. Res. 44:1676–1681.

Love, D.M., Jones, R.F., and Bradley, M. 1981. Characterization of Bacteroides species isolated from soft tissue infection in cats. J. Appl. Bacteriol. 50:567–575.

Love, D.N., Jones, R.F., and Calverley, A. 1984. Asaccharolytic black pigmented *Bacteroides* strains from soft tissue infection in cats. Int. J. Syst. Bacteriol. 34:300–303.

Mattick, J.S., Anderson, B.J., Mott, M.R., and Egerton, J.R. 1984. The isolation and characterization of the fimbriae of *Bacteroides nodosus*: Structural subunit and basal protein antigens. J. Bacteriol. 160:740–747.

Myers, L.L., Firehammer, B.D., Shoop, D.S., and Border, M.M. 1984. *Bacteroides fragilis*: A possible cause of acute diarrheal disease in newborn lambs. Infect. and Immun. 44:241–244.

Preez, J.H., Greeff, A.S., and Bothe, W.S. 1982. Pathology of the bovine udder parenchyma caused by asporogenous obligate anaerobic bacteria isolated from cases of bovine mastitis. J. S. Afr. Vet. Assoc. 53:157–159.

Roberts, D.S., and Egerton, H.S. 1969. The aetiology and pathogenesis of ovine foot-rot. II. The pathogenic association of *Fusiformis nodosus* and *F. necrophorus*. J. Comp. Pathol. 79:217–227.

Spais, A.G., and Arguroudis, S. 1982. Field evaluations of a combination of lincomycin and spectinomycin for treating footrot in sheep. Bull. Hell. Vet. Med. Soc. 33:363–370.

Stewart, D.J. 1977. Biochemical and biological studies on the lipopolysaccharide of *Bacteroides nodosus*. Res. Vet. Sci. 23:319–325.

Stewart, D.J. 1978. The role of various antigenic fractions of *Bacteroides nodosus* in eliciting protection against foot-rot in vaccinated sheep. Res. Vet. Sci. 24:14–19.

Thomas, J.H. 1958. A simple medium for the isolation and cultivation of *Fusiformis nodosus*. Aust. Vet. J. 34:411.

Thomas, J.H. 1963. A liquid medium for the growth of *Fusiformis nodosus*. Aust. Vet. J. 39:434–437.

Thorley, C.M., Calder, H.A.M., and Harrison, W.J. 1977. Recognition in Great Britain of *Bacteroides nodosus* in foot lesions of cattle. Vet. Rec. 100:387–389.

Walker, R.D., Richardson, D.C., Bryant, M.J., and Draper, C.S. 1983. Anaerobic bacteria associated with osteomyelitis in domestic animals. J. Am. Vet. Med. Assoc. 182:814–816.

18   The Genus *Staphylococcus*

The staphylococci are Gram-positive, nonmotile, facultatively anaerobic cocci that form grape-bunch-like clusters. The genus *Staphylococcus* is currently included with the genera *Micrococcus* and *Planococcus* in the family Micrococcacae. *Micrococcus* species are common in the environment and on the skin (particularly mammary glands) and frequently occur in specimens of milk and in swabs taken from epithelial surfaces. *Planococcus* organisms occur only in marine habitats. Staphylococci are normally found on the skin and mucosal surfaces of most warm-blooded animal hosts, and the parasite appears to be considerably adapted to the host (Kloos 1980).

There are at least 20 species of *Staphylococcus*, of which *S. aureus*, *S. epidermidis*, *S. intermedius*, and *S. hyicus* subsp. *hyicus* are of significance as causes of disease in animals. Table 18.1 details the characteristics that distinguish these disease-causing staphylococci from one another.

Other staphylococcal species from animals which have been reported recently include *S. caprae* and *S. gallinarum* from goats and chickens, respectively (Devriese et al. 1983), and *S. lentus* from sheep and goats (Kloos 1980). *S. simulans* is apparently the most common species found on cats (Cox et al. 1985).

Morphology and Staining Reactions of the Staphylococci.   The pathogenic staphylococci are perfectly spherical organisms of uniform size (0.8 μm). In pus the organisms frequently are grouped in irregular masses suggestive of clumps of grapes. This appearance inspired A. L. Ogston to adopt the generic name for the group from the Greek word *staphylo*, meaning "bunch of grapes"

(Figure 18.1). In fluid media the organisms usually appear singly, in small groups, or in short chains. They are nonmotile, do not form spores, and usually do not possess capsular substance in vitro. Polysaccharide capsules, however, are sometimes present on organisms in clinical material. Staphylococci are readily stained by the ordinary stains, and young cultures always are Gram-positive. Older cultures may lose the ability to retain Gram's stain.

Cultural and Biochemical Features of the Staphylococci.   Colonies of pathogenic staphylococci are porcelain white or yellowish orange when growing on solid media. The orange carotenoid pigment is best seen on a dry medium containing starch or fatty acids.

Colonies grown on blood agar are 1 to 3 mm in diameter after overnight incubation. They are smooth and round with a soft, butyrous consistency. Broth is uniformly and heavily clouded. Some strains are strongly hemolytic on cow-blood or sheep-blood agar, others are not. The hemolysis is the result of the presence of one or more different hemolysins. The alpha hemolysin produces complete hemolysis of rabbit, sheep, and bovine erythrocytes but has no effect on horse or human erythrocytes. The beta hemolysin is unique to animal strains; it is a sphingomyelinase C and produces incomplete hemolysis of sheep and bovine erythrocytes at 37°C.

After further storage at 4°C to 15°C, the incomplete hemolysis changes to complete hemolysis, namely *hot-cold hemolysis*. There is evidence that beta toxin causes complete or partial masking of alpha toxin (Marcia et al. 1976). When antibodies to beta toxin are present, the masking effect is neutralized and the alpha toxin is able to

Table 18.1. Laboratory recognition of the staphylococcal species of veterinary importance

Test or characteristic	S. epidermidis	S. aureus	S. intermedius	S. hyicus subsp. hyicus
Colony pigmentation	−	+	−	−
Coagulase production	−	+	+ (tube)*	+ (tube, usually delayed)
D-Mannitol fermentation	−	+	Delayed reaction	−
Hyaluronidase	−	+	−	+
Acetoin (Voges-Proskauer)	−	+	−	−
Beta galactosidase	−	−	+	−
Maltose fermentation	−	+	+ (weak)	−
Deoxyribonuclease	−	+	+	+

+ = positive reaction; − = negative reaction.
*Canine plasma should be used for strains of canine origin.

produce complete hemolysis. The delta hemolysin is a phospholipase and is active on human, rabbit, sheep, guinea pig, and horse erythrocytes. It migrates more slowly through agar than alpha hemolysin, so its effects take longer to be expressed.

The pathogenic staphylococci produce catalase, deoxyribonuclease, hyaluronidase, lysozyme, and coagulase. They also produce acetoin from glucose or pyruvate. They redden but frequently do not coagulate litmus milk. Most cultures form acid but no gas from glucose, maltose, lactose, sucrose, and mannitol. Nitrates usually are reduced. *S. aureus* produces phosphatase but not beta galac-

tosidase, and certain strains of this species produce a bacteriocin (staphylococcin), an antibiotic that inhibits some Gram-negative bacteria but does not inhibit Gram-positive bacteria (Gagliano and Hinsdill 1970). Many strains grow in the presence of 7.5 to 10 percent sodium chloride.

Staphylococci are among the most resistant of non-spore-bearing organisms. They resist dehydration, are relatively heat resistant, and tolerate common disinfectants better than most other bacteria.

Phage Typing of the Staphylococci. Phage typing is used extensively for studying the epidemiology of staphylococcal infections in humans. In the World Health Organization set, 22 phages are allocated into four groups (I, II, III, and IV) and four are unclassified (Parker 1983). Most strains from humans are lysed by the phages of one group only. Strains from cattle and other animal sources often cannot be typed satisfactorily according to the scheme devised for human strains. Strains from animals evidently have a high degree of host adaptation. *S. aureus* strains from goats have been shown to belong to phage group II and to the unclassified group (Adegoke et al. 1983).

Davidson (1961) has devised a phage-typing scheme for bovine staphylococci, but neither this scheme nor the one devised for human strains is suitable for typing *S. aureus* from dogs (Wang 1978). Schemes for typing strains from poultry have also been reported (Schimizu 1977, Thomas et al. 1972).

Figure 18.1. A stained film from a 24-hour-old culture of *Staphylococcus aureus* on slant agar showing the typical arrangement in grapelike clusters. × 940.

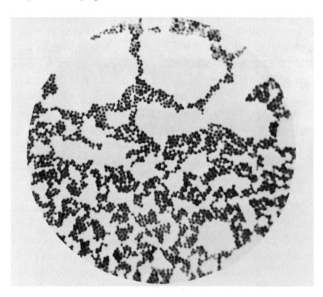

REFERENCES

Adegoke, G.O., Devriese, L.A., Godard, C., Fleurette, J., Brun, Y., and Ojo, M.O. 1983. Biotypes, serotypes and phage types of caprine strains of *Staphylococcus aureus*. Zentralbl. Bakteriol. Mikrobiol. Hyg. [A] 255:234–238.

Cox, H.A., Hoskins, J.D., Newman, S.S., Turnwald, G.H., Foil, C.S., Roy, A.F., and Kearney, M.T. 1985. Distribution of staphylococcal species on clinically healthy cats. Am. J. Vet. Res. 46:1824–1828.

Davidson, I. 1961. A set of bacteriophages for typing bovine staphylococci. Res. Vet. Sci. 2:396–407.

Devriese, L.A., Poutrel, B., Kilpper-Balz, R., and Schleifer, K.H. 1983. *Staphylococcus gallinarum* and *Staphylococcus caprae*, two new species from animals. Int. J. Syst. Bacteriol. 33:480–486.

Gagliano, V.G., and Hinsdill, R.D. 1970. Characterization of a *Staphylococcus aureus* bacteriocin. J. Bacteriol. 104:117–125.

Kloos, W.E. 1980. Natural populations of genus *Staphylococcus*. Annu. Rev. Microbiol. 34:559–592.

Marcia, D., Nagy, F., Vasiu, C., and Klemm, W. 1976. Studies on the intra- and inter-species relationships of bacterial hemolysins. Zentralbl. Veterinärmed. [B] 23:122–130.

Parker, M.T. 1983. The significance of phage-typing patterns in *Staphylococcus aureus*. In C.S.F. Easmon and C. Adlam, eds., Staphylococci and Staphylococcal Infections, vol. 1. Academic Press, London. Pp. 33–62.

Shimizu, A. 1977. Establishment of a new bacteriophage set for typing avian staphylococci. Am. J. Vet. Res. 38:1601–1605.

Thomas, C.L., Neave, F.K., Dodd. F.H., and Higgs, T.M. 1972. The susceptibility of milked and unmilked udder quarters to intra-mammary infection. J. Dairy Res. 39:113–131.

Wang, C.T. 1978. Bacteriophage typing of canine staphylococci. I. Typing by use of the international phage sets for human and bovine staphylococci. Jpn. J. Vet. Sci. 40:401–405.

Staphylococcus aureus

SYNONYM: *Staphylococcus aureus* biotype A and D

S. aureus was so named because of the yellow or gold color of its colonies; however, some strains are not pigmented or lose the trait on subculture. Those features that distinguish *S. aureus* from other common *Staphylococcus* species of veterinary significance are given in Table 18.1.

Antigens, Toxins, and Enzymes. The important components of the cell wall of *S. aureus* are its peptidoglycan ribitol, teichoic acids, and the precipitinogen protein A. The immunological specificities of *S. aureus* reside in the teichoic acid moieties, which are termed polysaccharides A and B. The teichoic acid complexes are covalently linked to the muramic acid mucopeptide of the cell wall. Protein A is a small basic protein (molecular weight 13,000) that reacts with the Fc fragments of IgG molecules and is antiphagocytic and fixes complement. More than 30 type-specific agglutinogens have been found on *S. aureus*, but these are not used routinely because of nonspecific clumping effects exhibited by the organisms.

Other antigens associated with the outer cell are several capsular antigens, which are antiphagocytic, and bound coagulase or clumping factor, which acts on fibrinogen, causing the cells to aggregate in plasma.

Staphylococci produce many extracellular toxins and enzymes, some of which can be important in the pathogenesis of disease. Those produced by *S. aureus* are listed in Table 18.2. The alpha hemolysin causes lysosomal

Table 18.2. Toxins and enzymes produced by *S. aureus*

Toxin or enzyme	Action
Toxins	
Alpha hemolysin	Hemolysis (sheep, rabbit); vasoconstriction and dermonecrosis
Beta hemolysin	Hot-cold hemolysis (sheep)
Gamma hemolysin	Weak hemolysis
Delta hemolysin	Dermonecrosis; destruction of leukocytes
Leukocidin	Leukocytic degranulation
Enterotoxin	Emesis and/or diarrhea
Enzymes	
Coagulase (free)	Clots purified fibrinogen in presence of CRF* from prothrombin
Hyaluronidase (spreading factor)	Hydrolyzes hyaluronic acid in intercellular ground substance
Deoxyribonuclease	Hydrolyzes DNA
Fibrinolysin (staphylokinase)	Dissolves clots by activation of plasminogen
Lipase	Hydrolyzes bactericidal lipids of skin
Protease	Hydrolyzes proteins

*Coagulase reacting factor.

disruption in leukocytes and is cytocidal for other cells; it is dermonecrotic when injected subcutaneously and is lethal for mice and rabbits when injected intravenously. It affects smooth muscle, leading to constriction, paralysis, and finally necrosis of smooth muscle cells in the walls of blood vessels. This hemolysin plays an important role in the pathogenesis of gangrenous mastitis (Brown and Sherer 1958). As mentioned earlier, the beta hemolysin is characteristic of *S. aureus* strains of animal origin but its role or significance in pathogenesis is unclear. Andersen (1963) has concluded that it is of little importance, but others (Naidu and Newbauld 1975) have observed that inflammatory and somatic cell responses of the mammary gland were related to the amount of beta hemolysin experimentally infused. The phospholipase action of the delta hemolysin is dermonecrotic.

Many strains of *S. aureus* produce one of five (A, B, C, D, and E) immunologically distinct enterotoxins. These heat-stable proteins range in molecular weight from 28,000 to 35,000. They cause gastroenteritis in humans but do not have any known role in the pathogenesis of staphylococcal disease in animals. They can be elaborated in milk, however, and hence it is possible that milk or milk products from cows with staphylococcal mastitis could cause food poisoning in humans (Crabtree and Litterer 1934, Minett 1938). *S. aureus* strains from chickens also produce enterotoxins D and C (Shiozawa et al. 1980).

Of the many enzymes produced, coagulase has been the most studied, although its role in pathogenesis is still unclear. It exists in two immunologically different forms: cell-bound and cell-free. Cell-free coagulase is a protein and exists in four antigenic types. Production of coagulase is related to the organism's ability to grow well in serum and to withstand antibacterial factors. Its ability to coagulate plasma appears to be irrelevant in cows because cows are deficient in the coagulase reacting factor (CRF), which is essential for coagulation to occur (Duthie and Lorenz 1952). Species with adequate levels of CRF can exhibit a small amount of intravascular clotting at the focus of infection (Blobel and Berman 1961).

Another enzyme, deoxyribonuclease, is usually present in coagulase-positive strains and can be used instead of coagulase as a criterion of potential virulence (Jasper 1973). Hyaluronidase, by degrading hyaluronic acid in the intercellular matrix, facilitates further spread of infection (Duran-Reynals 1942) and so conceivably contributes to virulence. Lipase production is important in skin invasion, and staphylococci that produce this enzyme are able to degrade bactericidal fatty acids on the skin surface. The Panton-Valentine (P-V) leukocidin is cytotoxic for bovine leukocytes but does not seem to be an important factor in virulence.

Epizootiology and Pathogenesis.   Colonization by *S. aureus* of the skin, nose, and oropharynx is frequent in healthy animals. Penetration and lesion production depend on a number of factors, such as maceration, skin trauma, the specific immune status of the animal, removal of other competing normal flora, the possession of lipase, and the existence of primary viral infections, which cause skin lesions that are subsequently invaded by staphylococci.

The important factors involved in staphylococcal survival, multiplication, and lesion production after initial invasion are (1) resistance to phagocytosis as mediated by protein A and capsular material; (2) intracellular survival in phagocytic cells—strains of *S. aureus* may have enhanced intracellular survival abilities; (3) coagulase-mediated resistance to serum antibacterial factor; (4) hyaluronidase production, which aids spread of the infection; (5) the production of alpha toxin; (6) the production of other leukocidins; (7) the development of delayed hypersensitivity; and (8) adhesion to epithelial cells within the cavities of bovine mammary glands (Frost et al. 1977).

Botryomycosis. *S. aureus* is usually found in pure culture in the peculiar disease of horses known as botryomycosis. The disease usually begins in the stump of the spermatic cord after castration of male animals. The infected cord becomes greatly enlarged and sclerotic. Small pockets of pus are found in the mass of newly formed tissue, and small granules resembling those of actinomycosis are found in the pus. When these granules are crushed, they yield masses of *S. aureus* embedded in a capsular material that is probably furnished by the host. Botryomycosis sometimes generalizes, in which case it is usually fatal (McFadyean 1919).

Mastitis. *S. aureus* is frequently found in suppurative lesions in cattle and is especially significant as a cause of mastitis. In many dairying regions it is the most common pathogen of the bovine udder. Modern systems of housing and milking cows have favored this pathogen, which usually enters the udder through the teat canal. The organism is an active colonizer of the tip of the teat. Transmission can also occur between cows by means of the milking machine or the hands of the milker. In a minority of cases the organism enters mammary tissue via wounds or lesions on the teat surface. After entry, the development, severity, and chronicity of the mastitis are related to such factors as the organism's adherence to the internal epithelial surfaces (Frost et al. 1977), the presence of antibody to alpha toxin, the number of neutrophils in the mammary secretion, the production of beta toxin and coagulase, the frequency of milking out (Thomas et al. 1972), and the ability of the organism to use nutrients within the udder and to multiply (Anderson 1976).

Phagocytosis and intracellular killing of *S. aureus* by leukocytes in the milk is inhibited by milk fat globules in the cells. Casein also inhibits intracellular killing (Paape and Guidry 1977, Russell et al. 1976). The inhibition by casein appears to be caused by a blocking of the bactericidal effects of the lactoperoxidase system and of histones. Although the efficiency of the intramammary phagocytic system can be reduced, it is still important in the mammary defense mechanism because subclinical *S. epidermidis* infection is known to lessen the susceptibility of the udder to infection by either *Streptococcus agalactiae* or *Escherichia coli*. This diminished susceptibility is related to the increased leukocyte counts produced in response to the presence of *S. epidermidis*.

Another important factor in the pathogenesis of staphylococcal mastitis is the delayed hypersensitivity reaction (Jones 1974). *S. aureus* does not always invade udder tissue, and the inflammation is apparently in part attributable to the immune response to the organism adherent to the internal duct and sinus epithelia.

S. aureus mastitis in cattle varies from subclinical to severely gangrenous. Most cases are of the subclinical chronic form, which, although quite inapparent, is of greatest economic significance because of losses in milk production.

Peracute gangrenous mastitis caused by *S. aureus* occurs in first-calf heifers in early lactation and results in the loss of large masses of udder tissue. The alpha toxin is important in the development of the gangrene seen in this disease (Brown and Sherer 1958). The toxin damages the blood vessels, resulting in ischemic coagulative necrosis of adjacent tissue. The skin becomes purplish over the affected area and may eventually slough off. Affected animals have a high fever and may die of toxemia within a day or two. Chronic staphylococcal mastitis results in induration of the udder, occasional clots, and an increased cellularity of the milk.

S. aureus also causes mastitis in sheep, goats, mares, sows, cats, and mink (Trautwein and Helmboldt 1966). The disease is usually acute but also occurs in a chronic form.

Tick pyemia of lambs. Tick pyemia occurs in Britain and Ireland and is associated with heavy infestations of the sheep tick, *Ixodes ricinus*, on 2- to 5-week-old lambs (Watson 1964). During feeding, the tick inoculates *S. aureus*, which is already on the skin surface, into the deeper tissues, where it multiplies. Acute septicemia or bacteremia is often produced along with toxemia, which rapidly kills the lamb. A less severe form of the disease results in abscesses in the kidneys, liver, joints, and the brain. *S. aureus* has also been implicated in the etiology of "facial" or "periorbital eczema" in sheep (Scott et al. 1980) and in dermatitis of unweaned lambs (Parker et al. 1983).

Purulent synovitis in poultry. Serious losses in chickens (Jungherr and Plastridge 1941) and turkeys (*bumble-foot*) from a purulent synovitis have been caused by *S. aureus*. The infection causes lameness, swellings on the feet, and occasionally spondylitis. The strains that cause these infections are of the same phage group as those found on the skin, and thus it is probable that the organism opportunistically enters birds whose resistance is compromised by such factors as concurrent viral infections or defects in husbandry.

Cutaneous staphylococcosis. Outbreaks of exudative dermatitis in young hairless rabbits and of subcutaneous abscesses in older animals have been caused by *S. aureus* (Okerman et al. 1984). A generalized staphylococcosis followed the superficial form in several cases. The organism is also associated with saddle boils, eczematoid dermatitis, and cellulitis of horses and with dermatitis-septicemia in 20-week-old broiler breeders (Froyman et al. 1982).

Porcine necrotizing staphylococcal endometritis. In pigs *S. aureus* is known to cause an endometritis charac-

terized by the accumulation of soft necrotic material on the surface of the endometrium and by the distention of the uterine horns and body with mural edema (Everitt et al. 1981). Abortions have also been attributed to the organism.

Immunity. Phagocytosis and intracellular killing are the key factors in the resistance of host animals to infection by *S. aureus*. Many of the enzymes, toxins, and capsular and cell wall components are antigenic, and antibodies are produced against them during infection. But because the basic lesion in staphylococcosis is an abscess that usually contains considerable quantities of pus, the organism is shielded from humoral antibodies. Furthermore, the presence of protein A allows *S. aureus* to bind immunoglobulin on its surface in such a way that surface receptors on phagocytes cannot attach to the organism to allow phagocytosis to proceed.

Repeated injections of heat-killed staphylococci will protect rabbits against otherwise fatal doses of *S. aureus*. Autogenous bacterins have been used with variable effects in animals with chronic infections (McDonald et al. 1972), and commercially available bacterins are widely used in mastitis control programs.

Toxoids that contain altered alpha toxin will stimulate production of antitoxin and are helpful in preventing acute gangrenous mastitis but have no apparent effect on the chronic form of the disease. Staphylococcal toxoid is made by treating filtrates with 0.3 percent formalin for a few hours. There is some evidence that intramammary infusion of vaccine is more effective than parenteral administration (McDowell and Watson 1974).

Live *S. aureus* vaccine has been shown to elicit better protection than killed vaccine against acute, experimentally produced mastitis in sheep (Watson and Kennedy 1981). Local immunization of cows by multiple intramammary infusions of heat-killed *S. aureus* resulted in an increased immunoglobulin content of the milk and enhanced phagocytosis and intracellular killing of *S. aureus* (Guidry et al. 1980).

The use of intramammary devices that stimulate a low grade leukocytosis has been shown to increase resistance of the mammary gland to invasion by *S. aureus*.

Diagnosis. Smears from abscesses, exudates, or deposits from centrifuged mastitic milk will reveal Gram-positive cocci. Culture on sheep-blood or cow-blood agar allows recognition of colonies of *Staphylococcus* or *Micrococcus* species. Heavily contaminated specimens should be cultured on selective media such as mannitol-salt or Columbia CNA agars. Tests for coagulase, deoxyribonuclease, acetoin, D-mannitol, and maltose fermentation are necessary for species identification (Table 18.1). Commercially available identification systems have greatly simplified the identification of staphylococci, although further research is needed on the adaptation of these systems to isolates from milk samples.

Antimicrobial Susceptibility. Plasmid-encoded, multiple antibiotic resistance is so common in strains of *S. aureus* from animals that antibiotic therapy must be based on results of susceptibility testing. Penicillin resistance caused by beta lactamase is found in a substantial proportion of the strains of *S. aureus* from animals (Biberstein et al. 1974, Jasper 1972). However, strains showing in vitro tolerance to penicillins, including cloxacillin, can exhibit responses in vivo after therapeutic administration of the antibiotic. It has been suggested that prior exposure to penicillin renders the organism more susceptible to killing by neutrophils (Craven et al. 1982).

Other antimicrobials to which *S. aureus* may be sensitive include chloramphenicol, lincomycin, spiromycin, erythromycin, rifampicin, and penicillin-resistant compounds such as oxacillin. These antibiotics exhibit minimal binding to purulent material and so should be effective in abscesses. Nitrofurantoin, fucidine, and 2-chloro-4-phenyl-phenol are effective for topical application (Kober 1977).

Dry cow therapy with high persistency antibiotic combinations has been shown to reduce by half new *S. aureus* intramammary infections during the dry period (Pankey et al. 1982).

REFERENCES

Andersen, A.A. 1963. Evaluation of a new bactericidal spray effective against *Staphylococcus aureus*. Appl. Microbiol. 11:239–243.

Anderson, J.C. 1976. Mechanisms of staphylococcal virulence in relation to bovine mastitis. Br. Vet. J. 132:229–245.

Biberstein, E.L., Franti, C.E., Jang, S.S., Ruby, A. 1974. Antimicrobial sensitivity patterns in *Staphylococcus aureus* from animals. J. Am. Vet. Med. Assoc. 164:1183–1186.

Blobel, H., and Berman, D.T. 1961. Further studies on the in vivo activity of staphylocoagulase. J. Infect. Dis. 108:63–67.

Brown, R.W., and Sherer, R.K. 1958. A study of the necrotizing action of staphylococci alpha toxin. Am. J. Vet. Res. 19:354–362.

Crabtree, J.A., and Litterer, W. 1934. Outbreak of milk poisoning due to a toxin-producing staphylococcus found in the udders of two cows. Am. J. Public Health 24:1116–1122.

Craven, N., Williams, M.R., and Anderson, J.C. 1982. Enhanced killing of penicillin-treated *S. aureus* by host defenses: Effects of amoxycillin, cloxacillin and nafcillin in vitro and in experimental mastitis. Comp. Immunol. Microbiol. Infect. Dis. 5:447–456.

Duran-Reynals, F. 1942. Tissue permeability and the spreading factors in infection. Bacteriol. Rev. 6:197–252.

Duthie, E.S., and Lorenz, L.L. 1952. Staphylococcal coagulase: Mode of action and antigenicity. J. Gen. Microbiol. 6:95–107.

Everitt, J.I., Fetter, A.W., Kenney, R.M., and Della-Ferra, M.A. 1981. Porcine necrotizing staphylococcal endometritis. Vet. Pathol. 18:125–127.

Frost, A.J., Wanasinghe, D.D., and Woolcock, J.B. 1977. Some factors affecting selective adherence of microorganisms in the bovine mammary gland. Infect. Immun. 15:245–253.

Froyman, R., Deruytiere, L., and Devriese, L.A. 1982. The effect of antimicrobial agents on an outbreak of staphylococcal dermatitis in adult broiler breeders. Avian Pathol. 11:521–525.

Guidry, A.J., Paape, M.J., Pearson, R.E., and Williams, W.F. 1980. Effect of local immunization of the mammary gland on phagocytosis and intracellular killing of *S. aureus* by polymorphonuclear neutrophils. Am. J. Vet. Res. 41:1427–1431.

Jasper, D.E. 1972. Antimicrobial susceptibility of staphylococci isolated from bovine mastitis. Calif. Vet. 26:12–15.

Jasper, D.E. 1973. Thermostable nuclease production by staphylococci in milk samples from bovine mastitis. Am. J. Vet. Res. 34:445–446.

Jones, R.L. 1974. The role of delayed-type hypersensitivity and cell-mediated immunity in bovine staphylococcal mastitis. Proc. Annu. Meet. U.S. Anim. Health Assoc. 78:143–149.

Jungherr, E., and Pastridge, W.N. 1941. Avian staphylococcosis. J. Am. Vet. Med. Assoc. 98:27–32.

Kober, U. 1977. Application of the staphylocide antibiotic Fucidine in small animal practice. Berl. Münch. Tierärztl. Wochenschr. 90:401–402.

McDonald, K.R., Greenfield, J., and McCausland, H.D. 1972. Remission of staphylococcal dermatitis by autogenous bacterin therapy. Can. Vet. J. 13:45–48.

McDowell, G.H., and Watson, D.L. 1974. Immunity to experimental staphylococcal mastitis: Comparison of local and systemic immunization. Aust. Vet. J. 50:533–536.

McFadyean, J. 1919. Botryomycosis. J. Comp. Pathol. Ther. 32:73–89.

Minett, F.C. 1938. Experiments on *Staphylococcus* food poisoning. J. Hyg. 38:623–637.

Naidu, T.G., and Newbauld, F.H.S. 1975. Significance of beta-hemolytic *Staph. aureus* as a pathogen to the bovine mammary gland. Zentralbl. Veterinärmed. [B] 22:308–317.

Okerman, L., Devriese, L.A.. Maertens, L., Okerman, F., and Godard, C. 1984. Cutaneous staphylococcosis in rabbits. Vet. Rec. 114:313–315.

Paape, M.J., and Guidry, A.J. 1977. Effect of fat and casein on intracellular killing of *Staphylococcus aureus* by milk leukocytes. Proc. Soc. Exp. Biol. Med. 155:588–593.

Pankey, J.W., Barker, R.M., Toomey, A., and Duirs, G. 1982. Comparative efficacy of dry-cow treatment regimens against *Staphylococcus aureus*. N.Z. Vet. J. 30:13–15.

Parker, B.N.J., Bonson, M.D., and Carroll, P.J. 1983. Staphylococcal dermatitis in unweaned lambs. Vet. Rec. 113:570–571.

Russell, M.W., Brooker, B.E., and Reiter, B. 1976. Inhibition of the bactericidal activity of bovine polymorphonuclear leukocytes and related systems by casein. Res. Vet. Sci. 20:30–35.

Scott, F.M.M., Fraser. J. and Martin, W.B. 1980. Staphylococcal dermatitis of sheep. Vet. Rec. 107:572–574.

Shiozawa, K., Kato, E., and Shimizu, A. 1980. Enterotoxigenicity of *Staphylococcus aureus* strains isolated from chickens. J. Food Protection 43:683–685.

Thomas, C.L., Neave, F.K., Dodd, F.H., and Higgs, T.M. 1972. The susceptibility of milked and unmilked udder quarters to intra-mammary infection. J. Dairy Res. 39:113–131.

Trautwein, G.W., and Helmboldt, C.F. 1966. Mastitis in milk due to *Staphylococcus aureus* and *Escherichia coli*. J. Am. Vet. Med. Assoc. 149:924–928.

Watson, D.L., and Kennedy, J.W. 1981. Immunization against experimental staphylococcal mastitis in sheep—Effect of challenge with a heterologous strain of *Staphylococcus aureus*. Aust. Vet. J. 57:309–313.

Watson, W.A. 1964. Studies on the distribution of the sheep tick (*Ixodes ricinus* L.) and the occurrence of enzootic staphylococcal infection of lambs in north-west Yorkshire and north-east Lancashire. Vet. Rec. 76:743–746.

Staphylococcus epidermidis

SYNONYM: *Staphylococcus albus*

S. epidermidis owes its name to its prevalence on human skin. It is also found on the normal skin, teat surfaces, hair, and superficial mucosa of a variety of animal species, but in numbers substantially less than those recorded for humans (Kloos et al. 1976).

Colonies of *S. epidermidis* are nonpigmented and nonhemolytic. Microscopically, *S. epidermidis* is indistinguishable from *S. aureus*. Its cell wall lacks protein A and contains glycerol instead of ribitol. Polysaccharide B is the form of its immunologically specific teichoic acid. It does not produce coagulase, deoxyribonuclease, or many of the other enzymes and toxins associated with *S. aureus*. Its differentiation from other staphylococci is shown in Table 18.1. A more extensive classification of *S. epidermidis* from intramammary infections can be found in the paper by Brown (1983).

Epizootiology and Pathogenesis. *S. epidermidis* is an opportunistic invader of low virulence. It has been isolated from a variety of lesions and sites on animals and is a common cause of wound infections and suture abscesses. Although its role as a pathogen in the mammary gland is unclear, it has the ability to cause mastitis, albeit of less severity and with a better prognosis and response to therapy than the mastitis caused by *S. aureus* (Osteras 1982). There is a substantial body of evidence that its presence on and within the teat is beneficial in that it stimulates release of phagocytic leukocytes that protect the gland against other potentially more virulent invaders.

Immunity. *S. epidermidis* is apparently readily phagocytosed and killed.

Antimicrobial Susceptibility. *S. epidermidis* is usually sensitive to penicillins, chloramphenicol, erythromycin, kanamycin, and tetracyclines.

REFERENCES

Brown, R.W. 1983. Biotypes of *Staphylococcus epidermidis* and *Micrococcus* spp. isolated from intramammary infections, reclassified into species of the genus *Staphylococcus* (*epidermidis, hyicus, xylosus*, and *scirui*). Cornell Vet. 73:109–116.

Kloos, W.E., Zimmerman, R.J., and Smith, R.F. 1976. Preliminary studies on the characterization and distribution of *Staphylococcus* and *Micrococcus* species on animal skin. Appl. Environ. Microbiol. 31:53–59.

Osteras, O. 1982. Prognosis for udder quarters infected with *Staphylococcus aureus* or *Staphylococcus epidermidis*. Nord. Vet. Med. 34:215–228.

Staphylococcus intermedius

SYNONYM: *Staphylococcus aureus* biotype E and F

First proposed by Hajek (1976), *S. intermedius* has since proved to be the most prevalent disease-producing *Staphylococcus* species in dogs and other carnivores (Cox et al. 1984, Phillips and Kloos 1981). It is probable that much of the earlier literature on *S. aureus* of canine origin was in fact referring to *S. intermedius*. Although showing little DNA homology, *S. aureus* and *S. intermedius* are phenotypically very similar.

The colonies of *S. intermedius* are not pigmented, are more convex than those of *S. aureus*, and vary greatly in the amount of hemolysis they produce (Kloos and Jorgensen 1985). The coagulase of *S. intermedius* is most active on canine plasma in the tube test, and little if any cell-bound coagulase is produced. *S. intermedius* can be differentiated from *S. aureus* by its lack of hyaluronidase, its failure to produce acetoin, its production of beta-galactosidase, and its delayed production of acid from mannitol (Table 18.1). It can also be recognized by the immunological specificity of the deoxyribonucleases produced (Gudding 1983). *S. intermedius* is not typable with either the human or bovine phage set (Samsonova et al. 1983).

Epizootiology and Pathogenesis. *S. intermedius* is a normal inhabitant of the nasopharynx of carnivora, and most lesions appear to be endogenous and opportunistic. It is the major pathogen of the canine skin, where such factors as trauma, dry skin, ectoparasitism, and matted, dirty hair can predispose an animal to invasion of the superficial and deeper layers of the skin by *S. intermedius*. A number of different clinical entities are produced, including skin-fold pyodermas that involve the face or genital-caudal area, impetigo, folliculitis, and furunculosis.

The role of *S. intermedius* in furunculosis in dogs has been rather neatly demonstrated by studies showing an increase in antibody to the deoxyribonuclease of *S. intermedius* but not to that of *S. aureus* (Ness 1984). Staphylococcal cellulitis of the deeper dermal layers is a frequent complication of demodectic mange. It is also found in the interdigital spaces of some breeds of dogs.

S. intermedius is a cause of external eye disease (Murphy et al. 1978) and or urinary tract infections in dogs (Clark 1974). In the case of urinary tract infections the production of phosphatase and urease by *S. intermedius* may play a role in calculus (struvite) formation. It also causes otitis externa and mastitis in bitches and can be found in a variety of other locations including the joints and uterus.

Not all canine isolates of staphylococci are *S. intermedius*, however. Contact with human sources of *S. aureus* has been shown to result in nasopharyngeal carriage of human strains by pet dogs (Live 1972). Some of these acquired infections have resulted in lesions in the same locations as those described for *S. intermedius* (Live 1985).

Immunity. Although the immune response to *S. intermedius* has not been studied, it is probably similar to that reported for *S. aureus*.

Diagnosis. *S. intermedius* can be distinguished from *S. aureus* by the failure of *S. intermedius* to produce acetoin and hyaluronidase and by its delayed fermentation of mannitol.

Antimicrobial Susceptibility. Penicillin resistance due to beta-lactamase production as well as resistance to a variety of other antibiotics has been reported (Love et al. 1981, Walser and Henschelchen 1983). Antimicrobial therapy thus must be based on the results of sensitivity testing.

REFERENCES

Clark, W.T. 1974. Staphylococcal infection of the urinary tract and its relation to urolithiasis in dogs. Vet. Rec. 95:204–206.

Cox, H.N., Newman, S.S., Roy, A.F., and Hoskins, J.D. 1984. Species of *Staphylococcus* isolated from animal infections. Cornell Vet. 74:124–135.

Guddig, R. 1983. Differentiation of staphylococci on the basis of nuclease properties. J. Clin. Microbiol. 18:1098–1191.

Hajek, V. 1976. *Staphylococcus intermedius*, a new species isolated from animals. Int. J. Syst. Bacteriol. 26:401–406.

Kloos, W.E., and Jorgensen, J.H. 1985. The Staphylococci. In E.H. Lennette, A. Balows, W.J. Hausler, and M.J. Shadomy, eds., Manual of Clinical Microbiology, 4th ed. American Society for Microbiology, Washington, D.C. Pp. 143–153.

Live, I. 1972. Differentiation of *Staphylococcus aureus* of human and of canine origins. Am. J. Vet. Res. 33:385–391.

Live, I. 1985. Specific and cross-reacting antigens of *Staphylococcus aureus* of human and canine origins. J. Clin. Microbiol. 21:43–45.

Love, D.N., Lomas, G., Bailey, M., Jones, R.F., and Weston, I. 1981. Characterization of strains of staphylococci from infections in dogs and cats. J. Small Anim. Prac. 22:195–199.

Murphy, J.M., Lavach, J.D., and Seserin, G.A. 1978. Survey of conjunctival flora in dogs with clinical signs of external eye disease. J. Am. Vet. Med. Assoc. 172:66–68.

Ness, E. 1984. Patterns of antibodies to staphylococcal DNAases in dog sera. J. Clin. Microbiol. 20:806–807.

Phillips, W.E., Jr., and Kloos, W.E. 1981. Identification of coagulase-positive *Staphylococcus intermedius* and *Staphylococcus hyicus* subsp. *hyicus* isolated from veterinary clinical specimens. J. Clin. Microbiol. 14:671–673.

Samsonova, T.M., Akatov, A.K., and Khatenener, M.L. 1983. Phage typing coagulase-positive staphylococci from various species of animals. Zh. Mikrobiol. Epidemiol. Immunobiol. 1:13–16.

Walser, K., and Henschelchen, O. 1983. Aetiology of acute mastitis in the bitch. Berl. Münch. Tierärztl. Wochenschr. 96:195–197.

Staphylococcus hyicus

SYNONYMS: *Micrococcus hyicus,*
   Staphylococcus epidermidis (*albus*)
   biotype 2

The eighth edition of *Bergey's Manual* does not list *S. hyicus* as a separate species, instead classifying it as biotype 2 of *S. epidermidis* (*albus*). Because the name *S. hyicus* now has widespread usage in the veterinary literature, we will use this name in the description of the organism and the disease it causes.

There are two subspecies of *S. hyicus: S. hyicus* subsp.

hyicus, the cause of exudative epidermitis of swine, and *S. hyicus* subsp. *chromogenes,* an organism of questionable virulence frequently isolated from mastitic milk. Since *S. hyicus* subsp. *chromogenes* apparently does not cause disease, it will be discussed only briefly at the end of this section.

Morphology and Staining Reactions. *S. hyicus* subsp. *hyicus* is a Gram-positive coccus (0.5 to 7.0 μm in diameter) that occurs as single cells, in pairs, and in short chains. There is no capsule (Underdahl et al. 1963).

Cultural and Biochemical Features. Colonies of *S. hyicus* subsp. *hyicus* on blood agar are creamy white, convex, and circular. They can become transparent on continued incubation. The organism hemolyses rabbit erythrocytes, but no hemolysis is seen on cow-blood or sheep-blood agar. Some strains produce coagulase (Underdahl et al. 1963). *S. hyicus* subsp. *hyicus* produces phosphatase, gelatinase, hyaluronidase, and deoxyribonuclease. Anaerobic growth occurs in thioglycollate broth. It does not ferment maltose. The organism produces enterotoxins that are serologically unrelated to those of *S. aureus* (Adesiyun et al. 1984). Protein A is present on strains isolated from swine (Phillips and Kloos 1981) but is not identical with that of *S. aureus.*

Antigens. *S. hyicus* subsp. *hyicus* shares antigens with *S. epidermidis* (Hunter et al. 1970). Most strains belong to one of three serotypes: ATCC19226, ZH1029, and ZH1037 (Hajsig 1984).

Phage typing. A Japanese study indicates that at least four bacteriophages can be isolated from *S. hyicus* subsp. *hyicus* (Kawano et al. 1983). Isolates from lesions exhibited two or more lysis patterns when tested with the four phage, whereas isolates from healthy pigs showed only one pattern.

Epizootiology and Pathogenesis. *S. hyicus* subsp. *hyicus* is highly contagious and easily spread from one group of pigs to another. Trading of animals has been shown to be an important factor in the spread of the disease, which usually occurs about 2 weeks after an infected animal has been brought onto clean premises (Stuker 1976). Piglets between 1 and 7 weeks old are usually affected, and both the morbidity and the mortality are highly variable.

The organism enters through breaks in the skin barrier. Such lesions can be initiated by the sharp teeth of piglets competing for feeding space. The disease produced varies in severity from a form in which the entire body becomes quickly covered with a moist, greasy exudate to a more chronic condition in which the onset is slower and the skin is more wrinkled. The lesions appear a few days after experimental exposure and may first be present as vesicles on hairless skin surfaces, the coronary bands, and behind

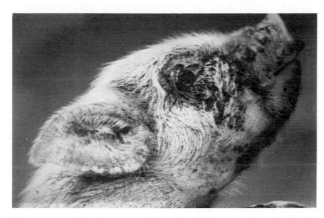

Figure 18.2. Lesions caused by *Staphylococcus hyicus* on the face of a piglet.

the ears. As the disease progresses over the body surface, the skin becomes thickened, and layers of the epidermis may peel off. Milder forms of the disease may appear as dandrufflike scaling or as reddish brown spots on the ears and other body areas (Figure 18.2). Pigs begin to recover about 14 days after the lesions appear and are fully recovered in 30 to 40 days. Histological examination of the skin of severely affected pigs reveals an accumulation of proteinaceous material, inflammatory cells, and bacteria over a parakeratotic layer (Mebus et al. 1968). At necropsy, the ureters are enlarged and the kidneys cystic because of debris that accumulates and blocks urinary flow.

A virulent form of the disease has been observed in which 50 percent of a group of month-old piglets died after becoming anorectic, febrile, and showing signs of excessive thirst (Portugal et al. 1979). The skin of the affected pigs showed extensive alopecia, fissures, and parakeratosis.

It has been suggested that the biotin requirement of affected swine is greatly increased by factors produced by *S. hyicus* subsp. *hyicus* and that biotin deficiency contributes to the lesions (Stuker and Glattli 1976). Interestingly, Luke and Gordon (1950) reported a good response to treatment with vitamin B supplements.

S. hyicus subsp. *hyicus* has also been isolated from the skin and from mange and udder lesions of cattle (Brown et al 1967, Devriese and Derycke 1979). Isolates from cattle usually lack protein A.

Diagnosis. Isolation of the causative organism can be made on the selective medium devised by Devriese (1977). This medium contains potassium thiocyanate (30 g/liter) and polysorbate 80 (10 ml/liter). Final laboratory diagnosis must be based on the characteristics listed in Table 18.1.

Immunity. Piglets born to sows that have been ac-

tively or passively immunized are resistant to challenge (Amptsberg 1978). Sow vaccination therefore is a useful means of controlling this disease. The specificity of the protective factors in immune serum has not yet been elucidated.

Antimicrobial Susceptibility. *S. hyicus* subsp. *hyicus* is sensitive to ampicillin, kanamycin, chloramphenicol, chloretetracycline, and nitrofurazone but is resistant to streptomycin, polymyxin B, and sulfa compounds (Underdahl et al. 1965).

Penicillin administered for 3 days to exposed pigs that had not yet shown lesions was effective in preventing exudative epidermitis. Once lesions have developed, however, antibiotic therapy is much less effective.

S. hyicus subsp. *chromogenes.* *S. hyicus* subsp. *chromogenes* is not pathogenic as far as is known. It is found predominantly on cattle and in milk samples (Devriese et al. 1978). Colonies are usually pigmented, and the organism produces enterotoxin(s) (Adesiyun et al. 1984). *S. hyicus* subsp. *chromogenes,* unlike *S. hyicus* subsp. *hyicus,* does not produce hyaluronidase and does not hydrolyze polysorbate (Devriese et al. 1978).

REFERENCES

Adesiyun, A.A., Tatini, S.R., and Hoover, D.G. 1984. Production of enterotoxin(s) by *Staphylococcus hyicus.* Vet. Microbiol. 9:487–495.

Amptsberg, G. 1978. Infection experiments with *Staphylococcus hyicus* in actively and passively immunized pigs. Berl. Münch. Tierärztl. Wocheschr. 91:201–206.

Brown, R.W., Sandvik, O., Sherer, R.K., and Rose, D.C. 1967. Differentiation of strains of *Staphylococcus epidermidis* isolated from bovine udders. J. Gen. Microbiol. 47:273–287.

Devriese, L.A. 1977. Isolation and identification of *Staphylococcus hyicus.* Am. J. Vet. Res. 38:787–792.

Devriese, L.A., and Derycke, J. 1979. *Staphylococcus hyicus* in cattle. Res. Vet. Sci. 26:356–358.

Devriese, L., Hajek, V., Oeding, P., Meyer, S.A., and Schleifer, K.H. 1978. *Staphylococcus hyicus* (Sompolinsky, 1953) comb. nov. and *Staphylococcus hyicus* subsp. *chromogenes* subsp. nov. Int. J. Syst. Bacteriol. 28:482–490.

Hajsig, D. 1984. *Staphylococcus hyicus* subsp. *hyicus:* Serotypes and susceptibility to some penicillins. Prax. Vet. 32:103–106.

Hunter, D., Todd, J.N., and Larkin, M. 1970. Exudative epidermitis of pigs. The serological identification and distribution of the associated *Staphylococcus.* Br. Vet. J. 126:225–229.

Kawano, J., Shimizu, A., and Kimura, S. 1983. Bacteriophage typing of *Staphylococcus hyicus* subsp. *hyicus* isolated from pigs. Am. J. Vet. Res. 44:1476–1479.

Luke, D., and Gordon, W.A.M. 1950. Observations on some pig diseases. Vet. Rec. 62:179–185.

Mebus, C.A., Underdahl, N.R., and Tweihaus, M.J. 1968. Exudative epidermitis. Pathogenesis and pathology. Pathol. Vet. 5:146–163.

Phillips, W.E., Jr., and Kloos, W.E. 1981. Identification of coagulase-positive *Staphylococcus intermedius* and *Staphylococcus hyicus* subsp. *hyicus* isolates from veterinary clinical specimens. J. Clin. Microbiol. 14:671–673.

Portugal, M.A., Loctatelli, J.C., Saliba, A.M., Rodrigues, A.J., and Calil, E.M. 1979. Exudative epidermitis of piglets. Biologico 45:89–95.

Stuker, G. 1976. Contribution to the epizootiology of exudative epidermitis: Spread of *Staphylococcus hyicus* by animal contact. Schweiz. Arch. Tierheilkd. 118:335–340.

Stuker, G., and Glattli, H.R. 1976. Relationship between biotin intake in piglets and the occurrence of exudative epidermitis. Schweiz. Arch. Tierheilkd. 118:305–306.

Underdahl, N.R., Grace, O.D., and Tweihaus, M.J. 1965. Porcine exudative epidermitis: Characterization of bacterial agent. Am. J. Vet. Res. 26:617–624.

Underdahl, N.R., Grace, O.D., and Young, G.A. 1963. Experimental transmission of exudative epidermitis of pigs. J. Am. Vet. Med. Assoc. 142:754–762.

19 The Genus *Streptococcus*

The generic name *Streptococcus* was first used by Rosenbach (1884) to describe a spherical bacterium that grew in chains which he had isolated from suppurative lesions in humans. Since then 29 separate species of *Streptococcus* have been described as well as a number of distinct and partially defined strains for which species status has not been established.

Streptococci cause a variety of diseases in humans and animals and are important saprophytes in milk and milk products. They are frequently present as parasites of the mucous membranes and intestines of animals and, given the appropriate conditions, can opportunistically produce disease.

The first systematic classification of the group was that of Sherman (1937), who divided the streptococci into pyogenic, viridans, lactic, and enterococcus groups. The pyogenic group included most of the pathogenic species; the viridans group was chiefly characterized by the production of alpha hemolysis or a greenish discoloration around colonies on blood agar; the lactic group was composed of strains associated with milk and having the ability to produce lactic acid in this substrate; and the enterococcus group included strains that resembled *S. faecalis,* an intestinal inhabitant. Although Sherman's classification is no longer used in its entirety, the tolerance tests he used to establish his primary divisions are still useful in classification. The present classification in *Bergey's Manual of Systematic Bacteriology,* vol. 2 (1986), is based partly on tolerance tests and partly on biochemical behavior.

Serologic grouping is also of great importance in the identification of the streptococci. The majority of these organisms possess a dominant serologically active carbohydrate (C substance), which is antigenically different from one species or group of species to another. Lancefield (1933), working with the precipitation test, used these antigenic differences to establish six groups (A to E and N), which were later found to correlate well with the groups in Sherman's (1937) classification. As a result many laboratories used the Lancefield grouping system as the principal identification method for the streptococci. Further serologic groups were added (F, G, H, K, L, M, O, P, Q, R, S, T, U, and V) as time passed, but no species designations were given to the organisms of these newer groups.

It later became apparent that although streptococci such as *S. bovis* and *S. faecalis* could share the same group antigen (D), they were physiologically and taxonomically quite different. Considerable physiological heterogeneity was observed among organisms of a number of the other Lancefield groups as well (Wilson and Miles 1975). The classification of the streptococci thus cannot be based solely on serologic grouping but must also include physiological and biochemical criteria.

The carbohydrate or polysaccharide antigen used in the Lancefield grouping system is located in the cell wall in the case of groups A, B, C, E, F, G, H, and K. In groups D and N these antigens are teichoic acids that lie between the cell wall and the cell membrane.

The carbohydrate antigens of groups B and C streptococci—the groups that contain the majority of the animal pathogens—are rhamnose-glucosamine and rhamnose-N-acetylgalactosamine polysaccharides, respectively. The chemical nature of the carbohydrates in the other groups were described by Deibel and Seeley (1974). DNA hybridization studies have recently indicated that streptococci of Lancefield groups C, G, and L are so closely related that their inclusion under the same specific name is justified (Farrow and Collins 1984). They therefore suggested that *S. zooepidemicus* be renamed *S. equi* subsp. *zooepidemicus.*

Streptococcal species are important causes of mastitis in cattle, of strangles and other diseases in horses, and of meningoencephalitis, arthritis, endocarditis, and cervical lymphadenitis in swine. Less frequently they have been associated with septicemia in chickens and with respiratory infections and other infections in kittens and puppies. The more common streptococci that produce diseases in animals are listed in Table 19.1.

Morphology and Staining Reactions of the Streptococci. Chains of cocci can be short (diplococci) or very long. Chain length depends on species differences and the medium on which the culture is growing. Typical chain

Table 19.1. Characteristics of the streptococci that cause disease in animals

Species or group	Disease	Hemolysis	Lancefield group	Fermentation of				Hydrolysis of		CAMP test
				Trehalose	Sorbitol	Lactose	Inulin	Sodium hippurate	Esculin	
S. agalactiae	Mastitis in cow, ewe, and goat	Narrow beta or absent	B	+	−	+	−	+	−	+
S. dysgalactiae	Mastitis in cow, ewe, and goat	Alpha	C	+	±	+	−	−	−	−
S. equi	Strangles in horse	Beta	C	−	−	−	−	−	−	
S. equisimilis	Cervicitis and abscesses in horse; arthritis in swine	Beta	C	+	−	±	−	−	−	
S. zooepidemicus	Mastitis in cow; cervicitis and metritis in mare; wound infections in horse	Beta	C	−	+	+	−	−	−	
S. bovis	Feedlot bloat	Absent	D	+	−	+	+	−	+	−
S. uberis	Mastitis in cow	Absent	Unknown	+	+	+	+	+	+	±
Group E (*S. infrequens*, *S. porcinus*)	Cervical lymphadenitis in swine	Beta (slow)	E	+	±	−	±	−		
Group G (*S. canis*)	Metritis, vaginitis in dog and cat; septicemia in puppies; abscesses in cat	Beta	G	+	−	+	−	−		−
Group L (rarely found)	Mastitis in cow; endocarditis in swine	Beta	L	+	−	+	−	±	−	−
S. suis type 1 (S)	Meningoencephalitis, septicemia, and arthritis in young pigs	Beta (horse blood)	D	+	−	+	+	−	−	−
S. suis type 2 (R)		Alpha	D	+	−	+	+	−	+	±

formation is best seen in fluid media; on solid media the chains become so entangled that they are difficult to distinguish.

The individual cells of streptococci are seldom perfectly spherical, and frequently there is considerable variation in the size and shape of the elements in a single culture. Sometimes the cells are flattened from side to side; more often they are elongated. In fact certain animal strains of streptococci can be so pleomorphic on primary isolation that they can be mistaken for short rods. Usually a few transfers on artificial media will bring forth the typical coccus form. Spores are never formed and, with rare exceptions, the organisms are nonmotile. A number of species form definite capsules when developing in tissues or in culture media containing blood serum. Such strains show 2 mucoid or matt-type of colony formation rather than the more usual smooth (glossy) or rough forms. Most streptococci are Gram-positive, but many Gram-negative forms are commonly found in old cultures. They are easily stained with all the usual dyes and are never acid-fast.

Cultural and Biochemical Features of the Streptococci. The streptococci are among the more fastidious bacteria with respect to nutritive requirements. They usually will not grow on meat extract media, and growth ordinarily is poor even on infusion media unless it is enriched by the addition of blood or serum. Horse-meat infusion agar, without enrichment, has proved to be an excellent medium for the isolation of animal strains of streptococci (Bruner 1949). Todd-Hewitt broth is also an excellent liquid medium. Most pathogenic streptococci grow well on a chemically defined medium (van de Rijn and Kessler 1980).

All streptococci produce small, delicate, translucent colonies about 1 mm in diameter on solid media. Heavy inoculations yield confluent growth that is nearly transparent. The surface of the growth is smooth and glistening, and the margins of individual colonies are perfectly circular. Deep colonies in agar usually are lenticular in shape. In softer media colonies can be globular and barely visible to the naked eye. Growth is often abundant in Todd-Hewitt broth. Strains that produce long chains quickly settle, resulting in a fluffy sediment at the bottom of the tube. Heavily encapsulated and short-chained strains remain in suspension much longer. All streptococci grow well in milk, and most strains produce lactic acid in this substrate.

Most streptococci grow readily under aerobic as well as anaerobic conditions, although a few strains grow only under anaerobic conditions. They are unique among aerobic bacteria in that they are unlikely to synthesize heme compounds. Thus they cannot synthesize cytochromes and are incapable of oxidative phosphorylation by means of a cytochrome-mediated electron-transport chain. Because of this the cytochrome inhibitor sodium azide is widely used in media for the selective isolation of streptococci from contaminated specimens.

Streptococci are catalase-negative and ferment sugars to dextrorotatory lactic acid. Only a few streptococci and none of the pathogenic types produce gas. The temperature growth range of streptococci varies from below 10°C to above 45°C. The pathogenic species are killed by temperatures below those used for pasteurization. Some of the milk-souring and intestinal species, however, are resistant to pasteurization temperatures; *S. thermophilus,* for instance, grows at 50°C.

Many of the pathogenic streptococci completely lyse horse erythrocytes. Colonies of the alpha (alpha hemolytic) or viridans group produce a narrow zone of discolored blood cells immediately surrounding the colony. This area can appear greenish.

REFERENCES

Bruner, D.W. 1949. Horsemeat-infusion agar medium. North Am. Vet. 30:243.

Deibel, R.H., and Seeley, H.W., Jr 1974. Family II: Streptococcaceae sp. nov. In R.E. Buchanan and N.E. Gibbons, eds., Bergey's Manual of Determinative Bacteriology, 8th ed. Williams & Wilkins, Baltimore. Pp. 490–509.

Farrow, J.A., and Collins, M.D. 1986. Taxonomic studies on streptococci of serological groups C, G, and L and possibly related taxa. Syst. Appl. Microbiol. 5:483–493.

Lancefield, R.C. 1933. A serological differentiation of human and other groups of hemolytic streptococci. J. Exp. Med. 57:571–595.

Rosenbach, F.J. 1884. Mikroorganismen bei den Wundinjektionskrankheiten des Menschen. J.F. Bergmann, Wiesbaden.

Sherman, J.M. 1937. The streptococci. Bacteriol. Rev. 1:1–97.

van de Rijn, I., and Kessler, R.E. 1980. Growth characteristics of group A streptococci in a new chemically defined medium. Infect. Immun. 27:444–448.

Wilson, G.S., and Miles, A. 1975. The streptococci. In W.W.C. Topley and G.S. Wilson, eds., Topley and Wilson's Principles of Bacteriology, Virology and Immunity, vol. 1, 6th ed. Arnold, London. Pp. 712–763.

Streptococcus agalactiae

SYNONYM: *Streptococcus mastitidis*

S. agalactiae is a common cause of bovine mastitis in the United States and in most areas of the world. It also causes mastitis in sheep and goats. The organism is less frequently a cause of bovine mastitis in Great Britain than in other countries, including the United States (Wilson and Salt 1978). The reasons for this disparity are not fully understood. In Denmark an eradication program (Olsen 1975) has reduced the infection rate to less than 1 percent in cows.

Morphology and Staining Reactions. *S. agalactiae*

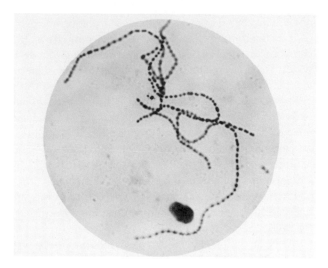

Figure 19.1. *Streptococcus agalactiae* on a stained film made from a sample of mastitis milk which had been incubated overnight at 37°C. Similar chains are often found in fresh udder secretions. Note that the chains consist of a series of paired organisms, a characteristic but not diagnostic feature. Gram's stain. × 1,050.

usually appears in the form of long chains in secretions from infected udders (Figure 19.1). In some samples these are numerous and easily found in stained films; in other cases the organisms may be so scarce that they can be located only with great difficulty even though the milk may be markedly altered in appearance. The organism is Gram-positive and is readily stained by all the ordinary stains.

Cultural and Biochemical Features. The most actively hemolytic strains produce hemolytic zones not more than 1 mm wide on blood agar; many strains produce only a trace of hemolysis on blood-agar plates, and others produce none. Some strains produce a slight greenish discoloration without hemolysis on blood-agar plates.

Growth in serum broth is granular or flocculent, the growth appearing in the bottoms of the tubes while the rest of the broth remains clear. *S. agalactiae* acidifies and coagulates litmus milk within 48 hours when incubated at 37°C. There is slight reduction of the litmus at the bottom of the tubes. At 10°C there is no observable growth after 5 days. It does not reduce methylene blue milk. In glucose broth the final pH is 4.4 to 4.7. It hydrolyzes sodium hippurate and regularly ferments glucose, trehalose, lactose, sucrose, and maltose; salicin is usually, but not always, fermented. It never attacks inulin, mannitol, sorbitol, and raffinose and does not hydrolyze esculin or gelatin. Many but not all strains of *S. agalactiae* produce a brick reddish growth on solid media, especially when the medium contains starch. About 90 percent of the *S.*

agalactiae strains tested by Gochnauer and Wilson (1951) produced hyaluronidase. *S. agalactiae* is killed by exposure to 60°C for 30 minutes and is destroyed by pasteurization. The mol% G + C of the DNA is 34.0 (Tm).

Christie, Atkins, and Muench-Petersen (1944) reported a lytic phenomenon produced by about 96 percent of the streptococci belonging to Lancefield serologic group B. Now referred to as the CAMP phenomenon (after the first letters of the authors' last names), it is a synergistic hemolysis produced by the sequential action of staphylococcal sphingomyelinase (beta toxin) and a ceramide- (*N*-acyl-sphingosine-) binding protein of *S. agalactiae* (Bernheimer et al. 1979). It is produced wherever the beta toxin of *Staphylococcus aureus* colonies has altered cow erythrocytes and sensitized them to the ceramide-binding protein of *S. agalactiae*. The combined action of both factors results in complete hemolysis (Figure 19.2). The CAMP phenomenon is now the basis of a widely used screening regimen for the presence of *S. agalactiae* in milk samples. Staphylococcal beta toxin can be incorporated in the primary isolation medium to allow presumptive recognition of the organism. A rapid tube test based on sheep erythrocytes sensitized with staphylococcal beta lysin has also been described (Phillips et al. 1980).

Antigens. The group antigen of *S. agalactiae*, is located in the cell wall and is a rhamnose-glucosamine polysaccharide. At least five type-specific antigens (S) have been described. They are composed of glucose-galactose-*N*-acetyl-glucosamine polysaccharide and are located on the outer envelope. The five antigens are designated 1a, 1b, 1c, 2, and 3. A protein antigen associated with the 1b antigen and designated 1bc can be lost or gained during the course of natural infection (Jensen 1980). These variations can be caused by antibodies produced in vivo. Two other antigenically related protein antigens that are sometimes present are designated R and X. In New York state *S. agalactiae* type 1a constitutes about 70 percent of all isolates; types 2 and 3 represent 17 and 10 percent, respectively. The type found varies in different areas (Norcross and Oliver 1976).

Epizootiology and Pathogenesis. The habitat of *S. agalactiae* is largely confined to the mammary gland of cows, sheep, and goats. Infection is spread between cows by the milker's hands or by contaminated milking equipment. Sometimes the mouths of calves can serve as a mode of transfer to the immature mammary glands of their comrades when they suckle each other. The organism enters through the end of the teat, and colonization of the gland is possibly favored by adhesion to the epithelium of the gland sinuses (Frost et al. 1977).

Multiplication of the organism on the surface of the teat and duct sinuses results in a slowly progressive inflamma-

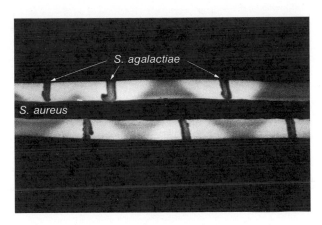

Figure 19.2. CAMP phenomenon produced by *Streptococcus agalactiae* on blood agar. The flare, or arrowhead, of complete hemolysis produced at the intersection of the *S. aureus* and *S. agalactiae* cultures constitutes a positive CAMP reaction.

tion and fibrosis of adjoining areas of the gland. The disease therefore begins insidiously and develops gradually. Older animals are more frequently affected. Excessive stripping can exacerbate the disease. Involution of secretory parenchyma and loss of productive capacity is in part caused by blockage of milk channels by inflammatory products.

The milk or udder secretion becomes altered in varying degrees, sometimes showing little or no abnormality and sometimes showing flakes, stringy masses of fibrin, blood, and thick purulent material. In many cases the degree of alteration of the milk varies; at one time it can be thick and purulent and at another practically normal. The inflammation in the udder causes the formation of new interstitial tissue, which changes the normally soft gland into a hard lump. The gland generally consists of indurated masses that cannot be seen but can be palpated.

The role of the CAMP phenomenon in the pathogenesis of mastitis has not been elucidated. Its lethal properties for rabbits and mice (Skalka and Smola 1981) suggest that it may have a cytotoxic action for mammary tissue.

The milk from affected quarters becomes alkaline and the leukocyte count usually exceeds 500,000/ml. In animals with advanced cases the secretion is much reduced in volume and is thin and watery.

Immunity. Serum antibody levels appear to have little protective effect against intramammary infection (Mackie et al. 1983). Furthermore, antibodies to the cellular antigens of *S. agalactiae* have been detected in the colostrum of first-calf heifers (Campbell and Norcross 1964) in the absence of any signs of disease. Thus cattle must undergo considerable exposure to the organism before they reach sexual maturity. Agglutinins for hematoxylin-stained *S.*

agalactiae can be detected in milk from infected cows by a milk ring test (Smith 1954). An enzyme-linked immunosorbent assay (ELISA) has also been used to measure antibody levels in milk (Logan et al. 1982) and as an aid in the detection of latent and subclinical carriers of infection.

Yokomizo and Norcross (1978) have shown that antibodies to *S. agalactiae* type 1a belonging to immunoglobulin classes IgA, IgG, and IgM are present in colostrum. Most of the protective activity appears to be associated with IgM and IgA classes, unlike the situation in human serum where protection is mediated by antibodies of the IgG subclass (Stewardson-Kreiger et al. 1977). Levels of IgA in the colostrum could be increased by previous intramammary vaccination; however, vaccination is not yet an effective means of controlling *S. agalactiae* infection in dairy herds. A fundamental problem that has yet defied solution is the short duration of the udder's immune response following infection and systemic priming (Logan et al. 1984).

Diagnosis. *S. agalactiae* can be difficult to demonstrate by direct staining of milk smears but is easier to find in smears of centrifuged sediment. Blood dextrose agar containing staphylococcal beta toxin allows presumptive recognition of colonies, the identity of which may then be confirmed by biochemical tests and commercially available latex agglutination or staphylococcal co-agglutination tests (Poutrel 1983).

Antimicrobial Susceptibility. *S. agalactiae* is sensitive to penicillin, ampicillin, erythromycin, chloramphenicol, cephalosporins, and tetracyclines. Berghash et al. (1983) detected strains resistant to tetracyclines and to beta-lactone antibiotics in dairy herds exposed to intensive antibiotic selection pressure from dry-cow therapy. Resistance to penicillin in that study, however, was low and possibly not of great therapeutic significance.

REFERENCES

Berghash, S.R., Davidson, J.N., Armstrong, J.C., and Dunny, G.M. 1983. Effects of antibiotic treatment of nonlactating dairy cows on antibiotic resistance patterns of bovine mastitis pathogens. Antimicrob. Agents Chemother. 24:771–776.

Bernheimer, A.W., Linder, R., and Avigad, L.S. 1979. Nature and mechanism of action of the CAMP protein of group B streptococci. Infect. Immun. 23:838–844.

Campbell, S.G., and Norcross, N.L. 1964. Antibodies against *Streptococcus agalactiae* in the colostrum of first-calf heifers. Am. J. Vet. Res. 25:993–997.

Christie, R., Atkins, F.E., and Muench-Petersen, E. 1944. A note on a lytic phenomenon shown by group B streptococci. Aust. J. Exp. Biol. Med. 22:197–200.

Frost, A.J., Warnasinghe, D.D., and Woolcock, J.B. 1977. Some factors affecting selective adherence of microorganisms in the bovine mammary gland. Infect. Immun. 15:245–253.

Gochnauer, T.A., and Wilson, J.B. 1951. The production of hyaluronidase by Lancefield's group B streptococci. J. Bacteriol. 62:405–414.

Jensen, N.E. 1980. Variation of type antigens of group B streptococci. III. Variation of the protein antigen Ibc. Acta Vet. Scand. 21:625–632.

Logan, E.F., Mackie, D.P., and Meneely, D.J. 1984. Immunologic features of consecutive intramammary infections with *Streptococcus agalactiae* in vaccinated and non-vaccinated heifers. Br. Vet. J. 140:535–542.

Logan, E.F., Meneely, D.J. and Mackie, D.P. 1982. Enzyme-linked immunosorbent assay for *Streptococcus agalactiae* antibodies in bovine milk. Vet. Rec. 110:247–249.

Mackie, D.P., Pollock, D.A., Meneely, D.J., and Logan, E.F. 1983. Clinical features of consecutive intramammary infections with *Streptococcus agalactiae* in vaccinated and non-vaccinated heifers.. Vet. Rec. 112:472–476.

Norcross, N.L., and Oliver, N. 1976. The distribution and characterization of group B streptococci in New York State. Cornell Vet. 66:240–248.

Olsen, S.J. 1975. A mastitis control system based upon extensive use of mastitis laboratories. In Proceedings of the International Dairy Federation Seminar on Mastitis Control, Reading University, England. Pp. 410–421.

Phillips, E.A., Tapsall, J.W., and Smith, D.D. 1980. Rapid tube CAMP test for identification of *Streptococcus agalactiae* (Lancefield group B). J. Clin. Microbiol. 12:135–137.

Poutrel, B. 1983. Comparative evaluation of commercial latex agglutination and coagglutination reagents for groups B, C and D mastitis streptococci. Am. J. Vet. Res. 44:490–492.

Skalka, B., and Smola, J. 1981. Lethal effect of CAMP-factor and UBERIS-factor, a new finding about diffusible exosubstances of *S. agalactiae* and *S. uberis*. Zentralbl. Bakteriol. Mikrobiol. Hyg. [A] 249:190–194.

Smith, I.M. 1954. The detection of agglutinins to *Str. agalactiae* strains using a milk ring test. J. Comp. Pathol 64:1–4.

Stewardson-Krieger, P.B., Albrandt, K., Nevin, T., Kretschmer, R.R. and Gotoff, S.P. 1977. Perinatal immunity to group B beta-hemolytic *Streptococcus* type Ia. J. Infect. Dis. 136:649–654.

Wilson, C.D., and Salt, G.F.H. 1978. Streptococci in animal disease. In F.A. Skinner and L.B. Quesnel, eds., Streptococci. Academic Press, New York. Pp. 143–156.

Yokomizo, Y., and Norcross, N.L. 1978. Bovine antibody against *Streptococcus agalactiae*, type IA, produced by preparturient intramammary and systemic vaccination. Am. J. Vet. Res. 39:511–516.

Streptococcus dysgalactiae

S. dysgalactiae causes an acute, severe mastitis. The organism differs from *S. agalactiae* only in minor cultural features. It belongs to Lancefield group C. The chains are usually short or medium in length, and colonies are usually nonhemolytic and often produce a distinct greenish discoloration. *S. dysgalactiae* does not always coagulate milk in 48 hours when incubated at 37°C. Methylene blue milk, however, is regularly reduced. The final pH in glucose broth varies between 5.3 and 5.0; it never goes below 5.0. *S. dysgalactiae* does not hydrolyze sodium hippurate, and this therefore is the best single test for differentiating *S. dysgalactiae* from *S. agalactiae*.

Epizootiology and Pathogenesis. Infection by this organism is much less frequent and more sporadic than infection by *S. agalactiae*. The organism occurs on the skin of the udder and elsewhere and in the mouth. It multiplies in wounds and sores and can enter the udder through sores that involve the teat orifice. Strains can vary in intramammary pathogenicity (Higgs et al. 1980). The mastitis produced is acute and painful, and the secretion is purulent and yellowish. *S. dysgalactiae* produces hyaluronidase, which can contribute to the invasiveness of *S. dysgalactiae* either alone or in synergy with *Actinomyces pyogenes*. In summer mastitis these two organisms are frequently found together. Damage to the affected quarter can result in complete loss of function.

Antimicrobial Susceptibility. *S. dysgalactiae* has an antibiotic susceptibility profile similar to that of *S. agalactiae*.

REFERENCE

Higgs, T.M., Neave, F.K., and Bramley, A.J. 1980. Differences in intramammary pathogenicity of four strains of *Streptococcus dysgalactiae*. J. Med. Microbiol. 13:393–399.

Streptococcus zooepidemicus

Widespread in a variety of animal species, *S. zooepidemicus* is a normal commensal of the skin, upper respiratory mucosa (Kasai et al. 1944), and tonsillar and associated pharyngeal lymphoid tissues of horses (Woolcock 1975). It produces either mucoid, matt, or glossy colonies surrounded by a wide zone of hemolysis on blood agar. It ferments lactose sorbitol and ribose but not trehalose or inulin. *S. zooepidemicus* belongs to group C of the Lancefield typing system and is closely related to *S. equi* and *S. equisimilis*.

Antigens. Strains of *S. zooepidemicus* belong to at least 15 serotypes, the type-specific antigen being proteinaceous and trypsin-labile (Moore and Bryans 1970). Another proteinaceous trypsin-resistant antigen that is pepsin-labile also has been found but is rare (Bryans and Moore 1972). It is found on *S. zooepidemicus* type 3.

All strains share with *S. equi* a trypsin- and acid-resistant R antigen, which is a protein with a molecular weight of about 82,000. This protein is immunologically reactive, and most horses carry serum antibodies to it (Timoney 1986). There are at least two other immunologically reactive proteins common to strains of *S. equi* and *S. zooepidemicus;* these have molecular weights of 31,000 and 56,000 (Timoney and Trachman 1985). These immunologically reactive proteins are of importance only in that antibody responses to them can cause confusion in the interpretation of assays of antibody responses to either *S. zooepidemicus* or *S. equi* infections in horses.

S. zooepidemicus strains also carry one of a number of different M proteins that are important in protective responses. These have not yet been fully characterized but are serologically different from the M protein of *S. equi*.

Epizootiology and Pathogenesis. *S. zooepidemicus* causes disease in many domestic animal species.

The disease in horses. *S. zooepidemicus* is by far the most common cause of wound infections and is also a routine secondary invader after viral infections of the upper respiratory tract of foals and young horses. It can cause a purulent nasal discharge and abscessation of submandibular lymph nodes in some cases in these animals. It can invade the umbilical stump of foals, causing omphalophlebitis, bacteremia, and polyarthritis. In mares it can cause cervicitis and endometritis. This can be a sequel to vulvar deformity or to injury during parturition. *S. zooepidemicus* can cause abortion when it is carried in the bloodstream to the placenta or enters the uterus from the distal genital tract (Dimock et al. 1947).

The disease in cows. Mastitis caused by *S. zooepidemicus* is usually acute and severe and is often found in small, handmilked herds on farms where the milker takes care of other species. The organism enters via a wound on the teat or via a damaged meatus. Arthritis sometimes occurs in association with mastitis caused by *S. zooepidemicus.*

The disease in other species. Fibrinous pleuritis, pericarditis, and pneumonia have been reported in lambs (Stevenson 1974). Mastitis with eventual severe gland atrophy has occurred in goats (Nesbakken 1975). Hand stripping after machine milking was believed to have spread the infection. Fatal septicemia in chickens caused by *S. zooepidemicus* has been reported (Peckham 1966).

Immunity. Most horses carry precipitating antibodies to *S. zooepidemicus* as a consequence of nasopharyngeal carriage of the organism. Antibodies and complement in uterine fluids have been shown to be effective in enhancing phagocytosis and clearance of the organism (Asbury et al. 1984).

Antimicrobial Susceptibility. *S. zooepidemicus* is sensitive to the same antimicrobials as *S. agalactiae.* A high frequency of gentamicin resistance has been noted in isolates from equine tissues and reproductive tracts (Welsh 1984).

REFERENCES

Asbury, A.C., Gorman, N.T., and Foster, G.W. 1984. Uterine defense mechanisms in the mare: Serum opsonins affecting phagocytosis of *Streptococcus zooepidemicus* by equine neutrophils. Theriogenology 21:375–385.

Bryans, J.T., and Moore, B.O. 1972. Group C streptococcal infections of the horse. In L.W. Wannamaker and J.M. Matsen, eds., Streptococci and Streptococcal Diseases. Academic Press, New York. Pp. 327–338.

Dimock, W.W., Edwards, P.R., and Bruner, D.W. 1947. Infections observed in equine fetuses and foals. Cornell Vet. 37:89–99.

Kasai, K., Nobata, R., and Rya, E. 1944. On the incidence of *Streptococcus hemolyticus* in the normal tonsils of horses and the typing of equine tonsillar streptococci. Jpn. J. Vet. Sci. 6:116–123.

Moore, B.O., and Bryans, J.J. 1970. Type specific antigenicity of group C streptococci from diseases of the horse. In J.T. Bryans and H. Gerber, eds., Proceedings of the 2d International Congress on Equine Infectious Diseases, Paris, 1969. Karger, Basel. Pp. 1–9.

Nesbakken, T. 1975. Chronic mastitis due to *Streptococcus zooepidemicus* as a problem in a flock of goats. Nord. Veterinärmed. Tidsskr. 87:188–191.

Peckham, M.C. 1966. An outbreak of streptococcosis (apoplectiform septicemia) in white rock chickens. Avian Dis. 10:413–421.

Stevenson, R.G. 1974. *Streptococcus zooepidemicus* infection in sheep. Can. J. Comp. Med. 38:243–250.

Timoney, J.F. 1986. Characteristics of an R antigen of *Streptococcus equi* and *Streptococcus zooepidemicus.* Cornell Vet. 76:49–60.

Timoney, J.F., and Trachman, J. 1985. Immunologically reactive proteins of *Streptococcus equi.* Infect. Immun. 48:29–34.

Welsh, R.D. 1984. The significance of *Streptococcus zooepidemicus* in the horse. Equine Pract. 6:6–16.

Woolcock, J.B. 1975. Epidemiology of equine streptococci. Res. Vet. Sci. 18:113–114.

Streptococcus uberis

Like *S. dysgalactiae*, *S. uberis* causes bovine mastitis, but it differs from *S. dysgalactiae* principally in the following details: It is nonhemolytic but can produce slight greenish discoloration on blood agar; it is salicin-, esculin-, and hippurate-positive. It does not react in the Lancefield grouping system. A few strains are CAMP-positive.

Epizootiology and Pathogenesis. *S. uberis* has been found in the rumen, rectum, feces, and on the lips and skin of cattle (Cullen and Little 1969). It multiplies in bedding. Infection of the udder is related to the amount of environmental contamination (King 1981): the disease is much more common in loosely housed cattle than in those on pasture.

The disease is usually acute but mild. More severe forms have been observed occasionally in which infection was caused by encapsulated variants of the organism. Control of this form of mastitis lies in improved environmental hygiene.

REFERENCES

Cullen, G.A., and Little, T.W.A. 1969. Isolation of *Streptococcus uberis* from the rumen of cows and from soil. Vet. Rec. 85:115–118.

King, J.S. 1981. *Streptococcus uberis:* A review of its role as a causative organism of bovine mastitis. II. Control of the infection. Br. Vet. J. 137:160–165.

Streptococcus equisimilis

S. equisimilis is beta hemolytic, although the zone of beta hemolysis is less than that produced by *S. zooepidemicus,* to which it is closely related. Colony morphology is similar to that of *S. zooepidemicus.* It produces acid from trehalose but not from sorbitol. In contrast to strains from cattle, swine, and humans, most equine strains do not ferment lactose.

Antigens. The group antigen (C) is located in the cell wall, and there are four subtypes within the group. Type-specific protein antigens also exist. A number of protein antigens are shared with *S. zooepidemicus* and *S. equi.*

Epizootiology and Pathogenesis. *S. equisimilis* is the most frequent cause of suppurative arthritis in pigs from birth to 6 weeks of age (Ross 1972). Infection is probably derived through the umbilicus from the genital tract of the sow, because group C streptococci are common in the vaginal secretions of sows. The disease is often confined to a single litter or to successive litters over a period of many months (Woods and Ross 1975b).

Clinical signs in piglets include loss of appetite, elevated temperature, roughened haircoat, lameness, and swelling of joints. Necrosis of the joint surfaces can lead to permanent joint damage.

S. equisimilis is rarely mentioned in association with disease in horses. Bazely and Battle (1940) found that about 10 percent of the streptococci in pathological material from horses were *S. equisimilis.* In a survey of equine tonsillar tissue and draining lymph nodes, Woolcock (1975) found that about 4 percent of the streptococci were *S. equisimilis.* The organism is occasionally isolated from cervicitis and from abscesses in the lymph nodes of the head of horses.

Immunity. A microtiter complement-fixation procedure has been developed for the detection of antibodies. In immune swine serums these antibodies are predominantly of the IgG class (Woods and Ross 1975a). Protection is not directly correlated with the antibodies, however, although their levels are a reliable measure of the immune status of groups of pigs. Extract vaccines and vaccines with adjuvants for immunization of piglets from 3 weeks of age onward have been shown to stimulate a protective immunity (Woods and Ross 1977).

REFERENCES

Bazely, P.L., and Battle, J. 1940. Studies with equine streptococci. I. A survey of beta-hemolytic streptococci in equine infections. Aust. Vet. J. 6:140–146.
Ross, R.F. 1972. In L.W. Wannamaker and J.M. Matson, eds., Streptococci and Streptococcal Diseases. Academic Press, New York. Pp. 339–346.
Woods, R.D., and Ross, R.F. 1975a. Purification and serological characterization of a type-specific antigen of *Streptococcus equisimilis.* Infect. Immun. 12:88–93.
Woods, R.D., and Ross, R.F. 1975b. Streptococcosis of swine. Vet. Bull. 46:397–400.
Woods, R.D., and Ross, R.F. 1977. Immunogenicity of experimental *Streptococcus equisimilis* vaccines in swine. Am. J. Vet. Res. 38:33–36.

Woolcock, J. 1975. Epidemiology of equine streptococci. Res. Vet. Sci. 18:113–114.

Streptococcus equi

S. equi is the cause of *strangles,* a severe purulent infection of the upper respiratory tract and draining lymph nodes of horses. The organism has also been isolated from abscessed lymph nodes of burros (Wisecup et al. 1967) and from humans with septicemia caused by the consumption of contaminated cheese.

Morphology and Staining Reactions. *S. equi* occurs in exudates and in fluid cultures in the form of long chains and occasionally in short chains. Sometimes the chains are surrounded by definite capsular material. The organism is readily stained with the usual dyes and is Gram-positive when cultures are young; old cultures retain Gram's stain poorly. Electron micrographs have revealed that the outer surface of the organism has a peach-fuzz-like coating of protein (Figure 19.3).

Cultural and Biochemical Features. The colonies are either mucoid or matt on primary isolation (Figure 19.4). Mucoid colonies are usually about 3 mm in diameter after 24 hours and adjacent colonies tend to run together. Matt colonies exhibit irregular surface folding and look dried out. This type of colony formation is a result of phage-controlled hyaluronidase action on the hyaluronic acid capsule (Spanier and Timoney 1977, Timoney et al. 1982). Hyaluronidase is released after about 10 hours of incubation. The hyaluronidase hydrolyzes the capsule, causing it to collapse and giving the colony a flattened, textured appearance.

An oxygen-sensitive streptolysin O-like hemolysin is produced that creates a wide zone of beta hemolysis around colonies on blood-agar plates. *S. equi* forms acid from glucose, sucrose, maltose, and galactose; it does not ferment lactose, sorbitol, or ribose nor will it acidify milk.

Antigens. *S. equi* carries the Lancefield group C carbohydrate antigen as well as a number of protein antigens, including the R and M antigens. The R antigen has a molecular weight of about 82,000 and is also found on *S. zooepidemicus* (Timoney 1986). The M antigen is an acid- and heat-resistant protein that occurs in acid extracts as a series of different-sized fragments, the most immunologically reactive of which have molecular weights of about 29,000–30,000, 37,000, and 41,000 (Timoney and Trachman 1985). The native M molecule occurs in a series of molecules with molecular weights between 52,000 and 60,000 (Galan and Timoney 1987). There is only one M protein type found among *S. equi* strains. It has an antiphagocytic function: it stimulates opsonizing antibodies, which are the basis of the so-called bactericidal

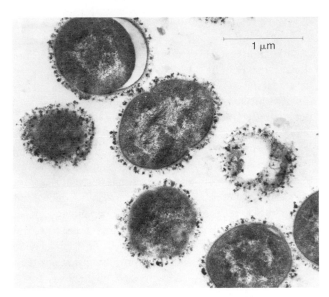

Figure 19.3. Electron micrograph of a section of *Streptococcus equi*. Note the typical Gram-positive cell wall and the peach-fuzz-like coating of protein surrounding it.

reaction of immune serum. Besides the R and M antigens, *S. equi* carries at least two other immunologically reactive proteins with molecular weights of 31,000 and 55,000. These proteins are also found on *S. zooepidemicus,* and horses infected with either *S. zooepidemicus* or *S. equi* produce antibody responses to them (Timoney and Trachman 1985).

Epizootiology and Pathogenesis. *S. equi* is an obligate parasite of members of the family Equidae. Transmission of the organism occurs through the oral or nasal routes,

Figure 19.4. Mucoid (smooth) and matt (wrinkled) colonies of *Streptococcus equi.*

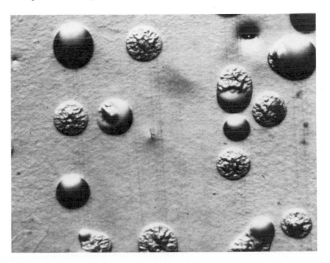

with ingestion of contaminated water or feed being the most common means by which the organism enters a new host. Inhalation of infective droplets can also be an effective mode of infection. Foals with infective nasal discharges sometimes infect the mammary gland of the mare during suckling and thereby initiate a purulent mastitis. Uterine infections of mares also occur.

Outbreaks are usually seen in large groups of horses held in close confinement and often begin soon after the introduction of a carrier or infected animal, which may itself have no overt signs of disease. The use of common feeding or drinking facilities greatly facilitates transmission, as do large numbers of flies. Flies feed on discharges and then carry the organism to new hosts. Because *S. equi* persists in discharges in the environment for only a few weeks, the most important factor in the interepizootic maintenance of infection is the infected horse.

The incubation period varies from 3 to 6 days to 3 weeks or longer. Some outbreaks of strangles are characterized by extended incubation periods and infection without overt clinical disease in a sizable proportion of infected animals. These animals can harbor the organism in the nasopharynx for weeks and exhibit only a slight nasal discharge. One report has documented a carrier state of many months' duration (Reif et al. 1982); however, such a situation appears to be unusual.

Matt-colony strains of *S. equi* have been associated with a less severe form of strangles (Mahaffey 1962), but this observation has not been substantiated (Timoney et al. 1984). Outbreaks of the disease have yielded both matt-colony and mucoid-colony strains from the same infected groups of horses, and the spectrum of severity of the lesions did not seem to be related to the colonial form of the isolate. Matt-colony and mucoid-colony strains also had similar M protein fragment profiles (Timoney et al. 1984) and were of approximately equal virulence.

S. equi attaches to epithelial cells after entry into the oropharynx (Srivastava and Barnum 1983) and then becomes interiorized. This phase of the pathogenesis is poorly understood. After passage through the mucosa, the organism is apparently carried in the lymph drainage to the submandibular and retropharyngeal lymph nodes, where it lodges and initiates abscess formation. The process by which polymorphonuclear leukocytes are attracted toward *S. equi* involves activation of the alternate complement pathway by cell wall peptidoglycan and, to a lesser extent, by M protein on the surface of the organism (Mukhtar 1985). Complement-derived chemotactic factors (C3a and C5a) are released and attract polymorphonuclear leukocytes. Some phagocytosis of *S. equi* cells then takes place; however, a powerful cytotoxin released by the organism damages many of the phagocytes, which quickly degenerate (Mukhtar 1985). The organism thus is able to multiply extracellularly and produce long chains.

Other factors that contribute to virulence and the ability to evade phagocytosis are the M protein and hyaluronic acid capsule and a high rate of intracellular survival, possibly resulting from the effect of the cytotoxin on the phagocytes.

Affected animals lose their appetites, exhibit a fever of 103° to 106°F, and develop a serous nasal discharge followed by a mucopurulent nasal discharge. The nasopharyngeal mucosa becomes inflamed and small abscesses can develop in the lymphoid follicles on the soft palate. The pharyngeal area becomes very painful and the animal stands with its head slightly lowered and extended anteriorly. Involvement of the submandibular lymph nodes is associated with swelling of the nodes and accumulation of lymph anterior to the nodes (Figure 19.5). The intermandibular area becomes greatly distended and the skin may exude serous fluid. Involvement of the retropharyngeal lymph nodes can result in obstruction of the airway and noisy, dyspneic, and labored respiration. Abscesses rupture about 1 to 2 weeks after the onset of the first signs and most animals recover quickly and completely after drainage of purulent material. Abscesses sometimes form in other areas of the body such as the thorax or abdomen (bastard strangles); rupture of such abscesses usually results in death of the animal.

A debilitating disease characterized by caseous abscesses in abdominal lymph nodes has been reported in burros (Wisecup et al. 1967). Cardiac failure has been reported to be caused by myocarditis associated with *S. equi* infection (Rubarth 1943). Laryngeal hemiplegia is a complication that can result from abscessation of the anterior cervical lymph node and involvement of the recurrent laryngeal nerve. Guttural pouch empyema can be a complication of abscessation of the anterior retropharyngeal lymph nodes, although abscesses in this area usually drain directly into the posterior pharynx and do not often extend into the guttural pouch.

Purpura hemorrhagica is another complicating aftermath of strangles and arises in a small percentage of animals that have recovered from the disease. Affected animals develop fever and edema of the dependent areas of the head and trunk and of the legs above the knee and hock. Punctate hemorrhages can also be found on the nasal mucosa and intestine. The primary lesion is a leukocytoclastic vasculitis characterized by necrosis of the walls of blood vessels. There is no evidence of thrombocytopenia.

The serums of affected animals carry immune complexes consisting of IgA and *S. equi* M protein (Galan and Timoney 1985b). Levels of serum IgA complexes are greatly elevated, and these elevations appear to involve an overgrowth of a specific IgA-producing clone rather than failure of hepatic clearance of IgA immunoglobulins. The M protein in immune complexes probably derives from purulent foci in which *S. equi* and its M antigen may be present in considerable quantity. Administration of strangles vaccine, however, has also triggered cases of purpura, suggesting that M protein in this form is capable of both selecting and stimulating the appropriate IgA-pro-

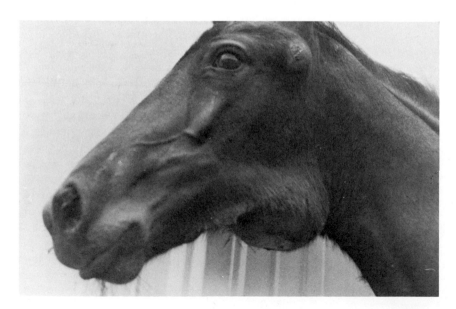

Figure 19.5. Strangles in a horse. Note the swelling in the submandibular area.

ducing clone and subsequently complexing with the antibody produced.

Immunity. The majority (70 percent) of animals are immune to further attacks of strangles after recovery from a first infection. However, a substantial proportion of animals (30 percent) can contract the disease a second time, and of these a small proportion can contract the disease more than twice (Todd 1910). Protection against the disease is primarily mediated by antibodies of the IgA and IgG subclasses locally produced in the nasopharynx. These antibodies are directed against an epitope (s) on a 41,000-dalton fragment and a 46,000-dalton fragment of the M protein and do not react with other acid-extracted fragments of the molecule (Galan and Timoney 1985a). In contrast, serum antibodies in the same animal react with a variety of M protein fragments. These observations have provided strong evidence for separation of the local and systemic immune responses of horses to *S. equi*.

Milk from mares that have recovered from strangles contains antibody that reacts with the 41,000-dalton fragment and so can provide the suckling foal with antibody protective for its nasopharynx (Galan et al. 1986).

Serum antibodies to *S. equi* can be measured by a variety of assays including the chain-length and bactericidal indices (Woolcock 1975), radioimmunoassay (Galan and Timoney 1985a), ELISA, (Reif et al. 1982), the mouse protection test (Bazely 1943), and the gel diffusion precipitin test. Mouse protection and bactericidal tests have been correlated with protection in horses (Bazely 1943); however, serum bactericidal or opsonic antibodies in vaccinated animals do not correlate well with protection in the field or in controlled challenge experiments in the laboratory (Timoney and Eggers 1985; Galan and Timoney 1985a).

Commercially available vaccines consisting of heat-inactivated bacterin or M-protein-rich extracts have been widely used in the field. Although effective in stimulating serum bactericidal antibodies, these vaccines apparently do not stimulate a useful level of nasopharyngeal antibody and so the level of protection stimulated in a horse population is disappointing. An avirulent, genetically modified strain of *S. equi* administered intranasally has recently been shown to stimulate local nasopharyngeal antibodies similar to those found in convalescent immune horses. Vaccinated horses were immune to subsequent experimental challenge with virulent *S. equi* (Timoney and Galan 1985). It therefore appears that an effective strangles vaccine must be able to stimulate a nasopharyngeal immune response.

Bacterin-type vaccines often cause undesirable local and systemic reactions consisting of edema, induration, stiffness, transient fever, and neutrophilia, effects that are probably due to cell wall peptidoglycan. M-protein-extract–type vaccines do not have these effects.

Antimicrobial Susceptibility. *S. equi* is very sensitive to penicillin, chloramphenicol, erythromycin, lincomycin, and tetracyclines. Many experienced clinicians, however, feel that antibiotics delay maturation and draining of abscesses (Ebert 1969) and may contribute to the incidence of bastard strangles (Bryans and Moore 1971). Use of penicillin is perhaps best reserved for prophylaxis of in-contact animals or for relief of life-threatening lesions such as abscesses and edema in retropharyngeal lymph nodes that are blocking the airway. Most animals with the disease recover quickly in the absence of antibiotic treatment and without consequence once the abscesses drain.

REFERENCES

Bazely, P.L. 1943. Studies with streptococci. V. Some relations between virulence of *S. equi* and immune response in the host. Aust. Vet. J. 19:62–85.

Bryans, J.T., and Moore, B.O. 1971. Group C streptococcal infections of the horse. In J.T. Bryans and H. Gerber, eds., Proceedings of the 3d International Congress on Equine Infectious Diseases. S. Karger, New York. Pp. 327–336.

Ebert, E.F. 1969. Some observations on equine strangles. Vet. Med. 64.71–73.

Galan, J.E., and Timoney, J.F. 1985a. Mucosal and nasopharyngeal immune responses of horses to protein antigens of *Streptococcus equi*. Infect. Immun. 47:623–628.

Galan, J.E., and Timoney, J.F. 1985b. Immune complexes in purpura hemorrhagica of the horse contain IgA and M antigen of *Streptococcus equi*. J. Immunol. 135:3134–3137.

Galan, J.E., and Timoney, J.F. 1987. Molecular analysis of the M protein of *Streptococcus equi* and cloning and expression of the M protein gene in *Escherichia coli*. Infect. Immun. 55.3181–3187.

Galan, J.E., Timoney, J.F., and Lengemann, F. 1986. Passive transfer of mucosal antibody to *Streptococcus equi* in the foal. Infect. Immun. 54:202–206.

Mahaffey, L.W. 1962. Respiratory conditions in horses. Vet. Rec. 74:1295–1313.

Muhktar, M.M. 1985. Chemotactic response of equine polymorphonuclear leukocytes to components of *Streptococcus equi*. Master's thesis, Cornell University, Ithaca, N.Y.

Reif, J.S., George, J.L., and Shideler, R.K. 1982. Recent developments in strangles research: Observations on the carrier state and evaluation of a new vaccine. Proc. Am. Assoc. Equine Practitioners 27:33–40.

Rubarth, S. 1943. Plotsliga dodsfall hos hast och deras samband med fokalinfektioner. Svend. Milit. Sailsk. Kvarthalsskr. 30:75–78.

Spanier, J., and Timoney, J.F. 1977. Bacteriophages from *Streptococcus equi*. J. Gen. Virol. 35:369–372.

Srivastava, S.K., and Barnum, D.A. 1983. Adherence of *Streptococcus equi* on tongue, cheek and nasal epithelial cells of ponies. Vet. Microbiol. 8:493–504.

Timoney, J.F. 1986. Characteristics of an R antigen of *Streptococcus equi* and *Streptococcus zooepidemicus*. Cornell Vet. 76:49–60.

Timoney, J.F., and Eggers, D. 1985. Serum bactericidal responses to *Streptococcus equi* of horses following infection or vaccination. Equine Vet. J. 17:306–310.

Timoney, J.F., and Galan, J.E. 1985. The protective response of the horse to an avirulent strain of *Streptococcal equi*. In Y. Kimura, S.

Kotami, and Y. Shiokawa, eds., Recent Advances in Streptococci and Streptococcal Disease. Reedbooks, Surrey, England. Pp. 294–295.

Timoney, J.F., and Trachman, J. 1985. Immunologically reactive proteins of *Streptococcus equi*. Infect. Immun. 48:29–34.

Timoney, J.F., Pesante, L., and Ernst, C. 1982. Hyaluronidase associated with a temperate bacteriophage of *Streptococcus equi*. In D. Schlessinger, ed., Microbiology 1982. American Society for Microbiology, Washington, D.C. Pp. 145–146.

Timoney, J.F., Timoney, P.J., and Strickland, K.L. 1984. Lysogeny and the immunologically reactive proteins of *Streptococcus equi*. Vet. Rec. 115:148–149.

Todd, A.G. 1910. Strangles. J. Comp. Pathol. Ther. 23:212–229.

Wisecup, W.G., Schroder, C., and Page, N.P. 1967. Isolation of *Streptococcus equi* from burros. J. Am. Vet. Med. Assoc. 150:303–306.

Woolcock, J. 1975. Immunity to *Streptococcus equi*. Aust. Vet. J. 51:554–559.

Streptococcus porcinus

SYNONYM: Group E streptococci
(*Streptococcus infrequens*)

Cervical lymphadenitis, a contagious disease of swine, was first shown to be associated with group E streptococci by Newsom (1937). He named this disease *swine strangles* because of its similarity to equine strangles.

Streptococci isolated from this disease produce small, elevated, entire colonies. Slowly developing beta hemolysis on horse-blood agar is visible in about 48 hours. Acid is produced from trehalose and, in the case of some strains, from sorbitol and inulin. The name *S. porcinus* has been designated for group E streptococci and other closely related organisms in groups P, U, and V isolated from pigs (Collins et al. 1984).

Antigens. Eight different serotypes (1 to 8) based on polysaccharide antigens have been described, but only types 2, 4, and 5 to 8 are currently recognized (Wessman et al. 1983). Type 4 is most frequently isolated from cases of cervical lymphadenitis. Strains from swine may lack the type antigen, are capsulated, and produce streptodornase and a streptokinase specific for porcine plasminogen (Ellis and Armstrong 1971).

Epizootiology and Pathogenesis. The disease is common in the swine-raising areas of the midwestern United States but appears to occur infrequently elsewhere. Swine between the ages of 9 weeks and $2\frac{1}{2}$ years are more susceptible than swine of other ages. Baby piglets are protected by colostral antibodies and perhaps by antibody secreted during lactation in the milk of the sow. Transmission occurs by nose contact and through contaminated drinking water or feces (Miller and Olsen 1983). The organism is carried in the tonsils and possibly in other sites in the carrier animal. Such animals can transmit the organism for 11 to 21 months. Shedding can also occur for long periods after clinical remission. *S. porcinus* can survive for extended periods in the soil (Schmitz and Olsen 1973).

Since the 1970s the disease has become less common in the United States, a decrease attributed to antimicrobial supplementation of feed. Miller and Olsen (1983) suggest, however, that changes in swine management may be a more important factor. These changes include housing of pigs in smaller groups and an "all-in, all-out" approach. Thus the animals commingle less during fattening and are less stressed because the social structure in the fattening pens is more stable.

The minimal infective dose of one group E strain for 12-week-old swine has been shown to be about 10^6 colony-forming units (Armstrong et al. 1970). The organism enters the mouth or nasal chambers, and entry is followed by a rise in temperature and leukocytosis 2 to 4 days later. Lymph node enlargement is evident in about 2 weeks, and abscessed nodes eventually drain to the surface about 6 weeks after this. The mandibular lymph nodes are most frequently abscessed, followed by the retropharyngeal and parotid nodes. The disease is frequently called *jowl abscessation* because of involvement of the mandibular lymph nodes. Condemnation losses when meat is inspected can be considerable. Affected animals are often not detected until this time.

Immunity. Antibodies are formed in about 7 days (Jenkins and Collier 1978a) in response to infection and can be detected by agglutination, precipitin, and passive hemagglutination tests (Wessman et al. 1970). Immunity can be passively transferred by means of serums from convalescent animals (Jenkins and Collier 1978b). Antibody to an antiphagocytic factor of the organism has been detected and shown to persist for at least 20 weeks (Wessman et al. 1977).

Immunity to cervical lymphadenitis can be stimulated by an oral, avirulent, group E vaccine strain (Englebrecht and Dolan 1968), although vaccination is not as effective in pigs less than 10 weeks old as in older pigs. Bacterins have been shown to be relatively ineffective in preventing abscessation, although they reduce the number and size of abscesses in affected pigs (Gosser and Olsen 1973, Shuman and Wood 1968).

Diagnosis. Procedures employing broth containing blood, azide, and crystal violet or penicillin and salt have been used for selective isolation of group E streptococci from tonsil swabs and biopsy specimens (Riley et al. 1973). The fluorescent-antibody technique, however, is reported to be the most effective procedure for detection of these organisms in tonsillar material (Riley et al. 1973, Schueler et al. 1973).

Antimicrobial Susceptibility. Group E streptococci are usually sensitive to penicillin, tetracycline, chloramphenicol, and nitrafurazone. Addition of 138 g of tetracycline per metric ton of food after weaning greatly reduces the frequency of abscessation (Miller and Olsen 1983).

REFERENCES

Armstrong, C.H., Boehm, P.N., and Ellis, R.P. 1970. Experimental transmission of streptococcal lymphadenitis (jowl abscess) of swine. Am. J. Vet. Res. 31:823–829.

Collins, M.D., Farrow, J.A.E., Katic, V., and Kandler, O. 1984. Taxonomic studies on streptococci of serological groups E, P, U, and V: Description of *Streptococcus porcinus* sp. nov. Syst. Appl. Microbiol. 5:402–413.

Ellis, R.P., and Armstrong, C.H. 1971. Production of capsular streptokinase and streptodornase by *Streptococcus* group E. Am. J. Vet. Res. 32:349–356.

Englebrecht, H., and Dolan, M. 1968. Vaccination of swine for jowl abscesses. Oral administration of group E streptococcus vaccine (live culture-modified). Vet. Med./Small Anim. Clin. 63:872–875.

Gosser, H.S., and Olsen, L.D. 1973. Failure to immunize swine against streptococcal lymphadenitis with autogenous bacterins. Am. J. Vet. Res. 34:129–130.

Jenkins, E.M., and Collier, J.R., 1978a. Immunity to Lancefield's group E *Streptococcus:* Flank inoculation of susceptible and immune swine. Am. J. Vet. Res. 39:325–328.

Jenkins, E.M., and Collier, J.R. 1978b. Immunity to Lancefield's group E streptococcus: Passive protection of swine. Am. J. Vet. Res. 39:1181–1183.

Miller, R.B., and Olsen, L.D. 1983. Frequency of joint abscesses in feeder and market swine exposed to group E streptococci and nursing pigs. Am. J. Vet. Res. 44:945–948.

Newsom, I.E. 1937. Strangles in hogs. Vet. Med. 37:137–138.

Riley, M.G.I., Morehouse, L.G., and Olsen, L.D. 1973. Detection of tonsillar and nasal colonization of group E streptococcus in swine. Am. J. Vet. Res. 34:1167–1169.

Schmitz, J.A., and Olsen, L.D. 1973. Duration of viability and the growth and expiration rates of group E streptococci in soil. J. Am. Vet. Med. Assoc. 162:55–58.

Schueler, R.L., Morehouse, L.G., and Olsen, L.D. 1973. A direct fluorescent antibody test for identification of group E streptococci. Can. J. Comp. Med. 37:327–329.

Shuman, R.D., and Wood, R.L. 1968. Swine abscesses caused by Lancefield's Group E streptococci. IV. Test of two bacterins for immunization. Cornell Vet. 58:21–30.

Wessman, G.E., Shuman, R.D., and Nord, N. 1970. Swine abscesses caused by Lancefield's group E streptococci. VI. Experimental application of hemagglutination tests for their detection. Cornell Vet. 60:286–296.

Wessman, G.E., Wood, R.L., and Nord, N. 1977. Detection of antibody to the antiphagocytic factor produced by group E streptococci. Cornell Vet. 67:81–91.

Wessman, G.E., Wood, R.L., and Nord, N.A. 1983. Identification of three new serotypes of group E streptococci isolated from swine. Cornell Vet. 73:307–313.

Streptococcus suis

Meningitis and septicemia in young pigs caused by a Lancefield group D streptococcus were first described in England by Elliott (1966). He proposed that the organism be named *S. suis* and observed that all strains belonged to one capsular type, which he designated type 1. Some years later capsular type 2 antigen was described on isolates from cases of meningitis in older pigs (Windsor and Elliott 1975). Since then disease caused by these strains of *S. suis* has been observed in most swine-raising areas of the world.

Morphology and Staining Reactions. *S. suis* produces Gram-positive, elongated diplobacilli that form short chains in fluid cultures.

Cultural and Biochemical Features. The colonies are flat, mucoid, weakly hemolytic, and about 1 to 2 mm in diameter. Some strains produce greenish discoloration in blood agar or an incomplete beta hemolysis and may exhibit a CAMP reaction (Erickson et al. 1984). *S. suis* usually ferments lactose, trehalose, and inulin. Esculin hydrolysis is variable and sorbitol is never fermented. It does not produce catalase and does not grow in 6.5 percent sodium chloride.

Antigens. Serotyping is based on the presence of the D cell wall antigen or on the possession of one of at least 8 capsular polysaccharide antigens (Perch et al. 1983). The cell wall antigen is a lipid-bound teichoic acid similar to other group D streptococcal cell wall antigens. The capsular polysaccharide antigens, designated 1 to 8, resemble those of group B streptococci isolated from cases of human neonatal meningitis (Elliott and Tai 1978). Capsular antigens 1 and 2 have also been designated S and R, respectively (de Moor 1963). Type 2 capsular polysaccharide has a molecular weight of at least 100,000 and elicits opsonizing antibody responses.

Epizootiology and Pathogenesis. *S. suis* is carried in the tonsils and nasal cavities of both normal and diseased pigs and is transmitted among herds mainly through the movement of infected animals (Clifton-Hadley and Alexander 1980). Capsular type 1 strains are usually isolated from diseased baby pigs, whereas type 2 strains—the most frequently observed in the field—are found in older pigs. At ambient temperatures the organism survives in feces for only about 8 to 10 days and is readily killed by disinfectants (Clifton-Hadley and Enright 1984).

Transmission is apparently by means of the respiratory and oral routes, although it is difficult to produce disease by experimental intranasal inoculation of type 2 strains (Elliott and Clifton-Hadley 1980). Type 1 strains appear to be much more invasive following intranasal inoculation.

Most outbreaks are observed in cold weather in intensive units of pigs aged 4 to 12 weeks. Weaning, regrouping, overcrowding, and poor ventilation are important predisposing factors. The tonsil carrier rate in weaned pigs may be as high as 50 percent during outbreaks and is much lower when no clinical disease is evident (Clifton-Hadley and Alexander 1980). Morbidity may be as high as 20 to 30 percent with mortality up to 8 percent.

Invasion of the regional lymph system apparently occurs from the palatine tonsils. The organism can remain localized in the mandibular lymph nodes or, in some pigs, can become rapidly invasive and cause septicemia, meningitis, and arthritis. Affected pigs may become blind. They show an elevated temperature, lassitude, incoordination, paddling movements, and tremors followed by paralysis, convulsions, and death. At necropsy there is a suppurative meningitis, polyarthritis, endocarditis, bronchopneumonia, and other lesions typical of generalized septicemia. In outbreaks in Nebraska bronchopneumonia was a conspicuous feature (Erickson et al. 1984).

Immunity. Although the capsular polysaccharide antigens are protective and elicit opsonizing antibodies (Elliott and Clifton-Hadley 1980), immune responses of pigs immunized with capsular polysaccharide are poor. The presence of serum opsonizing antibodies does not affect tonsillar carriage of the organism. Vaccination of sows with bacterins containing type 1 and 2 capsular antigens greatly reduces septicemic streptococcal disease in suckling piglets in endemic herds (Bercea et al. 1981). However, the disease has been reported to be self-limiting in self-contained herds, an effect caused by emerging population immunity. The effect of vaccination, therefore, has to be interpreted with caution.

Diagnosis. Isolation of alpha- or beta-hemolytic streptococci that react with group D or capsular typing antiserums and that do not grow in 6.5 percent sodium chloride is good evidence of the presence of *S. suis*. A technique based on formulation of immunoprecipitates in agar media enriched with antiserum has been devised for detection of *S. suis* colonies in slices of tonsil (Arends et al. 1984).

Antimicrobial Susceptibility. *S. suis* is sensitive to penicillin, ampicillin, chloramphenicol, and trimethoprim-sulfamethoxazole but is resistant to streptomycin and tetracycline (Sanford and Tilker 1982). The addition of penicillin to early weaning food is effective in controlling the disease but does not affect tonsillar carriage of the organism.

The Disease in Humans. *S. suis* is an important zoonosis, and many serious infections have been reported in persons whose jobs involve contact with pigs. The organism enters through cuts, abrasions, and possibly the conjunctiva. The disease in humans is similar to that in pigs. There can be meningitis, arthritis, septicemia, endophthalmitis, diarrhea, and petechiation. Patients can suf-

fer permanent hearing loss and vertigo after recovery (Clifton-Hadley 1983).

REFERENCES

Arends, J.P., Hartwig, N., Rudolphy, M., and Zanen, H.C. 1984. Carrier rate of *Streptococcus suis* capsular type 2 in palatine tonsils of slaughtered pigs. J. Clin. Microbiol. 20:945–947.

Bercea, I., Carol-Dimituir, E., Dobre, I., Nubert, V., and Girbacica, R. 1981. Streptococcus infection in swine. V. Emerging immunoprophylaxis in foci of streptococcosis. Lucr. Stint. Inst. Agron.–Nicolae Balcesca–Med. Vet. 24:51–53.

Clifton-Hadley, F.A. 1983. Review series: Zoonosis in practice. *Streptococcus suis* type 2 infections. Br. Vet. J. 139:1–5.

Clifton-Hadley, F.A., and Alexander, T.J.L. 1980. The carrier site and carrier rate of *Streptococcus suis* type II in pigs. Vet. Rec. 107:40–41.

Clifton-Hadley, F.A., and Enright, M.R. 1984. Factors affecting the survival of *Streptococcus suis* type 2. Vet. Rec. 114:584–586.

deMoor, C.E. 1963. Septicemic infection in pigs caused by haemolytic streptococci of new Lancefield groups designated R, S and T. Antonie Van Leeuwenhoek 29:272–278.

Elliott, S.D. 1966. Streptococcal infection in young pigs. I. An immunochemical study of the causative agent (PM streptococcus). J. Hyg. 64:205–212.

Elliott, S.D., and Clifton-Hadley, F.A. 1980 Streptococcal infection in young pigs. V. An immunogenic polysaccharide from *Streptococcus suis* type 2 with particular reference to vaccination against streptococcal meningitis in pigs. J. Hyg. 85:275–285.

Elliott, S.D., and Tai, J.Y. 1978. The type-specific polysaccharides of *Streptococcus suis*. J. Exp. Med. 148:1699–1702.

Erickson, E.D., Doster, A.R., and Pokorny, T.S. 1984. Isolation of *Streptococcus suis* from swine in Nebraska. Am. J. Vet. Res. 185:666–668.

Perch, B., Pedersen, K.B., and Henrickson, J. 1983. Serology of capsulated streptococci pathogenic for pigs: Six new serotypes of *Streptococcus suis*. J. Clin. Microbiol. 17:993–996.

Sanford, S.E., and Tilker, A.M.E. 1982. *Streptococcus suis* type II–associated diseases in swine: Observations of a one-year study. J. Am. Vet. Med. Assoc. 181:673–676.

Windsor, R.S., and Elliott, S.D. 1975. Streptococcal infection in young pigs. IV. An outbreak of streptococcal infection in weaned pigs. J. Hyg. 75:69–74.

Streptococcus canis (Lancefield Group G)

Group G streptococci are commonly found on the mucous membranes of dogs and cats. Closely related to the group C streptococci, they produce wide zones of beta hemolysis on horse-blood agar. Their important distinguishing characteristics are shown in Table 19.1.

Group G streptococci have been isolated from metritis and vaginitis in bitches (Hirsh and Wiger 1977) and from cases of septicemia in puppies. In cats they have been isolated from skin lesions, abscesses in mandibular lymph nodes (Figure 19.6), omphalophlebitis and septicemia in kittens, conjunctivitis, sinusitis, leg abscesses, and normal throats (Goldman and Moore 1973, Reitmeyer and Steele 1984). They have also been isolated from cattle (Clark et al. 1984). Genetic studies have shown that group G streptococci from animals are different from those in humans, and so it is unlikely that pet animals are a significant source of these organisms for their owners (Simpson et al. 1987).

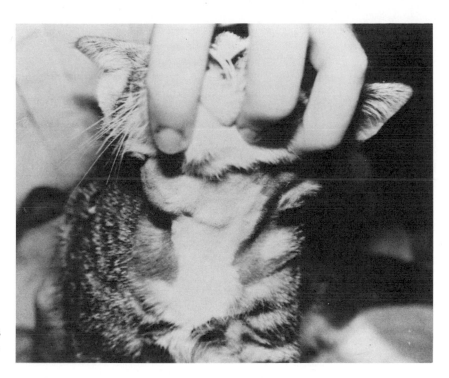

Figure 19.6. Mandibular lymphadenitis caused by *Streptococcus canis* in a cat. (Courtesy Patricia Blanchard.)

REFERENCES

Clark, R.B., Berrafati, J.F., Janda, J.M., and Bottone, E.J. 1984. Biotyping and exoenzyme profiling as an aid in the differentiation of human from bovine group G streptococci. J. Clin. Microbiol. 20:706–710.

Goldman, P.M., and Moore, T.D. 1973. Spontaneous Lancefield group G streptococcal infection in a random source cat colony. Lab Anim. Sci. 23:565–566.

Hirsh, D.C., and Wiger, N. 1977. The bacterial flora of the normal canine vagina compared with that of vaginal exudates. J. Small Anim. Pract. 18:25–30.

Reitmeyer, J.C., and Steele, J.H. 1984. The occurrence of beta-hemolytic streptococcus in cats. Southwestern Vet. 36:41–42.

Simpson, W.J., Robbins, J.C., and Cleary, P.P. 1987. Evidence for group A–related M protein genes in human but not animal-associated group G streptococcal pathogens. Microb. Pathogen. 3:339–350.

Streptococcus equinus

Always abundant in the feces of horses, *S. equinus* was first isolated from air, undoubtedly because of the presence of dried horse manure, once common in most cities. A striking characteristic of this organism is its inability to ferment lactose. It is closely related to *S. bovis*. It does not grow well in nor does it coagulate milk, and it does not grow at temperatures lower than 20°C. *S. equinus* is not known to be pathogenic for animals.

Streptococcus lactis

S. lactis has no pathogenic properties, but because of its omnipresence in milk and milk products, bacteriologists should be able to recognize it and differentiate it from other organisms that may be responsible for disease. *S. lactis* is the common milk-souring organism. In sour milk it usually occurs in short chains, whereas most pathogenic streptococci form long chains. This fact is of considerable differential value. In culture media, however, particularly those that contain serum, *S. lactis* can form long chains. It grows rapidly in milk. If litmus or other reducible dyes are present, the dye is reduced before coagulation occurs. It grows well over a wide range of temperatures. Reduction and coagulation of litmus milk will occur at temperatures as low as 10°C. It almost always attacks esculin.

The normal habitat of *S. lactis* has long been a mystery. Many workers have failed to find it in milk drawn aseptically from the udder; nor is it found in the mouths or intestines of cattle. It has been found on vegetation, however. Once established in a dairy it flourishes. Its heat resistance may be a factor in its persistence in those environments.

Streptococcus bovis

S. bovis is always present in the mouths and intestinal tracts of cattle and, because of fecal contamination, is usually present in milk, where it can be mistaken for *S. agalactiae*. Feedlot bloat in cattle is believed to be caused by excess production of capsular polysaccharide from sucrose by *S. bovis*. This polysaccharide increases the viscosity and the foaming properties of the contents of the rumen. Antibody to the capsular material is secreted in the saliva and may be a factor in the normal prevention of bloat (Horacek et al. 1977). The ability of *S. bovis* to multiply rapidly and to ferment certain dietary starches to lactic acid gives it considerable importance in the etiology of lactic acidosis.

S. bovis does not hydrolyze sodium hippurate but does attack esculin, characteristics that differentiate it from the streptococci that cause bovine mastitis.

REFERENCE

Horacek, G.L., Find, L.R., Tillinghast, H.S., Gettings, R.L., and Bartley, E.E. 1977. Agglutinating immunoglobulins to encapsulated *Streptococcus bovis* in bovine serum and saliva and a possible relation to feedlot bloat. Can. J. Microbiol. 23:100–106.

Nutritionally Variant Streptococci

Nutritionally variant streptococci that resembled the two viridans species *S. intermedicus* and *S. constellatus* have been isolated from corneal ulcers in horses (Higgins et al. 1984).

REFERENCE

Higgins, R., Biberstein, E.L., and Jang, S.S. 1984. Nutritionally variant streptococci from corneal ulcers in horses. J. Clin. Microbiol. 20:1130–1134.

20 The Genus *Erysipelothrix*

The genus *Erysipelothrix* contains the species *rhusiopathiae* and *tonsillarum*. Both organisms are small, Gram-positive rods and are widely distributed in the swine-raising areas of the world. *E. rhusiopathiae* is an important cause of disease in swine and poultry. *E. tonsillarum* is apparently an innocuous commensal of the tonsils of healthy swine (Takahashi et al. 1987).

Erysipelothrix rhusiopathiae

SYNONYMS: *Bacillus rhusiopathiae-suis,*
Bacterium erysipelatos-suum, Bacterium
rhusiopathiae, Erysipelothrix insidiosa,
swine rotlauf bacillus

E. *rhusiopathiae* is the cause of *swine erysipelas,* which has long been recognized as a destructive disease of young pigs in many parts of the world. A variety of disease forms are observed, including skin lesions (*diamond skin disease*), septicemia, polyarthritis, endocarditis, and abortion.

In addition to swine, *E. rhusiopathiae* has been found in lambs suffering from polyarthritis, in calves suffering from a similar disease, in turkeys and ducks (Reetz and Schulz 1978) suffering from acute septicemic infections, in wild and laboratory mice (Balfour-Jones 1935), in the tonsils and on the mucous membranes of apparently normal swine, in various decaying plant and animal tissues, on the skin of freshwater and saltwater fish, and in skin lesions in humans known as *erysipeloid.*

Morphology and Staining Reactions. E. *rhusiopathiae* cells are Gram-positive but are easily decolorized and stain unevenly. They are short (0.5 to 2.5 μm) and slender (0.3 μm). The rough form exhibits long filaments. There are no spores or flagella. The cell walls do not contain DL-diaminopimelic acid, a characteristic which distinguishes *E. rhusiopathiae* from *Listeria monocytogenes.*

Cultural and Biochemical Features. Colonies grown on solid media containing serum or blood are tiny, clear, and glistening. On blood agar there is first a greenish discoloration and later a definite clearing around the colonies. Colonies grown in stabs in gelatin take on a bottle-brush appearance in 3 to 4 days. *E. rhusiopathiae* does not liquefy gelatin but does produce hydrogen sulfide. Most strains ferment glucose, lactose, and galactose and form acid. Cultures are destroyed by exposure to moist heat at 55°C for 10 minutes. They are also phenol-resistant, a property that can be used for isolation from contaminated specimens. The mol% G +C is 36–40 (Tm).

Antigens. At least 22 serotypes have been described on the basis of cell wall peptidoglycans (Norrung 1979, Wood et al. 1978). According to Gledhill (1945), differences between serologic groups arise more from quantitative than from qualitative differences in the distribution of antigens on the organism. Serotypes are given arabic numerals (1–22), and subtypes are designated a, b, c, and so forth. Serotypes 1 and 2 are the ones most commonly found in cases of septicemia and in tonsils.

A study of the immunologically reactive surface proteins by Lachman and Deicher (1986) indicated that the major protein antigens have molecular weights of 78,000, 72,000, 68,000, and 48,000. A single immunologically reactive polysaccharide has a molecular weight of 14,000 to 22,000. The protective antigen is a glycolipoprotein that is sometimes associated with the peptidoglycans that confer serotypic specificity (White and Verwey 1970). The protective glycolipoprotein, however, is not serotype-specific. Serotype 2 live vaccine, for instance, has been shown to protect against other serotypes (Takahashi et al. 1984). Some antigens of *E. rhusiopathiae* cross-react with antigens in swine heart tissue (Bratberg 1981).

Epizootiology and Pathogenesis. The organism causes disease in a variety of domestic animal species.

The disease in swine. E. rhusiopathiae is rather resistant to drying, smoking, pickling, and salting. It has survived and maintained its virulence for 22 years in broth left at ambient temperature (Wellman 1955). The infection tends to remain endemic on farms where special soil conditions such as alkalinity favor its survival. This has been observed in the Sid area of Yugoslavia, where erysipelas is common in areas with alkaline soils but not in immediately contiguous areas with acid soils (Hajduk and Puhac 1974). Survival also can be quite prolonged in decaying carcasses and in water.

The source of the organisms that infect the first cases in outbreaks of erysipelas is uncertain. Many healthy swine carry the organism in their tonsils and reticuloendothelial tissues, and it is probable that stresses such as excessive heat and humidity or other predisposing factors cause impairment of the antibacterial defense mechanism with subsequent multiplication of the organism in the animal's body. In this situation infection is endogenous. The ubiquitous distribution of the organism in nature, however, suggests that a pig's habitat may also be an exogenous source of infection in some cases. In any event, once a pig becomes septicemic it sheds great numbers of organisms in its urine, feces, saliva, and vomitus, which leads to rapid spread among in-contact animals. Because the disease has been experimentally produced by the oral route of exposure and because the tonsil carrier state is so common among swine, it is likely that the majority of natural infections occur by the oral route. The disease can also be produced by skin scarification, however, suggesting that

skin scratches also contribute to spread of infection in groups of animals.

E. rhusiopathiae is a facultative intracellular parasite and exhibits a high rate of survival in pig neutrophils (Timoney 1970). It has been suggested that multiplication of the organism in and subsequent killing of phagocytes is the critical factor in determining the outcome of the infection (Ten Broeck 1920). Furthermore, there is evidence that the reticuloendothelial (RE) system becomes blocked in acute erysipelas in swine (von Jowtscheff 1961). This blocking effect may in fact be simply the depletion of viable phagocytes in the RE system.

The acute disease develops suddenly, producing high fever (106°F), prostration, conjunctivitis, and vomiting in some animals. Deep red to purple patches can appear on the skin, particularly on the ears, the abdomen, and the insides of the legs. The spleen and lymph nodes become enlarged and reddened and the mucosa of the stomach and small intestine acutely inflamed, hemorrhagic, and sometimes ulcerated. The kidneys generally develop cloudy swelling and often have ecchymotic hemorrhages. Mortality from this form of the disease is very high.

A less severe form of swine erysipelas is characterized by the formation of urticarial skin lesions that, in the beginning, consist of reddish or purplish rhomboidal blotches several centimeters in diameter, principally on the abdomen. These blotches have a diamond shape, from which the disease derives its common name, *diamond skin disease* (Figure 20.1). The urticarial areas later become necrotic. The affected skin dries into dense scabs, which finally peel off; a bleeding area develops if the scabs are removed too soon.

During the severe septicemic phase of erysipelas there is an increased level of serum glutamic oxaloacetic transaminase and a marked hypoglycemia of unknown origin (Dougherty et al. 1965). There is also increased erythrocyte destruction with a decrease in hemoglobin and packed cell volume. This effect has also been seen in experimental murine infections. Plasma acid phosphatase and hemoglobin levels rise rapidly together about 36

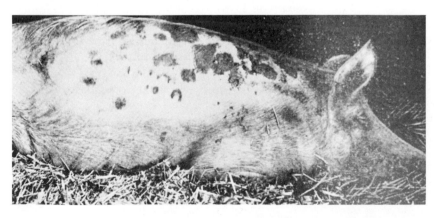

Figure 20.1. Diamond skin disease in a pig. The characteristic lesions of this type of swine erysipelas are visible. (Courtesy R. A. McIntosh.)

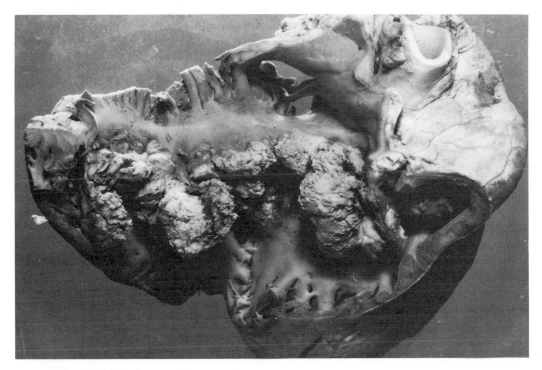

Figure 20.2. Subacute bacterial endocarditis (porcine). *Erysipelothrix rhusiopathiae* was isolated from the lesion. (Courtesy W. L. Boyd and H. C. H. Kernkamp.)

hours after experimental inoculation when the number of bacteria in the blood exceeds 10⁴/ml (Timoney and Shaw, unpublished data).

Nucleated erythrocytes appear in the late stages of the acute disease in pigs. At death the spleen is enlarged and pulpy—a condition that is consistent with hemolysis and stimulation of the hematopoietic system. Interestingly, *E. rhusiopathiae* has hemagglutinating activity for erythrocytes, and this has been shown to result in complement-dependent hemolysis after activation of the alternate complement pathway (Dinter et al. 1976). The hemagglutinating activity is probably related to the high neuraminidase activity of virulent strains (Muller 1971), which increases cell adhesiveness by removal of sialic acid residues, which, in turn, removes negative charges on the erythrocyte surface. Neuraminidase appears to have other important but as yet unknown roles in the disease process. Neutralizing antibodies to the enzyme are present in high titer in commercial swine erysipelas antiserum (Muller and Bohm 1977) and are protective for mice (Muller 1974). Also, the correlation between virulence and neuraminidase production is good in strains of *E. rhusiopathiae* (Krasemann and Muller 1975). It is also probable that neuraminidase activity is involved in the generalized coagulopathy that occurs about 36 hours after swine are inoculated with the organism, with formation of hyaline thrombi in blood vessels, thrombocytopenia, and sticking of fibrin in joints, heart valves, and muscle

(Wellman 1955). The high fever noted in erysipelas may be caused by the erysipelothrix endotoxin—a glycoprotein of molecular weight 31,700 (Leimbeck et al. 1975). This substance also produces a shock effect in swine.

The chronic form of the disease nearly always takes the form of a vegetative endocarditis (Figure 20.2). The heart valves, particularly the mitral valve, become eroded and so covered with fibrin deposits that their functioning is seriously impaired. Affected animals almost invariably die suddenly from this condition. Some strains of *E. rhusiopathiae* have been observed adhering to heart valves and endocardium (Bratberg 1981).

The arthritic form of the disease generally occurs spontaneously in older animals, although arthritis may be a sequel to the more acute forms of the disease. The joints become enlarged and painful; the animals are reluctant to move (Figure 20.3), their gait is stilted, and their growth is stunted. The synovial lining becomes hypertrophied, forming villous projections into the joint space (Figure 20.4). Erosions of the cartilage can result, and there is often a great increase in synovial fluid, which has a high content of neutrophils but is not grossly purulent. All diarthrodial joints can be affected, but arthritis is most noticeable in the limb joints.

In the early stages of the arthritis *E. rhusiopathiae* is readily cultured from affected joints. Later the organism is harder to isolate, and some of the joints that have become chronically arthritic are seemingly culturally nega-

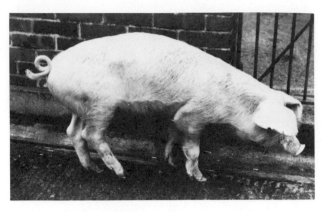

Figure 20.3. Erysipelothrix polyarthritis. Note the arched back, swollen right carpal region, and reluctance to bear weight on the right hind limb.

tive. This, together with the fact that the synovium in these cases is heavily infiltrated with mononuclear cells including many plasma cells (Figure 20.5), has inspired the thesis that the pathogenesis of the chronic disease has an immunological component (Collins and Goldie 1940). Further support for this theory includes an apparently higher incidence of and more severe form of arthritis in vaccinated swine after challenge (Freeman 1964, Neher et al. 1958) and the occurrence of autoantibody (rheumatoid factor) to complexed immunoglobulin in the serum and synovial fluid of some chronically arthritic swine (Sikes 1958, Timoney and Berman 1970a). Some

workers (Mercey and Bond 1977, Shuman et al. 1965), however, believe that vaccination has no effect on the incidence of arthritis. These observations, together with the gross and microscopic morphologic similarities that exist between the disease in pigs and rheumatoid arthritis in humans, led to the suggestion that erysipelothrix arthritis would be a useful model for the study of rheumatoid arthritis. However, erysipelothrix arthritis differs in some important ways from rheumatoid arthritis. Plasma cells in the synovium of arthritic pigs contain antibody to *Erysipelothrix*, and some arthritic synovial fluids contain higher antibody titers to the organism than companion serums (Timoney and Berman 1970a, 1970b). Levels of IgG immunoglobulins are higher in arthritic fluids than in serum—further evidence of local antibody synthesis and proof of the immunocompetence of the arthritic synovial tissue (Timoney and Yarkoni 1976). Unlike rheumatoid arthritis in humans, immune complexes seem to play a minor role in the pathogenesis of the disease in swine since there is no evidence of complement depletion (Timoney 1976a, 1976b) or of selective release of lysosomal enzymes (lysozyme, acid phosphatase) into joint fluids (Timoney 1976a, 1976b). The release of lysosomal enzymes might be expected to occur during phagocytosis of immune complexes. Instead, the cytoplasmic enzyme, lactic dehydrogenase, is present in amounts proportional to acid phosphatase levels—an indication of cell death and of a cytotoxic phenomenon. The cytotoxicity could be

Figure 20.4. Erysipelothrix arthritis in a stifle (*left*) and a shoulder joint (*right*). Note the hyperemia and hypertrophy of the synovial membranes and the villous projection extending onto the joint cartilage.

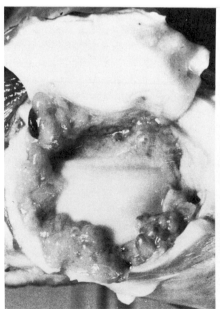
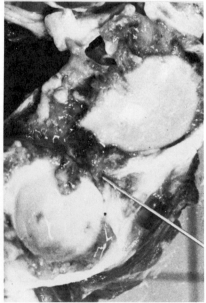

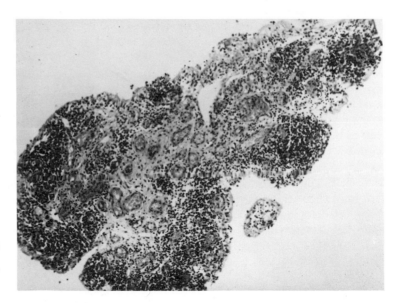

Figure 20.5. Erysipelothrix arthritis. A section of a hypertrophied villus showing cellular accumulations. These cells are mostly plasma and other mononuclear cells. × 110.

bacterial (Schulz et al. 1977) or immunological or both. The possibility that it is immunological must be invoked for arthritic joints that no longer contain viable *E. rhusiopathiae.*

Schulz et al. (1976) felt that fibrin deposition in the early stages is important in the pathogenesis of the chronic phase arthritis. They observed bacterial multiplication in the fibrin deposits (Schulz et al. 1977). It is possible that the chronicity and eventual apparent autonomicity of the arthritis is caused by erysipelothrix antigen that remains in organized fibrin deposits and continues to provoke a local immune response. Erysipelothrix antigens are known to persist in synovial tissue. White and Mirikitani (1976) demonstrated the persistence of a protein antigen, and Ajmal (1971), using the fluorescent antibody technique, observed antigen in synoviocytes of arthritic joints.

Many joints heal spontaneously with the disappearance of infection, but animals have been observed with both infected and healed joints at the same time (Timoney and Berman 1976b). This is a good indication of the need for the local presence of *E. rhusiopathiae* or its antigens in the maintenance of the local immune-inflammatory response. The rheumatoid factor seen in some arthritic synovial fluids is probably a response to complexes of erysipelothrix antigen and antibody. The rheumatoid factor occurs in swine hyperimmunized with erysipelas vaccines (Toshkov et al. 1968) and has also been produced in rabbits and guinea pigs immunized with complexes of killed *E. rhusiopathiae* cells and homologous IgG antibodies isolated from pig serum. It thus seems that the rheumatoid factor is not of primary importance in the pathogenesis of chronic erysipelas arthritis.

Much of the joint destruction seen in infected joints is undoubtedly a result of enzymes released from type A synoviocytes and from neutrophils attracted by *E. rhusiopathiae* or its products. The chemotactic stimulus in arthritic joints that are culturally negative is as yet unknown.

The disease in sheep. Polyarthritis caused by *E. rhusiopathiae* has been described in most sheep-raising areas of the world (Marsh 1931, Whitten 1952). The epizootiology of erysipelas in sheep is incompletely understood. The condition is seen in lambs beginning when they are 2 to 3 months old. Docking and castration wounds may be the route of entry in lambs. In older sheep the organism can enter shearing wounds from contaminated sheep-dip solution. The disease can also be contracted through umbilical infection, but this has not been proved. Affected animals develop a stiff gait and do not thrive although they eat well.

Animals with advanced cases often go down and have difficulty rising, but affected sheep seldom die of the disease. Lesions are not present in the visceral organs; in fact they are found nowhere except in some of the joints of the legs. One joint or several can be affected. The involved joint usually is swollen and the joint capsule is thickened. Granulation tissue develops on the inner surface of the capsule. The fluid is generally thin, but polymorphonuclear leukocytes are present in smears. The specific organism usually cannot be found in smears, but cultures are easily obtained.

The disease in cattle. In 1953 Moulton et al. reported an outbreak of arthritis in 6 of 20 calves in a herd involving the tibiotarsal, stifle, and carpal joints. *E. rhusio-*

pathiae was isolated from one of the infected joints. A case of bovine encephalomeningitis has also been attributed to this organism (Whaley et al. 1958).

The disease in birds. *E. rhusiopathiae* is pathogenic for turkeys, chickens, geese, ducks, mud hens, pigeons, parrots, quail, many small wild birds, and larger species often found in zoological parks. In the United States the turkey is most often and most seriously affected. The first outbreak was recognized by Beaudette and Hudson (1936).

Usually adult turkeys or birds nearing adult age are affected. They exhibit a cyanotic skin that is most obvious as a "blue comb." The birds become droopy, develop diarrhea, and die. Male birds frequently show the highest mortality. Lesions consist of massive hemorrhages and petechiae in the muscles of the breast and legs, also large hemorrhages from the various serous membranes, particularly those of the heart. Hemorrhages occur in the mucosa of the gizzard and the small intestine, and the contents of the intestine often are bloody. The liver and spleen ordinarily are congested and enlarged. The causative organism can be isolated easily from any of the tissues. In several reports of outbreaks in turkeys, it was noted that the first cases appeared within a few weeks after the birds came in contact with sheep or a sheep range. Erysipelas has also caused heavy losses in fattening ducks raised on free ranges that included large areas of standing water (Reetz and Schulz 1978).

The disease in laboratory animals. White mice and pigeons are highly susceptible to infection by inoculation and are commonly used in diagnostic work. They usually die 18 hours to 4 days after subcutaneous inoculation. Rabbits are not highly susceptible. Wayson (1927) has given a good account of a natural outbreak of this disease in wild mice, and Balfour-Jones (1935) has described an outbreak in laboratory mice.

The disease in aquatic animals. *E. rhusiopathiae* has been isolated from the spleen and liver tissue of caimans (*Caiman crocodilus*) and American crocodiles (*Crocodilus acutus*) (Jasmin and Baucom 1967). It also has produced an epizootic of septicemia in captive bottle-nosed dolphins (Geraci et al. 1966).

Immunity. Protective immunity against *E. rhusiopathiae* is mediated both by serum antibodies to the glycolipoprotein and by cell-mediated responses. The antigen responsible for the cell-mediated responses has not been identified.

Antibodies can be assayed by agglutination tests (Rice et al. 1952, Schoening et al. 1932, Timoney 1971), complement-fixation tests (Bercovich 1981), hemagglutination tests (Rhee and Lee 1971), and mouse protection tests (Sawada 1982).

A growth-agglutination test (*Wachstumsprobe*) is com-monly used in Europe (Wellman 1955). This test has been improved by Nielsen (1969), who incorporated the antibiotics of Wood's (1965) selective medium in the system to inhibit contaminants in the test serum.

Antibodies of both the IgG and the IgM isotypes are active in the growth-agglutination tests. Although a good correlation between mouse protection and growth agglutination titers has been found, there is no correlation between mouse protective antibody and protection of pigs after vaccination with live vaccine (Sawada 1979). This finding suggests that protection can be based on cell-mediated immune mechanisms as well as on serum antibody.

Immune serum is of value both for passive protection and for treatment. For therapy, 10 to 30 ml of serum is injected as soon as possible. The prophylactic dose of serum is 5 to 10 ml.

The first attenuated erysipelas vaccine was produced by Pasteur and Thuillier in 1883. Live attenuated vaccines that are currently available include the U.S. EVA (Erysipelas Vaccine Avirulent) (Gray and Norden 1955), the Swedish AV-R9 (Sandstedt and Lehnert 1944), and the German Dessan Spirovak strains. These vaccines stimulate protection for up to 8 months, and breeding stock should therefore be immunized at least once a year. Attenuated vaccines can also be administered in the drinking water (Ose et al. 1963) and as an aerosol (Mohlmann et al. 1972). In swine immunized by these routes there is a tonsillar blockade effect whereby the avirulent strain occupies colonization sites in the tonsils and prevents subsequent colonization by virulent strains; the avirulent strain stimulates an immune response as well. Because response to attenuated vaccines is adversely affected by maternal antibody, pigs vaccinated too early in life may not develop an immune response to the vaccine.

The feeding of medicated rations or rations contaminated with aflatoxin can also adversely affect immune responses, although Hopper (1981) found that feeding medicated rations to swine did not reduce the efficacy of live erysipelas vaccine. Use of live vaccine in pregnant swine is contraindicated because of the risk of abortion. In one incident the vaccine strain was recovered from aborted piglets 3 to 14 days after the sows were vaccinated (Henry 1979).

The immunity stimulated by attenuated strains is cell-mediated. Macrophages from mice immunized with EVA vaccine exhibit enhanced microbicidal activity for *E. rhusiopathiae* (Timoney 1969). The ability of mice to clear a challenge inoculum is present only so long as the vaccine strain persists in their tissues (Kuramasu et al. 1963). Presumably, the continued presence of the vaccine strain is necessary to maintain the cell-mediated immune response.

Killed vaccines are produced from cultures (serotype 2) designed for optimum production of the soluble protective glycolipoprotein antigen (White and Verwey 1970). Vaccines are formalinized and adsorbed to aluminum hydroxide. For long-term protection, this bacterin is injected subcutaneously in two doses 21 to 28 days apart. A single dose confers protection for up to 3 months and is usually sufficient for fattening swine vaccinated after weaning.

There has been considerable debate over the question of whether vaccination increases the frequency and severity of arthritis. In experiments a higher frequency of arthritis has been observed in vaccinated swine that subsequently were challenged with virulent organisms (Freeman 1964). Local infection by the organism undoubtedly is the primary cause of erysipelas arthritis. As discussed earlier, however, synovial tissue in this disease is immunocompetent; if the animal had previously been immunologically primed by exposure to *E. rhusiopathiae* antigen in the form of vaccine, it is reasonable to conclude that the response of immunocytes in the synovium to a second antigen exposure would be greater and there would be more severe tissue alteration. Vaccination thus might appear to increase the frequency of arthritis.

Diagnosis. The differentiation of acute swine erysipelas from hog cholera (swine fever) in the field is quite difficult, and even clinicians with much experience sometimes mistake one for the other. In cholera the affected animals are usually lethargic; in erysipelas they are usually bright and alert until shortly before death; erysipelas-affected animals frequently will continue to eat after they develop hyperthermia and other symptoms. Diarrhea is not as common in erysipelas as it is in cholera. The lesions often are not of great help in the differential diagnosis of these diseases. In erysipelas the spleen usually is slightly enlarged, tense, and bluish red in color, whereas in cholera it is usually unchanged or it may have one or more wedge-shaped infarcts along its margin. In erysipelas the mucosa of the stomach is often highly inflamed, showing a dark bluish red discoloration; this is not often found in cholera. The lymph nodes may or may not be congested in erysipelas, whereas they usually are hemorrhagic in cholera. Subserous hemorrhages of the epiglottis, trachea, kidneys, and urinary bladder can be found in both diseases but are ecchymotic in erysipelas and petechial in hog cholera.

Culturing blood from sick pigs usually results in isolation of *E. rhusiopathiae* in 18 hours, and there is a sensitive fluorescent antibody test that makes confirmation of hog cholera infection possible in a few hours. These diseases thus can be readily and rapidly distinguished by laboratory methods.

The growth-agglutination (*Wachstumsprobe*), mouse protection, complement-fixation, and agglutination tests have all been used for the serologic diagnosis of recent and chronic infections. Chronically affected animals often have titers in excess of 1:640 in the agglutination test. Many infected animals, however, do not have detectable agglutinins, yet are resistant to experimental infection. Moreover, the organism can persist in tissues with high antibody titers, such as synovial fluids (Timoney and Berman 1970a).

Antimicrobial Susceptibility. *E. rhusiopathiae* is very sensitive to penicillin G and ampicillin. Susceptibility to erythromycin, oxytetracyclines, and dihydrostreptomycin is variable, while all strains are resistant to kanamycin and sulfadimethoxazine (Takahashi 1983).

The Disease in Humans. Many cases of wound infection of the hands of humans have been reported. In Europe most of the human cases have been attributed to the handling of infected swine and pork, but some have occurred in fishermen and fish dealers who have had no contact with swine. The disease has also been observed in veterinarians, laboratory technicians, slaughterhouse personnel, and veterinary students (Klauder 1938, Morrill 1939, Wood 1975). The infection in humans is known as *erysipeloid* to distinguish it from human erysipelas, which is caused by a hemolytic *Streptococcus* species. The pathogen enters the body through small wounds or abrasions. The usual lesion is a localized, painful, purplish red swelling on a finger or arm. The center of the lesion eventually becomes pale and the superficial skin in this area may die and slough. There is no suppuration. A complication of erysipeloid is arthritis in nearby joints in about 5 percent of patients. Septicemia may occur on rare occasions.

REFERENCES

Ajmal, M. 1971. Experimental erysipelothrix arthritis. 1. Observations on specific-pathogen-free and gnotobiotic pigs following systematic administration of live *E. rhusiopathiae* or intra-articular injection of non-living *E. rhusiopathiae* cells or cell wall fragments. Res. Vet. Sci. 12:403–411.

Balfour-Jones, S.E.B. 1935. A bacillus resembling *Erysipelothrix muriseptica* isolated from necrotic lesions in the livers of mice. Br. J. Exp. Pathol. 16:236–243.

Beaudette, F.R., and Hudson, C.B. 1936. An outbreak of acute swine erysipelas infection in turkeys. J. Am. Vet. Med. Assoc. 88:475–488.

Bercovich, Z. 1981. Serological diagnosis of *Erysipelothrix rhusiopathiae:* A comparative study between the growth inhibition test and the complement fixation test. Vet. Q. 3:19–24.

Bratberg, A.M. 1981. Selective adherence of *Erysipelothrix rhusiopathiae* to heart valves of swine investigated in an *in vitro* test. Acta Vet. Scand. 22:39–45.

Collins, D.H., and Goldie, W. 1940. Observations on polyarthritis and an experimental erysipelothrix infection of swine. J. Pathol. Bacteriol. 50:321–353.

Dinter, Z., Diderholm, H., and Rockborn, G. 1976. Complement-fixation hemolysis following hemagglutination by *Erysipelothrix rhusiopathiae*. Zentralbl. Bakteriol. [Orig. A] 236:533–535.

Dougherty, R.W., Shuman, R.D., Mullenax, C.H., Witzel, D.A.,

Buck, W.B., Wood, R.L., and Cook, H.M. 1965. Physiopathological studies of erysipelas in pigs. Cornell Vet. 55:87–109.

Freeman, M.J. 1964. Effects of vaccination on the development of arthritis in swine with erysipelas: Clinical, hematologic, and gross pathologic observations. Am. J. Vet. Res. 25:589–598.

Geraci, J.R., Sauer, R.M., and Medway, W. 1966. Erysipelas in dolphins. Am. J. Vet. Res. 27:597–606.

Gledhill, A.W. 1945. The antigenic structure of *Erysipelothrix*. J. Pathol. Bacteriol. 57:179–189.

Gray, C.W., and Norden, C.J. 1955. Erysipelas vaccine avirulent (EVA)—A new agent for erysipelas control. J. Am. Vet. Med. Assoc. 127:506–510.

Hajduk, V., and Puhac, I. 1974. Pedological composition and pH of the soil as a factor in the epizootiology of erysipelas in swine within the territory of Sid. Vet. Glas. 28:369–372.

Henry, S. 1979. Swine abortion associated with the use of live erysipelas vaccine. J. Clin. Vet. Med. Assoc. 175:453–454.

Hopper, R.J. 1981. Efficacy of swine erysipelas vaccine given simultaneously with medicated rations. Vet. Med./Small Anim. Clin. 76:1345–1347.

Jasmin, A.M., and Baucom, J. 1967. *Erysipelothrix insidiosa* infections in the caiman (*Caiman crocidilus*) and the American crocodile (*Crocodile acutus*). Vet. Clin. Pathol. 1:173–177.

Klauder, J.V. 1938. Erysipeloid as an occupational disease. J.A.M.A. 111:1345–1348.

Krasemann, C., and Muller, H.E. 1975. The virulence of *Erysipelothrix rhusiopathiae* strains and their neuraminidase production. Zentralbl. Bakteriol. [Orig. A] 231:206–213.

Kuramasu, S., Imamura, Y., Sameshima, T., and Tajima, Y. 1963. Studies on erysipelosis. II. Changes in the characters of bacteria and in the response of mice after inoculation with the acriflavin-attenuated strain CHIRAN. Zentralbl. Veterinärmed. [B] 10:362–379.

Lachmann, P.G., and Deicher, H. 1986. Solubilization and characterization of surface antigenic components of *Erysipelothrix rhusiopathiae* T28. Infect. Immun. 52:818–822.

Leimbeck, R., Bohm, K.H., Ehard, H., and Schulz, L.-C. 1975. Studies of the toxic components of *Erysipelothrix rhusiopathiae*. II. Detailed characterization of an extracted endotoxin. Zentralbl. Bakteriol. [Orig. A] 232:266–286.

Marsh, H. 1931. The bacillus of swine erysipelas associated with arthritis in lambs. J. Am. Vet. Med. Assoc. 78:57–63.

Mercey, A.R., and Bond, M.P. 1977. Vaccination of pigs against *Erysipelothrix rhusiopathiae*. Aust. Vet. J. 53:600.

Mohlmann, H., Stohr, P., Schulz, V., and Michael-Meere, M. 1972. Investigation on the possibility of experimental aerogenic infection of pigs with erysipelas and its course. Arch. Exp. Veterinärmed. 26:1–9.

Morrill, C.C. 1939. Erysipeloid: Occurrence among veterinary students. J. Infect. Dis. 65:322–324.

Moulton, J.E., Rhode, E.R., and Wheat, J.D. 1953. Erysipelatous arthritis in calves. J. Am. Vet. Med. Assoc. 123:335–340.

Muller, H.E. 1971. Occurrence of neuraminidase in *Erysipelothrix insidiosa*. Pathol. Microbiol. 37:241–248.

Muller, H.E. 1974. The protection of mice by a specific anti-*Erysipelothrix insidiosa*-neuraminidase-antiserum against *Erysipelothrix insidiosa* infection. Med. Microbiol. Immunol. 159:301–308.

Muller, H.E., and Bohm, K.H. 1977. Neuraminidase neutralizing and precipitating antibodies in commercial erysipelas serum. Berl. Münch. Tierärztl. Wochenschr. 90:314–316.

Neher, G.M., Swenson, C.B., Doyle, L.P., and Sikes, D. 1958. The incidence of arthritis in swine following vaccination for swine erysipelas. Am. J. Vet. Res. 19:5–14.

Nielsen, N.C. 1969. The use of a selective medium in the growth-agglutination test for chronic *Erysipelothrix insidiosa* infections in swine. Acta Vet. Scand. 10:127–136.

Norrung, V. 1979. Two new serotypes of *Erysipelothrix rhusiopathiae*. Nord. Vet. Med. 31:462–465.

Ose, E.E., Barnes, L.E., and Berkman, R.N. 1963. Experimental evaluation of an avirulent erysipelas vaccine. J. Am. Vet. Med. Assoc. 143:1084–1089.

Reetz, G., and Schulz, L. 1978. Erysipelas infection of fattening ducks. Monatsschr. Vet. Med. 33:170–173.

Rhee, Y.O., and Lee, H.S. 1971. Serological studies on swine erysipelas antibodies using the passive haemagglutination (PHA) test and the tube agglutination test. Research Report of the Office of Rural Development, Korean Veterinary Service, no. 14. Pp. 17–22.

Rice, C.E., Connell, R., Byrne, J.L., and Boulanger, P. 1952. Studies of swine erysipelas. IV. Serological diagnosis in swine. Can. J. Comp. Med. 16:209–215.

Sandstedt, H., and Lehnert, E. 1944. Experience of swine erysipelas immunization in 1943. Sven. Vet. Tidskr. 56:189.

Sawada, T. 1982. Estimation of protective immunity of pigs inoculated with swine erysipelas live vaccine by passive mouse protection test. Jpn. J. Vet. Sci. 44:565–570.

Schoening, W.H., Creech, G.F., and Grey, C.G. 1932. A laboratory tube test and a whole blood rapid agglutination test for the diagnosis of swine erysipelas. North Am. Vet. 13:19–25.

Schulz, L.-C., Drommer, W., Ehard, H., Hertrampf, B., Leibold, W., Messow, C., Mumme, J., Trautwein, G., Ueberschar, S., Weib, R., and Winkelmann, J. 1977. The pathogenic significance of *Erysipelothrix rhusiopathiae* in the acute and chronic form of erysipelas arthritis. D.T.W. 84:107–111.

Schulz, L.-C., Ehard, H., Drommer, W., Seidler, D., Trautwein, G., Hertrampf, B., Giese, W., and Hazem, A.S. 1976. The pathogenic significance of the acute phase of erysipelas for the manifestation of chronic changes in organs: Comparative experimental studies in the pig, mouse and rat. Zentralbl. Veterinärmed. [B] 23:617–637.

Shuman, R.D., Wood, R.L., and Cheville, N.F. 1965. Sensitization by *Erysipelothrix rhusiopathiae (insidiosa)* with relation to arthritis in pigs. II. Pretreatment with dead cells of serotypes A and B and challenge with live homologous or heterologous cells. Cornell Vet. 55:387–396.

Sikes, D. 1958. A comparison of rheumatoid-like arthritis in swine with rheumatoid arthritis in man. Ann. N.Y. Acad. Sci. 70:717–723.

Takahashi, T. 1983. Antibiotic resistance of *Erysipelothrix rhusiopathiae* isolated from pigs with chronic swine erysipelas. Antimicrob. Agents Chemother. 25:385–386.

Takahashi, T., Fujisawa, T., Benno, Y., Tamura, Y., Sawada, T., Suzuki, S., Muramatsu, M., and Mitsuoka, T. 1987. *Erysipelothrix tonsillarum* sp. nov. isolated from tonsils of apparently healthy pigs. Int. J. Syst. Bacteriol. 37:166–169.

Takahashi, T., Sawada, T., Takagi, M., Seto, K., Kanzaki, M., Maruyama, T. 1984. Serotypes of *Erysipelothrix rhusiopathiae* strains isolated from slaughter pigs affected with chronic erysipelas. Jpn. J. Vet. Sci. 46:149–153.

Ten Broeck, C. 1920. Studies on *Bacillus murisepticus,* or the rotlauf bacillus, isolated from swine in the United States. J. Exp. Med. 32:331–343.

Timoney, J. 1969. The inactivation of *Erysipelothrix rhusiopathiae* in macrophages from normal and immune mice. Res. Vet. Sci. 10:301–302.

Timoney, J. 1970. The inactivation of *Erysipelothrix rhusiopathiae* in pig buffy-coat leukocytes. Res. Vet. Sci. 11:189–190.

Timoney, J. 1971. Antibody and rheumatoid factor in synovia of pigs with erysipelothrix polyarthritis. J. Comp. Pathol. 81:243–248.

Timoney, J.F. 1976a. Erysipelas arthritis in swine: Concentration of complement and third component of complement in synovia. Am. J. Vet. Res. 37:5–8.

Timoney, J.F. 1976b. Erysipelas arthritis in swine: Lysosomal enzyme levels in synovial fluids. Am. J. Vet. Res. 37:295–298.

Timoney, J.F., and Berman, D.T. 1970a. *Erysipelothrix* arthritis in swine: Serum-synovial fluid gradients for antibody and serum proteins in normal and arthritic joints. Am. J. Vet. Res. 31:1405–1409.

Timoney, J.F., and Berman, D.T. 1970b. *Erysipelothrix* arthritis in swine: Bacteriologic and immune-pathologic aspects. Am. J. Vet. Res. 31:1411–1421.

Timoney, J.F., and Yarkoni, U. 1976. Immunoglobulins IgG and IgM in synovial fluids of swine with *Erysipelothrix* polyarthritis. Vet. Microbiol. 1:467–474.

Toshkov, A., Toshkov, A., Stoev, I., Sokolova, E., and Karadjov, Y. 1968. Rheumatoid-like factors in the sera of swine hyperimmunized with *Erysipelothrix insidiosa*. C. R. Acad. Bulg. Sci. 21:1101–1103.

Von Jowtscheff, E. 1961. Zur Anwendung des Thorntestes bei gesunden und rotlaufkranken Schweinen. Monatsschr. Vet. Med. 16:216–218.

Wayson, N.E. 1927. An epizootic among meadow mice in California, caused by the bacillus of mouse septicemia or of swine erysipelas. U.S. Public Health Service Report No. 42. Pp. 1489–1493.

Wellman, G.G. 1955. Summaries of experiments in swine erysipelas in Germany. J. Am. Vet. Med. Assoc. 127:331–333.

Whaley, A.E., Robinson, V.B., Newberre, J.W., and Sipple, W.L. 1958. Bovine encephalo-meningitis associated with erysipelas infection. Vet. Med. 53:475–476.

White, R.R., and Verwey, W.F. 1970. Solubilization and characteriza-tion of a protective antigen of *Erysipelothrix rhusiopathiae*. Infect. Immun. 1:387–393.

White, T.G., and Mirikitani, F.K. 1976. Some biological and physico-chemical properties of *Erysipelothrix rhusiopathiae*. Cornell Vet. 66:152–163.

Whitten, L.K. 1952. A further note on lameness in sheep due to *Erysipelothrix rhusiopathiae*. Aust. Vet. J. 28:6–7.

Wood, R.L. 1965. A selective liquid medium utilizing antibiotics for isolation of *Erysipelothrix insidiosa*. Am. J. Vet. Res. 26:1303–1308.

Wood, R.L. 1975. Erysipelothrix infection. In W.T. Hubbert, W.F. McCulloch. and P.R. Schnurrenberger, eds., Diseases transmitted from Animals to Men, 6th ed. Charles C. Thomas, Springfield, Ill. Pp. 271–281.

Wood, R.L., Haubrich, D.R., and Harrington, R. 1978. Isolation of previously unreported serotypes of *Erysipelothrix rhusiopathiae* from swine. Am. J. Vet. Res. 39:1958–1961.

21 The Genus *Bacillus*

There are 22 species and 26 closely related taxa currently described in the genus *Bacillus,* but almost all are saprophytes and nonpathogenic for animals. The most pathogenic species is *B. anthracis,* the cause of anthrax in animals and humans and immortalized as the infectious agent upon which Koch based his famous postulates. *B. cereus* and *B. licheniformis* are occasionally isolated from cattle with bovine mastitis and from horses and cattle with suppurative lesions. These organisms have almost no invasive ability by themselves and multiply only in tissues weakened by injury or other infections.

Although *B. piliformis* carries the generic name *Bacillus,* there is no biochemical, genetic, or other evidence to support its inclusion in the genus. It is, however, an obligate intracellular parasite of a variety of mammalian species and resembles other members of the genus *Bacillus* in its production of resistant spores, so it will be included in this chapter.

Bacillus anthracis

B. anthracis causes the disease known as *anthrax* (in German, *milzbrand;* in French, *charbon*). Herbivorous animals are highly susceptible to infection by *B. anthracis*; carnivorous birds and reptiles are resistant. The disease is often fatal in humans, although they are not as susceptible as herbivores.

Morphology and Staining Reactions. The anthrax bacillus is a large, Gram-positive rod about 1 μm in diameter and 3 to 6 μm long. In cultures it forms long chains, which when unstained appear as solid filaments because the square ends of the individual cells fit very closely together (Figure 21.1). Long filaments are never seen in tissues, and the ends of the cells are rounded. Here the elements occur either individually or in short chains of two to five or six organisms and are regularly encapsulated, a single capsule enclosing as many organisms as remain in a chain (Figure 21.2). The capsules are well marked and can be readily stained. Spores are formed in abundance at 15° to 40°C when the organism is growing in the presence of air. Sporulation is inhibited by a high CO_2 tension such as occurs in dead carcasses; thus spores are rare in blood and internal organs. The spores are central to subterminal and nonswollen (Figure 21.1).

Cultural and Biochemical Features. *B. anthracis* grows well on most laboratory media exposed to atmospheric oxygen. Growth occurs at temperatures from 12° to 44°C, with optimum growth at 37°C. Anaerobic conditions result in meager growth. Spores germinate when exposed to 65°C for 15 minutes and change into the vegetative bacillary form.

On agar plates the anthrax organisms form surface colonies with a ground-glass appearance (Figure 21.3). The margins of these colonies are irregular and under low magnification resemble locks of wavy hair (Figure 21.4). It is for this reason that they are sometimes described as Medusa-head colonies, after the mythological creature whose flowing locks were changed to serpents. Deep colonies are small, ragged, and stringy. Other aerobic spore-forming bacilli whose surface colonies resemble *B. anthracis* form small, compact colonies in the depths of agar

Figure 21.1. *Bacillus anthracis* in a stained preparation from a 24-hour-old culture on solid media. Note the arrangement of cells in long chains and the development of spores in many of the organisms. × 896.

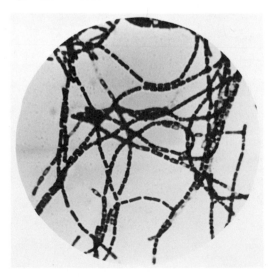

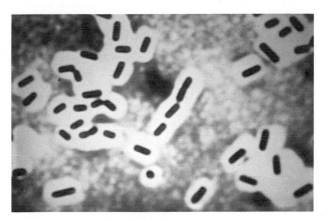

Figure 21.2. *Bacillus anthracis* in a bovine spleen. The polyglutamic acid capsule is clearly visible. × 864.

cultures and thereby can be distinguished from *B. anthracis*.

On 50 percent serum agar or brain heart infusion agar containing 0.5 percent sodium bicarbonate in an atmosphere of 65 percent CO_2, *B. anthracis* produces smooth, mucoid colonies and the organism is encapsulated. On blood agar, only a narrow zone of hemolysis is produced, in contrast to other anthracoid *Bacillus* species, which frequently produce a wide hemolytic zone.

Biochemically *B. anthracis* is much less active than other similar but nonpathogenic *Bacillus* species; it produces acid but no gas in glucose, sucrose, maltose, and salicin (Table 21.1).

B. anthracis is never motile. Alpha-glucosidase activity is increased in *B. anthracis* by incubation in 1 percent Triton X-100, whereas this activity is reduced in other anthracoid *Bacillus* species (Sadler et al. 1984).

The capsule is composed of polymers of D-glutamic acid residues and can also include some polysaccharide. Capsule production is plasmid-mediated (Uchida et al. 1985) and is enhanced by the presence of 0.7 percent bovine serum albumin. Virulent strains are always encapsulated. The spores resist steaming or boiling at 100°C for 5 minutes but are killed by autoclaving at 120°C for 20 minutes. They are also resistant to disinfectants such as 5 percent phenol or mercuric chloride. A 2 to 3 percent solution of formalin is effective if applied at a temperature of 40°C. A 0.25 percent solution is also effective when applied for 6 hours at 60°C. Spores have been shown to remain viable for more than 50 years (Umeno and Nobata 1938). Burlap feed bags can be disinfected by heating to 113°C for 30 minutes (Bryan 1953). Laboratory personnel should be aware that anthrax spores are not necessarily killed by the heat required to fix smears on microscope slides. The vegetative phase of *B. anthracis* is killed in 30 minutes at 60°C and is quickly destroyed by enzymic action and the effects of putrefactive bacteria in decaying carcasses.

Epizootiology and Pathogenesis. The major anthrax enzootic zones of the world are found in the tropics and subtropics—India, Pakistan, Africa, and South America, for example. The factors that determine this distribution

Figure 21.3 (*left*). A surface colony of *Bacillus anthracis* on agar photographed by transmitted light to show the ground-glass appearance. × 6.4.

Figure 21.4 (*right*). An impression preparation of *Bacillus anthracis* from a colony on a gelatin plate. The formation of long filamentous chains that lie parallel to each other accounts for the Medusa-head appearance of colonies. × 170.

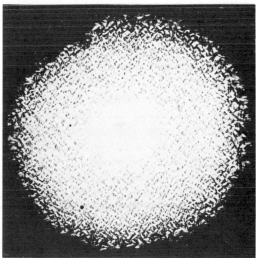
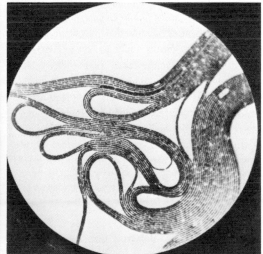

Table 21.1. Biochemical and other properties of *B. anthracis* and similar anthracoid *Bacillus* species

Property	*B. anthracis*	Other anthracoid *Bacillus* spp.
Motility	Nonmotile	Usually motile
Hemolysis	Absent or slight	Wide zone
Gamma phage susceptibility	Susceptible	Not susceptible
Penicillin (0.5 U/ml) sensitivity	Sensitive (most strains)	Resistant
Litmus milk coagulation and peptonization	Slow	Rapid
Gelatin hydrolysis	Slow	Rapid
Methylene blue reduction	Slow	Rapid
Salicin acid fermentation	Slow	Rapid
Lecithinase production	Absent or slight	Marked
Pathogenicity for guinea pigs, mice	Pathogenic	Nonpathogenic
Hydrolysis of *p*-nitro-phenyl alpha-D-glucoside in presence of 1 percent Triton X-100	Enhanced	Diminished

are related to the circumstances and conditions that allow sporulation of *B. anthracis* in discharges from carcasses and subsequent vegetative multiplication in the soil. The principal areas of enzootic anthrax are regions with alkaline soils with a high nitrogen level caused by decaying vegetation, alternating periods of rain and drought, and temperatures in excess of 15.5°C. Such areas have been described by van Ness (1965) as "incubator areas." The basis of the incubator area concept is that temporary accumulation of water causes vegetation to die and humus to increase when the temperature exceeds 15.5°C, thereby providing conditions for spore germination and vegetative multiplication. As the area dries out resporulation occurs. Cattle then gain access to these sites, graze down to ground level, and ingest the contaminated soils.

In the United States, endemic anthrax areas generally are found wherever there are soils rich in calcium and nitrogen, and with a periodic abundance of water. Many of these areas are found along the Sedalia Cattle Trail in Oklahoma and were first seeded with *B. anthracis* from dying cattle in the 1800s. Stern and van Ness (1955) reported the results of a 10-year survey of anthrax in the United States. From 1945 to 1954 losses among cattle, horses, mules, swine, and sheep were reported to be 17,604. These cases appeared in 3,447 outbreaks in 30 states. States reporting no cases were Arizona, Connecticut, Delaware, Idaho, Maine, New Hampshire, Rhode Island, Vermont, and West Virginia. States reporting 100 or more outbreaks were California (271), Illinois (205), Indiana (222), Iowa (133), Kansas (368), Louisiana (413), Missouri (267), New Jersey (114), Ohio (317), South Dakota (150), Tennessee (142), and Texas (288).

The incidence of anthrax in wild herbivores can be greatly increased by activities such as road building, fencing, and the provision of artificial watering points (Berry 1981). The alkaline gravel pits needed for road building provide man-made incubator areas for the organism.

Sources of infection for animals other than the soils of incubator areas also exist and in some regions are far more significant. In England, for instance, imported bone meals and vegetable proteins such as groundnut are an important source of infection for livestock. Wool and hair wastes, cleanings used in fertilizers, and tannery effluents can also be sources of infection.

Affected animals shed large numbers of the organism, and other animals in the group are thereby exposed; however, lateral contagion is not an important feature of anthrax outbreaks. Bloodsucking flies and carrion eaters can transmit or transport the anthrax organism (Cousineau and McClenaghan 1965).

Natural infection of animals can occur via the skin or respiratory tract but usually occurs by ingestion of spores, which germinate and produce vegetative bacilli, either in the mucosa of the throat or in the intestinal tract. The polyglutamic acid capsule formed on the surface of vegetative cells protects them from phagocytosis, lytic antibodies, and the bactericidal effect of the serum cationic peptide, PC III (Carroll and Martinez 1981). The organisms multiply in an edematous focus near the site of primary invasion and then spread through the lymphatic channels to lymph nodes, where multiplication continues. The organism eventually invades the bloodstream and is filtered out in the spleen until splenic clearance capacity is exceeded. Uncontrolled multiplication continues in the blood until the animal dies. At death, 80 percent of the organisms are in the blood and 20 percent are in the spleen, which is often greatly enlarged. Death of the animal results from the effects of the extracellular toxic complex released by the organism (Smith et al. 1955). The toxic complex, or holotoxin, consists of three protein fac-

Table 21.2. Components of the holotoxin of *B. anthracis*

Component	Properties
I (Edema factor)	Adenylate cyclase
II (Protective antigen)	Receptor binding molecule for EF and LF; immunogenic
III (Lethal factor)	Lethal for mice; depression of central nervous system; immunogenic

tors: edema factor (EF), protective antigen (PA), and lethal factor (LF) (Stanley and Smith 1961). These factors have also been named factors I, II, and III (Table 21.2). Edema factor is an adenylate cyclase that increases intracellular cyclic AMP concentrations after activation by cellular calmodulin (Leppla 1982). Protective antigen, the predominant protein produced, is plasmid-encoded and necessary for biological activity of EF and LF and is probably a receptor-binding molecule. The mode of action of LF is unknown. It causes depression of the central nervous system, and antibodies to it and to PA are protective. The net effect of the holotoxin is to damage and kill phagocytes, increase capillary cell permeability (Figure 21.5), damage the clotting mechanism, and inhibit the bactericidal effect of serum. Capillary thrombosis occurs and fluid leaks through damaged capillary endothelium. Blood pressure falls, and the animal lapses into shock. Because the toxic complex also blocks the opsonizing activity of the C3 factor of complement, phagocytosis is reduced. Animals with anthrax thus exhibit edema, shock, and hemorrhaging before death—effects that can be neutralized by specific antiserum. A lethal quantity

Figure 21.5. Anthrax in a mouse. Note the characteristic accumulation of gelatinous material (*arrow*) in the peritoneum. This is extravasated fluid that has clotted.

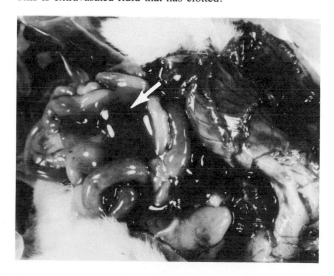

of toxin is elaborated some time before the organism attains the populations found in the blood and spleen after the animal dies (Smith et al. 1955). Antibiotic therapy must therefore be initiated early in the course of the infection before a lethal concentration of toxin has been elaborated.

The manifestations of the disease depend on the manner of infection. When it occurs through the respiratory or gastrointestinal tract with no visible evidence of a localization, its principal character is its sudden onset and rapidly fatal course. The peracute form that sometimes occurs in herbivores can terminate fatally in 1 or 2 hours, the acute form in less than 24 hours. The animals have a high fever, increased respiratory and cardiac rates, and congested mucosae. They are depressed and listless, and may bleed from body openings.

Localized anthrax is seen when infection has occurred through a wound in the skin. This form occurs naturally more often in humans than in any domestic animals. Recovery is more likely when the disease is localized than when it is septicemic. Localized infections often become generalized, however. Cases in grazing animals usually are acute or peracute, and most are fatal. Horses can exhibit signs of colic and edematous swellings of the throat, neck, and shoulders. In swine and dogs anthrax generally assumes a localized form with pharyngeal involvement and gastroenteritis. These animals are infected only by ingesting heavily contaminated food, either the raw meat of other animals that have died of anthrax or, in the case of swine, infected bone or meat meal given as a feed supplement. In these cases the organism apparently enters the tissues from the upper part of the digestive tract, probably through the tonsils, and the disease is manifested by an inflammatory edema of the tissues of the head and neck. Often these regions become greatly distorted and swollen, and suffocation can occur as a result of severe edema of the glottis. The infection occasionally localizes in the intestinal wall, the mesenteric lymph nodes, and the spleen of these animals.

A number of outbreaks of anthrax have occurred in mink, and mortality can be very high. The disease in this species is generally peracute and generalized and occurs when fresh meat from an infected carcass has been fed to the animals.

Generalized anthrax can easily be induced in susceptible animals by exposure to air-borne spores.

Immunity. Although the polyglutamic acid of the capsule protects the organism from phagocytosis, capsular antibodies are not protective. Effective vaccines must contain the protective antigen (PA) or the lethal factor (LF) or both. Antibodies to PA neutralize the effects of both LF and the edema factor (EF) by preventing their binding to receptor sites on cells. Toxic damage to leukocytes is also prevented and so the invading organism is rapidly phagocytosed and killed. Because the genes for PA synthesis have been cloned in *E. coli*, it should soon be technically feasible to obtain large amounts of this antigen for vaccine production.

The first vaccine against anthrax was made in 1879 by Pasteur, who discovered that cultivation at 43°C reduced the organism's virulence. The loss of virulence observed by Pasteur has recently been shown to be the result of the loss of a temperature-sensitive plasmid that encodes the genes for PA (Mikesell et al. 1983). Pasteur's vaccine was eventually superseded by spore vaccines with better keeping qualities. Spore vaccines were prepared from avirulent noncapsulated variants. Later refinement involved the addition of saponin to delay dissemination of the spores into the tissues and provide an adjuvant effect (Carbozoo vaccine).

The Sterne (Sterne 1937) vaccine is produced by growing virulent anthrax strains on 50 percent serum agar in an atmosphere of 10 to 30 percent CO_2.

Diagnosis. In many areas, anthrax is a notifiable disease; that is, state authorities must be informed of any reasonable suspicion of its presence. Diagnosis should be attempted by methods that release a minimum number of anthrax organisms into the environment. Exposure to atmospheric oxygen will allow the formation of spores, which will subsequently be extremely difficult to destroy. Samples of blood should be collected from a site such as an ear vein into a syringe and taken to the laboratory for preparation of smears for microscopic examination and for culture. Swabs or smears of local edematous lesions can also be examined.

Use of McFadyean's stain, as described by Parry et al. (1983), allows demonstration of the capsule, which stains pink, in contrast to the body of the organism, which stains blue. Spores are not usually seen in smears from specimens. A fluorescent antibody test is also available but is not particularly specific (Doyle et al. 1985). Capsular antigen in tissues or hides can be detected by an agar-gel precipitin technique (Ascoli's test), but this test, although very useful, is not absolutely specific.

There is little difficulty in culturing *B. anthracis* from fresh material. The characteristic ground-glass type nonhemolytic colonies can be grown on blood agar. The identity of the organism is confirmed by demonstration of (1) the production of capsules on brain heart infusion agar containing 0.5 percent sodium bicarbonate and incubated in 10 to 30 percent CO_2; (2) sensitivity to penicillin; (3) lack of motility, (4) increased alpha-glucosidase activity in 1 percent Triton X-100; (5) reaction with antiserum to protective antigen (Ristroph and Ivins 1983); (6) sensitivity to gamma bacteriophage (Brown and Cherry

1955); and, (7) inoculation of laboratory animals. Direct inoculation of guinea pigs with tissues, exudates, and the like, is a reliable method for diagnosing the disease provided the material does not contain other organisms such as clostridia, which are pathogenic in their own right. If viable anthrax organisms are present and if the animal does not die from other causes, it will usually die from anthrax 36 to 48 hours after subcutaneous injection. Occasionally death is as late as the fifth day after injection. Swarms of organisms will be found in the tissues of guinea pigs and mice, and there will be a gelatinous infiltration under the skin at the site of inoculation.

Isolation of *B. anthracis* from decomposing carcasses can be very difficult. Heating the specimen to 70°C for 10 minutes can be of help in the elimination of contaminating non-spore-bearing organisms. Dilutions of this material can then be inoculated into test animals. Capsular and protective antigen can be sought in tissue extracts by means of specific antiserums in agar gel precipitin tests. Rough, nonencapsulated dissociants that arise are then tested for loss of virulence by animal inoculation. Avirulent strains distinguished in this way are used for large-scale vaccine production throughout the world (Figure 21.6). One dose of vaccine given intradermally will protect an animal for 1 year.

Tests with alum-precipitated supernatant material from fermenter cultures have shown that they are also effective in immunizing cattle, sheep, and humans (Brachman et al. 1962, Jackson et al. 1957, Prokupek et al. 1981, Puziss and Wright 1963). This vaccine is the one currently used in humans. Antiserum can be effective in alleviating symptoms of anthrax and in prophylaxis; however, in many areas anthrax antiserum is no longer commercially available.

Antimicrobial Susceptibility. *B. anthracis* is very sensitive to penicillin G, ampicillin, sulfathiazole, chloramphenicol, and streptomycin. Gill (1982) described the use of depot preparations of penicillin in the control of an outbreak of anthrax in dairy cows. Doses of 2,500 mg procaine and 2,500 mg benethamine penicillin prevented development of new cases.

Disposal of Carcasses Infected with Anthrax. The carcasses of animals that die of anthrax should be completely burned or buried deeply in quick lime (calcium oxide). When carcasses have been opened and the parts scattered, the anthrax bacillus may sporulate, and the spores can remain viable in a contaminated area for many years.

The Disease in Humans. Cutaneous anthrax takes the form of an edematous swelling that is hot and painful at first but later becomes cold and painless. This type of lesion is known as a *malignant carbuncle.* Respiratory

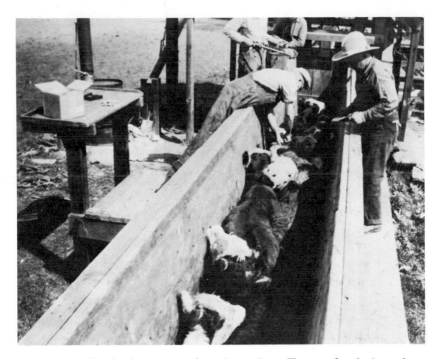

Figure 21.6. Vaccinating range cattle against anthrax. The use of such chutes for restraining semiwild range cattle is common. (Courtesy Jen-Sal Laboratories, Inc.)

infections can occur among employees of factories in which hides, wool, and hair contaminated with spores are processed. These infections are rapidly fulminating and are known as *woolsorters' disease*.

REFERENCES

Berry, H.H. 1981. Abnormal levels of disease and predation as limiting factors for wildebeest in the Etosha National Park. Madoqua 12:241–253.

Brachman, P.S., Gold, M., Plotkin, S.A., Fekety, F.R., Werrin, M., and Ingraham, N.R. 1962. Field evaluation of a human anthrax vaccine. Am. J. Public Health 52:632–645.

Brown, E.R. and Cherry, W.B. 1955. Specific identification of *Bacillus anthracis* by means of a variant bacteriophage. J. Infect. Dis. 96:34–39.

Bryan, H.S. 1953. The effect of dielectric heat on anthrax spores under feed-bag processing plant conditions. Am. J. Vet. Res. 14:328–330.

Carroll, S.F. and Martinez, R.J. 1981. Antibacterial peptide from normal rabbit serum. 3. Inhibition of microbial electron transport. Biochemistry 20:5988–5994.

Cousineau, S.G. and McClenaghan, R.J. 1965. Anthrax in bison in the northwest territories. Can. Vet. J. 6:22–24.

Doyle, R.J., Keller, K.F., and Ezzell, J.W. 1985. Bacillus. In E.H. Lennette, A. Balows, W.J. Hausler, and H.J. Shadomy, eds., Manual of Clinical Microbiology, 4th ed. American Society for Microbiology, Washington, D.C. Pp. 211–215.

Gill, I.J. 1982. Antibiotic therapy in the control of an outbreak of anthrax in dairy cows (correspondence). Aust. Vet. J. 58:214–215.

Jackson, F.C., Wright, G.G., and Armstrong, S. 1957. Immunization of cattle against experimental anthrax with alum-precipitated protective antigen or spore vaccine. Am. J. Vet. Res. 18:771–777.

Leppla, S.H. 1982. Anthrax toxin edema factor: A bacterial adenylate cyclase that increases cyclic AMP concentrations in eukaryotic cells. Proc. Natl. Acad. Sci. USA 79:7–9.

Mikesell, P., Ivins, B.E., Ristroph, J.D., and Dreier, T.D. 1983. Evidence for plasmid-mediated toxin production in *Bacillus anthracis*. Infect. Immun. 39:371–376.

Parry, J.A., Turnbull, P.C.B., and Gibson, J.R. 1983. A Colour Atlas of *Bacillus Species*. Wolfe Medical Publications, London.

Prokupek, K., Dvorak, R., and Polaecnk, R. 1981. Immunogenic effect of anthrax protective antigen. Vet. Med. 26:279–290.

Puziss, M., and Wright, G.G. 1963. Studies on immunity in anthrax. X. Gel-adsorbed protective antigen for immunization of man. J. Bacteriol. 85:230–236.

Ristroph, J.D. and Ivins, B.E. 1983. Elaboration of *Bacillus anthracis* antigens in a new defined culture medium. Infect. Immun. 39:483–486.

Sadler, D.F., Ezzell, J.W., Keller, K.F., and Doyle, R.J. 1984. Glycosidase activities of *Bacillus anthracis*. J. Clin. Microbiol. 19:594–598.

Smith, M., Keppie, J., and Stanley, J.L. 1955. The chemical basis of the virulence of *Bacillus anthracis*. V. The specific toxin produced by *B. anthracis* in vivo Br. J. Exp. Pathol. 36:460–466.

Stanley, J.L., and Smith, M. 1961. Purification of factor 1 and recognition of a third factor of the anthrax toxin. J. Gen. Microbiol. 26:49–66.

Stern, D.C., and van Ness, G.B. 1955. A ten-year survey of anthrax in livestock with special reference to outbreaks in 1954. Vet. Med. 50:579–588.

Sterne, M. 1937. The effects of different carbon dioxide concentrations on the growth of virulent anthrax strains. Pathogenicity and immunogenicity tests on guinea pigs and sheep with anthrax variants derived from virulent strains. Onderstepoort J. Vet. Sci. Anim. Indust. 9:49–67.

Uchida, I., Sekizaki, T., Hashimoto, K., and Terakado, N. 1985. Association of the encapsulation of *Bacillus anthracis* with a 60 megadalton plasmid. J. Gen. Microbiol. 131:363–367.

Umeno, S., and Nobata, R. 1938. On viability of anthrax spores. J. Jpn. Soc. Vet. Sci. 17:221–223. (English summary p. 87.)

van Ness, G., and Stein, C.D. 1956. Soils of the United States favorable for anthrax. J. Am. Vet. Med. Assoc. 128:7–9.

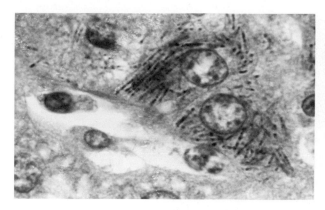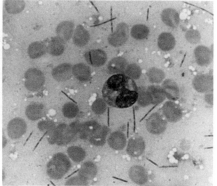

Figure 21.7. (*Left*) Clumps of *Bacillus piliformis* within mouse hepatocytes. Gomori's methenamine silver nitrate stain. (*Right*) The individual organisms in a smear from a liver. Giemsa stain. (From Fujiwara, 1978, courtesy of *Japanese Journal of Experimental Medicine.*)

Bacillus piliformis

SYNONYM: *Actinobacillus piliformis*

B. piliformis is the cause of *Tyzzer's disease,* an acute, fatal disease of laboratory rodents. The organism was first observed by Ernest Tyzzer (1917) in focal necrotic lesions of the livers of Japanese waltzing mice in a colony that was experiencing an epizootic of a highly fatal diarrheal disease. Since Tyzzer's report the disease has been noted in many parts of the world in laboratory and wild rodents but also in foals, puppies, gray foxes, snow leopard kittens, a lesser panda, coyotes, cats, and monkeys (see reviews by Fujiwara 1978, Schmidt et al. 1984). *B. piliformis* is the only Gram-negative, spore-bearing, motile, obligate, intracellularly parasitic bacterium ever described and there is almost no justification for its inclusion in the genus *Bacillus*.

Morphology and Staining Reactions. *B. piliformis* forms slender, Gram-negative rods 2 to 20 μm by 0.3 to 0.5 μm in size. These rods are formed in bundles within the cytoplasm of hepatic and intestinal epithelial cells (Figure 21.7). Subterminal spores are formed, but these are not easily seen in tissue sections. *B. piliformis* is motile by means of many peritrichous flagella (Figure 21.8).

Pleomorphic forms can also be seen. These can be beaded, banded, thickened, and short with occasional subterminal bulbous swellings (Ganaway et al. 1971).

Giemsa-stained organisms are bluish purple. Other stains commonly used to dye the organism are periodic acid–Schiff and the silver impregnation techniques such as Warthin-Starry.

Cultural and Biochemical Features. *B. piliformis* cannot be propagated outside of living cells. It grows well in the epithelial cells of chick embryos and in primary mono-layer cultures of adult mouse hepatocytes (Kawamura et al. 1983). In adult mouse hepatocytes, it produces plaguelike cytopathic effects. Maximal production of bacterial cells occurs in about 72 hours.

The obligate intracellular mode of replication of *B. piliformis* has greatly hindered biochemical and taxonomic studies. The spores are moderately heat resistant and sensitive to 0.3 percent sodium hypochlorite (Ganaway 1980).

Antigens. The antigenic proteins that are active in the complement-fixation test have been isolated from infected livers. These proteins have molecular weights of

Figure 21.8. Electron micrograph of *Bacillus piliformis* showing the peritrichous flagella. (From Fujiwara, 1978, courtesy of *Japanese Journal of Experimental Medicine.*)

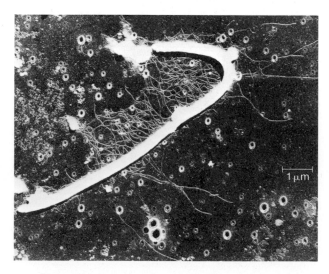

1 μm

about 52,000 and 66,000 (Orikasa et al. 1984). Organisms from mice and rats have been shown to be antigenically related (Fujiwara 1978), but organisms from hamsters or kittens did not cross-react with those from mice.

Epizootiology and Pathogenesis. Most healthy laboratory rodents are resistant to Tyzzer's disease. Outbreaks of disease are typically associated with stress or an inherited susceptibility. Enteritis is the form of the disease usually seen in suckling mice and probably results from ingestion of spores from dirty bedding. Local necrosis of the liver is characteristic in adult mice. Cortisone administration is useful for the detection of the inapparent disease and for enhancing experimental infections.

It is not known whether natural transmission occurs between different host species. Experimentally, material from hamsters, rats, kittens, and rabbits is infective for mice (Fujiwara 1978).

Tyzzer's disease has been observed in 3- to 4-week-old foals that died suddenly with no history of clinical illness (Harrington 1975). Gross findings included jaundice, focal areas of hepatic necrosis, and catarrhal enterocolitis. The organism was observed in hepatocytes at the margin of liver lesions. Other accounts of the disease in foals emphasize its acute onset with signs of diarrhea, elevated levels of serum sorbitol dehydrogenase, bilirubin, and amino aspartate transferase, recumbency, and shock (Brown et al. 1983, Yates et al. 1980). The incidence of infection in healthy foals is unknown.

Diarrhea and liver dysfunction associated with focal necrosis is also characteristic of the disease in other host species.

Immunity. Mice experimentally immunized with formalin-inactivated mouse liver emulsion are resistant to experimental challenge with *B. piliformis* from different host species. The protective properties of hyperimmune serum are in the IgG fraction (Fujiwara 1978). Antibodies bind to both the surface and the flagella of the organism. The effect of various stresses and corticosteroids on susceptibility to infection suggests that cell-mediated immunity can also be important in controlling infections.

Diagnosis. Tyzzer's disease can be diagnosed definitively only by demonstration of *B. piliformis* in cells adjacent to lesions. Smears or sections of lesions should be stained with Giemsa stain or by silver impregnation or fluorescent antibody techniques (Fujiwara 1978).

Antimicrobial Susceptibility. *B. piliformis* appears to be sensitive to penicillin, ampicillin, tetracyclines, neomycin, and erythromycin.

REFERENCES

Brown, C.M., Ainsworth, D.M., Personett, L.A., and Derksen, F.J. 1983. Serum biochemical and haematological findings in two foals with focal bacterial hepatitis (Tyzzer's disease). Equine Vet. J. 151:375–376.

Fujiwara, K. 1978. Tyzzer's disease. Jpn. J. Exp. Med. 48:467–480.

Ganaway, J.R. 1980. Effect of heat and selected chemical disinfectants upon infectivity of spores of *Bacillus piliformis* (Tyzzer's disease). Lab. Anim. Sci. 30:192–196.

Ganaway, J.R., Allen, A.M., and Moore, T.D. 1971. Tyzzer's disease. Am. J. Pathol. 64:717–732.

Harrington, D.D. 1975. Naturally occurring Tyzzer's disease (*Bacillus piliformis* infection) in horse foals. Vet. Rec. 96:59–63.

Kawamura, S., Taguchi, F., Ishida, T., Nakoyama, M., and Fujiwara, K. 1983. Growth of Tyzzer's organism in primary monolayer cultures of adult mouse hepatocytes. J. Gen. Microbiol. 129:277–283.

Orikasa, M., Iwase, I., Kozima, K., and Shimizu, F. 1984. Purification by sucrose density gradient zonal centrifugation and affinity column chromatography of antigenic substances from the livers of mice infected with Tyzzer's disease. J. Gen. Microbiol. 130:1757–1763.

Schmidt, R.E., Eisenbrandt, D.C., and Hubbard, G.B. 1984. Tyzzer's disease in snow leopards. J. Comp. Pathol. 94:165–167.

Tyzzer, E.E. 1917. A fatal disease of the Japanese waltzing mouse caused by a spore-bearing bacillus (*Bacillus piliformis* n. sp.) J. Med. Res. 37:307–338.

Yates, W.D.G., Hayes, M.A., Finell, G.R., and Chalmers, G.A. 1980. Tyzzer's disease in foals in western Canada. Can. Vet. J. 21:63.

the intestine, leading to a disease state termed *enterotoxemia*. The toxins may act on the intestinal mucosa or at other sites after distribution in the bloodstream. Wounds or injection sites of animals sometimes become infected with the invasive clostridia, producing gas gangrene, edema, and necrosis.

The invasive or enterotoxigenic clostridia that cause disease in animals are as follows:

22 The Genus *Clostridium*

The anaerobic spore-bearing organisms that are grouped in the genus *Clostridium* are generally similar in morphology and staining qualities. They are rather large, rod-shaped, and Gram-positive when young. The rods usually are straight with the exception of *C. spiroforme*, which has a curved or spiral form. Some species commonly appear in tissue fluids singly or in pairs, whereas others usually are found in long chains. The spores in most species are oval, are located somewhat centrally in the rod, and often are greater in diameter than the rod itself. Many species produce a characteristic range of short-chain acids as products of metabolism. The symptoms or lesions of the diseases produced by the different clostridial species are often sufficiently characteristic to allow a reliable diagnosis to be made. A total of 83 *Clostridium* species are officially recognized.

The clostridia can be divided into two groups on the basis of their disease-producing mechanisms. The first group consists of those species that have little or no ability to invade and multiply in living tissues. Such organisms owe their pathogenicity to the production of powerful toxins that are produced outside the body of the host or in localized areas within the body. The damage is almost wholly caused by the toxin. Two organisms of this group that are described herein are *C. tetani* and *C. botulinum*. The second and larger group consists of species that can invade and multiply in the tissues or the intestine of the host animal. These organisms in most cases also produce toxins, but the toxins are less potent than those of the first group. A number of these species elaborate their toxins in

C. perfringens	The cause of lamb dysentery, struck, and pulpy kidney disease in sheep and occasionally of malignant edematous infections in other species
C. haemolyticum	The cause of bacterial icterohemoglobinuria, or redwater, in cattle
C. novyi	The cause of black disease in sheep and occasionally of malignant edematous infections in other species
C. chauvoei	The cause of blackleg in cattle and sheep
C. septicum	The cause of braxy in sheep and of malignant edematous infections in other species
C. colinum	The cause of ulcerating enteritis, or quail disease, in young game birds, turkeys, and chickens
C. spiroforme	The cause of spontaneous and antibiotic-induced enterotoxemia in rabbits
C. villosum	The cause of subcutaneous abscesses in cats
C. difficile	The cause of antibiotic-induced enterocolitis in hamsters, rabbits, and guinea pigs and of naturally occurring enterocolitis in swine and foals

C. sporogenes, although not directly toxigenic or invasive, may be important in the etiology of cerebrocortical necrosis of ruminants as a consequence of its ability to produce thiaminase in the rumen and intestine (Shreeve and Edwin 1974).

The anaerobic spore-bearing bacteria cause animal diseases that are infectious without being contagious; that is, the diseases seldom if ever are transmitted directly from one animal to another. Most of these organisms live in the soil and intestine, and it is from the soil or from vegetation contaminated with intestinal contents that the infections are derived. Epizootics seldom occur, although they are possible when conditions are favorable for many animals to become infected simultaneously from the same source.

REFERENCE

Shreeve, J.E., and Edwin, E.E. 1974. Thiamase-producing strains of *Clostridium sporogenes* associated with outbreaks of cerebrocortical necrosis. Vet. Rec. 94:330.

The Toxin-Forming, Noninvasive Group

Clostridium tetani

SYNONYM: *Bacillus tetani*

The causative agent of tetanus is the best known of all anaerobic spore-bearing bacilli, principally because the symptoms of the disease are so well known and characteristic. The organism was isolated in impure culture by Nicolaier in 1884 from white mice that had been inoculated with garden soil. Five years later Kitasato (1889) obtained pure cultures by heating mixed cultures from infected wounds, thus destroying the ordinary bacteria of suppuration but leaving the heat-resistant tetanus spores. In the following year Von Behring and Kitasato (1890) published their classic work announcing the discovery of bacterial toxins, the first of which was that of *C. tetani*.

Morphology and Staining Reactions. *C. tetani* is a straight, slender rod 0.4 to 0.6 μm wide and 2 to 5 μm long. It most often occurs singly in both tissues and cultures, but sometimes the organisms form long filaments. In old cultures the rods and threads disappear, leaving the spherical spores. These spores are formed after 24 to 48 hours of incubation and appear in the ends of the rods, swelling them so they have the appearance of badminton rackets or drumsticks (Figure 22.1). In some media, spores are formed in abundance; in others, few spores are seen even after prolonged incubation. *C. tetani* in cultures

Figure 22.1. *Clostridium tetani* in a Gram-stained smear from a puncture wound on a dog. The terminal spores are characteristic. × 2,000.

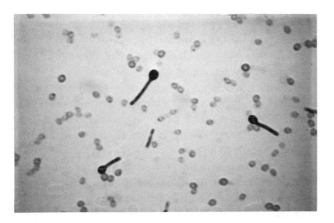

is Gram-positive when young, but after a few days most of the cells become Gram-negative. Young organisms are actively motile by means of peritrichous flagella.

Cultural and Biochemical Features. The tetanus organism grows on all the ordinary media if fairly good anaerobic conditions are maintained. It will grow in aerobic cultures in association with other aerobic organisms. Colonies of *C. tetani* in deep agar are fluffy, cottony spheres. When blood is present, hemolysis occurs. The organism slightly clouds broth but this clears by sedimentation. When *C. tetani* is grown in stabs in gelatin, a spike first develops along the stab; cottony filaments next extend from the stab at right angles into the medium, producing a brushlike effect; liquefaction and blackening of the medium then occur and gas bubbles form. *C. tetani* does not usually change litmus milk, although a soft clot may be formed. It softens coagulated blood serum and may blacken it if the culture is old, but the blood serum is not liquefied. It does not digest cooked-meat medium or brain medium, causing them instead to become turbid and produce a foul odor. *C. tetani* does not ferment carbohydrates, but the addition of glucose greatly favors growth in the simpler types of media. Growth occurs best at 37°C, although colonies will grow slowly at 20°C. Acetic, butyric, and propionic acids are the principal products of fermentation.

C. tetani can sometimes be isolated in pure culture from contaminated specimens by lightly inoculating a fresh blood-agar plate. After incubation for 24 hours, the plate should be checked for swarming, which will be evident as a thin veil of growth on the surface of the agar. Cells (Gram-positive rods) from the edge of the swarming area should be transferred to a tube of broth and to another blood plate containing 5 percent agar. After incubation an isolated colony can be picked for further characterization.

Resistance of the Organism. *C. tetani* spores are highly resistant to most sporicidal agents and techniques and when protected from light and heat remain viable for years. Some strains resist steaming at 100°C for 40 to 60 minutes. Five percent phenol destroys tetanus spores in 10 to 12 hours; the addition of 0.5 percent hydrochloric acid can reduce the time to 2 hours. Boiling kills the spores of most strains in 15 minutes. Autoclaving at 120°C for 20 minutes is also sporicidal.

Antigens and Serotypes. The serologic types of *C. tetani* have been categorized by Gunnison (1937) and Mandia (1955). A heat-stable glycopeptide antigen designated IV, V is shared by all strains, but a variety of different heat-labile flagellar or somatic antigens occurs. Smith (1975) listed nine serotypes of *C. tetani*.

Epizootiology and Pathogenesis. The organism of tetanus originally was found by Nicolaier in garden soils. Fildes (1925) in England examined 70 soil samples, including both cultivated and uncultivated soil, and found 33 to be positive for *C. tetani*. Sanada and Nishida (1965) have indicated that the higher the temperature applied to soil specimens the weaker the toxigenicity of *C. tetani* cultures isolated from them.

The organism is common in horse manure and has also been found in the feces of cows, sheep, dogs, chickens, rats, and guinea pigs. Human feces are sometimes infected with tetanus bacilli. TenBroeck and Bauer (1922) demonstrated the bacilli in the stools of 27 of 78 persons residing in Peking, and concluded that the organism must be living in the intestinal canal because some subjects who had existed on an almost sterile diet for more than a month continued to yield several million tetanus spores per stool.

Infections in all animals and humans can occur as a result of contamination of wounds or the umbilicus. Deep penetrating wounds, the depths of which become necrotic with reduced oxygen and lowered Eh, are the usual sites where *C. tetani* multiplies and subsequently produces toxin. Washed spores injected into healthy tissue do not set up tetanus in the inoculated host.

C. tetani produces three toxins: (1) tetanospasmin (neurotoxin) (2) hemolysin, and (3) a peripherally active nonspasmogenic toxin. The structural gene for tetanospasmin is on a plasmid (Finn et al. 1984). Tetanospasmin is responsible for the characteristic clinical features of tetanus, and antibodies to the toxin are protective. The hemolysin causes local tissue necrosis and creates more favorable conditions for multiplication of *C. tetani*. It is hemolytic for erythrocytes and lethal in laboratory animals when administered intravenously.

Tetanospasmin is produced initially as a single polypeptide chain with a molecular weight of about 150,000. This chain is cleaved into two subunits (molecular weights 100,000 and 50,000) by endogenous proteases. The subunits are held together by a disulfide bond and noncovalent interactions. The heavy and light chains are nontoxic when separated (Matsuda and Yoneda 1977). The toxin is destroyed by gastric juices, is heat resistant, and is poorly absorbed across mucous membranes. It is extremely potent—one lethal dose with 50 percent survival (LD_{50}) for mice is equivalent to 2×10^{-8}mg.

Van Heyningen and Mellanby (1971) showed that tetanospasmin binds specifically to gangliosides in nerve tissue. Gangliosides are chloroform- and water-soluble mucolipids containing sialic acid, stearic acid, sphingosine, galactose, acetylgalactosamine, and glucose. In nerve tissue the ganglioside is bound to the water-insoluble cerebrosides. Two molecules of ganglioside will bind to one molecule of toxin. The reaction is extremely difficult to reverse and the neutralizing antibody is ineffective once the toxin is bound. After it binds to gangliosides, the toxin travels along the nerve trunk to the spinal cord by retrograde axonal transport (Schwab et al. 1979).

The specific action of tetanospasmin appears to be that of preventing the release of glycine—the transmitter substance for the inhibitory nerve network in the spinal cord (Osborne and Bradford 1973). This network prevents contraction of one muscle when its opposite-acting counterpart contracts. The toxin thus causes continuous stimulation and tetanic spasm of groups of muscle. Other effects include a paralytic action on the peripheral nervous system as well as an inactivating effect on the inhibitory network in the central nervous system. There is also an inhibitory effect on protein synthesis in the brain. Neuromuscular activity favors migration of the toxin, which can migrate along both motor axons and sensory nerves (Habermann and Wellhöver 1972). There is preferential uptake of toxin via the ventral roots in the spinal cord. The toxin also accumulates selectively in the lumbar and cervical regions of the cord and in the gray matter of the postpontine area of the brain stem. When the toxin travels up a regional motor nerve in a limb, tetanus develops first in the muscles of that limb and then, as the toxin spreads upward, in the opposite limb and subsequently in the muscles of the trunk. This is known as *ascending tetanus*. The toxin can also circulate in the blood and lymph and produce tetanus first in the muscles supplied by the most susceptible motor nerve centers that serve the head and neck. The voluntary muscles of the forelimbs, the upper trunk, and later the hind limbs become involved. This form of tetanus is described as *descending* and is the form usually seen in humans and horses. In descending tetanus the first symptoms involve the nictitating membrane, which cannot be retracted, and the facial and jaw muscles, leading to *lockjaw* and *risus sardonicus* (Figure 22.2). The shorter the incubation period in tetanus, the worse the prognosis.

The action of the nonspasmogenic toxin is poorly defined. There is some evidence that it may play a role in the peripheral paralytic action of tetanus toxin.

The signs of tetanus are similar in all animals. They consist of chronic or tetanic spasms of the muscles (Figure 22.3). Sometimes these begin in the part of the body where the infected wound is located, but generally the disease extends to all parts.

Infections in horses occur most often as a result of nail wounds in the foot. In sheep the infection is seen most often after lambs are castrated or docked. In cattle it may be a puerperal infection that follows calving or it may follow dehorning, castration, and nose ringing of bulls.

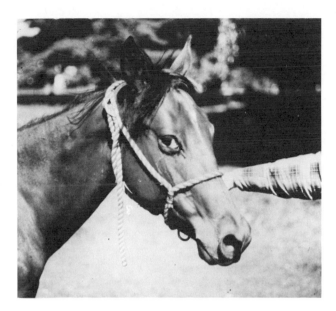

Figure 22.2. Tetanus in a horse. The membrana nictitans is visible and the nostrils are dilated because of tetanus of the facial muscles. (Courtesy W. Rebhun.)

Herd and Riches (1964) and Wallis (1963) reported outbreaks of idiopathic tetanus in groups of heifers and suggested that this condition was caused by an autointoxication resulting from massive multiplication of *C. tetani* in the forestomachs under certain unspecified conditions. In swine it is most frequently results from infection of castration wounds. The disease in dogs and cats also is a complication of wound infection (Mason 1964). In all animals

it can result from infection of trivial wounds. Umbilical infections of newborn animals often occur.

Immunity. Birds and other animals that are naturally resistant to tetanus have no antibodies in their tissues. The brain tissue of such animals, however, seems to have no affinity for the toxin, as was first demonstrated by Metchnikov (1898). The blood of most cattle contains neutralizing antibodies, and small amounts are found in the blood of sheep and goats. It has been suggested that this may come about from the activity of tetanus bacilli in the forestomachs of these ruminants. The blood of horses, dogs, pigs, and humans does not normally contain antitoxin. The brain tissues of all susceptible animals possess the power of binding with tetanospasmin in vitro.

Tetanus antitoxin prepared from the sera of hyperimmunized horses can be used to passively protect animals that have received accidental or surgical wounds. Usually 1,500 units will protect an animal for 2 to 3 weeks.

Vaccines against tetanus are made by incubating highly potent toxin with 0.4 percent formalin until the toxicity has been completely destroyed. The toxoid is then precipitated from solution with aluminum potassium sulfate (alum), and the washed precipitate is suspended in saline.

A single injection of toxoid will produce an appreciable degree of immunity, but experience has shown that it is best to give a second and a third dose at about 3-week intervals. Animals treated in this way will have sufficient antitoxin in their blood to protect them from natural infection for at least a year. Fessler (1966) recommends that horses should be given two toxoid injections 6 to 8 weeks

Figure 22.3. Tetanus in a pig. Tetanic spasms of the muscles manifested by rigidity of the parts is characteristic of tetanus in all animals. (Courtesy Jen-Sal Laboratories, Inc.)

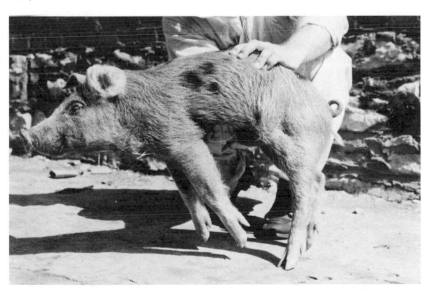

apart, followed by a booster dose 6 to 12 months later and then by annual booster injections. A similar regimen will be effective for other domestic animals. If the animal later receives a dangerous wound it is best to administer another dose at once. This will cause an immediate increase in antibodies. If the animal has not already received toxoid, the injection of toxoid is useless in an emergency because the initial production of antitoxin is too slow. It has been established that a simultaneous injection of tetanus antitoxin and toxoid will not significantly reduce the efficacy of the antitoxin but will markedly decrease the ability of the toxoid to produce active immunity. Passive protection of foals is best achieved by immunization of the mare before foaling. Many newborn foals, however, maintain protective titers (0.01 IU/ml serum) of antitoxin for 3 months after administration of 1,500 IU antitoxin shortly after birth (Liu et al. 1982).

Once symptoms of tetanus have appeared, the efficacy of the antitoxin is much less than when it is used prophylactically. In animals already suffering from the disease, the antitoxin is administered as soon as possible and preferably is given in a single intravenous and intracisternal dose of 100,000 to 200,000 units. Adequate treatment also includes large doses of penicillin. The therapeutic effectiveness of tetanus antitoxin is markedly reduced by simultaneous administration of cortisone (Chang and Weinstein 1957).

Diagnosis. The signs of tetanus are so characteristic that laboratory examination of specimens is rarely performed. When it is done, microscopic examination of smears from infected wounds may reveal the characteristic drumstick appearance of the organism and its spore. Contaminants in specimens may be removed by treatment with 50 percent ethanol for 1 hour. Toxin present in the wound may be demonstrated by surgically excising the necrotic tissue and homogenizing it in some saline. The homogenate is centrifuged and 0.2 ml is injected into the hind-leg muscle of each of four mice, two of which have been given antitoxin a few hours earlier. The mice are then observed for up to 3 days for the development of tetanus in the unprotected group. If a large amount of toxin is present, the mice may be found dead after a few hours.

Antimicrobial Susceptibility. *C. tetani* is sensitive to penicillin, tetracycline, and chloramphenicol. It is resistant to the aminoglycosides. Treatment of tetanus must include sedation with tubocurarine chloride (Booth and Pierson 1956) or other sedatives. Tranquilizers such as chlorpromazine hydrochloride, diazepam (7-chloro-1,3-dihydro-1-methyl-5-phenyl-2H-1, 4-benzodiazepin-2-one), and chlordiazepoxide [7-chloro-2-(methylamino)-5-phen-yl-3H-1,4-benzodiazepine 4-oxide] are also highly recommended in the treatment of tetanus (Femi-Pearse and Fleming 1965, Lowenthal and Lavalette 1966). Barbiturates are of value in the control of grand mal tetanic seizures.

REFERENCES

Booth, N.H., and Pierson, R.E. 1956. Treatment of tetanus with *d*-tubocurarine chloride. J. Am. Vet. Med. Assoc. 128:257–261.

Chang, T.W., and Weinstein, L. 1957. Effect of cortisone on treatment of tetanus with antitoxin. Proc. Soc. Exp. Biol. Med. 94:431–433.

Femi-Pearse, D., and Fleming, S.A. 1965. Tetanus treated with high dosage of diazepam. J. Trop. Med. Hyg. 68:305–306.

Fessler, J.F. 1966. Prophylaxis of tetanus in horses. J. Am. Vet. Med. Assoc. 148:399–404.

Fildes, P. 1925. Tetanus. I. Isolation, morphology and cultural reactions of *B. tetani*. Br. J. Exp. Pathol. 6:62–70.

Finn, C.W., Silver, R.P., Habig, W.H., Hardegree, M.C., Zon, G. and Garon, C.F. 1984. The structural gene for tetanus neurotoxin is on a plasmid. Science 224:881–884.

Gunnison, J.B. 1937. Agglutination reaction of the heat stable antigens of *Clostridium tetani*. J. Immunol. 32:63–74.

Habermann, E., and Wellhöver, H.H. 1972. Studies on the pathogenesis of tetanus with 125 I-labelled toxin. In Radioactive Tracers in Microbial Immunology. International Atomic Energy Agency, Vienna. Pp. 67–76.

Herd, R.P., and Riches, W.R. 1964. An outbreak of tetanus in cattle. Aust. Vet. J. 40:356–357.

Kitasato, S. 1889. Über den Tetanusbacillus. Z. Hyg. 7:225–233.

Liu, I.K.M., Brown, S.L., Kuo, J., Neeley, D.P., and Feeley, J.C. 1982. Duration of maternally derived immunity to tetanus and response in newborn foals given tetanus antitoxin. Am. J. Vet. Res. 42:2019–2022.

Lowenthal, M.N., and Lavalette, J. 1966. Chlordiazepoxide in the treatment of tetanus. J. Trop. Med. Hyg. 69:157–159.

Mandia, J.W. 1955. The position of *Clostridium tetani* within the serological schema for the proteolytic clostridia. J. Infect. Dis. 97:66–72.

Mason, J.H. 1964. Tetanus in the dog and cat. J. S. Afr. Vet. Med. Assoc. 35:209–213.

Matsuda, M., and Yoneda, M. 1977. Antigenic substructure of tetanus neurotoxin. Biochem. Biophys. Res. Commun. 77:268–274.

Metchnikov, E.L. 1898. Recherches sur l'influence de l'organisme sur les toxines. Ann. Inst. Pasteur (Paris) 12:81–90.

Osborne, R.H., and Bradford, H.F. 1973. Tetanus toxin inhibits amino acid release from nerve endings in vitro. Nature 244:157–158.

Sanada, I., and Nishida, S. 1965. Isolation of *Clostridium tetani* from soil. J. Bacteriol. 89:626–629.

Schwab, M.E., Suda, E., and Thoenen, H. 1979. Selective retrograde transsynaptic transfer of a protein tetanus toxin, subsequent to its retrograde axonal transport. J. Cell Biol., 82:798–810.

Smith, L. 1975. The Pathogenic Anaerobic Bacteria, 2d ed. Charles C Thomas, Springfield, Ill. Pp. 177–201.

TenBroeck. C., and Bauer, J.H. 1922. The tetanus bacillus as an intestinal saprophyte in man. J. Exp. Med. 36:261.

Van Heyningen, W.E., and Mellanby, J. 1971. Tetanus toxin. In S. Kadis, T.C. Monte, and S.J. Ajl, eds., Microbial Toxins, vol. 2A. Academic Press, New York. Pp. 69–108.

Von Behring, S., and Kitasato, S. 1890. Über das Zustandekommen der Dieptherid-Immunität und der Tetanus-Immunität bei Tieren. Dtsch. Med. Wochnschr. 16:1113–1114.

Wallis, A.S. 1963. Some observations on the epidemiology of tetanus in cattle. Vet. Rec. 75:188–191.

Clostridium botulinum

SYNONYM: *Bacillus botulinus*

C. botulinum is the source of a number of antigenically different potent neurotoxins that cause botulism, a disease characterized by flaccid paralysis and eventual death due to respiratory failure.

Botulism has been known for many years as a disease of humans and was given its name by Muller in 1870. The organism itself was discovered by Van Ermengem (1897), who studied an outbreak in Ellezelles, Belgium, in a group of people who ate an imperfectly smoked ham at a dinner. The organism was found in the ham and in the tissues of one of the persons who died of the disease. The toxigenic properties of the organism and the effects of the toxin on the nervous system were also recognized by Van Ermengem.

The disease is usually an intoxication, but toxin production in necrotic lesions of foals and horses is well documented (Swerczek 1980a, 1980b) and there are a few reports of wound infection in humans (Breukink et al. 1978, Hampson 1952). In general, the organism does not appear to generate toxin in the alimentary tract of animals but has been reported to do so in the crops of birds (Von Dinter and Kull 1954). Botulism in infants is now the most frequently encountered form of the disease in humans in the United States and is associated with intestinal colonization by the organism and subsequent elaboration and absorption of toxin (Marx 1978).

Morphology and Staining Reactions. The types within the species cannot be distinguished on a morphologic basis. All are relatively large rods that usually occur singly but may form short chains. They measure 0.5 to 0.8 μm in width and 3 to 6 μm in length. The organism is motile in young cultures, the cells having peritrichous flagella. Spores form readily and abundantly, are oval and centric and excentric (Figure 22.4). The organism is Gram-positive, but the cells in old cultures may appear Gram-negative.

Cultural and Biochemical Features. Colonies grown in deep agar are fluffy. Surface colonies are large and semitransparent with irregular edges. Media prepared from liver provide better growth than those prepared from muscle tissue. *C. botulinum* liquefies gelatin and produces acid and gas from glucose, levulose, and maltose. Acetic acid is a major metabolic product of all strains. It produces other fatty acids in amounts that vary according to strain; these include propionic, isobutyric, butyric, isovaleric, valeric, and isocaproic acids.

The nonproteolytic types (*C. botulinum*) acidify but do not coagulate milk. They do not liquefy coagulated blood

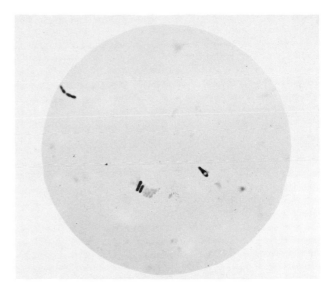

Figure 22.4. A culture of *Clostridium botulinum* in meat-piece medium incubated 48 hours at 37°C. × 1,040

serum or coagulated egg albumen, nor do they digest brain or meat medium. A narrow zone of hemolysis may be produced on horse-blood agar.

The proteolytic types (*C. parabotulinum*) slowly curdle milk and partially digest and darken the curd. When inoculated on coagulated blood serum or egg albumen, they digest and blacken the media and produce a putrefactive odor. They also digest and blacken brain or meat medium and emit putrefactive odors.

All organisms included in these species are strict anaerobes but are not otherwise fastidious in their growth requirements. They grow best at temperatures around 30°C but are capable of growing in a wide range of temperatures up to that of the body. The strains that are not proteolytic nevertheless give off a strong odor, which is suggestive of putrefaction but is not so powerful as that produced by the protein-liquefying types.

Resistance of the Organism. The spores are highly resistant and may withstand boiling for 30 minutes to several hours. Autoclaving at 120°C for 20 minutes is usually sufficient to kill most strains.

Serologic and Toxigenic Types. According to Mandia (1951) there are at least six serotypes of *C. botulinum* in his group II of proteolytic clostridia, and antigens are shared by some strains with *C. sporogenes* (Mandia and Bruner 1951). The antigenic configuration of strains bears no relationship to the toxin type produced, and because the toxin type is much more useful epidemiologically, strains of *C. botulinum* are classified according to the type

Table 22.1. Distribution, hosts, and diseases associated with *C. botulinum* strains

Strain	Distribution*	Hosts affected	Disease
A	North America (West)	Humans	Botulism
		Cattle, horses	Forage poisoning
		Chickens	Limberneck
		Mink	Botulism
B	North America (Midwest & East)	Humans	Botulism
		Cattle, foals and adult horses	Forage poisoning
	Europe	Chickens	Limberneck
		Mink	Botulism
		Foal	Shaker foal syndrome
C (1, 2)	North America	Ducks and other wild birds	Limberneck, western duck disease
	Australia		
	Canada	Humans	Botulism
	Europe	Mink	
D	South Africa	Cattle	Lamziekte
E	Soviet Union	Humans	Botulism
	North America (Great Lakes)		
F	Denmark	Humans	Botulism
	North America		
G	Argentina, Switzerland	Humans?	Botulism?

*Places where disease due to this strain has been reported.

of toxin produced. There are seven groups described on the basis of toxin type (Table 22.1).

Some strains of *C. botulinum* type C are culturally indistinguishable from strains of *C. novyi* type A (Holdeman and Brooks 1970) except for toxin production. Nontoxigenic cultures of *C. botulinum* type C, cured of phage, can be reinfected with specific phage and induced to produce alpha toxin of *C. novyi* type A, thus becoming indistinguishable from *C. novyi* type A (Eklund et al. 1974, Nakamura et al. 1983).

Toxigenicity in type D strains of *C. botulinum* has also been shown to require the presence of bacteriophage (Eklund et al. 1974). Types A, B, E, and F are probably saprophytes of soil and aquatic sediments. Types C and D appear to be obligate parasites of the intestinal tracts of mammals and birds and occur in soil or aquatic sediments only as transients. In general *C. botulinum* is most common in the northern hemisphere between the latitudes of 35° and 55°N.

Botulinum Toxin. The toxin is a protein with a molecular weight of about 150,000 daltons and comprises heavy chains (molecular weight 100,000) and light chains (molecular weight 50,000). It usually exists as a complex consisting of toxin molecules and a hemagglutinin moiety (molecular weight 500,000). The toxins of nonproteolytic strains, including types C, D, E, and G, and a few strains

of types B and F require exposure to proteolytic enzymes such as trypsin for full expression of toxic activity. The activated toxin may have a toxicity as high as 2.6×10^8 mouse LD_{50} per milligram of nitrogen.

Botulinum toxins may be produced at temperatures as low as 30°C, and complete absence of oxygen is not required for toxin synthesis. Only one toxin type is usually produced by a strain, although types C and D have been shown to produce multiple toxins (Smith 1977). Toxin is released during lysis of cells.

Epizootiology and Pathogenesis. Botulism almost always arises from ingestion of food contaminated with preformed toxin. The toxin may be elaborated in a decaying carcass that is ingested or indirectly causes contamination of another foodstuff. Fly larvae that develop on carcasses in which toxin has been produced can carry sufficient toxin to cause botulism in birds that feed on them. Another source is decaying vegetation at the edges of ponds and lakes, which may provide an environment for toxin synthesis. Aquatic birds such as ducks that feed in these areas can develop botulism. Offal and fish meats are other well-known sources of botulinum toxin for mink and foxes, respectively.

Aphosphorosis may cause cattle and sheep to develop a depraved appetite for decaying carcasses, and this in turn may lead to the occurrence of botulism (Theiler et al.

1927). Because of the lameness associated with the phosphorus deficiency, the disease in South Africa has been called *lamziekte* or the lame sickness. It occurs only in certain restricted areas on the range. A disease evidently the same as *lamziekte* occurs in certain parts of the Texas plains, where phosphorus deficiency exists and bone chewing is common. *C. botulinum* type D has been found in mud samples taken from lakes in the Zululand game parks of Africa (Mason 1968). Carcasses buried in the litter of broiler houses have resulted in outbreaks of botulism type C in broiler chickens (Haagsma and ter Laak 1977). Levels of toxin in such carcasses can reach 10^6 mouse LD_{50} per gram. In Holland botulism in cattle has been caused by brewers' grains contaminated by *C. botulinum* type B (Breukink et al. 1978).

Toxicoinfectious botulism is a form of the disease first observed on a wide scale in Kentucky, where *C. botulinum* produced toxin in necrotic areas of the body. Typically, 2- to 8-week-old foals are affected and, after absorption of toxin, show typical signs of the shaker foal syndrome—acute onset of dysphagia, tremors, weakness, and recumbency followed by death. Areas of necrosis colonized by *C. botulinum* include gastric ulcers, umbilical or lung abscesses, and wounds (Swerczek 1980a, 1980b).

The spores of *C. botulinum* are distributed far more widely than the occurrence of botulism would suggest. This is so because a combination of circumstances is necessary for occurrence of the disease. These are (1) contamination of a suitable substrate by the organism, (2) multiplication of the organism and production of its toxin, (3) survival of the toxin in the face of autolytic processes that might degrade it, and (4) ingestion of the toxin by susceptible animals.

After ingestion the toxin passes across the intestinal wall to the blood and the lymph. The hemagglutinin may serve to protect the toxin from the digestive processes before its passage into the bloodstream. Because ruminal bacteria inactivate substantial quantities of ingested toxin (Allison et al. 1976), the oral lethal dose for cattle and sheep is much larger than when the toxin is administered by other routes. This observation is important in relation to handling of diagnostic specimens of rumen contents for assay for toxin; these should be frozen until assays are performed.

Once in the bloodstream, the toxin is carried to the peripheral nervous system, where it apparently binds to gangliosides at the neuromuscular junction. The toxin then enters the nerve and binds to the inside surface of the nerve membrane, which becomes functionally changed so that vesicles containing acetylcholine are no longer able to meld to the membrane to release their stores of acetyl-

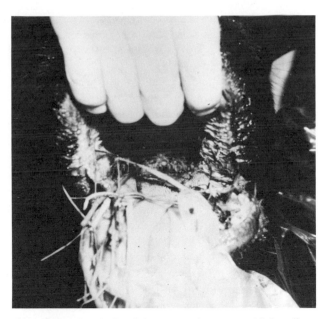

Figure 22.5. Paralysis of the tongue in a cow with botulism. Note the food material in the mouth, which the animal was unable to swallow.

choline. Botulinum toxin affects only cholinergic nerves of the peripheral nervous system, the blood-brain barrier protects the cholinergic nerves of the brain.

The external effect in an affected animal is flaccid paralysis, which when it progresses to involve the respiratory muscles will result in death. Disturbances in vision also occur, locomotion is difficult, the tongue often becomes paralyzed (Figure 22.5), swallowing becomes impossible because of pharyngeal paralysis, and respiratory paralysis finally terminates the disease. In poultry the wings, legs, and neck become paralyzed and the birds cannot retract the nictitating membrane (Figure 22.6). Posterior paralysis is a usual symptom in mink. Swine and

Figure 22.6. Limberneck in a duck. (Courtesy D. Mills.)

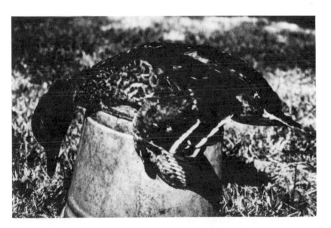

carnivorous animals are resistant to the effects of botulinum toxin. The disease (type C), however, has been reported in young dogs (Farrow et al. 1983) and in foxhounds (Barsanti et al. 1978).

Immunity. Homologous antitoxins protect animals very well against botulism. Because of the sporadic and infrequent occurrence of the disease in birds in many areas, however, vaccination is not a universally routine practice. In high-risk regions such as South Africa and Australia and in certain populations such as mink or zoo animals exposed to circumstances in which there is a high probability of toxin in their food or environment, vaccination with formalinized, alum-precipitated toxoids is practiced. These have been used successfully in immunizing mink (Appleton and White 1959), horses (White and Appleton 1969), cattle, sheep, pheasants, and ducks (Boroff and Reilly 1959). In some areas polyvalent toxoids are used for this purpose. In Australia nonimmune cattle and sheep are usually given a series of two injections and from then on a booster dose each year (Bennetts and Hall 1937, Larsen et al. 1955). In South Africa types C and D toxoids have been shown to be most effective in a vaccination program when the primary and secondary inoculations are made with vaccines presented in water and oil emulsion and subsequent booster inoculations are performed with aqueous solutions (Jansen et al. 1976).

Free toxin can be neutralized by the administration of polyvalent antitoxin. The response to antitoxin varies greatly depending on the amount of toxin bound and the toxin type. Antitoxin is not effective once the toxin becomes bound to nerve membranes. Efforts should also be made to empty the gastrointestinal tract of unabsorbed toxin by administration of purgatives.

Diagnosis. Diagnostic proof of botulism in animals centers on the demonstration of toxin in the serum, intestinal contents, and suspect foodstuffs. Toxin in the serum or filtered macerates of food or intestinal contents can be demonstrated by mouse inoculation. Mice passively protected with polyvalent antitoxin should also be inoculated. If toxin is present, only the unprotected mice should die. The levels of toxin in the serum of affected animals are about 20 mouse LD_{50} per milliliter or lower. In the case of samples of intestinal contents or foodstuffs, the sample should be trypsinized before inoculation so that precursor toxin can be activated.

Enzyme-linked immunosorbent assays (ELISAs) for the detection of type A, B, E and G toxins have been described (Dezfulian and Bartlett 1984, Lewis et al. 1981, Notermons et al. 1982), but these have not yet been applied to routine diagnosis. Because the spores of C. botulinum are ubiquitous, their presence in specimens has limited diagnostic value.

REFERENCES

Allison, M.J., Maloy, S.E., and Matson, R.R. 1976. Inactivation of *Clostridium botulinum* toxin by ruminal microbes from cattle and sheep. Appl. Environ. Microbiol. 32:685–688.

Appleton, G.S., and White, P.G. 1959. Field evaluation of *Clostridium botulinum* type C toxoids in mink. Am. J. Vet. Res. 20:166–169.

Barsanti, J.A., Walser, M., Hatheway, C.L., Bowen, J.M., and Crowell, W. 1978. Type C botulism in American foxhounds. J. Am. Vet. Med. Assoc. 172:809–813.

Bennetts, H.W., and Hall, H.T.B. 1937. The control of toxic paralysis (botulism) in sheep and cattle. J. Dept. Agric. W. Aust. 14:381–386.

Boroff, D.A., and Reilly, J.R. 1959. Studies of the toxin of *Clostridium botulinum*. V. Prophylactic immunization of pheasants and ducks against avian botulism. J. Bacteriol 77:142–146.

Breukink, H.J., Wagenaar, G., Wensing, T., Notermans, S., and Poulos, P.W. 1978. Food poisoning in cattle caused by ingestion of brewers grains contaminated with *Clostridium botulinum* type B. Tijdschr. Diergeneeskd. 103:303–311.

Dezfulian, M., and Bartlett, J.G. 1984. Detection of *Clostridium botulinum* type A toxin by enzyme-linked immunosorbent assay with antibodies produced in immunologically tolerant animals. J. Clin. Microbiol. 19:645–648.

Eklund, M.W., Poysky, F.T., Meyers, J.A., and Pelroy, G.A. 1974. Interspecies conversion of *Clostridium botulinum* type C to *Clostridium novyi* type A by bacteriophage. Science 186:656–658.

Farrow, B.R., Murrell, W.G., and Revington, M.C. 1983. Type C botulism in young dogs. Aust. Vet. J. 60:374–377.

Haagsma, J., and ter Laak, E.A. 1977. Aetiology and epidemiology of botulism in broiler fowls. Tijdschr. Diergeneeskd. 102:429–439.

Hampson, C.R. 1952. A case of probable botulism due to wound infection. J. Bacteriol 61:647.

Holdeman, L.V., and Brooks, J.B. 1970. Variation among strains of *Clostridium botulinum* and related clostrids. In M. Herzberg, ed., Proceedings of the First U.S.-Japan Conference on Toxic Microorganisms. Government Printing Office, Washington, D.C. Pp. 278–286.

Jansen, B.C., Knoetze, P.C., and Visser, F. 1976. The antibody response of cattle to *Clostridium botulinum* types C and D toxoids. Onderstepoort J. Vet. Res. 43:165–173.

Larsen, B.C., Nicholes, P.S., and Gebhardt, L.P. 1955. Successful immunization of mink with a toxoid against *Clostridium botulinum*, type C. Am. J. Vet. Res. 16:573–575.

Lewis, G.E., Jr., Kulinski, S.S., Metzger, P.W. Reichard, D.W., and Metzger, J.F. 1981. Detection of *Clostridium botulinum* type G toxin by ELISA. Appl. Environ. Microbiol. 42:1018–1022.

Mandia, J.W. 1951. Serological group II of the proteolytic clostridia. J. Immunol. 67:49–55.

Mandia, J.W., and Bruner, D.W. 1951. The serological identification of cultures of *Clostridium sporogenes*. J. Immunol. 66:497–505.

Marx, J.L. 1978. Botulism in infants: A cause of sudden death? Science 201:799–801.

Mason, J.H. 1968. *Clostridium botulinum* type D in mud of lakes of the Zululand Game Parks. J. S. Afr. Med. Assoc. 39:37–38.

Nakamura, S., Kimura, I., Yamakawa, K., and Nishida, S. 1983. Taxonomic relationships among *Clostridium novyi* types A and B, *Clostridium hemolyticum* and *Clostridium botulinum* type C. J. Gen. Microbiol. 129:1473–1479.

Notermons, S., Hogenaars, A.M., and Kozaki, S. 1982. The enzyme-linked immunoabsorbent assay (ELISA) for the detection and determination of *Clostridium botulinum* toxins A, B, and E. Methods Enzymol. 84:223–239.

Smith, C.D.G. 1977. Botulism: The organism, its toxins, the disease. Charles C Thomas, Springfield Ill. Pp. 113–141.

Swerczek, T.W. 1980a. Toxicoinfectious botulism in foals and adult horses. J. Am. Vet. Med. Assoc. 176:217–220.

Swerczek, T.W. 1980b. Experimentally induced toxicoinfectious botulism in horses and foals. Am. J. Vet. Res. 41:348–350.

Theiler, A., Viljoen, P.R., Green, H.H., du Toit, P.J., Meier, K., and Robinson, E.M. 1927. Lamsiekte. In 11th and 12th Annual Reports,

Director of Veterinary Education and Research, Union of South Africa, vol. 2. Pp. 819–821.

Van Ermengem, E. 1897. Über einen neuen anaeroben Bacillus und seine Beziehungen zum Botulismus. Z. Hyg. 26:1–56.

Von Dinter, Z. and Kull, K.-E. 1954. Über einen Ausbruch des Botulismus bei Fasanenküken. Nord. Vet. Med. 6:866–872.

White, P.G., and Appleton, G.S. 1969. Botulinum toxoid. J. Am. Vet. Res. Assoc. 137:652–653.

The Tissue-Invading and Enterotoxigenic Group

Clostridium perfringens

SYNONYM: *Bacillus aerogenen capsulatus,*
Bacillus phlegmonis emphysematosae,
Clostridium welchii, gas bacillus,
Welch's bacillus

C. perfringens was first isolated and described by Welch and Nuttall (1892) from a decomposing human cadaver in which the tissues were gaseous; they named it *Bacillus aerogenes capsulatus.* The organism was later named *Bacillus perfringens* by Veillon and Zuber (1898). In 1900 W. Migula termed it *Bacillus welchii,* the name by which it is best known to American workers. However, the name given by Veillon and Zuber clearly seems to have precedence and it has been used in recent editions of *Bergey's Manual;* hence it will be used here.

C. perfringens is widespread in the soil and is found in the alimentary tract of nearly all species of warm-blooded animals. It is frequently found as a postmortem invader from the alimentary tract in the tissues of bloating cadavers of animals. For this reason caution is necessary in drawing conclusions based on the presence of the organism in tissues collected after death. It is found more often in the so-called gas gangrene infections of humans than any other organism, although it generally is associated with other species of anaerobes in these processes. It also is found in malignant edemalike infections of animals, particularly sheep. Toxigenic varieties of the organism are involved in fatal toxemias in sheep, calves, young pigs, and humans. These varieties are divided into five types, A to E, on the basis of the production of four major lethal toxins.

Morphology and Staining Reactions. *C. perfringens* occurs as thick, straight-sided rods, either singly or in pairs, seldom in chains. The individual cells are about 1 μm wide and 4 to 8 μm long. The spores are oval and small enough not to cause much swelling of the rods. Spores do not form in highly acid media; hence they are unlikely to be found in media that contain fermentable carbohydrate. Strains vary in their ability to sporulate; sometimes it is difficult to find spores no matter what the nature of the culture medium. Sporulation in tissues is uncommon. In old cultures, *C. perfringens* is pleomorphic, appearing as clubbed types, ballooned cells, and filaments. Capsules are formed in tissues and in some types of culture media. There are no flagella. The organisms of young cultures retain Gram's stain; older organisms frequently decolorize.

Cultural and Biochemical Features. Colonies of *C. perfringens* on blood agar are surrounded by an inner zone of complete hemolysis and an outer zone of incomplete hemolysis. On egg-yolk agar, an opaque, whitish precipitate is formed within the medium as a result of the activity of lecithinase (phospholipase C). In deep agar the colonies are small and biconvex. In a tube containing glucose or other fermentable substrates, the medium is fragmented and even blown out of the tube by the abundant amounts of gas that are formed. *C. perfringens* rapidly liquefies gelatin but not coagulated egg medium or Loeffler's blood serum. It grows well in cooked-meat medium and produces considerable amounts of gas. The meat fragments are pinkish and not digested, and a sour odor is emitted. A very characteristic reaction, "stormy" fermentation, occurs in litmus milk. *C. perfringens* forms acid and gas from glucose, levulose, galactose, mannose, maltose, lactose, sucrose, xylose, trehalose, raffinose, starch, glycogen, and inositol. Some strains attack glycerol and inulin. The products of fermentation include acetic and butyric acids. The characteristics of *C. perfringens* and of the other tissue-invading clostridia are listed in Table 22.2.

Antigens and Toxins. Studies on serologic relationships have indicated considerable heterogeneity within the species. Cross-reactions due to common capsular antigens have been found, and the use of the quellung reaction and the agar-gel diffusion technique have demonstrated the sharing of common antigens among the five toxicogenic types. The production of four major toxins (alpha, beta, epsilon, and iota) is the basis for the classification of *C. perfringens.* These toxins are proteinaceous, enzymic in action, heat-labile, antigenic, and can be "toxoided" by the addition of chemicals that destroy their toxicity but not their antigenicity. The alpha toxin is a phospholipase and historically the first bacterial toxin for which the biochemical mode of action was elucidated (MacFarlane and Knight 1941).

The major toxins associated with the five *C. perfringens* types and the diseases produced by them are listed in Tables 22.3 and 22.4. Other less important toxins include hyaluronidase, deoxyribonuclease, collagenase, and proteinase. The site of action of phospholipase C is shown in Figure 22.7.

Epizootiology and Pathogenesis. *C. perfringens* is

Table 22.2. Characteristics of tissue-invading spore-bearing anaerobes

Morphologic and biochemical tests	C. perfringens	C. haemolyticum	C. novyi	C. chauvoei	C. septicum	C. colinum	C. villosum
Spores	Cent.	S.T.	S.T.	S.T.	S.T.	S.T.	S.T.
Motility	–	+	+	+	+	+	–
Deep agar colonies	Lenticular	Lenticular	Lenticular	Pin point	Fluffy lenticular	Fluffy lenticular	Fluffy
Milk	Stormy ferm.	Coagulation	0	Coagulation	Coagulation	Coagulation	Coagulation
Gelatin	Gas liq., black	Gas liq.	Gas liq., black	Gas liq.	Gas liq.	Gas liq.	Gas liq.
Glucose agar	Growth	Growth	Growth	No growth	Growth	Growth	No growth
Glucose	+	+	+	+	+	+	–
Lactose	+	–	–	+	+	–	–
Sucrose	+	–	–	+	–	+	–
Maltose	+	–	+	+	+	+	–
Galactose	+	–	–	+	+	–	–
Salicin	–	–	–	–	+	–	–
Pathogenic	+	+	+	+	+	+	+
Toxin formed	+	?	+	±	+	?	?
Liver surface smear	Single and short chains		Single and chains	Single	Single and filaments	Single and short chains	Not relevant

S.T. = subterminal; Cent. = central; 0 = no change.

Table 22.3. Characteristics of the major toxins of *C. perfringens*

Toxin	Properties	Mode of action	Effect in body
Alpha	Phospholipase C (lecithinase)	Hydrolyses lecithin complexes in mitochondria, cell membranes, blood phospholipids, and capillary endothelium	Hemolytic; leukocidal; increased capillary permeability due to endothelial damage; degeneration of muscle plasma membrane
Beta	Necrotizing, trypsin labile	Unknown	Necrosis of intestinal mucosa
Epsilon	Necrotizing and neurotoxic	Damages junctions between vascular endothelial cells of brain	Local liquefactive necrosis of brain tissue; necrosis of renal cortex; permeability of intestinal mucosa; increased perivascular edema produced in meninges and brain
Iota	Necrotizing, lethal; enzymic activation of prototoxin necessary	Unknown	Necrosis of intestinal mucosa

ubiquitous in nature and is part of the normal intestinal flora of healthy animals. Highly proteinaceous diets lead to great increases in populations of the organism in the gut. Type A strains are well adapted to survival in the soil, whereas type B, C, D, and E strains appear to be more highly adapted to the intestine. Also, type B and E strains have a much more distinct regional distribution than the other strains. *C. perfringens* is the most common cause of necrotizing myositis in horses as a sequel to contaminated wounds or injection sites.

C. perfringens type A. *C. perfringens* type A causes a disease known as *yellow lamb disease,* which occurs in California and Oregon during spring when nursing lamb populations are at a maximum (McGowan et al. 1958). Affected lambs are depressed, have pale mucous membranes, anemia, icterus, and hemoglobinuria, and die within 6 to 12 hours of showing symptoms. Alpha toxin is produced in the small intestine, is absorbed into the circulation, and causes massive intravascular hemolysis and capillary damage.

The disease has also been reported in captive wild goats (Russell 1970). A case of recurrent diarrhea in a dog associated with *C. perfringens* type A has been described (Carman and Lewis 1983). Enterotoxemia in mink caused by this type has also been reported (Macarie et al. 1980). *C. perfringens* type A enterotoxemia in horses characterized by high counts of *C. perfringens* type A (10^4–10^7 CFU/g), acute foul smelling diarrhea, depression, and death shortly after onset has been described by Weirup (1977).

Table 22.4. The diseases in animals caused by, and the major toxins of, *C. perfringens* types A, B, C, D, and E

Type	Disease	Distribution	Toxins			
			Alpha	Beta	Epsilon	Iota
A	Yellow lamb disease	California	+*	−	−	−
B	Lamb dysentery	Europe, South Africa	+	+*	+	−
	Hemorrhagic enteritis of sheep and goats	Middle East, Iran				
C	Necrotic enteritis (lambs, piglets, calves, chickens)	Worldwide	+	+*	−	−
	Struck (sheep)	England				
D	Enterotoxemia—overeating disease, pulpy kidney disease (sheep)	Worldwide	+	−	+*	−
E	Enterotoxemia (lambs and calves)	United States, England, Australia	+	−	−	+*

*The most important toxin in the disease process.

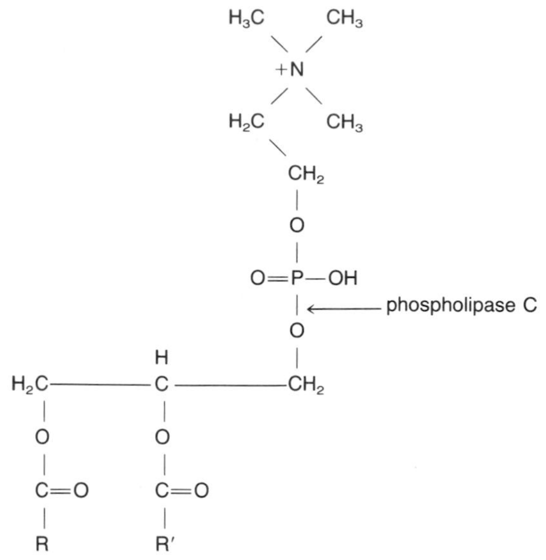

Figure 22.7. Site of action of phospholipase C of *Clostridium perfringens* on lecithin.

C. perfringens type B. Type B is usually found in the disease known as *lamb dysentery.* The disease in prevalent in the border country between England and Scotland, in Wales, and in South Africa and the Middle East. A similar disease was also described in Montana by Tunnicliff (1933). Lambs apparently become infected in the first days of life with type B strains derived from their dams or from the environment. The populations of the organism become large in those lambs getting great quantities of milk. Beta toxin is produced and causes hemorrhagic zones and ulceration of the small intestine. Affected lambs die in a few hours after showing signs of abdominal pain, lack of interest in suckling, and continuous bleating.

Hemorrhagic enteritis of sheep, goats, calves, and foals caused by *C. perfringens* type B has also been described (Buxton et al. 1978, Frank 1956) and has been reviewed by Roberts (1958).

C. perfringens type C. Type C causes *enterotoxemia* in a variety of animal species. Hemorrhagic and necrotic enteritis in calves (Griner and Bracken 1953) and lambs (Griner and Johnson 1954) has occasionally been shown to be caused by the toxins of *C. perfringens* type C. In lambs the disease resembles lamb dysentery. In calves the disease is usually seen in animals that are healthy and vigorous and less than a week old. The hemorrhagic enteritis is caused by the beta toxin, which can sometimes be demonstrated in fresh intestinal contents. This toxin is very labile and easily denatured by enzymatic action in the intestine, so a failure to demonstrate it is not significant from a diagnostic standpoint.

Piglets in the first week of life may exhibit an acute hemorrhagic enteritis with high mortality (Field and Gibson 1955). Severe enteritis with patches of necrosis on the mucosa involving mainly the jejunum is seen at postmortem examination. The disease is common in the United States, Denmark, and Britain and once established in a herd, tends to become enzootic. Outbreaks of type C exterotoxemia in chickens aged 6 to 12 weeks have also been described (Parish 1961, Roberts and Collings 1973). Affected birds exhibit weakness and dysentery. Beta toxin is apparently responsible for the intestinal lesions because it is found in the intestinal contents of affected birds. Predisposing causes of outbreaks include overcrowding and regrouping.

The disease of adult sheep called *struck* or *Romney Marsh disease* is also caused by *C. perfringens* type C. The organism is present in the soil of the Romney Marsh areas of England, and presumably most sheep in the area become infected. The disease is seen in early spring. For reasons as yet unknown, the organism multiplies in the abomasum and small intestine and produces beta toxin. The beta toxin causes necrosis of the mucosa of these regions. Dysentery or diarrhea are seldom present. In some cases, evidence of toxemia such as accumulation of fluid in the peritoneal and thoracic cavities is present without visible lesions in the intestinal tract. The beta toxin may be demonstrated in the fluids (Sterne and Thomson 1963).

C. perfringens type D. Type D causes *enterotoxemia* in sheep (*pulpy kidney disease, overeating disease*), a disease that is common in most sheep-raising areas of the world. The organism is found in the soil and in the digestive tracts of most healthy sheep. Intensive sheep-raising systems, including feedlots, are particularly prone to outbreaks of enterotoxemia. During periods when the sheep are fed high levels of concentrates, the organism multiplies in the intestine and can produce lethal quantities of toxin.

The important toxin in this disease is the epsilon toxin, which requires trypsin or chymotrypsin activation. The toxin has a permease effect on the intestinal mucosa that enhances its own absorption. After absorption the toxin causes foci of liquefactive necrosis, perivascular edema, and hemorrhages, especially in the meninges (Buxton et al. 1978). Receptor sites for the toxin are present on the vascular endothelium of the brain, where the toxin causes the intercellular junctions to break down and fluid to escape (Buxton and Morgan 1976). Hemorrhagic areas on the small intestine and petechiation of the endocardium can be present. A frequent lesion is subendocardial hemorrhage around the mitral valve. Hyperemia and degenerative changes are found in the kidney cortex, which becomes soft and friable (pulpy kidney) (Figure 22.8). Permeability changes affecting the vasculature of the serous surfaces of the peritoneum and pericardium are also reflected in effusions of straw-colored fluid into these cavities. Glucose is usually present in the urine in the bladder at death. Activated epsilon toxin has been shown to have a pressor activity, causing a rise in blood pressure apparently as a result of vasoconstriction (Sakurai et al. 1983). Death of the animal may be sudden or it may be preceded by dullness, retraction of the head, and convulsions with agonal struggling.

C. perfringens type D enterotoxemia has also been reported in calves (Griner et al. 1956). The disease is similar to that in sheep, but some calves may exhibit a sudden onset of bellowing, manic charging about, and eventual convulsions and death.

C. perfringens type E. Type E is believed to have caused hemorrhagic, necrotic enteritis of calves in Australia (Hart and Hooper 1967). Both the organism and its toxin are also sometimes found in sheep or bovine intestines at postmortem examination even though there are no signs of clostridial enterotoxemia (Sterne and Thomson 1963).

C. sordellii has been reported in association with *C. perfringens* in cases of enterotoxemia of sheep and lambs (Popoff 1984), but its contribution to the disease process was not determined. It is probable that its numbers in the intestinal contents were increased by the same conditions that promoted overgrowth of the toxigenic clone of *C. perfringens*.

Immunity. Type-specific alum-precipitated toxoids or formalinized toxoids are effective vaccines against the *C. perfringens* enterotoxemias. Type B and type C vaccines or antiserums will cross-protect because beta toxin is the important toxin in each. Either type B or type C antiserum thus can be used to passively protect against lamb dysentery. Piglets can be protected against type C necrotic enteritis by immunization of sows with type B or C toxoids (Ripley and Gush 1983).

Ewes should be vaccinated with either type B or type C vaccine in the fall and again a few weeks before lambing. Lambs will thereby be protected against lamb dysentery by colostral antibodies in the ewes' milk. Vaccination of ewes against type D enterotoxemia will similarly result in passive protection of lambs (Smith and Matsuoka 1959). Lambs should be vaccinated at about 10 days of age and again 2 to 6 weeks later (Kennedy et al. 1977). During an outbreak, toxoid and antiserum can be administered at the same time, followed by a booster inoculation of toxoid 4 weeks later (Parish 1961).

Diagnosis. *C. perfringens* type A is present in the muscles and organs of virtually all carcasses within a few

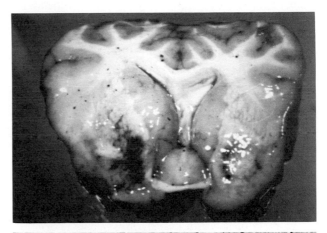

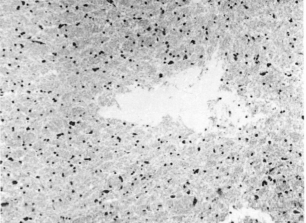

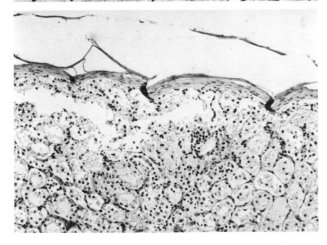

Figure 22.8. Lesions of enterotoxemia caused by *Clostridium perfringens* type D in a lamb. (*Top*) Lesions of malacia toward the ventral surface of each side of the cerebrum. The section of cerebrum (*middle*) shows an area of malacia; the section of kidney cortex (*bottom*) reveals necrosis of the tissues underlying the capsule. Middle and bottom photos × 370.

hours of death unless they have been rapidly chilled. Laboratory diagnosis of yellow lamb disease thus depends on demonstration of alpha toxin in the intestinal contents and bloodstream of fresh carcasses. Large numbers of *C. perfringens* type A will be found in the contents of the small intestine. Counts in this area normally are about 10^2/ml.

In lamb dysentery the presence of type B organisms or beta toxin in intestinal contents or tissues of neonatal lambs is good evidence of the disease.

Enterotoxemias in lambs and calves and struck in adult sheep are diagnosed in the laboratory by the demonstration of beta toxin in the intestinal contents and serous exudates, and high counts of type C organisms in the small intestine. Type C organisms are differentiated from type B strains by the production of epsilon toxin.

The mere presence of *C. perfringens* type D or of its epsilon toxin in the intestinal contents is insufficient evidence for a diagnosis of type D enterotoxemia. This is so because of the widespread occurrence of type D strains and because epsilon toxin may normally be present in the intestine but is not absorbed by the naturally resistant or immune animal (Sterne and Thomson 1963). Diagnosis of type D enterotoxemia must be based on (1) large numbers of *C. perfringens* type D in the intestine, (2) epsilon toxin in the small intestine, (3) type D organisms in the kidney and other parenchymatous organs at death, and (4) sugar in the urine. Sterne and Thomson (1963) pointed out that the simultaneous presence of epsilon toxin in the intestine and sugar in the urine is pathognomic for type D enterotoxemia.

The toxins of *C. perfringens* are detected and identified by serum-neutralization tests in mice and guinea pigs. The procedures are described by Carter (1984). Samples of the intestinal contents (small intestine) and other body fluids should be collected as soon after death as possible and 1 percent chloroform added as a preservative. Samples should be kept chilled during transport to the laboratory, where they are centrifuged. The supernatant (0.2 to 0.4 ml) then is injected intravenously into mice and intradermally into white skin areas of guinea pigs. Part of the sample should be treated with trypsin (1 percent trypsin powder, w/v) and left at room temperature for 1 hour to activate epsilon and iota toxins and destroy beta toxins. The enzyme-treated solutions are then injected into a second group of mice and pigs. If toxin is present, the mice die in 4 to 12 hours. Guinea pigs are observed for 48 hours for the development of necrotic lesions at the site of inoculation. Simultaneously or after toxic activity has been detected, a third group of animals is inoculated with the toxic supernatants that have been reacted with antiserums against types A, B, C, D, and E. The neutralization tests are read over 72 hours and interpreted according to the data in Table 22.5.

Table 22.5. Interpretation of serum neutralization tests for *C. perfringens* toxin

Antitoxin	Types neutralized	Toxins neutralized
Type A	Type A only	Alpha
Type B	Types A, B, C, and D	Alpha, beta, epsilon
Type C	Types A and C	Alpha, beta
Type D	Types A and D	Alpha, epsilon
Type E	Types A and E	Alpha, iota

Antimicrobial Susceptibility. *C. perfringens* is sensitive to penicillin G, tetracyclines, chloramphenicol, avoparcin, monensin, furazolidone, bacitracin, carbadox, erythromycin, lincomycin, clindomycin and virginiamycin. It is naturally resistant to the aminoglycosides (Kinsey and Hirsh 1978). Acquired resistance to tetracyclines and other antimicrobials used for growth promotion and disease prevention has been noted in strains from swine and poultry (Dutta and Devriese 1980). Penicillin-resistant strains have not been observed.

REFERENCES

Buxton, D., and Morgan, K.T. 1976. Studies of lesion produced in the brains of colostrum deprived lambs by *Clostridium welchii (Cl. perfringens)* type D toxin. J. Comp. Pathol. 86:435–447.

Buxton, D., Linklater, K.A., and Dyson, D.A. 1978. Pulpy kidney disease and its diagnosis by histological examination. Vet. Rec. 102:241.

Carman, R.J., and Lewis, J.C.M. 1983. Recurrent diarrhea in a dog associated with *C. perfringens* type A. Vet. Rec. 112:342–343.

Carter, G.R. 1984. Diagnostic Procedures in Veterinary Microbiology. Charles C Thomas, Springfield, Ill. Pp. 191–192.

Dutta, G.N., and Devriese, L.A. 1980. Susceptibility of *Clostridium perfringens* of animal origin to fifteen antimicrobial agents. J. Vet. Pharmacol. Ther. 3:227–236.

Field, H.I., and Gibson, E.A. 1955. Studies on piglet mortality. 2. *Clostridium welchii* infection. Vet. Rec. 67:31–34.

Frank, F.W. 1956. *Clostridium perfringens* type B from enterotoxemia in young ruminants. Am. J. Vet. Res. 17:492–494.

Griner, L.A., and Bracken, F.K. 1953. *Clostridium perfringens* (type C) in acute hemorrhagic enteritis of calves. J. Am. Vet. Med. Assoc. 122:99–102.

Griner, L.A., and Johnson, H.W. 1954. *Clostridium perfringens* type C in hemorrhagic enterotoxemia of lambs. J. Am. Vet. Med. Assoc. 125:125–127.

Griner, L.A., Aichelman, W.W. and Brown, G.D. 1956. *Clostridium perfringens* type D (Epsilon) enterotoxemia in Brown Swiss dairy calves. J. Am. Vet. Med. Assoc. 129:375–376.

Hart, B., and Hooper, P.T. 1967. Enterotoxaemia of calves due to *Clostridium welchii* type E. Aust. Vet. J. 43:360–363.

Kennedy, K.K., Norris, S.J., Bechenhauer, W.H., and White, R.G. 1977. Vaccination of cattle and sheep with combined *Clostridium perfringens* types C and D toxoid. Am. J. Vet. Res. 38:1515–1517.

Kinsey, P.B., and Hirsh, D.C. 1978. Obligate anaerobes in clinical veterinary medicine: Susceptibility to antimicrobial agents. J. Vet. Pharmacol. Ther. 1:63–68.

MacFarlane, M.G., and Knight, B.C.J.G. 1941. The biochemistry of bacterial toxins. I. The lecithinase activity of *Cl. welchii* toxins. Biochem. J. 35:884–902.

McGowan, B., Moulton, J.E., and Rood, S.E. 1958. Lamb losses associated with *Clostridium perfringens* type A. J. Am. Vet. Med. Assoc. 133:219–221.

Macarie, I., Cure, C., and Pop, A. 1980. Histopathology of natural *Clostridium perfringens* type A infection in mink. Lucr. Stiint. Inst. Agron.–Nicolae Balcescu–C 23:23–27.

Parish, W.E. 1961. Necrotic enteritis in the fowl. III. The experimental disease. J. Comp. Pathol. 71:405–413.

Popoff, M.R. 1984. Bacteriological examination in enterotoxemia of sheep and lamb. Vet. Rec. 114:324.

Ripley, P.H., and Gush, A.F. 1983. Immunization schedule for the prevention of infectious necrotic enteritis caused by *Clostridium perfringens* type C in piglets. Vet. Rec. 112:201–202.

Roberts, R.S. 1958. Clostridial diseases. In A.W. Stableforth and I.A. Galloway, eds., Diseases Due to Bacteria, Vol. 1. Academic Press, New York. Pp. 194–200.

Roberts, T.A., and Collings, D.F. 1973. An outbreak of type C botulism in broiler chicken. Avian Dis. 17:650–658.

Russell, W.C. 1970. Type A enterotoxemia in captive wild goats. J. Am. Vet. Med. Assoc. 157:643–646.

Sakurai, J., Nagahama, M., and Fujii, Y. 1983. Effect of *Clostridium perfringens* epsilon toxin on the cardiovascular system of rats. Infect. Immun. 42:1183–1186.

Smith, L., and Matsuoka, T. 1959. Maternally induced protection of young lambs against the *Epsilon* toxin of *Clostridium perfringens* using inactivated vaccine. Am. J. Vet. Res. 20:91–93.

Sterne, M., and Thomson, A. 1963. The isolation and identification of *Clostridia* from pathological conditions of animals. Bull. Off. Int. Epizoot. 59:1487–1498.

Tunnicliff, E.A. 1933. A strain of *Clostridium welchii* producing fatal dysentery in lambs. J. Infect. Dis. 52:407–412.

Veillon, M.M., and Zuber, W. 1898. Recherches sur quelques microbes strictement anaérobies et leur vole en pathologie. Arch. Med. Exp. Anat. Pathol. 10:517–545.

Welch, W.H., and Nuttall, G.H.F. 1882. A gas-producing bacillus (bacillus aerogenes capsulatus, nov. species) capable of rapid development in the blood-vessels after death. Johns Hopkins Hosp. Bull. 3:81–91.

Wicrup, M. 1977. Equine intestinal clostridiosis. An acute disease in horses associated with high intestinal counts of *Clostridium perfringens* type A. Acta Vet. Scand. (Suppl.) 62:1–182.

Clostridium haemolyticum

SYNONYMS: *Bacillus haemolyticus,*
Clostridium haemolyticus bovis,
Clostridium novyi type D, *Clostridium oedematiens* type D

C. haemolyticum is closely related to *C. novyi* and is the cause of a disease of cattle and occasionally of sheep commonly known as *red water disease*. It is also known as *hemorrhagic disease* and *infectious icterohemoglobinuria*. One case in a hog has been described by Records and Huber (1931). Because of its similarity to *C. novyi,* the organism has been called *C. novyi* type D (Oakley and Warrack 1959), a classification supported by DNA-DNA homology studies (Nakamura et al. 1983).

Morphology and Staining Reactions. *C. haemolyticum* is somewhat larger than most of the other tissue-invading anaerobic bacilli. It measures 1.0 to 1.3 μm in breadth and 3.0 to 5.6 μm in length. It has straight sides and rounded ends. It occurs singly as a rule but may form short chains in tissues and cultures. The spores are oval and are located subterminally. They cause bulging of the cells in which they lie. The cells are actively motile when young. Young cells are Gram-positive but rapidly lose their ability to retain this stain.

Cultural and Biochemical Features. Colonies grown in deep agar are lenticular at first and later become woolly. Little or no gas is formed unless fermentable sugar is added to the medium. When blood is present, it is rapidly hemolyzed. *C. haemolyticum* liquefies gelatin in 2 to 4 days, but it does not soften or liquefy coagulated serum and egg media. Cooked-meat medium and brain medium support good growth of *C. haemolyticum* but it does not digest the solids or blacken the medium unless iron salts are added; even in the presence of an abundance of iron salts the blackening is only slight. The organism does not affect milk. Glucose and levulose are the only carbohydrates it will ferment. These are actively destroyed with the evolution of both acid and gas. The organism forms large amounts of H_2S in liver medium and in media containing proteose-peptone. It reacts negatively to the methyl red and Voges-Proskauer tests, and it does not reduce nitrates. It forms large amounts of indole.

This organism is very exacting in its cultural requirements. Good anaerobic conditions are necessary, and the medium must contain tryptophan for optimum growth and toxin formation. Acetic, propionic, and butyric acids are the principal fermentation products.

Antigens and Toxins. *C. haemolyticum* and *C. novyi* type B have protein profiles on polyacrylamide gel electrophoresis which are indistinguishable (Cato et al. 1982). *C. haemolyticum* produces beta toxin only, whereas *C. novyi* type B produces both beta and alpha toxins. Alpha toxin in *C. novyi* has been shown to be phage mediated (Eklund et al. 1976), and the phage carrying the alpha toxin gene has been shown to be capable of transducing the trait to *C. haemolyticum* (Shallehm and Eklund 1980). It thus appears that *C. haemolyticum* and some types of *C. novyi* may differ only in phage-mediated traits. Beta toxin has a molecular weight of about 32,000 and is trypsin labile (Durakhashan and Lauerman 1981).

Epizootiology and Pathogenesis. The organism was initially thought to be restricted to the Rocky Mountain region of the United States, but it was later found in the delta parishes of Louisiana, along the Gulf of Mexico, in Florida, Central Mexico, and as far away as Wales, New Zealand, Rumania, Turkey, and South America. A closely related organism has been isolated from a similar disease in Chile (Smith 1954). The organism shows a predilection for alkaline water, and the disease is associated with pastures that contain swampy areas in which the pH remains at 8.0 or higher. It is believed that carrier animals may introduce the organism into uninfected areas (Safford and Smith 1954, Smith and Jasmin 1956).

In the United States the disease occurs principally during the summer and early fall months. The site of toxin production is the liver. There is good circumstantial evidence that the tissue destruction caused by the migration of liver flukes provides a suitable microenvironment for germination of the spores of *C. haemolyticum,* with subsequent multiplication and toxin synthesis. This phase of the pathogenesis is similar to that of *C. novyi* type B. The disease is unlikely to occur when fluke infestations are minimal. That damage to the liver is important in initiating bacterial multiplication and toxin synthesis is illustrated by an outbreak of bacillary hemoglobinuria that occurred 2 to 3 days after liver biopsies were performed on a group of cattle raised in an endemic area (Olander et al. 1966).

The beta toxin (phospholipase C) released in the liver causes massive intravascular hemolysis and capillary damage. Hemoglobin is passed in the urine, and there is hemorrhage into the lumen of the intestine as a result of local capillary destruction.

Affected animals stand apart from the rest of the herd. The animal will arch its back and tuck up its abdomen; it is difficult to make the animal move. Breathing is shallow, and there is grunting with each step. The temperature varies from 104° to 106°F in the early stages but becomes subnormal before death. The feces become deeply bile-stained or bloody. The urine is dark red or port-colored and clear but foamy. The color is due to large amounts of hemoglobin. There are no intact erythrocytes in the urine. Sugar is absent, but albumin tests yield strongly positive results.

At the time that hemoglobinuria appears, as much as 40 to 50 percent of the erythrocytes have been destroyed. The red cell count at this time may not be greater than $2,000,000/\mu l$ and the hemoglobin readings may be as low as 3.5 g/100 ml of blood. The leukocyte count increases, sometimes to as high as $30,000/mm^3$. Mortality is high, varying from 90 to 95 percent in untreated animals. Death is caused by anoxemia because of the wholesale destruction of erythrocytes.

The most characteristic lesion is the large infarct that is always found in the liver (Figure 22.9). This is a mass of necrotic tissue, varying from 5 to 20 cm in diameter, often mottled, and usually lighter in color than the normal liver tissue. The infarct may be located in any part of the organ and results from an occluding thrombosis of one of the branches of the portal vein. In the sinusoids of these areas great numbers of large rod-shaped bacteria containing subterminal or terminal spores may be found (Figure 22.10).

Extensive hemorrhages are found in the serous membranes, in the subcutaneous connective tissue, and in the

Figure 22.9. A massive infarct in a bovine liver caused by infection with *Clostridium hemolyticum.* This lesion is characteristic of redwater disease of cattle. (Courtesy E. Records.)

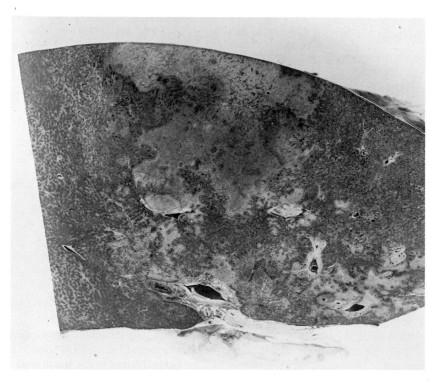

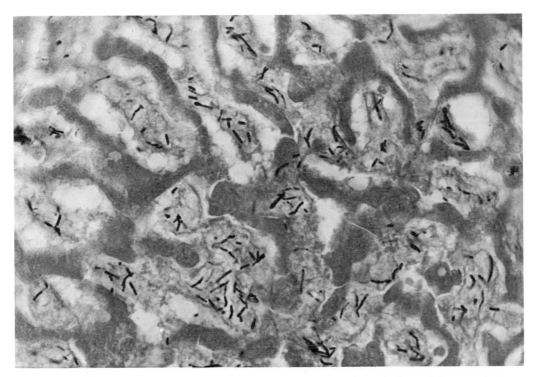

Figure 22.10. *Clostridium hemolyticum* in a characteristic liver infarct. A few of the organisms are beginning to form spores. × 750. (Courtesy E. Records.)

substance of the visceral organs. Acute degenerative changes occur in the organs, and the peritoneal and pleural cavities usually contain large quantities of hemoglobin-stained transudates. Besides the subserous hemorrhages that regularly occur in the intestinal wall, there is a severe hemorrhagic enteritis, the mucous membrane often being almost wholly undermined with extensive hemorrhage.

Rabbits, guinea pigs, and mice can be readily killed by cultures containing toxin. Subcutaneous injection leads to the formation of a hemorrhagic, edematous area at the point of inoculation with little or no gas formation. Intravenous inoculation of rabbits usually leads to death in 2 to 4 hours with widespread destruction of blood and hemoglobinuria.

Immunity. Alum-precipitated formalinized whole cultures of *C. haemolyticum* are used for immunization of cattle. Vaccination must be repeated every 6 to 12 months in endemic areas. Immunized animals produce agglutinating antibodies but little antitoxin. Immunity appears to be primarily antibacterial (Claus and Macheak 1965). Antiserum has been used for prophylaxis and therapy (Vawter and Records 1929). For therapy 500 to 1,000 ml must be given.

Diagnosis. *C. haemolyticum* can be cultured from and phospholipase C demonstrated in the liver lesion. Guinea pigs inoculated intramuscularly with homogenates of lesions die in 1 or 2 days.

Antimicrobial Susceptibility. *C. haemolyticum* is sensitive to penicillin G, ampicillin, chloramphenicol, and tetracyclines.

REFERENCES

Cato, E.P., Holdeman, L.V., and Moore, W.E.C. 1982. Electrophoretic study of *Clostridium* species. J. Clin. Microbiol. 15:688–702.

Claus, K.D., and Macheak, M.E. 1965. Nonantigenic nature of *Clostridium haemolyticum* toxoid. Am. J. Vet. Res. 26:353–356.

Durakhashan, H., and Lauerman, C.H. 1981. Some properties of beta toxin produced by *Clostridium hemolyticum* strain IRP135. Comp. Immunol. Microbiol. Infect. Dis. 4:307–316.

Eklund, M.W., Poysky, F.T., Peterson, M.E., and Meyers, J.A. 1976. Relationships of bacteriophages to alpha toxin production in *Clostridium novyi* types A and B. Infect. Immun. 14:793–803.

Nakamura, S., Kimura, I., Yamakawa, K., and Nishida, S. 1983. Taxonomic relationships among *Clostridium novyi* types A and B, *Clostridium haemolyticum* and *Clostridium botulinum* type C. J. Gen. Microbiol. 139:1473–1479.

Oakley, C.L., and Warrack, G.H. 1959. The soluble antigens of *Clostridium oedematiens* type D (*Cl. haemolyticum*). J. Pathol. Bacteriol. 78:543–551.

Olander, H.J., Hughes, J.P., and Biberstein, E.L. 1966. Bacillary hemoglobinuria: Induction by liver biopsy in naturally and experimentally infected animals. Pathol. Vet. 3:421–450.

Records, E., and Huber, M. 1931. Hemolyticus infection in a hog. J. Am. Vet. Med. Assoc. 78:863–865.

Safford, J.W., and Smith, L.D. 1954. A study of the epizootiology of bacillary hemoglobulinuria. In Proceedings of the 91st Annual Meeting of the American Veterinary Medical Association, Seattle, Wash. Pp. 159–162.

Shallehm, G., and Eklund, M.W. 1980. Conversion of *Clostridium novyi* type D (*Cl. hemolyticum*) to alpha toxin production by phages of *Cl. novyi* type A. FEMS Microbiol. Lett. 7:83–86.

Smith, L. 1954. Introduction to Pathogenic Anaerobes. University of Chicago Press, Chicago. Pp. 147.

Smith, L., and Jasmin, A.M. 1956. The recovery of *Clostridium hemolyticum* from the livers and kidneys of apparently normal cattle. J. Am. Vet. Med. Assoc. 129:68–71.

Vawter, L.R., and Records, E. 1929. Immunization of cattle against bacillary hemoglobinuria. J. Am. Vet. Med. Assoc. 75:210–214.

Clostridium novyi

SYNONYM: *Clostridium edematis,
Novy's Bacillus edematis maligni* II

C. novyi was first described by F. G. Novy in 1894, who isolated it from a guinea pig that had been inoculated with unsterilized milk protein. It was lost for many years until Weinberg and Séguin (1915) rediscovered it in gas gangrene infections in humans. It is similar to *C. septicum* in its cultural features and pathogenicity. There are three types: A, B, and C. The relationship of *C. novyi* type B, *C. haemolyticum,* and *C. botulinum* type C (Stockholm) and the involvement of bacteriophages in toxigenesis have been discussed earlier in this chapter. *C. novyi* type C is not toxigenic or pathogenic for animals.

Morphology and Staining Reactions. *C. novyi* is one of the largest of anaerobic bacilli. It measures 0.8 to 1.0 μm in breadth and is from 3 to 10 μm long. The rods usually are quite straight and the ends rounded. The spores generally are present in abundance, are located subterminally, and are oval. Organisms in young cultures are motile by peritrichous flagella and are Gram-positive. Those in older cultures usually lose this property.

Cultural and Biochemical Features. *C. novyi* is more strictly anaerobic than most of the other clostridia and requires cysteine in its reduced form. The reduced state can be maintained by the addition of 0.03 percent dithiothreitol to the medium. In deep agar cultures the colonies grow well, especially when glucose is present. The colonies vary in form, some being compact and slightly yellowish, others loose and woolly. The medium is disrupted by gas formation. On blood agar the colonies are surrounded by hemolytic zones. *C. novyi* liquefies gelatin but not coagulated blood serum or egg albumen. It reduces but does not coagulate litmus milk. Growth is poor in broth, most of it settling to the bottom, but good in cooked-meat medium. The meat fragments become reddish and a rancid smell is emitted. The organism forms acid and gas from glucose, levulose, maltose, xylose, starch, and glycerol, but it does not ferment lactose, sucrose, mannitol, dulcitol, inulin, or salicin. Principal fermentation products are acetic, propionic, and butyric

Table 22.6. Toxins and diseases produced by and hosts of *C. novyi*

Type	Toxins produced	Disease	Hosts
A	Alpha, gamma, epsilon	Gas gangrene Big head	Sheep and cattle Rams
B	Alpha, beta	Black disease	Sheep and cattle
C	—	Osteomyelitis*	Buffalo

*Of questionable etiological significance.

acids. Types A and B but not C produce a positive lecithinase reaction.

Antigens and Toxins. No detailed study of the serologic characteristics of *C. novyi* has been made. The organism shares somatic protein antigens with *C. haemolyticum.* The three immunologic types (A, B, and C) are based on the toxins produced (Oakley and Warrack 1959, Pomberton et al. 1971). These are listed in Table 22.6.

Epizootiology and Pathogenesis. *C. novyi* type A occurs in the soil and in the intestinal tract of herbivorous animals. It may multiply in wounds contaminated by soil and cause gas gangrene. In yearling rams, infections of the head and neck area result from wounds sustained in fighting and cause the condition known as *big head.*

After invasion toxins are synthesized and released. The alpha toxin produced by type A strains damages capillary endothelium at the site of invasion (Elder and Miles 1957) and in the brain after it is absorbed into the bloodstream. Muscle, the liver, and the heart are also damaged, as is evidenced by the elevation of intracellular enzymes such as lactic dehydrogenase and glutamic oxalacetic transaminase (Pomberton et al. 1971). Alpha toxins can be demonstrated in the lesions of affected animals (Williams 1962).

Black disease (necrotic hepatitis) of sheep and, to a lesser extent, of cattle occurs in Europe, Australia, New Zealand, and the United States. The disease is seen in areas infested with liver flukes. When pastures are heavily infested with *Fasciola hepatica,* liver damage from the migration of immature flukes creates suitable foci for germination of the spores of *C. novyi* type B in the liver. The organism multiplies, producing large amounts of alpha and lesser amounts of beta toxin, which circulate in the bloodstream. The effects of the alpha toxin leads to the death of the animal. On postmortem examination, necrotic areas are found near the surface of the liver. Extensive blood-stained edema occurs under the skin, hence the name *black disease.* Other effects of the alpha toxin are seen in the serous cavities, where straw-colored fluid accumulates as a result of endothelial damage.

Byrne and Armstrong (1948) reported two outbreaks of

an alimentary tract infection of Canadian cattle caused by *C. novyi*. The animals had atypical symptoms of blackleg infection. In the first outbreak, 21 of 47 animals died. In the second, use of a bacterin contining *C. novyi* limited deaths to 2 in a herd of 50 cattle. Bourne and Kerry (1965) have described cases of sudden death in sows from which *C. novyi* was isolated. The clinical signs and postmortem lesions resembled those seen in anthrax.

Immunity. Alum-precipitated formalinized whole broth cultures are effective when administered in two doses (Turner 1930). Vaccination is usually carried out a short time before expected heavy fluke activity. During an outbreak of black disease, hyperimmune serum can be administered for prophylaxis. Vaccination during this time will also reduce mortality after a lag of 10 days.

Diagnosis. The mere presence of *C. novyi* in liver tissue may not be sufficient evidence for a diagnosis of black disease because many healthy cattle and sheep in endemic areas harbor the organism in their livers (Jamieson 1949). Demonstration of alpha toxin in the lesion and in exudates, however, is excellent diagnostic proof (Sterne and Thomson 1963). The fluorescent antibody test is a rapid and reliable means of demonstrating the organism in smears from lesions (Batty et al. 1964).

Antimicrobial Susceptibility. *C. novyi* is sensitive to penicillin G, tetracycline, and chloramphenicol. The practicality of treatment is questionable because of the rapid course of the disease. Depot preparations of penicillin administered parenterally might be useful in cattle because the disease progresses more slowly in cattle than in sheep.

REFERENCES

Batty, I., Buntain, D., and Walker, P.D. 1964. *Clostridium oedematiens:* A cause of sudden death in sheep, cattle and pigs. Vet. Rec. 76:1115–1116.

Bourne, F.J., and Kerry, J.B. 1965. *Clostridium oedematiens* associated with sudden death in the pig. Vet. Rec. 77:1463–1464.

Byrne, J.L., and Armstrong, J.H.O. 1948. Blackleg with atypical symptoms caused by *Clostridium novyi*. Can. J. Comp. Med. 12:155–160.

Elder, J.M., and Miles, A.A. 1957. The action of the lethal toxins of gas gangrene clostridia on capillary permeability. J. Pathol. Bacteriol 74:133–145.

Jamieson, S. 1949. The identification of *Clostridium oedematiens* and an experimental investigation of its role in the pathogenesis of infectious necrotic hepatitis ("black disease") of sheep. J. Pathol. Bacteriol. 61:389–402.

Oakley, C.L., and Warrack, G.H. 1959. The soluble antigens of *Clostridium oedematiens* type D (*Cl. haemolyticum*). J. Pathol. Bacteriol. 78:543–551.

Pomberton, J.R., Matson, R.L., Claus, K.D., and Macheak, M.E. 1971. Changes in plasma enzyme levels of sheep infected with *Clostridium novyi,* type B. Clin. Chim. Acta 34:431–436.

Sterne, M., and Thomson, A. 1963. The isolation and identification of *Clostridia* from pathological conditions of animals. Bull. Off. Int. Epizoot. 59:1487–1498.

Turner, A.W. 1930. Black disease (infectious necrotic hepatitis) of sheep in Australia. Aust. Coun. Sci. Ind. Res. Bull. 46. Pp. 5–12.

Weinberg, M., and Séguin, P. 1915. Flore microbienne de la gangrène gazeuse. Le *B. fallox*. C. R. Seances Soc. Biol. Fil. 78:686–689.

Williams, B.M. 1962. Black disease of sheep: Observations on the disease in mid-Wales. Vet. Rec. 74:1536–1542.

Clostridium chauvoei

SYNONYMS: *Bacillus anthracis symptomatici, Bacillus carbonis, Bacillus chauvoei, Clostridium chauvei, Clostridium feseri*

C. chavoei is the cause of *blackleg* in ruminants. It occurs throughout the world and is a source of considerable economic loss. In cattle the disease is also called *blackquarter, quarter evil,* and *symptomatic anthrax.* The disease has been reported in swine (Clay 1960, Sterne and Edwards 1955) and in mink fed infected beef liver (Langford 1970) but rarely occurs in species other than ruminants. *C. chauvoei* is also the causative agent of parturient gas gangrene in sheep.

Morphology and Staining Reactions. *C. chauvoei* is seen in tissues and cultures as a straight, round-ended rod about 0.6 μm wide and from 3 to 8 μm long (Figure 22.11). It can be highly pleomorphic, however. It usually appears singly or in chains of three to five organisms in the peritoneal exudate of inoculated guinea pigs, a configuration that is useful in distinguishing it from *C. septicum* and other anaerobic bacilli, which usually occur in long chains and are frequently found in specimens from animals suspected of having blackleg. Spores are oval and appear excentrically, swelling the rods into lemon-shaped structures. Organisms in very young cultures are motile by means of peritrichous flagella. Pleomorphic cells stain somewhat unevenly. When young, the organisms are

Figure 22.11. A film from a brain-liver medium culture of *Clostridium chauvoei* incubated 48 hours at 37°C. × 1,545.

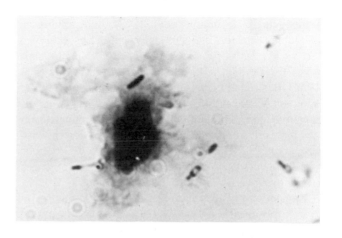

positive to Gram's stain but stain erratically after they are a few days old.

Cultural and Biochemical Features. *C. chauvoei* is a little more exacting in its cultural requirements than are most of the clostridia in the tissue-invading and enterotoxigenic group. It is strictly anaerobic and will not grow on ordinary glucose agar except when tissues are carried over in the inoculum. The addition of blood or tissue favors its growth in ordinary broth and agar. It will grow luxuriantly on all media made with a liver infusion base without enrichment. It has a high requirement for cysteine.

Colonies grown in deep agar are delicate and compact, being irregularly spherical. When blood is present, there is evidence of slight hemolysis, but definite zones are not formed around surface colonies. It usually does not grow in plain broth unless blood or tissue has been carried over with the inoculum. In liver broth the fluid becomes moderately clouded. It slowly liquefies gelatin containing a little serum, forming a few gas bubbles. Growth on coagulated blood serum and coagulated egg is poor, and there is no liquefaction. Cooked-meat medium becomes pinkish and the fluid slightly clouded. *C. chauvoei* grows well on liver-brain medium, a good medium on which to maintain cultures, and does not digest it. The organism forms acid and gas from glucose, levulose, galactose, maltose, lactose, and sucrose, but it does not ferment inulin, salicin, mannitol, glycerol, or dextrin. Cultures of this organism give off a characteristic odor, which experienced workers can use to identify the species. The principal fermentation products are butanol and acetic and butyric acids.

Antigens and Toxins. *C. chauvoei* strains have flagella antigens (designated by lower-case letters), somatic antigens (arabic numerals), and spore antigens (capital letters). Most strains share the same spore, somatic, and flagellar antigens (A:3:f). The spore antigen is shared with *C. septicum* (Moussa 1959).

The toxins produced include alpha toxin with hemolytic and necrotizing activity, hyaluronidase, and deoxyribonuclease (Jayaraman et al. 1962). Both soluble and insoluble protective antigens also occur. The soluble protective antigen is formed in conjunction with the alpha toxin from which it later dissociates (Veerpoort et al. 1966). It is found in the supernatant of fluid cultures after 17 hours (Claus and Macheak 1972). It is heat labile, pH sensitive, and nonagglutinogenic. An acid-extracted antigen that is rich in flagellar protein has also been shown to be protective (Stevenson and Stronger 1980). The number and characteristics of the protective antigen or antigens of *C. chauvoei* clearly require more definition.

Epizootiology and Pathogenesis. The organism of blackleg exists in the soil. Whether it multiplies there or whether it merely lives there in the spore form and multiplies in the intestinal canal of animals is not known. Once pastures or grazing grounds become infected, the disease reappears in susceptible animals year after year.

Spring and fall are the seasons of greatest occurrence of blackleg in the United States. In Europe the disease is frequent in the summer. The infection is most common on permanent pasture or wet bottomland, and certain pastures in a locality appear to be at especially high risk. Land cultivation diminishes this risk.

Cattle are susceptible between the ages of 6 months and 2 years. Fat, thriving animals are much more likely to develop blackleg than stock that are unthrifty.

The mode of entry in cattle is uncertain because in many cases of blackleg there are no external wounds that would explain entry of the organism into the animal. It appears that entry is by the oral route during grazing. The organism multiplies in the intestine and then passes into the lymphatic and blood circulation. Muscle and liver tissue are thereby seeded by the organism, which remains dormant until the muscle mass is altered or damaged in a way that provides the right milieu for its growth. Kerry (1964) has been able to demonstrate the organism in the livers and spleens of 20 percent of normal cattle, suggesting that the liver could serve as a source of the organism for dissemination to muscle. It has also been suggested (Shaw 1958) that the organism may enter via the alveoli when the deciduous teeth are lost and that this is the reason for the occurrence of the disease in cattle 6 months to 2 years old. Lesions in the throat and neck are easily explained by this mode of entry. The muscles of the neck, throat, back, and abdomen may occasionally be affected.

In sheep the disease often seems to be a wound infection, occurring after lambing, docking, and shearing. In Montana infection has been reported in pregnant ewes soon after they were shorn. The organism was recovered from edematous fetuses in these ewes (Butler and Marsh 1956). When the organism begins to multiply, the necrotizing, leukocidic, and spreading effects of alpha toxin and hyaluronidase promote the development of the typical myonecrosis. The affected area is dark reddish brown to black in color. It has a crepitant, spongy texture because of entrapped gas and is dry on the cut surface. Leukocyte and platelet counts decrease and the level of serum glutamic oxalacetic transaminase rapidly increases (Barnes 1963). Circulating toxin and tissue breakdown products lead to fatal toxemia with degenerative changes in the heart muscle and parenchymatous organs. In the later stages of the disease, there also is bacteremia. The animal if seen before death will appear dull and lame and it usually stands away from the herd. The affected area is first swollen, painful, and crepitant. Sensation later is lost and the skin becomes tighter. The animal dies in a day or two.

Immunity. Vaccines currently used consist of formalinized whole cultures or anacultures to which alum may be added to increase antigenicity. Protection depends on the presence of the heat-labile soluble protective antigen (Veerpoort et al. 1966). Some strains produce much more of this than others (Chankler and Gulasekhuram 1970). Some immunity can be produced from injection of heated washed cells, indicating that somatic antigens are also important in protection.

Immunizing horses with washed cultures of the blackleg organism results in a highly potent serum that is useful, if used in large amounts, in protecting valuable calves when blackleg is present in a herd and in treating cases that have already developed.

Diagnosis. The organism can be found in the heart, blood, liver, and peritoneal fluid. However, cultural identification should always be performed because other clostridia pathogenic for guinea pigs (e.g., *C. septicum*) can be secondary postmortem invaders of specimens of muscle. A fluorescent antibody technique that utilizes conjugates prepared from antiserums against *C. chauvoei* and *C. septicum* and labeled with contrasting fluorescent dyes can be routinely used to distinguish between the two organisms (Batty and Walker 1963).

Antimicrobial Susceptibility. *C. chauvoei* is sensitive to penicillin G, ampicillin, tetracycline, and chloramphenicol. Penicillin is effective in treating blackleg if administered systemically and locally into the lesion while the disease is still in the early stages (Aitken 1949). Butler and Marsh (1956) described similar results for sheep. A large amount of muscle may eventually slough away, however, and the wound will require prolonged treatment. Also, the animal's body condition deteriorates considerably, and recovery may be slow. The decision to treat thus must be carefully made.

REFERENCES

Aitken, W.A. 1949. Penicillin in blackleg. North Am. Vet. 30:441–442.

Barnes, D.M. 1963. Mechanisms of pathogenesis of clostridial myonecrosis. Ph.D. dissertation, University of Minnesota.

Batty, I., and Walker, P.D. 1963. Differentiation of *Clostridium septicum* and *Clostridium chauvoei* by the use of fluorescent-labelled antibodies. J. Pathol. Bacteriol. 85:517–521.

Butler, H.C., and Marsh, H. 1956. Blackleg of the fetus in ewes. J. Am. Vet. Med. Assoc. 128:401–402.

Chankler, H.M., and Gulasekhuram, J. 1970. An evaluation of characteristics of *Clostridium chauvoei* which possibly indicate a highly protective strain. Aust. J. Exp. Biol. Med. Sci. 48:187–197.

Claus, K.D., and Macheak, M.E. 1972. Characteristics and immuniz-

ing properties of culture filtrates of *Clostridium chauvoei*. Am. J. Vet. Res. 33:1031–1038.

Clay, H.A. 1960. A case of "blackquarter" in the pig. Vet. Rec. 72:265–266.

Jayaraman, M.S., Lal, R., and Dhanda, M.R., 1962. Toxin production by *Clostridium chauvoei*. Indian Vet. J. 39:481–484.

Kerry, J.B. 1964. A note on the occurrence of *Clostridium chauvoei* in the spleen and livers of normal cattle. Vet. Rec. 76:396–397.

Langford, E.V. 1970. Feed-borne *Clostridium chauvoei* infection in mink. Can. Vet. J. 11:170–172.

Moussa, R.S. 1959. Antigenic formulae for *Clostridium septicum* and *Clostridium chauvoei*. J. Pathol. Bacteriol. 77:341–350.

Shaw, I.G. 1958. Black-leg. Agriculture 65:138–141.

Sterne, M., and Edwards, J.B. 1955. Blackleg in pigs caused by *Clostridium chauvoei*. Vet. Rec. 67:314–315.

Stevenson, J.R., and Stronger, K.A. 1980. Protective cellular antigen of *Clostridium chauvoei*. Am. J. Vet. Res. 41:650–653.

Verpoort, J.A., Joubert, F.J., and Jansen, B.C. 1966. Studies on the soluble antigen and haemolysin of *Clostridium chauvoei* strain 64. S. Afr. J. Agric. Sci. 9:153–172.

Clostridium septicum

SYNONYMS: *Bacillus septicus, Vibrion septique;* probably Ghon-Sachs bacillus; also, erroneously, *Bacillus edematis, Bacillus edematis-maligni*

C. septicum was first identified by Pasteur and Joubert in 1877 from carcasses of animals thought to have died of anthrax. It is generally called the *malignant edema bacillus* and the condition produced in animals is termed *malignant edema*.

Morphology and Staining Reactions. *C. septicum* is a rather large rod similar in shape and size to the blackleg organism. It is 0.6 to 0.8 μm wide and 3 to 8 μm long. Usually it is straight and the ends are rounded. In cultures it often occurs singly or in short chains, but in animal exudates it appears in long chains. Its tendency to form long chains on the surface of the liver of inoculated guinea pigs is a feature by which it may be distinguished from *C. chauvoei*, which occurs singly or in very short chains. Organisms in young cultures show active motility because of peritrichous flagella. The spores are oval, occur excentrically, and swell the cells in which they are formed. It is Gram-positive but, like most of the other organisms of this group, the cells in old cultures usually decolorize. It dyes readily with all the usual stains.

Cultural and Biochemical Features. *C. septicum* grows readily in all ordinary media so long as good anaerobic conditions prevail. In its growth vigor it differs from the blackleg organism with which it is often confused, the latter being much more fastidious in its requirements than *C. septicum*.

Colonies of *C. septicum* grown in deep agar usually are cottony and filamentous. On blood agar plates the colonies are surrounded by hemolytic zones. The organism liquefies gelatin and forms a few gas bubbles in it. It lightly clouds plain infusion broth. *C. septicum* coagulates litmus milk and may form some gas in the curd, but it does not digest the curd. It also does not digest coagulated blood serum or coagulated egg albumen. There is good growth in meat medium and in brain-liver medium, but no digestion or darkening occurs. It forms acid and gas from glucose, levulose, galactose, maltose, lactose, and salicin but does not ferment sucrose and mannitol. Fermentation products are mainly acetic and butyric acids with small amounts of isobutyl, butyl, and ethyl alcohols.

Antigens and Toxins. Strains of *C. septicum* are serologically heterogeneous. By antigenic analysis of their somatic and flagellar agglutinogens they can be divided into six groups defined by two O and five H antigens (Moussa 1959). The possession of a common spore antigen renders the straight agglutination test useless as a means of distinguishing between *C. septicum* and *C. chauvoei,* but their toxins are specific. Protection against infection with *C. septicum* is afforded for the most part by immunization directed against alpha toxoid.

Epizootiology and Pathogenesis. *C. septicum* is common in soil and the intestinal tract of most animal species. After the death of the animal it frequently invades the body tissues from the intestine. This is especially true for ruminants.

In living lambs or sheep the organism may enter wounds, the umbilicus, or the abomasal lining. In the latter case the disease is known as *braxy* or *bradsot* and causes heavy mortality among yearling sheep in hilly areas of Great Britain, Ireland, Norway, Iceland, and the Faroe Islands. The circumstances that favor multiplication and invasion of the abomasal mucosa are not clear, although it is known that ingestion of frosted grass is frequently associated with the occurrence of braxy. It is possible that the icy feed material devitalizes the mucosa, allowing entry of the organism. Affected animals die suddenly without previously showing symptoms. The walls of the abomasum and the first part of the small intestine are edematous, hemorrhagic, and sometimes necrotic. The internal organs show only degenerative changes.

Wound infections in animals are known under the general name of *malignant edema.* Such infections are characterized by rapidly expanding swellings, which are soft and pit on pressure. The diseased animals show fever and other signs of intoxication, and most of them die within a few hours or within 1 to 2 days. The affected tissues are infiltrated with large quantities of gelatinous exudate, most of which is in the subcutaneous and intermuscular connective tissue. The muscular tissue is dark red, but unlike blackleg contains little or no gas. Infections in cattle sometimes strongly resemble blackleg. In recogni-

tion of this, the organism is referred to in German literature as the *parablackleg bacillus.* It is believed that in many cases cattle and sheep suffer from a mixed infection with blackleg and other anaerobic organisms and that the organism of blackleg in such cases often is overlooked because it grows more delicately than the others and is crowded out of cultures (Breed 1937).

C. septicum also causes infections in horses and swine, but swine are only slightly susceptible. In horses, contaminated injection sites are sometimes invaded by *C. septicum.* Although clostridial infections are rare in poultry, *C. septicum* infection has been recorded on a number of occasions in chickens (Helfer et al. 1969, Saunders and Bickford 1965). In a broiler flock infected with this organism, the birds showed varying degrees of depression, incoordination, inappetence, and ataxia. Mortality was about 1 percent.

C. septicum produces four toxins (alpha, beta, gamma, and delta), which are responsible for the tissue damage seen in braxy and malignant edema. The alpha toxin is a lecithinase and is necrotizing, lethal, and hemolytic. The beta toxin is a deoxyribonuclease and is leukocidal. The gamma and delta toxins have hyaluronidase and hemolysin activities, respectively. These toxins increase capillary permeability and cause myonecrosis and further spread of the infection along the fascial planes of muscle. The sytemic effects of the toxins and tissue breakdown products result in a fatal toxemia in 2 to 3 days.

Guinea pigs are very susceptible to inoculation with *C. septicum,* but the lesions cannot be distinguished from those of blackleg. A blood-tinged gelatinous exudate is found beneath the skin at the point of inoculation, and the muscular tissue is dark red. Gas is not usually present in the tissues. The peritoneal cavity often is moist and may have a little more fluid in it than normal. The liver is lighter than normal, having a semicooked appearance. Stained films from the liver surface show long, jointed chains of cells.

Immunity. Animals may be immunized with formalinized whole culture of *C. septicum* or toxoided alpha toxin. This usually produces lifelong immunity.

Diagnosis. If *C. septicum* is the dominant organism in the lesion or in fresh pathological material, it is probably the etiological agent. Once putrefaction has begun there is a good chance that *C. septicum* will be present anyway as a result of postmortem invasion from the intestine; thus the diagnosis is less certain. Specimens should also be carefully checked for *C. chauvoei.* If present, *C. chauvoei* should preferentially be considered the etiological agent (Sterne and Thomson 1963). The most rapid and efficient method for detection of *C. septicum* or *C. chauvoei* is the fluorescent antibody technique that employs antiserums conjugated with contrasting-colored fluorescent dyes (Batty and Walker 1963).

Antimicrobial Susceptibility. *C. septicum* is sensitive to penicillin G, ampicillin, and tetracycline. Tetracycline has been used in control of the disease in chickens (Saunders and Bickford 1965).

REFERENCES

Batty, I., and Walker, P.D. 1963. Fluorescent labelled clostridial antisera as specific reagents. Bull. Off. Int. Epizoot. 59:1499–1513.

Breed, F. 1937. A study of blackleg and its complications. J. Am. Vet. Med. Assoc. 90:521–528.

Helfer, D.H., Dickinson, E.M., and Smith, D.H. 1969. Case report—*Clostridium septicum* infection in a broiler flock. Avian Dis. 13:231–233.

Moussa, R.S. 1959. Antigenic formulae for *Clostridium septicum* and *Clostridium chauvoei*. J. Pathol. Bacteriol. 77:341–350.

Saunders, J.R., and Bickford, A.A. 1965. Clostridial infections of growing chickens. Avian Dis. 9:317–326.

Sterne, M., and Thomson, A. 1963. The isolation and identification of clostridia from pathological conditions of animals. Bull. Off. Int. Epizoot. 59:1487–1489.

Clostridium colinum

Peckham (1959) first associated a Gram-positive, spore-forming anaerobe with lesions of *ulcerative enteritis*, or *quail disease*. Earlier, a similar but incompletely described organism had been reported in lesions of the disease by Bass (1939). This organism was later fully characterized by Berkhoff et al. (1974) and named *C. colinum* (Berkhoff 1985).

Quail disease was so named because of the frequency with which it was seen in bobwhite quail. The disease also occurs in a wide variety of wild and domestic avian species.

Morphology and Staining Reactions. *C. colinum* occurs in tissues and cultures as a Gram-positive rod about 1 μm in width and 3 to 4 μm in length. It has oval, subterminal spores, but sporulation is infrequent. Peritrichous flagella are present, but motility is difficult to establish conclusively because the organism produces gas.

Cultural and Biochemical Features. *C. colinum* is difficult to culture on the usual media but grows readily on tryptose-phosphate-glucose-yeast agar or broth to which 8 percent sterile citrated horse plasma has been added. The colonies on agar are 1 to 3 mm in diameter, semiconvex with a filamentous margin, semitranslucent, grayish, and glossy. Some strains are beta hemolytic. *C. colinum* ferments fructose, glucose, maltose, sucrose, raffinose, and trehalose. Acetic and formic acids are the principal fermentation products. It does not produce indole, hydrogen sulfide, urease, catalase, or lecithinase.

Epizootiology and Pathogenesis. The ecology of *C. colinum* has not yet been elucidated. The disease has been described in such game birds as bobwhite quail, partridge, and grouse and in young domestic chickens and turkeys. Natural infection occurs probably by means of the oral route. Experimentally it has been shown that quail must ingest at least 10^6 organisms before they become ill with the disease (Berkhoff and Campbell 1974). Chickens are much more resistant, and the disease in this host has been observed only after outbreaks of coccidiosis or infectious bursal disease (Witter 1952). Overcrowding and poor sanitation have been noted to be predisposing causes in grouse (Le Dune 1935). The intestinal contents are infective (Witter 1952), and it must be presumed that *C. colinum* is shed in the feces. Quail that develop a chronic form of the disease have been shown to remain carriers of infection (Bass 1939).

After oral infection the organism enters the intestine and then passes into the portal circulation and lodges in the liver, where diffuse liver necrosis is produced. The necrosis is centrilobular or diffuse pinpoint to coagulative, and many bacteria are present (Berkhoff et al. 1974). The intestine becomes ulcerated along the lower third of its length. The ulcers vary from about 0.1 mm to 2 or 3 mm in diameter. In some birds extensive necrosis of the spleen occurs. A toxin has not been implicated in the pathogenesis of *C. colinum* lesions (Berkhoff et al. 1974). Birds may die in a day or two or linger for a week. Affected birds are inactive, sluggish, and anorexic. In the later stages they cannot move and die within a few hours. Chronically affected quail become emaciated and pass watery feces.

Diagnosis. The disease must be diagnosed by the isolation and identification of *C. colinum* from the lesions. No other diagnostic procedures are available yet. The incorporation of polymyxin B (25 μg/ml) in the isolation medium facilitates isolation from intestinal contents.

Antimicrobial Susceptibility. *C. colinum* is sensitive to tetracyclines, penicillin, bacitracin, and furacin. Streptomycin is apparently effective in control of the naturally occurring disease (Peckham 1972), although the organism is resistant to this antibiotic in vitro.

REFERENCES

Bass, C.C. 1939. Observation on the specific cause and nature of "quail disease" or ulcerative enteritis in quail. Proc. Soc. Exp. Biol. Med. 42:377–380.

Berkhoff, G.A. 1985. *Clostridium colinum* sp. nov. nom. rev., the causative agent of ulcerative enteritis (quail disease) in quail, chickens, and pheasants. Int. J. Syst. Bacteriol. 35:155–159.

Berkhoff, G.A., and Campbell, S.G. 1974. Etiology and pathogenesis of ulcerative enteritis ("quail disease"): The experimental disease. Avian Dis. 18:205–212.

Berkhoff, G.A., Campbell, S.G., Naylor, H.B., and Smith, L. 1974.

Etiology and pathogenesis of ulcerative enteritis ("quail disease"): Characterization of the causative anaerobe. Avian Dis. 18:195–204.

Le Dune, E.K. 1935. Ulcerative enteritis in ruffed grouse. Vet. Med. 30:394–395.

Peckham, M.C. 1959. An anaerobe, the cause of ulcerative enteritis, "quail disease." Avian Dis. 3:471–478.

Peckham, M.C. 1972. Ulcerative enteritis (quail disease). In M.S. Hofstad, B.W. Calnek, C.F. Helmboldt, W.M. Reid, and H.W. Yoder, Jr., eds., Diseases of Poultry, 6th ed. Iowa State University Press, Ames. Pp. 360–371.

Witter, J.F. 1952. Observations on apparent complications of coccidiosis in broiler flocks. In Proceedings of the 24th Annual Conference of Laboratory Workers in Pullorum Disease Control, University of Maine.

Clostridium spiroforme

C. spiroforme has been shown to be the cause of iota enterotoxemia of rabbits and other laboratory rodents (Borriello and Carman 1983).

Morphology and Staining Reactions. *C. spiroforme* has a characteristic loosely coiled, spiral form when cultured on blood agar (Figure 22.12). Cells measure 0.3 to 0.5 μm by 2 to 10 μm. In feces or cecal contents the spiral morphology is not so apparent; instead the organism has a semicircular shape. It is spore-bearing and Gram-positive, although smears of organisms made from culture media may be Gram-variable. Spores are terminal.

Cultural and Biochemical Features. Colonies (0.7 to 1.5 mm) on blood agar are whitish to brownish gray,

Figure 22.12. *Clostridium spiroforme* from a surface colony. Gram's stain. (From Carman and Borriello, 1983, courtesy of *Journal of Clinical Microbiology*.)

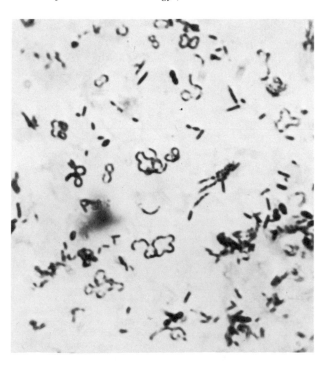

convex, circular, shining, and semiopaque to opaque.

Typically *C. spiroforme* produces acid only from glucose, lactose, and sucrose, but some strains also produce acid from cellobiose and salicin. The organism is nonhemolytic and nonmotile, does not produce lecithinase or lipase, does not hydrolyze gelatin, and does not reduce nitrates. The only fermentation product is acetic acid.

Toxins. In chopped-meat glucose medium strains of *C. spiroforme* isolated from rabbits with iota enterotoxemia produce a toxin neutralized by antiserum to *C. perfringens* type E iota toxin. Nontoxigenic strains apparently also exist, but these have not been found in diseased animals.

Epizootiology and Pathogenesis. *C. spiroforme* diarrhea occurs spontaneously in weanling rabbits but can also be induced in adult animals by the administration of antibiotics (Katz et al. 1978). In adults exposure to both clindamycin and *C. spiroforme* is necessary to induce disease (Carman and Borriello 1984). Rabbits with spontaneously occurring disease have high mean concentrations (10^6) of spores of *C. spiroforme* per gram of cecal contents, and iotalike toxin is present in cecal contents.

Affected rabbits quickly develop diarrhea, with perianal staining, and then die. At necropsy, the cecum is massively dilated with watery stool. There is necrosis of the surface epithelium and a prominent inflammatory infiltrate in the lamina propria.

Diagnosis. The presence of semicircular Gram-positive bacteria in the feces or cecal contents is not sufficient evidence for a diagnosis. Iotalike toxin must be demonstrated to confirm diarrhea caused by *C. spiroforme*. The assay for iota toxin has been described by Sterne and Batty (1975). The toxin is cytotoxic to Vero cells.

REFERENCES

Borriello, S.P., and Carman, R.J. 1983. Association of iota-like toxin and *Clostridium spiroforme* with both spontaneous and antibiotic-associated diarrhea and colitis in rabbits. J. Clin. Microbiol. 17:414–418.

Carman, R.J., and Borriello, S.P. 1984. Infectious nature of *Clostridium spiroforme*—mediated rabbit enterotoxemia. Vet. Microbiol. 9:497–502.

Katz, L., Lamont, J.T., Trier, J.S., Sonnenblick, E.B., Rothmon, S.W., Broitman, S.A., and Reith, S. 1978. Experimental clindamycin-associated colitis in rabbits. Gastroenterology 74:246.

Sterne, M., and Batty, I. 1975. Pathogenic Clostridia. Butterworth, London. Pp. 179.

Clostridium villosum

Love et al. (1979) first described *C. villosum* in smears and cultures from subcutaneous abscesses on fight wounds

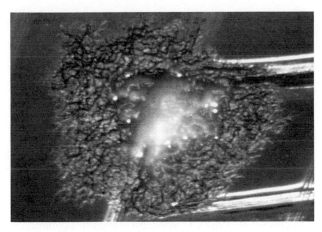

Figure 22.13. A colony of *Clostridium villosum* showing the typical rhizoid periphery, roughened surface, and raised center. × 10. (From Love et al., 1979, courtesy of *International Journal of Systematic Bacteriology.*)

in cats. The specific name is derived from the hairy, shaggy morphology of the colonies (Figure 22.13).

Morphology and Staining Reactions. The cells of *C. villosum* are rod-shaped with parallel sides and rounded ends and measure 0.6 μm by 4 to 6 μm. In older cultures and tissue smears, long, beaded, and fragmented filaments are common (Figure 22.14). The cells are Gram-positive but may lose this characteristic after 24 hours. There are no flagella. Surface colonies on solid media are about 0.5 mm at 24 hours and increase to about 5 mm at 3 days. The center of mature colonies is raised, convex, rough, and whitish to yellowish, and the periphery is rhizoid. Colonies adhere strongly to the agar, and there is no hemolysis on blood agar. Colonies in stabs are cottony. The spores are single, oval, and subterminal and cause a

Figure 22.14. *Clostridium villosum* in a smear of thoracic fluid from a cat. The filamentous form is typical. Gram's stain. × 1,120. (Courtesy D. Love.)

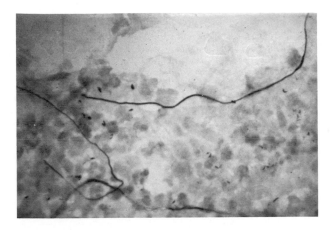

slight distention of the sporangium. They are produced sparingly only in old cultures.

Cultural and Biochemical Features. *C. villosum* is an obligate anaerobe that requires serum for growth. It grows well in cooked-meat medium supplemented with peptic digest of meat, 0.4 percent glucose, 0.1 percent cellobiose, 0.1 percent maltose, and 0.1 percent starch. *C. villosum* produces a delicate membrane near the surface of broth that contains chunks of organisms; these later settle onto the surface of meat particles. All strains liquefy gelatin weakly, produce ammonia, but do not ferment carbohydrates and are unreactive in other biochemical tests (Love et al. 1979). Fermentation products include acetic, isobutyric, butyric, isovaleric, lactic, methylmalonic, and succinic acids, but not propionic acid.

Epizootiology and Pathogenesis. Love et al. (1979) suggested that the organism is a component of the feline oral flora and enters bite wounds in association with other oral bacteria. The organism has also been isolated from 16 percent of cats with pyothorax (Love et al. 1982) and perhaps reaches the thorax through the airway from the oropharynx.

Diagnosis. *C. villosum* must be distinguished from *Nocardia asteroides* in smears of clinical specimens. The beaded and fragmented Gram-positive and Gram-variable form of *C. villosum* is easily mistaken for *N. asteroides;* however, results of aerobic and anaerobic culture, colony morphology, and the partial acid-fast reaction of *N. asteroides* allow definitive identification.

Antimicrobial Susceptibility. All strains of *C. villosum* are sensitive to penicillin, amoxicillin, carbenicillin, doxycycline, chloramphenicol, and erythromycin (Love et al. 1979).

REFERENCES

Love, D.N., Jones, R.F., and Bailey, M. 1979. *Clostridium villosum* sp. nov. from subcutaneous abscesses in cats. Int. J. Syst. Bacteriol. 29:241–244.
Love, D.N., Jones, R.F., Bailey, M., Johnson, R.S., and Gamble, N. 1982. Isolation and characterization of bacteria from pyothorax (empyaemia) in cats. Vet. Microbiol. 7:455–461.

Clostridium difficile

For many years *C. difficile* was regarded as a normal inhabitant of the intestinal tract. Its recognition as a significant pathogen did not come about until the late 1970s, when it was shown that clindamycin-induced enterocolitis in hamsters was associated with toxin-producing species of *C. difficile* (Bartlett et al. 1977). Since then the organism has been associated with a similar syndrome in rabbits

(Rehg and Shoung 1981), guinea pigs (Lowe et al. 1980) and humans (Bartlett et al. 1978). It has also been implicated in naturally occurring enterocolitis in swine (Jones and Hunter 1983), a Kodiak bear (Orchard et al. 1983), and foals (Jones et al. 1988).

Morphology and Staining Reactions. *C. difficile* is a large, nonencapsulated, Gram-positive rod (0.5 μm by 3 to 6 μm) that forms oval subterminal or terminal spores that lie within the walls of the parent cell. Flagella are present.

Cultural and Biochemical Features. On blood agar, colonies have a rhizoid edge and are nonhemolytic, large (2 to 4 mm), raised, translucent, and matt-surfaced. On egg-yolk agar there is no evidence of lecithinase or lipase production. The organism is a strict anaerobe. *C. difficile* hydrolyzes gelatin and actively growing cultures produce an odor similar to that of para-cresol. Only glucose and mannitol among the commonly used carbohydrates are fermented. The principal metabolic products are acetic, proprionic, isobutyric, butyric, isovaleric, valeric, and isocaproic acids.

Toxins. Two immunologically different toxins designated A and B have been identified from culture filtrates of *C. difficile*. Toxin A has a molecular weight of about 45,000, is a protein, is lethal to mice, and causes a fluid response in the ileal loop assay. Toxin B is a protein with a slightly lower molecular weight and is cytotoxic for Vero cells, lethal to mice, but inactive in the ileal loop assay (Lyerly et al. 1982).

Epizootiology and Pathogenesis. *C. difficile* has been observed in the feces of a variety of animals including household pets. It has also been found in the immediate environment of these animals. The presence of *C. difficile* in animals is not necessarily associated with antibiotic therapy, and the existence of naturally occurring cases suggests that there are circumstances other than antibiotic depression of normal flora that create the conditions that allow *C. difficile* to increase in numbers and subsequently produce toxin. The organism is also common in the feces of human infants but not in those of adults. Cases of disease in human adults exhibit a definite geographic and temporal clustering, which suggests that infection was acquired from the environment or contagion. In humans and laboratory animals production of disease usually requires both the presence of the organism and administration of an antibiotic to which *C. difficile* is resistant. The toxins produce a severe, often fatal, hemorrhagic ileitis or cecitis with ulceration, formation of a pseudomembrane, and watery and bloody diarrhea.

Diagnosis. Both *C. difficile* and its toxins can be detected in the feces and gut contents of affected animals. A procedure for the routine isolation of *C. difficile* on a selective medium containing brain-heart infusion agar, yeast extract, hemin, vitamin K, C cysteine hydrochloride, sodium formaldehyde sulfoxylate, cycloserine, and cefoxitin has been described by Borriello and Honour (1981).

Cytotoxin can be detected either by a tissue-culture serum neutralization assay or by an enzyme immunoassay (Laughon et al. 1984). *C. sordellii* antitoxin is commonly used to neutralize the cytotoxin of *C. difficile* because it has a similar immunospecificity.

Antimicrobial Susceptibility. *C. difficile* is sensitive to vancomycin, which is the antibiotic of choice in the treatment of cases of antibiotic-induced pseudomembrane colitis in humans.

REFERENCES

Bartlett, J.G., Chang, T.W., Gurowith, M., Gorbach, S.L., and Onderdonk, A.B. 1978. Antibiotic associated pseudomembranous colitis due to toxin producing clostridia. N. Engl. J. Med. 198:531–534.

Bartlett, J.G., Onderdonk, A.B., Cisneros, R.C., and Kasper, D.C. 1977. Clindamycin-associated colitis due to a toxin producing species of *Clostridium* in hamsters. J. Infect. Dis. 136:701–705.

Borriello, P.S., and Honour, P. 1981. Simplified procedure for the routine isolation of *Clostridium difficile* from faeces. J. Clin. Pathol. 34:1126–1127.

Jones, M.A., and Hunter, D. 1983. Isolation of *Clostridium difficile* from pigs. Vet. Rec. 112:253.

Jones, R.L., Shideler, R.K., and Cockerell, G.L. 1988. Association of *Clostridium difficile* with foal diarrhea. In Proceedings of the 5th International Conference on Equine Infectious Diseases, Lexington, Ky. The University Press of Kentucky, Lexington.

Laughon, B.E., Viscidi, R.P., Gdovin, S.L., Yolken, R.H., and Bartlett, J.G. 1984. Enzyme immunoassays for detection of *Clostridium difficile* toxins A and B in fecal specimens. J. Infect. Dis. 149:781–788.

Lowe, B.R., Fos, J.G., and Bartlett, J.G. 1980. *Clostridium difficile*-associated cecitis in guinea pigs exposed to penicillin. Am. J. Vet. Res. 41:1277–1279.

Lyerly, D.M., Lockwood, D.E., Richardson, S.H., and Wilkins, T.D. 1982. Biological activities of toxins A and B of *Clostridium difficile*. Infect. Immun. 35:1126–1127.

Orchard, J.C., Fekety, R., and Smith, J.R. 1983. Antibiotic-associated colitis due to *Clostridium difficile* in a Kodiak bear. Am. J. Vet. Res. 44:1547–1548.

Rehg, J.E., and Shoung, L.Y. 1981. *Clostridium difficile* colitis in a rabbit following antibiotic therapy for pasteurellosis. J. Am. Vet. Med. Assoc. 179:1296.

23 The Genus *Listeria*

There are five species in the genus *Listeria,* only one of which, *Listeria monocytogenes,* is pathogenic for warm-blooded animals and humans.

Listeria monocytogenes

SYNONYM: *Listerella monocytogenes*

Morphology and Staining Reactions. *L. monocytogenes* is a Gram-positive, non-acid-fast organism that occurs in the form of small rods 1 to 2 μm long (Figure 23.1). The rods frequently show slight clubbing and therefore a diphtheroid appearance. Coccoid elements are commonly found. When grown at 20° to 25°C organisms in young cultures are motile by means of peritrichous flagella and exhibit a tumbling motility. Spores are not produced. Gram-negative cells can usually be found in young cultures, and the organisms in old cultures may be almost entirely Gram-negative.

Cultural and Biochemical Features. *L. monocytogenes* grows on most of the ordinary laboratory media, although the growth is never abundant. In general, the gross features of cultures resemble those of streptococci. After 24 hours' incubation at 37°C deep colonies appear as minute points; surface colonies are small, flat, bluish-white, and transparent. The deep colonies are surrounded by narrow zones of hemolysis of the beta type (Figure 23.2), and this characteristic makes them conspicuous. The surface colonies seldom if ever exceed 1 mm in diameter and on clear solid media appear blue-green when illuminated obliquely. Cultures grown in stabs in gelatin

have the appearance of an inverted fir tree or a line of discrete colonies along the stab.

L. monocytogenes forms acid without gas from glucose, rhamnose, and salicin within 48 hours. It sometimes produces acid but no gas in 3 to 10 days in arabinose, galactose, lactose, maltose, sucrose, dextrin, sorbitol, and glycerol. The organism does not form H_2S or indole. Unlike *Erysipelothrix rhusiopathiae, L. monocytogenes* produces catalase, and this test is a simple method for differentiating these organisms. Nonpathogenic isolates of *L. monocytogenes* are nonhemolytic and do not hydrolyze rhamnose, features that distinguish them from pathogenic isolates. Also, most nonpathogenic isolates produce acid from xylose (Groves and Welshimer 1977).

Antigens. There are somatic (O) and flagellar (H) antigens expressed by *L. monocytogenes.* Fifteen O antigens (I–XV) and five H antigens (A–E) have been described (Paterson 1940, Seeliger 1975). Serotypes are assigned according to the antigenic formula and are given arabic numbers and lowercase letters. There are 7 serotypes and 14 subtypes. Cattle and sheep are commonly infected with serotypes 1 or 4.

Epizootiology and Pathogenesis. *L. monocytogenes* is ubiquitous in nature and in animal and human feces. It survives for years in soil (Bind et al. 1976), milk, silage, and feces (Dijkstra 1976). A major factor in survival is pH: at a pH of 5.0 or above the organism multiplies; below pH 5, survival of the organism is poor (Kahn et al. 1973).

Figure 23.1. A culture of *Listeria monocytogenes* from a serum-agar slant incubated for 18 hours at 37°C. × 1,000.

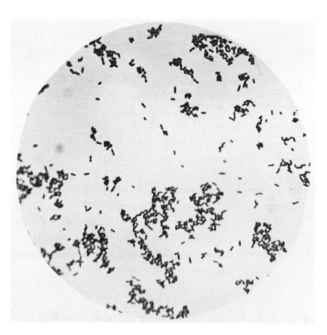

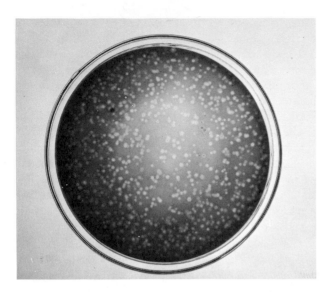

Figure 23.2. *Listeria monocytogenes* on a blood-agar plate incubated at 37°C for 24 hours. The colonies, not discernible in the photograph, are minute, and each is surrounded by a sharply defined but narrow zone of beta hemolysis.

This effect appears to be associated with the lactic microflora in low-pH silage (Gouet et al. 1977). *L. monocytogenes* is more heat-tolerant than most other non-sporulating bacteria and has been shown to survive pasteurization by the low-temperature holding process (Bearns and Girard 1958). Pasteurization is unlikely to be effective if the number of organisms exceeds 1,000/ml of milk. It has also been suggested that organisms within milk leukocytes may be more heat resistant than those that are extracellular (Fleming et al. 1985).

Because *L. monocytogenes* is widely distributed in soil, vegetation, and feces, most animals are exposed to the organism during their lifetimes. Large numbers of *L. monocytogenes* can be isolated from the feces of ruminants—a reflection of the animals' exposure to large quantities of contaminated herbage. The organism is also commonly found in the tissues, such as the tonsils of swine (Hohne et al. 1976), and the lymph nodes of apparently healthy animals (Hyslop 1976). Furthermore, many healthy animals are seropositive (Hyslop 1976). *L. monocytogenes* is common in poor-quality silage in which the pH is greater than 5.0, and ruminants fed such material are much more likely to develop listeriosis (Kruger 1963). The same serotype has been found in silage and in tissues of affected animals fed this silage. The association of listeriosis with silage in Iceland was so striking that the disease in that country has been named *Votheysveiki* (silage disease).

Intercurrent disease, climatic and other stresses, and pregnancy are important predisposing factors in the oc-currence of listeriosis. The disease thus is more common in sheep and cattle in winter and early spring. Viral damage to mucosal surfaces can also be a factor in allowing the organism to breach epithelial barriers. The organism is a facultative intracellular parasite, and stresses that diminish the host's cell-mediated immune competence may allow the parasite to escape from phagocytic cells and to multiply out of control and so cause disease.

L. monocytogenes produces no known toxins, and its hemolysins are unlikely to play a major role in the virulence of the organism. A high-molecular-weight component of the cell envelope is immunosuppressive, but this effect may not be of great importance as a virulence factor (Otokunefor and Galsworthy 1982).

The initial mode of entry of *L. monocytogenes* into an animal is usually ingestion, although infection has been demonstrated through the nasal mucosa and along branches of the trigeminal nerve (Charlton and Garcia 1977). Because entry into the dental terminals of the trigeminal nerve in sheep can cause an ascending neuritis and encephalitis, listeric encephalitis is most common in winter and early spring in sheep that are losing and cutting teeth (Barlow and McGorum 1985). Direct infection of the conjunctiva in cattle has occurred as a result of silage particles falling into the faces of browsing cattle (Morgan 1977). Keratoconjunctivitis in cattle caused by the organism has also been described (Pohjanvirta 1984).

Entry of the organism through the intestinal epithelial barrier into the tissues is not well understood. Experimental intestinal infections (Racz et al. 1976) have indicated that the organism can enter and multiply in ileal cells and then pass directly from cell to cell. Infected cells eventually degenerate. This degeneration is potentiated by neutrophils, which are attracted toward infected cells. Infection eventually involves the Peyer's patches and the liver. A bacteremic or septicemic phase may then develop, depending on the immune status of the animal.

In pregnant animals, the organism can localize in the placentomes and then enter the amniotic fluid. The fetus aspirates the organism, which multiplies and kills the fetus. Abortion results. Abortions in cattle usually occur in the second half of pregnancy; in sheep and goats abortions are seen at a late stage of gestation. Ingestion of pine needles is a known but poorly understood predisposing factor in listeria abortion in cattle (Stevenson et al. 1972).

Primary listeric septicemia is much more common in young than in adult ruminants, whereas in monogastric animals, septicemia is the most common form of listeriosis irrespective of age (Gray and Killinger 1966). Death may occur suddenly or after an illness of a few days' duration characterized by depression, dyspnea, slobbering, nasal discharge, and lacrimation. At necropsy

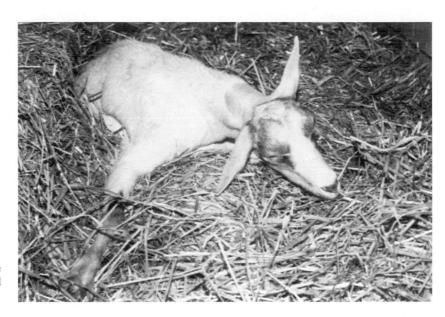

Figure 23.3. Listeriosis in a goat. The drooping right ear is a sign of right-sided facial paralysis.

focal necrosis of the liver, spleen, and abdominal lymph nodes are seen. Enteritis and occasionally myocardial necrosis occur. The pathogenesis of the focal hepatic necrosis has been studied by Siddique et al. (1978), who observed that *L. monocytogenes* enters hepatic cells by endocytosis, where it is initially found in a membrane-bound vesicle. The hepatic cell dies, leading to multiple necrotic foci in the parenchyma. This toxic effect is poorly understood. Phospholipase and lipase activities have been associated with some strains of *L. monocytogenes* (Leighton et al. 1976) and can cause cell membrane damage. Also, Watson and Lavizzo (1973) have described hemolytic and lipolytic antigens that are toxic for mouse macrophages and may be similar to the enzymes described above.

Meninogencephalitis is perhaps the most easily recognized form of listeriosis seen in domestic animals. The name *circling disease* was given by Gill (1931) to this disease in sheep in New Zealand. The disease has since been observed in cattle and sheep in many parts of the world. Affected animals may move in circles in one direction, may exhibit unilateral facial paralysis (Figure 23.3), eyelid spasticity, nystagmus, and difficulty in swallowing. Fever, blindness, and headpressing are also commonly observed. The disease progresses until the animal is completely paralyzed, and it dies within 2 or 3 days. During these later stages, many animals exhibit constant chewing motions.

In the encephalomyelitic form the cerebrospinal fluid can be cloudy because of an increased globulin and leukocyte content. The meninges can be congested. Usually the visceral organs show little or no evidence of disease.

Sections of the brains of such animals show polymorphonuclear and mononuclear foci in the white matter of the cerebrum and cerebellum and perivascular cuffing with mononuclear cells (Figure 23.4). Areas of malacia occur in the pons and medulla oblongata (Charlton 1977), with loss of parenchyma and accumulations of macrophages. Bacteria are not found in the macrophages, but

Figure 23.4. Brain tissue of a cow with listeriosis. The cells infiltrating the brain substance are both mononuclear and polymorphonuclear. There is marked perivascular cuffing. Hematoxylin and eosin stain. × 65. (Courtesy S. H. McNutt.)

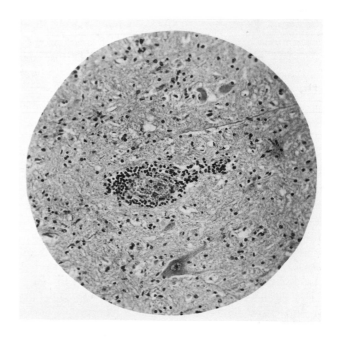

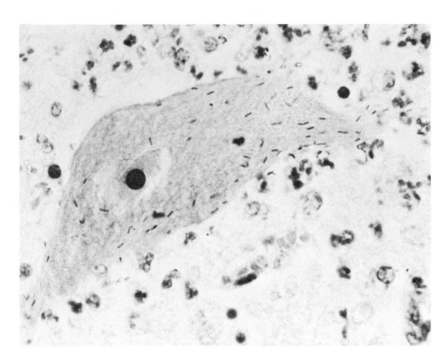

Figure 23.5. *Listeria monocytogenes* in a large neuron from an infected sheep. Giemsa stain. × 1,050. (From Charlton and Garcia, 1977, courtesy of *Veterinary Pathology.*)

rather are seen in neutrophils in the area. The malacia might result from phospholipase released by the organism, but the precise cause is unclear.

It has been suggested that glutamic acid decarboxylase produced by *L. monocytogenes* plays a role in the pathogenesis of encephalitic listeriosis (Shah et al. 1981). Its substrate, glutamic acid, is an excitatory neurotransmitter and the end-product, gamma-aminobutyric acid, acts as an inhibitory neurohormone in the central nervous system. The formation of these molecules in nerve cells could clearly cause severe disturbance and convulsions.

Charlton and Garcia (1977) have provided an excellent description of the histologic features of spontaneously occurring encephalitic listeriosis in sheep. Diffuse and focal intrafascicular and perineural accumulations of lymphocytes and plasma cells unilaterally involve the trigeminal nerve. Accumulations of *L. monocytogenes* in proximal parts of damaged cranial nerves and sometimes in intact nerve fibers suggests centripetal migration of the organism along the trigeminal nerve to the brain (Figure 23.5). Charlton and Garcia postulated that further dissemination within the brain probably occurs by means of intra-asconal movement. Other workers have also suggested that the organism may enter the brain after entry through the mucosa of the nasopharynx and upward migration along either the first cranial or the trigeminal nerve (Asahi et al. 1957). However, listeric encephalomyelitis also has been frequently observed as a sequel to and in conjunction with septicemia; hematogenous spread of the organism to brain tissue thus must also occur.

Listeriosis in chickens sometimes exhibits distinctive features (Gray 1958). Necrotic myocarditis may be observed, accompanied by fluid in the peritoneal and pericardial cavities, muscle edema, and focal necrosis of the liver. The septicemic disease is the form most often seen. Intercurrent diseases of bacterial, viral, and parasitic origin are important predisposing factors in the occurrence of listeriosis in poultry (Paterson 1940).

In horses, listeriosis usually appears in its septicemic form. Emerson and Jarvis (1968) described listeriosis in ponies. The symptoms were fever, mild colic, restlessness, depression, anorexia, jaundice, and reddish urine. McCain and Robinson (1975) described two cases of the septicemic disease. The organism was isolated from blood, liver, and skeletal musculature. Many apparently healthy horses are serologically positive (Mayer et al. 1975).

Listeriosis has been described in many other domestic and feral species, including rodents raised for food, for laboratory use, or for pelts. The disease is usually septicemic, but rabbits and chinchillas also have a characteristic hemorrhagic and necrotic metritis that may be associated with abortion (Gray and Killinger 1966). Central nervous system involvement is occasionally observed. Conjunctival instillation of *L. monocytogenes* results in a purulent conjunctivitis in rabbits and guinea pigs—the Anton reaction. The organism rapidly enters conjunctival epithelial cells and thereafter is indirectly chemotactic to neutrophils.

Immunity. Immunity to *L. monocytogenes* is cell-mediated by means of rapidly dividing, short-lived T lymphocytes (Mackaness 1964, North 1973). Antibody, often at high titers, is produced by clinically affected animals but does not play an important role in resolution of the disease (Hyslop 1976).

Antibodies may be detected by growth-inhibition (Schafer 1976), precipitin (Drew 1946, Seeliger 1961), complement-fixation (Schafer 1976), passive immunohemolysis (Bind et al. 1976), and hemagglutination tests (Von Sachse and Potel 1957). Because of cross-reactions with other organisms, a high rate of seropositivity in normal animals, and lack of antibody responsiveness in many clinically infected animals, antibody titers are seldom measured. No vaccines are in use in the United States. In the Soviet Union an avirulent strain (AUF) has been used in sheep and has been reported to give complete protection for 10 months (Selivanov et al. 1972).

Diagnosis. The encephalitic form of the disease is diagnosed by observation of the characteristic perivascular cuffing with mononuclear cells and focal necrosis in the pons, medulla, and anterior spinal cord. Brain tissue may be cultured directly on blood agar but should also be macerated in nutrient broth, stored at 4°C, and subcultured onto colistin–nalidixic acid agar (CNA agar) at weekly intervals if the direct culture is negative. The organism is difficult to demonstrate in cerebrospinal fluid of ruminants with encephalitis, possibly because it is confined to lesions in the brain parenchyma.

Inhibitory solid and fluid media containing nalidixic acid (40 µg/ml), trypaflavine (10 µg/ml), and serum have been developed and are excellent for isolation of the organism from contaminated specimens such as genital exudates, fetuses, feces, and the like.

The fluorescent antibody technique (Smith et al. 1960) is rapid, but false-positive results may occur because of cross-reacting antibodies in the conjugate. The occurrence of monocytosis is not useful in the diagnosis of listeriosis in ruminants because it is seen only in monogastric animals (Gray and Killinger 1966).

Antimicrobial Susceptibility. Ampicillin and benzyl penicillin G exert a bacteriostatic rather than a bactericidal action on *L. monocytogenes,* but both are often therapeutically effective (Macnair et al. 1968, Medoff et al. 1971). Treatment failures also occur. Intrathecal administration of ampicillin has been used for treatment of listeria meningitis in humans (Macnair et al. 1968). Olafson (1940) treated circling disease of ruminants with sulfonamides with some success. Penicillin and sulfanilamide (Jensen and Mackey 1949) and tetracyclines (Bennett et al. 1952) have been found to be effective in the early stages of listeriosis in animals. Penicillin and gentamicin in combination have a bactericidal effect on *Listeria* and may be

a more effective treatment than either antibiotic used alone (Mohan et al. 1977).

The Disease in Humans. Listeriosis in humans is a cause of abortion, perinatal infection, septicemia, and meningoencephalitis. Persons with underlying immunosuppressive disorders are especially at risk (Bottone and Sierra 1977) and usually exhibit a bacteremic form of the disease, which in some cases may be complicated by meningitis. In contrast to ruminants, in which the primary nervous lesion is encephalitis, the primary nervous lesion in humans involves the meninges. The source of infection for humans is not always clear, but statistics on human cases indicate that animal contact is not an important factor (Moore and Zehmer 1973). Human infections could result from consumption of milk or milk products because the organism can be shed from the bovine udder (Fleming et al. 1985, Hyslop 1976, Jasinska et al. 1969, Sipka et al. 1973). Vegetables contaminated with sheep manure have also been a source of infection for humans (Schlech et al. 1983).

REFERENCES

Asahi, O., Hosoda, T., and Akiyama, Y. 1957. Studies on the mechanism of infection of the brain with *Listeria monocytogenes.* Am. J. Vet. Res. 18:147.

Barlow, R.M., and McGorum, B. 1985. Ovine bilateral encephalitis: Analysis, hypothesis, and synthesis. Vet. Rec. 116:233–236.

Bearns, R.E., and Girard, K.F. 1958. The effect of pasteurization on *Listeria monocytogenes.* Can J. Microbiol. 4:55–61.

Bennett, I.L., Jr., Russell, P.E., and Derivaux, J.H. 1952. Treatment of *Listeria* meningitis. Antibiot. Chemother. 2:142–146.

Bind, J.L., Maupas, P., Chiron, J.P., and Raynaud, B. 1976. Passive immunohaemolysis applied to serological diagnosis of Listeriosis. In M. Woodbine, ed., Problems of Listeriosis. Leicester University Press, Leicester, England. Pp. 42–250.

Bottone, E.J., and Sierra, M.F. 1977. *Listeria monocytogenes:* Another look at the "Cinderella among pathogenic bacteria." Mt. Sinai J. Med. 44:42–59.

Charlton, K.M. 1977. Spontaneous listeric encephalitis in sheep. Electron microscope studies. Vet. Pathol. 14:429–434.

Charlton, K.M., and Garcia, M.M. 1977. Spontaneous listeric encephalitis and neuritis in sheep. Light microscope studies. Vet. Pathol. 14:297–313.

Dijkstra, R.G. 1976. Recent experiences on the survival times of *Listeria* bacteria in suspensions of brain, tissue, silage, faeces and in milk. In M. Woodbine, ed., Problems of Listeriosis. Leicester University Press, Leicester, England. Pp. 71–73.

Drew, R.M. 1946. Occurrence of two immunological groups within the genus *Listeria.* Studies based upon precipitation reactions. Proc. Soc. Exp. Biol. Med. 61:30–33.

Emerson, F.G., and Jarvis, A.A. 1968. Listeriosis in ponies. J. Am. Vet. Med. Assoc. 152:1645–1646.

Fleming, D.W., Cochi, S.L., MacDonald, K.L., Brondum, J., Hayes, P.S., Plikaytis, B.D., Holmes, M.B., Audurier, A., Broome, C.V., and Reingold, A.L. 1985. Pasteurized milk as a vehicle of infection in an outbreak of listeriosis. N. Engl. J. Med. 312:404–407.

Gill, D.A. 1931. "Circling" disease of sheep in New Zealand. Vet. J. 87:60–74.

Gouet, P., Girardeau, J.P., and Riou, Y. 1977. Inhibition of *Listeria monocytogenes* and maize—Influence of dry matter and temperature. Animal Feed Sci. Tech. 2:296–314.

Gray, M.L. 1958. Listeriosis in fowls—A review. Avian Dis. 2:296–314.

Gray, M.L., and Killinger, A.H. 1966. *Listeria monocytogenes* and listeric infections. Bacteriol. Rev. 30:309–382.

Groves, R.D., and Welshimer, H.J. 1977. Separation of pathogenic from apathogenic *Listeria monocytogenes* by three in vitro reactions. J. Clin. Microbiol. 5:559–563.

Hohne, K., Loose, B., and Seeliger, H.P.R. 1976. Recent findings of *Listeria monocytogenes* in slaughter animals of Togo (West Africa). In M. Woodbine, ed., Problems of Listeriosis. Leicester University Press, Leicester, England. Pp. 125–130.

Hyslop, N.St.G. 1976. Epidemiologic and immunological factors in listeriosis. In M. Woodbine, ed., Problems of Listeriosis. Leicester University Press, Leicester, England. Pp. 91–103.

Jasinska, S., Lewandowski, L., Sobiech, T., Adamczewski, T., and Radzimski, S. 1969. Environmental studies on the incidence of *Listeria monocytogenes* in endemic areas. Weterynaria (Wroclaw) 24:53–68.

Jensen, R., and Mackey, D.R. 1949. Listerellosis in cattle and sheep. J. Am. Vet. Med. Assoc. 114:420–424.

Khan, M.A., Seaman, A., and Woodbine, M. 1973. The pathogenicity of *Listeria monocytogenes*. Zentralbl. Bakteriol. [Orig. B] 224:355–361.

Kruger, W. 1963. Das Vorkommen von *Listeria monocytogenes* in dem verschiedenen Silogen und dessen ätiologische Bedeutung. Arch. Exp. Veterinärmed. 17:181–203.

Leighton, I., Threlfall, D.R., and Oakley, C.L. 1976. Phospholipase C activity in culture filtrates from *Listeria monocytogenes* Boldy. In M. Woodbine, ed., Problems of Listeriosis. Leicester University Press, Leicester, England. Pp. 239–241.

McCain, C.S., and Robinson, M. 1975. *Listeria monocytogenes* in the equine. In Proceedings of the 18th Annual Meeting of the American Association of Veterinary Laboratory Diagnosticians. Pp. 257–261.

Macnair, D.R., White, J.E., and Graham, J.M. 1968. Ampicillin in the treatment of *Listeria monocytogenes* meningitis. Lancet 1:16–18.

Mackaness, G.B. 1964. The immunological basis of acquired cellular resistance. J. Exp. Med. 120:105–120.

Mayer, H., Seeliger, H.P.R., Sichel, E., and Kinzler, M. 1975. Serological studies on listeriosis on horse farms. Berl. Münch. Tierärztl. Wochenschr. 88:345–347.

Medoff, G., Kunz, L.J. and Weinberg, A.N. 1971. Listeriosis in humans: An evaluation. J. Infect. Dis. 123:247–250.

Mohan, K., Gordon, R.C., Beaman, T.C., Belding, R.C., Luecke, D., Edmiston, C., and Gerhardt, P. 1977. Synergism of penicillin and gentamicin against *Listeria monocytogenes* in ex vivo hemodialysis culture. J. Infect. Dis. 135:51–54.

Moore, R.M. Jr., and Zehmer, R.B. 1973. Listeriosis in the United States, 1971. J. Infect. Dis. 127:610–611.

Morgan, J.H. 1977. Infectious keratoconjunctivitis in cattle associated with *Listeria monocytogenes*. Vet. Rec. 100:113–114.

North, R.J. 1973. Cellular mediators of anti-*Listeria* immunity as an enlarged population of short-lived, replicating T-cells: Kinetics of their production. J. Exp. Med. 138:342–355.

Olafson, P. 1940. Listeria encephalitis (circling disease) of sheep, cattle and goats. Cornell Vet. 30:141.

Otokunefor, T.V., and Galsworthy, S.B. 1982. Immunosuppression, nonspecific B-cell activation, and mitogenic activity associated with a high molecular weight component of *Listeria monocytogenes*. Can. J. Microbiol. 28:1373–1381.

Paterson, J.S. 1940. Experimental infection of the chick embryo with organisms of the genus *Listerella*. J. Pathol. Bacteriol. 51:437–440.

Pohjanvirta, R. 1984. Keratoconjunctivitis caused by *Listeria monocytogenes* in a herd of cattle. Suom. Elainlaakaril. 90:375–378.

Racz, P., Tenner, K., and Kaiserling, E. 1976. Epithelial phase in listeric infection. In M. Woodbine, ed., Problems of Listeriosis. Leicester University Press, Leicester, England. Pp. 173–179.

Schafer, I. 1976. Use of growth inhibition test in serodiagnosis of listeriosis in animals. Inaugural dissertation, Tierärztliche Hochschule, Hannover.

Schlech, W.F., Lavigne, P.M., and Bortolussi, R.A. 1983. Epidemic listeriosis—evidence for transmission by food. N. Engl. J. Med. 312:404–407.

Seeliger, H.P.R., ed. 1961. Listeriosis. S. Karger, Basel.

Seeliger, H.P.R. 1975. Serovars of *Listeria monocytogenes* and other *Listeria* species. In M. Woodbine, ed., Problems of Listeriosis. Leicester University Press, Liecester, England. P. 27.

Selivanov, A.V., Sedov, N.K. and Kotyleva, O.A. 1972. Duration and degree of immunity in sheep inoculated with "AUF" vaccine strain (of *Listeria monocytogenes*). Uch. Zap. Kazan. Vet. Inst. 112:123–126.

Shah, M.S., Siddique, I.H., and Dalvi, R.R. 1981. Studies on glutamic acid decarboxylase from *Listeria monocytogenes*. Can J. Comp. Med. 45:196–198.

Siddique, I.H., McKenzie, B.E., Sapp, W.J., and Rich, P. 1978. Light and electron microscopic study of the livers of pregnant mice infected with *Listeria monocytogenes*. Am. J. Vet. Res. 39:887–892.

Sipka, M., Stajner, B., and Zakula, S. 1973. Detection of *Listeria* in milk. Wien. Tierärztl. Monatsschr. 60:50–52.

Smith, C.W., Marshall, J.D. Jr., and Eveland, W.C. 1960. Identification of *Listeria monocytogenes* by the fluorescent antibody technique. Proc. Soc. Exp. Biol. Med. 102:842–845.

Stevenson, S.H., Jones, L.F., and Call, J.W. 1972. Pine needle (*Pinus ponderosa*) induced abortion in range cattle. Cornell Vet. 62:519–524.

Von Sachse, H., and Potel, J. 1957. Über Kreuzreaktionen zwischen Hämosensitinen aus Streptokokken und Listerien. Z. Immun. Exp. Ther. 114:472–485.

Watson, B.B., and Lavizzo, J.C. 1973. Extracellular antigens from *Listeria monocytogenes*. II. Cytotoxicity of hemolytic and lipolytic antigens of *Listeria* for cultured mouse macrophages. Infect. Immun. 7:753–758.

ated with disease in animals are *C. renale* and *C. pseudo-tuberculosis*. *C. bovis* is found as a commensal of cow udders and has been implicated on a few occasions as a cause of bovine mastitis. Other *Corynebacterium* species occasionally isolated from lesions in animals are *C. pilosum* from equine urine (Thomas and Gibson 1981) and *C. ulcerans* from bovine mastitis (Hart 1984).

The corynebacteria do not form spores, are not acid-fast, and are nonmotile; the species that are pathogenic for animals are facultative anaerobes.

REFERENCES

Hart, R.J.C. 1984. *Corynebacterium ulcerans* in humans and cattle in North Devon. J. Hyg. 92:161–164.

Keddie, R.M., and Bousfield, I.J. 1980. Cell wall composition in the classification and identification of coryneform bacteria. In F.A. Skinner, ed., Society of Bacteriology Symposium, Series 8. Academic Press, New York. Pp. 167–188.

Reddy, C.A., Cornell, C.P. and Fraga, A.M. 1982. Transfer of *Corynebacterium pyogenes* (Glage) Eberson to the genus *Actinomyces* as *Actimyces pyogenes* (Glaze) comb. nov. Int. J. Syst. Bacteriol. 32:783–789.

Thomas, R.J., and Gibson, J.A. 1981. *Corynebacterium pilosum* from a horse. Aust. Vet. J. 57:145–146.

Wegienek, J., and Reddy, C.A. 1982. Taxonomic study of "*Corynebacterium suis*" (Soltys and Spratling): Proposal of *Eubacterium suis* (nom. rev.) comb. nov. Int. J. Syst. Bacteriol. 32:218–228.

24 The Genera *Corynebacterium* and *Eubacterium*

The Genus *Corynebacterium*

The genus *Corynebacterium* contains a large number of species from a variety of habitats and includes some important human and animal pathogens. The basic criterion for inclusion in the genus used to be appearance. *Corynebacterium* organisms typically were pleomorphic, Gram-positive rods that stained irregularly and occurred in angular and palisade (fence of stakes) arrangements. Club-shaped swellings at one or both ends of the organism were also a characteristic—hence the name *Corynebacterium* ("club bacterium"). Studies of cell wall chemistry and DNA homology, however, have revealed that superficial morphologic appearance has been an inadequate taxonomic criterion for organisms historically placed in the genus, and most taxonomists believe that only those species whose cell walls contain meso-diaminopimelic acid, galactose, arabinose, and mycolic acids with chain lengths of 22 to 38 carbon atoms should be retained in the genus *Corynebacterium* (Keddie and Bousfield 1980). Many saprophytic and some pathogenic *Corynebacterium* species thus have been or are in the process of being transferred to other genera. Examples of transfers of animal pathogens are the reclassification of *C. equi* as *Rhodococcus equi* (see Chapter 25) and the transfer of *C. pyogenes* and *C. suis* to the genera *Actinomyces* (see Chapter 26) (Reddy et al. 1982) and *Eubacterium* (Wegienek and Reddy 1982), respectively.

C. diphtheriae, the cause of human diphtheria, is the type species, and other *Corynebacterium* species are often termed diphtheroid bacilli. The important species associ-

Corynebacterium renale Group: *C. renale*, *C. pilosum*, and *C. cystitidis*

SYNONYMS: *Bacillus pyelonephritidis bovis*, *Bacillus renalis bovis*

The *C. renale* group of organisms was formerly known as *C. renale* immunological types I, II, and III (Yanagawa et al. 1967). DNA homology studies and numerical analysis of phenotypic characters in the late 1970s revealed that these types were in fact three different species, and the organisms were renamed *C. renale* (type I), *C. pilosum* (type II), and *C. cystitidis* (type III) (Yanagawa and Honda 1978). These species can be distinguished biochemically by the characteristics listed in Table 24.1.

Of the *C. renale* group, *C. renale* is the most frequently isolated organism from cases of bovine cystitis, ureteritis, and pyelonephritis (Hiramune et al. 1970). Since it is probable that most of the literature published before *C. pilosum* and *C. cystitidis* were distinguished is actually about *C. renale*, the following descriptions will focus on this species with occasional references to the other two species as appropriate.

C. renale predominantly affects female animals, producing a diphtheritic inflammation of the bladder, ureters, kidney, pelvis, and, frequently, the kidney tissue itself. Lesions caused by this organism have been reported in

Table 24.1. Distinguishing characteristics of *Corynebacterium* species important in infectious diseases of domesticated animals

Characteristic	C. renale group			C. pseudotuberculosis (ovis)	C. bovis
	C. renale	C. cystitidis	C. pilosum		
Hemolysis	−	−	−	+	−
Catalase production	+	+	+	+	+
Liquefaction of inspissated serum	−	−	−	−	−
Casein hydrolysis	+	−	−	−	−
Pigment production	−	−	−	−	−
Metachromatic granules	+	+	+	+	−
Acid from glycose	+	+	+	+	−
Acid from xylose	−	+	−	−	−
Acid from starch	−	+	+	+	−
Nitrate reduction	+	−	+	±*	−
Urease production	+	+	+	+	−

+ = positive reaction; − = negative reaction.
*Most isolates from horses and cattle are positive.

cows and occasionally in horses and sheep. One case has been described in a dog (Olafson 1930). The disease is commonly known by several different names: *bacillary pyelonephritis* of cattle, *specific pyelonephritis* of cattle, and *infectious pyelonephritis* of cattle.

Morphology and Staining Reactions. *C. renale* is a rather large diphtheroid bacillus (0.5 by 1.3 to 2.6 μm). Individual organisms do not vary greatly in morphology, all being rather short, stumpy rods that are usually a little thicker at one end than at the other (Figure 24.1). In exudates and in cultures the organisms are found in clumps varying from a few cells to many hundreds. They are nonmotile, non-spore-bearing, and nonencapsulated. They are strongly Gram-positive. Bars and granules are sometimes seen when *C. renale* is stained with methylene

Figure 24.1. A film containing *Corynebacterium renale* from the urine of a naturally infected cow.

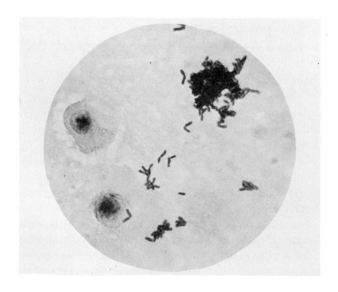

blue. Pili are present, but strains of *C. renale* can carry fewer pili than *C. pilosum* or *C. cystitidis*.

Cultural and Biochemical Features. Growth of *C. renale*, *C. pilosum*, and *C. cystitidis* in common laboratory media is enhanced by the addition of serum or blood. Colonies are opaque, ivory-colored, and dull, and the margins are uneven. The colonies of *C. pilosum* are cream-colored to pale yellow, circular, opaque, and about 1 mm in diameter. Those of *C. cystitidis* are white, entirely circular, semitranslucent, and pinpoint in size (Yanagawa et al. 1978).

When cultured in broth the organisms may produce slight clouding but most of the growth appears in the form of granular sediment. A characteristic reaction of *C. renale* is seen in litmus milk. It begins with the reduction of the litmus in the bottom of the tube, followed by the formation of a soft curd, which is slowly digested. The medium is alkaline at all times. The medium finally separates into a dark red fluid and a heavy sediment. The main differential characteristics of *C. renale* are presented in Table 24.1. The mol% G + C of the DNA lies between 52 and 60 depending on the source species.

Only *C. renale* produces caseinase, the enzyme responsible for the reaction in litmus milk. The action of caseinase is readily seen on skim-milk agar (Lovell 1946).

There is good growth on coagulated blood serum and gelatin, but *C. renale* produces no proteolysis. The organism also multiplies in sterile bovine urine, which becomes strongly alkaline because of the production of ammonia from urea.

Antigens. Each species in the *C. renale* group carries specific surface antigens, which were used by Yanagawa et al. (1967) in gel diffusion precipitin tests to establish immunological types I, II, and III. The pilus protein is antigenic and is different in each of the three species. The

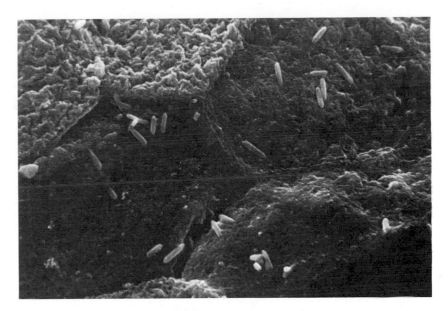

Figure 24.2. *Corynebacterium renale* attached to the mucous membrane of the urinary bladder of a mouse during an experimental infection. × 1,060. (From Honda and Yanagawa, 1978, courtesy of *American Journal of Veterinary Research.*)

pilus protein of *C. pilosum* has a molecular weight of 19,000.

Epizootiology and Pathogenesis. Given the rapidity with which strains of the *C. renale* group die out on laboratory media, it is probably safe to say that resistance to physical and chemical factors in natural environments is slight. Each species is highly adapted to the bovine and ovine urinary tract and is maintained there. Transmission occurs when contaminated droplets of urine are splashed on the vulvar area of a susceptible animal from an adjacent infected or carrier animal. Adherence to the vulvar epithellum appears to be pilus-mediated (Hayashi et al. 1985). Penetration and colonization of the urinary tract is aided by the ability of *C. renale* to adhere to aging epithelial cells of the bladder (Figure 24.2) (Sato et al. 1982). However, other predisposing factors such as pregnancy or parturition are required for disease to occur.

The epizootiology of each member of the *C. renale* group has distinctive features (Hiramune et al. 1970). *C. renale* is the most frequently isolated member from cases of pyelonephritis. It also is often found in healthy animals in diseased herds. *C. pilosum* occurs in the urine and vagina of approximately 4 percent of healthy cows and causes cystitis and pyelonephritis only very occasionally. It is much less virulent for mice and cows than *C. renale.*

C. cystitidis is widely distributed and causes severe hemorrhagic cystitis followed by pyelonephritis. It is never isolated from healthy cows but is carried as a commensal on the prepuce by more than 90 percent of bulls (Hiramune et al. 1975). Although well adapted to the urinary tract of male animals, it is poorly adapted to the female tract, where it causes severe disease after venereal transmission or infection via contaminated urine from an-

other female. In natural occurrences of the disease the urinary bladder is always involved, including one or both ureters in most cases and usually one or both kidneys (Boyd 1918). The walls of affected bladders are thickened and the mucosa is superficially ulcerated and covered with a slimy secretion mixed with shreds of tissue and fibrin. Petechiae and larger hemorrhages are usually present in the bladder wall, and small clots of blood often are found in the bladder contents. The affected ureters become enormously distended, and the mucosa usually contains necrotic areas or is necrotic in its entirety. The kidneys often are greatly enlarged, and in extreme cases most of the kidney substance can undergo necrosis. More often the kidney pelvis is enlarged, the papillae are necrotic, and abscesses form throughout the kidney structure. The content of the affected pelvis consists of a grayish, slimy, odorless exudate mixed with fibrin, small blood clots, necrotic tissue, and calcareous material.

Great numbers of the characteristic diphtheroid bacilli can be found both free and bound in the fragments of necrotic tissue in this exudate. These generally occur in clumps arranged in a palisade and radiating fashion. Quite often streptococci are also found in this exudate.

The urine, which is voided in small amounts at frequent intervals because of the bladder irritation, contains large quantities of albumin, leukocytes, fibrin, epithelial debris, and usually small bright red blood clots. The disease is rarely seen in sheep (Higgins and Weaver 1981), but a condition known as *ovine posthitis* (pizzle rot) of rams is believed to be caused by the irritating effect of the ammonia released by urease from *C. renale* in the prepuce.

Immunity. A number of serologic tests, including agglutination, indirect hemagglutination, and agar-gel diffusion (Hiramune et al. 1972), have been used for the detection of antibodies against *C. renale* in experimental studies. None is used for routine diagnostic purposes. A serum antibody response is present in cows with pyelonephritis and urethritis but not in those with cystitis alone (Hiramune et al. 1971). Organisms in urinary sediments from animals with upper urinary tract involvement are often coated with antibody (IgG), whereas organisms from animals in which only the lower tract is involved are not (Nicolet and Fey 1979). The antibody is probably derived from the plasma that accompanies the inflammatory exudate. The protective response of the host is, however, ineffective, and untreated animals seldom recover.

Diagnosis. The symptoms of pyelonephritis are quite characteristic in most cases. A sample of urine should be collected in a sterile bottle for laboratory confirmation. If it contains blood clots or bits of necrotic tissue, films can be made from these on slides and stained with Gram's technique. Characteristic clumps of short, stubby, Gram-positive organisms is presumptive evidence. If clumps are not present, the sample can be centrifuged and the sediment examined microscopically. The characteristics listed in Table 24.1 can be used for species identification. Healthy animals that are carriers of *C. renale* or *C. pilosum* have fewer than 100 organisms per milliliter of urine.

Antimicrobial Susceptibility. Organisms of the *C. renale* group are sensitive to penicillin, streptomycin, kanamycin, erythromycin and polymyxin B. *C. renale* and *C. cystitidis* are sensitive to tetracycline at a level of 10 μg/ml, whereas *C. pilosum* is resistant to this concentration. Penicillin in large doses is the antibiotic of choice in therapy and is often effective if administered before lesions have become far advanced (Morse 1948).

REFERENCES

Boyd, W.L. 1918. Pyelonephritis in cattle. Cornell Vet. 8:120.
Hayashi, A., Yanagawa, R., and Kida, H. 1985. Adhesion of *Corynebacterium renale* and *Corynebacterium pilosum* to epithelial cells of bovine vulva. Am. J. Vet. Res. 46:409–411.
Higgins, R.J., and Weaver, C.R. 1981. *Corynebacterium renale* pyelonephritis and cystitis in sheep. Vet. Rec. 109:256.
Hiramune, T., Inui, S., and Murase, N. 1972. Antibody response in cows infected with *Corynebacterium renale*, with special reference to the differentiation of pyelonephritis and cystitis. Res. Vet. Sci. 13:82–86.
Hiramune, T., Inui, S., Murase, N., and Yanagawa, R. 1971. Virulence of three types of *Corynebacterium renale* in cows. Am. J. Vet. Res. 32:237–242.
Hiramune, T.M., Murase, N., and Yanagawa, R. 1970. Distribution of the types of *Corynebacterium renale* in cows of Japan. Jpn. J. Vet. Sci. 32:235–242.
Hiramune, T.M., Narita, N., Murase, N., and Yanagawa, R. 1975. Distribution of *Corynebacterium renale* among healthy bulls with special reference to inhabitation of type III in the prepuce. Natl. Inst. Anim. Health Q. (Tokyo) 15:116–121.
Honda, E., and Yanagawa, R. 1978. Pili-mediated attachment of *Corynebacterium renale* to mucous membrane of urinary bladder of mice. Am. J. Vet. Res. 39:155–158.
Lovell, R. 1946. Studies on *Corynebacterium renale*. I. A systemic study of a number of strains. J. Comp. Pathol. Ther. 56:196–204.
Morse, E.V. 1948. Pyelonephritis. IV. Physiological and bacteriological studies of eight cases of pyelonephritis treated with penicillin. Cornell Vet. 38:273–285.
Nicolet, J., and Fey, H. 1979. Antibody-coated bacteria in urine sediment from cattle infected with *C. renale*. Vet. Rec. 105:301–303.
Olafson, P. 1930. Pyelonephritis in a dog due to *Corynebacterium renale*. Cornell Vet. 20:69–73.
Sato, H., Tanagawa, R., and Fukuyama, H. 1982. Adhesion of *Corynebacterium renale*, *Corynebacterium pilosum*, and *Corynebacterium cystitidis* to bovine urinary bladder epithelial cells of various ages and levels of differentiation. Infect. Immun. 36:1242–1245.
Yanagawa, R., and Honda, E. 1978. *Corynebacterium pilosum* and *Corynebacterium cystitidis*, two new species from cows. Int. J. Syst. Bacteriol. 28:209–216.
Yanagawa, R., Basri, H., and Otsuki, K. 1967. Three types of *Corynebacterium renale* classified by precipitin reactions in gels. Jpn. J. Vet. Res. 15:111–119.

Corynebacterium pseudotuberculosis

SYNONYMS: *Corynebacterium ovis*, Preisz-Nocard bacillus

C. pseudotuberculosis causes *caseous lymphadenitis*, a disease prevalent in sheep and goats in many parts of the world. It also causes disease in horses, camels, deer, mules, and, rarely, cattle and humans. The lesions produced in all species usually involve suppuration and necrosis of the lymph nodes.

Morphology and Staining Reactions. *C. pseudotuberculosis* is a pleomorphic rod that frequently is so short that it may be mistaken for a coccus. It sometimes occurs as a rod form in the caseous pus taken from lymph nodes. It forms no spores and is nonmotile. It retains Gram's stain but is not acid-fast.

Cultural and Biochemical Features. *C. pseudotuberculosis* grows on all the ordinary media, albeit slowly. Colonies take several days to reach maximum size at 37°C. When fully developed they have papilliform centers surrounded by concentric rings that parallel the irregular margin. The color is grayish or yellowish, and the surfaces are dull and dry. The colonies fragment easily when touched with a needle. Because of the high lipid content cell wall, entire smaller colonies can be pushed around the surface of the medium as if they were flakes of wax. *C. pseudotuberculosis* produces slight hemolysis on blood agar.

The biochemical reactions of *C. pseudotuberculosis* vary greatly. Isolates from cattle and horses reduce nitrate but those from sheep or goats rarely do (Biberstein et al. 1971). A phospholipase D is produced. The distinguishing features of *C. pseudotuberculosis* are given in Table 24.1.

Antigens and Toxins. Two serotypes have been described (Barakat et al. 1984). Serotype 1 predominates in sheep and goats but also occurs infrequently in cattle. Serotype 2 is found in buffalo and cattle. An exotoxin that is a phospholipase D (Carne and Onon 1978) is an important virulence antigen. It has a molecular weight of 31,000, and antibodies to it are protective. Its biological effects in vivo include intravascular hemolysis, necrosis, pulmonary edema, and shock (Hsu 1984). It produces synergistic hemolysis with the phospholipase C of *Rhodococcus equi*.

Antigens of *C. pseudotuberculosis* stimulate cellular immune responses including delayed-type hypersensitivity.

Epizootiology and Pathogenesis. In sheep and goats caseous lymphadenitis commonly spreads directly from an open abscess and enters a new host through a skin abrasion. Because *C. pseudotuberculosis* can survive briefly in the environment, spread can also occur indirectly, and animals can become infected from heavily contaminated resting areas, hay racks, and the like. Shearing wounds in sheep and butting abrasions in goats facilitate entry. Sometimes the organism penetrates the abraded buccal mucosae or is inhaled, subsequently producing pulmonary abscesses.

The distribution of lesions of ulcerative lymphagitis on the fetlocks of horses supports the contention that skin abrasions are important in this disease. However, the seasonal incidence of pectoral abscesses (*pigeon fever*) and other abscesses in horses suggests that in such instances the organism is borne by arthropods (Knight 1969).

Once *C. pseudotuberculosis* has gained entry into a host, it adopts the status of a facultative intracellular parasite. The following factors are thought to contribute to its ability to survive and produce abscesses in sheep and goats: the phospholipase D, which increases vascular permeability; a heat-stable pyogenic factor (Bull and Dickinson, 1935), which attracts leukocytes; and the presence of a large amount of surface lipid, (Carne et al., 1956), which is toxic for phagocytes. The lipid is also thought to allow the organism to survive unharmed in phagolysosomes of the host's phagocytic cells and to produce an abscess in the regional node or to be carried to another site. Caseous lymphadenitis is prevalent in sheep and goats in many parts of the world. Female goats and intact males have more abscesses than do castrated males. The prevalence of abscesses increases with the age of the animal (Ashfag and Campbell 1979). The disease is primarily a wound infection and starts with local inflammation at the site of entry of the organism, often going unnoticed and then proceeding to the regional lymph node, which slowly enlarges and becomes filled with pus.

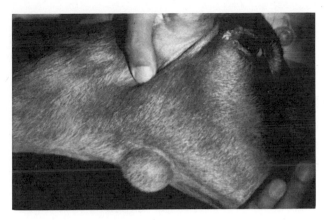

Figure 24.3. Lymphadenitis caused by *Corynebacterium pseudotuberculosis* in a goat.

The pus is greenish and odorless. Initially it may be thin, but eventually it is thick and caseous and may become arranged in concentric layers resembling an onion. The superficial nodes are often affected. Superficial nodes close to shearing wounds in sheep can be enlarged and abscessed, and in goats the superficial nodes of the head and neck are most often affected (Figure 24.3). In both species deep abscesses can be found in the lungs and the mediastinal or mesenteric lymph nodes. Animals that appear quite normal are often found at slaughter to be rather badly affected. Those that are not slaughtered eventually become emaciated and weak and die. The infection is therefore an important component of the thin ewe syndrome. In rams abscesses can be found in the scrotum (Williamson and Nairn 1980).

C. pseudotuberculosis is the cause of ulcerative lymphangitis in horses, a condition similar to cutaneous glanders (farcy) in horses. Nodules appear on the legs and break down to form ulcers, which exude a thick greenish pus that is usually mixed with blood. They are located most often around the fetlocks. These lesions fill with cicatricial tissue and heal after a time, but others appear nearby. Some cases heal spontaneously within a few weeks, but most progress slowly for months or even years. Spread of infection is through the lymph system. Hematogenous spread in two mares which resulted in abortion has also been reported (Brumbaugh and Ekman 1981).

Pigeon fever, another disease entity frequently seen in horses in California, is characterized by large painful abscesses in the pectoral, lower abdominal, and inguinal regions. The lesions typically occur in adult horses, develop slowly, and sometimes recur after opening and draining (Hughes and Biberstein 1959). Generalization sometimes occurs, resulting in death.

C. pseudotuberculosis is rarely isolated from cattle in the United States or Europe. Kitt (1890) found it in a cow with bronchopneumonia, and Hall and Stone (1916) found it in a calf. A considerable number of cases of so-called skin-lesion tuberculosis in Utah reportedly contained the organism (Daines and Austin 1932). A similar disease has recently been described in Kenya. Kariuka and Poulton (1982) described a series of isolates from buffalo and cattle in Africa.

Immunity. Antibodies are produced in response to infection with *C. pseudotuberculosis*. Investigators have used various serologic tests to detect the antibodies, to confirm the diagnosis, and to detect the inapparent carrier. These tests include bacterial agglutination, toxin neutralization in mice and rabbits, antihemolysin-inhibition tests (Zaki 1968), hemolysin (exotoxin) inhibition (Burrell 1980a), a double immunodiffusion technique for detection of antitoxin (Burrell 1980b), and an enzyme-linked immunosorbent assay (ELISA) based on detection of antibody to exotoxin (Maki et al. 1985). The ELISAs appear to have the most promise for the field detection of naturally infected animals.

Although researchers have used many biological agents, including killed and autogenous bacterins, in attempts to produce artificial immunity to *C. pseudotuberculosis,* none has yet been proved to give a high level of protection. As an aid in control, however, these agents reduce the number and size of abscesses. Commercially available vaccines consist of various combinations of whole cells, cell walls, and toxoids.

The use of aluminum hydroxide gel and saponin has been found to give a better immune response and to be less irritating than other adjuvants in *C. pseudotuberculosis* vaccines (Cameron and Bester 1984).

A toxoid vaccine has been shown to protect 3-month-old goats. Vaccinated does secreted colostral antibody that protected kids (Anderson and Nairn 1984). The facultative intracellular nature of this infection suggests that cell-mediated immunity and agents that stimulate its production, such as attenuated live vaccines, are likely to be necessary for protection against *C. pseudotuberculosis* (Ayers 1977).

Interestingly, lambs less than 1 month old developed a high level of protection when vaccinated with attenuated bovine tubercle bacillus of Calmette and Guerin (BCG) (Barakat 1979).

Diagnosis. The appearance of the lesions in sheep and goats is quite characteristic, and *C. pseudotuberculosis* can usually be isolated in large numbers from the abscesses without difficulty. The dry, scaly colonies, which cause hemolysis on blood-agar plates, are easily recognized. Animals devoid of abscesses of the superficial

lymph nodes but having abscesses deep in their body cavities still pose a great diagnostic challenge.

Antimicrobial Susceptibility. *C. pseudotuberculosis* is sensitive to penicillin, ampicillin, chloramphenicol, erythromycin, gentamicin, and tetracycline; however, in vivo responses are poor. The intracellular location of the organism together with the antibiotic binding properties of proteins in pus and the thick capsule that surrounds abscesses greatly favors survival of the parasite in the face of antimicrobial therapy. Antibiotics appear to have little value except in light, superficial infections (Maddy 1953).

The Disease in Humans. A few cases of *C. pseudotuberculosis* infection in humans have been reported. Localized adenopathy and hepatomegaly accompanied by fatigue and myalgia were noted in one patient (Lopez et al. 1966). Other reports include those of Battey et al. (1968) and Goldberger et al. (1981).

REFERENCES

Anderson, V.M., and Nairn, M.E. 1984. I. Role of maternal immunity in the prevention of caseous lymphadenitis in kids. II. Control of caseous lymphadenitis in goats by vaccination. In Les maladies de la chèvre, colloque international, Niort (France), 9–11 Oct. 1984. Institut National de la Recherche Agronomique, Paris. Pp. 601–609.

Ashfag, M.K., and Campbell, S.G. 1979. A survey of caseous lymphadenitis and its etiology in goats in the United States. Vet. Med./Small Anim. Clin. 74:1161–1165.

Ayers, J.L. 1977. Caseous lymphadenitis in goats and sheep: A review of diagnosis, pathogenesis, and immunity. J. Am. Vet. Med. Assoc. 171:1251–1254.

Barakat, A.A. 1979. Immunization against caseous lymphadenitis of sheep using attenuated bovine tubercle bacillus of Calmette and Guerin (BCG). Bull. Off. Int. Epiz. 91:679–692.

Barakat, A.A., Selim, S.A., Atef, A., Saber, M.S., Nafie, E.K., and El-Ebeedy, A.A. 1984. Two serotypes of *Corynebacterium pseudotuberculosis* isolated from different animal species. Rev. Sci. Tech. O.I.E. 3:151–163.

Battey, Y.M., Tonge, J.I., Horsfoll, W.E., and McDonald, I.R. 1968. Human infection with *Corynebacterium ovis*. Med. J. Aust. 2:540–543.

Biberstein, E.L., Knight, H.D., and Jang, S. 1971. Two biotypes of *Corynebacterium pseudotuberculosis*. Vet. Rec. 89:691–692.

Brumbaugh, G.W., and Ekman, T.L. 1981. *Corynebacterium pseudotuberculosis* bacteremia in two horses. J. Am. Vet. Med. Assoc. 178:300–301.

Bull, L.B., and Dickinson, C.G. 1935. Studies on infection by and resistance to the Preisz-Nocard bacillus. Aust. Vet. 11:126–138.

Burrell, D.H. 1980a. A hemolysis inhibition test for detection of antibody to *Corynebacterium ovis* exotoxin. Res. Vet. Sci. 28:190–194.

Burrell, D.H. 1980b. A simplified double immunodiffusion technique for detection of *Corynebacterium ovis* antitoxin. Res. Vet. Sci. 28:234–237.

Cameron, C.M., and Bester, F.J. 1984. An improved *Corynebacterium pseudotuberculosis* vaccine for sheep. Onderstepoort J. Vet. Res. 51:263–267.

Carne, H.R., and Onon, E. 1978. Action of *C. ovis* exotoxin on endothelial cells of blood vessels. Nature 271:246–248.

Carne, H.R., Wickham, N., and Kater, J.C. 1956. A toxic lipid from the surface of *Corynebacterium ovis*. Nature 178:701–702.

Daines, L.L., and Austin, S.H. 1932. A study of so-called skin-lesion and no-visible-lesion tuberculin-reacting cattle. J. Am. Vet. Med. Assoc. 80:414–433.

Goldberger, A.C., Lipsky, B.A., and Plorde, J.J. 1981. Suppurative granulomatous lymphadenitis caused by *C. ovis (pseudotuberculosis)*. Am. J. Clin. Pathol. 76:486–490.

Hall, I.C., and Stone, R.V. 1916. The diphtheroid bacillus of Preisz-Nocard from equine, bovine, and ovine abscesses. J. Infect. Dis. 18:195–208.

Hsu, T.-Y. 1984. Caseous lymphadenitis in small ruminants: Clinical, pathological, and immunological responses to *Corynebacterium pseudotuberculosis* and to fractions and toxins from the micro-organism. Diss. Abstr. Int. B 45:1396.

Hughes, J.P., and Biberstein, E.L. 1959. Chronic equine abscesses associated with *Corynebacterium pseudotuberculosis*. J. Am. Vet. Med. Assoc. 135:559–562.

Kariuka, D.P., and Poulton, J. 1982. Corynebacterial infection of cattle in Kenya. Trop. Anim. Health Prod. 14:33–36.

Kitt, T. 1890. Zur Kenntnis tuberculose ähnlicher Zustande der Lunge des Rhindes (eine bacillare käsige Pneumonie). Monatsschr. Prakt. Tierheilkd. 1:145.

Knight, H.D. 1969. Corynebacterial infections in the horse: Problems of prevention. J. Am. Vet. Med. Assoc. 155:446–451.

Lopez, J.F., Wong, F.M. and Quesada, J. 1966. *C. pseudotuberculosis*: First case of human infection. Am. J. Clin. Pathol. 46:562–567.

Maddy, K.T. 1953. *Corynebacterium pseudotuberculosis* infection in a horse. J. Am. Vet. Med. Assoc. 122:387.

Maki, L.R., Shan, S.H. Berstrom, R.C. and Stetzenbach, L.D. 1985. Diagnosis of *Corynebacterium pseudotuberculosis* infections in sheep, using an enzyme-linked immunosorbent assay. Am. J. Vet. Res. 46:212–214.

Williamson, P., and Nairn, M.E. 1980. Lesions caused by *C. pseudotuberculosis* in the scrotum of rams. Aust. Vet. J. 56:496–498.

Zaki, M.M. 1968. The application of a new technique for diagnosing *C. ovis* infection. Res. Vet. Sci. 9:489–493.

Corynebacterium bovis

Commonly found in the milk from healthy udders, *C. bovis* also occurs in the reproductive tracts of cows and bulls. It is widely believed to be a commensal of the udder, where it stimulates a low-grade leukocytosis that is protective against infection by more virulent pathogens such as *Staphylococcus aureus* (Brooks and Barnum 1984). However, it has occasionally been reported as a primary pathogen in outbreaks of mastitis (Cobb and Walley 1962, Counter 1981).

C. bovis exhibits classic coryneform morphology as described in the introduction to this chapter. Its distinguishing characteristics are listed in Table 24.1. It is lipophilic and requires enriched basal media for the study of fermentation reactions.

REFERENCES

Brooks, B.W., and Barnum, D.A. 1984. The susceptibility of bovine udder quarters colonized with *Corynebacterium bovis* to experimental infection with *Staphylococcus aureus* or *Streptococcus agalactiae*. Can. J. Comp. Med. 48:146–150.

Cobb, R.W., and Walley, J.K. 1962. *Corynebacterium* as a probable cause of bovine mastitis. Vet. Rec. 74:101–102.

Counter, D.E. 1981. Outbreak of bovine mastitis associated with *C. bovis*. Vet. Rec. 108:560–561.

The Genus *Eubacterium*

Eubacterium suis

SYNONYM: *Corynebacterium suis*

For convenience *E. suis* used to be classified as a *Corynebacterium* species because its cells resembled those of other corynebacteria. The organism has been recently assigned to the genus *Eubacterium* on the basis of its cultural and biochemical properties (Wegienek and Reddy 1982).

E. suis is a common cause of cystitis and pyelonephritis of breeding sows in Europe, Canada, and Australia. Although the organism has been reported to be a common preputial commensal of boars in the United States and Mexico (Pijoan et al. 1983), disease in sows has not yet been reported from these countries.

Morphology and Staining Reactions. In cultures *E. suis* is a pleomorphic, slim, Gram-positive rod (0.4 μm by 2.0 to 3.0 μm). It does not form spores and has no flagella. In smears from specimens the organism exhibits branching and patterns resembling Chinese letters.

Cultural and Biochemical Features. Optimum growth of *E. suis* occurs under anaerobic conditions at 37°C. Some growth also occurs in the presence of air. Colonies on blood agar are tiny, gray, and shiny after 24 hours. As they mature colonies enlarge to a diameter of 3 mm and are flattened, with a gray matt appearance. There is no hemolysis. Growth of *E. suis* in enriched broths such as tryptic soy is excellent. Urea enhances growth.

E. suis produces and forms acid from glucose, arabinose, xylose, and maltose. For more information see the review by Dagnall (1983).

Epizootiology and Pathogenesis. Most male pigs over 10 weeks old in enzootic areas carry *E. suis* in their prepuce. Infection is more widespread among pigs kept in large groups than in those left in comparative isolation (Jones and Dagnall 1984). The organism is rarely isolated from healthy females, and its survival in the vestibule of healthy sows is short-lived after mating (Jones 1984). The factors that predispose some sows to colonization and penetration of the urinary tract by *E. suis* are unknown.

Colonization and multiplication of *E. suis* in the bladder leads to cystitis. The production of ammonia clearly could be important in the pathogenesis of the hemorrhagic response of the bladder mucosa. Lesions can be focal or diffuse and, depending on the stage of the infection, hyperemic to fibrinopurulent with necrosis.

The urine contains clots of blood and purulent material. The infection is usually localized to the bladder, but in some animals it may ascend to the kidneys, causing ureteritis and pyelonephritis.

Diagnosis. The presence of blood and pus in the urine of breeding sows is suggestive of urinary tract infection by *E. suis* or other bacteria. Smears of urinary sediment or pus will show large numbers of Gram-positive, slender, coryneform organisms. Urine should be cultured aerobically and anaerobically on blood agar and on CNA agar containing 50 mg of metronidazole per milliliter (Dagnall and Jones 1982). Growth of Gram-positive, anaerobic, coryneform organisms is good presumptive evidence of the presence of *E. suis* (Jones 1984).

Treatment with penicillin of early cases of cystitis is usually effective. Attempts to cure preputial carriage by administration of antibiotics are likely to succeed only when boars are isolated in an environment free of the organism.

REFERENCES

Dagnall, G.J.R. 1983. *Corynebacterium suis:* An investigation of its laboratory characteristics, habitat and survival. Med. Lab. Sci. 40:194–199.

Dagnall, G.J.R., and Jones, J.E.T. 1982. A selective medium for the isolation of *Corynebacterium suis.* Res. Vet. Sci. 32:389–390.

Jones, J.E.T. 1984. Cystitis and pyelonephritis associated with *Corynebacterium suis* infection in sows. Vet. Annu. 24:138–142.

Jones, J.E.T., and Dagnall, G.J.R. 1984. The carriage of *Corynebacterium suis* in male pigs. J. Hyg. 93:381–388.

Pijoan, C., Lastra, A., and Leman, A. 1983. Isolation of *Corynebacterium suis* from the prepuce of boars. J. Am. Vet. Med. Assoc. 183:428–429.

Wegienek, J., and Reddy, C.A. 1981. Taxonomic study of "*Corynebacterium suis*" (Soltys and Spartling): Proposal of *Eubacterium suis* (novn. rev.) comb. nov. Int. J. Syst. Bacteriol. 32:218–228.

and Schaal, K.P. 1980b. Ribosomal ribonucleic acid similarities in the classification of *Rhodococcus* and allied taxa. J. Gen. Microbiol. 118:313–319.

Rhodococcus equi

SYNONYM: *Corynebacterium equi*

First described and named by Magnusson (1923) as the causative agent of a purulent pneumonia in foals in southern Sweden, *R. equi* was subsequently found in foals in Australia (Bull 1924), the United States (Dimock and Edwards 1932), and India (Rajagopalon 1937). At the same time the organism was isolated from the lymph nodes of pigs (Plum 1940), although its role in disease in this species is still controversial. It has been isolated from two cows with pyometra (Craig and Davies 1940), from a water buffalo that had aborted (Rajagopalon and Gopalakrishnan 1938), and from a sheep in Australia with chronic pneumonia (Roberts 1957).

Morphology and Staining Reactions. *R. equi* is a rather large organism that shows considerable pleomorphism, ranging from coccoid to bacillary forms. On solid media the form usually is coccoid; in fluids it usually is bacillary. Sometimes short chains are found in fluid media. Metachromatic granules can usually be demonstrated, especially in cultures grown in milk.

R. equi is Gram-positive, variably acid-fast, and stains readily with other dyes. It does not form spores. A lamellar polysaccharide capsule is usually present (Woolcock and Mutimer 1978).

Cultural and Biochemical Features. *R. equi* grows well on all the ordinary media. After 2 days' incubation, colonies on the surface of agar plates measure nearly 1 cm in diameter and are raised, moist, translucent, and regular in outline. At first they are white but soon become rose pink. Old cultures are distinctly pinkish, especially those developing on potato. The organism grows rather poorly in milk, which it does not coagulate or change in chemical composition. *C. equi* is catalase- and urease-positive, is usually cytochrome-c-negative, ferments no carbohydrates, reduces nitrate, does not form indole, and is not hemolytic. The organism, however, produces a phospholipase and a cholesterol oxidase that interact with the phospholipase D of *Corynebacterium pseudotuberculosis* (*ovis*), the beta toxin of *Staphylococcus aureus,* and the hemolysin of *Listeria monocytogenes* to completely hemolyze sheep, cattle, or rabbit erythrocytes (Fraser 1964) (Figure 25.1). This phenomenon has been used as the basis for a rapid presumptive test for the identification of *R. equi* (Prescott 1982).

Antigens. The polysaccharide capsule of *R. equi* exists in many different antigenic configurations. Prescott

---

25 The Genus *Rhodococcus*

The genus *Rhodococcus* belongs to the order Actinomycetales and consists of nine species of soil-associated bacteria that have in common the production of red pigment. *R. equi,* formerly known as *Corynebacterium equi,* has been transferred to the genus on the basis of studies in numerical taxonomy (Goodfellow et al. 1982), genetics (Modarski et al. 1980a, 1980b), chemistry (Barton and Hughes 1981, Minnikin and Goodfellow 1980), and ecology (Barton and Hughes 1982). Of the *Rhodococcus* species only *R. equi* has been reported to cause lesions in animals, including purulent pneumonia, mesenteric lymphadenitis, and arthritis in foals and lesions similar to tuberculosis in the cervical lymph nodes of swine and cattle. *R. equi* and the diseases it causes have been reviewed by Barton and Hughes (1980).

REFERENCES

Barton, M.D., and Hughes, K.C. 1980. *Corynebacterium equi:* A review. Vet. Bull. 50:65–80.

Barton, M.D., and Hughes, K.L. 1981. Comparison of three techniques for isolation of *Rhodococcus (Corynebacterium) equi* from contaminated sources. J. Clin. Microbiol. 13:219–221.

Barton, M.D., and Hughes, K.L. 1982. Is *Rhodococcus (Corynebacterium) equi* a soil organism? J. Reprod. Fert. (Suppl.) 32:481–489.

Goodfellow, M., Beckham, A.R., and Barton, M.D. 1982. Numerical classification of *Rhodococcus equi* and related actinomycetes. J. Appl. Bacteriol. 53:1207.

Minnikin, D.E., and Goodfellow, M. 1980. Lipid composition and identification of acid-fast bacteria. In M. Goodfellow and R.G. Board, eds., Microbiological Classification and Identification. Academic Press, London. Pp. 189–256.

Mordarski, M., Goodfellow, M., Szyba, K., Tkacz, A., Pulverer, G.,

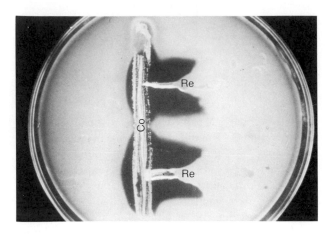

Figure 25.1. Synergistic effect of phospholipases produced by *Rhodococcus equi* (Re) and *Corynebacterium ovis* (Co). The erythrocytes in the cow-blood–agar plate are completely hemolyzed, as is apparent in the areas where the two organisms are close to each other. (From Prescott et al., 1982, courtesy of *Journal of Clinical Microbiology.*)

(1981) recognized seven capsular serotypes in a series of 97 North American strains. Another study of a larger number of strains from Japan and North America revealed even greater diversity (Nakazawa et al. 1983). Antigens of horses, pigs, and cattle extracted by hot acid have been studied by Bruner and Edwards (1941) and shown to be species-specific. They found that the majority of strains belonged to four groups and that these groups contained at least 14 serologic types. The group antigen was thought to be capsular. Cultures from the genital tracts of mares, from aborted equine fetuses, from foals with pneumonia, and from the submaxillar lymph nodes of pigs belonged to the same serologic group.

In North America about 60 percent of strains belong to capsular serotype 1 and 26 percent to capsular serotype 2 (Prescott 1981). In Japan, serotype 3 predominates in foals (Nakazawa et al. 1983).

Epizootiology and Pathogenesis. There is substantial evidence that *R. equi* is a soil organism and that animals acquire the infection from the soil (Barton and Hughes 1984, Robinson 1982). The organism is common in soil and in the gut contents and feces of herbivores grazing on soil that contains the organism; it is not present in the feces of penned animals that do not graze. The organism multiplies in voided feces, and numbers of *R. equi* in the environment are therefore magnified by fecal contamination.

R. equi is somewhat heat resistant, requiring exposure to 60°C for 1 hour before it is killed. It resists 2.5 percent oxalic acid for 1 hour, a treatment that can be used in the isolation of the organism from contaminated tissues. It also resists extremes of pH, 0.01 percent sodium azide, 0.5 percent formaldehyde, sunlight, and desiccation.

Prescott and co-workers (1984) have shown that *R. equi* populations correlate with the length of time farms have been used for horses. A critical factor in the occurrence of clinical disease in foals was the number of *R. equi* in the stable. Numbers of the organism in the pasture did not seem to be an important risk factor. Apparently, respiratory disease in foals requires exposure to large numbers of air-borne organisms, as can occur in a dusty atmosphere in the confined conditions of a stable. Isolates from diseased foals have predominantly the same capsular serotype as those occurring in the foals' environment (Prescott et al. 1984).

The route of infection in foals appears to be the respiratory tract, although some investigators (Bain 1963, Bull 1924) have maintained that intestinal lesions are the usual progenitors of pulmonary lesions. In a study by Johnson et al. (1983) experimentally induced intestinal lesions did not usually result in pulmonary lesions in weaned pony foals, a finding that argues against an intestinal source for naturally occurring pulmonary infections.

The circumstances or factors involved in the organism's penetration of the respiratory tract of young foals are not yet understood. *R. equi* pneumonia is endemic on some farms and sporadic on others. Most farms are free of the disease (Rooney 1966). After entry into the alveoli, the organism is phagocytosed by alveolar macrophages. Digestion of significant numbers of organisms requires the presence of immune serum (Zink et al. 1982). A massive infiltration of macrophages and multinucleate giant cells into the alveolar spaces then occurs. Foci of alveolar necrosis develop in which groups of bacteria-laden macrophages undergo degeneration (Johnson et al. 1983) (Figure 25.2). Because the organism is apparently able to survive within these macrophages, researchers have speculated that it is a facultative, intracellular parasite with a distribution in lymphatic tissue and macrophages (Cimprich and Rooney 1977, Knight 1969). The initial granulomatous response of the lung is followed by a massive invasion of polymorphonuclear neutrophils, thus giving rise to the typical suppurative bronchopneumonia with prominent abscesses (Figure 25.3).

The organism causes pneumonia in foals 2 to 5 months of age and older. The onset of the disease is insidious. Affected foals eventually may be anorectic, have a nasal discharge, and, less frequently, show signs of arthritis and diarrhea (Burrows 1968). Mortality is high (64 percent). Lymphadenitis is common and the lymph nodes may be abscessed. In contrast to strangles, the lymph nodes of the head are seldom involved.

Although pneumonia in foals is the most common dis-

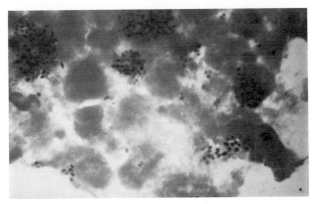

Figure 25.2. Impression smear of a lung of a foal infected with *Rhodococcus equi*. The characteristic clumps of organisms result from multiplication in alveolar macrophages. Gram's stain. (Courtesy John Prescott.)

ease entity with which *R. equi* is associated, the organism has also been found in internal abscesses with pleurisy in foals and in uterine infections in mares (Bruner and Edwards 1939). The organism has been isolated from two foals with enteritis, in which it was found in association with focal necrosis and thickening of the intestinal tract (Cimprich and Rooney 1977).

In swine the infection occurs in the submandibular and cervical lymph nodes. *R. equi* may be present by itself in apparently normal lymph nodes or in association with tubercle bacilli in nodes with typical lesions of tuberculosis (Cutchin 1943, Karlson et al. 1940). *R. equi* has also been recovered from pneumonic lungs of sheep (Addo and Dennis 1977), cattle (Holtman 1945), and from the lymph nodes of a cat (Jang et al. 1975).

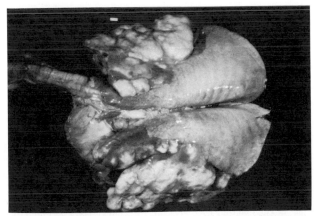

Figure 25.3. Appearance of the lungs of a foal after the animal was experimentally infected with *Rhodococcus equi*. The anterior and dependent areas of both lungs contain many abscesses. (Courtesy John Prescott.)

Lesions in Australian cattle that resembled those of tuberculosis yielded *R. equi* but no mycobacteria when cultured (McKenzie and Donald 1979).

Immunity. Protective immunity to *R. equi* is poorly understood but probably involves cell-mediated immune responses (Knight 1969, Prescott, Johnson, and Markham 1980). The presence of a surface component capable of inhibiting the bactericidal mechanisms of polymorphonuclear leukocytes has been detected (Ellenberger et al. 1984) and may in fact be responsible for the high rate of survival of *R. equi* in alveolar macrophages and polymorphonuclear leukocytes.

Antibody production as measured by precipitin reaction, complement fixation, agglutination, indirect hemagglutination, and enzyme-linked immunosorbent assay (ELISA) has been detected in the serums of naturally infected animals (Bull 1924, Hietala et al. 1985, Prescott et al. 1979).

R. equi antibody is present in the serum of normal mares and is passively transferred to their foals (Hietala et al. 1985). However, many affected animals or animals that have recently recovered from *R. equi* infections have very low levels of antibodies. Prescott et al. (1979) found that animals vaccinated with *R. equi* bacterin also produce only poor antibody responses. These workers obtained evidence that intestinal infections involving large numbers of organisms can stimulate immune responses that can be protective. Attempts to demonstrate a protective effect of leukocyte extracts (transfer factor) from mares that had positive skin tests to *R. equi* antigen have not been successful (Wilks et al. 1982).

Diagnosis. *R. equi* is usually recognized on the basis of the source of the isolate; the reaction to Gram's stain; pleomorphism; pinkish, mucoid, spreading colonies; catalase and urease positivity; and lack of fermentative activity in carbohydrates. The *equi* factors test of Prescott et al. (1982) is also of potential value as a supportive confirmatory test.

Transtracheal aspirates and subsequent culture and staining with Gram's stain are of great value in detection of infections in the earlier stages of lesion development when treatment is still potentially of value. Lymphocyte immunostimulation has been used successfully to detect infections in foals less than 2 months old (Prescott, Ogilvie, and Markham 1980), but this test is unlikely to become commonly available. A selective medium containing nalidixic acid, novobiocin, cycloheximide, and potassium tellurite (NANAT medium) is useful for the isolation of *R. equi* from contaminated samples (Woolcock and Mutimer 1980). Colonies of *R. equi* grown on this medium are black.

Antimicrobial Susceptibility. *R. equi* is sensitive to

penicillin G, doxycycline, erythromycin, lincomycin, gentamicin, neomycin, and streptomycin (Woolcock and Mutimer 1980). Woolcock and Mutimer (1980) concluded that erythromycin, streptomycin, and gentamicin should be effective if large doses are given intravenously. Combinations of erythromycin with rifampicin or penicillin have shown synergistic effects, as did a combination of penicillin and gentamicin (Prescott and Nicholson 1984). An increase in killing ability of 10-fold or greater was noted for the combinations over the antimicrobials used alone.

The Disease in Humans. Many cases of infection with *R. equi* have been reported in humans with AIDS or who are undergoing immunosuppressive therapy for malignant neoplasms (Berg et al. 1977, Williams et al. 1971). Pulmonary abscesses developed in all patients, some of whom were bacteremic. Almost all the patients had come in contact with animals.

REFERENCES

Addo, P.B., and Dennis, S.M. 1977. Ovine pneumonia caused by *Corynebacterium equi*. Vet Rec. 101:80.

Bain, A.M. 1963. *Corynebacterium equi* infections in the equine. Aust. Vet. J. 39:116–121.

Barton, M.D., and Hughes, K.L. 1984. Ecology of *Rhodococcus equi*. Vet. Microbiol. 9:67–76.

Berg, R., Chmel, H., Mayo, J., and Armstrong, D. 1977. *Corynebacterium equi* infection complicating neoplastic disease. Am. J. Clin. Pathol. 68:73–77.

Bruner, D.W., and Edwards, P.R. 1939. Classification of *Corynebacterium equi*. Ky. Agric. Exp. Sta. Bull. 414. Pp. 92–107.

Bull, L.B. 1924. Corynebacterial pyaemia of foals. J. Comp. Pathol. Ther. 37:294–298.

Burrows, G.E. 1968. *Corynebacterium equi* infection in two foals. J. Am. Vet. Med. Assoc. 152:1119–1124.

Cimprich, R.E., and Rooney, J.R. 1977. *Corynebacterium equi* enteritis in foals. Vet. Pathol. 14:95–102.

Cotchin, E. 1943. *Corynebacterium equi* in the submaxillary lymph nodes of swine. J. Comp. Pathol. Ther. 53:298–309.

Craig, J.F., and Davies, G.O. 1940. *Corynebacterium equi* in bovine pyometra. Vet. J. 96:417–419.

Dimock, W.W., and Edwards, P.R. 1932. Infections of fetuses and foals. Ky. Agric. Exp. Sta. Bull. 333.

Ellenberger, M.A., Kaeberle, M.L., and Roth, J.A. 1984. Effect of *Rhodococcus equi* on equine polymorphonuclear leukocyte function. Vet. Immunol. Immunopathol. 7:315–324.

Fraser, G. 1964. The effect on animal erythrocytes of combinations of diffusible substances produced by bacteria. J. Pathol. Bacteriol. 88:43–53.

Hietala, S.A., Ardans, A.A., and Sasome, A. 1985. Detection of *Corynebacterium equi*–specific antibody in horses by enzyme-linked immunosorbent assay. Am. J. Vet. Res. 46:13–15.

Holtman, D.F. 1945. *Corynebacterium equi* in chronic pneumonia of the calf. J. Bacteriol. 49:159–162.

Jang, S.S., Lock, A., and Biberstein, E.L. 1975. A cat with *Corynebacterium equi* lymphadenitis clinically simulating lymphosarcoma. Cornell Vet. 65:223–239.

Johnson, J.A., Prescott, J.F., and Markham, R.J.F. 1983. I. The pathology of *Corynebacterium equi* infection in foals following intrabronchial challenge. II. The pathology of experimental *Corynebacterium equi* in foals following intragastric challenge. Vet. Pathol. 20:440–449, 450–459.

Karlson, A.G., Moses, H.E., and Feldman, W.E. 1940. *Corynebacterium equi* (Magnusson, 1923) in the submaxillary lymph nodes of swine. J. Infect. Dis. 67:243–251.

Knight, H.D. 1969. Corynebacterial infections in the horse: Problems of infection. J. Am. Vet. Med. Res. 155:446–452.

McKenzie, R.A., and Donald, B.A. 1979. Lymphadenitis in cattle associated with *Corynebacterium equi*: A problem in bovine tuberculosis diagnosis. J. Comp. Pathol. 89:31–34.

Magnusson, H. 1923. Spezifische infektiose Pneumonie beim Fohlen: Ein neuer Eitererreger beim Pferde. Arch. Tierheilk. 50:22–38.

Nakazawa, M., Kubo, M., Sugimoto, C., and Isayama, Y. 1983. Serographing of *Rhodococcus equi*. Microbiol. Immun. 27:837–866.

Plum, N. 1940. On corynebacterial infections in swine: Preliminary report. Cornell Vet. 30:14–20.

Prescott, J.F. 1981. Capsular serotypes of *Corynebacterium equi*. Can. J. Comp. Med. 45:130–134.

Prescott, J.F. 1982. The susceptibility of isolates of *Corynebacterium equi* to antimicrobial drugs. J. Vet. Pharmacol. Ther. 4:27–31.

Prescott, J.F., and Nicholson, V.M. 1984. The effects of combinations of selected antibiotics on the growth of *Corynebacterium equi*. J. Vet. Pharmacol. Ther. 7:61–64.

Prescott, J.F., Johnson, J.A., and Markham, R.J.F. 1980. Experimental studies on the pathogenesis of *Corynebacterium equi* infection in foals. Can. J. Comp. Med. 44:280–288.

Prescott, J.F., Lastra, M., and Barksdale, L. 1982. Equi factors in the identification of *Corynebacterium equi* Magnusson. J. Clin. Microbiol. 16:988–990.

Prescott, J.F., Markham, R.J.F., and Johnson, J.A. 1979. Cellular and humoral immune response of foals to vaccination with *Corynebacterium equi*. Can. J. Comp. Med. 43:356–364.

Prescott, J.F., Ogilvie, T.H., and Markham, R.J.F. 1980. Lymphocyte immunostimulation in the diagnosis of *Corynebacterium equi* pneumonia of foals. Am. J. Vet. Res. 41:2073–2075.

Prescott, J.F., Travers, M., and Yager-Johnson, J.A. 1984. Epidemiological survey of *Corynebacterium equi* infections on five Ontario horse farms. Can. J. Comp. Med. 48:10–13.

Rajagopalan, V.R. 1937. Pneumonia in foals due to *Corynebacterium equi*. Indian J. Vet. Sci. 7:38–53.

Rajagopalan, V.R., and Gopalakrishnan, V.R. 1938. The occurrence of *Corynebacterium equi* in a she-buffalo. Indian J. Vet. Sci. 8:225–234.

Roberts, D.S. 1957. *Corynebacterium equi* infection in a sheep. Aust. Vet. J. 33:21.

Robinson, R.C. 1982. Epidemiological and bacteriological studies of *Corynebacterium equi* isolates from California farms. J. Reprod. Fertil. (Suppl.) 32:477–480.

Rooney, J.R. 1966. Corynebacterial infections in foals. Med. Vet. Prac. 47:43–45.

Wilks, C.R., Barton, M.D., and Allison, J.F. 1982. Immunity to and immunotherapy for *Rhodococcus equi*. J. Reprod. Fertil. (Suppl.) 32:497–505.

Williams, G.D., Flanigan, N.J., and Campbell, G.S. 1971. Surgical management of localized thoracic infections in immunosuppressed patients. Ann. Thorac. Surg. 12:471–482.

Woolcock, J.B., and Mutimer, M.D. 1978. The capsules of *Corynebacterium equi* and *Streptococcus equi*. J. Gen. Microbiol. 109:127–130.

Woolcock, J.B., and Mutimer, M.D. 1980. *Corynebacterium equi*: In vitro susceptibility to twenty-six antimicrobial agents. Antimicrob. Agents Chemother. 18:976–977.

Zink, M.C., Johnson, J.A., Prescott, J.F., and Pascal, P.J. 1982. The interaction of *Corynebacterium equi* and equine alveolar macrophages in vitro. J. Reprod. Fertil. (Suppl.) 32:491–496.

26 The Genus *Actinomyces*

Most species of *Actinomyces* produce a true mycelium that fragments into elements of irregular size and may exhibit angular branching. They are non-acid-fast, carboxyphilic, and nonmotile, usually growing as facultative anaerobes. The cell wall contains neither diaminopimelic acid nor arabinose.

The four species of *Actinomyces* that commonly cause disease in domesticated animals are *A. bovis, A. viscosus, A. suis,* and *A. pyogenes.* A new species, *A. hordeovulneris,* has been described in lesions caused by grass awns in dogs (Buchanan et al. 1984).

Actinomyces bovis

SYNONYMS: *Discomyces bovis, Nocardia bovis, Streptothrix actinomyces, Streptothrix israeli,* and others

A. bovis is the cause of the common disease of cattle known as *actinomycosis* and *lumpy jaw.* Human infections occasionally occur, the manifestations being similar to those in cattle. True actinomycosis of cattle usually affects the bony structures, particularly the mandible or lower jaw. Pulmonary actinomycosis in swine has been reported by Vawter (1946), and *A. bovis* has been isolated from the lungs of a cow (Biever et al. 1969).

In studies of equine poll evil and fistulous withers, which are inflammations of the supra-atloid and supraspinous bursa, respectively, Roderick et al. (1948) were able to isolate *A. bovis* and *Brucella abortus* regularly. *Brucella suis* has also been obtained from these lesions, and injections of either *B. abortus* or *B. suis* combined with *A. bovis* into the supraspinous bursa of experimental horses produces a bursitis that is apparently identical with that in field cases.

Morphology and Staining Reactions. In the so-called sulfur granules in the tissues, *A. bovis* is seen as a tangled mass of filaments around the periphery of which is a considerable mass of acidophilic capsular material. The filaments stain positively with Gram's stain and also retain the usual basophilic stains. When crushed granules are stained, a great diversity of forms resembling a mixed infection is seen. *A. bovis* can be cocci, rods of varying size, filaments, branching forms, club-shaped forms, or spiral (Figure 26.1). In cultures *A. bovis* usually appears in the form of diphtheroid bacilli when young (Figure 26.2); older cultures may show filaments of all kinds. When grown in an atmosphere of CO_2, *A. bovis* frequently takes the form of branching filaments and clubs (Figure 26.3).

Cultural and Biochemical Features. *A. bovis* is a facultative anaerobe and grows best in an atmosphere rich in CO_2 (10 to 15 percent). Under aerobic culture conditions colonies are subsurface. *A. bovis* is serophilic, catalase-negative, and requires a temperature of 37°C for growth. Loeffler's blood serum slants are good for isolation of *A. bovis* provided they are incubated in 10 to 15 percent CO_2. Growth is evident after 2 or 3 days in the form of fine colonies, which may easily be scraped off the medium. After 5 or 6 days' incubation at 37°C the colonies will have reached maximum size, about 0.5 mm in diameter. The condensation water at the bottom of the slant usually contains excellent growth in the form of a slimy deposit.

On blood-agar plates the colonies are small and non-hemolytic. *A. bovis* does not grow well in milk unless serum is added to it. In serum milk *A. bovis* does little to change the appearance of the medium. Sometimes the litmus is bleached in the bottom of the tube.

The organism will not grow in gelatin unless serum is added, and it does not liquefy serum gelatin. When grown in serum-containing broth under a petrolatum seal, *A. bovis* slowly ferments glucose, levulose, maltose, galactose, sucrose, and salicin without producing gas. The products of fermentation include acetic, formic, lactic, and succinic acids but not propionic acid.

The cell wall peptidoglycan contains alanine, glutamic acid, lysine, and aspartic acid. Arabinose does not occur. The mol% G + C of the DNA is 62 (Tm).

Serotypes. *A. bovis* belongs to group B of Slack and Gerencser's classification (1970) of *Actinomyces.* There are two serotypes, 1 and 2.

Epizootiology and Pathogenesis. The organism is apparently a normal and obligate parasite of the oropharynx and digestive tract. It opportunistically invades the deeper

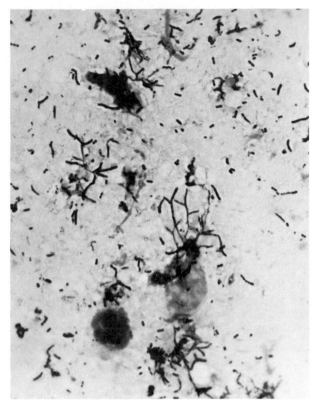

Figure 26.1. *Actinomyces bovis.* Branched filaments and coccoid bodies in actinomycotic pus. × 1,230. (Courtesy L. R. Vawter.)

tissues of the jaw through the dental alveoli or in association with entry of foreign materials such as pieces of wood or wire. In the mandible *A. bovis* produces a rarefying osteomyelitis (Figure 26.4). Characteristically, soft granulation tissue forms both in the mandible and along the lower esophagus and reticulum in those rare cases of visceral involvement. This tissue develops necrotic areas filled with pus, which may discharge to the surface through fistulous tracts. The connective tissue later hardens into dense tumorlike masses. A thick, mucoid, tenacious, greenish yellow, nonodorous pus is characteristic of the disease. The pus contains cheeselike granules up to 3 or 4 mm in diameter. These are the colonies of the organism and are commonly called *sulfur granules* (Figures 26.5 and 26.6).

If one examines these granules while they are fresh, the ray-fungus appearance can be easily discerned simply by pressing a clean cover glass on them. This is the most rapid way to make a definite diagnosis. The borders of the crushed granules show radiating, swollen, clublike filaments (Figure 26.7). As a general rule, the clublike forms are not seen in stained preparations of the pus, but they can be observed in histological sections.

Sulfur granules are found in the pus of actinobacillosis and also in those lesions that resemble actinomycosis which are caused by staphylococci. Fresh impression preparations show radiating clublike forms not unlike those of true actinomycosis. The sulfur granules in the

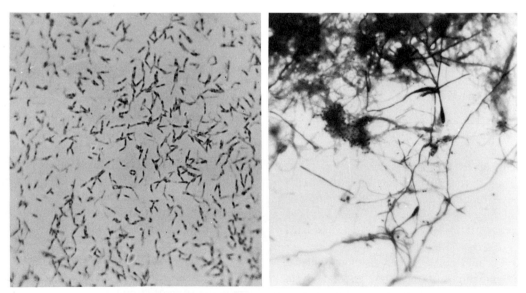

Figure 26.2 (*left*). Diphtheroid forms of *Actinomyces bovis* in a culture on Loeffler's blood serum incubated for 7 days at 37°C under increased CO_2 tension. × 980. (Courtesy L. R. Vawter.)
Figure 26.3 (*right*). *Actinomyces bovis* from a serum-broth culture incubated 6 days at 37°C. Clubs, filaments, and diphtheroid forms are present. × 980. (Courtesy L. R. Vawter.)

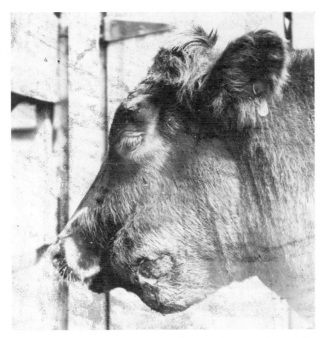

Figure 26.4. A cow with a case of true actinomycosis, involving the bone of the jaw and caused by *Actinomyces bovis*.

nonactinomycotic lesions usually are much smaller than those of true actinomycosis and frequently are so small that they are difficult to find on gross examination. The granules may be differentiated with stained preparations: true actinomycosis shows small Gram-negative rods; staphylococci show their typical morphology. When such

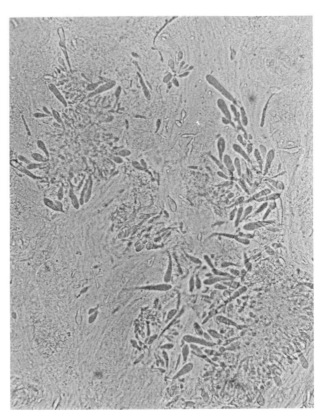

Figure 26.7. Sulfur granules of *Actinomyces bovis* showing clubs in the pus of a bone lesion. Unstained. × 490. (Courtesy L. R. Vawter.)

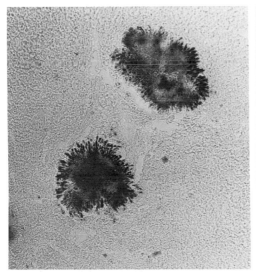

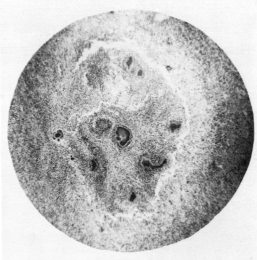

Figure 26.5 (*left*). Sulfur granules of *Actinomyces bovis* in the pus of a bone lesion. Picrofuchsin stain. × 330. (Courtesy L. R. Vawter.)
Figure 26.6 (*right*). Actinomycotic lesion with sulfur granules embedded in the pus in center of the lesion. Much of the actinomycotic nodule consists of granulation tissue. × 82.

examinations are made, the granules should be selected from the pus, washed, and crushed on clean slides; if the slide is made at random from the pus, no organism at all may be found. One can usually obtain the granules rather easily by placing some of the pus in a tube of broth or salt solution, shaking the tube to dissolve the mucin that holds the pus together, pouring the solution into a flat dish, and searching for the granules, which do not break up.

A. bovis infection occurs more commonly in cattle than in other animals, and lesions are seen most frequently in the bones of the face and jaw. Kimball et al. (1954) found *A. bovis* in the bovine testis, where it causes orchitis.

Actinomycosis also occurs in other animal species. Ryff (1953) described a case of encephalitis in a deer caused by *A. bovis*. Burns and Simmons (1952) reported a case of actinomycotic infection in a horse in which the intermandibular space was affected. Cases of actinomycosis in dogs have also been recorded. In one case *A. bovis* was isolated from lung tissue (Menges et al. 1953); in a second case the right cheek bones of the animal were involved (McGaughey et al. 1951); and in a third case the infection was localized in the osseous tissue of the mandible (Migliano and Stopiglia 1949).

Immunity. The mononuclear response and the granulomatous nature of the lesion suggests that cell-mediated immunity is important in the host response to infection. This has not been studied nor has any attempt been made to develop a vaccine.

Antimicrobial Susceptibility. *A. bovis* is sensitive to penicillin, streptomycin (Kingman and Palen 1951), tetracyclines (Lane et al. 1953), cephalosporin, lincomycin, and the sulfonamides. Because actinomycosis is sensitive to iodine, local lesions are treated with Lugol's solution, and sodium iodide is administered intravenously for internal infection.

Suter (1957) studied in vitro development of resistance of *A. bovis* to antibiotics and concluded that none resulted on exposure to erythromycin, carbomycin, and penicillin, whereas treatment with oxytetracycline, tetracycline, chloramphenicol, and dihydrostreptomycin produced a slow and moderate buildup of resistance.

REFERENCES

Biever, L.J., Roberstad, G.W., Van Steenbergh, K., Scheetz, E.E., and Kennedy, G.F. 1969. Actinomycosis in a bovine lung. Am. J. Vet. Res. 30:1063–1066.

Buchanan, A.G., Scott, J.L., Gerencser, M.A., Beaman, B.L., Jang, S., and Biberstein, E.L. 1984. *Actinomyces hordeovulneris* sp. nov., an agent of canine actinomycosis. Int. J. Syst. Bacteriol. 34:439–443.

Burns, R.H.G., and Simmons, G.C. 1952. A case of actinomycotic infection in a horse. Aust. Vet. J. 28:34–35.

Kimball, A., Twiehaus, M.J., Frank, E.R. 1954. *Actinomyces bovis* isolated from six cases of bovine orchitis: A preliminary report. Am. J. Vet. Res. 15:551–553.

Kingman, H.E., and Palen, J.S. 1951. Streptomycin in the treatment of actinomycosis. J. Am. Vet. Med. Assoc. 118:28–30.

Lane, S.L., Kutscher, A.H., and Chaves, R. 1953. Oxytetracycline in the treatment of orocervical fascial actinomycosis. J.A.M.A. 151:986–988.

McGaughey, C.A., Batemann, J.K., and Mackenzie, P.Z. 1951. Actinomycosis in the dog. Br. Vet. J. 107:428–430.

Menges, R.W., Larsh, H.W., and Habermann, R.T. 1983. Canine actinomycosis: A report of two cases. J. Am. Vet. Assoc. 122:73–78.

Migliano, M.F., and Stopiglia, A.V. 1949. Actinomycos of the mandible in a dog. Rev. Fac. Med. Vet. Univ. São Paulo 4:161–165.

Roderick, L.M., Kimball, A., McLeod, W.M., and Frank, E.R. 1948. A study of equine fistulous withers and poll evil. Am. J. Vet. Res. 9:5–10.

Ryff, J.F. 1953. Encephalitis in a deer due to *Actinomyces bovis*. J. Am. Vet. Med. Assoc. 122:78–80.

Slack, J.M., and Gerencser, M.A. 1970. Two new serological groups of *Actinomyces*. J. Bacteriol. 103:265–266.

Suter, L.S. 1957. In vitro development of resistance of *Actinomyces bovis* to antibiotics. Antibiot. Chemother. 77:285–288.

Vawter, L.R. 1946. Pulmonary actinomycosis in swine. J. Am. Vet. Med. Assoc. 109:198–203.

Actinomyces viscosus

The cause of periodontal disease and subgingival plaques in hamsters fed a high-carbohydrate diet (Jordan and Keyes 1964), *A. viscosus* causes abscessation in dogs (Bestetti et al. 1977). Infections by this organism probably have been frequently diagnosed as nocardiosis because of the lack of club formation in the sulfur granules found in the lesions.

Morphology and Staining Reactions. *A. viscosus* produces a diphtheroidal form that resembles *Corynebacterium* sp., and a filamentous form similar to that of *A. bovis*. The cells are Gram-positive. Both the diphtheroid and filamentous forms are found together in sulfur granules. They are non-acid-fast and nonmotile.

Cultural and Biochemical Features. Microcolonies on brain-heart–infusion agar incubated in CO_2 for 24 hours have a dense center with a filamentous fringe. After 3 to 4 days' incubation the colonies are circular, convex, smooth, glistening, and cream-colored to white. Rough colonies yield the filamentous form of the organism. In liquid media, a viscous rope forms when swirled. *A. viscosus* is catalase-positive, unlike other members of the genus. It reduces nitrate, produces H_2S in triple sugar–iron agar, and hydrolyzes esculin. The organism ferments glucose, resulting in the production of acetic, lactic, and succinic acids. It does not form gelatinase and urease. The mol% G + C of the DNA is 63.

Epizootiology and Pathogenesis. The habitat of *A. viscosus* is probably the oropharynx and digestive tract, where the organism is an obligate parasite. It opportunistically invades wounds in dogs, possibly as a result of the tendency of these animals to lick wounded areas or as a result of simple extension from the oropharyngeal area. Most infections are seen in large hunting dogs, and there is a consistent history of trauma to the infected sites. They frequently result in abscesses or pedunculated cysts around the head and neck. Love (1977) has described a case of ascites in the dog in which *A. viscosus* was isolated from the fluid. A case of *A. viscosus* infection in a cat has also been described (Bestetti et al. 1977) in which a suppurative granulomatous lesion was produced in the tail and anal area.

Granules found in the lesions consist of soft irregular masses of filaments and diphtheroidal forms in an acidophilic matrix (Sneath 1957). There are no clubs. Unlike *Nocardia asteroides*, *A. viscosus* does not disseminate in the body.

Diagnosis. Large amounts of purulent exudate must be cultured because the causative organism may be infrequent. It is important to include granules in attempts to culture the organism. These should be placed in thioglycollate broth. Because the lesions often involve skin areas, secondary contamination with other bacteria can complicate interpretation of the culture. Detailed biochemical testing of isolates will be necessary to identify an isolate as *A. viscosus* (Davenport et al. 1975). Its failure to grow on Sabouraud-dextrose agar distinguishes it from *Nocardia* species, which grow well on this medium.

Antimicrobial Susceptibility. *A. viscosus* is sensitive to penicillin, chloramphenicol, erythromycin, and the tetracyclines. High doses of penicillin given on a long-term basis is the therapy of choice (Attleberger 1983). Extensive fistulated lesions do not respond well to therapy.

REFERENCES

Attleburger, M.H. 1983. Subcutaneous and opportunistic mycoses, the deep mycoses, and the actinomycetes. In R.W. Kirk, ed., Current Veterinary Therapy 8. Philadelphia, W.B. Saunders. Pp. 1177–1180.
Bestetti, G., Buhlmann, V., Nicolet, J., and Frankhauser, R. 1977. Paraplegia due to *Actinomycetes viscosus* infection in a cat. Acta Neuropath. 37:231–235.
Davenport, A.A., Carter, G.R., and Patterson, M.J. 1975. Identification of *Actinomyces viscosus* from canine infections. J. Clin. Microbiol. 1:75–78.
Jordan, H.V., and Keyes, P.H. 1964. Aerobic gram-positive, filamentous bacteria as etiologic agents of experimental periodontal disease in hamsters. Arch. Oral Biol. 9:401–414.
Love, D.N. 1977. Isolation of an actinomycete resembling *Actinomyces viscosus* from the peritoneal fluid of a dog. Aust. Vet. J. 53:107–108.
Sneath, P.H.A. 1957. Some thoughts on bacterial classification. J. Gen. Microbiol. 17:184–200.

Actinomyces suis

Actinomycosis of the mammary gland of sows is a relatively common disease that has long been thought to be caused by *A. bovis*. Detailed investigations of isolations of *Actinomyces* sp. from swine, however, have indicated that they differ consistently in some important respects from classical *A. bovis* strains. Swine isolates produce granular colonies with filamentous offshoots, do not produce hydrogen sulfide, and may utilize adonitol, inulin, raffinose, and xylose; they also differ antigenically from *A. bovis* and *A. israelii* (Franke 1973; Grasser 1962, 1963). These authors have proposed therefore that the species *A. suis* be established for the organism commonly isolated from actinomycosis of the swine mammary gland. *Bergey's Manual of Systematic Bacteriology,* vol 2 (1986), gives this organism the status of *species incertae sedis*.

Morphology and Staining Reactions. Short, Gram-positive forms are present on initial isolation, giving rise to branched filaments on subculture. The cells in smooth colonies are of medium length and uniform thickness with variable staining characteristics. Cells from rough colonies exhibit long, curved, swollen V-shaped and Y-shaped forms with frequent branching.

Cultural and Biochemical Features. *A. suis* produces granular microcolonies with filamentous offshoots. As the colonies enlarge, smooth-rough and rough colonial forms may occur. On serum agar colonies of *A. suis* are white and on blood agar they are brown to reddish brown. *A. suis* is catalase-, indole-, gelatinase-, and hydrogen sulfide–negative; does not reduce nitrate; and ferments adonitol, inulin, raffinose, and xylose. In agar-gel precipitin tests the organism is antigenically different from *A. bovis*, *A. israelii*, *A naeslundii*, and *A. propionicus* (Franke 1973).

Epizootiology and Pathogenesis. Little is known about the habitat of *A. suis*, but it is likely that it is a parasite of the oropharynx of swine and opportunistically invades wounds on the mammary gland. The sharp teeth of piglets frequently cause superficial wounds of the mammary skin during suckling, and infection probably occurs in this way. After entry the organism produces a typical actinomycotic granuloma, resulting in enlargement, induration, and eventual escape of pus that contains typical sulfur granules.

Antimicrobial Susceptibility. *A. suis* is highly sensitive to penicillin, erythromycin, and chloramphenicol and less sensitive to chlortetracycline and streptomycin. It is resistant to polymyxin B (Franke 1971). Treatment is more likely to be successful when the lesions are less than fist size. If large lesions are present, surgical excision with antibiotic therapy is necessary but relapses are frequent (Bethke and Buschmann 1972).

REFERENCES

Bethke, M., and Buschmann, G. 1972. Comparison of treatments of actinomycosis in sows. D.T.W. 79:238–241.

Franke, F. 1971. The in vitro antibiotic sensitivity of microaerophilic actinomycetes isolated from actinomycotic mammary glands of sows. D.T.W. 78:574–576.

Franke, F. 1973. Aetiology of actinomycosis of the mammary gland of the pig. Zentrabl. Bakteriol. 223:111–124.

Grasser, R. 1962. Mikroaerophile Actinomyceten aus Gesaugeaktinoomykosen des Schweines. Zentralbl. Bakteriol. 184:478–492.

Grasser, R. 1963. Untersuchungen über fermentative und seroligische Eigenschaften mikroaerophiler Actinomyceten. Zentralbl. Bakteriol. 188:251–263.

Actinomyces pyogenes

SYNONYM: *Corynebacterium pyogenes*

The specific epithet *pyogenes* ("pus producer") is an apt name for this organism because it is frequently associated with the production of pus, particularly in ruminants. It is found in abscesses in cattle, sheep, goats, and swine, and occasionally in other animals, but it rarely affects humans.

Morphology and Staining Reactions. *A. pyogenes* most often occurs as small, slender, Gram-positive rods, which frequently are slightly curved and often clubbed at one end. The individual elements are usually short, and some strains form chains that are hard to distinguish from streptococci. Wide variation in morphology exists between different strains and between individual cells of a single pig strain. The organism is nonmotile and never forms a capsule.

Cultural and Biochemical Features. Ordinarily *A. pyogenes* does not grow on plain agar or in plain broth unless a considerable amount of blood, tissue, or tissue debris is carried over in the inoculum. However, a complex, chemically defined growth medium has been devised which allows good growth in the absence of serum or tissue extracts (Reddy et al. 1980). *A. pyogenes* grows readily in milk and on coagulated serum slants, where a trough of liquefaction develops along the lines of growth.

A few drops of blood or blood serum make all of the usual laboratory media favorable for the growth of this organism. In fluid media the growth is granular and sinks to the bottom of the tube.

A. pyogenes is hemolytic on blood-agar plates, and colonies are very small and translucent. After an 18-hour incubation at 37°C colonies can be easily overlooked, for at that time there is little evidence of hemolysis. After approximately 24 hours hemolysis begins to be evident, making the colonies conspicuous. The zones of hemolysis are exceedingly clear but always narrow, seldom exceeding 2 mm in diameter (Figure 26.8). Strains from swine produce more hemolysis than those of bovine origin.

Growth occurs best at body temperature. The minimum temperature for growth is about 24°C. The organism is

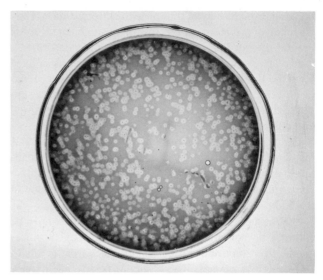

Figure 26.8. *Actinomyces pyogenes* on a blood-agar plate incubated for 36 hours at 37°C. The colonies appear as minute points surrounded by narrow zones of clear hemolysis. Blood plates incubated overnight can have numerous colonies on them, but the colonies are likely to be overlooked unless the plates are inspected with care because the hemolytic zones will have not appeared yet. At about 24 hours' incubation the hemolytic zones begin to appear, but they are not well developed until 36 hours.

aerobic and facultatively anaerobic. It does not produce indole, H_2S, and nitrites, but it does liquefy gelatin. Biochemically, *A. pyogenes* is very similar to *A. bovis* except that it is highly proteolytic and produces a hemolysin. Porcine strains are biochemically more active than bovine strains (Tainaka et al. 1983). An unusual strain associated with bovine mastitis has been described by Afnan (1970).

Antigens. Little is known about the antigens of *A. pyogenes*. Porcine and bovine strains share a common protein antigen, and there are at least three specific antigens unique to porcine or bovine strains. Specific antigens are protein, protein and carbohydrate, and carbohydrate alone (Tainaka et al. 1983). *A. pyogenes* also carries an antigen that cross reacts with *Mycobacterium paratuberculosis* (*johnei*).

Epizootiology and Pathogenesis. *A. pyogenes* is easily destroyed by heat, drying, and ordinary disinfectants. It survives and is maintained on the mucous membranes of cattle, sheep, swine, and other related species. It occurs in the tonsils, retropharyngeal lymph nodes, and the udders of apparently normal heifers (Natterman and Horsch 1977).

Entry of *A. pyogenes* into the deeper tissues requires an insult or a stress of some kind such as a wound or a primary viral or other bacterial infection. *A. pyogenes* is

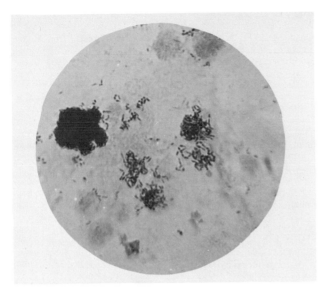

Figure 26.9. A film from vegetations of *Actinomyces pyogenes* on the heart valve of a calf. × 1,030.

therefore an opportunist that will enter wounds or abrasions of the skin; the umbilicus of calves; the reticulum of adult cattle injured by a foreign object; the teats of cattle punctured by biting flies; hooves or interdigital skin devitalized by maceration or *Fusobacterium necrophorum* infection; and the lungs of cattle, sheep, and swine devitalized by viral or pasteurella infection. The protease and hemolysin are probably important virulence factors (Kune et al. 1983). *A. pyogenes* can be found by itself or in association with other bacteria. It is also a common invader of the uterus post partum, where it is associated with endometritis or pyometra. *A. pyogenes* has been implicated as a cause of abortion in cattle (Hinton 1972) and seminal vesiculitis and lowered fertility in bulls and boars (Ogasa et al. 1980). It is a frequent cause of cardiac valvular vegetations in cattle (Figure 26.9).

A. pyogenes is a common invader of tail-bite lesions on swine, through which it frequently enters the bloodstream and lodges in the lungs, producing abscesses (Van Den Berg et al. 1981). It is also a frequent cause of septic arthritis in swine. Arthritis can appear after farrowing, suggesting that the uterus was the primary site of invasion of the bloodstream. Stiffness of gait, lameness, wasting, pneumonia, and posterior paralysis are sometimes seen. Chronic purulent pneumonia and joint infections of sheep resulting in acute lameness are frequently caused by *A. pyogenes*. Its presence is associated with the formation of large amounts of connective tissue and with pleurisy, which is accompanied by a foul-smelling pleural exudate.

Cameron and Britton (1943) described a form of *A.*

pyogenes infection in sheep fed large amounts of grain, especially barley, in which bilateral deep-seated chronic abscesses developed in the larynx. These abscesses were believed to be caused by abrasions resulting from gulping the grain. Affected lambs were dyspneic and there was high mortality.

In Europe mastitis in dairy cows and heifers caused by *A. pyogenes* has a marked seasonal incidence and is known as *summer mastitis*. Flies are thought to be important vectors of the organism, hence the high incidence at the height of the fly season. They are not the sole vectors, however. Control of populations of head flies (*Hydatea irritans*) has been shown to effectively reduce the frequency of summer mastitis (Tolle et al. 1983). In North America the seasonal incidence is not so marked, and transmission occurs by some other means or infection is precipitated by unknown factors that cause the commensal organism to proliferate and produce mastitis. *A. pyogenes* is often found with two other organisms, *Peptococcus indolicus* and *Streptococcus dysgalactiae*, but the role of *P. indolicus* in pathogenesis is unknown.

The disease can be sporadic or involve a number of animals in the herd. The affected quarters of udders usually suffer extensive permanent damage. *A. pyogenes* sometimes causes damage to the immature udders of young calves that are kept together and have developed the habit of suckling each other. Secondary infections of the joints in these animals can result in suppurative arthritis, which usually leads to death.

A. pyogenes has been associated with a number of cases of generalized lymphadenitis in cattle in Scotland. The animals had generalized abscessation of the lungs, joints, and subcutaneous tissues of the legs and lumbar region. *A. pyogenes* was isolated in pure cultures from the lesions (Cowie 1962).

A. pyogenes has also been implicated in the etiology of periodontal disease (*cara inchada*) of cattle in Brazil (Blobel et al. 1984). Abscesses caused by *A. pyogenes* usually develop slowly and often have heavy fibrous capsules. The pus may be thick, greenish white, and nonodorous or it may be thin and fetid, especially when other anaerobes are present.

Immunity. Little is known about immunity to *A. pyogenes*. It appears to be able to evade phagocytosis and intracellular killing. Antibody to the organism has been detected in an immunofluorescence test in the serum and cervical mucus of cattle. Many animals have evidence of serum antibodies but not of cervical mucus antibodies (Schulz et al. 1979). The presence of mucus antibodies may be a local immune response to infection in the reproductive tract. About 50 percent of pigs with abscesses from which *A. pyogenes* are isolated have serum antibodies to the organism (Hara 1980). Although many vaccines, toxoids, and antisera have been used to prevent and treat diseases caused by *A. pyogenes,* particularly summer mastitis, their efficacy is equivocal.

Diagnosis. One can best demonstrate the presence of *A. pyogenes* in inflammatory exudates by staining smears of the exudate and examining them for pleomorphic, Gram-positive rods and by making cultures on blood-agar plates. The culture should be incubated for not less then 36 hours at 37°C unless other organisms threaten to overrun the plate. The minute, distinctive colonies are surrounded by sharp, clear, narrow zones of hemolysis. These colonies should be picked up and transferred to blood-agar slants. The subcultures can be identified by their action on litmus milk and especially by their ability to liquefy solidified blood-serum slants. A failure to produce catalase and reduce nitrates are other identifying characteristics of *A. pyogenes.*

An immunodiffusion test for antibody to *A. pyogenes* protease appears to have value for diagnosis of infection in piggeries (Takeuchi et al. 1979).

Antimicrobial Susceptibility. *A. pyogenes* is sensitive to penicillin, ampicillin, chloramphenicol, erythromycin, sulfamethazine, sulfadoxine-trimethoprim, and tetracycline. Strains resistant to sulfonamides and trimethoprim have been observed.

The in vivo responses of *A. pyogenes* to antimicrobials are poor. The antibiotic-binding properties of proteins in pus together with the thick fibrous capsule of the abscess protect the organism from the effects of the antimicrobial.

Intramammary antibiotic prophylaxis of heifers and cows against summer mastitis is a highly successful procedure. The antibiotics used include semisynthetic penicillins such as oxacillin.

REFERENCES

Afnan, M. 1970. A new *Corynebacterium* sp. isolated from bovine mastitis. Vet. Rec. 86:229–230.

Blobel, M., Dobereiner, J., Lima, F.G.F., and Rosa, I.V. 1984. Bacterial isolations from "cara inchada" lesions of cattle. Pesqui. Vet. Bras. 4:73–77.

Cameron, H.S., and Britton, J.W. 1943. Chronic ovine laryngitis. Cornell Vet. 22:265–268.

Cowie, R.S. 1962. A generalized *Corynebacterium pyogenes* disease of cattle. Vet. Rec. 74:258.

Hara, F. 1980. A study on pig pyogenic infections. Results of clinical, pathological, bacteriological, and serological examinations of slaughtered pigs. Bull. Azabu Univ. Vet. Med. 1:187–202.

Hinton, M. 1972. Bovine abortion associated with *Corynebacterium pyogenes.* Vet. Bull. 42:753.

Kune, T., Tainaka, M., Saito, M., Hiruma, M., Nishro, S., Kashiwazaki, M., Mitani, K., and Nakajima, Y. 1983. Research on experimental *Corynebacterium pyogenes* infections in pigs. Kitasato Arch. Exp. Med. 56:119–135.

Natterman, H.S., and Horsch, F. 1977. Die *Corynebacterium-pyogenes*-infektion des Khindes. Arch. Exp. Veterinärmed. 31:405–413.

Ogasa, A., Yokoki, Y., Azuma, R., Takeuchi, S., and Ishii, Y. 1980. Defective spermatogenesis in boars infected with *C. pyogenes.* Jpn. J. Anim. Reprod. 26:115–119.

Reddy, C.A., Cornell, C.P., and Fraga, A.M. 1980. Chemically defined growth medium for *C. pyogenes.* Am. J. Vet. Res. 41:843–845.

Schulz, J., Von Aert, A., Dekeyser, P., and Vandeplassche, M. 1979. Immunofluorescence tests to detect antibody against *C. pyogenes* and streptococci in blood serum and vaginal mucus of cattle. Arch. Exp. Veterinärmed. 33:783–789.

Tainaka, M., Kume, T., Takeuchi, S., Nishio, S., and Saito, M. 1983. Studies on the biological and serological properties of *Corynebacterium pyogenes.* Kitasato Arch. Exp. Med. 56:105–117.

Takeuchi, S., Azuma, R., Nakajima, Y., and Suto, T. 1979. Diagnosis of *Corynebacterium pyogenes* infection in pigs by immunodiffusion test with protease antigen. Natl. Inst. Anim. Health Q. (Tokyo) 19:77–82.

Tolle, A., Franke, V., and Reichmuth, J. 1983. *Corynebacterium pyogenes* mastitis—Bacteriological aspects. D.T.W. 90:256–260.

Van Den Berg, J., Narucka, V., Nouws, J.F.M., Okma, B.D., Peelen, J.P.J., and Soethout, A.E.E. 1981. Lesions in slaughtered animals. II. Inflammation of the tail and embolic pneumonia in pigs. Tijdschr. Diergeneeskd. 106:407–410.

27 The Genus *Nocardia*

The nocardia are aerobic, nonmotile, Gram-positive organisms that can form mycelial masses that fragment into bacillary forms. Most are soil saprophytes. Some of the pathogenic species are partially acid-fast. Most species produce aerial hyphae. Colonies may be rough or smooth, of a soft to doughlike consistency, or compact and leathery. Some species produce blue, violet, red, yellow, orange, or green pigments on protein-rich media. There are 20 officially listed species, of which 4, *N. farcinica*, *N. asteroides*, *N. caviae*, and *N. brasiliensis*, have been isolated from lesions in animals. Gordon (1981) has proposed that *N. asteroides* be the type species.

Nocardia possess cell walls of type IV meso-diaminopimelic acid, arabinose, and galactose. Their mycolic acids are characteristically medium sized with 46 to 58 carbon atoms and include LCN-A, a lipid found only in members of the genus (Stanford 1983). They also have unique lipid-soluble, iron-binding nocobactins.

N. farcinica was formerly the type strain for *Nocardia* and was isolated by Nocard (1888) from cattle with bovine farcy on Guadelupe. In the 1970s investigators discovered that Nocard's original culture actually consisted of a *Nocardia* sp. and a *Mycobacterium* sp. Because it now appears that bovine farcy in West Africa, once widely thought to be due solely to *N. farcinica*, is usually caused by *Mycobacterium farcinogenes* or *M. senegalense* and not *N. farcinica* (Chamoiseau 1979), the disease is described in Chapter 28, "The Genus *Mycobacterium*." It should be stressed, however, that there is evidence that *N. farcinica* is still an important cause of farcy in Sudanese cattle (Shigidi et al. 1980).

REFERENCES

Chamoiseau, G. 1979. Etiology of farcy in African bovines: Nomenclature of the causal organisms *Mycobacterium farcinogenes* (Chamoiseau) and *Mycobacterium senegalense* (Chamoiseau) comb. nov. Int. J. Syst. Bacteriol. 29:407–410.

Gordon, R.E. 1981. A proposed new status for *Nocardia asteroides*. In K.P. Schaal and G. Pilnerer, eds., *Actinomycetes*. Zentralbl. Bakteriol. Mikrobiol. Hyg. (I. Abt.), Suppl. 2, pp. 3–6.

Nocard, M.E. 1888. Note sur la maladie des boeufs de la Guadeloupe connue sous le nom de farcin. Ann. Inst. Pasteur 2:293–302.

Shigidi, M.T.A., Mirgham, T., and Mura, M.T., 1980. Characterization of *Nocardia farcinica* isolated from cattle with bovine farcy. Res. Vet. Sci. 28:207–211.

Stanford, J.C. 1983. A simple view of nocardial taxonomy. J. Hyg. 91:369–376.

Nocardia asteroides

SYNONYMS: *Actinomyces asteroides, Cladothrix asteroides, Streptothrix eppingeri*

N. asteroides is an opportunistic pathogen that is being isolated with increasing frequency from cases of bovine mastitis and from granulomatous lesions of the subcutis and thoracic organs of dogs and cats. In humans the infection is often a complication of neoplasia or immunosuppression. The infection in animals has recently been reviewed by Beaman and Sugar (1983).

Morphology and Staining Reactions. *N. asteroides* forms long, filamentous, branching cells that tend to break into coccoid or bacillary forms after 4 days' incubation. It is Gram-positive, and some strains are acid-fast.

Cultural and Biochemical Features. The organism is aerobic and produces raised, heaped, folded granular colonies with irregular borders. Yellow-orange pigment formation is common. *N. asteroides* produces acid from D-fructose and D-glucose, dextrin, and mannose. It reduces nitrate and produces urease but not gelatinase. Its optimum growth temperature is 28° to 30°C. It does not hydrolyze casein.

Epizootiology and Pathogenesis. Because *N. asteroides* is a soil saprophyte, it is widely distributed in the environment. Entry of the organism occurs through wounds, ingestion, and inhalation. The cutaneous form of the disease is characterized by pyogranuloma formation and tracts that drain pus to the surface. Infection of the respiratory tract in dogs and cats results in pleural effusion and pyothorax. The exudate usually has the appearance of tomato soup. Sulfur granules may be uncommon.

Systemic nocardiosis in dogs is sometimes accompanied by pyrexia, emaciation, coughing, and nervous signs—signs indistinguishable from those of distemper. Such cases may in fact be mixed infections involving both distemper virus and *N. asteroides,* the latter being an opportunistic invader that has taken advantage of the immunosuppressive effects of the viral infection (Blake 1954). The bacterium has also been isolated from lesions in the central nervous system of dogs at necropsy (Rhoades et al. 1963) and from dogs with vertebral osteomyelitis (Mitten 1974). Nocardiosis is three times more likely in male dogs than in females, and those less than 2 years old are most commonly affected. Although *N. asteroides* is the most commonly identified species in these cases, *N. caviae* and *N. brasiliensis* have also occasionally been observed (Beaman and Sugar 1983). Ackerman (1982) has recently reviewed canine nocardiosis in considerable detail.

Feline nocardiosis is less common than the disease in dogs and has been reviewed by Frost (1959). Akun (1952) described cases involving the submandibular lymph gland, the pleura, and the lungs. Most cases involve the thoracic organs with subsequent systemic dissemination. Affected cats exhibit fever, anorexia, emaciation, and dyspnea. *N. caviae* infections have not been reported in cats.

In horses *N. asteroides* is an opportunistic infection of Arabian foals, in which it causes pulmonary and systemic infection. The disease has also been diagnosed in equine mandibles, where it was associated with bilateral anomalies of the inferior dentition (Tritschler and Romack 1965). Equine cases of pleuritis caused by *N. brasiliensis* have also been observed (Deem and Harrington 1980).

Numerous reports of bovine mastitis caused by *N. asteroides* exist (Fuchs and Boretius 1972; Pier et al. 1958, 1961). The organism is a common contaminant of the skin of the udder and has been found in bulk tank milk (Eales et al. 1964). Entry apparently occurs by means of contaminated infusion equipment used in treatment of other forms of mastitis. The organism then multiplies in the already devitalized tissue, producing a purulent granulomatous inflammation. Systemic signs may or may not be present. Diffuse fibrosis or discrete hard nodules may be felt in the affected areas. An enzootic of nocardia mastitis in a dairy herd in California was described by Pier et al. (1958). In this outbreak the disease was acute, and the animals had high fevers. Most cases developed soon after calving. Nocardia-infected cows should be culled because of permanent loss of mammary function and the risk of their becoming permanent shedders of the microorganism (Fuchs and Boretius 1972). *N. caviae* and possibly *N. brasiliensis* have also been isolated from cases of mastitis.

In goats *N. asteroides* has been observed in mycetomas, pulmonary infections, and in mastitis. The infection has also been described in swine (Gottschalk et al. 1971).

Immunity. Because the nocardia are facultative intracellular pathogens, it is probable that cell-mediated immunity is critical in protective immune responses. The evidence for this has been reviewed by Beaman and Sugar (1983).

Sensitized T lymphocytes have been shown to bind to and kill *N. asteroides* (Deem et al. 1983). Also, more virulent strains inhibit phagosome-lysosomal fusion and so have a greater potential for intracellular survival following phagocytosis. B lymphocytes are not important in the protective response. Pier et al. (1968) prepared a nocardial antigen from *N. asteroides* and claimed that it can be used in allergic, precipitin, and complement-fixation tests to detect present or previous nocardiosis in cattle. Salman (1982) described a skin test for detection of bovine mammary infections caused by *N. asteroides*.

Diagnosis. The organism appears as Gram-positive, branched, slender filaments (0.5 to 1.0 μm). It is partially acid-fast, a characteristic that is best demonstrated when alcohol is omitted from the staining procedure. Specimens must also be cultured, and the causative organism isolated and identified. Specimens of milk should not be refrigerated before culture, because refrigeration has been shown to reduce the chances of successful culture of *N. asteroides*.

Antimicrobial Susceptibility. In vitro drug sensitivity tests are not accurate guides to the treatment of nocardiosis. For instance, sulfonamides are inactive against most strains in vitro yet are very effective in therapy. Bach et al. (1973) observed great variability in the minimum inhibitory concentration of a wide variety of antimicrobials. They noted the marked synergy of erythromycin and ampicillin in vitro and reported minocycline was the most effective drug in vitro. Reports by Runyon (1951) and Strauss et al. (1951) indicate that sulfadiazine is effective in animal protection tests, but tetracycline, chloramphenicol, and streptomycin give only partial protection. Sapegin and Cormack (1956) treated two cases of canine nocardiosis with bis-*p*-chlorophenyldiguanidohexane and reported good clinical recovery. Others have indicated that benzalkonium chloride (Merkal and Thurston 1968) and the combination of cycloserine and sulfonamides (Hoeprich et al. 1968) are effective. Trimethoprimsulphamethoxazole, amikacin, and cephalosporins are also active against *N. asteroides* (Sugar et al. 1983).

REFERENCES

Ackerman, N. 1982. Canine nocardiosis. J. Am. Anim. Hosp. Assoc. 18:147–153.

Akun, R.S. 1952. Nokardiose bei zwei Katzen in der Turkei. D.T.W. 59:202–204.

Bach, M.C., Sabath, L.D., and Finland, M. 1973. Susceptibility of *Nocardia asteroides* to 45 antimicrobial agents in vitro. Antimicrob. Agents Chemother. 3:1–8.

Beaman, B.C., and Sugar, A.M. 1983. Nocardia in naturally acquired and experimental infection in animals. J. Hyg. 91:393–419.

Blake, W.P. 1954. A report of two canine cases of nocardiosis in Missouri. J. Am. Vet. Med. Assoc. 125:467–468.

Deem, D.A., and Harrington, D.D. 1980. *Nocardia brasiliensis* in a horse with pneumonia and pleuritis. Cornell Vet. 70:321–328.

Deem, R., Doughty, F., and Beaman, B.L. 1983. Immunologically specific direct T-lymphocyte–mediated killing of *Nocardia asteroides*. J. Immunol. 130:2401–2406.

Eales, J.D., Leaver, D.D., and Swan, J. 1964. Bovine mastitis caused by *Nocardia*. Aust. Vet. J. 40:321–324.

Frost, A.J. 1959. A review of canine and feline nocardiosis with the report of a case. Aust. Vet. J. 35:22–25.

Fuchs, H.W., and Boretius, J. 1972. Pathology, diagnosis, and pathogenesis of bovine mastitis caused by *Nocardia asteroides*. Arch. Exp. Veterinärmed. 26:683–700.

Gottschalk, A.F., Correa, C.N.M., Correa, W.M., and Campos, C.L.O.P. 1971. Isolamento de *Nocardia asteroides* de suino. Arq. Inst. Biol. São Paulo 38:167–171.

Hoeprich, P.D., Brandt, D., and Parker, R.H. 1968. Nocardial brain abscess cured with cycloserine and sulfonamides. Am. J. Med. Sci. 255:208–216.

Merkal, R.S., and Thurston, J.R. 1968. Susceptibilities of mycobacterial and nocardial species to benzalkonium chloride. Am. J. Vet. Res. 29:759–761.

Pier, A.C., Gray, D.M., and Fossatti, M.J. 1958. *Nocardia asteroides*—A newly recognized pathogen of the mastitis complex. Am. J. Vet. Res. 19:319–331.

Pier, A.C., Thurston, J.R., and Larsen, A.B. 1968. A diagnostic antigen for nocardiosis: Comparative tests in cattle with nocardiosis and mycobacteriosis. Am. J. Vet. Res. 29:397–403.

Pier, A.C., Willers, A.C., and Mejia, M.J. 1961. *Nocardia asteroides* as a mammary pathogen of cattle. II. The sources of nocardial infection and experimental reproduction of the disease. Am. J. Vet. Res. 22:698–703.

Rhoades, H.E., Reynolds, H.A., Rahn, D.P., and Small, E. 1963. Nocardiosis in a dog with multiple lesions of the central nervous system. J. Am. Vet. Med. Assoc. 142:278–280.

Runyon, E.H. 1951. *Nocardia asteroides:* Studies of its pathogenicity and drug sensitivities. J. Lab. Clin. Med. 37:713–720.

Salman, M.D. 1982. Determination of sensitivity and specificity of the *Nocardia asteroides* skin test for detection of bovine mammary infections caused by *N. asteroides* and *N. caviae*. Am. J. Vet. Res. 43:332–335.

Sapegin, G., and Cormack, G.R. 1956. Canine nocardiosis treated with Hibitane. North Am. Vet. 37:385–388.

Strauss, R.E., Kligman, A.M., and Pillsbury, D.M. 1951. The chemotherapy of actinomycosis and nocardiosis. Am. Rev. Tuberc. 63:441–448.

Sugar, A.M., Chabal, R.S., and Stevens, D.A. 1983. A cephalosporin active in vivo against *Nocardia:* Efficacy of cefotoxime in murine model of acute pulmonary nocardiosis. J. Hyg. 91:421–427.

Tritschler, L.G., and Romack, F.E. 1965. Nocardiosis in equine mandibles associated with bilateral anomalies of the inferior dentition. Vet. Med. 60:605–608.

28 The Genus *Mycobacterium*

Members of the genus *Mycobacterium* are strictly aerobic, non-spore-forming, curved or straight Gram-positive rods. Under some conditions, *Mycobacterium* organisms form filaments, but these fragment into rods or cocci when disturbed. Mycobacteria are acid-fast in that they resist the decolorization effect of acid-alcohol after they are stained with hot carbol-fuchsin. The lipid content of the cell wall is as high as 60 percent of the dry weight. This high lipid content is responsible for the hydrophobicity of mycobacteria in fluid media and for their slow growth and resistance to acids, disinfectants, antibodies, and desiccation. The lipid is composed of waxes and glycolipids containing high-molecular-weight mycolic acids, including trehalose 6,6′dimycolate ("cord factor").

The mycobacteria other than *M. tuberculosis* and *M. bovis* have been loosely classified on the basis of growth rate and pigment production into four groups (Runyon et al. 1974). Group 1 contains the photochromogenic strains that grow slowly and produce a yellow pigment only when exposed to light. This group contains such organisms as *M. ulcerans* and *M. marinum* (*balnei*), producer of skin ulcers, as well as *M. kansasii*, which is an acid-fast bacillus that can cause pulmonary disease in humans.

Group 2 includes the scotochromogenic strains such as *M. scrofulaceum* that grow slowly and form an orange-yellow pigment whether grown in light or dark. Although they frequently occur in children with adenitis, they are rarely found as independent causes of pulmonary disease and are usually considered to be saprophytes.

Group 3 contains the nonchromogenic strains that grow slowly, do not produce pigment, form smooth colonies, and are resistant to isoniazid. They are highly pleomorphic and produce filaments resembling those of *Nocardia*. They occasionally cause pulmonary disease in humans. Strains of *M. avium* are found in this group.

Group 4 is reserved for the rapid growers that mature in less than 1 week at 25°C or 37°C. Most of these belong to the *M. fortuitum* subgroup and to the *M. phlei* and *M. smegmatis* subgroups. *M. fortuitum* is pathogenic for humans and other animals and has been implicated in epizootics of bovine mastitis.

The species of mycobacteria can also be grouped as obligate parasites (*M. leprae* and *M. lepraemurium*), as facultative intracellular parasites (*M. avium, M. bovis, M. fortuitum, M. kansasii*, and *M. tuberculosis*), or as saprophytes (the majority of species including *M. phlei*).

The diseases produced by mycobacteria are known as tuberculosis, a term derived from the small granulomatous nodules or tubercles that are seen in advanced infections by *M. tuberculosis* or *M. bovis*.

M. bovis, M. avium, M. paratuberculosis, and *M. farcinogenes* are the most important disease-producing species in domestic animals. *M. tuberculosis*, the type species and principal cause of tuberculosis in humans and other primates is an occasional cause of tuberculosis in dogs, pigs, and cattle. *M. bovis* and *M. avium* are also pathogenic for humans, and the diseases they cause are therefore important zoonoses. In many developed countries, the zoonotic importance of *M. bovis* has been the stimulus for highly successful eradication programs that have reduced the prevalence of *M. bovis* infection in cattle populations to very low levels. *M. paratuberculosis* is the cause of Johne's disease, a debilitating disease of cattle characterized by chronic or intermittent diarrhea. In sheep and goats, *M. paratuberculosis* causes a slow loss of condition with diarrhea being present only in the terminal phase of the disease. *M. farcinogenes* is found only in tropical countries, where it causes bovine farcy (*farcin-de-boeuf*).

Mycobacterium species, such as *M. fortuitum* and *M. phlei*, are occasionally found in cutaneous lesions of animals or as opportunistic infections of the udder. *M. lepraemurium* is believed to be the cause of feline leprosy, a cutaneous granulomatous-type disease.

REFERENCE

Runyon, E.H., Wayne, S., and Kabucci, J. 1974. Mycobacteriaceae. In R.E. Buchanan and N.E. Gibbons, eds., Bergey's Manual of Determinative Bacteriology, 8th ed. Williams & Wilkins, Baltimore. P. 681.

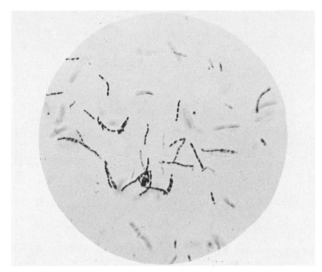

Figure 28.1. *Mycobacterium bovis,* from a culture on Dorset's egg medium incubated 6 weeks at 37°C. These long beaded forms are seen only in cultures. In tissues this type ordinarily stains solid. × 1,030.

Mycobacterium bovis

SYNONYM: *Mycobacterium tuberculosis* subspecies *bovis*

M. bovis causes tuberculosis in cattle, pigs, cats, horses, primates, dogs, sheep, and goats. It does not cause disease in birds.

Morphology and Staining Reactions. *M. bovis* is a short, relatively plump, Gram-positive rod in smears of tissue and is larger, slender, and beaded in preparations from culture media (Figure 28.1). It stains red (acid-fast) by the Ziehl-Neelsen staining technique. It does not produce spores and does not have flagella, fimbria, or capsules.

Cultural and Biochemical Features. The most frequently used media (Dorset, Stonebrinks) incorporate egg yolk, phosphate buffer, magnesium salts, sodium pyruvate, and occasionally amino acids. Glycerol is inhibitory and is therefore omitted from culture media (Collins and Lyne 1984). Primary cultures usually require from 3 to 4 weeks incubation at 37°C before colonies can be detected with the naked eye. The colonies appear first as minute dull flakes, which gradually thicken into dry, irregular masses that stand high above the surface of the medium. They are slightly yellow, but if exposed to light they slowly progress through shades of deep yellow to brick red. When cultures have become accustomed to growing on media, confluent growth develops over the entire surface. This has the appearance of rough, waxy blankets, which after several weeks' incubation become thick and wrinkled. Where this blanket reaches the margin of the medium's surface, it often crowds up the side of the glass container for an appreciable distance. Old, isolated colonies on solid media become so firm and so loosely attached to the medium that an inoculating loop can be used to skate them around. If the tubes are shaken vigorously, the dry growth often breaks loose and rattles.

In fluid media, growth is restricted to the surface (Figure 28.2) unless a wetting agent such as the nonionic detergent, Tween 80, is added (Collins and Lyne 1984). *M. bovis* is strictly aerobic and the optimum growth temperature is 37°C. It does not grow at 25°C, does not reduce nitrate, and is usually resistant to pyrazinamide. It does not reduce niacin and is sensitive to thiophene-2-carboxylic acid hydrazide (Sommers and Good 1985). It is destroyed by pasteurization and sunlight but is resistant to desiccation, acids, and alkalis.

Antigens. The lipid of the cell wall is composed of waxes, mycosides (glycolipids containing high-molecular-weight fatty acids) that are species specific, waxes D (mycolic acid, peptides, and polysaccharides), and cord factor (trehalose 6,6′-dimycolate). Waxes D contain N-acetylmuramyl dipeptide, which is a potent enhancer of humoral and cell-mediated immune responses.

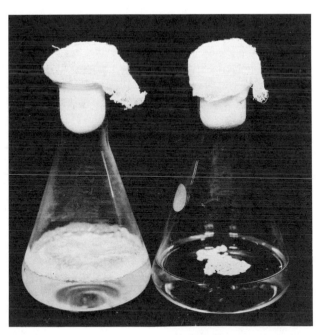

Figure 28.2 A growth of *Mycobacterium bovis* on broth. The culture in the flask on the right is about 2 weeks old; the other is about 2 months old. Growth appears as a dull, grayish white pellicle, which finally covers the surface of the fluid medium, becomes thick, opaque, and folded into creases, and pushes up on the sides of the flask at the margins. The fluid remains perfectly clear.

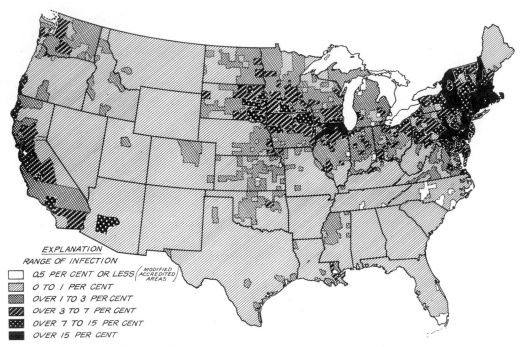

Figure 28.3. This map, which shows the extent of bovine tuberculosis in the United States in 1924, conveys a good idea of the distribution of the disease before its eradication.

A number of protein and polysaccharide antigens elicit agglutinin, complement-fixing, precipitating, and opsonic antibody responses, but these responses are low-level and apparently unimportant in protective immunity. Tuberculoprotein, or tuberculin, is a protein or polypeptide released into the medium by *M. bovis* that is active in the cutaneous delayed hypersensitivity reaction. Animals sensitized by *M. bovis* infection exhibit strong cutaneous delayed hypersensitivity when inoculated with tuberculin; this procedure is therefore a powerful aid in the detection of infected animals.

The antigen(s) involved in protective immune responses are not well defined but do not include tuberculin.

Epizootiology and Pathogenesis. *M. bovis* is present in cattle populations throughout the world, but its prevalence in the United States and in Great Britain and other European countries where intensive eradication programs have been in place for many years is very low (Thoen et al. 1979). In 1981 only 13 herds infected with *M. bovis,* comprising 4,000 animals, were detected in the United States. During 1972 to 1977 the greatest number of isolations were recorded in California, Texas, Illinois, Nebraska, Georgia, and Florida (Thoen et al. 1979). The low prevalence of *M. bovis* in 1981 in the United States contrasts with infection rates of greater than 15 percent in the Northeast, Midwest, and West in 1924, before the National Bovine Tuberculosis Eradication program took effect (Figure 28.3).

The principal route of transmission is aerogenous, although a small proportion of infections are milk borne, congenital, or sexually transmitted. Studies have shown that the walls and windows of barns housing infected cattle are contaminated with acid-fast bacilli (Jensen 1953). Dairy cattle traditionally have by far the greatest infection rates because of the ease with which the organism can be transmitted between animals in close proximity. Infected humans can shed the organism from open pulmonary lesions and can be a source of infection for cattle (Collins and Grange 1983). *M. bovis* survives for extended periods in shaded situations but quickly loses viability in sunlight and in feces (Duffield and Young 1985). Isolation of the organism from samples of an environment inhabited by infected badgers (*Meles meles*) suggests that feces can be a source of viable organisms but that survival in the environment is brief (Little, Naylor, and Wilesmith 1982). European badgers in Great Britain and opossums (*Trichosuris vulpecula*) in New Zealand have both been shown to be feral reservoirs of *M. bovis* infection for cattle (Julian 1981; Little, Swan, et al. 1982). The disease tends to be progressive in these species, and the organism is shed in feces (badger) or from draining sinus tracts (opossum).

Calves can be infected in utero or from the ingestion of milk from a tuberculous udder. Prepucial carriage of *M. bovis* has been recorded (Thoen et al. 1977) and suggests that venereal transmission is possible.

Although cattle are the natural primary hosts of *M. bovis,* horses, swine, cats, mink, and primates are also susceptible and can develop progressive disease. So, too, can captive wild ruminants in zoological parks. Sheep, goats, and dogs are relatively resistant to infection and birds are completely resistant.

M. bovis does not elaborate a toxin or other extracellular virulence factor. Although cord factor is present on virulent strains but not on avirulent strains, its role in virulence is not understood. It is believed to be important in stimulating granulomatous responses.

Following inhalation, the organism is deposited in an alveolar sac, where it is ingested by an alevolar macrophage. It slowly multiplies, eventually killing the phagocyte and then is reingested by macrophages of hematogenous origin that are drawn by the inflammatory response at the primary infection site. Organisms that escape are filtered from the regional lymphatic drainage by macrophages in the regional lymph nodes. Intracellular multiplication of the organism continues with subsequent carriage to the bloodstream through the efferent lymphatics and thoracic ducts. In this way, the infection can be disseminated to other body sites and back to the lungs. Unlike most bacteria, *M. bovis* can survive and grow intracellularly in macrophages. The organism has the ability to prevent fusion of the cell's lysosomes with the phagosome and thus avoid intracellular digestion and killing (Goren 1977). Sulfatides from *M. bovis* accumulate in the lysosomes, which then do not fuse with the cell's phagosomes. This "antifusion" effect prevents access of lysosomal enzymes to the bacteria in the phagosome.

Tubercles consisting of aggregations of macrophages, lymphocytes, and other leukocytes are formed at the primary site, in the regional lymph node, and at sites of secondary metastasis. To the naked eye they are translucent, pearly structures similar to small grains of tapioca. As growth of the tubercles continues, necrosis begins in their centers (Figure 28.4), and the pearl appearance gives way to yellowish white opaqueness. Generally about this time another type of cell appears in the lesion—giant cells of the Langhans type. These are formed from macrophages either by fusion or by continued growth and multiplication of nuclei without division of cytoplasm. They become quite large and conspicuous. Their cytoplasm is clear and their nuclei, numbering from 2 to 10 or more, are arranged in the form of a crescent, or half-circle, around the periphery of one side of the cell. Tubercle bacilli frequently can be seen lying within the cytoplasm of these cells. As the tuberculous mass grows and the necrotic center becomes larger and larger, macrophages and giant cells can generally be found just outside the advancing necrotic front.

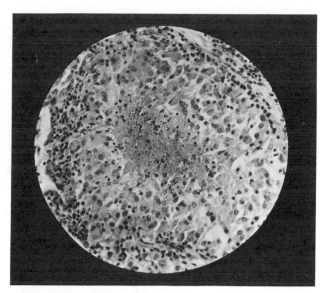

Figure 28.4. A tubercle in the lung of a rabbit caused by *Mycobacterium avium* very early in the course of the disease. The structure is typical of all primary tubercles regardless of the type of bacillus concerned. The central area of necrosis is surrounded by a layer of macrophages, which make up the great part of the field. The periphery of the lesion consists of fibroblasts and lymphocytes. Giant cells appear a little later near the margin of the necrotic area. × 110.

Old tuberculous masses can be very large. They can involve entire lung lobes and large areas of the liver and spleen, and they can cause lymph nodes to become 20 times as large as normal. The central parts of such lesions usually consist of very dry cheesy material in which calcium deposits often appear, so that they make a gritty sound when they are incised. Such lesions often become surrounded by dense connective tissue.

Lesions in cattle. In recently infected cattle the bronchial, mediastinal, submaxillary, and retropharyngeal nodes more often exhibit visible lesions than do the lungs, but this may well be because small pulmonary lesions are not readily found. The lung lesions usually take the form of caseocalcareous masses located in the anterior lobes. Some are so small that they can be overlooked; others involve entire lobes (Figure 28.5). Active lesions may show hyperemia around the periphery of the caseous masses. Old, inactive lesions may become very calcareous and heavily encapsulated. Tubercle bacilli are often difficult to demonstrate with microscopy, especially in the older lesions, but cultural methods and guinea pig inoculation usually succeed. Cows with pulmonary lesions may have a soft, moist cough.

Tuberculous pleuritis or peritonitis is relatively common where tuberculosis of cattle is prevalent. In this form of the disease large masses of smooth grapelike bodies

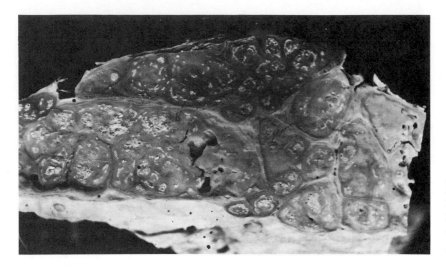

Figure 28.5. Advanced tuberculosis in the lung of a cow. The entire diaphragmatic lobe is involved in the tuberculous process. There is extensive necrosis and fibrosis. The necrotic tissue contains large amounts of calcareous material.

cover the serous surfaces. Often the lung tissue itself is not as seriously involved as the serous surface. In most cows with lung tuberculosis, however, the disease causes massive adhesions of the lungs to the chest wall, the fibrous tissue being so strong that the lungs can only be removed from the cavity by cutting. Less often involved in adult cattle are the liver, the spleen, and the mesenteric lymph nodes. Infection of the udder is found in less than 1 percent of cows with tuberculous pleuritis or peritonitis, even those with fairly advanced disease. In these animals the lesions, like those found elsewhere, may be nodular or they may involve large areas of tissue. When large areas are involved, bacilli are shed into the lactiferous ducts, and the milk from such animals may contain large numbers of organisms. Calves fed this milk will develop primary lesions in the abdominal cavity rather than the thorax. They can also be infected by inhalation. The lesions of tuberculosis in cattle were well described by Stamp (1944).

In some infected cattle, the organism may be present without visible pathology. Since the mid-1970s such latent infections account for about 4 percent of *M. bovis* isolations in the United States (Thoen et al. 1979).

Lesions in swine. *M. bovis* causes a progressive disease in swine, and lesions occur in the lymph nodes of the head, neck, and abdomen, reflecting entry through the digestive tract. Lesions are also found in the visceral organs and lungs, and large fluid-filled vesicles may be present in the spleen.

Lesions in horses. Tuberculosis lesions in horses occur in the pharyngeal region, mesentery, lungs, liver, and spleen. These lesions often resemble tumors and do show caseous necrosis (Figure 28.6).

Lesions in sheep and goats. The lesions in sheep and goats are mainly pulmonary, and the disease is progressive only in young kids.

Lesions in cats. Cats are highly susceptible to *M. bovis,* which they usually contract by drinking milk from tuberculous cows or by eating contaminated meat or offals. The lesions occur primarily in the abdominal organs and secondarily in the lungs and resemble those of lymphosarcoma (Orr et al. 1980).

Immunity. About 4 weeks after infection, cell-mediated responses become effective, resulting in enhanced intracellular killing of the organism. Spread of the infection in the body is reduced or halted. In some animals organisms at the primary invasion site and regional lymph node are completely eliminated. Activation of macrophages is by means of lymphokines released by T lymphocytes sensitized to antigens of *M. bovis.* The increased bactericidal activity of the macrophages is not specific and can be expressed against other bacterial intracellular pathogens. There is, however, also evidence for a specific lymphokine effect directed only against mycobacterium and which inhibits intracellular multiplication of the organism (Youmans 1975). Lymphokines from sensitized T lymphocytes are also responsible for the caseation necrosis observed within tubercles.

Immunity as described, although protective, often does not result in elimination of all organisms from the tissues, and so there is the possibility of future reactivation of the infection and shedding of the organism. Also, some animals fail to mount effective protective responses and go on to develop generalized tuberculosis, with wasting and eventual death.

The T lymphocyte remains sensitized for the life of the animal. Reinfection results in rapid activation of macrophages and destruction of the invading organisms, an effect known as the *Koch phenomenon.*

Antibodies formed during the infection can be measured by serologic tests including precipitation, complement fixation, and hemagglutination. They are usually

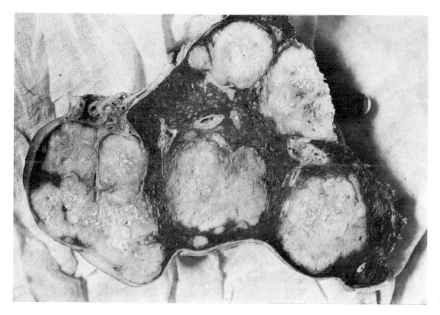

Figure 28.6. Tuberculosis of the spleen in a horse. Lesions in horses often resemble tumors, being white or gray, uniform in consistency, and lacking gross evidence of necrosis.

found in low titer in tuberculous animals and bear no relation to the state of resistance of the individual. These antibodies are not bactericidal in vivo, even in the presence of complement; although they do opsonize the tubercle bacilli and facilitate phagocytosis, this process merely enables the bacilli to enter cells, where they can multiply.

Many attempts at developing vaccines against *M. bovis* were made in the early years of the twentieth century. However, the lack of efficacy of these vaccines together with their potential to confuse interpretation of the tuberculin test has impeded the use of artificial immunization to control bovine tuberculosis.

Diagnosis. Because the lesions caused by *M. bovis* infection usually have a characteristic appearance at necropsy, tentative diagnosis of the disease is not difficult when combined with microscopic examination of sections and films stained by the Ziehl-Neelsen procedure. Bacteriological confirmation of the diagnosis is mandatory, however, because of its public health and statutory implications. Culture, isolation, and identification are the only certain methods by which the presence of *M. bovis* can be established. The procedures used are described in the *Manual of Standardized Methods for Veterinary Microbiology* (Cottral 1978) and elsewhere (Jenkins et al. 1985, U.S. Dept. of Agriculture 1974). Briefly, they involve transport of representative tissue samples in sodium borate to the laboratory, where the sample is homogenized, treated with 2 percent sodium hydroxide, neutralized with acid, and then inoculated onto Lowenstein-Jensen, acid egg, or Kirchner medium in which glycerol is replaced by sodium pyruvate (7.0 g/liter). The cultures are incubated at 37°C and examined once a week for 6 to 8 weeks. Final typing is based on sensitivity to thiophene

2-carboxylic acid hydrazide (TCH), pyrazinamide, and cycloserine; failure to reduce nitrate; and a microaerophilic oxygen preference (Jenkins et al. 1985). Lipid analysis to detect the specific lipid of *M. bovis* can also be performed (Jarnagin et al. 1983). Inoculation of guinea pigs, rabbits, and chickens has been used extensively in the past to differentiate *M. bovis* from *M. tuberculosis* and *M. avium* (Table 28.1).

Milk samples are difficult to decontaminate, but guinea pig inoculation is effective in detecting *M. bovis* in milk. The cream is removed and combined with the pellet formed after centrifugation and then injected into the thigh muscle. The animal is then examined each day and killed when it shows lymph node enlargement or local draining sinuses. If visible lesions do not appear after 6 weeks, the animal is killed and examined. Lesions detected at necropsy are examined microscopically for acid-fast organisms and cultured as described above.

Tuberculin tests. In vivo diagnosis of *M. bovis* infection is based on the delayed hypersensitivity reaction as evoked by the inoculation of tuberculin. Tuberculin derived from either *M. bovis* or *M. tuberculosis* can be used in the test, but tuberculin from *M. tuberculosis*, although more potent, is less specific than that of *M. bovis*.

The usual sites of inoculation in cattle are the skin of the

Table 28.1. Relative virulence for laboratory animals of the types of tubercle bacilli

Type	Guinea pig	Rabbit	Chicken
M. tuberculosis	+	±	0
M. bovis	+	+	0
M. avium	±	+	+

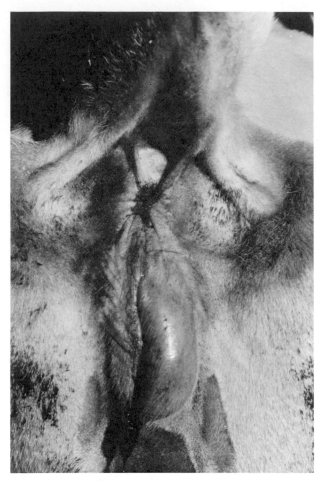

Figure 28.7. A positive intradermal tuberculin test in a cow. A firm, warm swelling is present at the injection site 72 hours after inoculation.

caudal fold (Figure 28.7), the lip of the vulva, or the side of the neck. The skin of the neck is the most sensitive site and demonstrates greatest swelling. The tuberculin is injected intradermally and the increase (if any) in skin thickness is measured after 72 hours.

Sources of error in the test include sensitization of the animal to mycobacterial species other than *M. bovis* or to *M. farcinogenes,* anergy or lack of responsiveness because the infection is too recent, old age, immunosuppression associated with calving, and desensitization associated with advanced generalized tuberculosis or with recent tuberculin administration.

The interpretation of the test is greatly enhanced when it is used as a comparative test. In this format, avian and mammalian tuberculins are injected into two sites, one above the other. The test is read at 72 hours, and the increases in skin thickness are entered on a nomograph, from which the reactor status of the animal is determined. The greater of the two reactions generally indicates the mycobacterial species causing the infection. Animals sen-

sitized by exposure to environmental mycobacteria, *M. paratuberculosis,* or to the mycobacteria involved in skin tuberculosis will respond to both mammalian and avian tuberculins and can only be distinguished by the comparative test.

The single intradermal and the comparative intradermal tests have been the basis of the highly successful eradication schemes of the United States, Great Britain, and many other countries. Slaughter of infected animals detected by these methods has almost eliminated *M. bovis* from cattle populations in these countries.

The intradermal test is also used for the detection of mycobacterial infection in other host species including pigs, chickens, dogs, and cats. In swine, the skin of the ear is usually injected, and the test is read at 72 hours. Chickens are tested by inoculating the skin of the wattle, and the test is read after 48 hours. BCG (Bacillus Calmette and Guerin) vaccine is sometimes used instead of tuberculin to detect hypersensitivity in dogs or cats (Hawthorne and Lander 1962).

Other modifications of the tuberculin test used in the past include the ophthalmic test, the thermal test, and the Stormont test (Kerr et al. 1946). Only the Stormont test is still used, albeit infrequently, as a means of detecting infected animals unreactive by the single or comparative intradermal tests. In the Stormont test, a single intradermal inoculation of mammalian tuberculin is given into the skin of the neck, followed by a second inoculation at the same site 7 days later. Animals unresponsive to one inoculation usually respond to the second. Thus, the test has value in problem herds in which the single or comparative tests are not detecting all the infected stock.

As an eradication program proceeds, the error rate of the tuberculin test increases. The number of reactors with no evidence of lesions at slaughter increases. Occasional failure of the test to detect an infected animal sometimes results in dramatic outbreaks of tuberculosis in herds that have long been free of infection and therefore have no acquired immunity to the disease.

Antimicrobial Susceptibility. *M. bovis* is sensitive to isoniazid, streptomycin, para-aminosalicylic acid, rifampicin, and thiacetozone. However, treatment of infected animals, with the possible exception of valuable animals in zoological parks, is not attempted because of the zoonotic implications.

REFERENCES

Collins, C.H., and Grange, J.M. 1983. The bovine tubercle bacillus. A review. J. Appl. Bacteriol. 55:13–59.

Collins C.M., and Lyne, P.M. 1984. Microbiologic Methods, 5th ed. Butterworths, London. Pp. 373–395.

Cottral, G.E., ed. 1978. Manual of Standardization Methods for Veterinary Microbiology. Cornell University Press, Ithaca, N.Y. P. 537.

Dubos, R.J., and Middlebrook, G. 1947. Media for tubercle bacilli. Ann. Rev. Tuberc. 56:333–345.

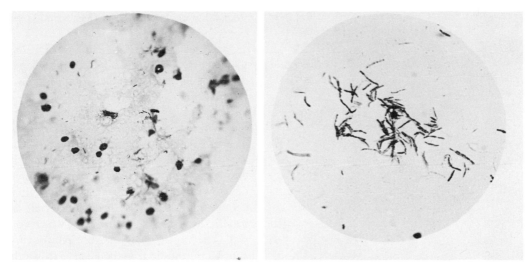

Figure 28.8. (*Left*) *Mycobacterium avium* from a liver lesion of a naturally infected chicken. × 360 (*Right*) *M. avium* from a culture on Dorset's egg medium which had been incubated for 6 weeks at 37°C. × 770.

Duffield, B.J., and Young, D.A. 1985. Survival of *Mycobacterium bovis* in defined environmental conditions. Vet. Microbiol. 10:193–197.

Goren, M.B. 1977. Phagocyte lysosomes: Interactions with infectious agents, phagosomes and experimental perturbations in function. Ann. Rev. Microbiol. 31:507–533.

Hawthorne, V.M., and Lander, I.M. 1962. Tuberculosis in man, dog and cat. Am. Rev. Respir. Dis. 85:858–869.

Jarnagin, J.L., Brennan, P.J., and Harris, S.K. 1983. Rapid identification of *Mycobacterium bovis* by a thin-layer chromatographic technique. Am. J. Vet. Res. 44:1920–1922.

Jenkins, P.A., Duddridge, L.R., Collins, C.H., and Yates, M.D. 1985. Mycobacteria. In C.H. Collins and J.M. Grange, eds., Isolation and Identification of Micro-organisms of Medical and Veterinary Importance. Society for Applied Microbiology, Technical Series no. 21. Academic Press, New York. Pp. 275–296.

Jensen, K.A. 1953. Second report of the Subcommittee of Laboratory Methods of the International Union against Tuberculosis. Bull. Int. Union Tuberc. 25:89–104.

Julian, A.F. 1981. Tuberculosis in the possum, *Trichosuris vulpecula*. In B.O. Ball, ed., Proceedings of the First Symposium on Marsupials in New Zealand. Zoology Publication, Victoria University of Wellington. Pp. 164–174.

Kerr, W.R., Lamont, H.G., and McGirr, J.C. 1946. Studies on tuberculin sensitivity in the bovine. Vet. Rec. 58:443–446.

Little, T.W.A., Naylor, P.F., and Wilesmith, J.W. 1982. Laboratory study of *Mycobacterium bovis* infection in badgers and calves. Vet. Rec. 111:550–557.

Little, T.W.A., Swan, C., Thompson, H.V., and Wilesmith, J.W. 1982. Bovine tuberculosis in domestic and wild animals in an area of Dorset. II. The badger population, its ecology and tuberculosis status. J. Hyg. 89:211–224.

Orr, C.M., Kelly, D.F., and Lucke, V.M. 1980. Tuberculosis in cats. A report of two cases. J. Small Anim. Pract. 21:247–253.

Sommers, H.M., and Good, R.C. 1985. Mycobacterium. In E.H. Lennette, A. Balows, W.J. Hausler, and H.J. Shadomy, eds., Manual of Clinical Microbiology, 4th ed. American Society for Microbiology, Washington, D.C. Pp. 216–248.

Stamp, J.T. 1944. A review of the pathogenesis and pathology of bovine tuberculosis with special reference to practical problems. Vet. Rec. 56:443–446.

Thoen, C.O., Himes, E.M., Richards, W.D., Jarnagin, J.L., and Harrington, R. 1979. Bovine tuberculosis in the United States and Puerto Rico: A laboratory summary. Am. J. Vet. Res. 40:118–120.

Thoen, C.O., Himes, E.M., and Stumpff, C.D. 1977. Isolation of *Mycobacterium bovis* from the prepuce of a herd bull. Am. J. Vet. Res. 38:877–878.

U.S. Dept. of Agriculture. 1974. Methods of Veterinary Mycobacteriology, rev. ed. Veterinary Services Services Laboratory, Animal and Plant Health Inspection Service, U.S. Dept. of Agriculture, Ames, Iowa.

Youmans, G.P. 1975. Relation between delayed hypersensitivity and immunity in tuberculosis. Am. Rev. Respir. Dis. 111:109–118.

Mycobacterium avium

M. avium belongs to group 3 of the Runyon classification and is often grouped with the closely related organism, *M. intracellulare*, as the *M. avium-intracellulare* complex. It produces disease primarily in birds and occasionally in pigs, cattle, sheep, and humans. Infection is common in swine in the corn belt of the midwestern United States and leads to economic losses in the packing plants when portions of carcasses with lesions have to be trimmed out. *M. avium* is also a common source of nonspecific hypersensitivity in the tuberculin test in cattle.

Morphology and Staining Reactions. *M. avium* is more variable in shape than *M. bovis* and may appear in the form of long beaded rods or as short, solid-staining forms (Figure 28.8). It is strongly acid- and alcohol-fast.

Cultural and Biochemical Features. Colonies grown on Dorset's egg or other solid media are usually visible in less than a week and are well developed at 2 weeks. They have a soft, moist consistency and are cream in color but sometimes become yellowish to pinkish with age and exposure to light. In liquid culture they show considerable mucoid sediment. Growth occurs at temperatures between 25°C and 42°C. *M. avium* reduces tellurite but not nitrate; it does not hydrolyze Tween 80 (Jenkins et al. 1985).

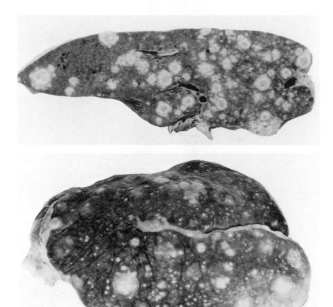

Figure 28.9. Tuberculosis of the liver in a chicken. Gross lesions in cut section (*top*). Lesions as seen from the surface (*bottom*).

Antigens. The *M. avium-intracellulare* complex is classified into a number of serotypes designated 1 to 21 on the basis of agglutination with serotype specific antiserums (Schaefer 1965). Serotypes 1 and 2 predominate among isolates from chickens and other birds, swine, and cattle (Thoen et al. 1979). Serotype 3 is also frequently found in cattle. The chemical nature of the agglutinin has not been determined.

Epizootiology and Pathogenesis. Birds are the natural hosts of *M. avium*. Serotypes 1, 2, and 3 are usually more virulent for chickens than other serotypes and generally cause mild disease or inapparent infections in hosts other than birds. The serotype of a strain, however, is not a good guide to its pathogenicity (Viallier and Viallier 1981).

Birds become infected by ingesting water or feed contaminated by feces or soil, in which the organism survives for long periods. Egg transmission also occurs and can therefore be a route by which the organism can enter previously uninfected flocks. Both domesticated and wild birds are susceptible, although ducks and geese are infected less often than other domestic species.

Tuberculosis in birds develops rather slowly and developed lesions are usually not seen in birds less than 1 year old. The disease therefore is not observed in intensively raised flocks that are left isolated from endogenous environmental sources of infection and slaughtered in the first year of life. Typically, the disease is seen in barnyard flocks that are kept for 2 to 3 years and in wild birds held in captivity.

The disease is manifested by loss of weight, weakness, listlessness, and eventual death. Lameness and wing drooping caused by bone and joint lesions are frequent. Lesions also occur in the intestinal tract, liver, and spleen. Ulcers can be found in any part of the intestine. They are readily found as tumorlike masses on the outside of the gut measuring up to 4 or 5 cm in diameter. When incised they are filled with caseous material, which is discharged through a relatively small ulcerated passage into the lumen of the intestine. Great masses of bacilli are ordinarily demonstrated with ease in this material, and it is these bacilli, discharged with the feces, which contaminate the soil. The organism is actively phagocytosed or endocytosed by intestinal epithelial cells (Mapother and Songer 1984).

Liver lesions are always found in infected birds (Figure 28.9). These appear as caseous areas, varying in size, distributed through all parts of the organ.

The spleen is generally enlarged, showing moderate to marked hypertrophy. Instead of being smooth, tuberculous spleens usually become nodular. When incised, the spleen may exhibit either a few large caseous masses or large numbers of very minute foci.

Infected joints are swollen and contain caseous material. Tubercle bacilli can be found in abundance in this material and, in fact, in all tuberculous lesions in birds.

Shedding of organisms does not occur for some months after infection, but a rapid buildup of contamination then occurs because of the extended survival of the organism in the environment.

The disease in swine. Swine are readily infected by *M. avium* and other related mycobacteria of Runyon's group 3, which are the common mycobacterial infections in this host in countries in which *M. bovis* eradication programs exist. Although birds, both wild and domestic, can be a source of infection for swine, many pigs that become infected have no contact with poultry. In some intensive indoor operations, lesions have been found in as many as 70 percent of pigs at slaughter (Ellesworth et al. 1980). The source of the infection in these populations has not been found, but there is good evidence that *M. avium* is maintained in the intestine of the pig and that this site and the tonsils can be sources of large numbers of organisms for 3 to 7 weeks after infection (Ellesworth et al. 1980).

Infected pigs develop caseocalcareous foci in the mandibular and mesenteric lymph nodes, and some animals develop granulomatous lesions in the intestinal mucosa or the tonsils. Young pigs (4 to 8 weeks) old are more susceptible than older animals. The organism apparently enters through the tonsils or the lining of the intestine. It passes into the bloodstream through the portal circulation, subsequently causing miliary lesions in the liver. From the liver, infection can spread through the hepatic vein to the lungs and spleen; however, fewer pigs have lesions in these organs than in the liver (Windsor et al. 1984).

The incidence of visible tuberculoid caseous lesions in swine at meat inspection varies between 1 and 3 percent, but this figure underestimates the true infection rate (Windsor et al. 1984).

The disease in cattle. M. avium causes minimal lesions in the lymph nodes of cattle but sensitizes the animal to avian and to a lesser extent to mammalian tuberculin and to johnin, a tuberculinlike extract of *M. paratuberculosis.* Infections of the mammary gland in which the organism was shed for an extended period yet no lesions were visible have been reported (Timoney 1939).

The disease in sheep, goats, dogs, and cats. Rare cases of progressive tuberculosis caused by *M. avium* have been reported in sheep, goats, dogs, and cats.

Immunity. The immune response of chickens has been shown to be both cell mediated and humoral when virulence of the infective strain is high or intermediate. Avirulent strains of the *M. avium-intracellulare* complex tend to stimulate a humoral response only (Tuboly 1979).

The cell-mediated response involves a spectrum of effects including activation of macrophages, inhibition of leukocyte migration, and the delayed hypersensitivity reaction. Avian tuberculin inoculated into the wattle is used to detect delayed hypersensitivity to *M. avium* in birds. The test is read at 48 hours. However, detection of agglutinating antibody appears to be a more reliable method of diagnosing infection (Baskaya et al. 1983). Cattle produce agglutinins and complement-fixing antibodies about 1 to 1.5 weeks after infection.

A variety of serologic tests including enzyme-linked immunosorbent assay (ELISA) (Thoen et al. 1979) and the tuberculin skin test have been used to detect infection in swine. The tuberculin skin test appears to be unreliable possibly because of the need to use tuberculin of the same serotype as that causing the infection but also because sensitization wanes quickly after infection in pigs. A pig mounts an effective protective immune response against the *M. avium* complex, and this is probably an important factor in the rapid loss of skin hypersensitivity that occurs after infection. There is therefore a poor correlation between skin reactions and postmortem findings in long-standing infections. In vitro correlates of cell-mediated immunity such as the lymphocyte stimulation index and the leukocyte migration–inhibition test have been shown to be more reliable in detecting subclinical infections in pigs (Bergman 1980), but these tests are not widely available.

Diagnosis. Smears or sections of typical lesions are stained by the Ziehl-Neelsen method and examined for the presence of acid-fast bacilli. Representative tissues are ground in sterile broth, treated with 2 percent sodium hydroxide to neutralize contaminants and inoculated onto Dorset's egg, Lowenstein-Jensen, or Middlebrook media. The cultures are incubated at 37°C and examined at 7-day intervals. Organisms of the *M. avium-intracellulare* complex produce visible colonies at between 1 and 2 weeks. Species identification is made on the basis of a combination of colonial appearance and biochemical, serologic, and animal pathogenicity studies. *M. avium* and related mycobacteria are catalase- and urease-negative, reduce tellurite but not nitrate, do not hydrolyze Tween 80, are sensitive to 5 percent NaCl, are usually nonpigmented, are agglutinated by specific antiserums, and may be pathogenic for chickens. The chicken bioassay is more reliable for isolates from avian sources than from mammalian tissues, which may be less virulent for chickens. The methodology of typing *Mycobacteria* species is outlined in more detail elsewhere (Jenkins et al. 1985, U.S. Dept. of Agriculture 1974).

Antimicrobial Susceptibility. Mycobacteria of the *M. avium-intracellulare* complex are generally resistant to isoniazid, rifampin, and aminoglycosides. Thus, the chemotherapy of infections by these organisms is difficult (Bailey et al. 1983).

The Disease in Humans. Infectivity for humans is very low. Infections are progressive, refractory to treatment, and often fatal (Kubin et al. 1966). Lesions in children occur in the cervical lymph nodes. Adults usually have pulmonary disease. *M. avium* is highly virulent for patients with acquired immunodeficiency syndrome (AIDS).

REFERENCES

Bailey, W.C., Albert, R.K., Davidson, P.T., Farer, L.S., Glassroth, J., Kendig, E., London, R.G., and Inseliman, L.S. 1983. Treatment of tuberculosis and other mycobacterial diseases. Am. Rev. Respir. Dis. 127:790–796.

Baskaya, H., Aydin, N., and Akay, O. 1983. Comparison of allergic and serologic methods for the diagnosis of avian tuberculosis. Vet. Fak. Tesi Dergisi Ankara Univ. 30:440–448.

Bergman, R. 1980. Cell-mediated immune response in pigs persistently infected with a *Mycobacterium avium* strain. Res. Vet. Sci. 28:315–320.

Ellesworth, S., Kirkbride, C.A., and Johnson, D.D. 1980. Excretion of *Mycobacterium avium* from lesions in the intestine and tonsils of infected swine. Am. J. Vet. Res. 41:1526–1530.

Jenkins, P.A., Duddridge, L.R., Collins, C.H., and Yates, M.D. 1985. Mycobacteria. In C.H. Collins and J.M. Grange, eds., Isolation and Identification of Micro-Organisms of Medical and Veterinary Importance. Society for Applied Bacteriology, Technical Series no. 21. Academic Press, New York. Pp. 275–296.

Kubin, M., Druml, J., Horak, Z., Lukavsky, J., and Vanek, C. 1966. Pulmonary and non-pulmonary disease in humans due to avian mycobacteria. I. Clinical and epidemiologic analysis of nine cases observed in Czechoslovakia. Am. Rev. Respir. Dis. 94:20–30.

Mapother, M.E., and Songer, J.G. 1984. In vitro interaction of *My-*

cobacterium avium with intestinal epithelial cells. Infect. Immun. 45:67–73.

Schaefer, W.D. 1965. Serologic identification and classification of the atypical mycobacteria by their agglutination. Am. Rev. Respir. Dis. (Suppl.) 92:85–93.

Thoen, C.O., Himes, E.M., Richards, W.D., Jarnagin, J.L., and Harrington, R. 1979. Bovine tuberculosis in the United States and Puerto Rico: A laboratory summary. Am. J. Vet. Res. 40:118–120.

Timoney, J.F. 1939. Avian tuberculosis in the cow. Vet. Rec. 51:191–196, 239–243.

Tuboly, S. 1979. Avian immune response to Mycobacterium avium strains of different virulence. Acta Vet. Acad. Sci. Hung. 27:245–252.

U.S. Dept. of Agriculture. 1974. Methods in Veterinary Mycobacteriology, rev. ed. Veterinary Services Laboratory, Animal and Plant Health Inspection Service, U.S. Dept. of Agriculture, Ames, Iowa.

Viallier, J., and Viallier, G. 1981. Avian mycobacterial infections due to Mycobacterium avium. Origin and serovars of 64 strains. Bull. Soc. Sci. Vet. Med. Comp. Lyon 83:287–290.

Windsor, R.S., Durrant, D.S., Burn, K.J., Blackburn, J.T., and Duncan, W. 1984. Avian tuberculosis in pigs: Miliary lesions in bacon pigs. J. Hyg., 92:129–138.

Mycobacterium tuberculosis

M. tuberculosis is the type species of the genus Mycobacterium and the most common cause of tuberculosis of humans and other primates. Infections of domestic animals by this species are usually instances of reverse zoonosis in which the owner or the attendant is the source of infection for the animal.

Dogs and members of the Psittacidae family (parrots, budgerigars) are most susceptible to M. tuberculosis and develop a progressive form of tuberculosis. Dogs often develop effusive pleurisy or peritonitis, and the organism is readily detected in the fluid.

In cattle and swine, M. tuberculosis causes minimal lesions in the lymph nodes and stimulates a transitory positive tuberculin reaction. There are a few reports of shedding of M. tuberculosis in the milk of cows naturally or experimentally infected with the organism (Lesslie 1968).

M. tuberculosis is similar in growth characteristics to M. bovis, although its growth is usually more luxuriant (eugonic). It prefers an oxygenated environment, in contrast to M. bovis, which is microaerophilic, and it reduces nitrate, hydrolyzes nicotinamide and pyrazinimide, and produces niacin. Unlike M. bovis, it is relatively avirulent for rabbits. The differentiation of M. bovis from M. tuberculosis is discussed in further detail by Collins and Grange (1983).

REFERENCES

Collins, C.M., and Grange, J.M. 1983. The bovine tubercle bacillus—A review. J. Appl. Bacteriol. 55:13–29.

Lesslie, I.W. 1968. Cross infections with mycobacterium between animals and man. Bull. Int. Union Tuberc. 41:285–288.

Mycobacterium paratuberculosis

SYNONYMS: Johne's bacillus,
  Mycobacterium enteritidis,
  Mycobacterium johnei

M. paratuberculosis is the cause of a chronic debilitating enteritis of cattle, sheep, goats, llamas, camels, and some wild ruminants. The disease is known as Johne's disease, paratuberculosis, chronic bacterial enteritis, chronic hypertrophic enteritis, and other local names. M. paratuberculosis grows very slowly and has a strict requirement for mycobactin, an iron-chelating agent. It is closely related to M. avium.

Morphology and Staining Reactions. M. paratuberculosis appears in both tissues and cultures as short, thick rods measuring about 0.5 by 1.0 μm. It is considerably smaller than any of the tubercle bacilli. In tissues and feces it commonly appears in clumps, some containing a great many organisms. This arrangement is an aid in its identification. It is strongly acid- and alcohol-fast and Gram-positive. It has neither spores nor capsules. In tissues it develops intracellularly in the macrophages and giant cells, which appear at the site of localization.

Cultural and Biochemical Features. Primary cultures of M. paratuberculosis grow more slowly than any other Mycobacterium species. The iron-chelating compounds, mycobactin P or J, extracted from M. phlei and M. paratuberculosis (laboratory adapted strain), respectively, must be supplied in the medium (3.0 μg/ml) for propagation of M. paratuberculosis. M. phlei itself incorporated in Dorset's egg medium can also serve as a source of mycobactin.

Mycobactin J is a better source of mycobactin than mycobactin P in that colonies appear sooner and in greater numbers when mycobactin J is used. (Merkal and McCullough 1982).

On a medium such as Herrold's, Smith's, or modified Dubos' with mycobactin added, growth at 37°C appears at between 6 and 8 weeks. The colonies are small, smooth, raised, and dull white with thin irregular margins. By 12 weeks, a colony diameter of 1 to 2 mm can be seen.

Growth can also be obtained in fluid media such as Smith's or modified Dubos'. Dry, rough, folded pellicles are formed on the surface after extended incubation. The addition of 0.4 percent sodium pyruvate accelerates the growth of many strains but inhibits a few (Merkal 1984).

Because the usual specimens for culture of M. paratuberculosis are intestinal or fecal, contaminating organisms must be removed by treatment with hexadecylpyridinium chloride (HPC) or 5 percent oxalic acid. HPC has less inhibitory effect on M. paratuberculosis than oxalic acid and now appears to be the decontaminant of choice (Merkal 1984).

M. paratuberculosis is rather inactive biochemically and identification is usually based on its slow growth and mycobactin dependence. Specific antiserums have been used to confirm identification (Jarnagin et al. 1975).

Pigmented strains have been isolated fron sheep (Taylor 1950) but are uncommon.

Organisms similar to *M. paratuberculosis* have been isolated from wood pigeons in Europe and from cases of Crohn's disease in humans (Merkal 1984). These organisms produce infections in calves and goats, respectively, that resemble paratuberculosis. They differ from classical *M. paratuberculosis* strains of bovine origin only in drug sensitivity (Merkal 1984).

M. paratuberculosis is resistant to acids and alkalies and remains viable in feces for at least 15 weeks at $-70°C$ (Richards and Thoen 1977). In atmospheric conditions it can survive in feces or soil for up to a year and even longer in water (Larsen et al. 1956). It is readily destroyed by moderate heat and by 5 percent formalin or 5 percent lysol (Gilmour 1985).

Antigens. At least 44 different antigens occur in *M. paratuberculosis* (Gunnarson and Fodstad 1979). Many antigens are shared with *M. avium* and with the BCG variant of *M. bovis*. At least one antigen (A) is unique to *M. paratuberculosis* and recognized by serums of infected animals. Polysaccharide antigens reactive in the complement-fixation test have been identified and shown to carry two antigenic determinants. The protective antigen(s) has not been characterized.

Epizootiology and Pathogenesis. *M. paratuberculosis* is enzootic throughout the world, but is more common in temperate zones and in wet climates. There is some evidence that cattle raised on alkaline soils are less susceptible to Johne's disease (Kopecky 1977, Smythe 1935). Jersey and shorthorn cattle are more susceptible than other breeds.

In the United States the prevalence of infected herds varies between 1 and 33 percent, but there are regions where infection is rare. Prevalence rates are higher in the Great Lakes and the northeastern United States than elsewhere in the country (Amstutz 1984). An overall herd infection rate of 4.3 percent for the period 1973 to 1978 has been recorded in the northeastern United States.

Infection is also widespread in sheep, goats, and the wild ruminant population and can be transmitted between host species. Pigs can also serve as intermediate hosts of *M. paratuberculosis* (Amstutz 1984).

The organism is transmitted in feces. Young animals are most susceptible, and therefore infections that later become Johne's disease are contracted during the first year of life. Calves suckling cows with clinical disease are at greater risk of becoming diseased (Gilmour 1985). In utero transmission is known to occur, but it is not known whether this can cause clinical disease later in life. Cattle infected as adults are usually resistant to the development of clinical disease (Rankin 1962). Male animals appear to be more susceptible and therefore the incidence of disease is higher in bulls. The role of semen in transmission has not been determined. The incidence of infection is higher in regions where the density of cattle is high and where cattle are confined (Hoffsis et al. 1983).

Usually once a herd is infected, most losses occur during a relatively short period, with new cases appearing from time to time. Typically, only about 1 in 20 animals develops obvious clinical disease. Subclinical infection, however, can cause greater economic losses (Amstutz 1984). Cattle seldom develop signs of Johne's disease after 5 years of age, and most cases appear in 2- and 3-year-old females. The disease most often becomes apparent in the early part of the first or second lactation period. The greatest losses occur among animals that are high producers; the stress of lactation breaks down the resistance of the animal to an infection that previously had been latent.

Once ingested, the organism penetrates the epithelium of the ileum and colon and is phagocytosed by macrophages. The organism lies directly in the cytoplasm or in lysosomes and is not seen in phagosomes as is the case with *M. tuberculosis* or *M. bovis*. Kubo et al. (1983) suggest that the triple-layered cell wall may be important in this unusual intracellular behavior of *M. paratuberculosis* in infected cattle. The organism is resistant to intracellular degradation (Bendixen et al. 1981) and can survive for weeks in bovine macrophages. Replication of the organism in the mucosa stimulates a granulomatous response in the caudal ileum. Lesions develop at this site a few months after infection and later involve the cecum and distal colon. In animals with advanced cases, lesions can be found throughout the intestine and regional lymph nodes. The lesions in the intestinal wall take the form of a thickening that may be very obvious or very slight. This thickening is caused by proliferation of great masses of epithelioid cells in the lower layers of the mucosa and the submucosa (Figure 28.10). Unlike tuberculosis there are no tubercles and no necrosis. The epithelium always remains intact, but it is often thrown into deep folds that cannot be flattened by stretching of the gut wall. The mesenteric lymph nodes never show great enlargement or necrosis, but they are often slightly enlarged. Sometimes the lymphatics on the serous surface of the affected bowel become filled with epithelioid cells, which convert the usually inconspicuous channels into glassy, tortuous cords along the mesenteric attachment. Numerous small acid-fast organisms can be easily demonstrated in films

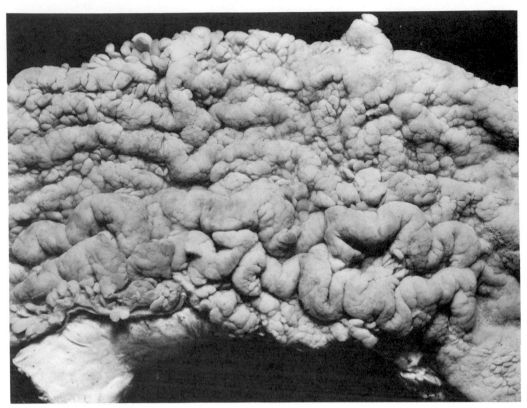

Figure 28.10. The mucous membrane of a portion of the ileum from an animal with Johne's disease. The wall is greatly thickened by large deposits of epithelioid cells in the subepithelial tissue of the mucosa. The irregular folds and plaques are characteristic. There is a complete absence of ulcers and necrosis.

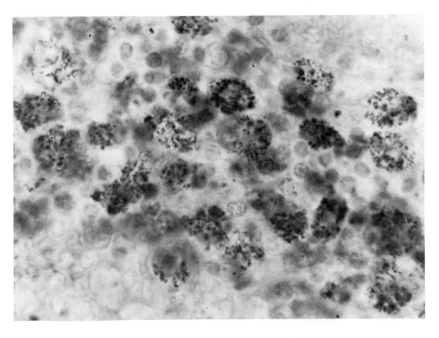

Figure 28.11. Epithelioid cells in the mucous membrane of an animal with rapidly progressing Johne's disease. The cells are packed with masses of *Mycobacterium paratuberculosis*. This preparation had been stained with the Ziehl-Neelsen technique for acid-fast bacteria. In preparations stained with hematoxylin and eosin these cells appear normal. × 890.

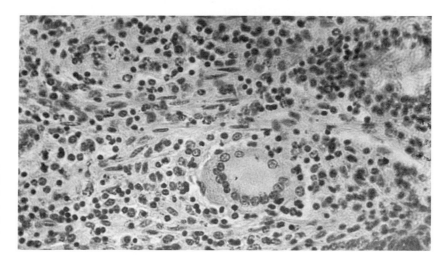

Figure 28.12. A section through the sub-epithelial tissue of the small intestine mucosa of an animal with acute Johne's disease, showing the epithelioid cells that infiltrate this tissue and cause thickening of the mucosa. A typical giant cell is shown. Hematoxylin and eosin stain. × 540.

made from scrapings from the cut surface of the thickened portion of the intestinal wall, or from that of the lymph nodes which drain the affected areas. The organisms are usually found in clumps, and many of them are located intracellularly. In sections, most of the organisms are present in the epithelioid cells (Figure 28.11). Large giant cells, of the type seen in tubercles, are usually conspicuous in sections (Figure 28.12).

Organisms can be carried in macrophages to the liver, spleen, uterus, udder and male reproductive organs, but lesions are uncommon at these sites.

Cattle with clinical disease have chronic or intermittent diarrhea and are emaciated (Figure 28.13), even though the appetite remains good, and generally unthrifty. Cows may improve during pregnancy but relapse after calving. In its final stages, Johne's disease is characterized by ventral and intermandibular edema (bottle jaw) and dysentery. Large numbers of organisms are shed in the feces at this stage. Loss of protein through the diseased mucosa and failure of absorption of ingested nutrients are important causes of the hypoalbuminemia associated with the disease. Immune phenomena (immune complex forma-

Figure 28.13. An advanced case of Johne's disease. The animal is emaciated, has a rough dry coat and harsh skin, is constantly scouring, and is so weak that it must brace its legs to keep from falling.

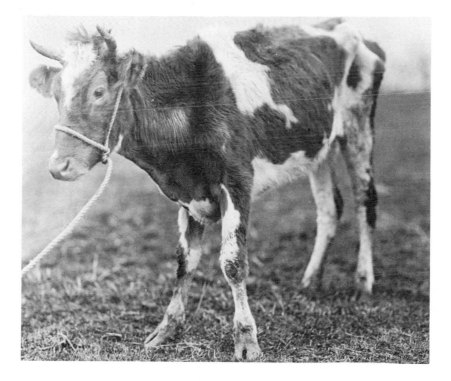

tion, local delayed hypersensitivity responses) also contribute to the diarrhea via release of histamine and other compounds that affect the permeability of the intestinal vasculature. Death may occur within a week of the onset of diarrhea, but many animals exhibit remissions and exacerbations over a long period before they die or are culled from the herd. A few animals recover completely. Affected herds have reduced fertility and an enhanced susceptibility to mastitis.

In sheep and goats diarrhea is not prominent but chronic wasting is characteristic. The disease can be more acute in these animals than in cattle but the lesions frequently are not conspicuous. There may be no observable thickening; instead, petechial hemorrhages may be seen. In goats granulomas have been observed in the mesentery (Lenghaus et al. 1977), although in some the thickening is marked and similar to that seen in cattle. A study by Stamp and Watt (1954) of the pathology of Johne's disease in sheep as it occurs in Scotland also indicated that the lesions vary from insignificant to characteristic masses of epithelioid and giant cells which may undergo encapsulation, necrosis, caseation, and calcification. They suggest that the pigmented variety of *M. paratuberculosis* is more virulent for sheep than is the classical strain. Nakamatsu et al. (1968) conducted a histopathological study on 45 naturally infected goats and determined that the lesions were located mainly in the intestines and regional lymph nodes.

Immunity. Most young animals raised under conditions of moderate exposure to *M. paratuberculosis* become infected but eventually develop a protective immunity. Only a small proportion of these become clinical cases later in life. The nature of the protective response has not been determined but probably involves cell-mediated immune responses (Gilmour 1985).

A variety of vaccines including attenuated strains (Doyle 1945, Wilesmith 1982), heat-killed bacterins, and virulent organisms suspended in oil and pumice powder (Vallee and Rinjard 1926) have been used to control the disease. There is widespread agreement that vaccines reduce both the number of clinical cases and the volume of shedding in an infected herd. Vaccination of calves and adults in combination with management procedures whereby calves are raised in noncontaminated surroundings eventually results in disappearance of the disease (Merkal 1984). Vaccination, however, sensitizes some animals to mammalian tuberculin and is a potential source of confusion in interpretating the results of tuberculin testing. Vaccination of lambs has been shown to be highly effective in control of Johne's disease (Sigurdsson 1960).

Diagnosis. Lack of reliable laboratory methods for the detection of latently infected animals is the greatest obstacle in the control of Johne's disease. All of the bacteriological or immunological procedures currently available have high error rates. False-positive results in immunological tests are due to cross-reactivity to related bacteria or to previous exposure to the organism. False-negative results can be due to tolerance or terminal anergy or the fact that the animal was in the early stages of infection before immune responses were elicited. Culture of the organism from an animal is the only certain means by which the infection can be established in an animal in the preclinical stages of the disease.

Serologic tests. ELISA, complement-fixation (CF), agar-gel immunodiffusion (AGID), crossed immunoelectrophoresis (CIE), radioimmunoassay (RIA), and immunoperoxidase (Nguyen and Buergelt 1983) procedures are used to detect antibodies to *M. paratuberculosis*. The reliability of all these tests increases as the disease progresses, and animals with severe clinical disease therefore usually give positive results. Absorption of serums with preparations of *M. phlei* improves the specificity of serologic tests for *M. paratuberculosis* by removing antibodies that are cross-reactive with other mycobacteria (Merkal 1984).

The CF and AGID tests are most widely used, and the AGID test has the particular advantage that it is simple to perform and the results are available within 24 hours. It is therefore an excellent and rapid method of establishing the presence of *M. paratuberculosis* infection in advanced cases of the disease (Sherman et al. 1984). The CIE test, although more sensitive, is more difficult to perform.

The AGID, CF, and CIE tests are also used to detect infection in sheep and goats but exhibit the same limitations as in cattle (Collins et al. 1984, Thomas 1983).

Allergic tests. Allergic tests are designed to measure delayed hypersensitivity responses to antigens of *M. paratuberculosis* in animals sensitized by infection. The tests used are the intradermal inoculation of johnin, the lymphocyte transformation test, and the macrophage migration and macrophage inhibition tests.

In the intradermal test, johnin, a protein purified from culture supernatants of *M. paratuberculosis,* is injected intradermally into the suspect animal. The test is read as an increase in skin thickness at 48 hours. The test is unreliable for a number of reasons including false-positive reactions in animals that have previously rid themselves of infection or that have been sensitized by other mycobacteria. False-negative reactions are common in animals that have become tolerant or anergic in advanced stages of the disease. Also, some animals with subclinical infections do not show skin test reactions. In goats, skin test reactivity is usually not observed until a year or more after the infection began (Collins et al. 1984).

The whole blood lymphocyte transformation test offers promise in early detection of infection (de Lisle and Duncan 1981, Milner et al. 1981) but has not been applied as a routine diagnostic procedure because it is difficult to perform.

Culture and isolation. Cultivation of *M. paratuberculosis* from feces, scrapings of rectal mucosa, or mesenteric lymph node biopsy specimens is the definitive means of establishing the presence of *M. paratuberculosis* in a herd. Specimens must be decontaminated in 9.75 percent hexadecylpyridinium chloride (HPC) for 30 minutes before inoculation onto Herrold's medium, Stuart's medium, or another mycobacterial medium enriched with mycobactin J (3 μg/ml). Cultures are incubated for 12 weeks at 37°C. Serologic identification of isolates can be performed with polyvalent and specific antiserums (Matthews et al. 1979).

The disadvantages of culture are the lengthy incubation times and its inability to detect *M. paratuberculosis* in animals with latent infections. Culture, however, is 100 percent specific and will detect the organism in all infected herds of more than 50 animals with an infection rate greater than 20 percent (Merkal 1984). A herd can be regarded as free from the disease once negative results are obtained from three fecal tests conducted at 6-month intervals on the entire herd (Argente et al. 1983).

Microscopic examination of fecal or mucosal smears. Positive diagnosis can be made in many cases by staining fecal samples. Small shreds of mucus should be sought and spread on new, chemically cleaned slides, which are then stained with the Ziehl-Neelsen technique. *M. paratuberculosis* is quite small and has a tendency to occur in clumps. It must be distinguished from larger acid-fast organisms, which are common in cattle feces.

Antimicrobial Susceptibility. *M. paratuberculosis* is sensitive to a combination of streptomycin sulfate and isoniazid or isoniazid and rifampin. These drugs, however, do not eradicate the organism from the infected tissues, although they do produce clinical improvement in diseased goats (Slocombe 1982, Zahinuddin and Sinha 1984).

REFERENCES

Amstutz, H.E. 1984. Bovine paratuberculosis: An update. Mod. Vet. Pract. 65:134–135.

Argente, G., Le Menec, M., Hillion, E., and Lagadic, M.A. 1983. Detection of paratuberculosis carriers: Faecal culture. Point Vet. 15:473–479.

Bendixen, P.H., Bloch, B., and Jorgensen, J.B. 1981. Lack of intracellular degradation of *Mycobacterium paratuberculosis* by bovine macrophages infected in vitro and in vivo: Light microscopic and electron microscopic observations. Am. J. Vet. Res. 42:109–113.

Collins, P., Davies, D.C., and Matthews, P.R. 1984. Mycobacterial infection in goats: Diagnosis and pathogenicity of the organism. Br. Vet. J. 140:196–201.

de Lisle, G.W., and Duncan, J.R. 1981. Bovine paratuberculosis, III.

An evaluation of a whole blood lymphocyte transformation test. Can. J. Comp. Med. 45:304–309.

Doyle, T.M. 1945. Vaccination against Johne's disease. Vet. Rec. 57:385.

Gilmour, N.J.L. 1985. *Mycobacterium paratuberculosis.* In Handbuch der bakteriellen Infektionen bei Tieren, Band V. VEB Gustav Fischer Verlag, Jena. Pp. 281–313.

Gunnarsson, E., and Fodstad, F.H. 1979. Analysis of antigens in *Mycobacterium paratuberculosis.* Acta Vet. Scand. 20:200–215.

Hoffsis, G.F., Dorn, C.R., and Bonham, J.B. 1983. A bovine practitioner survey of Johne's disease. Bovine Pract. 18:58–66.

Jarnagin, J.L., Champian, M.L., and Thoen, C.O. 1975. Seroagglutination test for identification of *Mycobacterium paratuberculosis.* J. Clin. Microbiol. 2:268–269.

Kopecky, K.E. 1977. Distribution of paratuberculosis in Wisconsin. J. Am. Vet. Med. Assoc. 170:320–324.

Kubo, M., Moriwaki, M., and Watase, H. 1983. Electron microscopic observations on the intestine of a cow with Johne's disease. Jpn. J. Vet. Sci. 45:259–262.

Larsen, A.B., Merka, R.S., and Vardaman, T.H. 1956. Survival time of *Mycobacterium paratuberculosis.* Am. J. Vet. Res. 17:549–551.

Lenghaus, C., Badman, R.T., and Gillick, J.C. 1977. Johne's disease in goats. Aust. Vet. J. 53:460.

Matthews, P.R.J., Brown, A., and Collins, P. 1979. The use of polyvalent antisera for the serotyping of mycobacteria. J. Appl. Bacteriol. 46:425–430.

Merkal, R.S. 1984. Paratuberculosis: Advances in cultural, serologic, and vaccination methods. J. Am. Vet. Med. Assoc. 184:939–943.

Merkal, R.S., and McCullough, W.G. 1982. A new mycobactin, mycobactin J from *Mycobacterium paratuberculosis.* Curr. Microbiol. 7:333–336.

Milner, A.R., Wilks, C.R., and Borland, R. 1981. In vitro responses of lymphocytes from cattle with advanced *Mycobacterium paratuberculosis* infection to homologous and heterologous antigens. Res. Vet. Sci. 31:93–99.

Nakamatsu, M., Fujimoto, Y., and Satoh, H. 1968. The pathological study of paratuberculosis in goats, centered around the formation of remote lesions. Jpn. J. Vet. Res. 16:103–117.

Nguyen, H.T., and Buergelt, C.D. 1983. Indirect immunoperoxidase test for the diagnosis of paratuberculosis. Am. J. Vet. Res. 44:2173–2174.

Rankin, J.D. 1962. The experimental infection of cattle with *Mycobacterium johnei.* IV. Adult cattle maintained in an infectious environment. J. Pathol. Bacteriol. 72:113–117.

Richards, W.D., and Thoen, C.O. 1977. Effect of freezing on the viability of *Mycobacterium paratuberculosis* in bovine feces. J. Clin. Microbiol. 6:392–395.

Sherman, D.M., Markham, R.J.F., and Bates, F. 1984. Agar gel immunodiffusion tests for diagnosis of clinical paratuberculosis in cattle. J. Am. Vet. Med. Assoc. 185:179–182.

Sigurdsson, B. 1960. A killed vaccine against paratuberculosis in sheep. Am. J. Vet. Res. 80:54–67.

Slocombe, R.F. 1982. Combined streptomycin isoniazid-rifampin therapy in the treatment of Johne's disease in a goat. Can. Vet. J. 23:160–163.

Smythe, R.H. 1935. The clinical aspects of Johne's disease. Vet. Rec. 15:85–86.

Stamp, J.T., and Watt, J.A. 1954. Johne's disease in sheep. J. Comp. Pathol. Ther. 64:26–39.

Taylor, A.W. 1950. Varieties of *Mycobacterium johnei* isolated from sheep. J. Pathol. Bacteriol. 63:333–336.

Thomas, G.W. 1983. Paratuberculosis in a large goat herd. Vet. Rec. 113:464–466.

Vallee, H., and Rinjard, P. 1926. Etudes sur l'entérite paratuberculeuse des bovidés. Rev. Gen. Méd. Vét. 35:1–9.

Wilesmith, J.W. 1982. Johne's disease: A retrospective study of vaccinated herds in Great Britain. Vet. J. 138:321–331.

Zahinuddin, M., and Sinha, R.P. 1984. Effect of antituberculous agents on *Mycobacterium johnei* in infected goats. Indian Vet. J. 61:574–577.

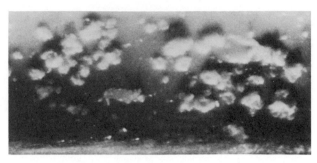

Figure 28.14. Colonies of *Mycobacterium farcinogenes* on Petragnani medium.

Mycobacterium farcinogenes

SYNONYMS: *Actinomyces farcinicus,*
    Actinomyces nocardii, Nocardia
    farcinica, Streptothrix farcinica,
    Streptothrix nocardii

M. farcinogenes is a causative agent of a disease of cattle in tropical countries known as *bovine farcy (farcin-de-boeuf)*. Nocard (1888) first described the disease and the causative agent.

The organism isolated by Nocard was named *Nocardia farcinica,* but the validity of this name is in doubt because of recent evidence from lipid analyses (Chamoiseau 1979, El Sanousi and Tag El Din 1986) which reveals that the agents of farcy in African bovines are *M. farcinogenes* and *M. senegalense* and that strains of these species have been misidentified as *N. farcinica* (Ridell et al. 1982). *M. farcinogenes* grows slowly, whereas *M. senegalense* is a fast grower.

Morphology and Staining Reactions. Stained specimens show filaments varying in length and averaging perhaps 0.3 μm in width. Branching is frequently seen. The filaments easily break into fragments, many of which resemble bacilli. These elements are Gram-positive, and most retain the acid-fast stain.

Cultural and Biochemical Features. Growth on solid media resembles that of many of the saprophytic actinomycetes common in soil. Growth occurs at 37°C in 15 to 20 days on Petragnani medium or modified Sauton's medium. Small ragged colonies with a pale halo later coalesce to form a tough, yellowish white, convoluted, raised wrinkled growth (Figure 28.14). The cell walls contain mycolates, ketomycolates, and methoxymycolates (Ridell et al. 1982).

Epizootiology and Pathogenesis. Little is known of the epizootiology and pathogenesis of bovine farcy. The occurrence of lesions on the limbs, particularly the prescapular area, suggests that the organism enters superficial wounds contaminated with soil or other environmental factors (Salih et al. 1978). Tick bites may also be a route of entry (Al Janabi et al. 1975). Entry is followed by a localized subcutaneous cellulitis (Figure 28.15) that spreads along local lymphatic channels to regional lymph nodes. The lesions may break through the skin, forming sinuses that communicate with cold abscesses. The disease is chronic; eventually lung involvement may occur, after which the animal becomes emaciated and dies. Cultures are easily obtained from the freshly opened nodules.

Immunity. There are no vaccines. Immunity is probably cell-mediated, but this aspect has not been studied.

Diagnosis. Smears made from pus are stained by Gram's and the Ziehl-Neelsen methods. The organism appears as masses of fine branching filaments, which tend to stain uniformly when the smear is taken from a young lesion. In many cases ovoid enlargements are seen along the course of the filaments, giving them a beaded appearance.

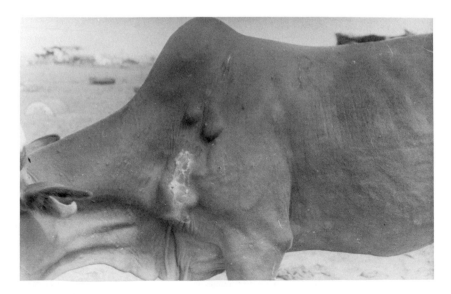

Figure 28.15. A cow with bovine farcy. The lesions involve the prescapular lymph node and lymphatics. (Courtesy S. M. El Sanousi.)

The diagnosis can be confirmed by inoculation of a guinea pig. The animal develops draining abscesses and usually dies within 10 to 20 days. Necropsy shows general emaciation and numerous tuberclelike nodules scattered over the surface of the peritoneum.

Antimicrobial Susceptibility. *M. farcinogenes* is sensitive to a combination of trimethoprim and sulfamethoxazole and to ampicillin, erythromycin, sulfonamides, minocycline, and amikacin. The later stages of farcy are difficult to treat successfully. Sodium iodide administered parenterally has been a recommended treatment for many years.

REFERENCES

Al Janabi, B.M., Branagan, D., and Danskin, D. 1975. The transstadial transmission of the bovine farcy organism, *Nocardia farcinica*, by the ixodid *Amblyomma variegatum* (Farbricius, 1974). Trop. Anim. Health Prod. 7:205–209.

Chamoiseau, G. 1979. Etiology of farcy in African bovines: Nomenclature of the causal organisms *Mycobacterium farcinogenes* Chamoiseau and *Mycobacterium senegalense* (Chamoiseau) comb. nov. Int. J. Syst. Bacteriol. 29:407–410.

El Sanousi, S.M., and Tag El Din, M.H. 1986. On the aetiology of bovine farcy in the Sudan. J. Gen. Microbiol. 132:1673–1675.

Nocard, M.E. 1888. Note sur la maladie des boeufs de la Guadeloupe connue sous le nom de farcin. Ann. Inst. Pasteur 2:293–302.

Ridell, M., Goodfellow, M., Minnikin, D.E., Megan, S., and Hutchinson, I.G. 1982. Classification of *Mycobacterium farcinogenes* and *Mycobacterium senegalense* by immunodiffusion and thin-layer chromatography of long-chain components. J. Gen. Microbiol. 128:1299–1307.

Salih, M.A.M., El Sanousi, S.M., and Tag El Din, M.H. 1978. Predilection sites of bovine farcy lesions in Sudanese cattle. Bull. Anim. Health Prod. Afr. 26:168–171.

The Saprophytic Acid-Fast Bacilli

A variety of species of saprophytic mycobacteria of Runyon's group 4 whose normal habitat is the soil and aquatic environments can be found as opportunistic invaders of the tissues of domestic animals. The frequency of occurrence and the species involved vary greatly from region to region. These mycobacteria are often inappropriately described as atypical "mycobacteria"—a description based on their lack of similarity to *M. tuberculosis*, which is historically the best characterized *Mycobacterium* species found in lesions of classical tuberculosis.

Examples of saprophytic mycobacteria that have been found in lesions in animals include *M. fortuitum, M. gordonae, M. intracellulare, M. kansasii, M. marinum, M. scrophulaceum,* and *M. xenopi.* Serotypes of *M. avium* are sometimes included with these species.

Identification of the saprophytic mycobacteria is based on speed of growth, pigment formation, optimum growth temperature, production of catalase and sulfatase, ability to reduce nitrates and tellurite, ability to hydrolyze Tween 80, and resistance to thiophene-2-carboxylic acid hydrazide (Jenkins et al. 1985).

Saprophytic mycobacteria have been found in cases of bovine mastitis (Richardson 1970) in which granulomatous lesions were produced. These infections are often iatrogenic, being introduced during infusion of antibiotics in oily vehicles for treatment or prophylaxis of other forms of bacterial mastitis. *M. intracellulare* is a frequent cause of caseous lymphadenitis in pigs, a condition also caused by *M. avium* (see "The Disease in Swine," under "*Myobacterium avium*"). A series of cases of cutaneous granulomas due to *M. fortuitum* and *M. phlei* has been described in cats (White et al. 1983). The lesions were sometimes fistulated and were found predominantly on the abdomen and thorax.

In calves, *M. fortuitum, M. intracellulare* (serotypes 8 and 9), *M. kansasii, M. marinum, M. scrofulaceum,* and *M. xenopi* stimulated sensitivity to tuberculin from *M. bovis* and *M. avium* following oral inoculation of live cultures. *M. fortuitum, M. intracellulare,* and *M. kansasii* caused microgranulomas in mesenteric lymph nodes (Jorgensen 1981). In some regions, sensitization of cattle to these antigens is an important cause of nonspecific reactions in routine tuberculin testing for *M. bovis* infection.

Diagnosis. Direct smears of lesions should be stained by the Ziehl-Neelsen method. Cultures are made on Lowenstein-Jensen or Stonebrinks medium or on blood agar.

REFERENCES

Jenkins, P.A., Duddridge, L.R., Collins, C.H., and Yates, M.D. 1985. Mycobacteria. In C.H. Collins and J.M. Grange, eds., Isolation and Identification of Micro-organisms of Medical and Veterinary Importance. Academic Press, New York. Pp. 275–296.

Jorgensen, J.B. 1981. Pathogenicity and immunogenicity of atypical mycobacteria for calves: A short summary. Rev. Infect. Dis. 3:979–980.

Richardson, A. 1970. Bovine mastitis associated with *Mycobacterium smegmatis* and an untypable mycobacterium. Vet. Rec. 86:497–498.

White, S.D., Ihrke, P.J., Stannard, A.A., and Jang, S. 1983. Cutaneous atypical mycobacteriosis in cats. J. Am. Vet. Med. Assoc. 182:1218–1222.

Acid-Fast Bacilli Associated with Ulcerative Lymphangitis (Skin Tuberculosis) in Cattle

Lesions of skin tuberculosis in cattle occur in the skin of the lower parts of the legs (Figure 28.16). Their frequent presence at these sites has led to the suggestion that the acid-fast organisms invade the host through wounds, abrasions, or scratches inflicted by thorny plants. The lesions first appear as nodules that seem to be attached to the skin but are actually located in the subcutaneous

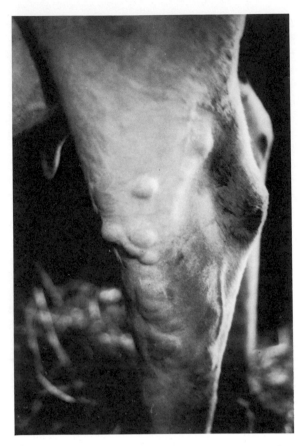

Figure 28.16. Acid-fast lymphangitis, or skin tuberculosis, of a cow. The nodules eventually soften and ulcerate through the skin.

tissue. These nodules usually soften and ulcerate through the skin. In the meantime, other nodules often appear along the course of the lymphatics. It is not uncommon to see animals with 4 to 5 to as many as 25 nodules, many of which have broken through the skin. After discharging their contents, the lesions usually heal. Sometimes instead of discharging the lesions coalesce, forming large dense masses consisting largely of connective tissue in which areas of suppuration occur. The pus may be fluid, pasty, or dry and also calcareous. The neighboring lymph nodes usually do not become involved, unlike the situation that invariably occurs in the presence of true tubercle infection.

The histological structure of these nodules resembles that of tuberculous tissue. Acid-fast bacilli that cannot be distinguished morphologically from bovine tubercle bacilli can be found in most cases, although usually they are not numerous. Mycobacteria have never been successfully cultured from these lesions (Hagan 1929), and only one successful attempt at transmission of the disease

with homogenized lesion material has been reported (Hedstrom 1949).

Because affected animals often react in the tuberculin test for *M. bovis* infection, reactor animals must be carefully examined for the presence of skin tuberculosis before a final interpretation of the results of the tuberculin test is made. Skin tuberculosis is therefore an important cause of nonspecific sensitization, since it is universally accepted that the disease is not caused by *M. bovis*.

Skin tuberculosis is found throughout the world but tends to have a localized distribution with areas of high prevalence restricted to specific farms.

REFERENCES

Hagan, W.A. 1929. Subcutaneous lesions which sometimes induce tuberculin hypersensitivities in cattle. Cornell Vet. 19:173–181.
Hedström, H. 1949. So-called skin tuberculosis in cattle. Collected papers from the State Veterinary Medicine Institute, Stockholm. P. 180.

Mycobacterium lepraemurium

First observed in rats in lesions that resembled human leprosy (Stefansky 1903), *M. lepraemurium* is an acid-fast bacillus that occurs in dense clumps within enlarged cells. It can be propagated in cell culture (Rees and Tee 1962) but not on cell-free culture media.

M. lepraemurium or a similar organism is the cause of feline leprosy, a granulomatous disease of the skin of the head and limbs of cats. In skin tests the organism of feline leprosy has antigens similar to those of *M. lepraemurium* (Leiker and Poelma 1974).

Epizootiology and Pathogenesis. Feline leprosy has been observed in domestic cats in the United States, Canada, Great Britain, New Zealand, Australia, and Holland. Cases in the United States and Canada occurred or orginated on the Pacific seaboard (McIntosh 1982, Snider 1971). In New Zealand most cases have been observed on the North Island (Thompsen et al. 1979).

Lesion homogenates from cats have been used to successfully produce lesions of leprosy in inoculated rats and mice (Lawrence and Wickham 1963, Leiker and Poelma 1974). Similarly, the disease has been transmitted back to cats from rats experimentally infected with lesion material from cats (Schiefer and Middleton 1983). Experimental infections in cats resulted in lesion production in from 2 to 6 months and a previously affected but cured cat was resistant to reinfection (Schiefer and Middleton 1983). Other evidence for the development of protective immunity includes the observation that the majority of cases are seen in cats less than 3 years old (McIntosh 1982, Thompsen et al. 1979).

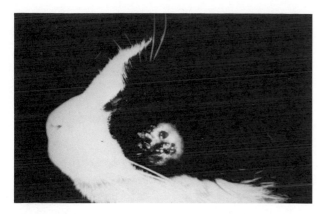

Figure 28.17. A lesion of feline leprosy on the face of a cat. Note the granulomatous character of the lesion.

Since most cases of feline leprosy in western Canada are observed about 2 to 6 months after summer, it has been suggested that the causative organism is transmitted by arthropod vectors active during summer (Schiefer and Middleton 1983). Similarly, case prevalence among cats in New Zealand increases during winter.

The granulomas can occur anywhere on the head (Figure 28.17) but are most noticeable on the skin of the head and limbs; they can also be found on the nasal mucosa.

The skin may ulcerate, and occasionally the subcutis and peripheral lymph nodes are affected (Thompsen et al. 1979). The cellular reaction consists of many macrophages, lymphocytes, and neutrophils. The macrophages contain large numbers of acid-fast organisms. Nerves are not involved in feline leprosy.

REFERENCES

Lawrence, W.E., and Wickham, N. 1963. Cat leprosy: Infection by a bacillus resembling *Mycobacterium lepraemurium*. Aust. Vet. J. 39:390–393.

Leiker, D.L., and Poelma, F.G. 1974. On the etiology of cat leprosy. Int. J. Lepr. 42:218–221.

McIntosh, D.W. 1982. Feline leprosy: A review of forty-four cases from western Canada. Can. Vet. J. 23:291–295.

Rees, R.J.W., and Tee, R.D. 1962. Studies on *Mycobacterium lepraemurium* in tissue culture. II. The production and properties of soluble antigens from *Myco. lepraemurium* in tissue culture. Br. J. Exp. Pathol. 43:480–487.

Schiefer, H.B., and Middleton, D.M. 1983. Experimental transmission of a feline mycobacterial skin disease (feline leprosy). Vet. Pathol. 20:460–471.

Snider, W.R. 1971. Tuberculosis in canine and feline populations. Am. Rev. Respir. Dis. 104:877–887.

Stefansky, W.K. 1903. Eine lepraähnliche Erkrankung der Haut und der Lymphdrusen bei Wanderratten. Zentralbl. Bakteriol., I. Abt. Orig. 33:481–487.

Thompsen, E.J., Little, P.B., and Cordes, D.O. 1979. Observations of cat leprosy. N. Z. Vet. J. 27:233–235.

29 The Genus *Dermatophilus*

In 1958 Austwick reviewed the histories of *streptotrichosis* (also known as *streptothricosis*), *mycotic dermatitis*, and *strawberry foot-rot* and concluded that the causal organisms were congeneric. He proposed that *Dermatophilus*, the earliest generic name, be used for them and recognized three species: *D. congolensis* from streptotrichosis in cattle, *D. dermatonomus* from mycotic dermatitis in sheep, and *D. pedis* from strawberry foot-rot in sheep. He also suggested that these organisms be assigned to the family Dermatophilaceae and placed in the order Actinomycetales. In 1964 Gordon studied members of the genus *Dermatophilus* and decided that all isolates could be accommodated in the species *D. congolensis*, with *D. dermatonomus* and *D. pedis* falling into synonymy. This conclusion was supported by the serologic studies of Roberts (1965). Accordingly, we will consider *D. congolensis* to be the cause of the diseases commonly known as cutaneous streptotrichosis, mycotic dermatitis, lumpy wool, strawberry foot-rot, and cutaneous actinomycosis.

REFERENCES

Austwick, P.K.C. 1958. Cutaneous streptothricosis, mycotic dermatitis and strawberry foot-rot and the genus *Dermatophilus* Van Saceghem. Vet. Rev. Annot. 4:33–48.
Gordon, M.A. 1964. The genus *Dermatophilus*. J. Bacteriol. 88:509–522.
Roberts, D.S. 1965. Cutaneous actinomycosis due to the single species *Dermatophilus congolensis*. Nature 206:1068.

Dermatophilus congolensis

SYNONYMS: *Actinomyces congolensis, Dermatophilus dermatonomus, Dermatophilus pedis, Nocardia dermatonomus, Polysepta dermatonomus, Polysepta pedis, Rhizobium pedis, Streptothrix bovis, Tetragenus congolensis*

First described by Van Saceghem in 1915 in the Belgian Congo, *D. congolensis* is the cause of cutaneous streptotrichosis in cattle, horses, sheep, goats, deer, elands, and rabbits. The disease is most common in Africa, but similar cases have been described in Europe, Australia, New Zealand, India, and North and South America (Ainsworth and Austwick 1973). It is widespread in the United States and Canada.

Morphology and Staining Reactions. *D. congolensis* forms characteristic narrow, tapering filaments with lateral branching at right angles. Septa develop in transverse horizontal and vertical planes and give rise to parallel rows of coccoid cells that form motile flagellate zoospores (Figures 29.1 and 29.2). Both the mycelia and spores are Gram-positive.

Cultural and Biochemical Features. The organism grows well at 37°C. Colonies grown on solid media are grayish white, becoming yellowish with age; they are smooth, moist, mucoid, and sometimes viscous and adherent to the medium. *D. congolensis* coagulates milk, usually liquefies gelatin slowly, and may produce a pellicle on liquid media. It ferments glucose and mannitol and produces acid. It attacks dextrin, galactose, levulose, and sucrose to varying degrees but does not attack arabinose, dulcitol, lactose, or sorbitol.

Antigens. All the strains of *D. congolensis* studied so far appear to have similar somatic antigens, hemolysins, and precipitinogens. Flagellar antigens exhibit considerable variability, but there is some sharing of flagellar antigen among isolates (Roberts 1965). The soluble antigens responsible for the delayed hypersensitivity reaction seem to be similar in a variety of isolates (Roberts 1965).

Epizootiology and Pathogenesis. *D. congolensis* causes infection of the skin of cattle, sheep, deer, and other species. It survives well in the environment and has been shown to occur in soil collected during the dry season (Bida and Dennis 1977). The infective form of the organism is the motile zoospore, which is released when infected skin becomes wet (Roberts 1963a). The life-span of the motile zoospore is only a few hours, but dried spores can survive for long periods. Infection is spread by contact, by the splashing effects of heavy rain, and by

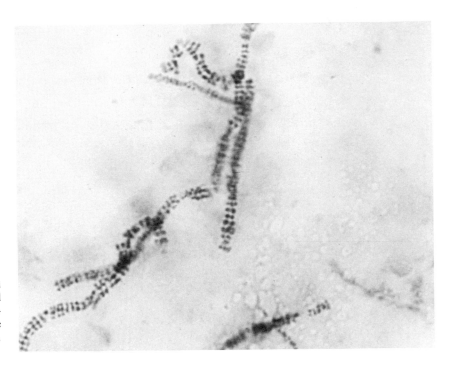

Figure 29.1. *Dermatophilus congolensis* in a smear from the skin of a horse affected with cutaneous streptotrichosis. The parallel rows of the coccoid cells formed in the filaments are characteristic. Giemsa stain. (Courtesy J. R. Saunders.)

insect activity. Infection is maintained on carrier animals, in which small lesions persist for long periods (Bida and Dennis 1977). The hair follicles are possible sites where infection persists in carrier cattle (Bida and Dennis 1977). There is a definite correlation between the incidence of cutaneous streptothricosis and wet weather—the disease

in tropical Africa is closely associated with the rainy season, and cases in deer and horses in New York State are more numerous after wet summers.

Besides rainfall, other predisposing environmental factors are the activities of ticks and bloodsucking flies and exposure to thorny bushes or overhanging tree branches

Figure 29.2. Electron micrograph of *Dermatophilus congolensis*. Note the flagella. × 26,800. (Courtesy I. Grinyer.)

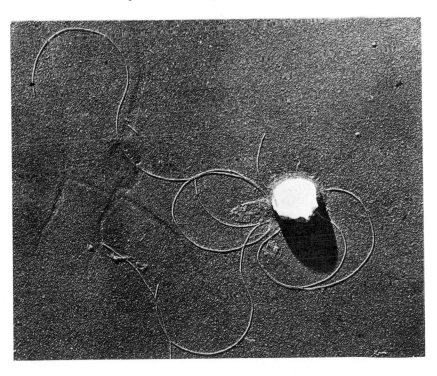

where cattle congregate. In some areas of Africa pecker birds are involved in the spread of infection.

Lumpy wool disease in sheep is more frequent during periods of mild wet weather, and strawberry foot-rot is similarly a disease seen during wet summers. Fine-wooled breeds are more severely affected (Smith and Austwick 1975). Gheradi et al. (1984) found, however, that the wax-suint ratio was more important than wool characteristics as a factor that predisposed the animals infection. Dipping can serve as a mode of spread of infection. Wilkinson (1979) showed that dipped sheep developed more lesions than undipped sheep and that wool production was lower.

The extent to which the disease occurs in cattle varies considerably in different parts of Africa. In East Africa the disease is of relatively little economic importance, but in Nigeria losses resulting from death or culling are substantial (Oduye and Lloyd 1971). In some herds 4 percent of cattle have to be culled because of the disease. Substantial losses also occur because of damage to hides and poor growth rates. Reproduction can be affected when the infection involves the perineal area (Ogwu et al. 1981).

Nutritional deficiency is believed to predispose animals to clinical infection (Lloyd 1971). The presence of infections such as rinderpest, lumpy skin disease, trypanosomiasis, histoplasmosis, strongylosis, and ectoparasitisms also increase the susceptibility of animals to dermatophilosis (see the review by Abu-Samra 1980).

Breed susceptibility has also been noted. White Fulani cattle, zebu, and exotic breeds (Bida and Dennis 1977) are susceptible, whereas N'Dome and Muturu breeds appear to be resistant (Amakiri 1977, Bida and Dennis 1977). European breeds and Brahman cattle are highly susceptible.

Entry of zoospores into the skin of a new host involves successful penetration of the hair or fleece, the sebaceous wax layer, and finally the stratum corneum epidermidis (Roberts 1963b).

The zoospores are chemotactically responsive to CO_2 diffusing out through the skin. They germinate and a hyphal branch penetrates the epidermis. The hyphae branch laterally and invade the hair or wool follicles. The dermis is not invaded. Neutrophils collect beneath the infected epidermis, and a serous exudate accumulates and leaks to the surface. A new layer of epidermis is formed as the older layer above deteriorates, a process that continues and eventually results in the formation of a thick scab. Infection of newly forming epidermis occurs from organisms already in the follicular sheath.

The restriction of *D. congolensis* to the epidermis is the result of a factor produced by the neutrophils that have gathered in the dermis (Roberts 1965). It is also probable that the basement membrane of the epidermis is a natural barrier to dermal invasion. Many affected animals in tropical areas show a severe, generalized form of the disease; the factors that contribute to generalization are not understood (Lloyd 1984). Healing of lesions eventually occurs, the time required depending on the onset of a delayed hypersensitivity to antigens of *D. congolensis*. This hypersensitivity results in an accelerated neutrophil response that curtails further invasion of the epidermis.

Streptotrichosis as it usually is seen in cattle, horses, deer, and, at times, sheep is characterized by small, confluent, raised, and circumscribed crusts composed of epidermal cells and coagulated serous exudate with embedded hairs on the skin of the back. The lesions can be local or they can be progressive and sometimes fatal. The disease is essentially an exudative dermatitis followed by extensive scab formation (Figure 29.3).

The first signs of mycotic dermatitis in sheep are the appearance of small areas of hyperemia, which persist for 10 to 14 days, followed by the formation of crusts. Masses of amber-colored crust may mat the wool fibers, but usually the crust separates from the skin surface and either remains as a zone of hardened exudate or is cast off. If the scab is removed from an active lesion, a concave, raw, and moist area is found on the skin. Progressive lesions can result in death and can cause serious losses in lambs. Dipping has been shown to predispose sheep to mycotic dermatitis, and routine dipping of infected flocks may be undesirable (Wilkinson 1979).

D. congolensis also causes strawberry foot-rot in sheep (Harriss 1948). The natural course of the disease in sheep begins with the appearance of dry scabs on the legs at any point between the coronet and the knee or hock. Papules preceding scab formation have not been observed. Me-

Figure 29.3. A horse with dermatophilosis (streptotrichosis).

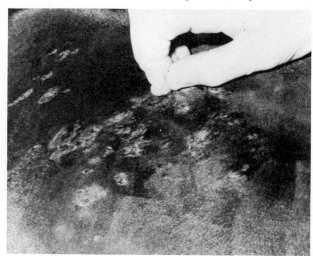

chanical injury to the skin from prickly plants probably precedes the formation of lesions. The local lesions show a tendency to spread until sometimes almost the entire skin area of the lower portions of the legs is involved. More often the lesions heal without further spread after they have reached 2 to 4 cm in diameter. The affected areas become denuded of hair or wool. When the areas are large, the exudate mats the hair and forms a hard, dry casing over the region. This usually can be stripped off easily, leaving a mass of granulation tissue that has the appearance of a strawberry, hence the common name of the disease. The lesions may remain for long periods but they usually heal within 5 to 6 weeks. The secondary infection rarely invades deeper structures, and the animal usually does not become lame. When lameness does occur, it is because the interdigital space has been invaded. There is little evidence of systemic reaction, although affected animals often do not gain weight as they should. The lesions usually heal without scar formation.

The disease usually appears 2 to 4 weeks after animals are placed on an infected pasture. The longest period between exposure and appearance of symptoms has been 98 days for lambs and 117 days for adult sheep. Mortality is very low but morbidity is high. Most of the sheep on infected pastures contract the disease.

Dermatophilosis in horses is usually sporadic in occurrence. Pascoe (1972), however, has described an unusual outbreak in Australia in which 68 of 278 horses involved had lesions on the coronets and pasterns. The disease was termed *aphis* or *greasy heel* and resembled the disease in England known as *mud fever*. *D. congolensis* was isolated from the lesions. Most horses recovered within 7 days.

Immunity. The immune response to *D. congolensis* involves both the formation of antibodies and the development of cell-mediated immunity, as evidenced by the delayed hypersensitivity reaction. Lloyd (1984) has provided an excellent review of the contributions of humoral immunity to host resistance to *D. congolensis*. Flagellar and somatic antibodies are produced and occur in the serum and milk of infected cows and on the skin surface after intradermal vaccination (Lloyd and Jenkinson 1981). Anamnestic responses have also been observed. Serum antibody, however, does not protect against clinical disease (Perreau and Chambrou 1966) although antibodies against the flagellar antigen of zoospores are immobilizing (Roberts 1964). These antibodies also appear to promote enhanced intracellular destruction of zoospores following their phagocytosis by sheep neutrophils (Roberts 1966b) and to increase the resistance of scarified skin to experimental infection.

The appearance of delayed hypersensitivity coincides with an accelerated infiltration of the lesion by neutrophils accompanied by decreased hyphal penetration of follicle sheaths and earlier healing (Roberts 1966a). The mechanism underlying this phenomenon is not understood. In sheep delayed hypersensitivity appears in 4 or 5 days, at just about the time acute primary infections show signs of being overcome (Roberts and Graham 1966).

Abu-Samra (1980) has demonstrated hypersensitive responses in rabbits, goats, sheep, donkeys, calves, and camels. These animals were relatively resistant to rechallenge 3 weeks after primary infection.

Failure of these responses to protect animals against severe generalized dermatophilosis have not been explained. Abu-Samra (1980) suggested that allergens introduced with the organism stimulate an allergic tuberculinlike hypersensitivity that exacerbates or potentiates *D. congolensis* infection. It is possible that allergens from fly and tick bites are important in the development of this hypersensitivity (Davis 1984).

Resistance to experimental infection has been demonstrated after intradermal or parenteral administration of vaccines prepared from *D. congolensis* (see the review by Lloyd 1984). Effective vaccines must contain live whole organisms. In a field trial in the southern region of Chad, young cattle appeared to be protected after intradermal vaccination with young live cultures (Provost et al. 1974). In another trial in a herd of Brahman and Brahman-cross cattle, vaccination with a live intradermal vaccine had little effect on the incidence rate, although it reduced the severity of disease (Blancou 1976).

This method of vaccination has been shown to be effective in stimulating specific antibodies in the stratum corneum epidermis (Lloyd and Jenkinson 1981). Because *D. congolensis* exhibits considerable variability of flagellar antigens (Roberts 1964), vaccines should contain the antigen of the field strains that predominate in the area where the vaccines are used.

Lloyd (1984) also pointed out that a successful vaccine must not only provide antibodies at the superficial level in the stratum corneum but must also stimulate antibodies with different antigenic specificity in the deep layers of the epidermis.

Diagnosis. Smears prepared from moistened scab material and stained with methylene blue or Gram's stain will usually reveal the typical branched filaments dividing both transversely and longitudinally. A fluorescent antibody technique has also been developed (Pier et al. 1964) and is particularly useful when the scabs have deteriorated as a result of secondary bacterial contamination. Polymyxin B in the isolation medium has been found to reduce the growth of contaminants (Abu-Samra and Walton 1977).

Antimicrobial Susceptibility. *D. congolensis* is sensitive in vitro to tetracyclines, chloramphenicol, penicillin, and streptomycin (Plowright, 1958). It is resistant to kanamycin, polymyxin B sulfate, bacitracin, and sulfonamides (Abu-Samra et al. 1976). For cattle, intramuscular penicillin (5,000 U/kg) for 5 days or 75,000 U/kg in a single injection is sometimes effective (Oduye 1975). Penicillin and streptomycin have a synergistic action against *D. congolensis* in sheep and have been shown to be effective in the treatment of lumpy wool disease (Roberts and Graham 1966). Others (LeRoux 1968, Shotts et al. 1969) have similarly shown that penicillin and streptomycin can produce marked improvement in cattle and sheep. Oduye (1975), however, warns that in West Africa, at least, antibiotic therapy is effective only in a limited number of cases.

According to Kammerlocher and Mammo (1965), griseofulvin administered orally with 1 percent gentian violet in potassium iodide has proved to be beneficial in cattle in Nigeria. Ilemobade (1984), also working in Nigeria, reported that a single dose of long-acting oxytetracycline resulted in a 90 percent cure rate in different grades of infection.

Chemical defleecing of sheep with cyclophosphamide (25 mg/kg) given in a drench has been found to be a valuable adjunct in therapy (McIntosh et al. 1971).

REFERENCES

Abu-Samra, M.T. 1980. The epizootiology of *Dermatophilus congolensis* infection (a discussion article). Rev. Elev. Méd. Vét. Pays Trop. 33:23–32.

Abu-Samra, M.T., and Walton, G.S. 1977. Modified techniques for the isolation of *Dermatophilus* spp. from infected material. Sabouraudia 15:23–27.

Abu-Samra, M.T., Imbabi, S.E., Mahgoub, E.S. 1976. *Dermatophilus congolensis:* A bacteriological, in vitro antibiotic sensitivity and histopathological study of natural infection in Sudanese cattle. Br. Vet. J. 132:627–631.

Ainsworth, G.C., and Austwick, P.K.C. 1973. Fungal Diseases of Animals, 2d ed. Commonwealth Agricultural Bureau, Slough, England. P. 22.

Amakiri, S.F. 1977. Electrophoretic studies of serum proteins in healthy and streptothricosis infected cattle. Br. Vet. J. 133:106–107.

Bida, S.A., and Dennis, S.M. 1977. Sequential pathological changes in natural and experimental dermatophilosis in Dunaji cattle. Res. Vet. Sci. 22:18–22.

Blancou, J. 1976. Bilan de sept années de prophylaxie de la Dermatophilose dans un troupeau de zébus Brahman. Rev. Elev. Méd. Vét. Pays Trop. 29:211–215.

Davis, D. 1984. Infection with *Dermatophilus congolensis* at a contact hypersensitivity site and its relevance to chronic streptothricosis lesions in the cattle of West Africa. J. Comp. Pathol. 94:25–32.

Gheradi, S.G., Harris, D.J., and Rolls, S.W. 1984. The association of fleece characteristics and susceptibility to dermatophilus. Anim. Prod. Aust. 15:357–360.

Harriss, S.T. 1948. Proliferative dermatitis of the legs ("strawberry foot-rot") in sheep. J. Comp. Pathol. Ther. 58:319–328.

Ilemobade, A.A. 1984. Clinical experiences in the use of chemotherapy of bovine dermatophilosis in Nigeria. Prev. Vet. Med. 2:83–92.

Kammerlocher, A.A., and Mammo, A.E. 1965. Evaluation of drugs effective against streptothricosis. Vet. Med. 60:65–68.

LeRoux, D.J. 1968. The treatment of "lumpy wool" *Dermatophilus congolensis* infection in merino sheep with streptomycin and penicillin. J. S. Afr. Vet. Med. Assoc. 39:87–88.

Lloyd, D.H. 1971. Streptothricosis in the domestic donkey (*Equus Asinus asinus*) I. Clinical observations and clinical pathology. Br. Vet. J. 127:572–581.

Lloyd, D.H. 1984. Immunology of dermatophilus: Recent developments and prospects for control. Prev. Vet. Med. 2:93–102.

Lloyd, D.M., and Jenkinson, D.M. 1981. Serum and skin surface antibody responses to intradermal vaccination of cattle with *Dermatophilus congolensis*. Ph.D. dissertation, University of London.

McIntosh, G.H., Smith, G.W., and Cunningham, R.B. 1971. Cyclophosphamide in the treatment of mycotic dermatitis of sheep. Aust. Vet. J. 47:542–546.

Oduye, O.O. 1975. Bovine cutaneous streptothricosis in Nigeria. World Anim. Rev. 16:13–17.

Oduye, O.O., and Lloyd, D.H. 1971. Incidence of bovine cutaneous streptothricosis in Nigeria. Br. Vet. J. 127:505–510.

Ogwu, D., Osori, D.I.K., and Kumi-Diaka, J. 1981. Bovine streptothricosis and reproduction in northern Nigeria: A case study. Theriogenology 15:469–475.

Pascoe, R.R. 1972. Further observations on *Dermatophilus* infections in horses. Aust. Vet. J. 48:32–34.

Perreau, P., and Chambrou, J. 1966. Immunology of bovine cutaneous streptothricosis in cattle. Vaccination trials. Rev. Elev. Méd. Vét. Pays Trop. 19:263–274.

Pier, A.C., Richard, J.L., and Farrell, E.F. 1964. Fluorescent antibody and cultural techniques in cutaneous streptothricosis. Am. J. Vet. Res. 25:1014–1020.

Plowright, W. 1958. Cutaneous streptothricosis of cattle in Nigeria. II. The aerobic actinomycete (*Nocardia* sp.) associated with the lesions. J. Comp. Pathol. Ther. 68:133–147.

Provost, A., Touade, M.M., Guillanme, Peleton, H., and Damsou, F. 1974. Vaccination tests against bovine dermatophilosis in the southern region of Chad. Bull. Epizoot. Dis. Afr. 22:223–229.

Roberts, D.S. 1963a. The release and survival of *Dermatophilus dermatonomus* zoospores. Aust. J. Agr. Res. 14:386–399.

Roberts, D.S. 1963b. Barriers to *Dermatophilus dermatonomus* infection on the skin of sheep. Aust. J. Agr. Res. 14:492–508.

Roberts, D.S. 1964. The host parasite relationship in infection with *Dermatophilus congolensis*. Ph.D. dissertation, University of London.

Roberts, D.S. 1965. Cutaneous actinomycosis due to the single species *Dermatophilus congolensis*. Nature 206:1068.

Roberts, D.S. 1966a. The influence of delayed hypersensitivity on the course of infection with *Dermatophilus congolensis*. Br. J. Exp. Pathol. 47:9–16.

Roberts, D.S. 1966b. The phagocytic basis of acquired resistance to infection with *Dermatophilus congolensis*. Br. J. Exp. Pathol. 47:372–382.

Roberts, D.S., and Graham, N.P.H. 1966. Control of ovine cutaneous actinomycosis. Aust. Vet. J. 42:74–78.

Shotts, E.B. Jr., Tyler, D.E., and Christy, J.E. 1969. Cutaneous streptothricosis in a bull. Am. Vet. Med. Assoc. J. 154:1450–1454.

Smith, L.P., and Austwick, P.K.C. 1975. Effect of weather on the quality of wool in Great Britain. Vet. Rec. 96:244–248.

Van Saceghem, P.R. 1915. Dermatose contagieuse (impetigo contagieux). Soc. Pathol. Exot. Bull. 8:354–359.

Wilkinson, F.C. 1979. Dermatophilosis of sheep, association with dipping and effects on production. Aust. Vet. J. 55:74–76.

30 The Genera *Mycoplasma* and *Ureaplasma*

The mycoplasmas are the simplest and tiniest self-replicatory prokaryotes and consist essentially of membrane-bound bags of protoplasm with ribosomes and a molecule of double-stranded DNA. They are separated from the Eubacteria in the class Mollicutes (soft skin), which contains the single order Mycoplasmatales. Within the order are the genera *Acholeplasma, Anaeroplasma, Mycoplasma, Spiroplasma,* and *Ureaplasma.*

There are more than 70 species of *Mycoplasma,* including a number of important pathogens of animals. The genus *Acholeplasma* comprises 10 species of poorly defined pathogenicity for animals and whose known importance is as contaminants of tissue culture and serums. *U. diversum* and *U. urealyticum* are the only species of *Ureaplasma. U. diversum,* as its name implies, consists of a variety of strains, some of which are pathogens of the bovine genitourinary tract. *U. urealyticum* is found only in humans. Other *Ureaplasma* strains as yet without specific epithets have been isolated from a variety of vertebrate hosts (Taylor-Robinson and Gourlay 1984). Members of the genus *Spiroplasma* are pathogens of plants and arthropods. The two *Anaeroplasma* species are anaerobic commensals of the rumens of sheep and cattle.

Mycoplasma and *Ureaplasma* species are unique among self-replicating organisms in the small size of their genomes (500 megadaltons). Thus their coding capacity is limited to less than 700 different proteins. The genomes of *Acholeplasma* species have slightly greater coding capacity, a reflection of their more complex metabolic capabilities including fatty acid biosynthesis, which absolves them of the requirement for sterols.

Another unusual feature of the mycoplasmas as a group is the low guanine and cytosine (G + C) content of their DNA. The G + C content of most species falls within the range of 25 to 34 mol% (Razin 1985).

The inherent simplicity of the mycoplasmas imposes on them a parasitic reliance on cells of higher species for a variety of complex biological compounds including lipids. They are therefore highly adapted parasites whose niche in vertebrate hosts is the mucosal surface of different body sites. Each species is adapted to a specific host, and in most instances, this adaptation results in a commensal-type existence. However, a number of *Mycoplasma* species cause serious diseases in domestic animals. In fact, the first observations of mycoplasmas were made by E. Nocard in 1891, who isolated the agent of contagious bovine pleuropneumonia, a debilitating disease of cattle. The term *pleuropneumonialike organism* (PPLO) was commonly used to describe mycoplasmas for many years thereafter.

The intimate association of mycoplasmas with the surface of the host cell and the tendency of exogenous proteins to bind to the mycoplasmal membrane may allow the parasite to evade the host's immune response by covering itself with host antigens. The incorporation of host cell antigens onto the mycoplasma membrane is termed *capping.* Conversely, mycoplasma protein antigens may become incorporated onto the surface of the host cell and thereby involve the host cell in a variety of deleterious immunological reactions intended for the parasite (Wise et al. 1978).

This chapter considers only the *Mycoplasma* and

Ureaplasma species that are known to cause disease in domestic animals. For information on the nonpathogenic species and on the acholeplasmas, see Razin and Freundt (1984), Rosendal (1982), and Tully and Whitcomb (1979). The general characteristics of the mycoplasmas are given next. Descriptions of individual species that infect domestic animals follow.

Morphology and Staining Reactions of the Mycoplasmas. The mycoplasmas are extremely pleomorphic and can appear as cocci, filaments, spirals, rings, globules, and granules. This plasticity is a result of the lack of a cell wall. The basic cell shape is the coccus; filament formation is a consequence of a fast growth rate in which genome replication precedes and outstrips cytoplasmic division. The filamentous form tends to be transient and changes eventually into chains of cocci.

The ability of mycoplasma cells to change shape is probably related to the presence of contractile proteins resembling actin (Neimark 1983), and the gliding motility exhibited by some mycoplasmas, including *M. gallisepticum,* may have its basis in this contractile material. *M. gallisepticum* also has a polar bleb that serves as a fulcrum during movement by virtue of its ability to adhere to surfaces.

The mycoplasmas are Gram-negative, but Gram's stain is not satisfactory in routine work with these organisms. They are stained pink or purple by the Giemsa, Castaneda, Dienes, or methylene blue methods. Phase contrast microscopy of films of broth cultures or fluids from specimens is a good procedure for visualizing the natural shape of the organism.

The mycoplasma membrane is trilaminar and lacks the skeletal support of peptidoglycan found in other bacterial cell walls. Its chemical structure is that of a typical cytoplasmic membrane, being composed of phospholipids, sterols, glycolipids, and proteins. Some *Mycoplasma* species, most notably *M. mycoides* subsp. *mycoides* are covered with a capsular polysaccharide. The internal structure of the mycoplasmal cell is simple and consists of ribosomes and a DNA strand. Some species have specialized tip structures or polar blebs that have a bundle of fibrils in their cores.

Cultural and Biochemical Features of the Mycoplasmas. Because mycoplasmas require cholesterol or related sterols for growth, this compound must be supplied in the medium. Serum is a commonly used source of this compound. Cholesterol functions as a regulator of membrane fluidity during changes in growth and temperature and is a necessary ingredient for membrane synthesis. Supplementary ingredients usually included in media are beef heart infusion, peptone, glucose, and yeast extract.

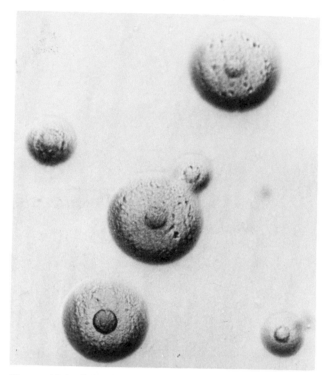

Figure 30.1. Colonies of *Mycoplasma gallinarum.* × 200. (From Hofstad and Doerr, 1956, courtesy of *Cornell Veterinarian.*)

Other substances added to mycoplasma media for the isolation and culture of specific strains include vaginal mucus (for *M. agalactiae* and *M. bovigenitalium*), avian allantoic fluid (for *M. capri*), and swine gastric mucin (for *Acholeplasma granularum*). Penicillin and thallium acetate (A4000) are also commonly added to media to inhibit other bacterial contaminants. Special media additives have been developed for work with avian mycoplasmas (Adler et al. 1974).

The optimum temperature for the growth of *Mycoplasma* species from animals is about 37°C. Primary cultures for fermentative mycoplasmas should be grown under conditions of anaerobiasis or in an atmosphere of 10 percent CO_2 and a pH of 7.6 to 8.0. The incubation time ranges from 3 to 7 days. The typical colonies are minute and have a fried egg appearance (Figure 30.1), consisting of a flat transparent ring surrounding a central granular area that is embedded in the agar. In liquid medium, growth appears as a faint clouding.

Mycoplasmas can also be propagated in embryonated eggs or in cell-culture systems, and many strains grow more profusely in these systems than in cell-free media. Chick embryo inoculation is particularly valuable for the growth of fastidious strains.

The fermentative mycoplasmas can utilize glucose as an energy source and form lactic acid as the major end product. Arginine degradation is the source of energy of nonfermentative strains. Electron transport does not involve quinones or cytochromes and is mediated by a truncated flavin-terminated chain. The mycoplasmas are catalase-negative.

Identification of the Mycoplasmas. Identification of isolates of *Mycoplasma* species is sometimes complicated by the presence of more than one species or strain in a specimen. Purification by picking and cloning must be performed before identification is attempted. Fermentation behavior is determined in broth containing phenol red glucose or arginine.

Colonies can be identified as to genus by sensitivity to paper disks impregnated with 0.02 ml of a 1.5 percent digitonin solution, by fermentation behavior and by formation of urease. *Mycoplasma* and *Ureaplasma* species are sensitive to digitonin, *Acholeplasma* species are not. *Ureaplasma* species produce urease. Other tests helpful in identification include hemolysis and hemadsorption, reduction of tetrazolium chloride, liquefaction of heat-aggregated serum, and requirement for coenzymes (Timms 1978).

Definitive species identification depends on growth inhibition tests based on specific antisera and monoclonal antibodies, colony immunofluorescence (epifluorescence) tests, complement-fixation tests, immunoperoxidase tests, and enzyme-linked immunosorbent assays (ELISAs) (Clark et al. 1963, Taylor-Robinson et al. 1963, Tully and Razin 1983). The use of species-specific DNA probes in colony hybridization tests is becoming increasingly important in identification (Taylor et al. 1985).

Mycoplasmas cannot synthesize purine bases or pyrimidines and so guanine, uracil, and thymidine must be obtained from the host. These essential precursors of nucleic acid synthesis are obtained from the host by means of endonucleases situated on the membrane surface (Minion and Goguen 1986).

For more detailed information on identification and characterization, see the excellent reviews in the books edited by Razin and Tully (1983) and Tully and Razin (1983).

Antimicrobial Susceptibility of the Mycoplasmas. With the exception of *M. hyopneumoniae* and *M. dispar,* mycoplasmas are resistant to beta lactam antibiotics that inhibit peptidoglycan synthesis. They are usually sensitive to chloramphenicol, nitrofurans, and tetracyclines. Some species are sensitive to macrolides including erythromycin and tylosin.

REFERENCES

Adler, H.E., Damassa, A.J., and Field, S.W. 1974. Factors influencing growth of *Mycoplasma synoviae.* Avian Dis. 18:568–577.

Clark, H.W., Bailey, J.S., Fowler, R.C. and Brown, T.M. 1963. Identification of Mycoplasmataceae by the fluorescent antibody method. J. Bacteriol. 85:111–118.

Hofstad, M.S., and Doerr, L. 1956. A chicken meat infusion medium enriched with avian serum for cultivation of an avian pleuropneumonialike organism, *Mycoplasma gallinarum.* Cornell Vet. 46:439–446.

Minion, F.C., and Goguen, J.D. 1986. Identification and preliminary characterization of external membrane-bound nuclease activities in *Mycoplasma pulmonis.* Infect. Immun. 51:352–354.

Neimark, H. 1983. Mycoplasma and bacterial proteins resembling contractile proteins: A review. Yale J. Biol. Med. 56:419–423.

Razin, S. 1985. Molecular biology and genetics of mycoplasmas (mollicutes). Microbiol. Rev. 49:419–455.

Razin, S., and Freundt, E.A. 1984. Biology and pathogenicity of mycoplasmas. Isr. J. Med. Sci. 20:749–1027.

Razin, S., and Tully, J.G., eds. 1983. Methods in Mycoplasmology, vol. 1: Mycoplasma Characterization. Academic Press, New York.

Rosendal, S. 1982. Canine mycoplasmas: Their ecologic niche and role in disease. J. Am. Vet. Med. Assoc. 180:1212–1214.

Taylor, M.A., Wise, K.S., and McIntosh, M.A. 1985. Selective detection of *Mycoplasma hyorhinis* using cloned genomic DNA fragments. Infect. Immun. 47:827–830.

Taylor-Robinson, D., and Gourlay, R.N. 1984. *Ureaplasma.* In N.R. Krieg and J.G. Holt, eds., Bergey's Manual of Systematic Bacteriology, vol. 1. Williams & Wilkins, Baltimore. Pp. 770–775.

Taylor-Robinson, D., Somerson, N.L., Turner, H.C., and Chanock, R.M. 1963. Serological relationships among human mycoplasmas as shown by complement fixation and gel diffusion. J. Bacteriol. 85:1261–1273.

Timms, L.M. 1978. *Mycoplasma synoviae:* A review. Vet. Bull. 48:187–198.

Tully, J.G., and S. Razin, eds. 1983. Methods in Mycoplasmology, vol. 2: Diagnostic Mycoplasmology. Academic Press, New York

Tully, J.G., and Whitcomb, R.F., eds. 1979. The Mycoplasmas, vol. 2: Human and Animal Mycoplasmas. Academic Press, New York.

Wise, K.S., Cassell, G.M., and Acton R.T. 1978. Selective association of murine T lymphoblastoid cell surface alloantigens with *Mycoplasma hyorhinis.* Proc. Natl. Acad. Sci. USA 75:4479–4483.

Mycoplasma Species of Cattle

At least 12 *Mycoplasma* species are found as commensals of bovine mucous membranes and as pathogens of the respiratory, ocular, mammary, or urogenital tissues (Table 30.1). *M. mycoides* is the type species of the genus *Mycoplasma* and contains two serologically different subspecies, *capri* and *mycoides.* The subspecies *mycoides* is of historic interest as the infectious agent that was the stimulus for development of government programs for animal disease control. The economic losses it cost the U.S. cattle industry following its importation in 1843 led to the formation in 1884 of the Bureau of Animal Industry of the U.S. Department of Agriculture. By 1892 the eradication program organized by the Bureau had resulted in disappearance of contagious bovine pleuropneumonia (CBPP) from U.S. cattle.

Table 30.1. *Mycoplasma* species affecting cattle

Species	Virulence	Disease produced (if any)
M. alkalescens	Moderate	Arthritis (calves), mastitis; preputial commensal
M. alvi	Low	None described; intestinal and vaginal commensal
M. arginini	Low	Respiratory, conjunctival, and vaginal commensal
M. bovigenitalium	Moderate	Mastitis, seminal vesiculitis, arthritis of calves; preputial commensal
M. bovirhinis	Low	Mastitis; respiratory commensal
M. bovis	High	Severe mastitis, arthritis, calf pneumonia; respiratory commensal
M. bovoculi	High	Conjunctivitis, keratoconjunctivitis
M. californicum	High	Acute mastitis
M. canadense	Moderate	Mastitis, arthritis of calves; respiratory and preputial commensal
M. dispar	Moderate	Bronchiolitis and alveolitis; respiratory commensal
M. mycoides subsp. *mycoides* (small colony type)	High	Contagious bovine pleuropneumonia (CBPP)
M. verecundum	Low	Conjunctivitis of calves; preputial commensal

Mycoplasma mycoides subspecies *mycoides* (small colony type)

SYNONYMS: *Asterococcus mycoides, Bovimyces pleuropneumoniae,* organism of contagious bovine pleuropneumonia

M. mycoides subsp. *mycoides* is the cause of a destructive disease of cattle which has been known to occur in Asia, Africa, and Australia for more than 200 years. The disease originated in central Europe in the second half of the seventeenth century and spread over the greater part of Europe during the Napoleonic wars. From there it was disseminated to South Africa, Australia, and the United States in exported cattle. It first entered the United States in a ship's cow purchased by Peter Dun, a milkman who had a dairy near South Ferry, New York. The infection spread rapidly from this cow to others in the city. Other importations of the organisms followed in 1847 and 1859. CBPP has not occurred in the United States since March 1892 and in Great Britain since 1898.

The disease is still enzootic in Africa and Asia (Lindley 1981).

Morphology and Staining Reactions. *M. mycoides* subsp. *mycoides* has a typical mycoplasmal morphology, as described on p. 296. Repeatedly branching filaments are formed and "rho" forms may be present. These are cells with an axial fiber and a terminal swelling.

Cultural and Biochemical Features. *M. mycoides* subsp. *mycoides* occurs as two types: a small colony type and large colony type. Colonies of the small colony (SC) type are not visible until after 3 days on 5 percent sheep-blood agar and attain a diameter no greater than 0.1 mm (Thigpen et al. 1983). Colonies of the large colony (LC) form are visible at 2 days and eventually attain a diameter of 0.4 to 0.7 mm. The SC form is isolated from cases of CBPP, whereas the LC form is commonly isolated from a variety of lesions in goats and seldom is found in cattle. LC strains can be differentiated from SC strains by their more vigorous casein proteolysis, sorbitol fermentation, hemolysis, heat stability, and digestion of heat-denatured serum.

Both colony types ferment glucose and mannose, reduce tetrazolium aerobically and anaerobically, do not hydrolyze arginine, and do not produce phosphatase.

Antigens. Galactan and several membrane proteins constitute the important antigens of *M. mycoides*. The subspecies can be distinguished serologically by agglutination, growth inhibition, metabolic inhibition, and immunofluorescence tests. The protein profiles of the subspecies are not identical, although similar.

The SC and LC types of *M. mycoides* subsp. *mycoides* are closely related serologically, although LC strains are closer to *M. mycoides* subsp. *capri* than are SC strains (Rodwell and Rodwell 1978).

The capsular galactan is produced in great quantity and is a potent precipitinogen. Antigalactan serum can be used in a precipitin test for CBPP.

The protective antigen(s) of *M. mycoides* subsp. *mycoides* have not been identified. Differences in protective antigens exist between LC and SC strains (Smith and Oliphant 1981).

Epizootiology and Pathogenesis. *M. mycoides* subsp. *mycoides* (SC) is an obligate parasite of cattle and water buffaloes and is transmitted by droplet inhalation. Close and prolonged contact is therefore required for successful transmission. The organism has been shown to survive in hay kept in the shade for at least 216 hours (Windsor and Masiga 1977a). Animals fed contaminated hay seroconverted and had lesions of CBPP at slaughter (Windsor and Masiga 1977b). Furthermore, the organism is shed in the urine and is transmitted across the placenta. Although other modes of transmission are possible, the most important factor in spread of CBPP is the closeness of contact between animals and opportunity for air-borne transmission (Lindley 1981). Infected cattle are thus the means by which the organism is maintained and carried from one region to another.

Animals that develop subclinical disease and those that recover are both important in the epizootiology of CBPP because they constitute a clinically inapparent reservoir of infection which can thus spread insidiously.

The natural disease spreads slowly, and morbidity in a herd may not peak for 7 to 8 months after introduction of the infection. The incubation period is related to strain virulence, the intensity of challenge, and the immune status of the host. Some animals may not show evidence of the disease until months after they contract the infection.

The disease can be quite acute, proving fatal within a week, or it can be chronic. Animals with acute disease exhibit extreme respiratory distress; those more chronically affected have a moist cough, high temperature, roughened coat, and nasal discharge and are reluctant to move. Calves may develop arthritis (Lindley 1981). Infected lung foci often become encapsulated, in which case the animal may appear to have recovered, but the sequestration can break down at any time, perhaps weeks or months later, with reappearance of signs and discharge of virulent material. The movement of such animals into new herds and the reopening of the lesions spreads the disease.

The pleural cavity of acutely infected animals contains a great deal of fluid—as much as 15 to 20 liters. The surface of the lung is inflamed and covered with a thin deposit of fibrin. The subpleural tissue is thickened and filled with fluid (Figure 30.2) that distends the interlobular septa. When the affected lobes are incised, these fluids run out, coagulating after a few hours' exposure to the air.

The pneumonia begins as nodules or foci, which spread until entire lobes are involved. These areas are hepatized and are bright red, brownish red, or grayish depending on the stage of the process. The surface of a cut section presents a marbled effect, the varicolored lobules being separated from each other by wide bands of infiltrated interlobular tissue (Figure 30.3). Necrosis occurs in animals with chronic disease, large portions of lung tissue often being necrotic and sequestered by connective tissue.

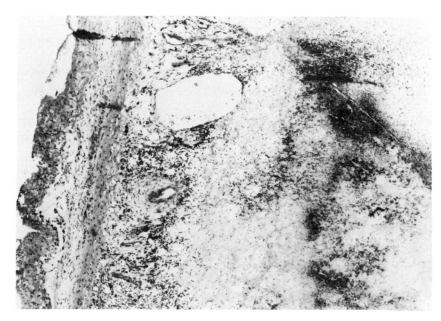

Figure 30.2. Micrograph of the greatly thickened pleura from a steer with contagious bovine pleuropneumonia. The thickening is due to severe edema and leukocyte infiltration. From the pleural lining inward, there are fibrin and leukocytes, edematous connective tissue infiltrated by leukocytes, dilated lymphatics, and then an area of necrotic edematous connective tissue and necrotic inflammatory cells. Hemotoxylin and eosin. × 105. (Courtesy Charles A. Mebus, Plum Island Animal Disease Center, U.S. Dept. of Agriculture.)

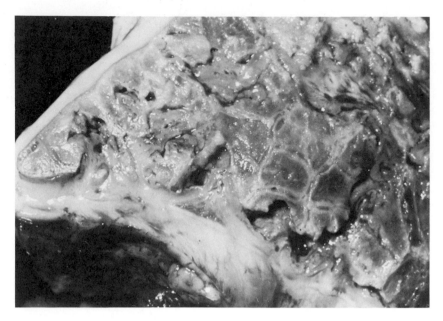

Figure 30.3. Cut surface of a lung from a steer affected with contagious bovine pleuropneumonia. The pleura is greatly thickened by connective tissue and the lung parenchyma is necrosed. The necrotic lobules are separated by zones of infiltrated interlobular tissue. (Courtesy D. A. Gregg, Plum Island Animal Disease Center, U.S. Dept. of Agriculture.)

Capsular galactan has a number of potent pathophysiological effects including the production of pulmonary edema, capillary thrombosis, collagen deposition (Buttery et al. 1980), and immunosuppression. Immunosuppression adversely affects phagocytosis and so the organism persists in the bloodstream. The bacteremia may result in localization in joints or in abortion, and there is a neutropenia and lymphocytosis (Sharma et al. 1978).

About 50 percent of exposed cattle develop clinical signs. The mortality varies from 10 to 90 percent. Animals that recover are unthrifty and may continue to carry and shed the organism for months. These animals are immune to reinfection (Windsor and Masiga 1977b).

The LC strains of *Mycoplasma mycoides* subsp. *mycoides* are rarely isolated from cattle and appear to be of low virulence for them. The LC strains are isolated mostly from goats and occasionally from sheep, in which they cause septicemia and lesions in the joints, peritoneum, mammary gland, lungs, and pleura (Cottew 1979, MacOwan 1984). In dairy goats mastitis is the most commonly observed effect of the infection. Milk from cases of mastitis is highly infectious for kids, which develop a highly fatal septicemia.

Immunity. The protective immune response of cattle to *M. mycoides* subsp. *mycoides* is poorly understood. Cell-mediated immune responses are active during the chronic phase of the disease and are probably of critical importance in protection. Humoral responses to membrane protein antigens and to capsular galactan are easily detected and measured by agglutination (stained antigen), precipitin, and complement-fixation tests.

Methods of artificial immunization have been used for many years in enzootic zones. The original vaccine involved the subcutaneous injection, usually in the tail, of pleural fluid. This method gave protection from the pulmonary disease, but reactions were often severe. It was eventually superseded by an attenuated vaccine, which although highly effective in the control of CBPP, was difficult to use in the field because of potency problems. These problems were solved in part by the development of protocols for lyophilization of the vaccine strain. Strain T1/44 is now widely used in Africa as a lyophilized vaccine and protects for about 18 months (Lindley 1979, 1981).

Diagnosis. *M. mycoides* can be visualized in fluids by dark-field or phase microscopy and isolated from tissues collected at necropsy. Cultures are made on agar containing serum, ox heart, and liver digest, penicillin, and thallium acetate (Tully 1974). A fluorescent antibody procedure is also available to detect the organism in tissues. Field detection of infected animals depends heavily on serologic methods. These include the complement-fixation test, which is particularly sensitive for the diagnosis of infections in the acute and the late chronic carrier stages. A negative test should be repeated after a month. An agar-gel diffusion precipitation test is also useful in detecting acute infection. It has special value in the slaughterhouse, where it can be used to reveal antigen in suspect lesions. An allergic skin test is the most reliable method of detecting chronic infection because the dominant immune response at this stage of the infection is cell-mediated (Roberts et al. 1973) and because circulating antigen combines with antibody in the plasma and so makes antibody detection more difficult. Gourlay (1965) has reported that in the late acute stage the complement-fixation and agar-gel tests detected 100 percent of CBPP cases, the slide-agglutination test 35 percent, and agar-gel test alone 21 percent.

A whole blood rapid-slide test for diagnosing CBPP which incorporates a stained antigen can be used in the field. A similar test based on serum is more reliable. The test fails to detect about 25 percent of acute cases and more than half of cases in the chronic phase.

REFERENCES

Buttery, S.H., Cottew, G.S., and Lloyd, L.C. 1980. Effect of soluble factors from *Mycoplasma mycoides* subsp. mycoides on the collagen content of bovine connective tissue. J. Comp. Pathol. 90:303–314.

Cottew, G.S. 1979. Caprine-ovine mycoplasmas. In J.G. Tully and R.F. Whitcomb eds., The Mycoplasmas, vol. 2: Human and Animal Mycoplasmas. Academic Press, New York. Pp. 103–132.

Gourlay, R.N. 1965. Comparison between some diagnostic tests for contagious bovine pleuropneumonia. J. Comp. Pathol. 75:97–109.

Lindley, E.P. 1979. Control of contagious bovine pleuropneumonia with special reference to the Central African empire. World Anim. Rev. 30:18–22.

Lindley, E.P. 1981. Contagious bovine pleuropneumonia. In M. Ristic and I. McIntyre, eds., Diseases of Cattle in the Tropics. Martinus Nijhoff, The Hague. Pp. 225–269.

MacOwan, K.J. 1984. *Mycoplasma mycoides* infections in ruminants: The current situation. Isr. J. Med. Sci. 20:854–858.

Roberts. D.H., Windsor, R.S., Masiga, W.N., and Kariavu, C. 1973. Cell-mediated immune response in cattle to *Mycoplasma mycoides* var. *mycoides*. Infect. Immun. 8.349–354.

Rodwell, A.W. and Rodwell, E.S. 1978. Relationship between strains of *Myoplasma mycoides* subsp. *mycoides* and *capri* studied by two-dimensional gel electrophoresis of cell proteins. J. Gen. Microbiol. 109:259–263.

Sharma, S.N., Vyos, C.B., Vyos, U.K., Chouhan, D.S., and Jatkar, P.R. 1978. Clinico-pathological studies on contagious caprine pleuro pneumonia. Indian J. Anim. Sci. 48:108–112.

Smith, G.R., and Oliphant, J.C. 1981. Observations on the antigenic differences between the so-called SC and LC strains of *Mycoplasma mycoides* subsp. *mycoides*. J. Hyg. 87:437–442.

Thigpen, J.E., Cottew, G.S., Yeats, F., McGhee, C.E., and Rose, D.L. 1983. Growth characteristics of large- and small-colony types of *Mycoplasma mycoides* subsp. *mycoides* on 5% sheep blood agar. J. Clin. Microbiol. 18:956–960.

Tully, J.G. 1974. The FAO/WHO programme on comparative mycoplasmology. Vet. Rec. 95:457–461.

Windsor, R.S., and Masiga, W.N. 1977a. Investigations into the epidemiology of contagious bovine pleuropneumonia. Bull. Anim. Health Prod. Afr. 25:357–363.

Windsor, R.S., and Masiga, W.N. 1977b. Investigations into the role of carrier animals in the spread of contagious bovine pleuropneumonia. Res. Vet. Sci. 23:224–229.

Mycoplasma alkalescens

M. alkalescens is moderately pathogenic for cattle and has been isolated from cases of mastitis (Bushnell 1984), abortion (Rosenfeld and Hill 1980), febrile arthritis in calves and from the prepuce and semen of bulls. Congenitally acquired infection of embryo-transplant calves has been observed in which the organism caused poly-arthritis and appeared to originate in the donor cow (Whitaker 1983). It is commonly found on the respiratory and urogenital mucosal surfaces of cattle, where it is a normal commensal (Bushnell 1984). Its occurrence in lesions is probably the result of opportunistic invasion. It grows slowly and sparsely on standard mycoplasma media and hydrolyzes arginine, producing an alkaline reaction.

REFERENCES

Bushnell, R.B. 1984. Mycoplasma mastitis. Vet. Clin. North Am. [Large Anim. Pract.] 6:301–312.

Rosenfeld, L.E., and Hill, M.W.M. 1980. The isolation of *Mycoplasma alkalescens* from cases of polyarthritis in embryo-transplant calves. Aust. Vet. J. 60:191–192.

Mycoplasma arginini

Named for its ability to hydrolyze arginine, *M. arginini* is a common commensal of mucosal surfaces of ruminants and has also been reported from a variety of other domestic species and pet animals. It has little or no virulence for cattle. One instance of its occurrence in bovine mastitis has been recorded (Bushnell 1984). Its role in respiratory disease of calves has not been proved, although it is commonly isolated from lesions in the respiratory tract of calves.

REFERENCE

Bushnell, R.B. 1984. Mycoplasma mastitis. Vet. Clin. North Am. [Large Anim. Pract.] 6:301–312.

Mycoplasma bovigenitalium

M. bovigenitalium was first isolated in England (Edward et al. 1947) from the genital tracts of heifers and from the seminal fluid of bulls. Since then it has been shown to occur worldwide (Doig 1981). A normal commensal of the urogenital tract, it can opportunistically invade the mucosa of the vulva, vagina, and uterus, where it causes granular vulvovaginitis (Afshar et al. 1966) and endometritis (Bushnell 1984). Its growth on media is markedly enhanced by the addition of DNA.

M. bovigenitalium is present in the vesicular gland secretions of the majority of apparently healthy pubescent bulls. Its persistence in some animals, however, has been associated with epidydimitis, vesiculitis, and lowered sperm motility. A local immune response to the organism also occurs and may be a factor in the lowered sperm motility observed. Because *M. bovigenitalium* is known to adhere to bovine spermatozoa, it could indirectly mediate agglutination of sperm when antibody to mycoplasma antigen is present. Its precise role in bovine infertility remains to be defined.

It is an undoubted, although infrequently opportunistic, cause of a mastitis that is characterized by firm, swollen, but relatively painless quarters, reduced milk flow, and a thick yellow secretion. The leukocyte count is increased and the organism can be demonstrated in stained smears of the secretion (Bushnell 1984, Stuart et al. 1960). Complement-fixing antibodies are produced locally and in the serum some weeks after infection. The disease has also been described in heifers and nonlactating cows (Counter 1978). Many affected cows suffer permanent loss of udder function.

The lesions in affected tissues are characterized by extensive accumulations of eosinophilic leukocytes.

REFERENCES

Afshar, A., Stuart, P., and Huck, R.A. 1966. Granular vulvovaginitis (nodular venereal disease) of cattle associated with *Mycoplasma bovigenitalium*. Vet. Rec. 78:512–519.

Bushnell, R.B. 1984. Mycoplasma mastitis. Vet. Clin. North Am [Large Anim. Pract.] 6:301–312.

Counter, D.E. 1978. A severe outbreak of bovine mastitis associated with *Mycoplasma bovigenitalium* and *Acholeplasma laidlawii*. Vet. Rec. 103:130–131.

Doig, P.A. 1981. Bovine genital mycoplasmosis. Can. Vet. J. 22:339–342.

Edward, D.G., Hancock, J.L., and Hignett, S.L. 1947. Isolation of pleuropneumonia-like organisms from the bovine genital tract. Vet. Rec. 59:329–330.

Stuart, P., Davidson, I., Slavin, G., Edgson, F.A., and Howell, D. 1960. Bovine mastitis caused by *Mycoplasma*. Vet. Rec. 75:59–64.

Mycoplasma bovirhinis

A common parasitic commensal of the bovine respiratory tract, *M. bovirhinis* has been reported from the United States, Europe, and Australia. Although most isolations have been made from animals with respiratory disease, the organism is frequently found on the respiratory mucosa of normal animals. *M. bovirhinis* is therefore not a primary pathogen (Dawson et al. 1966), and its as yet ill-defined role in respiratory disease is believed to be secondary to other agents. In one outbreak of calf pneumonia in Indiana, *M. bovirhinis* was recovered from 23 percent of specimens (Muenster et al. 1979).

REFERENCES

Dawson, P.S., Stuart, P., Darbishire, J.H., Parker, W.H., and McCrae, C.T. 1966. Respiratory disease in a group of intensively reared calves. Vet. Rec. 78:543–546.

Muenster, O.A., Ose, E.E., and Matsuoka, T. 1979. The incidence of *Mycoplasma dispar*, ureaplasma and conventional *Mycoplasma* in the pneumonic calf lung. Can. J. Comp. Med. 43:392–398.

Mycoplasma bovis

SYNONYMS: *Mycoplasma agalactiae* var. *bovis, Mycoplasma bovimastitidis*

M. bovis causes an acute, rapidly spreading mastitis in dairy herds. Found throughout the world, it causes more than 50 percent of incidents of mycoplasma mastitis and ranks next to *M. mycoides* subsp. *mycoides* in virulence for cattle.

M. bovis can be seen in Giemsa- or methylene blue–stained smears of milk and appears as ring or pleomorphic coccobacillary forms, tiny branched or beaded filaments, or amorphous clumps.

Epizootiology and Pathogenesis. *M. bovis* is frequently isolated from the respiratory mucosa of cattle. Calves in herds with a history of *M. bovis* mastitis are much more likely to carry the organism on their nasal mucosa than calves from nonmastitic herds (Bennett and Jasper 1977). The organism survives in milk for 63 days at 4°C and for 14 days at 20°C (Weinhus and Kirchhoff 1984). It also survives for extended periods on sponges used for cleaning udders before milking.

Poor husbandry and sanitation are therefore important in the spread of infection. Milking cows are often infected in all four quarters whereas dry cows are infected in only one or two. The organism is shed in the milk of affected cows in great numbers and may continue to be shed for an indefinite period after clinical recovery.

Systemic signs are usually absent, although some infected cows may develop a transient fever. A leukopenia may appear, however, and the mastitis is characterized by a sharp drop in milk production and extremely swollen udders that are not painful. The supramammary lymph nodes may be enlarged and firm. The secretion may be slightly yellow and, on standing, deposit a fine sediment on the bottom of the container. In some animals the milk is watery, with flakes and a few clots, and in others contains large yellow-white caseous chunks or pus. Cell counts in milk can be as high as 100 million/ml, and the neutrophil is the dominant cell. The California milk test (CMT) is usually 3+ a few days after infection. Casein nitrogen is greatly increased in contrast to most other forms of mastitis (Resmini and Ruffo 1969).

Affected quarters may contain nodules, abscesses, and purulent material in pockets and in plugs in the collecting ductules. The organism is present as discrete microcolonies in the affected gland (Kehoe et al. 1967). It has been suggested that the interaction of the immune defense in the gland with the organism is responsible for the tissue damage (Bennett and Jasper 1978). Lymphocytes and other mononuclear cells infiltrate a week after infection and the secretory parenchyma is replaced by granulation tissue, which in turn becomes fibrosed. Milk production therefore is permanently lost.

M. bovis has also caused severe arthritis and tendovaginitis in calves and cows (Jasper 1967) and in feedlot cattle (Hjerpe and Knight 1972). In some outbreaks there is an association with respiratory disease in calves (Moulton et al. 1956). It has also been isolated from the genital tract of normal cows (Jasper 1967).

Immunity. Systemic and local protective immune responses develop during convalescence. Local humoral and cell-mediated responses persist for about 1 year but protect only the quarter previously affected (Bushnell 1984). Colonization resistance in the respiratory tract of calves can be stimulated by a combination of intramuscular and intratracheal inoculations of *M. bovirhinis* antigen (Howard et al. 1977).

The following methods have been used to detect antibodies to *M. bovis*: complement fixation, growth and film inhibition, indirect hemagglutination, agar-gel diffusion, and single radial hemolysis. These tests have been reviewed by Boughton (1979).

Antimicrobial Susceptibility. Although *M. bovis* is sensitive to colistin, kanamycin, nitrofurazone, novobiocin, tetracycline, and tylosin, field experience suggests that treatment of affected quarters is unlikely to be effective.

REFERENCES

Bennett, R.H., and Jasper, D.E. 1977. Nasal prevalence of *Mycoplasma bovis* and IHA titers in young dairy animals. Cornell Vet. 67:361–373.

Bennett, R.H., and Jasper, D.E. 1978. Systemic and local immune responses associated with bovine mammary infections due to *Mycoplasma bovis*: Resistance and susceptibility in previously infected cows. Am. J. Vet. Res. 39:417–423.

Boughton, F. 1979. *Mycoplasma bovis* mastitis. Vet. Bull 49:377–387.

Bushnell, R.B. 1984. Mycoplasma mastitis. Vet. Clin. North Am. [Large Anim. Pract.] 6:301–312.

Hjerpe, C.A., and Knight, H.D. 1972. Polyarthritis and synovitis associated with *Mycoplasma bovimastitidis* in feedlot cattle. J. Am. Vet. Med. Assoc. 160:1414–1418.

Howard, C.J., Gourlay, R.N., and Taylor, L.H. 1977. Induction of immunity in calves to *Mycoplasma bovis* infection of the respiratory tract. Vet. Microbiol. 2:29–37.

Jasper, D.E. 1967. Mycoplasmas: Their role in bovine disease. J. Am. Vet. Med. Assoc. 151:1650–1655.

Kehoe, J.M., Norcross, N.L., Carmichael, L.E., and Strandberg, J.D. 1967. Studies of bovine *Mycoplasma* mastitis. J. Infect. Dis. 117:171–179.

Moulton, J.E., Boidin, A.G., and Rhode, E.A. 1956. A pathogenic pleuropneumonia-like organism from a calf. J. Am. Vet. Med. Assoc. 129:364–367.

Resmini, P., and Ruffo, G. 1969. Physico-chemical changes in milk of cows affected with *Mycoplasma* mastitis. Latte 43:720–722.

Weinhus, M., and Kirchhoff, H. 1984. Detection and survival of *Mycoplasma bovis* in milk. Berl. Münch. Tierärztl. Wochenschr. 97:269–271.

Mycoplasma bovoculi

SYNONYM: *Mycoplasma oculi*

M. bovoculi has been isolated from epizootics of infectious bovine keratoconjunctivitis in the United States, Canada, Europe, and the Ivory Coast. It is coccoid to coccobacillary and does not appear to form filaments.

Epizootiology and Pathogenesis. Infection of bovine eyes in enzootic areas appears to be widespread in spring and summer but the organism is cleared during winter (Rosenbusch and Knudtson 1980). Infection by *M. bovoculi* has been shown to increase ocular colonization of the eyes of cattle by *Moraxella bovis* (Friis and Pedersen 1979, Kelly et al. 1983) and *Moraxella ovis*. Severity of lesions after *M. bovoculi* infection is in part determined, therefore, by the presence or subsequent entry of organisms such as *Moraxella bovis*. Calves inoculated with *M. bovoculi* alone developed mild localized conjunctivitis and serous lacrimation, suggesting that *M. bovoculi* by itself is not highly pathogenic (Rosenbusch and Knudtson 1980).

An IgA protective antibody response develops after natural and experimental infection.

REFERENCES

Friis, N.F., and Pedersen, K.B. 1979. Isolation of *Mycoplasma bovoculi* from cases of infectious bovine keratoconjunctivitis. Acta Vet. Scand. 20:51–59.

Kelly, J.I., Jones, G.E., and Hunter, A.G. 1983. Isolation of *Mycoplasma bovoculi* and *Acholeplasma oculi* from outbreaks of infectious bovine keratoconjunctivitis. Vet. Rec. 112.482.

Rosenbusch, R.F., and Knudtson, W.U. 1980. Bovine mycoplasmal conjunctivitis: Experimental reproduction and characterization of the disease. Cornell Vet. 70:307–320.

Mycoplasma californicum

M. californicum ranks second in frequency of isolation from outbreaks of mycoplasma mastitis in California dairy herds (Jasper 1980). It has also been reported in Czechoslovakia and Ireland (Jurmanova et al. 1983, Mackie and Logan 1982). The mastitis is characterized by swelling of the udder and a watery yellow secretion with flakes, clots, pus, and a sandy sediment. The lesion is slow to resolve. The organism does not persist following clinical recovery.

Its cultural, morphologic, biologic, and serologic characteristics have been described by Jasper et al. (1981). The colonies are conical, smooth, and with a distinct center. They attain a size of about 0.3 mm after 3 days.

REFERENCES

Jasper, D.E. 1980. Prevalence of mycoplasmal mastitis in the western states. Calif. Vet. 4:24–26.

Jasper, D.E., Erno, H., Dellinger, J.D. and Christiansen C. 1981. *Mycoplasma californicum,* a new species from cows. Int. J. Syst. Bacteriol. 31:339–345.

Jurmanova, K., Hajkova, H., and Vedova, J. 1983. Further evidence of the involvement of *Mycoplasma californicum* in bovine mastitis in Europe (Czechoslovakia). Vet. Rec. 112:608.

Mackie, D.P., and Logan, E.F. 1982. Isolation of *Mycoplasma californicum* from an outbreak of bovine mastitis and the experimental reproduction of the disease. Vet. Rec. 110:578–580.

Mycoplasma canadense

M. canadense is found in the upper respiratory and urogenital tracts of cattle, where it is a normal commensal. It hydrolyzes arginine. It is occasionally isolated from cases of mastitis in the United States, Canada, and Europe (Dellinger et al. 1977, Gourlay et al. 1978). The mastitis is less severe and the infection less persistent than that caused by *M. bovis.* Although the mastitis responds to tetracycline therapy, the organism may continue to spread in an infected herd, and segregation of affected animals is necessary to control an outbreak. *M. canadense* has also been isolated from aborted bovine fetuses (Boughton et al. 1983).

REFERENCES

Boughton, E., Hopper, S.A., Gayford, P.J.R. 1983. *Mycoplasma canadense* from bovine fetuses (correspondence). Vet. Rec. 112:87.

Dellinger, J.D., Jasper, D.E. and Ilic, M. 1977. Characterization studies on mycoplasmas isolated from bovine mastitis and the bovine respiratory tract. Cornell Vet. 67:351–360.

Gourlay, R.N., Wyld, S.G., Bourke, N., and Edmonds, M. 1978. Isolation of *Mycoplasma canadense* from an outbreak of bovine mastitis in England. Vet. Rec. 103:74–75.

Mycoplasma dispar

A respiratory tract commensal of cattle, *M. dispar* forms coccoid cells and short filaments, and the colonies on primary culture lack the defined center typical of most *Mycoplasma* species. An extracellular capsule is present. *M. dispar* is a fastidious grower and enriched media such as GS, SP-4, or FF without penicillin should be used for its culture (Razin and Freundt 1984).

M. dispar is a primary pathogen in the lung of calves but is usually found with other organisms such as *Pasturella multocida, Ureaplasma* species, and viruses. The lesions caused are generally mild and consist of a bronchiolitis and alveolitis. The organism becomes closely associated with the bronchiolar cilia and inhibits the ciliary beat (Howard and Thomas 1974). There is epithelial necrosis and invasion of the bronchiolar wall by lymphocytes. Some infected animals may develop alveolar collapse.

The environmental conditions and stress that predispose an animal toward invasion of the deeper regions of the respiratory tract include regrouping, crowding, chilling, ammonia, fatigue, and change of feed (Stalheim 1983). Primary viral infections are also important in increasing the susceptibility of the tract to opportunistic invasion by *M. dispar.*

REFERENCES

Howard, C.J., and Thomas, L.H. 1974. Inhibition by *Mycoplasma dispar* of ciliary activity in tracheal organ cultures. Infect. Immun. 10:405–508.

Razin, S., and Freundt, E.A. 1984. *Mycoplasma.* In N.R. Kreig and J.G. Holt, eds., Bergey's Manual of Systematic Bacteriology, vol. 1. Williams & Wilkins, Baltimore. P. 755.

Stalheim, O.H. 1983. Mycoplasmal respiratory diseases of ruminants: A review and update. J. Am. Vet. Med. Assoc. 182:403–406.

Mycoplasma verecundum

M. verecundum lacks any outstanding biochemical features. It forms typical coccoid and filamentous cells. It is found in the prepuce of apparently healthy bulls and has also been isolated from the eyes of calves with conjunctivitis (Gourlay et al. 1974).

REFERENCE

Gourlay, R.N., Leach, R.H., and Howard, C.J. 1974. *Mycoplasma verecundum:* A new species isolated from bovine eyes. J. Gen. Microbiol. 81:475–484.

Mycoplasma Species of Goats and Sheep

The *Mycoplasma* species found in goats and sheep are listed in Table 30.2.

Mycoplasma agalactiae

SYNONYMS: *Anulomyces agalaxiae, Borrelomyces agalactiae, Capromyces agalactiae,* organism of contagious agalactia of sheep and goats

Contagious agalactia occurs in the Mediterranean countries of Europe, Portugal, Switzerland, North Africa, Australia, Asia, North and South America, and the Soviet Union. The causative organism, *M. agalactiae,* has typical mycoplasmal morphology. It does not metabolize glucose or hydrolyze arginine but does produce phosphatase and reduce tetrazolium.

Epizootiology and Pathogenesis. Transmission of *M.*

Table 30.2. *Mycoplasma* species affecting sheep and goats

Species	Hosts	Virulence	Disease produced (if any)
M. agalactiae	Sheep, goat	High	Contagious agalactia, arthritis, vulvovaginitis, conjunctivitis, pneumonitis
M. arginini	Wide host range	Low	Mucosal commensal
M. capricolum	Sheep, goat	High	Mastitis, polyarthritis, septicemia in kids
M. conjunctivae	Sheep, goat, chamois	Moderate	Keratoconjunctivitis
M. mycoides subsp. *capri*	Goat	High	Contagious caprine pleuropneumonia
M. mycoides subsp. *mycoides* (large colony type)	Sheep, goat	High	Septicemia, polyarthritis, mastitis, keratoconjunctivitis
M. ovipneumoniae	Sheep, goat	Low	Chronic pneumonia in association with *Pasteurella haemolytica*
M. putrefaciens	Goat	Moderate	Mastitis
Mycoplasma strain F38	Goat	High	Septicemia, contagious caprine pleuropneumonia

agalactiae occurs by ingestion and by direct entry into the test meatus. Because the organism has also been demonstrated in ear mites of affected goats, ectoparasites may play a role in transmission (Cottew and Yeats 1982).

Although the name of the disease suggests udder involvement, the mastitis that develops is usually secondary to a transient bacteremia that can affect males and females alike. The organism localizes in joints, the eyes, lungs, and pleura. The lesions in these sites tend to be chronic. The mastitis is characterized by an altered secretion that is greatly diminished. In some animals milk secretion may cease completely. Abortion may occur and chronically affected animals become weak and emaciated. Animals with subclinical cases can shed the organism in milk for months and can carry the organism from one farm to another (Perreau 1981). The organism can survive in the supramammary lymph nodes and thus be maintained between lactations.

Immunity. Clinical recovery is associated with the development of protective immunity. A live attenuated vaccine has been shown to be protective for goats (Foggie et al. 1970). A killed adjuvanated vaccine is used in eastern Europe. Antibodies detectable by the complement-fixation test and ELISA (Schaeren and Nicolet 1982) develop following a clinical infection and are used to detect flock infection and to determine the infection status of animals being shipped between regions or countries. However, the available serologic tests do not detect all carriers (Cottew 1984).

Antimicrobial Susceptibility. *M. agalactiae* is sensitive to erythromycin, oxytetracycline, and tylosin.

REFERENCES

Cottew, G.S. 1984. Overview of mycoplasmoses in sheep and goats. Isr. J. Med. Sci. 20:962–964.

Cottew, G.S., and Yeats, F.R. 1982. Mycoplasmas and mites in the ears of clinically normal goats. Aust. Vet. J. 59:77–81.

Foggie, A., Etheridge, J.R., Erdag, O., and Arisoy, F. 1970. Contagious agalactia of sheep and goats: Preliminary studies on vaccines. J. Comp. Pathol. 80:345–350.

Perreau, P. 1981. Epidémiologie et diagnostic des mycoplasmoses caprines. Bull. Group. Tech. Vét. 3:87–92.

Schaeren, W., and Nicolet, J. 1982. Micro-ELISA for detecting contagious agalactia in goats. Schweiz. Arch. Tierheilkd. 124:163–177.

Mycoplasma capricolum

M. capricolum causes septicemia, polyarthritis, conjunctivitis, and mastitis in sheep and goats. It forms coccobacillary and short filamentous rods, and colonies are large (1 to 3 mm in diameter). The requirement for cholesterol is lower than for other *Mycoplasma* species.

Epizootiology and Pathogenesis. Having been reported from the United States, France, England, Spain, Australia, India, and Zimbabwe, *M. capricolum* appears to be widely distributed. There is evidence that a similar but apparently less virulent organism is carried in the external ear of sheep and goats (Da Massa et al. 1984) and on the respiratory and genital mucosae of normal goats (Cottew and Yeats 1981). Colostrum or milk can be a source of infection for kids, in which a rapidly developing and fatal septicemia occurs. Transmission in older animals is not well understood but probably occurs by ingestion or inhalation. Carrier animals have been implicated in spread of the infection from one region to another.

The disease is acute and severe. An initial septicemia results in joint localization with a fibrinopurulent polyarthritis (Da Massa et al. 1984). Localization in the udder results in mastitis. Acute diffuse interstitial pneumonia has also been described (Perreau and Breard 1979), and the organism has been isolated from an outbreak of vulvovaginitis and balanoposthitis in a sheep flock in England (Jones 1983).

REFERENCES

Cottew, G.S. and Yeats, F.R. 1981. Occurrence of mycoplasmas in clinically normal goats. Aust. Vet. J. 57:52–53.
Da Massa, A.J., Brooks, D.L., and Holmberg, C.A. 1984. Pathogenicity of *Mycoplasma capricolum* and *Mycoplasma putrefaciens*. Isr. J. Med. Sci. 20:975–978.
Jones, G.E. 1983. Mycoplasmas of sheep and goats: A synopsis. Vet. Rec. 113:619–620.
Perreau, P., and Breard, A. 1979. La mycoplasmose caprine à *M. capricolum*. Comp. Immunol. Microbiol. Infect. Dis. 2:87–97.

Mycoplasma conjunctivae

M. conjunctivae has been isolated from outbreaks of conjunctivitis in sheep and goats in North America and Australia and is probably distributed in sheep and goat populations throughout the world (Cottew 1979). Coccoid to coccobacillary cells are formed. The colonies are greenish or olive (Barile et al. 1972).

Epizootiology and Pathogenesis. The habitat of *M. conjunctivae* has not been discovered, and little is known about transmission of the agent or the pathogenesis of the conjunctivitis. The organism is occasionally found in the respiratory tract.

REFERENCES

Barile, M.F., DelGiudice, R.A., and Tully, J.G. 1972. Isolation and characterization of *Mycoplasma conjunctivae* sp. n. from sheep and goats with keratoconjunctivitis. Infect. Immun. 5:70–76.
Cottew, G.S. 1979. Caprine-ovine mycoplasmas. In J.G. Tully and R.F. Whitcomb, eds., The Mycoplasmas, vol. 2: Human and Animal Mycoplasmas. Academic Press, New York. P. 103.

Mycoplasma mycoides subspecies *capri*
SYNONYMS: *Asterococcus mycoides* var. *capri, Capromyces pleuropneumoniae*

M. mycoides subsp. *capri* causes contagious pleuropneumonia (CCPP) in goats, a disease similar to CBPP in cattle and found in Africa, Asia, Australia, and Sweden (Jones 1983). Although a disease of considerable antiquity, there have been very few reports of the isolation of *M. mycoides* subsp. *capri* from cases of the disease in recent years (Cottew 1984, McMartin et al. 1980).

Rather, a CCPP-like disease has been observed in Europe, Africa, and Asia, where the causative agent was either *M. mycoides* subsp. *mycoides* (large colony type) or a *Mycoplasma* strain designated F38. Strain F38 was recovered from cases of CCPP in Kenya and Sudan. CCPP is therefore a disease entity that can be caused by three different *Mycoplasma* species. Caprine isolates of *M. mycoides* subsp. *mycoides* (large colony type), although capable of producing severe experimental disease in calves (Rosendal 1981), do not appear to be easily transmitted from goats to cattle, nor have goats ever been shown to be a source of contagion in outbreaks of contagious bovine pleuropneumonia.

Morphology and Staining Characteristics. The morphology of *M. mycoides* subsp. *capri* is typical of mycoplasmas, as described on p. 296. Oleic acid in the medium (50 μm/ml) enhances filament formation.

Cultural and Biochemical Features. The colonies attain a diameter of 1.5 to 2.5 mm after 3 days. Only minimal quantities of cholesterol are required for growth. *M. mycoides* subsp. *capri* metabolizes glucose, reduces tetrazolium, and hydrolyzes gelatin, coagulated serum, and casein.

Antigens. Capsular glucan is a major antigenic component. *M. mycoides* subsp. *capri* is more closely related serologically to the large colony type of *M. mycoides* subsp. *mycoides* than to the small colony strains of subspecies *mycoides* (Rodwell and Rodwell 1978).

Epizootiology and Pathogenesis. *M. mycoides* subsp. *capri* is transmitted by the respiratory route via inhalation of droplets. Because it produces hydrogen peroxide and inhibits the activity of epithelial cilia, the host is unable to clear the invading organism from its respiratory airways. The incubation period is about 6 to 10 days. Although close contact among goats is necessary for spread of infection, the morbidity may reach 100 percent and as many as 70 percent of affected animals may die. Migrating nomadic herds can carry the infection from one region to another (Okoh and Kaldas 1980). Affected animals develop a cough, lag behind the flock, and lie down, exhibiting labored respiration. There is a fever of 40.5° to 41.5°C. Animals with acute disease may die in a couple of days.

At necropsy there are many pea-sized yellow nodules throughout the lung parenchyma. In some animals these lesions are coalescent. There is pleuritis with deposits of fibrin on the pleura and accumulation of fluid in the pleural and pericardial cavities (arthritis may also be present). Animals with highly acute disease may show lesions only of septicemia. See the excellent review by McMartin et al. (1980) for further details on the epizootiology and pathogenesis of *M. mycoides* subsp. *capri*.

This organism is readily demonstrated in the tissues and

fluids of goats with acute cases but is difficult to find in chronic lesions.

Immunity. *M. mycoides* subsp. *capri* carries protective antigens that immunize the animal against other strains of subsp. *capri* but not against most small or large colony strains of *M. mycoides* subsp. *mycoides* (Smith and Oliphant 1982). Diagnostic serologic tests include a slide serum agglutination test with stained antigen and the complement-fixation test. These tests are not widely available and have not been well standardized (Cottew 1984). A vaccine adsorbed to aluminum hydroxide terpene has been successfully used in the field (Cecarelli and Fontanelli 1950).

Antimicrobial Susceptibility. *M. mycoides* subsp. *capri* is sensitive to tetracyclines, tiamulin, and tylosin.

REFERENCES

Cecarelli, A., and Fontanelli, E. 1950. The complement fixation test for the diagnosis of contagious agalactiae in sheep and goats. Zooprofilassi 5:409–418.
Cottew, G.S. 1984. Overview of mycoplasmoses in sheep and goats. Isr. J. Med. Sci. 20:962–964.
Jones, G.E. 1983. Mycoplasmas of sheep and goats: A synopsis. Vet. Rec. 113:619–620.
McMartin, D.A., MacOwan, K.J., and Swift, L.L. 1980. A century of classical contagious caprine pleuropneumonia: From original description to aetiology. Br. Vet. J. 136:507–511.
Okoh, A.E.J., and Kaldas, M.Y. 1980. Contagious caprine pleuropneumonia in goats in Gumel, Nigeria. Bull. Anim. Health Prod. Afr. 28:97–102.
Rodwell, A.W., and Rodwell, E.S. 1978. Relationships between strains of *Mycoplasma mycoides* subsp. *mycoides* and *capri* studied by two-dimensional gel electrophoresis of cell proteins. J. Gen. Microbiol. 109:259–263.
Rosendal, S. 1981. Experimental infection of goats, sheep, and calves with the large colony type of *Mycoplasma mycoides* subsp. *mycoides*. Vet. Pathol. 18:71–81.
Smith, G.R., and Oliphant, J.C. 1982. Some in-vitro characters of the subspecies of *Mycoplasma mycoides*. J. Hyg. 89:521–527.

Mycoplasma ovipneumoniae

Occuring on the mucosal surface of the respiratory and reproductive tracts of normal sheep and goats (Cottew and Yeats 1981), *M. ovipneumoniae* contributes to lesion development in the lower respiratory tract only as an opportunistic invader. Its morphology is poorly defined and the colonies are unusual in that they lack the distinct central area characteristic of most *Mycoplasma* species. They have a vacuolated appearance.

Epizootiology and Pathogenesis. The circumstances that lead to invasion of the respiratory tract by *M. ovipneumoniae* are not well defined. The organism has been isolated from pneumonic lungs in goats in Texas (Livingston and Gauer 1979) and from chronic proliferative interstitial pneumonia in sheep (Carmichael et al.

1972). Its role in disease production is probably as a synergist with other respiratory pathogens such as *Pasteurella haemolytica* (Jones et al. 1982).

REFERENCES

Carmichael, L.E., St. George, T.D., Sullivan, N.D., and Horsfall, N. 1972. Isolation, propagation and characterization studies of an ovine mycoplasma responsible for proliferative interstitial pneumonia. Cornell Vet. 62:654–679.
Cottew, G.S., and Yeats, F.R. 1981. Occurrence of mycoplasmas in clinically normal goats. Aust. Vet. J. 57:52–53.
Jones, G.E., Gilmour, J.S., and Rae, A.G. 1982. I. The effect of *Mycoplasma ovipneumoniae* and *Pasteurella haemolytica* on specific pathogen-free lambs. II. The effects of different strains of *Mycoplasmas ovipneumoniae* on specific pathogen-free and conventionally-reared lambs. J. Comp. Pathol. 92:261–266, 267–272.
Livingston, C.W., Jr., and Gauer, B.B. 1979. Isolation of *Mycoplasma ovipneumoniae* from Spanish and Angora goats. Am. J. Vet. Res. 40:407–408.

Mycoplasma putrefaciens

M. putrefaciens has been isolated from outbreaks of purulent mastitis of goats in California and France (Adler et al. 1980). The geographic distribution of the organism has not been defined. It produces mostly coccoid cells. A strong putrefactive odor emanates from broth cultures, hence the specific name of the organism. Cholesterol should be supplied at 1 µg/ml of medium.

Epizootiology and Pathogenesis. The ecological niche of *M. putrefaciens* in goats is not known. As few as 50 organisms will induce mastitis following intramammary infusion. The mastitis is unusual in that there is no clinical evidence of abnormality other than a drop in milk flow and the presence of inflammatory cells in the secretion (Adler et al. 1980). The mastitis is confined to the inoculated quarter, and the infection results in a protective immune response that persists for at least a year (Brooks et al. 1981).

REFERENCES

Adler, H.E., DaMassa, A.J., and Brooks, D.L. 1980. Caprine mycoplasmosis: *Mycoplasma putrefaciens*, a new cause of mastitis in goats. Am. J. Vet. Res. 41:1677–1679.
Brooks, D.L., DaMassa, A.J., and Adler, H.E. 1981. Caprine mycoplasmosis: Immune response in goats to *Mycoplasma putrefaciens* after intramammary inoculation. Am. J. Vet. Res. 42:1898–1900.

Mycoplasma strain F38

SYNONYM: *Mycoplasma capripneumoniae*

Mycoplasma strain F38 was first isolated from outbreaks of caprine contagious pleuropneumonia (CCPP) in Kenya in 1977. It also caused outbreaks in Sudan in 1981, where the disease is termed *Abu Nino,* and in Tunisia in 1984 (MacOwan 1984).

Strain F38 is antigenically distinct from *M. mycoides* subsp. *capri* and subsp. *mycoides* (large colony type) but cross-reacts in the growth precipitation test with all of the subspecies and strains of *M. mycoides* (Erno et al. 1983). On the basis of morphologic, biochemical, electrophoretic, and serologic studies, researchers have proposed that strain F38 has enough distinctive characteristics to justify the formation of a new species, *M. capripneumoniae* (El Tahir and Blobel 1984).

Epizootiology and Pathogenesis. The epizootiology and pathogenesis associated with strain F38 is apparently similar to that of *M. mycoides* subsp. *capri.* Indeed, most African outbreaks of CCPP in recent years have probably been caused by strain F38, not by *M. mycoides* subsp. *capri.* So far, there is no evidence that strain F38 has spread to other continents. Sheep do not appear to be susceptible.

In one study goats inoculated with strain F38 developed a severe disease indistinguishable from classical CCPP. The only difference noted was that edema was not produced at the site of inoculation as is usually the case with *M. mycoides* subsp. *capri* (MacOwan and Minette 1976). The organism was transmitted by contact between the inoculated and noninoculated goats in the group. In another study experimental infection of goats with strain F38 resulted in a septicemia with fever, anorexia, ptyalism, and dyspnea. The organism was present in the lung, liver, kidney, lymph, blood, and spleen. The lungs exhibited a serofibrinous pneumonia (Perreau et al. 1984).

Immunity. Sonicated, adjuvanated F38 has been successfully used to vaccinate goats (Rurangirwa, Masiga, and Muthomi 1981). Complement-fixing and passive hemagglutinating antibody is present in the serum of infected goats (MacOwan and Minette 1976, Muthomi and Rurangirwa 1983). The complement-fixation test is more specific for F38 infection.

Antimicrobial Susceptibility. Strain F38 appears to be susceptible to oxytetracycline, streptomycin, and tylosin (Hassan et al. 1984; Rurangirwa, Masiga, Muria, et al. 1981).

REFERENCES

El Tahir, M.S., and Blobel, H. 1984. Mycoplasmas in goats with contagious caprine pleuropneumonia. Zentralbl. Veterinärmed. [B] 31:51–57.

Erno, H., Leach, R.H., Salih, M.M. and MacOwan, K.J. 1983. The F38-like group, a new group of caprine mycoplasmas? Acta Vet. Scand. 24:275–286.

Hassan, S.M., El Harbi, M.S.M.A., and Bakr, M.I. 1984. Treatment of contagious caprine pleuropneumonia. Vet. Res. Comm. 8:65–67.

MacOwan, K.J. 1984. Role of mycoplasma strain F38 in contagious caprine pleuropneumonia. Isr. J. Med. Sci. 20:979–981.

MacOwan, K.J., and Minette, J.E. 1976. A mycoplasma from acute contagious caprine pleuropneumonia in Kenya. Trop. Anim. Health Prod. 8:91–95.

Muthomi, E.K., and Rurangirwa, F.R. 1983. Passive haemagglutination and complement fixation as diagnostic tests for contagious caprine pleuroponeumonia caused by F38 strain of mycoplasma. Res. Vet. Sci. 35:1–4.

Perreau, P., Breard, A., and Goff, C. 1984. Experimental infection of goats with type F38 mycoplasma strains (CCPP). Ann. Microbiol. 135A:119–124.

Rurangirwa, F.R., Masiga, W.N., Muria, D.N., Muthomi, E., Mulira, G., Kagumba, M., and Nandskha, E. 1981. Treatment of contagious caprine pleuropneumonia. Trop. Anim. Health Prod. 13:177–182.

Rurangirwa, F.R., Masiga, W.N., and Muthomi, E. 1981. Immunity to contagious caprine pleuropneumonia caused by F38 strain of mycoplasma. Vet. Rec. 109:310–311.

Mycoplasma Species of Swine

Four species of *Mycoplasma* infect pigs (Table 10.3), of which *M. hyopneumoniae* is the most important as a cause of disease.

Mycoplasma flocculare

M. flocculare has occasionally been isolated from lesions typical of mycoplasmal pneumonia of swine (Armstrong and Friis 1981). In some animals it was present with *M. hyopneumoniae.* Of low virulence, it is normally found as a commensal of the nasopharynx and eye of healthy swine.

The cells have a typical mycoplasmal morphology. The colonies are small (0.5 to 1.0 mm in diameter) and do not look like fried eggs. Colonies in broth form fluffy aggregates. *M. flocculare* is very fastidious and requires either A26 or FF medium for growth (Razin and Freundt 1984).

Table 30.3. *Mycoplasma* species affecting swine

Species	Virulence	Disease produced (if any)
M. flocculare	Low	Pneumonia; a commensal of the upper respiratory mucosa and eye
M. hyopneumoniae	High	Enzootic pneumonia
M. hyorhinis	Low	Arthritis, polyserositis, pneumonia; a commensal of the upper respiratory mucosa that can opportunistically invade the lungs
M. hyosynoviae	Moderate	Nonsuppurative polyarthritis; nasopharyngeal commensal

REFERENCES

Armstrong, C.H., and Friis, N.F. 1981. Isolation of *Mycoplasma floc-culare* from swine in the United States. Am. J. Vet. Res. 42:1030–1032.

Razin, S.H., and Freundt, E.A. 1984. Mycoplasmataceae. In N.R. Kreig and J.G. Holt, eds., Bergey's Manual of Systematic Bacteriology, vol. 1. Williams & Wilkins, Baltimore. Pp. 755–758.

Mycoplasma hyopneumoniae

SYNONYM: *Mycoplasma suipneumoniae*

M. hyopneumoniae causes enzootic pneumonia of pigs (EPP), a disease that has also been called virus pneumonia of swine, infectious pneumonia of pigs, and *Ferkelgrippe*. EPP occurs wherever swine are raised and causes severe economic hardship because of slowed weight gain and inefficient food conversion. Switzer (1973) has estimated that between 35 and 60 percent of swine slaughtered in the midwestern United States have lesions of EPP.

Morphology and Staining Characteristics. The cells have a typical mycoplasmal coccoid and short filamentous form. In liquid culture the organism appears as cocci on fine branching filaments or as globular structures (microcolonies).

Cultural and Biochemical Features. The colonies are tiny, convex (0.5 mm in diameter), and very slow growing. Since there is no distinct central area, there is no fried egg appearance. Primary cultures must be grown in complex broth media such as A26 or FF (Razin and Freundt 1984) in an atmosphere of 5 percent CO_2.

Epizootiology and Pathogenesis. *M. hyopneumoniae* lives only in the respiratory tract of pigs and survives briefly in the external environment. It was once believed that herds free of infection based on clinical and pathological criteria would remain free of the disease if no swine were added except those derived from EPP-free herds or those raised in isolation after being born by cesarian section. Experience in England, however, has indicated that EPP-free herds do experience breakdowns (Goodwin 1977, 1984) in which the origin of infection is unexplained but appears to be extraneous.

M. hyopneumoniae is spread in aerosols generated by infected pigs and can be transmitted in this way from sows to their piglets. It is also introduced into herds by the addition of infected stock. It is not transmitted across the placenta (Heitmann and Kirchhoff 1981). Pigs usually show signs of infection at 3 to 10 weeks of age. After an incubation period of 8 to 14 days, a transient diarrhea may develop, followed by a dry cough that may last for a few weeks or persist indefinitely. Affected pigs eat well but are unthrifty and are slow to gain weight. The worst affected may be severely stunted. Many infected animals may be clinically normal but have pronounced lung lesions at slaughter.

Following infection, the organism is found adhering to the bronchial and bronchiolar epithelial surfaces of the lungs, where it causes ciliostasis. By 4 to 6 weeks, the number of cells at these locations is maximal and thereafter the numbers decline as lesion severity increases (Amanfu et al. 1984). Lesion development appears partly to be associated with cell-mediated responses to the organism. Thymectomized pigs exhibit less prominent perivascular and peribronchiolar infiltrations of lymphocytes following infection than do nonthymectomized animals (Tajima et al. 1984).

The lesions of EPP are hepatized, purplish or grayish pneumonic areas in the apical and cardiac lobes of the lung. Histologically, the lung lesions are characterized by mononuclear cell accumulation and peribronchiolar lymphoreticular hyperplasia. An exudate consisting mainly of polymorphonuclear leukocytes is present in the alveoli and lumina of the terminal airways. Secondary bacterial invasions of pneumonic areas may occur.

Infected animals may continue to shed the organism, which persists in pulmonary lesions and draining lymph nodes. The lesions may be exacerbated by secondary invasions of a variety of opportunistic pathogens such as pasteurellae, *Bordetella bronchiseptica*, and *M. hyorhinis*.

Immunity. Recovered swine are resistant to reinfection, indicating that protective immunity does develop in EPP (Goodwin et al. 1969). The roles of local and cell-mediated immune responses have not been well defined, but presumably both are required for optimum protection. Vaccines prepared from formalinized whole cells, culture supernatant, and saline washes of cells and administered intramuscularly have been shown to protect swine against pneumonia (Ross et al. 1984). Complement-fixing, precipitating, and growth-inhibitory antibodies are produced some weeks after infection, but tests based on the presence of these antibodies are not reliable for the detection of infected individuals (Lloyd et al. 1984). Complement-fixing antibodies are probably not involved in resistance to infection (Stipkovitz et al. 1978).

Diagnosis. The indirect hemagglutination and CF tests are useful in the detection of infected herds (Schuller et al. 1977). Switzer (1973) observed that the complement-fixation test is positive in twice as many swine as have lesions of EPP at slaughter.

The organism may be demonstrated in Giemsa-stained touch preparations of lung lesions (Goodwin et al. 1967), where it appears in ring and bipolar forms. Touch preparations can also be examined by the more sensitive indirect immunofluorescent or immunoperoxidase procedures.

Almost 20 percent of normal lungs may reveal the presence of the organism by indirect immunofluorescence (Armstrong et al. 1984).

Complement-fixing antibodies are detectable about 5 weeks after nasal infection (Lloyd et al. 1984). Antibodies detectable by ELISA appear about 2 weeks after nasal infection (Piffer et al. 1984). Similarly, antibodies are detectable earlier by a tube latex agglutination test than by a CF test.

A variety of liquid media for the isolation of *M. hyopneumoniae* from lung tissue have been developed (Chenglee et al. 1982, Goodwin 1976, Li et al. 1982). The medium developed by Goodwin contains 30 percent serum, of which one-third by volume is rabbit antiserum to *M. hyorhinis*. This antibody suppresses growth of *M. hyorhinis*, a common secondary invader of lesions initiated by *M. hyopneumoniae*.

Besides the laboratory methods described above, herd diagnosis of EPP also relies heavily on the gross and microscopic pathological appearance of the lesions at slaughter and the clinical and epizootiological features of the disease in the herd.

Antimicrobial Susceptibility. *M. hyopneumoniae* is sensitive to doxycycline, kitasamycin, lincomycin, tiamulin, tetracycline, and tylosin. However, antibiotics are less effective therapeutically than prophylactically. Studies have shown that tetracycline will inhibit lesion development if administered at the time the pigs are infected but does not affect lesions if given later (Switzer 1973). Tiamulin in the feed has been shown to significantly improve weight gain and feed conversion efficiently in affected herds (Burch 1984).

REFERENCES

Amanfu, W., Weng, C.N., Ross, R.F., and Barnes, H.J. 1984. Diagnosis of mycoplasmal pneumonia of swine: Sequential study by direct immunofluorescence. Am. J. Vet. Res. 45:1349–1352.
Armstrong, C.H., Schiedt, A.B., Thacker, H.L., Runnels, L.J., and Freeman, M.J. 1984. Evaluation of criteria for the postmortem diagnosis of mycoplasmal pneumonia of swine. Can. J. Comp. Med. 48:278–281.
Burch, D.G.S. 1984. Tiamulin feed premix in the improvement of growth performance of pigs in herds severely affected with enzootic pneumonia. Vet. Rec. 114:209–211.
Chenglee, H., Tzinghua, C., and Hungshiao, C. 1982. A new inexpensive medium for cultivation of *Mycoplasma hyopneumoniae*. Rev. Infect. Dis. (Suppl.) 4:265.
Goodwin, R.F.W. 1976. An improved medium for the isolation of *Mycoplasma suipneumoniae*. Vet. Rec. 98:260–261.
Goodwin, R.F.W. 1977. Apparent reinfection of enzootic-pneumonia-free pig herds: Specificity of diagnosis. Vet. Rec. 101:419–421.
Goodwin, R.F.W. 1984. Apparent reinfection of enzootic-pneumonia-free pig herds: Early signs and incubation period. Vet. Rec. 115:320–324.
Goodwin, R.F.W., Hodgson, R.G., Whittlestone, P., and Woodhams, R.L. 1969. Immunity in experimentally induced enzootic pneumonia of pigs. J. Hyg. 67:193–208.
Goodwin, R.F.W., Pomeroy, A.P., and Whittlestone, P. 1967. Characterization of *Mycoplasma suipneumoniae*: A mycoplasma causing enzootic pneumonia of pigs. J. Hyg. 65:85–96.
Heitmann, J., and Kirchhoff, H. 1981. Transmission of mycoplasma from dam to fetus in the pig. Zentralbl. Veterinärmed. [B] 28:378–385.
Li, Y.L., Dong, Q.H., and Ziu, X.W. 1982. A study on liquid media for cultivation of *Mycoplasma hyopneumoniae*. I. Improvement of liquid media for *M. hyopneumoniae* (MSP). II. Infusion preparation and its effect on the growth of MSP. Chin. J. Vet. Med. 8:8–11.
Lloyd, L.C., Badman, R.T., Etheridge, J.R., McKechnie, K., and Iyer, H. 1984. Assessment of a complement fixation test to detect *Mycoplasma hyopneumoniae* infection in pigs. Aust. Vet. J. 61:216–218.
Piffer, I.A., Young, T.F., Petenate, A., and Ross, R.F. 1984. Comparison of complement fixation test and enzyme-linked immunosorbent assay for detection of early infection with *Mycoplasma hyopneumoniae*. Am. J. Vet. Res. 45:1122–1126.
Razin, S.H., and Freundt, E.A. 1984. Mycoplasmataceae. In N.R. Kreig and J.G. Holt, eds., Bergey's Manual of Systematic Bacteriology, vol. 1. Williams & Wilkins, Baltimore. Pp. 755–758.
Ross, R.F., Zimmermann-Erickson, B.J., and Young, T.F. 1984. Characteristics of protective activity of *Mycoplasma hyopneumoniae* vaccine. Am. J. Vet. Res. 45:1899–1905.
Schuller, V.W., Swoboda, R., and Baumgartner, W. 1977. Comparative investigations about some nonclinical diagnostic methods for the diagnosis of enzootic pneumonia. Wien. Tierärztl. Monatsschr. 64:236–241.
Stipkovitz, V.L., Laher, G., and Schuntze, E. 1978. Tiamulin, a new antibiotic for controlling enzootic pneumonia in swine. D.T.W. 85:464–466.
Switzer, W.P. 1973. Response of swine to *Mycoplasma hyopneumoniae* infection. J. Infect. Dis. 127:S59–S60.
Tajima, M., Yagihashi, T., Nunoya, T., Takeuchi, A., and Ohashi, F. 1984. *Mycoplasma hyopneumoniae* infection in pigs immunosuppressed by thymectomy and treatment with antithymocyte serum. Am. J. Vet. Res. 45:1928–1932.

Mycoplasma hyorhinis

M. hyorhinis is a normal inhabitant of the nasopharynx of swine and is also a common contaminant of cell and tissue cultures. Methods for its detection have been intensively studied for this reason.

It has a typical mycoplasmal morphology. Some strains cannot be cultivated on available cell-free media and are apparently inhibited by medium components. A number of serologic variants exist, but the significance of these in opportunistic disease production is unknown.

Epizootiology and Pathogenesis. Infection by *M. hyorhinis* develops during the first few weeks of life. Initial invasion of the respiratory tract is commonly subclinical. If the pigs are stressed, however, invasion of the bloodstream may sometimes occur, with subsequent localization of the organism on serous surfaces including the synovial membranes. The polyserositis caused by *M. hyorhinis* is characterized by a serofibrinous synovitis and arthritis, pericarditis, pleuritis, and peritonitis. The synovial membrane shows mild hyperemia and hypertrophy of the synovial villi associated with a yellowish coloration of the synovial membrane. Histopathologically, these changes are characterized by hypertrophy of the synovial villi, hyperplasia of synovial cells, and lymphocytic infiltration concentrated in nodular foci (Roberts et al. 1963). The synovial fluid is increased in volume and contains flecks of fibrin. Affected pigs are stiff and reluctant to stand or move. Recovery is slow but often is complete, without permanent damage to the joint. Complement-fixing antibodies develop within 2 weeks of infection and persist for at least 6 months (Ross et al. 1973).

M. hyorhinis is frequently isolated from the turbinates of pigs with atrophic rhinitis, where it is an opportunistic invader secondary to *Bordetella bronchiseptica* or *Pasteurella multocida* infection. It is also commonly found in the nasal cavities and in lung lesions of EPP in association with *M. hyopneumoniae*. Its presence complicates the isolation of *M. hyopneumoniae*. Some studies have shown that 70 percent of nasal swabs from pigs from herds with EPP were positive for *M. hyorhinis*. The isolation rate declined with increasing age.

Immunity. A healthy pig has a high level of natural resistance to invasion by *M. hyorhinis*. Resistance can be increased by immunization with inactivated vaccine (Androsik 1983).

Antimicrobial Susceptibility. *M. hyorhinis* is sensitive to lincomycin, tiamulin, and tylosin. Treatment is effective in the early stages of infection.

REFERENCES

Androsik, N.N. 1983. Immunological efficacy of inactivated vaccines against *Mycoplasma hyorhinis*. Vet. Nauka-Proizvodstvu 21:37–40.

Roberts, E.D., Switzer, W.P., and Ramsey, F.K. 1963. The pathology of *Mycoplasma hyorhinis* arthritis produced experimentally in swine. Am. J. Vet. Res. 24:19–31.

Ross, R.F., Dale, S.E., and Duncan, J.R. 1973. Experimentally induced *Mycoplasma hyorhinis* arthritis of swine: Immune response to 26th postinoculation week. Am. J. Vet. Res. 34:367–372.

Mycoplasma hyosynoviae

M. hyosynoviae is a common inhabitant of the nasopharynx of swine. In the United States it is often the cause of polyarthritis in weanling pigs.

The cell morphology is typical of the genus. A granular deposit and a surface pellicle are produced in broth culture. Strain differences as reflected by differences in protein profiles have been observed (Wreghitt et al. 1974).

Methods for its isolation and identification have been described (Gois and Taylor-Robinson 1972, Ross and Karman 1970). It requires sterols, does not ferment glucose or hydrolyze urea, and uses arginine. Its growth is enhanced under anaerobiasis, a property that is useful in its selective isolation from nasal cavities of pigs (Ogata et al. 1982).

Epizootiology and Pathogenesis. The principal reservoir of *M. hyosynoviae* is the adult carrier pig. The organism persists in the tonsil and is shed in the nasal and pharyngeal secretions (Ross and Spear 1973). Stress is an important predisposing cause of outbreaks, and there is a breed susceptibility: Hampshire swine develop a more severe disease following infection than do other breeds (Ross et al. 1971).

As a result of stress (regrouping, change of feed or housing, transport) the infection in the tonsil spreads into the bloodstream and then into the joints, causing synovitis, synovial effusion, and villous hypertrophy. There is minimal damage to cartilage. Affected swine become stiff and lame and have difficulty in rising. The organism is rapidly cleared from affected joints, and complete recovery usually occurs after a few weeks.

Diagnosis. The organism can be demonstrated only during the acute phase of the arthritis (Ross 1973). Complement-fixing antibodies develop about 10 days after infection. These antibodies are also present in pharyngeal carriers (Ross and Spear 1973).

Antimicrobial Susceptibility. *M. hyosynoviae* is sensitive to tiamulin, lincomycin, and tylosin. Tiamulin given intramuscularly has been shown to be an effective treatment for clinically affected pigs (Burch and Goodwin 1984).

REFERENCES

Burch, D.G.S., and Goodwin, R.F.W. 1984. Use of tiamulin in a herd of pigs seriously affected with *M. hyosynoviae* arthritis. Vet. Rec. 115:594–595.

Gois, M., and Taylor-Robinson, D. 1972. The identification and characterization of some porcine arginine-utilising mycoplasma strains. J. Med. Microbiol. 5:47–54.

Ogata, M., Kawamura, S., and Yamamoto, K. 1982. Selective isolation of *M. hyosynoviae* by anaerobic cultivation. Jpn. J. Vet. Sci. 44:725–733.

Ross, R.F. 1973. Pathogenicity of swine mycoplasmas. Ann. N.Y. Acad. Sci. 225:359–368.

Ross, R.F., and Karman, J.A. 1970. Heterogeneity among strains of *Mycoplasma granularum* and identification of *Mycoplasma hyosynoviae*, sp.n. J. Bacteriol. 103:707–713.

Ross, R.F., and Spear, M.L. 1973. Role of the sow as a reservoir of infection for *Mycoplasma hyosynoviae*. Am. J. Vet. Res. 34:373–378.

Ross, R.F., Switzer, W.P., and Duncan, J.R. 1971. Experimental production of *Mycoplasma hyosynoviae* arthritis in swine. Am. J. Vet. Res. 32:1743–1749.

Wreghitt, T.G., Windsor, G.D., and Butler, M. 1974. Flat gel polyacrylamide electrophoresis of porcine mycoplasmas. Appl. Microbiol. 28:530–533.

Mycoplasma Species of Poultry

At least nine *Mycoplasma* species have been identifed as either commensals or significant pathogens of poultry

Table 30.4. *Mycoplasma* species affecting poultry

Species	Host	Virulence	Disease produced (if any)
M. anatis	Duck	Low	Sinusitis; normal commensal of respiratory tract and cloaca
M. cloacae	Turkey	Low	Commensal of cloaca
M. columbinasale	Pigeon	Low	Mild respiratory disease; commensal of upper respiratory tract
M. columbinum	Pigeon	Low	Mild respiratory disease; commensal of upper respiratory tract
M. columborale	Pigeon	Low	Mild respiratory disease; commensal of upper respiratory tract
M. gallisepticum	Chicken, turkey, and other birds	High	Air sacculitis, sinusitis, arthritis, synovitis, encephalitis
M. iowae	Turkey	High	Embryo mortality, air sacculitis
M. meleagridis	Turkey	High	Air sacculitis, perosis, arthritis, salpingitis, synovitis
M. synoviae	Chicken, turkey	High	Synovitis

(Table 30.4). *M. anatis* has been isolated from a duck with sinusitis but appears to be relatively avirulent. It is a component of the normal respiratory and cloacal flora of ducks. *M. cloacae* is a normal commensal of the cloaca of turkeys. *M. columbinasale, M. columbinum,* and *M. columborale* are commensals of the upper respiratory tract of pigeons and can contribute to lesion development in the upper respiratory tract (Keymer et al. 1984). *M. gallisepticum* is an important respiratory pathogen of chickens and turkeys. *M. iowae* causes mortality in turkey embryos, and *M. meleagridis* and *M. synoviae* are associated with air sacculitis and synovitis, respectively, of older turkeys and chickens. Only the latter four pathogenic species are described in further detail in this chapter.

Mycoplasma gallisepticum

Found wherever poultry are raised intensively, *M. gallisepticum* is associated with the disease complex described as chronic respiratory disease (CRD) and observed in chickens, turkeys, pheasants, pigeons, partridges, and other domestic and wild birds. In turkeys the disease is also known as infectious sinusitis of turkeys (IST).

Morphology and Staining Characteristics. *M. gallisepticum* is ovoid with a characteristic polar bleb that serves as an adhesion organ.

Cultural and Biochemical Features. Colonies of *M. gallisepticum* have a classical fried egg morphology. The organism metabolizes glucose and reduces tetrazolium. There is no phosphatase or protease activity. Erythrocytes are agglutinated by most strains; attachment involves the polar bleb and glycophorin, a glycoprotein found on the surface of the erythrocyte and rich in sialic acid. Hemagglutination is inhibited by antiserum to *M. gallisepticum.* The organism is inactivated in infected eggs at 45°C for 12 to 14 hours (Yoder et al. 1977).

Epizootiology and Pathogenesis. *M. gallisepticum* is commonly spread by infectious aerosol, by contact, and by egg transmission following infection of the egg during formation in the ovary or passage through the oviduct. It has also been transmitted in contaminated virus vaccines. CRD may enhance the severity of infections by bacteria such as *Haemophilus gallinarum* and *Escherichia coli* or viruses such as infectious bronchitis virus.

The polar bleb and possibly capsular material mediate adhesion of *M. gallisepticum* to tracheal and bronchial epithelium (Tajima et al. 1982). The ciliostatic property of the organism is also of importance in its ability to colonize the lower respiratory tract and avoid removal by the mucociliary escalator.

CRD in chickens typically has a long incubation period (1 to 3 weeks) and a long course. It is accompanied by tracheal rales, nasal discharge, and coughing. Feed consumption is reduced, egg production may be lowered, and the birds lose weight. In chicks the disease may take the form of a simple coryza. Gross lesions of the respiratory tract give rise to mucoid to mucopurulent exudate in the trachea, bronchi, air sacs, and nasal passages. The oviducts are frequently involved. Instances of synovitis involving the synovial membranes of the joints, tendovaginal sheaths, and bursae have been noted. Microscopically, the mucous membranes are thickened, hyperplastic, and infiltrated with mononuclear cells.

In turkeys IST is characterized by swelling of the infraorbital sinuses. These are filled with a thick mucoid exudate. In some birds conjunctivitis and inflammation of the air sacs are observed. The disease runs a chronic course, and affected birds lose weight. The death rate usually is not high, but the failure to gain weight may cause considerable economic loss. The lesions are progressive and much more extensive than those of CRD, with severe involvement of the nasal passages, sinuses, lungs, and air sacs. Brain, synovial, and joint lesions have also been seen.

Immunity. Both cell-mediated and humoral immune responses develop following infection and contribute to protective immunity. Cell-mediated responses become evident at about 1 week and peak at about 7 weeks after infection (Chhabra and Goel 1981). Hemagglutinating antibodies also peak at about 7 weeks in serum and at 6 weeks in tracheal washings. Recovery coincides with the time of peak immune responsiveness.

Maternal antibodies confer very little protection against experimental challenge a few days after hatching (Lin and Kleven 1984b).

Both live and inactivated vaccines give partial protection against egg production losses, respiratory signs and lesions, and egg transmission (Kleven et al. 1984). Attenuated live vaccines (F, R, S6, and A5969) given intraconjunctivally or by aerosol routes are effective (Lin and Kleven 1984a). A temperature-sensitive mutant of *M. gallisepticum* (Ts100) has also been used to protect chicks (Lam and Lin 1984).

Diagnosis. The history, lesions observed, and cultural and serologic procedures are all used to establish the diagnosis. The rapid serum plate (RSA) and tube agglutination tests, the hemagglutination-inhibition (HI) test, the complement-fixation test, ELISA, electrophoresis of cell proteins, immunofluorescence, and immunoperoxidase techniques have been used for serologic diagnosis and identification of isolates. The rapid serum plate and hemagglutination-inhibition tests in particular have been widely and successfully used for detection of infection in eradication programs. These two tests and metabolic inhibition tests have been shown to be of comparable sensitivity (Nougayrede et al. 1984).

Antimicrobial Susceptibility. *M. gallisepticum* is sensitive to lincomycin, tetracyclines, tiamulin, and tylosin. Strains resistant to tylosin have been observed in Japan (Harada et al. 1984).

Antibiotic treatment of hatching eggs has proved to be an efficacious and practical method of producing chicks free from *M. gallisepticum*. Prewarmed eggs are immersed in chilled tylosin solution, and the antibiotic is drawn into the egg (Chalquest and Fabricant 1959).

REFERENCES

Chhabra, P.C., and Goel, M.C. 1981. Immunological response of chickens to *Mycoplasma gallisepticum* infection. Avian Dis. 25:279–293.

Chalquest, R.R., and Fabricant, J. 1959. Survival of PPLO injected into eggs previously dipped in antibiotic solutions. Avian Dis. 3:257–271.

Harada, Y. 1984. *Mycoplasma gallisepticum* and *M. synoviae* in breeding flocks and drug sensitivity of field isolates. J. Jpn. Vet. Med. Assoc. 37:93–99.

Keymer, I.F., Leach, R.H., Clarke, R.A., Bardsley, M.E., and McIntyre, R.R. 1984. Isolation of *Mycoplasma* spp. from racing pigeons (*Columba livia*). Avian Pathol. 13:65–74.

Kleven, S.H., Glisson, J.R., Lin, M.Y., and Talkington, F.D. 1984. Bacterins and vaccines for the control of *Mycoplasma gallisepticum*. Isr. J. Med. Sci. 20:989–991.

Lam, K.M., and Lin, W. 1984. Further studies on the immunization of chickens with temperature-sensitive *Mycoplasma gallisepticum* mutant. Avian Dis. 28:131–138.

Lin, M.Y., and Kleven, S.H. 1984a. Evaluation of attenuated strains of *Mycoplasma gallisepticum* as vaccines in young chickens. Avian Dis. 28:88–89.

Lin, M.Y., and Kleven, S.H. 1984b. Transferred humoral immunity in chickens to *Mycoplasma gallisepticum*. Avian Dis. 28:79–87.

Nougayrede, P., Toquin, D., Andral, B., and Guittet, M. 1984. Serological tests for avian mycoplasmosis: Rapid plate agglutination, haemagglutination inhibition and metabolic inhibition applied to *Mycoplasma gallisepticum* infection. Avian Pathol. 13:753–768.

Tajima, M., Yagihashi, T., and Miki, Y. 1982. Capsular material of *Mycoplasma gallisepticum* and its possible relevance to the pathogenic process. Infect. Immun. 36:830–833.

Yoder, H.W., Drury, L.N., and Hopkins, S.R. 1977. Influence of environment on airsacculitis: Effects of relative humidity and air temperature on broilers infected with *Mycoplasma synoviae* and infectious bronchitis. Avian Dis. 21:195–208.

Mycoplasma iowae

M. iowae has been associated with air sac lesions in turkey embryos and poults. Experimentally infected poults became depressed, displayed poor feathering, and had toe and leg deformities and pronounced stunting (Bradbury and Ideris 1982). All strains produce branching filaments that develop into chains of coccal, coccobacillary, and elongated cells. Antigenic variants occur among the different strains and may pose difficulties in serologic diagnosis of infection (Rhodes 1984).

REFERENCES

Bradbury, J.M., and Ideris, A. 1982. Abnormalities in turkey poults following infection with *Mycoplasma iowae*. Vet. Rec. 110:559–560.

Rhodes, K.R. 1984. Comparison of strains of *Mycoplasma iowae*. Avian Dis. 28:710–717.

Mycoplasma meleagridis

M. meleagridis produces air sacculitis and skeletal abnormalities in turkeys. The cells have typical mycoplasmal morphology but are encapsulated. Biotin stimulates growth. Strains of *M. meleagridis* appear to be similar morphologically and antigenically (Elmahi et al. 1982). The organism is transmitted in the egg as a result of infection of the oviducts; dipping eggs in antibiotic solution is an effective control measure.

REFERENCES

Elmahi, M.M., Ross, R.F., and Hofstad, M.S. 1982. Comparison of seven isolates of *Mycoplasma meleagridis*. Vet. Microbiol. 7:61–76.

Mycoplasma synoviae

M. synoviae is a cause of infectious synovitis and air sacculitis in chickens and turkeys. The broiler breeds are more susceptible to synovitis than the laying breeds. The disease causes losses through condemnations at meat inspection and poor weight gain. Infection by *M. synoviae* has become increasingly more important as the eradication of *M. gallisepticum* has progressed.

The morphologic and cultural features of *M. synoviae* are similar to those of *M. gallisepticum*. It ferments glucose and maltose, and most strains have a specific requirement for coenzyme I (nicotine adenine dinucleotide). There appears to be a single serotype that contains three subtypes. Some strains agglutinate erythrocytes (Weinack and Snoeyenbos 1976).

Epizootiology and Pathogenesis. *M. synoviae* is an obligate parasite of chickens and turkeys and is distributed widely wherever poultry are intensively raised. The most frequent source of infection is infected eggs, natural infection in this case being transmitted vertically. The organism is therefore a potential contaminant of vaccines propagated in eggs, and lateral spread can occur by this means. The organism is also shed from the respiratory tract of infected birds and can spread by contact or infectious aerosol to other birds kept nearby. Air sacculitis is most extensive at low ambient temperature regardless of humidity. At moderate ambient temperature the incidence is greater when humidity is low than when it is high (Yoder et al. 1977).

Invasion by the respiratory route usually results in air sac inflammation, whereas intravenous inoculation of the organism commonly results in synovitis. Lymphocytes have been shown to be necessary for the development of macroscopic lesions of synovitis (Kune et al. 1977). The form of the disease and the tissue tropism of strains appears to vary from one region to another, a phenomenon that has not been explained.

Mixed infections of *M. synoviae* and viruses such as infectious bronchitis virus result in more severe respiratory lesions. Vaccination with infectious bronchitis or Newcastle disease virus when *M. synoviae* infection is spreading therefore greatly increases the frequency and severity of air sac inflammation.

Clinical manifestations of infectious synovitis include swollen joints and tendon sheaths, which contain a creamy white viscid purulent exudate. The hocks, the feet, and the bursae on the breast are most commonly affected. A sign of air sacculitis is slight rales. The linings of the air sacs are thickened with a whitish yellow exudate. There may also be endocarditis, valvular lesions, and anemia. The anemia is probably caused by the hemolytic effect of hydrogen peroxide, which is produced by *M. synoviae* organisms that have adhered to the erythrocytes (Timms 1978).

Immunity. The presence of B lymphocytes is correlated with the development of resistance to lesions, whereas T lymphocytes are necessary for the development of macroscopic synovitis (Kune et al. 1977). A cell-mediated response develops during the second week of infection (Timms and Cullen 1974), and its effect in lesion development may be cytotoxic. Rheumatoid factor is produced during the course of the disease as a response to immunoglobulin complexed to *Mycoplasma* antigen.

Diagnosis. Infection is usually detected by the plate agglutination and hemagglutination-inhibition tests (Timms 1978). The organism can be isolated on media containing NAD and differentiated from *M. gallisepticum* by serologic methods using specific antiserums.

Antimicrobial Susceptibility. The organism is sensitive in vitro to lincomycin, nitrofuran (furaltadone), tetracyclines, tiamulin, and tylosin. When started early in the course of the disease, administration of antibiotics in feed or water is effective in reducing egg infection in breeder flocks and in controlling synovitis and air sac inflammation in broilers. The use of antibiotic solution for egg dipping and heating of eggs to 46°C before incubation are important in preventing vertical transmission of infection.

REFERENCES

Kune, K., Kawkuho, Y., Morita, C., Hayatsu, E., and Yoshioka, M. 1977. Experimentally induced synovitis of chickens with *Mycoplasma synoviae*: Effects of bursectomy and thymectomy on course of the infection for the first four weeks. Am. J. Vet. Res. 38:1595–1599.

Timms, C.M. 1978. *Mycoplasma synoviae*: A review. Vet. Bull. 48:187–198.

Timms, L., and Cullen, G.A. 1974. Detection of *M. synoviae* infection in chickens and its differentiation from *M. gallisepticum* infection. Br. Vet. J. 130:75–83.

Weinack, O.M., and Snoeyenbos, G.H. 1976. Serologic studies with *Mycoplasma synoviae* in experimentally inoculated chickens. Avian Dis. 20:253–259.

Yoder, H.W., Drury, L.N., and Hopkins, S.R. 1977. Influence of environment on air sacculitis: Effects of relative humidity and air temperature on broilers infected with *Mycoplasma synoviae* and infectious bronchitis. Avian Dis. 21:195–208.

Mycoplasma Species of Horses

Mycoplasmas including *M. arginini, M. equirhinis,* and *M. salivarium* are commonly found on the upper respiratory mucosa of horses, where they apparently live as harmless commensals. *M. felis* has been recovered from the thoracic cavity of a horse with pleuritis (Ogilvie et al. 1983). *M. equirhinis* has been found in bronchial secretions of horses with respiratory disease (Ammar et al. 1980), but its significance as a pathogen has not been established. It probably opportunistically multiplies following development of disease in the tract. Unidentified mycoplasmas cross-reactive with *M. mycoides* subsp. *mycoides* and similar to the large colony type have also been observed in the equine respiratory tract by Lemcke et al. (1981).

Mycoplasmas including *M. equigenitalium* have been detected in stallion semen, in which their presence is correlated with lower levels of glycerylphosphorylcholine, fructose, and total protein (Zgorniak-Nowosielska et al. 1984).

REFERENCES

Ammar, A., Kirchhoff, H., Heitmann, I., Meier, C., Fischer, J., and Deegen, E. 1980. Isolation and differentiation of mycoplasmas in bronchial secretions of horses with acute and chronic respiratory disease including serological investigations. Berl. Münch. Tierärztl. Wochenschr. 93:457–462.
Lemcke, R.M., Erno, H., and Gupta, U. 1981. The relationship of two equine mycoplasmas to *Mycoplasma mycoides.* J. Hyg. 87:93–100.
Ogilvie, T.H., Rosendal, S., Blackwell, T.E., Rotkowski, C.M., Julian, R.J., and Ruhnke, L. 1983. *Mycoplasma felis* as a cause of pleuritis in horses. J. Am. Vet. Med. Assoc. 182:1374–1376.
Zgorniak-Nowosielska, I., Bielanski, W., and Kosiniak, K. 1984. Mycoplasmas in stallion semen. Anim. Reprod. Sci. 7:343–350.

Mycoplasma Species of Cats

The two most commonly encountered mycoplasmas in cats are *M. felis* and *M. gateae.* These species were first observed in the saliva of cats by Cole et al. (1967). In their study and in subsequent studies *M. felis* has occasionally been associated with conjunctivitis and other diseases (Wilkinson 1980). *M. gateae* is a normal commensal of the feline oropharynx (Tan et al. 1977) but has the potential, albeit rarely expressed, to enter the bloodstream and cause polyarthritis (Moise et al. 1983). *M. arginini, M. arthritidis, M. feliminutum, M. gallisepticum,* and *M.*

pulmonis, have also been recovered from cat specimens (Tan et al. 1977).

REFERENCES

Cole, B.C., Golightly, L., and Ward, J.H.R. 1967. Characterization of mycoplasma strains from cats. J. Bacteriol. 94:1451–1458.
Moise, N.S., Crissman, J.W., Fairbrother, J.F., and Baldwin, C. 1983. *Mycoplasma gateae* arthritis and tenosynovitis in cats: Case report and experimental reproduction of the disease. Am. J. Vet. Res. 44:16–21.
Tan, R.J.S., Linn, E.W.. and Ishak, B. 1977. Ecology of mycoplasmas in clinically healthy cats. Aust. Vet. J. 53:151–518.
Wilkinson, G.T. 1980. Mycoplasmas of the cat. Vet. Ann. 20:145–150.

Mycoplasma Species of Dogs

As in other domestic animal species, most of the accessible mucous membranes of dogs are colonized by mycoplasmas. At least 11 species, including *M. arginini, M. canis, M. cynos, M. edwardsii, M. feliminutum, M. gateae, M. maculosum, M. opalescens,* and *M. spumans,* have been found, of which *M. canis* and *M. cynos* are potentially pathogenic for the genitourinary and respiratory tracts, respectively (Jang et al. 1984; Rosendal 1982). Although *M. canis* has been shown in experiments to produce orchitis, epididymitis, and purulent endometritis, a role for it in naturally occurring disease has not yet been convincingly established. However, its presence in pure culture in cases of urinary tract infection argues strongly for its involvement as a urinary tract pathogen (Jang et al. 1984). *M. cynos* has been isolated from dogs with bronchitis and distemper pneumonia, in which it was probably a secondary invader (Rosendal 1982). Mycoplasmas have also been isolated from canine cardiac lesions and from lesions of granulomatous colitis in boxers (Rosendal 1982).

REFERENCES

Jang, S.S., Ling, G.V., Yamamoto, R., and Wolf, A. 1984. Mycoplasmas as a cause of canine urinary tract infection. J. Am. Vet. Med. Assoc. 185:45–47.
Rosendal, S. 1982. Canine mycoplasmas: Their ecologic niche and role in disease. J. Am. Vet. Med. Assoc. 180:1212–1214.

The Genus *Ureaplasma*

Ureaplasmas occur on the mucous membranes of a wide variety of animal species (Taylor-Robinson and Gourlay 1984). Their ability to hydrolyze urea distinguishes them from members of the genus *Mycoplasma.* Other distinguishing features include their small colony size (15 to 60 μm in diameter), optimum pH (6.0), and low cell productivity (10^7/ml) in broth cultures. They do not hydrolyze arginine or ferment glucose. The genome size is between 4.1 and 4.8 × 10^8 daltons.

There are only two species, *U. diversum* and *U. urealyticum,* found in animals and humans, respectively. *U. diversum* contains a variety of strains that inhabit different animal hosts. New species within this group will likely emerge because the species designation was proposed for strains from cattle only and may not be valid for strains from other hosts.

Ureaplasma diversum

Strains of *U. diversum* are commonly found on the mucosae of ruminants, horses, poultry, swine, cats, and dogs.

Morphology and Staining Characteristics. The cells are coccoid and similar to other mycoplasmas. Filament formation occurs only in older cultures. A thin capsular layer is present.

Cultural and Biochemical Features. Ureaplasmas can be cultivated on essentially the same media as *Mycoplasma* species, but the medium must be adjusted to pH 6.0. On solid media the colonies are small and lack the typical fried egg appearance of other mycoplasmas. Urea is hydrolyzed and ammonia is produced. A reagent containing 0.05 M HEPES buffer and manganese sulfate is often added to the agar medium to aid in the detection of ammonia-producing colonies, which appear dark brown (Shepard and Lunceford 1976). Growth is optimum in an atmosphere of 10 percent CO_2 in nitrogen. *U. diversum* produces phosphatase and proteases including IgA'ase. Tetrazolium is not reduced. The mol% G + C of the DNA is 28.7 to 30.2. Restriction endonuclease analysis of the DNA of bovine and other animal strains suggests that the strains are distinct from one another (Harasawa et al. 1984).

Antigens. Three clusters of serologically similar bovine strains have been observed (Howard and Gourlay 1981). Strains from sheep and goats appear to be serologically homogeneous (Kotani et al. 1980). Feline strains belong to two groups, group 1 being much larger than group 2 (Koshimizu et al. 1979). Canine ureaplasmas form four serologic groups and avian ureaplasmas comprise one serologic group (Koshimizu et al. 1984).

Epizootiology and Pathogenesis. Each animal host is colonized by its own specifically adapted ureaplasmas (Howard 1984), which have a commensal relationship with the host. When an animal is diseased, ureaplasmas may become more numerous and invasive, and some

strains have been shown in experiments to be capable of causing mastitis or vulvitis in ewes (Ball and McCaughey 1982, Ball and Mackie 1985). Ureaplasmas have been associated with cuffing pneumonia of calves (Pirie and Allan 1975) and with vulvovaginitis in heifers and cows with a history of infertility (Thornber 1982). The organism is common in semen and in the prepuce of normal bulls, and the serotypes are the same as those occurring in the vagina of cows with vulvovaginitis and infertility (Truscott 1983). However, the most frequently isolated serotype from the vagina is not the most frequently observed strain in semen or the prepuce, suggesting that all bovine serotypes are not of equal virulence in the vagina. Reproductive failure of sows inseminated with boar semen containing ureaplasmas has also been reported (Stipkovits 1983).

Ureaplasmas have been observed in the urinary tract of grain-fed lambs with urinary calculi composed of magnesium ammonium phosphate, and their presence may have contributed to the formation of the calculi (Livingston et al. 1984).

Antimicrobial Susceptibility. Ureaplasmas are sensitive to chloramphenicol, erythromycin, lincomycin, tetracyclines, tiamulin, and tylosin. A combination of lincomycin, spectinomycin, and tylosin is effective against strains from bovine semen (Truscott and Ruhnke 1984).

REFERENCES

Ball, H.J., and McCaughey, W.J. 1982. Experimental production of vulvitis in ewes with a ureaplasma isolate. Vet. Rec. 110:581.

Ball, H.J., and Mackie, D.P. 1985. The experimental production of mastitis in ewes as a determinant of the virulence of ovine ureaplasma strains. Vet. Microbiol. 10:117–123.

Harasawa, R., Kotani, H., Razin, S., and Koshimizu, K. 1984. Genomic analysis of animal ureaplasmas by restriction endonucleases. Jpn. J. Vet. Sci. 46:737–740.

Howard, C.J. 1984. Animal ureaplasmas: Their ecological niche and role in disease. Isr. J. Med. Sci. 20:954–957.

Howard, C.J., and Gourlay, R.N. 1981. Identification of ureaplasmas from cattle using antisera prepared in gnotobiotic calves. J. Gen. Microbiol. 126:365–367.

Koshimizu, K., Kotani, H., Yamamoto, K., Magaribuchi, T., Harasawa, R., Ito, M., and Ogata, M. 1984. Serological analysis of ureaplasmas isolated from various animals. Isr. J. Med. Sci. 20:950–953.

Koshimizu, K., Magaribuchi, T., and Ito, M. 1979. Serological typing of ureaplasmas of feline origin. Jpn. J. Vet. Sci. 41:545–549.

Kotani, H., Nagatomo, H., and Ogata, M. 1980. Isolation and serological comparison of ureaplasmas from goats and sheep. Jpn. J. Vet. Sci. 42:31–40.

Livingston, C.W., Jr., Calhoun, M.C., Gauer, B.B., and Baldwin, B.C., Jr. 1984. Effect of experimental infection with ovine ureaplasma upon the development of uroliths in feedlot lambs. Isr. J. Med. Sci. 20:958–961.

Pirie, H.M., and Allan, E.M. 1975. Mycoplasmas and cuffing pneumonia in a group of calves. Vet. Rec. 97:345–349.

Shepard, M.C., and Lunceford, C.D. 1976. Differential agar medium (A7) for identification of *Ureaplasma urealyticum* (human T mycoplasmas) in primary cultures of clinical material. J. Clin. Microbiol. 3:613–625.

Stipkovits, L. 1983. Reproductive failure of sows in association with ureaplasma infection. Arch. Exp. Vet. 37:453–459.

Taylor-Robinson, D., and Gourlay, R.N. 1984. The mycoplasmataceae. In N.R. Kreig and J.G. Holt, eds., Bergey's Manual of Systematic Bacteriology, vol. 1. Williams & Wilkins, Baltimore. Pp. 770–774.

Thornber, P.M. 1982. Ureaplasma association with bovine infertility in south-west Scotland (correspondence). Vet. Rec. 11:591.

Truscott, R.B. 1983. Ureaplasma serotypes associated with the bovine urogenital tract. Can. J. Comp. Med. 47:471–591.

Truscott, R.B., and Ruhnke, H.L. 1984. The effect of antibiotics against bovine mycoplasmas and ureaplasmas. Can. J. Comp. Med. 48:171–174.

31 The Rickettsiaceae

In *Bergey's Manual of Systematic Bacteriology* (1984) a group of small (less than 0.5 μm in diameter), rod-shaped coccoid, and often pleomorphic microorganisms that occur intracellularly as elementary bodies, but may occasionally be extracellular, are placed in the order Rickettsiales. The rickettsias are true bacteria with typical structure and most of the typical bacterial enzymes. They are usually nonfilterable and Gram-negative and can be cultivated outside the host only in living tissues, embryonated chicken eggs, and, rarely, in media containing body fluids. They are associated with reticuloendothelial vascular cells or with erythrocytes in vertebrates and also in invertebrates, which may act as vectors. Rickettsias cause diseases in humans and animals but seldom kill invertebrate hosts.

The Family Rickettsiaceae

The rickettsias are a group of small bacteria commonly found in the tissues of arthropods. In 1909 Howard Ricketts described the bacterium that causes Rocky Mountain spotted fever in humans. He demonstrated that the disease is transmitted to humans by ticks, principally the Rocky Mountain wood tick, *Dermacentor andersoni*, and showed that the infection occurs commonly in the tick, the human infections being merely incidental. During Ricketts's studies of a similar infection, typhus, in 1910 he contracted the disease and died. Another scientist, Von Prowazek, who was one of the early workers in this field, also died of typhus, and in 1916 Roberto Da

Rocha-Lima named the causative agent of louse-borne typhus fever *Rickettsia prowazekii*. It is the type species of the group.

Morphology and Staining Reactions. Rickettsias are small bacteria with a typical cell wall; nearly all measure less than 0.5 μm in diameter. Some exhibit a great deal of pleomorphism, whereas others are quite uniform in size and shape. Most occur in groups in the cytoplasm of the parasitized cells, although they sometimes occur intranuclearly. They stain poorly with ordinary dyes, but stain well with May-Grünwald-Giemsa, Gimenez, and Macchiavello stains. With Macchiavello and Gimenez stains the rickettsias appear bright red against a blue (Macchiavello) or greenish (Gimenez) background. *Rickettsia tsutsugamushi* cannot be successfully stained by Macchiavello stain; a modification of the standard Gimenez staining procedure is required. With the modified Gimenez staining procedure *R. tsutsugamushi* organisms appear reddish black against a green background. With Gram's stain they are negative.

Cultural and Biochemical Features. Most species of rickettsias have been cultivated successfully in tissue culture, which is a good medium for study of their growth requirements. A few species, including *R. melophagi*, a nonpathogenic form found in the sheep ked, *Melophagus ovinus*, have been cultivated in special lifeless laboratory media, but none of the pathogenic forms except *R. quintana* has been cultivated in the absence of living cells. The pathogenic forms can readily be propagated in chicken embryos and in cell cultures. Although they may be grown on the chorioallantois of the developing chick embryo, a more successful method, devised by Cox (1941), consists of cultivation in the yolk sac of a developing chick embryo. Rabinowitz et al. (1948) demonstrated that *R. prowazekii* could be grown by inoculation of the yolk sac of dead embryos. In this case 3-day-old embryos were killed by chilling. Upon reincubation at 37°C, living cells were demonstrated for as long as 16 days, and apparently the rickettsias grew in these cells.

Rickettsias can exchange adenosine diphosphate (ADP) for host adenosine triphosphate (ATP) by an unusual transport system similar to that of mitochondria. When stored at 0°C, rickettsias lose their biological activity because of the progressive loss of nicotinamide adenine dinucleotide (NAD). These properties—including toxicity, hemolytic activity, infectivity, and respiratory activity—can be restored by subsequent incubation with NAD. Purified rickettsias may also lose their biological activity if they are starved by incubation for several hours at 36°C. This loss of activity can be prevented by the addition of glutamate, pyruvate, or ATP. During the starvation process the ATP level falls to zero; the level rises when glutamate is added.

Rickettsias may be preserved in the lyophilized state for several months or in infected tissues stored at −20°C or lower.

Epizootiology and Pathogenesis. The rickettsias appear to be well-established parasites of arthropods (Huff 1938). Some are transmitted transovarially in ticks but do not seem to be pathogenic for them. Certain types are pathogenic for the body louse. They also appear to be well adapted to mammals, especially smaller mammals such as rodents, which may constitute a reservoir of infection in nature. When intraperitoneally inoculated into male guinea pigs, many varieties of rickettsias will produce a febrile reaction within 7 to 12 days, which may be accompanied by orchitis. The disease in the guinea pig is often not fatal. Other laboratory animals such as dogs, cats, rabbits, rats, and mice are more resistant and may show no fever or other reaction to injection, although the organism may become established and persist for months. According to Price (1953), guinea pigs that are infected intraperitoneally with a strain of rickettsia of low virulence are protected against a simultaneous injection of a highly virulent strain, if the less virulent strain is given in a concentration about 10 to 30 times that of the more virulent one. This is known as the rickettsial-interference phenomenon. Infection with Q fever, scrub typhus, and epidemic typhus protects guinea pigs against a virulent strain of spotted fever under the same conditions.

The rickettsias cause a number of diseases in humans and animals. These infections are discussed below under the headings "Animal Rickettsial Diseases" and "Human Rickettsial Diseases."

Immunity. Recovery from an attack of rickettsial disease usually confers a solid and lasting immunity. Vaccines are now being prepared by injection of the yolk sac of developing chicken embryos with inactivated organisms. The rickettsiae are concentrated by a process of grinding, washing, and centrifugation and are then purified by the removal of yolk lipids and tissue debris (Craigie 1945). The infected yolk sac material usually is inactivated in formalin before the concentration procedure is started. Craigie (1945) claims that the ethyl ether used in the process is bactericidal for rickettsias. Antibodies after vaccination are initially IgM, and later IgG.

Diagnosis. The diagnosis of rickettsial diseases is based on recovery of the causative agent from acute-phase blood specimens or selected tissues from infected vertebrate hosts, or on findings of a fourfold or greater increase in agglutinin or complement-fixing antibody titer in the convalescent-phase serums as compared with the acute-phase serum. Tissues from dead or live ticks are examined for rickettsias by means of a hemolymph test or immunofluorescence test.

Guinea pig and chicken embryo inoculations are usually employed to isolate rickettsias. At present the complement-fixation test seems to be the most accurate way to differentiate the various types (Bengston and Topping 1942). Several agglutination and toxin-neutralization systems have been developed for research purposes. Each species has group-specific antigens that do not cross-react with antiserums to other groups; although the rickettsias of the spotted fever and typhus fever groups share common antigens, they cross-react in the complement-fixation test only with other members of their respective groups.

The most reliable serologic results are obtained with ether-extracted antigens prepared from yolk sacs of embryonated chicken eggs containing a maximum growth of rickettsiae (Stoenner et al. 1962). Except for *R. akari*, members of the spotted fever group achieve maximum growth in 5-day-old embryos inoculated with a dose calculated to destroy most embryos by the fourth day after inoculation into the yolk sac. Inoculated eggs are incubated at 33.5°C for 48 hours after embryo death before yolk sacs are harvested. Maximum yields of *R. prowazekii* and *R. typhi* are achieved in 5-day-old embryos maintained at 36.5°C whose yolk sacs were inoculated with a dose calculated to cause death in 60 to 70 percent of the embryos between the eighth and ninth days after inoculation. Maximum growth of *Coxiella burnetii*, the causative agent of Q fever, is obtained when given as an inoculum producing 50 percent embryo mortality 7 to 8 days after inoculation. Yolk sacs are harvested from surviving embryonated eggs and from embryos not dead for more than 6 hours. Yolk sacs infected with rickettsial organisms are stored at $-20°$ to $-70°C$ for subsequent antigen preparation.

Ether extraction of infected yolk sacs is used for the preparation of rickettsial antigens. Yolk sacs are emulsified in a Waring blender with sufficient 0.66 M phosphate-buffered saline, pH 5.8, to make a 20 percent suspension. The material is held overnight at $4°C$ after the addition of enough formalin to make a 0.2 percent concentration. This suspension is mixed with 1.5 volumes of ether in a separatory funnel, shaken several times during the day, and allowed to separate overnight at $4°C$. The aqueous phase containing the antigen is removed and residual ether is removed by vacuum. Antigen activity is then assayed by cross-box titration against three specific antiserums with adequate controls to evaluate anticomplementary activity. This activity can sometimes be removed by one or more additional ether extractions.

According to Van der Scheer et al. (1947), soluble antigens can be prepared from infected yolk sacs by ether extraction, followed by treatment with benzene and precipitation with sodium sulfate. Complement fixation with this antigen does not always distinguish between European and murine typhus.

In 1915 Weil and Felix found that the serum of patients with typhus fever agglutinated certain strains of *Proteus* bacteria. Apparently these *Proteus* strains possess somatic (O) antigens in common with the rickettsias. This reaction (Weil-Felix) is not specific, but it has proved useful in serologic diagnosis and identification of rickettsial infections.

The identification of *R. rickettsii* in a film from the gut tissues of the Rocky Mountain wood tick, *Dermacentor andersoni*, can be established by means of the fluorescent antibody technique. The indirect fluorescent antibody method has been used to demonstrate *R. tsutsugamushi* in smears of serum from patients with scrub typhus. Some cross-reactions are observed with the fluorescent antibody technique because some rickettsial organisms share common antigens.

The cultivation of live rickettsias in the laboratory is hazardous, particularly during centrifugation and when infected animals are handled. Laboratory and animal personnel should be vaccinated and facilities should be adequate for the isolation and study of these pathogens.

Antimicrobial Susceptibility. Streptomycin, kanamycin, chlortetracycline, chloramphenicol, oxytetracycline, ampicillin, and para-aminobenzoic acid (PABA) have

been reported to be highly effective in the treatment of rickettsial diseases (Fellers 1952, Haig et al. 1954, Ley and Smadel 1954).

REFERENCES

Bengston, I.A., and Topping, N.H. 1942. Complement-fixation in rickettsial diseases. Am. J. Public Health 32:48–58.

Cox, H.R. 1941. Cultivation of rickettsiae of the Rocky Mountain spotted fever, typhus and Q fever groups in the embryonic tissues of developing chicks. Science 94:399–403.

Craigie, J. 1945. Application and control of ethyl-ether–water interface effects to the separation of rickettsiae from yolk sac suspensions. Can. J. Res. 23 (Sect. E):104–114.

Fellers, F.X. 1952. Outbreak of Q fever; Treatment with aureomycin and chloramphenicol. U.S. Armed Forces Med. J. 3:665–671.

Haig, D.A., Alexander, R.A., and Weiss, K.E. 1954. Treatment of heartwater with terramycin. J. S. Afr. Vet. Assoc. 25:45–48.

Huff, C.G. 1938. Studies on the evolution of some disease-producing organisms (rickettsiae, spirochaetes, and protozoa). Q. Rev. Biol. 13:196–206.

Ley, H.L., Jr., and Smadel, J.E. 1954. Antibiotic therapy of rickettsial diseases. Antibiot. Chemother. 4:792–802.

Price, W.H. 1953. Interference phenomenon in animal infections with rickettsiae of Rocky Mountain spotted fever. Proc. Soc. Exp. Biol. Med. 82:180–184.

Rabinowitz, E., Aschner, M., and Grossowicz, N. 1948. Cultivation of *Rickettsia prowazekii* in dead chick embryos. Proc. Soc. Exp. Biol. Med. 67:469–470.

Stoenner, H.G., Luckman, D.B., and Bell, E.J. 1962. Factors affecting the growth of rickettsias of the spotted fever group in fertile hens' eggs. J. Infect. Dis. 110:121–128.

Van der Scheer, J., Bohnel, E., and Cox, H.R. 1947. Diagnostic antigens for epidemic typhus, murine typhus and Rocky Mountain spotted fever. J. Immunol. 56:365–375.

Animal Rickettsial Diseases

The rickettsias afflicting domestic animals compose a heterogeneous group (Table 31.1) whose members share only a few common traits. The morphologic and staining characteristics of these infectious agents are similar. Vectors are involved in the transmission of the disease, and intermediate hosts definitely exist for six of the animal rickettsial diseases. Except for contagious ophthalmia, caused by *Colesiota conjunctivae*, the disease in the natural hosts principally involves pathological changes in the blood vascular system. The effects of *C. conjunctivae* are limited to the conjunctival sac. Certain of these diseases have been studied extensively in their natural hosts, but their limited host ranges are a handicap. Each organism is thought to be immunologically distinct. None has been cultivated in embryonated hens' eggs, and only *Cowdria ruminantium*, *Ehrlichia equi*, and *E. phagocytophilia* cause disease or infection in laboratory animals.

There is no evidence that any of the animal rickettsial organisms listed in this section produces disease in hu-

Table 31.1. Animal rickettsial diseases

Disease	Geographic distribution	Causative organism	Major vectors	Natural hosts: cell or tissues affected	Suggested experimental and diagnostic test hosts	Suggested laboratory diagnostic tests*
Heartwater	Eastern and southern Africa, Caribbean	*Cowdria ruminantium*	*Amblyomma hebraeum, A. variegatum,* and other *Amblyomma* spp.	Sheep, cattle, goats, and some wild ungulates: vascular endothelium	Bluetongue-immune sheep, goats, and mice	Vascular and cerebral brain smears; capillary flocculation test
Tick-borne fever (pasture fever)	Great Britain, Norway, Finland, The Netherlands, India	*Ehrlichia phagocytophilia*	*Ixodes ricinus*	Cattle, sheep, bison, and wild ungulates: primarily granulocytes	Cattle, sheep, guinea pig, mice, and goats	Febrile-phase blood smears; smears better than complement fixation
Benign bovine ehrlichiosis ("nopi," "nofel")	Northern and central South Africa, Middle East, Sri Lanka	*Ehrlichia bovis*	*Hyalomma excavatum* and other *Hyalomma* spp.	Cattle: lymphocytes and monocytes	Cattle, sheep, and monkeys	Febrile-phase blood smears; necropsy tissues, lungs, liver, and spleen
Benign ovine ehrlichiosis	North and central Africa	*Ehrlichia ovina*	*Rhipicephalus bursa*	Sheep: lymphocytes and monocytes	Sheep	Same
Canine ehrlichiosis	Worldwide	*Ehrlichia canis*	*Rhipicephalus sanguineus*	Domestic and wild canids, humans: lymphocytes and monocytes	Babesia-free dogs	Direct blood smears; smears from buffy coat superior

Disease	Geographic distribution	Agent	Vector	Hosts and cells	Hosts	Diagnosis
Equine ehrlichiosis	California and Illinois (USA), Israel	Ehrlichia equi	Ornithodoros erraticus (Israel)	Horses and burros: primarily granulocytes	Horses, donkeys, sheep, goats, dogs, monkeys, and cats	Febrile-phase blood smears; buffy coat smears better
Potomac horse fever	USA, Europe	Ehrlichia risticii	None identified	Horses and ponies: monocytes	Horses, ponies	Blood leukocyte smears; fluorescent antibody, Giemsa
Bovine petechial fever (ondiri disease)	Kenya, Tanzania	Cytoecetes ondiri	—	Cattle and sheep: primarily granulocytes	Cattle and sheep	Blood or spleen tissue smears
Contagious ophthalmia	Africa, Australia, New Zealand, Europe, North and South America	Colesiota conjunctivae	Flies	Sheep, cattle, goats swine, and chickens: conjunctival epithelium and monocytes	Sheep, cattle, goats, swine, and chickens	Epithelial conjunctival smears
Jembrana	Indonesia	—	—	Cattle and buffalo	Cattle	Hepatic and spleen smears
Salmon poisoning syndrome	Northwestern USA	Neoricketsia helminthoeca, Elokomin fluke fever agent	Nanophyes salmincola	Dogs and wild canids: reticuloendothelial system, lymph nodes	Dogs and black bears	Presence of fluke eggs in feces; smear preparations from mandibular lymph

Modified from a table supplied by Herbert G. Stoenner, Rocky Mountain Laboratory, Hamilton, Mont.
*Smears usually stained with Giemsa, Macchiavello, and/or Levediti stain.

mans. *E. equi* does produce infection in nonhuman primates (rhesus, macaques, and baboons) (Lewis et al. 1975).

REFERENCE

Lewis, G.E., Jr., Huxsoll, D.L., Ristic, M., and Johnson, A.J. 1975. Experimentally induced infection of dogs, cats, and nonhuman primates with *Ehrlichia equi,* etiologic agent of equine ehrlichiosis. Am. J. Vet. Res. 36:85–88.

Heartwater Disease

Heartwater disease is caused by *Cowdria (Rickettsia) ruminantium*. The organism was first described by Cowdry (1925a, 1925b), who was working in South Africa at the time. It is the cause of a disease of cattle, sheep, goats, and some wild ungulates which is commonly called *heartwater* because one of the characteristics of the disease is hydropericardium. This disease occurs in eastern and southern Africa—it has long been known in South Africa—and in the Caribbean. It is associated with the bont tick (*Amblyomma hebraeum*), *A. variegatum,* and other *Amblyomma* species, which are the transmitting agents (Alexander 1931, Camus and Barre 1982, Uilenberg 1981). Certain breeds of cattle are more susceptible and some indigenous breeds are resistant.

Excellent review articles on heartwater are available (Camus and Barre 1982, Uilenberg 1981).

Epizootiology and Pathogenesis. Although several kinds of tick occur in the heartwater districts, apparently the bont tick and other *Amblyomma* species are the only vectors. Larval ticks retain the infection through the molts to the adult form, but the parasite is not transmitted through the egg to the next generation (transtadial transmission).

The disease can be transmitted by inoculation with blood taken from sick animals during the early febrile period, but transmission is not always achieved. The route of injection is important. The preferred route is intravenous inoculation; the subcutaneous route has been used with less success. Ingestion usually fails. It is clear that the disease is naturally transmitted solely through the activities of the *Amblyomma* ticks.

A. maculatum Koch, a tick residing in the United States, transmitted *C. ruminantium* to healthy goats in experimental studies (Uilenberg 1982). A potential danger thus exists of the disease gaining access to the American mainland from the Caribbean, where the disease and *A. maculatum* are known to occur (Uilenberg 1982).

Affected ruminants develop a high fever and show gastrointestinal and nervous signs. The disease can assume a peracute form characterized by high fever, sudden collapse, and death, or it can be mild or even abortive. In the more common acute form a rise in temperature occurs with leukopenia and a decrease in eosinophils, followed by a depression and loss of appetite, although some animals may continue to eat and ruminate. Nervous signs are first manifested by a high-stepping and unsteady gait, followed by progressive signs of encephalitis including chewing movements, twitching eyelids, walking in circles, aggressive and blind charges into objects, and a final collapse with attendant convulsions, galloping movements, and twitching muscles.

Animals that die with the peracute form rarely have gross lesions. Hydropericardium is not always seen in sheep with the acute form, and the absence of pericardial fluid in cattle is not uncommon. Mucous membranes are congested. Edema of the lungs is a constant finding. The peritoneal and pleural cavities contain excessive fluid, with a variable amount of hemorrhage usually present on the serous membranes of the abdominal viscera and heart. The spleen and lymph nodes, particularly in cattle, are enlarged. The liver is usually enlarged and hemorrhagic, and distention of the gallbladder is common. A transparent fluid often infiltrates the mucosa of the abomasum. Patches of ramiform congestion and diffuse hyperemia of the small intestine, particularly in cattle, produce so-called zebra markings. Capillaries can be occluded by swollen epithelial cells containing masses of rickettsiae.

The principal microscopic changes are lymphostasis in all organs and perivascular leukocytic infiltration in the liver and kidney and occasionally in the adrenal glands.

A high mortality is often reported in cattle, sheep, and goats, except in those that are indigenous. The organism infects a variety of feral ungulates without necessarily causing overt disease.

Immunity. Cross-immunity tests in goats have demonstrated that a strain of *C. ruminantium* from Nigeria and two strains from South Africa are completely cross-protective (Winkelhoff and Uilenberg 1981). Serviceable protection persists for at least 9 months and probably longer. Under field conditions animals have continuous exposure to ticks, so repeated subclinical infections produce adequate protection against disease.

Calves up to 3 weeks old are quite resistant to heartwater disease and can be rendered actively immune by infection with serum from infected animals or vaccine made from infected tick nymphae (Bezuidenhout 1981). This procedure is practiced in certain heavily infected areas of South Africa, where the possible loss of a few young calves through the use of live vaccine is preferred to larger losses of older calves from natural infection (Neitz and Alexander 1945).

Diagnosis. Diagnosis is established by demonstration of rickettsias in tissue smears from animals with suspect cases or by reproduction of the disease in sheep or in goats; the latter are often used as experimental or diagnostic animals. Ilemobade and Blotkamp (1978) reported that the subcutaneous injection of brain homogenate from animals dying or dead of heartwater consistently produced the disease in susceptible goats. In attempting to diagnose heartwater, clinicians should use brain homogenate, whole blood, and lung macrophages as test materials from field cases. Specimens taken 2 to 4 days after the onset of fever give the best results. After the animal's temperature has returned to normal, blood may not be infectious. Blood should be obtained in sterile containers, and inoculated intravenously into test animals as defibrinated blood immediately after withdrawal. If field material cannot be inoculated promptly into sheep, white mice inoculated intraperitoneally will preserve the organism for 90 days and permit later injection of sheep (Haig 1952). An incubation period in mice is required for a successful transfer. Consequently, spleens of infected mice are harvested between 14 and 21 days after inoculation, and the suspension is injected intravenously into susceptible sheep. *C. ruminantium* cannot be maintained by serial passage in mice.

C. ruminantium is quite labile and survives in blood for only a few hours at room temperature. It is known to survive for 2 years at −70°C. After rapid freezing at −85°C and −196°C, with or without 10 percent dimethyl sulfoxide, a Nigerian isolate remained highly virulent for months, killing all the goats and sheep inoculated with the frozen stabilized suspensions (Ilemobade et al. 1975). Rickettsias lose their staining properties rapidly in unfixed tissues.

Bluetongue immune sheep should be used for the reproduction of the disease because many cattle and sheep harbor bluetongue virus, which may confuse the diagnosis. There is a distinct difference in incubation period, however: bluetongue virus produces signs in 5 days, whereas *C. ruminantium* requires 11 days. Regardless of the test animal used, the diagnosis should be confirmed by demonstrating the rickettsial organisms in endothelial cells of test animals sacrificed 2 to 4 days after the onset of illness.

Vascular scrapings and smears from cerebral gray matter (Figure 31.1) yield equally good results after the preparations are air-dried, fixed with methanol, and stained with Giemsa stain. Areas rich in capillaries are sought with low power. Under high power or oil immersion the organisms appear dark blue in the cytoplasm, whereas the nuclei of the endothelial cells are purple. The organism may be coccoid (0.3 μm in diameter), bacillary (0.3 by 0.5 μm), or diplococcoid (Figure 31.1).

A capillary flocculation test for diagnosis of heartwater disease uses antigen prepared from infective cattle brain or goat brain (Ilemobade and Blotkamp 1976). Antibodies are detected 1 to 2 weeks after clinical recovery, but unfortunately persist for only 1 to 4 weeks. Consequently, the test has its limitations.

Clinicians can obtain an early diagnosis during the febrile stage by culturing leukocytes and identifying inclusion bodies by Giemsa and direct fluorescent antibody staining and by electron microscopy (Sahu et al. 1983). An early diagnosis enhances successful treatment with antibiotics.

Andreasen (1974) propagated *C. ruminantium* in *Amblyomma* tick cells in vitro, and the culture material produced heartwater in a susceptible sheep.

Antimicrobial Susceptibility. Studies by Haig et al. (1954) indicated that oxytetracycline and chlortetracycline are effective therapeutic agents. Oxytetracycline as a soluble powder in the drinking water has been used successfully in the treatment of sheep, goats, and cattle. Doxycycline (100 mg/ml) given intramuscularly to sheep at a dose of 2 mg/kg of body weight protected them against heartwater (Immelman and Dreyer 1982).

Control of ticks on sheep by dipping in benzene hexachloride helps prevent the disease (Marsh 1958).

Dithiosemicarbazone given to immune sheep had a slightly deleterious effect on their immunity to *C. ruminantium*.

REFERENCES

Alexander, R.A. 1931. Black lung in ruminants. In 17th Annual Report by the Director of Veterinary Services, Union of South Africa. P. 89.

Andreasen, M.P. 1974. Multiplication of *Cowdria ruminantium* in monolayer of tick cells. Acta Pathol. Microbiol. Immunol. Scand. [B] 82:455–456.

Bezuidenhout, J.D. 1981. The development of a new heartwater vaccine using *Amblyomma hebraeum* nymphae infected with *Cowdria ruminantium*. In G.B. Whitehead and J.D. Gibson, eds., Tick Biology and Control. Proceedings of an International Conference, Auspices of Tick Research Unit, Rhodes University, Grahamstown, South Africa. Pp. 41–45.

Camus, E., and Barre, N. 1982. La cowdriose (heartwater)—Revue générale des connaissances. Publ. F-94704, Institut d'Elevage et de Médecine Vétérinaire des Pays Tropicaux, Maisons-Alfort, France.

Cowdry, E.V. 1925a. Etiology of heartwater: Observation of a rickettsia, *Rickettsia ruminantium*, in tissues of infected animals. J. Exp. Med. 42:231–252.

Cowdry, E.V. 1925b. Etiology of heartwater: *Rickettsia ruminantium* in tissues of ticks transmitting disease. J. Exp. Med. 42:253–274.

Haig, D.A. 1952. Note on the use of the white mouse for the transport of strains of heartwater. J. S. Afr. Vet. Med. Assoc. 23:167–170.

Haig, D.A., Alexander, R.A., and Weiss, K.E. 1954. Treatment of heartwater with Terramycin. J. S. Afr. Vet. Med. Assoc. 25:45–48.

Ilemobade, A.A., and Blotkamp, J. 1976. Preliminary observations on the use of the capillary flocculation test for the diagnosis of heartwater (*Cowdria ruminantium* infection). Res. Vet. Sci. 21:370–372.

Ilemobade, A.A., and Blotkamp, J. 1978. Heartwater in Nigeria. II. The isolation of *Cowdria ruminantium* from live and dead animals and

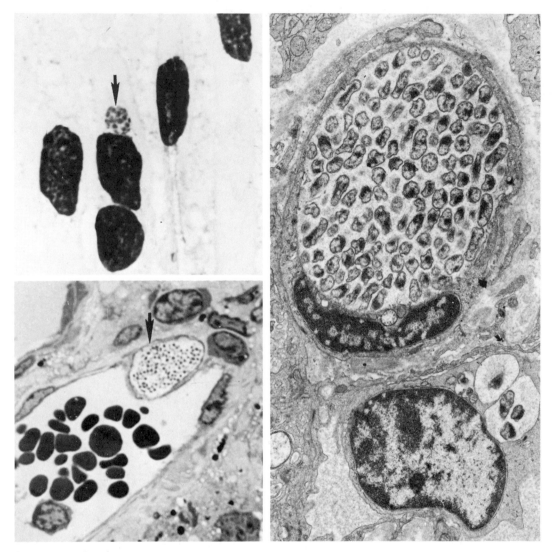

Figure 31.1. *Cowdria ruminantium* in sheep. In brain smear (*top left*). Giemsa stain. × 1,160. In choroid plexus (*bottom left*), araldite section 0.5 μm thick. × 1,160. In a distended endothelial cell (*right*), a colony of organisms is seen completely obstructing the lumen of the capillary. In an adjoining capillary (*at the bottom*), a monocyte has organisms in a cytoplasmic vacuole. × 7,750. (Courtesy J. D. Smith.)

the importance of routes of inoculation. Trop. Anim. Health Prod. 10:39–44.

Ilemobade, A.A., Blotkamp, J., and Synge, B.A. 1975. Preservation of *Cowdria ruminantium* at low temperatures. Res. Vet. Sci. 19:337–338.

Immelman, A., and Dreyer, G. 1982. The use of doxycycline to control heartwater in sheep. J. S. Afr. Vet. Assoc. 53:23–24.

Marsh, H. 1958. Infectious diseases of sheep. Adv. Vet. Sci. 4:163–209.

Neitz, W.O., and Alexander, R.A. 1945. Immunization of cattle against heartwater and the control of the tick-borne disease, redwater, gallsickness, and heartwater. Onderstepoort J. Vet. Res. 20:137–158.

Sahu, S.P., Dardiri, A.H., and Wool, S.H. 1983. Observation of *Rickettsia ruminantium* in leukocytic cell cultures from heartwaterinfected goats, sheep, and cattle. Am. J. Vet. Res. 44:1093–1097.

Uilenberg, G. 1981. Heartwater disease. Curr. Top. Vet. Med. Anim. Sci. 6:345–360.

Uilenberg, G. 1982. Experimental transmission of *Cowdria ruminantium* by the Gulf Coast tick *Amblyomma maculatum:* Danger of introducing heartwater and benign African theileriasis onto the American mainland. Am. J. Vet. Res. 43:1279–1282.

Winkelhoff, A.J., and Uilenberg, G. 1981. Heartwater: Cross immunity studies with strains of *Cowdria ruminantium*. Trop. Anim. Health Prod. 13:160–164.

Tick-Borne Fever

SYNONYM: Pasture fever

Foggie (1951) described tick-borne fever in sheep and proposed the name *Ehrlichia (Rickettsia) phagocytophilia* for the organism. The organism infects sheep, cattle, goats, and wild ungulates. Following an acute attack, the infection may persist up to 2 years in the surviving animal. The disease has been described in Great Britain, Norway, Finland, The Netherlands, and India.

Tick-borne fever is characterized by a sudden rise in temperature and the persistence of a fluctuating fever for 3 to 5 days in cattle and for 10 days in sheep. Milk production drops in dairy cows and may never fully recover. Febrile relapses can occur 2 to 4 weeks after the initial attack. In some outbreaks sheep and cattle in the later stages of gestation have aborted.

Sometimes clinical disease is complicated by concurrent infection with *Babesia,* by viral diarrhea infection, or by cobalt deficiency. Concurrent infections of *E. phagocytophilia* with *Listeria monocytogenes* (Groenstoel and Oeveras 1980), parainfluenza 3 virus (Batungbacal and Scott 1982b), or *Pasteurella haemolytica* (Gilmour et al. 1982) produces a more severe disease in experimental lambs than either agent alone. Suppression of the humoral immune system by *E. phagocytophilia* (Batungbacal and Scott 1982a) may play a role in the more severe dual infections. The lymphocytopenia probably results from a depletion of circulating B lymphocytes (Batungbacal et al. 1982).

The infecting agents recovered from sheep and cattle are different strains of the same organism. They produce more severe disease in their respective natural hosts. The incubation period varies from 4 to 8 days after exposure to infected ticks (*Ixodes ricinus*) and from 5 to 12 days after inoculation with infective blood.

Immunity. All evidence suggests that strains of *E. phagocytophilia* are immunologically heterogenous. There is little or no apparent cross-immunity between the Scottish and Finnish strains of *E. phagocytophilia.* In one study experimental cattle and sheep were given successive injections with 11 Finnish strains, and some animals reacted to 6 different strains (Tuomi 1966). Virulent strains appeared to be more immunogenic than mild strains.

Woldehiwet and Scott (1982a, 1982b) found that infection induced a primary antibody response characterized by an initial production of IgM antibodies followed by IgG antibodies but that immune animals produced IgM antibodies for long periods. This is believed to be due to the carrier state. Sheep were resistant to reinfection when their reciprocal complement-fixing antibody titers were higher than 24. In sheep challenged when their complement-fixing antibody titers were lower than 24, a few *E. phagocytophilia* organisms appeared in the blood, with or without fever.

In nature repeated attacks, exclusive of relapses, are seldom seen. Reinfection from repeated tick bites pre-

sumably occurs and confers adequate immunity during the same tick season; however, tick-borne fever can recur in the same animal during subsequent tick seasons.

The complement-fixation test was used to assess antigenic relationships between three ovine strains of *E. phagocytophilia.* Cross-reactions suggested that the strains share common antigens, and quantitative differentiation by the complement-fixation test was possible (Woldehiwet and Scott 1982a, 1982b).

Diagnosis. The ideal time to take blood specimens for demonstration or isolation of *E. phagocytophilia* is during the initial febrile period when large numbers are in the circulation. Some sheep remain carriers for 2 years, but most animals rid their tissues of demonstrable organisms within a month. Blood smears may be made immediately or later from a citrated blood specimen. The organism usually remains viable for 7 days at 4°C and survives for several months at −70°C.

Either Giemsa or May-Grünwald-Giemsa stains are excellent for demonstration of the organism in blood smears. The fluorescent antibody method can be used, but offers no advantage in ease of technique or certainty of diagnosis. The organisms have a predilection for granulocytes, but monocytes can be infected. At the peak of infection 50 percent or more of the granulocytes can be infected with virulent strains, whereas other strains can infect 6 percent. At least 100 cells should be examined before a blood smear is called negative.

The pleomorphism of *E. phagocytophilia* is apparent in stained preparations, even in the same cell (Figure 31.2). The deep-purple-staining coccoid or rod-shaped body usually situated at the periphery of the cell is about 0.5 μm in diameter. The larger, homogeneously staining body more deeply situated in the cell cytoplasm is 1.3 by 2 μm and often appears to fragment into smaller irregularly shaped bodies. The rounded or oval masses, termed *morula,* contain numerous distinct bodies that stain a deeper blue or purple than the surrounding matrix.

Intravenous inoculation of infective defibrinated blood into susceptible sheep or cattle is another means of diagnosis. A definitive diagnosis requires that the granulocytes in blood smears from test animals contain the characteristic organism.

REFERENCES

Batungbacal, M.R., and Scott, G.R. 1982a. Suppression of the immune response to clostridial vaccine by tick-borne fever. J. Comp. Pathol. 92:409–413.

Batungbacal, M.R., and Scott, G.R. 1982b. Tick-borne fever and concurrent parainfluenza-3 virus infection in sheep. J. Comp. Pathol. 92:415–428.

Batungbacal, M.R., Scott, G.R., and Burrells, C. 1982. The lymphocytopenia in tick-borne fever. J. Comp. Pathol. 92:403–407.

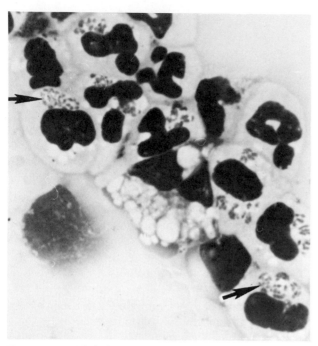

Figure 31.2. *Ehrlichia phagocytophilia* in granulocytes of a leukocyte concentrate. May-Grünwald-Giemsa stain. × 1,400. (Courtesy J. Tuomi.)

Foggie, A. 1951. Studies on the infectious agent of tick-borne fever in sheep. J. Pathol. Bacteriol. 63:1–15.

Gilmour, N.J., Brodie, T.A., and Holmes, P.H. 1982. Tick-borne fever and pasteurellosis in sheep (correspondence). Vet. Res. 111:512.

Groenstoel, H., and Oeveras, J. 1980. Listeriosis in sheep. Tick-borne fever used as a model to study predisposing factors. Acta Vet. Scand. 21:533–545.

Tuomi, J. 1966. Studies in epidemiology of bovine tick-borne fever in Finland and a clinical description of field cases. Ann. Med. Exp. Biol. Fenn. Vol. 44 (Suppl. 6).

Woldehiwet, Z., and Scott, G.R. 1982a. Immunological studies on tick-borne fever in sheep. J. Comp. Pathol. 92:457–467.

Woldehiwet, Z., and Scott, G.R. 1982b. Differentiation of strains of *Cytoecetes phagocytophilia*, the causative agent of tick-borne fever, by complement-fixation. J. Comp. Pathol. 92:475–478.

Bovine and Ovine Ehrlichiosis

Benign bovine and ovine ehrlichiosis is limited geographically to the Middle East, Sri Lanka, and North and South Africa. Little is known about this disease in cattle and in sheep, but *Ehrlichia bovis* and *E. ovina* are considered to be different strains of the same organism (Lewis 1976).

Epizootiology and Pathogenesis. *E. bovis* is transmitted to cattle by ticks of the genus *Hyalomma,* whereas *E. ovina* is transmitted to sheep by the tick *Rhipicephalus bursa.* A 10 percent suspension of spleen tissue, lung tissue, or blood taken during the febrile stage is used to transmit the organism to its natural host. The incubation period in sheep and cattle is approximately 12 days.

The disease is rarely fatal in either cattle or sheep. Both species show a fluctuating fever of several weeks' duration. The most significant lesion is excessive pericardial fluid, similar to heartwater fever in sheep. Other consistent changes are lymphadenopathy and splenomegaly. Cattle and sheep may remain carriers for 10 months.

Immunity. Chronic infections may persist for 10 months in sheep and cattle. Animals that recover develop a solid immunity against challenge with the homologous organism, although the duration of immunity is unknown.

Diagnosis. The organisms can be readily demonstrated in blood smears from animals in the febrile stage. Tissues from the lungs, liver, and spleen are also suitable for *Ehrlichia* demonstration.

These rickettsias are found in the cytoplasm of the circulating monocytes and monocytelike cells in the lungs, liver, and spleen. The monocytes in the blood smear usually gather at the edge of the preparation. They frequently assemble in round colonies 2 to 10 μm in diameter and also in closely packed granules 0.5 to 1.0 μm in diameter. With Giemsa stain they appear similar to *E. phagocytophilia*. Initial bodies, 3 by 6 μm, stain a homogenous red and later separate into elementary bodies that appear purple with May-Grünwald-Giemsa stain. A thorough search should be made of smears because the percentage of monocytes with organisms is usually low.

REFERENCE

Lewis, G.E. 1976. Equine ehrlichiosis: A comparison between *E. equi* and other pathogenic species of *Ehrlichia*. Vet. Parasitol. 2:61–74.

Canine Ehrlichiosis

Canine ehrlichiosis has been reported in North and East Africa, India, Sri Lanka, Aruba, and the United States. Three species are recognized to cause the disease in dogs: *Ehrlichia canis, E. equi,* and *E. platys.* Once considered a rare disease in the United States, canine ehrlichiosis now is diagnosed more frequently in endemic areas owing to increased transport of infected animals and ticks and to greater recognition of the disease by veterinarians and dog owners (Hibler et al. 1986). *E. canis* often occurs in dogs infected with *Babesia canis* because both rickettsias are transmitted by the brown dog tick, *Rhipicephalus sanguineus.* Jackals, foxes, wolves, coyotes, and other wild canids are also susceptible. An excellent review article on canine ehrlichiosis has been written by Hibler et al. (1986).

Epizootiology and Pathogenesis. As noted above, *E. canis* is transmitted to dogs by the tick *R. sanguineus.*

Lung, liver, or spleen tissue as a 10 percent suspension

or blood taken during the febrile stage of infective dogs produces the disease in susceptible dogs 7 to 21 days after parenteral injection.

Dogs can remain carriers for at least 29 months after an acute attack (Ewing and Philip 1966) and constitute a constant reservoir for the infection in nature. Unfortunately, carrier dogs may become donors of whole blood used for therapeutic purposes in veterinary hospitals. There is evidence that this has occurred despite efforts to ensure that the donor was free of the disease. Inoculation of puppies with donor blood is the only known means to detect carriers. Obviously, the same problem exists with other diseases in which the organism persists in the animal's bloodstream after the signs of illness are gone.

E. canis can persist in adult *R. sanguineus* ticks for 155 days after detachment, as engorged nymphs, from a dog in the acute phase of ehrlichiosis. Infected but unfed ticks may be more important than the chronically infected carrier dog as a natural reservoir of *E. canis* (Lewis et al. 1977).

The signs of canine ehrlichiosis are generally mild or inapparent and include fever, anorexia, dyspnea, purulent oculonasal discharge, slight weight loss, and lymph adenopathy. Typically, dogs recover in 1 to 2 weeks after their onset. During the acute stage, ticks are often found on the dogs. Hematological abnormalities can be present, but bleeding episodes do not occur. The dogs remain infected with persisting hematological abnormalities. A recurrence of signs can occur after apparent recovery.

Dogs with chronic illness show depression, weight loss, pale mucous membranes, abdominal tenderness, and bleeding tendencies (Greene and Harvey 1984). Epitaxis is typical of the chronic phase. Pulmonary and ocular signs may occur. During the acute or chronic phase nervous signs may result from mononuclear cell infiltration in the meninges and hemorrhage from thrombocytopenia. An arched back, severe pain in the neck or the back, unilateral or bilateral paraparesis, cranial nerve deficits, and convulsions are commonly associated with neurological ehrlichiosis.

In the terminal stages kidney function is reduced (Price and Sayer 1983). Infective bitches can have reproductive problems including bleeding, inability to conceive, abortion, and neonatal death.

Signs associated with *E. equi* infection in dogs are not as severe as those occurring with *E. canis* infection. The causative agent of experimental infectious cyclic thrombocytopenia in dogs is *E. platys*. Although it does not produce natural disease and infects platelets rather than leukocytes, it is similar morphologically to *E. canis*.

At necropsy the gross pathological changes of canine ehrlichiosis include anemia, hyperactive bone marrow, petechiae of the lungs, and enlarged spleen, liver, and lymph nodes. Less commonly observed changes are hemorrhages and ulcers in the intestinal tract, hydrothorax, and pulmonary edema.

The histological lesion in the bone marrow of dogs with severe pancytopenia consists of hypoplasia, depletion of megakaryocytes, and often loss of normal sinusoidal architecture (Buhles et al. 1975). Dogs chronically infected, but without severe pancytopenia, have normocellular marrow.

Immunity. Animals that recover from an acute attack usually are immune to reinfection. Nyindo (1976) suggested that the elimination of *E. canis* from a carrier dog renders it susceptible to reinfection. Others suggested that there may be a correlation between a high antibody titer, as determined by the indirect fluorescent antibody test, and protection in the dog (Smith et al. 1976). Persistence of the organism in recovered dogs can be demonstrated by splenectomy, with the ensuing appearance of *E. canis* in the circulating monocytes.

In experimental studies Kakoma et al. (1977) found that cell-mediated responses developed in the majority of the dogs, but that they declined and disappeared in most dogs by 19 to 21 weeks after infection. Serum antibody titers, as measured by the indirect fluorescent antibody test, increased with time and remained at significant levels. It is interesting that lymphocytes from dogs infected with *E. canis* were shown to be toxic for autologous monocytes. Neither immune serum and complement nor anticanine globulin had any observable effect on cytotoxicity. The monocytotoxicity bore a temporal relationship to the thrombocytopenia. The authors also suggested that T lymphocyte activation accompanying ehrlichiosis contributes to the pathogenesis of the disease; the specific immune elimination of parasitized monocytes is antibody independent (van Heerden and Immelman 1979).

E. canis, *E. equi*, and *E. platys* show no cross-protection in dogs.

Diagnosis. *E. canis* organisms can be recovered from the blood of infected dogs for long periods. They are demonstrated most readily 2 or 3 days after the onset of fever until the clinical signs end. If direct blood smears are negative, smears of the buffy coat of heparinized or citrated blood samples may be positive. During the febrile period, *E. canis* can be demonstrated in biopsy material taken from the lung, liver, or spleen. As there are insufficient data on the survival of the organism, fresh test material should be injected promptly into susceptible dogs.

With the development of an indirect fluorescent antibody test for *E. canis* it is possible to detect the organism in smears of midgut tissues of *R. sanguineus* (Smith et al. 1976). The test is also used to detect and titrate antibodies in the serum of dogs infected with *E. canis* (Ristic et al. 1972).

Stephenson and Osterman (1977) developed another diagnostic test for this disease: a tissue-culture system that uses canine peritoneal macrophages. The cultures are well established in 6 days and are maintained for at least 30 days. Infected cells can be detected by 60 hours after inoculation with *E. canis,* and replication is evident by 12 to 18 days.

E. canis has the same morphologic and staining characteristics as *E. bovis* and *E. ovina*. Because ehrlichiosis, particularly in the dog, is often complicated by concurrent infections with *Babesia,* a thorough search should also be made for the latter organism in the erythrocytes.

Antimicrobial Susceptibility. Certain drugs, such as broad-spectrum antibiotics, employed successfully in the treatment of Rocky Mountain spotted fever and salmon poisoning disease, can alter the course of canine (and presumably ovine and bovine) ehrlichiosis, but do not prevent the development of the carrier stage.

Price and Dolan (1980) prefer to use imidocarb deproprionate at dosages of 5–7 mg/kg of body weight given intramuscularly twice at an interval of 14 days. They found it was as effective as tetracycline hydrochloride in alleviating clinical signs and was better at reducing the number of carriers. It also had the further advantage of controlling concurrent babesiosis.

In treating 20 dogs with erhlichiosis, van Heerden and Immelman (1979) found that doxycycline was effective even in those animals that had not responded to treatment with oxytetracycline.

The Disease in Humans. Since 1986 human infections by an organism similar to *E. canis* have been diagnosed in the eastern, southern, and midwestern United States. Clinical features included fever, headache, anorexia, myalgia, and leukopenia; a rash like that of Rocky Mountain spotted fever is generally not present. Diagnosis is made on the basis of the indirect fluorescent antibody test on paired serums.

REFERENCES

Buhles, W.C., Jr., Huxsoll, D.L., and Hildebrandt, P.K. 1975. Tropical canine pancytopenia: Role of aplastic anaemia in the pathogenesis of severe disease. J. Comp. Pathol. 85:511–521.
Ewing, S.A. 1969. Canine ehrlichiosis. Adv. Vet. Sci. 13:331–353.
Ewing, S.A., and Philip, C.B. 1966. Discovery of an *Ehrlichia*-like disease agent in Oklahoma (USA) dogs and its relationship to *Neorickettsia helminthoeca*. Am. J. Vet. Res. 27:67–69.
Greene, C.E., and Harvey, J.W. 1984. Canine ehrlichiosis. In C.E. Greene, ed., Clinical Microbiology and Infectious Diseases of the Dog and Cat. W.B. Saunders, Philadelphia. Pp. 545-561.
Hibler, S.C., Hoskins, J.D., and Greene, C.E. 1986. Rickettsial infections in dogs. II. Ehrlichiosis and infectious cyclic thrombocytopenia. Compend. Cont. Ed. Pract. Vet. 8:107–114.
Kakoma, I., Carson, C.A., Ristic, M., Huxsoll, D.L., Stephenson, E.H., and Nyindo, M.B.A. 1977. Autologous lymphocyte-mediated cytotoxicity against monocytes in canine ehrlichiosis. Am. J. Vet. Res. 38:1557–1559.
Lewis, G.E., Jr., Ristic, M., Smith, R.D., Lincoln, T., and Stephenson, E.H. 1977. The brown dog tick, *Rhipicephalus sanguineus,* and the dog as experimental hosts of *Ehrlichia canis.* Am. J. Vet. Res. 38:1953–1955.
Nyindo, M.B.A. 1976. Immune responses to *Ehrlichia canis* and *Ehrlichia equi* in experimentally-infected dogs and ponies. Diss. Abstr. Int. B Sci. Eng. 36:4334.
Price, J.E., and Dolan, T.T. 1980. A comparison of the efficacy of imidocarb depropionate and tetracycline hydrochloride in the treatment of canine ehrlichiosis. Vet. Rec. 107:275–277.
Ristic, M., Huxsoll, D.L., Weisiger, R.M., Hildebrandt, P.K., and Nyindo, M.B.A. 1972. Serological diagnosis of tropical canine pancytopenia by indirect immunofluorescence. Infect. Immun. 6:226–231.
Smith, R.D., Sells, D.M., Stephenson, E.H., Ristic, M., and Huxsoll, D.L. 1976. Development of *Ehrlichia canis,* causative agent of canine ehrlichiosis in the tick *Rhipicephalus sanguineous* and its differentiation from a symbiotic rickettsia. Am. J. Vet. Res. 37:119–126.
Stephenson, E.H., and Osterman, J.V. 1977. Canine peritoneal macrophages: Cultivation and infection with *Ehrlichia canis.* Am. J. Vet. Res. 38:1815–1819.
van Heerden, J., and Immelman, A. 1979. The use of doxycycline in the treatment of canine ehrlichiosis. J. S. Afr. Vet. Assoc. 50:241, 243–244.

Equine Ehrlichiosis

Equine ehrlichiosis occurs as a distinct entity in horses located in California and Illinois, United States. There have been 46 naturally occurring cases in California through 1980 (Madigan and Gribble 1982). Gunders and Gottlieb (1977) collected ticks from burros in Israel which transmitted a granulocyte-inhabiting parasite believed to be a rickettsial organism that may have caused disease. It is not known if the organism was *Ehrlichia equi,* the causative agent of equine ehrlichiosis.

Epizootiology and Pathogenesis. No arthropod has yet been incriminated as the vector of *E. equi* except for the cases in Israel, in which the tick *Ornithodoros erratius* was found on burros parasitized with a granulocyte-inhabiting organism similar to *Rickettsia*. As Gunders and Gottlieb (1977) did not claim the organism was *E. equi,* further studies are necessary to establish the identity of the disease agent.

Infective blood produces equine ehrlichiosis in experimental horses. Horses less than 2 years old usually do not show clinical signs other than fever. Dogs, sheep, and goats develop a mild or inapparent infection after parenteral injection, and the organism can be demonstrated in the cytoplasm of the granulocytes.

Knowledge of this disease has been derived from the 46 natural cases and from experimental disease produced in horses and burros (Gribble 1969, Stannard et al. 1969). In experimental cases the incubation period ranged from 1 to 9 days, with a mean of 2.5 days with fresh blood and 6.5 days with frozen blood.

The disease is characterized by fever, depression, anorexia, edema of the legs, and ataxia. Hematological changes are thrombocytopenia, elevated plasma icterus index, decreased packed cell volume, and marked leukopenia involving lymphocytes and then granulocytes. Subcutaneous edema of the legs appears first at the metacarpal and metatarsal regions and can ascend to the radius and 6 to 8 inches above the hock.

At necropsy edema and petechial and ecchymotic hemorrhages are found in the subcutaneous tissues, fascia, and epimysium of the legs distal to the elbow and stifle joints. Carcasses are frequently jaundiced, and orchitis is often seen in mature males. Some horses have excessive fluid in the peritoneal cavity and pericardial sac. Histologic examination shows vasculitis of small arteries and veins which involves swelling of endothelial and smooth muscle cells, thromboses, and perivascular infiltrations of monocytes and lymphocytes. The vessels in the testes, ovaries, legs, and pampiniform plexus are principally affected.

Immunity. Current evidence suggests that one attack confers immunity (Madigan and Gribble 1982). Horses recovered from experimental disease withstood challenge with infectious blood given 2.5 to 20 months later. This evaluation was based on the lack of clinical signs and of organisms in circulating granulocytes.

Diagnosis. As with other ehrlichioses, blood specimens are taken preferably during the febrile period, usually 3 to 5 days after its onset. The best smears are made with fresh blood, but citrated blood samples in sterile tubes maintained at 4°C can be used for later examination. Fresh blood is preferred for inoculation into susceptible horses, but defibrinated blood sealed in glass ampules and stored at −70°C remains infectious, although the incubation period is prolonged.

The diagnosis is based on the demonstration of rickettsias in the granulocytes contained in blood smears from natural and experimental cases. With Giemsa or Wright-Leishman stain the inclusion bodies appear deep blue to pale blue-gray. They may vary from small darkly stained bodies 0.2 μm in diameter to large granular bodies 5 μm in diameter, which represent a cluster of smaller bodies. The percentage of parasitized granulocytes varies with the stage of the disease, with a mean maximum of 36 percent.

E. equi found in equine pheripheral leukocytes has the same structure as other agents of the genus *Ehrlichia* (Sells et al. 1976). A great variation in size is observed. Lewis (1976) believes *E. equi* is a different strain of *E. canis* and *E. phagocytophilia*.

Antimicrobial Susceptibility. The best agent for the treatment of the 46 cases in California was oxytetracycline (Madigan and Gribble 1982).

REFERENCES

Gribble, D.H. 1969. Equine ehrlichiosis. J. Am. Vet. Med. Assoc. 155:462–469.

Gunders, A.E., and Gottlieb, D. 1977. Intra-erythrocytic inclusion bodies of *Psammomys obesus* naturally transmitted by *Ornithodoros erraticus* (small race). Refu. Vet. 34:5–9.

Lewis, G.E., Jr. 1976. Equine ehrlichiosis: A comparison between *E. equi* and other pathogenic species of *Ehrlichia*. Vet. Parasitol. 2:61–74.

Madigan, J.E., and Gribble, D.H. 1982. Equine ehrlichiosis: Diagnosis and treatment. A report of 46 clinical cases in California, USA. Proc. Annu. Conv. Am. Assoc. Equine Pract. 27:305–312.

Sells, D.M., Hildebrandt, P.K., Lewis, G.E., Jr., Nyindo, M.B.A., and Ristic, M. 1976. Ultrastructural observations on *Ehrlichia equi* organisms in equine granulocytes. Infect. Immun. 13:273–280.

Stannard, A.A., Gribble, D.H., and Smith, R.S. 1969. Equine ehrlichiosis: A disease with similarities to tick-borne fever and bovine petechial fever. Vet. Rec. 84:149–150.

Potomac Horse Fever

SYNONYMS: Acute equine diarrhea syndrome, equine monocytic ehrlichiosis, Potomac fever of horses

In the summer of 1978 Potomac horse fever, an acute disease of horses and ponies, was first recognized in Maryland, with most cases located in Montgomery County. More recently the disease has been found in Pennsylvania, Virginia, Wisconsin, Idaho, Ohio, Oklahoma, and Colorado in the United States and also in Europe. The disease occurs only in the summer months. The causative agent is a newly described parasite named *Ehrlichia risticii* (Holland, Weiss, et al. 1985), which is closely related to *E. sennetsu* and to a lesser degree to *E. canis*, the type species of the genus. There is no serologic relationship to *E. equi*.

Cultural Features. Two groups of investigators (Holland et al. 1984; Holland, Ristic, et al. 1985; Rikihisa and Perry 1984) reported the successful cultivation of *E. risticii*. The agent reproduces well in human histiocytes, as determined on smears of cultured cells prepared by modified Giemsa and fluorescent antibody staining techniques (Rikihisa and Perry 1984, Rikihisa et al. 1984) and in primary cultures of canine blood monocytes that caused disease in an experimental pony (Holland et al. 1984; Holland, Ristic, et al. 1985) (Figure 31.3).

Epizootiology and Pathogenesis (Knowles et al. 1984, Whitlock et al. 1984). Epidemiological evidence suggests that Potomac horse fever is not contagious. Because it occurs only in the warm summer months and is caused by an *Ehrlichia* agent, in all likelihood the disease is transmitted by a tick. The disease has been transmitted by direct transfer of infective blood to susceptible experimental horses and ponies, so only sterile needles and syringes should be used for injections.

Potomac horse fever is characterized by loss of appetite, depression, fever, leukopenia, explosive diarrhea, dehydration, and terminal shock. The severity of the clinical signs ranges from transient fever and depression with-

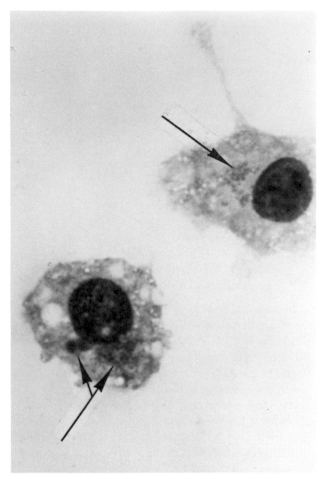

Figure 31.3. *Ehrlichia risticii* in the cytoplasm of cultured canine blood monocytes. Giemsa stain. × 1,800. (Courtesy Cynthia Holland.)

out diarrhea, to hypovolemic shock, diarrhea, and death. Colic of variable severity occurs in a few horses, and these horses usually develop diarrhea and seem to have a higher incidence of laminitis. Laminitis occurs in 20 to 30 percent of clinical cases. Horses with laminitis rarely survive. In 60 to 70 percent of the horses that do survive, recovery is complete. It has been postulated that further field and experimental studies will show that inapparent infections are not uncommon.

Laboratory findings usually include a white blood cell count of 2000–5000/μl and packed cell volumes of 40 to 65 percent or higher, depending on the severity of diarrhea. The plasma protein concentration is often elevated because of the dehydration and hemoconcentration that occur early in the disease process.

At necropsy severe petechial and ecchymotic hemorrhages are found in fat at the heart base, along coronary vessels, and on the endocardium and adventitial surfaces of the ascending and thoracic aortas. The lungs are congested and occasionally consolidated. The liver is mottled and slightly swollen. The gastrointestinal tract shows ulceration of the mucosal surface of the glandular and pyloric regions, regional patchy areas of congestion in the duodenum, fluid contents with some mucus in the small intestine, and focal areas of congestion and watery contents in the cecum and colon. Vesicles on oral mucosa have been seen in three cases.

Microscopic pathological changes occur in various organs. Necrotizing enterocolitis occurs, with the most severe alterations in the cecal and colonic segments. Vasculitis is seen in the smaller blood vessels, and microscopic thrombi in veins and arteries, especially in cecal and colonic regions. Pneumonia occasionally occurs. There is hemorrhage and disruption of architectural arrangements in the liver. Lymphoidal depletion occurs within the lymph nodes and spleen.

Investigators first reproduced the disease in horses by using a large volume of infective blood obtained from naturally infected horses in the acute stages of the disease (Rikihisa and Perry 1984, Rikihisa et al. 1984, Whitlock et al. 1984). The agent has been serially transferred with whole blood more than 30 times in horses (Whitlock et al. 1984). Koch's postulates were fulfilled by other investigators: Holland and co-workers (1984, 1985) isolated the organism in cultured blood monocytes from an experimentally infected pony, maintained the organism through successive passages in primary canine blood monocyte cultures, and then reproduced the disease in a susceptible pony by inoculating it with an infected canine blood monocyte culture. The intracytoplasmic agent was then reisolated from this diseased pony, which had typical lesions at necropsy (Holland et al. 1984; Holland, Ristic, et al. 1985).

Immunity. There is some field evidence that recovered horses are immune to subsequent exposures. Perhaps more significant is the observation that experimental horses that recover develop antibodies and are resistant to a challenge dose of infective blood (Whitlock et al. 1984). Immunity studies can now be extended because the etiology has been ascertained (see discussion under "Diagnosis").

A bacterin prepared from cell-free morulae of *E. risticii* has given a high level of protection against experimental infection and is being field-tested in clinical trials (Ristic et al. 1988).

Diagnosis. Diagnostic tests for Potomac horse fever include the use of the Giemsa stain or the fluorescent antibody technique to demonstrate the organism in dried blood smears or buffy coat smears from potentially infected horses (Rikihisa and Perry 1984). The use of cell cultures such as human histiocytes (Rikihisa and Perry 1984) or canine monocytes (Holland et al. 1985) for the cultivation of the agent provides another approach to diagnosis. Paired serum samples can also be used to demonstrate a rising antibody titer to *E. risticii* in those cases for which a quick diagnosis is not imperative.

In cases of diarrhea in horses, salmonellosis must be considered in the differential diagnosis. *Salmonella* organisms can be readily grown on artificial media and quickly identified. Colitis X is more difficult to distinguish from Potomac horse fever, but colitis X appears to be more fulminating than Potomac horse fever and the horse usually has a history of stress (Whitlock et al. 1984).

Antimicrobial Susceptibility. Given that other *Ehrlichia* organisms can often be controlled with appropriate doses of antibiotics, a variety of antibiotics have been tried in horses with Potomac horse fever. So far, tetracyclines are giving the best results, but more study must be done. Correction of the dehydration is important. The amount of fluid replacement depends on laboratory and clinical evaluations. Other forms of supportive treatment are indicated (Knowles et al. 1984).

Unfortunately, it is impossible to predict the outcome. Some horses with mild cases never recover, whereas others with more alarming early signs recover nicely. Any sign of laminitis indicates a poor prognosis.

REFERENCES

Holland, C.J., Johnson, P., Baker, G., and Goetz, T. 1984. Causative agent of Potomac horse fever (communication). Vet. Rec. 115:554.

Holland, C.J., Ristic, M., Cole, A.I., Johnson, P., Baker, G., and Goetz, T. 1985. Isolation, experimental transmission, and characterization of causative agent of Potomac horse fever. Science. 227:522–524.

Holland, C.J., Weiss, E., Burgdorfer, W., Cole, A.I., and Kakoma, I. 1985. *Ehrlichia risticii* sp. nov.: Etiological agent of equine monocytic ehrlichiosis (synonym, Potomac horse fever). Int. J. Syst. Bacteriol. 35:524–526.

Knowles, R.C., Shook, J.C., Roble, M.G., Whitlock, R.H., and Davidson, J.P. 1984. Acute equine diarrhea syndrome (AEDS)—A situation report. Proc. U.S. Anim. Health Assoc. Pp. 353–357.

Rikihisa, Y., and Perry, B.D. 1984. Causative agent of Potomac horse fever. Vet. Rec. 115:554.

Rikihisa, Y., Perry, B.D., and Corres, D. 1984. Rickettsial link with acute equine diarrhea. Vet. Rec. 115:390.

Ristic, M., Holland, C.J., and Goetz, T.E. 1988. Evaluation of a vaccine for equine monocytic ehrlichiosis (syn., Potomac horse fever). In Proceedings of the 5th International Conference on Equine Infectious Diseases, Lexington, Ky., October 1987. Univ. of Kentucky Press, Lexington. (In press.)

Whitlock, R.H., Palmer, J.E., Tablin, F., Acland, H.M., Jenny, A., and Ristic, M. 1984. Potomac horse fever: Clinical characteristics and diagnostic features. In Proceedings of the American Association of Veterinary Laboratory Diagnosticians. Pp. 88–97.

Bovine Petechial Fever
SYNONYM: Ondiri disease

Reported in Kenya and Tanzania, bovine petechial fever has been recognized only in cattle and sheep of the highland areas of Kenya. The involvement of an invertebrate host in the disease cycle has not been established. *Cytoecetes ondiri,* the causative agent, has all the characteristics of a rickettsial animal pathogen.

A recent search of the literature yielded no new significant information since the seventh edition of this textbook was written.

Epizootiology and Pathogenesis. Clinical bovine petechial fever develops in exotic breeds of cattle. Sahiwal crosses and Borans are susceptible, where Ayrshires and Herefords are resistant to experimental inoculation with *C. ondiri.*

The disease is characterized by fever, petechiae, and depression. Initially, eosinophils disappear and the number of lymphocytes is reduced; the number of neutrophils then falls (Snodgrass 1975a). Latent infections can occur: the blood from some experimentally infected cattle or sheep can be infective for up to 4 weeks after clinical signs end.

Snodgrass (1975c) found that multiplication of *C. ondiri* occurs within 24 hours after inoculation into sheep or cattle, probably in the spleen, because the organism could not be demonstrated in other tissues until later. During the period of greatest concentration of the organism in the tissues, organisms could be demonstrated in the circulating leukocytes. The spleen always had the greatest number of organisms, based on titrations in susceptible sheep.

Immunity. Snodgrass (1975c) reported that effective immunity to challenge with homologous and heterologous strains was observed in cattle and to homologous strains in sheep. Sheep challenged with heterologous strains usually were susceptible. The duration of immunity was not ascertained.

Diagnosis. The clinical signs and necropsy findings are similar to those of several other diseases; diagnosis therefore depends on the demonstration of the presence of the organism. This can usually be done directly in blood or spleen tissue smears prepared with Giemsa stain. Parasitemia can sometimes be absent when signs first appear. In these cases animal inoculations are required to verify a presumptive diagnosis (Snodgrass 1975b).

Antimicrobial Susceptibility. Gloxazone is more effective than tetracycline in the treatment of ondiri disease in sheep, and it is also efficacious in infected cattle (Snodgrass 1976).

REFERENCES

Snodgrass, D.R. 1975a. Clinical response and apparent breed resistance in bovine petechial fever. Trop. Anim. Health Prod. 7:213–218.
Snodgrass, D.R. 1975b. Diagnosis of bovine petechial fever. Vet. Rec. 96:132–133.
Snodgrass, D.R. 1975c. Pathogenesis of bovine petechial fever. Latent infections, immunity, and tissue distribution of *Cytoecetes ondiri*. J. Comp. Pathol. 85:523–530.
Snodgrass, D.R. 1976. Chemotherapy of experimental bovine petechial fever. Res. Vet. Sci. 20:108–109.

Contagious Ophthalmia

Strains of *Colesiota conjunctivae* produce conjunctivitis in sheep, cattle, goats, swine, and chickens and have been reported on all continents except Asia and Antartica. Flies apparently play a role in its transmission.

The relationships among these conjunctival agents in livestock have not been well established. The strains are host specific and not transferable among livestock. Consequently, some investigators contend that *C. conjunctivae* occurs only in sheep and the rickettsias that infect the conjunctivae of other livestock should be given another generic name. In this respect Rizvi (1950) reported a conjunctivitis in young goats caused by *Rickettsia conjunctivae*. Certain features of its morphologic and staining characteristics differed from *C. conjunctivae*.

Pathogenesis. The severity of the disease ranges from mild cases of purulent conjunctivitis with recovery within a week to severe cases with keratitis, vascularization, and occasionally corneal ulceration which persist longer. Most severely affected eyes eventually heal without residual blemish.

Saline washings from the eyes of sheep in the acute phase of the disease are an excellent source of material for transmission of the disease to experimental animals. The disease is reproduced by instilling the conjunctival washings into the eyes of susceptible animals of the same species. The incubation period is 2 to 4 days in the instilled eye; the opposite eye becomes infected 3 to 4 days later.

Immunity. In sheep, immunity persists for 3 months, but after 8 months approximately 10 percent of the animals are again susceptible. The carrier stage persists in some sheep for over a year, and that fact coupled with the loss of immunity in others may account for the survival of the organism in the flock. Immunity in animals other than sheep has not been thoroughly studied.

Diagnosis. Epithelial scrapings from the inner surface of the conjunctiva are made with a scalpel until a tinge of blood appears. The material is spread on a slide, air-dried, fixed with methanol, and stained. The viability of the organism is unknown, but it should be considered labile. The organisms do not survive desiccation.

In Giemsa-stained smears several types of inclusions are observed. Many polymorphonuclear leukocytes are observed in smear preparations taken early in the disease. Most of the organisms are found in the cytoplasm and appear as purplish red, small (0.2 by 0.5 μm) ovoid or short rod-shaped organisms. As recovery ensues, lymphocytes and monocytes replace the polymorphonuclear leukocytes. At this stage irregular extracellular organisms, 0.8 by 1.4 μm, that stain unevenly appear as triangles, imperfect rings, and horseshoe-shaped clusters.

Antimicrobial Susceptibility. Chloramphenicol given to sheep reduces the severity of the disease and also the number of cases of ulcerative keratitis. Riboflavin in daily 15-mg doses is also effective (Marsh 1958).

REFERENCES

Marsh, H. 1958. Infectious diseases of sheep. Adv. Vet. Sci. 4:163–209.
Rizvi, S.W.H. 1950. Transmission of *Rickettsia conjunctivae* to goats. J. Am. Vet. Med. Assoc. 117:409–411.

Jembrana

Budiarso and Hardjosworo (1976) described a highly fatal disease in Bali cattle and buffalo which killed an estimated 60,000 animals in Indonesia within 3 years (Teuscher et al. 1981). Examination of hepatic and splenic smears prepared with Giemsa or Macchiavello stain revealed intracellular organisms resembling rickettsias. On the basis of studies in male guinea pigs, Jembrana disease was suggested to be a rickettsiosis. Other investigators suggested that the disease may be caused by a virus (Teuscher et al. 1981). Plant poisoning and photosensitization have also been proposed as possible causes (Teusher et al. 1982). Clearly, more research must be done before the cause of Jembrana is established.

Pathogenesis. The disease is characterized by anorexia, fever, nasal discharge, increased salivation, and anemia. Bali disease may be a late sporadic form of Jembrana and is characterized by a fever episode followed by inflammation of the head (rhinitis), with erosions as the most frequent sequela (Teuscher et al. 1981).

At necropsy the gross changes consist of a somewhat generalized lymphadenopathy, splenomegaly, hemorrhages, edema, ulceration of the mucous membranes, probable disturbances of coagulation, and sometimes thrombosis. Hematological examinations show leukopenia, anemia, and abnormal lymphocytes. Multifocal infiltrations by lymphoid cells are seen in most organs, especially the lung, heart, liver, and kidney. The brain shows edema and vascular changes such as thrombosis and hemorrhages (Teuscher et al. 1981).

REFERENCES

Budiarso, I.T., and Hardjoswaro, S. 1976. Jembrana disease in Bali cattle. Aust. Vet. J. 52:97.

Teuscher, E., Ramachandran, S., and Hardins, H.P. 1981. Observations on the pathology of "Jembrana disease" in Bali cattle. Zentralbl. Veterinärmed. [A] 28:608–622.

Teuscher, E., Ramachandran, S., and Hardins, H.P. 1982. Is "Bali disease" in cattle a late complication of "Jembrana disease"? Zentralbl. Veterinärmed. [A] 29:547–556.

Salmon Poisoning

SYNONYM: Salmon disease

Salmon poisoning occurs in western Oregon, northwestern California, and southwestern Washington in the United States, and in India. It affects several members of the family Canidae: dogs, foxes, and coyotes are known to be susceptible. House cats, mink, raccoons, and swine apparently are resistant. The disease in the United States has long been associated with the eating of fluke-infested salmon and trout from streams that flow into the Pacific Ocean. Although the disease has the appearance of an infection, it was long regarded as a poisoning or intoxication. Several facts about this disease indicated that it was more than a simple intestinal parasitism (see discussion under "Epizootiology and Pathogenesis), and Philip et al. (1954a) proposed the name *Neorickettsia helminthoeca* for the agent resembling rickettsias which is associated with the fluke infestation and plays an important role in the disease among mammals (Philip 1933; Philip, Hadlow, et al. 1954; Philip, Hughes, et al. 1954).

A series of papers by a group at Washington State University described a second agent, immunologically distinct from *N. helminthoeca* and called the Elokomin fluke fever agent, as a part of the salmon poisoning syndrome (Farrell et al. 1973; Frank, McGuire, Gorham, and Davis 1974; Frank, McGuire, Gorham, and Farrell 1974; Sakawa et al. 1973). It causes a less severe disease in dogs, with recovery ensuing in dogs with experimental disease, whereas dogs infected with *N. helminthoeca* have a high mortality.

Epizootiology and Pathogenesis. *N. helminthoeca* is transmitted to susceptible animals by means of an intestinal fluke, the encysted form of which occurs in the musculature of fish of the family Salmonidae. Chapin (1926) studied this fluke and named it *Nanophytes salmincola*. It is also known as *Troglotrema salmincola*. When parasitized fish are eaten by susceptible carnivores, the adult flukes develop in the intestines. Ova escaping from these

animals infect a small snail, *Goniobasis plicifera* var. *silicula,* which in turn infects the fish. The limited distribution of this snail apparently is the factor that controls the spread of the disease.

Simms et al. (1932) and Simms and Muth (1933) were successful in transmitting the disease to dogs by intraperitoneal injection of blood or of ground, washed flukes from infected dogs, by injection of metacercaria from parasitized fish, and by feeding fluke-infected trout and salmon. The signs produced were the same as those seen in the naturally contracted disease.

Donham et al. (1926) failed to produce salmon poisoning with ocean-caught salmon in which no encysted flukes could be found. The same species taken in fresh water in the salmon poisoning area contained metacercaria and produced salmon poisoning when fed to dogs. A survey of the streams of the region showed only one species of snail occurring where fish infection existed. This was the species shown to be the intermediate host of the fluke. Parasitized fish included the Chinook, silverside, and chum (or dog) salmon, the brook (or speckled) trout, the cutthroat (or mountain) trout, the rainbow trout, and the steelhead trout. Other types of fish occurring in the region were not infected.

It had been assumed that smoke-treated salmon were not dangerous to dogs, but Farrell et al. (1968) reported signs resembling salmon poisoning in dogs after the ingestion of uncooked, smoke-treated salmon that harbored *N. helminthoeca*.

The first sign of disease in dogs is a slight rise in body temperature. Within 24 hours there is a complete loss of appetite and marked depression, and the temperature rises to 104° to 107°F. The animal appears dejected and apathetic. After several days the temperature usually decreases. A slight purulent discharge can occur from the eyes during the fourth to sixth day of illness. The eyelids and adjacent tissues become edematous about this time, giving the eyes a sunken appearance. Beginning about the fourth or fifth day, persistent vomiting usually occurs. This is accompanied by a rapid loss of body weight. The animals become avid for water, but most of it is lost by further vomition. Diarrhea usually begins about the fifth to seventh day. In the beginning the diarrheal discharge frequently is tinged with blood, and later it is heavily impregnated with blood. After a day or two of diarrhea, many animals appear to improve, but often only temporarily. Finally the temperature falls to subnormal. At this time the animal is so emaciated and weak that it can hardly stand.

Signs of illness usually appear on the sixth or eighth day after the parasitized fish are eaten. A few animals show signs as early as the fifth day or as late as the twelfth day.

Most untreated dogs die within 6 to 10 days after the appearance of signs. Simms et al. (1931) observed recovery in only 4 dogs in a series of 102.

At necropsy hemorrhagic inflammation of the intestine is the most characteristic lesion. The inflammatory reaction can be observed throughout the bowel, or it can be limited to certain regions. In many cases the entire bowel is lined with bloody exudate; in others the contents are merely blood-tinged. Ulceration is seen in a few cases. The ulcers often are superficial and range in size from barely visible to 2 to 3 cm in diameter. Flukes and fluke eggs can be found in the intestinal contents in large numbers. As many as 200,000 parasites have been recovered from a single dog.

Gross changes are found in the lymphocytic tissues. Variable enlargement of the ileocecal, mesenteric, portal, and internal iliac lymph nodes is common. The predominant and most consistent microscopic finding in the lymph nodes is a decrease in the number of mature lymphocytes accompanied by a proliferation of the reticuloendothelial elements in both the cortex and medulla. Similar changes are found in the tonsils, thymus, and lymphoid tissues of the spleen and intestinal tract. Coccobacillary bodies are present in the numerous reticular cells, either clustered in morulalike masses or diffusely scattered in the cytoplasm. They are often numerous in the histiocytes of the intestinal villi. Some are seen as free bodies, as though released by cell disintegration (Cordy and Graham 1950).

Follicles of the spleen rarely contain necrotic foci, but often show central hemorrhage. Flukes are found embedded in the villi or duodenal glands of the intestinal tract with no evidence of inflammatory response. Small foci of macrophages and neutrophils, often necrotic, are frequently found in the connective tissue of the lamina propria. Cellularity of the propria can also be increased, principally with plasma cells and neutrophils. Centrolobular lipidosis of the liver is common in foxes, but rare in dogs. Both foxes and dogs show a moderate mononuclear infiltration of the liver interlobular connective tissue. Occasionally, a few small hemorrhages are observed beneath the bladder epithelium. An accumulation of mononuclear and neutrophil leukoctyes in small areas causes a slight thickening of the alveolar walls of the lungs. A monocytic leptomeningitis is most intense over the cerebellum. Exudative and proliferative cellular changes in the sheaths of the small and medium-sized vessels in the cerebrum and focal collections of glia of mesenchymal cells (glial nodules) are commonly observed lesions.

Immunity. Dogs that recover from salmon poisoning are solidly immune for long periods and perhaps for life. Simms et al. (1932) found it possible to immunize dogs solidly by the simultaneous injection of virulent blood and hyperimmune serum. Shaw and Howarth (1939) showed that feeding dogs parasitized salmon and curing the resultant disease with sulfanilamide resulted in strong immunity.

Dogs that recover from the Elokomin fluke fever agent are fully susceptible to *N. helminthoeca* and usually succumb to infection. The reverse is also true; thus no cross-immunity develops between the two agents.

Diagnosis. Although the signs of illness are characteristic, the most certain method of diagnosis is a search for fluke eggs in the feces of the patient. In most cases the eggs are so numerous that a microscopic examination of the fecal material adhering to the rectal thermometer will result in a diagnosis. These eggs appear in the feces of dogs on the fifth to seventh day after ingestion of infected fish. They are oval and measure 75 to 80 μm in length and 45 to 55 μm in breadth. There are no embryos in the eggs recovered directly from feces. When the eggs are stored in cool water, embryonation occurs in 75 to 90 days.

Microscopic examination reveals intracytoplasmic microorganisms that resemble rickettsias and are sometimes pleomorphic; they are found particularly in the reticuloendothelial cells of lymphoid tissues of infected canids. One can readily obtain suitable material for this purpose by aspirating cells from the mandibular lymph node with a syringe or by performing a biopsy. Tissue smears require fixation with methanol prior to staining. Blood drawn during the febrile stage contains the organism but not in sufficient number for detection by direct microscopic examination. The organisms are about 0.3 μm in diameter and Gram-negative; they appear purple with Giemsa, pale bluish with hematoxylin, red or blue with Macchiavello, and dark brown or black with Levaditi stain. They occur in plaques or loose groups in the cells, often nearly filling the cytoplasm (Figure 31.4).

The organism can be transmitted to susceptible dogs by the inoculation of infective blood or spleen taken during the acute phase of the disease. The organisms are labile, but they will survive for at least 6 months in fresh-frozen tissue stored at −70°C and will withstand lyophilization. *N. helminthoeca* has been cultivated in canine monocytes (Frank, McGuire, Gorham, and Davis 1974).

Sakawa et al. (1973) used a complement-fixation test to show a serologic distinction between *N. helminthoeca* and the Elokomin fluke fever agent. A direct fluorescent antibody test can also be applied to distinguish the same two agents (Kitao et al. 1973).

Antimicrobial Susceptibility. Coon et al. (1938) showed that sulfanilamide, administered to dogs during the early febrile period, brought about rapid recovery from the disease. This was confirmed by Shaw and Howarth (1939) and by Cordy and Graham (1950), who

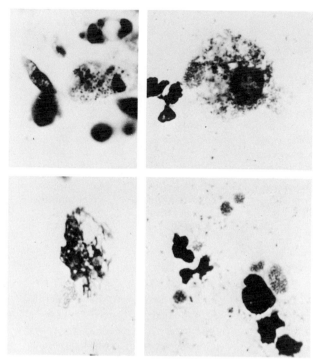

Figure 31.4. *Neorickettsia helminthoeca* in lymph node aspirations. Coccobacillary bodies (*top left and right*) diffusely scattered in the cytoplasm of reticular cells; bacillary bodies (*bottom left*) in a disintegrating macrophage; morulalike clusters (*bottom right*) free and in a macrophage. Giemsa stain ✕ 800. (From Farrell et al., 1968, courtesy of *Journal of the American Veterinary Medical Association.*)

also showed sulfamerazine and sulfamethazine to be effective. They found that penicillin and chlortetracycline were equally effective but streptomycin was ineffective. Philip et al. (1954b) highly recommended the use of either chlortetracycline or oxytetracycline as therapy for salmon poisoning.

REFERENCES

Chapin, E.A. 1926. A new genus and species of trematode, the probable cause of salmon-poisoning in dogs. North Am. Vet. 7(4):36–37.

Coon, E.W., Myers, F.C., Phelps, T.R., Ruehle, O.J., Snodgrass, W.B., Shaw, J.N., Simms, B.T., and Bolins, F.M. 1938. Sulfanilamide as a treatment of salmon poisoning in dogs. North Am. Vet. 19(9):57–59.

Cordy, D.R., and Graham, J.R. 1950. The pathology and etiology of salmon disease in the dog and fox. Am. J. Pathol. 26:617–637.

Donham, C.R., Simms, B.T., and Miller, F.W. 1926. So-called salmon poisoning in dogs (progress report). J. Am. Vet. Med. Assoc. 68:701–715.

Farrell, R.K., Dee, J.F., and Ott, R.L. 1968. Salmon poisoning in a dog fed kippered salmon. J. Am. Vet. Med. Assoc. 152:370–371.

Farrell, R.K., Leader, R.W., and Johnston, S.D. 1973. Differentiation of salmon poisoning disease and Elokomin fluke fever: Studies with the black bear (*Ursus americanus*). Am. J. Vet. Res. 34:919–922.

Frank, D.W., McGuire, T.C., Gorham, J.R., and Davis, D.W. 1974.

Cultivation of two species of *Neorickettsia* in canine monocytes. J. Infect. Dis. 129:257–262.

Frank, D.W., McGuire, T.C., Gorham, J.R., and Farrell, R.K. 1974. Lympho-reticular lesions of canine neorickettsiosis. J. Infect. Dis. 129:163–171.

Kitao, T., Farrell, R.K., and Fukada, T. 1973. Differentiation of salmon poisoning disease and Elokomin fluke fever: Fluorescent antibody studies with *Rickettsia sennetsu*. Am. J. Vet. Res. 34:927–928.

Philip, C.B. 1933. Rocky Mountain spotted fever. Investigation of sexual transmission in the wood tick *Dermacentor andersoni*. Public Health Rep. 48:266–272.

Philip, C.B., Hadlow, W.J., and Hughes, L.E. 1954. Studies of salmon poisoning disease of canines. I. The rickettsial relationships and pathogenicity of *Neorickettsia helminthoeca*. Exp. Parasitol. 3:336–350.

Philip, C.B., Hughes, L.E., Locker, B., and Hadlow, W.J. 1954. Salmon poisoning disease of canines. II. Further observations on etiologic agent. Proc. Soc. Exp. Biol. Med. 87:397–400.

Sakawa, H., Farrell, R.K., and Mori, M. 1973. Differentiation of salmon poisoning disease and Elokomin fluke fever: Complement fixation. Am. J. Vet. Res. 34:923–925.

Shaw, J.N., and Howarth, C.R. 1939. Immunity to salmon poisoning follows treatment of affected dogs with sulfanilamide. North Am. Vet. 20(5):67–68.

Simms, B.T., and Muth, O.H. 1933. Salmon poisoning. In Proceedings of the 5th Pacific Scientific Congress. Pp. 2949–2960.

Simms, B.T., Donham, C.R., and Shaw, J.N. 1931. Salmon poisoning. Am. J. Hyg. 13:363–391.

Simms, B.T., McCapes, A.M., and Muth, O.H. 1932. Salmon poisoning: Transmission and immunization experiments. J. Am. Vet. Med. Assoc. 81:26–36.

Human Rickettsial Diseases

The human rickettsial diseases, with some exceptions, are clinically similar. They are characterized by fever, rashes or dark blotches resulting from lesions of the blood vessels, and nervous symptoms. They can be divided into five groups on the basis of clinical data, insect vectors, locality, serology, and other factors (Table 31.2). Both humans and animals, wild and domestic, are susceptible to diseases of all five groups, and various biting insect vectors may transmit each type.

Typhus Fever

Typhus is found in central Europe, South and Central America, Asia, Africa, the Soviet Union, and the United States. Mortality may be as low as 5 percent or as high as 70 percent. The blood of patients is infectious, but the organisms have not been seen in the blood.

The European type, the classic form of typhus, is transmitted by the human body louse, *Pediculus humanus corporis*. The reservoir of infection is not known. It is not transmitted transovarially in lice, and infected lice usually die within 2 weeks. The disease may be maintained in endemic form by mild infections, or possibly humans may be asymptomatic carriers. It has spread to the Atlantic

Table 31.2. Human rickettsial diseases

Disease group	Geographic distribution	Causative organism	Major vectors	Primary natural hosts	Suggested experimental hosts
I. Spotted fever group					
Rocky Mountain spotted fever	North and South America	*Rickettsia rickettsii*	*Dermacentor andersoni* *D. variabilis* *Rhipicephalus sanguineus* *Amblyomma americanum* *A. cajennense*	Many species of feral mammals, chiefly rodents; dogs; birds	Male guinea pigs, *Microtus* sp., and fertile hens' eggs
Russian tick typhus	Siberia	*R. siberica*	*Dermacentor nuttalli* *D. silvarum* *D. marginatus* *D. pictur* *Haemaphysalis concinna* *H. punctata*	Many species of feral mammals, chiefly rodents	Male guinea pigs and fertile hens' eggs
Rickettsialpox	Soviet Union, North America	*R. akari*	*Allodermanyssus sanguineus*	*Mus* spp. and *Rattus* spp.	Mice and fertile hens' eggs
North Queensland tick typhus	Australia	*R. australis*	*Ixodes holocyclus*	Small marsupials and rats	Mice and fertile hens' eggs
Fievre boutonneuse	Mediterranean area of Africa and Europe	*R. conori*	*Rhipicephalus sanguineus*	Dogs and small feral mammals	Male guinea pigs and fertile hens' eggs
South African tick-bite fever	South Africa		*Rhipicephalus appendiculatus*		
Indian tick-bite typhus	India		*Haemaphysalis leachi*		
Kenya fever	Africa		*Amblyomma hebraeum*		
II. Typhus fever group					
Epidemic typhus (European type)	Worldwide (colder climates)	*R. prowazekii*	*Pediculus humanus corporis* *Amblyomma variegatum* *Hyalomma* spp.	Humans (cattle, sheep and goats?)	Male guinea pigs, cotton rats, and fertile hens' eggs
Murine typhus	Worldwide (warmer climates)	*R. typhi*	*Xenopsylla cheopis*	*Rattus norvegicus*	Male guinea pigs and fertile hens' eggs
New typhus member	North America	*R. canada*	*Haemaphysalis leporispalustris*	Humans and rabbits	Rabbits and fertile hens' eggs

Table 31.2.—*continued*

Disease group	Geographic distribution	Causative organism	Major vectors	Primary natural hosts	Suggested experimental hosts
III. Scrub typhus	Eastern and southern Asia, islands of southwest Pacific	*R. tsutsu-gamushi*	*Leptotrom-bidium akamushi* *L. deliensis*	Many species of small feral mammals, chiefly rodents	Mice, cotton rats, and fertile hens' eggs
IV. Q fever	Worldwide	*Coxiella burneti*	Chiefly airborne, also found in many species of ticks	Cattle, sheep, goats, and many species of feral mammals	Guinea pigs, hamsters, and fertile hens' eggs
V. Trench fever	Europe, North Africa, Mexico, North America	*R. quintana*	*Pediculus humanus corporus*	Humans and voles	Laboratory-reared body lice, voles

Modified from a table supplied by Herbert G. Stoenner, Rocky Mountain Laboratory, Hamilton, Mont.

seaboard of the United States, where it appears in a mild form sometimes called *Brill's disease* (Zinsser 1934). Brill's disease also occurs in Europe; Murray et al. (1951), after studying 26 cases in Yugoslavia, which is a louse-borne typhus zone, supported Zinsser's hypothesis that humans are the interepidemic reservoirs of epidemic typhus fever.

Murine typhus, which prevails in the southern United States and in Mexico, is a disease associated with rats (Maxcy 1926). It is transmitted to humans by the oriental rat flea, *Xenopsylla cheopis*, and the spined rat louse, *Polyplax spinulosa*. In an epidemic it may be transmitted from person to person by the human louse.

The European type is caused by *Rickettsia prowazekii*, while the murine type is caused by *R. typhi*. A third type, caused by *R. canada*, is marked by a febrile illness in humans that resembles human Rocky Mountain spotted fever (Bozeman et al. 1970). The three organisms may be differentiated by the complement-fixation test.

REFERENCES

Bozeman, F.M., Elisberg, B.L., Humphries, J.W., Runcik, K., and Palmer, D.P., Jr. 1970. Serologic evidence of *Rickettsia canada* infection of man. J. Infect. Dis. 121:367–371.

Maxcy, K.F. 1926. Clinical observations on endemic typhus (Brill's disease) in southern United States. Public Health Rep. 25:1213–1220.

Murray, E.S., Psorn, T., Djakovic, P., Djakovic, S., Sielski, S., Broz, V., Ljupsa, F., Gaon, J., Pavlevic, K., and Snyder, J.C. 1951. Brill's disease. IV. Study of 26 cases in Yugoslavia. Am. J. Public Health 41:1359–1369.

Zinsser, H. 1934. Varieties of typhus virus and epidemiology of American form of European typhus fever (Brill's disease). Am. J. Hyg. 20:513–532.

Rocky Mountain Spotted Fever

Clinically, Rocky Mountain spotted fever resembles typhus. In recent years the incidence of human disease has increased in endemic areas in the eastern and western United States. There appear to be at least three forms of the disease: (1) the eastern form, which occurs in the eastern United States, is less frequently fatal, and is transmitted by the American dog tick, *Dermacentor variabilis;* (2) the more frequently fatal western form, which occurs in the Rocky Mountain area and is transmitted by the sheep tick *D. andersoni;* and (3) the Brazilian form (São Paulo typhus), which is transmitted by the tick *Amblyomma cajennense*. The ticks probably maintain the disease among dogs, rabbits, field mice, sheep, and the like, by their bites, and in the western form, at least, transmit the infectious agent to their progeny (Philip 1933). The rickettsias of spotted fever are usually called *Rickettsia rickettsii*.

Among domestic animals, the disease is most important in the dog. Sexton et al. (1976) surveyed Mississippi dogs for Rocky Mountain spotted fever antibodies and for tick parasites infected with rickettsias of the spotted fever group. Of 116 serum samples, 53 (46 percent) had complement-fixing antibody titers greater than 1 : 8, as compared with only 1 (5 percent) of 21 samples from a group of dogs from metropolitan Chicago. *R. rickettsii* was demonstrated in only 1 of 129 *D. variabilis* ticks removed from Mississippi dogs, whereas 167 (19 percent) of 884 *Rhipicephalus sanguineus* ticks from these dogs harbored spotted fever rickettsias. The clinical and clinicopathological changes and the pathogenesis of experimental studies with *R. rickettsii* in dogs have been described by Keenan et al. (1977a, 1977b) and by Hibler et al. (1985).

Clinical signs of Rocky Mountain spotted fever in dogs vary considerably, and most cases are seen during the summer (Hibler et al. 1985). Fever (102.2° to 105.8°F), anorexia, vomiting, diarrhea, and depression can occur within 2 to 3 days after attachment of infected ticks. Engorged ticks are not always found during the initial examination, but conjunctivitis, mucopurulent oculonasal discharge, and a nonproductive cough are frequently seen. Weight loss, dehydration, lymphadenopathy, and muscle or joint tenderness can occur. Early skin lesions include edema and hyperemia of the lips, pinnae, prepuce, scrotum, and other dependent portions of the body. Abdominal tenderness or paralumbar hyperesthesia are common findings.

Petechial and ecchymotic hemorrhages of ocular, oral, and genital mucous membranes and nonpigmented skin sometimes develop after the early manifestations of Rocky Mountain spotted fever (Greene et al. 1985). Evidence of epistaxis, melena, and hematuria frequently accompanies the hemorrhages. Retinal hemorrhages and anterior uveitis are common in dogs with bleeding problems. Severely affected male dogs often develop scrotal edema, hyperemia, hemorrhages, and epididymal swelling. In the late stages of the disease the previously hyperemic or edematous portions of the body can undergo necrosis and sloughing.

Death in severely affected dogs usually results from complications in the cardiovascular, nervous, or urinary systems (Greene et al. 1985). Rapid onset of a hemorrhagic diathesis that leads to shock and cardiovascular collapse can occur as a result of disseminated intravascular coagulation and thrombocytopenia. Acute renal failure can develop from renal hypoperfusion, hypotension, and circulatory collapse (Walker and Mattern 1979). Neurological signs of generalized cerebral involvement include lethargy, confusion, stupor, convulsions, coma, and ultimately death, resulting from disseminated, rapidly progressive meningoencephalitis. Paraparesis, ataxia, and signs of spinal cord involvement can also occur.

Hematological findings usually include mild leukopenia at the onset of fever, followed by moderate leukocytosis with a left shift or a stress leukogram (Greene et al. 1985). The longer the duration of clinical signs before diagnosis, the more pronounced the leukocytosis will be. Toxic neutrophils may be noted during rickettsemia.

Thrombocytopenia is present in most dogs at the time of initial examination. Platelet counts of less than 75,000 cells/μl are common, particularly if petechiae are observed. Mild normocytic, normochromic anemia may be present in dogs with slight blood loss, and the results of a direct Coombs' test may be positive.

Biochemical abnormalities often include increased serum glucose levels and increased activities of serum aspartate transaminase, alanine transaminase, and alkaline phosphatase (Greene et al. 1985). Hyponitremia, hypochloremia, and metabolic acidosis are occasionally seen. Prolonged prothrombin time, activated partial thromboplastin time, and elevated fibrin degradation products can be evident in dogs with coagulation defects, thereby indicating acute or end-stage disseminated intravascular coagulation. The blood urea nitrogen increases in the terminal stages of illness, corresponding to oliguria and renal failure. Proteinuira and hematuria can be present. Cerebrospinal and synovial fluids are often normal; however, increased protein and polymorphonuclear or mononuclear cells may be present.

R. conori infection occurred in a young dog from Tunisia. The dog had fever and loss of appetite and also vomited. It responded favorably to daily intramuscular injection of 400 mg of oxytetracycline for 1 week (Clerc and Lecomte 1974).

Other rickettsial diseases that may be included in the spotted fever group are fievre boutonneuse (Marseilles fever), Kenya fever, South African tick-bite fever, rickettsialpox, Bullis fever, North Queensland tick typhus, Indian tick-bite fever, and Russian tick typhus.

REFERENCES

Clerc, B., and Lecomte, R. 1974. Rickettsiosis in a dog. Rec. Med. Vet. 150:189–192.

Greene, C.E., Burgdorfer, W., Cavagnolo, R., Philip, R.N., and Peacock, M.G. 1985. Rocky Mountain spotted fever in dogs and its differentiation from canine ehrlichiosis. J. Am. Vet. Med. Assoc. 186:465–472.

Hibler, S.H., Hoskins, J.D., and Greene, C.E. 1985. Rickettsial infections in dogs. I. Rocky Mountain spotted fever and *Coxiella* infections. Compend. Cont. Ed. Pract. Vet. 7:856–866.

Keenan, K.P., Buhles, W.C., Jr., Huxsoll, D.L., Williams, R.G., and Hildebrandt, P.K. 1977a. Studies on the pathogenesis of *Rickettsia rickettsii* in the dog: Clinical and clinicopathologic changes of experimental infection. Am. J. Vet. Res. 38:851–856.

Keenan, K.P., Buhles, W.C., Jr., Huxsoll, D.L., Williams, R.G., Hildebrandt, P.K., Campbell, J.M., and Stephenson, E.H. 1977b. Pathogenesis of infection with *Rickettsia rickettsii* in the dog: A disease model for Rocky Mountain spotted fever. J. Infect. Dis. 135:911–917.

Philip, C.B. 1933. Rocky Mountain spotted fever. Investigation of sexual transmission in the wood tick *Dermacentor andersoni*. Public Health Rep. 48:266–272.

Sexton, D.J., Burgdorfer, W., Thomas, L., and Norment, B.R. 1976. Rocky Mountain spotted fever in Mississippi: Survey for spotted fever antibodies in dogs and for spotted fever group rickettsiae in dog ticks. Am. J. Epidemiol. 103:192–197.

Walker, D.H., and Mattern, W.D. 1979. Acute renal failure in Rocky Mountain spotted fever. Arch. Intern. Med. 139:443–448.

Scrub Typhus

SYNONYMS: Mite typhus, tsutsugamushi
disease

Scrub typhus, which resembles typhus clinically, is found principally in Japan, Malaya, and the islands of the South Pacific. The common transmitting agent, *Leptotrombidium akamushi,* is much like the American "chigger." Rodents serve as a reservoir for the disease (Ahlm and Lipschutz 1944). The causative agent is *Rickettsia tsutsugamushi.*

REFERENCE

Ahlm, C.E., and Lipschutz, J. 1944. Tsutsugamushi fever in southwest Pacific theater. J.A.M.A. 124:1095–1100.

Trench Fever

SYNONYMS: Five-day fever, shin bone fever,
Wolhynian fever

Trench fever occurred in World War I in the armies in France, Mesopotamia, and Salonika (Arkwright et al. 1919–1920). According to Jacobi (1942), it appeared in World War II in the German army in Russia. Usually it produces a high fever of the relapsing type, and the most constant symptom is pain in the legs. Natural transmission is through the human body louse, *Pediculus humanus corporis.* The cause is *Rickettsia quintana.*

REFERENCES

Arkwright, J.A., Bacot, F., and Duncan, L. 1919–1920. Association of rickettsia with trench fever. J. Hyg. 18:76.

Jacobi, J. 1942. Über die Reaktionsfähigkeit und das Neutralisationsvermogen der lebenden menschlichen Haut. Münch. Med. Wochenschr. 89:615.

Q Fever

SYNONYM: Nine-mile fever

Q fever is a febrile disease of humans resembling influenza. It is an acute and specific rickettsial infection of variable severity and duration. Its clinical course is characterized by sudden onset, severe headache, malaise, and patchy infiltration of the lungs. It is distinguished from most other human rickettsial diseases by the failure of patients to develop a rash.

Q fever was first described as a human disease in 1937

in Queensland, Australia, and its etiologic agent was named *Rickettsia burnetii* by Australian workers (Burnet and Freeman 1937, Derrick 1937, 1939). Davis and Cox (1938) recovered a rickettsia from infected ticks at Nine-Mile Creek, Montana, which upon subsequent study proved to be *R. burnetii.* In *Bergey's Manual of Systematic Bacteriology* (1984) this organism is now called *Coxiella burnetii.* The disease appears to be quite common all over the world, usually masquerading as "flu" or atypical pneumonia. The fever may also be associated with hepatitis, pericarditis, meningitis, arthritis, orchitis, epididymitis, phlebitis, esophagitis, and arteritis.

C. burnetii is a bipolar rod, measuring 0.2 by 1.0 μm (Figure 31.5). It occurs intracellularly in the cytoplasm of infected cells and possibly extracellularly in infected ticks. Some observations suggest the existence of a smaller, filterable stage, but its true nature has not been identified. Strains newly isolated from animals and ticks are characteristically in phase I, which means they react only with antibodies in late convalescent-phase serums. With

Figure 31.5. Smear of yolk sac culture of embryonated hen's egg showing *Coxiella burnetii.* Macchiavello stain. × 1,290. (Courtesy Herbert G. Stoenner, Rocky Mountain Laboratory, Hamilton, Mont.)

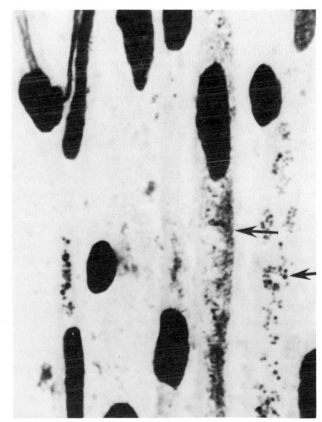

repeated passage in embryonated chicken eggs the organisms convert to phase II, which means they react with antibodies of early convalescent-phase serums.

The phase I *C. burnetii* antigen isolated by phenol extraction is a complex lipopolysaccharide molecule containing substances similar to lipopolysaccharides from other Gram-negative bacteria (Schramek and Brezina 1976). Phase I *C. burnetii* are more resistant to phagocytosis than are phase II organisms (Kazar et al. 1975, Kishimoto and Walker 1976).

The prevalence of infection with *C. burnetii* among domestic animals is determined by examination of serums with the complement-fixation, capillary-tube agglutination, or radioisotope precipitation (RIP) tests. These techniques measure different kinds of antibodies, so complete agreement cannot be expected. Complement-fixing antibodies are associated with 19S macroglobulins, whereas RIP antibodies seem to occur in the 7S gamma globulins. Furthermore, the rate of antibody response to *C. burnetii* and the persistence of antibodies vary in different animal species. The RIP test is the most sensitive and will detect antibodies for longer periods after the infection has occurred than do other tests. Infection rates among herds of dairy cattle are most easily determined by testing individual or pooled milk samples by the capillary-tube test.

Q fever is essentially an occupational disease, being limited almost entirely to livestock attendants, farm residents, and laboratory personnel. Most human cases are associated with infected dairy cows, sheep, or goats (Hall et al. 1982, McKelvie 1982, Meiklejohn et al. 1981). According to Derrick (1944), it is a natural infection of certain wild animals, especially bandicoots in Australia, and is transmitted in nature by ticks. These ticks spread the infection to livestock, which sometimes develop a mild illness. Ticks become infected by feeding on infected livestock. It is possible that feces deposited on the skins of the animals by the infected ticks are a source of infection for humans. Infection also occurs in other domestic animals such as dogs, cats, donkeys, and domestic fowl, as well as in pigeons. The organisms have been demonstrated in the wool or hair, in birth fluids, in the feces, in the milk, and in the placental tissues and aborted fetuses from naturally infected sheep, cattle, and goats. *C. burnetii* produces only mild or inapparent illness in domestic animals in most instances, but these animals act as reservoirs of the organism. Its importance as a cause of abortion in sheep, goats, and cattle has recently been revealed (Quignard et al. 1982, Russo and Malo 1981). Herd-to-herd transmission among cattle has been demonstrated (Reed and Wentworth 1957). Dairy farmers and meat packers from areas where there is evidence of Q fever infection in the milk-producing livestock show

serum antibodies against *C. burnetii* (Kitze et al. 1957). Infection in a dairy herd may be followed by excretion of rickettsiae in the milk for as long as 32 months (Grist 1959), and the udder is the primary site of localization of *C. burnetii* (Schaal 1982).

Epidemiological evidence also points to the spread of infection by the inhalation of dust contaminated with infected secreta or excreta of diseased animals or ticks. The fact that outbreaks of Q fever in people who have no contact with livestock sometimes follow dust storms adds weight to this theory (Spicer et al. 1977). The organism has also been found in sheep, goat, and cow milk, where it may survive ordinary pasteurization. It is claimed that exposure to a temperature of 145°F for 30 minutes will kill *C. burnetii*, whereas 143°F for the same period of time is not sufficient (Enright et al. 1957).

The disease rarely spreads from person to person, although this mode of transmission has been reported. The role of ticks in the spread of Q fever in humans is uncertain, but six strains of ticks common in various parts of the world have been shown to harbor *C. burnetii*. Certainly the infectious cycle is not entirely dependent on arthropod transmission. Liebisch (1976), in Germany, observed that the two peaks in the prevalence of Q fever in humans (April and September) correspond to periods of activity of adult *Dermacentor marginatus*. Soviet investigators (Pchelkina and Korenberg 1974) suggested that Q fever is transmitted by the ticks *Ixodes persulcatus* and *I. trianguliceps* to cattle and sheep in the Udmurt Republic, Soviet Union. The virulence of the organism can be enhanced by residence in the tick *Alveonasus canestrinii* (Pautov and Morozov 1974). Although antibodies to *C. burnetii* have been detected in birds, their role in transmission is unclear. On occasion brucellosis and Q fever have occurred in the same cows.

Vaccination may have some value in the control of the disease among occupationally exposed individuals and among infected livestock (Wentworth 1955). Extended studies by Biberstein et al. (1974, 1977) employed a phase I formalin-inactivated Q fever vaccine, which proved effective in the immunization of dairy cattle. Furthermore, the field trials indicated vaccination greatly reduced the shedding of the organism in the milk of dairy cows. Sadecky and co-workers (Sadecky and Brezina 1977, Sadecky et al. 1975) also showed that the administration of a formalin-inactivated phase I *C. burnetii* vaccine in naturally infected ewes and cows eliminated the shedding of the organism in the milk. Because a similar type of vaccine produced by German investigators failed to reduce the total number of milk shedders in 886 dairy cows, they concluded that protection of humans cannot be achieved by vaccination of infected cattle (Schmittdiel et al. 1981). These conflicting reports pose a dilemma that only continued research and vaccine trials can solve. Because goats and sheep are often used in medical research, Ruppanner et al. (1982) have recommended that a *C. burneti* vaccination program be developed for goats and sheep. Formalin-inactivated epidemic typhus and Q fever vaccines administered as a mixture have produced an immunity to both organisms in guinea pigs and humans (Morris et al. 1967).

Results of oral chemotherapy studies in cows and guinea pigs suggest that in some cases chlortetracycline may suppress rather than eradicate the Q fever agent (Behymer et al. 1977).

REFERENCES

Behymer, D., Ruppanner, R., Riemann, H.P., Biberstein, E.L., and Franti, C.E. 1977. Observation on chemotherapy in cows chronically infected with *Coxiella burnetii* (Q fever). Folia Vet. Lat. 7:64–70.

Biberstein, E.L., Crenshaw, G.L., Behymer, D.E., Franti, C.E., Bushnell, R.B., and Riemann, H.P. 1974. Dermal reactions and antibody responses in dairy cows and laboratory animals vaccinated with *Coxiella burnetii*. Cornell Vet. 64:387–406.

Biberstein, E.L., Riemann, H.P., Franti, C.E., Behymer, D.E., Ruppanner, R., Bushnell, R., and Crenshaw, G. 1977. Vaccination of dairy cattle against Q fever (*Coxiella burnetii*): Results of field trials. Am. J. Vet. Res. 38:189–193.

Burnet, F.M., and Freeman, M. 1937. Experimental studies on the virus of "Q" fever. Med. J. Aust. 2:299–305.

Davis, G.E., and Cox, H.R. 1938. A filter-passing infectious agent isolated from ticks. I. Isolation from *Dermacentor andersoni*, reactions in animals, and filtration experiments. Public Health Rep. 53:2259–2267.

Derrick, E.H. 1937. "Q" fever, new fever entity: Clinical features, diagnosis and laboratory investigation. Med. J. Aust. 2:281–299.

Derrick, F.H. 1939. *Rickettsia burneti*: Cause of "Q" fever. Med. J. Aust. 1:14.

Derrick, E.H. 1944. The epidemiology of Q fever. J. Hyg. 43:357–361.

Enright, J.B., Sadler, W.W., and Thomas, R.C. 1957. Pasteurization of milk containing the organisms of Q fever. Am. J. Public Health 47:695–700.

Grist, N.R. 1959. The persistence of Q-fever infection in a dairy herd. Vet. Rec. 71:839–841.

Hall, C.J., Richmond, S.J., Caul, C.E., Pearce, N.H., and Silver, I.A. 1982. Laboratory outbreak of Q fever acquired from sheep. Lancet 1:1004–1006.

Kazar, J., Skultetyova, E., and Brezina, R. 1975. Phagocytosis of *Coxiella burneti* by macrophages. Acta Virol. 19:426–431.

Kishimoto, R.A., and Walker, J.S. 1976. Interaction between *Coxiella burneti* and guinea pig peritoneal macrophages. Infect. Immun. 14:416–421.

Kitze, L.K., Hiemstra, H.C., and Moore, M.S. 1957. Q fever in Wisconsin. Serologic evidence of infection in cattle and in human beings and recovery of *C. burneti* from cattle. Am. J. Hyg. 65:239–247.

Liebisch, A. 1976. Role of indigenous ticks (Ixodidae) in the epidemiology of "Q" fever in Germany. D.T.W. 83:274–276.

McKelvie, P. 1982. Q fever in a Queensland meatworks. Med. J. Aust. 112:590–593.

Meiklejohn, G., Reimer, L.G., Graves, P.S., and Helmick, C. 1981. Cryptic epidemic of Q fever in a medical school. J. Infect. Dis. 144:107–113.

Morris, J.A., Wisseman, C.L., Aulidio, C.G., Jackson, E.B., and Smadel, J.E. 1967. Combined epidemic typhus and Q-fever vaccine: Adjuvant effect of *Coxiella burneti*. Proc. Soc. Exp. Biol. Med. 125:1216–1220.

Pautov, V.N., and Morozov, Yu.I. 1974. Izuchenie antigennoi struktury vak ts innogo shtamma M-44 rikketsii Berneta. Zh. Mikrobiol. Epidemiol. Immunobiol. 8:29–32.

Pchelkina, A.A., and Korenberg, E.I. 1974. Gumoral'nyi immunitet pri Ku-rikketsioze u koz raznogo vozrasta. Zh. Mikrobiol. Epidemiol. Immunobiol. 5:123–124.

Quignard, H., Geral, M.F., Pellerin, J.L., Milton, A., and Lautie, R. 1982. La fièvre Q chez les petits ruminants. Enquête épidémiologique dans la région Midi pyrénées. Rev. Méd. Vet. 133:413–422.

Reed, C.F., and Wentworth, B.B. 1957. Q fever studies in Ohio. J. Am. Vet. Med. Assoc. 130:458–461.

Ruppanner, R., Brooks, D., Morrish, D., Spinelli, J., Franti, C.E., and Behymer, D.E. 1982. Q fever hazards from sheep and goats used in research. Environ. Health 37:103–110.

Russo, P., and Malo, N. 1981. La fièvre Q dans le département de la Vienne. Cinétique des anticorps et avortement. Rev. Méd. Vet. 157:585–589.

Sadecky, E., and Brezina, R. 1977. Vaccination of naturally infected ewes against Q-fever. Acta Virol. 21:89.

Sadecky, E., Brezina, R., Kazar, J., Schramek, S., and Urvolgyi, J. 1975. Immunization against Q-fever of naturally infected dairy cows. Acta Virol. 19:486–488.

Schaal, E.H. 1982. Zur Euterbesiedlung mit *Coxiella burneti* beim Q-Fieber des Rindes. In Proceedings of the 12th World Congress on Diseases of Cattle, Utrecht, The Netherlands, vol. 2. Pp. 1069–1074.

Schmittdiel, E., Bauer, K., Steinbrecher, H., and Justl, W. 1981. Untersuchungen zur Beeinflussung der Ausscheidung von *Coxiella burneti* durch Q Fieber-Infizierte Rinder nach der Vakzinierung. Tierärztl. Umsch. 36:159–160.

Schramek, S., and Brezina, R. 1976. Characterization of an endotoxic lipopolysaccharide from *Coxiella burneti*. Acta Virol. 20:152–158.

Spicer, A.J., Crowther, R.W., Vella, E.E., Bengtsson, E., Miles, R., and Pitzolis, G. 1977. Q fever and animal abortion in Cyprus. Trans. R. Soc. Trop. Med. Hyg. 71:16–20.

Wentworth, B.B. 1955. Historical review of the literature on Q fever. Bacteriol. Rev. 19:129–149.

sions do have appendages and the organisms infect cattle but not deer or sheep.

3. *Aegyptianella*. The parasites form inclusions (0.3 to 3.9 μm in diameter) in erythrocytes, and infect only birds and some poikilothermic animals.

4. *Haemobartonella*. The parasites are within or on erythrocytes. Ring forms are rare or absent in blood preparations, which stain intensely by Romanowsky methods.

5. *Eperythrozoon*. The organisms are on erythrocytes and in plasma. Ring forms are common in blood preparations stained by Romanowsky methods.

32 The Anaplasmataceae

The Anaplasmataceae are obligate parasites found within or on erythrocytes or free in the plasma of various wild and domestic vertebrates. No demonstrable multiplication occurs in other tissues.

In blood smears prepared with Giemsa stain, the organisms appear as rod-shaped, spherical, coccoid, or ring-shaped bodies staining reddish violet and measuring 0.2 to 0.4 μm in diameter. They can occur in short chains or in irregular groups. Each organism has a membrane with an internal structure resembling that of the rickettsias. They multiply by binary fission and have not been cultured. The organisms are Gram-negative. They are transmitted by arthropods, and parenteral inoculation of any infective blood-containing tissue can cause infection. Disease can occur, but the usual result is long-term persistence with accompanying resistance to clinically demonstrable reinfection. Anemia is the most prominent feature. The infection occurs throughout the world. The organisms usually respond to the tetracyclines but not to penicillin or streptomycin.

Bergey's Manual of Systematic Bacteriology (1984) lists the following five genera in the family Anaplasmataceae:

1. *Anaplasma*. The parasites form inclusions (0.3 to 1.0 μm in diameter) in erythrocytes. Several parasites may be found in each inclusion. No appendages to the inclusions are observed. The organisms infect ruminants only.

2. *Paranaplasma*. Member organisms have the same characteristics as *Anaplasma* species except that the inclu-

The Genus *Anaplasma*

In the course of their classical work on piroplasmosis (babesiasis), or Texas fever of cattle, conducted between 1883 and 1897, Smith and Kilborne observed and described small coccuslike bodies located near the periphery of many of the red blood cells in animals suffering from the disease. They interpreted these bodies as a stage in the life cycle of the Texas fever parasite. It is clear today that these small bodies were not piroplasms and that Smith and Kilborne were dealing with animals that suffered from two diseases simultaneously, anaplasmosis and piroplasmosis. In 1910 Theiler differentiated the two diseases, but because both occurred in the same regions of South Africa, many disagreed with Theiler and continued to look upon the small marginal bodies either as artifacts or as piroplasms. The matter was not fully resolved until the 1930s when anaplasmosis was found to be prevalent in most of the southern and many of the northern states of the United States—regions that are now free of or have never been known to be affected by piroplasmosis.

Anaplasma marginale

The name *Anaplasma marginale* was given to the organism by Theiler. The word *Anaplasma* means "without plasma" (cytoplasm) and refers to the fact that the parasite seems to consist of nothing but a bit of chromatic material without any evidence of cytoplasm. The specific epithet is derived from the fact that these bodies are characteristically located near the periphery of the red blood cells and thus appear, in smears, as if on the margin of cells.

The parasite is widely distributed throughout the tropics, Africa, the Middle East, some parts of southern Europe, Latin America, and the Far East.

Morphology and Staining Reactions. The parasites of anaplasmosis are seen in the red blood cells as minute, deeply staining points usually located near the margin of the cell. If prepared with Giemsa stain, they are deep red. With other stains they are likely to be so dark that no color is distinguished; however, a one-step toluidine blue staining technique has proved useful for rapid detection of *Anaplasma* species in erythrocytes in the field or laboratory (Rogers and Wallace 1966).

With Romanowsky-type stains, these organisms appear in the erythrocytes as dense, homogenous, bluish purple, round structures, 0.3 to 1.0 μm in diameter. Electron microscopy reveals that these structures are inclusions separated from the cytoplasm of the erythrocyte by a limiting membrane. Each inclusion contains from one to eight subunits, or initial bodies, (Lotze 1946). These are the actual parasitic bacteria, each measuring 0.3 to 0.4 μm in diameter. They are dense aggregates of fine granular material embedded in an electron-lucid plasma. Each bacterium is enclosed in a membrane and the inclusion is surrounded by a double membrane.

The organism (initial body) enters the erythrocyte by causing invagination of the cytoplasmic membrane and subsequent formation of a vacuole. In the vacuole the initial body multiplies by binary fusion and forms an inclusion. Thus, the formation of the inclusion body, which is most frequently observed during the acute and convalescent phases of infection, represents only a phase in the developmental cycle of the initial body. Spores or resistant stages are not formed. The adenosine triphosphate and glutathione concentrations of erythrocytes remain essentially unchanged, regardless of the intensity of infection, and only a small quantity of methemoglobin occurs in parasitized erythrocytes. Histochemical analysis of parasites reveals DNA, RNA, protein, and organic iron.

The inclusions are spherical, and ordinarily there is but one per cell, although two or more may be seen in some cells. In the early stages of the disease, before the temperature rises, few or no parasites can be found. When the febrile period begins, the percentage of infected cells can reach 25 percent or even more than 50 percent. If the animal recovers, the number of cells containing the marginal bodies diminishes rapidly until none can be found microscopically. The blood of recovered animals is infectious for many years and probably for life; hence it is probable that a few bodies are present indefinitely, but too few to be observed.

Espana et al. (1959) employed phase-contrast and electron microscopy in studying hemolyzed erythrocytes from cattle infected with *A. marginale*. They found ring, match, comet, and dumbbell-like forms in natural and experimental infections. They also observed that the organism is motile.

Bedell and Dimopoullos (1962, 1963) reported that infectivity of *A. marginale* is destroyed by exposure to 60°C for 50 minutes and by sonic energy treatments for 90 minutes when the blood is maintained at 30° to 35°C. Storage of heparinized and infected *A. marginale* bovine erythrocytes in glycerol for 4.5 years at −70°C did not alter the infectivity or the virulence of the parasite (Summers and Matsuoka 1970). A concentration of 4 M dimethyl sulfoxide prevents lysis of bovine erythrocytes when they are subjected to rapid freezing and thawing. This procedure also enhances the infectivity of infected erythrocytes (Love 1972).

In a study of two isolates of *A. marginale* the molecular weights of the proteins ranged from less than 14,000 to more than 200,000 (Barbet et al. 1983).

Epizootiology and Pathogenesis. Many species of ticks have been shown to be capable of transmitting anaplasmosis. Most of these probably are mechanical rather than biological carriers, but several are biological carriers (Boynton 1928, 1929), including *Boophilus (Margaropus) annulatus, Dermacentor occidentalis*, and *D. andersoni*, all of which occur in the United States. In these species the infective agent passes through the egg into the next generation. Freidhoff and Ristic (1966) demonstrated *A. marginale* in the gut contents and in the Malpighian tubes of engorged *D. andersoni* nymphs with the fluorescent antibody technique and reported that the anaplasmas multiplied in the Malpighian tubes by binary fission. A peroxidase-antiperoxidase technique can also be used to demonstrate the parasite (Staats et al. 1982).

At least seven species of horseflies (Tabanidae) have been shown to be mechanical carriers, and certain mosquitoes, such as *Aedes* and *Anopheles* species, have also been incriminated. The stable fly (*Stomoxys calcitrans*) and the horn fly (*Haematobia irritans*) apparently seldom, if ever, act as transmitters.

The fact that deer are susceptible to anaplasmosis indicates that they may constitute an important reservoir of infection in areas where they occupy the same range land as cattle (Christensen et al. 1960, Osebold et al. 1959).

An important means of transmission is through the use of common surgical instruments that have not been thoroughly disinfected after being used on an animal. Reese (1930) showed that anaplasmosis can easily be carried on a lancet for drawing blood if it is merely wiped after being used on an infected animal. Outbreaks have occurred in herds after dehorning operations, the drawing of blood samples, castrations, and minor operations. In areas where anaplasmosis occurs, veterinarians should be exceedingly cautious in carrying out these mass operations to avoid spreading this disease to many animals from a few, or even one, carrier animal.

Uterine transmission has also been reported, and Davis et al. (1970) demonstrated that *A. marginale* has the ability to infect via the ocular route.

Although the specific host for anaplasmas appears to be cattle, they have been found in American deer (Boynton and Woods 1940), water buffalo, bison, African antelopes, gnu, blesbok, duiker, elk, and camels. Sheep and goats can develop a submicroscopic infection. The African buffalo is not susceptible.

As in piroplasmosis, young animals are quite resistant. Cases in calves less than a year old are rare, although in infected territories many calves become infected without signs of illness and become immune carriers. The natural resistance of young calves is removed by splenectomy. The marginal bodies appear in great numbers in such animals; hence they are suitable for diagnostic purposes.

In older animals the disease can be acute or chronic. In natural infections the period of incubation ranges from 20 to 40 days. Experimentally, signs of illness can be produced much earlier by inoculation with large doses of acutely infected blood. Those affected with the acute form may die within 2 or 3 days after the appearance of the first signs of illness. The disease begins with a fever of 105° to 107°F. After a day or two, signs of anemia and icterus appear, and about this time the temperature falls to normal and even subnormal as death approaches. The mucous membranes are pale and yellowish, as are the thin-skinned parts of the body. Urination is frequent, but the urine is not blood-tinged, as it often is in piroplasmosis. The animal is usually constipated; the feces are dark, often blood-stained, and covered with mucus. Abortions have been observed, particularly in the early and middle trimesters of gestation.

Animals with chronic cases live longer, are weak, become progressively emaciated, and show icterus and anemia. The red blood cell count may fall from a normal of about 7×10^6 to less than $1 \times 10^6/\mu l$; the hemoglobin can be less than g/dl.

Mortality is quite variable. It can be greater than 50 percent or less than 5 percent. Losses are greatest in hot weather and in older animals.

The principal lesions are those associated with blood destruction, anemia, and icterus. The spleen is enlarged, and the pulp is dark and soft. The blood appears as if diluted with water. A catarrhal enteritis is common. There may be a few petechiae on the heart wall and on the mucosa of the urinary bladder. The lymph nodes are swollen and edematous. The liver shows marked icterus, with the bile channels engorged and the gallbladder distended with dark green, mucilaginous bile. Kreier et al. (1964) reported that the anemia in *Anaplasma*-infected animals is caused by intensive erythrophagocytosis initiated by parasitic damage to red blood cells and by anti-erythrocytic autoantibody. Buening (1974) found that during the parasitemic stage of anaplasmosis in calves, serum lipids fell and gamma globulin increased.

Testicular degeneration and libido loss were observed in experimentally infected bulls (Swift et al. 1979).

Hadani et al. (1982) reported that eperythrozoonosis caused suppression of *A. marginale* disease in a splenectomized calf until the *Eperythrozoon teganodes* infection was controlled with neoarsphenamine.

Immunity. Animals that recover from anaplasmosis remain carriers for long periods and probably for life. Such animals are relatively resistant to reinfection. Signs of illness are seldom seen in calves less than a year old. Young calves can be inoculated with virulent blood, especially during the winter when the disease is naturally not so severe as it is in the hot months, and made immune thereafter. Because they become permanent carriers and because the number of vectors is great, however, such animals are a danger to any nonimmune animals with which they come in contact.

In cattle infected with *A. marginale,* IgG and IgM antibodies are found during the acute and convalescent phases of the infection. Erythrocytes from acutely infected cattle yield two distinct antigens, a nonsedimentable one (NS) and a sedimentable one (S). The NS antigen is active in the gel precipitation system, and the S anitgen is a suspension of initial bodies. Carson et al. (1977) utilized the leukocyte migration–inhibition test as an index for cell-mediated immunity. The response increased greatly in cattle given virulent anaplasmas or attenuated anaplasmas.

Immunity in adult cattle persists even after the latent infection is eliminated with imidocarb dihydrochloride treatment (Roby et al. 1974). This suggests that latency is not the sole means for protection.

Various inactivated and attenuated vaccines have been developed in attempts to provide cattle with protection against natural disease with *A. marginale*. Inactivated vaccines yield increased resistance and clearly reduce losses to the disease (Brock 1963, McHardy and Simpson 1973, Richey et al. 1977a). Osorno et al. (1975) used an attenuated strain produced in sheep, and vaccination protected cattle exposed to natural disease, whereas the attenuated vaccine developed by Zaraza and Kuttler (1976) protected most of the immunized cattle against challenge with virulent organisms. The use of either type of vaccine may complicate control of the disease because it prevents differentiation of vaccinated and infected cattle by serologic tests (Brock 1963). Ristic and Carson (1977)

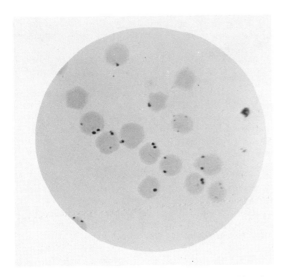

Figure 32.1. *Anaplasma marginale* organisms in a blood smear from a cow with acute anaplasmosis. Giemsa stain. × 770.

reviewed the methods of immunoprophylaxis against bovine anaplasmosis, particularly the use of attenuated *A. marginale*.

Diagnosis. Finding the characteristic marginal bodies in the red blood cells makes the diagnosis conclusive. The examiner must be cautious in this identification and not confuse such structures as basophilic stippling and the Howell-Jolly bodies, seen in severe anemias, with anaplasmas. Artifacts resembling these bodies also are often seen. The examinations should be made only on good films that are well prepared with Giemsa stain (Figure 32.1). Ristic et al. (1957) detected *A. marginale* by means of fluorescein-labeled antibody.

In using splenectomized calves to diagnose anaplasmosis, Gates et al. (1957) noted that blood obtained from cattle whose serums showed a high complement-fixation titer had a much lower degree of infectivity than that of other cattle. It should also be noted that the splenectomized cow is even more susceptible to infection than the splenectomized calf (Roby et al. 1961). Splenectomized, disease-free calves are suitable for location of carrier animals. The complement-fixation test is also used to detect the disease and, according to Price et al. (1954), is highly accurate. The antigen is obtained from the blood of infected splenectomized calves (Franklin et al. 1963, Price et al., 1952).

Boynton and Woods (1935) reported a simple test that seems to have some value in the diagnosis of anaplasmosis. The blood is allowed to clot, and a little clear serum is obtained. Two drops are added to 2 ml of distilled water in a tube. The serum of normal animals does not cloud the water; that of animals affected with anaplasmosis causes an immediate clouding, and after the tube stands overnight, a white precipitate covers the bottom. Animals with acute anaplasmosis and recently recovered carriers give this reaction. The test depends on the precipitation of euglobulin, which appears to be present in increased amounts in this disease.

Ristic and co-workers have used a gel diffusion test (Ristic and Mann 1963) and a capillary-tube agglutination test (Ristic 1962). Ristic claims that the latter test is as accurate as the complement-fixation test and is simpler, faster, and more economical than gel diffusion and complement fixation in detecting anaplasmosis. A card system is used by some diagnosticians as a rapid, practical, economical, and portable procedure for the diagnosis of anaplasmosis (Amerault and Roby 1977). This modified agglutination test is a direct conglutination reaction with some animals.

Antimicrobial Susceptibility. Numerous investigators around the world have been actively studying a variety of chemotherapeutic agents. These substances have been used to treat clinical cases and to eliminate the organism from carrier animals. According to Splitter and Miller (1953), infection in anaplasmosis carriers can be eradicated by treatment with oxytetracycline (11 mg/kg of body weight each day in single or divided doses for 12 to 14 days) or chlortetracycline (33 mg/kg of body weight each day in single doses for 16 days). Pearson et al. (1957) used intramuscular injections of tetracycline at the rate of 11 mg/kg of body weight daily for 10 consecutive days. Aralen hydrochloride, 5 percent sterile aqueous solution, has been approved for the parenteral treatment of anaplasmosis in cattle, and Roby et al. (1968) have recommended dithiosemicarbazone. Kuttler (1972) combined appropriate levels of dithiosemicarbazone and oxytetracycline to eliminate *A. marginale* in splenectomized calves. Roby (1972) and Roby and Mazzola (1972) showed that imidocarb rapidly causes clearance of the organism from the blood, and it has been used effectively in the field to treat and control the disease. Adult carrier cattle are given 5 mg/kg of body weight subcutaneously or intramuscularly at 14-day intervals to eliminate the parasite. Two or three doses usually suffice. Other drugs, such as chloramphenicol, rolitetracycline, and dithiosemicarbazone (in combination with pytetracycline), presumably can accomplish the same objective. Latent infections have been eliminated by feeding chlortetracycline, 1.1 mg/kg of body weight, in the ration for 120 days (Richey et al. 1977b).

Ristic et al. (1958) reported that the relapse that ordinarily follows splenectomy in *Anaplasma*-infected calves does not occur in those animals previously treated with cortisone.

Eradication programs have entailed continual testing and stray-dipping of imported cattle, or the selection of uninfected replacement heifers from infected dams. Such selection is made on the basis of a complement-fixation test conducted 30 to 60 days after weaning; those heifers with negative test results are segregated into groups.

REFERENCES

Amerault, T.E., and Roby, T.O. 1977. Card test: An accurate and simple procedure for detecting anaplasmosis. World Anim. Rev. 22:34–38.

Barbet, A.F., Anderson, L.W., Palmer, G.H., and McGuire, T.C. 1983. Comparison of proteins synthesized by two different isolates of *Anaplasma marginale*. Infect. Immun. 40:1068–1074.

Bedell, D.M., and Dimopoullos, G.T. 1962. Biologic properties and characteristics of *Anaplasma marginale*. I. Effects of temperature on infectivity of whole blood preparations. Am. J. Vet. Res. 23:618–625.

Bedell, D.M., and Dimopoullos, G.T. 1963. Biologic properties and characteristics of *Anaplasma marginale*. II. The effects of sonic energy on the infectivity of whole blood preparations. Am. J. Vet. Res. 24:278–282.

Boynton, W.H. 1928. Observations on *Anaplasma marginale* (Theiler) in cattle of California. Cornell Vet. 18:28–48.

Boynton, W.H. 1929. Studies on anaplasmosis in cattle with special reference to (1) the susceptibility of calves born to recovered cows, and (2) the length of time recovered animals may remain carriers. Cornell Vet. 19:387–395.

Boynton, W.H., and Woods, G.M. 1935. A serum reaction observed in anaplasmosis. J. Am. Vet. Med. Assoc. 87:59–63.

Boynton, W.H., and Woods, G.M. 1940. Anaplasmosis among deer in the natural state. Science 91:168.

Brock, W.E. 1963. Anaplasmosis—An up-to-date look at transmission, diagnosis and immunization. Proc. Am. Vet. Med. Assoc. 100:258–261.

Buening, G.M. 1974. Hypolipodemia and hypergammaglobulinemia associated with experimentally induced anaplasmosis in calves. Am. J. Vet. Res. 35:371–374.

Carson, C.A., Sells, D.M., and Ristic, M. 1977. Cell-mediated immune response to virulent and attenuated *Anaplasma marginale* administered to cattle in live and inactivated forms. Am. J. Vet. Res. 38:173–179.

Christensen, J.F., Osebold, J.W., Harrold, J.B., and Rosen, M.N. 1960. Persistence of latent *Anaplasma marginale* infection in deer. J. Am. Vet. Med. Assoc. 136:426–427.

Davis, H.E., Dimopoullos, G.T, and Roby, T.O. 1970. Anaplasmosis transmission: Inoculation by the oral route. Res. Vet. Sci. 11:594–595.

Espana, C., Espana, E.M., and Gonzolez, D. 1959. *Anaplasma marginale*. I. Studies with phase contrast and electron microscopy. Am. J. Vet. Res. 20:795–805.

Franklin, T.E., Heck, F.C., and Huff, J.W. 1963. Anaplasmosis complement-fixation antigen production. Am. J. Vet. Res. 24:483–487.

Freidhoff, K.T., and Ristic, M. 1966. Anaplasmosis. XIX. A preliminary study of *Anaplasma marginale* in *Dermacentor andersoni* (Stiles) by fluorescent antibody technique. Am. J. Vet. Res. 27:643–646.

Gates, D.W., Madden, P.A., Martin, W.H., and Roby, T.O. 1957. The infectivity of blood from anaplasma infected cattle as shown by calf inoculation. Am. J. Vet. Res. 18:257–260.

Hadani, A., Guglielmone, A.A., and Anziani, O.S. 1982. A case of apparent suppression of *Anaplasma marginale* infection by eperythrozoonosis (*Eperythrozoon teganodes*). Vet. Parasitol. 9:267–272.

Kreier, J.P., Ristic, M., and Schroeder, W. 1964. Anaplasmosis. XVI. The pathogenesis of anemia produced by infection with *Anaplasma*. Am. J. Vet. Res. 25:343–352.

Kuttler, K.L. 1972. Efficacy of oxytetracycline and a dithiosemicarbazone in the treatment of bovine anaplasmosis. Res. Vet. Sci. 13:536–539.

Lotze, J.C. 1946. Further observations on the nature of anaplasma. Proc. Heminthol. Soc. Wash. 13:56–57.

Love, J.N. 1972. Cryogenic preservation of *Anaplasma marginale* with dimethyl sulfoxide. Am. J. Vet. Res. 33:2557–2560.

McHardy, N., and Simpson, R.M. 1973. Attempts at immunizing cattle against anaplasmosis using a killed vaccine. Trop. Anim. Health Prod. 5:166–173.

Osebold, J.W., Christensen, J.F., Longhurst, M.M., and Rosen, M.N. 1959. Latent *Anaplasma marginale* infection in wild deer demonstrated by calf inoculation. Cornell Vet. 49:97–115.

Osorno, M.B., Solana, P.M., Perez, J.M., and Lopez, T.R. 1975. Study of an attenuated *Anaplasma marginale* vaccine in Mexico—Natural challenge of immunity in an enzootic area. Am. J. Vet. Res. 36:631–633.

Pearson, C.C., Brock, W.E., and Kliewer, I.O. 1957. A study of tetracycline dosage in cattle which are anaplasmosis carriers. J. Am. Vet. Med. Assoc. 130:290–292.

Price, K.E., Brock, W.E., and Miller, J.G. 1954. An evaluation of the complement-fixation test for anaplasmosis. Am. J. Vet. Res. 15:511–516.

Price, K.E., Poelma, L.J., and Faber, J.E. 1952. Preparation of an improved antigen for anaplasmosis complement-fixation tests. Am. J. Vet. Res. 13:149–151.

Reese, C.W. 1930. The experimental transmission of anaplasmosis by *Rhipiciphalus sanguineus*. North Am. Vet. 11(9):17–20.

Richey, E.J., Brock, W.E., Kliewer, I.O., and Jones, E.W. 1977a. Low levels of chlortetracycline for anaplasmosis. Am. J. Vet. Res. 38:171–172.

Richey, E.J., Brock, W.E., Kliewer, I.O., and Jones, E.W. 1977b. Resistance to anaplasmosis after elimination of latent *Anaplasma marginale* infections. Am. J. Vet. Res. 38:169–170.

Ristic, M. 1962. A capillary tube-agglutination test for anaplasmosis—a preliminary report. J. Am. Vet. Med. Assoc. 141:588–594.

Ristic, M., and Carson, C.A. 1977. Methods of immunoprophylaxis against bovine anaplasmosis with emphasis on the use of the attenuated *Anaplasma marginale*. In E.A. Wells, ed., Workshop on Hemoparasites (Anaplasmosis and Babesiosis), Cali, Columbia, 1975. Pp. 105–132.

Ristic, M., and Mann, D.K. 1963. Anaplasmosis. IX. Immunoserologic properties of soluble *Anaplasma* antigens. Am. J. Vet. Res. 24:478–482.

Ristic, M., White, F.H., Green, J.H., and Sanders, D.A. 1958. Effect of cortisone on the mechanism of anaplasma immunity in experimentally infected calves. I. Hematological and immunoserological studies. Am. J. Vet. Res. 19:37–43.

Ristic, M., White, F.H., and Sanders, D.A. 1957. Detection of *Anaplasma marginale* by means of fluorescein-labeled antibody. Am. J. Vet. Res. 18:924–928.

Roby, T.O. 1972. The inhibitory effect of imidocarb on experimental anaplasmosis in splenectomized calves. Res. Vet. Sci. 13:519–522.

Roby, T.O., and Mazzola, V. 1972. Elimination of the carrier state of bovine anaplasmosis with imidocarb. Am. J. Vet. Res. 33:1931–1933.

Roby, T.O., Amerault, T.E., Mazzola, V., Rose, J.E., and Ilemobade, A. 1974. Immunity in bovine anaplasmosis after elimination of *Anaplasma marginale* infections with imidocarb. Am. J. Vet. Res. 35:993–995.

Roby, T.O., Amerault, T.E., and Spindler, L.A. 1968. The inhibitory effect of a dithiosemicarbazone on acute infections of *Anaplasma marginale*. Res. Vet. Sci. 9:494–499.

Roby, T.O., Gates, D.W., and Mott, L.O. 1961. The comparative susceptibility of calves and adult cattle to bovine anaplasmosis. Am. J. Vet. Res. 22:982–985.

Rogers, T.E., and Wallace, W.R. 1966. A rapid staining technique for *Anaplasma*. Am. J. Vet. Res. 27:1127–1128.

Splitter, E.J., and Miller, J.G. 1953. The apparent eradication of the anaplasmosis carrier state with antibiotics. Vet. Med. 48:486–488.

Staats, J.J., Kocan, K.M., Hair, J.A., and Ewing, S.A. 1982. Immunocytochemical labeling of *Anaplasma marginale* Theiler in *Dermacentor andersoni* Stiles with peroxidase-antiperoxidase technique. Am. J. Vet. Res. 43:979–983.

Summers, W.A., and Matsuoka, T. 1970. Infectivity of *Anaplasma marginale* after long-term storage in bovine blood. Am. J. Vet. Res. 31:1517–1518.

Swift, B.L., Reeves, J.D., III, and Thomas, G.M. 1979. Testicular degeneration and libido loss in beef bulls experimentally inoculated with *Anaplasma marginale*. Theriogenology 11:277–290.

Zaraza and Kuttler. 1976. Rev. Inst. Colomb. Agropecu. 11:363.

Anaplasma ovis

Anaplasmosis of sheep was described in South Africa in 1926, and in 1955 Splitter et al. reported a diseased flock of sheep in Kansas. In 1981 an Idaho sheep flock was investigated because of an obscure debilitating condition (Magonigle et al. 1981). Routine blood examination revealed marginal bodies in the erythrocytes identical in appearance with *A. marginale*, together with extracellular forms characteristic of *Eperythrozoon ovis*. Splenectomized calves inoculated with this sheep blood did not develop evidence of *A. marginale* infection. It seems probable that the infecting organism was *A. ovis*.

An organism identified as *A. ovis* was recovered from sheep originating in the Rocky Mountain area of the United States (Splitter et al. 1956). The organism produced variable degrees of subclinical anemia in sheep and goats. Cattle could not be infected with the parasite, nor did it produce any detectable immunity against *A. marginale* in these animals. Kreier and Ristic (1963) experimentally infected two Virginia white-tailed deer (*Dama virginiana*) with *A. ovis*.

Electron microscopy studies of erythrocytes infected with *A. ovis* have revealed a membrane-enclosed body, usually marginally located, and filled with two initial bodies (Jatkar, 1969).

REFERENCES

Jatkar, P.R. 1969. Electron microscopic study of *Anaplasma ovis*. Am. J. Vet. Res. 30:1891–1892.

Kreier, J.P., and Ristic, M. 1963. Anaplasmosis. VII. Experimental *Anaplasma ovis* infection in white-tailed deer (*Dama virginiana*). Am. J. Vet. Res. 24:567–572.

Magonigle, R.A., Eckblad, W.P., Lincoln, S.D., and Frank, F.W. 1981. *Anaplasma ovis* in Idaho sheep. Am. J. Vet. Res. 42:199–201.

Splitter, E.J., Anthony, H.D., and Twiehaus, M.J. 1956. *Anaplasma ovis* in the United States. Experimental studies with sheep and goats. Am. J. Vet. Res. 17:487–491.

Splitter, E.J., Twiehaus, M.J., and Castro, E.R. 1955. Anaplasmosis in sheep in the United States. J. Am. Vet. Med. Assoc. 127:244–245.

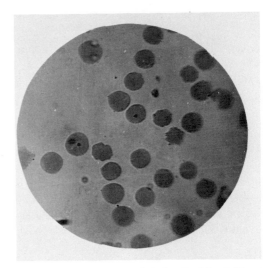

Figure 32.2. *Anaplasma centrale* in bovine blood. Two typical parasites are seen as sharply staining dots near the center of the red blood cells. Poikilocytosis and anisocytosis are present as a result of anemia. Giemsa stain. × 770.

Anaplasma centrale

Theiler (1912), in his studies that led to the differentiation of the anaplasmas from the piroplasmas, distinguished two kinds of anaplasmas: the marginal bodies, already described, which are the only bodies found in anaplasmosis in the United States; and central bodies, which are identical in appearance to the marginal bodies, but are characteristically located in the central part of red blood cells (Figure 32.2). The central bodies are now called *Anaplasma centrale*.

Theiler showed that animals that had recovered from an infection with blood containing the central bodies could still be infected with blood containing the marginal bodies. He also noted that the disease caused by *A. centrale* was much milder than that caused by *A. marginale*. Schmidt (1937) reported that in South Africa adult cattle coming from Europe were first injected with blood containing *A. centrale* and later with *A. marginale*, and the first and milder infection gave some protection against the more severe second disease. In Australia, where immunization with *A. centrale* is practiced, it was found that citrated calf blood infected with this parasite retains its effectiveness for 254 days when frozen in 1-ml doses and maintained at −72° to −80°C (Turner, 1944).

REFERENCES

Schmidt, H. 1937. Anaplasmosis in cattle. J. Am. Vet. Med. Assoc. 90:723–736.

Theiler, A. 1912. Weitere Untersuchungen über die Anaplasmosis der Rinder und deren Schutzimpfung. Z. Infekt. Haustiere 11:193–207.

Turner, A.W. 1944. The successful preservation of *Anaplasma centrale* at the temperature of solid carbon dioxide. Aust. Vet. J. 20:295–298.

The Genus *Paranaplasma*

There are two species of *Paranaplasma*: *P. caudatum* and *P. discoides*. These organisms have the same characteristics as *Anaplasma* species except the inclusions have appendages. The organisms are infective for cattle but not deer or sheep. All isolations of *P. caudatum* have been from mixed infections of *A. marginale* and *P. discoides* (Ristic and Kreier 1974).

REFERENCE

Ristic, M., and Kreier, J.P. 1974. Family III. Anaplasmataceae. In R.E. Buchanan and N.E. Gibbons, eds., Bergey's Manual of Determinative Bacteriology, 8th ed. Williams & Wilkins, Baltimore. P. 906.

The Genus *Aegyptianella*

Aegyptianella pullorum

A. pullorum is the causative agent of aegyptianellosis in birds. Natural infections have been described in chickens, geese, ducks, turkeys, guinea fowls, pigeons, quail, and ostriches. Certain wild birds have been infected experimentally. The disease has been found in South Africa, Indochina, and the Balkans and probably exists in most subtropical and tropical countries. The principal features of infection with *A. pullorum* have been reviewed by Ristic and Kreier (1974).

Chickens are naturally infected with *A. pullorum* by the tick *Argas persicus*. Experimental infection can be achieved by parenteral injection or by scarification with infected blood. The disease is frequently associated with fowl spirochetosis. Native fowl rarely suffer an acute disease, but newly introduced stock can die within a few days with diarrhea, anorexia, a high temperature, and paralysis. The epizootiology has been reviewed by Goethe (1976).

In blood smears prepared with Giemsa stain, the infected hosts's erythrocytes exhibit many inclusions that are reddish violet with a diameter of 0.3 to 3.9 μm. In larger inclusions clearly defined, smaller, round organisms (initial bodies) can be seen. The organisms can be found free in the plasma and in phagocytic cells. The infectivity can be preserved for 5 years by freezing in liquid nitrogen (Goethe and Hartman 1979). The organism has not been cultured in vitro. The organisms are sensitive to dithiosemicarbazones and tetracyclines.

There are other species that eventually may be placed in this genus, but their true identity or relationship to *A. pullorum* has not been established. They are *Tunetella emydis*, *Sogdianella moshkovskii*, *Aegyptianella carpani*, and other organisms that have been reported in a number of domestic and wild birds.

REFERENCES

Goethe, R. 1976. New aspects of the epizootiology of aegyptianellosis in poultry. In J.K. Wilde, ed., Tick-Borne Diseases and Their Vectors. Proceedings of an International Congress. University Press, Edinburgh. Pp. 201–204.

Goethe, R., and Hartman, S. 1979. The viability of cryopreserved *Aegyptianella pullorum* Carpani, 1928, in the vector *Argas (Persicargas) walkerae* Kaiser and Hoogstraal, 1969. Z. Parasitenkd. 58:189–190.

Ristic, M., and Kreier, J.P. 1974. Genus III. *Aegyptianella*. In R.E. Buchanan and N.E. Gibbons, eds., Bergey's Manual of Determinative Bacteriology, 8th ed. Williams & Wilkins, Baltimore. P. 909.

The Genus *Haemobartonella*

Most species of *Haemobartonella* are infectious, but the disease they cause usually is not apparent except in the case of *H. felis* infection in cats. Treatment with organic arsenical substances, such as thiacetarsamide sodium and antimony-arsenic compounds, is effective, but the disease is refractory to sulfa compounds.

Haemobartonella muris

SYNONYM: *Bartonella muris*

The organism *H. muris* was first described in 1921 in Germany. It was isolated from laboratory rats that had been infected with trypanosomes. This organism is found in and on the surface of the red blood cells. According to Peters and Wigand (1955), *H. muris* prepared by Giemsa stain shows mostly coccoid forms, in contrast to *Bartonella bacilliformis*, which shows mostly rod shapes. Electron microscopy studies of *H. muris* do not show structural details, cell walls like those of bacteria, or flagella. Thin sections reveal a spherical or ellipsoidal agent, 0.35 to 0.70 μm in size (Tanaka et al. 1965). The organism is nonmotile and increases by binary fission, but apparently does not multiply outside the host's blood. It is transmitted by lice and is found throughout the world.

H. muris usually will not cause infection in rats unless the animals are infected with trypanosomiasis, are given certain blood-destroying agents, or are splenectomized. It is of great interest that rats in many parts of the world, including the United States, carry this organism latently.

This can be demonstrated by the fact that removal of the spleen often leads to prompt development of the disease. It appears that the spleen, possibly through a protective activity of its reticuloendothelial system, is able to hold the disease in abeyance. The disease is manifested by a rapidly developing anemia and by the appearance of the organism in the blood. The animals can die, or they can recover in a few days. Other animals susceptible to infection with *H. muris* are mice, hamsters, and rabbits. The organism resists penicillin and streptomycin, but is quite sensitive to chlortetracycline, oxytetracycline, and tetracycline. Chloramphenicol has little, if any, effect (Peters and Wigand 1955).

REFERENCES

Peters, D., and Wigand, R. 1955. Bartonellaceae. Bacteriol. Rev. 19:150–155.
Tanaka, H., Hall, W.T., Sheffield, J.B., and Moore, D.H. 1965. Fine structure of *Haemobartonella muris* as compared with *Eperythrozoon coccoides* and *Mycoplasma pulmonis*. J. Bacteriol. 90:1735–1749.

Haemobartonella canis

SYNONYM: *Bartonella canis*

In 1928 an organism was described in Germany which was believed to be the cause of an infectious anemia of dogs. The organism was similar to other species of *Haemobartonella*. Workers in other countries have more recently seen the same organism; but because none has succeeded in culturing it, its relationship to the other *Haemobartonella* species has not been proved. The disease appears to be rather mild when it occurs. The organism has also been seen in blood smears from dogs with parvovirus disease (Harvey 1982); the concurrent infection may contribute to a more severe disease. Some dogs with ehrlichiosis are concurrently infected with *H. canis*.

Knutti and Hawkins (1935) in the United States encountered the condition in splenectomized, bile fistula dogs. Spontaneous periods of anemia, associated with excess bile production, were regularly associated in some dogs with the appearance in the blood of bodies resembling haemobartonellae (Figure 32.3). Simple splenectomy would not regularly produce the disease, but the inoculation of dog's blood containing the haemobartonellae into splenectomized animals was regularly followed by anemia and the appearance of the parasite. *H. canis* was transmitted to splenectomized dogs by all stages of the tick *Rhipicephalus sanguineus*. There was stage-to-stage as well as transovarial transmission (Seneviratna et al. 1973).

Haemobartonellosis in the dog has been reviewed by West (1979).

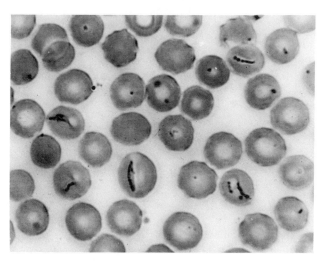

Figure 32.3. *Haemobartonella canis* in the blood of an infected dog. Giemsa stain. × 1,070. (Courtesy M. M. Benjamin and W. V. Lumb, *Journal of the American Veterinary Medical Association*.)

REFERENCES

Harvey, J.W. 1982. *Haemobartonella canis* in the blood of dogs with parvovirus disease. J. Small Anim. Pract. 23:800–801.
Knutti, R.E., and Hawkins, W.B. 1935. Bartonella incidence in splenectomized bile fistula dogs. J. Exp. Med. 61:115–125.
Seneviratna, P., Weerasinghe, N., and Ariyadasa, S. 1973. Transmission of *Haemobartonella canis* by the dog tick, *Rhipicephalus sanguineus*. Res. Vet. Sci. 14:112–114.
West, H.J. 1979. Haemobartonellosis in the dog. J. Small Anim. Pract. 20:543–549.

Haemobartonella felis

Feline infectious anemia was first reported by Flint and Moss (1953). It is described as an acute, subacute, or chronic infectious disease of domestic and wild cats. When acute, it is characterized by fever, a marked hemolytic anemia, anorexia, depression, and rapid weight loss (Harvey 1982). Although *H. felis* is rarely the cause of primary disease in cats, it occurs concurrently with feline leukemia virus infection and secondarily to disorders that lower the host's immune response.

The laboratory disease in cats was described by Harvey and Gaskin (1977) as a mild disease, but all inoculated nonsplenectomized cats in their study became carriers. Attempts to induce relapses of clinical disease in stressed, chronically infected cats failed, and these results were not anticipated because stress usually causes a relapse with this class of organisms (Harvey and Gaskin 1978).

Blood smears offer the best diagnostic aid. The parasites occur as small round dots, short rods, or coccoids that sometimes are in chains. The rods are 0.2 to 0.5 μm wide and 0.9 to 1.5 μm long and the coccoids are 0.1 to 0.8 μm in diameter. These organisms do not have a rigid cell wall, but possess a double limiting membrane. They frequently occur attached to or partly embedded in the erythrocyte membrane, which may be eroded at the point of contact. The parasites appear deep purple with Giemsa stain. Fluorescent antibody or acridine orange may reveal the organism when it cannot be seen with Giemsa stain. The organism has not been cultured in vitro.

The infection can be transmitted orally or by parenteral injection (Harvey and Gaskin 1977). Intrauterine infection can occur, and the infection can be spread by biting during cat fights. Transmission by arthropods has not been established, and the organism is rather host specific. Carriers do exist. The disease appears to be widespread in the United States.

Various chemotherapeutic agents, such as chloramphenicol, tetracycline, oxytetracycline, and thioacetarsamide sodium (Sauerwein and Graber 1982) are effective in suppressing the disease.

REFERENCES

Flint, J.C., and Moss, L.C. 1953. Infectious anemia in cats. J. Am. Vet. Med. Assoc. 122:45–48.
Harvey, J.W. 1982. *Haemobartonella canis* in the blood of dogs with parvovirus disease. J. Small Anim. Pract. 23:800–801.
Harvey, J.W., and Gaskin, J.M. 1977. Experimental feline haemobartonellosis. J. Am. Anim. Hosp. Assoc. 13:28–38.
Harvey, J.W., and Gaskin, J.M. 1978. Feline haemobartonellosis: Attempts to induce relapses of clinical disease in chronically infected cats. J. Am. Anim. Hosp. Assoc. 14:453–456.
Sauerwein, G., and Graber, A. 1982. Zur Behandlung der Hemobartonellose der Katze mit Thioacetarsamid-Natrium (Caparsolate). Kleintierpraxis 27:323–326, 328.

Haemobartonella bovis

SYNONYM: *Bartonella bovis*

Donatien and Lestoquard (1934) reported *Haemobartonella* in the blood of cattle in France. Lotze and Yiengst (1942) found similar forms in cattle in the United States. Since these organisms were found in animals infected with anaplasmosis, the American workers were uncertain whether they represented a stage of the life cycle of *Anaplasma marginale*. Later Lotze and Bowman (1942) found them in an anaplasma-free calf shortly after it had been splenectomized. It is clear, therefore, that *H. bovis* is not necessarily associated with anaplasmosis. Usually few parasites are found in the blood, but they may become much more numerous during the incubation period following inoculation with anaplasmas. There is no evidence that *H. bovis* is of any economic importance.

The organism was first cultivated in the yolk sac of an embryonated hen's egg and then in a medium containing yolk, bovine serum, and calf spleen extract. Culture forms were coccal and often arranged in long chains, and

they produced high agglutination titers in inoculated cattle (Rodriguez et al. 1975).

Haemobartonellae are also found in goats (Mukherjee 1952), but appear to be of little economic importance.

REFERENCES

Donatien, A., and Lestoquard, F. 1934. La prémunition et les vaccinations prémunitives dans la pathologie vétérinaire. Bull. Soc. Pathol. Exot. 27:652–654.
Lotze, J.C., and Bowman, G.W. 1942. The occurrence of *Bartonella* in cases of anaplasmosis and in apparently normal cattle. Proc. Helminthol. Soc. Wash. 9:71–72.
Lotze, J.C., and Yiengst, M.J. 1942. Studies on the nature of anaplasma. Am. J. Vet. Res. 8:312–320.
Mukherjee, B.N. 1952. Bartonella in goats. Indian Vet. J. 28:343–351.
Rodriguez, O.N., Espaine, L., Rodriguez, P., and Jurasek, V. 1975. Aislamiento de elementors cocobaciliformes en los cultvos de *Hemobartonella bovis* (Donatien y Lestoquard, 1934). Folia Vet. 19:233–242.

Haemobartonella tyzzeri

The organism *H. tyzzeri* was found by Weinman and Pinkerton (1938) in splenectomized guinea pigs from Colombia. The parasite can be transmitted to splenectomized *Haemobartonella*-free guinea pigs by intraperitoneal injection (Groot 1942).

REFERENCES

Groot, H. 1942. *Haemobartonella tyzzeri* in Colombia. Proc. Soc. Exp. Biol. Med. 51:279.
Weinman, D., and Pinkerton, H. 1938. A bartonella of the guinea pig. Ann. Trop. Med. Parasitol. 32:215–224.

The Genus *Eperythrozoon*

Differentiation of members of the genus *Eperythrozoon* from *Haemobartonella* species is often difficult and perhaps arbitrary in some instances (Kreier and Ristic 1974). Two distinguishing features of eperythrozoa are that they often occur as ring forms and that they can be found with equal frequency on the erythrocytes and in the plasma; by contrast, haemobartonellae rarely assume a ring form and almost never occur free in the plasma. Swarmlike clusters of ring-shaped eperythrozoa are sometimes seen on the surface of erythrocytes (Figure 32.4), and rod-shaped forms can partially or entirely encircle a blood cell. In fresh preparations examined by dark-field and phase microscopy the organism appears pleomorphic, surrounded by a single limiting membrane, and with no cell wall, nucleus, or other organelles. Typical of the family Anaplasmataceae, the organism has not been cultured in cell-free media. Some species have been transmitted by ar-

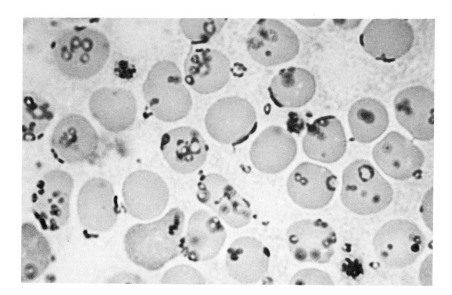

Figure 32.4. *Eperythrozoon suis* in the blood of an infected pig. Romanowsky stain. × 2,225. (Courtesy A. Savage and J. M. Isa, *Cornell Veterinarian.*)

thropods. Infective blood readily produces the disease upon parenteral inoculation. Splenectomy in the animal host activates latent infection with most species. The growth of the organism is inhibited by tetracyclines and arsenicals, but the disease is refractory to sulfa compounds.

REFERENCE

Kreier, J.P., and Ristic, M. 1974. Genus V. *Eperythrozoon.* In R.E. Buchanan and N.E. Gibbons, eds., Bergey's Manual of Determinative Bacteriology, 8th ed. Williams & Wilkins, Baltimore. P. 912.

Eperythrozoon coccoides

The organism *E. coccoides* was described by Dinger in 1929 as a blood parasite of mice. The characteristics of *H. muris* and *E. coccoides* correspond in nearly every respect, except for some minor differences in morphology. Giemsa staining of both organisms generally shows a preponderance of coccoid forms for *H. muris* and ring-shaped bodies for *E. coccoides*. Like *H. muris*, *E. coccoides* is nonmotile and appears not to multiply outside the host blood. It is ubiquitous and is transmitted by lice. Rats, hamsters, and rabbits are also subject to infection.

Ott and Stauber (1967) observed mice that were infected with malaria and also with *E. coccoides*. The malarial infection had a low-level, chronic course producing infrequent deaths. When the eperythrozoa were eliminated through treatment with oxophenarsine hydrochloride (arsenoxide), the malarial infection assumed an acute course always ending in death.

Glasgow et al. (1974) reported that the organism inhibited the interferon response in mice during the first 3 weeks after infection. By 6 weeks the production of interferon in response to Newcastle disease virus returned to normal. Furthermore, the clearance of parasitemia was correlated with the appearance of circulating neutralizing antibody.

Like *H. muris*, *E. coccoides* is resistant to penicillin and streptomycin but is sensitive to chlortetracycline, oxytetracycline, and tetracycline. The effect of chloramphenicol is minimal at best (Peters and Wigand 1955). Gledhill et al. (1965) studied a mouse colony that had a history of long-established infection with *E. coccoides* and claimed that the organisms were eliminated by regular insecticidal treatments designed to reduce infestation with lice and fleas.

REFERENCES

Dinger, J.E. 1929. Näheres über das *Eperythrozoon coccoides.* Zentralbl. Bakteriol. [Orig. A] 113:503–509.
Glasgow, L.A., Murrer, A.T., and Lombardi, P.S. 1974. *Eperythrozoon coccoides*. II. Effect on interferon production and role of humoral antibody in host resistance. Infect. Immun. 9:266–272.
Gledhill, A.W., Niven, J.S.F., and Seamer, J. 1965. Elimination of *Eperythrozoon coccoides* infection from mouse colonies. J. Hyg. 63:73–78.
Ott, K.J., and Stauber, L.A. 1967. *Eperythrozoon coccoides:* Influence on course of infection of *Plasmodium chabaudi* in mouse. Science 155:1546–1548.
Peters, D., and Wigand, R. 1955. Bartonellaceae. Bacteriol. Rev. 19:150–155.

Eperythrozoon suis

Splitter and Williamson (1950) found an eperythrozoon in swine associated with a clinical entity known as *ana-*

plasmosislike disease and *icteroanemia*. They saw the organism in three separate outbreaks. Since then ictero-anemia has been found to be rather widespread in the United States (Adams et al. 1959, Biberstein et al. 1956). It has also been described in western Germany, where it is associated with louse infestations (Hoffman and Saalfeld 1977). The causative agent has been named *Eperythrozoon suis*. A second species, which apparently is a nonpathogenic blood parasite, has been named *E. parvum;* it is a common parasite of swine in the midwestern United States and can be confused with *E. suis*. *E. suis* is frequently found in the blood of swine in enzootic areas.

Most young pigs become infected during the summer and remain immune, latent, clinically unrecognized carriers. The clinical disease depends on the number of parasites that develop in the blood following infection. In most swine, parasitic attacks are mild and cause no visible damage. Pigs heavily infected with *E. suis* show inappetence, lassitude, weakness, anemia, and often icterus. The infection in sows apparently has no effect on reproductive performance.

Diagnosis is made by finding small, ring-shaped bodies on the erythrocytes of diseased pigs. Splitter (1958) found a complement-fixation test useful in diagnosing icteroanemia in swine. He employed an antigen prepared from CO_2-precipitated erythrocytes heavily parasitized with *E. suis*. Smith and Rahn (1975) used an indirect hemagglutination test for the diagnosis of *E. suis* infection in swine.

The exact mode of transmission is not known, but insect vectors such as flies and lice seem to play a role. Berrier and Gouge (1954) reported a case of transmission in utero.

REFERENCES

Adams, E.W., Lyles, D.I., and Cockrell, K.O. 1959. Eperythrozoonosis in a herd of purebred Landrace pigs. J. Am. Vet. Med. Assoc. 135:226–228.

Berrier, H.H., and Gouge, R.E. 1954. Eperythrozoonosis transmitted in utero from carrier sows to their pigs. J. Am. Vet. Med. Assoc. 124:98–100.

Biberstein, E.L., Barr, L.M., Larrow, L.L., and Roberts, S.J. 1956. Eperythrozoonosis of swine in New York State. Cornell Vet. 46:288–297.

Hoffman, R., and Saalfeld, K. 1977. Outbreak of an *Eperythrozoon suis* infection on a pig fattening farm. D.T.W. 84:7–9.

Smith, A.R., and Rahn, T. 1975. An indirect hemagglutination test for the diagnosis of *Eperythrozoon suis* infection in swine. Am. J. Vet. Res. 36:1319–1321.

Splitter, E.J. 1958. The complement-fixation test in diagnosis of eperythrozoonosis in swine. J. Am. Vet. Med. Assoc. 132:47–49.

Splitter, E.J., and Williamson, R.L. 1950. Eperythrozoonosis in swine. A preliminary report. J. Am. Vet. Med. Assoc. 116:360–364.

Eperythrozoon wenyoni

Neitz (1940) reported the presence of *E. wenyoni* in cattle in South Africa. This organism is observed with other bovine blood organisms, which together cause a mixed infection. Lotze and Yiengst (1941) observed eperythrozoonosis in the United States in cattle experimentally infected with *Anaplasma marginale*. Mirzabekov (1974), in Russia, described the disease in conjunction with *Babesia bigemina*. Hinaidy (1973), in Austria, described the organism in a steer with severe *B. divergens* infection. The infection has also been reported in Holland (Wensing et al. 1974), New Zealand (Sutton et al. 1977), England (Purnell et al. 1976), Colombia, and Ireland (Poole et al. 1976)—in some instances associated with clinical signs of illness. Although the economic importance of *E. wenyoni* is unknown, infection in calves is believed to be significant at times. Finerty et al. (1968) prepared an antigen by ultrasonic disruption of purified suspensions of *E. wenyoni* and found that it was specific when used in passive hemagglutination tests to detect naturally occurring eperythrozoonosis in calves.

REFERENCES

Finerty, J.F., Hidalgo, R.J., and Dimopoullos, G.T. 1968. Disk electrophoretic separation of soluble preparations of *Plasmoduim lophurae* and *Anaplasma marginale*. Am. J. Vet. Res. 30:43–45.

Hinaidy, H.K. 1973. Die Gastrointestinal Helminthen des Rindes in Österreich. Wien. Tierärztl. Monatsschr. 60:364–366.

Lotze, C.J., and Yiengst, M.J. 1941. Eperythrozoonosis in cattle in the United States. North Am. Vet. 22:345–346.

Mirzabekov, K.D. 1974. Experimental eperythrozoonosis (in cattle). Veterinariia 6:68–69.

Neitz, W.O. 1940. Eperythrozoonosis in cattle. Onderstepoort J. Vet. Res. 14:9–28.

Poole, D.B.R., Cutler, R.S., Kelly, W.R., and Collins, J.D. 1976. *Eperythrozoon wenyoni* anaemia in cattle. Vet. Rec. 99:481.

Purnell, R.E., Brocklesby, D.W., and Young, E.R. 1976. *Eperythrozoon wenyoni* a possible cause of anaemia in British cattle. Vet. Rec. 98:411.

Sutton, R.H., Charleston, W.A.G., and Collins, G.H. 1977. *Eperythrozoon wenyoni*—A blood parasite of cattle. A first report in New Zealand. N.Z. Vet. J. 25:8–9.

Wensing, T., Nouwens, G., Schotman, A.J.H., Vernooy, J., and Zwart, D. 1974. Effect of *Eperythrozoon wenyoni* on the glucose level and acid-base balance of bovine blood in vivo and in vitro. Tijdschr. Diergeneeskd. 99:136–142.

Eperythrozoon ovis

Neitz (1937) reported that *E. ovis* causes illness in sheep that are not splenectomized. This disease of lambs has considerable mortality; postmortem features include anemia, enlarged soft spleen, and an excess of pericardial fluid. More recently, Sonoda et al. (1977) observed the disease in some adult sheep that had fever, anemia, cardiac palpitation, tachypnea, and hemoglobinuria. In southern Australia Sheriff et al. (1966) found that the majority of anemias in young sheep and the majority of outbreaks of ill-thrift are caused by *E. ovis* infection. They also reported that the severity of the disease may depend on complicating factors. Experimental and natural diseases have been observed in goats with *E. ovis* (Daddow 1979a, 1979b).

Daddow and Dunlop (1976) monitored the disease in a national outbreak among sheep in Australia. The complement-fixation test (Daddow 1977) and blood smears were used to determine the presence of infection in ewes and their lambs. The ewes appeared to be the main source of infection for their lambs, and the infection could be spread by mosquitoes (Daddow 1980) and possibly sand flies. The complement-fixation test is a valuable diagnostic procedure for herds. Diagnosis can also be made using an indirect immunofluorescent antibody test (Ilemobade and Blatkamp 1978).

Sutton and Jolly (1973) studied the effects of *E. ovis* in sheep under experimental conditions. Infection in lambs was characterized by a hypochromic anemia with one-half the normal hemoglobulin content. In lambs maintained on pasture, growth was retarded; normal growth was observed in housed sheep fed without restriction.

Sutton (1977) found that the incubation period is inversely proportional to the infecting dose. Infected sheep have low blood glucose levels and corresponding increased blood lactic acid levels. The acidosis and hypoglycemia associated with infection could potentially be serious in pregnant ewes and in poorly fed sheep.

Additional work by Sutton (1978) showed that the main pathological features of experimental *E. ovis* infection were an increase of spleen weight by up to 250 percent at the peak of parasitemia and an increase in liver weight by 36 percent. Hemosiderin was present in the kidneys, livers, and spleens of all infected sheep at the peak and late stages of parasitemia. Control sheep had hemosiderin in the spleen only. On the basis of these findings, intravascular hemolysis appears to be the predominant mode of red cell removal. Although not observed histologically, some erythrophagocytosis by the spleen and liver probably occurs in the course of the infection.

Neitz (1937) reported that antimony-arsenic compounds are valuable in treating the infection. Spirotrypan forte is effective but sometimes quite toxic and expensive, so it is not recommended for field use (Sheriff 1973).

REFERENCES

Daddow, K.N. 1977. A complement fixation test for the detection of eperythrozoon infection in sheep. Aust. Vet. J. 53:139–143.

Daddow, K.N. 1979a. The transmission of a sheep strain of *Eperythrozoon ovis* to goats and the development of a carrier state in the goats. Aust. Vet. J. 55:605.

Daddow, K.N. 1979b. The natural occurrence in a goat of an organism resembling *Eperythrozoon ovis*. Aust. Vet. J. 55:605–606.

Daddow, K.N. 1980. *Culex annulirostris* as a vector of *Eperythrozoon ovis* infection in sheep. Vet. Parsitol. 7:313–317.

Daddow, K.N., and Dunlop, L.B. 1976. Eperythrozoon infection in sheep. Queensland J. Agric. Anim. Sci. 33:233–236.

Ilemobade, A.A., and Blatkamp, C. 1978. *Eperythrozoon ovis*. I. Serological diagnosis of infection by the indirect immunofluorescent antibody test. Tropenmed. Parasitol. 29:307–310.

Neitz, W.O. 1937. Eperythrozoonosis in sheep. Onderstepoort J. Vet. Res. 9:9–30.

Sheriff, D. 1973. The effect of Spirotrypan on *Eperythrozoon ovis* in sheep. Vet. Rec. 93:288–289.

Sheriff, D., Clapp, K.H., and Reid, M.A. 1966. *Eperythrozoon ovis* infection in South Australia. Aust. Vet. J. 42:169–176.

Sonoda, M., Takahashi, K., Tamura, T., and Koiwa, M. 1977. Clinical and haematological observation on spontaneous and experimental cases of *Eperythrozoon* infection in sheep. J. Jpn. Vet. Med. Assoc. 30:374–379.

Sutton, R.H. 1977. The effects of *Eperythrozoon ovis* infection on the glucose level and some acid-base factors in the venous blood of sheep. Aust. Vet. J. 53:478–481.

Sutton, R.H. 1978. Observations on the pathology of *Eperythrozoon ovis* infection in sheep. N.Z. Vet. J. 26:224, 229–230.

Sutton, R.H., and Jolly, R.D. 1973. Experimental *Eperythrozoon ovis* infection of sheep. N.Z. Vet. J. 21:160–166.

Eperythrozoon felis

Seamer and Douglas (1959) described a new blood parasite in cats in England and called it *E. felis*. Because the differences between *Haemobartonella* and *Eperythrozoon* species are minor, it is possible that they were dealing with haemobartonellosis.

REFERENCE

Seamer, J., and Douglas, S.W. 1959. A new blood parasite of British cats. Vet. Rec. 71:405–408.

33 The Chlamydiaceae

The name Chlamydiaceae was suggested by Smadel (1943) to designate a family of agents that share many characteristics not possessed by viruses. The chlamydias are small bacteria that live as obligate parasites of cells. They have RNA and DNA as well as an elaborate multiplication cycle that takes place inside the cell. The nature of this cycle together with differences in antigenic structure distinguishes the chlamydias from the rickettsias. Unlike the latter, the chlamydias are cytochrome-free and lack adenosine triphosphate (ATP). Their genome size is about 660 megadaltons, and they have a Gram-negative-type cell wall.

The genus *Chlamydia* can be separated into two species, *C. trachomatis* and *C. psittaci* (Page 1968). This separation is based on relatively stable morphologic and chemical characteristics of the organisms rather than on their presumed natural hosts or tissue preferences or on the specific serology of their cell wall antigens. Attempts to classify these bacteria by host specificity or serology have led to great confusion in the past. Included in this group are the agents of psittacosis, ornithosis, pneumonitis, conjunctivitis, sporadic bovine encephalomyelitis, polyarthritis, placentopathy, enteritis, enzootic ovine abortion, and enzootic bovine abortion.

The agents of all these diseases contain a common group antigen. They are susceptible to some chemotherapeutic and antibiotic agents. Most are capable of producing pneumonitis in mice and can be cultured in the yolk sac of chick embryos. The infectious particles are elementary bodies, 0.3 μm in diameter. They have the same developmental cycle, and each contains RNA and DNA in the same relative amounts at different growth stages.

They can vary in the specificity of cell wall antigens, toxins, and species-differentiating biochemical properties. In studies of four purified strains of *C. psittaci* (one bovine and three ovine) and one purified strain of *C. trachomatis,* the number of polypeptides varied between 17 and 20. Two polypeptides predominated and comprised approximately one-third of the total protein in each of the five strains. In another study Charton et al. (1976) found that two strains of *C. psittaci* had 16 principal polypeptides, with 9 located in the envelope. Of the five glycopeptides, one was isolated from the envelope and the others from the nucleus.

Bedson and Bland (1932, 1934) studied the development of the psittacosis agent in the tissues of animals. They observed that early in the course of infection reticulate bodies appeared in the macrophages of the spleen and in the epithelial cells of the lungs, intestine, liver, and kidneys. At first these bodies appeared homogeneous, but later they became granular. Eventually they resolved into spherical masses of distinctly stained elementary bodies.

The elementary bodies can be characteristically stained with Giemsa, Macchiavello, or Castaneda stain. When these bodies are fully formed, the cells that contain them rupture, discharging showers of infective elementary bodies into the tissue fluids. This developmental cycle is characteristic of all members of this group. Fluorescent antibody studies have confirmed that the granular material in the plaques consists of psittacoid protein (Donaldson et al. 1958). These observations were corroborated by electron microscopy studies of thin sections of infected mammalian cells in culture (Friis 1972).

Chlamydias have an affinity for epithelial cells of

mucous membranes; with these cells or mouse fibroblasts (L cells), attachment and penetration seems to involve a heat-labile surface component on the elementary bodies and a trypsin-sensitive receptor on the host cells. On HeLa cells sialic residues also appear to serve as receptors. The elementary bodies enter by a phagocytic process, creating a phagosome or inclusion in which the microcolony develops. The uptake of chlamydias by macrophages or granulocytes presumably does not depend on specific attachment mechanisms.

Within a few hours after host cell entry the elementary bodies begin to undergo changes in their cell envelope, and the central condensate disperses to form a more homogeneous cytoplasm in which strands of nucleic acid and ribosomes are observed. The resulting reticulate bodies continue to grow (up to 1 μm), and 10 to 15 hours after infection binary fission commences. At 20 to 30 hours after infection some reticulate bodies develop a central condensation of cytoplasmic contents, become smaller, and become typical elementary bodies. Most of the reticulate bodies continue to replicate until the host cell cytoplasm is almost filled by the colony. The transformation of the elementary body into the reticulate body involves marked changes in structure and composition of the cell membrane. Little is known about the cell release mechanism of the elementary bodies, but the host cells in cell culture die and autolyze 40 to 60 hours after infection.

The elementary body membrane is rigid, is resistant to sonic vibration, is relatively impermeable to macromolecules, contains hemagglutinin, and has an inner layer of hexagonally arranged subunits. After the elementary body enters the phagosome its envelope quickly loses its rigidity, and the subunit layer is disrupted and disappears. The cell membrane of the reticulate body is fragile: it is easily disrupted and is highly permeable to macromolecules. It does not contain hemagglutinin or a subunit layer. Reticulate bodies are not infectious.

C. trachomatis organisms that are associated either with mouse pneumonitis or trachoma, inclusion conjunctivitis, or lymphogranuloma venereum of humans have compact intracytoplasmic microcolonies; these microcolonies produce sufficient quantities of glycogen to be detectable by staining with iodine and are inhibited by sodium sulfadiazine (Becker 1974). In contrast, the members of *C. psittaci* frequently associated with psittacosis, meningopneumonitis, guinea pig conjunctivitis, bovine encephalomyelitis, feline pneumonitis, or caprine pneumonitis have diffuse microcolonies that fail to produce glycogen or to exhibit susceptibility to sodium sulfadiazine. Except for the 6BC parakeet strain, which is glycogen-negative but sulfadiazine sensitive, all strains isolated from many animal species are readily separated into one of the two species, *C. trachomatis* or *C. psittaci.*

Until we obtain more concrete information regarding the epidemiology of the chlamydias and develop more specific tests for and information about how they cause the disease(s) in various hosts, the above scheme for recognition of the two species, as proposed by Page (1968) is logical and acceptable. It has been reviewed and approved by a majority of the members of the Subcommittee on the Chlamydiaceae (Taxonomy Committee, American Society of Microbiology) and will be used in this book. Some of the diseases caused by various strains of *C. psittaci* are listed in Table 33.1, with emphasis on the diseases in domestic animals. The review article by Pienaar and Schutte (1975) provides more detailed information and additional references on chlamydial diseases in animals and in humans.

REFERENCES

Becker, Y. 1974. Recent studies on the agent of trachoma: Biology, biochemistry, and immunology of a prokaryotic obligate parasite of eukaryocytes. Prog. Med. Virol. 16:1.

Bedson, S.P., and Bland, J.O.W. 1932, 1934. A morphological study of psittacosis virus with the description of a developmental cycle. The development forms of psittacosis virus. Br. J. Exp. Pathol. 13:461–466, 15.243–247.

Charton, A., Faye, P., Gueslin, M., Solsona, M., and Layee, C. 1976. Chlamydia infections of ruminants (cattle, sheep, goat): Experimental studies. II. Polypeptide composition of elementary bodies of strains from various sources. Bull. Acad. Vet. 49:401–408.

Donaldson, P., Davis, D.E., Watkins, J.R., and Sulkin, S.E. 1958. The isolation and identification of ornithosis infection in turkeys by tissue culture and immunocytochemical staining. Am. J. Vet. Res. 19:950–954.

Friis, R.R. 1972. Interaction of L cells and *Chlamydia psittaci:* Entry of the parasite and host responses to its development. J. Bacteriol. 110:706.

Page, L.A. 1968. Proposal for the recognition of two species in the genus *Chlamydia* Jones, Rake and Stearns, 1945. Int. J. Syst. Bacteriol. 18:51–66.

Smadel, J.E., Wall, M.J., and Gregg, A. 1943. An outbreak of psittacosis in pigeons, involving the production of inclusion bodies, and transfer of the disease to man. J. Exp. Med. 78:189–203.

Psittacosis and Ornithosis

Psittacosis is a disease that occurs in birds belonging to the parrot family (Psittacidae). Ornithosis is the same disease but occurs in a variety of nonpsittacine birds. Formerly it was thought that in humans ornithosis was much milder than psittacosis, but this is not always true (Meyer and Eddie 1953). The disease contracted from pigeons generally is milder than that contracted from parrots or parakeets, but that contracted from turkeys is as severe as any of psittacine origin. The agent causing these diseases

Table 33.1. Chlamydial diseases caused by *C. psittaci*

Disease manifestation	Geographic distribution	Natural hosts	Recommended experimental hosts	Epidemiological aspects
Psittacosis (humans)	Worldwide	Humans, wild and domestic fowl	Embryonated hens' eggs, mice, guinea pigs, wild and domestic birds	Principally transmitted from birds to humans, but human-to-human transmission occurs as aerosol infection. Also associated with cases of lymphogranuloma venereum and abortions in humans.
Psittacosis, ornithosis (birds)	Worldwide	Wild and domestic fowl	Same	Endemic in psittacine and columbidine birds and probably in water fowl. Carriers exist in all fowl.
Placentopathy Enzootic ovine abortion	Scotland, England, Hungary, Germany, France, United States	Sheep	Embryonated hens' eggs, guinea pigs, sheep, cattle, pigeons, and sparrows	Endemic in sheep. Ticks and/or insects may play a role in transmission. Perhaps pigeons, sparrows, and other domestic animals as well.
Bovine abortion and infertility	Worldwide	Cattle	Embryonated hens' eggs, guinea pigs, sheep, and cattle	Periodically endemic in California and Oregon (USA) cattle. Ticks and/or insects may play a role in transmission as well as sheep and other domestic animals.
Abortions in other domestic animals	United States, Spain	Pigs, goats, horses, rabbits, mice	Embryonated hens' eggs, guinea pigs, and respective natural hosts for each *C. psittaci* isolate	Placentopathy not widely observed in these species. Interspecies disease relationships not well known.

	Geographic distribution	Natural host	Experimental host	Remarks
Sporadic bovine encephalomyelitis	Australia, Canada, Germany, South Africa, United States	Cattle, dogs, buffalo	Embryonated hens' eggs, guinea pigs, hamsters, cattle, and dogs	Endemic in cattle in USA. Little known about the infection in dogs.
Pneumonitis				
Feline	Worldwide	Cats, humans?	Embryonated hens' eggs, mice, cats, hamsters, and guinea pigs	Endemic in the domestic cat. Transmitted by aerosol and infective excretions from cat to cat.
Ovine	Probably worldwide	Sheep	Embryonated hens' eggs, mice, guinea pigs, sheep	Probably endemic in sheep-raising areas of USA. Sheep-to-sheep transmission.
Bovine	Czechoslovakia, Italy Japan, United States	Cattle	Embryonated hens' eggs, mice, guinea pigs, and cattle	Endemic. Cattle-to-cattle transmission.
Caprine	Probably worldwide	Goats	Goats, embryonated hens' eggs, guinea pigs	Endemic.
Canine	United States	Dogs, budgerigars, humans?	Dogs, budgerigars, embryonated hens' eggs, guinea pigs	Only one natural case in dog reported.
Equine	Australia, West Germany, Finland	Horse	Embryonated hens' eggs, horse	Endemic in horses.
Murine	United States	Mice	Mice, embryonated hens' eggs, guinea pigs	Endemic in certain mouse colonies.

Table 33.1.—*continued*

Disease manifestation	Geographic distribution	Natural hosts	Recommended experimental hosts	Epidemiological aspects
Conjunctivitis Guinea pig	Worldwide	Guinea pigs	Guinea pigs, embryonated hens' eggs	Endemic as a conjunctivitis in some colonies. May be transmitted transovarially.
Hamster	Worldwide	Hamsters	Hamsters, embryonated hens' eggs, guinea pigs	Endemic as conjunctivitis in some hamster colonies.
Ovine	Worldwide	Sheep	Cell culture	Endemic in some flocks.
Polyarthritis Ovine	United States (principally intermountain area)	Sheep	Sheep, turkeys, guinea pigs, embryonated hens' eggs	Endemic in lambs in intermountain area of USA. Transmission from sheep to sheep; intestinal carriers may cause polyarthritic disease.
Bovine	United States	Cattle	Cattle, guinea pigs, embryonated hens' eggs	Calf-to-calf transmission.
Equine	United States, Spain	Horses	Embryonated hens' eggs, horses	Little known.
Enteritis Snowshoe hare and muskrat	Canada, Wisconsin (USA)	Snowshoe hares and muskrats	Snowshoe hares, muskrats, embryonated hens' eggs	Muskrat may be principal reservoir in nature.
Bovine	Worldwide	Cattle	Cattle, guinea pigs, embryonated hens' eggs, mice.	Endemic cattle. Many intestinal carriers.

generates a toxin that apparently is largely responsible for the virulence of the strain.

Psittacosis in the United States occurs principally in green Amazon parrots and in shell parakeets. In the tropics it occurs widely in many kinds of parrots and parakeets. Ornithosis was first reported in the domestic pigeon (Pinkerton and Swank 1940). Subsequently it has been found in this species in many U.S. cities, such as New York City, (Smadel et al. 1943) Baltimore (Davis and Ewing 1947), and Chicago (Zichis et al. 1946). Meyer and Eddie (1932–1933) reported a human case of ornithosis contracted from a flock of chickens, and Wolins (1948) reported a number of cases contracted from domestic ducks. Haagen and Mauer (1938) identified the agent in a sea bird, the fulmar petrel, which is eaten by the inhabitants of the Faroe Islands. The domestic turkey is also a possible reservoir of ornithosis.

The disease has attracted wide attention from time to time because of human epidemics. During one outbreak in Paris in 1893, Nocard isolated a bacterium belonging to the *Salmonella* groups which he regarded as the causative agent. It was commonly accepted as such until the pandemic in Europe and the United States in the winter of 1929–1930, during which it was shown that Nocard's organism was not commonly present but that a psittacoid agent could regularly be isolated. The *Salmonella psittacosis* described by Nocard is now known to have been *S. typhimurium,* a chance contaminant.

The outbreak in humans which occurred in 1929–1930 was traced to green Amazon parrots imported from South America. In 1930 rigid restrictions on the importation of these birds into the United States were instituted to prevent a recurrence of the incident. In a 1932 survey Meyer et al. (1935) discovered that the disease was well established in southern California in shell parakeets (lovebirds). They found that more than 1,100 aviaries, containing more than 100,000 birds, engaged in breeding as a "backyard industry" in that region and that nearly half of these premises were infected. In 1933 the interstate quarantine regulations were amended to control interstate shipment of psittacine birds in order to prevent infected birds from being shipped out of the region where the disease was enzootic. Through the efforts of health authorities, the incidence of the disease has been greatly reduced in the enzootic region. In addition, approximately 98 percent of psittacine birds are introduced into the United States from Public Health Service–approved treatment centers. This program has markedly reduced the transmission of bird and human psittacosis from imported psittacine birds.

From 1929 through 1942, 380 human cases of psittacosis (including ornithosis) were reported to the U.S. Public Health Service (Dunnahoo and Hampton 1945). Of

these, 170 occurred during the epidemic of 1929–1930 and 210 occurred later; 80 deaths were recorded, of which 33 occurred during the epidemic. The number of cases of psittacosis in humans dropped off sharply when the government established restrictions on the trade in psittacine birds. These restrictions were lifted in 1953, and the incidence of human infections has again risen as a result of an increased incidence of psittacosis in pet birds (Fitz et al. 1955, Sigel et al. 1953). From 1963 to 1973 the average number of cases of human psittacosis was 46 per year. During 1974, 163 cases were reported, the majority of which occurred in employees of turkey-processing plants (Durfee 1975).

From the public health viewpoint the most serious reservoir of infection in the United States is the domestic turkey. Irons et al. called attention to this in 1951 when they reported 22 human cases, with 3 deaths, among 78 employees in a small turkey-dressing plant in Texas. Others have since reported outbreaks in Texas, Nebraska, Oregon, California, Michigan, Wisconsin, Minnesota, Ohio, and New Jersey. The disease is widespread in turkeys in the United States and undoubtedly exists in many other areas where it has not yet been recognized. Turkey ornithosis has been identified in Canada but, according to the published literature, not in any other part of the world.

Two outbreaks of psittacosis occurred in individuals associated with duck-processing plants in England (Palmer et al. 1981).

Morphology and Staining Reactions. The disease can be produced by filtrates made from organs of diseased birds (Bedson et al. 1930). *C. psittaci* is filterable only through rather coarse filters. Membrane studies indicate that its particulate size is between 0.2 and 0.3 μm, which is large enough for the elementary bodies to be visible under the light microscope. The coccoid bodies found in the lesions of parrots, mice, and humans are about this size. A general relationship exists between the concentration of these bodies and virulence, and it is known that they are the infectious agents. These bodies were identified and described at about the same time by Levinthal (1930) in Germany, by Coles (1930) in England, and by Lillie (1930) in the United States, and therefore became known as *LCL bodies.*

The fluorescent antibody technique has been used to prove that the LCL bodies contain RNA and DNA. The LCL bodies are Gram-negative, nonmotile organisms that multiply within the cytoplasm by a developmental cycle unique among bacteria (see discussion at beginning of chapter). Microscopic examination of wet-cell preparations by phase microscopy or of stained preparations by regular light microscopy shows clusters of organisms of various sizes in the cytoplasm of many host cells. The small infectious form, which is 0.3 μm in diameter, appears purple with Giemsa stain, red with Macchiavello and Gimenez stains, and blue with Castaneda stain. The large noninfectious form, 1 μm in diameter, is blue with Giemsa and Macchiavello stains and purple with Castaneda stain. Phase-contrast microscopy avoids time-consuming staining procedures, and it also eliminates staining artifacts. By either method it is difficult to distinguish intracellular mycoplasmas from chlamydias, so procedures other than smear preparations should be included to make a positive diagnosis.

Ultrastructural analyses of infected cell cultures and cells of the intestinal mucosa of newborn calves have revealed four distinct morphologic forms of chlamydial development: elementary bodies, dispersing forms, reticulate bodies, and condensing forms that proceed to form elementary bodies (Todd and Storz 1975, Todd et al. 1976).

Culture. The elementary bodies can be propagated rather easily in a number of ways. Yanamura and Meyer (1941) reported successful culture of the agent in tissue fragments suspended in various fluids, in tissue fragments spread over the surface of serum agar slants, and in the yolk sac of developing chick embryos when the agent was introduced by a technique developed by Cox (1938) for the propagation of rickettsias. The elementary body will also develop on the chorioallantoic membrane and in the allantoic cavity of the chick embryo. Because infected cells rupture and discharge their content of elementary bodies, it is possible to obtain suspensions comparatively free from extraneous yolk sac materials. These suspensions can be used for agglutination and complement-fixation tests. Various strains produce a cytopathic effect in mammalian cell cultures (Pinkerton and Swank 1940). (For more information about cell culture, see "Diagnosis.")

Resistance of the Organism. The cell walls of chlamydiae contain a considerable amount of lipid, which makes them susceptible to lipid solvents and detergents. Consequently, a 1:1,000 dilution of quaternary compound (alkyldimethylbenzylammonium chloride) is an effective disinfectant for laboratory and hospital use. Phenol, in contrast, is a poor disinfectant. The organisms resist acid and alkali. They are rapidly destroyed by heat, but the time it takes to die is related to the amount of protective cellular material present.

Epizootiology and Pathogenesis. In both birds and mammals psittacosis and ornithosis apparently are transmitted largely by means of infected droplets. Davis et al. (1957) were unable to find any evidence that the organism was ever transmitted vertically through the eggs of birds. A considerable number of infections in laboratory personnel have occurred. In many cases these individuals actually handled the infected birds, but a considerable number

became infected without any direct contact, and air-borne infection seems to have been the only possible route (Badger 1930, McCoy 1930). An investigation of a turkey-dressing establishment revealed that most of the infections occurred in people who worked in areas where an aerosol was created by the machinery (Irons et al. 1951). Rivers and Schwentker (1934) found that monkeys could easily be infected by inhalation, but fully virulent material failed to infect when injected subcutaneously or intramuscularly. A number of volunteers among laboratory workers were immunized by parenteral injection of the fully virulent psittacosis agent without adverse results.

The ornithosis agent has been isolated from several species of poultry ectoparasites, suggesting that this may also be a vector-borne infection.

The virulence of psittacosis and ornithosis agents varies greatly. In many outbreaks among animals the disease was recognized only after human attendants became ill from it, and in others, only by the recognition of antibodies. Some outbreaks, however, have exhibited high mortalities among both birds and human contacts. In birds the disease generally is manifested by inappetence, great depression, nasal and eye discharges, and severe diarrhea. Recovered birds usually continue to eliminate the agent in their discharges for a long time.

Mortality varies widely according to species, age, and virulence of the agent. In young psittacine birds it can be as high as 75 to 90 percent. In young pigeons it can be nearly as high. In turkeys it generally is much lower, but can be as high as 25 percent. The attack rate in most species is significant. In humans, before the advent of antibiotics, mortality varied between 10 percent and 30 percent, averaging about 20 percent. These cases were of parrot origin. Current mortality is much lower because the disease can be effectively treated with antibiotics if diagnosed early.

The disease in psittacine birds. Generally speaking, older birds with psittacosis show few or no signs of illness. It is the younger birds that are most likely to develop acute and fatal infections, and they are the principal spreaders of the disease. The incubation period in parrots varies widely from a few days to several weeks. In young birds the course of illness is short—3 to 7 days. In older birds it is usually chronic. Affected birds refuse feed, are soiled with yellowish green diarrheal feces, and have mucopurulent nasal discharges; often their eyes are pasted shut with exudate. Usually they become greatly dehydrated and emaciated before death. Those that recover almost always continue to eliminate the organism in their discharges for long periods. It is these birds that keep the disease alive by infecting the younger birds of the flock. Parrots and parakeets that are convalescent carriers remain completely well or can at times suffer from transient diarrhea. The carrier state is often discovered only when the pet owners develop psittacosis.

The lesions vary in different species of birds, but the general pattern is the same. In psittacine birds splenomegaly is generally seen. The liver is enlarged and frequently has necrotic foci. Sometimes it is covered with a layer of fibrin. The air sacs are inflamed, and the lesion varies from mild clouding to the presence of caseous masses of exudate. Fibrinous pericarditis is common. All birds with acute cases show a severe enteritis characterized by bloody diarrhea.

The disease in nonpsittacine birds. Affected adult pigeons can be listless, have no appetite, show nasal and eye discharges, and suffer from diarrhea. According to Coles (1930), who was the first to describe ornithosis in pigeons, this disease should be suspected in any bird with conjunctivitis. The incubation period is 5 to 9 days.

Diseased squabs are weak and show signs similar to those of adults; most die. Many of the adult pigeons recover, become convalescent carriers, and serve as sources of infection to fanciers and to those who feed and fondle these birds in city parks and squares. The incidence in pigeons may be very high. The lesions are similar to those described for psittacine birds, except splenomegaly usually does not occur in nonpsittacine birds.

In many of the outbreaks in turkeys the virulence of the infection is low (Bankowski and Page 1959), the losses are not serious, and the disease is likely to be undiagnosed. Graber and Pomeroy (1958) showed that strains from such outbreaks can cause human infections. On the other hand, the disease can be serious, with mortalities in well-developed turkeys running as high as 25 percent. The signs of the disease often resemble those of fowl cholera or erysipelas. The birds become apathetic, eat poorly, show depression, and develop diarrhea. The diarrheic feces are fluid, often contain blood, and generally cause matting of the feathers around the vent. Many birds become greatly emaciated.

Outbreaks in ducks in the United States have generally been inapparent; the disease has been recognized either because of human contact cases or by serologic or cultural procedures.

A few cases of ornithosis in chickens have been reported, but the disease has been inapparent.

The disease in goose flocks has been economically significant in Hungary (Szemeredy and Sztojkov 1973). In 1972 it caused 15 to 55 percent mortality among goslings between 12 and 45 days old in several flocks.

Ornithosis has also been present in an inapparent form in geese, gray herons, and pheasants and has been identified in the petrels of the Faroe Islands. Page (1976) investigated the involvement of wildlife in an epornosis of domestic turkeys and found antibodies in blackbirds, sparrows, and one of four mourning doves, but no *C. psittaci* organisms were isolated.

The disease in laboratory animals. Parrots that have not previously suffered from the disease are readily infected by inoculation parenterally, orally, or by the respiratory route. Java sparrows and reed birds are readily infected by contact and by inoculation. Adult chickens are not readily infected, but young birds can easily be infected by inoculation. White mice are highly susceptible and are commonly used for diagnostic purposes. Intraperitoneal injection with agents from psittacine birds causes infection, but injection with agents from nonpsittacine birds frequently fails. Ornithosis agents are best inoculated intracerebrally. Guinea pigs, rabbits, and monkeys can be infected by inoculation, but the disease in these species often is not fatal.

Immunity. After recovery from the active disease, birds usually harbor the chlamydias for long periods. During this time they possess a marked resistance to reinfection, as might be expected. The organism tends to remain in mammals also for considerable periods after clinical recovery, and it has been suggested that immunity to this disease is always due to the harboring of latent infection, but this has not been substantiated.

Neutralizing antibodies are not always demonstrable in animals immune to chlamydias and are seldom present in great concentration. Nevertheless, animals that have received chlamydias intramuscularly without production of disease are protected against intratracheal inoculations that produce pneumonia in nonimmunized animals.

Mice and pigeons can be partially immunized by several injections of inactivated chlamydias (Bedson 1938, Hughes 1947), but the protection is not great enough to be useful. Direct complement-fixing antibody titers can be obtained in turkeys that have been vaccinated intratracheally, intramuscularly, or subcutaneously with live ornithosis agents of low virulence prepared from yolk sac and mouse tissue suspensions. The presence of these titers in the vaccinated turkeys, however, cannot be equated to resistance to infection by a highly virulent ornithosis isolate (Bates et al. 1965). Adding concentrated suspensions of *Bordetella pertussis* to a bacterin of *C. psittaci* has afforded significant protection to turkeys (Page 1975). Because *B. pertussis* organisms selectively stimulate T lymphocytes, cell-mediated immunity probably has an important part in the immunity to *C. psittaci.*

Diagnosis. The clinical picture may suggest psittacosis or ornithosis, but seldom can a positive diagnosis be made without confirmation by laboratory tests.

Animal inoculations. Experienced workers have been successful in isolating the agent by inoculating chick embryos in the chorioallantoic cavity or the yolk sac (Hudson et al. 1955), but the most effective way of recovering the agent is by mouse inoculation (Rivers and Berry 1935). Intraperitoneal injection of filtrates of sputum or unfiltered sputum from an infected human usually kills the mice in 5 to 14 days, and occasionally as late as 30 days—unless other organisms present in the sputum kill the animals prematurely. If any of the mice sicken after the fourth or fifth day, they should be destroyed and examined for the characteristic focal necrosis of the liver. Impression smears are made from the liver tissue, and a search is done for the elementary bodies of psittacosis. If the mice are still living after 30 days, they should be injected with the known psittacosis agent to determine whether they may have developed immunity from an infection that did not become apparent. A 20 to 40 percent suspension of suspect tissues can be used for transfer to experimental animals.

This method is efficient for detection of the disease in humans or in birds of the parrot family, but the pigeon agent usually does not kill mice or produce the liver lesions. One can usually recover the organism from these birds, however, by inoculating the mice intracerebrally instead of intraperitoneally. The pigeon agent is more highly virulent for pigeons than the parrot agent, which usually produces only inapparent infections in pigeons (Meyer and Eddie 1932–1933).

The diagnostician and research worker should be aware that mouse and guinea pig colonies may be naturally infected with chlamydias. The murine pneumonitis strain of *C. trachomatis* has been isolated from the lungs of mice from many colonies. The organisms are demonstrated by repeated passage of homogenized lung suspensions from carrier mice into normal mice by aerosol exposure. Infected mice eventually develop a diffuse pneumonitis, and the organisms are readily demonstrated in lung smear

preparations. Guinea pigs may be naturally infected with *C. psittaci*, which manifests itself as a conjunctivitis and is readily transmitted by contact.

All strains of *Chlamydia* can be isolated and propagated in the yolk sacs of embryonated hens' eggs. Depending on the source of inoculum, proper treatment must be performed to rid the inoculum of bacteria or mycoplasmas, which usually grow well in the egg. If bacterial contaminants are suspected, the test material should be ground in a phosphate-buffered saline solution (pH 7.2) containing 1 mg/ml each of streptomycin sulfate, vancomycin, and kanamycin. This markedly reduces bacterial contamination without affecting the chlamydia population.

Normally, the inoculum is a 10 percent suspension that is injected into the yolk sacs of 5- to 7-day-old embryonated hens' eggs; the embryos usually die 5 to 12 days later. The capillaries of infected eggs are not sharply outlined when candled. Infected embryos and yolk sac membranes are congested and frequently hemorrhagic. Stained smears of yolk sac membranes show the presence of chlamydiae (Figure 33.1). An antigen prepared from an infected yolk sac fixes complement in the presence of a positive chlamydial antiserum in the complement-fixation test. This result constitutes a positive diagnosis. If no embryos die in the first passage, three blind passages of yolk sac material harvested 10 to 14 days after inoculation with no specific embryo deaths are required to conclude that the avian tissue homogenate did not contain *C. psittaci*.

Cell cultures. Most strains of *C. psittaci* propagate in cultured cells and produce sufficient cell destruction to show plaque formation (Piraino 1969). Intracellular microcolonies (plaques) can be seen 2 to 7 days after inoculation. The presence of chlamydias can be demonstrated

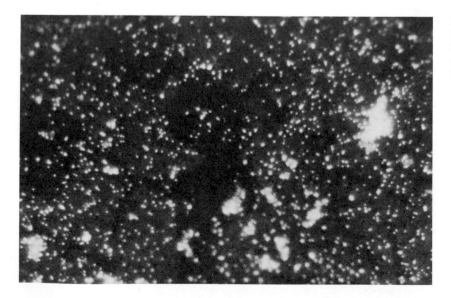

Figure 33.1. Chlamydial elementary bodies of ovine abortion strain B-577 propagated in the yolk sac of an embryonated hen's egg. Smear reacted with fluorescent antibodies. × 3,000. (Courtesy J. Storz.)

in two ways: (1) by the direct fluorescent antibody test, and (2) by use of the tissue-cultured preparation as an antigen in the complement-fixation test. The fluorescent antibody test is reputedly more sensitive for their identification in cell cultures, but not in smear preparations from yolk sac and other animal tissues.

Chlamydial agents multiply in cell cultures derived from various tissues of different hosts. A few such cell cultures are human embryonic skin, muscle, or lung (Page 1968), chick embryo (Rivers and Schwentker 1934), and most cells of the McCoy line (Tanami et al. 1961). When a cytopathic effect occurs, it is mediated by the release of lysosomal enzymes into the host cytoplasm during the late stages of chlamydial development (Szemeredy and Sztojkov 1973).

Serologic tests. All members of *Chlamydia* contain a group-specific antigen that is a lipopolysaccharide. The antigen is resistant to phenol, heat, and various proteinases but inactivated by lecithinase and periodate. Antigens may be prepared in a variety of ways (Lennette and Schmidt 1970) to test for the group-specific antigen. Some of the techniques used are the following: the direct complement-fixation test, which is used principally for detection of complement-fixing antibodies in avian serums (normal rooster serum must be added as a test component to make the test workable); the indirect complement-fixation test; the capillary-tube agglutination test; gel diffusion techniques; and the hemagglutination test (Barron et al. 1965). These test procedures are described in the textbook by Lennette and Schmidt (1970).

The cell walls of chlamydias contain a mosaic of antigens that are distinct from the group-specific antigen. The cell wall antigens are often shared within a group of strains affecting a certain class of animals (human, mammal, and avian strains), and some antigens cross animal classes. Consequently, no precise serologic classification of chlamydial strains is possible at present.

The complement-fixation test can be used to confirm the presence of the disease in flocks, but it has been shown that carrier birds of all species do not always react to this test and recent infections may not be detected. Complement-fixing antibodies usually appear in birds and mammals within 7 to 10 days after infection. Some animals with intestinal infection may have no detectable complement-fixing antibodies. The level of a titer reflects the antigenic properties and recentness of infection, but it may not reflect current infection. The serologic diagnosis of infection thus requires demonstration of a fourfold rise in complement-fixing antibody titer using paired serums. If 80 percent or more of the individuals in a group have a demonstrable titer and half have titers of 1 : 64 or greater, this constitutes reasonable proof that the group of animals is currently infected with chlamydias. The agar-gel diffusion test has been used as an adjunct to the complement-fixation test because antibodies can be detected in serums of pigeons which are negative by the latter test, thus demonstrating differing kinetics of precipitating and complement-fixing antibody formation (Ismael et al. 1975). The modified direct complement-fixation test appears to be more sensitive than the direct complement-fixation and agar-gel diffusion tests (Grimes and Page 1978).

The direct and indirect enzyme-linked immunosorbent assays (ELISAs) are sensitive methods for detection of antibody in birds. The indirect method has the added advantage of detecting IgM antibody, which indicates birds that are latent carriers (Smeer et al. 1983).

Serum neutralization, plaque reduction, and toxin neutralization. In the serum-neutralization test the chick embryo is protected from death by the neutralization of the infective particle with the specific antiserum prior to inoculation. In the toxin-neutralization test the early death of mice inoculated intravenously with large numbers of organisms is prevented by the injection of specific antitoxin. The mechanism of the plaque-reduction test is similar to the serum-neutralization test in the hen's egg, except cell cultures are used as the indicator system for detecting chlamydial activity. In these three tests high-titered antiserums must be used. The use of all three tests for comparative studies of chlamydias can reveal variations in cell wall antigens responsible for infectivity and provide a means to establish serotypes among some strains of *C. psittaci.*

Antimicrobial Susceptibility. Unlike viruses, the psittacosis lymphogranuloma group shows definite susceptibility to some of the sulfonamides and antibiotics. In a study by Heilman and Herrell (1944), large doses of penicillin saved the majority of mice inoculated with the psittacosis agent; most of them developed inapparent infections, which made them resistant to later injections of the same strain. Several researchers have demonstrated that the same thing is true of the disease in humans. Meiklejohn et al. (1946) showed that penicillin inhibits growth of this agent in tissues but is ineffective in eggs. Early and Morgan (1946) found that sulfadiazine in food protects mice from death when the mice are inoculated with the psittacosis agent, but most of the animals become carriers. Streptomycin, however, is not effective. Sulfadiazine also protects chick embryos from some strains but is ineffective against others.

Many of the antibiotics exert an influence on agents of the ornithosis group, but it appears that most are incapable of completely eliminating the chlamydiae from victims of the disease. The most successful drugs are tetracycline compounds (Cox 1955): chloramphenicol, rifampicin, nalidixic acid, and 5-fluorouracil. These agents must be given in rather high concentrations in the feed to accomplish sterilization. Lower doses reduce mortality, but leave many carriers. Davis and Delaplane (1958) found that a concentration of chlortetracycline of 200 g/metric ton in an all-mash ration is required to eliminate the ornithosis agent from 3-week-old poults. Experimentally infected adult turkeys, treated for 2 to 3 weeks with 200–400 g/metric ton of mash, failed to yield organisms.

In view of the initially low rate of psittacosis infection in most wild or uncrowded captive psittacines, group treatment with 0.5 percent chlortetracycline in dry pelleted feed for 45 days is practical, effective, and economically feasible, and might be considered an adequate safeguard against psittacosis (Arnstein et al. 1968). Haass (1973), in southwest Germany, however, reported that the widely recommended antibiotic feeding of imported psittacine birds is an inadequate control method since there is an increasing number of positive isolations of *C. psittaci* from cage birds.

Chlortetracycline can be very successful in treating human infections, providing the diagnosis is made early and the treatment is carried on for a considerable time at a high dosage. Too small a dosage and too short a treatment time result in relapses.

The Disease in Humans. The disease in humans is characterized by fever, headache, and pneumonia. The pneumonia is an atypical, patchy, bronchopneumonia that cannot be clinically differentiated from virus-induced pneumonia. *C. psittaci* has been demonstrated in left atrial or valve biopsy specimens from 7 of 27 patients with acquired valvular heart disease, suggesting that the organism may be the cause of some cases of valvular heart disease (Ward and Ward 1974).

The disease is seldom conveyed from person to person, although it can be if precautions against droplet infection are not taken. Ordinarily the disease in humans is derived from the considerable reservoir that exists in birds, in which it often occurs as a latent disease. In recent years the majority of diagnosed human cases in the United States occurred in individuals associated with infected turkeys.

REFERENCES

Arnstein, P., Eddie, B., and Meyer, K.F. 1968. Control of psittacosis by group chemotherapy of infected parrots. Am. J. Vet. Res. 29:2213–2227.

Badger, L.F. 1930. Psittacosis outbreak in a department store. Public Health Rep. 45:1403–1409.

Bankowski, R.A., and Page, L.A. 1959. Studies of two epornitics of ornithosis caused by agents of low virulence. Am. J. Vet. Res. 20:935–940.

Barron, A.L., Jakay-Roness, Z., and Bernkopf, H. 1965. Hemagglutination of chicken erythrocytes by the agent of psittacosis. Proc. Soc. Exp. Biol. Med. 119:377–381.

Bates, H.A., Pomeroy, B.S., and Reynolds, D.P. 1965. Ornithosis: Experimental immunofluorescent studies. Avian Dis. 9:220–226.

Bedson, S.P. 1938. A study of experimental immunity to the virus of psittacosis in the mouse with special reference to persistence of infection. Br. J. Exp. Pathol. 19:353–366.

Bedson, S.P., Western, G.T., and Levy Simpson, S. 1930. Observations on etiology of psittacosis. Lancet 1:235–236.

Coles, A.C. 1930. Micro-organisms in psittacosis. Lancet 1:1011–1012.

Cox, H.R. 1938. Studies of a filter-passing infectious agent isolated from ticks. V. Further attempts to cultivate in cell-free media. Suggested classification. Public Health Rep. 53:2241–2247.

Cox, H.R. 1955. Chemotherapy of psittacosis. In R. Beaudette. Psittacosis: Diagnosis, Epidemiology, and Control. Rutgers University Press, New Brunswick, N.J. Pp. 137.

Davis, D.E., and Delaplane, J.P. 1958. The effect of chlortetracycline treatment of turkeys affected with ornithosis. Am. J. Vet. Res. 19:169–173.

Davis, D.J., and Ewing, C.L. 1947. Recovery of ornithosis virus from pigeons in Baltimore, Maryland. Public Health Rep. 62:1484–1488.

Davis, D.E., Delaplane, J.P., and Watkins, J.R. 1957. The role of turkey eggs in the transmission of ornithosis. Am. J. Vet. Res. 18:409–413.

Dunnahoo, G.L., and Hampton, B.C. 1945. Psittacosis. Occurrence in the United States and report of 97 percent mortality in a shipment of psittacine birds while under quarantine. Public Health Rep. 60:354–357.

Durfee, P.T. 1975. Psittacosis in humans in the United States, 1974. J. Infect. Dis. 132:604–605.

Early, R.L., and Morgan, H.R. 1946. Studies on the chemotherapy of viruses in the psittacosis-lymphogranuloma venereum group. III. Effect of certain chemotherapeutic agents on the growth of psittacosis virus (6 BC strain) in tissues cultures and eggs. IV. Effect of certain chemotherapeutic agents on psittacosis virus (6 BC strain) infections in mice. J. Immunol. 53:151–156, 251–257.

Fitz, R.H., Meiklejohn, G., and Baum, M.D. 1955. Psittacosis in Colorado. Am. J. Med. Sci. 229:252–261.

Graber, R.E., and Pomeroy, B.S. 1958. Ornithosis (psittacosis): An epidemiological study of a Wisconsin human outbreak transmitted from turkeys. Am. J. Public Health 48:1469–1483.

Grimes, J.E., and Page, L.A. 1978. Comparison of direct and modified direct complement-fixation and agar-gel diffusion methods in detecting chlamydial antibody in wild birds. Avian Dis. 22:422–430.

Haagen, E., and Mauer, G. 1938. Die Psittakose in Deutschland. Zentralbl. Bakteriol. [Orig. A] 143:81–82.

Haass, K. 1973. Critical survey of the psittacosis situation in south western Germany. Tierärztl. Umsch. 28:625–628.

Heilman, F.R., and Herrell, W.E. 1944. Penicillin in the treatment of experimental ornithosis. Proc. Mayo Clin. 19:204–212.

Hudson, C.B., Bivins, J.A., Beaudette, F.R., and Tudor, D.C. 1955. Use of the chicken embryo technique for diagnosis of psittacosis in avian hosts, with epidemiological notes. J. Am. Vet. Med. Assoc. 126:111–117.

Hughes, D.L. 1947. Ornithosis (psittacosis) in a pigeon flock. J. Comp. Pathol. Ther. 57:67–76.

Irons, J.V., Sullivan, T.D., and Rowen, J. 1951. Outbreak of psittacosis (ornithosis) from working with turkeys or chickens. Am. J. Public Health. 41:931–937.

Ismael, A.S., Krauss, H., and Geissler, H. 1975. Detection of group-specific precipitating chlamydial antibodies in chlamydia infection in poultry. Berl. Münch. Tierärztl. Wochenschr. 88:21–24.

Lennette, D.A., and Schmidt, N.J. 1970. Diagnostic Procedures for Viral and Rickettsial Diseases, 4th ed. American Public Health Association, New York.

Levinthal. 1930. Klin. Wochenschr. 9:654.

Lillie, R.D. 1930. Psittacosis: Rickettsia-like inclusions in man and in experimental animals. Public Health Rep. 45:773–778.

McCoy, G.W. 1930. Accidental psittacosis infection among the personnel of the hygienic laboratory. Public Health Rep. 45:843–845.

Meiklejohn, G., Wagner, J.C., and Beveridge, G.W. 1946. Studies on the chemotherapy of viruses in the psittacosis-lymphogranuloma group. I. Effect of penicillin and sulfadiazine on ten strains in chick embryos. J. Immunol. 54:1–8.

Meyer, K.F., and Eddie, B. 1932–1933. Latent psittacosis infections in shell parrakeets. Proc. Soc. Exp. Biol. Med. 30:484–488.

Meyer, K.F., and Eddie, B. 1953. Characteristics of a psittacosis viral agent isolated from a turkey. Proc. Soc. Exp. Biol. Med. 83:99–101.

Meyer, K.F., Eddie, B., and Stevens, I.M. 1935. Recent studies on psittacosis. Am. J. Public Health 25:571–579.

Page, L.A. 1968. Proposal for the recognition of two species in the genus Chlamydia Jones, Rake and Stearns, 1945. Int. J. Syst. Bacteriol. 18:51–66.

Page, L.A. 1975. Studies on immunity to chlamydiosis in birds, with particular reference to turkeys. Am. J. Vet. Res. 36:597–600.

Page, L.A. 1976. Observations on the involvement of wildlife in an epornitic of chlamydiosis in domestic turkeys. J. Am. Vet. Med. Assoc. 169:932–935.

Palmer, S.R., Andrews, B.E., and Major, R. 1981. A common-source outbreak of ornithosis in veterinary surgeons. Lancet 2:798–799.

Pienaar, J.G., and Schutte, A.P. 1975. Occurrence and pathology of chlamydiosis in domestic and laboratory animals: A review. Onderstepoort J. Vet. Res. 42:77–89.

Pinkerton, H., and Swank, R.L. 1940. Recovery of virus morphologically identical with psittacosis from thiamin-deficient pigeons. Proc. Soc. Exp. Biol. Med. 45:704–706.

Piraino, F. 1969. Plaque formation in chick embryo fibroblast cells by chlamydia isolated from avian and mammalian sources. J. Bacteriol. 98:475–480.

Rivers, T.M., and Berry, G.P. 1935. A laboratory method for the diagnosis of psittacosis in man. J. Exp. Med. 61:205–207.

Rivers, T.M., and Schwentker, F.F. 1934. Louping ill in man. J. Exp. Med. 60:211–225.

Sigel, M.M., Cole, L.S., and Hunter, O. 1953. Mounting incidence of psittacosis. Am. J. Public Health 43:1418–1422.

Smadel, J.E. 1943. Atypical pneumonia and psittacosis. J. Clin. Invest. 22:57–65.

Smadel, J.E., Wall, M.J., and Gregg, A. 1943. An outbreak of psittacosis in pigeons, involving the production of inclusion bodies, and transfer of the disease to man. J. Exp. Med. 78:189–203.

Smeer, N., Busche, R., Krauss, H., and Weiss, R. 1983. Untersuchungen über den Zusammenhang zwischen Antikörperstatus und Infektionsgeschehen bei Ornithose und Salmonellose von Reisetauben. Berl. Münch. Tierärztl. Wochenschr. 96:234–238.

Stephenson, E.H., and Storz, J. 1975. Antigenic analysis of dense centered forms of chlamydial isolates of animal origin by gel diffusion. Am. J. Vet. Res. 36:881.

Szemeredy, G., and Sztojkov, V. 1973. Disease caused by Bedsonia in goose flocks. Magy. Allatorv. Lapja 28:554–557.

Tanami, Y., Pollard, M., and Starr, T.J. 1961. Replication pattern of psittacosis virus in a tissue culture system. Virology 15:22–29.

Todd, W.J., and Storz, J. 1975. Ultrastructural cytochemical evidence for the activation of lysosomes in the cytocidal effect of Chlamydia psittaci. Infect. Immun. 12:638–646.

Todd, W.J., Doughri, A.M., and Storz, J. 1976. Ultrastructural changes in host cellular organelles in the course of the chlamydial developmental cycle. Zentralbl. Bakteriol. [Orig. A] 236:359–373.

Ward, C., and Ward, A.M. 1974. Acquired valvular heart disease in patients who keep pet birds. Lancet 2:734–736.

Wolins, W. 1948. Ornithosis (psittacosis), a review with a report of eight cases resulting from contact with the domestic Pekin duck. Am. J. Med. Sci. 216:551–564.

Yanamura, H.Y., and Meyer, K.F. 1941. Studies on the virus of psittacosis cultivated in vitro. J. Infect. Dis. 68:1–15.

Zichis, J., Shaughnessy, H.J., and Lemke, C. 1946. Isolation of psittacosis-like viruses from Chicago pigeons. J. Bacteriol. 51:616–617.

Enzootic Ovine Abortion

SYNONYMS: Enzootic abortion of ewes, ovine virus abortion

Enzootic ovine abortion is caused by *C. psittaci*. It affects pregnant ewes, causing them to abort in late pregnancy. The clinical signs of the disease are indistinguishable from those of ovine vibriosis. This form of the disease occurs in Europe and the United States and causes marked economic losses.

Enzootic ovine abortion was recognized as an infectious disease by Stamp et al. (1950) in Scotland. The disease has since been diagnosed in England, Germany, France, and Hungary. A disease that had been observed for several years in Montana, United States, was recognized as being caused by an agent of the psittacosis-lymphogranuloma-trachoma group (Young et al. 1958). When the agent was compared with the agent that causes the European disease, they were found to be identical (Studdert and McKercher 1968b). In some countries enzootic abortion and toxoplasmosis are the most common causes of abortion in sheep.

C. psittaci causes a variety of diseases in sheep. Schachter et al. (1974) used the plaque-reduction test to show that ovine chlamydial isolates can be separated into two types: type 1 isolates are usually associated with ovine abortion and intestinal infection, whereas type 2 isolates cause polyarthritis and conjunctivitis.

The ovine abortion agent is a typical member of the psittacosis-lymphogranuloma-trachoma group, exhibiting a morphology that conforms to the general characteristics of the group.

Culture. The agent grows readily and in high concentration in the yolk sacs of embryonated hens' eggs 5 to 7 days old. The growth of the embryos is retarded, and they succumb before hatching. Chlamydias injected into the chorioallantoic cavity cause some embryos to die.

Various mammalian cell cultures will support the replication of strains of the enzootic ovine abortion agent: diploid cells from the lungs and myocardium of sheep embryos (Pankova et al. 1977), suspensions of hamster embryo cells (Saint-Aubert and Mougeot 1975), and McCoy and HeLa 229 cells (Rodolakis and Chancerelle 1977). The plaque assay method in McCoy cells is highly sensitive and reproducible (Rodolakis and Chancerelle 1977).

When *C. psittaci* (var. *ovis*) is cultured in *Hyalomma* tick embryo cells, the antigen is detected by direct immunofluorescence for 30 to 45 days after inoculation (Shatkin et al. 1977). Not all strains produce a cytopathic effect on monolayer cultures. In some instances it may be necessary to stain the cultures to enhance observation of the cytoplasmic inclusions.

Epizootiology and Pathogenesis. The disease can readily be transmitted to susceptible pregnant ewes by inoculation. Pregnant ewes acquire elementary bodies from aborting ewes and abort themselves a few weeks later (Blewett et al. 1982). The persistence of the agent in feces may explain how the disease carries over from one lambing season to the next. The susceptibility of pigeons and sparrows to the enzootic ovine abortion agent suggests another means of transmission to sheep and a reservoir for it in nature. It has been suggested that ticks or insects or both may play some role in its transmission. Susceptible sheep, placed on pastures on which the disease occurs one season, seldom show any evidence of the disease the following season (Tunnicliff 1958). Venereal transmission by infected rams is probably another means of transmission.

Abortions occur from midgestation to late pregnancy. Retention of the placenta is frequent, and a vaginal discharge is seen for several days following lambing or abortion. The aborted fetuses can be mummified or normal in appearance. The cotyledons are dark red or clay-colored. The ewe is visibly ill and has fever of 2° or 3°F higher than normal, lasting for up to 1 week. The genital organs quickly return to normal, and subsequent fertility is not impaired. Experimentally infected sheep react with a febrile response beginning about 3 days after inoculation. Abortions occur at least 56 days following injection or feeding of the infectious agent.

The mortality in the ewes is virtually nil, although many lambs can be lost. In the ewe, inflammation and necrosis of the placentoma is observed. The affected fetus shows hepatopathy, occasionally edema, ascites, vascular congestion, and tracheal petechiae. Histological changes in the fetus have been described by Djurov (1972).

Associated neonatal complications such as weak lambs showing nervous signs or pneumonia can occur in flocks (Schutte and Pienaar 1977). In flocks where ovine abortion occurs, epididymitis and orchitis in rams is observed. The organism has been isolated from the genital tract of two neonatal lambs after the clinical onset of epididymitis (Rodolakis and Bernard 1977).

Weanling white mice may be killed by intranasal inoculation of infective yolk sac material. Large doses sometimes kill adult mice when they are administered intracerebrally or intravenously. Some of these mice die as a result of intoxication from the toxin within a few hours following inoculation. Others die after a few days of infection.

Febrile reactions can be produced in guinea pigs by intraperitoneal injections, but these animals seldom die of the infection. Animals killed during the febrile reaction show enlarged friable livers containing minute necrotic areas, splenic enlargement, and little else (Parker 1960). Guinea pigs are the laboratory animal of choice for the isolation of ovine chlamydias because these animals are more susceptible than chick embryos or mice.

Strains of the enzootic ovine abortion agent produce abortions in sheep under natural conditions (Storz 1966). A strain of the enzootic bovine abortion agent also has been incriminated in the production of disease and abortions of sheep (Studdert and McKercher 1968a). The goat enzootic abortion agent caused abortion in an experimental ewe and also in two experimental cows (McCauley and Tieken 1968). The enzootic ovine abortion agent causes experimental disease in pigeons and a lethal disease in sparrows under experimental conditions (Page 1966). A sheep strain of *C. psittaci* that was isolated from a naturally occurring case of pneumonia caused abortion in experimental ewes, but the disease differed from a typical ovine abortion agent infection (Studdert and McKercher 1968a).

Parenteral injection of bovine or ovine chlamydial agents into rams produced seminal vesiculitis with a granulomatous response that was limited mostly to interstitial tissues (Eugster et al., 1971). Excretion of chlamydias in the semen continued until the experimental rams were slaughtered 8 to 22 days after inoculation. During the acute febrile stage the organism was isolated from the blood and somatic organs. Complement-fixing antibodies rose sharply 1 week after inoculation, reaching peak titers of 128 to 512. The number of leukocytes in the semen increased during the experiment, and the two rams receiving the calf polyarthritis strain of *C. psittaci* had pus in the the semen. The frequency of secondary morphologic abnormalities of spermatozoa increased by 20 days after injection.

Immunity. A single infection solidly immunizes ewes for their normal life expectancy (McEwan and Foggie 1956, McEwan et al. 1955). The presence of complement-fixing antibody resulting from the presence of chlamydia group antigen in a subclinical or clinical infection ameliorates the clinical response and can prevent abortion in sheep following inoculation with the enzootic bovine abortion agent. The immunity conferred by the antibody is relative because a large challenge dose can cause ewes to abort (Studdert and McKercher 1968b).

The disease can be readily controlled by vaccination of all young ewes with a formalinized vaccine made from the infected yolk sacs of embryonated eggs. Commercial vaccine for this purpose is available. The disease has been successfully controlled in some European flocks by vaccination of the young ewes prior to first bleeding. Sheep infected with toxoplasmosis do not respond well to enzootic abortion vaccine because of immunosuppression (Buxton et al. 1981).

Diagnosis. It is difficult to make a definite clinical diagnosis because chlamydial abortion and vibriosis exhibit essentially the same clinical signs. Flocks in which vibrios cannot be found should be suspected of harboring the psittacoid agent. The diagnosis can be verified by inoculating stomach contents of aborted fetuses or placental tissues into the yolk sac of embryonated eggs or guinea pigs. The complement-fixation test will give evidence of infection with an agent of the group.

Other serologic tests have been recommended to reinforce the diagnosis of ovine abortion. They include the hemagglutination test (Faye et al. 1973), immunofluorescence test (Russo et al. 1977), agar-gel precipitation test (Sadowski and Truszcynski 1977), and a complement-fixation micromethod (Saint-Aubert et al. 1975).

The elementary bodies generally can be identified in Giemsa-stained smears of cotyledons of aborting ewes. After some experience this method can be used as a diagnostic procedure.

Antimicrobial Susceptibility. Like other members of the psittacosis-lymphogranuloma-trachoma group, the enzootic ovine abortion agent is sensitive to penicillin and some of the sulfonamides but is unaffected by streptomycin and para-aminobenzoic acid. It is highly sensitive to chloramphenicol, erythromycin, and the tetracyclines.

Long-acting oxytetracycline (20 mg/kg of body weight given intramuscularly) has been used in the treatment of enzootic abortion of ewes. Greig et al. (1982) found that on a few farms this treatment caused a significant reduction in abortions. On some farms the dose, given 14 to 64 days before parturition, reduced the prevalence of abortions, and another injection at 6 to 8 weeks before parturition and again 3 weeks after parturition reduced abortions further.

The Disease in Humans. There is no evidence that the enzootic ovine abortion agent has produced human disease, but care should be exercised in handling material from animals infected with this agent because of the potential health hazard of the *Chlamydia* species to humans.

REFERENCES

Blewett, D.A., Gisemba, F., Miller, J.K., Johnson, F.W., and Clarkson, M.A. 1982. Ovine enzootic abortion: The acquisition of infection and consequent abortion within a single lambing season. Vet. Rec. 111:499–501.

Buxton, D., Reid, H.W., Finlayson, J., Pow, I., and Anderson, I. 1981. Immunosuppression in toxoplasmosis: Studies in sheep with vaccines for chlamydial abortion and louping-ill virus. Vet. Rec. 109:559–561.

Djurov, A. 1972. Histological changes in the foetus in ovine enzootic abortion. Zentralbl. Veterinärmed. [B] 19:578–587.

Eugster, A.K., Ball, L., Carroll, E.J., and Storz, J. 1971. Experimental genital infection of bulls and rams with chlamydial (psittacosis) agents. In Sixth International Meeting on Diseases of Cattle, Philadelphia, Pa. Pp. 327–332.

Faye, P., Charton, A., Layee, C., Mage, C., and Joisel, F. 1973. Comparison of various serological techniques on the same serum samples, using antigens prepared from the same strain of *Chlamydia ovis* (the agent of ovine abortion). Bull. Acad. Vet. 46:57–60.

Greig, A., Linklater, K.A., and Dyson, D.A. 1981. Long-acting oxytetracycline in the treatment of enzootic abortion of ewes. Vet. Rec. 111:445.

McCauley, E.H., and Tieken, E.L. 1968. Psittacosis-lymphogranuloma venereum agent isolated during an abortion epizootic in goats. J. Am. Vet. Med. Assoc. 152:1758–1765.

McEwan, A.D., and Foggie, A. 1956. Enzootic abortion in ewes. Prolonged immunity following the injection of adjuvant vaccine. Vet. Rec. 68:686–690.

McEwan, A.D., Dow, J.B., and Anderson, R.D. 1955. Enzootic abortion in ewes: An adjuvant vaccine prepared from eggs. Vet. Rec. 67:393–394.

Page, L.A. 1966. Interspecies transfer of psittacosis-LGV-trachoma agent: Pathogenicity of two avian and two mammalian strains for eight species of birds and mammals. Am. J. Vet. Res. 27:397–407.

Pankova, G.E., Zalkind, S., Karavaev, Yu., Semenova, E.N., and D'yakonov, L.P. 1977. Sensitivity of diploid cell lines to *Chlamydia*. Veterinariya 7:39–41.

Parker, A.M. 1960. Contagious bovine pleuropneumonia: Production of complement fixing antigen and some observations on its use. Am. J. Vet. Res. 21:243–245.

Rodolakis, A., and Bernard, K. 1977. Isolation of *Chlamydia ovis* from genital organs of rams with epididymitis. Bull. Acad. Vet. 50:65–69.

Rodolakis, A., and Chancerelle, L. 1977. Plaque assay for *Chlamydia psittaci* in tissue samples. Ann. Microbiol. (Paris) 128B:81–85.

Russo, P., Vitu, C., Lambert, M., and Giauffret, A. 1977. Application of an immunofluorescence technique to the serological diagnosis of chlamydia infection of sheep and goats. Bull. Acad. Vet. 50:415–424.

Sadowski and Truszcynski. 1977. Evaluation of the agar gel precipitation test for the detection of chlamydia antibodies in cattle and sheep sera. Bull. Vet. Inst. Pulawy 21:1–6.

Saint-Aubert, G., and Mougeot, H. 1975. Growth of *Chlamydia psittaci* var. *ovis* in cell cultures, and practical applications. Rev. Med. Vet. 126:1323–1331.

Saint-Aubert, G., Fayet, M.T., and Valette, L. 1975. Micromethod of complement fixation in the diagnosis of ovine chlamydia infections, and its use in practice. Rev. Med. Vet. 126:787–800.

Schachter, J., Banks, J., Sugg, N., Sung, M., Storz, J., and Meyer, K.F. 1974. Serotyping of *Chlamydia*. 1. Isolates of ovine origin. Infect. Immun. 9:92–94.

Schutte, A.P., and Pienaar, J.G. 1977. Chlamydiosis in sheep and cattle in South Africa. J. S. Afr. Vet. Assoc. 48:261–265.

Shatkin, A.A., Beskina, S.R., Medvedeva, G.I., and Grokhovskaya, I.M. 1977. Culture of the agent of ovine enzootic abortion in hyalomma tick embryo cells. Med. Parazitol. (Mosk.) 4:420–423.

Stamp, J.T., McEwan, A.D., Watt, J.A.A., and Nisbet, D.I. 1950. Enzootic abortion in ewes. I. Transmission of the disease. Vet. Rec. 62:251–254.

Storz, J. 1966. Psittacosis-lymphogranuloma infection of sheep. Antigenic structures and interrelations of PL agents associated with polyarthritis, enzootic abortion, intrauterine and latent intestinal infections. J. Comp. Pathol. 76:351–362.

Studdert, M.J., and McKercher, D.G. 1968a. Bedsonia abortion in sheep. I. Aetiological study. Res. Vet. Sci. 9:48–56.

Studdert, M.J., and McKercher, D.G. 1968b. Bedsonia abortion in sheep. III. Immunological studies. Res. Vet. Sci. 9:331–336.

Tunnicliff, E.A. 1958. Ovine virus abortion. Proc. U.S. Livestock Sanit. Assoc. 62.261–265.

Young, S., Parker, H., and Firehammer, B.D. 1958. Abortion in sheep due to a virus of the psittacosis-lymphogranuloma group. J. Am. Vet. Med. Assoc. 133:374–379.

Bovine Abortion and Infertility

Specific strains of *C. psittaci* cause pregnant domestic cows to abort during late gestation and have also been isolated from bulls with the seminal vesiculitis syndrome (Storz et al. 1968).

Chlamydial abortion was first reported in the United States and occurs principally in California and in the adjoining far western states. It is endemic in California and Oregon cattle. *C. psittaci* has for many years been widely recognized as the cause of foothill abortion in cattle in California (McKercher 1969). However, the detection of *Borrelia burgdorferi* in cases of this disease and in fetuses of cattle raised on foothill rangeland has raised doubt as to the importance of chlamydia in the etiology of foothill abortion (Lane et al. 1985, Osebold et al. 1987). The disease has also been reported in Germany, Italy, and Spain. It is now recognized as a disease of worldwide occurrence. The seminal vesiculitis syndrome in bulls occurs in the same areas as enzootic bovine abortion.

Evidence exists that a neonatal disease in calves associated with herd abortions is transmitted in utero and in some instances by infected colostrum (Blanco-Loizelier and Page 1974). Prenatal and postnatal losses in nine herds as a result of chlamydial infection were described by Ehret et al. (1973).

Schachter et al. (1975) serotyped chlamydial isolates of bovine origin using the plaque-reduction method and obtained results similar to those for isolates of ovine origin. Type 1 included isolates from bovine abortion and enteric infections. Type 2 isolates were associated with polyarthritis or encephalomyelitis. Chlamydial isolates causing abortions or intestinal infections in cattle and sheep are closely related antigenically, as are those isolates producing polyarthritis, encephalomyelitis, and conjunctivitis.

Morphology. Chlamydias isolated from cases of bovine abortion share the properties of all strains of *C. psittaci*. The strain that Storz et al. (1968) isolated from seminal vesiculitis was indistinguishable from the California enzootic bovine abortion strain by the neutralization test.

A bull injected intravenously with a strain of *C. psittaci* that had been recovered from the joint of a calf with polyarthritis developed a seminal vesiculitis similar to the disease in rams described in the previous section on enzootic abortion in ewes (Eugster et al. 1971). The organism persisted in the semen after the bull recovered from acute disease.

Culture. Strains of *C. psittaci* from cases of bovine abortion have the same cultural characteristics of the enzootic ovine abortion strains.

Epizootiology and Pathogenesis. Abortion is readily produced in susceptible pregnant cows. Natural disease can be spread by ingestion of infected tissues, and venereal transmission is another likely route because the bull can harbor the organism in the semen (McKercher et al. 1966). The tick *Ornithodoros coriaceous* (McKercher et al. 1980) and/or insects may play a role in the transmission of the agent in a herd. Reindeer may be another source of infection for cattle: Neuvonen (1976) reported an incidence of disease of 21 percent (63 or 291) in a group of reindeer that had complement-fixing antibody titers of 1 : 16 or greater.

The persistence of the agent in feces indicates that some animals remain carriers; it may also explain how the disease persists in a herd.

The agent usually produces a febrile reaction in susceptible cows of all ages. After a latent period of a few months, during which *C. psittaci* propagates in the fetus, pregnant animals abort. The disease affects pregnant heifers primarily, and the abortion losses are likely to be as high as 60 percent in these animals (Jubb and Kennedy 1970). The delivery of the aborted fetuses is uneventful, and the placenta is not retained.

Aborted fetuses in natural and experimental disease show distinctive and similar pathological changes (Jubb and Kennedy 1970). The fetuses are usually full term and die during delivery or shortly thereafter, but some premature calves survive the disease.

Gross lesions are limited to the aborted fetus and the fetal membranes (Jubb and Kennedy 1970). The latter are usually thick and edematous. Pale and anemic fetuses usually show petechial hemorrhages of the skin and mucous membranes. Subcutaneous tissues are wet and edematous. Straw-colored peritoneal and pleural fluid is present. In some animals the liver is swollen and nodular as a result of chronic passive congestion. Petechial hemorrhages are often seen in trachea, tongue, thymus, and lymph nodes. Lymphoid tissues are enlarged with associated lymph stasis. Tiny gray foci that are difficult to see without proper lighting are irregularly scattered in all tissues. Granulomatous lesions can be present in any organ. The characteristic histological lesion is a diffuse or focal reticuloendothelial hyperplasia that can be seen in all organs, but the spleen, thymus, and lymph nodes are most likely to be severely affected.

The seminal vesiculitis syndrome is often found during examination of bulls for breeding soundness and is more common among younger bulls. Ball and his co-workers (1964) characterized this condition as a chronic inflammation of the seminal vesicles, accessory sex glands, epididymides, and testicles. Affected bulls have inferior semen quality, and some have atrophic testicles. The incidence in a herd can reach 10 percent.

Injection of pregnant cows with chlamydias from bovine abortion of enzootic ovine abortion produces a disease similar to that observed in the field. In a study by Lincoln et al. (1969) a thin, yellowish vaginal discharge—a sign of impending abortion—occurred in 6 of 12 inoculated heifers that aborted. The elementary bodies were frequently demonstrated in stained smears of this vaginal discharge. It was further observed that pathological changes also occurred in the internal iliac lymph nodes. Because these nodes drain the genital organs, the lesions are probably the result of the inflammatory process in the gravid uterus, where the bovine agent localizes after a short initial infectious stage in the blood. Omuri et al. (1960) have induced endometritis by intrauterine inoculation of nonpregnant cows with a C. psittaci strain.

Guinea pigs are the laboratory animal of choice for isolation and study of enzootic bovine abortion agents. Embryonated hens' eggs and mice are also susceptible. These hosts show the same general signs as described for the enzootic ovine abortion agent.

A strain of C. psittaci isolated from a bull with seminal vesiculitis produced interstitial orchitis and epididymitis, testicular degeneration, and granulomas adherent to the tunica vaginalis propria in inoculated male guinea pigs (Storz et al. 1968). In contrast, uninoculated control male guinea pigs failed to show genital lesions.

Immunity. All field strains of Chlamydia from cases bovine abortion that have been compared by neutralization tests are immunologically identical. This helps explain, in part, the field experience of various investigators and clinicians who have noted that a single exposure to the agent affords protection against this disease for the rest of the animal's life. In experimental studies Lincoln et al. (1969) found that the presence of complement-fixing antibodies and intestinal chlamydial infection seemingly had no influence on the experimental production of enzootic bovine abortion disease in pregnant heifers. No vaccine is currently recommended for the control of this disease.

The seminal vesiculitis syndrome is observed most frequently in young bulls. After the animals recover, they might be solidly immune, but there is no experimental evidence to support this conjecture.

Diagnosis. A positive diagnosis requires isolation and identification of C. psittaci. In making a clinical and pathological diagnosis, one must be careful to differentiate this disease from that caused by Brucella abortus or by Borrelia burgdorferi (Lane et al. 1985). Granulomatous lesions can be present in any organ of enzootic bovine abortion fetuses, and those in the kidney are similar to those found in brucellosis, although the bronchopneumonia characteristics of fetal brucellosis are absent (Jubb and Kennedy 1970). Cultural examinations for Brucella and Campylobacter are indicated in herds experiencing abortions. The cultural, microscopic, and serologic

procedures previously described in this chapter should be used for the isolation or identification of C. psittaci.

The Disease in Humans. There is no evidence that the chlamydial bovine abortion strains have caused disease in humans, but the possibility certainly exists. Page and Smith (1974) experimentally produced abortion in a pregnant cow with a strain of C. psittaci isolated from aborted human placental tissue.

REFERENCES

Ball, L., Griner, L.A., and Carroll, E.J. 1964. The bovine seminal vesiculitis syndrome. Am. J. Vet. Res. 25:291–302.

Blanco-Loizelier, A., and Page, L.A. 1974. Unusual forms of chlamydiosis in Spanish livestock. Abstr. Annu. Meet. Am. Soc. Microbiol. 74:73.

Ehret, W.J., Schutte, A.P., Pienaar, J.G., and Henton, M.M. 1973. Chlamydiosis in a beef herd. J. S. Afr. Vet. Assoc. 46:171–179.

Eugster, A.K., Ball, L., Carroll, E.J., and Storz, J. 1971. Experimental genital infection of bulls and rams with chlamydial (psittacosis) agents. In 6th International Meeting on the Diseases of Cattle, Philadelphia, Pa. Pp. 328–332.

Jubb, K.V., and Kennedy, P.C. 1970. Pathology of Domestic Animals, 2d ed. Academic Press, New York.

Lane, R.S., Burgdorfer, S.F., Hayes, S.F., and Barborer, A.G. 1985. Isolation of a spirochete from the soft tick, Ornithodoros coriaceus: A possible agent of epizootic bovine abortion. Science 230:85–87.

Lincoln, S., Kwapien, R.P., Reed, D.E., Whiteman, C.E., and Chow, T.L. 1969. Epizootic bovine abortion: Clinical and serologic responses and pathologic changes in extra genital organs of pregnant heifers. Am. J. Vet. Res. 30:2105–2113.

McKercher, D.G. 1969. Cause and prevention of epizootic bovine abortion. J. Am. Vet. Med. Assoc. 154:1192–1196.

McKercher, D.G., Wada, E.M., Ault, S.K., and Theis, J.H. 1980. Preliminary studies on transmission of Chlamydia to cattle by ticks (Ornithodoros coriaceus). Am. J. Vet. Res. 41:922–924.

McKercher, D.G., Wada, E.M., Robinson, E.A., and Howarth, J.A. 1966. Epizootiologic and immunologic studies of epizootic bovine abortion. Cornell Vet. 56:433–450.

Neuvonen, E. 1976. Occurrences of antibodies to group specific chlamydia antigen in cattle and reindeer sera in Finnish Lapland. Acta Vet. Scand. 17:362–369.

Omuri, T., Ishii, S., and Matumoto, M. 1960. Miyagawanellosis of cattle in Japan. Am. J. Vet. Res. 21:564–573.

Osebold, J.W., Osburn, B.I., Spezialetti, R., Bushnell, R.B., and Stott, J.L. 1987. Histopathologic changes in bovine fetuses after repeated reintroduction of a spirochete-like agent into pregnant heifers: Association with epizootic bovine abortion. Am. J. Vet. Res. 48:627–633.

Page, L.A., and Smith, P.C. 1974. Placentitis and abortion in cattle inoculated with chlamydiae isolated from aborted human placental tissue. Proc. Soc. Exp. Biol. Med. 146:269–275.

Schachter, J., Banks, J., Sugg, N., Sung, M., Storz, J., and Meyer, K.F. 1975. Serotyping of Chlamydia: Isolates of bovine origin. Infect. Immun. 11:904–907.

Storz, J., Carroll, E.J., Ball, L., and Faulkner, L.C. 1968. Isolation of a psittacosis agent (Chlamydia) from semen and epididymis of bulls with seminal vesiculitis syndrome. Am. J. Vet. Res. 29:549–555.

Placentopathy in Other Domestic Animals

Placentopathy in the goat, pig, rabbit, and mouse caused by C. psittaci is not widely observed in the United States. The character of the disease in these species is similar to enzootic ovine abortion. Comparative studies of the strains of *C. psittaci* that cause placentopathy in domestic animals have not been conducted.

McCauley and Tieken (1968) documented an instance of epizootic psittacosis abortion in goats. A chlamydial organism was isolated from an aborted goat fetus in an outbreak that caused a 12 percent abortion rate in a California flock of 216 milk goats. The incidence decreased markedly after penicillin therapy was given to the pregnant goats. This isolate of *C. psittaci* caused abortion in two experimental pregnant cows and one experimental pregnant ewe. Since then, an accurate delayed hypersensitivity skin test has been developed for the diagnosis of chlamydiosis in goats. The test uses purified chlamydias from yolk sac or McCoy cells (Rodolakis et al. 1977).

In two outbreaks of abortion among mares in Spain, chlamydiae were isolated by chick embryo passage from the liver and spleen of fetuses, and a similar strain was isolated from the synovial fluid of horses with polyarthritis. Horses with polyarthritis had specific complement-fixing antibodies, but aborting mares did not. The agents were morphologically similar to *C. psittaci* (Blanco-Loizelier et al. 1976–1977).

REFERENCES

Blanco-Loizelier, A., Marcotegui Jaso, M.A., and Delgado Casado, I. 1976–1977. Clamidiosis equina (aborto y poliartritis clamidial en equinos). An. Inst. Nac. Invest. Agrar. Ser. Hig. Sanid. Anim. (Madr.) 3:105–123.
McCauley, E.H., and Tieken, E.L., 1968. Psittacosis-lymphogranuloma venereum agent isolated during an abortion epizootic in goats. J. Am. Vet. Med. Assoc. 152:1758–1765.
Rodolakis, A., Dufrenoy, J., and Souriav, A. 1977. Allergic diagnosis of abortive chlamydial infection in the goat. Ann. Rech. Vét. 8:213–219.

Sporadic Bovine Encephalomyelitis

SYNONYM: Buss disease; abbreviation, SBE

Sporadic bovine encephalomyelitis affects cattle, particularly those less than 3 years old, and is characterized by encephalitis, fibrinous pleuritis, and peritonitis. It occurs sporadically and is caused by an agent belonging to the psittacosis-lymphogranuloma-trachoma group. So far as is known, cattle and buffalo are affected. It has been suspected that human infections occur, but the evidence is inconclusive. Dogs apparently are susceptible, but little is known about the disease in this species.

The disease was first recognized and described in Iowa by McNutt (1940). It has since been diagnosed in Texas, California, South Dakota, Minnesota, and Missouri. Schoop and Kauker (1956) described a disease in Ger-

many that was caused by a psittacoid agent that may be the same as the SBE agent. An outbreak was described in South Africa (Tustin et al. 1961) and in Canada (Bannister et al. 1962). The disease is also present in Australia. Except for a report that *C. psittaci* was isolated from the brain of two encephalitic buffalo calves (Ognyanov et al. 1973), there have no been no new reports on this type of chlamydial disease since 1962.

It is conceivable that the organism causing SBE would fall into the serotype 2 classification of Schachter et al. (1975).

Morphology. The causative agent of SBE is a typical member of the psittacosis-lymphogranuloma-trachoma group. In morphology and growth characteristics in embryonated eggs, and its serology, it is difficult to differentiate from other members of *Chlamydia*.

Culture. The agent reproduces readily in the yolk sac of chick embryos. We have seen no report of its cultivation in tissue cultures.

Epizootiology and Pathogenesis. The mode of transmission of SBE is wholly unknown. The disease does not appear to be highly transmissible, but this may be a misconception, because many mild or inapparent cases occur. Often it appears on a single farm with no other recognized cases nearby. Frequently only a small number of cases occur in a herd containing many other presumably susceptible animals. The disease can be transmitted to calves through the milk of infected dams (Enright et al. 1958, McNutt and Waller 1940).

SBE is manifested by profound depression. Fever occurs early in the course of the disease and lasts until recovery or death ensues. Inappetence, weakness, emaciation, and prostration are characteristic. A clear mucoid discharge from the nose and eyes frequently occurs. A staggering gait is often seen, and some animals tend to walk or stagger in circles. The principal joints can be swollen and tender. A mild diarrhea is sometimes present. Opisthotonos occurs occasionally. The disease appears to spread slowly, and many exposed animals seem to escape infection, although this may be more apparent than real. As a rule, only a few animals in a herd show illness.

With experimental inoculation, the incubation period varies widely from 4 to 27 days. In the naturally transmitted disease it is not known, but apparently it is fairly long. The disease is said to have a course of 1 to 3 weeks. Enright et al. (1958) presented evidence that there are many mild or inapparent cases; these obviously have a much shorter course. From 40 to 60 percent of the clinically sick animals die; however, because many others are infected with the agent without showing detectable signs of illness, mortality is really much lower.

The gross lesions are not conspicuous. Often the body

cavities contain more than the usual amount of fluid, in which strings of fibrin can be found. The brain usually appears normal, but shows microscopic evidence of a severe and diffuse meningoencephalitis. The meningitis is most severe at the base of the brain.

The disease is readily produced in young calves by intracerebral or subcutaneous inoculation. Horses, sheep, swine, and mice are not susceptible to inoculation. Guinea pigs inoculated intraperitoneally usually die in 4 to 5 days with a fibrinous peritonitis. Hamsters are also susceptible.

Immunity. No observations on the solidity and duration of immunity to SBE have been reported. It is probable that one experience with this disease is sufficient to protect the animal thereafter.

Diagnosis. The diagnosis is not easy because the signs of illness are often vague. Evidence of encephalitis, combined with a stiff awkward gait, and the presence of pleuritis, peritonitis, and sometimes pericarditis are indicative. Isolation of the agent by the inoculation of yolk sacs of embryonated eggs is generally successful and convincing.

Appropriate staining procedures can reveal elementary bodies in the cytoplasm of mononuclear cells in the exudates in the meninges, in the mononuclear cells of serosa membranes, and in microglia of nodules. The elementary bodies are not numerous, and often embryonated hens' eggs, guinea pigs, or hamsters are inoculated to demonstrate their presence.

Antimicrobial Susceptibility. The agent is very sensitive to most of the antibiotics (except streptomycin).

The Disease in Humans. Enright et al. (1958) reported that 51 of 481 samples of human serums collected from persons who had had contact with cattle in California fixed complement with an antigen made from the McNutt strain of the SBE agent. Several of these individuals described clinical syndromes of persisting headache and stiff neck lasting about a week, followed by complete recovery. These data provide circumstantial evidence of infection in humans, but certainly not conclusive proof.

REFERENCES

Bannister, G.L., Boulanger, P., Gray, D.P., Chapman, C.H., Avery, R.J., and Corner, A.H. 1962. Sporadic bovine encephalomyelitis in Canada. Can. J. Comp. Med. Vet. Sci. 26:25–32.

Enright, J.B., Sadler, W.W., and Robinson, E.A. 1958. Sporadic bovine encephalomyelitis in California. Proc. U.S. Livestock Sanit. Assoc. 62:127.

McNutt, S.H. 1940. A preliminary report on an infectious encephalomyelitis of cattle resembling listerella infection. Vet. Med. 35:228–230.

McNutt, S.H., and Waller, E.F. 1940. Sporadic bovine encephalomyelitis. Cornell Vet. 30:437–448.

Ognyanov, D.D., Panova, M., Pavlov, N., Arnaudov, S., and Minchev, S. 1973. Neorickettsial encephalomyelitis in buffalo calves. Vet. Sbirka (Bulg.) 70:13–15.

Schachter, J., Banks, J., Sugg, N., Sung, M., Storz, J., and Meyer, K.F. 1975. Serotyping of Chlamydia: Isolates of bovine origin. Infect. Immun. 11:904–907.

Schoop, G., and Kauker, E. 1956. Infektion eines Rinderbestandes durch ein Virus der Psittalosis-Lymphogranuloma-Gruppe. D.T.W. 23:233–235.

Tustin, R.C., Mare, J., and Van Herrden, A. 1961. A disease of calves resembling sporadic bovine encephalomyelitis. J. S. Afr. Vet. Med. Assoc. 32:117–123.

Feline Pneumonitis

SYNONYM: Feline chlamydiosis

Feline pneumonitis is an infection of the respiratory tract and conjunctiva of domesticated cats caused by *C. psittaci*. Baker (1944) showed that it is caused by an agent that can be naturally transmitted from cat to cat and, experimentally, from cats to white mice. Later in the same year Hamre and Rake (1944) showed that the agent belongs to the psittacosis-lymphogranuloma-trachoma group. The disease is found throughout the world.

Morphology. Baker (1944) found that the agent of feline pneumonitis usually failed to pass through Berkefeld N filters. Lung tissue of affected animals contained bodies similar to those of *C. psittaci*, and large numbers could be produced in the yolk sac membrane of developing chick embryos by inoculation of the agent into the sac. Dense structures or plaques appeared in the lungs of mice and hamsters, which suggested that the agent was undergoing a developmental cycle, now recognized as characteristic of this group of chlamydial agents. Centrifugation at 10,000 rpm for 30 minutes caused sedimentation of numerous elementary bodies from suspensions derived from yolk sac membranes. The supernatant fluid lost most of its pathogenicity for mice, but this was regained when the suspensions were shaken and the elementary bodies were resuspended.

Cultural and Biochemical Features. The agent is readily propagated in the yolk sac of developing chick embryos (Baker 1944). Embryonic deaths occur on the second or third day after inoculation of 5-day-old embryos, and numerous elementary bodies are found in the cytoplasm of the cells from the yolk sac membrane. The organism also develops when infective material is dropped on the chorioallantoic membrane of 10-day-old embryos. The membranes become thickened, but the embryos are not affected by this method of inoculation. Some isolates replicate in cell culture.

The feline pneumonitis agent hemagglutinates mouse erythrocytes only. Differential centrifugation shows that the activity is found in particles distinct from the elementary bodies.

Resistance of the Organism. The organism is destroyed when heated at 50°C for 30 minutes and at 60°C for 10 minutes. It is not completely inactivated, but its pathogenicity is reduced by heating at 45°C for 30 minutes or for 50°C for 10 minutes. Lung suspensions in 50 percent glycerol lose most of their disease-producing power in 30 days. Suspensions of yolk sac material retain their activity for at least a week at room temperature and for at least a month at 4°C. In the lyophilized state the agent retains its activity for 6 months or longer, but there is a significant loss in titer. Storage at −70°C preserved infectivity in most instances.

Antigens and Toxins. The group and specific antigens of the feline pneumonitis agent are located in the cell wall. When the cell walls are isolated by treatment of the elementary bodies with deoxycholate and trypsin, the group antigen is found in the deoxycholate extract and the specific antigens remain in the cell wall (Jenkin et al. 1961).

Yerasimides (1960) described a strain isolated from a case of acute feline catarrhal conjunctivitis. A neutralization test showed a one-sided relationship because antiserum to Baker's virus did not neutralize Yerasimides's isolate, but equal cross-neutralization occurred with antiserum produced by Yerasimides's isolate. These antiserums were specially prepared for these tests, and these data demonstrate a close, but not complete, antigenic relationship.

Hamre and Rake (1944) showed that the elementary bodies of feline pneumonitis, like those of several other diseases of this group, produce an endotoxin that in large doses ($>10^8$ ID$_{50}$) kills mice within 12 to 24 hours after intravenous injection.

Epizootiology and Pathogenesis. Feline pneumonitis is contagious. The natural disease in cats evidently is transmitted by contact with infected excretions and by air droplet infection. The disease in mice and guinea pigs does not transmit naturally from animal to animal.

Affected animals usually do not die, but they become greatly debilitated, and recovery is slow. In the beginning the disease is manifested by fever and inappetence. A mucopurulent discharge appears in the eyes and nose, and the animal coughs and sneezes a great deal. In most animals signs of pneumonia are not detected. The period of incubation ranges from 6 to 10 days, and the illness usually continues for about 2 weeks, after which there is gradual improvement. Much weight is lost during the time when signs are most obvious. It is usually at least a month before the affected animals regain their original body weight. Unless the disease is complicated by other factors, mortality is low.

Lesions are confined principally to the upper respiratory tract and the conjunctival membranes. The mucosa of these regions are reddened, swollen, and covered with exudate. Pneumonic lesions may be found after the animal is euthanized during the period of acute signs. These lung lesions disappear promptly as recovery begins. The consolidated portions are pinkish gray. The bronchial nodes are not noticeably enlarged. Histological sections of the pneumonic areas show alveoli filled with an exudate consisting largely of monocytic and polymorphonuclear leukocytes. Occasional areas of necrosis are found, but in general the epithelium of the air passages is intact. Elementary bodies are found in the cytoplasm of the monocytic cells. Cello (1971) reported that significant involvement of the lung is rare in the cat.

C. psittaci has been identified as a cause of gastritis in cats, and in experimentally infected cats organisms isolated from clinical gastritis produce signs and lesions similar to those produced by the respiratory strains (Gaillard et al. 1984, Hargis et al. 1983). Chlamydias have also been isolated from a cat with peritonitis (Dickie and Sniff 1980).

Investigators have been able to transmit the chlamydias of this disease to white mice, hamsters, guinea pigs, and rabbits by inoculating them with infective material intranasally while they are under light anesthesia—a technique that has been used successfully in work with the influenza viruses. Using doses 10 to 50 times greater than were needed to infect by the nasal route, Baker (1944) was unable to infect mice by parenteral injection. Hamre and Rake (1944), however, using much larger doses of yolk sac material, were successful in producing infections by intracerebral and intraperitoneal injection.

The disease in adult guinea pigs and in rabbits is manifested by fever and pneumonia, but the animals do not die. Young guinea pigs, hamsters, and mice exhibit the same signs of illness, but the disease usually is fatal: mice die on the second or third day, hamsters on the third or fourth day, and the young guinea pigs on the fifth to seventh day.

Immunity. Cats convalescent from feline pneumonitis do not always have demonstrable serum-neutralizing antibodies or complement-fixing antibodies in their serums. Much remains to be learned about immunity to the feline pneumonitis agent in the domestic cat (Baker 1971, Bittle 1971, Cello 1971). Studies, in pathogen-free cats, of immunity to various strains of the feline pneumonitis agent are needed to clarify the degree and duration of immunity.

On the basis of our limited knowledge of feline pneumonitis immunity in cats and of immunity to psittacoid agents, it is reasonable to assume that the resistance of cats to the feline pneumonitis agent may be partial and transitory. Apparent remissions and exacerbations of the disease in an individual animal may represent recovery and reinfection rather than activation of a latent infection (Cello 1971). Furthermore, some of the presumed recurrent infections of *C. psittaci* may be caused by a feline respiratory viral pathogen. We know that carriers of *C. psittaci* exist as do carriers of such viruses as feline calicivirus and feline rhinotracheitis virus, and this obviously leads to considerable confusion in diagnosis. Cello (1971) found that mycoplasmosis of the conjunctival sac, nasal passages, and sinuses often develops in cats that have had chlamydial infections. This could also lead to the erroneous impression that the original infection had developed into a chronic state or that it had recurred. Such misdiagnosis will occur unless attempts to isolate the agent are performed completely and precisely.

In experimental trials McKercher (1949) found that inactivated elementary body suspensions of the feline pneumonitis agent were relatively ineffective in producing immunity in kittens and in mice. Mitzel and Strating (1977) tested a commercially available modified live chlamydial vaccine and found that the vaccine afforded some protection, although not complete, and that *C. psittaci* could be isolated from tissues of 34 percent of the vaccinated cats 3 days after challenge by the aerosol route. In other vaccine trials the majority of cats had complete protection 1 year after vaccination, and the balance had a serviceable immunity (Kolar and Rude 1981).

In 1971 at an American Veterinary Medical Association Colloquium on Selected Feline Infectious Diseases, a panel of experts evaluated the only modified hen's egg–propagated vaccine for immunization of domestic cats against feline pneumonitis (Expert Panel 1971). The vaccine stimulated complement-fixing antibodies. The duration of immunity and the degree of protection were unknown. Later studies by Mitzel and Strating (1977) suggested some degree of protection with this type of vaccine. At a recent meeting another panel of experts recommended that cell-cultured attenuated virus vaccine be given to cats at 8 weeks and 12 months of age and once a year thereafter (Rude et al. 1985). Care should be exercised in administering the vaccine because ocular contamination can cause inflammation. Its use in pregnant cats was not recommended because the relevant data were limited. The panel recognized that *C. psittaci* of cats is only one of many feline respiratory pathogens. Consequently, vaccine efficacy in a respiratory outbreak may be questioned at times.

Diagnosis. The clinical diagnosis is exceedingly difficult because many pathogens have been isolated from animals with signs of respiratory illness similar to those described for feline pneumonitis. Only by isolation and

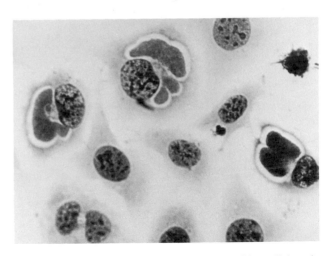

Figure 33.2. Mouse L cells infected with the chlamydial strain of feline pneumonitis. Large inclusions are present in the cytoplasm, and the nuclei of cells are dislocated. Giemsa stain. × 730. (Courtesy J. Storz.)

identification of the agent is it possible to differentiate *C. psittaci* from other respiratory and conjunctival pathogens in the cat, such as feline rhinotracheitis virus, feline calicivirus, and feline reoviruses. Of course, concurrent infections with one or more of these pathogens do occur.

The agent reproduces in guinea pigs, producing a febrile reaction, and the complement-fixation test has been used to demonstrate the presence of antibodies. Demonstration of large microcolonies (2 to 12 μm in diameter) of elementary bodies (Figure 33.2) in various stages of development in Giemsa-stained conjunctival cells from a cat is a reliable and accurate diagnostic feature of feline pneumonitis (Cello 1971).

Antimicrobial Susceptibility. The feline pneumonitis agent is susceptible to certain antibiotics. Tetracyclines will free diseased animals of infection; the problem is to keep them free (Cello 1971).

The Disease in Humans. Schachter et al. (1969) isolated a chlamydial organism from conjunctival scrapings of a man with acute follicular keratoconjunctivitis. The patient owned two cats, one of which had clinical manifestations of feline pneumonitis. Chlamydial isolates from the two cats and their owners had the same characteristics as *C. psittaci*. The human isolate produced typical, acute, inclusion-positive conjunctivitis in experimental cats. This suggests that certain strains of feline and human *C. psittaci* with an affinity for the conjunctiva may produce disease in both humans and domestic cats.

REFERENCES

Baker, J.A. 1944. A virus causing pneumonia in cats and producing elementary bodies. J. Exp. Med. 79:159–172.

Baker, J.A. 1971. Comments on feline pneumonitis. J. Am. Vet. Med. Assoc. 158:941–942.

Bittle, J.L. 1971. Comments on feline pneumonitis. J. Am. Vet. Med. Assoc. 158:942–943.

Cello, R.M. 1971. Microbiological and immunological aspects of feline pneumonitis. J. Am. Vet. Med. Assoc. 158:932–938.

Dickie, C.W., and Sniff, E.S. 1980. Chlamydia infection associated with peritonitis in a cat. J. Am. Vet. Med. Assoc. 176:1256–1259.

Expert Panel. 1971. Report of the panel of the Colloquium on Selected Feline Infectious Diseases. J. Am. Vet. Med. Assoc. 158:835–843.

Gaillard, E.T., Hargis, A.M., Prieur, D.J., Evermann, J.F., and Dhillon, A.S. 1984. Pathogenesis of feline gastric chlamydial infection. Am. J. Vet. Res. 45:2314–2321.

Hamre, D.M., and Rake, G. 1944. A new member of the lymphogranuloma-psittacosis group of agents. J. Infect. Dis. 74:206.

Hargis, A.M., Prieur, D.J., and Gaillard, E.T. 1983. Chlamydial infection of the gastric mucosa in twelve cats. Vet. Pathol. 20:170–178.

Jenkin, H.M., Ross, M.R., and Moulder, J.W. 1961. Species-specific antigens from the cell walls of the agents of meningopneumonitis and feline pneumonitis. J. Immunol. 86:123–127.

Kolar, J.R., and Rude, T.A. 1981. Duration of immunity in cats inoculated with a commercial feline pneumonitis vaccine. Vet. Med. Small Anim. Clin. 76:1171–1173.

McKercher, D.G. 1949. Immunization studies in cats against *Miyagawanella felis*. Thesis, Cornell University, Ithaca, N.Y.

Mitzel, J.R., and Strating, A. 1977. Vaccination against feline pneumonitis. Am. J. Vet. Res. 38:1361–1363.

Rude, R., Barndt, R., Grant, W., Scott, F., Storz, J., and Williams, J. 1985. Feline chlamydiosis: Stalking elusive prey. Panel discussion. Veterinary Medicine Publishing Co., Lenexa, Kans.

Schachter, J., Ostler, H.B., and Meyer, K.F. 1969. Human infection with the agent of feline pneumonitis. Lancet 1:1063–1065.

Yerasimides, T.G. 1960. Isolation of a new strain of feline pneumonitis virus from a domestic cat. J. Infect. Dis. 106:290–296.

Pneumonitis and Conjunctivitis in Other Animals

In general, pneumonitis and conjunctivitis in sheep, cattle, goats, dogs, and mice are characterized by a conjunctival and nasal discharge, lethargy, anorexia, labored breathing, signs of penumonia, and fever. Diarrhea may occur. The diseases are rarely fatal, and their severity is largely determined by secondary bacterial infections, or in some instances by viral or mycoplasmal pathogens of the respiratory tract. A lethal pneumonia in animals such as mice can be produced by serial passage in young animals infected by the intranasal route.

The pulmonary lesions of experimental psittacoid infections are characterized by an intense neutrophilic response, whereas viral infections are proliferative (Jubb and Kennedy 1970). Copious mucoid exudates of tracheobronchitis can be present, with red, lobular consolidation in the anterior lobes of the lung. The histological lesion is an exudative bronchopneumonia of the bronchioles with extension into adjacent alveoli. Demonstration of elementary bodies in smears or in histological sections is difficult. Diagnosis should emphasize the demonstration of elementary bodies in experimentally inoculated hosts—in smears of yolk sac, mouse lung, or guinea pig peritoneal exudate—or of a rising serum titer with paired serum samples.

The strains isolated from a given animal species with pneumonitis can produce experimental pneumonia by intratracheal inoculation in the homologous species. In some instances these strains produce disease in another organ system such as the genital tract of the homologous species. Occasionally, a strain that produces a characteristic disease in one species can do likewise in another mammal. One can conclude only that *C. psittaci* organisms contain a specific antigen(s) in their structure that has a selective cell tropism for one or more animal hosts and that this dictates the nature of the disease. Many animals remain carriers, thereby serving as sources of infection for susceptible animals.

Various colonies of guinea pigs are chronically infected with *C. psittaci* organisms that produce conjunctivitis. These organisms are also transmitted transovarially (Storz 1961). *C. psittaci* has been isolated from diseased conjunctiva of hamsters (Murray 1964). Because guinea pigs and hamsters are used for diagnostic and research studies of *C. psittaci,* the worker must be aware of possible latent psittacoid infections in colonies of these species.

Presumably, the strains of *C. psittaci* that cause pneumonia and conjunctivitis are serotype 2.

In sheep and goats. An agent was described by McKercher (1953) that caused pneumonia in sheep. An ovine pneumonic strain of *C. psittaci* studied by Studdert and McKercher (1968) produced abortion in ewes, but the disease differed from typical enzootic abortion of ewes. Dungworth (1963) produced experimental pneumonitis in lambs with an ovine abortion strain, and experimental abortions in ewes infected with an ovine pneumonitis strain were reported by Page (1966). Abortion and pneumonia in sheep are caused by similar chlamydial agents, although some serotypic differences exist between ovine pneumonic and abortion strains. A pneumonic condition of goats in Japan may be caused by *C. psittaci;* the agent was transmissible to many other domestic animals.

Follicular conjunctivitis, sometimes with complicating eye lesions, occurs commonly in sheep. Storz et al. (1967) isolated *C. psittaci* from sheep with follicular conjunctivitis in three different herds (Figure 33.3). The isolates were specifically related to strains of *C. psittaci* that cause polyarthritis. Some of the sheep with follicular conjunctivitis also had signs of polyarthritis. Parenteral injection of conjunctival *C. psittaci* resulted in follicular conjunctivitis and polyarthritis in lambs. Cooper (1974) described the transmission of *C. psittaci* isolated from keratoconjunctivitis of New Zealand sheep.

No vaccines are available for sheep and goats. Various antibiotics are effective chemotherapeutic agents.

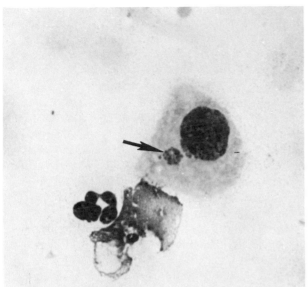

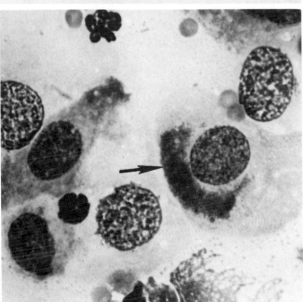

Figure 33.3. Early (*top*) and mature (*bottom*) chlamydial inclusions in conjunctival cells of infected sheep. Giemsa stain. × 1,300. (Courtesy J. Storz.)

In cattle. Bovine strains of *C. psittaci* are responsible for pneumonitis in cattle in Czechoslovakia (Gmitter 1960) and for pneumoenteritis in cattle in Italy (Messieri 1959) and in Japan (Omuri et al. 1960). The disease has also been described in the United States.

U.S. (Werdin 1973) and German (Baumann 1974, Stellmacher et al. 1974) investigators studied the etiology of calf pneumonia, with emphasis on the effects of *C. psittaci* in experimental calves. The *C. psittaci* isolates from natural cases produced respiratory signs and patho-

logical changes of varying intensities in experimental animals, and the organism was reisolated from the respiratory tract in all cases and from the intestinal tract in some.

In dogs. At a dog pound in Fort Collins, Colorado, more than half of 119 dogs contained group-specific chlamydial antibodies, with the greatest incidence in older male dogs. In a serologic survey for chlamydial antibodies in laboratory dogs, 7.6 percent (77 of 1,007 random samples) had complement-fixing antibody titers between 1 : 5 and 1 : 40, and 10 of the 15 colonies in the test had dogs with antibodies (Weber et al. 1977).

Fraser et al. (1969) described respiratory signs of illness in a dog that had access to an aviary in which psittacosis occurred. There is strong evidence that the dog as well as three persons associated with the aviary had psittacosis. *C. psittaci* can also cause nervous manifestations in conjunction with pneumonic signs, or chronic keratitis alone.

Maierhofer and Storz (1969) described clinical and serologic responses in dogs inoculated parenterally with a chlamydial strain isolated from a sheep with polyarthritis. The affected dogs had fever, anorexia, signs of depression, pneumonia, incoordination, muscle and joint pain, and diarrhea. The chlamydial agent was isolated from somatic organs, including the brain and portions of the intestinal tract, and also from joints. Complement-fixing group-specific antibodies were produced with maximum titers 21 to 28 days after inoculation and were still detectable 1 year later.

In horses. In serologic surveys of horse populations in Finland (Neuvonen and Estola 1974) and West Germany (Schmatz et al. 1977) complement-fixing antibodies were found in enough animals to indicate that *C. psittaci* is a common infection. Evidence of the organism has also been found in horses in Australia. Its importance as a disease entity still has not been established. *C. psittaci* has been isolated from the nasal tract of two horses with acute respiratory disease, but transmission trials in horses were not performed with these isolates (Moorthy and Spradbrow 1978).

REFERENCES

Baumann, G. 1974. Fluorescent histological demonstration of experimental bedsonia (chlamydia) infections in the calf. Arch. Exp. Veterinärmed. 28:847–867.
Cooper, B.S. 1974. Transmission of a chlamydia-like agent isolated from contagious conjunctivo-keratitis of sheep. N.Z. Vet. J. 22:181–184.
Dungworth, D.L. 1963. The pathogenesis of ovine pneumonia. III. Placental infection by pneumonitis virus. J. Comp. Pathol. Ther. 73:68–75.
Fraser, G., Norval, J., Withers, A.R., and Gregor, W.W. 1969. A case history of psittacosis in the dog. Vet. Rec. 85:54–58.

Gmitter, J. 1960. Large viruses, probably of the neorickettsial group isolated from cattle with respiratory diseases in Slovakia. Sb. Cesk. Akad. Ved Vet. Med. 5:475–489.

Jubb, K.V., and Kennedy, P.C. 1970. Pathology of Domestic Animals, 2d ed. Academic Press, New York.

McKercher, D.G. 1953. Feline pneumonitis. II. The effect of antibiotics on the experimental infection. Science 115:543–548.

Maierhofer, C.A., and Storz, J. 1969. Clinical and serologic responses in dogs inoculated with the chlamydial (psittacosis) agent of ovine polyarthritis. Am. J. Vet. Res. 30:1961–1966.

Messieri. 1959. Atti Soc. Ital. Sci. Vet. 8:702.

Moorthy, A.R.S., and Spradbrow, P.B. 1978. *Chlamydia psittaci* infection of horses with respiratory disease. Equine Vet. J. 10:38–42.

Murray, E.S. 1964. Guinea pig inclusion conjunctivitis virus. I. Isolation and identification as a member of the psittacosis-lymphogranuloma-trachoma group. J. Infect. Dis. 114:1–12.

Neuvonen, E., and Estola, T. 1974. Occurrence of antibodies to group specific chlamydia antigen in Finnish sheep, cattle, and horse sera. Acta Vet. Scand. 15:256–263.

Omuri, T., Ishii, S., and Matumoto, M. 1960. Miyagawanellosis of cattle in Japan. Am. J. Vet. Res. 21:564–573.

Page, L.A. 1966. Interspecies transfer of psittacosis-LGV-trachoma agent: Pathogenicity of two avian and two mammalian strains for eight species of birds and mammals. Am. J. Vet. Res. 27:397–407.

Schmatz, H.D., Schmatz, S., Weber, A., and Sailer, J. 1977. Complement fixing chlamydiae antibodies in serum samples of horses, cattle, sheep, dogs, cats and wild ruminants. Berl. Münch. Tierärztl. Wochenschr. 90:74–76.

Stellmacher, H., Baumann, G., and Ilchmann, G. 1974. Studies on the aetiology of enzootic pneumonia of the calf, with special reference to bedsonia organisms. Monatsschr. Vet. 29:539–544.

Storz, J. 1961. The diaplacental transmission of psittacosis lymphogranuloma group viruses in guinea pigs. J. Infect. Dis. 109:129–146.

Storz, J., Pierson, R.E., Marriott, M.E., and Chow, T.L. 1967. Isolation of psittacosis agents from follicular conjunctivitis of sheep. Proc. Soc. Exp. Biol. Med. 125:857–860.

Studdert, M.J., and McKercher, D.G. 1968. Bedsonia abortion of sheep. I. Aetiological studies. Res. Vet. Sci. 9:48–56.

Weber, A., Krauss, H., and Schmatz, H.D. 1977. Seroepidemiological investigations for complement fixing chlamydial antibodies in beagles. Z. Versuchstierkd. 19:270.

Werdin, R.E. 1973. Studies on the pathogenesis and pathology of chlamydial pneumonia in calves. Diss. Abstr. Int. B Sci. Eng. 33:5569–5570.

Ovine Polyarthritis

Polyarthritis in sheep was first observed in Wisconsin by Mendlowski and Segre (1960) and further described as an arthritic disease caused by a chlamydial agent (Mendlowski et al. 1960). The disease was found to be widespread in the intermountain area of the United States (Storz et al. 1960).

Culture. The ovine polyarthritis psittacoid agent is readily cultivated in embryonated hens' eggs (Mendlowski et al. 1960). Guinea pigs, turkeys, and lambs readily grow the organisms (Page 1966).

Epizootiology and Pathogenesis. The main habitat for the polyarthritis agents of sheep may be the intestinal tract. Infections producing polyarthritis are systemic, and chlamydiae can be isolated from many tissues.

The disease affects lambs up to 6 months old. The principal feature of the disease is lameness, and a few animals become permanently lame. There is also depression, reluctance to move, and conjunctivitis. Tetanuslike spasms can be seen occasionally. The morbidity is high, and the mortality is 3 to 7 percent as a rule.

At necropsy a constant finding is a serous to serofibrinous or fibrinous synovitis. The subcutaneous and adjacent periarticular tissues are edematous with clear fluid that extends around tendon sheaths. Surrounding muscles are hyperemic and edematous, and petechial hemorrhages appear in the fascia. The viscera can show changes associated with systemic infection and histological changes indicative of inflammation of soft tissues, including the central nervous system.

The experimental disease in 5- to 6-month-old lambs is similar to the naturally occurring disease (Storz et al. 1965).

The ovine polyarthritis agent produced a severe polyarthritis in the leg joints of sheep and in the hock joint of turkeys (Page 1966). It failed to affect mice inoculated intraperitoneally or pigeons inoculated intracerebrally, but caused disease in guinea pigs inoculated intraperitoneally. Both the pigeon ornithosis and sheep polyarthritis agents produced aerosacculitis in intraperitoneally inoculated turkeys. These observations may be important to our understanding of natural interspecies transfer.

Immunity. The isolates of *C. psittaci* from the intestinal tract and affected joints of polyarthritic lambs are antigenically identical but differ from enzootic ovine abortion isolates from the same flock or other flocks with enzootic ovine abortion (Storz 1966).

Convalescent sheep that are injected with ovine polyarthritis strains of *C. psittaci* do not develop polyarthritis, although they harbor the organism 21 days after challenge (Storz et al. 1965).

The natural disease is limited to lambs, so it is a self-limiting disease in this respect. Whether an age factor is responsible or this is a common disease with ensuing protection after recovery is unknown, but the latter is probably true.

Diagnosis. Examination of wet mounts of joint exudates with a phase-contrast microscope often reveals numerous mononuclear cells whose cytoplasm contains elementary bodies. As this is a systemic infection, the organism can be isolated from hens' eggs or from the visceral tissues, feces, or joint exudate of guinea pigs or turkeys.

The psittacoid organisms are principally responsible for polyarthritis in lambs, although mycoplasmas have been incriminated.

The Disease in Humans. Caution must be exercised because the turkey can be readily infected with the ovine polyarthritis agent and many human cases are derived from infected turkeys.

REFERENCES

Mendlowski, B., and Segre, D. 1960. Polyarthritis in sheep. I. Description of the disease and experimental transmission. Am. J. Vet. Res. 21:68–73.
Mendlowski, B., Kraybill, W.H., and Segre, D. 1960. Polyarthritis in sheep. II. Characterization of the causative virus. Am. J. Vet. Res. 21:74–80.
Page, L.A. 1966. Interspecies transfer of psittacosis-LGV-trachoma agent: Pathogenicity of two avian and two mammalian strains for eight species of birds and mammals. Am. J. Vet. Res. 27:397–407.
Storz, J. 1966. Psittacosis-lymphogranuloma infection of sheep. Antigenic structures and interrelations of PL agents associated with polyarthritis, enzootic abortion, intrauterine and latent intestinal infections. J. Comp. Pathol. 76:351–362.
Storz, J., McKercher, D.G., Howarth, J.A., and Staub, O.C. 1960. The isolation of a viral agent from epizootic bovine abortion. J. Am. Vet. Med. Assoc. 137:509–514.
Storz, J., Shupe, J.L., Marriott, M.E., and Thornley, W.R. 1965. Polyarthritis of lambs induced experimentally by a psittacosis agent. J. Infect. Dis. 115:9–18.

Bovine Polyarthritis

Polyarthritis in calves has been recognized for years. In this species it is caused by certain bacteria, including *Mycoplasma* and *Chlamydia*. Bovine psittacoid polyarthritis occurs in the United States.

Epizootiology and Pathogenesis. Chlamydial infection in calves is severe, causing high mortality. Some affected calves are weak at birth, implying intrauterine infection. The infant calves have a fever and develop anorexia, reluctance to move or stand, and swelling of the joints in 2 to 3 days. Death ensues 2 to 12 days after signs of illness first appear. The limb joints are most severely affected, with the synovial structures distended with a turbid yellowish fluid and strands of fibrin adhering to the synovium. The surrounding subcutaneous and adjacent periarticular tissues are edematous, with an extension around the tendon sheaths. Muscles around the joints are edematous and hyperemic, and petechial hemorrhages appear in the fascia. The visceral organs can show changes attributable to systemic infection.

The natural and experimental diseases in calves are similar (Storz, Shupe, et al. 1966). In the experimental disease chlamydiae are recovered from the blood within 18 hours after intra-articular inoculation. The *C. psittaci* organisms persist in the blood for 6 days. The organism is also readily isolated from the joint fluids by inoculation of the yolk sacs of embryonated hens' eggs.

The guinea pig and embryonated hens' egg are excellent laboratory hosts.

Immunity. Little is known about the immunity, but a calf is probably protected against reinfection if it recovers from polyarthritic psittacoid infection.

The bovine polyarthritic psittacoid strains are antigenically related to each other and to the ovine polyarthritic psittacoid strains, but apparently are different from bovine abortion psittacoid strains (Storz, Shupe, et al. 1966). A close relationship also exists between one bovine polyarthritis psittacoid strain and one guinea pig psittacoid strain that causes inclusion conjunctivitis and systemic infection.

Diagnosis. The same diagnostic procedures apply for ovine and bovine psittacoid polyarthritis. In bovine polyarthritis other infectious agents must be sought as well. Certain bacterial organisms such as *Escherichia coli* and streptococci cause polyarthritis in calves, and occasionally the former is present with *C. psittaci* in the joint exudate. Mycoplasmas frequently cause polyarthritis in calves, but cytopathogenic viruses have not been isolated (Storz, Smart, et al. 1966).

The Disease in Humans. There are no reports of this agent causing disease in humans, but one should exercise caution in handling calves with polyarthritis.

REFERENCES

Storz, J., Shupe, J.L., Smart, R.A., and Thornley, R.W. 1966. Polyarthritis of calves: Experimental induction by a psittacosis agent. Am. J. Vet. Res. 27:987–995.
Storz, J., Smart, R.A., Marriott, M.E., and Davis, R.V. 1966. Polyarthritis of calves: Isolation of psittacosis agents from affected joints. Am. J. Vet. Res. 27:633–641.

Equine Polyarthritis

Chlamydial polyarthritis was diagnosed in a newborn foal (McChesney et al. 1974). The disease was characterized by fever, leukocytosis, conjunctivitis, depression, and polyarthritis. Most joints in all four limbs were swollen, contained large amounts of fluid, and were sensitive to pressure. Clinical recovery was complete after treatment with penicillin and tetracycline.

The diagnosis was confirmed in the laboratory by the demonstration of *C. psittaci* in chick embryo yolk sacs that had been inoculated with infective joint fluid.

A case of equine polyarthritis was diagnosed in Spain (Blanco-Loizelier et al. 1976–1977).

REFERENCES

Blanco-Loizelier, A., Marcotegui-Jaso, M.A., and Delgado-Casado, I. 1976–1977. Clamidiosis equina (aborto y poliartritis clamidial en equinos). An. Inst. Nac. Invest. Agrar. Ser. Hig. Sanid. Anim. (Madr.) 3:105–123.

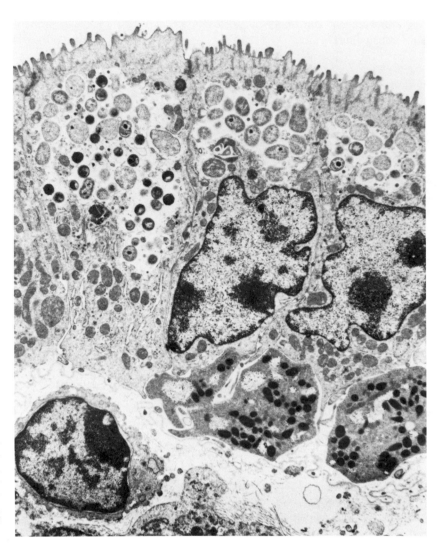

Figure 33.4. *Chlamydia*-infected enterocytes of a calf with dense-centered, infectious forms and intermediate and reticulated developmental forms. Microvilli and terminal web of enterocytes are altered. Macchiavello stain. × 13,650. (From Doughri et al., 1974, courtesy of *American Journal of Veterinary Research*.)

McChesney, A.E., Becerra, V., and England, J.J. 1974. Chlamydial polyarthritis in a foal. J. Am. Vet. Med. Assoc. 165:259–261.

Bovine Enteritis

Pneumoenteritis of calves is one of the limiting factors in a successful veal operation. In all likelihood there is no single pathogenic organism responsible for this disease. Certain respiratory viruses may be responsible, and pneumoenteritis reputedly also occurs as a psittacoid disease in cattle in Italy (Messieri 1959) and in Japan (Omuri et al. 1960).

York and Baker (1951) described an agent isolated from the intestinal tract of calves, which they named *Miyagawanella bovis,* and later suggested it may produce enteritis in colostrum-deprived calves. *C. psittaci* is commonly present in the feces of many animals in infected herds, and a high percentage of herds in New York State harbor this fecal organism and also have antibodies to it.

A comparable herd situation likely exists in other parts of the United States and also in other countries. Because there is a close antigenic relationship between many intestinal strains of *C. psittaci* and many strains that cause enzootic ovine abortion, enzootic bovine abortion, or ovine and bovine psittacoid polyarthritis, the intestinal-carrier strains may explain, in part, the epidemiology of psittacoid disease in domestic ruminants.

In experimental studies in newborn colostrum-deprived or colostrum-treated Hereford calves infected orally with a bovine chlamydial strain, Doughri et al. (1974) described clinical and pathological changes associated with the disease (Figure 33.4). Gross lesions were found in the abomasum and the intestinal tract, with the terminal portion of the ileum most severely affected. There were edema, petechial hemorrhage, and epithelial erosion and ulceration. Histological features included desquamation of surface epithelium, central lacteal dilatation, occlusion, and dilatation of Lieberkuhn's glands as well as infiltration of the lamina propria by neutrophils and mononuclear cells.

REFERENCES

Doughri, A.M., Young, S., and Storz, J. 1974. Pathological changes in intestinal chlamydial infection of newborn calves. Am. J. Vet. Res. 35:939–944.

Messieri. 1959. Atti Soc. Ital. Sci. Vet. 8:702.

Omuri, T., Ischii, S., and Matumoto, M. 1960. Miyagawanellosis of cattle in Japan. Am. J. Vet. Res. 21:564–573.

York, C.J., and Baker, J.A. 1951. A new member of the psittacosis-lymphogranuloma group of viruses that causes infection in calves. J. Exp. Med. 93:587–603.

Cat-Scratch Disease in Humans

SYNONYMS: Benign lymphoreticulosis, cat-scratch fever; abbreviation, CSD

Cat-scratch disease of humans is commonly associated with a history of contact with a cat, and cat owners frequently ask veterinarians about measures that can be taken to minimize transmission of the causative agent from cats suspected of carrying it. The description of CSD is included with the discussion of pathogenic chlamydias because the causative organism is a bacterium that at one time could not be easily cultured in vitro and because it was once thought to belong to the genus *Chlamydia*.

Morphology and Staining Reactions. The CSD bacterium is a small, pleomorphic, Gram-negative, non-acid-fast bacillus that is found consistently in areas of acute inflammation in recently affected lymph nodes (Wear et al. 1983). The organism is stained by Warthin-Starry silver stain and by Brown-Hopps tissue Gram stain (Hadfield et al. 1985). Organisms stained by the latter technique are only about 0.2 μm in diameter as compared with a diameter of about 0.5 μm when stained by the Warthin-Starry method.

Culture. English et al. (1988) reported successfully culturing the agent of CSD in an aerobic liquid medium consisting of a biphasic brain-heart infusion solution incubated at 30° to 32°C. Gerber et al. (1985) isolated on blood agar an organism that was morphologically similar to the CSD bacterium but that was Gram-positive. The organisms cultured in biphasic brain-heart infusion appear to lack cell walls.

Epidemiology and Pathogenesis. CSD is observed predominantly in children between the ages of 2 and 12 years, and most cases occur in the late summer and autumn. Almost all patients have come in contact with a cat. (Carithers 1985). The exact role of the cat as a source of the CSD agent is unclear; the organism may be a commensal of the skin, paw, or mouth of the animal. Cats implicated as sources of infection are healthy and are usually less than a year old.

Inoculation often results from a scratch but can arise from a puncture wound (Carithers 1985). Conjunctival entry occurs in the manifestation of CSD known as Parinaud's oculoglandular syndrome and is probably effected by the patient's own hand. Soon after the patient is scratched, a pink or red macule develops at the site of inoculation; it later forms a vesicle. The vesicle ruptures, encrusts, and then develops into a small papule a few millimeters to 1 cm in diameter which persists for some weeks. The CSD bacillus is present in the papule. Regional lymphadenopathy becomes evident about 2 to 3 weeks after the scratch was inflicted. The gland is swollen and painful, and fever and other systemic signs may be present. Regional lymphadenopathy is usually unilateral and involves the axillary, cervical, or trochlear lymph glands. The nodes remain enlarged for a long time, and a significant proportion (12 percent) of affected lymph nodes suppurate.

Diagnosis. CSD bacteria can be detected in smears or sections of biopsy material collected in the early stages of lesion development. Warthin-Starry silver stain is effective for microscopic visualization of the organism, which is seen as pleomorphic rods (3 by 0.5 μm) to small coccoid forms 1 μm or less in diameter. The bacteria tend to be extracellular and are distributed as microcolonies in necrotic debris in the center of focal abscesses (Miller-Catchpole et al. 1986, Wear et al. 1983).

A skin test (Hanger-Rose) based on an antigen extracted from heat-treated pus is of great value in the diagnosis of CSD (Daniels and MacMurray 1952). The test is highly specific, with a false-negative rate of only about 1 percent (Carithers 1985).

Antimicrobial Susceptibility. The antimicrobial susceptibility of the CSD bacterium is unknown. Antibiotics do not appear to shorten the course of the disease or to prevent suppuration.

REFERENCES

Carithers, H.A. 1985. Cat-scratch disease: An overview based on a study of 1200 patients. Am. J. Dis. Child. 139:1124–1133.

Daniels, W.B., and MacMurray, F.G. 1952. Cat scratch disease; nonbacterial regional lymphadenitis: A report of 60 cases. Ann. Int. Med. 37:697–713.

English, C.K., Wear, D.J., Margileth, A.M., Lissner, C.R., and Walsh, G.P. 1988. Cat-scratch disease. Isolation and culture of the bacterial agent. J.A.M.A. 259:1347–1352.

Gerber, M.A., MacAlister, T.J., Ballow, M., Sedgwick, A.K., Gustafson, K.B., and Tilton, R.C. 1985. The aetiological agent of cat-scratch disease. Lancet 1:1236–1239.

Hadfield, T.L., Malaty, R.H., VanDellan, A., Wear, D.J., and Margileth, A.M. 1985. Electron microscopy of the bacillus causing cat-scratch disease. J. Infect. Dis. 152:643–645.

Miller-Catchpole, R., Variakojis, D., Vardiaman, J.W., Lowe, J.M., Carter, J. 1986. Cat scratch disease: Identification of bacteria in seven cases of lymphadenitis. Am. J. Surg. Pathol. 10:276–281.

Wear, D.J., Margileth, A.M., Hadfield, T.L., Fischer, G.W., Schlogel, C.J., and King, F.M. 1983. Cat-scratch disease: A bacterial infection. Science 221:1403–1405.

Part II The Pathogenic Fungi

34 Classification and Morphology of the Fungi

Fungi are eukaryotic, nonphotosynthetic, filamentous or unicellular organisms, most of which grow on nonliving materials as saprophytes. They derive nutrition through absorbtion and require both carbon and nitrogen sources. They do not produce flagella, are either haploid or dikaryotic, and exhibit meiotic division. Fungi reproduce asexually by means of specialized, differentiated parts of the thallus or sexually by means of spores formed from the product of fusion of parent haploid nuclei and subsequent meiosis. The sexual phase of the pathogenic fungi is rarely seen during routine clinical mycological work.

Classification. Fungal classification is based on the mode of asexual and sexual spore production and on the morphologic characteristics of these structures, the colonies, and their constituent hyphae. Identification of some fungi, such as yeasts, requires study of certain biochemical and physiological characteristics. The B vitamin requirements of some *Trichophyton* species are also helpful in identification.

The kingdom Fungi (Mycetae) contains six divisions (phyla). These are the Chitridomycota, the Zygomycota, the Ascomycota, the Basidiomycota, the Deuteromycota (Fungi Imperfecti) and the Mycophycophyta. Only the Zygomycota, Ascomycota, Basidiomycota and Deuteromycota contain genera of veterinary importance.

The Zygomycota are characterized by their formation of zoospores or sporangia during asexual reproduction. Sexual reproduction results in zygospores. The hyphae are coenocytic. Examples of genera in this phylum are *Mucor* and *Rhizopus*.

The Ascomycota reproduce asexually by means of conidia. Sexual reproduction occurs in an ascus, a saclike structure that eventually contains eight ascospores (Figure 34.1). The hyphae are septate. *Arthroderma, Nannizzia, Aspergillus, Penicillium, Ajellomyces,* and *Emmonsiella* are examples of genera in this phylum. The genera *Arthroderma* and *Nannizzia* were established for those *Trichophyton* and *Microsporum* species in which a sexual stage (perfect state or teleomorph) in the life cycle has been observed.

The Deuteromycota are often called Fungi Imperfecti because their life cycle is not yet completely defined and a sexual stage has not been observed. The hyphae are septate. Most of the Deuteromycota probably belong in the Ascomycota. Examples of genera in this phylum are *Candida, Cryptococcus, Microsporum, Trichophyton, Sporothrix,* and *Cladosporium*.

Morphology. Because mycology is still very much a descriptive science, visible morphologic features constitute a significant component of the evidence used in identification. The following explanations of commonly used terms in veterinary mycology will prove useful for the next three chapters on specific and opportunistic fungal infections of animals.

Hypha	A single vegetative filament that may contain a number of cells joined end to end.
Mycelium	A mass of hyphae.
Yeast	A unicellular growth form of a fungus.
Septate	Divided by cross-walls, or septums.
Coenocytic	Having few or no septums.

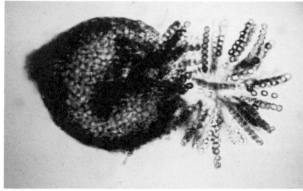

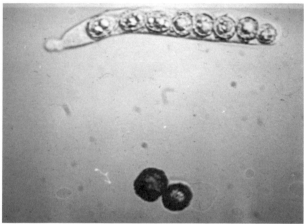

Figure 34.1. (*Top*) Asci being released from an ascocarp. (*Bottom*) Close-up of the eight ascospores in the ascus. The photographs were taken by means of Nomarski interference micrography.

Conidium   A cell that is the product of asexual multiplication.

Spore   A cell that is usually the product of sexual multiplication. However, the term sporangiospore is applied to the asexual propagule of the *Zygomycota*.

There are at least six kinds of conidia, each of which is named according to its mode of production:

Arthroconidia   A conidium formed by fragmentation of a hypha, e.g., *Coccidioides immitis*.

Aleurioconidia   A conidium produced as a swelling of the end of a hypha, e.g., *Trichophyton* spp.

Anneloconidium   A conidium produced from a specialized cell that carries a ringlike

scar for each conidium released, e.g., *Scopulariopsis* spp.

Blastoconidium   A conidium produced as a bud from a parent cell, e.g., *Candida* spp.

Phialoconidium   A conidium produced from within a specialized flask-shaped cell (phialid), e.g., *Phialophora* spp.

Poroconidium   A conidium released through a pore of a specialized cell, e.g., *Drechslera* spp.

The typical fungus exists only in either a filamentous (mold) or a single-cell (yeast) form. Some of the important pathogenic fungi such as *Blastomyces dermatitidis* or *Histoplasma capsulatum* can exist in either mold or yeast forms and are therefore said to be dimorphic. The yeast form is found in deeper tissue or in cultures grown at 37°C in an atmosphere of enriched CO_2. In cultures kept at lower temperatures or in the environment, the filamentous mold form is produced.

The filaments, or hyphae, of molds are usually about 2 to 10 μm in diameter and may be several centimeters long. The hypha lengthens by growth at the tip. The hyphae of most fungi also produce side branches. The more evolved fungi such as the Ascomycota and the Deuteromycota exhibit regular septums along their length. Dark pigments may also be present. Fungi that are pigmented in this way are known as dematiacious fungi. The conidia or sporangiospores also are frequently pigmented with a variety of different colored pigments.

The fungi are nucleated organisms with a definite separation of the chromosomes from the cytoplasm. The DNA content is usually five to ten times that of typical bacteria. Also present are a well-developed endoplasmic reticulum and ribosomes, a Golgi apparatus, mitochondria, and storage granules that contain glycogen or lipid.

The cytoplasm is enclosed by the cytoplasmic membrane which is composed of phospholipids, proteins, glycoprotein, and sterols. The proteins are inserted in a bilayer of phospholipid in which two phospholipid molecules are joined by their lipophilic regions and with their hydrophilic regions facing outward on each side of the bilayer (Singer and Nicolson 1972). The cytoplasmic membrane controls both movement of solutes into and out of the fungal cell and cell wall synthesis.

The fungal cell wall consists of polysaccharides such as cellulose, beta-glucans, and chitin arranged in microcrystalline arrays that confer strength and shape to the fungus (Bartnicki-Garcia 1970). Other polysaccharides known as amorphous homopolysaccharides and protein polysaccharides have a bonding function and, more important, carry the antigenic determinants of the cell wall. In addition, they have a variety of enzyme functions in relation to hyphal penetration of tissue. The surface of the fungal cell wall consists of these amorphous glycoproteins (Ballau 1976).

Some yeasts such as *Cryptococcus neoformans* have thick, acidic polysaccharide capsules that are antiphagocytic and have a number of effects on the immune defense mechanisms of the hosts as well. Because they lie to the outside of the cell wall, these capsules mask the antigenic determinants of the cell wall.

The cell wall chemistry of the yeast phase of dimorphic fungi is quite different from that of the mycelial phase (Oujezdsky et al. 1973). However, the biochemical

mechanisms that underlie the changes seen in dimorphism are poorly understood.

REFERENCES

Ballau, C.D. 1976. Structure and biosynthesis of the mannan component of the yeast cell envelope. Adv. Microbiol. Physiol. 14:93–102.

Bartnicki-Garcia, S. 1970. Cell wall composition and other biochemical markers in fungal phylogeny. In J.B. Harborne, ed., Phytochemical Phylogeny. Academic Press, New York. P. 81.

Singer, S.J., and Nicolson, G.L. 1972. The fluid mosaic model of the structure of cell membranes. Science 175:720–722.

Oujezdsky, K.B., Grone, S.N., and Szaniszolo, P.J. 1973. Morphological and structural changes during the yeast-to-mold conversion of *Phialophora dermatitis*. J. Bacteriol. 113:468–472.

35 The Dermatomycoses

The most frequent causes of superficial mycoses in domestic animals are members of the genera *Microsporum* and *Trichophyton*. These organisms are often referred to as *dermatophytes* because of their association with the skin. They are unique among the pathogenic fungi both because they cause contagious infections and because they are dependent on keratin as a nutrient source; they are among the very few microorganisms that can hydrolyze this substance.

The dermatophytes have considerable zoonotic importance because humans can be infected by all the common species found in animals. Their growth on feathers, hair, nails, and skin elicit host responses manifested in a variety of diseases. These diseases are commonly referred to as *ringworm* (from the circular nature of the lesion) or *tinea* (from the Latin word for the clothes moth, whose feeding habits result in circular holes in woollen cloth).

At least 15 species of *Microsporum* and 21 species of *Trichophyton* have been described (Ajello 1974), but only a few of these are commonly involved in cases of animal ringworm, and some, although keratinophilic, are not known to cause disease. Table 35.1 lists the *Microsporum* and *Trichophyton* species that commonly affect domestic animals.

REFERENCES

Ainsworth, G.C., and Austwick, P.K.C. 1973. Fungal Diseases of Animals, 2d ed. Commonwealth Agricultural Bureaux, Farnham Royal, England, Pp. 10–34.

Ajello, L. 1974. Natural history of the dermatophytes and related fungi. Mycopathol. Mycol. Appl. 53:93–110.

General Characteristics of the Genera *Microsporum* and *Trichophyton*

Morphology. Both *Microsporum* and *Trichophyton* species produce colonies that have a variety of textures, pigments, and rates of growth—characteristics that are valuable in identification. Both produce fine, branching, septate hyphae and varying numbers of macroconidia and microconidia. The macroconidia are large and multilocular (Figure 35.1) with either rough (*Microsporum*) or smooth (*Trichophyton*) walls.

The macroconidia of *Microsporum* species are concentrated toward the center of the colony and are found on the periphery in *Trichophyton* species. Other microscopic features such as chlamydoconidia or spiral hyphae can be present and are useful in identification.

Cultural and Biochemical Features. Good growth occurs on media (such as Sabouraud agar) that contain glucose, neopeptone, and agar. Chloramphenicol and cyclohexamide can be added to inhibit bacterial contaminants and saprophytic fungi, as in Mycobiotic or Mycosel agars. A selective and differential medium (Dermatophyte Test Medium) is also available which changes from yellow to red when dermatophytes are growing and producing alkali on it. Potato dextrose agar that contains potato extract is useful for identification studies because it promotes sporulation, in contrast to Dermatophyte Test Medium, which tends to inhibit it.

Incubation of *Microsporum* and *Trichophyton* organisms is performed at 30°C. The exception is material obtained from bovine samples suspected to contain *T. verrucosum*; these preparations should be incubated at 37°C. A humid environment must be provided and the incubation time can be as long as 3 or 4 weeks because of the slow growth of some dermatophytes.

A series of seven media (*Trichophyton* media) that contain different B vitamins and other growth factors is used for identification of some of the *Trichophyton* species. *T. verrucosum*, the common cause of bovine ringworm, requires inositol and thiamine, and *T. equinum*, a cause of ringworm in horses, requires nicotinic acid for growth. However, a variety (*autotrophicum*) of *T. equinum* in Australia and New Zealand does not require nicotinic acid.

Epizootiology and Pathogenesis. *Microsporum* and *Trichophyton* species are classified as geophilic, zoophilic, or anthropophilic dermatophytes on the basis of their natural habitat. Geophilic dermatophytes (*M. gypseum, M. nanum*) live in the soil and resist the degrading effects of soil bacteria by means of antibacterial substances in their cell walls. Zoophilic dermatophytes (*M. canis, M. distortum, T. gallinae, T. verrucosum, T. equi-*

Table 35.1. The common dermatophyte species affecting animals

Host animal	Dermatophyte
Horse	*T. equinum**
	T. mentagrophytes
	T. verrucosum
	M. gypseum
	M. canis
Ox	*T. verrucosum**
	T. mentagrophytes
	T. equinum
Sheep†	*M. canis*
	T. mentagrophytes
Pig	*M. nanum**
	M. gypseum
Poultry	*M. gallinae** (*T. gallinae*)
	T. simiae
Dog	*M. canis**
	M. gypseum
	T. mentagrophytes
	M. audouini
Cat	*M. canis**
	M. gypseum
	T. mentagrophytes

*The most common dermatophyte species.
†Rarely infected by dermatophytes.
Note: A more exhaustive list of species of dermatophytes found in animals is given in Ainsworth and Austwick (1973).

num) are specialized parasites of the skin of animals and are not known to live in soil as saprophytes. Several of these organisms are readily transmitted from animals to humans. Anthropophilic dermatophytes (*T. mentagrophytes* var. *interdigitale, T. tonsurans, M. audouini*) are parasites of human skin and can survive briefly in the soil.

Animal infections by geophilic dermatophytes are contracted by exposure to contaminated soil. These infections are sporadic and do not spread readily between animals. An important factor in the infectivity of soil is the presence of hair. For instance, soil-derived infections of dogs by *M. gypseum* occur only in situations where hair and macroconidia are present together in the soil (Kushida 1978). The infections are observed in autumn after the fungus multiplies on the hair during the summer. In Australia, moist atmospheric conditions and the activities of biting insects have been associated with outbreaks of *M. gypseum* infection in horses (Pascoe and Connole, 1974).

Infections by zoophilic dermatophytes are seen mostly in young, sexually immature animals that are kept in close contact. High humidity and environmental temperature, traumatization of the neck and shoulder areas by collars or chains, and poor nutrition are common predisposing factors (Pascoe 1979). Abrasions from harness straps, brushes, and self-grooming activities are therefore important influences in the occurrence and transmission of zoophilic dermatophyte infections. Lesions in cats and dogs thus are common on the head and paws.

Survival of the conidia (arthrospores) of zoophilic dermatophytes on the interior surfaces of buildings depends on the availability of moisture. The conidia are highly resistant to freezing but extremely susceptible to desicca-

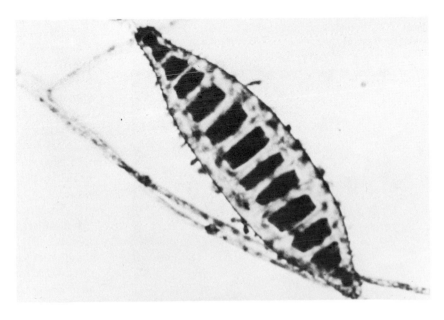

Figure 35.1. A multilocular macroconidium *Microsporum canis* showing the rough surface typical of the genus. × 880.

tion and also to temperatures greater than 50°C (Hoshimoti and Blumenthal 1978). Conidia of *T. verrucosum* that contaminate buildings are probably the most important means by which the infection is maintained from one season to the next. In the case of *M. canis*, carrier cats and dogs are a very important source of infection for other animals. The conidia of *T. equinum* have been observed to remain infective for 3 years (Krivanec et al. 1978).

Both *Microsporum* and *Trichophyton* species enter the skin through abrasions. The conidium germinates and hyphae appear within the stratum corneum and invade the walls of the hair follicles. They then emerge into the follicular canal and grow downward between the hair cuticle and wall of the follicle. The hyphal tip penetrates into the hair cortex by dissolving the keratin and by mechanical pressure. Massive hyphal and conidial (arthrospore) formation then occur in the peripilar space and to a lesser extent in the cortex (Hutton et al. 1978). As the hair grows, the fungal elements are carried out of the hair follicle and above the surface of the skin. Many of these hairs fall out or are broken off.

In endothrix infections the hyphae and conidia are located within the hair, whereas in ectothrix infections the conidia are located on the hair (Figure 35.2). All of the common dermatophyte infections of animals are of the ectothrix type. The conidia of *Trichophyton* species tend to form linear chains on the hair.

Extensive hyphal growth and spore formation also occurs in the stratum corneum of the epidermis and a hyperkeratosis soon develops. The fungal invasion spreads centrifugally from the point of initial invasion, resulting

Figure 35.2. Ectothrix conidia (arthrospores) of *Trichophyton mentagrophytes* on the exterior of a hair from an infected rat. × 400.

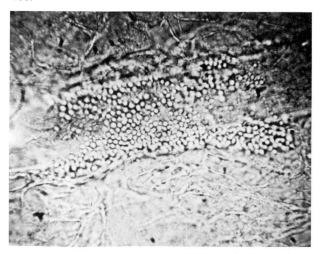

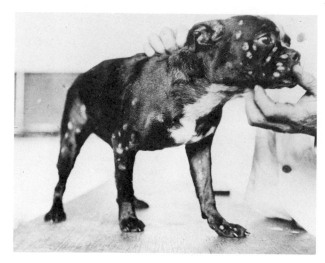

Figure 35.3. Ringworm in a dog. (Courtesy H. J. Milks and H. C. Stephenson.)

in a ring-shaped lesion. Because the greatest inflammatory response is at the zone of recent fungal invasion, the circular nature of the lesion is emphasized. The dermatophytic fungi do not invade the living areas of the skin, although their presence in the dead layers does provoke an active inflammatory response beneath the stratum malpighii. They show a preference for the hairy body surfaces. The hairs become brittle and appear dry and lusterless. The skin of affected areas becomes scaly and harsh and crusts form. In cats and dogs the lesions are most common on the head, elbows, and paws (Figure 35.3). In cattle the lesions involve principally the head and neck. In horses friction areas such as the saddle girth are usually affected. The lesions in cats can be difficult to detect and may be present as a faint scurfiness in the fur resembling cigarette ashes.

Generally speaking, ringworm thrives best in young animals and in older ones that have been devitalized by disease or malnutrition. It is seen more often in stabled animals than in those on pasture and more often in winter than in summer. Ringworm infection that has become widespread in groups of calves will often clear up spontaneously in the spring several weeks after the animals have been turned out into the sunshine. This may be a result of better nutrition or it may be the result of the direct influence of the light. Ultraviolet light has proved useful in the treatment of many forms of ringworm.

Immunity. *Microsporum* and *Trichophyton* species possess both group- and species-specific antigens that are highly allergenic and elicit a state of delayed hypersensitivity (Jadassohn et al. 1935). Precipitins and complement-fixing antibodies appear about 30 to 80 days after infection in some animals but are usually present in low titer. In addition most animal serums contain a nonantibody antifungal factor that restricts the growth of dermatophytes to the stratum corneum (Grappel et al. 1974).

Dermatophyte infection can result in the development of resistance to reinfection. This resistance can be local and such that reinfection of the original infection site is of restricted duration and severity. *T. verrucosum* antigen apparently persists at the site of original infection in cattle or stimulates formation of persisting sensitized immunocytes, which give rise to an immediate skin reaction at this site when an extract of the fungus is injected intravenously (Lepper 1972). Immunity is always associated with the development of delayed hypersensitivity, which appears in cattle 14 days after infection with *T. verrucosum* (Lepper 1972). It disappears on healing of the lesions but is recalled within 2 days after reinfection. This memory persists for at least a year. *T. equinum* infection in horses produces a strong stable immunity lasting at least 3 to 4 years (Pascoe 1976). The strength of the immunity depends on the length and severity of clinical disease (Sarkisov and Petrovich 1976).

Live vaccines prepared from the mycelium of *T. verrucosum* have been successfully used in cattle (Florian et al. 1964, Kielstein and Richter 1970, Naess and Sandvik 1981). Sarkisov and Petrovich (1976) showed that a *T. verrucosum* vaccine gave protection for 3 to 5 years. This was confirmed by Krdzalic et al. (1978), who used LTF-130 vaccine to produce similar effects. These workers found that this vaccine was also effective when used therapeutically and produced remissions within a few weeks of administration.

Diagnosis. Direct microscopic examination and culture of skin scrapings and hairs from the periphery of suspect lesions is necessary to confirm a clinical diagnosis of dermatophyte infection. The steps involved in the laboratory diagnosis of ringworm are shown in Figure 35.4. Detection of lesions in cats and dogs can be greatly enhanced by preliminary screening with ultraviolet light from a Wood's lamp. An apple green fluorescence is produced by hairs invaded by *M. canis, M. distortum,* or *M. audouini.* Fluorescent hairs can be removed with a forceps and examined microscopically. A toothbrush can also be used to check the coats of animals for dermatophytes. Skin scrapings are placed in a drop of 20 percent potassium hydroxide solution, gently warmed, and examined under the microscope with reduced lighting. Preparations stained with periodic acid–Schiff (PAS) stain are more reliable and easier to interpret than potassium hydroxide preparations because the fungal elements stain a deep red. However, the latter method is simpler and more suited to the practice laboratory. Hyphae and conidia can be present both in infected skin scales and on hairs.

Specimens for culture should be transported in an envelope or petri dish. Sealed glass containers are unsuitable because moisture can permit growth of contaminating bacteria and fungi. The specimens should be placed on Dermatophyte Test Medium, on Mycobiotic (or Mycosel) agar, and on Sabouraud dextrose agar. Plates should be incubated at 30°C. If *T. verrucosum* is suspected, the incubation temperature should be 37°C. A moist atmosphere must be maintained during incubation, which should be continued for 1 to 4 weeks if necessary.

Culture of specimens is necessary not only to allow

Figure 35.4. Laboratory diagnosis of ringworm.

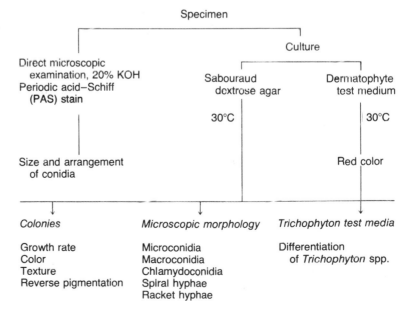

direct microscopic confirmation of the diagnoses but also to allow identification of the dermatophyte. The elements present in skin scrapings are usually not characteristic enough to permit definitive identification. Immunological methods are not typically used for detection of dermatophyte infections of animals.

Antimicrobial Susceptibility. Both *Trichophyton* and *Microsporum* species are sensitive to 0.5 µg/ml of griseofulvin, an antibiotic produced by *Penicillium griseofulvum*. Griseofulvin is highly effective in the treatment of dermatophyte infections in cats (Kaplan and Ajello 1959), chinchillas (Belloff 1967), and cattle (Andrews and Edwardson 1981, Lauder and O'Sullivan 1958). The antibiotic is administered orally in fine particle size for up to 6 weeks and becomes incorporated into the keratin in the skin and hair. Treated animals are therefore refractory to reinfection for a number of weeks after treatment is discontinued (Huddleston 1973). Griseofulvin binds to intracellular lipids and interferes with DNA synthesis so that fungal cells are unable to divide normally. It thus has a fungistatic effect. Teratogenic effects in pregnant cats have also been observed (Scott et al. 1975).

Miconazole and other imidazoles such as clotrimazole and enilconazole damage fungal membrane function and structure by inhibiting ergosterol synthesis. Miconazole thus is commonly incorporated into ointments for topical application to ringworm lesions. Oral administration of ketoconazole to dogs and cats (10 mg/kg of body weight for 20 days) is highly effective in the treatment of ringworm (de Keyser and van den Brande 1983).

Preparations that contain oils, povidone, iodine, sulfur, captan, salicylic acid, sodium caprylate, and a variety of other drugs are also used as treatment for ringworm. Chinchillas with ringworm have been treated with iodochlorohydroxyquinoline (Hayes 1956). Natamycin has been successfully used in a topical application for treatment of horses with *T. equinum* infection (Oldenkamp 1979). Thiabendazole has been shown to inhibit *T. verrucosum* infection in cattle when applied topically (Krivanec et al. 1978).

Formaldehyde vapor or 2.5 percent lime sulfur solution can be used as a disinfectant for contaminated tack or other fomites or surfaces (Pascoe 1979).

REFERENCES

Andrews, A.H., and Edwardson, J. 1981. Treatment of ringworm in calves using griseofulvin. Vet. Rec. 108:498–500.
Belloff, G.B. 1967. The feeding of griseofulvin in treatment of trichophytosis (ringworm) in chinchillas. Vet. Med. 62:438–440.
de Keyser, H., and van den Brande, M. 1983. Ketoconazole in the treatment of dermatomycosis in cats and dogs. Vet. Q. 5:142–144.

Florian, E.L., Nemeseri, L., and Lovas, G. 1964. Active immunization of calves against ringworm. Magy. Allatorv. Lapja 19:529–530.
Grappel, S.F., Bishop, C.T., and Blank, F. 1974. Immunology of dermatophytes. Bacteriol. Rev. 38:222–250.
Hayes, F.A. 1956. Treatment of ringworm in chinchillas. J. Am. Vet. Med. Assoc. 128:193–195.
Huddleston, W.A. 1973. The treatment of bovine ringworm. Vet. Rec. 92:123.
Hoshimoti, T., and Blumenthal, H.J. 1978. Survival and resistance of *Trichophyton mentagrophytes* arthrospores. Appl. Environ. Microbiol. 35:274–277.
Hutton, R.D., Kerbs, S., and Yee, K. 1978. Scanning electron microscopy of experimental *Trichophyton mentagrophytes* infection in guinea pig skin. Infect. Immun. 21:247–253.
Jadassohn, W., Schaaf, F., and Laetsch, W. 1935. Antigenanalytische Untersuchungen an Trichophytinen. Arch. Dermatol. Syphilol. 171:461–468.
Kaplan, W., and Ajello, L. 1959. Oral treatment of spontaneous ringworm in cats with griseofulvin. J. Am. Vet. Med. Assoc. 135:253–261.
Kielstein, P., and Richter, W. 1970. Prophylaxis of bovine ringworm on large farms by active immunisation (preliminary communication). Monatsh. Veterinärmed. 25:334–337.
Krdzalic, P., Stojicevic, S., and Bresjanac, D. 1978. Feasibility of immunizing large herds of cattle against ringworm (using Russian LTF–130 vaccine). Vet. Glas. 32:343–349.
Krivanec, K., Dvorak, J., and Hanak, F. 1978. Dermatophytosis in cattle caused by *Trichophyton equinum*. Zentralbl. Veterinärmed. [B] 25:356–362.
Kushida, T. 1978. Studies on dermatophytosis in dogs. III. An experimental study on some factors for establishment of infection with *Microsporum gypseum* of soil origin. Jpn. J. Vet. Sci. 40:1–7.
Lauder, I.M., and O'Sullivan, J.G. 1958. Ringworm in cattle. Vet. Rec. 70:949–951.
Lepper, A.W.D. 1972. Experimental bovine *Trichophyton verrucosum* infection. Res. Vet. Sci. 13:105–115.
Naess, B., and Sandvik, O. 1981. Early vaccination of calves against ringworm caused by *Trichophyton verrucosum*. Vet. Rec. 109:199–200.
Oldenkamp, E.P. 1979. Treatment of ringworm in horses with natamycin. Equine Vet. J. 11:36–38.
Pascoe, R.R. 1976. Studies on the prevalence of ringworm among horses in racing and breeding stables. Aust. Vet. J. 52:419–421.
Pascoe, R. R. 1979. The epidemiology of ringworm in racehorses caused by *Trichophyton equinum* var. *autotrophicum*. Aust. Vet. J. 55:403–407.
Pascoe, R.R., and Connole, M.D. 1974. Dermatomycosis due to *Microsporum gypseum* in horses. Aust. Vet. J. 50:380–383.
Sarkisov, A.K., and Petrovich, S.V. 1976. Immunity of horses to spontaneous and experimental ringworm caused by *Trichophyton equinum*. Veterinarii 11:39–40.
Scott, F.W., de Lahunta, A., Schultz, R.D., Bistner, S.I., and Riis, R.C. 1975. Teratogenesis in cats associated with griseofulvin therapy. Teratology 11:79.

The Genus *Microsporum*

Microsporum canis

PERFECT STATE: *Nannizzia otae*

M. canis is distributed throughout the world and causes almost all ringworm cases in cats and about 70 percent of cases in dogs. The natural host of this dermatophyte is probably the cat, but a wide variety of animals, including humans, can be infected. Siamese and Persian cats appear to be more susceptible than other breeds.

The disease appears as small scabby areas on any part of the body but is seen most frequently on the ears, face, neck, and tail. These areas do not appear to cause much irritation, nor do they have any appreciable effect on the general health of the animal. The hair is not shed, especially in cats. If the disease affects an individual of a long-haired breed and occurs on parts that are especially well covered with fur, the lesions may be overlooked until the disease has spread over a considerable part of the body. Such cases resist treatment, and animals so affected readily infect other cats, dogs, and often human beings with whom they come in contact. Rebell et al. (1956) found that kittens react to experimental infection with *M. canis* by producing only a minimal inflammatory response, which reaches a peak in about 28 days and then regresses. In humans the disease can appear on the scalp, or circinate lesions may appear on the relatively hairless parts of the body. There are records of the disease being transmitted indirectly by human agency from one cat to another.

REFERENCE

Rebell, G., Timmons, H.F., Lamb, J.H., Hicks, P.K., Groves, F., and Coalson, R.E. 1956. Experimental *Microsporum canis* infections in kittens. Am. J. Vet. Res. 17:74–78.

Microsporum gypseum

PERFECT STATES: *Nannizzia gypsea,*
  Nannizzia incurvata

M. gypseum commonly occurs in the soil throughout the world and causes sporadic infections in many different animal hosts. The typical colonial appearance and macroconidia are shown in Figure 35.5. Macroconidia can contaminate the skin and hair from contact with soil in the absence of any disease. *M. gypseum* causes about a quarter of all canine ringworm cases in the United States and about 1 percent of cases in cats. It causes the majority of equine ringworm cases in the southern United States.

There are at least two perfect states of *M. gypseum* in which a sexual phase in the life cycle has been seen: *Nannizzia gypsea* and *N. incurvata*. The epizootiological significance of these two species in relation to animal disease is not known.

REFERENCE

Menges, R.W. 1954. Histoplasmin sensitivity in animals. Cornell Vet. 44:21–31.

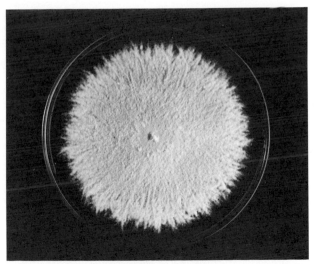

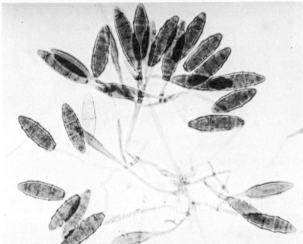

Figure 35.5. *Microsporum gypseum.* (*Top*) Cultural appearance on Sabouraud glucose agar. (*Bottom*) Macroconidia. × 315. (From Menges, 1954, courtesy of *Cornell Veterinarian.*)

Microsporum nanum

PERFECT STATE: *Nannizzia obtusa*

M. nanum occurs on swine in the United States, Australia, New Zealand, Kenya, and Cuba. Although the infection was not reported in the United States until 1964, it must have been present before then because the fungus is common in the soil in many regions. Lesions begin as small circular areas that gradually enlarge in a circular fashion until they cover much of the animal's body. Most have a somewhat roughened although not obviously raised surface that is covered with thin brown crusts that are easily removed. The crusts can cover the area uniformly, or they can be more prominent at the periphery, forming a band that clearly outlines the infected area. Other lesions have few brown crusts but have a red cast or

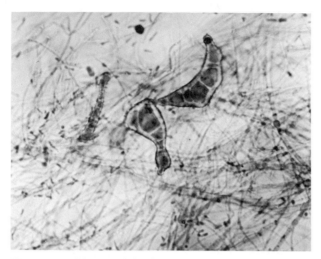

Figure 35.6. Macroconidia of *Microsporum distortum* showing their characteristic shapes. × 400.

a brown, speckled appearance. There is no alopecia, pruritus, or general involvement, and lesions can be hidden by dirt and easily overlooked. Hyphae are the only fungal elements usually found in lesions. *M. nanum* has been isolated from cases of ringworm in humans.

Microsporum distortum

M. distortum has been reported only in Australia, New Zealand, and the United States (Ajello 1974). Infections in cats and dogs have occasionally been reported, but the most important host appears to be primates in laboratory colonies. The macroconidia have bizarre shapes that are highly characteristic (Figure 35.6).

REFERENCE

Ajello, L. 1974. Natural history of the dermatophytes and related fungi. Mycopathol. Mycol. Appl. 53:93–110.

Microsporum audouini

M. audouini is the most common of the anthropophilic *Microsporum* species and is the primary agent of tinea capitis in children. Puppies and monkeys can be infected from human cases and can therefore serve as sentinels of infection in human communities. These infections are usually seen in animals from economically depressed urban areas. The circular lesions are single or scattered, and are accompanied by loss of hair, scaling, and some erythema.

Microsporum gallinae
SYNONYMS: *Achorion gallinae,* *Trichophyton gallinae*

Favus (or *white comb*) of fowl, particularly chickens and turkeys, is a disease of minor importance in Europe and the United States. It also occurs in wild birds and has been reported in humans and dogs. It appears as small white patches on the comb, usually of male birds (Figure 35.7). These enlarge and coalesce, so that finally the comb is covered with a dull white, moldy layer several millimeters thick. The disease usually is self-limiting, healing after several months if untreated. Scutula are not found on the comb lesions, but occasionally the disease extends into the feathered parts, in which case typical shields are formed. As long as the disease is limited to the comb, the health of the bird is little affected. When the feathered portions are involved, however, the bird becomes emaciated and may die.

The Genus *Trichophyton*

Trichophyton verrucosum
SYNONYMS: *Trichophyton album,* *Trichophyton discoides, Trichophyton faviforme, Trichophyton ochraceum*

T. verrucosum survives for years in farm buildings. Muende and Webb (1937) found visible colonies growing on semidried fecal material over a period of 3 to 4 weeks in a stable in England.

Ringworm of cattle is a very common disease, especially in young animals kept indoors during winter. The causative agent is easily demonstrated, but the lesions are so characteristic that demonstration of the fungus is unnecessary for diagnosis. Hairs plucked from the margins of the lesions and examined microscopically have large, ectothrix conidia (arthrospores). The fungus grows slowly and is often overgrown by contaminants. It requires thiamine and inositol for growth.

The lesions are usually found on the face, particularly around the eyes, and also occur on the neck and shoulders. They consist of raised, dry, crusty, grayish white masses from which a few broken hairs protrude. The disease spreads rapidly among calves kept under crowded conditions in damp, dark housing. Infections of the face, wrists, and hands are frequent in humans who have contact with infected stock.

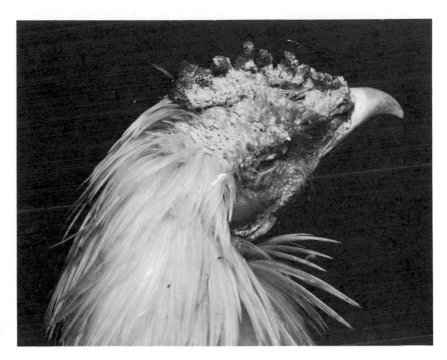

Figure 35.7. Lesions of favus in a chicken. This condition is caused by *Microsporum (Trichophyton) gallinae*.

REFERENCE

Muende, I., and Webb, P. 1937. Ringworm fungus growing as a saprophyte under natural conditions. Arch. Dermatol. 36:987–990.

Trichophyton equinum and *T. equinum* var. *autotrophicum*

Ringworm of horses is occasionally a common skin disease in large stables. The disease spreads readily, principally through the use of common grooming tools, harnesses, and blankets. Outbreaks can be controlled only by treatment of the affected animals and by thorough disinfection of all stable equipment. The disease is most common in autumn and winter, and the majority of cases are observed during periods of high humidity (Pascoe 1979).

Lesions appear on parts of the body where harness or blanket straps rub the skin. The face, breast, croup, flanks, and back where the saddle and saddle girth rub are the areas most often involved. Areas subject to abrasion from buckles are especially likely to be affected. The hair on these areas breaks off and much of it comes out, leaving semibald patches. The skin becomes progressively thickened and covered with flaky crusts. The underlying skin is dry and has a dull luster. Bacterial infections often complicate the picture, making the areas moist and reddened. The disease in horses is not debilitating and the principal damage is the temporary disfigurement of the coat. If untreated the disease can spread over large areas. A case of infection by this species has been recorded in a dog (Goldberg 1965).

REFERENCES

Goldberg, H.C. 1965. Brush technique for detection of fungus diseases. J. Am. Vet. Med. Assoc. 147:845.
Pascoe, R.R. 1976. Studies on the prevalence of ringworm among horses in racing and breeding stables. Austral. Vet. J. 52:419–421.

Trichophyton mentagrophytes
SYNONYMS: *Trichophyton granulosum, Trichophyton gypseum, Trichophyton quinckeanum*

PERFECT STATES: *Arthroderma benhamiae, Arthroderma vanbreuseghemii*

T. mentagrophytes commonly infects mice, rats, dogs, cats, rabbits, chinchillas, and guinea pigs in laboratory colonies (Figure 35.8). It is seen occasionally in horses, cows, muskrats, opossums, squirrels, and foxes and rarely in swine (Ginther and Ajello 1965). Mice infected with this species have transmitted it to cats, in which the lesions most commonly occur around the paws and on the ears. Wild rodents appear to be the natural reservoir of the zoophilic variant *T. mentagrophytes* var. *mentagrophytes*. The zoophilic variant has granular and red-pig-

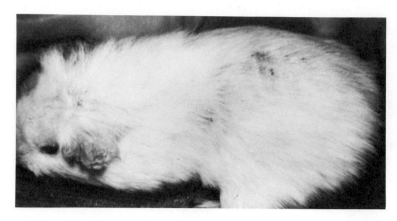

Figure 35.8. *Trichophyton mentagrophytes* infection in a laboratory guinea pig.

mented colonies, whereas the variant found in humans (*T. mentagrophytes* var. *interdigitalis*) produces white downy colonies. *T. mentagrophytes* var. *mentagrophytes,* with *T. rubrum,* is the prime cause of athlete's foot in humans in the United States (Ajello 1974).

The zoophilic strains isolated from animals frequently change to the white downy form upon prolonged subcultivation. Humans directly infected by the zoophilic form from contact with animals develop typical ringworm.

REFERENCES

Ajello, L. 1974. Natural history of the dermatophytes and related fungi. Mycopathol. Mycol. Appl. 53:93–110.

Ginther, O.J., and Ajello, L. 1965. The prevalence of *Microsporum nanum* infection in swine. J. Am. Vet. Med. Assoc. 146:361–365.

36 The Systemic Mycoses

The systemic mycoses are a group of truly pathogenic fungi that invade the internal organs following hematogenous carriage from the lungs. The majority of infections are clinically inapparent. The systemic mycoses differ from the opportunistic mycoses described in Chapter 37 in being inherently invasive in healthy subjects, in having a unique tissue form, and in having restricted geographic distribution. They include *Blastomyces dermatitidis*, *Coccidoides immitis*, *Histoplasma capsulatum*, *H. farciminosum*, and *Paracoccidioides (Blastomyces) brasiliensis*. *P. brasiliensis* is not a significant pathogen of animals.

The Genus *Blastomyces*

The genus *Blastomyces* is included in the phylum Ascomycota. Although the generic name *Ajellomyces* has been applied to the perfect state of *Blastomyces dermatitidis*, we call this fungus by its older name.

Blastomyces dermatitidis
PERFECT STATE: *Ajellomyces dermatitidis*

B. dermatitidis causes *North American blastomycosis*, a chronic granulomatous and suppurative mycotic infection that occurs occasionally in humans and animals. The lesions may be confined to the skin and subcutaneous tissue, or the disease may be generalized. The organisms appear as yeastlike bodies in infected tissues, but in cultures they produce a mycelial growth (dimorphism).

B. dermatitidis is common in the eastern and central United States and in Canada. Sporadic isolations have been reported from Africa, Europe, and the Middle East. Blastomycosis was first recognized in dogs by Meyer (1912). Since then the organism has been reported in dogs (Newberne et al. 1955, McDonough and Kuzman 1980), in a horse (Benbrook et al. 1948), in cats (Jasmin et al. 1969, Nasisse et al. 1985), in a sea lion (Williamson et al. 1959), and in humans.

Morphology and Staining Characteristics. *B. dermatitidis* has a spherical, thick-walled, budding, yeastlike form in tissue or exudates and in culture at 37°C. The cells are 7 to 15 μm in diameter, with single buds resembling those found in exudates or tissues. They are positive for periodic acid–Schiff stain and stain well with silver impregnation techniques. The mycelial form seen at 25°C consists of fine, septate hyphae that carry small pear-shaped aleurioconidia (2 to 4 μm in diameter).

Cultural Features. *B. dermatitidis* grows well on common laboratory media, where it becomes wrinkled, waxy, and yeastlike at 37°C. At 25°C it develops slowly as a typical moldlike filamentous fungus. The colonies are white-buff to brown and may be either furrowed or smooth. They are very slow growing and do not attain full development for 3 weeks or more.

Antigens. The antigens of *B. dermatitidis* are poorly defined. Yeast cell walls carry a species-specific antigen (Lancaster and Sprouse 1976). Many antigens are shared with other systemic mycoses.

Epizootiology and Pathogenesis. Blastomycosis is more prevalent in the middle Atlantic, south central, and St. Lawrence and Ohio–Mississippi River Valley states. There is no evidence that the disease is contagious, and no proof that it is transmitted from person to person or from animal to animal. There has been much speculation over whether its presence in soil is a source of infection. Denton et al. (1961) isolated *B. dermatitidis* from a soil sample that came from a tobacco-stripping barn in Lexington, Kentucky, that had sheltered a dog that died of blastomycosis 2 years previously. In 1964 it was recovered from 10 of 356 soil samples collected in an endemic area in Augusta, Georgia (Denton and DiSalvo 1964). In Wisconsin enzootic areas are located where the soil is sandy and acidic (Archer et al. 1987), and most dogs with blastomycosis are from areas in the state that are close to rivers or dams, where the soil is wet and organic matter is abundant. The organism appears to be a self-sufficient saprophyte, capable of thriving in nature. The yeast phase of the organism seems to be the infective phase and survives for only a short time in soil (McDonough et al. 1965). Ajello (1967) remarked that elucidation of the habitat of *B. dermatitidis* presents one

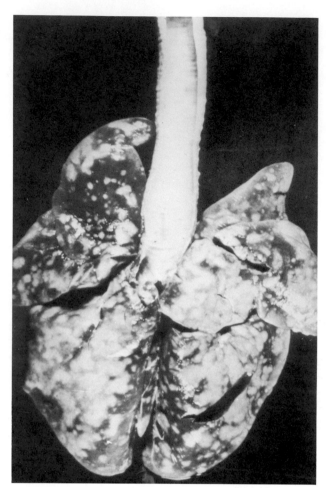

Figure 36.1. Lesions of *Blastomyces dermatitidis* in the lungs of a dog.

of the greatest ecological challenges in microbiology.

The organism most commonly enters an animal through the respiratory tract. In dogs the lungs are most frequently infected and show the most extensive lesions (Figure 36.1). A chronic granulomatous lesion develops which may metastasize to other sites such as the eye, skin, and subcutis. The lungs are dotted with miliary nodules. The animal slowly loses condition and has a chronic cough, shortness of breath, and irregular pyrexia. Lameness may also be present. Cutaneous blastomycosis in dogs can occur as a primary skin infection in the form of papulopustules. Lesions can also appear in the spleen, liver, kidneys, lungs, and intestines. Ocular involvement has been observed in some dogs (Simon and Helper 1970), as has secondary amyloidosis of the kidneys, liver, and spleen (Sherwood et al. 1967).

Systemic blastomycosis has been described in Siamese cats (Jasmin et al. 1969); because most reported cases in cats have occurred in this breed, there may be a breed

susceptibility. A case of disseminated blastomycosis in a cat has been described in detail by Nasisse et al (1985). This case had a pyogranulomatous chorioretinitis with large numbers of yeast cells within the tapetum.

Immunity. Protective immunity in blastomycosis appears to be cell-mediated. Animals that develop clinically apparent systemic disease rarely recover. The relentless progression of the disease suggests that the infection itself may be immunosuppressive. Depression of lymphocyte responsiveness has been observed in cases of acute canine blastomycosis (Legendre and Backer 1982).

Complement-fixing antibodies can be demonstrated in the serums of animals with extensive or progressive infection but not in the serums of animals with localized cutaneous lesions. However, neither this nor any other serologic procedure is reliable for diagnosis or surveys.

Diagnosis. The characteristic spherical, thick-walled budding yeast 8 to 20 μm in diameter in tissues, exudates, or tracheal aspirates is easily recognized (Figure 36.2). However, yeast cells can be difficult to find in some specimens. On Sabouraud dextrose agar at room temperature, *B. dermatitidis* grows as white to tan mold that produces round to oval conidia ranging in size from 3 to 5 μm. Such cultures can be confused with unusual isolates of *Histoplasma capsulatum* and with some *Chrysosporium* species that bear small conidia (Kaufman and Standard 1978). Definitive identification in this situation requires conversion to the typical tissue (yeast) form, which may be difficult with some strains. Alternatively, the antigen produced by the mycelial form can be identified by immunodiffusion using standard antiserums prepared against the A precipitin (Kaufman et al. 1973).

Antimicrobial Susceptibility. *B. dermatitidis* is sensitive to amphotericin B (0.4–0.8 μg/ml) 5 fluorocytosine (25 μg/ml), 2-hydroxystilbamidine, ketoconazole, and stilbamidine. Only ketoconazole and amphotericin B are of low enough toxicity for long-term systemic use.

The Disease in Humans. In humans the disease may occur as the cutaneous form, with the initial lesion appearing on the exposed skin surface following trauma. Systemic infection is usually pulmonary in origin but may result from metastasis of a cutaneous lesion. The disease extends mainly by the hematogenous route. Although the disease can be transmitted from dogs to humans through bites, most cases in humans are contracted from the environment.

REFERENCES

Ajello, L. 1967. Comparative ecology of respiratory mycotic disease agents. Bacteriol. Rev. 31:6–24.
Archer, J.R., Trainer, D.O., and Schell, R.F. 1987. Epidemiologic

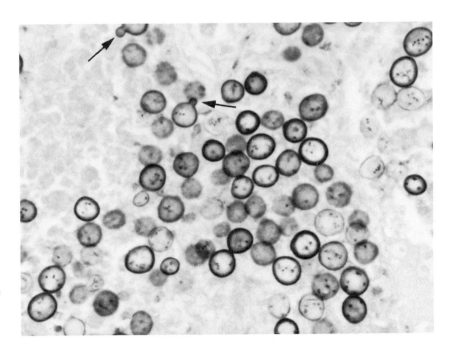

Figure 36.2. Cells of *Blastomyces dermatitidis* in the lung of a dog. The yeast cells are thick-walled and replicate by budding (*arrows*). Gomori-methanamine-silver stain. × 1500. (Courtesy J. Saunders.)

study of canine blastomycosis in Wisconsin. J. Am. Vet. Med. Assoc. 190:1292–1295.

Benbrook, E.A., Bryant, J.B., and Saunders, L.Z. 1948. A case of blastomycosis in the horse. J. Am. Vet. Med. Assoc. 112:475–78.

Denton, J.F., and DiSalvo, A.F. 1964. Isolation of *Blastomyces dermatitidis* from natural sites at Augusta, Georgia. Am. J. Trop. Med. Hyg. 13:716–722.

Denton, J.F., McDonough, E.S., Ajello, L., and Ausherman, R.J. 1961. Isolation of *Blastomyces dermatitidis* from soil. Science 133:1126–1127.

Jasmin, A.M., Carroll, J.M., and Baucom, J.N. 1969. Systemic blastomycosis in Siamese cats. Vet. Med. 64:33–37.

Kaufman, L., and Standard, P. 1978. Improved version of the exoantigen test for identification of *Coccidioides immitis* and *Histoplasma capsulatum* cultures. J. Clin. Microbiol. 8:42–45.

Kaufman, L., McLaughlin, D.W., Clark, M.J., and Blumer, S. 1973. Specific immunodiffusion test for blastomycosis. Appl. Microbiol. 26.244–247.

Lancaster, M.V., and Sprouse, R.F. 1976. Isolation of a purified skin test antigen from *Blastomyces dermatitidis* yeast-phase cell wall. Infect. Immun. 14:623–625.

Legendre, A.M., and Becker, P.U. 1982. Immunologic changes in acute canine blastomycosis. Am. J. Vet. Res. 43:2050–2053.

McDonough, E.S., and Kuzman, J.F. 1980. Epidemiological studies on blastomycosis in the state of Wisconsin. Sabouraudia 18:173–183.

McDonough, E.S., Van Prooien, R., and Lewis, A.L. 1965. Lysis of *Blastomyces dermatitidis* yeast-phase cells in natural soil. Am. J. Epidemiol. 81:86–93.

Meyer, K.F. 1912. Blastomycosis in dogs. Proc. Pathol. Soc. Philadelphia 15:10.

Nasisse, N.P., Van Ee, R.T., and Wright, B. 1985. Ocular changes in a cat with disseminated blastomycosis. J. Am. Vet. Med. Assoc. 187:629–631.

Newberne, J.W., Neal, J.E., and Heath, M.K. 1955. Some clinical and microbiological observations on four cases of canine blastomycosis. J. Am. Vet. Med. Assoc. 12:220–223.

Sherwood, B.F., LeMay, J.C., Castellanos, R.A. 1967. Blastomycosis with secondary amyloidosis in the dog. J. Am. Vet. Med. Assoc. 150:1377–1381.

Simon, J., and Helper, L.C. 1970. Ocular disease associated with blastomycosis in dogs. J. Am. Vet. Med. Assoc. 157:922–925.

Williamson, W.M., Lombard, L.S., and Getty, R.E. 1959. North American blastomycosis in a northern sea lion. J. Am. Vet. Med. Assoc. 135:513–515.

The Genus *Coccidioides*

Coccidioides immitis

C. immitis was originally thought to be a protozoon. The form that occurs in the lesions resembles an oocyst of a coccidium, and it is from this resemblance that the generic name was derived.

The fungus is the causative agent of an influenzalike disease of considerable importance in humans, especially among those living in the valleys of central and southern California. Most patients recover in 3 to 6 weeks. The fungus also occurs in Arizona and Texas in the United States and in Argentina, Paraguay, Bolivia, Guatemala, Honduras, Venezuela, Colombia, and Mexico. Most of the early cases of human infection originated in the valley of the San Joaquin River, and the disease became well known as the *San Joaquin Valley disease, valley fever,* and *desert fever.* Coccidiodomycosis has also been documented in dogs, burros, swine, sheep, horses, a monkey, a gorilla, a chinchilla, a llama, a tapir, and several species of wild rodents (Maddy 1959b).

Morphology and Staining Reactions. As it occurs in purulent material and granulation tissue from lesions, the fungus appears as spherical bodies (known as spherules or sporangia) that vary from 10 to 80 μm in diameter. The wall is double-contoured and highly refractile (Figure

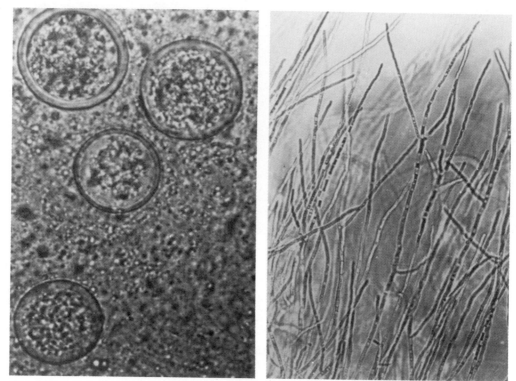

Figure 36.3 (*left*). Several spherules of *Coccidioides immitis* contained in pus expressed from a lesion in a lymph node. × 550. (From Stiles et al., 1933, courtesy of *Journal of the American Veterinary Medical Association*.)

Figure 36.4 (*right*). Mycelium of *Coccidioides immitis* in a hanging drop preparation from a culture. × 210. (From Stiles et al., 1933, courtesy of *Journal of the American Veterinary Medical Association*.)

36.3). The protoplasm is finely granular. In many of the larger spherules a number of endospores can be seen as spherical bodies varying from 2 to 5 μm in diameter. Mycelium is rarely observed in the tissues.

When tissues are cultured on solid media, protoplasmic

shoots appear from the spherules. These develop into hyphae, and soon a well-developed mycelium is formed. The hyphae branch extensively and exhibit well-marked septa (Figure 36.4). In time, aerial hyphae appear and a white woolly colony is formed (Figure 36.5). Micro-

Figure 36.5. (*Left*) A single colony of *Coccidioides immitis* growing on a solid medium. Note the cottonlike appearance. × 2. (*Right*) Coccidioidal granuloma in a bovine lymph node. The lesions vary in size and strikingly resemble those of tuberculosis. Their centers are caseous. Note the hemorrhages and the encapsulation. About × 2. (From Stiles et al., 1933, courtesy of *Journal of the American Veterinary Medical Association*.)

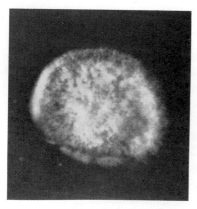 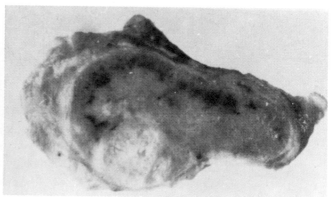

scopically, numerous chlamydoconidia and several arthroconidia can be seen. The spherical structures found in tissues are never present in cultures unless they are incubated under special conditions (Breslau and Kubota 1964) or in special media (Northey and Brooks 1962).

Cultural and Biochemical Features. *C. immitis* will grow on all the common media of the bacteriological laboratory. When cultures on solid media are incubated at 20°C, growth does not appear for 3 or 4 days, but at 37°C it is usually evident within 24 hours. The colonies are circular, silvery gray, and slightly raised. The mycelium penetrates deeply into the medium, so that the colonies cannot be removed except by digging out the medium. After a few days the cultures have a whitish, moldy appearance because of the development of short aerial hyphae. In some tubes the hyphae are abundant and from 2 to 3 mm long; in others they may be scarce and short. In old cultures the medium develops a brownish discoloration but the growth remains white.

Antigens. The antigens of *C. immitis* are known as coccidioidins and can be prepared from supernatants of mycelial cultures or from in vitro cultured mature spherules (Levine et al. 1969). Mycelial and spherulin coccidioidins contain at least 26 and 12 antigens, respectively. There are both common and specific antigens in each preparation. Some of the antigens are rich in mannose and peptide components (Anderson et al. 1971).

Spherulin coccidioidin appears to be more reactive and sensitive for cutaneous hypersensitivity testing than does mycelial coccioidin. Either antigen seems to be suitable for use in the complement-fixation test, although spherulin is less specific (Huppert et al. 1977).

Epizootiology and Pathogenesis. The enzootic region in the United States is the desert country of the southwest and the San Joaquin Valley of California. These areas are in the lower Sonoran life zone, an ecologically distinct area characterized by low rainfall occurring in one or two seasonal periods, high ambient temperature, and vegetation composed largely of cactus and creosote bushes. Enzootic zones also occur in Central and South America.

Desert rodents infected with *C. immitis* inhabit the ground beneath the vegetation and may excrete large numbers of spherules in their feces, which then germinate and multiply vegetatively in nearby soil after rain falls. When the ground dries, large numbers of arthroconidia are produced and released. These are readily spread to surrounding areas by the wind. Animals grazing these areas or dogs that sniff in the area of rodent burrows may inhale large numbers of arthroconidia. Most animals that live in the enzootic zone are exposed and infected during their lifetimes, but few develop serious disease.

The disease is not transmitted from animal to animal.

Maddy (1959a) conducted a 2-year study of a site in Arizona where a dog had acquired *C. immitis* infection. Soil samples collected from areas some distance from rodent burrows were negative but were positive when taken directly from the burrows. Most of the samples that yielded *C. immitis* were collected during September through December, when fall rains supplied moisture needed for growth of the fungus. Fifty dogs (Reed and Converse 1966) were exposed in an area where coccidioidomycosis was known to exist, and 29 (58 percent) became infected. Most cases developed in the cool months of the year, in contrast to the warm seasonal pattern of infection reported for humans. Archaeological sites in enzootic zones also exhibit high concentrations of *C. immitis*—an effect of past nutrient (midden) enrichment of the soils of such areas (Walch et al. 1961).

Although direct transmission is unlikely, bedside transmission of coccidioidomycosis between humans through growth on fomites has been reported in a hospital epidemic that involved six persons (Eckman et al. 1964).

The disease in cattle. Coccidioidomycosis in cattle (Stiles et al. 1933) is a benign disease that ordinarily involves only the posterior mediastinal and bronchial lymph nodes. In a few diseased animals small granulomatous lesions have been found in the lungs and in the submaxillary, retropharyngeal, and mesenteric lymph nodes. The affected glands are enlarged and contain a yellowish, glutinous pus, similar to that of tuberculosis (see Figure 36.5). The abscess wall consists of granulation tissue (Figure 36.6). Some degree of calcification is shown by 15 percent of the lesions. Infections are clinically inapparent.

Most cases of bovine coccidiodomycosis are seen in the inland valleys of California. Cases also occur in enzootic areas of Arizona, New Mexico, and other parts of the southwestern United States.

The disease in horses. Generalized coccidioidomycosis in a horse has been described (Zontine 1958). The main clinical features were a course of 4 months, severe progressive emaciation, variable temperature, moderate anemia, pronounced leukocytosis, edema of the lower parts of the legs, and a peculiar attitude of the front feet. At necropsy it was found that the animal had died of recent abdominal hemorrhage resulting from a ruptured liver. Granular abcesses of various sizes were seen scattered throughout the lungs (Figure 36.7), spleen, and liver. Other cases have been observed in horses and in a pony (De Martini and Riddle 1969).

The disease in sheep. Coccidioidomycosis in a sheep has also been described (Beck et al. 1931). Since then a number of similar reports have appeared. The lesions resemble those in cattle.

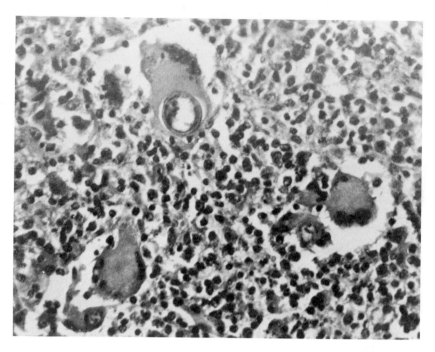

Figure 36.6. Section of a coccidioidal granuloma in a bovine lymph node showing granulation tissue and several giant cells, one of which contains a spherule. × 400. (From Stiles et al., 1933, courtesy of *Journal of the American Veterinary Medical Association.*)

The disease in swine. Infection of pigs raised near Tucson, Arizona, has been reported (Prchal and Crecelius 1966). Lesions occurred as granulomas in the bronchial lymph nodes and were found to contain *C. immitis.*

The disease in dogs. More cases of coccidioidomycosis have been described in dogs than in any other domestic animal (Farness 1940, Reed 1956). Boxers and Doberman pinschers appear to be more susceptible than other breeds. Cases have been reported from Arizona, California, Iowa, Kansas, Texas, and Quebec. In general, gran-

ulomatous lesions involve the lungs as the primary site, but they are also seen in the pleura, liver (Figure 36.8), spleen, kidneys, brain, and bones (Figure 36.9). The picture grossly resembles tuberculosis. In affected animals partial anorexia, vomition, and distress or collapse after eating are frequent. The disseminated form occurs frequently in dogs and usually produces a progressive fatal disease. Ocular lesions in dogs appear as iritis and uveitis. They have been described by Angell et al. (1987).

The disease in cats and chinchillas. Coccidioidomy-

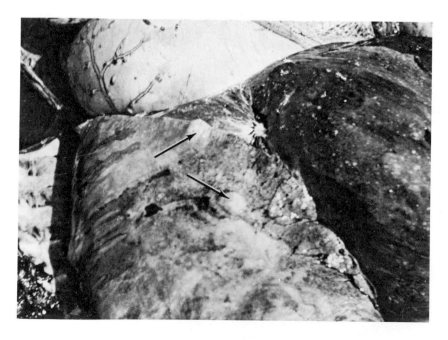

Figure 36.7. Coccidioidomycosis in a horse. Note the raised nodules of coccidioidal granulomata (*arrows*) on the surface of the lung. The largest nodule measured 3 cm in diameter. (From Rehkemper, 1959, courtesy of *Cornell Veterinarian.*)

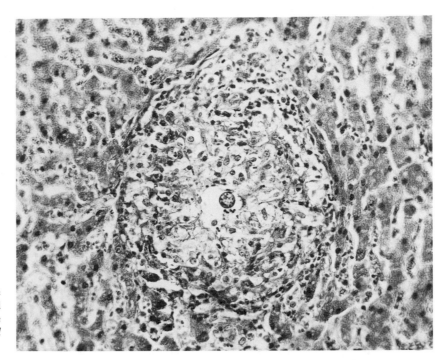

Figure 36.8. Coccidioidal granuloma in the liver of a dog showing a central spherule and surrounding epithelioid cells. (From Hage and Moulton, 1954, courtesy of *Cornell Veterinarian*.)

cosis has been described in two cats in Arizona (Reed et al. 1963). One animal developed an abscess on the hip, and histological sections of the subcutaneous tissue, lungs, and thoracic lymph nodes all showed *C. immitis*. In the second cat granulomas were found in the liver and kidneys in addition to the sites listed for the first victim. A case apparently involving only the eye has also been described (Angell et al. 1985).

Coccidioidomycosis in a chinchilla has been reported

by Jasper (1953). The disease was similar to that seen in dogs.

Immunity. Resistance to *C. immitis* is cell-mediated. Infection is followed by development of delayed skin hypersensitivity, lymphocyte transformation, and migration inhibition of macrophages. Resistance can be transferred from immunized mice by means of T lymphocytes (Beaman et al 1977).

Cell-mediated immunity is usually severely impaired in

Figure 36.9. The lumbar vertebrae and pelvis of dog showing coccidioidal lesions. (From Hage and Moulton, 1954, courtesy of *Cornell Veterinarian*.)

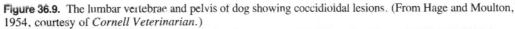
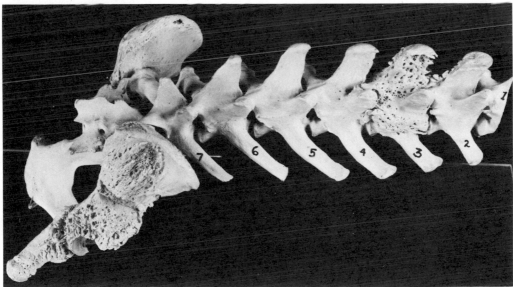

cases of disseminated coccidiodomycosis. It is not known whether this effect is secondary to the disseminated fungal growth or is based on a primary genetic inability to mount a cell-mediated response to the antigens of *C. immitis*.

Antigens from spherules are protective, and there appears to be only one antigenic type. Killed arthroconidia have also been used to successfully vaccinate dogs (Castleberry et al. 1965).

Diagnosis. Coccidioidin, a product made from filtrates of broth cultures, is used for diagnostic purposes. The complement-fixation test based on several serum samples also is useful, especially to indicate the progress of the disease. Complement-fixing antibodies persist much longer than precipitating antibodies and are therefore more useful for diagnosis of chronic infections. The fluorescent antibody technique applied with absorbed conjugates can be used to detect *C. immitis* in clinical materials (Kaplan and Clifford 1964). The agar-gel diffusion test with soluble spherule antigens is recommended for the detection of *C. immitis* antibody in serum samples from animals with suspect cases (Landay et al. 1970). Precipitins appear early after infection but do not persist.

Demonstration of the fungus either in the lesions or by cultural means provides a definitive diagnosis. The fungus may be converted to the spherule form by culture at 35°C in Converse medium in an atmosphere of 50 percent CO_2 (Converse 1955).

An exoantigen test developed by Kaufman and Standard (1978) can be used for rapid identification of suspect cultures. This test is based on the reaction in agar gel of extracts from the fungal mycelium with specific precipitating antiserum to the TP and F antigens of *C. immitis*.

Anitmicrobial Susceptibility. *C. immitis* is sensitive to amphotericin B and to ketoconazole, 5–10 mg/kg of body weight, given twice a day. However, euthanasia is usually recommended for pets with disseminated coccidiomycosis.

The Disease in Humans. Primary pulmonary coccidioidomycosis in humans may be subclinical or clinical. Annual infection rates have been estimated at 35,000 to 100,000. The subclinical type occurs with minimal manifestations and is often overlooked. Patients with more severe cases show low-grade fever and other signs of pulmonary disease. Some may develop a hypersensitivity, indicated by erythema several weeks later. The coccidioidin skin test becomes positive within about 3 weeks after exposure or within days after symptoms appear. A small percentage of primary infections disseminate to the internal organs, meninges, bones, and joints.

REFERENCES

Anderson, K.L., Wheat, R.W., and Conant, N.F. 1971. Fractionation and composition studies of skin test active components of sensitins from *Coccidioides immitis*. Appl. Microbiol. 22:296–297.

Angell, J.A., Merideth, R.E., Shively, J.N., and Sigler, R.L. 1987. Ocular lesions associated with coccidioidomycosis in dogs: 35 cases (1980–1985). J. Am. Vet. Med. Assoc. 190:1319–1322.

Angell, J.A., Shively, J.N., Merideth, R.E., Reed, R.E., and Jamison, K.C. 1985. Ocular coccidioidomycosis in a cat. J. Am. Vet. Med. Assoc. 187:167–168.

Beaman, L., Pappagianis, D., and Benjamini, E. 1977. Significance of T cells in resistance to experimental murine coccidioidomycosis. Infect. Immun. 17:580–584.

Beck, M.D., Traum, J., and Harrington, E.S. 1931. Coccidioidal granuloma. J. Am. Vet. Med. Assoc. 78:490–499.

Breslau, A.M., and Kubota, M.Y. 1964. Continuous in vitro cultivation of spherules of *Coccidioides immitis*. J. Bacteriol. 87:468–472.

Castleberry, M.W., Converse, J.L., Sinski, J.T., Lowe, E.P., Pakes, S.P., and Del Favero, J.E. 1965. Coccidioidomycosis: Studies of canine vaccination and therapy. J. Infect. Dis. 115:41–48.

Converse, J.L. 1955. Growth of spherules of *Coccidioides immitis* in a chemically defined liquid medium. Proc. Soc. Exp. Biol. Med. 90:709–711.

De Martini, J.C., and Riddle, W.E. 1969. Disseminated coccidioidomycosis in two horses and a pony. J. Am. Vet. Med. Assoc. 155:149–156.

Eckmann, B.H., Schaefer, G.L., and Huppert, M. 1964. Bedside interhuman transmission of coccidioidomycosis via growth on fomites. Am. Rev. Respir. Dis. 89:175–185.

Farness, O.J. 1940. Coccidioidal infection in a dog. J. Am. Vet. Med. Assoc. 97:263–264.

Hage, T.J., and Moulton, J.E. 1954. Skeletal coccidioidomycosis in dogs. Cornell Vet. 44:489–500.

Huppert, M., Krushow, I., Vukovich, K.R., Sun, S.H., Rice, E.H., and Kutner, L.J. 1977. Comparison of coccidoidin and spherulin in complement fixation tests for coccidioidomycosis. J. Clin. Microbiol. 6:33–37.

Jasper, D.E. 1953. Coccidioidomycosis in a chinchilla. North Am. Vet. 34:570–571.

Kaplan, W., and Clifford, M.K. 1964. Production of fluorescent antibody reagents specific for the tissue form of *Coccidioides immitis*. Am. Rev. Respir. Dis. 89:651–658.

Kaufman, L., and Standard, P. 1978. Improved version of the exoantigen test for identification of *Coccidioides immitis* and *Histoplasma capsulatum* cultures. J. Clin. Microbiol. 8:42–45.

Landay, M.E., Pash, R.M., and Millar, J.W. 1970. Spherules in the serodiagnosis of coccidioidomycosis. J. Lab. Clin. Med. 75:197–205.

Levine, H.B., Cobb, J.M., and Scalarone, G.M. 1969. Spherule coccidioidin in delayed dermal sensitivity reaction of experimental animals. Sabouraudia 7:20–23.

Maddy, K.T. 1959a. A study of a site in Arizona where a dog apparently acquired a *Coccidioides immitis* infection. Am. J. Vet. Res. 20:642–646.

Maddy, K.T. 1959b. Coccidioidomycosis in animals. Vet. Med. 54:233–242.

Northey, W.T., and Brooks, L.D. 1962. Studies on *Coccidioides immitis*. J. Bacteriol. 84:742–746.

Prchal, C.J., and Crecelius, H.G. 1966. Coccidioidomycosis in swine. J. Am. Vet. Med. Assoc. 148:1168–1169.

Reed, R.E. 1956. Diagnosis of disseminated canine coccidioidomycosis. 128:196–201.

Reed, R.E., and Converse, J.L. 1966. The seasonal incidence of canine coccidioidomycosis. Am. J. Vet. Res. 27:1027–1030.

Reed, R.E., Hoge, R.S., and Trautman, R.J. 1963. Coccidioidomycosis in two cats. J. Am. Vet. Med. Assoc. 143:953–956.

Rehkemper, J.A. 1959. Coccidioidomycosis in the horse: A pathologic study. Cornell Vet. 49:198–211.

Stiles, G.W., Shahan, M.S., and Davis, C.L. 1933. Coccidioidal granuloma in cattle in Colorado. J. Am. Vet. Med. Assoc. 82:928–930.

Walch, H.A., Prinbow, J.F., Wyborney, V.J., and Walch, R.K. 1961. Coccidioidomycosis in San Diego County and the involvement of transported topsoil in certain cases. Am. Rev. Respir. Dis. 84:359–363.

Zontine, W.J. 1958. Coccidioidomycosis in the horse—A case report. J. Am. Vet. Med. Assoc. 132:490–492.

The Genus *Histoplasma*

The genus *Histoplasma* belongs to the phylum Ascomycota. There are two species of importance as causes of disease in humans and animals, *H. capsulatum* and *H. farciminosum*.

Histoplasma capsulatum

PERFECT STATE: *Ajellomyces capsulatus*

H. capsulatum was first described by Darling (1906) in the tissues of inhabitants of the Canal Zone. Its fungal nature was demonstrated by De Monbreun (1934), who cultured the fungus from a human case. Since then, histoplasmosis has been described in a wide variety of species in many parts of the world. The majority of cases are subclinical, inapparent infections.

Morphology and Staining Characteristics. *H. capsulatum* is a small (about 1 to 3 μm in diameter), oval, yeastlike fungus in tissues (Figure 36.10) and in media incubated at 37°C and can be stained by Giemsa, periodic acid–Schiff, or hematoxylin and eosin methods. At 30°C small, pear-shaped microconidia are produced. In old cultures or under adverse conditions *H. capsulatum* produces diagnostic macroconidia—round, thick-walled structures 7 to 15 μm in diameter and covered with evenly spaced tubercles.

Cultural Features. Cultures made on Sabhi, Sabour-

Figure 36.10. Hypercellular bone marrow of a horse containing many *Histoplasma capsulatum* organisms. Hematoxylin and eosin stain. × 390. (From Panciera, 1969, courtesy of *Cornell Veterinarian*.)

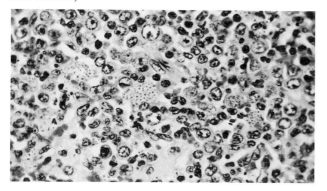

aud, or Mycobiotic agars at 30°C should be held for up to 10 weeks because some strains grow very slowly. In culture at room temperature colonies are usually fluffy and tan to whitish. The yeast phase is produced at 37°C on brain-heart infusion agar with glutamine. Tissue culture can also be used to convert *H. capsulatum* to the yeastlike phase (Larsh et al. 1965a).

Antigens. The cell wall of the yeast cell contains protective antigens and antigens reactive in complement fixation. The protein moiety of cell wall glycoprotein may be important in the detection of delayed hypersensitivity to the organism. Filtrates of mycelial cultures (histoplasmin) contain this high-molecular-weight protein (Sprouse et al. 1969). Polysaccharide (mannose, glucose) antigens are active in serum antibody tests.

Epizootiology and Pathogenesis. Enzootic areas in the United States include the Mississippi, Ohio, and St. Lawrence river valleys. The organism is found throughout the world wherever appropriate conditions are available. The natural reservoir of the fungus is soil (Larsh et al. 1956b), which when enriched with bird or bat droppings in enzootic areas supports large populations of *H. capsulatum*. For instance, the soil of chicken houses and yards located in enzootic regions frequently contains high concentrations of the organism (Ibach et al. 1954). Because chickens themselves have too high a body temperature to support growth of the organism in their tissues, they do not get the disease. Urban starling-blackbird roosts may harbor *H. capsulatum* and contribute significantly to the prevalence of cutaneous sensitivity to histoplasmin among children residing or attending school near the roosts (Di Salvo et al. 1969, Tosh et al. 1970).

Emmons (1958) reported that dung from bats was responsible for the constant saprophytic infestation of soil in certain premises he investigated, and Shacklette et al. (1967) recovered the organism from the liver and spleen of bats. Subsequent investigations (Di Salvo et al. 1969) concerning the role of bats in the spread of histoplasmosis have shown that they harbor *H. capsulatum,* that their feces contain the organism, and that caves they inhabit are heavily contaminated with the fungus (Shacklette et al. 1967). It seems likely that bats seed the soil with infected feces and that *H. capsulatum* may then be transmitted by air from these foci. Naturally infected bats have been found in Alabama, Arizona, Maryland, Oklahoma, and Texas.

Entry into the body is by means of air-borne conidia into the lung, where phagocytosis occurs. Infection can then spread or disseminate throughout the reticuloendothelial system by means of migrating mononuclear cells that contain the parasite. However, most infections are clinically inapparent. Primary lesions are often located in

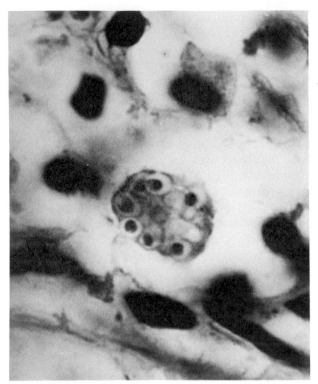

Figure 36.11. *Histoplasma capsulatum* yeast cells in the macrophage of a dog with a natural infection. × 2,800. (Courtesy J. W. Osebold, Oregon Agricultural Experiment Station.)

the lungs. Severe systemic infections are associated with splenomegaly, hepatomegaly, leukopenia, anemia, and emaciation. Ulcerations of the intestine can occur and result in diarrhea. The central nervous system, kidneys, bone marrow, and skin are frequently involved in clinical cases. The organism is packed within mononuclear phagocytic cells in great numbers (Figure 36.11).

Dogs are the most commonly infected domestic animal. The disease is characterized by a chronic debilitating digestive disturbance with enlarged abdomen, hepatomegaly, lymphadenopathy, and ascites. A chronic cough, irregular pyrexia, and dyspnea frequently are present. (Schwabe 1954).

The communicability of *H. capsulatum* from dog to dog has been established, and although there is no proof of a relationship between the disease in dogs and that in humans, an infected dog must be considered a potential source of disease for humans because it can disseminate the organism by saliva, vomitus, feces, and urine (Cole et al. 1963).

In cats disseminated histoplasmosis is less common than in dogs and is characterized by anemia, weight loss,

lethargy, fever, anorexia, and interstitial lung disease (Clinkenbeard et al. 1987).

Spontaneous infections have also been found in cattle, a horse, a pig, a woodchuck, a skunk, an opossum, a gray fox, a ferret, and a monkey, but the incidence of the disease in these animals is low. Histoplasmin sensitivity has been observed in sheep, cattle, a pig, and chickens.

A spontaneous outbreak of histoplasmosis has been described in guinea pigs (Correa and Pacheco 1967). Adult animals showed a chronic disease with progressive emaciation and lameness of the hind legs. Guinea pigs less than 3 months old died in 2 to 4 weeks, having ruffled fur, great dorsal curvature, and sometimes closed eyelids and catarrhal conjunctivitis. At necropsy the principal lesions were ulcerative gastritis, hemorrhagic and catarrhal enteritis, and enlarged spleen and mesenteric lymph nodes.

Immunity. Recoveries from localized infections are common and are associated with the development of cell-mediated and humoral immunity. With recovery, antibody titers tend to wane, but the delayed hypersensitivity reaction persists and so the skin test with histoplasmin remains positive (Loosli et al. 1954). Hemagglutination, complement-fixation, agar-gel precipitin (Kaufman 1980), and sensitized latex particle tests are available for measuring antibody titers. Complement-fixation titers are low in asymptomatic infections and become increasingly elevated as the infection progresses to severe disease.

H. capsulatum shares H or H and M precipitinogens with *H. capsulatum* var. *duboisii* and *H. farciminosum* (Kaufman and Standard 1978). This cross-reactivity limits the value of the exoantigen test (Kaufman and Standard 1978) for identification of *Histoplasma* isolates in areas such as Africa where all three strains occur.

Diagnosis. Smears stained by periodic acid–Schiff or silver impregnation and cultures on Emmon's modified Sabouraud agar of lesions, peritoneal fluid, cerebrospinal fluid, tracheal aspirates, bone marrow, and other tissues are prepared. The organism is often difficult to culture from specimens at 37°C, and it may be necessary to culture specimens on blood agar at 30°C to obtain mycelial growth. Smears can also be examined by the fluorescent antibody technique (Kaufmann and Kaplan 1963).

Complement-fixation tests with yeast or mycelial antigens and immunodiffusion tests are used for serologic diagnosis. Skin testing with histoplasmin is not useful diagnostically because of cross-reactions with other fungi.

Although isolation of a hyphomycete that bears tuberculate macroconidia is suggestive of *H. capsulatum*, several saprophytic *Arthroderma, Chrysosporium,* and *Sepedonium* species grossly and microscopically resemble the mycelial form of *H. capsulatum*. They can be distinguished by the exoantigen test (Kaufman and Standard 1978).

Antimicrobial Susceptibility. *H. capsulatum* is sensitive to amphotericin B, ethyl vanillate, ketoconazole, miconazole, nystatin, and sulfonamides (Hansen and Beene 1951). Amphotericin B is not recommended for treatment of acute histoplasmosis.

REFERENCES

Clinkenbeard, K.D., Cowell, R.L., and Tyler, R.D. 1987. Disseminated histoplasmosis in cats: 12 cases (1981–1986). J. Am. Vet. Med. Assoc. 190:1445–1448.

Cole, C.R., Farrell, R.L., Chamberlain, D.M., Prior, J.A., and Saslaw, S. 1963. Histoplasmosis in animals. J. Am. Vet. Med. Assoc. 122:471–473.

Correa, W.M., and Pacheco, A.C. 1967. Naturally occurring histoplasmosis in guinea pigs. Can. J. Comp. Med. Vet. Sci. 31:202–206.

Darling, S.T. 1906. A protozoon general infection producing pseudotubercules in the lungs and focal necrosis in liver, spleen and lymph nodes. J. Am. Vet. Med. Assoc. 46:1283–1285.

De Mombreun, W.A. 1934. The cultivation and cultural characteristics of Darling's *Histoplasma capsulatum*. Am. J. Trop. Med. 14:93.

Di Salvo, A.F., Ajello, L., Palmer, J.W., and Winkler, W.G. 1969. Isolation of *Histoplasma capsulatum* from Arizona bats. Am. J. Epidemiol. 89:606–614.

Emmons, C.W., Klite, P.D., Baer, G.M., and Hill, W.B. 1966. Isolation of *Histoplasma capsulatum* from bats in the United States. Am. J. Epidemiol. 84:103–109.

Hansen, A.E., and Beene, M.L. 1951. Sensitivity studies in vitro with *Histoplasma capsulatum* to various potential therapeutic agents. Proc. Soc. Exp. Biol. Med. 77:365–366.

Ibach, M.J., Larsh, H.W., and Furclow, M.L. 1954. Epidemic histoplasmosis and airborne *Histoplasma capsulatum*. Proc. Soc. Exp. Biol. Med. 85:72–74.

Kaufman, L. 1980. Serodiagnosis of fungal diseases. In N.R. Rose and H. Friedman, eds., Manual of Clinical Immunology. American Society of Microbiology, Washington, D.C. P. 563.

Kaufman, L., and Kaplan, W. 1963. Serological characterization of pathogenic fungi by means of fluorescent antibodies. J. Bacteriol. 85:986–991.

Kaufman, L., and Standard, P. 1978. Improved version of the exoantigen test for the identification of *Coccidioides immitis* and *Histoplasma capsulatum* cultures. Curr. Microbiol. 1:135–137.

Larsh, H.W., Hinton, A., and Cozad, G.C. 1956a. Natural reservoir of *Histoplasma capsulatum*. Am. J. Hyg. 63:18–27.

Larsh, H.W., Hinton, A., and Silberg, S.L. 1956b. Conversion and maintenance of *Histoplasma capsulatum* in tissue culture. Proc. Soc. Exp. Biol. Med. 93:612–615.

Loosli, C.J., Procknow, J.J., Tanxi, F., Grayston, J.T., and Combs, L.W. 1954. Pulmonary histoplasmosis in a farm family. A 3-year follow-up. J. Lab. Clin. Med. 43:669.

Panciera, R.J. 1969. Histoplasmic (*Histoplasma capsulatum*) infection in a horse. Cornell Vet. 59:306–312.

Schwabe, C.W. 1954. Present knowledge of systemic mycoses in dogs: A review. Vet. Med. 49:479–486.

Schacklette, M.H., Hansclever, H.F., and Miranda, E.A. 1967. The natural occurrence of *Histoplasma capsulatum* in a cave. 2. Ecological aspects. Am. J. Epidemiol. 86:246–251.

Sprouse, R.F., Goodman, N.L., and Larsh, H.W. 1969. Fractionation, isolation and chemical characterization of skin test active components of histoplasmin. Sabouraudia 7:1–4.

Tosh, F.E., Doto, I.L., Beecher, S.B., and Chin, T.D.Y. 1970. Relationship of starling-blackbird roosts and endemic histoplasmosis. Am. Rev. Respir. Dis. 101:283–288.

Histoplasma farciminosum

SYNONYMS: *Blastomyces farciminosa, Cryptococcus farciminosus, Endomyces farciminosa, Histoplasma farciminosa, Saccharomyces equi, Saccharomyces farciminosus*

H. farciminosum is the causative agent of *epizootic lymphangitis,* or pseudofarcy, of horses and mules. A few cases have been reported in cattle, but these animals are not highly susceptible. The infection is endemic in countries bordering the Mediterranean. It is also found in central and southern Africa and in parts of Asia and the Soviet Union. The disease was very prevalent during the Boer War, and cases were brought back to England after its conclusion. Outbreaks have commonly been associated with wartime when horses were gathered in large numbers for military purposes.

The organism was first demonstrated in pus by Rivolta in 1873 but was not successfully cultivated until 1896 by Tokishiga in Japan.

Morphology and Staining Reactions. In pus the organism appears as a double-contoured yeastlike oval or ovoid body, measuring 2.5 to 3.5 by 3 to 4 μm. The cytoplasm is granular, and bits of cytoplasm can be seen extruding from a break in the cell wall, forming buds from which daughter cells arise. In cultures the organism produces both hyphae and ascospores. Although the fungus cells are Gram-positive, structural details are best seen in fresh, unstained preparations.

Cultural and Biochemical Features. *H. farciminosum* is strongly aerobic. It has been successfully cultivated on a variety of media, but growth is slow and usually not evident for 1 to 3 weeks or longer. The organism can be grown on plain nutrient agar and broth and on coagulated egg medium or serum medium. On solid media, growth appears in the form of small grayish white granules that look dry and may become leatherlike in structure. In liquid media, growth generally occurs in the form of scanty, granular sediment. Sugar media are not fermented.

H. farciminosum is characteristically sterile in its mycelial form. These cultures can be identified by the type of exoantigen produced (Kaufman and Standard 1978).

Epizootiology and Pathogenesis. In areas where the disease is enzootic, new cases are most frequent in fall and winter. Although a soil phase has not been demonstrated, there is considerable indirect evidence that such a phase exists. Lesions are common on the lower limbs of horses, and removal of infected animals is not effective in eradicating the disease from a region. Yeast cells can be transferred between animals by direct and indirect contact, and infection enters through wounds.

An ulcer forms some weeks after entry of the fungus. The regional lymph channels become enlarged and appear as tortuous cords beneath the skin. The swollen nodes soften and rupture, forming craterlike ulcers from which a thick pus exudes. When mucosal lesions occur, they are most likely to be found in the nasal passages, but there are records of their occurrence on the genitalia and of the venereal transmission of the disease from stallions to mares.

Keratitis, conjunctivitis, sinusitis, and pneumonia (Bennett 1931) can also occur in some infected animals. The pneumonia is of the interstitial type, with infiltrations of lymphocytes followed by monocytes. Syncytia and giant cells appear, and the organism can be seen in these. Multiplication of yeast cells leads to extensive destructive changes and death of the animal.

Typical epizootic lymphangitis runs a chronic course for as long as a year. There is considerable loss of condition and animals are unable to work. Most animals, however, eventually develop a solid immunity and recover.

Immunity. Cell-mediated immunity is believed to be important in resistance to infection. Infected animals exhibit a delayed hypersensitivity reaction to a filtrate of culture supernatant of *H. farcinimosum*.

Diagnosis. The characteristic double-walled Gram-positive yeast cells can be demonstrated in smears of exudates. The fluorescent antibody test (Fawi 1969) is an effective and accurate diagnostic method. Bacterial contaminants in exudates may be suppressed by the addition of penicillin (500 μm/ml) to the specimen before culture on nutrient or serum agar.

Antimicrobial Susceptibility. *H. farcinimosum* is sensitive to iodides and ketoconazole.

REFERENCES

Bennett, S.C.J. 1931. Cryptococcus pneumonia in Equidae. J. Comp. Pathol. Therap. 44:85–105.

Fawi, M.T. 1969. Fluorescent antibody test for the serodiagnosis of *Histoplasma farciminosum* infections in Equidae. Br. Vet. J. 125:231–234.

Kaufman, L., and Standard, P. 1978. Improved version of the exoantigen test for the identification of *Coccidioides immitis* and *Histoplasma capsulatum* cultures. Curr. Microbiol. 1:135–137.

37 The Opportunistic Fungal Infections

In this chapter we describe a number of fungal diseases in which infection characteristically is opportunistic. The causative fungi are either environmental saprophytes or mucosal commensals that normally are not invasive. However, given a variety of circumstances, such as damage to mucosae, wounds, exposure to overwhelming numbers of conidia, immunosuppression, immunodeficiency, and antibiotic suppression of normal bacterial flora, these fungi may enter the tissues and cause disease. Some of these infections may be acquired in the hospital (nosocomial) or from veterinary procedures such as intramammary infusion (iatrogenic). However, the majority of opportunistic fungal infections in animals are endogenous or derived from the animal's feed or its environment.

In the first half of the chapter we describe opportunistic infections caused by specific fungal species. The remainder of the chapter deals with opportunistic fungal infections of specific tissues, organs, or organ systems that characteristically are caused by any of a variety of different fungal species.

The Genus *Aspergillus*

The genus *Aspergillus* belongs to the phylum Ascomycota and contains many saprophytic species that are very common in the air and soil and in animal feed. Some of these species can opportunistically cause disease in animals under conditions of stress, excessive exposure to fungal contamination, or prolonged antibiotic or corticosteroid therapy. *Aspergillus flavus* and *A. parasiticus* produce aflatoxins in moldy feed, which when ingested, cause acute or chronic aflatoxicosis in swine, cattle, and poultry. In cattle various species have been found to be associated with abortions. Cases of pulmonary and cutaneous aspergillosis have also been reported in cattle (Davis and Schaefer 1962), generalized infection has been recorded in lambs (Gracey and Baxter 1961), and aspergilli have been associated with abortion in mares (Hensel et al. 1961), persistent diarrhea in foals (Ludvall and Romberg 1960), and pulmonary disease in cats (Pakes et al. 1970). Bovine abortion, rumenitis and gastritis, mastitis, and equine guttural pouch mycosis caused by fungi including *Aspergillus* species are described in detail later in this chapter.

Aspergillus fumigatus

One of the most important disease-producing *Aspergillus* species is *A. fumigatus,* a common cause of respiratory disease of poultry and of penguins in captivity.

Morphology and Staining Reactions. The most characteristic feature of *A. fumigatus* is the swollen expansion of the tips of certain of the aerial hyphae that bear the conidia (Figures 37.1 and 37.2). These expansions carry small papillae (phialides) on which the conidia are borne externally. The conidia are dark green and are responsible for the color of the colony. The hyphae are nonpigmented, branched, and septate. They stain deep red with periodic acid–Schiff and dark brown to black with silver impregnation techniques.

Cultural and Biochemical Features. Growth is rapid on Sabouraud agar at 30°C. Woolly colonies appear that enlarge and contain greenish specks. These are the masses of conidia. Later, the entire colony is covered with a thick, matted mycelial growth that is greenish and dusty.

Antigens. *Aspergillus* species carry galactomannan, protein antigens that stimulate immediate and delayed type hypersensitivity, and humoral antibodies. Both species-specific and group-specific antigens occur (Piechura et al. 1983).

Epizootiology and Pathogenesis. *A. fumigatus* is introduced into poultry flocks in feeds and in moldy litter. The fungus is widely scattered in nature and can readily multiply in feeds that become wet or are stored in a damp room. Outbreaks are produced by the inhalation of conidia from such sources. Air-borne conidia can also penetrate sound and cracked eggs in the incubator (Wright et al. 1960). Aspergillosis has been reported in chickens, pigeons, turkeys, ducks, geese, canaries, mynah birds, and many species of wild birds. So far as is known all birds are susceptible. The disease is known as brooder pneumonia and sometimes occurs in epizootic form, causing heavy

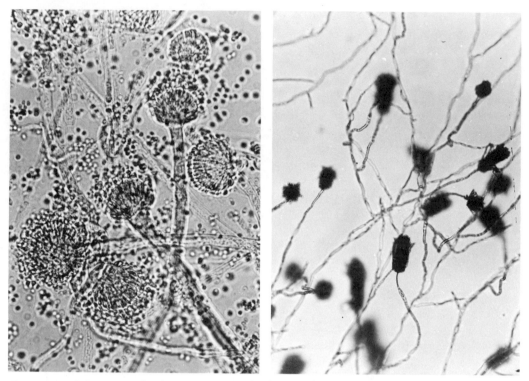

Figure 37.1 (*left*). *Aspergillus fumigatus,* an unstained preparation showing mycelium, fruiting bodies, and free conidia. The straight, stiff stalks are aerial hyphae. The bulbous expansions at their free tips contain papillalike processes (phialides) that bear long chains of highly refractile green conidia. The photograph was made from a bit of culture removed from a solid medium and immersed in a clearing solution. The majority of the conidia have broken loose from their attachments. × 550.

Figure 37.2 (*right*). The aerial hyphae and the fruiting bodies of *Aspergillus fumigatus* in a Henrici slide preparation. × 55.

losses. Unlike most of the other opportunistic fungi that produce deep-seated disease, *A. fumigatus* infects young birds more often than older ones. Outbreaks in hatcheries have been seen in day-old chicks, although the classical disease usually does not appear before the birds are 5 days old (Clark et al. 1954).

The infection is limited to the upper air passages and sometimes the mouth, lungs, and air sacs. In these locations the mold has access to air and vegetates readily. Tuberclelike bodies containing giant cells and lymphocytes form and quickly caseate. These caseous lesions may be seen in the lungs, and the walls of the air sacs are thickened. Sometimes the air sacs are lined with greenish areas because of the presence of large numbers of conidia. In other cases the air sacs are not uniformly thickened; instead, many small, whitish bodies of dense composition are present. Hyphae in many of these lesions may be recognized by crushing them with a little 10 percent potassum hydroxide. In the green areas the conidia are readi-

ly found. In denser lesions it is difficult or impossible to find evidence of the mold except by cultural means.

Encephalitic aspergillosis has been described in very young poults in which the fungus invaded the eggs during incubation and infected the embryos (Raines et al. 1956).

Austwick et al. (1960) described seven cases of pulmonary aspergillosis in lambs, one of them subclinical. *A. fumigatus* was recovered from all lung lesions. It has also been recovered from amniotic fluid of ewes and from the skin and lungs of fetal sheep (Leash et al. 1968). Jasmin et al. (1968) isolated the organism from pneumonic lesions in captive alligators (*Alligator mississippiensis*). It has also been found in calves and horses.

Antimicrobial Susceptibility. Experimentally, amphotericin B has shown strong antifungal action against *A. fumigatus* (Evans and Baker 1959); however, isolates from clinical cases have been reported to be resistant (Utz et al. 1977). It is sensitive to ketoconazole.

REFERENCES

Austwick, P.K.G., Gitter, M., and Watkins, C.V. 1960. Pulmonary aspergillosis in lambs. Vet. Rec. 72:19–21.

Clark, D.S., Jones, E.E., Crowl, W.B., and Ross, F.K. 1954. Aspergillosis in newly hatched chicks. J. Am. Vet. Med. Assoc. 124:116–117.

Davis, C.L., and Schaefer, W.B. 1962. Cutaneous aspergillosis in a cow. J. Am. Vet. Med. Assoc. 141:1339–1343.

Evans, J.H., and Baker, R.D. 1959. Treatment of experimental aspergillosis with amphotericin B. Antibiot. Chemother. 9:209–213.

Gracey, J.F., and Baxter, J.T. 1961. Generalized *Aspergillus fumigatus* infection in a lamb. Br. Vet. J. 117:11–14.

Hensel, L., Bisping, W., and Schimmelpfennig, H. 1961. Aspergillusabort beim Pferde. Berl. Münch. Tierärztl. Wochenschr. 74:290–293.

Jasmin, A.M., Carroll, J.M., and Baucom, J.N. 1968. Pulmonary aspergillosis of the American alligator (*Alligator mississippiensis*). Am. J. Vet. Clin. Path. 2:93–95.

Leash, A.M., Sachs, S.D., Abrams, J.S., and Limbert, R. 1968. Control of *Aspergillus fumigatus* infection in fetal sheep. Lab. Anim. Care 18:407–409.

Ludvall, R.L., and Romberg, P.F. 1960. Persistent diarrhea in colts. J. Am. Vet. Med. Assoc. 137:481–483.

Pakes, S.P., New, A.E., and Benbrook, S.C. 1970. Pulmonary aspergillosis in a cat. J. Am. Vet. Med. Assoc. 151:950–953.

Piechura, J.E., Huang, C.J., Cohen, S.H., Kidd, J.M., Kurup, V.P., and Calvanico, N.J. 1983. Antigens of *Aspergillus fumigatus*. Immunology 49:657–665.

Raines, T.V., Kuzdas, C.D., Winkel, F.H., and Johnson, B.S. 1956. Encephalitis in turkeys. A case report. J. Am. Vet. Med. Assoc. 129:435–436.

Utz, C.J. 1977. The current status of chemotherapeutic agents for the systemic mycoses. In A.M. Beemer, A. Ben-David, M.A. Klingberg, E.S. Kuttin, eds., Host-Parasite Relationships in Systemic Mycoses, part 2. S. Karger, Basel. Pp. 124–135.

Wright, M.L., Anderson, G.W., and Epps, N.A. 1960. Hatchery sanitation as a control measure for aspergillosis in fowl. Avian Dis. 4:369–379.

The Genus *Cryptococcus*

Cryptococcus neoformans

SYNONYMS: *Cryptococcus hominis, Torula histolytica*

PERFECT STATE: *Filobasidiella neoformans*

Cryptococcosis is a subacute or chronic mycotic infection of animals and humans caused by *C. neoformans*. The organism frequently attacks the tissues of the nervous system, but lesions can also be found in the lungs, skin, lymph glands, and other tissues. The disease has been reported from all parts of the world. In the United States cryptococcosis has been reported in horses, cattle, sheep, goats, a pig, dogs, cats, foxes, mink, ferrets, koala bears, cheetahs, a civet cat, guinea pigs, monkeys and humans (Barron 1955, Holzworth 1952, Pounden et al. 1952, and Seibold et al. 1953).

Morphology and Staining Reactions. *C. neoformans* grows as a yeast at room temperature and at 37°C. It is spherical or ovoid, thick-walled, single or budding, and refractile and measures from 3 to 25 μm in diameter (Figure 37.3). It develops capsules but usually no mycelium. Variants that have lost their capsules are avirulent. Capsules are better developed in infected tissue than in culture and can be visualized in wet preparations by negative staining with India ink. Mucin stains such as alcian blue or mucicarmine allow presumptive identification of the organism in sections of infected tissue.

Cultural and Biochemical Features. *C. neoformans* grows rapidly on Sabouraud glucose agar under aerobic conditions at 37°C but not 40°C. The colony is flat or slightly heaped, shiny, moist or mucoid, with smooth edges. The color is cream at first, later becoming brown. Growth is inhibited by factors in serum and by cycloheximide. The genus is characterized by inositol assimilation and urease production. *C. neoformans* does not reduce nitrate but can probably acquire nitrogen from urea, creatinine, and peptones.

Antigens. There are five serotypes of *C. neoformans*, A, B, C, D, and AD. Serotype B is found in southern California, and serotype A occurs everywhere else in the United States. Serotyping is based on the capsular polysaccharide, which is a high-molecular-weight polymer with a linear alpha-(1,3)-linked mannose backbone that is substituted with nonreducing D-xylosyl and D-glucosyluronic acid groups. O-Acetylation varies with the serotype. The most heavily O-acetylated serotype is serotype D.

Epizootiology and Pathogenesis. *C. neoformans* is distributed throughout most of the world. It flourishes in bird manures, especially that of pigeons, and utilizes as nutrient the abundant supply of creatinine in this material. It does not fare so well in soil, where it probably survives in its sexual, hyphal form.

Most cases of cryptococcosis result from inhalation of the fungus, but direct invasion of the skin or entry through the teat meatus in cows and goats also frequently occur. In its desiccated form or as a basiodiospore of the sexual phase it is small enough (1 μm) to penetrate the lower reaches of the respiratory tract. The vast majority of infections are subclinical, and disease occurs only in individuals with an underlying deficit in cell-mediated immunity.

The disease is slow to develop and predominantly involves the central nervous system. The organism's tropism for nervous tissue is probably related to its ability to metabolize nitrogen-containing substances of low molecular weight such as urea, uric acid, and creatine, which are relatively plentiful in the cerebrospinal fluid. The organism continues to grow extracellularly in tissue and causes pressure atrophy of surrounding areas. The great mass of capsular material may give affected tissue a gelatinous appearance. There is little inflammatory response.

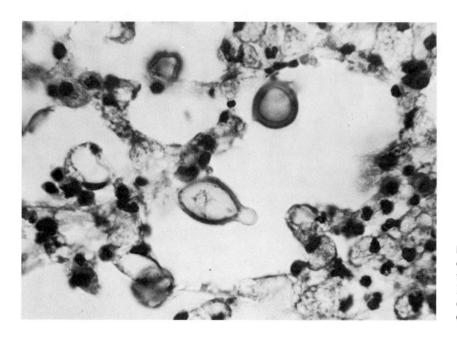

Figure 37.3. Micrograph showing a round cell of *Cryptococcus neoformans* with a thick capsule in the upper part of the field. Below is an oval cell in the process of budding. × 790. (From Holzworth, 1952, courtesy of *Cornell Veterinarian.*)

Encephalitis or a chronic respiratory condition may herald the disease in dogs. Cases have been accompanied by pulmonary, generalized, and intraocular involvement. The usual pathological findings are a granulomatous destructive process involving nasal mucosa and turbinates, facial sinuses, adjacent osseous structures, and meninges. Primary pulmonary lesions with secondary meningitis can also occur (Price and Powers 1967).

Cryptococcosis in cats (Fischer 1971, Holzworth 1952) has also been characterized by lesions in the central nervous system and granulomas involving the eye, sinuses, and nasal septum. There may be a chronic ocular and nasal discharge. Lesions of the skin of the nose and head have also been observed (Medleau et al. 1985) (Figure 37.4).

Laws and Simmons (1966) have reported a case of cryptococcosis in a sheep in which organisms were present in the leptomeninges, brain, mucosa of the nose and maxillary sinuses, and lungs. Clinically the sheep had swollen maxillary sinuses, mucoid nasal discharge, dyspnea, coughing, and anorexia.

In cattle, outbreaks of cryptococcic mastitis with regional lymph node involvement have occurred (Barron 1955, Innes et al. 1952). The subject is described in more detail in the section "Mycotic Mastitis" later in this chapter.

In horses, respiratory disease accompanied by obstructive growths in the nasal passages and lesions on the lip have been caused by *C. neoformans.*

Immunity. Noncapsulated strains of *C. neoformans* are avirulent. The capsular polysaccharide has a number of distinctly different effects on immune-mediated clearance and on the immune response. These effects include inhibition of phagocytosis, decomplementation of serum by activation of the alternate complement pathway, suppression of leukocyte migration, adsorption of protective opsonins, and depression of antibody synthesis (Murphy and Cozad 1972). Inhibition of phagocytosis is apparently by a passive mechanism wherein the surface of the organism is not recognized by the phagocyte. Depression of antibody synthesis is associated with an increase in numbers of suppressor cells that prevents proliferation of differentiated T and B cell clones.

The crucial determinant in protection against invasion of tissue by *C. neoformans* is a competent cell-mediated immune response. The fungus can be killed both following ingestion by phagocytes and, more important, by soluble factors released by monocytes and macrophages drawn in the course of the inflammatory response to the invading cryptococci (Kalina et al. 1974). This phase of the immune response is deficient in individuals with T lymphocyte macrophage disorders.

Fromtling and Shadomy (1982) provide a good review of immunity to cryptococcosis.

Diagnosis. Spinal fluid and material from lesions should be spread in a drop of India ink and examined microscopically. *C. neoformans* appears as a large transparent halo surrounding a cell, which may carry a single bud. No other similar capsulated organism is known to invade the nervous system in animals.

In culture a moist, creamy, spreading growth appears in a few days at 30°C. Capsule development is slow and is

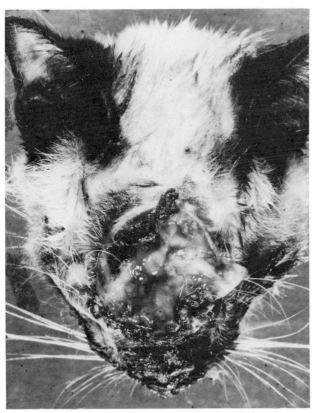

Figure 37.4. Lesion caused by *Cryptococcus neoformans* on the head of a cat. (Courtesy Joseph Kowalski.)

not optimal for some days more. Chloramphenicol or other broad-spectrum antibiotics should be included in the medium to inhibit bacterial contaminants. Nonpathogenic *Cryptococcus* species can be differentiated by a failure to grow at 37°C, a lack of pathogenicity for mice, and a failure to produce urease.

A selective medium that permits recovery of *C. neoformans* from heavily contaminated materials has been devised (Shields and Ajello 1966). It contains creatinine as a nitrogen source, diphenyl and chloramphenicol as mold and bacterial inhibitors, and *Guizotia abyssinica* seed (nigerseed) extract as a specific color marker. Phenoloxidase in the cryptococcal cell wall converts caffeic acid in the nigerseed extract to a brown pigment.

Pigeons and mice are very susceptible to experimentally induced infections of *C. neoformans*. Intracerebral or intraperitoneal inoculation of specimens containing *C. neoformans* will cause death in 3 to 18 days. Pigeons and mice both show signs of central nervous system disturbance before death.

Immunological methods are of little value in diagnosis, although a sensitized latex particle test is available for detection of capsular antigen in cerebrospinal and other fluids. Tests for antibody are unreliable.

Antimicrobial Susceptibility. *C. neoformans* is sensitive to amphotericin B, ketoconazole, and miconazole. Isolates vary in their sensitivity to 5-flucytosine (5FC).

An aqueous solution of hydrated lime and sodium hydroxide has been used to disinfect contaminated pigeon coops (Walter and Coffee 1968).

The Disease in Humans. In humans *C. neoformans* may produce a cutaneous form of disease in which healing sometimes occurs spontaneously after several weeks; a pulmonary disease with unilateral or bilateral lesions and a low-grade pneumonia; or a central nervous disease in which symptoms suggestive of a subacute or chronic meningitis, abscess, or brain tumor appear. Meningitis may follow the cutaneous form, or it may occur as a primary condition. Hepatitis has also been reported (Procknow et al. 1965). Approximately 50 percent of cases of cryptococcosis in humans are observed in patients with impaired immune responses due to such causes as Hodgkin's disease or immunosuppressive therapy.

REFERENCES

Barron, C.N. 1955. Cryptococcosis in animals. J. Am. Vet. Med. Assoc. 127:125–132.

Fischer, C.A. 1971. Intraocular cryptococcosis in two cats. J. Am. Vet. Med. Assoc. 158:191–198.

Fromtling, R.A., and Shadomy, H.J. 1982. Immunity in cryptococcosis: An overview. Mycopathologia 77:183–190.

Holzworth, J. 1952. Cryptococcosis in a cat. Cornell Vet. 42:12–15.

Innes, J.R.M., Siebold, H.R., and Arentzen, W.P. 1952. The pathology of bovine mastitis caused by *Cryptococcus neoformans*. Am. J. Vet. Res. 13:469–475.

Kalina, M., Kletter, T., and Aronson, M. 1974. The interaction of phagocytes and the large-sized parasite *Cryptococcus neoformans*: Cytochemical and ultrastructural study. Cell Tiss. Rec. 152:165–169.

Laws, L., and Simmons, G.C. 1942. Cryptococcosis in a sheep. Aust. Vet. J. 42:321–323.

Medleau, L., Hall, E.J., Goldschmidt, M.H., and Irby, N. 1985. Cutaneous cryptococcosis in three cats. J. Am. Vet. Med. Assoc. 187:169–170.

Murphy, J.W., and Cozad, G.C. 1972. Immunological unresponsiveness induced by cryptococcal capsular polysaccharide assayed by the hemolytic plaque technique. Infect. Immun. 5:896–899.

Pounden, W.P., Amberson, E.M., and Jaeger, A.B. 1952. A severe mastitis problem associated with *Cryptococcus neoformans* in a large dairy herd. Am. J. Vet. Rec. 13:121.

Price, R.A., and Powers, R.D. 1967. Cryptococcosis in a dog. J. Am. Vet. Med. Assoc. 150:988–983.

Procknow, J.J., Benfield, J.R., Rippon, J.W., Diener, C.F., and Archer, F.L. 1965. Cryptococcal hepatitis presenting as a surgical emergency. J. Am. Vet. Med. Assoc. 191:269–274.

Siebold, H.R., Roberts, C.S., and Jordan, E.M. 1953. Cryptococcosis in a dog. J. Am. Vet. Med. Assoc. 122:213–214.

Shields, A.B., and Ajello, L. 1966. Medium for selective isolation of *Cryptococcus neoformans*. Science 151:208–209.

Walter, J.E., and Coffee, E.G. 1968. Control of *Cryptococcus neoformans* in pigeon coops by alkalinization. Am. J. Epidemiol. 87:173–177.

The Genus *Candida*

The genus *Candida* belongs to the class Deuteromycetes, subclass Blastomycetidae (imperfect yeasts). The Blastomycetidae are yeastlike fungi, with or without pseudohyphae, that produce blastoconidia and rarely produce a true mycelium. *Candidiasis* is a general term applied to disease caused by *Candida* species, usually *C. albicans*.

Candida albicans
SYNONYM: *Monilia albicans*

Morphology and Staining Reactions. Young cultures of *C. albicans* consist of oval, budding, yeastlike cells that measure 3.0 by 4.0 μm. *C. albicans* produces thick-walled chlamydoconidia when grown on corn meal agar. Most other species of *Candida* do not. Yeastlike cells in the process of budding as well as fragments of septate mycelium are present in lesions. Pseudohyphae formed from buds on blastoconidia that continue to elongate are frequently seen in culture (Figure 37.5). The segments of pseudohyphae usually are 5 to 10 μm long, are constricted at the ends, and have the appearance of links of sausages.

Figure 37.5. An unstained preparation from a deep colony of a *Candida* sp. on agar showing pseudohyphae and the yeastlike blastoconidia that arise at the ends of filaments and at mycelial nodes. Surface colonies of *Candida* species consist largely of yeastlike cells. A pseudomycelium is produced only under conditions of reduced O₂ tension. Both pseudomycelia and yeastlike blastoconidia are found in lesions. × 500.

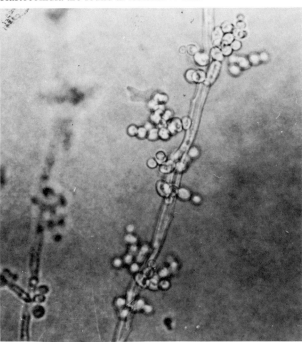

All forms of *C. albicans* stain well with periodic acid–Schiff and methanamine silver stains. Germ tubes are produced on serum agar.

Cultural and Biochemical Features. On Sabouraud agar, *C. albicans* forms soft creamy colonies that are highly convex and appear in 24 to 48 hours when incubated at 30°C. Growth is aerobic. *C. albicans* uses carbohydrates in an oxidative and fermentative pattern. It forms acid and gas from glucose, levulose, maltose, and mannose. A little acid but no gas is formed from sucrose and galactose. It does not attack lactose, raffinose, and inulin.

Antigens. The important antigenic determinants in *Candida* species are glycoproteins and polysaccharides such as mannans and glucans on the surface of the cell wall. The antigenic specificity of the mannans depends on the length of the polysaccharide side chains and the glycosidic linkages that they contain. There are at least two serotypes of *C. albicans* that differ in the position and number of their glycosidic linkages.

All *Candida* species share a common antigen. Individual species differ in their content of heat-stable polysaccharide and heat-labile glycoprotein antigen.

Epizootiology and Pathogenesis. *C. albicans* is a minor constituent of the normal flora of the skin and mucosal surfaces of all domesticated animals. It can opportunistically increase in numbers and become invasive in animals whose normal bacterial flora has been disturbed by prolonged antibiotic therapy and abnormal nutrition. Stresses that compromise immune defenses also predispose animals toward outbreaks of candidiasis. Examples of such stresses include overcrowding in substandard housing.

Candidiasis (thrush) in birds—chickens, pigeons, turkeys, pheasants, and grouse—is common and can cause significant losses. Lesions involve the mouth, crop, proventriculus, and gizzard and consist of whitish circular areas or elongated patches along the crests of folds in the mucosa. These areas become confluent and rather large and finally slough off, leaving superficial ulcers. Epizootics in very young birds can cause heavy mortality. Infections also occur in older birds but are less severe. Beemer et al. (1973) detected venereal candidiasis in geese.

Systemic candidiasis has been reported in feedlot cattle (McCarty 1956). The clinical signs included dyspnea, pneumonia, nasal discharge, diarrhea, and wasting. In calves, following prolonged antibiotic therapy, *C. albicans* has caused lesions in the rumen, liver, lungs, brain, and kidneys (Cross et al. 1970). Candidiasis has been reported in piglets on an artificial diet (McCrea and Osborne 1957) and in older pigs (Baker and Cadman 1963). Affected animals exhibit a white pseudomembrane on the tongue, esophagus, and stomach. They vomit and show rapid wasting. Cutaneous candidiasis has been described in dogs and cats (Kral and Uscavage 1960, Litwack 1966). The role of *C. albicans* in mastitis, abortion, keratitis, and rumenitis is described in the section "Opportunistic Fungal Disease of Multiple Etiology" later in this chapter.

Immunity. Cell-mediated immunity is critical in host resistance to candidiasis. Although antibody is effective in passive protection and in therapy, most cases in humans do not occur in patients with deficiencies in antibody production. There is some evidence that antigen-antibody complexes may in fact inhibit the cell-mediated immune system in mucocutaneous candidiasis in humans. Little is known about the immune response of domestic animals to *Candida* species. Enzootic venereal candidiasis in geese has been controlled by vaccination (Beemer et al. 1973).

The mechanisms of host resistance to *C. albicans* in humans have been reviewed by Diamond (1981).

Diagnosis. Mere culture and isolation of a *Candida* species from a specimen is not evidence for diagnosis of candidiasis. The organism must be demonstrated in sections, scrapings, and squash mounts of lesion material. In tissue the organism has the form of round or oval budding cells and septate hyphae.

C. albicans can be identified by the production at 30°C of chlamydoconidia on corn meal agar containing 1 percent Tween 80 (Dalmau plate). The inoculated area of the plate should be protected by a coverslip during the incubation period. Another presumptive test for the identification of *C. albicans* is its ability to form a germ tube when incubated for 3 hours in serum at 37°C. *C. albicans* is lethal for mice when injected intravenously. Commercially available carbohydrate assimilation tests provide a rapid and economical means of identifying clinical isolates.

Antimicrobial Susceptibility. *Candida* species are sensitive to amphotericin B, ketoconazole, miconazole, and nystatin. Haloprogin and nystatin are used topically in treating lesions on the skin or mucosae.

REFERENCES

Baker, E.D., and Cadman, L.P. 1963. Candidiasis in pigs in northwestern Wisconsin. J. Am. Vet. Med. Assoc. 142:763–767.

Beemer, A.M., Kuttin, E.S., and Katz, Z. 1973. Epidemic venereal disease due to *Candida albicans* in geese in Israel. Avian Dis. 17:639–649.

Cross, R.F., Moorhead, P.D., and Jones, J.E. 1970. *Candida albicans* infection of the forestomachs of a calf. J. Am. Vet. Med. Assoc. 157:1325–1330.

Diamond, R.D. 1981. Mechanisms of host resistance to *Candida albicans*. In D. Schlessinger, ed., Microbiology—1981. American Society for Microbiology, Washington, D.C. Pp. 200–204.

Kral, F., and Uscavage, J.P. 1960. Cutaneous candidiasis in a dog. J. Am. Vet. Med. Assoc. 136:612–615.

Litwack, M. 1966. Candicidin therapy for mycotic dermatoses in dogs and cats. J. Am. Vet. Med. Assoc. 148:23–25.

McCarty, R.T. 1956. Moniliasis as a systemic infection in cattle. Field case reports. Vet. Med. 51:562–564.

McCrea, M.R., and Osborne, A.D. 1957. A case of "thrush" (candidiasis) in a piglet. J. Comp. Pathol. Ther. 67:342–344.

The Genus *Sporothrix*

The genus *Sporothrix* contains only one species of importance as an opportunistic fungal pathogen: *S. schenckii*. The perfect state of *S. schenckii* has not been determined with certainty, but there is evidence that it may be a *Ceratocystis* sp. (Mariat 1977). If so, then its correct affiliation would be to the phylum *Ascomycota*.

Sporothrix schenckii

SYNONYMS: *Sporotrichum beurmonsis, Sporotrichum schenckii*

PERFECT STATE: *Ceratocystis stenoceras*

S. schenckii was first described in the United States in a human. It is now known to be widely distributed and has been observed in horses, donkeys, mules, cattle, a pig, dogs, cats, fowl, camels, rats, and mice. Records of sporotrichosis in animals far outnumber those in humans (Ainsworth and Austwick 1959).

Morphology and Staining Reactions. *S. schenckii* is a dimorphic fungus, growing in a yeast form in tissue and in culture at 37°C, but as a filamentous fungus at 30°C. At 30°C it forms fine (1.5 μm in diameter), septate branching hyphae that carry ovoid sympoduloconidia either on short support hyphae or directly on the sides of the main hyphae. A thick-walled, darkly pigmented, triangular chlamydoconidium may also be formed. In pus the organism is very difficult to demonstrate microscopically. The characteristic form in tissue is a cell resembling an elongated yeast, sometimes described as cigar-shaped. The cells vary in length from 2 to 10 μm and in breadth from 1 to 3 μm.

Cultural and Biochemical Features. *S. schenckii* grows on all the ordinary laboratory media, but solid media are more productive than liquid ones. Maltose favors growth. Good growths are obtained on potato-dextrose agar, where the characteristic brownish black pigment is best seen.

Small, whitish filamentous colonies appear on potato-dextrose agar slants on the second day of incubation at 30°C. These gradually enlarge and darken until finally the color is almost black. The surface is woolly because of the short aerial hyphae. Old cultures develop convoluted, wrinkled surfaces.

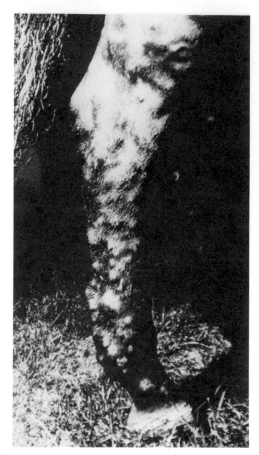

Figure 37.6. Sporotrichosis of the right hind limb of a horse. Note the extensive nodule formation and thickening of the fetlock area resulting from subcutaneous fibrosis and lymph stasis.

On Mycobiotic agar the growth is similar to that on potato but the colonies remain whitish in color. They adhere because the mycelium penetrates the medium. S. Schenckii slowly liquefies gelatin.

Yeastlike colonies appear at 37°C in 10 percent CO_2 on blood agar and have a creamy consistency.

Antigens. Cell wall glycoproteins are the major antigens of *S. schenckii*. Mannose and rhamnose are the important sugars in the polysaccharides of the cell wall.

Epizootiology and Pathogenesis. *S. schenckii* is a common saprophyte on dead plant material such as sphagnum moss. Most cases in humans are therefore found in forestry workers, gardeners, and miners who handle timber props left under damp conditions underground. The conidia are also common in the soil. The organism enters through skin wounds, the usual sites being the hands, feet, and head. Horses (Figure 37.6) and dogs are much more commonly infected than other animals.

A lesion begins as a small reddish nodule that may exude a thin seropurulent fluid. Infection then spreads by means of the lymphatic channels. Nodules form along these channels and ulcerate to the surface, discharging a thick pale yellow pus. The lymph nodes are also enlarged. The subcutaneous tissues of the limb may become thickened because of accumulated lymph fluid, whose return to the general lymphatic circulation is restricted by lesions in the lymph channels. Dissemination to other tissues is rare in horses but sometimes occurs in dogs. Transmission between cats and from cats to humans is possible.

The organism is sparse in lesions and is usually found intracellularly in macrophages. It is pleomorphic and exhibits multiple budding. The typical cigar-shaped form may not always be easy to find.

The lesions contain microabscesses and granulation tissue with lymphocytes, plasma cells, and giant cells. There may be extensive fibrosis.

Immunity. There is both a humoral and cell-mediated response to infection. Agglutinins to the yeast form rise during infection. Complement-fixing antibodies are present in about 50 percent of cases, and a rapid rise in titer suggests a favorable prognosis. Filtrates of old fluid cultures (sporotrichin) will give specific delayed-type hypersensitivity reactions in infected animals.

Diagnosis. The tiny spherical and cigar-shaped yeast bodies of *S. schenckii* in tissues and pus are best observed by the fluorescent antibody technique (Kaplan and Ochoa 1963) and by the periodic acid–Schiff staining procedure. These methods are rapid but must be supported by culture of specimens on brain-heart infusion or Mycobiotic agar slants at 37°C in 10 percent CO_2 and at 30°C or room temperature. The typical colonies are seen after about 1 week; initially they are white and glabrous, becoming brown as they age. The yeast phase is produced at 37°C and differentiates *S. schenckii* from infections by other *Sporotrichum* species and *Sporothrix* species, which occasionally have caused lesions in the subcutaneous tissues of humans.

Diagnosis can also be confirmed by intraperitoneal inoculation of mice with tissue macerates or exudates. Mice develop peritonitis, and the cigar-shaped and pleomorphic budding yeast forms are abundant in the peritoneal exudate a week after inoculation.

Anitmicrobial Susceptibility. *S. schenckii* is sensitive to miconazole and ketoconazole and is moderately sensitive to amphotericin B (2–23 μg/ml). Intravenous or oral potassium iodide has been used successfully for treatment of horses, although treatment failures have been frequent. Griseofulvin has also been recommended for horses.

REFERENCES

Ainsworth, G.C., and Austwick, P.K.C. 1959. Fungal Diseases of Animals. Commonwealth Bureau, Farnham Royal, England. P. 26.

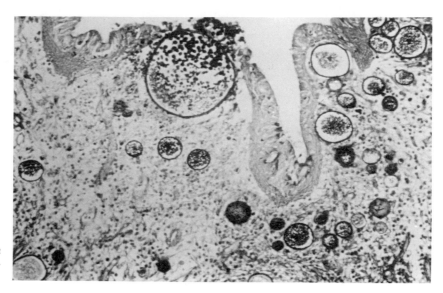

Figure 37.7. Sporangia of *Rhinosporidium seeberi* in a nasal polyp. The mature sporangia are filled with endospores.

Kaplan, W., and Ochoa, A.G. 1963. Application of the fluorescent antibody technique to the rapid diagnosis of sporotrichosis. J. Lab. Clin. Med. 62:835–841.

Mariat, F. 1977. Taxonomic problems related to the fungal complex *Sporothrix schenckii/Ceratocystis* spp. In K. Iwata, ed., Recent Advances in Medical and Veterinary Mycology. University Park Press, Baltimore. P. 265.

The Genus *Rhinosporidium*

The genus *Rhinosporidium* contains only one species, *R. seeberi,* a cause of chronic infection of the nasal and ocular mucosa which is characterized by polypoid growths. The disease is seen mainly in humans, horses (Myers et al. 1964, Smith and Frankson 1961), mules (Saunders 1948), and cattle (Saunders 1948) and to a lesser extent in goats, dogs (Niño and Freine 1964), and waterfowl (Faln and Herin 1957).

The fungus can be demonstrated microscopically in tissues or in exudates from polyps, in which it is seen as white specks. These specks are the sporangia, about 300 to 400 μm in diameter and filled with thousands of endospores (Figure 37.7). The latter are about 5 μm in diameter and leave the ripe sporangia by means of an exit pore. Hyphae have been seen in cavitary lesions.

Epizootiology and Pathogenesis. *R. seeberi* has not been cultured, and its ecology and mode of transmission are not understood. The infection is endemic in India and Sri Lanka but occurs only sporadically in the southern United States, South Africa, South America, Japan, and parts of Europe. There appears to be a positive correlation between the amount of water contact and the frequency of occurrence of the infection; however, ocular infections are common in dry, dusty areas of Texas, suggesting that the infective stage can also be dust-borne.

The polypoid lesions can be pedunculated or sessile. They are less than 3 cm in diameter and pinkish, consisting of fibromyxomatous tissue that is heavily vascular and bleeds easily. Affected animals may have a unilateral mucopurulent nasal discharge. Lesions have also been found in the conjunctival sac, ears, vagina, and other external parts of the body.

Diagnosis. Diagnosis is made by finding the giant sporangia in the polyps. Treatment consists of surgical removal of the polyp and cautery of its base.

REFERENCES

Faln, A., and Herin, V. 1957. Deux cas de Rhinosporidiose nasale chez une oie et un canard sauvages à astradia (ruand-urundi). Mycopathologia 8:54–61.

Myers, D.D., Simon, J., and Case, M.T. 1964. Rhinosporidiosis in a horse. J. Am. Vet. Med. Assoc. 145:345–347.

Niño, F.L., and Freine, R.S. 1964. Existencia de un foco endemico de Rhinosporidiosis en la provincia del Chao. V. Estudio de nuevas observaciones y consideraciones finales. Mycopathol. Mycol. Appl. 24:92–102.

Saunders, L.Z. 1948. Systemic fungus infections in animals. A review. Cornell Vet. 38:213–238.

Smith, H.A., and Frankson, M.C. 1961. Rhinosporidiosis in a Texas horse. Southwest Vet. 15:22–24.

Opportunistic Fungal Diseases of Multiple Etiology

The remainder of this chapter discusses opportunistic fungal infections involving any of a variety of different fungal genera and species. The varied etiology emphasizes the contaminative and opportunistic nature of these diseases.

Mycotic Abortion

Fungal infections of the placenta are a well-known and important cause of abortion in cattle. One survey found that fungal infection accounted for 13.4 to 24.9 percent of all abortions investigated annually in a large area of southern England between 1959 and 1966 (Hugh-Jones and Austwick 1967). In the United States about 5 percent of bovine abortions are caused by fungi (Leash et al. 1968). In Switzerland mycotic placentitis is the most common form of infectious abortion in cattle (Stuker and Ehrensperger 1983). Fungal abortions have also been reported in swine, horses (Hensel et al. 1961), and sheep (Leash et al. 1968).

Etiology. The primary fungal pathogens known to cause mycotic abortion are *Aspergillus fumigatus,* other *Aspergillus* species, *Candida tropicalis, Cephalosporium* species, *Mortierella wolfii, Mucor pusillus, Petriellidium boydii,* and *Torulopsis glabrata.*

Mortierella wolfii is the most important cause of bovine mycotic abortion in New Zealand (Carter et al. 1973). It has also been found in aborted bovine fetuses in the United States (Wohlgemuth and Knudtson 1977). Because it is relatively difficult to culture and isolate from specimens, its importance may have been underestimated.

Epizootiology and Pathogenesis. The majority of fungal abortions in cattle occur in winter and spring, the time when cattle are fed hay, silage, and other conserved feeds (Ainsworth and Austwick 1955, Williams et al. 1977). Part of the high incidence of fungal abortions in winter, however, can be explained by the greater number of calves born at this time. In the northeastern United States and in England mycotic abortions peak in January and February, and the majority occur during the last trimester of pregnancy. The abortion rate for English cattle fed hay in cowsheds was much higher than that for animals kept in loose housing systems (Williams et al. 1977). There is therefore circumstantial evidence that prolonged exposure to spores in feed is important in the epizootiology of mycotic abortion.

According to Bendixen and Plum (1929), infection takes place by the respiratory or alimentary route. Subsequent hematogenous spread leads to placental infection. The ability of blood-borne spores to produce placental infection has been demonstrated experimentally (Cordes et al. 1972, Pier et al. 1972). Mycotic pneumonia associated with mycotic abortion occurs frequently (Cordes et al. 1964, Donnelly 1967) and suggests that infection initially enters the respiratory tract—a conclusion supported by the much higher incidence of mycotic abortion in cattle tied close to their feed in cowsheds and thereby continuously exposed to potentially high local concentrations of fungal spores in the air they inspire. However, spores in the feed may also enter the bloodstream from the intestine (Angus et al. 1972).

Initial germination of spores in the bovine placenta is stimulated by a carbohydrate-containing substance of low molecular weight in the placental tissue (Conbel and Eades 1973). Fungal growth in the placenta leads to areas of infarction in the caruncles. The fetal membranes become infiltrated with gelatinous lemon yellow masses. Hyphae proliferate in the arterial walls of the cotyledons and sometimes in the eyelid or the skin of the fetus, where necrotic plaques are produced (Figure 37.8). Serous fluid accumulates in the fetal peritoneum and pericardium. Abortion eventually occurs because of impaired placental circulation.

There is evidence that not all placental fungal infections result in abortion and that a viable fetus may be born of infected dams (Williams et al. 1977). The amount of placental damage is probably critical in determining whether the fetus will die and abortion ensue.

The cotyledons are usually necrotic and dry, and portions of the maternal carnucles may remain adherent to the fetal villi (Figure 37.9). Although endometritis is present in mycotic abortion, the subsequent reproductive performance of the cows is usually unaffected. Cows apparently do not continue to carry the infection in their reproductive tracts.

Diagnosis. Fungal elements in fetal stomach contents and in the placenta (Figure 37.10) are diagnostic and can be demonstrated by direct microscopic examination and by culture on Sabouraud medium. Mycotic placentitis is usually accompanied by hyphae in the fetal stomach contents (Williams et al. 1977). There is no reliable method of diagnosing mycotic placentitis before abortion occurs.

Because animals develop precipitin responses to the antigens of *A. fumigatus* when exposed by a variety of routes, a positive reaction to the antigens of this fungus is not particularly informative. Moreover, the multiplicity of fungal agents that can cause mycotic placentitis makes selection of antigens for use in serologic testing difficult.

Stuker and Ehrensperger (1983) and Pepin (1983) provide good reviews of the problems involved in the diagnosis of mycotic placentitis.

Antimicrobial Susceptibility. Although most of the agents found in cases of mycotic placentitis are sensitive to ketoconazole and amphotericin B, the lack of a suitable diagnostic test to detect infection before abortion precludes consideration of their use in therapy.

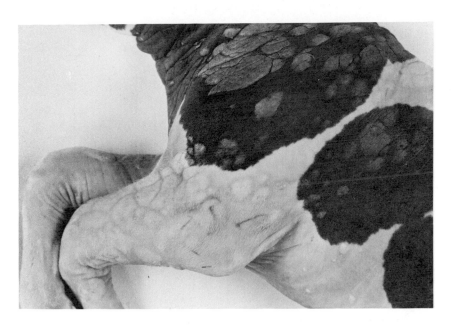

Figure 37.8. Lesions on the skin of a fetus aborted because of *Aspergillus* sp. infection. (Courtesy Kenneth McEntee.)

REFERENCES

Ainsworth, G.C., and Austwick, P.K.C. 1955. A survey of animal mycoses. Vet. Rec. 67:88.

Angus, K.W., Gilmour, N.J.L., and Dawson, C.O. 1972. Alimentary lesions in cattle: A histological and cultural study. J. Med. Microbiol. 6:207–213.

Bendixen, H.C., and Plum, N.S. 1929. *Aspergillus fumigatus* and *Absidia ramosa*. Acta Pathol. Microbiol. Scand. 6:252–322.

Carter, M.E., Cordes, D.O., Di Menna, M.E., and Hunter, R. 1973. Fungi isolated from bovine mycotic abortion and pneumonia with special reference to *Mortierelli wolfii*. Res. Vet. Sci. 14:201–206.

Conbel, M.J., and Eades, S.M. 1973. The effect of soluble extracts of bovine placenta on the growth of fungi implicated in bovine mycotic abortion. Br. Vet. J. 129:125–129.

Cordes, D.O., DiMenna, M.E., and Carter, M.E. 1972. Mycotic pneumonia and placentitis caused by *Mortierella wolfii*. Vet. Pathol. 9:131–141.

Cordes, D.O., Dodd, D.C., and O'Hara, P.J. 1964. Bovine mycotic abortion. N.Z. Vet. J. 12:95.

Donnelly, W.J.C. 1967. Systemic bovine phycomycosis: A report of two cases. Ir. Vet. J. 21:82–87.

Hensel, L., Bisping, W., and Schimmelpfennig, H. 1961. Aspergillusabort beim Pferde. Berl. Münch. Tierärztl. Wochenschr. 74:290–293.

Hugh-Jones, M.E., and Austwick, P.K.C. 1967. Epidemiological studies on bovine mycotic abortion. Vet. Rec. 81:273–275.

Leash, A.M., Sachs, S.D., Abrams, J.S., and Limbert, R, 1968. Control of *Aspergillus fumigatus* infection in fetal sheep. Lab. Anim. Care, 18:407–409.

Pepin, G.A. 1983. Bovine mycotic abortion. Vet. Annu. 23:79–90.

Pier, A.C., Cysewski, S.J., and Richard, J.L. 1972. Mycotic abortion

Figure 37.9. A placenta aborted because of *Aspergillus* sp. infection. The fetal cotyledons on the lower half have areas of necrosis and adherent tissue from the maternal caruncle. (Courtesy John King.)

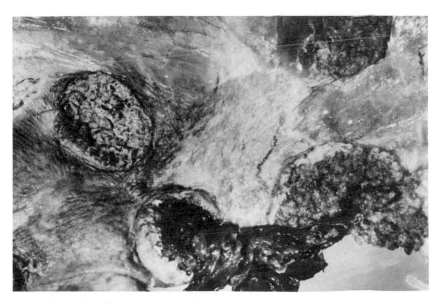

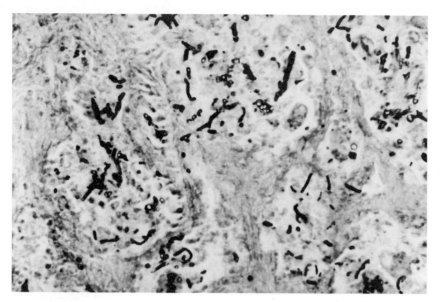

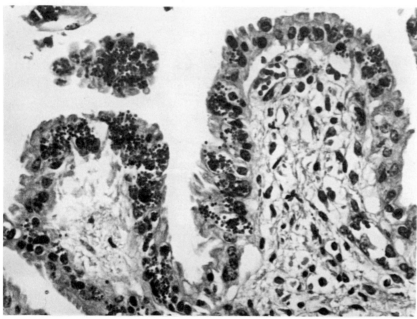

Figure 37.10. (*Top*) A section of placenta from an animal with mycotic abortion. Note the many hyphal segments. × 400. (Courtesy Clyde Boyer.) (*Bottom*) A section of bovine placenta showing trophoblasts distended by cells of *Candida albicans.* × 360. (Courtesy George L. Foley.)

in ewes produced by *Aspergillus fumigatus:* Intravascular and intrauterine inoculation. Am. J. Vet. Res. 33:349–356.

Stuker, G., and Ehrensperger, F. 1983. Significance and diagnosis of fungal abortion in cattle. In Proceedings of the 3d International Symposium of the World Association of Veterinary Laboratory Diagnosticians, June 13–15. Pp. 91–96.

Williams, B.M., Shreeve, B.J., Hebert, C.N., and Swire, P.W. 1977. Bovine mycotic abortion: Some epidemiological aspects. Vet. Rec. 100:382–385.

Wohlgemuth, K., and Knudtson, W.U. 1977. Abortion associated with *Mortierella wolfii* in cattle. J. Am. Vet. Med. Assoc. 171:437–438.

Mycotic Mastitis

Fungal mastitis is usually caused by yeastlike fungi, and its prevalence is closely correlated with the use of intramammary antibiotic therapy. In some herds yeasts cause 1 to 4 percent of subclinical cases and up to 25 percent of clinical cases of mastitis (Mehnert et al. 1964).

Etiology. The majority of organisms isolated from cases of fungal mastitis in the United States belong to the genera *Candida, Cryptococcus,* and *Trichosporon* (Farnsworth 1977, Richard et al. 1980). In other parts of the world, genera such as *Pichia* and *Torulopsis* can be important. The following are the more common genera and species that have been reported: *Aspergillus fumigatus, Candida albicans, C. albidus, C. guilliermundi, C. krusei, C. norvegensis, C. parakrusei, C. parapsilosis, C. pseudotropicalis, C. stellatoidea, C. trop-*

icalis, Cryptococcus neoformans, Geotrichum candidum, Petriellidium boydii, Pichia species, *Rhodotorula* species, *Torulopsis* species, and *Trichosporon cutaneum.*

Epizootiology and Pathogenesis. In the United States *Candida tropicalis* is the most commonly isolated yeast from cases of bovine mastitis. Yeasts are normal commensals of the skin of the udder and teats and may be introduced into the teat sinus on instruments or in intramammary infusions. Trauma to the end of the teat or irritating teat dips have also been incriminated as factors that predispose a cow to yeast invasion (Giesecke et al. 1968). Epizootics of yeast mastitis have been traced to the use of intramammary antibiotic preparations that were contaminated with yeasts (Beck 1957, Loken et al. 1959). The disease occurred in a herd a few days after it had been treated for *Streptococcus agalactiae* infection (Farnsworth and Sorensen 1972). Many yeast infections of the mammary gland have been associated with the administration of home-produced infusions or the use of the same cannula or syringe to infuse a number of quarters. Moreover, Farnsworth (1977) noted that the use of single-dose antibiotic preparations from disposable tubes is much less likely to be associated with fungal mastitis. Thus there is compelling evidence that many cases of yeast mastitis are iatrogenic.

The disease can also occur in cows with no history of antibiotic administration (Stuart 1951). This suggests that other unknown factors may be involved in the pathogenesis of the disease. Yeasts may occasionally colonize the teat canal or the teat and gland cisterns without causing disease. If a bacterial mastitis should occur, these yeasts may multiply and invade the damaged parenchyma, causing a secondary fungal mastitis. Commensal bacteria on and in the udder probably inhibit yeast multiplication, and their removal by antibiotics likely allows the yeast to multiply.

Mastitis caused by *Cryptococcus neoformans* is often associated with soiling of the barn by pigeon feces. The fungus has infected udders by way of contaminated distilled water used to prepare intramammary infusions for dry cow therapy (Sipka and Petrovic 1975). Infection by this species is more severe than that by other fungi, and milk production is often permanently lost when the secretory parenchyma is replaced by granulation tissue (Innes et al. 1952). Many affected cows must eventually be culled for economic reasons.

The severity of mycotic mastitis is related to the number of organisms that enter the gland, the genus of fungus involved, and its ability to grow at 40°C (Topolko 1968). *Candida* species, *Trichosporon* species, and other similar yeasts in sufficient numbers cause severe local inflammation, swelling, fever, loss of milk production, and a great-ly increased leukocyte count in the milk. Most of these infections are cleared in 1 to 2 weeks, and udder function returns to normal. Some cows continue to shed the causative organism for 6 to 12 months.

The variety of genera and species implicated in this disease certainly emphasizes the importance of the primary contaminative aspect of its epizootiology. Consistent with this is the fact that infection does not secondarily spread from quarter to quarter or from cow to cow.

Diagnosis. Farnsworth and Sorensen (1972) have reported that 2 percent of Minnesota dairy cattle with clinically normal udders shed yeasts in their milk. Mere isolation of yeasts therefore is not proof of their etiologic significance in cases of mastitis. More convincing evidence is the presence of large numbers of a single yeast species that grows well at 37°C in conjunction with a history of previous antibiotic infusion. Milk samples should be cultured on both blood and Sabouraud agars at 37°C. The Sabouraud agar should contain antibiotics such as penicillin and streptomycin to inhibit bacteria, which grow faster than yeast colonies, thereby tending to obscure them.

Antimicrobial Susceptibility. Most yeast species are sensitive to amphotericin B, 5-flucytosine, ketoconazole, miconazole (Van Damme 1983), natamycin, and nystatin. Antifungal agents are generally toxic for the mammary gland and may cause as much or more damage as the yeast infection itself, which often clears up spontaneously in a few days. Less toxic antifungal agents such as ketoconazole, miconazole, pimaricin, and undecylenic acid may provide more satisfactory therapy.

REFERENCES

Beck, C.G. 1957. Mycotic mastitis. Mich. State Coll. Vet. 17:82–88.

Farnsworth, R.J. 1977. Significance of fungal mastitis. J. Am. Vet. Med. Assoc. 170:1173–1174.

Farnsworth, R.J., and Sorensen, D.K. 1972. Prevalence and species distribution of yeast in mammary glands of dairy cows in Minnesota. Can. J. Comp. Med. 36:329–332.

Giesecke, W.H., Nel, E.E., and von den Heever, C.W. 1968. Blastomycotic mastitis. J. S. Afr. Vet. Med. Assoc. 3:69–85.

Innes, J.R.M., Siebold, H.R., and Arentzen, W.P. 1952. The pathology of bovine mastitis caused by *Cryptococcus neoformans*. Am. J. Vet. Res. 13:469–475.

Loken, K.I., Thompson, E.S., Hoyt, H.H., and Ball, R. 1959. An infection of the bovine udder with *Candida tropicalis*. J. Am. Vet. Med. Assoc. 134:401–403.

Mehnert, B., Ernst, K., and Gedek, W. 1964. Yeasts as causes of mastitis. Zentrbl. Veterinärmed. [A] 11:97–121.

Richard, J.C., McDonald, J.S., Fichtner, R.E., and Anderson, A.J. 1980. Identification of yeasts from infected bovine mammary glands and their experimental infectivity in cattle. Am. J. Vet. Res. 41:1991–1994.

Sipka, M., and Petrovic, D. 1975. Gehäuftes Auftreten von Hefemastitiden beim Rind. Zentrbl. Veterinärmed. [B] 22:353.

Stuart, R. 1951. An outbreak of bovine mastitis from which yeasts were isolated and attempts to reproduce the condition experimentally. Vet. Rec. 63:314.

Topolko, S. 1968. Učestalost Kvasnica u vimenu krava i eksperimentalna istrazivanja gijivičnog mastitisa. Vet. Arh. 38:242–244.

Van Damme, D.M. 1983. Use of miconazole in treatment for bovine mastitis. Vet. Med./Small Anim. Clin. 78:1425–1427.

Mycotic Rumenitis and Gastritis

Mycotic infections of the bovine stomach are caused mainly by fungi of the class Phycomycetes (phylum Zygomycota) and by the yeast *Candida albicans*. The frequency of these fungal diseases has increased greatly with the increased use of antibiotics for prophylaxis and therapy and with the advent of systems of husbandry that include the feeding of concentrates.

Etiology. The following organisms have been identified in cases of mycotic rumenitis and gastritis: *Absidia* species, *Aspergillus* species, *Candida albicans, Mucor* species, and *Rhizopus* species.

Epizootiology and Pathogenesis. The fungi involved in lesions of bovine rumenitis or gastritis are common contaminants of the animals' feed and of the normal gastrointestinal contents. They become opportunistic invaders of the stomach mucosa given the appropriate predisposing conditions. Prolonged antibiotic treatment, for example, by reducing the normal bacterial flora, diminishes the controlling effect of the latter on fungal multiplication. Since bacterial stimulation of epithelial renewal is also reduced, the mucosa is more susceptible to fungal invasion. Furthermore, antibiotics may even stimulate the growth of some fungi, including *Candida* species (Mills 1967, Seelig 1966).

Mycotic gastritis associated with antibiotic administration is seen most often in calves. In older cattle the disease is more often associated with rumenitis caused by excess acid from consumption of larger than usual quantities of grain or concentrates. The pH of the rumen contents drops as low as 3.5, and the normal protozoal fauna and bacterial flora are destroyed. The rumenal mucosa, particularly in the ventral sacs, becomes ulcerated and is then invaded by fungi from the gastric contents.

The fungal hyphae penetrate the mucosa, infiltrate the walls of blood vessels, and form thrombi that obstruct blood flow. Such obstruction may lead to ischemic infarction and necrosis of neighboring tissue. Gross lesions in the rumen, omasum, or abomasum consist of circumscribed areas of necrosis surrounded by a zone of congestion (Figures 37.11 and 37.12). The stomach may also adhere to other organs such as the liver and diaphragm. Histologically, lesions are characterized by necrosis, congestion, and occlusion of blood vessels by thrombi and fungal hyphae. Hyphae and other fungal elements are also present in the necrotic tissue (Neitzke and Schiefer 1974).

Affected animals exhibit rumen atony, anorexia, and depression and excrete foul-smelling feces (Lock 1975). There is no effective treatment.

Diagnosis. Microscopic evidence of fungal elements in lesions provides good support for a diagnosis of mycotic rumenitis or gastritis. However, phycomycetes in lesions of calves are not readily cultured (Gitter and Austwick 1957). The ubiquitous presence of fungi in the

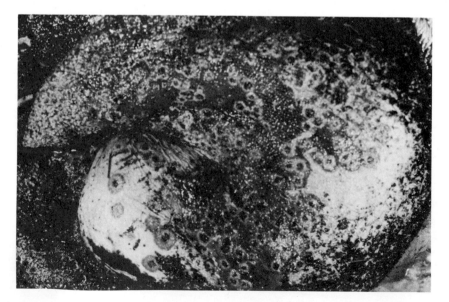

Figure 37.11. Lesions of mycotic rumenitis in a cow. (Courtesy John King.)

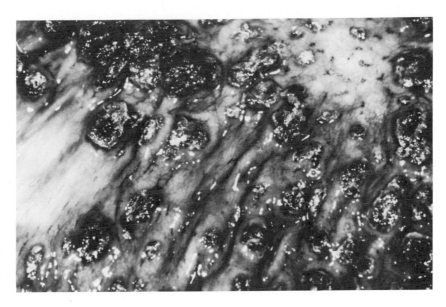

Figure 37.12. Lesions of mycotic abomasitis in a cow. Note the raised circular lesions with depressed necrotic centers. (Courtesy John King.)

digesta and on the mucosal surface further confounds the interpretation of cultural findings.

REFERENCES

Gitter, M., and Austwick, P.K.C. 1957. The presence of fungi in abomasal ulcers of young calves: A report of seven cases. Vet. Rec. 69:924–928.
Lock, T.F. 1975. Mycotic rumenitis in cattle. Vet. Med./Small. Anim. Clin. 70:197–198.
Mills, J.H.L. 1967. Systemic candidiasis in calves on prolonged antibiotic therapy. J. Am. Vet. Med. Assoc. 150:862–869.
Neitzke, J.P., and Schiefer, B. 1974. Incidence of mycotic gastritis in calves up to 30 days of age. Can. Vet. J. 15:139–143.
Seelig, M.S. 1966. The role of antibiotics in the pathogenesis of *Candida* infections. Am. J. Med. 40:887–917.

Mycotic Keratitis

A variety of saprophytic, commensal, and pathogenic fungi have been isolated from ocular lesions in animals and humans. They include *Aspergillus* species, *Blastomyces dermatitidis*, *Candida* species, *Cryptococcus neoformans*, *Drechslera* species, *Fusarium* species, and *Penicillium* species.

Mycotic keratitis usually results from corneal injury, which allows opportunistic entry of fungal cells into the corneal stroma. It can also result, in a minority of cases, from dissemination to the eye of a systemic infection by *B. dermatitidis* or *C. neoformans*.

Opportunistic fungal invasion may be suspected if a primary bacterial infection does not respond to prolonged antibiotic therapy. Combined antibiotic-corticosteroid medication is particularly likely to be associated with secondary fungal invasion of the cornea. As the cornea un-

dergoes fungal invasion it slowly becomes opaque and ulcerates (Figure 37.13). The ulcer is often accompanied by characteristic endothelial plaques in the center of the cornea. If hypopyon is present, it is generally sterile.

Diagnosis. Mycotic keratitis may be misdiagnosed as bacterial infection or a squamous cell carcinoma. Material should be scraped from the edge of the ulcer on the anesthetized cornea and stained by Gram's, Giemsa, and periodic acid–Schiff methods. Hyphae, blastoconidia, and pseudohyphae may be observed in this material. Fungal identification requires culture of specimens and isolation of the causative fungus.

Antimicrobial Susceptibility. The fungi present in cases of mycotic keratitis are likely to be sensitive to ketoconazole and miconazole and possibly to amphotericin B, nystatin, pimaricin, and potassium iodide.

Figure 37.13. Mycotic keratitis in a horse. Note the extensive opacity and formation of scar tissue.

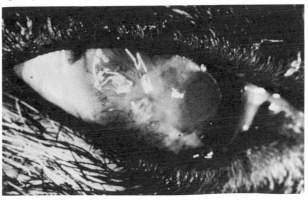

Guttural Pouch Mycosis

Infection of the guttural pouch by *Aspergillus fumigatus,* other *Aspergillus* species, and *Mucor* species is occasionally found in stabled horses and may be associated with damage to the internal carotid artery or nerves that pass close to the guttural pouch. Infections are found most often on the left side but can occur bilaterally. They apparently arise from inhalation of spores in moldy feed.

Affected horses may have a unilateral nasal discharge, epistaxis, and dysphagia caused by involvement of the pharyngeal branch of the vagus or the glossopharyngeal nerves. Diagnosis is based on detection of hyphal elements in tissue and exudates. Treatment involves ligation of the internal carotid artery to prevent epistaxis, surgical removal of mycelium, and oral administration of ketoconazole or intravenous administration of sodium iodide (Owen and McKelvey 1979).

REFERENCE

Owen, R.R., and McKelvey, W.A.C. 1979. Ligation of the internal carotid artery to prevent epistaxis due to guttural pouch mycosis. Vet. Rec. 104:100–101.

Mycetomas (Maduromycosis and Chromomycosis)

Mycetomas are tumorlike lesions caused by opportunistic, localized, chronic fungal infections. They typically involve the cutaneous and subcutaneous tissues of the legs and feet and are characterized by excessive granulation tissue that contains abscesses. The causative fungi are present in the lesions in the form of granules. Mycetomas are most common in tropical and subtropical areas.

The term *maduromycosis* is derived from the Indian province of Madura, where mycetomas were first described in humans. The term *chromomycosis* has been specifically applied to mycetomas caused by darkly pigmented (dematiacious) fungi.

Etiology. The following species are most often involved in mycetomas: *Cladosporium* species, *Curvularia geniculata, Fonsecaea pedrosoi, Helminthosporium* species, *Petriellidium boydii (Allescheria boydii),* and *Phialophora* species.

Epizootiology and Pathogenesis. The fungi that cause mycetomas are saprophytes of the soil and decaying vegetation and enter the skin through small wounds. Bridges (1957) observed that most cases of maduromycotic mycetomas in the United States are seen in the southern regions. He reported three cases in dogs and one in a horse and identified *Curvularia geniculata* as the causative

agent affecting the feet of one of the dogs. The genus *Curvularia* is closely related taxonomically to *Helminthosporium,* another genus that has been associated with the disease. Brodey et al. (1967) described a case of eumycotic (maduromycotic) mycetoma in a coonhound that had been used for hunting in Virginia and Pennsylvania. Clinically the dog had intermittent lameness and a progressively enlarged swelling in the right shoulder. *C. geniculata* was identified as the causative agent. Cases of eumycotic mycetoma in dogs have been reported (Jang and Popp 1970). In one animal the lesion was in the abdominal region, and in the other the spleen and portions of the gastric and duodenal walls were involved. *Petriellidium boydii,* an ascomycete, was isolated from both cases.

Brachycladium spiciferum was identified as a cause of maduromycosis in a cat, a horse, and a dog (Bridges and Beasley 1960). Generally, the clinical signs consisted of chronic inflammation with formation of nodular granulomatous masses in the foot of the cat, the skin of the head and body of the horse, and the prescapular lymph node of the dog. Pigmented colonies of fungus could be seen as brown to black specks in the lesions from the dog and the horse. Colonies of fungus were easily found in stained smears of pus taken from draining sinuses of the cat's foot.

Maduromycotic nasal granulomas have also been recorded on bovine nasal mucosa (Bridges 1960, Roberts et al. 1963). Cases have been observed in Louisiana, Texas, and Colorado. The disease is similar to snoring disease of cattle in India. Growth appears on the turbinate bones, causing the animal to sneeze and rub its nostrils on any available object. After several months a thick mucous discharge may block the nasal passages to the point where breathing is difficult. Microscopically there is an eosinophilic granulomatous proliferation of the nasal mucosa and submucosa accompanied by the appearance of deep epithelial crypts, Langhans' giant cells, and thinwalled chlamydoconidia. In some areas segmented hyphal elements also can be seen. A *Helminthosporium* species is believed to be the cause of snoring disease in American cattle.

Chromomycosis is rare in animals. Natural infection in a horse and a dog has been described by Simpson (1966). The mycetomas in this condition contain small (6 to 12 μm) dark single or clustered bodies. The causative fungi—*Curvularia* species, *Fonsecaea* species, and *Phialophora* species—are slow growing.

Diagnosis. Maduromycotic mycetomas are recognized by the presence of granules (100 to 300 μm) composed of compact masses of hyphae, chlamydoconidia in pus, and granulation tissue (Figure 37.14). The granules of

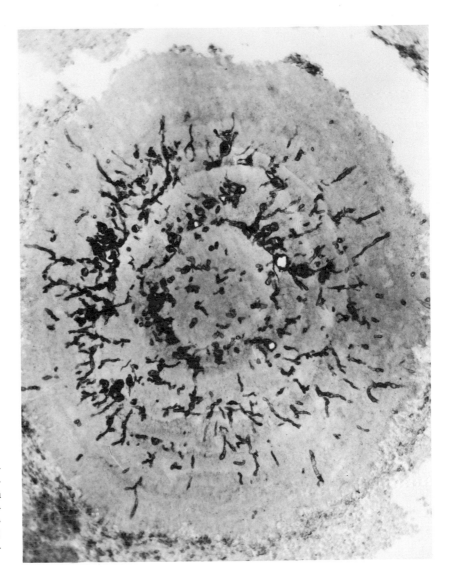

Figure 37.14. A large laminated acidophilic body from a case of bovine maduromycosis. It contains many chlamydoconidia and hyphae. The white holes represent microchlamydoconidia that extend to both surfaces of the section. Gridley fungus stain. × 190. (From Bridges, 1960, courtesy of *Cornell Veterinarian*.)

chromomycotic mycetomas are much smaller (6 to 12 μm) and do not contain hyphae. Identification of the causative fungi can be performed following culture and isolation on Sabouraud agar that contains a broad-spectrum antibiotic to inhibit bacterial contaminants. Incubation must be continued for 2 to 3 weeks because most of the fungi that cause mycetomas are very slow growing.

Antimicrobial Susceptibility. *Cladosporium* species, *Petriellidium boydii, Phialophora* species, and other dematiacious fungi are sensitive to ketoconazole and miconazole, but there are no reports of the use of these agents to treat mycetomas in animals.

REFERENCES

Bridges, C.H. 1957. Maduromycotic mycetomas in animals: *Curvularia geniculata* as an etiologic agent. Am. J. Pathol. 33:411–427.

Bridges, C.H. 1960. Maduromycosis of bovine nasal mucosa (nasal granuloma of cattle). Cornell Vet. 50:468–484.

Bridges, C.H., and Beasley, J.N. 1960. Maduromycotic mycetomas in animals—*Brachycladium spiciferum* Brainer as an etiologic agent. J. Am. Vet. Med. Assoc. 137:192–201.

Brodey, R.S., Schryver, H.S., Deubler, M.J., Kaplan, W., and Ajello, L. 1967. Mycetoma in a dog. J. Am. Vet. Med. Assoc. 151:442–451.

Jang, S.S., and Popp, J.A. 1970. Eumycotic mycetoma in a dog caused by *Allesheria boydii*. J. Am. Vet. Med. Assoc. 157:1071–1076.

Roberts, E.D., McDaniel, H.A., and Carbrey, E.A. 1963. Maduromycosis of the bovine nasal mucosa. J. Am. Vet. Med. Assoc. 142:42–48.

Simpson, J.G. 1966. A case of chromoblastomycosis in a horse. Vet. Med. 61:1207–1209.

Phaeohyphomycosis

Phaeohyphomycosis is the name applied to a disease caused by various species of dematiacious fungi whose tissue form consists of septate, dark-walled hyphae. Unlike maduromycosis, granules are not present in the lesions.

The disease is rare in animals (Kaplan et al. 1975). *Cladosporium* species, *Curvularia* species, and *Drechslera spicifera* are the most frequently encountered causative agents. Isolates of *Drechslera* organisms have been erroneously identified as *Helminthosporium* species. *Drechslera* organisms produce sympoduloconidia, whereas the conidia of *Helminthosporium* are borne on straight conidiophores of a definite length.

Horses infected with *D. spicifera* had lesions consisting of multiple cutaneous plaques 1 to 3 cm in diameter on various parts of the body. The lesions were black, denuded, and covered with small pustules and papules. The fungus in these lesions was in the form of individual and small groups of darkly pigmented septate hyphae (Kaplan et al. 1975). In horses and cats the lesions are localized in the subcutaneous tissues (Muller et al. 1975).

Kaplan et al. (1975) reported that Iodovet detergent applied frequently to lesions resulted in clinical improvement.

REFERENCES

Kaplan, W., Chandler, F.W., Ajello, L., Ganthier, R., Higgins, R., and Cayouette, P. 1975. Equine phaeomycosis caused by *Drechslera spicifera*. Can. Vet. J. 16:205–208.

Muller, G.H., Kaplan, W., Ajello, L., and Padhye, A.A. 1975. Phaeohyphomycosis caused by *Drechslera spicifera* in a cat. J. Am. Med. Assoc. 166:150–154.

Part III The Virales

---

38 The Viruses

Quite understandably the early bacteriologists believed that all contagious and infectious diseases were caused by bacteria, except for a few that were known to be caused by higher fungi and protozoa. But time showed that bacteria and other known disease-producing agents could not be identified with many diseases. Eventually it was learned that some of these infective fluids retained their ability to produce disease after they had been forced through fine-pored clay filters that retained all ordinary bacteria. This fact indicated that agents smaller than bacteria were capable of causing infectious diseases. For more than 40 years (1892 to 1935) this was about all that was known of such agents, which became known as filter-passing or filterable viruses. The adjective *filterable* is not used now because it is known that not all viruses are small enough to be filterable and some well-known bacteria can be made to pass through so-called bacteria-proof filters. The word *virus* now connotes a series of characteristics, among which filter passing is only one probable feature.

The first known virus was that of the tobacco mosaic disease (Figure 38.1). It was demonstrated by a Russian, Iwanowski (1892). Loeffler and Frosch (1898), in Germany, demonstrated that foot-and-mouth disease of cattle was caused by an agent that readily passed bacteria-proof filters and could not be seen with the microscope. Sanarelli (1898) proved that a highly contagious rabbit tumor (myxomatosis) was caused by a virus. In the years that have elapsed since these early discoveries, many viruses and virus diseases have been found or differentiated.

D'Herelle (1922) described the first of a series of viruses, which he named *bacteriophages* because they para-sitized bacterial cells, causing them to swell and burst. The ease with which these agents could be studied greatly stimulated research on viruses, and many of the observations on bacteriophages have been applicable to the viruses that infect plant and animal cells. An even greater stimulus to the study of viruses was the announcement by Stanley (1935) that he had successfully extracted a crystalline nucleoprotein with all the properties of the virus from tobacco plants affected with mosaic disease. The virus research field has been very active and productive in recent years because of the introduction of a number of new techniques. A new science of virology has been formed, staffed by individuals trained in biochemistry, genetics, electron microscopy, microbiology, immunology, biophysics, statistics, and/or pathology.

Terms Commonly Used by Virologists

Virion: The complete infective virus particle. It may be identical to the nucleocapsid. More complex virions include the nucleocapsid plus the surrounding envelope.

Capsid: The protein shell that encloses the nucleic acid core (genome).

Nucleocapsid: The capsid together with the enclosed nucleic acid.

Structure units: The basic units of similar structure in the capsid. They may be individual polypeptides.

Capsomeres: Morphologic units seen on the surfaces of isometric virus particles. They represent clusters of structure units.

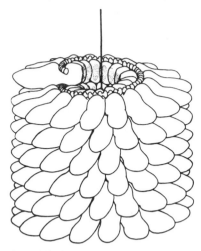

Figure 38.1 A model of tobacco mosaic virus with 2,130 elongated capsomeres, consisting of protein molecules, arranged around a hollow core. The helical coil embedded in the capsomeres represents the viral nucleic acid. (From Franklin et al., 1963, courtesy of Williams & Wilkins.)

Primary nucleic acid structure: The spatial arrangement of the complete nucleic acid chain. For example, is the nucleic acid single- or double-stranded, circular or linear, branched or unidirectional?

Tertiary nucleic acid structure: The fine spatial detail in the helix, such as super-coiling, breakage points, deletions, gaps, catenation, and regions of strand separation.

Envelope: The outer coat some viruses acquire as they penetrate or are budded from the nuclear or cytoplasmic membrane. Envelopes always contain altered host-cell membrane components.

Peplomers: Morphologic units composed of structural units embedded in the envelope.

Complementation: A general term to describe situations where mixed infections result in enhanced yields of one or both viruses in the mixture.

Translation: The mechanism by which a particular base sequence in messenger RNA produces a specific amino acid sequence in a protein.

Transcription: The means by which specific information encoded in a nucleic acid chain is transferred to messenger RNA.

Transcapsidation: A form of complementation in which two viruses "hybridize"; for example, an adenovirus capsid is spontaneously transferred to SV-40 nucleoids (or DNA).

Helper virus: Certain viruses are defective and require a closely related "helper" virus to complete their replication.

Defective virus: Functionally deficient particles in some aspect of replication; may interfere with replication of normal virus.

Pseudovirions: Normal-appearing particles under an electron microscope which are formed when the capsid sometimes erroneously encloses host nucleic acid. They do not replicate.

Viroids: A class of infectious agents, occurring in plants and perhaps in animals, that are smaller than viruses and consist of a short strand of ribonucleic acid without a capsid.

The Biological Nature of Viruses

From the time that viruses were discovered until Stanley initiated a new series of investigations on their nature, little had been learned about them. They were known for what they could do, not for what they were. The only criterion for their recognition was their ability to produce signs of disease in plants or animals and, in some cases, to form certain foreign bodies (inclusion bodies) within parasitized cells. Many speculated that a whole host of living beings, too small to be seen with the microscope and many perhaps leading a wholly saprophytic existence, might exist. There were no ways by which such a hypothesis could be proved or disproved. Gradually it became generally accepted that viruses could not be propagated like most bacteria in artificial culture media devoid of living cells—that viral growth and multiplication occurred only in living cells. Whether viruses were living or nonliving entities was a subject of considerable controversy until approximately three decades ago. Some virologists still speak of *live* and *killed* viruses. A Dutchman, Beijerinck (1899), started the controversy with his idea of a *contagium vivum fluidum*, a form of life that, if it existed, would certainly be different from anything known, since it would be noncellular. A still more unorthodox idea appeared—that viruses might be nonliving autocatalytic chemical agents that could instigate abnormal metabolic activities in the cells they attacked, one of the products of such abnormal activity being more of the instigating substance, which then became available in increased quantity for repeating the process in other cells of the same individual or, if it could escape to another host, for causing in it the same chain of events.

Life in the higher plants and animals generally is easily detectable by a series of well-known criteria. When it comes to determining life in very primitive beings, which probably are at a subcellular level, the usual distinctions fail. Unless new distinctions are made, we must regard viruses as nonliving agents. The basic structure of a virus is shown in Figure 38.2. It is perfectly clear that a strand of nucleic acid, which forms the core of a virus, is a

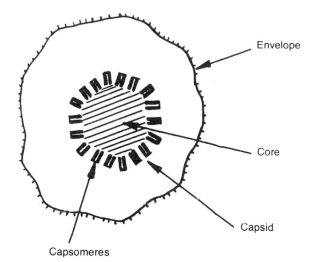

Envelope

Core

Capsid

Capsomeres

Figure 38.2. A diagram of a complete virus particle, or virion. The core is either RNA or DNA. (From R. W. Horne, courtesy of *Scientific American*.)

macromolecule with a definable chemical structure that can perform essential functions of living things in a suitable environment. This macromolecule can replicate and can also direct the synthesis of proteins. The newly formed nucleic acid and proteins are then assembled to form a complete virus particle. While the controversy was still raging in 1945, McFarlane Burnet suggested that epidemiologists and public health workers think of viruses as microorganisms. Lwoff and Tournier (1966) made it clear that viruses differ from other living things, including microorganisms, by five characters: (1) mature virus particles (virions) have only one type of nucleic acid, either DNA or RNA, whereas microorganisms possess both types, (2) virions are unable to grow or undergo binary fission; (3) virions make use of the ribosomes of their host cell; (4) virions are reproduced solely from their nucleic acid; other agents grow from the integrated sum of their constituents and reproduce by division; and (5) viruses lack genetic information for the synthesis of essential cellular systems such as that responsible for the production of energy with high potential. As our knowledge of viruses increased, it was shown that Lwoff's concepts did not encompass all discoveries; for example, the satellite viruses (Lwoff and Tournier 1966) cannot reproduce from their own nucleic acid, and neither the nucleic acid nor the virions are infectious. Even some bacteria such as chlamydiae with some ribosomes also are dependent on host-cell ribosomes.

The "contagious-living-fluid" concept is no longer tenable. Although there are many differences among virologists on other points, all now agree that viruses are particulate in nature; that is, they can be filtered out of

suspensions with appropriate filters, and they can be centrifuged out of suspensions with ultracentrifuges. Virus particles have been photographed with the electron microscope and their morphology and size accurately determined.

Animal and bacterial viruses contain either RNA or DNA, but not both, whereas plant viruses have RNA. Release of the nucleic acid from its protein outer coat involves lysis of the capsid by a detergent such as sodium dodecyl sulfate and further treatment of the nucleic acid with Pronase and phenol. Viruses from various groups, such as enterovirus, yield infectious RNA by such treatment, and members of Papovaviridae and the bacteriophages have yielded infectious DNA. Infectious RNA and infectious DNA are inactivated by their respective enzymes (ribonuclease or deoxyribonuclease), whereas the infectivity of intact particles is not affected by such treatment. On the other hand, antiserum produced for intact particles readily neutralizes the virion as the antibodies react with the antigens of the protein coat, but fails to inactivate free viral infectious nucleic acid. Purified DNA is not immunogenic, but DNA complexes containing appreciable protein not readily dissociated from DNA are antigenic and produce precipitating and C^1-fixing antibodies in rabbits.

Some viruses are toxic, as evidenced by the peracute death of mice within a few hours after parenteral injection of concentrated suspensions of influenza virus. At necropsy these animals show no pathological lesions except marked vascular congestion. In most viral diseases the inflammatory response usually is characterized by an infiltration of mononuclear cells and lymphocytes, whereas polymorphonuclear leukocytes predominate in the lesions of acute bacterial diseases. In many viral diseases pathogenic bacteria play an important role as secondary invaders of ectodermal tissues, so polymorphonuclear leukocytes invade the infected tissues after the mononuclear cells.

Classification and Nomenclature of Viruses

With the rapid advances in virology since the mid-1960s, virologists are producing a reasonable classification and nomenclature of viruses, including vertebrate, invertebrate, plant, and bacterial viruses. The responsibility for this task lies in the hands of the International Committee on the Taxonomy of Viruses (ICTV), which was established at the Ninth International Congress of Microbiology. The committee has approved a number of rules with the purpose of establishing uniformity and standardized terminology. Because many virologists other than members of the committee were involved in the task, the final product represented a consensus but by no means unanimity.

Many virus groups were proposed for consideration at the International Congress of Virology in Hungary in 1971. As taxonomy is a dynamic, ever-changing scheme, Figures 38.3 and 38.4 show the latest changes established by the ICTV on recommendation of its Vertebrate Virus Subcommittee. Detailed characterization data of virus groups usually are published in *Intervirology*, the official journal of the Virology Section of the International Association of Microbiological Societies. Viruses have been separated into families on the basis of their physical, chemical, and biological characteristics. For all virus groups family names now have been established, and these end in *idae*. Names of genera end with the word *virus*, and members of each genus share certain common characteristics. In general an effort has been made to provide for a latinized binomial nomenclature, and existing latinized names are to be retained if possible. Each virus-group description must include a designated type species, its taxonomic position (genus or family), its main characteristics, a list of viruses in the group, and a file of probable or possible members belonging in the group. The description should also include cryptograms for the groups and its individual viruses. Each cryptogram should contain (1) type of nucleic acid, strandedness of nucleic acid, molecular weight of nucleic acid (in millions), and percentage of nucleic acid in virus particle; (2) outline of virus particle and outline of nucleocapsid; and (3) kinds of host infected and kinds of vector. A proposed classification for viruses should be based on the features cited in the cryptogram and, in addition: (1) the presence or absence of an envelope; (2) certain measurements: for helical viruses, the diameter of the nucleocapsid; for cubical viruses, the triangulation number and the number of capsomeres; (3) the symmetry of the nucleocapsid (helical, cubical, or binal); and (4) certain characteristic biological and biophysical features. Ultimately, the classification undoubtedly will include comparisons of the nucleotide sequences of the viral nucleic acids homology (genetic relatedness) and nearest neighbor analyses.

Figure 38.5 is a diagram illustrating the shapes and relative sizes of animal viruses of the major families.

The key reference for virus nomenclature are the current Report of the International Committee on Taxonomy of Viruses, *Classification and Nomenclature of the Viruses* (Matthews 1982), and current specialty group and culture collection publications. The chapter on virus tax-

onomy written by Murphy (1985) is also an excellent reference.

DNA Viruses

Parvoviridae. Currently, the members of the family Parvoviridae are the only known viruses with single-stranded DNA. The prototype virus is *Parvovirus* RV. These small DNA viruses, 18 to 22 nm in diameter, are divided into two genera. The genus *Parvovirus* includes the Kilham rat virus, the X14 virus of rats, hamster osteolytic H viruses, minute virus of mice, porcine parvovirus, human parvovirus, infectious feline panleukopenia virus, and its closely related mink enteritis virus. Other members in the genus are avian parvovirus, canine parvovirus, minute virus of canines, hemorrhagic encephalopathy virus, and bovine parvovirus. The adeno-associated viruses 1, 2, 3, and 4 constitute the genus *Dependovirus*. The DNA liberated from adeno-satellites by conventional procedures acts like double-stranded nucleic acid; but the DNA within the virion stains with acridine orange and reacts with formaldehyde, as single-stranded DNA within the satellite particles exists as positive and negative complementary strands in separate particles. Upon extraction of DNA the positive and negative strands unite to form double-stranded DNA helix. The adenovirus satellites are defective and require an adenovirus "helper" to complete replication. Members of the *Parvovirus* genus are nondefective and replicate without assistance from another virus. The single-stranded DNA inside and outside of all particles indicates that the strands have a similar polarity. The icosahedral particles probably have 32 capsomeres, 2 to 4 nm in diameter, with a buoyant density in cesium chloride of 1.4 g/ml and a molecular mass of 1.4×10^6 daltons. The nonenveloped particles are acid- and heat-stable and ether-resistant. The mol% G + C of the DNA is 39. The viruses in this genus have three major polypeptides.

Viral replication occurs in the nucleus, and intranuclear inclusion bodies are formed.

Papovaviridae. The family Papovaviridae has two genera: *Polyomavirus* and *Papillomavirus*. The type species for the genus *Polyomavirus* is *Polyomavirus* m-1 (murine). Other viruses in the genus are simian vacuolating virus (SV40), rabbit-vacuolating virus, K virus, and also the virus associated with leukoencephalopathy in man. The viruses contain double-stranded, cyclic DNA (Figure 38.6) with a mol% G + C of 41 to 49. The icosahedral particles, 45 nm in diameter and with 5-3-2 symmetry, have a buoyant density in cesium chloride of 1.34 g/ml, a molecular mass of 3×10^6 daltons, and a sedi-

Figure 38.3. Taxonomy of DNA animal viruses*

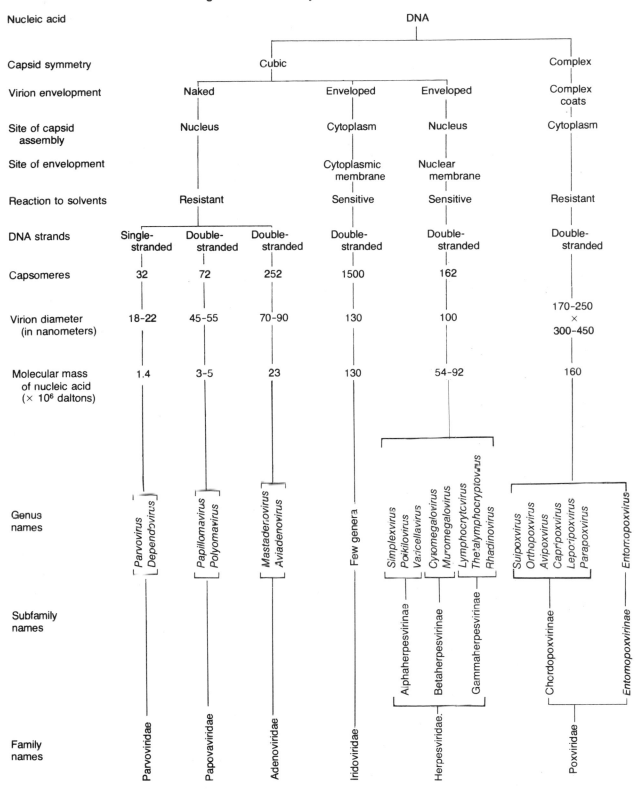

*A new proposed DNA family is the Hepadnaviridae, which includes pathogens with properties similar to the hepatitis B viruses.

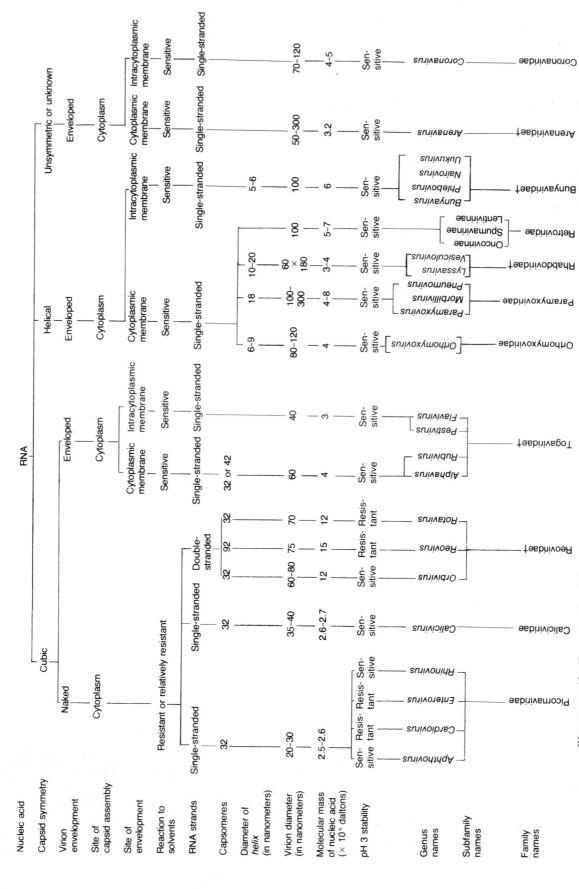

Figure 38.4. Taxonomy of RNA animal viruses*

*New proposed families are the Birnaviridae, which includes the two-segment ds RNA viruses, and the Filoviridae, which includes Marburg and Ebola viruses.
†Arboviruses included; cytoplasmic polyhedrosis viruses included in Reoviridae.

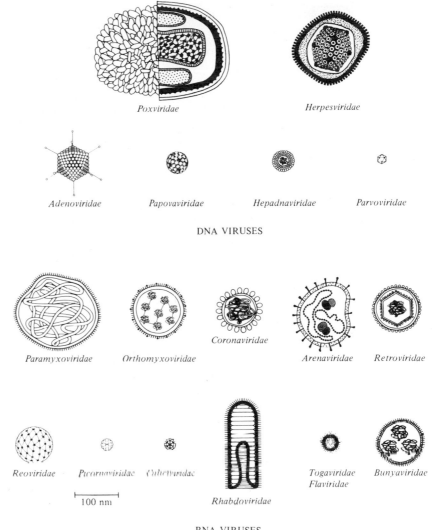

Poxviridae   *Herpesviridae*

Adenoviridae   *Papovaviridae*   *Hepadnaviridae*   *Parvoviridae*

DNA VIRUSES

Paramyxoviridae   *Orthomyxoviridae*   *Coronaviridae*   *Arenaviridae*   *Retroviridae*

Reoviridae   *Picornaviridae*   *Caliciviridae*   *Rhabdoviridae*   *Togaviridae Flaviridae*   *Bunyaviridae*

100 nm

RNA VIRUSES

Figure 38.5 Shapes and relative sizes of animal viruses of the major families (bar = 100 nm). From White and Fenner, 1986, courtesy of Academic Press.

mentation rate of 240S. The nonenveloped capsid has 72 capsomeres in a skew arrangement. There are five to seven structural proteins. The particles are acid- and heat-stable and ether-resistant. The viruses are assembled in the nucleus with the formation of intranuclear inclusion bodies. Some are oncogenic under certain conditions, but inapparent infections are the rule in most hosts. Several viruses hemagglutinate by reacting with neuraminidase sensitive receptors.

The *Papillomavirus* S-1 (Shope papillomavirus) is the type species for the genus *Papillomavirus*. Other members of the genus are rabbit oral papilloma, human papilloma, canine papilloma, canine oral papilloma, and bovine papillomaviruses. Probable members include papillomata of horses, monkeys, sheep, goats, and other species. Members of this genus contain double-stranded,

cyclic DNA with a mol% G + C of 49. The nonenveloped icosahedral particles, 55 nm in diameter and with 5–3–2 symmetry, have a molecular mass of 5×10^6 daltons, a buoyant density in cesium chloride of 1.34 g/ml, a sedimentation rate of 280 to 300S, and 72 capsomeres in a skew arrangement. The virions are ether-resistant and heat- and acid-stable.

The viruses replicate in the nucleus and cause papillomata in many animal hosts. Several viruses hemagglutinate by reacting with neuraminidase-sensitive receptors.

Adenoviridae. The genus *Mastadenovirus* includes a rather large number of viruses represented by the type species, *Adenovirus* h-1 (human). Other members of the genus include human types 2 to 35, 25 simian, 2 canine, 10 bovine, porcine, murine, avian, and other mammalian

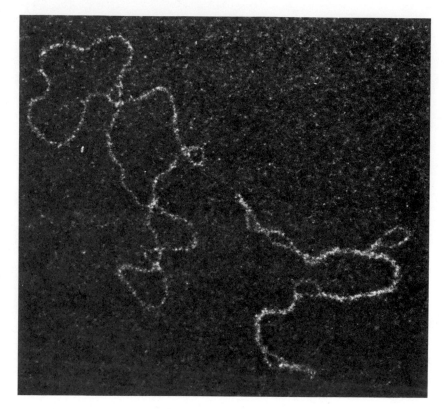

Figure 38.6. Electron micrograph of SV-40 DNA circular molecules. DNA molecules were picked up on 20-Å-thick carbon-aluminum film and spread by the aqueous technique. The DNA samples were imaged by tilted beam dark-field electron microscopy. Final magnification was 230,600. The length of both the relaxed form II SV-40 DNA (*left*) and that of the superhelical form I SV-40 DNA (*right*) was 1,500 nm. (Courtesy George Ruben and Ray Wu, Section of Biochemistry, Molecular and Cell Biology, Cornell University, Ithaca, N.Y. Reprinted with permission from *Biochemistry,* 15 (1976):738. Copyright by the American Chemical Society.)

adenoviruses from sheep, horse, and opossum. The genus *Aviadenovirus* covers the adenoviruses involving pathogens of various avian species. These double-stranded DNA viruses, 70 to 90 nm in diameter, have a mol% G + C of 48 to 57. Isometric nonenveloped particles with icosahedral symmetry have 252 capsomeres, 7 nm in diameter, arranged in a 5-3-2 axial symmetry. The vertex capsomeres carry a filamentous projection that is antigenically distinct from that of other capsomeres of the particle. The virions have a molecular mass of 23×10^6 daltons, a buoyant density in rubidium chloride of 1.34 g/ml, and a sedimentation rate of 795S. The particles are ether-resistant and heat- and acid-stable.

The virus replicates in the nucleus, where it causes intranuclear inclusion bodies. Some viruses hemagglutinate red blood cells of various species. Some adenoviruses are oncogenic in hamsters. A common antigen shared by all mammalian adenoviruses differs from a corresponding antigen of avian strains.

Iridoviridae. The type species of the single genus in the family Iridoviridae is *Iridovirus* t-1 (tipula iridescent virus). Other members are *Sericesthis iridescent* virus and *Chilo iridescent* virus; probable members are *Aedes iridescent* virus and other iridescent viruses of the mosquito. Other members include *Lymphocystis* virus of fish, African swine fever virus, *Amphibian cytoplasmic* virus,

and Gecko virus. The viruses contain approximately 15 percent double-stranded DNA (a single molecule) with a molecular mass of 130×10^6 daltons and a mol% G + C of 29 to 32. The icosahedral particles, 130 nm in diameter, have an icosahedral edge length of approximately 85 nm and a sedimentation rate of 2,200S. The complex particle contains several proteins, and the outer icosahedral shell contains approximately 1,500 capsomeres. Members in the genus have an envelope and are sensitive to solvents. The site of capsid assembly and envelopment is in the cytoplasm and virions are released by budding or cell destruction.

Herpesviridae. The family Herpesviridae is divided into three subfamilies: Alphaherpesvirinae (prototype virus: human herpes simplex), Betaherpesvirinae (prototype virus: human cytomegalovirus), and Gammaherpesvirinae (prototype virus: Epstein-Barr virus). The family contains an exceedingly large number of viruses involved in the production of disease. The type species is *Herpesvirus* h-1 (herpes simplex virus). Other members are *Herpesvirus simiae* (B virus), *Herpesvirus T* (of marmosets), perhaps two herpesviruses of *Cercopithecus*, herpesvirus of patos monkeys, herpesvirus of saimiri, *Herpesvirus cuniculi* (virus III of rabbits), pseudorabies virus, infectious bovine rhinotracheitis virus, varicella virus, equine rhinopneumonitis and other related equine herpesviruses, malignant catarrhal fever virus of cattle, bovine ulcerative mammillitis (Allerton) virus, feline rhinotracheitis virus, canine herpesvirus, Epstein-Barr virus (associated with infectious mononucleosis and Burkitt lymphoma), Marek's disease virus, avian infectious laryngotracheitis, avian herpesviruses of pigeons, parrots, owls, and cormorants, herpesvirus associated with lymphosarcoma in the African clawed frog, snake herpesvirus, cytomegaloviruses affecting various species including humans, porcine inclusion body rhinitis virus, sheep pulmonary adenomatosis (jaagsickte) virus, duck plague virus, and fish viruses.

Most animal pathogens have been assigned to either a subfamily or genus. Examples of some of the important animal herpesvirus that have been assigned to genera are as follows: *Simplexvirus*, bovine mammillitis and B virus; *Poikilovirus*, pseudorabies, equine rhinopneumonitis; *Muromegalovirus*, murine megalovirus; *Lymphocryptovirus*, baboon herpesvirus, chimpanzee herpesvirus; *Thetalymphocryptovirus*, Marek's disease herpesvirus, turkey herpesvirus; and *Rhadinovirus*, herpesvirus ateles, herpesvirus saimiri.

The herpesviruses contain linear double-stranded DNA with terminal reiterations and internal repetition of terminal sequences; the mol% G + C of the DNA is 57 to 74. The viruses have a molecular mass of 54 to 92 $\times 10^6$ daltons, and the nucleocapsid, 100 nm in diameter with more than 20 structural proteins, shows cubic and icosahedral symmetry with 162 hollow and elongated capsomeres that are usually hexagonal, but sometimes pentagonal in cross-section. Lipid membrane surrounding the capsid is 150 nm in diameter and sometimes has an Fc receptor. The particles are sensitive to lipid solvents and also are acid-labile. The particle DNA content is approximately 7 percent of its weight, and it has a buoyant density in cesium chloride of 1.27–1.29 g/ml. The development begins in the nucleus, and the particle is completely formed by the addition of protein membranes as the virus passes into the cellular cytoplasm.

Intranuclear inclusion bodies are formed by these viruses. A few contain hemagglutinins. Viruses in this group cause a broad variety of infectious diseases ranging in character from acute catarrhal disease to oncogenic disease.

Poxviridae. The Poxviridae family is divided into two subfamilies: Chordopoxvirinae, which contains six genera of mammalian viruses, and Entomopoxvirinae, consisting of one genus of insect viruses.

Member viruses in the genera of the subfamily Chordopoxvirinae are as follows. *Orthopoxvirus* includes vaccinia, variola, alastrim, cowpox, horsepox, catpox, ectromelia, rabbitpox, monkeypox, buffalopox, and cam-

elpox. *Avipoxvirus* includes turkeypox, canarypox, fowlpox, quailpox, lovebirdpox, sparrowpox, starlingpox, and pigeonpox. *Capripoxvirus* includes sheeppox, goatpox, and lumpy skin disease virus. *Leporipoxvirus* includes myxoma viruses, rabbit fibroma, hare fibroma, and squirrel fibroma. *Parapoxvirus* includes contagious pustular dermatitis of sheep (orf), sealionpox virus, bovine papular stomatitis, and pseudocowpox viruses. *Suipoxvirus* includes swinepox. It is interesting to note that no poxvirus has been described in the dog. Many important animal pathogens in this group cause fatal disease and serious economic losses.

The symmetry of the capsid of these largest vertebrate viruses is unknown. The poxviruses contain 5 to 7.5 percent double-stranded DNA in linear form with a molecular mass of 160×10^6 daltons. The mol% G + C of the nucleic acid is 35 to 40. Brick-shaped or ovoid complex particles, 170 to 250 by 300 to 450 nm have a buoyant density in cesium chloride varying from 1.1–1.33 g/ml. The particles have characteristic surface patterns and lateral bodies and some poxviruses have an envelope. Some poxviruses are known to contain RNA polymerase. There is a nucleoprotein antigen common to all members, and members of Chordopoxvirinae also have other antigens in common and can recombine genetically. All poxviruses exhibit nongenetic reactivation and replicate in cytoplasmic foci.

Hepadnaviridae (proposed family). The family Hepadnaviridae, if formally accepted, would include viruses similar to hepatitis B–type viruses found in humans, woodchucks, ground squirrels, red-bellied squirrels, and Pekin ducks. No genera have been proposed.

RNA Viruses

A group of more than 350 viruses, called the arbovirus group, have interesting ecological cycles involving vertebrate hosts and arthropods, which serve as vectors in the transmission of the viruses to humans and domestic and wild animals. Many arboviruses are pathogenic in vertebrate hosts. As our knowledge of these viruses has advanced and our system of virus classification has improved, it has been possible to place many arboviruses into one of five RNA virus families: Reoviridae, Togaviridae, Bunyaviridae, Rhabdoviridae, and Arenaviridae.

Picornaviridae. The family Picornaviridae now has four genera: *Aphthovirus*, *Cardiovirus*, *Enterovirus*, and *Rhinovirus*. Member viruses in the genus *Enterovirus* are the three poliovirus serotypes; Coxsackie A and B viruses; human ECHO viruses; bovine, porcine, murine, and simian enteroviruses; Nodamura virus; avian encephalomyelitis; duck hepatitis virus; and human hepatitis A virus. The genus *Rhinovirus* includes human (more than 90 serotypes), bovine, and equine rhinoviruses. The genus *Aphthovirus* contains seven foot-and-mouth disease serotypes. The genus *Cardiovirus* has only one virus, that of encephalomyocarditis, which rarely infects humans.

Member viruses contain single-stranded RNA in linear form. The molecular mass of RNA is 2.5 to 2.6×10^6 daltons, and the mol% G + C is 40 to 54. Virions are isometric, nonenveloped, and 20 to 30 nm in diameter, with icosahedral symmetry (T = 3, 32 capsomeres probably). Virions are assembled in cytoplasm. The viruses have four major polypeptides. Rhinoviruses have a buoyant density in cesium chloride of 1.34–1.35 g/ml. Infectivity is ether-resistant. Enteroviruses and encephalomyocarditis virus are acid-stable, and rhinoviruses and foot-and-mouth disease virus are acid-labile. Enteroviruses and some rhinoviruses are stabilized against heat inactivation by magnesium chloride. Many viruses hemagglutinate. Replication involves translation of large precursor polyproteins and posttranslational cleavage into functional polypeptides. Replication and assembly take place in the cytoplasm, and the virus is released by cell destruction. There are very important human and animal pathogens in this family.

Caliciviridae. The family Caliciviridae has a single genus, *Calicivirus*, which includes vesicular exanthema viruses of swine, sea lions, and fur seals as well as feline caliciviruses. These viruses cause disease in their respective hosts.

Member viruses contain single-stranded RNA with a molecular mass of about 2.6 to 2.7×10^6 daltons and a mol% G + C of 46. Virions are isometric, nonenveloped, and 35 to 40 nm in diameter, with icosahedral symmetry (probably T = 3). Buoyant density in cesium chloride is 1.36 to 1.39 g/ml. Virions contain only one major structural polypeptide and two minor polypeptides. Infectivity is ether-resistant, and stability at acid pH is variable (generally labile at pH 3). The 32 capsomeres are cup-shaped.

Replication and assembly occur in the cytoplasm and particles are released upon cell destruction.

Reoviridae. The family Reoviridae has been expanded considerably in the last few years and now includes many important animal pathogens, particularly in the genera *Orbivirus* and *Rotavirus*. The three mammalian serotypes in the genus *Reovirus* have been associated with respiratory and enteric diseases of animals, most often as inapparent infections.

This is the only family with animal viruses that contain double-stranded RNA, which is arranged in 10 linear segments. Molecular mass of these segments varies from 0.3 to 3.0×10^6 daltons, and total genome is 15×10^6 (reovirus) or 12×10^6 daltons (orbivirus and rotavirus). The mol% G + C is 42 to 44. Virions are isometric, nonenveloped, and 75 nm (reovirus), 60 to 80 nm (orbivirus), or 70 nm (rotavirus) in diameter. There are 6 to 10 major structural polypeptides, and the viruses carry a transcriptase and other enzymes. Virions have a double capsid shell, and the structure of outer capsid layer is indistinct. The inner capsids of orbiviruses and rotaviruses have icosahedral symmetry (T = 3 plus complex secondary symmetry). Virions are assembled in cytoplasm. Buoyant density in cesium chloride is 1.36 g/ml. Infectivity is resistant (reoviruses) or partly resistant (orbiviruses) to ether treatment; infectivity is resistant (reoviruses and rotaviruses) or sensitive (orbiviruses) to acid conditions. Intracytoplasmic inclusion bodies are formed by many viruses. Reoviruses and rotaviruses hemagglutinate.

Important diseases caused by organisms in the genus *Orbivirus* are African horsesickness, bluetongue in sheep and cattle, Colorado tick fever, and epizootic hemorrhagic disease of deer. Viruses in the genus *Rotavirus* cause diseases such as human infantile diarrheal disease, rotavirus diarrheal disease of neonatal calves, foals, piglets, kittens, and puppies; and epizootic diarrhea of infant mice. Infectious pancreatic necrosis virus of trout and infectious bursal disease virus of chickens, previously placed in this family, are provisionally placed in a new family, Birnaviridae.

Togaviridae. There are four genera in the family Togaviridae: *Alphavirus*, *Rubivirus*, *Pestivirus*, and *Flavivirus*. Member viruses contain single-stranded RNA in linear form. The molecular mass of RNA is 3 or 4×10^6 daltons, and the mol% G + C is 48 to 51. Virions are either isometeric and enveloped, 60 nm (alphaviruses and rubiviruses), or 40 nm (flaviviruses and pestiviruses), in diameter, including envelope and surface projections. They have three to four structural polypeptides, one or two of which are glycosylated. Icosahedral symmetry has been proved for capsid of alphaviruses only (T = 3 or T = 4). Virions are assembled in cytoplasm by budding from host cell membranes. Buoyant density in cesium chloride is 1.25 g/ml. Infectivity is ether-sensitive and variably sensitive to acid conditions. Alphaviruses and flaviviruses replicate in vertebrate and arthropod hosts; rubiviruses and pestiviruses have no invertebrate host. Virions act as hemagglutinin. There are a large number of viruses assigned to this family. Only members that are significant pathogens in humans, animals, or both are listed here. In the genus *Alphavirus*, eastern, western, and Venezuelan equine encephalitides and Sindbis virus are worthy of mention. Yellow fever; dengue 1–4; Japanese

B, Murray Valley, Russian spring-summer, and St. Louis encephalitides; louping ill; Israel turkey meningoencephalitis; and West Nile fever viruses are important pathogens in the genus *Flavivirus*. In the genus *Rubivirus* are rubella and possibly equine arteritis viruses. Members of the genus *Pestivirus* cause two important diseases in domestic animals: bovine virus diarrhea and hog cholera.

Orthomyxoviridae. The well-characterized viruses in the Orthomyxoviridae constitute three types—A, B, and C—and are all classified in the genus *Orthomyxovirus*. The member viruses contain single-stranded RNA in eight segments. The molecular mass of RNA segments varies from 1.1×10^5 to 1×10^6 daltons, and total genome is 4×10^6 daltons. The mol% G + C is 41 to 43. Virions are spherical, elongated, or filamentous and are 80 to 120 nm in diameter; filaments may reach several nanometers in length. The viruses have seven to nine major polypeptides, including a transcriptase. Virions consist of a unit-membrane envelope modified with viral M protein that has two types of precise projections, hemagglutinin and neuraminidase, and helically symmetrical ribonucleocapsid, 6 to 9 nm. Viral ribonucleocapsid accumulates in the nucleus, and virions are formed by budding from plasma membrane. Buoyant density in sucrose is 1.19–1.21 g/ml. Infectivity is sensitive to ether, acid, and heat. Viruses hemagglutinate by attachment to neuraminidae-sensitive receptors, except for influenza C, which does not have demonstrable neuraminidase. Recombination is common between influenza A viruses. Antigenic variation is frequent as drifts and shifts occur. An RNA-dependent RNA polymerase is associated with purified virions.

The Orthomyxoviridae include viruses of types A, B, and C. Type A viruses include human influenza, porcine influenza, equine influenza, and avian influenza. Types B (B/Lee/40) and C(C/Taylor/1233/47) are human-influenza serotypes. Influenza A viruses have fifteen hemagglutinin variant types, and nine neuraminidase types are recognized. Strains from different species may share these antigens. Hemagglutinin and neuraminidase differences in influenza B virus distinguish antigenic variants, but no types are specified. Influenza C strains show hemagglutinin variants, but no types have been specified. Influenza A viruses cause respiratory infections of pigs, horses, and birds. The orthomyxoviruses are sensitive to dactinomycin.

Paramyxoviridae. The family Paramyxoviridae consists of three genera: *Paramyxovirus*, *Morbillivirus*, and *Pneumovirus*. Viruses in this family contain single-stranded RNA in unsegmented linear form. The molecular mass of RNA is 4 to 8×10^6 daltons, and the G + C is 48 to 52. Virions are spherical or pleomorphic and 100 to 300 nm in diameter. There are five to seven major polypeptides including a transcriptase and a neurominidase (except morbilliviruses). Virions consist of a unit-membrane envelope with surface projections containing a single, helically symmetric ribonucleocapsid, 18 nm in diameter. Virions are formed in the cytoplasm by budding from the cytoplasmic membrane. The buoyant density in cesium chloride is 1.23 g/ml. Virions are sensitive to acid, ether, and heat. Viruses in the genus *Paramyxovirus* hemagglutinate by attachment to neuraminidase-sensitive receptors. The paramyxoviruses are resistant to dactinomycin.

Viruses in the genus *Paramyxovirus* include Newcastle disease virus, mumps virus, parainfluenza viruses 1–4, turkey paramyxovirus, and Yucaipa virus. There are four important pathogens in the genus *Morbillivirus*: measles virus, canine distemper virus, rinderpest virus, and peste de petite ruminant virus. The respiratory syncytial viruses and pneumonia virus of mice are members of the genus *Pneumovirus*.

Rhabdoviridae. Members of the family Rhabdoviridae contain 2 percent single-stranded RNA with a molecular mass of 3 to 4×10^6 daltons and with a mol% G + C of approximately 42. The helical nucleocapsid, 10 to 20 nm in diameter is surrounded by a shell to which is closely applied an envelope with 10-nm spikes. The viruses have four to five major polypeptides, including a transcriptase. The whole particle is bullet-shaped, measuring 60 by 180 nm, and has a buoyant density in cesium chloride of 1.2 g/ml. Infectivity is destroyed by ether and acid. Some viruses hemagglutinate by means of the surface projection glycoprotein, and antigenic relationships exist between some members. Most members multiply in arthropods as well as vertebrates.

The type species is *Rhabdovirus* b-1 (vesicular stomatitis virus). Other members are cocal, Hart Park, Kern Canyon, Flanders, and rabies viruses, and also viruses of fish, bats, flies, and plants.

Retroviridae. The family Retroviridae has been divided into three subfamilies: Oncovirinae, Spumavirinae, and Lentivirinae. The viruses contain single-stranded RNA in linear form. The molecular mass of RNA is 5 to 7×10^6 daltons consisting of two subunits of equal size. The mol% G + C is 47 to 57. Virions are complex, enveloped, and about 100 nm in diameter. Virions consist of a unit-membrane envelope with surface projections (knobs), an inner shell with icosahedral symmetry, and a central core or nucleocapsid, probably with helical symmetry. Virions are assembled by budding through cytoplasmic and plasma membranes after the formation of inner structures in the cytoplasm. Buoyant density in cesium chloride is 1.18 g/ml. Infectivity is destroyed by ether, acid, and heat. All viruses contain a number of major polypeptides, including an antigenically specific, RNA-dependent DNA polymerase (reverse transcriptase); and replication of viral RNA involves a DNA provirus, which is integrated into host DNA. Many viruses cause neoplastic diseases, especially leukemias, sarcomas, mammary carcinomas, and degenerative diseases.

Members of Oncovirinae include many murine leukemia and sarcoma viruses, feline leukemia and sarcoma viruses, and tumor pathogens from many other species, including rats, guinea pigs, cattle, pigs, monkeys, baboons, chickens, and reptiles. Visna and maedi viruses of sheep are in the subfamily Lentivirinae. In the subfamily Spumavirinae are the foamy viruses of primates, cats, hamsters, cattle, and humans.

Bunyaviridae. All viruses in the family Bunyaviridae are arboviruses that contain single-stranded RNA in three or four linear segments. There are four genera: *Bunyavirus*, *Phlebovirus*, *Nairovirus*, and *Uukuvirus*. The total genome has a molecular mass of 6×10^6 daltons and consists of three molecules of circular, negative-sense single-stranded RNA. The viruses have four major polypeptides, including a transcriptase. Virions are spherical, enveloped, and 90 to 120 nm in diameter. Virions consist of a unit-membrane envelope with surface projections, which may be randomly placed or clustered in arrays with icosahedral symmetry, containing helically symmetrical ribonucleocapsids with circular configuration, 5 to 6 nm in diameter. The viruses exhibit hemagglutination via one of the two surface-projection glycoproteins. Virions are formed by budding from intracytoplasmic (primarily Golgi) membranes. Buoyant density in potassium tartrate is 1.20 g/ml. Infectivity is destroyed by ether, acid, and heat. Virus particles hemagglutinate.

Important diseases in this family are Nairobi sheep disease, sandfly fever, Rift Valley fever, and Crimean hemorrhagic fever.

Arenaviridae. Members of the only genus, *Arenavirus*, in the family Arenaviridae contain single-stranded RNA in linear segments. Molecular mass of four large RNA segments varies from 2.1, 1.7, 1.1, and 0.7×10^6 daltons; one to three small RNA segments are about 0.03×10^6 daltons. Virions are spherical or pleomorphic and 50 to 300 nm in diameter. Virions consist of a unit-membrane envelope with surface projections containing varying numbers of ribosome particles (20 to 25 nm) either free in the interior or, less commonly, connected by a linear structure. Virions are formed by budding from plasma membrane. Buoyant density in cesium chloride is 1.19–1.20 g/ml. Infectivity is sensitive to ether, acid, and heat. Most viruses have a limited rodent host range in

nature, in which maintenance is by persistent infection with viruria. All viruses share a group-specific antigen determined by the immunofluorescence test and in some instances by the complement-fixation test.

Important diseases caused by viruses in this family include lymphocytic choriomeningitis, Bolivian and Argentinian hemorrhagic fever, and Lassa fever.

Coronaviridae. Member viruses contain single-stranded RNA. The molecular mass of RNA is 4 to 5×10^6 daltons. Virions are spherical or pleomorphic and 70 to 120 nm in diameter. They consist of a unit-membrane envelope with unique, definitive, bulbous projections; the interior structure is not fully resolved, but probably is a loose, helically symmetrical nucleocapsid. The viruses have four to six structural polypeptides, two of which are glycosylated. Virions are formed budding from intracytoplasmic membranes. Buoyant density in sucrose in 1.18 g/ml. Infectivity is sensitive to ether, acid, and heat.

Viruses in the family Coronaviridae cause a variety of illnesses. Infectious bronchitis virus causes a respiratory disease in chickens. Coronaviruses have been implicated in disease processes in cattle, pigs, dogs, humans, cats, and possibly horses. One member causes bluecomb disease in turkeys.

Viroids. A new class of infectious agents, viroids are smaller than viruses. Viroids exhibit the characteristics of nucleic acids in crude extracts. They are insensitive to heat and organic solvents but sensitive to nucleases and do not appear to possess a protein coat. Viroids are small, naked infectious molecules of circular single-stranded RNA with extensive internal base pairing and a molecular mass of 75,000 to 100,000 daltons. The tight folding of the RNA and the closed circle presumable protect viroids from extracellular nucleases. These agents cause five separate plant diseases and may cause disease in humans and animals, although this is only speculative at present.

Instrumentation Used to Determine Size and Morphology of Viruses

Electron Microscopy

Electron micrographs are photographs made with an electron microscope (Figure 38.7). This instrument of magnification uses beams of electrons instead of light rays and electromagnetic fields instead of lenses of glass or quartz. Because the beams of electrons cannot be seen with the eye, the images are projected on a fluorescent plate, which renders them visible just as x-rays can be seen on a fluoroscope. The micrographs are the images secured on photographic plates.

With an electron microscope, images with sharp defini-

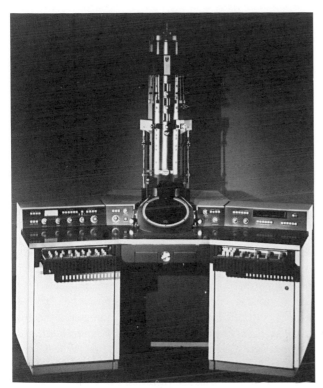

Figure 38.7. Electron microscope. Philips Model 302. (Courtesy Philips Electronic Instruments, Inc., Mahwah, N.J.)

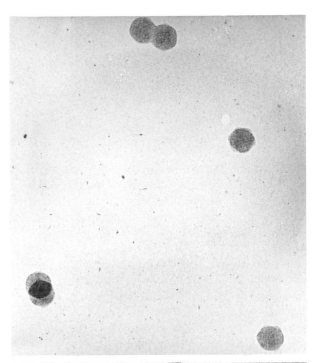

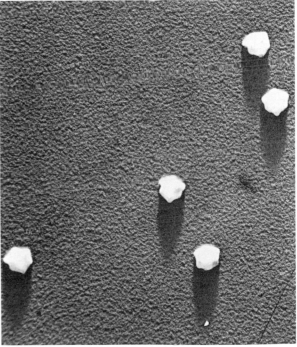

Figure 38.8. Electron micrographs of air-dried particles of the tipula iridescent virus. × 52,000. (*Top*) Unshadowed particles. (*Bottom*) Metallic shadowed particles. (From Robley C. Wiiliams and Kenneth M. Smith, courtesy of *Biochimica et Biophysica Acta.*)

tion can be secured at magnifications as high as 1:1,000,000 by enlarging electron micrographs. The advantages of this instrument can be seen when it is compared with the best optical equipment, in which resolution is difficult to obtain with magnifications greater than 1,200 diameters.

The objects from which electron micrographs are made usually are mounted on very thin collodion films supported on fine metallic screens. Because the density of many of the very small particles is not great, the early micrographs were not clear. This was remedied by the work of Williams and Wyckoff (1945), who introduced metallic shadowing into the process (Figure 38.8). Their innovation not only provided the needed contrast but also made possible the introduction of a third dimension into the photographs. The prepared films are dried and then introduced into a small chamber, which is evacuated. They are carefully oriented with reference to a focal point, where a small particle of the shadowing metal (silver, gold, chromium, etc.) is placed. The metal is then heated by an electric current until it is vaporized. In the vacuum the vaporized metal molecules are dispersed in every direction, lodging on the first surfaces encountered. Because the films on the collodion membranes are deliberately oriented at an angle to the source of the metallic

Table 38.1 The approximate size of virus units in comparison with other well-known molecules and other microorganisms

	Micrometers		Micrometers
Staphylococcus aureus	0.8 to 1.0	St. Louis encephalitis virus	0.025
Chlamydia organisms	0.3	Louping ill virus	0.015–0.020
Vaccinia virus	0.20	Foot-and-mouth disease virus	0.023
Pseudorabies virus	0.12	Poliomyelitis virus	0.025
Vesicular stomatitis virus	0.176 by 0.069	Serum globulin	0.0063
Fowl plague virus	0.080	Serum albumin	0.0056
Rift Valley fever virus	0.030	Egg albumin	0.004

dispersion, the metal film is deposited on any particles in this film, and there are "shadows" on the side of the particles where the metallic molecules are prevented from reaching the surface by the height of the particles. These shadows give a realistic idea of the third dimension of the particles.

The negative staining technique that employs the use of phosphotungstic acid is excellent for studying structures of viruses with the electron microscope. The phosphotungstate permeates the virus particle as a cloud and clearly shows the surface structure by virtue of negative staining. It also enters the core of noninfectious particles without nucleic acid. Thus it is possible to study the development of virus particles at different stages of replication.

Thin sections of infected animal tissues or pellets of centrifuged cells from infected cell cultures have also advanced our knowledge of virus structure. Unless special precautions are taken in preparation of specimens, electron micrographs may cause one to overestimate the diameter of viruses.

The size of some animal viruses, in comparison with some other microorganisms and protein molecules, is indicated in Table 38.1. It is customary in measuring such small objects to use the *nanometer* (nm) as the unit of measure, this unit being 0.001 of a micrometer (μm). By such a scale the elementary bodies of chlamydiae measure about 0.3 μm, or 300 nm. In the table, micrometers are used as the unit to avoid confusion. Particles with a twofold difference in diameter have an eightfold difference in volume.

Ultrafiltration

Because the pore size of silica filters (Pasteur, Berkefeld) is not the sole factor that determines whether particles in suspension will be passed, such filters have been discarded as a means of determining the approximate size of virus elements. To avoid the absorbing properties of silica filters, Bechhold as early as 1907 introduced the use of collodion membranes as filters for virus suspen-sions. Many years later, Elford (1931) and Bauer and Hughes (1934–1935) standardized such filters (gradocol membranes) so that they might be used for determining the approximate size of virus particles. By the use of membranes of differing pore sizes, it was possible to determine the approximate diameter of the elements of many viruses. The size of the limiting average pore diameter multiplied by 0.64 yields the diameter of the virus particle. Later, when other methods of determining particle size were discovered, it was found that the membrane filters had given reasonably accurate results. Early studies for estimation of size by filtration often underestimated the size.

Ultracentrifugation

The ordinary laboratory centrifuges, operating at full speed, rarely spin faster than 4,000 revolutions per minute (rpm). At this rate most bacteria and larger particles with a specific gravity heavier than the fluids in which they are suspended gravitate rapidly to the bottoms of the tubes that contain them. Most virus particles, being much more minute, are thrown down at a very much slower rate—so slow, in fact, that it is not possible to remove most of them from suspensions in this way. More successful are the angle centrifuges in which the tubes are held at an angle while spinning; here sedimenting particles have to travel only a short distance before they come in contact with the fluid-glass interface. For sedimenting the smaller virus particles, ultracentrifuges are needed. These are instruments of several types which can be operated at speeds of 60,000 rpm and more with centrifugal forces up to 200,000 times the force of gravity. One of them is described by Bauer and Pickels (1936). These instruments have been used to determine physical characteristics of virus elements, as well as of other minute bodies such as albumin molecules. The approximate size can be calculated from data yielded by the sedimentation constants. The agreement between these calculations and the data derived from filtration studies is very good. It was known before the electron microscope was developed that different viruses varied in size, some being only a little larger than protein molecules and others as large as some of the smaller bacteria.

Ionizing Radiation

A beam of charged particles such as high-energy electrons, alpha particles, or deuterons passing through a virus causes a loss in primary ionization. The release of these ions within the virion inactivates particle infectivity, antigenicity, and hemagglutinins.

By ascertaining the number of ionizations per unit volume or area required to inactivate 63 percent of the infectivity of the viral preparation, one can determine the average sensitive volume or area per ionization. This is the point at which there has been an average of one hit per sensitive target, according to the Poisson distribution, so the volume or area per ionization is equivalent to volume or area of the sensitive unit measured. Thus, knowledge of the volume or area permits calculation of the diameter or area of the infective unit in the virus particle. In the same way it is possible to measure the sizes of complement-fixing antigens and hemagglutinins.

Ultraviolet rays and x-rays inactivate viruses. The inactivating dose varies for different viruses.

Determination of Viral Morphology

The morphology of viruses is determined principally by electron microscopy and x-ray diffraction.

The capsids of animal viruses are arranged in two forms of symmetry, cubic and helical. All cubic symmetry in animal viruses is characteristic of an icosahedron with its 5-3-2 pattern of rotational symmetry. The arrangement of capsomeres to comply with icosahedral symmetry is limited. This limitation in its simplest form can be expressed by the formula

$$N = 10 (n - 1)^2 + 2$$

where N represents the number of capsomeres and n signifies the number of capsomeres on one side of each equilateral triangle. The icosahedron has 20 equilateral triangular faces with 12 vertices (see Figure 43.1, of an adenovirus), although the face (30 in number) of the Picornaviridae members may be a rhombus, thus changing the formula to

$$N = 30 (n - 1)^2 + 2$$

The triangulation number can also be used to group viruses with icosahedral symmetry. The number of capsomeres (morphologic units) is expressed by the formula

$$M = 10T + 2$$

One class has values of 1, 4, 9, 16, and 25; a second class, values of 3 and 12; and a third class, values of 7, 13, 19, and 21.

Properties of Viral Components

Nucleic Acid

The viral nucleic acid carries the genetic information for the replication of the virus. The type of nucleic acid can be determined by various means, using the intact virus particle or the free nucleic acid. The enzyme digestion test with free virus nucleic acid constitutes a method reliable for determining the nucleic acid type. The type of nucleic acid and its strandedness can be determined by fixing smears of purified virus with an alcohol fixation followed by staining with acridine orange (pH 4.0, dye concentration 0.01 percent). Double-stranded viruses, either RNA or DNA, stain red in the fluorescent microscope. Uranyl acetate is a specific stain for DNA while having no affinity for RNA. This stain is often used in electron microscopy preparations for this purpose. Density-gradient centrifugation in cesium salts also is used to differentiate RNA from DNA.

The viral nucleic acids are physically fragile once removed from their capsid protection, making it difficult to study their structure. It is possible now to examine many nucleic acid molecules in the electron microscope without disrupting them. The molecules are spread in a special inert protein monofilm so their complete contour lengths can be measured accurately. In most viruses the nucleic acids are linear, but in some the molecule takes the form of a circle. Papovaviridae have a double-stranded circle, often hypercoiled (Figure 38.9). By using linear densities of approximately 2×10^6 daltons (1 dalton equals the mass of one hydrogen atom) per micrometer for double-stranded forms and half that amount for single-stranded forms, the molecular mass of viral genomes can be calculated from direct measurements.

A finding of great interest and significance cited the presence of a DNA polymerase in RNA viruses that synthesizes DNA from an RNA template. Thus, it has been demonstrated that an RNA virus can make DNA.

Protein

Viral proteins have several important functions. They determine the antigenicity of the virus and are very much

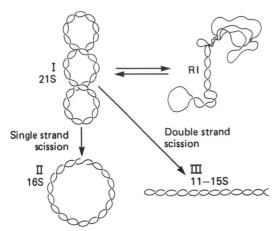

Figure 38.9. Forms of DNA of *Papovavirus* SV-40 and sedimentation coefficients in neutral sucrose gradients: supercoiled (I), nicked (II), linear (III), and replicative intermediate (RI). Linear DNA is formed by restriction endonucleases, which cleave both strands of the DNA at a single site. The RI shows two forks, three branches, and no ends, as seen in electron microscopy. (From E. Jawetz, J. L. Melnick, and E. A. Adelberg, *Review of Medical Microbiology,* 13th ed. Copyright 1978 by Lange Medical Publications, Los Altos, Calif.)

involved in the immunogenic process; thus they are of great interest to those who produce vaccines. In addition, these proteins determine the relatedness of viruses and thus are important to the diagnostician. The proteins also protect the viral genome against inactivation by nucleases in tissues, participate in the adsorption of the virus particle to a susceptible cell, and serve as they provide structural symmetry to the virus. Viral protein as such is not pathogenic.

The structural proteins of viruses have been extensively studied, including those of poliovirus. Despite some knowledge of the structural arrangement and chemical composition from poliovirus protein, there is little known about the binding of its RNA to the protein. Polypeptides of purified poliovirus particles obtained by treatment with detergents were analyzed by polyacrylamide gel electrophoresis. Four polypeptides were found to exist in poliovirus. Other analyses suggested that these polypeptides exist as precursors of the infectious virus in cells and become assembled with the viral RNA to form the virion.

In addition to the structural proteins, other virus specific proteins are formed in an infected cell (e.g., the virus-specific enzyme, thymidine kinase, in herpes- and vaccinia-infected cells).

Lipids

Lipids are found in viruses that have an envelope. Viruses containing essential lipids are ether-sensitive and

chloroform-sensitive. Certain poxviruses are ether-resistant and chloroform-sensitive, but this is the only virus family showing this distinction among certain of its members.

The study of viral lipids presents real problems because their distinction from contaminating host cell lipids associated with virus particles is difficult. In general the lipids are added to the virus particle as it matures or buds through the cell or nuclear membrane. In the process the host membranes are incorporated into the complete virus particle. The host membrane of the virus-infected cell differs from a noninfected cell. For example, the limiting membrane of orthomyxoviruses contains neuraminidase, an enzyme not found in normal cell membranes. Another RNA virus whose lipid envelopes have been studied with interesting results is the SV-5, a simian parainfluenza virus. The lipid content of its envelope is related to the nature of its host substrate. The SV-5 virions grown in monkey cells or in baby hamster kidney cells have a lipid composition similar to the plasma membrane composition of the cell in which the virus replicated. The proposed structure of the envelope of Sindbis virus, an arbovirus in the family Togaviridae, is depicted in Figure 38.10. In the case of a DNA virus, such as a herpesvirus, which is assembled as a nucleocapsid within the nucleus, the nucleocapsid contacts the nuclear membrane, whose inner membrane thickens and becomes electron-dense. The nucleocapsid is progressively enveloped by the thickened membrane and finally "buds" off as an enveloped virion in the perinuclear cisterna of the cell. Nucleocapsids can also bud off into nuclear vacuoles which seem to be continuous with the cisterna. The enveloped nucleocapsid is released from the cell by (1) the incorporation of some virions within the cytoplasmic vacuole formed by the out-

Figure 38.10. Proposed structure of Sindbis virus, an arbovirus. (After Harrison and others. From E. Jawetz, J. L. Melnick, and E. A. Adelberg, *Review of Medical Microbiology,* 13th ed. Copyright 1978 by Lange Medical Publications, Los Altos, Calif.)

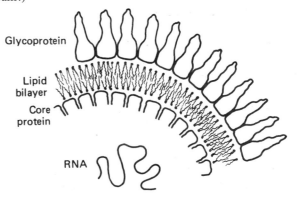

er lamella of the nuclear envelope and sequestration of it from the cytoplasm to the outside of the cell and (2) movement through the cisternae of the endoplasmic reticulum to the cell exterior. In the late stages of infection unenveloped virions appear as breaks in the nuclear membrane occur.

Carbohydrates

The viral envelope contains carbohydrates as well as lipids, principally as glycoproteins. The glycoproteins are important parts of viral antigenic determinants. Their synthesis is controlled by the viral and host cell genome.

Hemagglutination

The hemagglutination phenomenon was described independently by Hirst (1941) and by McClelland and Hare (1941) as a property of human influenza virus. A wide variety of animal viruses can agglutinate red blood cells of various animals and under a variety of conditions. Hemagglutination and hemadsorption are now widely used in both the diagnostic and experimental laboratory to assay for virus and antibody. This test is also a model for host-virus interactions. Hemagglutination is a virus property useful in classifying these organisms. The same can be said for the hemadsorption test, which is a useful manifestation of the hemadsorption phenomenon. This method has been used to demonstrate some viruses in tissue cultures. The erythrocytes added to such a culture cause red cell clumping at the sites of viral activity.

Certain Physical and Chemical Characteristics of Viruses

Effects of Heat and Cold

Most viruses are inactivated by heating at 56°C for 30 minutes, although some resist this treatment.

The ideal way to preserve viruses in the laboratory is storage at low temperatures, preferably −60°C or lower. All virus preparations stored under dry ice refrigeration must be tightly stoppered, as the liberated CO_2 will lower the pH of poorly buffered virus suspensions and inactivate viruses sensitive to acid conditions. Lyophilization is another means by which many viruses can be preserved in the dry state for long periods of time at 4°C. Heat-resistant viruses withstand lyophilization reasonably well, but there usually is some loss in titer during the process.

Enveloped viruses are less stable than those without an envelope, even at −90°C, and do not withstand repeated freezing and thawing. The addition of dimethyl sulfoxide (DMSO) in concentrations above 5 percent provides enveloped viruses with greater stability when maintained at very low temperatures.

Inactivation by Vital Dyes

Vital dyes such as toluidine blue, neutral red, and acridine orange penetrate many viruses to varying degrees. The dyes combine with the viral nucleic acid, and when exposed to light, inactivation results. These dyes do not penetrate some viruses, such as poliovirus; thus, inactivation does not occur. Other viruses, such as adenoviruses and reoviruses, are moderately susceptible, while still others, such as *Herpesvirus* and vaccinia virus, are readily susceptible. When poliovirus is grown in the presence of a vital dye and in the absence of light, dye penetrates the nucleic acid and the virus is then susceptible to photodynamic inactivation. The protein-coat antigen is not affected by this process.

Effect of pH

Practically all viruses are stable between pH 5 and pH 9. A notable exception is foot-and-mouth disease virus, which is readily inactivated at pH 6.

Electrostatic forces play an important role in hemagglutination reactions. Sometimes a variation of a few tenths of a pH unit may determine a negative or positive reaction.

Stabilization by Salts

Many viruses, such as poliovirus, can be stabilized by molar concentrations of salts. The mechanism is unknown. Viruses are preferentially stabilized by certain salts. Certain members of the Picornaviridae family and reoviruses are stabilized by 1 M magnesium chloride. The orthomyxoviruses and paramyxoviruses stabilize in the presence of 1 M magnesium sulfate, while 1 M sodium sulfate stabilizes herpes simplex virus.

This phenomenon can be utilized to rid certain polio preparations of viral adventitious agents such as SV-40, foamy virus, and herpes B virus, which are susceptible to heating in 1 M magnesium chloride, whereas this treatment has no adverse effects on the infectivity of poliovirus.

Antibiotic Sensitivity

With one exception, antibiotics and the sulfonamides, used so successfully in the treatment of bacteria, have no effects on viruses. The antibiotic rifampin readily inactivates bacterial RNA. It is active against poxviruses, presumably acting against the RNA polymerase of the particle, which is essential to poxvirus replication.

Metabolic analogues or antibiotics that interfere with DNA or RNA synthesis will inhibit viral replication. They also adversely affect RNA and DNA synthesis of the host cell. Consequently most are too toxic for use as viral chemotherapeutic agents.

Chemical Inactivants

Several classes of organic compounds react with viruses. Aldehydes and ethylene oxide or imine react with primary valence bonds, while others such as urea, phenol, detergents, guanidine, and lipid solvents affect mainly salt linkages or secondary valence bonds. Organic solvents such as ether and chloroform readily inactivate viruses with an envelope.

Phenol and hexylresorcinol are excellent protein denaturants that strip protein from some viruses, releasing the infectious nucleic acid, which usually contains sufficient RNase to slowly inactivate the acid.

Formaldehyde, ethylene oxide, acetylethylenimine, and glycidaldehyde are alkylating agents used for virus inactivation. Formaldehyde has been commonly employed to inactivate viruses for vaccine use. It reacts with amino, guanidyl, and amide groups of the viral protein and with non-hydrogen-bonded amino groups of the purine and pyrimidine bases of the nucleic acid. Ethylene oxide in a humid atmosphere is an effective virucide. Acetylethylenimine is an effective inactivant for foot-and-mouth disease virus vaccine because its kinetic curve for inactivation is essentially first-order, without tailing, and inactivation takes place in 24 to 48 hours without destruction of the virus immunizing properties; any excess can be neutralized with sodium thiosulfate. Organic iodine compounds are relatively ineffective against viruses because small amounts of organic matter rapidly deplete the active iodine.

Scott (1979) reported on the activity of selected virucides against certain feline viruses that include a feline parvovirus, a feline calicivirus, and a feline herpesvirus which can be considered as representative of their respective virus families. The former two viruses are known to be quite resistant because they do not contain an envelope. The information is given in Table 38.2.

Replication of Viruses

Viruses are highly parasitic and require living cells to furnish the energy, the enzymes for metabolic activity,

and the low-molecular-weight precursors for viral protein and nucleic acid. Viruses contain the essential genetic material for their replication in the host cell. The number of enzymes and structural antigens produced in the cell is a function of the size of the viral genome.

Viral replication was first observed in bacteriophages (D'Herelle 1922). The bacterial system is relatively easy to prepare and manipulate, and the growth cycle is short, being measured in minutes, whereas animal viruses take many hours to complete their growth cycle. Also, the assay of bacteriophages is more accurate and simple.

With the advent of improved methods of in vitro cultivation of animal cells, in assay for virus content and for study of biophysical, biochemical, and biological characteristics of viruses, many of the steps of interaction between animal viruses and tissue cells have been elucidated. The principal studies involving the adsorption of viruses to specific receptor sites have been done with the orthomyxoviruses. The receptor sites for these viruses are mucopolysaccharides on the cell surface. Viral adsorption can be prevented by the pretreatment of the host cells with an enzyme (receptor destroying enzyme, RDE) from *Vibrio cholerae*, which destroys the mucopolysaccharide receptors involved in the hemagglutination reaction. This procedure has been extensively used in the study of cell receptor sites. Viruses that contain lipid in their structure are released continuously from the cells. In contrast, viruses without lipid are released in large numbers at the time of cell lysis (burst process), similar to bacteriophages.

The replication of RNA and DNA viruses, in general, is similar, but differences do exist. The following two sections describe replication of an RNA and a DNA virus.

RNA Virus Replication

The replication of foot-and-mouth disease virus (FMDV), which contains a single-stranded RNA genome, has been studied in great detail, beginning with the process of infection and ending with the release of viral progeny. Moreover, the stage of the cycle dealing with the replication of viral RNA has been accomplished in a cell-free system. The complete growth cycle takes place in the cytoplasm, a known characteristic of all RNA viruses whose replication has been studied in any detail. Further, all steps of the cycle apparently are independent of the cellular DNA genome.

Infection of pig kidney cell cultures by FMDV is a two-step process involving adsorption and penetration. Adsorption of virus requires calcium ions and is temperature-dependent with an activation energy of 6,000 calories per mole. The cells appear to possess between 30 and 100

Table 38.2. Activity of virucides against feline viruses

Virucide	Manufacturer's recommended dilution	Dilution of virucide tested*	Percent of viral activity†		
			Feline panleukopenia virus (Parvovirus)	Feline Calicivirus	Feline viral rhinotracheitis virus (Herpesvirus)
I. *Alcohols*					
Methyl alcohol	78%	35%	−	−	+ + +
Ethyl alcohol	70%	50%	−	+	NT
Isopropyl alcohol	70%	50%	−	±	NT
Lysol spray	U	1/2	−	±	+ + +
Pentacresol	U	1/2	−	±	+ + +
II. *Coal and Wood Tars*					
Creolin	1/21	1/16	−	+ + +	+ + +
Hexachlorophene	3%	1/2 (1.5%)	NT	−	NT
Pine oil	1/180	1/180	NT	−	NT
III. *Iodines*					
Povidone-iodine	U	1/2	±	+ +	+ + +
GSI	1/64	1/64	−	−	+ + +
Hi-Sine	1/256	1/256	−	−	+ + +
Iodophor	1/640	1/640	−	−	+ + +
IV. *Phenolics*					
Amerse	1/32	1/32	−	+ + +	+ + +
Lysol solution	1/32	1/32	−	+ + +	+ + +
Lysol spray	U	1/2	−	±	+ + +
Matar	1/256	1/256	−	+ + +	+ + +
1-Stroke Environ	1/256	1/256	±	+ + +	+ + +
O-Syl	1/32	1/32	−	+ + +	NT
V. *Quaternary Ammonium Compounds (Cationic Detergents)*					
A-33	1/64	1/64	−		+ + +
Hi-TOR	1/256	1/256	−	−	+ + +
Omega	1/256	1/256	−	−	NT
Roccal-D	1/200	1/200	−	−	+ + +
VI. *Soaps (Anionic Detergents)*					
Klomine	5%	5%	NT	±	NT
Silk Floss	U	1/2	−	+ + +	+ + +
Super Green	1/42	1/42	NT	−	+ + +
VII. *Miscellaneous*					
Household chlorine bleach	1/32	1/32	+ + +	+ + +	+ + +
Formaldehyde	4%	4%	+ + +	+ + +	+ + +
Glutaraldehyde	2%	1%	+ + +	+ + +	+ + +
Hydrogen peroxide	3%	1/2 (1.5%)	+	+	NT
Nolvasan	1/128	1/128	−	−	+ + +

−, The concentration of virus was not affected.
±, 10 to 99 percent virus inactivated.
+, 99 to 99.9 percent virus inactivated.
+ +, 99.9 to 99.99 percent virus inactivated.
+ + +, >99.99 percent virus inactivated.
NT, No test.
U, Undiluted.
*Exposed to virus dilutions for 10 minutes at room temperature.
†After treatment with virucide.

receptor sites for virus. At low temperature (2 to 4°C) the virus remains attached without penetration and can be released by certain chemicals. At higher temperatures (37°C) the attached virus penetrates the cell by a first-order reaction with an activation energy of 24,000 calories per mole. The half-time of penetration at 37°C of 30 seconds allows infection of 90 percent of the cells within 3 minutes. Virus attaches itself to dead cells, but does not penetrate them. Following engulfment by the cell, the virion fragments into infectious RNA, and virus protein subunits appear within the cytoplasm. The fact that the host range of the disease is not widened by infection with free FMDV-RNA is further proof that cellular engulfment of the virion occurs.

Within 30 minutes after infection, cellular protein synthesis is decreased by 50 percent and followed by bursts of virus-specific protein as a result of translation by viral RNA. The first burst occurs 60 minutes after infection. It can be inhibited by guanidine and has a temporal correspondence with the expected synthesis of FMDV-specific RNA polymerase. Appreciable amounts of polymerase can be extracted from the cell after 2 hours, with a peak activity of 3.5 hours after infection. The viral infection–associated antigen (VIA) appears to be enzymatically inactive FMDV-specific RNA polymerase because its antibody inhibits polymerase activity. The VIA-RNA polymerase antigen is formed before virions and only when virus replicates in cells, indicating that it is translated from noncapsid cistrons of the viral genome.

The nature of the second burst is unknown, but the third one coincides with viral maturation. In the interim between the first and third burst of virus-specific protein, single-stranded viral RNA molecules (+ strands) presumably are synthesized from the viral RNA in replicate form. More recently it has been demonstrated that C-type particle RNA tumor viruses contain an enzyme, DNA polymerase, that synthesizes DNA from the viral RNA template, thus representing an early event in the replication of RNA tumor viruses and that the newly formed DNA serves as the template for viral RNA synthesis or more likely for a complementary DNA strand. The latter transcribes for viral RNA. Actinomycin D inhibits DNA-dependent RNA synthesis and thus inhibits the multiplication of DNA viruses, and also a few RNA viruses such as Rous sarcoma virus and RNA myxoviruses. The exact mechanism for this inhibition of RNA viruses is unclear, but perhaps the answer lies in the above explanation for the C-type particle RNA viruses.

The synthesis of viral capsid proteins apparently occurs at the same time. Subsequently the proteins form procapsids or empty protein shells. In some unknown manner the viral genome is incorporated in the procapsids to form the virion that represents maturation. The FMDV particles are released when the cell undergoes lysis.

DNA Virus Replication

The replication of adenoviruses has been thoroughly studied. Adsorption, penetration, and uncoating of a DNA virus such as an adenovirus are similar to that described for FMDV, an RNA virus. After uncoating, the viral DNA migrates to the nucleus, where a viral DNA strand is transcribed into specific messenger RNA that is translated to synthesize virus-specific proteins (such as tumor antigen) and enzymes necessary for the biosynthesis of viral DNA. Host cell DNA synthesis is initially elevated but becomes suppressed as the cell manufactures viral DNA. Messenger RNA transcribed during the late stage of cellular infection migrates to the cytoplasm, where translation into viral capsid protein occurs. The capsid protein is transported to the nucleus, where it incorporates the viral DNA to form a mature virus particle. The virions are released after cell lysis.

Infectious viral DNA also has been synthesized in vitro by means of a DNA template molecule from the bacterial virus X-174, which can occur as a single- or double-stranded particle. In the presence of a monomer mixture used for polymerization this covalently close circular viral DNA template (+) is copied by purified DNA polymerase with the formation of linear (−) strand complementary to the (+) circle that the joining enzyme converts into a covalent duplex circle similar to that which occurs in vivo.

Genetics of Animal Viruses

A vast amount of knowledge about genetics has been derived from studies of bacterial viruses. Two major advances since the early 1960s have made possible meaningful studies of animal viruses. The development of accurate and sensitive plaque assay procedures in cell culture systems permitted the quantitation of viral infectivity. Through the study of biophysical, biochemical, and biological characteristics of many animal viruses many stable genetic markers were observed which were amenable to experimental manipulation, were easy to recognize, and resulted from single mutations. Some markers that are used include plaque size, pathogenicity, specific viral induced antigens, drug resistance, and inability to grow at a higher temperature. These mutations may occur spontaneously or arise after treatment with a mutagen.

Conditional-lethal mutants are noninfective under a set

Table 38.3. Types and characteristics of interactions between animal viruses

Type of interaction	Viability of parental viruses	Some progeny different from parental virus	Progeny genetically stable	Example
I. Genetic				
A. Recombination	Active + active	Yes	Yes	Influenza virus, herpesvirus
B. Cross-reactivation	Active + inactive	Yes	Yes	Influenza virus
C. Multiplicity reactivation	Inactive + inactive	Yes	Yes	Vaccinia virus
II. Nongenetic				
A. Phenotypic mixing	Active + active	Yes	No	Picornaviruses
B. Genotypic mixing	Active + active	Yes	No	Paramyoxiviruses
C. Interference	Active + active	No	Yes	Coxsackieviruses
	Defective + active	No	Yes	Satellite + adenovirus
D. Enhancement	Active + active	No	Yes	Newcastle disease virus + para-influenza virus
E. Complementation	Active + inactive	No	Yes	Poxviruses
	Active + defective	No*	Yes	(a) Rous-associated virus (RAV) + Rous sarcoma virus (RSV)†
				(b) Murine leukemia virus (MLV) + murine sarcoma virus (MSV)†
				(c) SV-40 + adenovirus
				(d) Adenovirus + satellite
	Defective + defective	No*	Yes	PARA (SV-40–adenovirus) + adenovirus

*In those cases in which the helper virus is supplying the coat (RSV-RAV, MSV-MLV, PARA-ademovirus), the progeny defective virus will be antigenically different if a heterologous helper virus is present and transcapsidation or pseudotype formation occurs.
†Shares certain similarities with an extreme form of phenotypic mixing.
Slightly modified from E. Jawetz, J. L. Melnick, and E. A. Adelberg, *Review of Medical Microbiology,* 13th ed., Lange Medical Publications, Los Altos, Calif., 1978.

of conditions termed *nonpermissive* but yield normal infectious progeny under conditions termed *permissive*. These mutants may be either host range (hr) mutants or temperature-sensitive (ts) mutants. Ts mutants have been isolated from nearly all animal viruses. They grow at low temperatures (permissive) but not at high temperatures (nonpermissive). At a nonpermissive temperature the particles are defective because an altered amino acid sequence in some essential virus-specified protein renders that protein incapable of functioning. Hr mutants replicate and form plaques in one kind of cell (permissive), whereas abortive infection occurs in another cell type (nonpermissive). With hr bacterial virus mutants the permissible cell carries a transfer RNA that recognizes the altered nucleic acid base sequence as a codon and inserts an amino acid, thus forming a functional polypeptide. It is conceivable such a mechanism also operates in the hr mutants of animal viruses.

When more than one virus particle infects the same cell, they may interact in various ways; these types of interactions are given in Table 38.3. In genetic interaction some progeny emerge which are genetically different from either parent. Several types of viral interaction can occur simultaneously under the proper conditions. The true viral genetic reactions are recombination, cross-reactivation, and multiplicity reaction, as their progeny are genetically stable and some differ from their parents.

Recombination occurs when some progeny with traits not found together in either parent are produced. It is thought that nucleic acid strands break, resulting in the recombination of a part of the genome from one parent with part of the genome from the second parent. Recombinant progeny are stable and yield like progeny upon replication. Recombination has been demonstrated with polio and influenza viruses.

Cross-reactivation takes place between the genome of an infectious particle and the genome of an inactivated virus particle. Certain markers of the inactivated parent are rescued in viable progeny as a result of combination between a portion of the inactivated particle genome and the genome of the active particle. None of the progeny has the same characteristics as the inactivated parent. This phenomenon can be used to produce desirable vaccine strains, as was done with influenza virus.

Multiplicity reactivation involves the combination between the genomes of two inactive particles in the same cell, which results in the production of a viable genome that can replicate. None of the progeny is identical with either parent. This phenomenon has been demonstrated with vaccinia virus.

Phenotypic mixing has been demonstrated with some of the viruses in the *Enterovirus* group. It involves random incorporation of the genome of one virus such as poliovirus into the capsid of another heterologous virus such as Coxsackie virus. A stable genetic change does not occur as the phenotypically mixed parent will produce progeny with a capsid homologous to the genotype because protein synthesis is controlled by the viral genome. In this instance the phenotypically mixed parent would have a Coxsackie virus capsid, but its progeny would have a poliovirus capsid.

Genotypic mixing is characterized by a single virus particle that produces progeny of two distinct parental types. This is probably an accidental incorporation of two genomes in a single capsid. This unstable genetic change has been seen in the study of the orthomyxoviruses.

Complementation is the interaction between two viruses (one or both may be defective or inactive) which permits replication of either one or both of them. Neither the phenotype nor the genotype of the virus changes, and the progeny are like the parents. Different types of complementation between viruses are indicated by the following examples: (1) active fibroma virus provides the stimulation for an uncoating enzyme necessary for the genomal release of inactive myxoma virus; (2) active adenovirus provides the production of the coat protein that is required by defective SV-40 (PARA) virus; (3) active adenovirus may provide some essential gene product that induces replication of the defective adeno satellite virus; and (4) viable Rous-associated virus probably supplies genetic material for the replication of defective Rous sarcoma virus particles (Isaacs et al. 1957), and murine leukemia virus likewise serves as a "helper" for its defective murine sarcoma virus particles.

Interference

Investigators have noted that simultaneous injection of two viruses into a host may result in interference of one of the two viruses. This phenomenon may occur, wholly or in part, between two viruses of different antigenicity, between two strains of the same virus with differences in virulence, or between inactivated and virulent particles of the same virus. The phenomenon is discussed in detail by Vilches and Hirst (1947), who cite many examples. Monkeys infected with lymphocytic choriomeningitis fail to become paralyzed when given poliovirus. Distemperoid (ferret distemper virus) or egg-adapted distemper virus interferes with the multiplication of virulent distemper virus in dogs. Inactivated influenza virus inter-

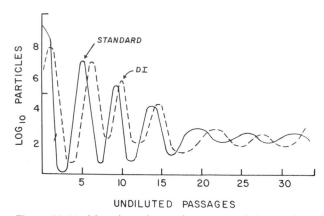

Figure 38.11. Many investigators have reported that continued passages of animal viruses in cell culture produced a cyclic variation in viral titers. Huang showed that this variation is due to defective particles (DI). (Courtesy Alice S. Huang. Reproduced, with permission, from the *Annual Review of Microbiology*, volume 27. © 1973 by Annual Reviews, Inc.)

feres with virulent influenza virus. The protective action in these cases cannot be due to antibodies because ample time had not elapsed for antibody formation. One plausible mechanism is the finding by Isaacs et al. (1957). These investigators described a macromolecular substance that they named *interferon*. In other instances of interference, interferon is not demonstrated. It is believed that the initial virus may alter either the host-cell surface or its metabolic pathways, or possibly the production of defective particles (DI) may cause interference of the superimposing virus. Many investigators have reported that continued passage of animal viruses in cell culture produced a cyclic variation in viral titers. Huang (1973) showed that this variation is due to defective particles (Figure 38.11). There is an intracellular accumulation of nucleocapsids in cells when the largest amount of defective particles is synthesized by the cells. There also may be other unknown factors that affect the relative proportions of defective and standard particles during continuous passages. In this cyclic viral production the DI particles lag slightly behind those representing standard virions. It is interesting to speculate on how these observations would relate to pathogenesis and the appearance and disappearance of clinical signs during certain diseases. In any instances of viral interference the process is generally short-lived, as cell susceptibility recurs soon after the disappearance of interfering virus or interferon.

The discovery of the interferons and their potential use in the treatment and prevention of viral diseases has created much excitement and considerable study. These virus inhibitors can be produced by cells in animals or in culture after infection with viruses. Appreciable quantities appear after maximum viral production in the host animal but before circulating antibodies appear, suggesting an important role for interferon in the body defenses against viral infection. The cells of the reticuloendothelial system seem to provide most of the interferon, although most cells of the body are believed to contribute to its production.

Interferon is a protein which is usually heat-labile, acid-stable at pH 2, nondialyzable, trypsin-sensitive, nonneutralizable by virus, and weakly antigenic (exception in natural bovine interferon, which is acid-labile). It is effective as an antivirus substance on cells from the host species from which it was produced; thus, it is species-specific. It is not virus-specific. As a matter of fact, interferon can be produced in vitro in cultures of cells when stimulated with viruses (particularly when double-stranded RNA is produced during replication) or synthetic double-stranded polynucleotides; and also by cells in the intact animal (in vivo) with viruses, rickettsiae, bacterial endotoxins, synthetic anionic polymers, or polynucleotides. After stimulation of animals with various interferon inducers, different classes of interferon are demonstrable, as evidenced by one with a molecular mass of 8.5×10^4 daltons which appears 2 hours after induction, whereas one with a molecular mass of 3.4×10^4 daltons appears at 18 hours. The cellular events of the induction and action of interferon are presented in schematic summary in Figure 38.12.

The use of interferon and interferon inducers in the prevention and treatment of disease has tremendous potential, but many important problems must be recognized and solved before their general use in humans and animals. The effectiveness of exogenous interferon in preventing disease or reducing its severity, if given early enough in the disease, has been demonstrated. Exogenous interferon is very costly to produce, and although interferon-inducers offer the greatest hope in controlling certain virus infections, they often are toxic in therapeutic doses, and nontoxic antilogues that are efficacious and reasonable in cost must be developed. The half-life of exogenous interferon is very short, and frequent injections are required to maintain effective prophylactic levels.

Enhancement, or dual infection, is the antithesis of interference. Dual infection of single cells with viruses producing intranuclear (herpes simplex virus) and cytoplasmic (vaccinia virus) inclusions was demonstrated by Syverton and Berry (1947). This suggests that interference may not take place between viruses that require different pathways for their replication. Another mechanism may be concerned with the activity of one virus that inhibits the formation of interferon. Parainfluenza virus reduces autoinhibition by Newcastle disease virus, a very

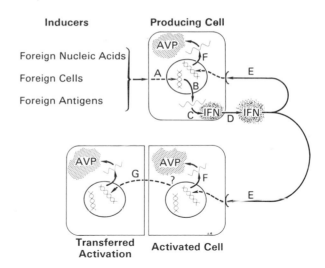

Figure 38.12. Cellular events of the induction, production, and action of interferon (IFN). Inducers of IFN react with cells to derepress the IFN gene(s) (*A*). This leads to the production of mRNA for IFN (*B*). The mRNA is translated into the IFN protein (*C*) that is secreted into the extracellular fluid (*D*), where it reacts with the membrane receptors of cells (*E*). The IFN-stimulated cells derepress genes (*F*) for effector proteins (AVP) that establish antiviral resistance and other cell changes. The activated cells also stimulate contacted cells (*G*) by a still unknown mechanism to produce AVP. (Courtesy Samuel Barron.)

potent interferon producer. Often coinfection enhances the production of one of the two viruses involved with the emergence of progeny similar to the parents.

Exaltation of disease may result when dual infection occurs in a host. For example, in dogs given canine distemper and infectious canine hepatitis viruses simultaneously, a more severe disease results than in dogs given either virus alone (Gillespie et al. 1952).

Chemotherapy of Viral Infections

The control of disease is based on measures that promote good health, immunization, and treatment. The first two criteria have proved to be successful against many viruses and are responsible for the reduced incidence of serious diseases such as canine distemper, hog cholera, rinderpest, feline panleukopenia, and many other infectious viral diseases of domestic animals. With very few exceptions at present, treatment of viral diseases consists of amelioration of signs rather than reduced replication of the virus.

There are two major deterrents to the effective treatment of viral disease. The first, and perhaps the most important, is the strict parasitic relationship of the virus and its host cell. It is quite clear that a virus depends on the metabolism of the host cell for its replication, and the majority of virus inhibitors act against cellular processes. A useful virus inhibitor must prevent completion of the viral growth cycle in the infected cell without causing lethal damage of the uninfected cells. This desired effect can be achieved by a compound that acts directly on a component of the virus or on a viral product, such as a virus-specific enzyme that is essential for successful replication. With the finding of virus-specific enzymes, the outlook for viral chemotherapy has brightened considerably. Inhibitors that prevent adsorption or penetration of the cell without damaging it are also being sought. The second problem involves the nature and pathogenesis of viral diseases and the attendant problem of early and accurate diagnosis. Many viral diseases may be recognized too late for effective treatment with a virus inhibitor. In other instances, success depends on the availability of safe and effective virus inhibitors.

Amantadine, a symmetrical amine, inhibits certain members of the *Orthomyxovirus* and *Paramyxovirus* groups, pseudorabies virus (a herpesvirus), and Rous sarcoma virus by blocking the penetration of the virus. It has no effect on adsorption of the virus. When administered prophylactically, it is very effective in protecting experimental animals and humans against influenza A strains. Therapeutic treatment has little or no effect on the course of the disease.

Many viruses of the Picornaviridae family are inhibited in cell culture systems by guanidine and hydroxybenzylbenzimidazole (HBB). These compounds interfere with the synthesis of viral RNA polymerase, thus preventing the formation of viral protein and viral RNA. After the RNA polymerase is formed, neither drug can prevent viral replication. The inhibitory effect can also be overcome by dilution with fresh tissue culture medium. The therapeutic action of the two drugs with marked structural difference presumably is similar but not identical, as some viruses can be inhibited by one drug but not the other. In some instances HBB and guanidine have a synergistic effect. Unfortunately, there is no protection by either drug in experimental animal infections. This may be due, wholly or in part, to the rapid production of drug-resistant mutants.

Thiosemicarbazones were shown to inhibit the growth of poxviruses. Later, isatin beta-thiosemicarbazone (methisazone) and its N-methyl derivative were shown to have greater protective capacity in experimental animals. These compounds also are an effective prophylactic for smallpox in humans if given within 24 to 48 hours after exposure. The drug is virus-specific without any effect on normal cell metabolism. There is normal synthesis of viral DNA and of the two enzymes (thymidine kinase and DNA polymerase) concerned in DNA synthesis. The synthesis of many, but not all, of the 20 or more soluble viral antigens that are formed during normal viral growth is inhibited, resulting in the formation of immature, noninfectious particles. Mutants resistant to this drug have been isolated.

Actinomycin D (dactinomycin) inhibits the replication of DNA viruses and some RNA viruses, such as Rous sarcoma virus and some orthomyxoviruses. The drug inhibits DNA-dependent RNA synthesis by a mechanism that is not clear.

The antibiotic rifampin shows a preferential inhibition of bacterial RNA polymerase. Poxviruses carry their own RNA polymerase for synthesizing viral messenger RNA, and this antibiotic was very effective against smallpox virus in tissue-culture studies by inhibiting the viral polymerase but not materially affecting cellular polymerase.

Analogues of purine and pyrimidine bases may inhibit both RNA and DNA synthesis. Iododeoxyuridine (IUDR) has been used topically with success in the treatment of corneal lesions caused by herpes simplex, a DNA virus. It cannot be used routinely for systemic infections because it is too toxic. Under heroic circumstances, massive near-lethal doses have been administered in cases of herpesvirus encephalitis with complete recovery ensuing. In tissue-culture studies of papovavirus-infected or herpesvirus-infected cells, IUDR arrests the synthesis of the virion but not the viral components, because large amounts of viral antigen have been found in the cells. Electron microscopic examination reveals immature virus particles in large numbers. Other halogenated deoxyuridines such as 5-fluoro-2'-deoxyuridine (FUDR), and 5-bromo-2'-deoxyuridine (BUDR), as well as IUDR, inhibit replication of members of the major DNA virus groups by producing an improperly functioning nucleic acid. Drug-resistant mutants of some viruses have emerged in the presence of IUDR or BUDR.

The activity of a purine or pyrimidine analogue can be enhanced by incorporation of ribose or deoxyribose into its molecule. The action of riboside or deoxyribose can be directed preferentially toward the inhibition of RNA or DNA. Ribosides of halogenated benzimidazoles are more selective inhibitors of influenza virus replication than the free benzimidazoles or their deoxyribosides.

The size of the halogen atom of the halogenated pyrimidine analogue determines the nature of its viral inhibitory action. The size and shape of 5-bromouracil (BU) is very similar to that of thymine, and 5-fluorouracil (FU) is similar to uracil. Thus, BU can inhibit DNA bacteriophage but has no effect on the RNA tobacco mosaic virus. FU inhibits RNA virus, and its action is reversed by the addition of uridine but not by the thymidine. In the study of specific virus inhibitors this reversion technique involving the addition of analogous normal metabolic compounds is essential to the proof of drug specificity, rather than inhibition caused by drug toxicity. Certain protein inhibitors have been useful in the study of viral replication. Cycloheximide, para-fluorophenylalanine, and puromycin inhibit synthesis of viral and cell protein. Consequently, they can interrupt the cycle of viral replication at various stages. Because they also inhibit cell-protein synthesis, these drugs are not viral chemotherapeutic candidates.

Virazole is a synthetic nucleoside that appears to inhibit an early step in viral replication involving the synthesis of viral nucleic acid, either DNA or RNA. As such, it has a broad spectrum of possibilities as an antivirus drug. Although not completely free of toxic reactions, it is sufficiently nontoxic to be used by the aerosol or parenteral routes. It has been licensed in several European countries but not in the United States. It is contraindicated during pregnancy.

Disodium phosphonoacetate is a promising, stable, nontoxic antivirus drug that selectively inhibits DNA-dependent DNA polymerase essential to DNA replication. The inhibition appears to be specific for the viral enzyme of several herpesviruses with little effect on cellular DNA synthesis.

Host Response

Viruses are completely dependent on the living cell for their survival and replication. The alterations caused by viruses in cells are regulated by the cell-virus relationships. Some viruses produce little or no alteration in the biochemical mechanisms of the cell. This phenomenon represents the ultimate in parasitism, because the virus and cell perform their physiological functions for survival with no adverse structural effects on each other. Other viruses have a severe effect, resulting in pathological changes. As a result of the marked dependence of viruses on cell functions for replication, many new techniques have been developed and refined for the study of host-virus relationships. Advances in electron microscopy permit the study of many ultrastructural features of cell tissue invaded by virus. Immunofluorescence enhances pathogenesis studies, allowing investigators to study the pattern of viral infections in various hosts and in tissue and organ cultures. Improved tissue-culture methods are used to excellent advantage in assaying virus for pathogenesis studies. Histochemistry and radioautography also are being used for studies of this nature. Both standard and phase microscopy provide the means for correlating the gross lesions of viral disease with the molecular level processes.

Pathogenesis

The induction of infection by viruses varies markedly, depending on the viral tropism, cell susceptibility, the means of transmission, and the site of body contact.

As a rule, the initial site of contact is in cells of exposed surfaces of various body systems, including the reproductive, digestive, and respiratory tracts and also the skin. In some instances, but not all, initial viral replication occurs in these primary sites of contact and adsorption. In some instances viral replication is limited to these superficial tissues. After a sufficient concentration of virus has been attained, it spreads to other cells in neighboring tissues. Prime examples of this type are parainfluenza in dogs and in cattle, rotavirus infection in many species, and influenza in pigs and in horses. This localized process also operates in certain viral skin diseases such as molluscum contagiosum, pseudocowpox, and papilloma. From initial infection sites, some viruses may disseminate through the lymph and the bloodstream to remote areas in the body, where replication occurs and pathological lesions are formed. Herpes infection in humans and animals constitutes a good example of this type of pathogenesis.

In other instances the virus gains entrance to the body through superficial tissues without replication, invades the macrophages, leukocytes, and other cellular elements in the bloodstream, and is then transported to various tissues throughout the body with adsorption and replication of virus occurring in other fixed, susceptible cells. Canine distemper is an excellent example (Figure 38.13). In neurotropic cases of canine distemper, virus also penetrates the blood-brain barrier with viral antigen appearing first in meningeal macrophages, long after viremia occurs, and then in perivascular cells, ependymal cells, and later in glial and neuronal cells of the brain(Appel 1969).

In the case of arthropod-borne viruses, transmission of the disease depends on insect vectors, which inject the virus through a bite. The virus invades the bloodstream and replicates in cells of the endothelial lining of lymph and blood vessels.

A variety of mechanisms operate in the successful adsorption of viruses to cells. Proper receptor sites on cell surfaces are essential to virus adsorption. Certain orthomyxoviruses contain a surface enzyme necessary for union with specific receptors at definite loci on the cell surface. Specific receptor sites also are involved in cell-enterovirus union. Phagocytosis of attached virus by the cell occurs when the viral nucleic acid is released from its

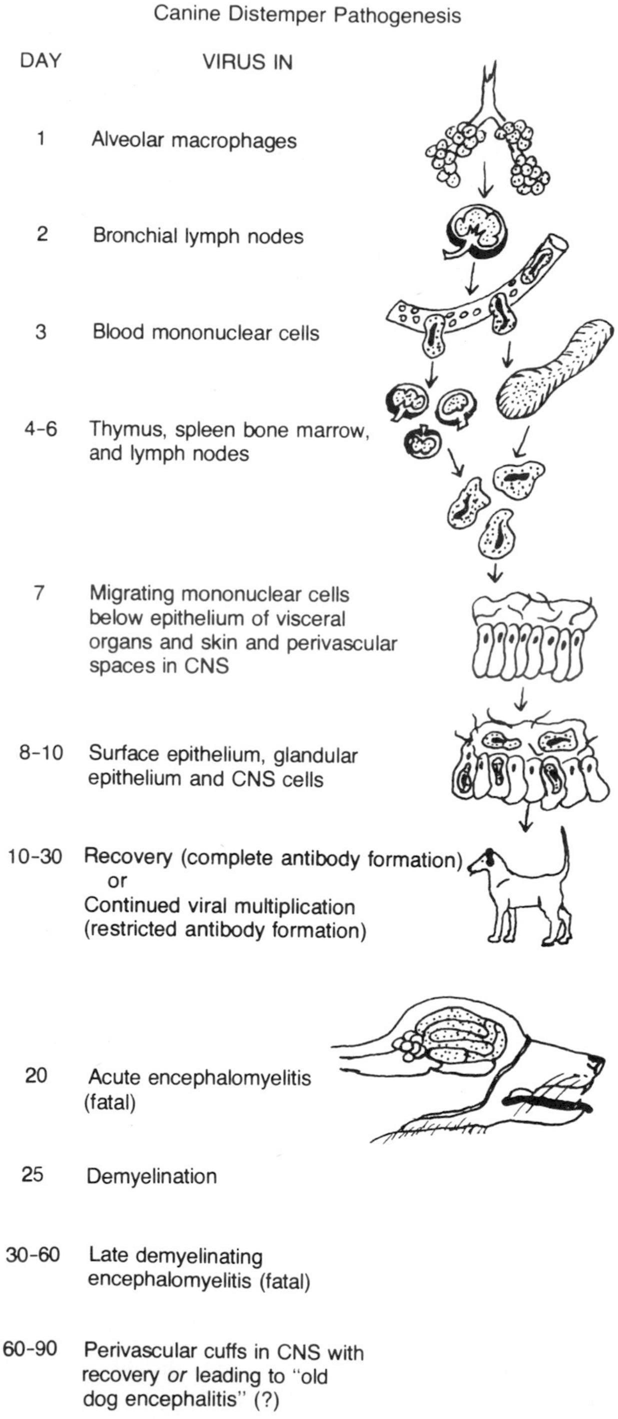

Canine Distemper Pathogenesis

DAY	VIRUS IN
1	Alveolar macrophages
2	Bronchial lymph nodes
3	Blood mononuclear cells
4-6	Thymus, spleen bone marrow, and lymph nodes
7	Migrating mononuclear cells below epithelium of visceral organs and skin and perivascular spaces in CNS
8-10	Surface epithelium, glandular epithelium and CNS cells
10-30	Recovery (complete antibody formation) or Continued viral multiplication (restricted antibody formation)
20	Acute encephalomyelitis (fatal)
25	Demyelination
30-60	Late demyelinating encephalomyelitis (fatal)
60-90	Perivascular cuffs in CNS with recovery or leading to "old dog encephalitis" (?)

Figure 38.13. Schematic illustration of canine distemper pathogenesis. (Drawing by Cynthia J. Holmes. Modeled from similar schemata by E. Jawetz, J. L. Melnick, and E. A. Adelberg, with modifications by M. Appel.)

protein coat, permitting the nucleic acid to direct the cellular activity essential to its successful replication (described under "Replication of Viruses" earlier in this chapter).

Cells in an animal host at different ages may vary in their susceptibility to viruses, producing diverse disease pictures. Infectious bovine rhinotracheitis virus in neonatal calves causes a generalized disease with the most dramatic lesions occurring in the anterior portion of the digestive tract, but with generalized pustular lesions in most body systems. In contrast, lesions in the anterior portion of the digestive tract in older calves or young adults do not occur, and lesions are likely to be confined to one body system (Baker et al. 1960). Less dramatic differences are seen with experimental foot-and-mouth disease in the avian host, but prominent heart lesions and the highest virus titers in this organ occur in the 14-day-old chicken embryo, whereas lesions and the higher virus titers occur in the gizzard muscle of the 1-day-old chick (Gillespie 1955). This finding demonstrates a remarkable difference in cell susceptibility of the developing avian host to foot-and-mouth disease virus within 8 days.

The effective transmission of viruses from one host to another is essential in the pathogenesis of any viral disease. This subject is covered in Chapter 39, "Epidemiology of Viral Infections."

Pathology

The various routes of viral transport within the body serve as a means to establish infection in the cells for which each virus has an affinity or tropism. The nature of the infection (and disease) is determined by the degree of parasitism, the number and type of cells involved in the virus-host relationship, and the nature of viral replication within the cell.

The intracellular processes leading to degeneration and necrosis manifest themselves in many different pathological changes in cells. Viral infections are usually characterized by vacuolation, ballooning degeneration, syncytium formations, hypertrophy, and hyperplasia. Nucleolar displacement, margination of nuclear chromatin, and the production of cytoplasmic or intranuclear inclusions are changes at the cellular level. The degree, nature, and type of cellular involvement determine the severity and nature of the disease. In some instances no clinical signs or lesions are associated with the infection, while in others severe disease with resulting host death ensues. In most viral infections the initial stages of pathogenesis are clinically inapparent, and in some diseases signs of illness do not occur until late in the acute stages, often when antibodies are first demonstrable.

Inclusion Bodies. In many viral diseases round to oval bodies may be found in the cytoplasm or within the nuclei of affected cells. These have long been known to pathologists as *inclusion bodies*. They are indicative of virus in the cell. Some are so characteristic in appearance and staining qualities that they are of diagnostic importance. They are not used as often for diagnosis as they once were because better methods are now available in most cases. The Negri body, found in certain nerve cells of animals suffering from rabies, is an inclusion body still commonly sought as a means of quick diagnosis of that disease.

Inclusion bodies have not been detected in some viral diseases, and in others their presence is not constant. Most inclusion bodies stain with acid dyes. A few are basophilic, and others are basophilic and Feulgen positive in their early stages and acidophilic later. The inclusion bodies of trachoma in humans, of psittacosis in humans and animals, and of some related diseases of the psittacosis-lymphogranuloma-trachoma group are quite different from and should not be confused with those of viral infections. They are described in Chapter 33.

The eosinophilic cytoplasmic inclusions vary in size (up to 20,000 nm in diameter) in different diseases and in variant cases of the same disease. There may be only one body within a single cell, or there may be several such bodies. Some may be large and others much smaller. Some appear to be quite hyaline, but most are granular, and some contain distinctly stained "inside" bodies.

Two types of intranuclear inclusions can be distinguished. Cowdry (1934) refers to them as A- and B-types. The *Type A inclusions* are found in nuclei in which there is evidence of severe disruption of the chromatic structure. The chromatin fragments are displaced to the margin of the nuclear membrane (margination). The inclusion body, or bodies, usually lie near the center of the nucleus and appear as amorphous or granular, generally acid-staining material. The affected tissue often shows cells with bodies in different stages of development; that is, fully developed bodies may be seen in some cells and much smaller ones in neighboring cells. The *Type B inclusions* may vary in size, but they are more circumscribed, there is no margination of chromatin, and the nucleus presents a less disorganized appearance than in the other type. Type A bodies are found in such diseases as infectious canine hepatitis, canine distemper, and pseudorabies. A good example of the Type B inclusion is the Joest body found in Borna disease.

Some of the earlier workers regarded inclusion bodies as the infective agent; some regarded them as protozoa; others thought them to be aggregates of minute parasites embedded in capsular or other hyaline material. When filtration experiments demonstrated that the viruses of many diseases obviously were much smaller than the inclusion bodies seen in those diseases, researchers tended to regard them as specific degeneration products of the cell substance. More recently, however, evidence has accumulated that some of the bodies contain aggregates of virus elementary bodies.

Borrel (1904) studied the inclusions, known as *Bollinger bodies*, found in pox of fowls. These are rather large structures that occur in the cytoplasm of infected epithelial cells. Microscopically, minute spherical corpuscles were detected within the larger body, which, when crushed, released smaller bodies. These are now known as *Borrel bodies*. Borrel bodies may be separated from affected tissues by crushing, by tryptic digestion, and by differential centrifugation. After many washings these bodies can induce fowlpox; that is, they contain virus. Borrel bodies can be specifically agglutinated by the serum of animals that have recovered from the disease or have been immunized against it. They are regarded as the virus particles, or *elementary bodies*. A similar condition can be demonstrated in several other viral diseases.

It has now been established that the intranuclear inclusion bodies may contain virus. It has not been proved that all inclusion bodies are virus carriers. It is possible, of course, that some are specific degenerative structures and others are essentially virus aggregates.

Inflammatory Response. The inflammation that accompanies viral infections is usually secondary to the primary cellular alterations. There is little to distinguish viral infections based on the character of the inflammatory response. Edema is often observed as an early and persistent feature, but the reason for its occurrence is unknown. The early cellular response to most viral infections is mononuclear and lymphocytic.

Polymorphonuclear leukocytes are commonly found in bacterial infections, but the initial and, in many instances, the whole reaction to viruses depends on mononuclear cells, including macrophages, lymphocytes, and plasma cells. Inflammation is found in most viral diseases but not in all of them. In louping ill of sheep, Purkinje cells undergo complete necrosis before any infiltration is observed. In rabies, neuronal cells are completely destroyed, and yet there is often no inflammatory response.

When secondary bacterial infection does occur in viral diseases, infiltration of polymorphonuclear leukocytes is presumably a response to cell degeneration and necrosis. The leukocytes predominate in the lesions of infectious bovine rhinotracheitis infection, where massive necrosis is observed. Perivascular infiltration with lymphocytes is especially characteristic of various types of viral encephalitis, such as the equine encephalomyelitides. The lymphocytic pleocytosis in the cerebrospinal fluid usually distinguishes aseptic meningitis from purulent meningitis.

Secondary bacterial infection often complicates viral diseases, especially respiratory and skin diseases and particularly the former. Many potential bacterial pathogens may reside on the skin, such as *Streptococcus* and *Staphylococcus* species, and in the respiratory tract, such as *Pasteurella* and *Streptococcus* species. The initial damage to the superficial cells of these structures by the virus provides the necessary conditions for the rapid invasion and multiplication of the bacterial pathogens, whose influence changes the nature and character of the disease to an acute pyogenic infection that is often responsible for the high morbidity and mortality rates encountered in many viral epidemics. This sequence of events is characteristic for most viral respiratory diseases of domestic animals.

Viral infections of cells cause chromosome damage with derangement of the karyotype. Most changes are random in nature. Breakage, fragmentation, and rearrangement of the chromosomes occur most frequently. Abnormal chromosomes and changes in their number also are observed. Cell cultures infected with, or transformed to malignancy by certain adenoviruses, such as infectious canine hepatitis virus, exhibit such changes as well as random chromosomal abnormalities and fragmentation. Certain viruses, such as herpes simplex virus in the Chinese hamster cell, cause chromosome breaks that are not random in distribution. Replication of the virus is necessary for induction of the chromosome aberrations. As yet, chromosome alterations cannot assist in the identification of virus-infected or virus-transformed cells.

Constitutional Effects. Many viral infections are recognized by a number of nonspecific constitutional disturbances including fever, myalgia, anorexia, malaise, and headache. These signs are attributed to a number of factors such as absorption of degradation products from injured cells, viral toxicity, vascular abnormalities producing circulatory disturbances, degree of viremia, and other less specific factors. Usually the mechanism that leads to the production of signs of disease, and certainly death, in viral diseases is unknown. Vascular shock, viral toxicity, and functional failure of one or more vital organs are believed to account for death.

Immunopathic Viral Diseases

Certain viruses cause chronic diseases. The presently accepted hypothesis holds that the immunological response of the host to persisting viruses in these diseases causes the formation of circulating virus-antibody complexes, which results in cellular alterations with the production of disease. This mechanism apparently exists in lymphocytic choriomeningitis in mice. If adults are rendered immunologically compromised by immunosuppressive drugs, irradiation, or antiserum produced against the lymphoid elements of the mouse, no illness is produced after inoculation with the virus. The virus replicates and persists until immunocompetence is reestablished, at which time the mouse becomes ill. Infection of newborn mice before they become immunocompetent results in a lifetime viral infection without illness. Age plays a definite role in the persistence of certain viruses, this fact may be related to the development of immunocompetence. Other notable examples that may have a similar basic mechanism include Aleutian disease of mink and equine infectious anemia. These are characterized by persisting virus and by pathological alterations of blood vessels and kidneys not unlike those seen in certain connective-tissue disorders of humans.

Latent Viral Infections

A few decades ago only a limited number of viruses were believed to persist in a latent state in the host. Now the vast majority of viruses are known to persist, a phenomenon that has been determined through new and refined techniques for the detection of incomplete and complete virus. In some viral diseases the agent may be transmitted vertically from mother to progeny, and horizontal transmission is not necessary—an ideal situation for the perpetuation of the parasite.

Many viral diseases occur as inapparent (or silent) infections in the human or animal populations. Such infections are important in the epidemiology and immunity of a given population. In many instances these inapparent viral infections end with the elimination of the parasite from the host. In others, especially in subclinical infections, this does not occur, but results in the phenomenon known as latent infection. With some diseases such as lymphocytic choriomeningitis in mice and Rous sarcoma infection in chickens, the virus persists, but antibody does not develop, and the animal remains a virus carrier for an indefinite period. In other diseases caused by herpesviruses, adenoviruses, and varicella zoster virus, virus persists after the initial infection despite the production of antibody. The basic nature of latent infection with these viruses is not always understood. However, some members of the Herpesviridae are known to survive within certain cells of the buccal mucous membranes, lymph nodes, or local sensory ganglia. The virus persists as a complete virion in latent form in the local sensory ganglia for extended periods of time. Reactivation follows stimulation by physical, nutritional, or endocrine alterations. An interesting observation was made in a tissue-culture system which may explain the pathogenesis of some reactivated latent diseases (Hoggan et al. 1961). Certain variants of *Herpesvirus* induce the formation of syncytia by which adjacent cells can be invaded by virus through interconnecting cytoplasmic channel ways. By this route virus avoids contact with antibody.

Occult (or masked) virus may account for the long duration of immunity attributed to such diseases as canine distemper, but presently there is no adequate way to detect this type of virus. In the case of certain tumor viruses such as Shope papilloma virus, the course of the infection is long, and eventually the virus becomes occult. The phenomenon of masked virus occurs with other DNA viruses such as polyoma, SV-40, and human adenoviruses 12 and 18. With polyoma, the antigenic components for the virus become undetectable, and there is no evidence of virus or viral genome in the transformed cells. It has been postulated that SV-49–induced transformed cells carry the viral genome in a noninfectious state, and on rare occasions a parasitized cell produces infectious virus. On the other hand, certain RNA tumor viruses such as Rous sarcoma virus and feline leukemia viruses persist in transformed cells. Defective Rous sarcoma virus can produce transformed cells in culture. For example, cells may grow in culture for many generations despite replication of a virus. Usually only a small proportion of the cells is infected with virus. This may be likened to slow viral infections in a natural host which are characterized by a prolonged incubation period lasting months or years, during which time the virus replicates with progressive destruction of tissue, as occurs in diseases like visna, maedi, Aleutian disease, and equine infectious anemia. In some virus cell-culture systems the cell continues to survive despite viral replication in that cell, thus resembling a moderate viral infection. In these virus-carrier cultures the virus seems to be under some control; perhaps interferon is responsible in some instances. By various means, the virus can be released in these cultures by cell crowding, lowering the temperature, or medium exhaustion. Although cell cultures have helped to increase our knowledge of viral latency, the results must be viewed with caution, as they may apply to the natural host where defense mechanisms are in operation which are lacking in an in vitro system.

Natural and Acquired Resistance in Viral Diseases

Natural Resistance. It is clear that mechanisms for resistance to viral infections involve more than the production of circulating antibodies. This became apparent from viral and bacterial resistance studies with hypogammaglobulinemia patients, from absence of an antibody response in certain congenital viral infections, and from the role of antibodies in the protection of animals against the production of tumors by oncogenic viruses.

Innate susceptibility or resistance are terms commonly used in discussing so-called natural resistance (or susceptibility) of a given species to a particular viral infection. This may also apply to the marked variation in resistance of individual members of an animal species to a given virus. The mechanisms of innate resistance are poorly understood, but they may operate at the level of the cell or organism (host). The route of viral entry also is a factor.

At the cellular level, adsorption of the virus to the cell receptors is the first and perhaps most important factor in cellular resistance or susceptibility. With some pathogens, such as poliovirus, other human enteroviruses, and phage-resistant strains of *Escherichia coli,* cellular resistance is caused by the failure of adsorption and not the ability of the nucleic acid to replicate in cells. Actually, little is known about intracellular factors affecting the susceptibility of cells to viral infection, but such things as pH, temperature, interferon, and genetics can play a role.

Two generally recognized forces operating at the organism level are the blood-brain barrier and the reticuloendothelial system.

At present, an effective experimental approach to the study of innate resistance to viral infections can only be made in "inbred" mouse colonies or perhaps in chicken flocks. These animal lines may differ markedly in their mechanisms of resistance to certain viral diseases. Susceptibility of mouse lines to St. Louis encephalitis and louping ill viruses was correlated with the level of viral multiplication in the mouse brain. The Princeton Rockefeller Institute mice were highly resistance to 17D strain of yellow fever virus, and this observation (Sabin 1952) extended to the other group B arboviruses but not the group A arboviruses. In the intact animal it is sometimes possible to produce resistance by transfer of macrophages from resistant to susceptible animals. Macrophages also play the same role in infectious hepatitis of mice. Unfortunately, this does not seem to be the case with mousepox, where macrophages apparently had no influence on the susceptibility of mice to this disease. Selective breeding for resistance to one viral disease does not insure resistance to others.

Natural selection in a population plays an important role in the history (ecology) of a viral disease. Most diseases as we know them represent such a situation, where adjustment of the host and virus occur over a long period. An excellent opportunity for the study of innate resistance occurred in Australia three decades ago when virulent myxoma virus was introduced into a previously unexposed, highly susceptible wild rabbit population. Initially the case-mortality rate was 90 percent but within 7 years fell to 25 percent under standardized conditions.

Other environmental factors known to operate in disease resistance include age, ambient temperature, and a poorly developed thermal regulating mechanism of most species at time of birth. Neonatal animals are often highly susceptible to viruses during the first weeks of life. Consequently, neonatal animals are often used for study of viruses. Certainly dogs are more susceptible to canine distemper and canine herpesvirus during the first 1 to 2 weeks of life. Fortunately, maternal antibodies are conferred to the progeny from immune dams, counteracting this highly susceptible period. Temperature also may have an effect on the viral multiplication, antibody response, and interferon production of the organism. The aged often are more susceptible to viral infections, for reasons unknown.

Acquired Resistance. Acquired resistance (or immunity) is obtained by contact with the antigens of infectious agents, and specific antibodies to these substances play an important role in the resistance of the host organism. There are two main segments in the immune response, namely, (1) the production and effects of humoral antibodies, and (2) cell-mediated immunity generated by cells of the reticuloendothelial system.

Immunity in a considerable proportion of all virus diseases is absolute and relatively long-lasting. This is quite different from that found in bacterial diseases, where immunity is relative and usually short-lived. Such solid and lasting immunities do not occur in all viral diseases; in fact in many, especially those which affect superficial structures such as herpes infections and foot-and-mouth disease, it is solid but not long lasting.

The prolonged solid immunity found in many viral diseases cannot be explained with certainty. When antigens come in contact with tissues, antibodies are produced, and these usually may be recognized by a variety of established methods. If the antigen is contained in a parasitic or pathogenic organism that multiplies and retains its position in the body for a considerable period of time, antibodies will be stimulated as long as the stimulus remains. If it is a nonviable antigen that is quickly eliminated from the body, antibody formation quickly ceases and the blood titer is soon lost. The same thing ordinarily happens when an animal recovers from an infection. How then can continued virus-neutralizing power be maintained, as it is in many viral diseases, long after all evidence of the diseases has disappeared?

No definite answer can be given to this question at present. The fact that viruses develop only intracellularly whereas bacteria usually develop in the body fluids may be responsible for the difference. In these cases viruses may find it possible to continue to exist in certain cells of the recovered host as latent or occult virus in spite of the fact that the body fluids contain virus-neutralizing antibodies. Such an individual may have little or no ability to infect others because the neutralizing antibodies bathing the infected cells prevent the escape of virus into any of the secretions or excretions of the body under most circumstances, but might not prevent the passage of virus through intercellular bridges to other susceptible cells of the same individual. In viral diseases it is at least theoretically possible that many individuals will continue to harbor the virus as long as they live. Such individuals would be expected to show continuous production of antibodies especially if the virus persisted in cells involved in antibody production and continued to stimulate a solid immunity to reinfection. This theory is supported by Poppensiek and Baker (1951), who showed that virus in the urine and immunity persisted in dogs that recovered from infectious canine hepatitis.

Rivers et al. (1929) inoculated rabbit cornea with vaccinia virus and then maintained the viability of the corneal cells by submerging them in antivaccinal plasma. They found that corneal lesions developed in spite of the virus-neutralizing antibodies in the plasma. When the vaccinia virus was first mixed with the plasma before the addition of the corneal tissue, the tissue did not become infected. These experiments prove that viruses may develop in cells that are bathed with antiviral substances. Such experiments serve to explain the frequent clinical experiences indicating that viral antiserum may be useful as preventive agents but are usually useless in treating already existing disease.

Another interesting possibility was pointed up by the findings of van Bekkum and colleagues (1959) with animals that had recovered from foot-and-mouth disease. This is a disease in which immunity is relatively short-lived and in which it has always been believed that virus disappears even though these animals did not transmit the disease to susceptible cattle kept in close contact with them. Convalescing animals apparently continued to produce a small amount of virus for a long period, the amount being too small to cause infection by ordinary contacts.

Passive Immunity. Specific hyperimmune serums are useful against a number of animal viral diseases. When these serums are administered before infection occurs, or perhaps very early in the course of the infection before the virus has been widely disseminated, they are fairly effective. The protection given by such serums usually is complete and solid, but it is of short duration. It is not safe to depend on passive immunity lasting for more than 1 to 2 weeks. Additional doses can be given to prolong this protection. Antiserum is often used to protect susceptible animals during critical periods. If the passively immunized animal comes in contact with virus during the period of protection, active immunization often occurs.

In general, it is useless to administer antiserums to animals that exhibit well-marked signs of viral infections. In these cases, the virus has already reached the susceptible cells, where it is beyond the reach of the antibodies.

Hyperimmune antiserums are used effectively in combating hog cholera and feline panleukopenia. They may be used in many more viral diseases, but in some either they are impracticable or ineffective, or better methods of protection are available.

In *maternal immunity* temporary immunity is conferred by the mother to her progeny. This is very important in many viral diseases, as neonatal infections are often fatal. Certainly this is true for many human and animal viruses. In general, there is a quantitative relationship between the serum titer of the dam at birth and the duration of the passive protection for the progeny. For example, the duration of maternal protection for puppies against canine distemper and infectious canine hepatitis viruses, in general persists from 4 to 15 weeks. Obviously, dams with the highest serum antibody titers confer protection to their progeny for the longest period of time. Most domestic animals receive the major portion of their maternal antibody through the colostrum; thus it is important for them to nurse well in the first 24 to 48 hours of life. For more information about maternal immunity, see the section on immunity to canine distemper in Chapter 52.

Active Immunization. The methods of actively immunizing against virus infections fall into four categories: (1) the use of fully virulent virus alone, (2) the use of virulent virus and antiserum simultaneously, (3) the use of vaccines made from attenuated virus, and (4) the use of inactivated virus. A list of virus vaccines licensed by the United States Department of Agriculture for animal use in the United States is provided in Tables 38.4 and 38.5.

Fully virulent virus. When fully virulent virus is used, it is introduced by a route different from that of natural transmission. This is a relatively dangerous method because the virulent material does not always behave predictably, and at best it is undesirable to spread virulent material to premises where it did not formerly exist. When it is used, *all susceptible stock* on the same premises should be treated, preferably at the same time; otherwise there is danger of producing an epizootic among the unprotected animals. This method is seldom used now, but it formerly was employed in the United States for the control of some animal diseases, including contagious ecthyma of sheep

and infectious laryngotracheitis and infectious bronchitis of chickens.

Virus and antiserum simultaneously. The best-known example of the use of virulent virus and antiserum simultaneously is in hog cholera. In this method of immunization, the antiserum is depended on to lessen the viral effect so the animal suffers only a mild or inapparent infection.

Attenuated virus. Attenuated viruses for immunization purposes are generally made by adapting them to hosts other than the one on which the vaccine is to be used. In many cases this increases the virulence for the new host but reduces it for others. The first virus vaccine, the rabies vaccine of Pasteur (1885), was of this type. It was produced by passing virulent virus through a series of rabbits. Finally when the virus had developed great virulence for the rabbit, it was found that it had lost most of its pathogenicity for other animals and humans. This attenuated virus thus could be used to stimulate antibodies that would protect against the more virulent strains. Other examples of such attenuated virus vaccines are the ferret-adapted virus vaccine for canine distemper, the mouse-brain vaccines for yellow fever of humans and the horsesickness of Africa, and the vaccines for rinderpest, canine distemper, and rabies made by cultivating the viruses in fertile hens' eggs. Viruses adapted to rabbits, hens' eggs, or tissue-cultured cells are called *lapinized, avianized,* or *tissue-cultured* vaccines, respectively.

The propagation of viruses in cell cultures from tissues of the same or alien hosts usually results in their attenuation for the natural host by the simple procedure of numerous transfers in cultures. More recently the selection of temperature-sensitive mutants and their repeated transfer through a susceptible cell system at 32°C has resulted in sufficient attenuation to use the altered virus as a safe and efficacious virus vaccine. Another genetic manipulation now being used experimentally to produce attenuated virus is recombination. Cell-cultured attenuated virus vaccines now are used to protect individuals against many diseases, and they are rapidly replacing attenuated virus vaccines produced in vivo. Tissue-cultured vaccines are usually simpler and cheaper to produce and also easier to assay for virus content because most viruses cause a cytopathogenic effect in cell cultures or provide some other indicator of their concentration. They are approved only after the vaccine is determined to be safe and efficacious.

The major concern in the production of attenuated virus vaccines in vivo and in vitro is the problem of latent virus and/or mycoplasma contamination. The latter seems to be easier to detect, but it is quite difficult to control. Latent viruses in both systems confront our medical professions with major problems. There is a slow but gradual shift

Table 38.4. Inactivated (killed) virus vaccines licensed in 1986 for immunization of domestic animals in the United States*

Disease	For use in	Preparation method
Avian encephalomyelitis	Chickens	Chicken embryo
Avian parainfluenza 3 infection	Turkeys	Chicken embryo
Avian paramyxovirus infection	Pigeons	Chicken embryo
Avian reovirus infection	Chickens	Cell culture
Avian tenosynovitis	Chickens	Cell culture
Bovine parainfluenza 3 infection	Cattle	Cell culture
Bovine rhinotracheitis	Cattle	Cell culture
Bovine virus diarrhea	Cattle	Cell culture
Bovine warts	Cattle	Infected tissue
Bursal (Gumboro) disease	Chickens	Cell culture or chicken embryo
Canine adenovirus type 2 infection	Dogs	Cell culture
Canine coronavirus infection	Dogs	Cell culture
Canine parvovirus infection	Dogs	Cell culture
Eastern, western, and Venezuelan encephalomyelitis	Horses	Cell culture
Equine influenza	Horses	Cell culture or chicken embryo
Equine rhinopneumonitis	Horses	Cell culture
Feline calicivirus infection	Cats	Cell culture
Feline leukemia	Cats	Cell culture
Feline panleukopenia	Cats	Cell culture
Feline rhinotracheitis	Cats	Cell culture
Fox encephalitis	Foxes	Cell culture
Infectious bronchitis	Chickens	Chicken embryo
Mink enteritis	Mink	Cell culture
Newcastle disease	Chickens	Chicken embryo
Pseudorabies (Aujeszky's disease)	Swine	Cell culture
Rabies	Dogs, cats, sheep, cattle, and horses	Cell culture or infected tissue
Sendai virus infection	Rodents	Chicken embryo
Swine parvovirus infection	Swine	Cell culture
Vesicular stomatitis	Cattle	Cell culture

*Many licensed veterinary biological products contain more than one immunizing component to protect against two or more infectious agents. Complete directions for use and appropriate cautions are provided on the label of each product.

This table was compiled from information provided by the Biologics Licensing and Standards Staff, Veterinary Services, Animal and Plant Health Inspection Service, U.S. Dept. of Agriculture. (Courtesy D. Long.)

from primary or secondary animal cell cultures to diploid- or stable-line cell cultures for the production of veterinary and human virus vaccines. These lines and bovine fetal serum are carefully monitored for all known non-cytopathogenic viruses and also mycoplasmas. In addition, critical cytologic studies, including karyography, possible reversion to virulence, and oncogenic capabilities, are made before approval is given for the production of virus vaccines in these cell lines.

The duration of the immunity conferred by vaccines containing active virus depends on the peculiarities of the virus itself. When the natural disease confers a solid and long-lasting immunity, attenuated virus vaccines generally provide solid protection but for a lesser period of time.

Inactivated virus. The word "inactivated" is used in virus terminology to avoid the use of the word "killed," which is commonly used in bacteriology. The implications with respect to life are thus avoided. Viruses may be inactivated with heat, chemicals, ultraviolet rays, ultrasonic vibration, and other processes that commonly destroy life in higher forms. Care must be exercised to be certain that inactivation is complete (Elford 1931).

There are those who do not believe that fully inactivated virus vaccines can induce useful immunity in animals. These people have thought, and some recent knowl-

Table 38.5. Attenuated virus vaccines licensed in 1986 for immunization of domestic animals in the United States*

Disease	For use in	Preparation method
Avian encephalomyelitis	Chickens	Chicken embryo
Bluetongue	Sheep	Cell culture
Bovine coronavirus infection	Cattle	Cell culture
Bovine parainfluenza 3 infection	Cattle	Cell culture
Bovine respiratory syncytial virus infection	Cattle	Cell culture
Bovine rhinotracheitis	Cattle	Cell culture
Bovine rotavirus infection	Cattle	Cell culture
Bovine virus diarrhea	Cattle	Cell culture
Bursal (Gumboro) disease	Chickens	Cell or chicken embryo
Canine adenovirus type 2 infection	Dogs	Cell culture
Canine coronavirus infection	Dogs	Cell culture
Canine distemper	Dogs	Cell culture
Canine hepatitis	Dogs	Cell culture
Canine parainfluenza	Dogs	Cell culture
Canine parvovirus infection	Dogs	Cell culture
Duck virus enteritis (plague)	Ducks	Chicken embryo
Duck virus hepatitis	Ducks	Chicken embryo
Equine rhinopneumonitis	Horses	Cell culture
Equine viral arteritis	Horses	Cell culture
Feline calicivirus infection	Cats	Cell culture
Feline panleukopenia	Cats	Cell culture
Feline rhinotracheitis	Cats	Cell culture
Fowl laryngotracheitis	Chickens	Cell culture or chicken embryo
Fowl pox	Chickens, turkeys, and pigeons	Cell culture or chicken embryo
Infectious bronchitis	Chickens	Chicken embryo
Marek's disease	Chickens	Cell culture
Mink distemper	Mink	Cell culture
Newcastle disease	Chickens	Chicken embryo
Ovine ecthyma	Sheep	Cell culture or infected tissue
Porcine rotavirus infection	Swine	Cell culture
Pseudorabies (Aujeszky's disease)	Swine	Cell culture
Rabies	Dogs and cats	Cell culture
Tenosynovitis (viral arthritis)	Chickens	Cell culture or chicken embryo
Transmissible gastroenteritis	Swine	Cell culture
Venezuelan equine encephalomyelitis	Horses	Cell culture

*Many licensed veterinary biological products contain more than one immunizing component to protect against two or more infectious agents. Complete directions for use and appropriate cautions are provided on the label of each product.

This table was compiled from information provided by the Biologics Licensing and Standards Staff, Veterinary Services, Animal and Plant Health Inspection Service, U.S. Department of Agriculture. (Courtesy D. Long.)

edge of the nature of viruses lends plausibility to their beliefs, that the so-called inactivated viruses generally contain some infective virions. It is possible that inactivation may prove to be a reversible phenomenon, that inactivated agents can be reactivated in some degree by contact with susceptible cells. It has been conclusively demonstrated many times that so-called inactivated viruses really have contained a very small fraction of active virus, a portion of which has much greater resistance to the inactivating agent than most of the virus particles (Bachrach et al. 1957, Elford 1931).

Today most virologists accept the concept that it is

possible to induce adequate immunity with wholly inactivated viruses. To be effective such vaccines must contain relatively large amounts of virus protein, because there can be no increase of viral antigen in the body such as that which occurs when active virus is used. It is often difficult to produce vaccines with sufficient protein to provide satisfactory antigenic stimulus, and it is believed that this has been the reason for many failures. Moreover, inactivated virus cannot supply continuing stimulation; hence the induced immunity may be initially solid but cannot last unless repeated immunizations are made. This leads to two concern: (1) reaching the patients a sufficient number of times and (2) possible hypersensitivity to repeated administration of foreign proteins. Further, some inactivated virus vaccines have induced hypersensitivity to subsequent infection. The inactivated virus vaccines for eastern and western equine encephalomyelitis and for feline panleukopenia are examples of excellent biologics.

Replication of foot-and-mouth disease virus produces an enzyme (VIA) detectable in the agar-gel diffusion test (Cowan and Graves 1966). Serums from animals given inactivated FMD virus fail to show this enzyme antibody. It is possible that this phenomenon may be used to test other inactivated virus vaccines for infectious virions.

Other Procedures for Improving Vaccines and Their Use. Manufacturers are using chemical and physical means such as zonal centrifugation to eliminate nonviral proteins in an effort to reduce adverse reactions.

There also is great activity by virologists to transfer foreign genes into *E. coli* or eukaryotic cells using plasmids, bacteriophages, or mammalian viruses as vectors. By this approach it is possible to produce large and pure amounts of desirable biologically active proteins such as interferon and virus subunit protein. The subunit vaccines produced in a vector such as vaccinia offer considerable promise since the incorporated genes carry only the message to produce the proteins that provide protection against one or more diseases and not the genes of the virion responsible for production of disease (Mackett et al. 1985, Perkus et al. 1985). The vaccinia vector has other advantages in domestic animals such as cattle since the vaccinia recombinant virus produces only a localized reaction and does not spread to susceptible contact cattle, can be given successfully at least five times within short periods of time, and produces good neutralizing antibody to the vaccinia virus and the immunogens produced by the foreign genes during viral replication (Gillespie et al. 1986). Improved promoters as they are developed can be inserted into a recombinant vaccinia virus to enhance the immunological response. Consequently, this system has great promise and undoubtedly will be used in the future

to immunize domestic animals against viruses and other infectious disease agents.

Improved adjuvants and the use of liposomes also will play an important role in the production of improved safe and efficacious inactivated virus vaccines.

More attention is being paid to the type of immunoglobulins involved in protection and their location in the body to make the best use of a biological product for host protection. For example, it may make more sense to administer a vaccine by the aerosol route to protect against respiratory viral diseases, by the oral route for enteric diseases. In essence, we are making use of our knowledge of immunology and pathogenesis to enhance the effectiveness of a biological product.

Cross-Immunity in Viral Infections

It has been pointed out that antigenicity is a property of the protein fraction of the virus moiety, the innocuous portion that protects the nucleic acid.

As known for a long time with bacteria, there are antigenic relationships and similarities among viruses. These do not necessarily mean that common pathogenic factors exist, or that the agents are biologically related. The literature contains a number of examples. One of the most intriguing of these is the relationship that exists between measles in humans, distemper in dogs, and rinderpest in cattle (Adams and Imagawa 1957, Polding et al. 1959). The protection conferred by measles virus in dogs against virulent distemper virus is based on the anamnestic response (Gillespie and Karzon 1960). The protection conferred by bovine virus diarrhea virus in pigs against virulent hog cholera is based on a similar phenomenon (Sheffy et al. 1962).

Viral Resistance

In general, viruses seem to possess about the same degree of resistance to heat, drying, and many chemical agents as the vegetative forms of most bacteria. Moist heat at 55 to 60°C for 30 minutes usually inactivates viruses; yet it has been shown that a very small residuum of active foot-and-mouth disease virus remains after exposure at these temperatures. This same situation exists for some other viruses. Drying is destructive to most viruses; yet there are some that survive very long periods of ordinary drying. Freeze drying, or lyophilization, is one of the best methods of preserving viruses for long periods. Another method is the storage of viruses at −60°C or lower.

Viruses respond to chemical disinfectants in the same way as vegetative forms of bacteria, but there are important differences. Most viruses are wholly unaffected by concentrations of most antibiotics that will inhibit and destroy bacteria. In most tissue culture work it is standard practice to incorporate such substances as penicillin, streptomycin, or mycostatin in the culture media to restrain the growth of bacteria and molds and to allow unrestricted growth of viruses.

Viruses, it should be remembered, are usually present in necrotic tissue fragments and mixed with coagulable proteins that may serve as effective protective coatings, delaying access of chemicals to the active agents. Because strongly alkaline solutions are effective tissue solvents, it has been believed that they were particularly effective agents in chemical disinfection. Two percent lye solution has been used for many years in disinfection following outbreaks of foot-and-mouth disease, apparently with complete success. Recently it has been found in laboratory experiments that this solution is not very effective with this virus, and with the virus of vesicular stomatitis. The virtue of the lye probably has resided not so much in its virucidal properties as in its solvent and detergent properties, because these expose the virus particles, dilute them, and remove them from the environment. (See the section on chemical inactivants earlier in this chapter.)

Most viruses are well preserved in strong solutions of glycerol (50 to 100 percent). Such concentrations dehydrate the cells that contain virus and tend to prevent their autolysis.

REFERENCES

Adams, J.M., and Imagawa, D.T. 1957. Immunological relationship between measles and distemper viruses. Proc. Soc. Exp. Biol. Med. 96:240–244.

Appel, M.J.G. 1969. Pathogenesis of canine distemper. Am. J. Vet. Res. 30:1167–1182.

Bachrach, H.L., Breese, S.S., Jr., Callis, J.J., Hess, W.R., and Patty, R.E. 1957. Inactivation of foot-and-mouth disease virus by pH and temperature changes and by formaldehyde. Proc. Soc. Exp. Biol. Med. 95:147–152.

Baker, J.A., McEntee, K., and Gillespie, J.H. 1960. Effects of infectious bovine rhinotracheitis–infectious pustular vulvovaginitis (IBR-IPV) virus on newborn calves. Cornell Vet. 50:156–170.

Bauer, J.H., and Hughes, T.P. 1934–35. Preparation of graded collodion membranes of Elford and their use in study of filterable viruses. J. Gen. Physiol. 18:143–162.

Bauer, J.H., and Pickels, E.G. 1936. A high speed vacuum centrifuge suitable for the study of filterable viruses. J. Exp. Med. 64:503–528.

Bechhold. 1907. Zeitschr. Phys. Chem. 60:257.

Beijerinck. 1899. Zentrbl. Bakt., II Abt. 5:27.

Bekkum, van, J.G., Frenkel, H.S., Fredericks, H.H.J., and Frenkel, S. 1959. Observations on the carrier state of cattle exposed to foot-and-mouth disease virus. Tjdschr. Diergeneeskd. 84:1159–1163.

Bernheimer, A.W., and Schwartz, L.L. 1965. Lysis of bacterial protoplasts and spheroplasts by staphylococcal α-toxin and streptolysin S. J. Bact. 89:1387–1392. (Original: Anderson, Hopps, Barile, and Bernheimer. 1965. J. Bact. 60:1387.)

Borrel. 1904. C. R. Soc. Biol. (Paris). 57:642.

Cowan, K.M., and Graves, J.H. 1966. A third antigenic component associated with foot-and-mouth disease infection. Virology 30:528–540.

Cowdry, E.V. 1934. The problem of intranuclear inclusions in virus diseases. Arch. Pathol. 18:527–542.

D'Herelle. 1922. The Bacteriophage: Its Role in Immunity. English trans. Williams & Wilkins, Baltimore.

Elford, W.J. 1931. A new series of graded collodion membranes suitable for general bacteriological use, especially in filterable virus studies. J. Pathol. Bact. 34:505–521.

Franklin, Klug, Caspar, and Holmes. 1963. Seventeenth Annual Symposium on Fundamental Cancer Research. Williams & Wilkins, Baltimore.

Gillespie, J.H. 1955. Propagation of type C foot-and-mouth disease virus in eggs and effects of the egg-cultivated virus in cattle. Cornell Vet. 45:170–179.

Gillespie, J.H., and Karzon, D.T. 1960. A study of the relationship between canine distemper and measles in the dog. Proc. Soc. Exp. Biol. Med. 105:547–551.

Gillespie, J.H., Geissinger, C., Scott, F.W., Higgins, W.P., Holmes, D.F., Perkus, M., Mercer, S., and Paoletti, E. 1986. Response of dairy calves to vaccinia viruses that express foreign genes. J. Clin. Microbiol. 23:283–388.

Gillespie, J.H., Robinson, J.I., and Baker, J.A. 1952. Dual infection of dogs with distemper virus and virus of infectious canine hepatitis. Proc. Soc. Exp. Biol. Med. 81:46–51.

Hirst, G.K. 1941. The agglutination of red cells by allantoic fluid of chick embryos infected with influenza virus. Science 94:22–23.

Hoggan, M.D., Roizman, B., and Roane, P.R., Jr. 1961. Further studies of variants of herpes simplex virus that produce syncytia or pocklike lesions in cell cultures. Am J. Hyg. 73:114–122.

Huang, A.S. 1973. Defective interfering viruses. Annu. Rev. Microbiol. 27:101–117.

Isaacs, A., Lindenmann, J., and Valentine, R.C. 1957. Virus interference. II. Some properties of interferon Proc. Roy. Soc. Ser. B. 174.268–273. (Original: Isaacs and Lindenmann. 1957. Proc. Roy. Soc. 147:258.)

Iwanowski, G. 1892. Bull. Acad. Imp. Science, St. Petersburg, 3d ser. 35:67.

Loeffler, G., and Frosch, L. 1898. Berichte der Kommission zur Erforschung der Maulund Klavenseuche bei dem Institut für Infektionskrankheiten in Berlin. Zentrbl. Bakt., I Abt. 23:371–395.

Lwoff, A., and Tournier, P. 1966. The classification of viruses. Annu. Rev. Microbiol. 20:45–74.

McClelland, L., and Hare, R. 1941. The adsorption of influenza virus by red cells and a new in vitro method of measuring antibodies for influenza virus. Can. J. Public Health 32:530–538.

Mackett, M., Hilma, T., Rose, J.K., and Moss, B. 1985. Vaccinia virus recombinants: Expression of VSV genes and protective immunization of mice and cattle. Science. 227:433–435.

Matthews, R.E.F. 1982. Classification and nomenclature of the viruses (Fourth Report of the ICTV). Intervirology. 17:1–199.

Murphy, F.A. 1985. Virus taxonomy. In B.N. Fields, D.M. Knipe, R.M. Chanock, J.L. Melnick, B. Roizman, R.E. Shope, eds., Virology. Raven Press, New York. Pp. 7–25.

Pasteur, 1885. C. R. Acad. Sci. 101:765.

Perkus, M.E., Piccini, A., Lipinskas, B.R., and Paoletti, E. 1985. Recombinant vaccinia virus: Immunization against multiple pathogens. Science 229:981–984.

Polding, J.B., Simpson, R.M., and Scott, G.R. 1959. Links between canine distemper and rinderpest. Vet. Rec. 71:643–645.

Poppensiek, G.C., and Baker, J.A. 1951. Persistence of virus in urine as factor in spread of infectious hepatitis in dogs. Proc. Soc. Exp. Biol. Med. 77:279–281.

Rivers, T.M., Haagen, E., and Muckenfuss, R.S. 1929. A study of vaccinal immunity in tissue cultures. J. Exp. Med. 50:673–685.

Sabin, A. B. 1952. Proc. Natl. Acad. Sci. USA 38:540.

Sanarelli, G. 1898. Das myxomatogene Virus: Beitrag zum Studium der Krankheitserreger ausserhalb des Sichtbaren. Zentrbl. Bakt., I. Abt. 23:865–873.

Scott, F.W. 1979. Feline infectious diseases—Practical viricidal disinfectants. Proc. Annu. Meet. Am. Anim. Hosp. Assoc. 46:105–107.

Sheffy, B.E., Coggins, L., and Baker, J.A. 1962. Relationship between hog cholera virus and virus diarrhea virus of cattle. Proc. Soc. Exp. Biol. Med. 109:349–352.

Stanley, W. 1935. Science. 81:644.

Syverton, J.T., and Berry, G.P. 1947. Multiple virus infection of single host cells. J. Exp. Med. 86:145–152.

Vilches, A., and Hirst, G.K. 1947. Interference between neurotropic and other unrelated viruses. J. Immunol. 57:125–140.

White, D. O., and Fenner, F. 1986. Medical Virology, 3d ed. Academic Press, New York.

Williams, R.C., and Wyckoff, R.W.G. 1945. Electron shadow micrography of the tobacco mosaic virus protein. Science 101:594–596.

39 Epidemiology of Viral Infections

The epidemiology of viral diseases is an exceedingly fascinating area of microbiology because of the unique biochemical, biophysical, and biological characteristics of viruses. With their highly parasitic nature and small size, viruses are more difficult to recognize in nature than other microorganisms, although modern cell-culture and molecular biological techniques, as well as improved methods of purification, concentration, and visualization, have made their detection easier. Our better knowledge of the host spectrum of viruses has also aided in their detection, which still relies heavily on the effects that viruses produce in various animals. Our knowledge of the epidemiology and ecology of viral diseases thus has grown at a rate commensurate with our technological advancements in animal virology. Consequently, a meaningful program in viral epidemiology requires a well-equipped laboratory with personnel capable of performing modern virus isolation and serologic procedures.

According to Shope (1965) periodicity and seasonal prevalence are two features characteristic of most viral diseases, but these are incompletely understood. The terms "distemper years," "hog cholera years," "foot-and-mouth disease years," and the like, are expressions that reflect the periodicity of viral diseases. These years of significant disease are thought to be due to increased virulence or invasiveness of the virus or to the fluctuating ratio of immune to susceptible animals in a population. Virus and host thus both play a major role in the periodicity of disease. Certain viral diseases do have a seasonal prevalence—canine distemper occurs more frequently in the fall and winter. When arthropod vectors are involved in the transmission of viruses, such as the arboviruses, disease occurs during the summer in temperate zones.

For many years epidemiologists limited their studies of an outbreak of a disease to the time it first appeared in a single host species until it disappeared from that population, treating each outbreak as an episode. More recently, epidemiologists have broadened their interests by concerning themselves with the natural history of viral diseases, seeking more information about the location and survival of the virus during the interepidemic phase. The epidemiology of animal viral diseases is generally less complex and less difficult to study than that of human viral diseases. Farm animals and pets usually do not travel beyond limited geographic areas, and contact with many animals from other areas is the exception rather than the rule. Our greatest disease problems in veterinary medicine are usually associated with the movement of animals from one location to another where animals from many sources are assembled. Even wild animals, except certain birds and bats, tend to reside within a limited territory; thus exposure to various disease agents is restricted. This situation does produce a more susceptible population and leads to more explosive outbreaks when an agent is introduced into a virgin population. For example, rather severe outbreaks of canine distemper with high morbidity and mortality in dogs of all ages have been reported in isolated arctic communities. Obviously, it is simpler to study the natural history of a disease in a virgin population than in a population in various stages of immunity; thus animal models are often used to enhance our knowledge of the epidemiology of certain human viral diseases. Of course, many viruses produce infection and disease in animals and humans under natural conditions, and these particular infections are of great interest in both human and veterinary medicine.

Persistence of Virus in Nature

The persistence of a virus in nature depends on two major factors; (1) the biophysical and biochemical characteristics of a virus which permit it to retain its infectiousness outside of its natural host(s), and (2) its biological characteristics that facilitate persistence in one or more hosts for varying periods of time. If failure occurs on both counts, the virus passes into oblivion.

Knowledge of the biophysical and biochemical characteristics of viruses is important in the assessment of their ability to survive outside the body of their natural host(s). It soon becomes apparent in most instances that the chances for viral survival outside these host(s) are rather meager. Most viruses cannot withstand severe environmental conditions. The majority are destroyed in strong alkali or acid solutions, or even in strong salt solutions. Viruses with a lipid coat are quickly inactivated by fat solvents. Exposure to high temperatures for a relatively short time destroys viral infectivity. Certain viruses are quickly inactivated by direct sunlight. On the other hand, many viruses can live for a long time in well-buffered media or in tissue at exceedingly low temperatures ($-60°C$ and lower) and also in a dried state at regular refrigeration temperature.

The successful spread and perpetuation of virus in the host are the principal mechanisms by which a viral species is maintained in nature. Several epidemiological models explain this success. These are discussed in subsequent sections of this chapter.

Virus Transmission

According to Shope (1965) the epidemiology of clinically apparent viral illnesses can be classified as intermittent or nonintermittent. Intermittent diseases constitute no good evidence for the existence of a continuous chain of animal-to-animal infection, either by contact or by a vector or intermediate host. Nonintermittent viral diseases apparently are maintained by contact infections, which are either clinical or subclinical infections. In addition, indigenous viral infections occur in nature and produce disease in more susceptible hosts. As our knowledge of animal viral diseases has improved, it has become apparent that viruses can readily exist in hosts as a persisting or occult virus, or even as a virogene, representing a potential source of virus in nature and not necessarily requiring a broad host spectrum to enhance its perpetuity.

Direct Species-to-Species Transmission

Infections transferred by direct contact between one animal and another of the same species are usually done so by salivary, aerosol, or fecal contamination. Examples of diseases spread this way are common—vesicular exanthema, transmissible gastroenteritis, and hog cholera in swine; virus diarrhea in cattle; avian bronchitis in chickens; and hepatitis in mice. We know little about these diseases in our wildlife, but some viruses, such as the one that causes virus diarrhea in deer, likely appear in closely related species and are not limited to a single species.

Subclinical infections often play an important role in maintaining the chain of transmission.

Most of the diseases in this epidemiological group result in long-lasting immunity. It was once believed that these viruses did not persist in a host; but it is now known that most of them do remain under certain conditions, serving as probable links in any subsequent chain of infection.

Virus Carriers: Recovered Animals

Many animal viral infections are transmitted by virus carriers. After initially infecting an individual, the virus persists in superficial tissue, where it can readily be eliminated in various body excretions. Viruses that typically persist in recovered animals are members of such families as Adenoviridae, Herpesviridae, Picornaviridae, and Poxviridae, to mention a few. Animals that are virus carriers are a source of potential infection to all susceptible species.

Some of the diseases caused by this group such, as herpes simplex, are characterized by clinical relapses that usually occur after a stress of some sort, such as another infection. Immunity and infection coexist in delicate balance in these persisting viral infections. In an interesting experiment Good and Campbell (1948) precipitated latent herpes simplex encephalitis in rabbits by anaphylactic shock, a severe form of stress.

Arthropod-Borne Transmission

Four principal cycles are involved in the transmission of the arboviruses: (1) arthropod to humans (urban yellow fever is an example); (2) arthropod–lower vertebrate cycle with tangential infection of humans and other higher vertebrates (examples are jungle yellow fever and equine encephalomyelitis); (3) arthropod-arthropod cycle with occasional infection of lower vertebrates and humans (an example is Colorado tick fever); and (4) lower vertebrate–arthropod cycle with infection of domestic animals (African horsesickness is a prime example; another probable one is turkey meningoencephalitis, although essential insect transmission has not been completely proved).

In arthropod-arthropod transmission the virus may travel from the adult arthropod to its offspring by transovarian passage, thus not involving a vertebrate host. Often the virus produces little or no disease in the arthropod host, but persists in an infective form in the host, which then serves for the rest of its life as a reservoir for the infection. In contrast, most vertebrate hosts infected with arboviruses show severe disease, which terminates quickly in survival or death. Survival results in the formation of excellent long-term immunity. In some arbovirus infections the presence of the virus in the vertebrate is temporary and short, the host therefore plays a minor role in perpetuating the agent in nature.

Accidental Infection

Two well-known viral diseases are transmitted by animal bites. The first is rabies, a disease of considerable historical importance. Its epidemiology is discussed at length in Chapter 53. Rabies virus has a broad host spectrum, and the primary means of transmission is a bite by an infected carnivorous animal or by an infected bat. The second disease is monkey B-virus infection in humans, caused by a bite from an infected monkey that shows no evidence of illness. In humans this disease manifests clinically as encephalitis and is often fatal.

Certain diseases can readily be produced by the accidental infection with a viral contaminant in a vaccine or by blood transfusion from virus carriers to susceptible individuals. These diseases, obviously caused by human actions, can be prevented by use of sterile techniques in the vaccination of animals and by strict control in the production and testing of biologicals. When fresh animal tissues (including blood) are used in therapy, certain hazards such as persisting microbes, must be considered. Equine infectious anemia virus and some blood protozoan agents are readily transmitted by these means.

Indigenous Viral Infections

Animals with indigenous viral infections have three main features, namely, (1) inapparent infection, (2) persisting virus, and (3) infection at an early age. The healthy carriers never show disease and yet serve as the means of perpetuating and transmitting the viruses that they carry. Some notable examples include lymphocytic choriomeningitis in mice, viral encephalitides in birds and in rodents, malignant catarrhal fever in cattle, and African swine fever.

Immunological tolerance may be an important characteristic of lymphocytic choriomeningitis, an indigenous infection in mice. Mice are infected in utero and as sucklings by their clinically well mothers. Through the excreta of latently infected mice, humans can contract clinical disease. Indigenous viral encephalitides in birds and in rodents can play important roles in the epidemiology of these viruses, from which frank disease develops in other hosts, such as horses and humans, through the medium of the arthropod that has contact with indigenous virus hosts. In bovine malignant catarrhal fever, cattle are the disease

(indicator) host of a virus carried as a silent infection by wildebeests and possibly by sheep. African swine fever is an indigenous viral infection in the wart hog, yet it is usually a highly acute and fatal disease in domestic swine.

The Case for the Virogene and the Oncogene

During bacteriophage replication bacteria in the prophage stage may lose the prophage for reasons as yet unknown, may remain in the prophage stage, or may develop from the prophage to the vegetative form with phage maturation and eventual lysis. It is believed that a comparable prophage stage exists for animal viruses, which Luria (1950) has called "parasitism at the genetic level." Shope (1965) has called it "masked virus," and the terms "occult" or "virogene" have also been suggested. The existence of this viral stage is most difficult to prove, especially when it cannot be reactivated into an infective form. A number of viruses can cause animal tumors, and presumably the agent becomes integrated into the genetic apparatus of the parasitized cell. Although the virus may lose its infectivity under these circumstances, it still can elicit the formation of specific antiviral antibodies.

The first notable example of this phenomenon involved the Shope papilloma rabbit virus. In naturally infected cottontail rabbits active virus could usually be demonstrated in the papillomas, yet no infective virus could be shown in papillomas induced by the cottontail virus in domestic rabbits. Viral antigen was demonstrated in these noninfective domestic rabbit papillomas (Shope 1937) and also in the carcinomas arising from them (Kidd et al. 1936). This noninfective antigenic virus was called "masked virus" by Shope.

Other oncogenic DNA viruses such as the polyoma and certain adenoviruses behave in a similar manner. Infective virus often is not demonstrable in polyoma-induced tumors in hamsters (Habel and Atanasiu 1959). Similarly, Huebner et al. (1963) failed to isolate infective virus from tumors induced by adenovirus types 12 and 18 in hamsters or by adenovirus type 12 in rats; however, antigens that produce antibodies capable of reacting with type-specific viral antigens of a given serotype were demonstrated in the tumor mass. The studies of Black et al. (1963) with simian virus (SV-40), hamster tumors, or with cells transformed in culture gave similar results, causing the investigators to conclude that the noninfective antigen is synthesized by information from the SV-40 viral genome integrated in the tumor and in cells transformed in vitro. Thus, we have four examples of DNA viruses that cause tumors that are usually free of infective virus but contain viral antigen(s).

Epidemiology of Tumor Viruses

Mammals and birds exhibit a number of virus-induced tumors, many of which have a structure similar to certain tumors in humans. Our limited knowledge of virus-induced tumors suggests that they sometimes are vertically transmitted, thus limiting the epidemiological means by which they may ultimately be controlled. The principal control measure appears to be the use of drugs that enhance the replication of specific viral enzymes.

The Bittner mouse virus that causes mammary carcinoma is an interesting epidemiological model. Virus is present in the milk and other tissues of certain strains of mice. The virus can remain dormant for the life of the infected mouse, but can readily be transmitted to its nursing offspring. Usually, mammary carcinoma develops in the infected adults at a certain stage of hormonal function, and the animals subsequently die.

Certain tumor viruses such as those that cause murine, avian, and feline leukemia can be transmitted directly from the dam to the progeny in utero and also from infected animals to uninfected ones. Some investigators have speculated that the virus is transferred in the ovum and perhaps even in the sperm. These viruses can persist within the cells for the life of an individual without disease manifestation. Why leukemias or sarcomas or both develop in some individuals harboring the agent and not in others is unknown. This close association of the virus with the genetic apparatus of the cell and its ability to persist for a long time assures the continued existence of the viral parasite as long as its natural hosts do not become extinct.

Certain superficial tumors such as fibromas and papillomas of rabbits and some domestic animals can be transmitted surgically and presumably by certain insects as well. For example, there is definite field evidence that the rabbit fibroma is transmitted in nature by a flying, biting insect (Shope 1965). Rabbit papilloma also appears to be insect transmitted in cottontail rabbits.

Epidemiological study of animal tumors has become rather extensive. There is considerable interest now in these diseases, particularly those for which good virus assay and serologic methods exist. The etiology of some human tumors is known, so epidemiological success in this area has been achieved. Currently most of our basic knowledge of tumor epidemiology has been developed with animal models of known viral etiology.

Epidemiology of Chronic and Degenerative Diseases

Chronic and degenerative diseases are caused by agents called slow viruses. The incubation period is, as a rule, extremely long in the natural host, and virus can be isolated from the tissues of these infected animals for a long time. Strong evidence exists that some of these diseases are autoimmune conditions with lesions resulting from the combined action of antigen, antibody, and complement.

Little is known about the transmission of slow viruses. Is vertical transmission or horizontal transmission the main mechanism for their spread from one individual to another? Are vectors required for their transmission? Do they have a narrow or broad host spectrum? How long do they persist in the host? Answers to these questions about the nature of these viruses are essential to an understanding of their ecology.

Eradication of Viral Diseases

In veterinary medicine test and removal has been the principal method used to eradicate certain viral diseases. Foot-and-mouth disease (FMD), a prime example, has been eliminated in certain countries bordered by nations free of the disease or by navigable waters. It is remarkable that this success has often been achieved by testing and removing the afflicted ruminant species and pigs in infected herds with no particular attention paid to other domesticate or wild animals susceptible, to some degree, to FMD virus. In Great Britain, where the disease has frequently occurred, reinfection of the population usually has been traced to virus in an animal product from a country where the disease is enzootic. Yet the virus does persist in recovered animals and in animals given attenuated virus vaccine, or in animals vaccinated with inactivated virus vaccine and subsequently exposed to infective virus. Consequently, a test-and-removal program seems the only reasonable approach to eradication of any viral disease with latency and vertical transmission as features.

Hog cholera has been eradicated from Canada and the United States by the test-and-removal method. Since this disease affects only domestic and wild pigs with no positive proof that the virus infects other animals naturally, it was reasonable, on the basis of the Canadian experience, to expect the U.S. program also to be successful. This proved to be the case despite the complexity of the pig-industry, which involves frequent and rapid movement of hogs over long distances.

Vaccination has proved helpful in preventing and controlling hog cholera, but not in eradicating it. Inactivated virus vaccine is not a very good biologic and has never completely controlled the disease. Attenuated virus vaccine helped to control the disease but led to latency and chronicity in certain animals, so its use was abandoned.

In certain arbovirus diseases insects are true biological vectors and are essential to disease perpetuation in humans and animals. If these vectors are removed from the environment where susceptible animals or humans reside, disease is eliminated. Of course the eradication of insects is a formidable task whose execution is usually neither feasible nor practical.

The elimination of viral disease from a country by vaccination has not been too successful. Inactivated virus vaccines generally provide insufficient immunity to prevent replication of virus in a vaccinated animal, even though disease may not occur. Attenuated virus vaccines provide greater immunity and usually prevent the residence of virulent (street) virus in the animal, but often the attenuated virus is transmitted to susceptible animals. After repeated transfer in nature, attenuated virus can become virulent again and produce acute or chronic disease, depending on its nature. A notable exception is the virus that causes rinderpest in cattle. Properly attenuated rinderpest vaccines prevent the virus from producing disease or transmitting it to susceptible hosts and cause a blind-ended infection in the vaccinated animal. This ideal vaccine leads to disease eradication when a large percentage of the population is vaccinated in a unified, country-wide campaign. Theoretically, it should be possible to abolish

canine distemper because excellent biologicals that do not spread the disease are available. A well-organized nationwide campaign—with strictly enforced quarantine and vaccination procedures—would be required to eliminate a virulent agent that spreads as readily in a susceptible population as does the distemper virus. At best it would be difficult to control in pets in an era when international travel is so common and dogs often accompany their owners.

REFERENCES

Black, Rowe, Turner, and Huebner. 1963. Proc. Natl. Acad. Sci. USA 50:1148.

Good, R.A., and Campbell, B. 1948. The precipitation of latent *Herpes simplex* encephalitis by anaphylactive shock. Proc. Soc. Exp. Biol. Med. 68:82–87.

Habel, K., and Atanasiu, P. 1959. Transplantation of polyoma virus induced tumor in the hamster. Proc. Soc. Exp. Biol. Med. 102.99–102.

Huebner, Rowe, Turner, and Lane. 1963. Proc. Natl. Acad. Sci. USA 50:379.

Kidd, J.G., Beard, J.W., and Rous, P. 1936. Serological reactions with a virus causing rabbit papillomas which become cancerous. I. Tests of the blood of animals carrying the papilloma. II. Tests of the blood of animals carrying various epithelial tumors. J. Exp. Med. 64:63–78, 79–96.

Luria, S.F. 1950. Bacteriophage: An essay in virus reproduction. Science 111:507–511.

Shope, R.E. 1937. Immunization of rabbits to infectious papillomatosis. J. Exp. Med. 65:219–231.

Shope, R.E. 1965. Transmission of viruses and epidemiology of viral infections. In F.L. Horsfall and I. Tamm, eds., Viral and Rickettsial Infections of Man, 4th ed. J.P. Lippincott, Philadelphia. Pp. 385–494.

40 Laboratory Diagnosis of Viral Infections

Ideally, disease is diagnosed at the clinical level by means of history, physical examination, and the signs of illness in a single patient or herd. The veterinarian, especially the small-animal practitioner, often resorts to fluoroscopy, radiography, surgery, and other specialized procedures to facilitate a proper diagnosis, and most cases can be adequately diagnosed in this manner. With the availability of more specialized equipment and increased knowledge, more veterinary practitioners are using laboratory examinations involving such disciplines as pathology, microbiology, physiology, and biochemistry. Many laboratory procedures today are simple, rapid, accurate, and inexpensive, and constitute ideal diagnostic tests. Many veterinary practices have a small laboratory for such tests. An occasional case may demand more sophisticated equipment and a specialized diagnostic approach that requires the services of a state or university veterinary diagnostic laboratory. Biological specimens for this purpose must be properly prepared, stored, and sent to the laboratory. The importance of specimen preparation and handling cannot be overemphasized because a poor specimen often elicits (and deserves) a poor answer.

Many viral diseases have rather characteristic features that permit identification at the clinical and pathological level. With some viral diseases, however, the veterinarian may find it necessary to establish a diagnosis either by virus identification or by serologic methods. Isolation of the virus often requires a few days or weeks, and most serologic tests require the use of paired serums taken 2 to 3 weeks apart. Until the 1970s diagnosis of viral diseases required too much time, but that situation is rapidly changing with the introduction, development, and availability of rapid diagnostic techniques that provide specific and accurate results. Examples of such procedures are the enzyme-linked immunosorbent assay (ELISA) and direct and indirect immunofluorescent antibody and complement-fixation tests.

There are a number of excellent books, journal articles, and monographs devoted to the laboratory diagnosis of viral diseases. The most desirable sources, which give excellent, authoritative, and up-to-date coverage, are the multiauthor books edited by Cottral (1978) and by Lennette (1985). The former volume deals with standardized methods for veterinary microbiology.

Isolation of Viruses

The effort and cost involved in virus etiological diagnosis requires careful selection of case material as well as proper collection and handling of the specimen. As a rule, virus isolation is desirable for the following purposes: (1) to identify a virus of concern in a herd health program; (2) to point out a possible public health problem, such as rabies; (3) to establish the viral etiology of a disease not previously encountered in a practice; (4) to determine the immunological type of a given virus when epidemics such as foot-and-mouth disease occur; and (5) to pinpoint the exact agent when serologic test methods fail because the agent shares common antigens with other viruses.

Isolation of a virus from a diseased animal does not necessarily mean that the isolate is the cause of the disease. Many viruses, including pathogens, persist in animals for a long time and tend to confuse the diagnosis. Some of these viruses, such as bovine enteroviruses, are of the orphan type, that is, they are not proven pathogens. A knowledge of clinical and epidemiological patterns for the various viruses is useful in assessing the significance of a viral isolate from a diseased animal. The occasional isolation of more than one virus from a patient can be a difficult problem if both isolates are known pathogens. One virus may be causing an inapparent infection while the other is responsible for the clinical signs of illness. A knowledge of the signs produced by each virus is important to establish the primary disease agent. If both viruses produce comparable signs, the diagnosis becomes academic unless it is known that the patient may have had previous contact with one or both agents. A rising titer with paired serums to one virus and not the other would be strong evidence of which virus is responsible for the present illness. Obviously, the diagnosis would be missed if antibody (serologic) studies were done only for the virus causing the inapparent infection.

Collection of Clinical Material

The ideal time to collect biological material for virus isolation is during the acute stage of illness before antibodies form. Many diagnostic laboratories supply the appropriate containers for storing tissue or serum samples for viral diagnosis. Obviously, every veterinarian should have a supply in stock.

Various materials such as blood, nasal swabs, nasopharyngeal swabs, feces, urine, pus, vesicular fluid, skin lesions, spinal fluid, and biopsy and autopsy specimens arc used for the isolation of viruses. The particular biological specimens required for diagnosis of a specific disease are included in the description of the disease in this textbook, in the section on diagnosis.

Some general guidelines exist for the proper selection of tissues for virus isolation. Virus is usually excreted in the nasal or pharyngeal secretions of animals in the acute stages of respiratory illnesses. Virus can be demonstrated in the fluid of vesicular lesions or in the scabs of pox lesions. Many generalized catarrhal diseases have a viremic state, and the virus can be readily isolated from the blood; virtually all body excretions contain virus during the acute stage of illness. Diseases of the central nervous system often present a problem, but an attempt should be made to isolate the virus from the blood and the brain of animals that die of the disease.

It is most important to obtain tissue specimens from animals immediately after death—in some instances an owner may agree to sacrifice a moribund animal, which further enhances virus isolation. Often a blood sample can be used for serologic tests and for virus isolation at the same time, but an aliquot of blood must be placed in two separate containers—one each for serologic testing and virus isolation.

Naturally, tissue specimens should be taken with sterile instruments in a sterile manner. If virus distribution in the tissues is a concern, separate sterile instruments must be used for procuring each tissue sample.

The biophysical and biochemical properties of viruses vary markedly. Many viruses are heat-sensitive and acid-sensitive, and great care must be exercised in handling specimens. In particular, fresh tissues must be used and then frozen to $-60°C$ or lower immediately after harvesting. The less time spent in attempted isolations with these tissues in cell cultures or test animals the better. If there is no alternative, the tissue specimens can be placed in a freezer at $-20°C$ until dry ice is obtained for transport to the laboratory. A wide-mouthed thermos jug or a polystyrene-insulated carton, filled with dry ice after the specimens are inserted, is used for shipment. If dry ice is not available, 50 percent glycerol can be used, but one must

remember that certain viruses remain viable longer than others in this solution. Small pieces of tissue, fecal material, or mucus are placed in a vial, and the vial is filled with 50 percent glycerol and stored at $6°C$. Tight, sterile screw-cap vials often are used for storage of suspect tissues and fluids. If fluid specimens are stored in dry ice, the vials should be airtight as the gaseous phase of dry ice is CO_2, which changes the pH of fluids and inactivates pH-labile viruses. When vials are not airtight, they should be placed in a sealed, airtight plastic bag.

Some laboratories do not operate over a weekend, so it is wise to ship the biological material during the early part of the week unless other arrangements are made.

Preparation of Specimens

Susceptible animals, cell cultures, and embryonated hens' eggs are used as substrates for virus isolation. Fluid specimens that are bacteria-free can be inoculated directly or after dilution with a buffered solution (pH 7.2 to 7.6).

Solid tissues are prepared as 10 to 20 percent suspensions, with a buffered solution (pH 7.2 to 7.6) as diluent. This suspension is lightly centrifuged to remove the coarse particles that tend to plug the inoculating equipment and often are toxic to cells in the test system. The supernatant fluid is used as the inoculum after centrifugation at 2,000 rpm for 10 minutes.

Certain test inocula such as feces, oral and nasal swabs, insects, and some infected tissues contain bacteria, which should be eliminated before inoculation. Several procedures are used for this purpose, but for various reasons they do not always succeed. Ether is bactericidal, but may not be harmful to the virus under consideration. In such instances 10 to 15 percent ether can be added to the test suspension for 1 to 2 hours, then removed prior to inoculation of test suspension in a test system. Antibiotics are used, and a mixture of penicillin (1,000 U/ml) and streptomycin (100 mg/ml) is most commonly employed in media, although the test material can be pretreated with higher levels of antibiotics if necessary to eliminate the contaminating organism. The dye proflavine is often used to inactivate microbes in fecal and throat specimens photodynamically, as it has little or no effect on enteroviruses or rhinoviruses. The specimen is treated with 10^{-4} M proflavine for 1 hour at pH 9 at $37°C$, after which the dye is removed by cation resins. The photosensitized bacterial and fungal contaminants are inactivated when exposed to light. Microbes also can be removed by mechanical means such as ultrafiltration and differential centrifugation. Earthenware, porcelain, and asbestos filters are used for this purpose, but virus concentration is reduced by adsorption to these materials. Differential centrifugation

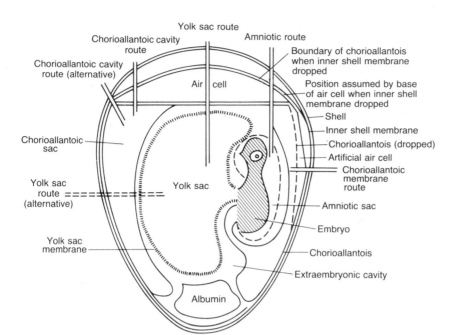

Figure 40.1. Various routes of inoculation into an embryonating hen's egg for the propagation of viruses.

is a convenient and excellent method to remove many bacteria from a heavily contaminated specimen of the smaller viruses. For viruses smaller than 100 nm, centrifugation at 18,000 rpm for 20 minutes in a 6-inch rotor will sediment the bacteria but not the virus. With specimens containing a minimal amount of virus, centrifugation at 40,000 rpm for 60 minutes in a 6-inch rotor concentrates most viruses in a small gelatinous pellet at the bottom of the tubes. The supernatant of such runs contains less than 1 percent of the original virus. The pellet is then resuspended in a small volume of buffered solution.

Isolation of Viruses in Embryonated Hens' Eggs

The marked progress in virology since the 1950s has been due, in part, to the use of the chicken embryo as a medium for the propagation of viral agents. Most viruses under natural conditions are relatively host-specific. Moreover, they show a definite predilection for groups of highly specialized cells of the host—for example, those constituting nerve tissue and epithelial tissue. Although growing readily in these tissues, they fail to grow in all or most others of the body. This affinity, one of the unique properties of viruses, is known as tissue tropism. Although many viruses show marked host specificity and tissue tropism, the great majority of these can be adapted by various procedures to foreign hosts. Most viruses are

capable of growing in chicken embryo tissues because of their ability to alter their tropism and to adapt to new host species and because the cells and the extraembryonic membranes of the developing chicken embryo, like most embryonic tissues, lack a high degree of specialization. Viruses grown in chicken embryo tissues frequently attain a much higher concentration than in the tissues of the natural host.

A variety of methods are available for the inoculation of the chicken embryo, and detailed procedures are described in the seventh edition of *Hagan and Bruner's Infectious Diseases of Domestic Animals*. The methods listed below are the ones most commonly used. Although there are a number of techniques for inoculating by each of the routes listed, the ones most widely used are depicted in Figure 40.1.

Yolk Sac Inoculation. The large elementary-body agents and the rickettsiae grow readily in the yolk sac membranes of 5- to 7-day-old fertilized chicken eggs. Although many of the smaller viruses are also inoculated by the yolk sac route, they invade the embryo and multiply in the body tissues rather than in the yolk sac tissues.

Chorioallantoic Cavity Inoculation. Influenza and the Newcastle disease viruses, and most other viral agents that cause respiratory infections, grow readily in the entodermal cells of the chorioallantoic sac wall of the 8- to 11-day-old embryonated hen's egg and are liberated into the chorioallantoic fluid. The encephalomyelitis viruses and the mumps virus also multiply readily when inoculated by this route.

Chorioallantoic Membrane Inoculation. Some viruses such as canine distemper virus and poxviruses produce lesions on the dropped membrane of 7- to 10-day-old chicken embryos. The pox lesions are discrete and can be counted with considerable accuracy. In contrast, the lesions caused by canine distemper virus are less clearly defined, but it is possible to distinguish a positive membrane from the uninoculated control membrane.

Amniotic Sac Inoculation. Inoculation of the amniotic sac is used principally for the isolation of the influenza virus from throat washings. From 7 to 15 days of age, chicken embryos during the course of their development swallow the amniotic fluid, thereby bringing the inoculated virus it contains into contact with the tissues of the respiratory and intestinal tract, where multiplication presumably occurs. The amniotic route of inoculation is used also for the isolation of the encephalomyelitis viruses.

Intravenous Inoculation. The intravenous route of inoculation of 12- to 14-day-old chicken embryos is not practiced to any extent but has been used for adaptation and replication of some strains of foot-and-mouth disease virus.

Isolation of Viruses in Tissue Culture

Advances in methods of cell culture have provided the virologist with highly valuable tools for isolation and propagation of viruses. Knowledge of the techniques of cell cultivation and maintenance is, therefore, a prerequisite to the study of viruses. Cell cultures are the most widely used methods for isolation of viruses from clinical material. Evidence of viral replication in cell cultures takes a variety of forms, such as cytopathic effects, viral interference, hemadsorption and hemagglutination, and the presence of fluorescent antigen, or complement-fixing antigen.

Usage of the following terms has been recommended by the Committee on Terminology of the Tissue Culture Association. Two methodological approaches—monolayer cell culture and suspended tissue or organ culture—have been developed to isolate viruses. Cell culture denotes the growing of cells in vitro, including the culture of single cells. In monolayer cultures cells are no longer organized into tissues and a single layer of cells attaches to a glass or plastic surface. In suspended tissue or organ cultures suspended tissues, or a whole organ or parts of an organ, are grown or maintained in vitro in a way that allows differentiation and preservation of their architecture or function or both. Suspension culture denotes a type of culture in which cells multiply while suspended in medium. A primary culture is a tissue culture started from material taken directly from an animal. It is regarded as

primary until it is subcultured for the first time. It then becomes a cell line, which is said to have become established when it demonstrates the potential to be subcultured indefinitely in vitro. Diploid cell line denotes a cell line in which, arbitrarily, at least 75 percent of the cells have the same karyotype as the normal cells of the species from which the cells were originally obtained. A diploid chromosome number is not necessarily equivalent to the diploid karyotype because a cell may lose one type of chromosome and acquire another type; thus the karyotype of the cell has changed, but the diploid number of chromosomes remains the same. Such cells should be referred to as pseudodiploid.

Primary cultures are prepared from a variety of human and animal tissues and are routinely employed in the cultivation of many viruses. Primary cultures are often preferred because of their increased susceptibility to viruses. On the other hand, lack of uniformity in susceptibility among different batches of cells and the possible presence of occult viruses are some of the inherent dangers of their use. Certain viruses such as some human coronaviruses replicate only in organ cultures.

Only under special circumstances can cell lines be grown continuously without changes in karyotype. Usually the conditions of culture select out variants in the cell population. These may differ radically from the predominant cell type in a primary culture. Most established cell lines used today are of this selected type, although diploid or pseudodiploid cell lines are increasingly being used. Freezing large batches of these cell lines permits work with cells of constant characteristics. In addition, cell lines offer the advantages of availability and rapid growth. One disadvantage is the attention required to keep them free of contaminants.

Viruses do not propagate outside living, actively metabolizing cells. While the body of the natural or experimental host provides the conditions necessary for viral multiplication, the tissue-culture system must be manipulated to assure optimal viral-growth conditions in the test tube or flask. It is therefore necessary to consider the cell, its nutritional requirements, its susceptibility to viruses, as well as the virus itself when working with cell-culture systems. Because the conditions necessary for viral multiplication are intimately associated with, and dependent on, the maintenance of viable cells, a sizable formulary of media has been devised to suit the growth requirements of various cell types. All media contain the following general substances in varying combinations and amounts: (1) balanced salt solutions—Earle's, Hanks', and Tyrode's solutions, to mention only a few; (2) "fortification substances"—lactalbumin hydrolysate, embryo extracts, amniotic fluid, vitamins, hormones, amino acids, minerals, and yeast extract; (3) serums—human, horse, dog, calf, rabbit, sheep, and other species free of inhibitors, viruses, and/or antibodies to the virus under study; and (4) antibiotics—penicillin, streptomycin, nystatin, tetracyclines, and many others used in doses that control microbial contamination but are not toxic to tissue-cultured cells.

Cell-culture work was plagued with contamination by unwanted bacteria and molds until the introduction of antibiotics, which allowed many more workers to prepare satisfactory tissue cultures in mass quantities. Contamination is still, however, one of the major hazards; for this reason strict aseptic technique is necessary.

The many techniques of tissue culture used in virus cultivation are modifications of five basic methods.

Suspended-cell method. The suspended-cell method is an old and still-employed method for the production of virus for foot-and-mouth disease.

Plasma-clot cell method. A film of plasma, often chicken plasma, is layered onto a glass surface and induced to clot by the addition of embryo extract. Into this matrix are placed tissue fragments (explants), which adhere and proliferate. With this method one can observe the cellular proliferation and can measure the growth of the explants. Growth of viruses in such cultures can be determined by several methods: (1) sampling the virus in the liquid or cellular phase of the culture and inoculating laboratory hosts known to be susceptible to infection, (2) noting the effect on cellular metabolism (i.e., inhibition of certain metabolic pathways), (3) observing cell death (necrosis), (4) testing for hemagglutinins, and (5) examining cells and purified fluids with the electron microscope.

Monolayer cell culture. Microtiter sterile plastic assay plates are by far the most widely used cultures in virology. They are prepared from trypsin-dispersed tissues and consist of small clumps of cells and single cells derived from the tissue suited for growth of a particular virus: kidney, testicle, skin, tumor, and other tissues. The tissues are finely minced with scissors, washed with saline to remove blood cells and tissue debris, and placed in a trypsin solution that is constantly stirred with a magnetic device. When the cells are dispersed (the time depends on the temperature of trypsinization and the type of tissue being prepared), they are lightly centrifuged, washed with media two or three times to remove the trypsin, filtered through several layers of cheesecloth, diluted to contain sufficient cells per milliliter to ensure good growth (the amount depends on the cell type), and placed in the wells of the assay plate with a dispensing pipette or syringe. The cell suspensions prepared from kidney fragments produce luxuriant monolayer cultures on any clean, stationary glass or plastic surface—petri dish, assay plate, test tube, or bottle. Cultures prepared in this way are used for virus isolations, titrations, neutralization tests, and for studying the growth of viruses in cells.

Direct cell culture. The procedure followed for direct cell culture is the same as described for monolayer cell cultures. Tissues are taken at autopsy or by biopsy from the diseased animal for the production of monolayer cell cultures to enhance the possibility of virus isolation when little virus is likely to be present in the tissues. As little trypsin as possible should be used because it inactivates some viruses.

Organ culture. Used for the inoculation of suspect viral material, organ cultures can be made directly from diseased tissues, as indicated in the previous paragraph. Organ cultures contain the differentiated tissues characteristic of a given organ. Some viruses—such as certain human coronaviruses—require a specialized cell for replication that is not present in a monolayer cell culture from the same organ. The viruses usually studied in organ cultures are the respiratory viruses. The cultures used are derived from embryonic respiratory tissues, and the emphasis is on viral propagation and its cytomorphological effects in the in vitro differentiated tissues. Organ cultures are used principally in research studies because the technique is time-consuming and tedious at present. Investigators of the pathogenesis and immunity of viral diseases will continue to use this method in future studies.

Detection of Viral Replication. The most characteristic change in virus-infected cultures is a degeneration or necrosis in their cellular elements (Figure 40.2). These cytopathic changes (cytopathic effect, or CPE) are visible with a light microscope, and first involve individual cells and then spread to all susceptible cells in a culture. The effect of the virus on the cells depends on the type of virus and cell. With certain viruses, such as herpesvirus (infectious bovine rhinotracheitis), canine and human adenoviruses, poliovirus, vesicular stomatitis virus, and foot-and-mouth disease virus, the cells become granular, round up into degenerated clumps, and finally drop from the glass surface, leaving islands of clear spaces. Eventually all the cells of a culture may become infected. In some infections the cells tend to clump together in aggregates to form "giant cells," which are syncytial formations of multinucleate cells. Such cells are characteristic of canine distemper, mumps, and measles viruses, parainfluenza viruses, and syncytium-forming viruses of monkeys, humans, cattle, and cats (Figure 40.3). In such infected cultures the virus is liberated into the fluids bathing the cells, although with certain viruses the con-

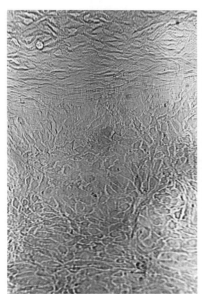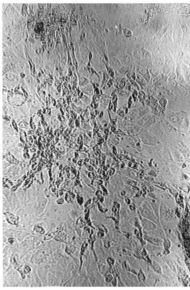

Figure 40.2. (*Left*) Uninoculated feline kidney cell culture. (*Right*) Cytopathic effect induced by a virus in feline kidney cell culture. May-Grünwald-Giemsa stain. × 82. (From F. Scott, C. Csiza, and J. Gillespie, 1970, courtesy of *American Journal of Veterinary Research.*)

centration of virus at any time in the growth cycle may be higher within the cell (cell-associated virus) than in the tissue-culture fluid. Certain tumor viruses cause a loss-of-contact inhibition, and the cells tend to pile upon each other, forming a plaque. The characteristic cytopathic effect produced by some viruses, along with the patient's clinical history, permits a rapid presumptive diagnosis. Because some viruses replicate without producing a cytopathic effect, other means are used for their identification in cell cultures.

Some viruses such as feline panleukopenia virus produce intranuclear inclusion bodies, which can be readily observed after May-Grünwald staining (Figure 40.4). Since there is no significant destruction of the cell layer, staining of cover-slip cultures offers a means of diagnosis. The diagnostician can demonstrate virus antigen by immunofluorescent staining with a specific conjugate (Figure 40.5) or a vital stain such as May-Grünwald. When an organism such as a noncytopathic strain of virus diarrhea–mucosal disease virus produced absolutely no cell alterations, a fluorescent antibody conjugate or the viral interference test with a cytopathogenic strain of virus diarrhea–mucosal disease virus can be used to assist in identification. In the interference test the noncytopathogenic strain interferes with a precalculated amount of cytopathogenic virus (usually 100 $TCID_{50}/0.1$ ml) and prevents the production of a cytopathic effect, often manifested as a plaque (Figure 40.6).

Some viruses, such as members of the Orthomyxoviridae and Paramyxoviridae families cause hemag-glutination and/hemadsorption. The hemadsorption phenomenon can be used for virus detection by adding 0.15 ml of a 0.25 percent suspension of red blood cells directly to washed test tube cell cultures and incubating at 37°C for

Figure 40.3. Cytopathic effects caused by a bovine syncytium-forming virus. The characteristic syncytium formation with marked vacuolation and numerous cytoplasmic inclusion bodies is clearly demonstrated. Cover-slip preparation colored with May-Grünwald-Giemsa stain. × 1,250.

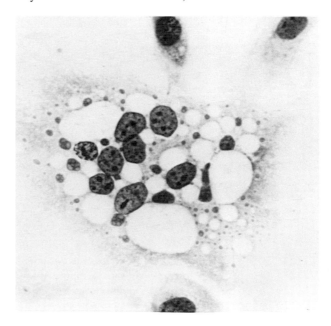

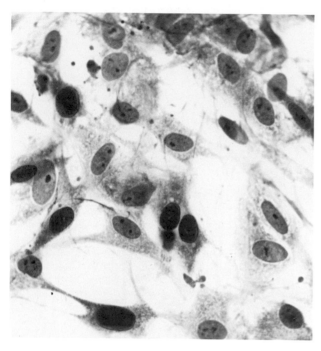

Figure 40.4. Cowdry type A intranuclear inclusion bodies produced by feline panleukopenia virus in tissue-cultured feline kidney cells. May-Grünwald stain. × 370. (Courtesy C. Geissinger and E. Tompkins.)

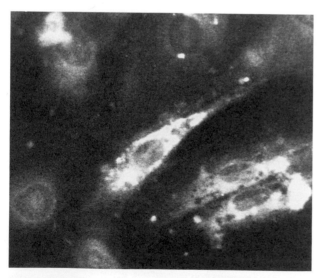

Figure 40.5. Immunofluorescence test. Specific cytoplasmic fluorescence (*white area*) in a cell culture infected with virus diarrhea–mucosal disease virus and stained with MD-VD antiglobulin conjugate. × 1,060. (Courtesy R. Schultz.)

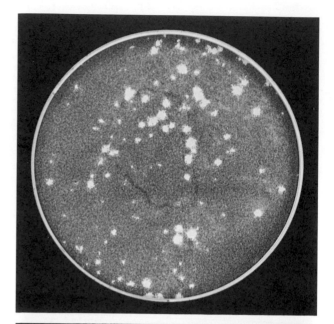

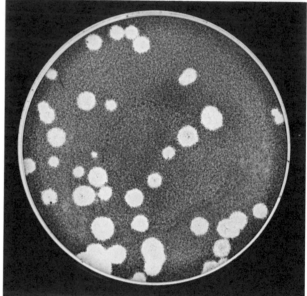

Figure 40.6. (*Top*) Plaques produced in NL-111 rabbit kidney cells by a field isolate of equine herpesvirus 1. (*Bottom*) Plaques produced in NL-111 rabbit kidney cells by a modified live-virus vaccine strain of equine herpesvirus 1. (Courtesy D. Holmes and M. Kemen.)

48 to 72 hours. In cultures containing virus the red blood cells are adsorbed to the infected cell sheets (Figure 40.7).

Virus can be produced in large quantities, as required for vaccines or complement-fixing antigens, by using sheets of cells grown in bottles. By using protein-free media (such as Parker-Morgan media 199), the operator can harvest virus in large quantities by withdrawing the fluid when the maximum yield is expected. Once the immunizing dose is established, the fluid can be harvested chemically to produce a vaccine or, if the agent has been adequately attenuated, diluted properly to contain sufficient virus to immunize.

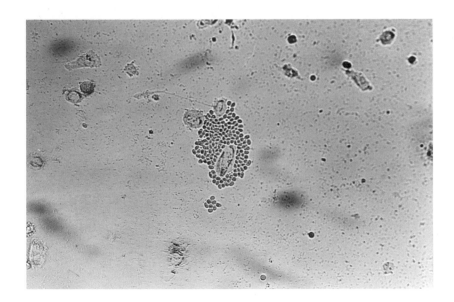

Figure 40.7. Hemadsorption (clumping) of chicken red blood cells in a culture of Vero cells inoculated with mumps virus. × 260. (Courtesy R. Schultz.)

Isolation of Viruses In Animals

Proper selection of a susceptible host for the isolation of a virus is essential to a diagnosis by this means. Sometimes age is important; suckling animals are more likely to develop recognizable infection than older animals. It is not a good idea to use an animal more than once for virus isolation, as subclinical infections could cause a false-negative result. The best chance for successful propagation of a new viral agent is in the natural host, something that can be readily done in veterinary medicine as opposed to human medicine.

Often, however, the natural host is a large animal, a fact that reduces its usefulness in achieving quick and easy solutions because of relatively high cost of such an animal, space limitations, and the problems of finding a source of the animal, obtaining it in sufficient numbers, and handling the animal. The researcher then studies the effects of the virus in many other hosts, particularly in caged laboratory animals such as mice, hamsters, guinea pigs, rats, cats, and rabbits. Sometimes adaptation to an unnatural host requires the use of a special virus strain; sometimes altering virus transfers between natural and unnatural hosts makes it possible to select viral particles that can be maintained in serial passage in the new host. The laboratory animal of choice, if one is available, for isolation of a virus is given under each viral infection discussed in this book. The inoculation route in a laboratory host is critical with certain viruses. If the virus is unknown, the most successful inoculaion route is one directly into the organ or tissue where the virus produces lesions in the natural host; for example, suspect brain material from encephalitic animals would be inoculated intracerebrally into suckling and older mice.

The source of animals is exceedingly important, as latent viruses occur in many animal colonies. To counteract this problem in part, researchers have established animal colonies by using cesarean-delivered animals as breeding stock. One can be reasonably certain that the cesarean-delivered animal is not harboring a viral agent that is transmitted horizontally; but this assumption cannot be made in the case of vertically transmitted viruses, such as the RNA (type C) endogenous viruses. Consequently, there is little chance of establishing a colony free of all viruses or their viral genomes. Of course the problem of latent viruses also applies to the chick embryo and tissue culture as well. Mycoplasmas and other microbes constitute a similar problem in all three virus isolation systems. At best, one can hope to establish a colony that is well defined and can be monitored for diseases that can be positively identified. Isolation procedures should be used to help maintain these colonies as pathogen-free stock.

With the introduction of the chick-embryo technique, and particularly tissue-culture techniques, animal inoculations are seldom used for diagnosis of viral infections. They are still essential for viral research studies, however, so the student should have some knowledge of their use and the associated problems.

Intracerebral Inoculation. The intracerebral route of inoculation in mice is used to isolate neurotropic viruses. Suckling or recently weaned mice (3 to 4 weeks old) or, occasionally, guinea pigs and rabbits are used for this purpose. The inoculum should be virtually free of bacteria because the brain has little resistance to such agents. Mice are lightly anesthetized with ether before injection of 0.03 ml of test inoculum, with a sharp 27-gauge, 0.25-inch needle, above the orbital ridge directly into the brain. Control mice are given a comparable amount of sterile buffered physiological salt solution to activate any latent brain virus such as lymphocytic choriomeningitis virus that might exist in the test mice.

After inoculation, all mice should be observed daily for signs of illness for approximately 30 days. Any mice that die during this period should be autopsied, with sterile techniques, to isolate microbes from the brain and heart blood. Negative cultures rule out contamination with bacteria, fungi, and mycoplasmas, assuming the proper media were used to isolate these agents. Brain tissue should also be retained for additional viral testing, if required, to establish the diagnosis. Careful observation is made for macroscopic lesions. In viral encephalitides, macroscopic brain lesions usually are lacking, but microscopic lesions are quite pronounced. If the control mice given sterile buffered physiological salt solution develop nervous mainfestations, the test is declared void and other test mice are sought if the infection is viral. If all the mice appear healthy at 30 days, they are sacrificed and examined carefully for lesions.

Intranasal Inoculation. As a rule the mouse is the animal of choice for the isolation of pneumotropic viruses. Occasionally ferrets are used but are generally avoided because they are difficult to handle. The mouse is anesthetized in a covered jar containing cotton soaked with ether, and 0.05 ml of test material is applied to the nares with a fine pipette. If properly anesthetized, the mouse will inhale the fluid preparation with no difficulty; otherwise it will discharge the fluid. Too much anesthestic or fluid inoculum causes death.

Most respiratory diseases have a short incubation, so a 14-day observation period for signs of illness is usually adequate. Mice that die are examined carefully at autopsy for lesions, especially of the respiratory tract. If the test mice show signs of respiratory illness, some are sacrificed. Some lungs are harvested for future virus studies; others are used for macroscopic and microscopic study of the lesions. Surviving mice are sacrificed and examined at autopsy at the end of the observation period. Although virus may have replicated in the mouse lung, no pneumonic lesions are produced in first passage. Depending on the virus, it may be possible to detect it by various means such as the hemagglutination phenomenon. Subsequent passages of infective mouse lungs in mice may select a viral population that does cause pneumonia. The number of mouse transfers required varies with the virus and also with the strain of virus.

Intraperitoneal Inoculation. This route is commonly used for isolation of agents in guinea pigs, particularly chlamydial and rickettsial organisms. Mice are also used but less frequently. The peritoneal cavity of the guinea pig is particularly effective at destroying most nonpathogenic bacterial organisms present in feces of various domestic animals; consequently, it is an effective filter to eliminate most bacteria from fecal specimens not treated with antibiotics.

The peritoneal cavity of each guinea pig is inoculated directly with a 0.5-inch, 24- to 25-gauge needle and a syringe with 0.5 ml of the lightly centrifuged test suspension. Daily temperatures and observations are recorded for all animals, which are maintained in a temperature-controlled environment. The guinea pig's thermal-regulating mechanism is sensitive to a marked rise in room temperature, and its normal temperature range is exceeded at 38° to 39.5°C. This becomes especially important when a rise in body temperature may be the only indication of infection. If the guinea pigs sicken, the appropriate tests on spleen, blood, and peritoneal cavity lining or fluid are made for possible bacterial contamination. Tissues, usually from the spleen, also are selected for further study of the pathogenic agent. Quite often guinea pigs recover from active infection, which is a distinct advantage for serologic studies.

Serologic Diagnosis of Viral Diseases

The immunological response of an animal to natural or planned viral infection can be detected and measured by many serologic procedures. There are two indispensable elements in any serologic test: the antigen and the antibody. The viral antigen(s) may be detected, identified, and quantified by testing against a number of specific antibody preparations. Conversely, the antibody in the serum of a recovered or vaccinated animal can be identified and quantitated by testing against a number of prepared viral antigens.

At present most diagnostic tests performed in a virological laboratory are serologic. The most widely used methods are serum neutralization, complement fixation, enzyme-linked immunosorbent assay (ELISA), and hemagglutination-inhibition. Others include hemadsorption, hemadsorption-inhibition, precipitation, agglutination, immunodiffusion, radioimmunoassay, indirect hemagglutination, and flocculation tests. The procedures with the greatest potential for quick and accurate diagnoses of viral diseases are the direct and indirect fluorescent antibody tests (FAT) involving immunofluorescence

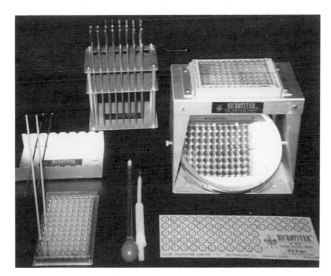

Figure 40.8. Most of the equipment (produced by Cooke Engineering Co., Alexandria, Va.) essential for performing virological and serologic microtiter plate tests. (Courtesy R. Schultz and D. Holmes.)

and the ELISA. A fluorescent virus precipitin test (FVPT) for the serologic identification of small particulate antigens such as virus is probably as sensitive as any serologic test (Foster et al. 1975). It is rapid and reliable, and only a single fluorescent conjugate is needed to detect many viruses. Cottral (1978) and Lennette and Schmidt (1979) have discussed most of these tests in detail.

Takatsy (1955) described the use of spiral loops in serologic and virological micromethods, and Sever (1960) utilized the microtechnique for virological and serologic investigations in the United States. With accurately calibrated equipment for measuring small volumes available commercially (Figure 40.8), microserologic techniques have been developed for the diagnosis of viral diseases in the United States and elsewhere. At present, microtests for the hemagglutination-inhibition, complement-fixation, gel-diffusion, and neutralization procedures (Figure 40.9) and, more recently, the ELISA are used in viral serologic diagnosis (Casey, 1970); they give results comparable to the macromethods. The microtests are preferred because they save time, space, and reagents.

The ELISA (Figure 40.10) is an exceedingly sensitive method for detecting antigen and antibody. Automation with appropriate equipment has minimized operator involvement, increased productivity, and furnished precise answers. The test's accuracy, simplicity, and low cost allow the diagnostician and epidemiologist to test large numbers of serum samples for antibody in a short time. Consequently, it is the test of choice for antigen-antibody systems that can be adapted to the automated procedure. In addition to the direct system, an indirect ELISA microplate test has been devised as a diagnostic and surveillance tool to aid in the control of animal disease (Saunders et al. 1977).

With most serologic methods, antibody titers are expressed as the reciprocal of the highest serum dilution causing a positive observable antigen-antibody reaction. In procedures such as the neutralization test, which is based on inhibition of viral replication by specific antibody, the level (titer) can be expressed as the neutralization index (alpha test procedure) or as the highest dilution that protects 50 percent of the test host against a precalculated virus dose (beta test procedure). The 50 percent end-

Figure 40.9. Results of a microtiter serum neutralization (SN) test with an accompanying virus titration using a feline herpesvirus antigen-antibody system. In the SN test 100 $TCID_{50}$ of virus was used against varying twofold dilutions of serum. After appropriate incubation at 37°C the nutrient fluid was discarded and cell layers in the plate were rinsed with saline, fixed with methanol, and stained with Giemsa. The stained wells (*dark*) indicate lack of viral cytopathic effect; the clear wells lack cells as a result of viral cytopathic activity. (Courtesy D. Holmes and R. Schultz.)

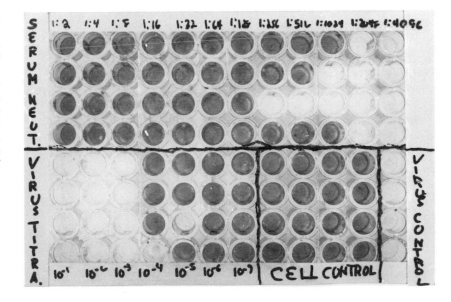

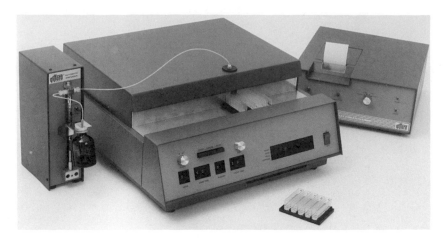

Figure 40.10. An automated system for performing the enzyme-linked immunosorbent assay procedure. (Courtesy Gilford Instrument Laboratories, Inc., Oberlin, Ohio.)

points for the beta test procedure can be calculated by the method of Karber (1931).

To perform satisfactory serologic tests, one should collect blood samples in sterile sealed units, preferably the B-D Vacutainer (without additive); available from Becton-Dickinson Company, Rutherford, N.J.). The specimens should be allowed to clot at room temperature for a few hours before overnight refrigeration. The following day the serum is decanted from the clot into a sterile centrifuge tube. The sample is centrifuged at 2,500 rpm for 20 to 30 minutes and the serum removed and placed in a sterile vial without disturbing the red cells. The non-hemolyzed serum sample can be frozen at $-10°$ to $-20°C$ and shipped immediately, under refrigeration, or sent later with a second sample drawn from the same animal. Under no circumstances should the blood sample be frozen before the serum is harvested from the collected specimen. Proper labeling of each sample, with its source and the date obtained, is essential for a correct diagnosis.

Diagnosis of Viral Diseases by Electron Microscopy

Improvements in the electron microscope and new techniques such as negative-staining with phosphotungstic acid in the preparation of specimens have enabled veterinarians to diagnose enteric viral diseases that were previously undetectable. Electron microscopy was used by Mebus (1969), who found virus particles about 65 nm in diameter in the feces of calves with acute diarrhea. About four years later medical virologists described similar particles in infants and young children with acute diarrhea. Now the examination of excretions, secretions, and solid tissues for virus particles has become routine in some diagnostic laboratories, especially in research facilities, where attempts are being made to establish virus particles as a possible cause of an epidemic.

The method of preparing specimens for electron microscopy causes some concentration of virus; a viral concentration of 10^5 particles per milliliter is just detectable, 10^6 particles provides a greater degree of detection, 10^8 particles permits a rapid diagnosis (Flewett, 1978). Diagnosis of the most important viruses causing acute diarrhea in any species is possible if the particles have a characteristic morphology (Figures 40.11, 40.12, and 40.13). The sensitivity and accuracy of the diagnosis can be enhanced by mixing known viral antiserums with the suspect viral specimen. This procedure is known as the immune electron microscopy technique. In a positive reaction virus particles are bound together by antibody, producing clumps (Figure 40.14). This technique provided the breakthrough in the identification of human hepatitis A virus, which defied the efforts of many talented and experienced investigators for years.

Preparing fecal specimens for examination is easy but time-consuming (Flewett 1978). An experienced worker can check, at most, 40 specimens in one day. Consequently, other diagnostic procedures such as tissue culture, ELISA, crossed electrophoresis, or complement fixation, in which 400 specimens can be processed at the same time, are superseding electron microscopy; yet it is still used to verify a diagnosis in doubtful cases, particularly when mixed viral infection may be responsible for enteric disease. Numerous viruses, such as rotaviruses, parvoviruses, coronaviruses, caliciviruses, adenoviruses, astroviruses, and enteroviruses (e.g., hepatitis A virus), have been demonstrated in stool specimens. Some—rotaviruses, parvoviruses, coronaviruses (Figures 40.11, 40.12, and 40.13), caliciviruses, and adenoviruses—are definitely responsible for disease in domestic animals.

The electron microscope definitely plays an important

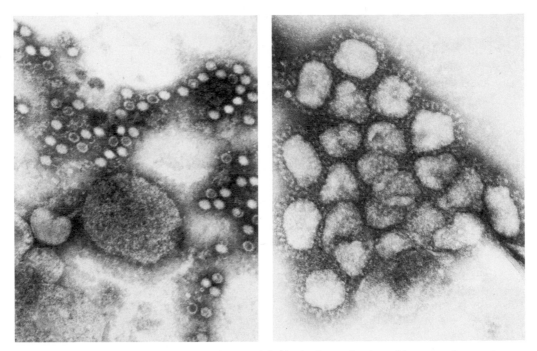

Figure 40.11 (*left*). Canine parvovirus. Virus particles in the feces of a dog with a natural case of acute diarrhea. × 127,000. (Courtesy Helen Greisen.)

Figure 40.12 (*right*). Canine coronavirus. Virus particles in the feces of a dog with a natural case of acute diarrhea. × 122,000. (Courtesy Helen Greisen.)

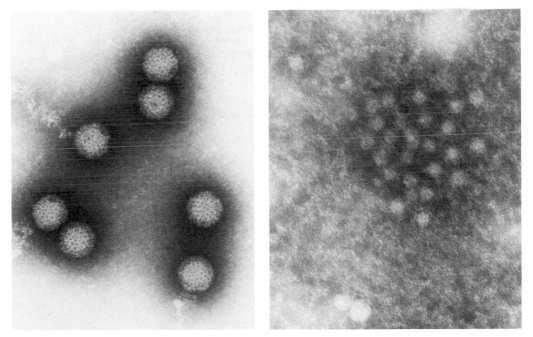

Figure 40.13 (*left*). Canine rotavirus. Virus particles isolated in Vero cells from a dog with acute diarrhea. × 127,000. (Courtesy Helen Greisen.)

Figure 40.14 (*right*). Human hepatitis A virus (enterovirus). Particles in infected spleen, demonstrated by immune electron microscopy. Note the fuzzy outline of the particles caused by the antigen-antibody interaction. × 154,000. (Courtesy M. Frey.)

Table 40.1. Characteristics of viral respiratory infections of cattle*

	Infectious bovine rhinotracheitis (IBR) (respiratory form only)†	Parainfluenza 3 (PI-3) infection†	Bovine rhinovirus (BRH) infection
Agent	Infectious bovine rhinotracheitis virus, a bovine herpesvirus	Bovine parainfluenza 3 virus	Bovine rhinovirus, 2 serotypes
Known geographic distribution	Worldwide	Worldwide	Germany, USA, England (probably worldwide)
Incubation, natural infection	4 to 5 days	5 to 10 days	2 to 4 days
Age	Any, usually in young stock	Any	Any
Signs	Respiratory form only—varies markedly in severity as a herd infection. Characterized by high fever, depression, inappetence, and copious mucopurulent exudate initially followed by nasal ulcers, necrosis of muzzle and nostril wings, dyspnea, mouth breathing, conjunctivitis, coughing, and sometimes bloody feces. WBC mostly normal	Seldom occurs in calves. In adult cattle respiratory signs encompass those associated with a fibrinous pneumonia such as coughing, difficult breathing, extended neck, foamy saliva	Serous nasal discharge, temperature, coughing, depression, dyspnea
Course of disease	Some of the cattle with the respiratory form show acute disease and then die, but most are sick for only a few days	4 to 7 days, occasionally longer	Approximately 1 week
Morbidity	In USA varies from 10 to 35 percent in cattle population	High in infected herds	Probably high
Mortality	Varies but in U.S. feedlots the average mortality is 10 percent	Varies markedly, but can be moderate in cattle shipped during cold weather	Little or none
Pathologic findings	Highly inflamed mucous membranes of upper respiratory tract with shallow erosions with a glary, fetid mucopurulent exudate. These lesions may be found in the pharynx, larynx, trachea, and larger bronchi. Sometimes patchy purulent pneumonia. Ulceration and inflammation of the abomasal mucosa is found, and catarrhal enteritis may occur	Lesions confined principally to respiratory tract. White fibrinous mass on lung surface. Lungs may be solid and heavy, filling the thoracic cavity. Cut sections show deep red and grayish lobules separated by interlobular tissue, greatly thickened by infiltration of coagulated exudate on serous surface	Principal lesions occur in nasal passages. A pneumonia in calves can occur after experimental intratracheal inoculation
Inclusions	Intranuclear inclusion bodies occur in epithelial cells of respiratory tract	Intracytoplasmic inclusion bodies in nasal and bronchial epithelial and alveolar macrophages that show marked fluorescence with specific antibody conjugate	None reported in cattle or in cell culture

Bovine adenovirus (BAV) infection	Bovine virus diarrhea (BVD)	Malignant catarrhal fever (MCF)	Bovine reovirus (BRE) infection	Bovine respiratory syncytial virus (BRSV) infection
Bovine adenovirus—9 serotypes	BVD virus, antigenic variants	A bovine herpesvirus	Bovine reovirus—3 serotypes	Bovine respiratory syncytial virus
USA, England, Hungary, Japan	Worldwide	Africa, most countries of south and central Africa, North America, Europe	Probably worldwide	Europe, Asia, and North America
Several days	6 to 9 days	Unknown. Experimental infection in cattle 10 to 44 days	Few days	3 to 4 days
Usually in calves	Any	Any	Any	Any
Signs associated with a pneumoenteritis	In clinical cases, diphasic temperature reaction, usually a dry, harsh, nonproductive cough and a watery conjunctivitis, no dyspnea, excessive salivation with erosions in oral cavity, mucoid and sometimes blood-tinged diarrhea, and bluish discoloration of muzzle. Abortions. Leukopenia often followed by leukocytosis	Initially, a fever lasting 1 to 2 days coinciding with inappetence and depression. Then inflammation of nasal passages, oral cavity, and eyes occurs. Difficult breathing follows and fibrinopurulent pneumonia may occur. Nervous signs develop early in most cases with either stupor or excitement	Usually inapparent infection. Presently recognized as a mild respiratory infection	Fever, nasal discharge, coughing, respiratory distress, and occasional lacrimation. Diarrhea, decreased milk production, and abortions may occur
Weeks in some instances	Usually subclinical, few days as a rule; occasionally chronic, persisting for months	Varies markedly. Sometimes death in 24 hours; usually 5 to 14 days	Unknown	Varies, usually 1 to 2 weeks
High in infected herds	Moderate to high	Low; usually only 1 to 2 cows in herd will show signs	Believed high	High
Low to moderate in infected herds	Low to high	Extremely high	Little or none	Low
Varying degrees of pneumonia with proliferative bronchiolitis with necrosis and bronchiolar occlusion causing alveolar collapse. Lesions may persist for weeks	The lesions are not confined to the respiratory tract; in fact the principal lesions are found in the oral cavity, digestive tract, and lymphatic system	Dark, swollen glassy membranes of turbinates and nasal sinuses covered with fibrin shreds and purulent excretion with shallow ulcers under this mass. Similar lesions seen in larynx, trachea, bronchi, and sometimes bronchopneumonia. Swollen head and lymph nodes. Inflammation and erosion of abomasum and small intestine sometimes occurs. Meninges congested and hemorrhagic. Nonpurulent encephalitis	Interstitial pneumonia and lymphadenitis of regional nodes	Bronchitis, bronchiolitis, interstitial pneumonia, multinucleation of alveolar and epithelial cells, and destruction of ciliated respiratory epithelium
Intranuclear inclusion bodies in bronchiolar epithelium, septal cells, bronchial lymph nodes, and endothelial cells	None	Inconclusive. Some investigators report nerve-cell intranuclear inclusion bodies; others, cytoplasmic inclusion bodies in epithelial cells	Unknown but should be present in bronchiolar epithelium	None

Table 40.1.—*continued*

	Infectious bovine rhinotracheitis (IBR) (respiratory form only)†	Parainfluenza 3 (PI-3) infection†	Bovine rhinovirus (BRH) infection
Other natural hosts	None known; goats can be experimentally infected	PI-3 virus has been isolated from humans, water buffalo, horses, and monkeys	None reported
Propagation	Cell culture; CPE in kidney cells from cattle, pigs, dogs, sheep, goats, and horses	Replicates in many types of cell cultures from many species, causing CPE and hemadsorption. Causes syncytia and cytoplasmic and intranuclear inclusion bodies	CPE produced in bovine kidney cell cultures at 33°C
Carrier state	Virus may persist for weeks; latency an important feature	Known to persist in lungs for at least 18 days	Unknown
Diagnosis	Sometimes possible on basis of history and character of the disease. Virus isolation from exudate of nasal passage in cell culture. SN, FA, CF, gel diffusion tests	Virus readily isolated from nasal exudate in cell culture. HI, HA-I, FA, and SN tests	Difficult clinically. Virus isolation in cell culture. SN test
Immunity	Long-term serviceable immunity	Maternal immunity apparently confers protection. The degree and duration of active immunity is yet to be determined with certainty	Status vague, immunity may be incomplete
Prophylaxis	Inactivated and attenuated virus vaccines	Inactivated vaccines, one incorporating PI-3 virus and *Pasteurella* sp., appear to be effective in controlling field disease	No vaccine available
Treatment	Antibiotic therapy and supportive measures	Antibiotic therapy is useful, as bacteria play an important role in the pathogenesis of the disease. Warm and dry quarters and supportive measures are important	Antibiotic therapy may be useful; supportive treatment

*See Table 40.6 for description of Rift Valley fever in sheep and cattle; the disease is less severe in cattle.
†In addition to virus, *Pasteurella* organisms are usually involved in this disease.
Abbreviations: CPE = cytopathic effect; SN = serum neutralization; FA = fluorescent antibody; CF = complement fixation; HI = hemagglutination inhibition; HA = hemadsorption; HA-I = hemadsorption inhibition.

Bovine adenovirus (BAV) infection	Bovine virus diarrhea (BVD)	Malignant catarrhal fever (MCF)	Bovine reovirus (BRE) infection	Bovine respiratory syncytial virus (BRSV) infection
Not determined	Sheep, goats, swine, and also white-tailed and mule deer	Sheep and African wildebeests	May infect humans and other animals; not known for certain	Antibodies have been found in cats, dogs, sheep, goats, and horses, denoting infection but unproved disease
Cell culture of calf kidney or testes	Cell cultures derived from bovine tissues. Some strains produce CPE; others do not	Cell culture of thyroid or adrenal glands	Cell culture—produces CPE in bovine kidney, pig kidney, and monkey kidney	Cell culture of several bovine tissues. CPE enhanced by addition of diethyl-aminoethyl-dextran, trypsin, thrombin, or plasmin
21 days known but probably longer	In animals with chronic cases, virus usually persists in the blood	Unknown	Up to 1 month	Unknown
Isolation in calf testes cell cultures from exudate of nasal passages or from feces; SN, HI, and agar-gel tests	Clinical signs, but more specifically upon lesions in severe cases; may be confused with rinderpest, malignant catarrhal fever, and certain respiratory diseases. Isolation of virus from blood or excretions and selected tissues in cell culture. Noncytopathogenic strains are identified in culture by exaltation, interference, or FA tests. SN and agar-gel tests	Clinical diagnosis is possible when sporadic cases with nervous and eye manifestations occur in a herd	Virus is isolated from nasal passages and conjunctiva in cell culture. SN, HI tests	Positive diagnosis depends on virus isolation, immunofluorescence, seroconversion in paired serum samples, or demonstration of typical lung lesions at necropsy
Duration of immunity presently unknown	Complete and long-lasting immunity in most cattle to a given variant. Complicated situation at present	Uncertain	No evidence of maternal immunity. Degree and duration of active immunity unknown	Recovery from BRSV infection confers partial immunity. Subsequent exposures to BRSV cause mild or inapparent disease
None	Attenuated virus vaccine available; do not use in pregnant cows	None. Keep sheep and wildebeests away from cattle if possible	None at present	Inactivated and modified live-virus vaccines confer partial or complete protection
Antibiotics to assist in control of bacterial invaders; supportive measures	Supportive measures	None	Antibiotics may be useful in controlling secondary bacterial infections such as *Pasteurella* organisms	Antibiotic therapy to control secondary bacterial disease; supportive measures

Table 40.2. Characteristics of viral respiratory infections of cats

	Rhinotracheitis (FVR)	Calicivirus infection (FPI)	Reovirus infection (FRI)
Agent	Feline herpesvirus 1	Calicivirus; 1 serotype and 1 serologic variant known	Reovirus serotypes 1 and 3
Known geographic distribution	USA, Canada, Europe, New Zealand	USA, Europe, Australia, New Zealand, Japan	USA
Incubation, natural infection	Several days	Usually 1 to 3 days shorter than for FVR	4 to 19 days
Age	Any	Any	Any
Signs	Sneezing and coughing, sometimes paroxysmal; salivation, ocular and nasal exudation, oral breathing, fever, inappetence, weight loss; pregnant females occasionally abort; fatal generalized infection in some newborn kittens; sinusitis, ulcerative keratitis, panophthalmitis in chronic infections. Leukocytosis when accompanied by bacterial infection	Asymptomatic to severe, depending on virus strain. Conjunctivitis, ocular discharge often unilateral, rhinitis, sneezing, depression, inappetence, dyspnea, rales, other abnormal lung sounds, and pneumonia; fever, often diphasic; ulcers on tongue and hard palate, preceded by salivation; mortality in newborn cats. Early transient lymphopenia in some cases.	Generally mild, with lacrimation, photophobia, serous conjunctivitis, gingivitis, and depression; nasal discharge and fever rarely. WBC mostly normal; no leukopenia
Course of disease	Usually 2 to 4 weeks	Average of 7 to 10 days	1 to 29 days
Morbidity	High	High	About 50 percent among contact controls
Mortality	Low in adults	Variable; up to 30 percent in experimental infections	Low

	Rhinotracheitis (FVR)	Calicivirus infection (FPI)	Reovirus infection (FRI)
Pathological findings	Necrotizing conjunctivitis, rhinitis, and tracheitis associated with intranuclear inclusions; sinusitis, resorption of turbinates in chronic infections; in some cases, patchy or general consolidation in anterior lung lobes characterized by necrotizing bronchiolitis and proliferation of alveolar septal cells; secondary bacterial or mycotic infections may occur*	Conjunctivitis, rhinitis, ulcers of the tongue and palate, patchy bronchopneumonia. Alternately dark and pale red banding of spleen associated with calicivirus infection in some cats	Conjunctivitis
Inclusions	Intranuclear inclusions in respiratory epithelial cells, nictitating membrane, tongue, and tonsils	None	Paranuclear cytoplasmic inclusions
Other natural hosts	None known	None known	Reovirus 1 and 3 isolated from many mammals
Propagation	Culture of cells of feline origin	Culture of cells of feline origin	Culture of feline and bovine kidney cells
Carrier state	Yes	Yes	Not determined
Diagnosis	Demonstration of intranuclear inclusions early in course of infection, cell-culture isolation, SN, HA, HI, FA tests	Cell-culture isolation, SN, FA tests	Cell-culture isolation, SN, HI tests
Immunity	Weak, transient	Many serotypes; heterologous protection likely	Not determined, but likely
Prophylaxis	Attenuated virus vaccine	Attenuated virus vaccine (1 serotype)	None
Treatment	Antibiotics indicated for secondary invaders, supportive measures	Antibiotics indicated for secondary invaders, supportive measures	Symptomatic

*Experimental intravenous inoculation results in necrosis in growth regions of all bones, focal necrosis in adrenal glands and liver, and, in pregnant females, placental necrosis, fetal death, and abortion.
See Table 40.1 for key to abbreviations.

Table 40.3. Characteristics of viral respiratory infections of horses

	Equine herpesvirus (EHV) infections (equine rhinopneumonitis)	Equine influenza (EI)
Agent	Equine herpesvirus 1, 2, and 3. EHV-1 has two subtypes. Subtype 1 (also known as EHV-4) causes abortions and nervous manifestations. Subtype 2 produces respiratory disease in weanlings. EHV-2 causes no known disease. EHV-3 produces lesions typical of coital exanthema.	Equine influenza virus. Two types designated A/Equi-1/Praha/56 and A/Equi-2/Miami/63
Known geographic distribution	USA, Europe, Australia (probably worldwide)	Worldwide
Incubation, natural infection	*Weanling disease*—a few days *Abortion disease*—3 to 4 weeks	1 to 3 days
Age	Any	Any
Signs	*Weanling disease*—mild febrile reaction accompanied by rhinitis or nasal catarrh; usually in fall of year. Sometimes a leukopenia in weanlings *Abortion disease*—infection in mares causes abortion (usually between 6 and 10 months of pregnancy) with no other signs, but cases of nervous disease may occur	Coughing is most common sign of illness. High temperature, inappetence, mental depression, photophobia, lacrimation, cloudy cornea, nasal catarrh, swollen lymph nodes of head. If pneumonia develops, horse usually dies from bacterial infection
Course of disease	Foals usually recover in 8 to 10 days	1 to 3 weeks, sometimes longer
Morbidity	Very high in foals in infected herds; varies from 10 to 90 percent on stud farms	Highly contagious with high morbidity
Mortality	No mortality in weanlings. Occasionally in mares with nervous manifestations, but loss of foals through abortions may be high	Usually does not exceed 5 percent
Pathologic findings	*Weanlings*—Reddening of mucous membranes of upper air passages with a collective mucopurulent exudate *Aborting mares*—CNS lesions in mares showing nervous disease *Aborted fetuses*—Multiple focal liver necrosis, petechial hemorrhages in heart muscle and in capsules of spleen and liver; lung edema	Principal lesions in fatal cases are extensive edema of lungs or a bronchopneumonia with pleurisy; hydrothorax; gelatinous infiltrations around larynx and in the legs; swollen lymph nodes
Inclusions	Intranuclear inclusion bodies are found in hepatic cells, and also in epithelial cells and endothelial cells of various organs of aborted fetuses	None
Other natural hosts	None known	Only members of equine family

Equine rhinovirus infection (ERI)	Equine parainfluenza infection (EPI)	African horsesickness (AHS)
2 equine rhinovirus serotypes; possibly a third serotype	Parainfluenza virus. Limited information about virus and the disease	Equine orbivirus (Reoviridae). Nine distinct immunological types
North America, South America, Africa	USA and Canada	Africa, Middle East, parts of Asia
3 to 7 days	Few days	Probably 7 to 9 days
Any, mostly young, animals	Any. Usually occurs in young horses	Any
Fever, anorexia, serous, followed by mucopurulent nasal discharge, cough	Mucopurulent discharge and other signs referable to respiratory tract, fever	Acute form characterized by respiratory signs with death resulting from severe edema in the lungs. There is fever, labored breathing, coughing, severe dyspnea, and copious foamy nasal discharge. Chronic cases also include heart distress coupled with edema of head and neck tissues
About 1 week	4 to 7 days, sometimes longer	3 to 5 days average, may be longer
Infected stables— high morbidity	Moderate to high in limited surveys	Usually high; spreads very rapidly
Low	Low	25 to 95 percent
Marked pharyngitis, lymphadenitis, abscesses in submaxillary lymph nodes	Insufficient information	Depends upon severity of case. *In acute type* thoracic cavity contains liters of fluid and lungs are distended. A yellowish fluid separates interlobular tissue from alveolar portions. The lung surfaces are wet and fluid runs from cut surface. Pericardial sac may have excess fluid and subendocardial hemorrhages usually are present. Some fluid is present in abdominal cavity, the liver is swollen, and intestines reddened. *In chronic form* edema of head and neck; hydropericardium and hydropic degeneration of myocardium. Lungs and thoracic cavity have moderate edema
None	Unknown	Unknown—should be present in bronchiolar epithelium
None known	Unknown	Zebras, dogs, angora goats, mules, donkeys

Table 40.3.—*continued*

	Equine herpesvirus (EHV) infections (equine rhinopneumonitis)	Equine influenza (EI)
Propagation	EHV-1 has been adapted to hens' eggs. Replicates and produces CPE in cell cultures of fetal horse kidney, lamb kidney, and rabbit kidney	Embryonated hen's egg is best. Cell cultures of monkey kidney more susceptible than bovine, equine, or human kidney cells. Madin-Darby dog kidney cell line often used
Carrier state	Latency has been demonstrated	Suggested that some horses remain carriers for months
Diagnosis	Clinical diagnosis of respiratory disease is difficult; aborting disease less complicated. Intranuclear inclusion bodies help establish diagnosis. Virus can be isolated from affected tissues in cell culture. SN, CF, precipitation tests	Usually can be diagnosed in an outbreak on basis of history, clinical signs, and lesions. Virus isolated from nasal exudate in hens' eggs or cell culture. SN and HI tests
Immunity	Probably transitory immunity, lasting few years. EHV-1, subtypes 1 and 2 cross-protect to some degree. EHV-1 and EHV-3 exhibit very little homology or cross-protection	Solid immunity to natural disease for 1 year
Prophylaxis	Attenuated virus vaccines or inactivated virus vaccines are recommended. None apparently provide complete protection. A vaccine with both EHV-1 subtypes provides greater protection	Two types of inactivated vaccine available. Yearly vaccination required
Treatment	None	Antibiotic therapy indicated to control bacterial infection. Supportive measures

See Table 40.1 for key to abbreviations.

Equine rhinovirus infection (ERI)	Equine parainfluenza infection (EPI)	African horsesickness (AHS)
Rabbits, guinea pigs, monkeys, and humans susceptible to intranasal instillation. Culture of cells of many animal species	Cell culture	Cell culture of baby hamster, bovine kidney, and others with production of CPE and cytoplasmic inclusion bodies; suckling mice
At least 1 month	Unknown	*Culicoides* (midges) are probable vectors. Direct transmission does not occur
Isolation of virus in cell culture from nasal excretions. SN test	Isolation of virus in cell culture. SN, HA-I, HA, HI, CF tests	May be confused with other diseases, especially when first occurring in virgin territory. Laboratory diagnosis required by virus isolation from infective blood or tissues inoculated intracerebrally into suckling mice. SN, CF, agar-gel, FA, HI tests; HI and SN used for virus serotyping
Limited knowledge. Evidence of maternal immunity and active immunity protection	Unknown	Apparent excellent immunity to homotypic serotype
No vaccine available, although one is needed	No vaccine available	Multiple mouse-brain virus vaccine available. Given annually. Stable nonvaccinated horses at night
Antibiotic therapy to help control bacterial invaders	Antibiotic therapy may be useful. Supportive measures and good nursing in warm, dry quarters	No treatment is effective

Table 40.4. Characteristics of viral respiratory infections of dogs

	Canine distemper (CD)	Infectious canine hepatitis (ICH)
Agent	Canine distemper virus	Canine adenoviruses 1 and 2; canine 2 causes its major effects in the respiratory tract
Known geographic distribution	Worldwide	Worldwide
Incubation, natural infections	4 to 6 days	5 to 9 days
Age	Any	Any
Signs	Some infections are inapparent; principal signs in others may be respiratory, enteric, or nervous or a combination of them. Respiratory signs include watery discharge from eyes and nose, which may become mucoid in 24 hours; diphasic temperature; and pneumonia may develop as a result of bacterial infection. Leukopenia followed sometimes by leukocytosis	*Classic hepatic form* (type 1) characterized by fever, intense thirst, sometimes edema of extremities, diarrhea, vomiting, intense pain, serous nasal discharge. *Respiratory form* (type 2) characterized by 1- to 3-day fever, harsh and dry hacking cough, serous nasal discharge sometimes becoming purulent, muscular trembling, depression, dyspnea. In hepatic form there is a leukopenia, but in respiratory form total WBC are variable
Course of disease	Usually 2 to 3 weeks; may last longer in few cases	*Hepatic form*—2 weeks. *Respiratory form*—5 to 28 days
Morbidity	High	High
Mortality	Varies markedly in outbreaks, usually related to brain involvement. Probably averages 20 percent in clinical cases	10 to 25 percent overall; especially high in puppies
Pathological findings	Viremic disease with affinity for epithelial cells thus capable of producing a wide variety of lesions. There is a virus-induced giant cell pneumonia which may be complicated by bacterial infection causing a purulent bronchopneumonia. There may be enteritis, encephalitis, vesicular and pustular skin lesions, atrophied and gelatinous thymus gland, eye lesions, urinary and reproductive system lesions	*Hepatic form*—characterized by edema and hemorrhage. Fibrinous peritonitis with blood-tinged fluid in cavity, hydrothorax, marked thickening of gall bladder, swollen liver, lung edema, uveitis. *Respiratory form*—moderate to severe pneumonic changes. Proliferative, adenomatous changes are seen in lungs of dogs with infection for 10 days
Inclusions	Cytoplasmic and/or intranuclear inclusion bodies in many epithelial cells; particularly seen in bronchi, bladder, renal pelvis, and glial cells	*Hepatic form*—intranuclear inclusion bodies in hepatic and endothelial cells. *Respiratory form*—intranuclear inclusion bodies in bronchial epithelium, alveolar septal cells, and turbinate epithelium
Other natural hosts	Principally members of canine family	Foxes (often show nervous disease), wolves, coyotes, bears; raccoons?

Canine parainfluenza (SV-5)	Canine reovirus infection (CRI)	Canine herpesvirus (CHV) infection
Parainfluenza 2 virus (SV-5)	Canine reovirus 1 and 2	Canine herpesvirus
USA	USA, Japan	USA, Canada, Great Britain, continental Europe
2 to 3 days	Uncertain	3 to 8 days in puppies
Any	Any	Any
Sudden onset, copious nasal discharge, fever, and coughing. If *Bordetella bronchiseptica* and *Mycoplasma* sp. are involved, a dry cough persists for weeks	Experimental dogs from conventional sources showed elevated temperature and respiratory signs and pneumonia. Sometimes causes enteritis. Germ-free dogs became infected without signs of illness	*Puppies*—labored breathing, abdominal pain, yellowish green stool, anorexia, and possible death following acute disease *Older dogs*—vaginitis and mild rhinitis
1 to 7 days; weeks in cases with complications	Not well studied	In 1- to 2-week-old puppies 1 to 2 days; older dogs—unknown
Low to moderate	Low to moderate	Low to moderate
Low	Low	High in 1- to 2-week-old puppies; negligible in older dogs
Usually no gross lesions except petechial hemorrhages in respiratory tract. Microscopic catarrhal changes are present in lower and upper respiratory tract and also in regional lymph nodes	Pneumonia and enteritis	*Puppies*—disseminated focal necrosis and hemorrhages found in virtually all internal organs, especially kidney. Lungs are diffusely pneumonic. Meningoencephalitic lesions frequently seen but without nervous signs
Unknown	Unknown	Intranuclear inclusion bodies in cells in areas of necrosis are found
Monkeys, humans, dogs, perhaps others	Unknown, may infect humans and other animals	Not known

Table 40.4.—*continued*

	Canine distemper (CD)	Infectious canine hepatitis (ICH)
Propagation	Cell culture-primary and cell lines from various dog tissues support the replication and show CPE. Embryonated hens' eggs with adapted strains. Suckling mice, suckling hamsters, ferrets, and many other species are susceptible	Canine, ferret, and swine kidney monolayer cell cultures
Carrier state	Footpads—4 to 6 weeks Brain—at least 49 days in some nervous cases of dogs	Urine—39 weeks Kidney—unknown Tonsils—unknown
Diagnosis	Demonstration of inclusion bodies constitutes a presumptive diagnosis. Isolation of virus constitutes a positive diagnosis—this can be done in dog macrophage cultures. FA and SN tests are excellent methods	Demonstration of intranuclear inclusion bodies. Isolation of virus from pathological lesions in cell culture; SN, FA, and CF tests
Immunity	Long-term durable immunity to natural disease. Maternal protection may persist for 15 weeks	Solid and long lasting, perhaps life. Cross-protection between types 1 and 2 virus
Prophylaxis	Excellent vaccines are available; for maximum protection yearly vaccination is advised	Inactivated and attenuated virus vaccines
Treatment	Antibiotic therapy recommended for control of bacterial disease; supportive measures	Antibiotics indicated for bacterial invaders, especially respiratory form; supportive measures

See Table 40.1 for key to abbreviations.

Canine parainfluenza (SV-5)	Canine reovirus infection (CRI)	Canine herpesvirus (CHV) infection
Replicates with CPE and cytoplasmic inclusion bodies in kidney cultures of dog, rhesus monkey, and human embryos. Replicates in amniotic cavity of hens' eggs without death	Produces CPE in dog kidney cell culture	Dog kidney cell culture
Unknown	Spleen—3.5 weeks	Turbinates—3 weeks Kidney—unknown Nasal—3 weeks
Clinically difficult. Virus isolation with respiratory exudates in cell cultures; HA, HA-I, HI, SN, FA tests	Isolation of virus from nasal exudate or feces in cell culture	Focal renal hemorrhages not seen in CD and ICH. Intranuclear bodies must be differentiated from ICH intranuclear inclusions. Virus can be isolated from many tissues of dead puppies in dog kidney cell cultures. SN, CF tests
Dogs infected naturally or by intranasal route are completely protected. Duration of immunity is low so it has little significance in natural protection	Unknown	Duration of immunity unknown, but puppies from immune mothers are temporarily resistant
Various vaccines that combine SV-5 with a virulent B. bronchiseptica are available. Another vaccine also includes canine adenovirus type 2. All administered intranasally	None	No vaccine available
Antibiotic therapy is indicated to control secondary invaders; supportive measures and good nursing	Antibiotics may be indicated; supportive measures	Supportive measures and especially warm environment for puppies

Table 40.5. Characteristics of viral respiratory infections of swine

	Swine influenza (SI)	Pseudorabies (PR)
Agent	Swine influenza A virus	Pseudorabies virus, a herpesvirus
Known geographic distribution	Worldwide	Worldwide
Incubation, natural infection	A few hours to several days	4 to 7 days, occasionally longer
Age	Any	Any
Signs	Whole herds seem ill at once. Disease begins with fever, extreme weakness, prostration, anorexia. Swine exhibit muscular stiffness and pain. Some show lung edema and bronchopneumonia and usually die. Coughing also is observed	Pruritis does not occur. Signs in sows usually are mild. Characterized by fever, depression, vomition, respiratory signs, and abortions. In suckling and recently weaned pigs the above signs are more severe
Course of disease	2 to 6 days	4 to 8 days
Morbidity	High	May be high
Mortality	Usually less than 4 percent, but may go to 10 percent	Young pigs—high Older pigs—very low
Pathological findings	Principal lesions are in the lungs. Thick, mucilaginous exudate in the bronchioles and bronchi cause atelectasis while remainder is usually pale because of interstitial emphysema. In some cases pneumonia develops and involves the areas in which atelectasis	The gross lesions are not extensive; in fatal cases cellular infiltrations and necrosis occur in various parts of nervous system as seen in microscopic sections. Animals may die before virus reaches and causes lesions in anterior part of cord and brain

first occurred. Regional nodes are swollen and wet. Spleen is enlarged, and there is hyperemia of stomach mucosa

Inclusions	None	Intranuclear inclusion bodies are not found in swine
Other natural hosts	Humans	Cattle, cats, dogs, sheep, rats; horses?
Propagation	Intra-amniotic and intra-allantoic inoculation of 10- to 12-day-old embryonated hens' eggs Various cell cultures useful for cultivation and assay	Chick embryos. Cell culture of chick, rabbit, guinea pig, dog, and monkey tissues
Carrier state	Infected pigs can transmit virus to contact pigs. Domestic fowl may disseminate the virus	Animals that exhibit no visible signs can transmit the virus
Diagnosis	Embryonated hens' eggs with respiratory exudates. SN, FA, HI, CF, HA-I tests	More difficult in swine than other animals unless nervous signs occur. Virus can be isolated from lesions by inoculating into brain of rabbits; SN test
Immunity	Believed to be immune after disease but not all investigators agree. Maternal immunity lasts for as long as 13 to 18 weeks	Long lasting, perhaps life
Prophylaxis	No vaccine available now; previous one not effective	Inactivated and attenuated virus vaccines available. Keep swine separated from cattle. Rat control
Treatment	Antibiotic therapy. Dry, warm quarters beneficial	None

See Table 40.1 for key to abbreviations.

Table 40.6. Characteristics of viral respiratory infections of sheep and goats

	Adenomatosis (sheep)	Parainfluenza virus (PIV) infection (sheep)	Rift Valley fever (RVF) (sheep)
Agent	Retrovirus	Parainfluenza 3 virus. Closely related to bovine and human PI-3 viruses, but not identical	Rift Valley fever virus, arbovirus (Bunyaviridae)
Known geographic distribution	Europe, Peru, Iceland, South Africa, India, Israel, USA	USA, Australia	Africa, Middle East
Incubation, natural infection	Very long	Unknown	1 to 3 days
Age	Any	Any	Any
Signs	Signs are seen only in sheep over 6 months of age. As air spaces in lungs become obliterated the animals become dyspneic and emaciated	Signs referrable to respiratory tract with production of pneumonia	Fever, prostration, rapid course, some vomiting, also show purulent nasal discharge and bloody stools. Ewes abort sometimes without other signs. Severe leukopenia
Course of disease	When sheep become dyspneic, they die in a few days to several months from anoxia	Usually 1 week; longer in some cases	2 weeks
Morbidity	Low	Common and widespread in USA	High
Mortality	High	Low	*Lambs*—high, often 95 to 100 percent *Ewes*—probably less than 20 percent *Cattle*—less than 10 percent
Pathological findings	Proliferation of cells in lung-supporting tissues with gradual filling of alveoli causing lung consolidation. Recognized as primary lung carcinoma that may metastasize	A fibrinous type of pneumonia	Most characteristic lesion is focal necrosis of the liver. Other lesions are principally hemorrhages in lymph nodes, gastric and intestinal mucosa, endocardium, and epicardium

	Adenomatosis (sheep)	Parainfluenza virus (PIV) infection (sheep)	Rift Valley fever (RVF) (sheep)
Inclusions	Unknown	Unknown	Intranuclear inclusion bodies in liver
Other natural hosts	None known	Unknown	Cattle and humans
Propagation	Unknown except in sheep	Sheep kidney cell cultures	Cell cultures of chick, rat, mouse, human, lamb, and hamster. Replicates in embryonated hens' eggs. In white mice
Carrier state	Carriers do exist	Unknown	Unknown
Diagnosis	Typical lesions at necropsy	Isolation of virus from respiratory exudates in cell culture. SN, HA, HA-I, HI tests	Clinical signs and history highly suggestive. Massive liver focal necrosis characteristic. Inoculation of white mice with liver and other infected tissues causes prompt fatal infection. CF, agar-gel, HI tests
Immunity	Animals with signs of illness do not recover	Maternal immune protection exists. Little known about active immunity	Long-term, durable immunity in animals and humans that recover
Prophylaxis	Remove affected sheep from flock	Inactivated, attenuated, and subunit vaccines have been developed	Live-virus vaccines are available but not safe in young lambs or pregnant cattle and ewes. Inactivated vaccines also avaliable. Move animals into mountains away from mosquito vectors if possible
Treatment	None	Antibiotic therapy, but it may not be feasible or practical	No effective treatment

See Table 40.1 for key to abbreviations.

Table 40.7. Characteristics of viral respiratory infections of chickens

	Newcastle disease (ND)	Avian infectious bronchitis (avian IB
Agent	Paramyxovirus	Coronavirus
Known geographic distribution	Worldwide	Worldwide
Incubation, natural infection	4 to 14 days	2 to 4 days
Age	Any	Any
Signs	Outbreaks vary in intensity—older birds may have inapparent infection, but chicks usually show marked respiratory distress and nervous manifestations appear in a varying percentage a few days later. When nervous signs occur, the death rate is high. In laying birds respiratory signs occur accompanied by a marked reduction to complete cessation in egg production	Severity of respiratory signs is age-dependent, with chicks showing greatest effects, including listlessness, depression, rales, gasping. In laying flocks egg production drops dramatically, and full production is not usually achieved until next laying period or later
Course of disease	6 to 8 days with respiratory disease; with CNS involvement usually longer	6 to 18 days
Morbidity	High	High
Mortality	Low to high depending on incidence of birds with nervous manifestations	Chicks—25 percent Older birds—none to low
Pathological findings	Gross lesions not particularly striking. Fluid or mucous in the trachea, cloudy air sac membranes. Spleen may be enlarged. Typical viral encephalitic lesions in birds with nervous signs	Mucoid or caseous plugs overlying highly inflamed bronchi and sometimes in nasal passages. Chicks that die usually have fibrinopurulent exudate in lower trachea and larger bronchi
Inclusions	None seen	None

Laryngotracheitis (LT)	Fowlpox	Avian influenza (AI)
Laryngotracheitis virus, an avian herpesvirus	Fowlpox virus	Avian influenza A virus
Worldwide	Worldwide	USA, Canada, Europe, South America, Asia
2 days	Several days	3 to 5 days
Any	Any	Any
Highly contagious. Respiratory signs include mouth breathing, gurgling and rattling sounds, nasal exudate in some birds	As a rule, the pox lesions are confined to head; occasionally they are limited to oral cavity and trachea causing a respiratorylike disease	Mucoid nasal discharge, fever, edema of head and neck, lethargy, bluish black discoloration of combs and wattles; rapid deaths
5 to 6 days in individual 3 to 4 weeks as a flock	Most birds recover in 3 to 4 weeks	A few hours to 3 days
Approaches 100 percent in susceptible flocks	High in affected flocks	High
Depends on time of year and stage of production. Young birds in warm weather have low mortality. In heavy layers during winter months may be high	Low to moderate	As a rule, high in chickens
Lesions confined to larynx, trachea, and bronchi and characterized by a reddened petechiated, slimy exudate containing blood. Sometimes exudate is caseous forming a plug that occludes trachea causing suffocation and death	In respiratory form, the infraorbital sinus is involved and greatly distended as a result of a yellowish or brownish caseous exudate. In mouth and trachea there are whitish cankerlike lesions that tend to ulcerate	Usually not numerous. Petechial hemorrhages in heart, gizzard, proventriculus, and body cavity serosa. Principal organs may show cloudy swelling and petechial hemorrhages. By microscopic examination, there is a diffuse encephalitis
Intranuclear inclusion bodies in epithelial cells of tracheal lesions	Cytoplasmic inclusions in swollen epithelial cells are termed Bollinger bodies	None

Table 40.7.—*continued*

	Newcastle disease (ND)	Avian infectious bronchitis (avian IB)
Other natural hosts	Turkeys, pheasants, ducks, geese, and many other species are naturally infected	None
Propagation	Readily propagated in embryonated hens' eggs and produces a CPE and also replicates in cell cultures of chick origin. Cytoplasmic and intranuclear inclusions occur in cell cultures	Causes dwarfing and curling of chick embryos. CPE in chicken embryo kidney cultures
Carrier state	Perhaps as long as 1 month	At least 7 weeks
Diagnosis	Chicks with respiratory and nervous signs suggest the disease is Newcastle disease; in this instance it must be distinguished from avian influenza. Virus isolation from nasal exudate or with lesions. Can be isolated in hens' eggs. SN, HI tests useful in diagnosis	Difficult to distinguish from Newcastle unless nervous signs are observed, then it can be diagnosed as Newcastle. In older birds must be distinguished from other respiratory infections requiring cultural tests for virus and bacteria. SN, FA, ELISA, agar-gel tests
Immunity	Immunity persists for years	Immune for at least 6 to 8 months after infection
Prophylaxis	Vaccines are available. Caution should be exercised in their use in laying flocks	Complicated by multiple serotypes, although attenuated virus vaccines are available and apparently useful
Treatment	Replacement of laying flock at appropriate time may be required to prevent infection of susceptible young stock	Often flocks are disposed of after disease if vaccination is not feasible or desirable

See Table 40.1 for key to abbreviations.

Laryngotracheitis (LT)	Fowlpox	Avian influenza (AI)
Occasionally pheasants	Turkeys, pheasants, canaries, and some wild birds	Turkeys (main host in USA and Canada), pheasants, and certain wild birds
Chicken embryos	Chorioallantoic membrane of hens' embroynated eggs. Cell cultures derived from chick embryo tissues	Embryonated hens' eggs and in certain cell cultures
Yes, for months after infection and serve as source for future infections	Some recovered birds are carriers	Unknown
As flock becomes diseased, diagnosis can be made by signs and lesions. Inoculation of two susceptible and two resistant birds with trachea exudate provides positive diagnosis	Typical skin pox lesions—or by demonstration of Bollinger bodies in wet preparations. Virus isolation in hens' eggs or cell culture. SN, HI, CF, agar-gel tests	Exceedingly high mortality accompanied by peracute deaths highly suggestive. Confirmation by virus isolation and serology. HI test best
Long-term and complete	Long-term and complete	Solidly immune for several months at least
Conjunctivally administered vaccine strain 146 provides durable immunity after production of conjunctivitis without permanent damage, but carriers may exist	Attenuated fowlpox vaccines available	No vaccine available in USA
Flock disposal may be indicated	In some instances flock disposal may be desirable	Flock disposal may be indicated

role in the modern well-equipped diagnostic laboratory. However, electron microscopy clearly has its limitations: it is not a sensitive method for detecting small concentrations of virus and obviously can never supplant virus isolation in cell culture or in animals.

Differential Diagnosis of Viral Respiratory Diseases

The differential diagnosis of infectious diseases of domestic animals offers the student and veterinary practitioner one of their greatest challenges, yet also contributes to their frustrations. This is especially true of the respiratory diseases, principally those of viral origin. Their manifestations are so similar that differential diagnosis is possible only through laboratory procedures ranging from simple cytologic examination to the isolation of the agent(s). Some viral respiratory diseases are further complicated by secondary infections with opportunist bacterial pathogens or even another virus. A clinical diagnosis can be no more than a calculated guess, as the problem in domestic animals is similar in complexity to the common cold in humans.

As an aid to the practitioner in the proper selection of biological materials for diagnosis of respiratory infections, major characteristics of the principal respiratory viral infections of domestic animals are listed in Tables 40.1 to 40.7. Some of the data in Table 40.1 (American Veterinary Medical Association 1968) and Table 40.2 (American Veterinary Medical Association 1971) were extracted from information developed by the respective panels of the American Veterinary Medical Association Symposia. The practitioners on these panels believed that this type of table would be useful to the student and the veterinarian as a summary of respiratory complexes and as an aid in differential diagnosis.

REFERENCES

American Veterinary Medical Association. 1968. Panel, Bovine Respiratory Disease Supplement. J. Am. Vet. Med. Assoc. 152:713.

American Veterinary Medical Association. 1971. Panel, Feline Infectious Diseases Report. J. Am. Vet. Med. Assoc. 158:835.

Casey, H.L. 1970. Experience at the National Communicable Diseases Center with microserological technique for the diagnosis of viral disease. Health Lab. Sci. 7:233–236.

Cottral, G.E., ed. 1978. Manual of Standardized Method for Veterinary Microbiology. Cornell University Press, Ithaca, N.Y.

Flewett, T.H. 1978. Electron microscopy in the diagnosis of infectious diarrhea. J. Am. Vet. Med. Assoc. 173:538–541.

Foster, L.G., Peterson, M.W., and Spendlove, R.S. 1975. Fluorescent virus precipitin test. Proc. Soc. Exp. Biol. Med. 150:155–160.

Lennette, D.A., and Schmidt, N.J. 1979. Diagnostic Procedures for Viral and Rickettsial Infections, 4th ed. American Public Health Association, New York.

Lennette, E.H., ed. 1985. Laboratory Diagnosis of Viral Infections. Marcel Dekker, New York.

Mebus, C.A., Underdahl, N.R., Rhodes, W.B., and Twiehaus, M.J. 1969. Calf diarrhea (scours) reproduced with a virus from a field outbreak. Univ. Nebr. Res. Bull. 233:1–16.

Saunders, G.C., Clinard, E.H., Bartlett, M.L., and Sanders, W.M. 1977. Application of the indirect enzyme-labeled antibody micro-test to the detection and surveillance of animal diseases. J. Infect. Dis. 136:258–262.

Sever, J.L. 1962. Application of a microtechnique to viral serological investigations. J. Immunol. 88:320–329.

Takatsy, G. 1955. The use of spiral loops in serological and virological micro-methods. Acta Microbiol. Hung. 3:191–195.

Viruses are divided into two major groups by the International Committee on Taxonomy of Viruses, depending on whether they contain ribonucleic acid (RNA) or deoxyribonucleic acid (DNA). The viruses that contain DNA constitute six families: Parvoviridae, Papovaviridae, Adenoviridae, Iridoviridae, Poxviridae, and Herpesviridae.

41 The Parvoviridae

The family Parvoviridae consists of three genera (Bachmann et al. 1979, Kurstak and Tijssen 1981, Siegl 1976):

Parvovirus. Type species: Parvovirus r–1 (rat virus). Members of the genus, *Parvovirus* infect vertebrates, encapsidate only the plus strand of DNA, and replicate without the aid of a helper virus, but they do require a mitotic cell for replication. This genus includes a number of important pathogens for animals.

Dependovirus (adeno-associated virus [AAV]). Type species: AAV-1 Adeno-associated viruses, isolated from vertebrates, require a helper virus in order to replicate, and both strands of the replicative form of the DNA are encapsidated separately. While a number of these viruses have been isolated from animals, none as yet have been shown to be pathogens.

Densovirus. Members of the genus *Densovirus* have been isolated only from invertebrates, and thus are not discussed in this text.

The parvoviruses contain linear, single-stranded DNA with a molecular mass of 1.5 to 2.2×10^6 daltons. Hairpin structures occur at both the 5′ and 3′ ends. Nucleic acid makes up 19 to 32 percent of the weight of the virion (Bachmann et al. 1979).

Proteins constitute 63 to 81 percent of the weight of the virion. Three polypeptides (VP-1, VP-2, and VP-3) usually can be demonstrated from the mature virion, and it is believed these are all derived from a common sequence. Virions contain 62 to 72 individual protein molecules. The polypeptides identified from various parvoviruses are listed in Table 41.1.

Parvoviruses do not have envelopes and therefore do not contain lipids or carbohydrates. The virions are cube-shaped, are 18 to 26 nm in diameter, and have a central core, 14 to 17 nm, which contains the nucleic acid. The nucleocapsids are composed of 32 capsomeres, each 3 to 4 nm in diameter, arranged in icosahedral symmetry. The morphology of parvoviruses is illustrated in the electron micrograph of the feline parvovirus in Figure 41.1.

Parvoviruses are resistant to many environmental and chemical agents. They are stable over a wide pH range (3 to 9) and over a wide temperature range (e.g., resistant to 56°C for 60 minutes) and are resistant to lipid solvents and disinfectants. They are susceptible to ultraviolet light and are inactivated by aldehydes (formaldehyde, glutaraldehyde), beta propiolactone, hydroxylamine, and oxidizing agents such as sodium hypochlorite (Bachmann et al. 1979, Brown 1981, Scott 1980). They may remain infectious in contaminated fecal material for months or even years.

The replication of parvoviruses has been reviewed by Kurstak and Tijssen (1981). Members of the genus *Parvovirus* apparently do not code for enzymes required for replication, but rather rely on the enzymes in the replicating cell to perform this function. Replication occurs only in the late S-phase of cell division. *Adeno-associated viruses* do not need replicating cells, but they do need a helper virus. Parvoviruses are adsorbed to the cell within minutes and penetrate the cell intact. The DNA appears to be released into the nucleus during the uncoating process.

Transcription of the DNA occurs within the nucleus of the cell, the mRNA is transported to the cytoplasm where protein synthesis occurs, then the proteins are transported

Table 41.1. Molecular mass (in kilodaltons) of viral proteins (VP) of parvoviruses

Virus	Protein				References
	VP-1	VP-2	VP-3	VP-4	
Feline parvovirus (FPV)	77.5–79.5	63.0–63.5	61.5–63.0	50.0–55.0	Carman and Povey (1983)
	73.1	60.3	39.6	—	Johnson et al. (1974)
Canine parvovirus (CPV)	77.5–79.5	63.0–63.5	61.5–63.0	50.0–55.0	Caman and Povey (1983)
	85.0	70.0	67.0	50.0	Surleraux and Burtonboy (1984)
Mink enteritis virus (MEV)	77.5–79.5	63.0–63.5	61.5–63.0	50.0–55.0	Carman and Povey (1983)
Bovine parvovirus (BPV)	85.5	77.0	67.0	—	Johnson and Hoggan (1973)
Aleutian disease virus (ADV)	89.1	77.6	—	—	Bloom et al. (1980)
Minute virus of mice (MVM)	83.3	64.3	61.4	—	Tattersall et al. (1973)

back to the nucleus where assembly and maturation of the virion occurs.

The complete growth cycle for parvoviruses occurs within 20 to 24 hours. After a brief latent period, viral antigens appear in the cytoplasm by about 6 hours after infection and in the nucleus about 3 hours later. Mature infectious virions are released from the cell as it is destroyed by the virus during replication.

A major characteristic of the replication of parvoviruses is the production of Cowdry type A intranuclear inclusion bodies. As intranuclear replication proceeds, the nuclear membrane thickens, and a halo or clear, non-

staining area develops both around the nucleolus and inside the nuclear membrane. The change in the nuclear material results in a large acidophilic mass that constitutes most of the nucleus (Figure 41.2).

The individual members of the genus *Parvovirus*, their hosts, and the diseases produced in animals are listed in Table 41.2. The type species is the Kilham rat virus (RV). The most significant pathogens of domesticated animals are feline parvovirus, canine parvovirus, porcine parvovirus, mink enteritis virus, and Aleutian disease virus of mink. Mink enteritis virus is considered a biological variant of feline parvovirus. Many investigators believe that canine parvovirus is a mutant of feline parvovirus or mink enteritis virus. Other pathogens include the bovine parvovirus, goose parvovirus, and gastroenteritis virus (Norwalk agent) of humans. Other members of the genus include the minute virus of canines and several rodent viruses such as the H viruses (H-1 and H-3), X-14, and minute virus of mice.

Figure 41.1. Electron micrograph of feline parvovirus particles showing a mixture of complete and empty capsides. × 92,500.

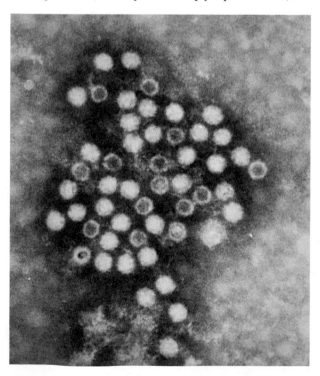

REFERENCES

Bachmann, P.A., Hoggan, M.D., Kurstak, E., Melnick, J.L., Pereira, H.G., Tattersall, P., and Vago, C. 1979. Parvoviridae: Second report. Intervirology 11:248–254.

Bloom, M.E., Race, R.E., and Wolpenbarger, J.B. 1980. Characterization of Aleutian disease virus as a parvovirus. J. Virol. 35:836–843.

Brown, T.T., Jr. 1981. Laboratory evaluation of selected disinfectants as virucidal agents against porcine parvovirus, pseudorabies virus, and transmissible gastroenteritis virus. Am. J. Vet. Res. 42:1033–1036.

Carman, P.S., and Povey, R.C. 1983. Comparison of the viral proteins of canine parvovirus-2, mink enteritis virus and feline panleukopenia virus. Vet. Microbiol. 8:423–435.

Johnson, F.B., and Hoggan, M.D. 1973. Structural proteins of HADEN virus. Virology 51:129–137.

Johnson, R.H., Siegl, G., and Gautschi, M. 1974. Characteristics of feline panleucopenia virus strains enabling definitive classification as parvoviruses. Arch. Gesam. Virusforsch. 46:315–324.

Kurstak, E., and Tijssen, P. 1981. Animal parvoviruses: Comparative aspects and diagnosis. In E. Kurstak and C. Kurstak, eds., Compara-

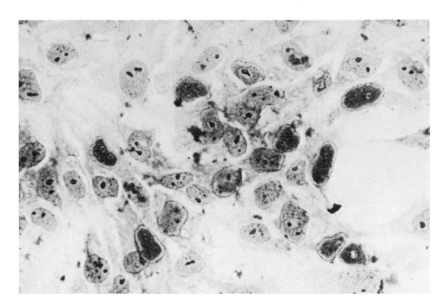

Figure 41.2. Mink cell cultures infected with feline parvovirus showing intranuclear inclusion bodies in several cells. Note the thickened nuclear membrane, the halo (or clear area) inside the nuclear membrane, and the dark-staining mass in the center of the nucleus of each infected cell. May-Grünwald-Giemsa stain. × 440.

tive Diagnosis of Viral Diseases, vol 3. Academic Press, New York. Pp. 3–65.

Scott, F.W. 1980. Virucidal disinfectants and feline viruses. Am. J. Vet. Res. 41:410–414.

Siegl, G. 1976. The parvoviruses. Virol. Monogr. 15:1–109.

Surlcraux, M., and Burtonboy, G. 1984. Structural polypeptides of a canine parvovirus. Arch. Virol. 82:233–240.

Tattersall, P., Crawford, L.V., and Shatkin, A.J. 1973. Replication of the parvovirus MVM. II. Isolation and characterization of intermediates in the replication of the viral deoxyribonucleic acid. J. Virol. 12:1446–1456.

The Genus *Parvovirus*

Feline Panleukopenia

SYNONYMS: Cat "distemper," cat plague, feline ataxia, feline infectious enteritis, feline parvovirus infection, gastroenteritis, granulocytosis, show plague, viral enteritis; abbreviations: FP, FPL

Table 41.2. Animal diseases caused by viruses in the Parvoviridae family, genus *Parvovirus*

Hosts	Virus	Name of disease produced	Type of disease
Cats	Feline parvovirus (FPV)	Feline panleukopenia	Enteritis, teratogenesis
Dogs	Canine parvovirus (CPV)	Canine parvovirus infection	Enteritis, myocarditis
	Minute virus of canines (MVC)	None	None
Pigs	Porcine parvovirus (PPV)	Porcine parvovirus infection	Mummified or aborted fetus
Cattle	Bovine parvovirus (BPV; HADEN virus)	Bovine parvovirus infection	Enteritis, reproductive disease
Geese	Derzsy's disease virus (DDV)	Goose hepatitis	Enteritis, influenza, myocarditis
Mink	Mink enteritis virus (MEV)	Mink enteritis	Enteritis
	Aleutian disease virus (ADV)	Aleutian disease	Plasmacytosis, hypergammaglobulinemia, respiratory disorders
Rabbits	Rabbit parvovirus (RPV)	None	None
Rodents	Rat virus (RV)	Cerebellar ataxia	Teratogenesis
	H-1 virus		Teratogenesis
	H-3 virus		Teratogenesis
	X-14 virus		Teratogenesis
	Minute virus of mice (MVM)		Neurological disorders
Humans	Gastroenteritis virus of man (GVM; Norwalk agent)	Gastroenteritis	Gastroenteritis

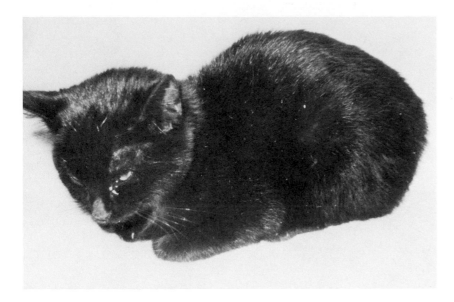

Figure 41.3. Characteristic attitude of a kitten with typical feline panleukopenia. Note the hunched-up appearance with the head down between the paws. The chin may rest on the floor. The third eyelids are usually prominent.

Feline panleukopenia is a highly contagious viral disease of domestic and exotic cats characterized by sudden onset, fever, anorexia, depression, leukopenia, vomiting and diarrhea, dehydration, and often high mortality. In unvaccinated populations FP is the most devastating disease of cats known.

Character of the Disease. The incubation period for FP can range from 2 to 7 days but is usually 4 or 5 days. The severity of illness in cats infected with feline panleukopenia virus varies from a completely subclinical or asymptomatic disease to one that is rapidly fatal and resembles acute poisoning. For convenience, clinical signs can be discussed under six headings.

Peracute form. FP may progress so rapidly that the owner claims the cat shows signs of acute poisoning. In these animals illness develops rapidly with severe depression progressing within hours to coma and death. Vomiting may occur, but the cat usually dies before diarrhea and dehydration have time to develop. The animal's temperature is usually dramatically subnormal. Mortality in the peracute form approaches 100 percent.

Acute, or typical, form. In the typical case of FP there is a sudden onset of clinical signs. The cat may have a temperature of 104°F (40°C) or higher and show severe depression and complete anorexia. Vomiting usually occurs, and severe, fetid diarrhea may develop within 24 to 48 hours. Blood and casts may be passed in the feces. Continued vomiting and diarrhea cause severe dehydration and electrolyte imbalances.

Cats with FP often assume a typical attitude, as shown in Figure 41.3. The cats are hunched with their heads between their paws, and they often hang their heads over a water or food dish. They frequently act as if they would like to drink and may even take a lap or two of milk or water, but they are unable or reluctant to swallow. The coat becomes rough and dull, and the skin loses its elasticity due to dehydration. The third eyelids often appear prominent. The abdomen is tender, and palpation elicits signs of pain. The mesenteric nodes are enlarged, and the gastrointestinal tract contains excess gas and liquid. A subnormal temperature indicates a grave prognosis; coma and death follow in a few hours.

Mortality in the acute form of FP may vary from 25 to 90 percent. Death may occur within the first 5 days of illness in uncomplicated cases, or after 5 days in complicated cases. If the cat survives approximately 5 days of illness and if secondary complications such as bacterial infections, severe dehydration, or chronic enteritis from concurrent infections do not occur, then recovery should be fairly rapid. It will take several weeks for the cat to regain its lost weight and former condition.

Subacute, or mild, form. A cat with the subacute form of FP will not eat and is mildly depressed. Temperature may be slightly elevated, and abdominal palpation usually reveals gas in the intestines. Illness lasts for 1 to 3 days, and recovery is usually rapid and uncomplicated.

Subclinical form. FP can occur without clinical signs. Pregnant cats may show no signs of illness and later abort or give birth to kittens with neonatal FP with one or more of its many manifestations. Serologic and experimental studies indicate that the subclinical form of FP is quite common in certain outbreaks. This is the usual form of the disease in germ-free kittens or in kittens reared in extremely clean environments, such as isolation units, where pathogenic intestinal flora are absent.

Neonatal form. Kittens infected during late gestation or the first few days after birth either die suddenly without any particular signs or develop ataxia at 2 or 3 weeks of age, when they become ambulatory (deLahunta 1971). The ataxia is a symmetrical incoordination, exemplified by rolling or tumbling as the cat tries to walk, by an involuntary twitching of the head, or by swaying of the body. There is a wide stance with the tail held high and stiff for balance. The gait is hypermetric, as the feet are raised unusually high. These ataxic kittens are alert and strong. If they are coordinated enough to eat, they will grow; but the ataxia will persist throughout life with little if any improvement or compensation.

Infection earlier in gestation, with or without clinical signs of FP in the queen, may result in fetal death with subsequent resorption, abortion, mummification, or stillbirth.

"Chronic" form. Although the diagnosis of chronic FP has been made occasionally by clinicians and pathologists, most cases of chronic, persistent leukopenia, usually with anemia and often with enteritis, are due to leukemia virus infection. Sporadic cases of chronic enteritis with severe leukopenia have been investigated in several catteries and appear to be infectious, but the etiological agent has not been identified. Some cases have been tentatively diagnosed as chronic FP, but serologic and virologic monitoring of the catteries involved does not support this diagnosis.

Properties of the Virus. FP is caused by feline panleukopenia virus (FPV), a small (20–24 nm), highly stable, nonenveloped, single-stranded DNA virus classified in the *Parvovirus* genus of the Parvoviridae family. FPV has the biochemical and biophysical properties of a typical parvovirus, as discussed above. Three major viral proteins and a fourth minor protein have been reported to make up the virion (see Table 41.1).

FPV is resistant to most commercial disinfectants, including those containing alcohols, phenols, and quaternary ammonium compounds (Scott 1980). It is susceptible, however, to a 1:32 or stronger dilution of commercial sodium hypochlorite (5.6 percent as household bleach). Sodium hypochlorite may be combined with certain detergents or disinfectants, although caution must be exercised to avoid toxic chlorine fumes. FPV is also inactivated by 2 percent glutaraldehyde and 4 percent formaldehyde. For many years formaldehyde was used to inactivate FPV from tissue and cell culture suspensions of virulent virus in order to prepare inactivated vaccines.

There is only one serotype of FPV, but there is a variation in virulence among various strains. The virus that causes mink enteritis (MEV) is antigenically identical to FPV (Gorham et al. 1965, Parrish et al. 1982). Canine parvovirus (CPV) is related to FPV and MEV antigenically, but it does have antigenic and biological properties that are distinct (Parrish et al. 1982).

FPV is partially deficient and requires an actively dividing cell to complete its replicative cycle. This property limits the cells that can be infected in vivo and thus the clinical disease produced (Carlson and Scott 1977). The replicative cycle is short; mature infectious virions appear within 20 to 24 hours after the initial cell infection. The virion is adsorbed to the host cell within minutes, and a large portion of the adsorbed virions penetrate the cell. Uncoating of the viral protein appears to occur either as the virion enters the nucleus or within the nucleus. Transcription, protein synthesis, assembly, and virion maturation for the various parvoviruses have been studied in some detail, and a summary has been presented by Kurstak and Tijssen (1981).

The first microscopic changes observed in stained FPV-infected cell cultures are an altered staining pattern of the nuclear mass, a margination of the nucleoli, and a thickening of the nuclear membrane. As replication progresses, there is a margination of chromatin, and a clear zone, or "halo," appears around the nucleoli and inside the nuclear membrane. At this stage a clear eosinophilic Cowdry type A intranuclear inclusion body is evident (Figure 41.2). During the next 8 to 12 hours the cytoplasm shrinks around the nucleus to give a dark-staining, pyknotic cell mass. By 24 hours the virions have been released from the cell, and only cell debris remains.

Epizootiology and Pathogenesis. FP occurs worldwide wherever domestic or exotic cats are found. It probably was the cause of the great cat plagues of ancient times. Because of the extreme resistance of the virus to environmental conditions, contaminated premises remain a source of infection for years after a clinical case occurs there.

The incidence of clinical FP varies, depending on the percentage of immune cats in the population, the virulence of the particular strain of virus, and the virulence of intestinal bacteria in the infected cats. Virtually 100 percent of susceptible cats on a premise that come in contact with an infected cat or contaminated environment will become infected with virus. Some will have a subclinical infection, others a mild infection, others a serious disease. There tends to be a seasonal incidence (Reif 1976), which coincides with the buildup of a susceptible population as young kittens lose their maternally derived immunity.

The exact time of year when this higher incidence occurs depends on the seasonal breeding for that locality. However, FP can and does occur at any time of the year.

In susceptible kittens morbidity from FP usually is extremely high. Mortality varies but is usually high. It may range from 25 percent to as high as 90 percent but usually averages around 50 percent.

Although FP is predominantly a disease of young kittens 2 to 4 months old, it can affect cats of all ages. Older cats, however, are more likely to have subclinical or mild infections, compared with more severe disease in kittens. There is no sex predilection for this disease.

The domestic cat is the primary host of FPV, but all members of the family Felidae are believed to be susceptible. Although the disease has been studied extensively in domestic cats, only limited studies of FP in nondomestic cats have been reported. Cockburn (1947) summarized several outbreaks in a zoological garden which caused high mortality in young cats (tigers, leopards, wildcats, lynxes, servals, leopard cats, tiger cats, ocelots, cheetahs, and a lyra cat). FPV has been isolated from lions, leopards, snow leopards, tigers, and panthers that died of the disease (Studdert et al. 1973; F. Scott, unpublished data). Torres (1941) reported an outbreak in wild felines in a Brazilian zoo from which he experimentally transmitted FP to domestic cats. Species involved were *Felis maracaja, F. pardalis, F. concolor, F. onca,* and other unspecified felids.

Mink (family Mustelidae) are susceptible to FPV and MEV but have subclinical infections with CPV (Barker et al. 1983). Ferrets can be infected in utero or neonatally (Kilham et al. 1967). Skunks are relatively resistant to FPV (Barker et al. 1983). Little information is available concerning the susceptibility to FPV of other Mustilidae such as otters, weasels, and badgers.

In the family Procyonidae the raccoon is highly susceptible to FPV and MEV (Barker et al. 1983; Gillespie and Scott 1973; F. Scott, unpublished data). Other Procyonidae such as the ringtail and the coatimundi are susceptible to FPV (Johnson and Halliwell 1968; F. Scott, unpublished data).

Nair et al. (1964) reported an outbreak of gastroenteritis, presumably FP, in a group of captive civet cats (family Viverridae) in India, with a 50 percent mortality.

Until the worldwide pandemic of canine parvovirus in 1977–1978, canids were generally believed to be resistant to FPV. Infection of dogs with FPV is abortive, with limited replication and no shed of the feline virus. The origin of the canine strain of parvovirus is not known, but it is generally assumed to be a mutant from CPV or MEV. Red foxes can be infected with FPV but may not show signs of illness (Barker et al. 1983).

FPV is usually transmitted by direct contact of susceptible cats with infected cats; during the acute phase of the illness virus is present in all body secretions and excretions. Contaminated food and water dishes, cages, bedding, litter boxes, rugs, and soil can harbor virus to infect a susceptible cat for many months, perhaps years. Virus can be transmitted on contaminated clothing, shoes, and hands of people. The rapid spread of the related canine parvovirus throughout the world probably occurred in this way. Aerosol transmission may also occur, especially if a cat is coinfected with respiratory viruses so that it sneezes. Insects and parasites, especially fleas, can transmit the virus as mechanical vectors (Torres 1941).

The pathogenesis of FPV infection depends on the state of mitotic activity of the various tissues within the body (Carlson and Scott 1977, Carlson et al. 1977). Virus enters the cat via the oral route, and primary infection occurs in the lymphoid tissues of the oral pharynx. The regional lymph nodes then become infected. Within 24 hours after ingesting virus, the cat is viremic, with FPV distributed throughout the body. The epithelial crypt cells of the ileum and jejunum are particularly susceptible to FPV. Cytolytic replication of the virus in these cells destroys the epithelial lining of the crypts, which results in ballooned, debris-filled crypts and shortened, blunted villi. If the mitotic rate of the crypt cells is low, as in gnotobiotic kittens, the virus destroys only an occasional crypt cell and does not produce gross or microscopic lesions of the intestine. Other tissues with rapidly dividing cells (thymus, bone marrow, lymph nodes) are affected by the cytolytic replication of the virus.

Virus persists in the blood of an infected cat until approximately 7 days after exposure (approximately the third day of illness), when neutralizing antibodies appear. The antibody titer increases rapidly and reaches its maximum by 14 days after exposure. With the appearance of antibody, virus in various tissues gradually disappears. It may persist intracellularly, where it is protected from antibodies, for several weeks, months, or even years in certain tissues such as the kidney (Csiza, deLahunta, et al. 1971). However, shed of infectious virus is not a common finding in cats recovered from FP. Generally, by 3 weeks after the illness, cats no longer shed infectious virus in the feces, urine, or other secretions or excretions. Virus shed from chronically infected tissues is quickly neutralized by antibody in these tissues or excretions. However, virus can be recovered from feces of a small percentage of recovered cats for several weeks after recovery.

If a susceptible pregnant cat becomes infected with FPV, the virus readily invades the uterus and crosses the placenta to infect the fetus (Csiza, Scott, et al. 1971). Infection spreads throughout the fetus and crosses the blood-brain barrier to infect the cerebellum and other tissues within the central nervous system. The results depend on the stage of gestation at the time of infection. The possibilities include abortion, stillbirths, early neonatal deaths, or teratological changes, especially cerebellar hypoplasia. Evidence suggests that hydrocephalus may result from FPV infection during mid-gestation (Csiza, Scott, et al. 1971).

In utero or neonatal infection can result in cell damage in the retina, leading to retinal dysplasia, but without loss of visual acuity (MacMillan 1974, Percy et al. 1975). MacMillan (1974) reported focal retinal lesions in 31 percent of kittens with naturally occurring cerebellar degeneration and ataxia due to FPV, compared with less than 2 percent in the general feline population.

Infection of queens during the first half of gestation can result in death of one or more fetuses, with total resorption of both fetuses and placental membranes if abortion does not occur. Later in gestation resorption of fluids from the dead fetus results in a dehydrated or mummified fetus and placenta that may be retained until term. Susceptible queens infected during the latter half of gestation may give birth to litters containing normal healthy kittens, stillborn kittens, partially autolyzed fetuses, and mummified fetuses.

Infection of the uterus and the fetuses occurs only when completely susceptible queens contract acute infection. Queens that have had a previous infection have neutralizing antibodies that protect the fetuses. Similarly, litters subsequent to an FPV-affected litter will not experience problems from FPV.

Immunity. The immune response to FPV infection is rapid and solid. Cats that have recovered from natural infection are immune for life. After experimental infection with FPV, humoral virus neutralizing antibodies appear in the serum by 6 or 7 days. The titer increases rapidly and reaches a maximal level within 14 days after infection. In active infection, antibody titers persist for long periods, probably for life. A cat that recovers from clinical FP does not need to be vaccinated for the rest of its life.

Diagnosis. The diagnosis of FP is based on history, clinical signs, and the presence of leukopenia; it can be confirmed by gross and microscopic changes and by various laboratory tests (Carpenter 1971, Cotter 1980, Gillespie and Scott 1973, Greene 1984, Ott 1983, Scott 1987).

Clinical diagnosis. The history, especially age, vaccination records, and contact with strange cats within the past 2 weeks (e.g., boarding kennel, hospital, or adoption shelter), often points to a diagnosis of FP. A sick, unvaccinated cat, less than a year old, should be highly sus-

pected of having FP. A history of vaccination does not rule out the possibility of FP, however. Maternally derived immunity can interfere with vaccination and leave a kitten susceptible to FP after that immunity has waned (Scott et al. 1970), especially if the kitten was last vaccinated when less than 12 weeks old. An older cat, vaccinated as a kitten and without periodic revaccinations, may lose its immunity after a few years. How common an occurrence this is remains unknown.

Laboratory diagnosis. The most characteristic finding in FP is the leukopenia, which occurs in almost all FPV-infected cats, even if they do not show clinical signs. There is usually a direct correlation between the severity of the leukopenia and the severity of the disease. This leukopenia is characterized by a progressive drop in circulating white blood cells 1 to 2 days before the development of clinical signs, with a precipitous drop on the day of the crisis. The leukocyte count usually is 4,000–8,000/dl in subclinical infections and less than 4,000/dl in clinical infections. Counts below 2,000/dl warrant a guarded prognosis. Due to the extreme reduction in neutrophils, relative lymphocytosis may occur, but as the disease progresses the lymphocytes may disappear also. A count of 0–200 leukocytes/dl of blood is not unusual. If the cat survives for approximately 5 days after the onset of signs, the total leukocyte count rebounds dramatically (with a marked left shift), often exceeding the upper normal limit in another 3 to 4 days (Schalm et al. 1975, Scott et al. 1970).

The diagnosis of FP can be confirmed by viral isolation, identification of viral antigen in tissues with immunofluorescence tests, serologic tests, or pathological changes. Virus can be isolated in cell cultures. Swabs should be taken from the pharynx or from the rectum, placed in viral transport medium and refrigerated, and then submitted to a diagnostic laboratory that is equipped to do feline virus isolations. The best tissues to submit from autopsied animals are from the spleen, thymus, ileum, or mesenteric lymph node. These samples should be placed in sterile vials, refrigerated, and either transmitted directly to the laboratory or shipped by overnight delivery under refrigeration. Electron microscopic examination of fecal samples for typical parvovirus particles also confirms the diagnosis.

For the serologic diagnosis of FP, virus neutralization or enzyme-linked immunosorbent assay (ELISA) with paired serum samples can be used. One serum sample is taken during the acute phase of the disease and a second sample is taken 2 weeks later.

Treatment. Panleukopenia normally causes high mortality, but with diligent treatment and good nursing care it can be reduced. The main objective is to keep the animal alive and in reasonably good health until the natural defense mechanisms—the rebound in white cells and the appearance of antibody—can take over. Serum antibodies usually appear about 3 to 4 days after the first signs of disease, and 2 to 3 days later the total white cell count rebounds sharply. If the cat can be maintained without complications for 5 to 7 days, the chances of recovery are usually good.

More specifically, the object of treatment is to correct and prevent abnormalities such as vomiting, diarrhea, and dehydration, and to prevent secondary bacterial infections.

The most important aspect of treatment is to restore and maintain fluid and electrolyte balances. To prevent the loss of fluids, one should give antiemetics and anticholinergic drugs. For replacement of fluids, 5 percent dextrose in saline, lactated Ringer's solution, or 5 percent dextrose in electrolyte replacer solution (formulated for replacement of electrolytes lost in vomiting and diarrhea) is indicated. Fluid should be administered intravenously (or subcutaneously as a poor second choice) at the rate of 11–33 ml/kg of body weight every 12 hours. Whole-blood transfusions, 22 ml/kg, can be highly beneficial (Cotter 1980, Ott 1983).

Kraft (1973) reported that animals with FP showing severe coagulation disturbances responded best when treated with heparin (100 U/kg) administered intravenously two or three times daily in combination with whole-blood transfusions or with electrolyte solutions.

Broad-spectrum antibiotics are used in all cases, since secondary bacterial infections are common. The antibiotics are administered parenterally until gastroenteritis is controlled. Then they may be administered orally for a total of 5 days.

Other supportive treatment should be administered as indicated. All food should be withheld until the gastroenteritis is controlled; strained baby foods or other highly palatable foods can then be fed in small quantities several times a day.

Secondary viral respiratory infections are common complications, since the stress of FP may trigger a latent respiratory virus infection, or there may have been dual infections from simultaneous exposure to two or more viruses. This dual infection is more severe than if either of the viruses had infected the cat alone. Secondary viral infections should be treated as indicated.

There is no treatment that is beneficial for cats with ataxia from FPV-induced cerebellar degeneration during neonatal FP.

Pathological Changes. The pathological changes in FP have been described by Carlson et al. (1977), Jubb and Kennedy (1970), Langheinrich and Nielsen (1971), Leasure et al. (1934), and Rohovsky and Griesemer (1967).

Gross findings. Cats that die of FP are gaunt and dehydrated, as evidenced at autopsy by sticky, dry tissues and sunken, soft eyes. There is usually evidence of diarrhea and vomiting.

The gross pathological changes in FP may be relatively mild and not noticed by the casual observer. Careful observation usually shows changes in the small intestine, primarily the ileum and jejunum (Figure 41.4). The intestine is usually dilated and edematous with a turgid,

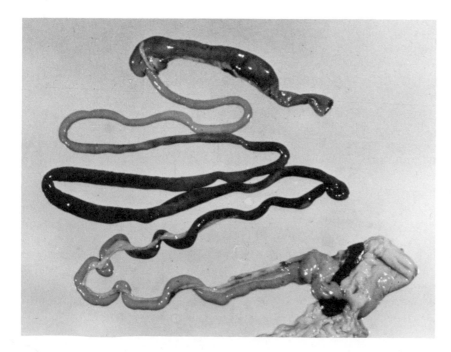

Figure 41.4 Gross pathological changes in the intestinal tract of a cat with feline panleukopenia. Note the turgid, hoselike appearance of the intestine, and the dark, hemorrhagic jejunum. The ileum often has extensive lesions as well.

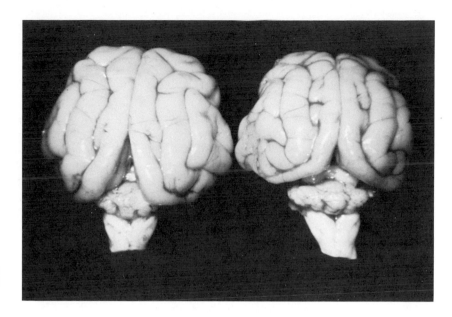

Figure 41.5. Cerebellar hypoplasia in two 8-week-old littermate kittens that had shown ataxia since 2 weeks of age.

hoselike appearance. Often hyperemia or petechial hemorrhages or both can be noted on the serosal and mucosal surfaces. The feces are scant and watery, with a fetid odor and a yellowish gray appearance. The mesenteric lymph nodes are edematous and may be hemorrhagic.

Kittens suffering from feline ataxia due to FPV have a gross reduction in the size of the cerebellum (Csiza, Scott, et al. 1971; deLahunta 1971) (Figure 41.5).

Kittens with FPV-induced hydrocephalus have an enlarged cranium with enlarged cerebral hemispheres due to dilated lateral and third ventricles. The cerebral cortex is thinned from increased pressure of the cerebrospinal fluid.

Newborn kittens that die of FP usually have minimal gross pathological changes. The main lesion is degeneration of the thymus. Hemorrhagic encephalopathy occasionally may be observed.

Histopathological findings. The histopathological changes are primarily restricted to tissues undergoing active cell mitosis. The most consistent and striking lesions are in the epithelium of the crypts of the small intestine, especially the ileum and jejunum. These crypts are ballooned and filled with debris. The epithelial cells lining the crypts are degenerating or may be sloughed off entirely (Figure 41.6). The villi are shortened due to sloughing of the tips. The bone marrow and the lymphoid tissues

Figure 41.6. Histopathological appearance of the small intestine of a cat with feline panleukopenia. Note the enlarged, ballooned crypts devoid of epithelial cells, and the shortened, blunted, fused villi.

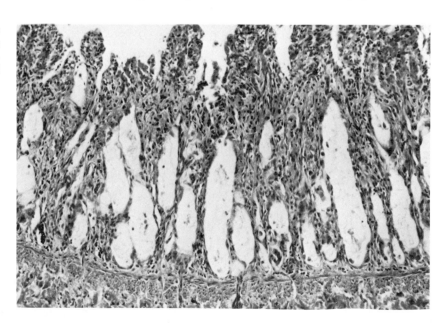

such as the mesenteric lymph nodes, spleen, and thymus, have markedly reduced cellular elements. Vessels in all organs usually are devoid of leukocytes. The liver often has a dissociation of hepatic cells. Intranuclear inclusion bodies may be observed, especially in the crypt epithelial cells of the small intestine early in the disease.

Disseminated intravascular coagulation has been reported in cases of FP in domestic cats and in *Felis sylvestris* (Hoffman 1973, Kraft 1973). Numerous microthrombi may occur in peripheral blood vessels in renal medulla and cortex, liver, heart, lungs, and occasionally in other organs.

In FPV-induced cerebellar hypoplasia there is a decrease or absence of the granular cells of the cerebellum. The Purkinje cells are decreased in number and scattered. There is no correlation between the degree of hypoplasia and the clinical signs exhibited (deLahunta 1971).

Tissues of newborn kittens with FP have widespread intranuclear inclusion bodies, especially in the heart (Csiza, deLahunta, et al. 1971).

Prevention and Control. FP is entirely preventable with proper immunization. Several excellent vaccines are available to immunize cats against FP. These vaccines are effective, inexpensive, and confer long-lasting immunity. FP vaccines are usually combined with feline viral rhinotracheitis and feline calicivirus vaccines, and sometimes with vaccines for feline chlamydiosis and rabies. Considerable information has been published concerning types of vaccines and vaccination recommendations (Bittle et al. 1970, 1982; Gorham et al. 1965; Greene 1984; Scott 1983, 1987; Scott and Gillespie 1971). Immunization against panleukopenia should be started at the first visit, or at 8 or 9 weeks of age, whichever comes first. Vaccine should be administered at 4-week intervals until the kitten is at least 12 and preferably 14 weeks of age.

The choice of inactivated or modified live-virus vaccine depends on the clinician's preference and on any special circumstances. Inactivated vaccines are safe and can be given to any cat, even a pregnant queen. Two doses are usually required initially, and annual or biannual revaccinations should be given. Modified live-virus vaccines produce high titers with a single dose after maternally derived immunity has been lost and theoretically should give longer protection. Modified live-virus vaccines produce protection faster than inactivated vaccines, usually within 1 or 2 days. They definitely are indicated where exposure to FPV is imminent, such as in adoption shelters or veterinary hospitals. Modified live-virus vaccines must not be given to pregnant queens.

Both types of vaccine produce immunity for long periods. Because the exact duration of immunity is not known, annual revaccinations are recommended for maximum protection. This is especially pertinent for indoor-dwelling cats that usually are not exposed to street viruses. Cats that have recovered from clinical FP or subclinical FPV infection are immune for life.

Maternally derived immunity must be considered in establishing a vaccination program, since it is the most common cause of vaccine failure. There is a direct correlation between the titer of the queen at the time of parturition and the duration of passive immunity acquired through the colostrum by the kitten. This passive immunity, if present in sufficient quantities, not only protects the kitten against virulent virus but also interferes with vaccination. Thus vaccination must be done after the kitten has lost all or most of its maternally derived immunity.

Exotic felids should be vaccinated according to the same schedule as that for domestic cats (Fowler 1983, Laughlin 1980). Contrary to earlier recommendations, modified live-virus vaccines can be used.

FPV is an extremely resistant virus. Thus, one must pay strict attention to the disinfectant used to clean contaminated areas. A 1:20 to 1:32 dilution of sodium hypochlorite (household bleach) is an effective and inexpensive disinfectant for inactivation of FPV (Scott 1980).

The Disease in Humans. Because FPV does not infect human cells, there are no known public health risks from either the virus or from cats infected with it.

REFERENCES

Barker, I.K., Povey, R.C., and Voigt, D.R. 1983. Response of mink, skunk, red fox and raccoon to inoculation with mink virus enteritis, feline panleukopenia and canine parvovirus and prevalence of antibody to parvovirus in wild carnivores in Ontario. Can. J. Comp. Med. 47:188–197.

Bittle, J.L., Emrich, S.A., and Gauker, F.B. 1970. Safety and efficacy of an inactivated tissue culture vaccine for feline panleukopenia. J. Am. Vet. Med. Assoc. 157:2052–2056.

Bittle, J.L., Grant, W., and Scott, F.W. 1982. Current canine and feline immunization guidelines. J. Am. Vet. Med. Assoc. 181:332–335.

Carlson, J.H., and Scott, F.W. 1977. Feline panleukopenia. II. The relationship of intestinal mucosal cell proliferation rates to viral infection and development of lesions. Vet. Pathol. 14:173–181.

Carlson, J.H., Scott, F.W., and Duncan, J.R. 1977. Feline panleukopenia. I. Pathogenesis in germfree and specific pathogen-free cats. Vet. Pathol. 14:79–88.

Carpenter, J.L. 1971. Feline panleukopenia: Clinical signs and differential diagnosis. J. Am. Vet. Med. Assoc. 158:857–859.

Cockburn, A. 1947. Infectious enteritis in the Zoological Gardens, Regent's Park. Vet. J. 103:261–262.

Cotter, S.M. 1980. Feline panleukopenia. In R.W. Kirk, ed., Current Veterinary Therapy, vol. 7. W.B. Saunders, Philadelphia. Pp. 1286–1288.

Csiza, C.K., deLahunta, A., Scott, F.W., and Gillespie, J.H. 1971. The pathogenesis of feline panleukopenia virus in susceptible newborn kittens. II. Pathology and immune fluorescence. Infect. Immun. 3:838–846.

Csiza, C.K., Scott, F.W., deLahunta, A., and Gillespie, J.H. 1971. Feline viruses. XIV. Transplacental infections in spontaneous panleukopenia of cats. Cornell Vet. 61:423–439.

deLahunta, A. 1971. Comments on cerebellar ataxia and its congenital transmission in cats by feline panleukopenia virus. J. Am. Vet. Med. Assoc. 158:901–906.

Fowler, M.E. 1983. Immunoprophylaxis in nondomestic carnivores. In R.W. Kirk, ed., Current Veterinary Therapy, vol. 8. W.B. Saunders, Philadelphia. Pp. 1129–1131.

Gillespie, J.H., and Scott, F.W. 1973. Feline viral disease. Adv. Vet. Sci. Comp. Med. 17:163–200.

Greene, C.E. 1984. Feline panleukopenia. In C.E. Greene, ed., Clinical Microbiology and Infectious Diseases of the Dog and Cat. W.B. Saunders, Philadelphia. Pp. 479–489.

Gorham, J.R., Hartsough, G.R., Burger, D., Lust, S., and Sato, N. 1965. The preliminary use of attenuated feline panleukopenia virus to protect cats against panleukopenia and mink against mink enteritis. Cornell Vet. 55:559–566.

Hoffman, R. 1973. Disseminated intravascular coagulation in spontaneous panleukopenia in domestic and wild cats. (In German.) Berl. Münch. Tierärztl. Wochenschr. 86:72–74.

Johnson, R.H. 1965. Feline panleukopenia. I. Identification of a virus associated with the syndrome. Res. Vet. Sci. 6:466–471.

Johnson, R.H., and Halliwell, R.E.W. 1968. Natural susceptibility to feline panleukopenia of the coati-mundi. Vet. Rec. 82:582.

Jubb, K.V.F., and Kennedy, P.C. 1970. Pathology of domestic animals, 2d ed., vol. 2. Academic Press, New York. Pp. 131–134.

Kilham, L., Margolis, G., and Colby, E.D. 1967. Congenital infections of cats and ferrets by feline panleukopenia virus manifested by cerebellar hypoplasia. Lab. Invest. 17:465–480.

Kraft, W. 1973. Thrombelastogram of healthy domestic cats and the treatment of disseminated intravascular coagulation in panleukopenia. (In German.) Berl. Münch. Tierärztl. Wochenschr. 86:394–396.

Kurstak, E., and Tijssen, P. 1981. Animal parvoviruses: Comparative aspects and diagnosis. In E. Kurstak and C. Kurstak, eds., Comparative Diagnosis of Viral Diseases. III. Vertebrate Animal and Related Viruses, part A: DNA viruses. Academic Press, New York. Pp. 3–65.

Langheinrich, K.A., and Nielsen, S.W. 1971. Histopathology of feline panleukopenia: A report of 65 cases. J. Am. Vet. Med. Assoc. 158:863–872.

Laughlin, D.C. 1980. Immunization of exotic cats. In R.W. Kirk, ed., Current Veterinary Therapy, vol. 7. W.B. Saunders, Philadelphia. Pp. 1258–1261.

Leasure, E.E., Lienhardt, H.F., and Taberner, F.R. 1934. Feline infectious enteritis. North Am. Vet. 15:30–34.

MacMillan, A.D. 1974. Retinal dysplasia and degeneration in the young cat: Feline panleukopenia virus as an etiological agent. Ph.D. dissertation, University of California, Davis.

Nair, K.P.D., Iyer, R.P., and Venugopalan, A. 1964. An outbreak of gastroenteritis in civet cats. Indian Vet. J. 41:763–765.

Ott, R.L. 1983. Systemic viral diseases. In P.W. Pratt, ed., Feline Medicine, 1st ed. American Veterinary Publications, Santa Barbara, Calif. Pp. 85–139.

Parrish, C.R., Carmichael, L.E., and Antczak, D.F. 1982. Antigenic relationships between canine parvovirus type 2, feline panleukopenia virus and mink enteritis virus using conventional antisera and monoclonal antibodies. Arch. Virol. 72:267–278.

Percy, D.W., Scott, F.W., and Albert, D.M. 1975. Retinal dysplasia due to feline panleukopenia virus infection. J. Am. Vet. Med. Assoc. 167:935–937.

Reif, J.S. 1976. Seasonality, natality and herd immunity in feline panleukopenia. Am. J. Epidemiol. 103:81–87.

Rohovsky, M.W., and Griesemer, R.A. 1967. Experimental feline infectious enteritis in the germfree cat. Pathol. Vet. 4:391–410.

Schalm, D.W., Jain, N.C., and Carroll, E.J. 1975. Veterinary Hematology, 3d ed. Lea & Febiger, Philadelphia. Pp. 679–682.

Scott, F.W. 1980. Virucidal disinfectants and feline viruses. Am. J. Vet. Res. 41:410–414.

Scott, F.W. 1983. Feline immunization. In R.W. Kirk, ed., Current Veterinary Therapy, vol. 8. W.B. Saunders, Philadelphia. Pp. 1127–1129.

Scott, F.W. 1987. Feline panleukopenia. In J. Holzworth, ed., Diseases of the Cat, vol. 1. W.B. Saunders, Philadelphia. Pp. 182–193.

Scott, F.W., and Gillespie, J.H. 1971. Immunization for feline panleukopenia. Vet. Clin. North Am. 1(2):231–240.

Scott, F.W., Csiza, C.K., and Gillespie, J.H. 1970. Maternally derived immunity to feline panleukopenia. J. Am. Vet. Assoc. 156:439–453.

Studdert, M.J., Kelly C.M., and Harrigan, K.E. 1973. Isolation of panleukopenia virus from lions. Vet. Rec. 93:156–159.

Torres, S. 1941. Infectious feline gastroenteritis in wild cats. North Am. Vet. 22:297–299.

Canine Parvovirus Infection

SYNONYMS: Canine parvovirus 1 (CPV-1) infection, canine parvovirus 2 (CPV-2) infection, minute virus of canines (MVC) infection

Canine parvovirus 1 produces a common subclinical enteric infection in dogs but causes no known disease. Canine parvovirus 2, apparently nonexistent in the dog population before 1977, causes the most severe canine enteric disease, a serious systemic infection with hemorrhagic enteritis as the main sign. CPV-2 may produce myocarditis with sudden death in 4- to 8-week-old pups. Review articles on canine parvovirus infection include those by Carmichael and Binn (1981), Greene (1984), and Pollock and Carmichael (1983a).

Character of the Disease. There are two main syndromes associated with CPV-2 infection in the dog. The first is acute enteritis, and the second is myocardial disease. The severity of clinical disease varies from subclinical (with no outward signs of illness) to acute, severe, fatal infection.

Clinical signs of acute CPV enteritis are similar to those in cats with feline parvovirus and include vomiting (often severe and protracted), anorexia, diarrhea, and rapid dehydration. Signs are especially severe in pups. The feces are generally light gray or yellow-gray at the onset of disease; however, fluid stools, either streaked with blood or frankly hemorrhagic, may be present as the initial sign and may persist until recovery or death.

Some animals vomit frequently and have diarrhea, sometimes projectile and hemorrhagic, until they die; others have only a loose stool and recover uneventfully. Temperatures ranging from 104° to 106°F are observed in some animals, especially pups; however, there may be little, if any, elevation of temperature in older dogs. Sudden "shock like" death may occur in some puppies as early as 2 days after the onset of illness.

A common feature of CPV disease is leukopenia, especially during the first 4 to 5 days of illness. Total leukocyte counts less than 100/dl have been recorded; however, counts of 500–2,000/dl are more common at the peak of illness.

During initial outbreaks of CPV infections, a sudden occurrence of myocardial disease was observed in litters of pups (Hayes et al. 1979, Jezyk et al. 1979, Mulvey et al. 1980). Until a particular population of dogs becomes immune either through natural infection or vaccination, myocardial disease from CPV is common. Two forms of the disease occur. The first is characterized by sudden death in otherwise healthy-appearing puppies less than 8 weeks of age (Greene 1984). Approximately 70 percent of puppies in an affected litter will develop this acute syndrome and will die after a short episode during which they may cry, show signs of respiratory distress, and attempt to vomit. Mucous membranes may be pale, and the extremities may feel cool. Any stress such as exercise or even eating may precipitate a cardiac crisis. Examination of puppies just before death reveals severe cardiac arrhythmias.

The surviving 30 percent of pups from an affected litter usually develop subacute heart failure weeks or months later (Greene 1984). These pups have subclinical arrhythmias for a time, then decompensating heart failure. Even pups that survive this phase of the disease usually are exercise intolerant and eventually die of progressive heart failure up to 27 months after the initial parvovirus infection.

The original isolates of CPV-1 were associated with diarrhea in dogs. More information is required to establish CPV-1's importance as a pathogen in canines. Many investigators think that CPV-1, unlike CPV-2, generally produces only subclinical infection.

Properties of the Virus. Two parvoviruses infect the intestinal tract of dogs. CPV-1, first isolated from feces of dogs by Binn et al. (1970), has the classic properties of a parvovirus, is common in dogs, but, as far as is known, produces only subclinical infections.

The second antigenic type of parvovirus in the dog, CPV-2, was associated with a fatal hemorrhagic enteritis in dogs that swept worldwide in 1978. A number of investigators identified a parvovirus associated with this zoonotic and recognized the similarity of the disease to feline panleukopenia (Appel et al. 1979, Carmichael et al. 1980, Eugster et al. 1978, Pletcher et al. 1979). CPV-2 appears to have the same biochemical and physical properties as CPV-1 but is antigenically distinct from CPV-1. CPV-2 is similar in antigenicity to feline parvovirus and mink enteritis virus, although there are differences in host susceptibility and in DNA sequencing (Carman and Povey 1983; Parrish and Carmichael 1983; Parrish, Carmichael, and Antczak 1982.).

The canine parvoviruses contain a single-stranded DNA core surrounded by a nonenveloped protein capsid 20 to 25 nm in diameter. The nucleic acid codes for three main proteins and a fourth protein found in lesser amounts (Carman and Povey 1983, Surleraux and Burtonboy 1984). These proteins and their reported molecular masses are listed in Table 41.1. Proteins of similar size were identified from the three closely related parvoviruses, CPV-2, mink enteritis virus, and feline parvovirus. Canine parvoviruses replicate in the nucleus of mitotic cells, producing Cowdry type A intranuclear inclusions and a cytolytic effect with cell destruction, as described above for feline parvovirus. Nondividing cells are resistant to infection.

Epizootiology and Pathogenesis. CPV-2 was not evident in the dog population before 1977 (Carmichael et al. 1980, Thomas et al. 1984). Within months of its first identification, CPV-2 spread throughout the world and is now considered ubiquitous. When a susceptible dog population is exposed to CPV-2, nearly 100 percent of the dogs become infected within days. Perhaps 75 percent of infections are subclinical, but clinical infections may be severe, with mortality being high. In one study of CPV-2 in a colony of dogs, 29 of 34 infections were subclinical (Parrish, Oliver, and McNiven 1982). Carrier dogs apparently shed virus in the feces periodically. This fact, combined with the extreme resistance of the virus in the environment, makes CPV-2 infection endemic in a population once the initial episode occurs. Sporadic cases occur in nonvaccinated pups once they have lost their passive maternal immunity.

The incidence of cardiomyopathy may be high when CPV infection occurs in newborn pups of susceptible dams. Once breeding-age dogs became immune through natural infection or vaccination, however, the incidence of cardiomyopathy decreases substantially, since neonatal pups—the only susceptible age group at risk for CPV-induced cardiomyopathy—carry protective passive immunity.

The incidence of CPV-1 infection has not been accurately established. The virus has been isolated from many dogs with no clinical disease and from dogs with clinical disease due to other infections. It is believed to be widespread.

The dog and other members of the canid family are susceptible to CPV-2. Coyotes were not infected before 1979, but after 1982 more than 70 percent of serum samples from wild coyotes contained antibodies against CPV-2 (Thomas et al. 1984).

Barker et al. (1983) tested the susceptibility of several species to feline, canine, and mink parvoviruses. Raccoons were highly susceptible to the feline parvovirus and mink enteritis virus, but apparently had only subclinical infections with seroconversion and shedding of virus when infected with CPV-2. Red foxes were susceptible to all three viruses, but showed no clinical signs, whereas striped skunks did not shed virus or show signs of illness. Antibody titers to CPV-2 were reported in 86 percent of coyotes, 79 percent of wild red foxes, 22 percent of wild raccoons, and 1 percent of wild skunks.

Severe parvovirus infection has been reported in three South American canids—maned wolf (*Chrysocyon brachyurus*), bush dog (*Speothos venaticus*), and crab-eating fox (*Cerdocyon thous*) (Fletcher et al. 1979, Mann et al. 1980). In all likelihood, all canids are susceptible to CPV-2 infection and, under appropriate conditions of stress, will develop clinical disease.

CPV-2 is transmitted by the fecal-oral route or by direct dog-to-dog contact. Extremely large quantities of the virus are shed in the feces of infected dogs during acute phase of infection. The resistant virus may be transmitted on shoes, hands, and clothing of people. This is the most likely method by which the infection was spread worldwide in such a short time.

Virus usually enters the dog by the oral route, and the initial infection may occur in the tonsils. It then spreads by means of the lymphatics to produce a primary viremia, which results in infection of all mitotic cells in the body. Virus is present in the thymus on day 1, the germinal centers of the lymph nodes and the spleen by day 2 or 3, and the intestine by day 3 to 4 (Macartney et al. 1984). CPV-2 causes necrosis of the crypt epithelium in the small intestine, often with extensive loss of the epithelial cells and dilatation of the remaining crypts. In advanced cases the epithelium regenerates, and inflammatory cells may infiltrate the lamina propria. Intranuclear inclusion bodies may be present in epithelial cells, but only rarely are they observed, especially if formalin is used as a fixative. Inclusion bodies are more readily observed if tissue specimens are fixed with a hard fixative.

Fecal excretion of CPV begins about 3 days after infection and reaches its peak between days 4 and 7; the amount of virus shed decreases sharply after day 7 (Macartney et al. 1984). This decrease follows by 1 to 2 days the appearance of viral neutralizing antibody in the serum.

Gross and microscopic lesions of CPV-2 infection in dogs are similar to those produced in cats with the feline parvovirus (Cooper et al. 1979, Eugster et al. 1978, Pletcher et al. 1979). The jejunum and ileum are the primary tissues involved; the lymphatic tissue and bone marrow may also be affected. The virus destroys the rapidly dividing crypt epithelium in the small intestine with resulting ballooning of the crypts and shortening, blunting, and fusion of villi.

If puppies from nonimmune bitches become infected in utero or within a few weeks after birth, myocardial disease may occur (Meunier et al. 1984). Virus may persist in cardiac fibers in a latent form, then multiply and cause necrosis of myofibers after the myocytes multiply into multinucleated cells around 3 to 8 weeks (Greene 1984).

Immunity. A rapid and effective humoral virus-neutralizing antibody response occurs in dogs infected with CPV. Antibodies appear in the serum within 5 days after infection, and antibody titers rise rapidly to high levels (Meunier et al. 1985, Nara et al. 1983, Pollock 1982). The initial antibody is IgM; IgG antibody titers appear within a few days. Secretory IgA and IgM antibodies are present in the intestinal tract. Dogs that recover from natural infection, whether clinical or subclinical, are solidly protected against clinical disease. Antibody titers appear to persist for long periods in recovered dogs.

Diagnosis. A clinical diagnosis of canine parvovirus infection in the acute intestinal form is based on clinical findings and hematological results. Laboratory findings of CPV in the feces, seroconversion of antibody titers to the virus, or microscopic lesions in tissues of animals with fatal cases confirm the diagnosis.

Leukopenia commonly occurs in the acute intestinal disease form and is usually lymphopenia rather than neutropenia (Greene 1984). The severity of the leukopenia frequently parallels the severity of the clinical disease. Total leukocyte counts may be 500–2,000 cells/dl. If dogs survive for a few days, total leukocyte counts rebound and leukocytosis results. However, hematological changes are not as consistent with CPV infection as with feline parvovirus infection, and dogs may experience severe clinical disease without significant leukopenia. Other hematological and biochemical findings are usually not diagnostic of the acute intestinal form of CPV infection.

Laboratory confirmation is usually done by identification of the virus itself or of viral protein in the feces. The hemagglutination (HA) test with porcine erythrocytes will identify CPV protein. Electron microscopic (EM) examination of feces can reveal the presence of parvovirus, which, if consistent with clinical signs, can be taken as confirmation of the clinical diagnosis in most cases. However, one cannot distinguish between CPV-1 and CPV-2 with electron microscopy, and therefore the mere presence of parvovirus particles in the feces is in itself not diagnostic of clinical parvovirus infection. Fecal samples for HA or EM examination should be taken as early in clinical disease as possible, cooled in the refrigerator, then submitted to the diagnostic laboratory in a cooled polystyrene shipping carton that contains cold packs.

Serologic assays for CPV antibodies by virus neutralization (VN) or hemagglutination-inhibition (HI) tests can be performed on acute and convalescent paired serum samples. A rise in antibody titer of at least fourfold confirms an active infection. A single acute sample also confirms a recent infection if the assay is run specifically for anticanine parvovirus IgM antibodies.

The diagnosis of myocardial disease caused by CPV-2 is based on the presenting clinical signs of heart insufficiency in the young puppy together with backup laboratory and diagnostic procedures. Echocardiography, ultrasonic cardiography, or radiography should be used to identify cardiac involvement. Clinical chemistry studies showing increased enzyme activities such as those of aspartate aminotransferase (AST), serum glutamic-oxaloacetic transaminase (SGOT), lactic dehydrogenase (LDH), and creatinine phosphokinase (CPK) suggest heart muscle involvement (Greene 1984).

Treatment. No specific antiviral drugs have proved effective against CPV. Treatment therefore involves extensive fluid and supportive therapy to allow sufficient time for an effective antibody response. Administration of lactated Ringer's solution or other appropriate fluid is a must in severe cases of enteritis.

A study by Ishibashi et al. (1983) suggested that hyperimmune serum treatment in dogs within the first 4 days after infection may result in a less severe disease with an increased recovery rate.

Antibiotic treatment in CPV infection is controversial. In most cases it appears that antimicrobial agents are not warranted and in fact may harm the normal intestinal flora. Certainly antibiotics cannot be used in place of adequate fluid and supportive therapy.

The course of clinical disease in myocardial parvovirus infection is usually so rapid that treatment is ineffective. Treatment of unaffected littermates will not prevent cardiac involvement.

Prevention and Control. The prevention and control of CPV infection relies primarily on an effective immunization program; but disinfection, animal movement control, and husbandry practices also must be considered, especially in kennels and adoption shelters.

There are four basic types of vaccines available: inactivated and modified live-virus feline parvovirus vaccines, and inactivated and modified live-virus canine parvovirus vaccines. There has been extensive research on these vaccines and their use in protecting dogs (Appel et al. 1979; Carmichael et al. 1983; Pollock and Carmichael 1982a, 1982b, 1983a, 1983b). A summary of these four types of vaccines has been published by Greene (1984).

Passive, maternally derived antibodies protect puppies against CPV infection, but they also interfere with CPV vaccines. The antibody titer in the pup depends on the antibody titer in the dam; the higher the titer in the dam, the longer the period of interference in the pup. This period of interference may last as long as 16 to 18 weeks. Any vaccination program must therefore take these maternally derived antibody titers into consideration.

No one immunization schedule will fit all circumstances and protect all puppies. Generally, vaccinations should begin at about 6 weeks of age and be repeated at 4-week intervals until the puppies are at least 16 weeks old. Many commercial vaccines are combined with antigens for one or more of the following: canine distemper virus, adenovirus, parainfluenza virus, rabies virus, *Leptospira* species, and *Bordetella bronchiseptica*.

In kennels and adoption shelters, both an adequate disinfection program and proper vaccination schedules must be maintained to control CPV-2. Disinfectants such as commercial bleach or one of the aldehyde preparations will inactivate the virus in the environment and should be routinely used to decontaminate cages, floors, and food and water dishes. Good husbandry will prevent the contact of infected and susceptible dogs and the mechanical spread of virus.

The Disease in Humans. There is no evidence that humans can be infected with canine parvovirus.

REFERENCES

Appel, M.J.G., Scott, F.W., and Carmichael, L.E. 1979. Isolation and immunisation studies of a canine parvo-like virus from dogs with haemorrhagic enteritis. Vet. Rec. 105:156–159.

Barker, I.K., Povey, R.C., and Voigt, D.R. 1983. Response of mink, skunk, red fox and raccoon to inoculation with mink virus enteritis, feline panleukopenia and canine parvovirus and prevalence of antibody to parvovirus in wild carnivores in Ontario. Can. J. Comp. Med. 47:188–197.

Binn, L.N., Lazar, E.C., Eddy, G.A., and Kajima, M. 1970. Recovery and characterization of a minute virus of canines. Infect. Immun. 1:503–508.

Carman, P.S., and Povey, R.C. 1983. Comparison of the viral proteins of canine parvovirus-2, mink enteritis virus and feline panleukopenia virus. Vet. Microbiol. 8:423–435.

Carmichael, L.E., and Binn, L.N. 1981. New enteric viruses in the dog. Adv. Vet. Sci. Comp. Med. 25:1–37.

Carmichael, L.E., Joubert, J.C., and Pollock, R.V.H. 1980. Hemagglutination by canine parvovirus: Serologic studies and diagnostic applications. Am. J. Vet. Res. 41:784–791.

Carmichael, L.E., Joubert, J.C., and Pollock, R.V. 1983. A modified live canine parvovirus vaccine. II. Immune response. Cornell Vet. 73:13–29.

Cooper, B.J., Carmichael, L.E., Appel, M.J., and Greisen, H. 1979. Canine viral enteritis. II. Morphologic lesions in naturally occurring parvovirus infection. Cornell Vet. 69:134–144.

Eugster, A.K. 1980. Studies on canine parvovirus infections: Development of an inactivated vaccine. Am. J. Vet. Res. 41:2020–2024.

Eugster, A.K., Bendele, R.A., and Jones, L.P. 1978. Parvovirus infection in dogs. J. Am. Vet. Med. Assoc. 173:1340–1341.

Fletcher, K.C., Eugster, A.K., Schmidt, R.E., and Hubbard, G.B. 1979. Parvovirus infection in maned wolves. J. Am. Vet. Med. Assoc. 175:897–900.

Greene, C.E. 1984. Canine viral enteritis: Canine parvoviral infection. In C.E. Greene, ed., Clinical Microbiology and Infectious Diseases of the Dog and Cat. W.B. Saunders, Philadelphia. Pp. 437–453

Hayes, M.A., Russell, R.G., and Babiuk, L.A. 1979. Sudden death in young dogs with myocarditis caused by parvovirus. J. Am. Vet. Med. Assoc. 174:1197–1203.

Ishibashi, K., Maede, Y., Ohsugi, T., Onuma, M., and Mikami, T. 1983. Serotherapy for dogs infected with canine parvovirus. Jpn. J. Vet. Sci. 45:59–66.

Jezyk, P.F., Haskins, M.E., and Jones, C.L. 1979. Myocarditis of probable viral origin in pups of weaning age. J. Am. Vet. Med. Assoc. 174:1204–1207.

Macartney, L., McCandlish, I.A., Thompson, H., and Cornwell, H.J. 1984. Canine parvovirus enteritis. 1. Clinical, haematological and pathological features of experimental infection. 2. Pathogenesis. 3. Scanning electron microscopical features of experimental infection. Vet. Rec. 115:201–210, 453–460, 533–537.

Mann, P.C., Bush, M., Appel, M.J.G., Beehler, B.A., and Montali, R.J. 1980. Canine parvovirus infection in South American canids. J. Am. Vet. Med. Assoc. 177:779–783.

Meunier, P.C., Cooper, B.J., Appel, M.J., and Slauson, D.O. 1984. Experimental viral myocarditis: Parvoviral infection of neonatal pups. Vet. Pathol. 21:509–515.

Meunier, P.C., Cooper, B.J., Appel, M.J., and Slauson, D.O. 1985. Pathogenesis of canine parvovirus enteritis: The importance of viremia. Vet. Pathol. 22:60–71.

Mulvey, J.J., Bech-Nielsen, S., Haskins, M.E., Jezyk, P.F., Taylor, H.W., and Eugster, A.K. 1980. Myocarditis induced by parvoviral infection in weanling pups in the United States. J. Am. Vet. Med. Assoc. 177:695–698.

Nara, P.L., Winters, K., Rice, J.B., Olsen, R.G., and Krakowka, S. 1983. Systemic and local intestinal antibody response in dogs given both infective and inactivated canine parvovirus. Am. J. Vet. Res. 44:1989–1995.

Parrish, C.R., and Carmichael, L.E. 1983. Antigenic structure and variation of parvovirus type-2, feline panleukopenia virus, and mink enteritis virus. Virology 129:401–414.

Parrish, C.R., Carmichael, L.E., and Antczak, D.F. 1982. Antigenic relationships between canine parvovirus type 2, feline panleukopenia virus and mink enteritis virus using conventional antisera and monoclonal antibodies. Arch. Virol. 72:267–278.

Parrish, C.R., Oliver, R.E., and McNiven, R. 1982. Canine parvovirus infections in a colony of dogs. Vet. Microbiol. 7:317–324.

Pletcher, J.M., Toft, J.D., Frey, R.M., and Casey, H.W. 1979. Histopathologic evidence for parvovirus infection in dogs. J. Am. Vet. Med. Assoc. 175:825–828.

Pollock, R.V.H. 1982. Experimental canine parvovirus infection in dogs. Cornell Vet. 72:103–119.

Pollock, R.V.H., and Carmichael, L.E. 1982a. Dog response to inactivated canine parvovirus and feline panleukopenia virus vaccines. Cornell Vet. 72:16–35.

Pollock, R.V.H., and Carmichael, L.E. 1982b. Maternally derived immunity to canine parvovirus infection: Transfer, decline and interference with vaccination. J. Am. Vet. Med. Assoc. 180:37–42.

Pollock, R.V.H., and Carmichael, L.E. 1983a. Canine viral enteritis. Vet. Clin. North Am. [Small Anim. Pract.] 13(3):551–566.

Pollock, R.V.H., and Carmichael, L.E. 1983b. Use of modified live feline panleukopenia virus vaccine to immunize dogs against canine parvovirus. Am. J. Vet. Res. 44:169–175.

Surleraux, M., and Burtonboy, G. 1984. Structural polypeptides of a canine parvovirus. Arch. Virol. 82:233–240.

Thomas, N.J., Foreyt, W.J., Evermann, J.F., Windberg, L.A., and Knowlton, F.F. 1984. Seroprevalence of canine parvovirus in wild coyotes from Texas, Utah, and Idaho (1972 to 1983). J. Am. Vet. Med. Assoc. 185:1283–1287.

Bovine Parvovirus Infection

SYNONYM: Hemadsorbing enteric (HADEN) virus infection

Bovine parvovirus (BPV) is a ubiquitous enteric virus of cattle which generally produces a subclinical infection in calves but may possibly produce fetal infection and reproductive failure in susceptible pregnant cows.

Character of the Disease. After an incubation period of 1 to 2 days, diarrhea is the main sign of illness in calves infected with BPV. Initially, feces may be watery; then they may become mucoid. Calves may be listless, but they usually will continue to drink milk. Fever may be as high as 105.8°F. Although most calves recover without serious side effects, some calves may be stunted. BPV has been isolated from calves with conjunctivitis and from those with both respiratory and enteric disease (Storz and Bates 1973; Storz, Leary, et al. 1978).

The role of BPV in reproductive disease has not been fully evaluated. Virus has been isolated from aborted fetuses, and when susceptible pregnant dams were inoculated with BPV, abortion with viral infection of the placenta and fetus occurred (Storz, Young, et al. 1978). In a study of reproductive problems in dairy cattle, 75 percent of cattle with a history of reproductive disease (embryonic mortality, abortion, anestrus, and metritis) had antibody titers to BPV, whereas only 28 percent of cattle without a history of reproductive problems were seropositive (Barnes et al. 1982). BPV may play a far more significant role in reproductive disease in cattle than previously believed.

Properties of the Virus. The first bovine parvovirus was isolated from the enteric tract of normal calves by Abinanti and Warfield (1961), although it was not classified as a parvovirus until later (Storz and Warren 1970). This isolate has been designated the prototype virus. Several isolates have been made from clinically normal cattle, from calves with diarrhea, and from calves with mixed infections of enteroviruses, coronaviruses, adenoviruses, and adeno-associated viruses (Storz, Leary, et al. 1978). BPV isolates have the typical properties of parvoviruses. They contain single-stranded DNA, are approximately 23 nm in diameter, are nonenveloped and resistant, and require mitotic cells for replication. Most strains are antigenically identical to the prototype virus, type 1, but one isolate from Japan appears to possess some antigenic differences (Inaba et al. 1973). All BPV isolates that have been checked are distinct antigenically from parvoviruses of other species.

BPV hemagglutinates erythrocytes from humans, dogs, and guinea pigs (Abinanti and Warfield 1961, Bachmann 1971). It replicates in the nucleus of dividing cells, producing Cowdry type A intranuclear inclusion bodies. Cytolysis of infected cells occurs during viral replication.

Detailed studies on the biochemical properties of BPV have not been reported, but one could reasonably assume that they would not differ appreciably from those of other parvoviruses such as feline and canine parvoviruses.

Epizootiology and Pathogenesis. BPV is ubiquitous in cattle, which are the only known hosts. Studies indicate that the incidence of antibodies to BPV in cattle may be as high as 60 to 85 percent (Abinanti and Warfield 1961, Barnes et al. 1982, Storz et al. 1972). It appears that most calves are infected before they reach adulthood.

Large quantities of virus are shed in the feces. The fecal-oral route thus is the common path of transmission. Like other resistant parvoviruses, BPV withstands environmental conditions, and contaminated premises will harbor infectious virus for long periods of time.

Detailed pathogenetic studies have not been conducted. However, after oral or intravenous exposure to virus, calves contained virus in epithelial cells of the jejunum, ileum, and cecum. Infected calves were viremic with virus isolated from many tissues, including those in spleen, adrenals, lymph nodes, thymus, and heart muscle. Because BPV requires mitotic cells for replication, its pathogenesis appears to be similar to that for mild or subclinical infections with canine and feline parvoviruses.

Immunity. Calves infected with BPV develop a rapid immune response, with antibodies appearing in their serum 5 to 7 days after infection (Liggitt et al. 1982; Storz, Leary, et al. 1978). It is safe to predict that recovered cattle will have solid and long-lasting immunity. Likewise, maternal immunity transferred to offspring through the colostrum should affect the incidence and epidemiology of this disease in calves.

Diagnosis. BPV infection is diagnosed by isolation and identification of the virus in the laboratory and/or confirmation of seroconversion. Because of the numerous agents that can produce enteritis in calves or cause reproductive problems in cattle, clinical diagnosis of BPV is usually not possible.

Identification of parvovirus in feces of calves with diarrhea by electron microscopy is the fastest method of laboratory diagnosis. Virus can also be isolated in cell cultures from feces or aborted fetuses, and viral antigen can be detected in tissues by immunofluorescence. Demonstration of seroconversion or a rise in antibody titer to BPV in acute and convalescent paired serum samples confirms BPV infection.

Detailed pathological studies of BPV-infected calves have not been reported. Brief studies indicate few if any gross changes. Microscopic changes are most prominent in the distal small intestine, where infection of epithelial cells of the crypts and villi results in cell loss. Infection of cells results in production of intranuclear inclusion bodies.

Treatment. Treatment of BPV infection is symptomatic because there are no antiviral compounds effective against parvoviruses. Neonatal calves with BPV-induced diarrhea should be given electrolyte and fluid therapy as indicated.

Prevention and Control. There are no vaccines for BPV, and specific control measures are not used in most herds. Water and feed pails in calf-rearing operations should be treated with a disinfectant such as sodium hypochlorite or glutaraldehyde.

The Disease in Humans. There are no known public health concerns with BPV.

REFERENCES

Abinanti, F.R., and Warfield, M.S. 1961. Recovery of a hemadsorbing virus (HADEN) from the gastrointestinal tract of calves. Virology 14:288–289.

Bachmann, P.A. 1971. Properties of a bovine parvovirus (brief report). Zentralbl. Vet. Med. 18B:80–85.

Barnes, M.A., Wright, R.E., Bodine, A.B., and Alberty, C.F. 1982. Frequency of bluetongue and bovine parvovirus infection in cattle in South Carolina dairy herds. Am. J. Vet. Res. 43:1078–1080.

Inaba, Y., Kurogi, H., Takahashi, E., Sato, K., Tanaka, Y., Goto, Y., Omori, T., and Matumoto, M. 1973. Isolation and properties of bovine parvovirus type 1 from Japanese calves. Arch. Gesam. Virusforsch. 42:54–66.

Liggitt, H.D., DeMartini, J.C., and Pearson, L.D. 1982. Immunologic responses of the bovine fetus to parvovirus infection. Am. J. Vet. Res. 43:1355–1359.

Storz, J., and Bates, R.C. 1973. Parvovirus infection in calves. J. Am. Vet. Med. Assoc. 163:884–886.

Storz, J., and Warren, G.S. 1970. Effect of antimetabolites and actinomycin D on the replication of HADEN, a bovine parvovirus. Arch. Gesam. Virusforsch. 30:190–194.

Storz, J., Bates, R.C., Warren, G.S., and Howard, T.H. 1972. Distribution of antibodies against bovine parvovirus 1 in cattle and other animal species. Am. J. Vet. Res. 33:269–272.

Storz, J., Leary, J.J., Carlson, J.H., and Bates, R.C. 1978. Parvoviruses associated with diarrhea in calves. J. Am. Vet. Med. Assoc. 173:624–627.

Storz, J., Young, S., Carroll, E.J., Bates, R.C., Bowen, R.A., and Keney, D.A. 1978. Parvovirus infection of the bovine fetus: Distribution of infection, antibody response, and age-related susceptibility. Am. J. Vet. Res. 39:1099–1102.

Porcine Parvovirus Infection

Porcine parvovirus (PPV) is a ubiquitous virus of swine that produces subclinical infections in adult and young animals and severe reproductive failure in pregnant sows and gilts. These reproductive failures are characterized by embryonic death with resorption, resulting in small litters, and by fetal infection with subsequent death, resulting in fetal mummification.

The first report of a possible association between PPV and reproductive failure in swine was by Cartwright and Huck (1967) in England. Subsequent reports of a similar association came from many parts of the world (Johnson

1973, Mayr et al. 1968, Mengeling 1972, Rodeffer et al. 1975). The first experimental reproduction of PPV disease was by Joo et al. (1976) and by Mengeling and Cutlip (1976).

Mengeling (1981, 1986) has provided comprehensive reviews of PPV infection.

Character of the Disease. In postnatal pigs acute infection is usually subclinical even though virus may replicate to high titers in tissues containing rapidly dividing cells (Brown et al. 1980). Viral replication is especially significant in lymphoid tissues (Cutlip and Mengeling 1975). The intestinal crypt cells are not involved in PPV as they are with many of the other parvoviruses, but there may be transient leukopenia during the acute stage (Joo et al. 1976, Mengeling 1981, Mengeling and Cutlip 1976). Brown et al. (1980) summarized PPV infection in postnatal pigs: "PPV infection of susceptible swine, other than pregnant females, has no harmful effect and will probably go unnoticed" (p. 1223).

The only significant disease produced by PPV is maternal reproductive failure (Mengeling 1981). Depending on when in gestation infection occurs, "dams may return to estrus, fail to farrow despite being anestrus, farrow few pigs per litter, or farrow a large proportion of mummified fetuses" (p. 356). Dams show no signs of disease other than a decrease in abdominal girth as the fetuses die and the fluids are resorbed. Other signs of reproductive failure such as infertility, abortion, stillbirths, neonatal deaths, and reduced neonatal viability may occasionally be observed. There is no evidence of reproductive disease in the boar.

Properties of the Virus. Porcine parvovirus is a typical member of the genus *Parvovirus* in the family Parvoviridae. All isolates studied to date are antigenically identical to each other, but PPV is antigenically distinct from the other parvoviruses that infect domestic animals and humans.

The biochemical and biophysical properties of PPV have been studied by several workers, including Cartwright et al. (1969), Mayr et al. (1968), Mengeling (1972), Siegl et al. (1971). This virus is a single-stranded DNA, nonenveloped resistant organism approximately 20 to 25 nm in diameter. It has cubic symmetry and has 32 capsomeres on the virion.

Replication of PPV is typical of that of other parvoviruses. It requires a mitotic cell because the genome does not code for all the necessary proteins. Replication occurs in the nucleus of the infected cell, and the cell is destroyed by cytolysis in the process of replication and release of virions (Shahrabadi et al. 1982).

Like other parvoviruses, PPV is extremely stable and persists on infected premises for months or years after an active infection. The virus is resistant to most common disinfectants (Brown 1981).

PPV hemagglutinates erythrocytes of several species, and guinea pig erythrocytes are most commonly used in the assay (Mengeling 1981).

Epizootiology and Pathogenesis. Porcine parvovirus is ubiquitous in the pig population, and therefore the exposure rate is high. The most common route of infection is oronasal in postnatal piglets and transplacental in fetuses (Mengeling 1981). During the acute phase postnatal pigs shed large quantities of virus in the feces, but once the immune response occurs, shedding of virus ceases. Chronic shedders of virus have not been demonstrated.

After exposure of postnatal pigs to PPV, viremia develops usually by day 2 and lasts for 4 to 5 days. Many tissues contain virus, with the highest titers in the lymphoid tissues. There are no detectable changes in the T and B lymphocytes, no gross or microscopic lesions are evident, and infected nonpregnant pigs do not show any clinical signs of disease (Brown et al. 1980, Cutlip and Mengeling 1975).

When pregnant susceptible sows or gilts become infected, viremia occurs during the acute infection. Virus readily crosses the placenta to infect one or more of the embryos or fetuses, but such infection often requires 10 to 14 days after exposure of the dam before it occurs. The stage of gestation at the time of infection determines the effect on the fetuses or embryos. If infection occurs before mid-gestation (56 days), the conceptus will become infected and die. If the conceptus is less than 30 days' gestation (embryo) when infected, it will be resorbed. A conceptus between 30 and 70 days' gestation (fetus) when infected will die and mummify. Most fetuses beyond 70 days of age at the time of infection develop an immune response and survive with no ill effects. An occasional stillbirth or neonatal death will occur with fetuses infected during late gestation (Mengeling 1978, 1981, 1986; Mengeling and Paul 1981; Mengeling et al. 1975, 1980; Thacker et al. 1981).

Immunity. Pigs infected with PPV develop an effective immune response with high titers of virus-neutralizing antibodies. Recovered swine are probably solidly immune for life.

Diagnosis. A tentative clinical diagnosis of PPV infection in a herd of breeding swine is usually possible on the basis of clinical signs of reproductive failure with resorptions but not abortions, small litter size without fetal anomalies, and a large number of mummified fetuses in litters of otherwise healthy sows and gilts. Confirmation requires laboratory identification of PPV in the fetuses, or the identification of seroconversion to PPV.

PPV can be identified by immunofluorescent microscopy of fetal tissues, or by virus isolation in cell cultures from tissues of recently infected fetuses and occasionally from mummified fetuses. Demonstration of seroconversion to PPV by determining antibody titers in acute and convalescent serums confirms the diagnosis. Usually by the time the reproductive disease is evident, however, the dam already has a high titer. A single serum sample from the dam is of little value since the incidence of PPV is very high. Demonstration of antibody to PPV in presuckling serums or body fluids of newborn or stillborn piglets also confirms the diagnosis (Mengeling 1981).

Treatment. Since infection in postnatal pigs is subclinical, treatment is not indicated.

Prevention and Control. Both inactivated and modified live-virus vaccines will protect sows against PPV reproductive disease (Mengeling et al. 1979, Paul and Mengeling 1980). Therefore, sows and gilts should be vaccinated before breeding. Two doses of inactivated vaccine should be given 2 to 4 weeks apart, starting 4 to 8 weeks before breeding. A single booster vaccination should be given 2 to 6 weeks before subsequent breedings. Inactivated vaccines may be combined with other antigens such as those for *Leptospira* or pseudorabies virus. Maternally derived immunity will not interfere with vaccination of gilts that are approaching breeding age (Paul et al. 1982).

Modified live-virus vaccines have been developed for experimental studies (Paul and Mengeling 1980, 1984). If available commercially, these should solidly immunize swine with a single dose given at least a few weeks prior to breeding. Protection should be of long duration.

If breeding sows and gilts have not been vaccinated, they should not be introduced into an enzootic area of PPV near or during pregnancy.

The use of disinfectants, such as sodium hypochlorite, that are effective against parvoviruses is recommended where possible in breeding facilities (Brown 1981). Since the virus is extremely stable in the environment, facilities, equipment, and food and water containers should be disinfected before introduction of a new batch of pigs.

The Disease in Humans. There is no evidence of infection in humans.

REFERENCES

Brown, T.T. 1981. Laboratory evaluation of selected disinfectants as virucidal agents against porcine parvovirus, pseudorabies virus, and transmissible gastroenteritis virus. Am. J. Vet. Res. 42:1033–1036.

Brown, T.T., Paul, P.S., and Mengeling, W.L. 1980. Response of conventionally raised weanling pigs to experimental infection with a virulent strain of porcine parvovirus. Am. J. Vet. Res. 41:1221–1224.

Cartwright, S.F., and Huck, R.A. 1967. Viruses isolated in association with herd infertility, abortions and stillbirths in pigs. Vet. Rec. 81:196–197.

Cartwright, S.F., Lucas, M., and Huck, R.A. 1969. A small haemagglutinating porcine DNA virus. I. Isolation and properties. J. Comp. Pathol. 79:371–377.

Cutlip, R.C., and Mengeling, W.L. 1975. Experimentally induced infection of neonatal swine with porcine parvovirus. Am. J. Vet. Res. 36:1179–1182.

Johnson, R.H. 1973. Isolation of swine parvovirus in Queensland. Aust. Vet. J. 49:157–159.

Joo, H.S., Donaldson-Wood, C.R. and Johnson, R.H. 1976. Observations on the pathogenesis of porcine parvovirus infection. Arch. Virol. 51:123–129.

Mayr, A., Bachmann, P.A., Siegl, G., Mahnel, H., and Sheffy, B.E. 1968. Characterization of a small porcine DNA virus. Arch. Gesam. Virusforsch. 25:38–51.

Mengeling, W.L. 1972. Porcine parvovirus: Properties and prevalence of a strain isolated in the United States. Am. J. Vet. Res. 33:2239–2248.

Mengeling, W.L. 1978. Prevalence of porcine parvovirus-induced reproductive failure: An abattoir study. J. Am. Vet. Med. Assoc. 172:1291–1294.

Mengeling, W.L. 1981. Porcine parvovirus infection. In A.D. Leman, R.D. Glock, W.L. Mengeling, R.H.C. Penny, E. Scholl, and B. Straw, eds., Diseases of Swine, 5th ed. Iowa State University Press, Ames. Pp. 352–365.

Mengeling, W.L. 1986. Porcine parvovirus infection. In A.D. Leman, B. Straw, R.D. Glock, W.L. Mengeling, R.H.C. Penny, and E. Scholl, eds., Diseases of Swine, 6th ed. Iowa State University Press, Ames. Pp. 411–424.

Mengeling, W.L., and Cutlip, R.C. 1976. Reproductive disease experimentally induced by exposing pregnant gilts to porcine parvovirus. Am. J. Vet. Res. 37:1393–1400.

Mengeling, W.L., and Paul, P.S. 1981. Reproductive performance of gilts exposed to porcine parvovirus at 56 or 70 days of gestation. Am. J. Vet. Res. 42:2074–2076.

Mengeling, W.L., Brown, T.T., Paul, P.S., and Gutekunst, D.E. 1979. Efficacy of an inactivated virus vaccine for prevention of porcine parvovirus-induced reproductive failure. Am. J. Vet. Res. 40:204–207.

Mengeling, W.L., Cutlip, R.C., Wilson, R.A., Parks, J.B., and Marshall, R.F. 1975. Fetal mummification associated with porcine parvovirus infection. J. Am. Vet. Med. Assoc. 166:993–995.

Mengeling, W.L., Paul, P.S., and Brown, T.T. 1980. Transplacental infection and embryonic death following maternal exposure to porcine parvovirus near the time of conception. Arch. Virol. 65:55–62.

Paul, P.S., and Mengeling, W.L. 1980. Evaluation of a modified live-virus vaccine for the prevention of porcine parvovirus-induced reproductive disease in swine. Am. J. Vet. Res. 41:2007–2011.

Paul, P.S., and Mengeling, W.L. 1984. Oronasal and intramuscular vaccination of swine with a modified live porcine parvovirus vaccine: Multiplication and transmission of the vaccine virus. Am. J. Vet. Res. 45:2481–2485.

Paul, P.S., Mengeling, W.L., and Pirtle, E.C. 1982. Duration and biological half-life of passively acquired colostral antibodies to porcine parvovirus. Am. J. Vet. Res. 43:1376–1379.

Rodeffer, H.E., Leman, A.D., Dunne, H.W., Cropper, M., and Sprecher, D.J. 1975. Reproductive failure in swine associated with maternal seroconversion for porcine parvovirus. J. Am. Vet. Med. Assoc. 166:991–992.

Shahrabadi, M.S., Lynch, J., Cho, H.J., and Marusyk, R.G. 1982. Studies on the multiplication of a porcine parvovirus. Vet. Microbiol. 7:117–125.

Siegl, G., Hallauer, C., Novak, A., and Kronauer, G. 1971. Parvoviruses as contaminants of permanent human cell lines. II. Physiochemical properties of the isolated viruses. Arch. Gesam. Virusforsch. 35:91–103.

Thacker, B.J., Leman, A.D., Hurtgen, J.P., Sauber, T.E., and Joo, H.S. 1981. Survey of porcine parvovirus infection in swine fetuses and their dams at a Minnesota abattoir. Am. J. Vet. Res. 42:865–867.

Aleutian Disease in Mink

SYNONYMS: Hypergammaglobulinemia, plasmacytosis; abbreviation, AD

Aleutian disease is an immunological disorder caused by persistent parvovirus infection and is characterized by genetic predisposition, persistent viremia, pronounced plasmacytosis, hypergammaglobulinemia, and progressive immune complexes. The increased susceptibility of genetically defined types of mink appears to be associated with an inherited dysfunction of the protective mechanism comparable to the Chédiak-Higashi syndrome in humans and in cattle.

The disease, originally seen in 1946, was first described by Hartsough and Gorham (1956). It is considered the most important infectious disease plaguing the mink industry (Shen et al. 1981). The history of the disease has been reviewed by Gorham et al. (1965) and by Porter et al. (1980). The term *Aleutian disease* was coined because the disease has a predilection for the recessive Aleutian genotype of mink. This genotype is a mutant coat color that first appeared in Oregon in 1941, and the gun-metal or "blue mink" color was called "Aleutian" because it resembled the pelt color of the Aleutian fox.

Character of the Disease. AD is a chronic, progressive disease of high mortality and morbidity characterized by anorexia, weight loss, lethargy, polydipsia, and hemorrhage. It has a long incubation period, and death usually occurs in a few to many months. Compared with that for Aa and AA genotypes, the mortality rate is five to eight times higher in mink with the recessive aa Aleutian genotype (Gorham et al. 1965).

Ocular lesions manifested as uveitis and iridocyclitis with cellular infiltration of the limbus are common in mink affected with AD (Hadlow 1982). These lesions probably result from the deposition of immune complexes.

Properties of the Virus. Several workers independently reported in 1962 that AD is caused by a virus (Gorham et al. 1965, Karstad and Pridham 1962, Trautwein and Helmboldt 1962). Several isolates have been made and their properties and pathogenicities evaluated. Most of these studies found that the virus has many properties like those of parvoviruses (Bloom et al. 1980, Porter et al. 1980, Yoon et al. 1975).

The size of AD virus particles ranges from 22 to 25 nm. The virus is nonenveloped and has cubic symmetry; the capsid contains 32 capsomeres. The density of the complete virions in cesium chloride is 1.40 to 1.43. The nucleic acid is single stranded DNA, with 4.8 kilobase pairs (Mayer et al. 1983).

Studies have indicated that three main proteins are coded for by the genome (Aasted et al. 1984, Mayer et al. 1983, Porter et al. 1980), although there is no agreement on the sizes of these proteins. Aasted et al. (1984) and van Dawen et al. (1983) indicated that there were two viral structural proteins of molecular mass 85,000 and 75,000 daltons, while Bloom et al. (1980) found two proteins of 89,100 and 77,600 daltons. A third nonstructural protein of 71,000 daltons was detected by Aasted et al. (1984). Other studies have reported that the individual polypeptides were much smaller, in the range of 20,000 to 35,000 daltons (Porter et al. 1980). Aasted et al. (1980) suggested that during infection the Aleutian disease virus (ADV) proteins were changed to smaller, highly antigenic polypeptides.

ADV is resistant to detergents, lipid solvents, and most disinfectants, but it is susceptible to some halogen derivatives (iodophor and sodium hypochlorite) as well as 2 percent glutaraldehyde (Shen et al. 1981). The virus is heat stable and is inactivated slowly at 56°C.

Cultivation. Specific morphologic alterations are produced by ADV in cultures of mink testis, mink kidney cells, or Crandell feline kidney cells (Basrur et al. 1963, Hahn et al. 1977, van Dawen et al. 1983). Virus apparently grows to higher titers at 31.8°C than at 37°C.

Epizootiology and Pathogenesis. Mink are the primary host for ADV, but certain other species of Mustelidae can be infected. Kenyon et al. (1978) studied the host range of a number of mustelids and viverrids. They found that ranch mink (*Mustela vision*), domestic ferrets (*Mustela putorius*), weasels (*Mustela erminea*), fisher (*Martes pennanti*), American marten (*Martes americana*), and striped skunks (*Mephitis mephitis*) had an immunological response to injection with ADV which was similar to that of mink with AD. AD lesions were present in ferrets and striped skunks, in addition to mink. Marten had an increased lymphocyte response in splenic red pulp, but weasels and fisher had no lesions of AD. Ten other species of Mustelidae and Viverridae had no immune response or lesions.

The disease is readily produced in genetically susceptible mink. Although Aleutian mink develop lesions more quickly and die sooner after injections, other genotypes are also susceptible (Trautwein and Helmboldt 1962). The virus can be serially transferred in mink (Gorham et al. 1964).

Both vertical and horizontal transmission occurs on infected mink ranches (Bazeley 1976, Gorham et al. 1965, Porter et al. 1980). Infection is persistent, with virus shed in the saliva, feces, and urine (Gorham et al. 1964, Shen et al. 1981). Thus, one or more of every litter of kits from an infected dam usually becomes infected. Virus is transmitted horizontally between infected and susceptible mink by contact, through bites, or by indirect fecal and urinary contamination (Shen et al. 1981). Aerosol transmission may also occur (Porter et al. 1980).

While viral replication occurs relatively quickly after exposure, with virus first being detected in gut and kidney by day 3 to 6 (Aasted and Bloom 1983), clinical disease or lesions may not develop until approximately 1 month after infection (Porter et al. 1980). The pathogenicity of ADV varies with different strains (Hadlow et al. 1983).

Two distinct forms of infection occur in mink. The first is an unapparent, nonprogressive infection that does not result in clinical AD and is not fatal, but the mink are persistently infected. The second type is a progressive immunological disease with persistent infection and immune complex–mediated glomerulonephritis and arteritis (An and Ingram 1977, 1978). Overproduction of antibody against ADV results in hypergammaglobulinemia, but this antibody is nonneutralizing. The virus is lymphotrophic and can persist in both B and T lymphocytes for long periods (Roth et al. 1984). Lethal changes arise during one of the hypergammaglobulinemia episodes. The gamma globulin level may reach 11 g/dl, and the virus circulates as infectious antigen-antibody complexes that are deposited in the renal glomeruli and in arteries and cause severe inflammatory lesions (Porter et al. 1980).

At necropsy the kidneys are enlarged, pale yellow, and mottled; the liver may be slightly enlarged and mottled. Animals that die in the early stages of the disease may have an enlarged spleen and lymph nodes (Gorham et al. 1965). Histological alterations are characterized by marked plasmacytosis of the lymph nodes, spleen, liver, and kidneys; marked rise in serum gamma globulin; hepatic degeneration with bile duct proliferation; and smudging of glomerular basement membranes (Helmboldt and Jungherr 1958). The severity of lesions is related to the degree of hypergammaglobulinemia. In one-fourth of natural cases there are vascular lesions consisting of segmental periarteritis and fibrinoid degeneration of small and medium-sized arteries.

Overt signs of Aleutian disease are not seen in naturally or experimentally infected ferrets (Porter et al. 1982). The infection produces a systemic proliferation of lymphoid elements in association with a hypergammaglobulinemia. Natural subclinical infection also occurs in ferrets maintained on ranches where AD is found in mink.

Immunity. Although plasmacytosis and hypergammaglobulinemia are characteristic of the disease, there is no evidence of natural or acquired immunity. The majority of the increased immunoglobulin in affected mink is IgG, but IgA levels are also markedly elevated in the serum of ADV-infected mink (Porter et al. 1984). IgM

levels are elevated about 6 days after infection, reach maximal levels by 15 to 18 days, and return to normal by 60 days. The first anti-ADV antibody to appear is IgM, and virus-specific IgM can persist for at least 85 days.

Gamma globulin from infected mink fails to neutralize virus, but circulating infectious antigen-antibody complexes do occur; these complexes are deposited in the renal glomeruli, in blood vessel walls, and in the eye. In one study counterelectrophoresis and complement fixation were reliably specific for AD antibody, whereas immunofluorescence was less reproducible. Immunofluorescence complement fixation was four to eight times more sensitive than regular or modified counterelectrophoresis but was limited by background staining and anticomplementary activity when used to detect small amounts of antibody in undiluted serums (Crawford et al. 1977).

Diagnosis. The diagnosis of AD can be established in several ways: (1) demonstration of serum antibodies against ADV, (2) a series of positive iodine agglutination tests of increasing activity, (3) clinical signs, and (4) typical lesions at necropsy.

Several tests, including immunofluorescence, complement fixation, counterelectrophoresis, radioimmunoassay, and ELISA, have been used to detect antiviral antibodies against ADV (Aasted and Bloom 1983, Porter et al. 1980). Virus-neutralization tests are not effective assays. Counterelectrophoresis, although not as sensitive as other tests, is practical and reliable for routine use. ELISA in one study did not reveal the nonprogressive form of the disease in subclinically infected mink and therefore was not considered a reliable screening test (Wright and Wilkie 1982). Radioimmunoassay was found to be more sensitive than other antibody assays (Aasted and Bloom 1983). The iodine test reveals an increase in gamma globulin, a decrease in albumin, an increase in total serum proteins, and a change in the A:G ratio (Gorham et al. 1964). The cytoplasmic inclusion bodies of Aleutian disease stain strongly by the periodic acid–Schiff method, which differentiates them from distemper inclusions.

Treatment. There is no effective treatment for AD.

Prevention and Control. No vaccine is available to protect mink against AD. Karstad et al. (1963) produced an inactivated vaccine by treating tissues of infected mink with 0.3 percent of formalin at 37°C. Vaccinated mink maintained in contact with infected mink failed to contract the disease, but they succumbed to injection with infective tissue suspension—even after vaccination with three doses.

Mink that have AD antibody also harbor the virus. By eliminating mink with AD antibody from a ranch,

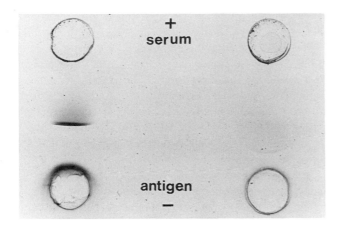

Figure 41.7. Counterimmunoelectrophoresis test for Aleutian disease. The positive antigen-antibody system is on the left, as indicated by the line of identity between the two wells, whereas the negative one is on the right. The positive (+) and the negative (−) signs indicate the presence of an electrical system. (From Tizard, 1977, courtesy of W.B. Saunders Co.)

breeders may eliminate the infection; counterimmunoelectrophoresis (Figure 41.7) is extremely useful in identifying these animals (Cho and Greenfield 1978).

The Disease in Humans. ADV is not known to cause infection in humans.

REFERENCES

Aasted, B., and Bloom, M.E. 1983. Sensitive radioimmune assay for measuring Aleutian disease virus antigen and antibody. J. Clin. Microbiol. 18:637–644.

Aasted, B., Avery, B., and Cohn, A. 1984. Serological analyses of different mink Aleutian disease virus strains. Arch. Virol. 80:11–22.

An, S.H., and Ingram, D.G. 1977. Detection of inapparent Aleutian disease virus infection in mink. Am. J. Vet. Res. 38:1619–1624.

An, S.H., and Ingram, D.G. 1978. Transmission of Aleutian disease from mink with inapparent infections. Am. J. Vet. Res. 39:309–313.

Basrur, P.K., Gray, D.P., and Karstad, L. 1963. Aleutian disease (plasmacytosis) of mink. III. Propagation of the virus in mink tissue cultures. Can. J. Comp. Med. 27:301–306.

Bazeley, P.L. 1976. The nature of Aleutian disease in mink. I. Two forms of hypergammaglobulinemia as related to method of disease transmission and type of lesion. J. Infect. Dis. 134:252–270.

Bloom, M.E., Race, R.E., and Wolfinbarger, J.B. 1980. Characterization of Aleutian disease virus as a parvovirus. J. Virol. 35:836–843.

Cho, H.J., and Greenfield, J. 1978. Eradication of Aleutian disease of mink by eliminating positive counterimmunoelectrophoresis test reactors. J. Clin. Microbiol. 7:18–22.

Crawford, T.B., McGuire, T.C., Porter, D.D., and Cho, H.J. 1977. A comparative study of detection methods for Aleutian disease viral antibody. J. Immunol. 118:1249–1251.

Gorham, J.R., Leader, R.W., and Henson, J.B. 1964. The experimental transmission of a virus causing hypergammaglobulinemia in mink: Sources and modes of infection. J. Infect. Dis. 114:341–345.

Gorham, J.R., Leader, R.W., Padgett, G.A., Burger, D., and Henson, J.B. 1965. Some observations on the natural occurrence of Aleutian disease. In D.C. Gajdusek, ed., Slow, Latent, and Temperate Virus Infections. U.S. Government Printing Office, Washington, D.C. Pp. 279–285.

Hadlow, W.J. 1982. Ocular lesions in mink affected with Aleutian disease. Vet. Pathol. 19:5–15.

Hadlow, W.J., Race, R.E., and Kennedy, R.C. 1983. Comparative pathogenicity of four strains of Aleutian disease virus for pastel and sapphire mink. Infect. Immun. 41:1016–1023.

Hahn, E.C., Ramos, L., and Kenyon, A.J. 1977. Properties of Aleutian disease virus assayed with feline kidney cells. Arch. Virol. 55:315–326.

Hartsough, G.R., and Gorham, J.R. 1956. Aleutian disease in mink. Natl. Fur News 28:10–11.

Helmboldt, C.F., and Jungherr, E.L. 1958. The pathology of Aleutian disease in mink. Am. J. Vet. Res. 19:212–222.

Karstad, L., and Pridham, T.J. 1962. Aleutian disease of mink. I. Evidence of its viral etiology. Can. J. Comp. Med. 26:97–102.

Karstad, L., Pridham, T.J., and Gray, D.P. 1963. Aleutian disease (plasmacytosis) of mink. II. Responses of mink to formalin-treated diseased tissue and to subsequent challenge with virulent inoculum. Can. J. Comp. Med. 27:124–128.

Kenyon, A.J., Helmboldt, C.F., and Nielson, S.W. 1963. Experimental transmission of Aleutian disease with urine. Am. J. Vet. Res. 24:1066–1067.

Kenyon, A.J., Kenyon, B.J., and Hahn, E.C. 1978. Protides of the Mustelidae: Immunoresponse of mustelids to Aleutian mink disease virus. Am. J. Vet. Res. 39:1011–1015.

Mayer, L.W., Aasted, B., Garon, C.F., and Bloom, M.E. 1983. Molecular cloning of the Aleutian disease virus genome: Expression of Aleutian disease virus antigens by a recombinant plasmid. J. Virol. 48:573–579.

Porter, D.D., Larsen, A.E., and Porter, H.G. 1980. Aleutian disease of mink. Adv. Immunol. 29:261–286.

Porter, D.D., Porter, H.G., Suffin, S.C., and Larsen, A.E. 1984. Immunoglobulin classes of Aleutian disease virus antibody. Infect. Immun. 43:463–466.

Porter, H.G., Porter, D.D., and Larsen, A.E. 1982. Aleutian disease in ferrets. Infect. Immun. 36:379–386.

Roth, S., Kaaden, O.R., van Dawen, S., and Moennig, V. 1984. Aleutian disease virus in B and T lymphocytes from blood and spleen and in bone marrow cells from naturally infected mink. Intervirology 22:211–217.

Shen, D.T., Leendertsen, L.W., and Gorham, J.R. 1981. Evaluation of chemical disinfectants for Aleutian disease virus of mink. Am. J. Vet. Res. 42:838–840.

Tizard, I.R. 1977. An Introduction to Veterinary Immunology. W.B. Saunders, Philadelphia.

Trautwein, G.W., and Helmboldt, C.F. 1962. Aleutian disease of mink. I. Experimental transmission of the disease. Am. J. Vet. Res. 23:1280–1288.

van Dawen, S., Kaaden, O.R., and Roth, S. 1983. Propagation of Aleutian disease parvovirus in cell line CCC clone 81. Arch. Virol. 77:39–50.

Wright, P.F., and Wilkie, B.N. 1982. Detection of antibody in Aleutian disease of mink: Comparison of enzyme-linked immunosorbent assay and counterimmunoelectrophoresis. Am. J. Vet. Res. 43:865–868.

Yoon, J.W., Dunker, A.K., and Kenyon, A.J. 1975. Characterization of Aleutian mink disease virus. Virology 64:575–580.

42 The Papovaviridae

Viruses in the Papovaviridae family are small (42 to 55 nm), nonenveloped, stable organisms with double-stranded DNA. The term *papovavirus* was coined by Melnick (1962) for the first viruses described in this group—human *papilloma* (or wart virus), mouse *polyomavirus*, and *vacuolating* virus (simian virus 40, or SV-40).

The family Papovaviridae comprises two genera, the division based on the size of member viruses' genomes and the diameter of their capsids (Lancaster and Olson 1981, Melnick et al. 1974): (1) *papillomavirus*, small (50 to 55 nm), nonenveloped DNA viruses that produce papillomatosis (warts) in animals and humans; and (2) *Polyomavirus*, small (42 to 45 nm) DNA viruses that are nonpathogenic for the most part in their natural host, although they can produce tumors in newborn rodents.

Because the viruses in the genus *Polyomavirus* do not cause diseases in domestic animals, this chapter covers only the diseases caused by the genus *Papillomavirus*.

The Genus *Papillomavirus*

The papillomaviruses contain double-stranded cyclic DNA with a mass of about 5×10^6 daltons, which is sufficient to code for about 300,000 daltons of protein (Lancaster and Olson 1981).

Up to 10 polypeptides can be identified from papillomaviruses. The major polypeptides range in size from 50,000 to 63,000 daltons (Lancaster and Olson 1978, Spira et al. 1974). Immunological cross-reactivity does not occur between papillomaviruses of different animal species, although these viruses apparently do share a common internal antigen (Jenson et al. 1980). Several of them hemagglutinate erythrocytes by reacting with neuraminidase-sensitive receptors.

The viruses studied in this genus are small icosahedral virions, 53 nm in diameter. The capsid is composed of 72 capsomeres in a skew arrangement. The buoyant density in cesium chloride is 1.34 g/ml.

Because papillomaviruses are nonenveloped, they do not contain lipids or carbohydrates and are quite resistant to environmental conditions. They are ether-resistant, acid-stable, and heat-stable. Although it has not been determined yet, it is likely that they would be relatively resistant to disinfectants.

Papillomaviruses do not reproduce readily in cell cultures (Lancaster and Olson 1981, Taichman et al. 1984); consequently, details of their replication are sketchy. Viral replication and assembly of the virions occur in the nucleus. Infection of cells cause transformation of these cells, resulting in tumor or wart formation. Papillomaviruses have a predilection for epithelial cells, and usually infection is not only species-specific but also restricted to certain defined epithelial tissues (Smith and Campo 1985).

A number of species-specific papillomaviruses of animals and humans are listed in Table 42.1. Several serotypes of virus have been identified for some viruses, especially the bovine papillomavirus.

The type species of the genus *Papillomavirus* is the Shope papillomavirus. Other members of the genus are the rabbit oral papillomavirus, human papillomaviruses, canine papillomavirus, canine oral papillomavirus, and six serotypes of bovine papillomaviruses. Additional members include the viruses causing papillomata of horses, sheep, goats, deer, hamsters, monkeys, and other species.

The principal viruses in the genus are oncogenic, especially in newborn or young animals. Nucleic acid extracted from these viruses is oncogenic. Subacute, latent, and chronic infections are commonly produced by these viruses. Papillomas, or common warts, occur in many species of animals. They seem to be most frequent in humans, cattle, dogs, and rabbits. All of these tumors contain filterable agents with which tumors can be induced in other individuals. They appear to have a high degree of host specificity, and some of them even have specificities for particular kinds of epithelium within a single host. Warts occur in epizootic form in herds of cattle and in kennels of dogs. All varieties are most prevalent in the young of the species.

Table 42.1. Papillomaviruses of animals and humans

Virus	Hosts	Disease produced	Primary site
Bovine papillomavirus			
BPV-1	Cattle	Fibropapilloma	Skin
BPV-2	Cattle	Fibropapilloma	Skin
BPV-3	Cattle	Papilloma	Skin
BPV-4	Cattle	Papilloma	Gut
BPV-5	Cattle	Fibropapilloma	Teats
BPV-6	Cattle	Papilloma	Udder
Equine papillomavirus	Horses	Papilloma	Skin
Caprine papillomavirus	Goats	Fibropapilloma	Skin
Ovine papillomavirus	Sheep	Fibropapilloma	Skin
Canine oral papillomavirus	Dogs	Papilloma	Oral mucosa
Canine papillomavirus	Dogs	Papilloma	Skin
Shope rabbit papillomavirus	Rabbits	Papilloma	Skin
Rabbit oral papillomavirus	Rabbits	Papilloma	Oral mucosa
Pig papillomavirus?	Pigs	Papilloma	Genitals
Deer fibromavirus	Deer	Fibroma	Skin
Elk papillomavirus	Elk	Fibropapilloma	Skin
Mouse papillomavirus	Mice	Papilloma	Skin
Chaffinch papillomavirus	Birds	Papilloma	Skin
Human papillomavirus, 8 serotypes	Humans	Papilloma	Skin, mucosa

Compiled from information in Hunt 1984, Jarrett et al. 1984, Lancaster and Olson 1982.

REFERENCES

Hunt, E. 1984. Infectious skin diseases of cattle. Vet. Clin. North Am. [Large Anim. Pract.] 6(1):155–174.

Jarrett, W.F., Campo, M.S., O'Neil, B.W., Laird, H.M., and Coggins, L.W. 1984. A novel bovine papillomavirus (BPV-6) causing true epithelial papillomas of the mammary gland skin: A member of a proposed new BPV subgroup. Virology 30:255–264.

Jenson, A.B., Rosenthal, J.D., Olson, C., Pass, F., Lancaster, W.D., and Shah, K. 1980. Immunologic relatedness of papillomaviruses from different species. J. Natl. Cancer Inst. 64:495–500.

Lancaster, W.D., and Olson, C. 1978. Demonstration of two distinct classes of bovine papilloma virus. Virology 89:372–379.

Lancaster, W.D., and Olson, C. 1981. Papovavirus infections of vertebrate animals. In E. Kurstak and C. Kurstak, eds., Comparative Diagnosis of Viral Diseases, vol. 3. Academic Press, New York. Pp. 69–98.

Lancaster, W.D., and Olson, C. 1982. Animal papillomaviruses. Microbiol. Rev. 46:191–207.

Melnick, J.L. 1962. Papova virus group. Science 135:1128–1130.

Melnick, J.L., Allison, A.C., Butel, J.S., Eckhart, W., Eddy, B.E., Kit, S., Levine, A.J., Miles, J.A.R., Pagano, J.S., Sachs, L., and Vonka, V. 1974. Papovaviridae. Intervirology 3:106–120.

Smith, K.T., and Campo, M.S. 1985. The biology of papillomaviruses and their role in oncogenesis. Anticancer Res. 5:31–47.

Spira, G., Estes, M.K., Dressman, G.R., Butel, J.S., and Rawls, W.E. 1974. Papovavirus structural polypeptides: Comparison of human and rabbit papilloma viruses with simian virus 40. Intervirology 3:220–231.

Taichman, L.B., Breitburd, F., Croissant, O., and Orth, G. 1984. The search for a culture system for papillomavirus. J. Invest. Dermatol. 83:2s–6s.

Bovine Papillomatosis

SYNONYMS: Fibropapillomatosis, infectious papilloma, warts

Bovine papillomatosis is a common viral disease of the skin of young cattle, manifested as benign tumors or warts. Papillomas or fibropapillomas may also occur on teats and udders of cows, the penis of bulls, in the alimentary tract, the larynx, the urinary bladder, and the eye.

Skin warts frequently occur in calves and young stock less than 2 years old, most often in the winter when the animals are closely housed. Warts on the teats and udders of cows and on the penis of bulls occur frequently in mature cattle. Outbreaks of laryngeal papillomas have been reported, as have urinary bladder papillomas and ocular papillomas. These are seen less frequently than common skin warts.

There is some evidence that one or more of the bovine papillomaviruses may also be involved in equine sarcoids (Lancaster and Olson 1981). BPV-1 DNA has been isolated from naturally occurring equine sarcoids (Amtmann et al. 1980, Trenfield et al. 1985). The horse is susceptible to experimental inoculation with BPV-1 and BPV-2 (Lancaster and Olson 1982, Olson and Cook 1951). Experimental tumors can be induced in hamsters and rabbits with BPV-1 and BPV-2 (Lancaster and Olson 1982).

Character of the Disease. The clinical findings in cattle with various forms of papillomatosis have been reviewed by Hunt (1984), Kahrs (1981), and Lancaster and Olson (1982). The incubation period may range from 3 to 8 weeks or longer. The papillomas appear first as small nodular epidermal growths, which develop slowly for a time and then often grow rapidly into dry, horny, whitish, cauliflowerlike masses that finally fall off as a result of dry necrosis of their bases. Sometimes hundreds of these masses occur on a calf at the same time. Their size varies from small ones no larger than a pea to confluent masses several inches in diameter.

The papillomas may take several forms, each affecting a different area of the body. Susceptible areas include the skin, the teats and udder, the penis of bulls, the pharynx, the urinary bladder, and the gastrointestinal tract.

The most common is the skin form, which occurs primarily in young cattle.The head, especially the region about the eyes (Figure 42.1), is most frequently involved, but warts may appear on the sides of the neck and, less

commonly, on other parts of the body. They usually do not occur on the legs. Such warts have been seen along the sides of the neck beginning at points where blood samples have been drawn from the jugular vein, an indication that an infected bleeding needle has been the transmitting agent. Warts have also been found in the nasal openings of many animals in the same herd, apparently transmitted by the fingers of persons who have held the animal, or by a bull lead used in restraint. They may appear around the site of dehorning, tattooing, or ear tagging. Outbreaks of perianal papillomas have been reported in heifers, apparently as a result of transmission by rectal examination for pregnancy (Tweddle and White 1977).

The skin form is most often seen during the winter months in calves or yearling heifers and often subsides once the animals are turned out to pasture in the spring.

There also is an atypical cutaneous form, which can be differentiated from the typical cutaneous fibropapilloma by the lack of the fibromatous dermal component (Barthold et al. 1974). Experimental attempts at transmission and immunization of this virus have failed.

Skin warts generally regress spontaneously without causing any harm. In purebred show cattle, however, their unsightly appearance and their potential contagiousness prevent showing and sale. In young animals affected with many of these tumors, the general growth rate may be retarded. The greatest economic losses are from damage to the hides of slaughtered animals.

The papillomas that develop on the teats and udders of milking cows or on the penis of breeding bulls often are pedunculated and large enough to interfere with milking

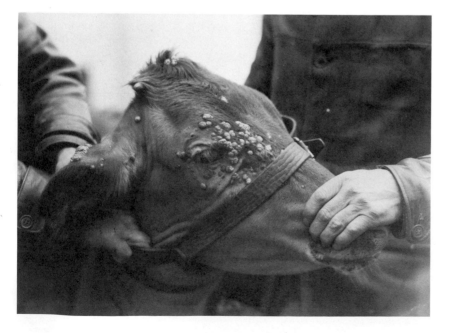

Figure 42.1. Bovine papillomatosis (warts).

or breeding. These papillomas tend to persist and do not regress spontaneously as readily as do skin papillomas.

Properties of the Virus. The causative viruses are typical members of the genus *Papillomavirus*. At least six serotypes of bovine papillomavirus (BPV) have been reported (Table 42.1, Hunt 1984, Jarrett et al. 1984, Lindholm et al. 1984). These six serotypes are divided into two subgroups, based on the type of lesion they produce. Serotypes BPV-1, BPV-2, and BPV-5 belong to subgroup A and produce fibropapillomas; BPV-3, BPV-4, and BPV-6 are classified in subgroup B and produce true epithelial papillomas (Jarrett et al. 1984).

The biophysical and biochemical properties of BPV are included in the general discussion of the genus *Papillomavirus* at the beginning of the chapter.

Epizootiology and Pathogenesis. The mode of natural transmission of warts is unknown, but is assumed to be by direct contact of infected animals or by abrasions from inanimate objects contaminated with virus. Crops of warts may appear at the site of dehorning or tattooing, around ear tags, around the nose after using contaminated bull leads, or along lesions produced by barbed wire (Blood et al. 1983). There are indications that transmission from animal to animal may occur through handling by people and through needles used for bleeding. Presumably they may be transmitted by friction between warty and normal animals or by rubbing against contaminated feed bunks. Often, the same pens may contain animals with extensive crops of warts and others of about the same age with few or none. Bagdonas and Olson (1953) studied an extensive wart epizootic in a large herd of beef cattle in a feedlot and discussed possible alternative routes of transmission of the disease. Tattooing an identification number in the ears causes a high incidence at this site in herds infected with the virus.

Papillomas commonly occur in dairy cattle, with the tumors usually appearing only on the teats. These cause difficulty in milking and evidently are spread in the milking process. Another rather common bovine papilloma, seen on the end of the penis of bulls and in the vagina of cows, may be spread during breeding (McEntee 1950).

The bovine papillomaviruses have a predilection for the basal cells of the epithelium. In the process of replication these viruses cause excessive growth of the epithelium to form the characteristic benign tumor or "wart." The details of the histopathological appearance of the various forms of bovine papillomas and fibropapillomas have been described (Fujimoto and Olson 1966, Jarrett et al. 1980).

Immunity. After several months the lesions of bovine papillomatosis usually regress spontaneously, presumably from a gradual development of an effective immune response. Once cattle eliminate these skin warts they appear to be resistant to reinfection. However, the incidence of cutaneous warts on the teats in older cattle appears to increase with age (Blood et al. 1983, Meischke 1979).

Diagnosis. The diagnosis of bovine papillomatosis is usually made from the presenting clinical signs, because the structure of the papillomas or fibropapillomas on the skin or mucosal membranes is easily observed and identified. The diagnosis can be confirmed by biopsy and histopathological examination of the tissues. The viral type involved can be determined by serologic assays for specific antibody, although this is not commonly done nor is it generally necessary (Hunt 1984).

Treatment. Common warts of cattle are generally self-limiting and require no treatment, except in severe cases or in show cattle. Genital fibropapillomas may interfere with breeding and may therefore require treatment.

Surgical removal of single or a limited number of pedunculated fibropapillomas may be indicated, especially in genital or teat involvement. Cryosurgery also may be effective. Clinical experience indicates that surgical removal of one or a few warts often results in the regression of the remaining warts in a few weeks. It is postulated that antigen is released and the immune response stimulated.

Autogenous vaccines may hasten the regression of cutaneous warts. A portion of the fibropapilloma is removed and submitted to a laboratory equipped to prepare autogenous vaccines. The tissue is minced and the virus inactivated with 0.4 percent formalin or other inactivant, the preparation clarified, then checked for sterility. The prepared vaccine is administered to the affected cattle intradermally, 1.5 to 2.0 ml once a week for 3 weeks (Hunt 1984).

Pearson et al. (1958) found that autogenous vaccines made from bovine tissues were effective against general body surface tumors in 87 percent of a large group of cattle, and nonautogenous bovine tissue vaccines protected 76 percent. Teat wart vaccines were successful in only 4 of 12 cases. Unvaccinated control cattle showed little change in their wart load, while vaccinated cattle showed wart regression.

It should always be kept in mind that most warts eventually regress spontaneously; therefore the success of all treatment methods should be assessed with caution.

Prevention and Control. Commercial wart vaccines are available. Cattle given three injections of a formalin-inactivated bovine papillomavirus vaccine produced significant levels of precipitating antibody similar to that produced by infection with papillomavirus (Barthold et al. 1976). Although such vaccines may be beneficial in some outbreaks, in many cases little or no protection apparently is produced. This may be due at least in part to the multiple serotypes of virus involved. Autogenous vaccines, as described under "Treatment," appear to be more effective in reducing the incidence of fibropapillomas in an affected herd.

Management practices on affected premises may reduce the number of cases. Sharp objects or abrasive elements should be eliminated, and the interchange of halters, ropes, and brushes should be prevented. Affected cattle should be segregated (Hunt 1984). Affected premises and objects can be decontaminated with appropriate disinfectants, but attempts to control papillomatosis in an entire herd are not practical because of the chronic nature of the infection.

The Disease in Humans. Early literature suggested possible transmission of bovine warts to humans, but recent investigations indicate that human and bovine viruses do not cross-infect (Lancaster and Olson 1981).

REFERENCES

Amtmann, E., Müller, H., and Sauer, G. 1980. Equine connective tissue tumors contain unintegrated bovine papilloma virus DNA. J. Virol. 35:962–964.

Bagdonas, V., and Olson, C. 1953. Observations on the epizootiology of cutaneous papillomatosis (warts) of cattle. J. Am. Vet. Med. Assoc. 122:393–397.

Barthold, S.W., Koller, L.D., Olson, C., Studer, E., and Holtan, A. 1974. Atypical warts in cattle. J. Am. Vet. Med. Assoc. 165:276–280.

Barthold, S.W., Olson, C., and Larson, L.L. 1976. Precipitin response of cattle to commercial wart vaccine. Am. J. Vet. Res. 37:449–451.

Blood, D.C., Radostits, O.M., and Henderson, J.A. 1983. Diseases caused by viruses and chlamydia, II: Papillomatosis. In Veterinary Medicine, 6th ed. Bailliere Tindall, London. Pp. 838–840.

Fujimoto, Y., and Olson, C. 1966. The fine structure of the bovine wart. Pathol. Vet. 3:659–684.

Hunt, E. 1984. Infectious skin diseases of cattle. Vet. Clin. North Am [Large Anim. Pract.] 6(1):155–174.

Jarrett, W.F.H., Campo, M.S., O'Neil, B.W., Laird, H.M., and Coggins, L.W. 1984. A novel bovine papillomavirus (BPV-6) causing true epithelial papillomas of the mammary gland skin: A member of a proposed new BPV subgroup. Virology 136:255–264.

Jarrett, W.F.H., McNeil, P.E., Laird, H.M., O'Neil, B.W., Murphy, J., Campo, M.S., and Moar, M.H. 1980. Papilloma viruses in benign and malignant tumors of cattle. Viruses in naturally occurring cancers. Cold Spring Harbor Conf. Cell Prolif. 7:215–222.

Kahrs, R.F. 1981. Fibropapillomatosis. In Viral Diseases of Cattle. Iowa State University Press, Ames. Pp. 121–126.

Lancaster, W.D., and Olson, C. 1981. Papovavirus infections of vertebrate animals. In E. Kurstak and C. Kurstak, eds., Comparative Diagnosis of Viral Diseases, vol. 3. Academic Press, New York. Pp. 69–98.

Lancaster, W.D., and Olson, C. 1982. Animal papillomaviruses. Microbiol. Rev. 46:191–207.

Lindholm, I., Murphy, J., O'Neil, B.W., Campo, M.S., and Jarrett, W.F. 1984. Papillomas of the teats and udder of cattle and their causal viruses. Vet. Rec. 115:574–577.

McEntee, K. 1950. Fibropapillomas of the external genitalia of cattle. Cornell Vet. 40:304–312.

Meischke, H.R.C. 1979. A survey of bovine teat papillomatosis. Vet. Rec. 104:28–31.

Olson, C., Jr., and Cook, R.H. 1951. Cutaneous sarcoma-like lesions of the horse caused by the agent of bovine papilloma. Proc. Soc. Exp. Biol. Med. 77:281–284.

Olson, C., Segre, D., and Skidmore, L.V. 1960. Further observations on immunity to bovine cutaneous papillomatosis. Am. J. Vet. Res. 21:233–242.

Pearson, J.K.L., Kerr, W.R., McCartney, W.D.J., and Steele, T.H.J. 1958. Tissue vaccines in the treatment of bovine papillomas. Vet. Rec. 70:971–973.

Trenfield, K., Spradbrow, P.B., and Vanselow, B. 1985. Sequences of papillomavirus DNA in equine sarcoids. Equine Vet. J. 17:449–452.

Tweddle, N.E., and White, W.E. 1977. An outbreak of anal fibropapillomatosis in cows following rectal examinations. Aust. Vet. J. 53:492–495.

Equine Papillomatosis

Skin warts in horses and mules (Figure 42.2) have long been recognized, although they do not appear to be as common as those affecting cattle. They appear most commonly on the nose and around the lips as small, elevated, horny masses that vary in number from a few to several hundred. Usually they remain quite small, but occasionally they may be large, especially when there are few of them. Generally they are not larger than 1 cm in diameter (Fulton et al. 1970, Pascoe 1984, Theilen 1983).

Cook and Olson (1951) studied the transmissibility of equine warts and also some of the characteristics of the virus. They had no difficulty in infecting horses, but they did not succeed in infecting calves, lambs, dogs, rabbits, and guinea pigs. Some degree of immunity was produced by experimental infections. Natural infections produced solid immunity.

Congenital papillomas occur on the skin of the head, neck, back, and croup of newborn foals and are present at birth (Attwell and Summers 1977, Garma-Avina et al. 1981, Njoko and Burwash 1972, Pascoe 1984, Schueler 1977). "The surface of the wart is comprised of numerous villose-like projections attached to the base. These are soft with a rubbery consistency. Pinkish at birth, the growths rapidly darken" (Pascoe 1984, p. 36). Congenital papillomas of foals are believed to be caused by infection from equine papilloma virus in utero (Pascoe 1984, Schueler 1977).

REFERENCES

Attwell, R.B., and Summers, P.M. 1977. Congenital papilloma in a foal. Aust. Vet. J. 53:299.

Cook, R.H., and Olson, C., Jr. 1951. Experimental transmission of cutaneous papilloma of the horse. Am. J. Pathol. 27:1087–1097.

Fulton, R.E., Doane, R.W., and MacPherson, L.W. 1970. The fine structure of equine papillomas and the equine papilloma virus. J. Ultrastruct. Res. 30:328–343.

Garma-Avina, A., Valli, V.E., and Lumsden, J.H. 1981. Equine congenital cutaneous papillomatosis: A report of 5 cases. Equine Vet. J. 13:59.

Njoko, C.O., and Burwash, W.A. 1972. Congenital cutaneous papilloma in a foal. Cornell Vet. 62:54.

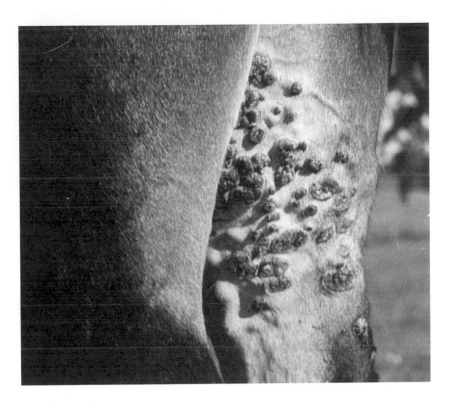

Figure 42.2. Papillomas on the leg of a mule. (Courtesy W. Cameron and C. Milton.)

Pascoe, R.R. 1984. Infectious skin diseases of horses. Vet. Clin. North Am. [Large Anim. Pract.] 6(1):27–46.

Schueler, R.L. 1977. Congenital equine papillomatosis. J. Am. Vet. Med. Assoc. 162:640.

Theilen, G.H. 1983. Papillomatosis (warts). In N.E. Robinson, ed., Current Therapy in Equine Medicine. W.B. Saunders, Philadelphia.

Caprine and Ovine Papillomatosis

Warts in goats are not common, but they rarely may occur on the skin, teats, or udder (Mullowney and Baldwin 1984, Smith 1981). They may be spread by milking. One outbreak affecting nearly an entire herd of milking goats was reported by Davis and Kemper (1936). The warts were located on various parts of the skin, and closely resembled those that occur in cattle. Although no transmission experiments were attempted, it was clear that the warts were infectious because they spread to many animals in the same herd. The herd was not in contact with cattle or other species of animals. It was believed that the disease had been introduced into the herd by purchased animals.

Papillomas in sheep are less common than in cattle. Ovine papillomavirus has been identified in these lesions by electron microscopy, and the virus can be transmitted experimentally (Gibbs et al. 1975, Jensen and Swift 1979). Lesions may occur on the face, legs, or on hairy skin; the papillomas, however, are usually hairless (Mullowney 1984).

REFERENCES

Davis, C.L., and Kemper, H.E. 1936. Common warts (papillomata) in goats. J. Am. Vet. Med. Assoc. 88:175–179.

Gibbs, E.P.J., Smale, C.J., and Lauman, M.J.P. 1975. Warts in sheep. J. Comp. Pathol. 85:327–334.

Jensen, R., and Swift, B.L. 1979. Diseases of Sheep. Lea & Febiger, Philadelphia.

Mullowney, P.C. 1984. Skin diseases of sheep. Vet. Clin. North Am. [Large Anim. Pract.] 6(1):131–142.

Mullowney, P.C., and Baldwin, E.W. 1984. Skin diseases of goats. Vet. Clin. North Am. [Large Anim. Pract.] 6(1):143–154.

Smith, M.C. 1981. Caprine dermatologic problems: A review. J. Am. Vet. Med. Assoc. 178:724-729.

Canine Papillomatosis

SYNONYMS: Canine oral papillomatosis, canine warts

Benign epithelial growths or papillomas, commonly called warts, are not uncommon in young dogs. The tumors usually are found around the lips and in the mouths, where they may cause serious inconvenience. The condition is highly contagious, often spreading through an entire kennel. A second canine papillomavirus causes cutaneous papillomas. These viral infections have been reviewed by Calvert (1984).

M'Faydean and Hobday (1898) and Penberthy (1898) demonstrated that the oral warts in dogs were infectious, and later the cause was shown to be a virus (Calvert 1984, Chambers et al. 1960, Watrach et al. 1969).

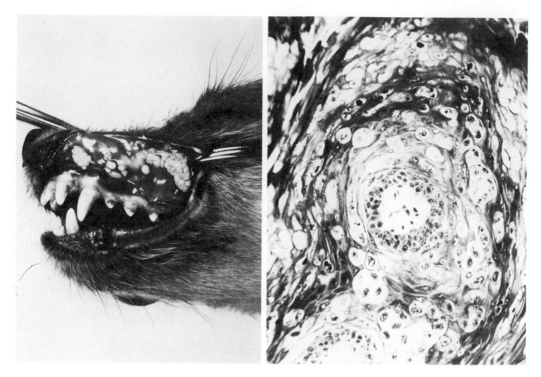

Figure 42.3. Canine oral papillomatosis. (*Left*) Warts in a puppy's mouth 66 days after injection of a Berkefeld filtrate of tumor emulsion. In this case the incubation period was 33 days. (*Right*) Transverse section of a papilla of an actively growing wart. The inner core of Malpighian cells is approximately normal in size. They are surrounded by the enlarged, vacuolated wart cells. × 132. (From De Monbreun and Goodpasture, 1932, courtesy of *American Journal of Pathology*.)

Character of the Disease. The warts of canine oral papillomatosis begin around the lips, generally as smooth whitish elevations that later develop a roughened surface and appear as typical papillomas (Figure 42.3). Usually following the first one or two tumors, a secondary crop appears on the insides of the cheeks, the hard palate, the soft palate, the tongue, and even on the walls of the pharynx. The tumors, which look like cauliflowers, may interfere considerably with mastication. After 1 to 5 months without any treatment they disappear spontaneously, although some tumors may persist for up to 24 months (Calvert 1984).

Affected dogs may be reluctant to eat and may have halitosis from the necrotizing tumors, bouts of hemorrhage from the mouth from trauma, and ropy oral discharge (Calvert 1984).

Ocular papillomatosis is not as common as oral papillomatosis. Cutaneous papillomas are uncommon in the United States but are reportedly common in racing greyhounds in Australia (Davis et al. 1976).

Properties of the Virus. Detailed studies on the biochemical characteristics of the canine papillomaviruses have not been reported to date, since it has been impossible to cultivate these viruses in cell cultures. Transmission and epidemiological studies indicate that at least two distinct types of papillomaviruses are involved. One type, canine oral papillomavirus (COPV), is involved in oral and lip warts, and probably also in ocular warts that are occasionally encountered in the dog (Hare and Howard 1977, Tokita and Konishi 1975). COPV replicates in the nucleus of the cell in closely packed crystalline arrays, with virion diameters of 47 to 53 nm and with 72 morphologic units on the surface. It is a typical papillomavirus morphologically (Watrach et al. 1969). The second type is associated with cutaneous warts (Calvert 1984, De Monbreun and Goodpasture 1932, Olson 1963). Watrach (1969) reported that the virus particles observed in canine cutaneous warts were indistinguishable from those of COPV, and that these particles were closely packed into crystalline arrays within the nucleoplasm. The particles measured 45 to 53 nm in diameter, and their morphology was identical to that of other papillomaviruses.

Epizootiology and Pathogenesis. The oral papillomavirus infects the dog, and similar warts caused by a papillomavirus morphologically identical to COPV have been reported in coyotes (Grieg and Charlton 1973). Attempts at experimental transmission to other species have been unsuccessful. Transmission of canine papillomaviruses is presumed to be through direct contact of infected and susceptible dogs. Tissue suspensions from oral papillomas are infectious to other dogs when inoculated into oral or conjunctival mucosa.

The incubation period is generally from 4 to 6 weeks (De Monbreun and Goodpasture 1932, Konishi et al. 1972, M'Faydean and Hobday 1898). Once tumors start to develop, the period until the first sign of regression in one study (Chambers et al. 1959) was 4 to 8 weeks for 65 percent of the affected dogs, and 9 to 21 weeks for 35 percent of the dogs. The incubation period for the ocular form of disease is longer (6 to 9 weeks) (Calvert 1984), while the incubation period for the cutaneous form in Australia was reported to be 4 to 7 weeks, with regression occurring on the average at 59 days after tumor formation (Davis et al. 1976).

The method of spread of virus from the initial site of infection to the multiple sites is not known. It could be via viremia, or via superficial routes.

Immunity. Puppies are immune to reinfection with COPV once the papillomas start to regress (Konishi et al. 1972). In experimental infections, puppies were resistant to reinfection of the oral mucosa 3 weeks after the original inoculation (Chambers et al. 1960).

Diagnosis. The diagnosis is generally based entirely on the presenting clinical appearance. Histopathological examination will confirm a suspicious case.

Treatment. Most oral papillomas regress spontaneously and therefore do not need treatment. However, when the masses interfere with swallowing, breathing, or mastication, surgical removal is indicated. Cryosurgery may prevent the spread of virus to new sites (Calvert 1984).

Autogenous vaccines prepared from an excised tumor mass may speed the regression of other papillomas, but controlled studies to substantiate this fact have not been done. Because most papillomas regress spontaneously anyway, the efficacy of autogenous vaccines is difficult to evaluate.

Prevention and Control. Commercial canine papillomavirus vaccines are not available. Autogenous formalin-inactivated vaccines may be helpful in immunizing unaffected dogs at risk.

Dogs with active oral (and possibly cutaneous) papillomas should be segregated from susceptible dogs.

The Disease in Humans. There is no evidence of any transmission of the canine papillomaviruses to humans.

REFERENCES

Calvert, C.A. 1984. Canine viral and transmissible neoplasms. In C.E. Greene, ed., Clinical Microbiology and Infectious Diseases of the Dog and Cat. W.B. Saunders, Philadelphia. Pp. 461–478.

Chambers, V.C., Evans, C.A., and Weiser, R.S. 1960. Canine oral papillomatosis: Immunologic aspects of the disease. Cancer Res. 20:1083–1093.

Davis, P.E., Huxtable, C.R.R., and Sabine, M. 1976. Dermal papillomas in the racing greyhound. Aust. J. Dermatol. 17:13–16.

De Monbreun, W.A., and Goodpasture, E.W. 1932. Infectious oral papillomatosis of dogs. Am. J. Pathol. 8:43–56.

Grieg, A.S., and Charlton, K.M. 1973. Electron microscopy of the virus of oral papillomatosis in the coyote. J. Wildl. Dis. 9:359.

Hare, C.L., and Howard, E.B. 1977. Canine conjunctivocorneal papillomatosis: A case report. J. Am. Anim. Hosp. Assoc. 13:688–690.

Konishi, S., Tokita, H., and Ogata, H. 1972. Studies on canine oral papillomatosis. I. Transmission and characterization of the virus. Jpn. J. Vet. Sci. 34:263–268.

M'Faydean, J., and Hobday, F. 1898. Note on the experimental transmission of warts in the dog. J. Comp. Pathol. 11:341–344.

Olson, C. 1963. Cutaneous papillomatosis in cattle and other species. Ann. N.Y. Acad. Sci. 108:1042–1056.

Penberthy, J. 1898. Contagious warty tumors in dogs. J. Comp. Pathol. 11:363–366.

Tokita, H., and Konishi, S. 1975. Studies on canine oral papillomatosis. II. Oncogenicity of canine oral papilloma virus to various tissues of the dog with special reference to eye tumor. Jpn. J. Vet. Sci. 37:109–120.

Watrach, A.M. 1969. The ultrastructure of canine cutaneous papilloma. Cancer Res. 29:2079–2084.

Watrach, A.M., Hansen, L.E., and Meyer, R.C. 1969. Canine papilloma: The structural characterization of oral papilloma virus. J. Natl. Cancer Inst. 43:453–458.

Rabbit Papillomatosis

Two kinds of virus-induced papillomas occur in rabbits. The rabbit cutaneous papilloma, commonly known as the Shope papilloma, occurs on the skin and is never found on the mucous membranes of the mouth. The other papilloma occurs on the oral mucosa and is never found on the skin.

Character of the Disease. Cutaneous warts are common among wild rabbits of the midwestern United States (Lancaster and Olson 1982, Shope 1933). An infected animal usually has from 1 to 10 of these tumors, but occasionally hundreds of small warts may cover almost the entire body surface. Even when the lesions are numerous, they have little effect on the general health of the rabbit. These naturally occurring tumors are tall, thin, horny structures, usually grayish or even black. Hunters sometimes refer to such animals as "horned" rabbits when the warts occur on the head. The sides of the neck, the shoulders, the abdomen (Figure 42.4), and the inside of the thighs are the sites of predilection.

The oral papillomas are small, gray-white, sessile or pedunculated nodules found usually on the under surface of the tongue, occasionally on the gums, and rarely on the floor of the mouth. They often are multiple and sometimes

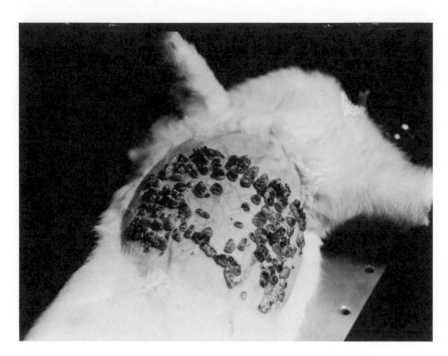

Figure 42.4. Rabbit papillomatosis. Warts on the scarified skin of the abdomen were produced experimentally. The rabbit had been inoculated about 1 month previously. (From Shope, 1933, courtesy of *Journal of Experimental Medicine*.)

quite numerous. The larger ones have cauliflowerlike surfaces and may be as large as 5 mm in diameter and 4 mm in height. The smaller ones usually are smooth and domelike. Microscopically they are typical papillomas, the epithelial cells being swollen and vacuolated. In the cells near the surface, intranuclear inclusion bodies are found in about 10 percent of the lesions in the domestic rabbit (Barthold and Olson 1974, Parsons and Kidd 1943).

Properties of the Virus. Shope (1933) showed that the common wart of the western wild cottontail rabbit was infectious and that the infectious agent was a virus. There are two types: the cottontail rabbit papillomavirus, or Shope papillomavirus, and the oral papillomavirus of rabbits. Both are typical members of the *Papillomavirus* genus (Barthold and Olson 1974, Lancaster and Olson 1982, Parsons and Kidd 1943, Spira et al. 1974), but the viruses of these tumors are not related to each other serologically, and neither immunizes against the other.

The biophysical and biochemical properties of the rabbit papillomaviruses are similar to those discussed earlier under "The Genus *Papillomavirus*."

Epizootiology and Pathogenesis. Because animals can easily be infected through superficial scarifications of the skin, it is presumed that natural infections occur through direct contact between infected and susceptible animals.

Experimentally the disease may be easily transmitted by inoculating scarified skin areas with filtered or unfiltered tumor tissue. Tumors can be transmitted in series in the wild cottontail rabbit (*Sylvilagus floridanus*), but those produced in domestic rabbits (*Oryctolagus cuniculus*) by such inoculations are not transmissible although otherwise typical. If the tumor-bearing domesticated rabbits are kept for long periods (200 days or more), a considerable number of the benign papillomas become malignant carcinomas (Rous and Beard 1935). The same is true of tumors produced by inoculation of members of the hare genus (*Lepus*), such as the jack rabbit and the snowshoe hare (Kidd and Rous 1940). In rabbit or hare species in which the virus is foreign, there apparently is virus variation, which leads to malignancy.

Oral papillomas are benign growths on the oral mucosa of domestic rabbits (Dominguez et al. 1981, Parsons and Kidd 1943, Sundberg et al. 1985). They are readily transmitted by filtrates to other domestic rabbits, to the cottontail rabbit and the jack rabbit of the midwestern United States, and to the snowshoe rabbit of the North, although they apparently do not occur naturally in any but the domestic species. Fibromas can be induced experimentally in neonatal hamsters (Sundberg et al. 1985).

Immunity. Shope (1933, 1937) proved that rabbits carrying experimentally produced cutaneous papillomas are partially or wholly immune to reinfection, and also that the serums of such animals can partially or completely neutralize the virus in vitro.

After recovery from oral papillomatosis, animals are solidly immune to reinfection for at least several months. There is no immunological relation with the Shope papilloma. Animals affected with one type of tumor can readily be infected with the other, and animals solidly immune to one type as a result of regression are fully susceptible to the other.

REFERENCES

Barthold, S.W., and Olson, C. 1974. Papovavirus-induced neoplasia. In E.C. Melby and N.H. Altman, eds., Handbook of Laboratory Animal Science, vol. 2. CRC Press, Cleveland. Pp. 70–75.

Dominguez, J.A., Corella, E.L., and Aurio, A. 1981. Oral papillomatosis in two laboratory rabbits in Mexico. Lab. Anim. Sci. 31:71–73.

Kidd, J.G., and Rous, P. 1940. A transplantable rabbit carcinoma originating in a virus-induced papilloma and containing the virus in masked or altered form. J. Exp. Med. 71:813–838.

Lancaster, W.D., and Olson, C. 1982. Animal papillomaviruses. Microbiol. Rev. 46:191–207.

Parsons, R.J., and Kidd, J.G. 1943. Oral papillomatosis of rabbits: A virus disease. J. Exp. Med. 77:233–250.

Rous, P., and Beard, J.W. 1935. The progression to carcinoma of virus-induced rabbit papillomas (Shope). J. Exp. Med. 62:523–548.

Shope, R.E. 1933. Infectious papillomatosis of rabbits. J. Exp. Med. 58:607–624.

Shope, R.E. 1937. Immunization of rabbits to infectious papillomatosis. J. Exp. Med. 65:219–231.

Spira, G., Estes, M.K., Dreesman, G.L., Butel, J.S., and Rawls, W.E. 1974. Papovavirus structural polypeptides: Comparison of human and rabbit papilloma viruses with simian virus 40. Intervirology 3:220–231.

Sundberg, J.P., Junge, R.E., and Shazly, M.O. 1985. Oral papillomatosis in New Zealand white rabbits. Am. J. Vet. Res. 46:664–668.

Genital Papillomas of Pigs

Papillomas in the genital region of boars were described by Parish (1961). These warts were transmissible by scarification or injection into the genital skin of adult boars and appeared 8 weeks after injection. Cytoplasmic inclusion bodies were observed in the lesions.

This agent, presumably a papillomavirus, is inactivated readily by heat, and survival at 4°C and −20°C is poor. It is resistant to ether. Neutralizing antibodies can be detected in the serums of hyperimmunized pigs and rabbits, but not in those of convalescent pigs. Animals that recover from the infection are resistant to challenge. Antigen can be demonstrated with the agar-gel immunodiffusion assay or the conglutination complement-absorption test (Parish 1962)

REFERENCES

Parish, W.E. 1961. A transmissible genital papilloma of the pig resembling condyloma acuminatum of man. J. Pathol. 81:331–345.

Parish, W.E. 1962. An immunological study of the transmissible genital papilloma of the pig. J. Pathol. 83:429–442.

43 The Adenoviridae

The Adenoviridae family contains two genera, *Mastadenovirus* and *Aviadenovirus* (Horwitz 1985a, Norrby et al. 1976). Adenoviruses of the *Mastadenovirus* genus commonly affect both animals and humans, with many species having multiple serotypes of adenoviruses that produce infections within that species. Many adenoviruses produce mild or subclinical respiratory diseases, and some produce mild or subclinical intestinal infections, but a few produce severe systemic disease. There are a number of adenoviruses of birds, and these are classified in the *Aviadenovirus* genus.

The term *adenovirus* was coined because the virus that eventually was placed in this family was first isolated from cell cultures of tonsils and adenoidal tissue surgically removed from children (Enders et al. 1956, Horwitz 1985a).

More than 40 serotypes of human adenoviruses have been recognized (Horwitz 1985b). These are divided into four subgroups on the basis of their ability to agglutinate rhesus monkey and rat red blood cells. There is some correlation between this method of grouping and immunological groupings, based on cross-reactions with serums from volunteers inoculated with various members of the group. Hemagglutination-inhibition and neutralization tests have also demonstrated antigenic relationships among members of the four respective hemagglutinating groups, although cross-reactions are generally of low level and vary with the virus strain and method employed. Other members of the genus *Mastadenovirus* include 2 canine, 16 simian, 9 bovine, 4 porcine, 6 ovine, 1 (possibly 2) equine, and 2 mouse adenovirus serotypes. Members of the *Aviadenovirus* genus include 11 fowl, 4 tur-

key, and 3 goose serotypes (McFerran 1981). Adenoviruses also have been isolated from the black bear (Pursell et al. 1983). There is little reaction between human and nonprimate serotypes of adenoviruses (Willimzik et al. 1981).

In general, the members of this family especially the human adenoviruses, have been well characterized; and excellent reviews are available (Cabasso and Wilner 1969; Horwitz 1985a, 1985b; McFerran 1981; Pereira 1959; Philipson 1984; Taylor 1977; Wigand et al. 1982). The virions contain double-stranded DNA with a molecular mass of 23×10^6 daltons. Isometric, nonenveloped particles have icosahedral symmetry, 70 to 90 nm in diameter, with 252 capsomeres, each 7 nm in diameter (Figure 43.1). Twelve vertex capsomeres ("pentons") are antigenically distinct from the other 240 capsomeres ("hexons"). Each penton carries a filamentous projection or fiber. The virions are resistant to solvents such as ether but are inactivated by many disinfectants. They have a density of 1.34 g/ml in cesium chloride. Viral assembly takes place in the nucleus of the cell, where inclusion bodies are seen. A common antigen shared by all mammalian strains differs from the corresponding antigen of avian strains. Some viruses hemagglutinate cells of various species.

Under certain conditions some adenoviruses are oncogenic. They produce a rather characteristic cytopathological pattern in monolayer cell cultures, with marked rounding of cells that form aggregates in grapelike clusters. The host specificity is relatively narrow, and persistence of the virus in the natural host is quite common.

The important diseases in this family are respiratory and ocular disease in humans and other species and infectious canine hepatitis (Table 43.1).

Laboratory diagnosis of adenovirus infections has been reviewed by Cooney (1985).

REFERENCES

Cabasso, V.J., and Wilner, B.I. 1969. Adenoviruses of animals other than man. Adv. Vet. Sci. Comp. Med. 13:159–217.
Cooney, M.K. 1985. Adenoviruses. In E.H. Lennette, ed., Laboratory Diagnosis of Viral Infections. Marcel Dekker, New York. Pp. 135–146.
Enders, J.F., Bell, J.A., Dingle, J.H., Francis, T., Jr., Hilleman, M.R., Huebner, R.J., and Payne, A.M.M. 1956. "Adenoviruses": Group name proposed for new respiratory-tract viruses. Science 124:119–120.
Horne, R.W., Brenner, S., Wildy, P., and Waterson, A.P. 1959. The icosahedral form of an adenovirus. (Letter to the editor.) J. Molec. Biol. 1:84–86.
Horwitz, M.S. 1985a. Adenoviruses and their replication. In B.N. Fields, D.M. Knipe, R.M. Chanock, J.L. Melnick, B. Roizman, and R.E. Shope, eds., Virology. Raven Press, New York. Pp. 433–476.
Horwitz, M.S. 1985b. Adenoviral diseases. In B.N. Fields, D.M. Knipe, R.M. Chanock, J.L. Melnick, B. Roizman, and R.E. Shope, eds., Virology. Raven Press, New York. Pp. 477–495.

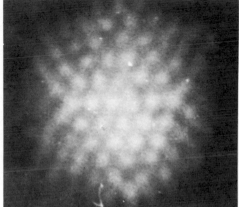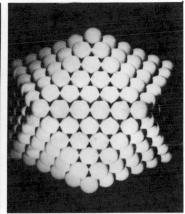

Figure 43.1. (*Left*) Electron micrograph of an adenovirus, an icosahedral virus. It is embedded in phosphotungstate, magnified about 1 million diameters. (*Right*) Model of the figure on the left showing how the particles, 252 surface subunits (capsomeres), are arranged with icosahedral symmetry. (From Horne et al., 1959, courtesy of *Journal of Molecular Biology*.)

McFerran, J.B. 1981. Adenoviruses of vertebrate animals. In E. Kurstak and C. Kurstak, eds., Comparative Diagnosis of Viral Diseases, vol. 3. Academic Press, New York. Pp. 101–165.

Norrby, E., Bartha, A., Boulanger, P., Dreizin, R.S., Ginsberg, H.S., Kalter, S.S., Kawamura, H., Rowe, W.P., Russell, W.C., Schlesinger, R.W., and Wigand, R. 1976. Adenoviridae. Intervirology 7:117–125.

Pereira, H.G. 1959. Adenoviruses. Br. Med. Bull. 15:225–230.

Philipson, L. 1984. Structure and assembly of adenoviruses. Curr. Top. Microbiol. Immunol. 109:1–52.

Pursell, A.R., Stuart, B.P., Styer, E., and Case, J.L. 1983. Isolation of an adenovirus from black bear cubs. J. Wildl. Dis. 19:269–271.

Taylor, P.E. 1977. Adenoviruses: Diagnosis of infections. In E. Kurstak and C. Kurstak, eds., Comparative Diagnosis of Viral Diseases, vol. 1. Academic Press, New York. Pp. 85–170.

Wigand, R., Bartha, A., Dreizin, R.S., Esche, H., Ginsberg, H.S., Green, M., Hierholzer, J.C., Kalter, S.S., McFerran, J.B., Pettersson, U., Russell, W.C., and Wadell, G. 1982. Adenoviridae: Second report. Intervirology 18:169–176.

Willimzik, H.F., Kalter, S.S., Lester, T.L., and Wigand, R. 1981. Immunological relationship among adenoviruses of humans, simians, and nonprimates as determined by the neutralization test. Intervirology 15:28–36.

The Genus *Mastadenovirus*

Infectious Canine Hepatitis

SYNONYMS: Canine adenovirus 1 infection, fox encephalitis, hepatitis contagiosa canis, Rubarth's disease; abbreviation, ICH

Infectious canine hepatitis is a highly contagious disease of domestic and wild canids caused by canine adenovirus type 1 (CAV-1). It was originally described by Rubarth (1947) as an acute disease of young dogs with severe hepatitis, edema of the gallbladder, tonsillitis, multifocal vasculitis, and hemorrhage (Baker et al. 1950, Cabasso, 1962, Wigton et al. 1976). Many infections are subclinical, but in unvaccinated dogs they may result in severe systemic disease primarily involving the liver. Routine vaccination has made this formerly common disease relatively rare.

The disease affects dogs, foxes, and other canids such as coyotes and wolves (Chaddock 1948, Greene 1984). It also occurs in bears (Collins et al. 1984). Serum samples in 95 percent of a population of wolves (*Canis lupis*) in Alaska had antibodies to CAV-1 (Stephenson et al. 1982). Bolin et al. (1958) found neutralizing antibodies in the blood of a wild raccoon. The disease in foxes, known as fox encephalitis (Green et al. 1930), can be readily transmitted to dogs. The experimental disease in the dog was described in detail by Green and Shillinger (1934). That the disease occurred naturally in dogs was soon recognized. Rubarth (1947) in Sweden published a detailed account of the disease, and it was he who supplied the name *infectious canine hepatitis*, by which it is now generally known. Rubarth also recognized that the disease was the same as that which American authors had been discussing for some years under the name fox encephalitis infection of dogs.

Canine adenovirus type 1 (strain Utrecht) was the first canine adenovirus officially recognized. The canine virus Toronto A26/61 of Ditchfield et al. (1962) is now regarded as a distinct virus, canine adenovirus type 2 (CAV-2), rather than a variant of CAV-1 (Darai et al. 1985, Hamelin et al. 1984, Whetstone 1985). These two viruses differ in biophysical properties, DNA restriction profiles, and in the antigens responsible for complement fixation, hemagglutination, and neutralization. CAV-2 also has a marked predilection for respiratory tissue, whereas CAV-1 has less effect on the respiratory system.

Character of the Disease. The hepatic form in dogs is the classic form of ICH and originally was very widespread, probably occurring wherever dogs were numerous. In Stockholm between 1928 and 1946, Rubarth (1947) diagnosed 190 cases, which constituted 3.4 percent of all the canine fatalities he observed. Before vaccination was routine, the disease was common in the British Isles, Denmark, Norway, Australia, and North Ameri-

Table 43.1. Diseases of domestic animals caused by viruses in the Adenoviridae family

Common name of virus	Natural hosts	Type of disease produced
Infectious canine hepatitis virus (canine adenovirus type 1)	Dogs	Hemorrhagic and hepatitic
Canine adenovirus type 2	Dogs	Respiratory
Bovine adenoviruses, types 1–9	Cattle	Variety of clinical syndromes—conjunctivitis, pneumonia, pneumoenteritis, diarrhea, polyarthritis (weak calf syndrome)
Porcine adenoviruses, types 1–4	Swine	Type 4 usually is the only pathogen causing diarrhea and/or meningoencephalitis
Ovine adenoviruses, types 1–6	Sheep	Respiratory and enteritic, usually mild or inapparent unless complications arise
Equine adenovirus type 1	Horses	Pneumonia; Arabian foals seem most susceptible
Turkey adenoviruses, types 1–4	Turkeys	Respiratory disease and occasionally enteritis in poults; marble spleen disease
Avian adenoviruses, types 1–11	Chickens (domestic)	Respiratory illness, enteric disease, egg-drop syndrome, aplastic anemia, atrophy of bursa of Fabricius

ca. ICH is now a relatively uncommon disease of dogs in the United States, although the incidence of antibodies in dogs is very high. Infections that do occur in unvaccinated dogs may be severe and may result in an unusually high death rate. The relatively high incidence of the mildly pathogenic respiratory virus CAV-2 may also be responsible in part for the decrease in clinical ICH.

The disease occurs at all times of the year. It is most frequent in young, unvaccinated dogs but has been seen in all age groups. Puppies, shortly after weaning, seem most susceptible, and in them mortality is highest.

The course of the disease may be peracute, with dogs becoming moribund within hours of the first signs of clinical illness (Greene 1984). These cases may resemble poisonings. The course of the disease frequently runs 5 to 7 days, unless complications occur (Greene 1984).

In typical cases of ICH the affected animal develops a biphasic febrile response (103° to 106°F), becomes apathetic, and loses its appetite but frequently shows intense thirst. Some dogs exhibit edema of the head, neck, and lower portion of the abdomen. Vomiting and diarrhea are common. Many animals manifest pain by moaning, especially when pressure is exerted on the abdominal wall. Hepatomegaly usually is present.

During the early febrile response, a blood count will disclose leukopenia, the leukocytes usually numbering 2,500/dl or less.

Common signs are transient opacity of the cornea, due to edema, and anterior uveitis. These ocular changes may be the only signs in subclinical infection, or they may appear 10 to 15 days after vaccination with an attenuated strain of CAV-1. The most common change observed by the clinician is corneal edema, the classic "blue eye" (Figure 43.2). This cloudiness starts at the limbus and proceeds rather rapidly throughout the entire cornea, producing a cornea that may be up to three times its normal thickness. Involvement may be unilateral or bilateral. The conjunctiva may be edematous and inflamed, resulting in pain, blepharospasm, photophobia, and a watery ocular discharge (Curtis and Barnette 1973). The Afghan hound appears to have a predilection for eye lesions from CAV-1 infection (Curtis and Barnett 1981). Visible ocular lesions may persist for weeks or months, and microscopic changes may persist for many months (Curtis and Barnett 1973).

The mucous membranes are usually pale, and petechiae or ecchymotic hemorrhages may appear on the gums or other mucous membranes. The tonsils are acutely in-

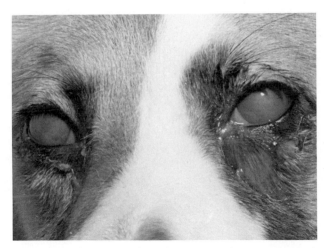

Figure 43.2. Corneal opacity of both eyes of an experimental dog following intravenous inoculation with an attenuated canine adenovirus serotype 1 strain, classic infectious canine hepatitis virus. (Courtesy L. E. Carmichael.)

flamed and enlarged. The heartbeat is often accelerated, and the respiratory rate increased. Albuminuria occurs in many cases.

The encephalitic form of CAV-1 infection (fox encephalitis) occurs among wild foxes, but losses are seen principally on fur ranches and may amount to 15 or 20 percent of the ranch population. The disease appears suddenly; in many cases animals are found dead before any signs have been observed. Loss of appetite may be noted for a day or two before other signs appear. Violent convulsions are often the initial sign, followed by a lethargic state in which the animal wanders about aimlessly and blindly and which may be interrupted by more convulsions. At the outset of the disease a watery nasal discharge is common, and sometimes there is a similar discharge from the eyes. The feces become soft and filled with mucus; sometimes there is profuse diarrhea in which blood streaks are common (Green et al. 1930).

The disease in foxes runs a very rapid course. It may be as short as 1 hour and usually is less than 24 hours, but a few cases may last as long as 3 days. Foxes that succumb to this disease generally have lost little weight because of the rapidity of its course.

Properties of the Virus. CAV-1 has biochemical and biophysical properties typical of those for other adenoviruses. Electron micrographs of the virus particles reveal rigid icosahedrons with 252 subunits (capsomeres) that constitute the capsid (Davies et al. 1961). The diameter is estimated at 75 to 80 nm.

The nucleic acid of CAV-1 is double-stranded DNA. Restriction enzyme mapping of the nucleic acid reveals

that it is distinct from that of CAV-2 (Darai et al. 1985, Hamelin et al. 1984).

CAV-1 survives well when frozen or dried. It is inactivated in 24 hours by 0.2 percent formalin but survives for days in 0.5 percent phenol (Surden et al. 1959). It is inactivated at 50°C after 150 minutes, or at 60°C in 3 to 5 minutes. It is ether- and chloroform-resistant and survives between pH 3 and 9 at room temperature. Many commercial disinfectants will inactivate the virus.

The virus hemagglutinates chicken red blood cells at 4°C and pH 7.5 to 8 (Fastier 1957). It also hemagglutinates rat and human type O blood cells at pH 6.5 to 7.5 (Espmark and Salenstedt 1961). Viral hemagglutination is inhibited by antibody.

A group complement-fixing antigen is shared by CAV-1 and other adenoviruses (Carmichael and Barnes 1961, Kapsenberg 1959). Complement fixation and precipitin reactions are unilateral between CAV-1 and human adenovirus types, because human adenovirus antiserums react with both human and canine virus types, but CAV-1 antiserum fails to react with the human adenovirus antigens. No cross-neutralization occurs between CAV-1 and certain other adenovirus types (Kapsenberg 1959). Interferon is not produced by CAV-1 in dog kidney cell cultures, nor is the virus sensitive to interferon.

Cultivation. Cabasso and co-workers (1954) reported successful cultivation of this virus in roller-tube cultures of dog kidney cells, in which specific cytopathogenic effects are produced (Figure 43.3). The virus can be carried indefinitely in such cultures. Since then, the virus has been isolated and maintained in a variety of cell cultures in the laboratory.

Epizootiology and Pathogenesis. CAV-1 is transmitted by direct contact of infected and susceptible dogs, by contact with urine-contaminated environment, or by contact with contaminated fomites, such as feed and water dishes. This disease, unlike canine distemper, is not transmitted by droplet infection but rather by more or less direct contact (Baker et al. 1950). Susceptible dogs, kept in cages separated from those of infected dogs by no more than 6 inches, have remained uninfected. Infection readily occurs orally with infective materials, including saliva on the fingertips. The respiratory form of adenovirus infection (CAV-2), in contrast to the classic form, may be conveyed by aerosol transmission (Swango et al. 1970). Poppensiek and Baker (1951) showed that CAV-1 is liberated in the urine during the acute phase of disease and for many months afterward in some dogs. Urine undoubtedly is the source of infectious virus for most outbreaks.

The incubation period for dogs infected with CAV-1 is

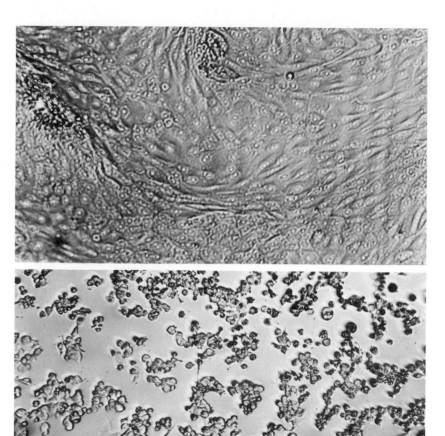

Figure 43.3. Roller-tube cultures of canine renal cortex. (*Top*) Uninoculated control showing solid sheet of epithelial cells. (*Bottom*) Epithelial cells 3 days after inoculation with 10^4 cell-culture inoculation doses of infectious canine hepatitis virus. × 90. (From Fieldsteel, courtesy of *American Journal of Veterinary Research.*)

short. Baker et al. (1950) reported that after intravenous inoculation dogs showed signs in 2 or 3 days; after subcutaneous inoculation, in 3 or 4 days; after being fed virus, in 4 to 6 days. When susceptible dogs were allowed natural contact with infected ones, susceptible dogs usually developed signs in 6 to 9 days.

The progress of this disease is much more rapid than that of distemper. Most dogs have either recovered or are dead within 2 weeks, and many succumb within a few days. Mortality varies according to the age of the dog and may range from 10 to 25 percent.

In natural infection CAV-1 localizes and replicates in the tonsil. It then spreads to the regional lymph nodes, through the lymphatics to the bloodstream, and is finally disseminated throughout the body. A diagram of the time sequence of events in the pathogenesis is given by Greene (1984). The main target areas for viral replication and pathological damage are the liver, kidney, eye, and endothelium of several organs.

For several days after infection and until antibody ap-

pears in the circulation, tissue injury is caused by cytolysis as the virus replicates. The predilection of CAV-1 for endothelial cells (Figure 43.4) results in cytolysis and vascular damage, with petechial and ecchymotic hemorrhages. The principal pathological process in the vascular system is one of virus-induced disseminated intravascular coagulation (DIC) (Wigton et al. 1976). Several hemostatic changes, including thrombocytopenia, altered platelet activity, prolonged prothrombin time, depressed factor VIII activity, and increased fibrin-fibrinogen degradation products, occur in ICH.

If the direct viral damage to the liver is sufficient, acute hepatic necrosis can result in severe disease and even death. Acute damage to the renal glomeruli can occur. The pathogenesis of renal lesions has been studied in some detail (Wright and Cornwell 1983, Wright et al. 1981).

After antibody appears (about day 7 after infection), virus is cleared from the circulation; but infectious virus may persist within tissues such as the renal tubules for

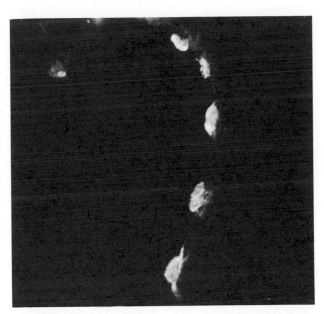

Figure 43.4. Section of vessel in a dog infected with canine adenovirus type 1 (infectious canine hepatitis virus) showing viral infection in vascular endothelial cells. Stained with fluorescent antibody. × 125. (Courtesy L. E. Carmichael and M. Appel.)

many months, with infectious virus shed in the urine (Poppensiek and Baker 1951). In the process of virus removal, immune complexes of virus and antibody can occur in the serum (Morrison and Wright 1976) or in tissues such as the kidney or the eye. Immune-complex glomerulonephritis, consisting of deposits of IgG, IgM, C3, and viral antigen, appears 5 to 10 days after infection and persists for as long as 40 days (Wright and Cornwell 1983, Wright et al. 1981).

Ocular lesions associated with ICH have been recognized since the classic description of the disease by Rubarth (1947). The pathogenesis of these lesions has been studied in detail (Carmichael 1964, 1965; Carmichael et al. 1975; Curtis and Barnett 1973, 1981, 1983). Keratouveitis, which is a manifestation of type III or Arthus-type hypersensitivity, develops.

Autopsy findings in animals that succumb to the hepatic form are rather characteristic. Because of the rapid progress of the disease, there is no evidence of emaciation. Edema of the subcutaneous tissues frequently occurs, and fluid is found in the peritoneal cavity in more than half the cases. This fluid may be clear, but more often it is blood-tinged; and usually it appears to consist almost wholly of blood. Upon exposure to the air this bloody exudate often coagulates. A fibrinous exudate is usually found among the intestinal loops even when there is no fluid in the cavity. Hydrothorax occurs only occasionally. Sometimes subserosal hemorrhages are seen in the stomach, intestines, gallbladder, and diaphragm. The liver may not be greatly changed in appearance, but usually it is somewhat swollen and light in color. The capsule is stiff, and the lobules appear more prominent than normal. Generally the gallbladder wall is markedly edematous. The thickened wall may be hemorrhagic, in which case the whole sac may appear black or reddish black. The gallbladder mucosa is normal in appearance, but fibrinous deposits are usually found in the vicinity of the organ. The spleen seems normal or slightly enlarged. The intestines may appear normal, but the contents are often mixed with blood. Edema of the lungs may be present, but pneumonia is absent.

The principal histological changes are found in the liver and endothelial cells. The blood content is increased, and the larger vessels are greatly dilated. The distended sinusoids cause pressure on the liver cells. The endothelial cells of the sinusoids and Kupffer cells are greatly swollen and are degenerating. Nuclear inclusions occur to a varying degree in the liver cells, as well as in the lining cells of the sinusoids, the Kupffer cells, and the endothelial cells of the veins. Rubarth (1947) considered the primary damage to be in the endothelial cells; circulatory disturbances were of secondary importance. In the brain, serous effusions frequently occur under the pia mater, and there are cellular infiltrations around the blood vessels. The endothelial cells of the blood vessels often are swollen and degenerating, and many of the smaller veins are filled with such cells. Inclusion bodies are usually found in these cells. The picture is that of nonpurulent encephalitis.

Inclusion bodies (Cowdry and Scott 1930) can be found readily in most cases, but sometimes they are not numerous. They occur in the endothelial cells of the spleen, lymph nodes, vascular system of the brain, sinusoids of the liver, and less commonly elsewhere. They may be found in detached endothelial cells in the small blood vessels, especially in the brain and in the glomeruli of the kidneys. They are always intranuclear and acidophilic. The chromatic material of the affected nuclei breaks down and marginates, leaving a clear central area in which the inclusion bodies may be found. Usually there is but one inclusion body in each nucleus, but multiples are occasionally seen. They may be round or oval. They may be found in tissue sections or in touch preparations of fresh liver tissue (Davis and Anderson 1950).

The disease can be reproduced in dogs and foxes by inoculation but it is innocuous for ferrets. It does not affect mink or the ordinary small laboratory mammals. Dogs, raccoons, and ferrets do develop interstitial ker-

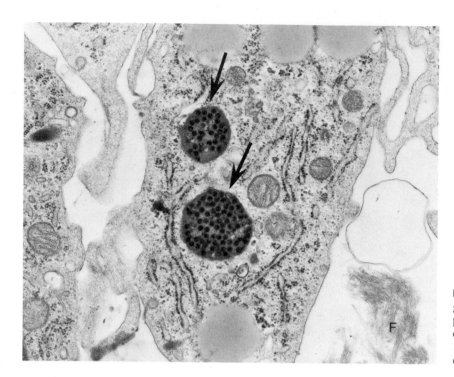

Figure 43.5. Double membrane body aggregates (immune complexes) in the cytoplasm of a macrophage composing a portion of the keratic precipitate. Note fibrin (*F*). × 13,000. (From Carmichael et al., 1975, courtesy of *Cornell Veterinarian*.)

atitis. Carmichael et al. (1975) reported that CAV-1 antibody complexes caused severe anterior uveitis with corneal edema (Figure 43.5). The response to such immune complexes was similar to the spontaneously occurring disease. Similar immune complexes have been found in the serum of experimental dogs during the acute stage of the disease, when serum antibody titers were low (Morrison and Wright, 1976).

Nearly all foxes that show signs die. The spread of the disease in breeding pens is rather slow, and usually not more than 5 percent of the animals contract it. The disease persists for many years on fox farms, reappearing annually. Losses over a period of years may be great.

Gross lesions in foxes consist of hemorrhages in various parts of the body. These hemorrhages are rather large in some cases and are small or absent in others. Large hemorrhages into the brain or spinal cord explain the paralytic signs often seen in this disease. Large hemorrhages into the lungs sometimes occur.

Although the name *fox encephalitis* suggests that the disease is caused by a neurotropic virus, this is not the case. The disease in foxes is generalized, involving primarily the endothelial system, especially the endothelial linings of the smaller blood vessels. Injuries to these cells result in hemorrhage and in cellular degeneration. As the nervous system is very susceptible to this form of damage, the signs are largely referable to it. Nuclear inclusion bodies can be readily demonstrated in endothelial cells of

various organs and in epithelial cells of the liver. These inclusions are identical in appearance with those found in dogs.

Immunity. CAV-1 protects dogs against itself and against CAV-2 (Toronto A26/61) and CAV-2 protects dogs against itself and against CAV-1 (Appel et al. 1975). Consequently, presently available vaccines for ICH protect dogs against both types of canine adenovirus.

One attack of this disease confers solid, permanent immunity. Immune animals may nevertheless shed virus in their urine for long periods of time. There is no cross-immunization between infectious hepatitis and canine distemper. Rubarth (1947) in Sweden and several workers in the United States, in studies prior to the routine use of vaccines against ICH, found that a considerable number of puppies with no history of the disease were nevertheless resistant to infectious hepatitis by virtue of neutralizing antibodies. This indicated that the virus was considerably more prevalent in dogs than the number of cases indicated.

Poppensiek (1952) showed that it was possible to protect susceptible puppies by passively immunizing them with homologous hyperimmune serum, and that solid, active immunity could be produced with serum and virus administered simultaneously. These dogs generally shed virus in their urine, as did animals with the natural disease; hence they were hazardous to nonprotected puppies with which they came in contact.

As with canine distemper, virus neutralization is the only serologic test that indicates immunity. Other tests may be used for diagnosis, but complement-fixing antibodies do not persist long after initial infection, whereas neutralizing antibodies remain for a long time. Most dogs have high levels of neutralizing antibodies at least 3.5 years after vaccination and at least 5.5 years after experimental infection.

The results obtained by Carmichael et al. (1962) with maternal immunity to ICH in puppies are remarkably but predictably similar to those obtained with distemper because the antibody half-life for both viruses is 8.5 days. Appel et al. (1975) suggested a practical way to overcome maternal immune interference. In their experiments, 4-week-old puppies with ICH maternal antibody titers ranging from 10^2 to $10^{2.4}$ were inoculated with their respiratory strain DK_{12} (closely related to Toronto A26/61) by the oronasal route. Virus was found in pharyngeal swabs 4 to 7 days after exposure, and when serum antibody titers of 1:10 were reached, a sudden increase in antibody occurred, suggesting the production of an active immunity presumably due to persisting virus replication. These antibody levels remained, and when some puppies were challenged at 14 weeks of age with canine adenovirus type 1 and the homotypic virus, the puppies showed no signs of illness, nor could virus be isolated from pharyngeal swabs or blood.

Diagnosis. A presumptive diagnosis of ICH can be made on the basis of clinical signs and supporting clinicopathological findings. The diagnosis can be confirmed by virus isolation in cell cultures, by demonstration of a rise in antibodies against CAV-1 by one of several serologic tests, or by the characteristic gross and microscopic lesions at necropsy.

Clincally ICH is difficult to distinguish from other infectious diseases of the dog, principally canine distemper (CD). ICH and CD vary in their signs of illness, but there is sufficient overlap that a positive diagnosis is difficult.

In the early stages of ICH marked neutropenia and lymphopenia are noted (Greene 1984). There are also marked thrombocytopenia and abnormal platelet activity, increased prothrombin time, and depressed factor VIII activity (Wigton et al. 1976), all of which translate into increased coagulation time (Poppensiek 1952). Hepatic necrosis results in elevated levels of liver enzymes, including alanine aminotransferase (ALT), aspartate aminotransferase (AST), and serum alkaline phosphatase (SAP) (Greene 1984). Bilirubinuria, but not bilirubinemia, is often present; and hypoglycemia may be present.

At necropsy the hepatic form of ICH in dogs can be readily distinguished from CD. The characteristic liver and gallbladder lesions and the effusions that occur in the body cavities with hepatic ICH distinguish it from CD. Intranuclear inclusion bodies are found in tissues infected with ICH, whereas CD has intracytoplasmic inclusion bodies—this readily differentiates the two viral diseases, regardless of the disease form of ICH. ICH, like CD, can be transmitted to susceptible dogs and foxes; but, unlike CD, the CAV-1 virus is not transmissible to ferrets.

The diagnostic methods used in dogs are applicable to the disease in foxes. In general, the acute course and the pronounced nervous signs make the clinical diagnosis easier in this species than in dogs.

A number of serologic tests can be used to identify antibodies in serum. The virus-neutralization test is the most specific. Rubarth (1947) found that the complement-fixation test could be used for diagnosing ICH. Hemagglutination-inhibition can be utilized (Espmark and Salenstedt 1961). Enzyme-linked immunosorbent assay (ELISA) is now available (Noon et al. 1979).

Field strains of CAV-1 readily produce a cytopathic effect in monolayer cultures of primary or secondary dog kidney cells. This method offers a convenient and excellent way of diagnosing the disease, as the tissue-cultured virus can be readily recognized by its characteristic adenovirus type of cytopathic effect, its ability to hemagglutinate erythrocytes from several animal species, its production of intranuclear inclusion bodies in tissue-cultured cells, and its neutralization with immune and convalescent ICH serum.

Treatment. Treatment for ICH is basically symptomatic and supportive. Unless complications occur, and if the initial hepatic necrosis is not too severe, dogs will recover. No specific antivirus therapy has been proved effective, although an interferon inducer, polyinosinic-polycytidylic acid, was shown experimentally to reduce the mortality from ICH even though interferon could not be detected (Wooley et al. 1974).

Fluid therapy is essential in severe cases. An indwelling intravenous catheter should be inserted with caution so as to prevent local hemorrhage, and replacement fluids administered by slow intravenous drip as indicated (Greene 1984). Fresh whole blood may be beneficial in counteracting the effects of disseminated intravascular coagulation caused by CAV-1. Synthetic Vitamin K is of questionable value (Greene 1984). Hypertonic glucose infusions should be administered to counteract hypoglycemia, its possible association with neurological signs, and the general comatose state in animals with severe cases.

Prevention and Control. Inactivated and attenuated CAV-1 and CAV-2 vaccines are available to immunize dogs against ICH (Bass et al. 1980, Fishman and Scarnell 1976, Wilson et al. 1977). These should be administered with canine distemper vaccines and other vaccines as indicated by the manufacturer.

CAV-1 has been attenuated by transfer in dog, ferret, or pig kidney culture. Some strains of the attenuated CAV-1 vaccine can cause corneal opacity and uveitis, with persistent problems of interstitial keratitis, corneal edema, and secondary glaucoma (Appel et al. 1973; Curtis and Barnett 1973, 1981, 1983). To overcome this adverse effect, many commercial vaccines now contain an attenuated strain of CAV-2 instead of CAV-1 to protect against ICH (Appel et al. 1975, Bass et al. 1980).

Passive temporary maternal immunity to CAV-1 is acquired by newborn puppies through the colostrum (Carmichael et al. 1962, Winters 1981). Because the adenovirus vaccines are given to puppies with an unknown maternal immunity for ICH or CD, they should be administered when puppies are 8 to 10 weeks old or whenever the animals are first presented, and then again 4 weeks later.

Attenuated CAV-1 is eliminated from the urine of vaccinated dogs. Susceptible dogs that come in contact with the attenuated virus will be immunized without signs of illness.

Foxes that recover from the natural infection are permanently immune thereafter, and it is possible to immunize with hyperimmune homologous serum and with vaccine (Chaddock 1948). Hyperimmune serum is used principally to stop outbreaks. Formalinized tissue vaccines have been used successfully in foxes. Some manufacturers of vaccine for dogs also recommend the vaccine for foxes.

The Disease in Humans. The virus of canine hepatitis does not infect humans. The agent of virus-induced infectious hepatitis of humans was compared by Bech (1959) with CAV-1 in many ways, and no antigenic relation between them could be detected. There appears to be cross-reactivity between CAV-1 and human adenoviruses when the complement-fixation test is used (Carmichael and Barnes 1961). This has resulted in erroneous conclusions that CAV-1 infected humans. With the neutralization test, only human adenovirus 8 cross-reacts with CAV-1.

REFERENCES

Appel, M., Bistner, S.I., Menegus, M., Albert, M.D., and Carmichael, L.E. 1973. Pathogenicity of low-virulence strains of two canine adenovirus types. Am. J. Vet. Res. 34:543–550.

Appel, M., Carmichael, L.E., and Robson, D.S. 1975. Canine adenovirus type 2–induced immunity to two canine adenoviruses in pups with maternal antibody. Am. J. Vet. Res. 36:1199–1202.

Baker, J.A., Richards, M.G., Brown, A.L., and Rickard, C.G. 1950. Infectious hepatitis in dogs. In Proceedings of the 87th Annual Meeting of the American Veterinary Medical Association. Pp. 242–248.

Bass, E.P., Gill, M.A., and Beckenhauer, W.H. 1980. Evaluation of a canine adenovirus type 2 strain as a replacement for infectious hepatitis vaccine. J. Am. Vet. Med. Assoc. 177:234–242.

Bech, V. 1959. Canine hepatitis virus: Attempts to find relationship with human hepatitis. Proc. Soc. Exp. Biol. Med. 100:135–137.

Bolin, V.S., Jarnevic, N., and Austin, J.A. 1958. Infectious canine hepatitis virus studies with special reference to passage of raccoon tissue cultures. Proc. Soc. Exp. Biol. Med. 98:414–418.

Cabasso, V.J. 1962. Infectious canine hepatitis virus. Ann. N.Y. Acad. Sci. 101:498–514.

Cabasso, V.J., Stebbins, M.R., Norton, T.W., and Cox, H.R. 1954. Propagation of infectious canine hepatitis virus in tissue culture. Proc. Soc. Exp. Biol. Med. 85:239–245.

Carmichael, L.E. 1964. The pathogenesis of ocular lesions of infectious canine hepatitis. I. Pathology and virological observations. Pathol. Vet. 1:73–95.

Carmichael, L.E. 1965. The pathogenesis of ocular lesions of infectious canine hepatitis. II. Experimental ocular hypersensitivity produced by the virus. Pathol. Vet. 2:344–359.

Carmichael, L.E., and Barnes, F.D. 1961. Serological comparisons between infectious canine hepatitis virus and human adenovirus types. Proc. Soc. Exp. Biol. Med. 107:214–218.

Carmichael, L.E., Medic, B.L.S., Bistner, S.I., and Aquirre, G.D. 1975. Viral-antibody complexes in canine adenovirus type 1 (CAV-1) ocular lesions: Leukocyte chemotaxis and enzyme release. Cornell Vet. 65:331–351.

Carmichael, L.E., Robson, D.S., and Barnes, F.D. 1962. Transfer and decline of maternal infectious canine hepatitis antibody in puppies. Proc. Soc. Exp. Biol. Med. 109:677–681.

Chaddock, T.T. 1948. Infectious canine hepatitis as it occurs in the dog experimentally. Auburn Vet. 5:11–12, 34, 36–39.

Collins, J.E., Leslie, P., Johnson, D., Nelson, D., Peden, W., Boswell, R., and Draayer, H. 1984. Epizootic of adenovirus infection in American black bears. J. Am. Vet. Med. Assoc. 185:1430–1432.

Cowdry, E.V., and Scott, G.H. 1930. A comparison of certain intranuclear inclusions found in the livers of dogs without history of infection with intranuclear inclusions characteristic of the action of filtrable viruses. Arch. Pathol. 9:1184–1196.

Curtis, R., and Barnett, K.C. 1973. The ocular lesions of infectious canine hepatitis. 1. Clinical features. 2. Field incidence. J. Small Anim. Pract. 14:375–389, 737–745.

Curtis, R., and Barnett, K.C. 1981. Canine adenovirus–induced ocular lesions in the Afghan hound. Cornell Vet. 71:85–95.

Curtis, R., and Barnett, K.C. 1983. The "blue eye" phenomenon. Vet. Rec. 112:347–353.

Darai, G., Rosen, A., Delius, H., and Flugel, R.M. 1985. Characterization of the DNA of canine adenovirus by restriction enzyme analysis. Intervirology 23:23–28.

Davies, M.C., Englert, M.E., Stebbins, M.R., and Cabasso, V.J. 1961. Electron microscopic structure of infectious canine hepatitis (ICH) virus—A canine adenovirus. Virology 15:87–88.

Davis, C.L., and Anderson, W.A. 1950. The rapid diagnosis of contagious canine hepatitis by touch preparation of fresh liver tissue. Vet. Med. 45:435–437.

Ditchfield, J., MacPherson, L.W., and Zbitnew, A. 1962. Association of a canine adenovirus (Toronto A26/61) with an outbreak of laryngotracheitis ("kennel cough"): A preliminary report. Can. Vet. J. 3:238–247.

Espmark, J.A., and Salenstedt, C.R. 1961. Hemagglutination-inhibition test for titration of antibodies against hepatitis contagiosa canis (infectious canine hepatitis). Arch. Gesam. Virusforsch. 11:64–72.

Fastier, L.B. 1957. Studies on the hemagglutinin of infectious canine hepatitis virus. J. Immunol. 78:413–418.

Fishman, B., and Scarnell, J. 1976. Persistence of protection after vaccination against infectious canine hepatitis virus (CAV/1). Vet. Rec. 99:509.

Green, R.G., and Shillinger, J.E. 1934. Epizootic fox encephalitis. VI. A description of the experimental infection in dogs. Am. J. Hyg. 19:362–391.

Green, R.G., Ziegler, N.R., Green, B.B., and Dewey, E.T. 1930. Epizootic fox encephalitis. I. General description. Am. J. Hyg. 12:109–129.

Greene, C.E. 1984. Infectious canine hepatitis. In C.E. Greene, ed., Clinical Microbiology and Infectious Diseases of the Dog and Cat. W.B. Saunders, Philadelphia. Pp. 406–418.

Hamelin, C., Marsolais, G., and Assaf, R. 1984. Interspecific differences between the DNA restriction profiles of canine adenoviruses. Experientia 40:482.

Kapsenberg, J.G. 1959. Relationship of infectious canine hepatitis virus to human adenovirus. Proc. Soc. Exp. Biol. Med. 101:611–614.

Morrison, W.I., and Wright, N.G. 1976. Detection of immune complexes in the serum of dogs infected with canine adenovirus. Res. Vet. Sci. 21:119–121.

Noon, K.F., Rogul, M., Binn, L.N., et al. 1979. An enzyme-linked immunosorbent assay for the detection of canine antibodies to canine adenoviruses. Lab. Anim. Sci. 29:603–609.

Poppensiek, G.C. 1952. Proceedings of the 89th Annual Meeting of the American Veterinary Medical Association. P. 288.

Poppensiek, G.C., and Baker, J.A. 1951. Persistence of virus in urine as factor in spread of infectious hepatitis in dogs. Proc. Soc. Exp. Biol. Med. 77:279–281.

Rubarth, S. 1947. An acute virus disease with liver lesion in dogs (hepatitis contagiosa canis): A pathologico-anatomical and etiological investigation. Acta Pathol. Microbiol. Scand. 69(Suppl.):1–222.

Stephenson, R.O., Ritter, D.G., and Nielsen, C.A. 1982. Serologic survey for canine distemper and infectious canine hepatitis in wolves in Alaska. J. Wildl. Dis. 18:419–424.

Surdan, C., Cure, C., Dumitriu, E., and Wegener, M. 1959. Investigations concerning the relationship of silver fox virus encephalitis to infectious canine hepatitis of Rubarth. Acta Virol. 3:115–124.

Swango, L.J., Wooding, W.L., Jr., and Binn, L.N. 1970. A comparison of the pathogenesis and antigenicity of infectious canine hepatitis virus and the A26/61 virus strain (Toronto). J. Am. Vet. Med. Assoc. 156:1687–1696.

Whetstone, C.A. 1985. Should the criteria for species distinction in adenoviruses be reconsidered? Evidence from canine adenoviruses 1 and 2. Intervirology 23:116–120.

Wigton, D.H., Kociba, G.J., and Hoover, E.A. 1976. Infectious canine hepatitis: Animal model for viral-induced disseminated intravascular coagulation. Blood 47:287–296.

Wilson, J.H.G., Hermann-Dekkers, W.M., Leemans-Dessy, S., and de Meijer, J.W. 1977. Experiments with an inactivated hepatitis leptospirosis vaccine in vaccination programs for dogs. Vet. Rec. 100:522–554.

Winters, W.D. 1981. Time dependent decreases of maternal canine virus antibodies in newborn pups. Vet. Rec. 108:295–299.

Wooley, R.E., Brown, J., Scott, T.A., Lukert, P.D., and Crowell, W.A. 1974. Effect of polyinosinic-polycytidylic acid in dogs experimentally infected with infectious canine hepatitis virus. Am. J. Vet. Res. 35:1217–1219.

Wright, N.G., and Cornwell, H.J. 1983. Experimental canine adenovirus glomerulonephritis: Histological, immunofluorescence and ultrastructural features of the early glomerular changes. Br. J. Exp. Pathol. 64:312–319.

Wright, N.G., Nash, A.S., and Cornwell, H.J. 1981. Experimental canine adenovirus glomerulonephritis: Persistence of glomerular lesions after oral challenge. Br. J. Exp. Pathol. 62:183–189.

Canine Adenovirus 2 Infection

SYNONYMS: Canine infectious tracheobronchitis, infectious canine laryngotracheitis virus infection, kennel cough, Toronto A26/61 virus infection; abbreviations, CIT, CITB

Canine adenovirus type 2 (CAV-2) is one of several viruses involved in the respiratory disease complex of dogs known as canine infectious tracheobronchitis or kennel cough. It is one of the most common respiratory pathogens in dogs. Although many infections are mild or even subclinical, in combination with other viruses or bacteria a significant disease syndrome usually occurs. Clinical disease tends to be prolonged, but mortality is quite low. Reviews include those of Appel (1981) and Thayer (1984).

Figure 43.6. Canine adenovirus type 2 in bronchial epithelial cells of a dog, 6 days after aerosol exposure. Stained with fluorescent antibody. × 120. (Courtesy M. Appel and I. Parkinson.)

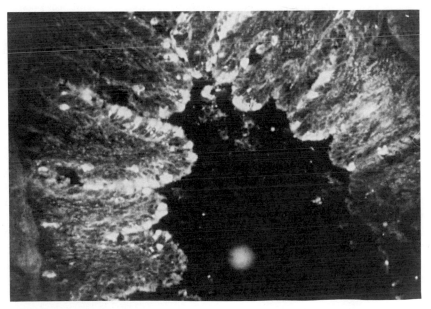

Character of the Disease. Infectious canine tracheobronchitis is a mild to inapparent respiratory disease of young dogs, usually occurring in kennels, adoption shelters, or pet shops where puppies are assembled. Signs generally include rhinitis, pharyngitis, tonsillitis, and tracheobronchitis (Appel et al. 1973). The original type 2 strain of canine adenovirus (Toronto A26/61) was isolated from a dog with respiratory illness (Ditchfield et al. 1962). This virus has a strict affinity for the epithelial cells lining the respiratory tract (Figure 43.6) and fails to produce hepatitis in dogs (Swango et al. 1970). The severity of clinical disease varies with different isolates, from inapparent to relatively severe respiratory disease (Appel et al. 1973, Fairchild et al. 1969, Swango et al. 1970). In dogs infected by parenteral inoculation, the infection is generally inapparent. Bacteria, especially *Bordetella bronchiseptica,* frequently increase the severity of the disease, especially when an epizootic occurs in a group of puppies (Bemis et al. 1977).

The incubation period is generally 3 to 5 days. Some dogs may have a mild fever for a short time. Tonsillitis may be present for a few days. The disease may vary in severity from a harsh, dry hacking cough of 6 to 7 days' duration to a fatal pneumonia. Other signs include depression, anorexia, dyspnea, muscular trembling, and serous nasal discharge. In some dogs the nasal discharge may become mucopurulent. Vomiting occurs in some animals, and some have soft, mucoid feces. Dogs with a harsh, dry cough have less lung involvement than dogs with a soft, moist, pulsating cough. The leukocyte counts are variable and inconclusive.

Properties of the Virus. CAV-2 has properties typical of other adenoviruses in the genus *Mastadenovirus.* The DNA is distinct from that of CAV-1 (Hamelin et al. 1984, Whetstone 1985). CAV-2 cross-reacts antigenically with CAV-1.

Epizootiology and Pathogenesis. CAV-2 has a predilection for respiratory epithelial cells. Viral replication produces a "severe necrotizing and proliferative bronchitis and bronchiolitis," which can result in bronchiolitis obliterans (Castleman 1985). The virus and viral antigen may be identified in animals with interstitial pneumonia and may be recovered from the lungs for 2 to 8 days after inoculation (Castleman 1985).

The gross lesions apparently are confined to the respiratory tract. There is atelectasis and congestion of the lungs with varying degrees of consolidation sharply demarcated from normal tissue. Congestion and hemorrhages of the bronchial lymph nodes are seen in most dogs. There are no gross lesions in the liver or gallbladder, as is characteristic of the hepatic disease in dogs caused by CAV-1.

Histological studies reveal moderate to severe pneumonic changes in dogs infected with virulent strains of virus (Bass et al. 1980, Castleman 1985, Emery et al. 1978). Cowdry type A intranuclear inclusion bodies may occur in the bronchial epithelium, alveolar septal cells, and turbinate epithelium. Proliferative, adenomatous changes are seen in the lungs 10 days after infection ensues. The bronchial lymph nodes are congested and edematous. Intranuclear inclusion bodies in the liver and marked edema and hemorrhage in the gallbladder are lacking in CAV-2 infections.

In studies with CAV-2, corneal opacities were not seen in experimental dogs after infection (Appel et al. 1973, Bass et al. 1980). Corneal opacities are known to occur in a small percentage of dogs given attenuated CAV-1 vaccine, or in those that have naturally contracted infectious canine hepatitis.

Diagnosis. Canine infectious tracheobronchitis is easily diagnosed by its clinical signs, but identification of CAV-2 as the causative virus requires laboratory tests. Nasal or pharyngeal swab samples or tracheal wash samples can be submitted to the diagnostic laboratory for virus isolation. The virus is easily isolated and identified in cell cultures.

Paired serum samples can be assayed for antibody titers to CAV-2. Several tests, including virus neutralization and ELISA, are available to measure antibodies.

Treatment. CIT caused by CAV-2 is generally a mild, self-limiting disease of 7 to 10 days' duration which does not require specific therapy (Thayer 1984). A warm environment and rest is usually sufficient for natural recovery if systemic signs are not present. Central nervous system—suppressing antitussives can be used to suppress the dry, hacking cough.

Antibiotics have no effect on CAV-2, but secondary bacterial infections may have to be treated with antibiotics, especially if systemic signs are present. Parenteral antibiotics often are ineffective (Odio et al. 1975), but aerosol or intratracheal administration of kanamycin sulfate (250 mg), gentamicin sulfate (50 mg), or polymyxin B sulfate (166,666 international units) twice a day for 3 days may be beneficial in ameliorating clinical signs (Bemis and Appel 1977, Thayer 1984).

Prevention and Control. Attenuated and inactivated vaccines are available for immunization of dogs against CAV-2 infection (Bass et al. 1980, Cornwell et al. 1982, Glickman and Appel 1981, Studdert 1984. Both the CAV-2 and the heterotypic CAV-1 or ICH virus strains provide solid protection against clinical disease caused by CAV-2. Routine vaccination programs for dogs should include immunization against this virus. Puppies should be vaccinated at 8 to 10 weeks of age (or on the first visit to the veterinary hospital) and again 4 weeks later. Annual revaccination is recommended.

The Disease in Humans. There is no indication that humans can be infected with CAV-2.

REFERENCES

Appel, M. 1981. Canine infectious tracheobronchitis (kennel cough): A status report. Compend. Cont. Ed. Pract. Vet. 3:70–77.

Appel, M., Bistner, S.I., Menegus, M., Albert, M.D., and Carmichael, L.E. 1973. Pathogenicity of low-virulence strains of two canine adenovirus types. Am. J. Vet. Res. 34:543–550.

Appel, M., Carmichael, L.E., and Robson, D.S. 1975. Canine adenovirus type 2-induced immunity to two canine adenoviruses in pups with maternal antibody. Am. J. Vet. Res. 36:1199–1202.

Bass, E.P., Gill, M.A., Beckenhauer, W.H. 1980. Evaluation of a canine adenovirus type 2 strain as a replacement for infectious canine hepatitis vaccine. J. Am. Vet. Med. Assoc. 177:234–242.

Bemis, D.A., and Appel, M.J.G. 1977. Aerosol, parenteral, and oral antibiotic treatment of Bordetella bronchiseptica infections in dogs. J. Am. Vet. Med. Assoc. 170:1082–1086.

Bemis, D.A., Greisen, H.A., and Appel, M.J.G. 1977. Pathogenesis of canine bordetellosis. J. Infect. Dis. 135:753–762.

Castleman, W.L. 1985. Bronchiolitis obliterans and pneumonia induced in young dogs by experimental adenovirus infection. Am. J. Pathol. 119:495–504.

Cornwell, H.J., Koptopoulos, G., Thompson, H., McCandlish, I.A., and Wright, N.G. 1982. Immunity to canine adenovirus respiratory disease: A comparison of attenuated CAV-1 and CAV-2 vacines. Vet. Rec. 110:27–32.

Cornwell, H.J., Paterson, S. D., McCandlish, I.A., Thompson, H., and Wright, N.G. 1983. Immunity to canine adenovirus respiratory disease: Effect of vaccination with an inactivated vaccine. Vet. Rec. 113:509–512.

Ditchfield, J., MacPherson, L.W., and Zbitnew, A. 1962. Association of a canine adenovirus (Toronto A26/61) with an outbreak of laryngotracheitis ("kennel cough"): A preliminary report. Can. Vet. J. 3:238–247.

Emery, J.B., House, J.A., and Brown, H.R. 1978. Cross-protective immunity to canine adenovirus type 2 by vaccination. Am. J. Vet. Res. 39:1778–1785.

Fairchild, G.A., Medway, W., and Cohen, D. 1969. A study of the pathogenicity of a canine adenovirus (Toronto A26/61) for dogs. Am. J. Vet. Res. 30:1187–1193.

Glickman, L.T., and Appel, M.J. 1981. Intranasal vaccine trial for canine infectious tracheobronchitis (kennel cough). Lab. Anim. Sci. 31:397–399.

Hamelin, C., Marsolais, G., and Assaf, R. 1984. Interspecific differences between the DNA restriction profiles of canine adenoviruses. Experientia 40:482.

Odio, W., Van Laer, E., and Klastersky, J. 1975. Concentrations of gentamicin in bronchial secretions after intramuscular and endotracheal administration. J. Clin. Pharmacol. 15:518–524.

Studdert, V.P. 1984. Kennel cough and canine adenovirus vaccines in Australia. Aust. Vet. J. 61:198–199.

Swango, L.J., Wooding, W.L., Jr., and Binn, L.N. 1970. A comparison of the pathogenesis and antigenicity of infectious canine hepatitis virus and the A26/61 virus strain (Toronto). J. Am. Vet. Med. Assoc. 156:1687–1696.

Thayer, G.W. 1984. Canine infectious tracheobronchitis. In C.E. Greene, ed., Clinical Microbiology and Infectious Diseases of the Dog and Cat. W.B. Saunders, Philadelphia. Pp. 430–436.

Whetstone, C.A. 1985. Should the criteria for species distinction in adenoviruses be reconsidered? Evidence from canine adenoviruses 1 and 2. Intervirology 23:116–120.

Bovine Adenovirus Infection

Bovine adenoviruses are a group of nine antigenically distinct viruses of the *Mastadenovirus* genus in the family Adenoviridae which infect cattle and produce mild or subclinical respiratory disease and, on occasion, enteric infection. Klein (1962) first isolated two bovine adenoviruses, now known as types 1 and 2, from cattle during a search for viruses responsible for the production of poliovirus antibodies. A serotype antigenically distinct from types 1 and 2 was isolated in England from the conjunctiva of a healthy cow (Darbyshire 1968), and it is now recognized as bovine adenovirus (BAV) type 3. Other strains have been isolated in Hungary from calves and lambs with diarrhea and still others from calves with pneumoenteritis (Aldasy et al. 1965). Nine serotypes are now recognized; others will probably be identified as studies progress. A strain of ovine adenovirus, isolated from naturally infected sheep and closely related to bovine adenovirus type 2, produced pneumoenteritis in experimental calves (Belak et al. 1977). Serologic surveys indicate widespread BAV infections in cattle (Lehmukhul et al. 1979.

Character of the Disease. BAV infection is common in cattle in many countries, including the United States, Japan, Hungary, England, and Germany. Various serotypes cause a variety of clinical signs such as conjunctivitis, pneumonia, pneumoenteritis, diarrhea, and polyarthritis (weak calf syndrome). Types 3, 4, and 5 are the ones usually incriminated in the production of disease in the United States (Corio et al. 1975, Lehmkuhl et al. 1975, McClurkin and Coria 1975, Mattson et al. 1977). Bovine adenoviruses have been isolated repeatedly from natural cases of pneumoenteritis in calves in which mortality was significant (Aldasy et al. 1965, Reed et al. 1978, Thompson et al. 1981). The disease was reproduced with many of these isolates in colostrum-deprived calves and in susceptible calves 2 to 16 weeks old.

Bovine adenoviruses have been incriminated as a cause of abortion and weak newborn calves (Bartha and Mate 1983, Ignatov and Pavlov 1978, Stauber and Card 1978).

Bovine adenovirus type 5 causes mild, self-limiting disease, characterized by marked pyrexia, polyarthritis, and occasional diarrhea, in colostrum-deprived calves (Cutlip and McClurkin 1975, McClurkin and Coria 1975). Natural disease is enhanced by cold weather and by other agents such as viral diarrhea virus. The signs of illness and necropsy findings were similar in both natural and experimental disease, according to Darbyshire (1968). In experimental disease clinical signs referable to the respiratory and digestive tracts were observed 7 days after intranasal or intratracheal injection of virus. At necropsy varying degrees of consolidation, collapse, and emphysema of the lungs were most prominent 7 days after exposure to the virus, but these lesions had persisted for at least 3 months. Histological features were proliferative bronchiolitis with necrosis and bronchiolar occlusion, resulting in alveolar collapse. Nuclear inclusion bodies were found in the bronchiolar epithelium, septal cells, and bronchial lymph nodes.

Properties of the Virus. Bovine adenoviruses have biochemical and biophysical properties consistent with those of other *Mastadenovirus* members. The different serotypes have been reviewed by Mohanty (1978).

Considerable interest in bovine adenovirus type 3 (BAV-3) and its oncogenic capability has led to detailed studies of its properties. In tests with purified virus in a cell line derived from calf kidney (CKT1), viral DNA synthesis was initiated after 24 hours and its rate was greatest after about 40 hours (Niiyama et al. 1975). Viral maturation occurred several hours later. Purified virus was separated into four discrete bands (representing complete, incomplete, empty, and degraded virions) in cesium chloride. The virus is similar in morphology and size to human and avian adenoviruses. The DNAs of bovine adenoviruses have been compared by DNA sequencing and restriction analysis (Belak et al. 1983, Hu 1984, Hu et al. 1984). There is a 25 percent homology between DNA of BAV-3 and human adenovirus type 5. Complete virions contain at least 10 polypeptides (Niiyama et al. 1975).

Types 1 and 2 agglutinate rat erythrocytes, and type 2 also agglutinates mouse erythrocytes. Neither serotype agglutinates red blood cells of chicks, guinea pigs, cattle, sheep, or humans (type O) (Klein 1962). Sheep isolates similar to BAV-2 can be differentiated by both restriction endonuclease mapping and hemagglutination tests (Belak et al. 1983).

Cultivation. After inoculation with bovine adenoviruses, calf kidney and calf testes cell monolayers of primary and stable cell cultures show a cytopathic effect characteristic of the adenovirus group.

Type 3 virus induced tumors when inoculated into newborn hamsters, but the virus was not recovered (Darbyshire 1968). Serotypes 1 and 2 failed to produce infection in suckling and adult hamsters, chicken embryos, guinea pigs, hamsters, or rabbits (Klein 1962).

Adult hamsters immunized with type 3 virus rejected tumor transplants from suckling hamsters with bovine adenovirus type 3 tumors, whereas transplants were readily made in nonimmune adult hamsters.

Epizootiology and Pathogenesis. Bovine adenoviruses are primarily transmitted by direct contact of infected and susceptible cattle, or by contact with their contaminated excretions. From experimentally infected calves, virus could be recovered from the conjunctiva, nose, and feces for 10 to 21 days after onset of infection. Aerosol transmission may occur; entry of virus is probably through the mouth or respiratory tract. Transplacental infection may also occur, as bovine adenoviruses have been repeatedly isolated from bovine fetuses (Batha and Mate 1983).

Infection probably begins in the lymphoid tissue of the oropharynx or in the epithelial cells of the respiratory tract and may spread to the intestinal epithelium and produce enteritis. Virus may spread down the respiratory tree or through the bloodstream to infect the lung and produce pneumonia. Infection of the conjunctival epithelium can result in conjunctivitis or keratoconjunctivitis.

Immunity. The mechanism of neutralization of virus by antibody is complex, but the type-specific determinants exposed on the virion must play a critical role (Willcox and Mautner 1976). Calves inoculated with bovine adenoviruses develop neutralizing antibodies in 10 to 14 days. Heterotypic responses are not observed. These antibody levels are maintained for at least 10 weeks. Precipitating antibodies appear in 3 weeks with no diminution of titer at 10 weeks (Darbyshire 1968). At necropsy of two young calves with diarrhea and dehydration that failed to respond to therapy, foci of necrosis were found in the abomasum and rumen of each calf, and the intestinal tract contained grayish, turbid fluid. Intranuclear inclusion bodies found in endothelial vessels of the abomasum, rumen, adrenal cortical sinusoids, and renal glomeruli, and also in intestinal epithelial cells contained adenovirus particles (Bulmer et al. 1975).

Complement-fixing (CF) antibodies were not always present, but CF antigen was found in various tissues, particularly in the upper respiratory tract, of calves infected with type 3 (Darbyshire 1968). Hemagglutinating antibodies reached a maximum level 7 days after intranasal exposure with type 1 virus, a level that was maintained for at least 6 weeks (Darbyshire 1968). The duration of immunity in cattle to BAV-3 after two intranasal administrations of attenuated virus 6 weeks apart was at least 21 months. Before challenge with virulent virus, local and systemic antibodies were detected in the animals (Zygraich et al. 1976). It is reasonable to anticipate that immunity after vaccination or natural disease will be strong and long-lasting. Submucosal application of the virus induces the production of interferon, which undoubtedly also plays some role in adenovirus immunity.

Diagnosis. BAV infections cannot be distinguished clinically from infections with other bovine viruses that produce respiratory signs and, frequently, diarrhea as well. Consequently a positive diagnosis requires laboratory isolation and identification of virus, or the identification of seroconversion to one of the serotypes of BAV (Kahrs 1981).

The best material for virus isolation is exudate from nasal passages and conjunctiva or feces of acutely ill cattle. Virus is regularly recovered in tissue cultures from trachea and lungs. The isolate can be identified by the characteristics listed under "Properties of the Virus." The ability of most serotypes to hemagglutinate rat erythrocytes provides an especially convenient and quick identification. The demonstration of a rising titer with paired serums utilizing serum neutralization, agar-gel immunodiffusion (AGID), complement fixation, passive hemagglutination, fluorescent antibody, hemagglutination inhibition, or ELISA also is an excellent way to diagnose the disease. Messner et al. (1983) developed a dual-antigen AGID test for detecting antibodies for the two subgroups of bovine viruses. In the serotyping of isolates no cross-reactions are noted in the neutralization test.

Treatment. There is no specific treatment for BAV infection in cattle. Antibiotics should be given to help control secondary bacterial invaders, and appropriate supportive measures should be applied.

Prevention and Control. There is considerable activity and interest in the production of inactivated and attenuated virus vaccines for the prevention and control of BAV infection. Present evidence suggests that these vaccines for either BAV-1 or BAV-3, usually in combination with vaccines for infectious bovine rhinotracheitis or bovine parainfluenza 3, are safe and very effective for a considerable time against homologous virus (Haralambiev 1975, Rondhuis 1975, Zygraich 1975). Rondhuis (1975) believes oil adjuvant vaccines are superior, but considerably more work must be done to prove his arguments. Present evidence suggests that cattle will also have a large number of serotypes, with no suggestion of cross-protection among them. It seems unlikely that vaccination will ever play a prominent role in the control of the disease unless researchers find that a very limited number of serotypes are the significant pathogens, or that cross-protection does occur with some of the nine serotypes.

A general characteristic of this adenovirus group is the persistence of the virus, which also makes control of these diseases more difficult. Good management, health care, and housing can reduce the severity of the disease; but prevention is difficult, if not impossible, until a practical and economic vaccination program becomes a reality. No vaccines are licensed in the United States at this time.

The Disease in Humans. The relation between bovine adenoviruses and infection in humans has not been established. There is no reported evidence of disease in humans caused by bovine adenoviruses, but serum-neutralizing antibodies to types 1 and 2 have been found in humans. There is no cross-reaction between these two bovine serotypes with antiserums to human adenoviruses 1 through 18.

REFERENCES

Aldasy, P., Csontos, L, and Bartha, A. 1965. Pneumo-enteritis in calves caused by adenoviruses. Acta Vet. Hung. 15:167–175.

Bartha, A., and Mate, S. 1983. Transplacental transmission of bovine adenoviruses. Comp. Immunol. Microbiol. Infect. Dis. 6:189–192.

Belak, S., Berencsi, G., Rusvay, M., Lukacs, K., and Nasz, X. 1983. DNA structure, and hemagglutination properties of bovine adenovirus type 2 strains which bypass species specificity. Arch. Virol. 77:181–194.

Belak, S., Palfi, V., Szekeres, T., and Tury, E. 1977. Experimental infection of calves with an adenovirus isolated from sheep and related to bovine adenovirus type 2. I. Clinical and virological studies. Zentralbl. Veterinärmed. 24:542–547.

Bulmer, W.S., Tsai, K.S., and Little, P.B. 1975. Adenovirus infection in two calves. J. Am. Vet. Med. Assoc. 166:233–238.

Coria, M.F., McClurkin, A.W., Cutlip, R.C., and Ritchie, A.E. 1975. Isolation and characterization of adenovirus type 5 associated with weak calf syndrome. Arch. Virol. 47:309–317.

Cutlip, R.C., and McClurkin, A.W. 1975. Lesions and pathogenesis of disease in young calves experimentally induced by a bovine adenovirus type 5 isolated from a calf with weak calf syndrome. Am. J. Vet. Res. 36:1095–1098.

Darbyshire, J.H. 1968. Bovine adenoviruses. J. Am. Vet. Med. Assoc. 152:786–792.

Haralambiev, H. 1975. The immunological response of calves after submucosal application of a live vaccine against parainfluenza-3 and adenovirus. (Brief report.) Arch. Exp. Veterinärmed. 29:397–400.

Hu, S.L. 1984. Restriction analysis and homology studies of the bovine adenovirus 7 genome. J. Virol. 51:800–803.

Hu, S.L., Hays, W.W., and Potts, D.E. 1984. Sequence homology between bovine and human adenoviruses. J. Virol. 51:604–608.

Ignatov, G., and Pavlov, N. 1978. Isolation of adenovirus type 1 from aborted cattle fetuses. (In Bulgarian.) Vet. Med. Nauki 15:82–88.

Ignatov, G., and Popov, G. 1978. Density gradient and ultrastructure of bovine adenovirus type 1. (In Bulgarian.) Vet. Med. Nauki 15:95–99.

Kahrs, R.F. 1981. Adenoviruses. In R.F. Kahrs, ed., Viral Diseases of Cattle. Iowa State University Press, Ames. Pp. 61–70.

Klein, M. 1962. The relationship of two bovine adenoviruses to human adenoviruses. Ann. N.Y. Acad. Sci. 101:493–497.

Lehmkuhl, H.D., Smith, M.H., and Dierks, R.E. 1975. A bovine adenovirus type 3: Isolation, characterization, and experimental infection in calves. Arch. Virol. 48:39–46.

Lehmkuhl, H.D., Smith, M.H., and Gough, P.M. 1979. Neutralizing antibody to bovine adenovirus serotype 3 in healthy cattle and cattle with respiratory tract disease. Am. J. Vet. Res. 40:580–583.

McClurkin, A.W., and Coria, M.F. 1975. Infectivity of bovine adenovirus type 5 recovered from a polyarthritic calf with weak calf syndrome. J. Am. Vet. Med. Assoc. 67:139–141.

Messner, A., Hinaidy, B., and Burki, F. 1983. Bovine adenoviruses. V. Diagnostic efficiency of dual-antigen immunodiffusion test using two different group-reactive antigens in parallel. Zentralbl. Veterinärmed. [B] 30:762–774.

Mohanty, S.B. 1978. Bovine respiratory viruses. Adv. Vet. Sci. Comp. Med. 22:83–109.

Niiyama, Y., Igarashi, K., Tsukamoto, K., Kurokawa, T., and Sugino,

W. 1975. Biochemical studies on bovine adenovirus type 3. I. Purification and properties. J. Virol. 16:621–633.

Reed, D.E., Wheeler, J.G., and Lupton, H.W. 1978. Isolation of bovine adenovirus type 7 from calves with pneumonia and enteritis. Am. J. Vet. Res. 39:1968–1971.

Rondhuis, P.R. 1975. Bovine adenoviruses: A review of vaccination experiments. Dev. Biol. Stand. 28:493–500.

Stauber, E., and Card, C. 1978. Experimental intraamniotic exposure of bovine fetuses with subgroup 2, type 7 adenovirus. Can. J. Comp. Med. 42:466–472.

Thompson, K.G., Thomson, G.W., and Henry, J.N. 1981. Alimentary tract manifestations of bovine adenovirus infections. Can. Vet. J. 22:68–71.

Willcox, N., and Mautner, V. 1976. Antigenic determinants of adenovirus capsids. II. Homogeneity of hexons, and accessibility of their determinants, in the virion. J. Immunol. 116:25–29.

Zygraich, N. 1975. Trivalent vaccines against bovine respiratory viral infections. Dev. Biol. Stand. 28:482–488.

Zygraich, N., Vascoboinic, E., and Huygelen, C. 1976. Immunity studies in calves vaccinated with a multivalent live respiratory vaccine composed of I.B.R., parainfluenza 3 and bovine adenovirus type 3. Dev. Biol. Stand. 33:379–383.

Equine Adenovirus Infections

Equine adenoviruses are common viruses of horses which generally produce asymptomatic or mild respiratory infections. In Arabian foals with combined immunodeficiency disease, inherited as a simple autosomal recessive defect, severe fatal pneumonia usually results from equine adenovirus (EAdV) infection (Coggins 1979, Parryman et al. 1978, Studdert 1978). Various investigators have isolated an adenovirus from animals with pneumonia (Henry and Gagnon 1976, Konishi et al. 1977, McChesney et al. 1973, Thompson et al. 1976, Whitlock et al. 1975). In one instance 28 Arabian and 3 non-Arabian foals less than 3 months old developed a disease characterized by pneumonia, lymphopenia, and intermittent fever; 27 Arabian foals and 1 non-Arabian foal died, and 1 Arabian and 2 non-Arabian foals recovered (McChesney et al. 1973).

Experimental studies of equine adenoviruses in specific-pathogen–free foals were conducted by Gleeson et al. (1978). In these immunocompetent foals clinical disease consisted of conjunctivitis, upper respiratory tract disease, and pneumonia. At necropsy, gross and microscopic lesions of bronchopneumonia with interstitial pneumonia, tracheitis, rhinitis, and conjunctivitis were present.

Edington et al. (1984) isolated EAdV from two of three animals with cauda equina neuritis. EAdV has been isolated from foals with diarrhea (Corrier et al. 1982, Studdert and Blackney 1982). The virus isolated by Studdert and Blackney had different hemagglutinating properties than EAdV-1, and it was not neutralized by antiserum to EAdV-1. They proposed that this fecal EAdV be designated EAdV-2. Seventy-seven percent of 339 equine serum samples tested contained neutralizing antibodies to EAdV-2.

Studdert et al. (1974) made antigenic comparisons of seven strains of EAdV from the United States, Germany, or Australia by the serum-neutralization and hemagglutination-inhibition methods. The seven equine strains were closely related. Further, these investigators found antibodies to EAdV in 73 percent of 631 equine serum samples tested. This finding indicates that EAdV infection is common in horses and suggests that only in unusual cases do clinical signs accompany the infection.

In experimental studies with EAdV neonates developed clinical signs that included fever, nasal and ocular discharge, and dyspnea (McChesney et al. 1974). Older foals were less affected, and colostrum-fed foals had milder illness than colostrum-deprived foals. Neonatal foals that were euthanatized during acute illness had lesions that included hyperplasia, swelling, necrosis, and intranuclear inclusions in epithelial cells of the respiratory tract. Virus was recovered from most experimentally infected foals.

Strains of EAdV have been isolated in cultures of fetal or horse kidney cells or of equine fetal dermis cells. The cytopathic alterations in cell culture were characteristic of adenoviruses, and examination by electron microscopy confirmed the presence of adenovirus particles and equine adeno-satellite viral particles (Dutta 1975). Other characteristics of the isolate also were typical of adenoviruses (Fatemie-Nainie and Marusyk 1979, Harden 1974, Konishi et al. 1977).

An experimental inactivated vaccine has been studied (Lew et al. 1979), but commercial vaccines for EAdV infections are not available.

REFERENCES

Coggins, L. 1979. Viral respiratory disease. Vet. Clin. North Am. [Large Anim. Pract.] 1(1):59–72.

Corrier, D.E., Montgomery, D., and Scutchfield, W.L. 1982. Adenovirus in the intestinal epithelium of a foal with prolonged diarrhea. Vet. Pathol. 19:564–567.

Dutta, S.K. 1975. Isolation and characterization of an adenovirus and isolation of its adenovirus-associated virus in cell culture from foals with respiratory tract disease. Am. J. Vet. Res. 36:247–250.

Edington, N., Wright, J.A., Patel, J.R., Edwards, G.B., and Griffiths, L. 1984. Equine adenovirus 1 isolated from cauda equina neuritis. Res. Vet. Sci. 37:252–254.

Fatemie-Nainie, S., and Marusyk, R. 1979. Biophysical and serologic comparison of four equine adenovirus isolates. Am. J. Vet. Res. 40:521–528.

Gleeson, L.J., Studdert, M.J., and Sullivan, N.D. 1978. Pathogenicity and immunologic studies of equine adenovirus in specific-pathogen-free foals. Am. J. Vet. Res. 39:1636–1642.

Harden, T.J. 1974. Characterization of an equine adenovirus. Res. Vet. Sci. 16:244–250.

Henry, J.N., and Gagnon, A.N. 1976. Adenovirus pneumonia in an Arabian foal. Can. Vet. J. 17:220–221.

Konishi, S.I., Harasawa, R., Mochizuki, M., Akashi, H., and Ogata, M. 1977. Studies on equine adenovirus. I. Characteristics of an adenovirus isolated from a thoroughbred colt with pneumonia. Jpn. J. Vet. Sci. 39:117–125.

Lew, A.M., Smith, H.V., and Studdert, M.J. 1979. Development and preliminary testing of an inactivated equine adenovirus vaccine. Am. J. Vet. Res. 40:1707–1712.

McChesney, A.E., England, J.J., and Rich, L.J. 1973. Adenoviral infection in foals. Am. J. Vet. Res. 162:545–549.

McChesney, A.E., England, J.J., Whiteman, C.E., Adcock, J.L., Rich, L.J., and Chow, T.L. 1974. Experimental transmission of equine adenovirus in Arabian and non-Arabian foals. Am. J. Vet. Res. 35:1015–1023.

Parryman, L.E., McGuire, T.C., and Crawford, T.B. 1978. Maintenance of foals with combined immunodeficiency: Causes and control of secondary infections. Am. J. Vet. Res. 39:1043–1047.

Studdert, M.J. 1978. Primary, severe, combined immunodeficiency disease of Arabian foals. Aust. Vet. J. 54:411–417.

Studdert, M.J., and Blackney, M.H. 1982. Isolation of an adenovirus antigenically distinct from equine adenovirus type 1 from diarrheic foal feces. Am. J. Vet. Res. 43:543–544.

Studdert, M.J., Wilks, C.R., and Coggins, L. 1974. Antigenic comparisons and serologic survey of equine adenoviruses. Am. J. Vet. Res. 35:693–699.

Thompson, D.B., Spradbrow, P.B., and Studdert, M. 1976. Isolation of an adenovirus from an Arab foal with a combined immunodeficiency disease. Aust. Vet. J. 52:435–437.

Whitlock, R.H., Dellers, R.W., and Shively, J.N. 1975. Adenoviral pneumonia in a foal. Cornell Vet. 65:393–401.

Porcine Adenovirus Infections

Porcine adenoviruses are widespread viruses of swine that generally produce asymptomatic infections but may be associated with pneumonia, enteritis, kidney lesions, transplacental infections, and encephalitis (Derbyshire 1986, Narita et al. 1985, Sanford and Hoover 1983). Porcine adenovirus (PAV) infections have been reviewed by Derbyshire (1986).

Porcine adenovirus was first isolated from a rectal swab of a 12-day-old piglet with diarrhea (Haig et al. 1964). Subsequently, porcine adenoviruses were derived from various tissues of normal pigs at slaughter, rectal swabs of healthy pigs, and from the brain of a 10-week-old pig with encephalitis (Darbyshire et al. 1966, Kasza 1966, Köhler and Apodaca 1966, Mahnel and Bibrack 1966, Mayr et al. 1967). Serologic surveys indicate the incidence of PAV infection in swine is quite widespread. In one survey in Canada 15 percent of serum samples from adult swine with respiratory disease had antibodies against porcine adenoviruses (Dea and El Azhary 1984). In another survey the incidence of infection in the pig populations of Hungary and Bulgaria was found to be approximately 20 percent (Genov and Bodon 1976).

At present, there are four recognized serotypes of porcine adenoviruses (Derbyshire 1986, Derbyshire et al. 1975). Reference antiserums against human adenoviruses types 1 to 31 do not neutralize PAV serotypes 1, 2, and 3, whereas neutralizing antibodies to the three PAV serotypes can be found in serum from normal sows (Haig et al. 1964). It appears that many strains are of relatively low pathogenicity, and usually serotype 4 is isolated in natural cases of diarrhea or encephalitis. This serotype produced meningoencephalitis in gnotobiotic pigs (Edington et al. 1972).

Studies of enteritis experimentally induced by PAV strain 6618 (type 3) in hysterotomy-derived, colostrum-deprived pigs found that virus was present in the altered epithelial cells 1 to 16 days after inoculation, and viral antigen could be detected in these cells for up to 45 days (Coussement et al. 1981, Ducatelle et al. 1982). After an incubation period of 3 to 4 days, all inoculated pigs had diarrhea. Villi of the terminal jejunum and ileum were shortened, and epithelial cells were destroyed by the virus.

The porcine adenoviruses have all the morphological and biochemical characteristics of the other adenoviruses (Genov and Bodon 1976). The strains usually replicate in primary cell cultures of embryonic and piglet kidney, rabbit kidney, porcine embryonic lung, or porcine embryonic testes and also in the stable cell line PK-15. The cytopathology is characteristic of adenoviruses, with typical intranuclear inclusion bodies produced in infected cells.

REFERENCES

Coussement, W,. Ducatelle, R., Charlier, G., and Hoorens, J. 1981. Adenovirus enteritis in pigs. Am. J. Vet. Res. 42:1905–1911.

Darbyshire, J.H., Jennings, A.R., Dawson, P.S., Lamont, P.H., and Omar, A.R. 1966. The pathogenesis and pathology of infection in calves with a strain of bovine adenovirus type 3. Res. Vet. Sci. 7:81–93.

Dea, S., and El Azhary, M.A. 1984. Prevalence of antibodies to porcine adenovirus in swine by indirect fluorescent antibody test. Am. J. Vet. Res. 45:2109–2112.

Derbyshire, J.B. 1986. Porcine adenovirus infection. In A.D. Leman, B. Straw, R.D. Glock, W.L. Mengeling, R.H.C. Penny, and E. Scholl, eds., Diseases of Swine, 6th ed. Iowa State University Press, Ames. Pp. 321–324.

Derbyshire, J.B., Clarke, M.C., and Collins, A.P. 1975. Serological and pathogenicity studies with some unclassified porcine adenoviruses. J. Comp. Pathol. 85:437–443.

Ducatelle, R., Coussement, W., and Hoorens, J. 1982. Sequential pathological study of experimental porcine adenovirus enteritis. Vet. Pathol. 19:179–189.

Edington, N., Kasza, L., and Christofinis, G.J. 1972. Meningo-encephalitis in gnotobiotic pigs inoculated intranasally and orally with porcine adenovirus 4. Res. Vet. Sci. 13:289–291.

Genov, I., and Bodon, L. 1976. Vurkhu tipiziraneto i razprostranenieto na adenovirusi po svine. Vet. Med. Nauki 13:31–38.

Haig, D.A., Clarke, M.C., and Pereira, M.S. 1964. Isolation of an adenovirus from a pig. J. Comp. Pathol. 74:81–84.

Kasza, L. 1966. Isolation of an adenovirus from the brain of a pig. Am. J. Vet. Res. 27:751–758.

Köhler, H., and Apodaca, J. 1966. Über die Erkennung von Adenovirus-Infektionen in Schweinenieren-Primärkulturen mit Hilfe histologischer Verfahren. Zentralbl. Bakteriol. I. Abt. Orig. 199:338–349.

Mahnel, H., and Bibrack, B. 1966. Isolierung von Adenoviren aus Zellkulturen von Nieren normaler Schlachtschweine. Zentralbl. Bakteriol. I. Abt. Orig. 199:329–338.

Mayr, A., Bibrack, B., and Bachmann, P. 1967. Züchtung von Schweineadenoviren in Kälbernierenkulturen. Zentralbl. Bakteriol. I. Abt. Orig. 203:59–68.

Narita, M., Imada, T., and Fukusho, A. 1985. Pathologic changes caused by transplacental infection with an adenovirus-like agent in pigs. Am. J. Vet. Res. 46:1126–1129.

Sanford, S.E., and Hoover, D.M. 1983. Enteric adenovirus infection in pigs. Can. J. Comp. Med. 47:396–400.

Ovine Adenovirus Infection

Ovine adenovirus serotypes produce mild or inapparent infection associated primarily with the respiratory tract, but occasionally with the intestinal tract as well. Six serotypes have been isolated and identified (Adair et al. 1982, 1985; Belak et al. 1980; McFerran et al. 1971; Sharp et al. 1974).

Ovine adenovirus 4 infection in specific-pathogen–free lambs (Rushton and Sharpe 1977, Sharp et al. 1976) failed to elicit clinical signs, but pathological changes referable to the respiratory and alimentary tracts were discernible. In all likelihood this infection may predispose the host to more serious infections. Belak et al. (1976) reported on a natural outbreak of adenovirus disease in suckling and fattening lambs which caused pneumoenteritis with heavy mortality on two large farms. One ovine serotype from this epizootic produced a similar disease in 3-week-old experimental lambs (Palya et al. 1977). Chronic progressive interstitial pneumonia can be caused by adenovirus infection (Zhelev et al. 1979). On the farm that raised only sheep, a virus was isolated from 6- to 8-week-old Merino lambs with mild respiratory signs of illness that was similar, if not identical, to BAV-2 infection (Belak et al. 1975) but different from that caused by known ovine serotypes.

Experimental infection with serotype 6 in lambs resulted in mild fever 4 to 8 days after exposure, upper respiratory signs, and lower respiratory tract infection (Cutlip and Lehmkuhl 1983; Lehmkuhl and Cutlip 1984a, 1984b).

REFERENCES

Adair, B.M., McFerran, J.B., and McKillop, E.R. 1982. A sixth species of ovine adenovirus isolated from lambs in New Zealand. Arch. Virol. 74:269–275.

Adair, B.M., McKillop, E.R., and McFerran, J.B. 1985. Serologic classification of two ovine adenovirus isolates from the central United States. Am. J. Vet. Res. 46:945–946.

Belak, S., Palfi, V., and Palya, V. 1976. Adenovirus infection in lambs. I. Epizootiology of the disease. Zentralbl. Veterinärmed. [B] 23:320–330.

Belak, S., Palfi, V., and Tury, E. 1975. Experimental infection of lambs with an adenovirus isolated from sheep and related to bovine adenovirus type 2. I. Virology studies. Acta Vet. Acad. Sci. Hung. 25:91–95.

Belak, S., Vetesi, F., Palfi, V., and Papp, L. 1980. Isolation of a pathogenic strain of ovine adenovirus type 5 and a comparison of its pathogenicity with that of another strain of the same serotype. J. Comp. Pathol. 90:169–176.

Cutlip, R.C., and Lehmkuhl, H.D. 1983. Experimental infection of lambs with ovine adenovirus isolate RTS-151: Lesions. Am. J. Vet. Res. 44:2395–2402.

Lehmkuhl, H.D., and Cutlip, R.C. 1984a. Experimental infection of lambs with ovine adenovirus isolate RTS-151: Clinical, microbiological, and serologic responses. Am. J. Vet. Res. 45:260–262.

Lehmkuhl, H.D., and Cutlip, R.C. 1984b. Characterization of the serotypes of adenovirus isolated from sheep in the central United States. Am. J. Vet. Res. 45:562–566.

McFerran, J.B., Nelson, R., and Knox, E.R. 1971. Isolation and characterisation of sheep adenoviruses. Arch. Gesam. Virusforsch. 35:232–241.

Palya, V., Belak, S., and Palfi, V. 1977. Adenovirus infection in lambs. II. Experimental infection of lambs. Zentralbl. Veterinärmed. [B] 24:529–541.

Rushton, B., and Sharp, J.M. 1971. Pathology of ovine adenovirus type 4 infection in SPF lambs: Pulmonary and hepatic lesions. J. Pathol. 121:163–167.

Sharp, J.M., McFerran, J.B., and Rae, A. 1974. A new adenovirus from sheep. Res. Vet. Sci. 17:268–269.

Sharp, J.M., Rushton, B., and Rimer, R.D. 1976. Experimental infection of specific pathogen-free lambs with ovine adenovirus type 4. J. Comp. Pathol. 86:621–628.

Zhelev, V., Ognyanov, D., Angelov, A.K., Karadzhov, Y.A., and Panova, M. 1979. Chronic progressive interstitial pneumonia in sheep (adenovirus pneumonia). (In Bulgarian.) Vet. Med. Nauki 16:78–87.

Other Mammalian Adenovirus Infections

Adenoviruses have been isolated from a number of vertebrate species and studied (McFerran 1981). Two serotypes of murine adenoviruses occur in some mouse colonies. They infect a large percentage of the mice in these colonies, and adenovirus is eliminated in the urine over extended periods. Suckling mice inoculated by various routes suffer fatal infection with disseminated pathological lesions, particularly in the brown fat, heart, and adrenals.

The opossum adenovirus was isolated from the kidney cell culture of this species. As adenoviruses commonly persist as latent viruses in the kidneys of various species, investigators using animal kidney cell cultures must be aware of this situation. The ability of the opossum isolate to produce disease has not been determined.

There are at least 16 recognized serotypes of simian adenoviruses (McFerran 1981). Most adenoviruses from nonhuman primates have been isolated from normal animals or cell cultures from normal animals, but some isolates have been associated with clinical disease of the respiratory tract, conjunctiva, or intestinal tract.

An adenovirus was isolated from the large intestine of two goats that died from *peste des petits ruminants* in separate outbreaks. The two isolates were considered to be serotypes different from the sheep and cattle types (Gibbs et al. 1977).

REFERENCES

Gibbs, E.P., Taylor, W.P., and Lawman, M.J. 1977. The isolation of adenoviruses from goats affected with peste des petits ruminants in Nigeria. Res. Vet. Sci. 23:331–335.

McFerran, J.B. 1981. Adenoviruses of vertebrate animals. In C. Kurstak and E. Kurstak, eds., Comparative Diagnosis of Viral Diseases, vol. 3. Academic Press, New York. Pp. 101–165.

The Genus *Aviadenovirus*

Avian Adenovirus Infections

SYNONYMS: Egg-drop syndrome (EDS), fowl adenovirus infections, hemorrhagic enteritis (HE), inclusion body hepatitis (IBH), marble spleen disease (MSD)

Adenoviruses are common infectious agents of poultry and other avian species throughout the world. Various diseases are attributed to the 12 avian adenovirus serotypes (McFerran 1981, McFerran and Connor 1977, Winterfield 1984) now known to exist. Ten serotypes have been established in the United States (Calnek and Cowen 1975, Calnek et al. 1982), and in all likelihood all serotypes are present.

Respiratory disease, clinical or subclinical, is a common manifestation of many of the avian serotypes (McFerran 1981, Mustaffa-Babjee and Spradbrow 1975). Multifocal interstitial or diffuse pneumonia can occur (Dhillon et al. 1982, Dhillon and Winterfield 1984). Pulmonary congestion and edema, as well as splenomegaly and hepatomegaly, can occur with marble spleen disease (Domermuth et al. 1982). Death in pheasants infected with MSD virus is caused by pulmonary edema (McFerran 1981).

Inclusion body hepatitis, first recorded by Helmboldt and Frazier (1963), produces a sudden increase in mortality of birds 5 to 7 weeks old; few birds appear to be sick (Grimes et al. 1977, McFerran 1981). Findings include hemorrhages, pale and friable livers, hepatomegaly, and anemia. Intranuclear inclusion bodies are present in hepatocytes. Many strains of avian adenovirus can produce hepatitis, but the pathogenicity for the liver varies among strains (Lee et al. 1978). Viral hepatitis with necrosis and intranuclear inclusions occurred in goslings (8 to 28 days old) in a closed breeding flock (Riddell 1984).

Egg-drop syndrome-1976 (EDS'76) is a clinical disease of fowl characterized by soft- or thin-shelled eggs, or eggs with no shells at all, in birds that are otherwise healthy (McFerran 1984, van Eck et al. 1976, Yamaguchi et al. 1981). Apparently a change in the sodium pump mechanism of the epithelial cells in the uterine mucosa increases the sodium concentration and decreases the concentration of potassium, calcium, magnesium, and glucose in the uterine fluid (van Eck and Vertommen 1984). Birds experimentally infected with the EDS'76 strain of adenovirus laid abnormal eggs 10 to 24 days after infection (Taniguchi et al. 1981). In these birds the uterus was edematous, and the epithelial cells, which contained intranuclear inclusion bodies and adenovirus particles, were undergoing degeneration and desquamation.

EDS'76 virus is indistinguishable antigenically from hemagglutinating adenovirus of ducks (Gulka et al. 1984). The duck virus is extremely widespread and indigenous in waterfowl and other aquatic birds (Gulka et al. 1984). Experimental infection of laying hens with a field isolate of the duck virus was nonpathogenic but protected the birds against subsequent infection from the pathogenic adenovirus 127 (Brugh et al. 1984).

Hemorrhagic enteritis virus of turkeys can produce infection in chickens, with intranuclear inclusion bodies, but the infection is usually subclinical (Beasley and Clifton 1979). Hemorrhagic enteritis and hepatitis of suspected adenovirus etiology has been reported in captive American kestrels (Sileo et al. 1983).

Avian adenoviruses as well as avian reoviruses have been incriminated in tenosynovitis and leg weakness (Jones et al. 1981, McFerran 1981, Takase et al. 1983). The exact role of these adenoviruses in this condition is not known. Atrophy of the bursa of Fabricius (Mustaffa-Babjee and Spradbrow 1975) and the hemorrhagic-aplastic anemia syndrome (Rosenberger et al. 1975) are other conditions attributed to avian adenovirus infection. Limited observations suggest the adeno-associated viruses (parvoviruses) coinfect many chickens that carry adenoviruses (Yates et al. 1977). Quail bronchitis, an acute, highly fatal respiratory disease of young quail, is caused by an avian adenovirus identical to the F1 virus (McFerran 1981). Quail that recover from experimental disease are resistant to natural disease, but reinfection does occur despite the presence of neutralizing antibody (Olson 1950).

The physical and chemical characteristics of the avian adenoviruses are typical of other adenoviruses (Cabasso and Wilner 1969). However, avian adenoviruses lack a common complement-fixing antigen shared by all mammalian adenoviruses. The DNA molecules of 17 strains (11 serotypes) of avian adenoviruses have been characterized and compared by restriction endonuclease mapping (Zsak and Kisary 1984). The 11 serotypes can be divided into 5 groups. At least 14 structural proteins and 3 core proteins have been identified from avian adenovirus type

1 (Li et al. 1984a, 1984b). Both short and long fibers have been identified and their respective polypeptides characterized.

Avian adenoviruses can be isolated in cell cultures or embryonated eggs. Chicken embryos infected with quail bronchitis virus become curled or dwarfed after one or a few serial passages (Olson 1950). The cytopathic effect of avian adenoviruses in chicken embryo kidney (Taylor and Calnek 1962) or liver (Defendi and Sharpless 1958) cell cultures is characteristic of the adenovirus group. A microneutralization test (with chicken kidney monolayers as an indicator), an immunodiffusion test, and various ELISAs can be used to facilitate immunity and serotyping determinations (Calnek et al. 1982, Grimes and King 1977a, Mockett and Cook 1983, Piela and Yates 1983). Hemagglutinating activity of an oncogenic strain (Phelps) of avian adenovirus is a function of complete and incomplete particles, and this characteristic facilitates the study of disease in birds (Mishad et al. 1975).

Solid, long-lasting immunity is conferred with monovalent virus. No cross-protection is conferred among heterologous serotypes 1, 2, and 3 (Winterfield et al. 1977). Maternal antibodies confer temporary protection to young chicks (Grimes and King 1977b, Otsuki et al. 1976, Winterfield et al. 1977). Polyvalent vaccines produced lower virus-neutralizing antibody titers on occasion when compared with chickens given monovalent vaccines (Winterfield et al. 1977). Their vaccines were effective and safe, and vaccine virus was not shed beyond 28 days after vaccination.

Because the duck adenovirus contaminant in Marek's vaccine may have caused the egg-drop syndrome in many European flocks, along with the problem of high incidence and latent infection characteristic of adenoviruses, an inactivated vaccine is in use in these breeder flocks, with probable success.

REFERENCES

Beasley, J.N., and Clifton, S.G. 1979. Experimental infection of broiler and leghorn chickens with virulent and avirulent isolates of hemorrhagic enteritis virus. Avian Dis. 23:616–621.

Brugh, M., Beard, C.W., and Villegas, P. 1984. Experimental infection of laying chickens with adenovirus 127 and with a related virus isolated from ducks. Avian Dis. 28:168–178.

Cabasso, V.J., and Wilner, B.I. 1969. Adenoviruses of animals other than man. Adv. Vet. Sci. Comp. Med. 13:159–217.

Calnek, B.W., and Cowen, B.S. 1975. Adenoviruses of chickens: Serologic groups. Avian Dis. 19:91–103.

Calnek, B.W., Shek, W.R., Menendez, N.A., and Stiube, P. 1982. Serological cross-reactivity of avian adenovirus serotypes in an enzyme-linked immunosorbent assay. Avian Dis. 26:897–906.

Defendi, V., and Sharpless, G.R. 1958. The RPL12 lymphomatosis virus in chicken embryo and in chicken embryo tissue culture. J. Natl. Cancer Inst. 21:925–939.

Dhillon, A.S., and Winterfield, R.W. 1984. Pathogenicity of various adenovirus serotypes in the presence of Escherichia coli in chickens. Avian Dis. 28:147–153.

Dhillon, A.S., Winterfield, R.W., Thacker, H.L., and Feldman, D.S. 1982. Lesions induced in the respiratory tract of chickens by serologically different adenoviruses. Avian Dis. 26:478–486.

Domermuth, C.H., van der Heide, L., and Faddoul, G.P. 1982. Pulmonary congestion and edema (marble spleen disease) of chickens produced by group II avian adenovirus. Avian Dis. 26:629–633.

Grimes, T.M., and King, D.J. 1977a. Serotyping avian adenoviruses by a microneutralization procedure. Am. J. Vet. Res. 38:317–321.

Grimes, T.M., and King, D.J. 1977b. Effect of maternal antibody on experimental infections of chickens with a type-8 avian adenovirus. Avian Dis. 21:97–112.

Grimes, T.M., King, D.J., Kleven, S.H., and Fletcher, O.J. 1977. Involvement of a type-8 avian adenovirus in the etiology of inclusion body hepatitis. Avian Dis. 21:26–38.

Gulka, C.M., Piela, T.H., Yates, V.J., and Bagshaw, C. 1984. Evidence of exposure of waterfowl and other aquatic birds to the hemagglutinating duck adenovirus identical to EDS-76 virus. J. Wildl. Dis. 20:1–5.

Helmboldt, C.F., and Frazier, M.N. 1963. Avian hepatic inclusion bodies of unknown significance. Avian Dis. 7:446–450.

Jones, R.C., Guneratne, J.R., and Georgiou, K. 1981. Isolation of viruses from outbreaks of suspected tenosynovitis (viral arthritis) in chickens. Res. Vet. Sci. 31:100–103.

Lee, K.P., Henry, N.W., and Rosenberger, J.K. 1978. Comparative pathogenicity of six avian adenovirus isolants in the liver. Avian Dis. 22:610–619.

Li, P., Bellett, A.J., and Parish, C.R. 1984a. Structural organization and polypeptide composition of the avian adenovirus core. J. Virol. 52:638–649.

Li, P., Bellett, A.J., and Parish, C.R. 1984b. The structural proteins of chick embryo lethal orphan virus (fowl adenovirus type 1). J. Gen. Virol. 65:1803–1815.

McFerran, J.B. 1981. Adenoviruses of vertebrate animals. In E. Kurstak and C. Kurstak, eds., Comparative Diagnosis of Viral Diseases, vol. 3. Academic Press, New York. Pp. 101–165.

McFerran, J.B. 1984. Egg drop syndrome 1976. In M.S. Hofstad, H.J. Barnes, B.W. Calnek, W.M. Reid, and H.W. Yoder, Jr., eds., Diseases of Poultry, 8th ed. Iowa State University Press, Ames. Pp. 516–523.

McFerran, J.B., and Connor, T.J. 1977. Further studies on the classification of fowl adenoviruses. Avian Dis. 21:585–595.

Mishad, A.M., McCormick, K.J., Stenback, W.A., Yates, V.J., and Trentin, J.J. 1975. Hemagglutinating properties of CELO, an oncogenic avian adenovirus. Avian Dis. 19:761–772.

Mockett, A.P., and Cook, J.K. 1983. The use of an enzyme-linked immunosorbent assay to detect IgG antibodies to serotype-specific and group-specific antigens of fowl adenovirus serotypes 2, 3, and 4. J. Virol. Methods 7:327–335.

Mustaffa-Babjee, A., and Spradbrow, P.B. 1975. Characteristics of three strains of avian adenoviruses isolated in Queensland. I. Biological properties. Avian Dis. 19:150–174.

Olson, N.O. 1950. A respiratory disease (bronchitis) of quail caused by a virus. Proc. U.S. Livestock Sanit. Assoc. 54:171–174.

Otsuki, K., Tsubokura, M., Yamamoto, H., Imamura, M., Sakaga, Y., Saio, H., and Hosokawa, D. 1976. Some properties of avian adenoviruses isolated from chickens with inclusion body hepatitis in Japan. Avian Dis. 20:693–705.

Piela, T.H., and Yates, V.J. 1983. Comparison of enzyme-linked immunosorbent assay with hemagglutination-inhibition and immunodiffusion tests for detection of antibodies to a hemagglutinating duck adenovirus in chickens. Avian Dis. 27:724–730.

Riddell, C. 1984. Viral hepatitis in domestic geese in Saskatchewan. Avian Dis. 28:774–782.

Rosenberger, J.K., Klopp, S., Eckroade, R.J., and Krauss, W.C. 1975. The roles of the infectious bursal agent and several avian adenoviruses in the hemorrhagic-aplastic-anemia syndrome and gangrenous dermatitis. Avian Dis. 19:717–729.

Sileo, L., Franson, J.C., Graham, D.L., Domermuth, C.H., Rattner, B.A., and Pattee, O.H. 1983. Hemorrhagic enteritis in captive American kestrels (*Falco sparverius*). J. Wildl. Dis. 19:244–247.

Takase, K., Maruyama, T., Nonaka, F., and Yamada, S. 1983. Isolation of fowl adenovirus from tendons and tendon sheaths of chickens with leg weakness. Jpn. Vet. Sci. 45:517–518.

Taniguchi, T., Yamaguchi, S., Maeda, M., Kawamura, H., and Horiuchi, T. 1981. Pathological changes in laying hens inoculated with the JPA-1 strain of egg drop syndrome-1976 virus. Natl. Inst. Anim. Health Q. 21:83–93.

Taylor, P.J., and Calnek, B.W. 1962. Isolation and classification of avian enteric cytopathogenic agents. Avian Dis. 6:51–58.

van Eck, J.H., and Vertommen, M. 1984. Biochemical changes in blood and uterine fluid of fowl following experimental EDS'76 virus infection. Vet. Q. 6:127–134.

van Eck, J.H.H., Davelaar, F.G., Van Den Heuvel-Plesman, T.A.M., Van Kol, N., Kouwenhoven, B., and Guldie, F.H.M. 1976. Dropped egg production, soft shelled and shell-less eggs associated with appearance of precipitins to adenovirus in flocks of laying fowls. Avian Pathol. 5:261–272.

Winterfield, R.W. 1984. Adenovirus infections of chickens. In M.S. Hofstad, H.J. Barnes, B.W. Calnek, W.M. Reid, and H.W. Yoder, Jr., eds., Diseases of Poultry, 8th ed. Iowa State University Press, Ames. Pp. 498–506.

Winterfield, R.W., Fadly, A.M., and Hoerr, F.J. 1977. Immunization of chickens against adenovirus infection. Poult. Sci. 56:1481–1486.

Yamaguchi, S., Imada, T., Kawamura, H., Taniguchi, T., and Kawakami, M. 1981. Pathogenicity and distribution of egg-drop syndrome-1976 virus (JPA-1) in inoculated laying hens. Avian Dis. 25:642–649.

Yates, V.J., Rhee, Y.O., and Fry, D.E. 1977. Serological response of chickens exposed to a type 1 avian adenovirus alone or in combination with the adeno-associated virus. Avian Dis. 21:408–414.

Zsak, L., and Kisary, J. 1984. Grouping of fowl adenoviruses based upon the restriction patterns of DNA generated by BamHI and HindIII. Intervirology 22:110–114.

Turkey Adenovirus Infections

Adenoviruses of turkeys fall into three classes: fowl adenoviruses, turkey adenoviruses, and the virus of turkey hemorrhagic enteritis (McFerran 1981). Adenovirus infection may cause respiratory illness, marble spleen disease, or enteric disease in turkey poults. Various investigators have isolated virus from birds with respiratory illness. In some instances the isolate produced no signs of illness (Simmons et al. 1976, Sutjipto et al. 1977) or only mild illness (Cheville and Sato 1977) in experimental poults. With another isolate identified as turkey type 1, respiratory signs were severe in day-old poults, and the mortality was 50 percent (Blalock et al. 1975). Itakura and Carlson (1975) produced hemorrhagic enteritis in two turkeys. Silim and Thorsen (1981) studied virus distribution and antibody formation in turkeys with hemorrhagic enteritis virus infection. Clinically, the affected young turkeys showed bloody diarrhea. Birds died acutely. At necropsy birds had a large number of dark red, bloody clots in the intestinal tract, many petechiae in the mucous membrane of small intestine and cecum, and atrophy of the spleen (Fujiwara et al. 1975). Characteristic histological changes were acute hemorrhagic enteritis, degenerative changes of lymphatic tissue, and proliferation of reticuloendothelial cells with intranuclear inclusion bodies in these cells throughout the host. Virus particles in these cells were characteristic of adenoviruses. Turkeys can be protected by a modified live-virus vaccine against hemorrhagic enteritis (Fadly and Nazerian 1984).

Marble spleen disease has been described in young poults and ring-necked pheasants (Iltis et al. 1977). Morphologically the virus was consistent with that of an avian adenovirus. MSD virus antigen showed a cross-reaction with antiserum to turkey adenovirus serotypes TA-1 and TA-2.

Easton and Simmons (1977) made an antigenic analysis of several turkey respiratory adenoviruses by reciprocal neutralization kinetics. These viruses were placed into four serologic groups. Certain surveys have showed that there has been widespread exposure of the U.S. turkey population to these viruses.

REFERENCES

Blalock, H.G., Simmons, D.G., Muse, K.E., Gray, J.G. and Derieux, W.T. 1975. Adenovirus respiratory infection in turkey poults. Avian Dis. 19:707–716.

Cheville, N., and Sato, S. 1977. Pathology of adenoviral infection in turkeys (*Meleagris gallopavo*) with respiratory disease and colisepticemia. Vet. Pathol. 14:567–581.

Easton, G.D., Jr., and Simmons, D.G. 1977. Antigenic analysis of several turkey respiratory adenoviruses by reciprocal-neutralization kinetics. Avian Dis. 21:605–611.

Fadly, A.M., and Nazerian, K. 1984. Efficacy and safety of a cell-culture live virus vaccine for hemorrhagic enteritis of turkeys: Laboratory studies. Avian Dis. 28:183–196.

Fujiwara, H., Tanaami, S., Yamaguchi, M., and Yoshino, T. 1975. Histopathology of hemorrhagic enteritis in turkeys. Natl. Inst. Anim. Health Q. 15:68–75.

Iltis, J.P., Daniels, S.B., and Wyand, D.S. 1977. Demonstration of an avian adenovirus as the causative agent of marble spleen disease. Am. J. Vet. Res. 38:95–100.

Itakura, C., and Carlson, H.C. 1975. Electron microscopic findings of cells with inclusion bodies in experimental hemorrhagic enteritis of turkeys. Can. J. Comp. Med. 39:299–304.

McFerran, J.B. 1981. Adenoviruses of vertebrate animals. In E. Kurstak and C. Kurstak, eds., Comparative Diagnosis of Viral Diseases, vol. 3. Academic Press, New York. Pp. 101–165.

Silim, A., and Thorsen, J. 1981. Hemorrhagic enteritis: Virus distribution and sequential development of antibody in turkeys. Avian Dis. 25:444–453.

Simmons, D.G., Miller, S.E., Gray, J.G., Blalock, H.G., and Colwell, W.M. 1976. Isolation and identification of a turkey respiratory adenovirus. Avian Dis. 20:65–74.

Sutjipto, S., Miller, S.E., Simmons, D.G., and Dillman, R.C. 1977. Physicochemical characterization and pathogenicity studies of two turkey adenovirus isolants. Avian Dis. 21:549–556.

Several reviews have appeared in the literature on these viruses (Coggins 1974; Flügel 1985; Granoff 1969; Hess 1971, 1981a, 1981b; Hess and Poinar 1985; Kelly 1985; Viñuela 1985; Willis 1985; Willis et al. 1985).

As mentioned earlier, the iridoviruses are rather large. The diameter of FLDV ranges from 130 to 300 nm (Hess 1981b) and the diameter of ASFV ranges from 175 to 215 nm (Breese and DeBoer 1966, Carrascosa et al. 1984, Viñuela 1985). The biophysical and biochemical characteristics for members of this family can be found in Chapter 38.

REFERENCES

Breese, S.S., Jr., and DeBoer, C.J. 1966. Electron microscope observations of African swine fever virus in tissue culture cells. Virology 28:420–428.
Carrascosa, J.L., Carazo, J.M., Carrascosa, A.L., García, N., Santisteban, A., and Viñuela, E. 1984. General morphology and capsid fine structure of African swine fever virus particles. Virology 132:160–172.
Coggins, L. 1974. African swine fever virus: Pathogenesis. Prog. Med. Virol. 18:48–63.
Devauchelle, G., Stoltz, D.B., and Darcy-Tripier, F. 1985. Comparative ultrastructure of Iridoviridae. Curr. Top. Microbiol. Immunol. 116:1–21.
Flügel, R.M. 1985. Lymphocystis disease virus. Curr. Top. Microbiol. Immunol. 116:133–150.
Granoff, A. 1969. Viruses of amphibia. Curr. Top. Microbiol. Immunol. 50:107–137.
Gut, J.P., Anton, M., Bingen, A., Vetter, J.M., and Kirn, A. 1981. Frog virus 3 induces a fatal hepatitis in rats. Lab. Invest. 45:218–228.
Hess, R.T., and Poinar, G.O., Jr. 1985. Iridoviruses infecting terrestrial isopods and nematodes. Curr. Top. Microbiol. Immunol. 116:49–76.
Hess, W.R. 1971. African swine fever virus. Virol. Monogr. 9:1–33.
Hess, W.R. 1981a. African swine fever: A reassessment. Adv. Vet. Sci. Comp. Med. 25:39–69.
Hess, W.R. 1981b. Comparative aspects and diagnosis of the iridoviruses of vertebrate animals. In E. Kurstak and C. Kurstak, eds., Comparative Diagnosis of Viral Diseases, vol. 3. Academic Press, New York. Pp. 169–202.
Kelly, D.C. 1985. Insect iridescent viruses. Curr. Top. Microbiol. Immunol. 116:23–35.
Viñuela, E. 1985. African swine fever virus. Curr. Top. Microbiol. Immunol. 116:151–170.
Willis, D.B. 1985. Iridoviridae. Curr. Top. Microbiol. Immunol. 116:1–21.
Willis, D.B., Goorha, R., and Chinchar, V.G. 1985. Macromolecular synthesis in cells infected by frog virus 3. Curr. Top. Microbiol. Immunol. 116:77–106.

44 The Iridoviridae

Viruses belonging to the Iridoviridae family are relatively large organisms with icosahedral shape, envelopes, and double-stranded DNA. They replicate entirely within the cytoplasm of the cell (Hess 1981b, Willis 1985).

Scientists do not agree on the classification of all viruses that potentially could belong to the Iridoviridae family. In earlier classification schemes only a single genus, *Iridovirus,* was listed for this family; however, at the 1982 meeting of the International Committee on Taxonomy of Viruses, five genera were established for the family (Table 44.1) (Willis 1985). The names Iridoviridae and *Iridovirus* are derived from the viruses isolated from insects with iridesent disease. Viruses in this family are also referred to as the *icosahedral cytoplasmic deoxyriboviruses,* abbreviated ICDV (Hess 1981b).

At present, African swine fever virus (ASFV) is the only animal virus included in this family which causes disease in a domestic animal species. Some researchers believe that the biochemical and biophysical properties of ASFV do not fit into any of the present DNA virus families and that the properties are more like those of poxviruses than those of iridoviruses (Viñuela 1985). Other members of the Iridoviridae family are fish lymphocystis disease virus (FLDV), gecko virus of reptiles, at least 32 small and large iridescent insect viruses, several viruses infecting isopods and nematodes, and the amphibian cytoplasmic virus frog virus 3 (Devauchelle et al. 1985, Hess 1981b, Hess and Poinar 1985, Kelly 1985, Willis 1985, Willis et al. 1985). Frog virus 3 has been shown to produce acute degenerative hepatitis in rats (Gut et al. 1981).

African Swine Fever
SYNONYMS: East African swine fever,
Montgomery's disease, wart hog disease;
abbreviation, ASF

African swine fever is an acute, highly fatal viral disease of domesticated swine of European breeds. The signs and lesions are much like those of hog cholera. Montgomery (1921) first described ASF from Kenya in East Africa, where it has been recognized since 1910. Until 1957 ASF

Table 44.1. Genera in the family Iridoviridae

Vernacular name	Scientific name	Type species
Small iridescent insect virus	*Iridovirus*	*Tipula* iridescent virus (type 1)
Large iridescent insect virus	*Chloriridovirus*	Mosquito iridescent virus (type 2)
Amphibian icosahedral deoxyribovirus	*Ranavirus*	Frog virus 3 (FV-3)
Fish lymphocystis disease virus	*Lymphocystivirus*	Flounder lymphocystis disease virus (FLCDV)
African swine fever virus	—	African swine fever virus, Kenya strain

Compiled from information in Willis 1985.

was not known to occur in any part of the world other than East Africa. In that year the disease was found in Portugal (Ribeiro et al. 1958). At first thought to be hog cholera, it was finally recognized to be ASF. Before it was stamped out, 433 herds comprising more than 16,000 pigs had become infected. In 1959 disease was found in Spain, and in 1960 it recurred in Portugal. The disease was widespread in Cuba in 1971 but was successfully eradicated, although it occurred again in 1979 and was eradicated in May 1980. In 1978 the disease was introduced into Brazil, the Dominican Republic, and Haiti. Its presence in Latin America, a Caribbean island, and Europe constitutes a threat to the swine industry in Europe, Central America, Mexico, Canada, and the United States.

Character of the Disease. In the early outbreaks of ASF, a severe, highly fatal, hemorrhagic disease occurred with signs and lesions quite similar to hog cholera. With the passage of time following the establishment of ASF in a susceptible pig population, subacute and chronic forms of the disease became important (Hess 1981).

The incubation period in experimental infections is 2 to 5 days, often somewhat longer in natural infections (McDaniel 1981, Schlafer and Mebus 1984). The onset of illness is characterized by a sudden rise in temperature and a loss of appetite. Infected pigs may be found dead or may show some or all of the following signs: labored breathing; depression; weakness; bloody feces; incoordination; reddish discolorations on ears, snout, fetlock, and flanks; coughing; and, occasionally, a sticky ocular discharge. A common finding is extensive hemorrhage. Unlike swine with hog cholera, pigs with ASF may continue to eat until death, which usually occurs 4 to 7 days after the onset of signs, with an exceedingly high mor-

tality as a rule. A day or two before death the temperature falls rapidly. Pregnant sows usually abort 5 to 8 days after infection (Schlafer and Mebus 1984).

Properties of the Virus. The morphology of ASFV has been reported in several studies (Breese and DeBoer 1966, Carrascosa et al. 1984). In electron micrographs of thin sections of cells, the mature virus particles have a hexagonal outer membrane, 175 to 225 nm in diameter, separated by a clear region from a dense nucleoid (Breese and DeBoer 1966). Virus particles are made up of several concentric structures arranged in an overall icosahedral shape (Carrascosa et al. 1984). In Figure 44.1 collapsed particles appear to be icosahedral capsids, suggesting cubic symmetry (Almeida et al. 1967).

Extraction of infectious nucleic acid from ASFV and direct characterization by ultraviolet light and by reaction with RNase and DNase have proved that it is a DNA virus (Adldinger et al. 1966). The DNA has a contour length of about 58 nm and a density in cesium chloride of 1.7 g/ml. The DNA apparently contains terminal cross-links similar to those in poxvirus DNA (Viñuela 1985).

Multiple viral proteins are present in the virion of ASFV. Letchworth and Whyard (1984) reported that at least 37 different viral proteins were involved in immunoprecipitin antigen-antibody reactions. Tabarés et al. (1980a) identified at least 34 polypeptides ranging in molecular mass from 9,500 to 243,000 daltons, including six structural proteins (VP172, VP162, VP146, VP73, VP34, and VP23.5). The major protein, VP73, appears to be located in the envelope, and the four larger structural proteins appear to react as antigens in natural infections (Tabarés et al. 1980b).

The virus contains a lipid membrane, yet is more stable

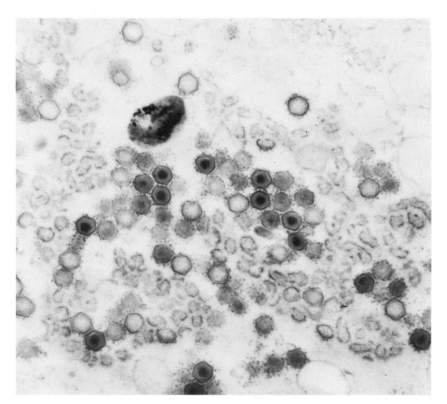

Figure 44.1. African swine virus particles (strain Lisbon 57) in a pig kidney cell culture. × 27,900. (Courtesy S. S. Breese, Plum Island Animal Disease Center, U.S. Dept. of Agriculture.)

than most enveloped viruses. It is inactivated in 30 minutes at 44°C and in 10 minutes at 60°C; thus it is less heat-resistant than hog cholera virus. The virus survives for years when dried at room temperature or frozen in skin or muscle tissue. It is resistant to most disinfectants, but is inactivated by 1 percent formaldehyde in 6 days, by 2 percent sodium hydroxide in 24 hours, and by chloroform and other lipid solvents.

The virus particles appear to be formed in the cell cytoplasm, and they bud out from the cell membrane, many acquiring an added layer (Breese and DeBoer 1966). Hemagglutination of red blood cells is not reported, but hemadsorption of pig red blood cells is seen in cultures of pig marrow or buffy coat (Hess 1981, Malmquist and Hay 1960) (Figure 44.2).

There are several serotypes in Africa, but probably only one in Europe. Specific and group antigens are demonstrated by the complement-fixation, gel diffusion, and other tests. The complement-fixation test is group-reactive, but the hemadsorption-inhibition test is specific (Malmquist 1963).

Cultivation. ASFV can be cultivated in chick embryos, in tissue cultures consisting of bone marrow cells or buffy coat cells of swine blood, or in several primary cell cultures or cell lines. Most strains of virus produce hemadsorption followed by cytopathic effects in bone marrow or leukocyte cultures (Hess 1981).

Wardley and Wilkinson (1978) observed a high rate of infection and complete destruction within 2 or 3 days of monocytes in cell cultures derived from pig bone marrow, whereas the macrophages in culture had only a low level of infection and survived to form persistently infected cultures. These observations help to explain the persistence of virus in the pig.

Results of a microplaque assay and conventional plaque assay were reproducible and reliable in titering the virus, but approximately 0.9 log lower in sensitivity in virus detection than results of the hemadsorption test (Pan et al. 1978).

Epizootiology and Pathogenesis. Domestic pigs in Africa may contract the infection from carrier wart hogs (*Phacochoerus* spp.), bush pigs (*Potamochoerus* spp.), and giant forest hogs (*Hylochoerus* spp.) by ingestion of infective material from feeding garbage, or by the bite of an infected tick (Hess 1981). Carrier animals may liberate the virus, particularly during farrowing and other periods of stress. Thereafter, infection is by contact and through fomites. Infected premises remain infective for long periods.

A different cycle of transmission has developed in Europe, where the disease became less virulent and chronically infected pigs perpetuated the infection. This also is true in Brazil and other Latin American countries.

Virus has been recovered from the ticks of the genus

tion with virulent virus, the organism appears in all the major blood fractions and is associated with equivalent numbers of both erythrocytes and leukocytes (Wardley and Wilkinson 1977). Ninety percent of the virus is in the erythrocytes. Of the leukocyte subpopulations, virus is associated with lymphocytes and possibly neutrophils. Virus infects the megakaryocytes and thrombocytes, producing acute thrombocytopenia 4 to 5 days after the onset of fever (Edwards et al. 1985). There is good correlation between the thrombocytopenia and the occurrence of hemorrhage.

Maurer et al. (1958) found few differences in the lesions caused by ASF, compared with those of hog cholera. The primary lesions in cases of fatal ASF are in the spleen, which is greatly enlarged, friable, and reddish black (Figure 44.3), in the lymphatic tissues (Figures 44.4, 44.5, 44.6) with their characteristic hemorrhages, and in the walls of the arterioles and capillaries. A marked difference is the karyorrhexis of the lymphocytes, which occurs in ASF but not in hog cholera.

After ASF is introduced into a susceptible pig population, the acute form of the disease is dominant. With the passage of time, coupled in some instances with introduction of "attenuated" virus vaccine, the chronic form of the disease predominates. Under these circumstances pigs develop a chronic pneumonia (Figure 44.7). The pathogenesis of this chronic pneumonia was studied by

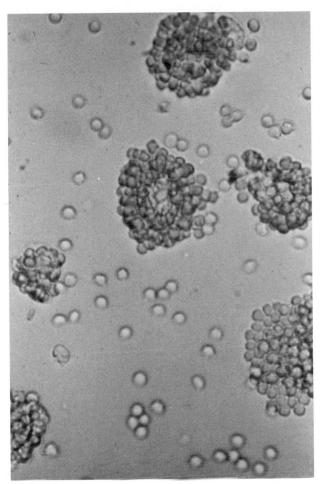

Figure 44.2. Hemadsorption of red blood cells in virus-infected cell cultures used for diagnosis of African swine fever. (Courtesy J. J. Callis and staff, Plum Island Animal Disease Center, U.S. Dept. of Agriculture.)

Ornithodoros, indicating that ticks may play a role in the spread of ASF (Hess 1981).

Outbreaks of ASF in several countries appear to start with the feeding of garbage containing infected pork scraps, or following the importation of chronically infected pigs. The virus can survive in feces, urine, and blood, and therefore mechanical transmission is possible (Hess 1981).

ASF sometimes behaves in European swine in about the same way as it does in native African swine in that surviving animals have a persisting viremia for long periods even though they appear well (DeTray 1957, Edwards et al. 1985). European pigs that show no signs of the disease after inoculation nevertheless may become virus carriers with persistent viremia. These persistently viremic pigs have complement-fixing and precipitating antibodies but not virus-neutralizing antibodies. After infec-

Figure 44.3. Acute African swine fever. The spleen is greatly enlarged, friable, and reddish black. (Courtesy D. A. Gregg, Plum Island Animal Disease Center, U.S. Dept. of Agriculture.)

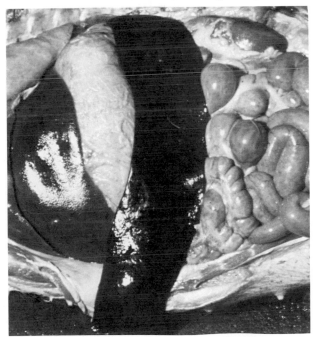

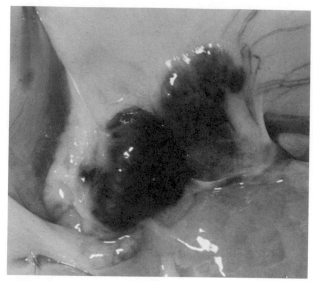

Figure 44.4. Acute African swine fever. The hepatogastric lymph node is enlarged and reddish black. (Courtesy D. A. Gregg, Plum Island Animal Disease Center, U.S. Dept. of Agriculture.)

Moulton et al. (1975). Interalveolar septa become thickened by accumulation of lymphocytes and monocytes, and focal areas of lymhocytes and macrophages appear in the lungs. Necrosis soon develops in these foci, which then become calcified. The calcified areas are surrounded by mononuclear cells, including plasma cells, and fibrous tissue. The viral antigen was seen mainly in the macrophages and cell debris in alveolar walls and lumens (Pan et al. 1975), suggesting that the virus replicated in the cytoplasm of alveolar macrophages, which subsequently degenerated and released the virus.

    Hypergammaglobulinemia, accompanied by hypo-

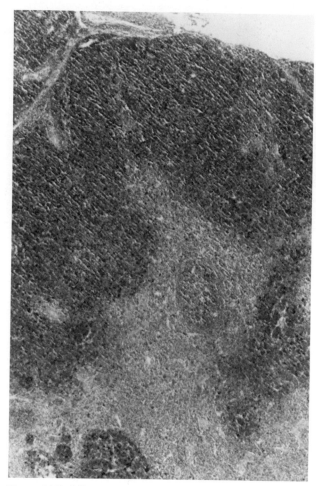

Figure 44.5. Micrograph of a section of lymph node from a pig with acute African swine fever. There is extensive hemorrhage in the cortical part of the node. Hematoxylin and eosin stain. (Courtesy C. A. Mebus, Plum Island Animal Disease Center, U.S. Dept. of Agriculture.)

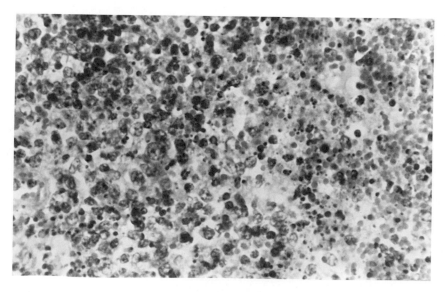

Figure 44.6. Micrograph of the cellular stroma in a lymph node from a pig with acute African swine fever. The right side of the photograph has many erythrocytes characteristic of hemorrhage. In the center of the photograph are numerous pyknotic nuclei. (Courtesy C. A. Mebus, Plum Island Animal Disease Center, U.S. Dept. of Agriculture.)

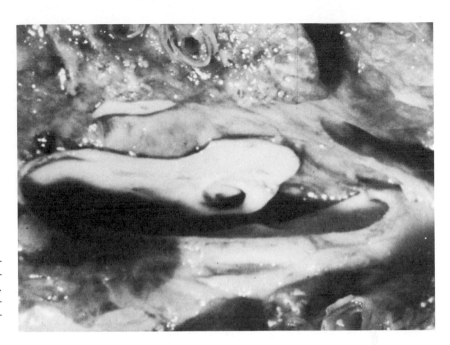

Figure 44.7. Lung lesion in chronic African swine fever. Note the lobular distribution and whitish necrotic appearance. (Courtesy D. A. Gregg, Plum Island Animal Disease Center, U.S. Dept. of Agriculture.)

albuminemia, occurs in chronic ASF. Sufficient protein changes occur in the serum of most chronically infected swine to give a positive iodine agglutination test (Pan et al. 1974). IgG immunoglobulin is bound to intracytoplasmic inclusion bodies in some degenerating macrophages, indicating that antibody against ASF viral antigen(s) excluded from blood circulation or produced by local immunocytes (or both) reacts with viral antigen at intramacrophage and extramacrophage levels, resulting in the formation of insoluble antigen-antibody (AG-AB) complexes. The participation of complement in the immune complex is evident in the early stage of the pneumonia but less evident in the subsequent extensive, progressive necrotic processes.

Immunity. Immunity to homologous strains seems to be transient. Pigs that recover from the disease often carry the virus in the bloodstream for months. Attenuated strains have been used as vaccines in Spain and Portugal, but vaccinated pigs may carry the virus despite the presence of antibody. The cellular immune mechanism is not impaired by ASFV infection, as demonstrated by the leukocyte migration–inhibition test and the development of delayed hypersensitivity, but viremia does persist in the pigs (Shimizu et al. 1977).

Diagnosis. Definitive clinical diagnosis of ASF is nearly impossible (Hess 1981b) because of the disease's similarity to hog cholera and other chronic diseases. Laboratory confirmation is essential.

ASF must be differentiated from hog cholera. This can be done by virus isolation or by demonstration of a rising serum titer, using the hemadsorption-inhibition, complement-fixation, or immunofluorescence test (Heuschele and Hess 1973).

Enzyme-linked immunosorbent assay (ELISA) is an extremely sensitive test for ASFV antigen (Hamdy et al. 1981, Wardley et al. 1979). This rapid, automated procedure is especially useful when a large number of serums must be tested (Callis 1979).

Because ASF is so difficult to differentiate from hog cholera in the field, many countries in which hog cholera now exists have broadened and improved their hog cholera vaccination program. This is not as simple as it sounds because attenuated hog cholera vaccines may produce a chronic disease that, under certain conditions, stunts growth and causes some pigs to become virus carriers.

Treatment. There is no known treatment or cure for ASF (Hess 1981b). Replication of ASFV is inhibited in cell cultures by certain antiviral compounds, including disodium phoshonoacetate (PAA) and iododeoxyuridine (IDU) (Gil-Fernández et al., 1979).

Prevention and Control. As yet, a satisfactory vaccine has not been developed despite concerted research efforts in several places throughout the world. The nature of this disease precludes development of a successful vaccine unless some novel approach to immunity to viral, chronic, and degenerative diseases is found.

Present control of the disease is based on early reporting and rapid diagnosis followed by immediate slaughter of all infected and exposed swine coupled with strict quarantine in the infected area. This approach has been successful in certain European countries and Cuba in recent years, and it is likely to be the control method used if the disease is ever introduced into the United States.

Because the United States imports some processed pork products, control officials are concerned about the effects of processing on the presence of ASFV in these products. Virus has been recovered from dried salami and pepperoni sausages, but not after the required curing period (McKercher et al. 1978). Partially cooked canned hams did not contain virus.

The Disease in Humans. This virus is not known to cause disease in humans.

REFERENCES

Adldinger, H.K., Stone, S.S., Hess, W.R., and Bachrach, H.L. 1966. Extraction of infectious deoxyribonucleic acid from African swine fever virus. Virology 30:750–752.

Almeida, J.D., Waterson, A.P., and Plowright, W. 1967. The morphological characteristics of African swine fever virus and its resemblance to *Tipula* iridescent virus. Arch. Gesam. Virusforsch. 20:392–396.

Breese, S.S., Jr., and DeBoer, C.J. 1966. Electron microscope observations of African swine fever virus in tissue culture cells. Virology 28:420–428.

Callis, J.J. 1979. African swine fever: A review. In Proceedings of the 12th Inter-American Meeting, Curaçao, Netherlands Antilles. Pan American Health Organization, Washington, D.C. Pp. 39–42.

Carrascosa, J.L,. Carazo, J.M., Carrascosa, A.L., García, N., Santisteban, A., and Viñuela, E. 1984. General morphology and capsid fine structure of African swine fever virus particles. Virology 132:160–172.

DeTray, D.E. 1957. Persistence of viremia and immunity in African swine fever. Am. J. Vet. Res. 18:811–816.

Edwards, J.F., Dodds, W.J., and Slauson, D.O. 1985. Megakaryocytic infection and thrombocytopenia in African swine fever. Vet. Pathol. 22:171–176.

Gil-Fernández, C., Páez, E., Vilas, P., and Gancedo, A.G. 1979. Effect of disodium phosphonoacetate and iododeoxyuridine on the multiplication of African swine fever virus in vitro. Chemotherapy 25:162–169.

Hamdy, F.M., Colgrove, G.S., de Rodriguez, E.M., Snyder, M.L., and Stewart, W.C. 1981. Field evaluation of enzyme-linked immunosorbent assay for detection of antibody to African swine fever virus. Am. J. Vet. Res. 42:1441–1443.

Hess, W.R. 1981. Comparative aspects and diagnosis of the iridoviruses of vertebrate animals. In E. Kurstak and C. Kurstak, eds., Comparative Diagnosis of Viral Diseases, vol. 3. Academic Press, New York. Pp. 169–202.

Heuschele, W.P., and Hess, W.R. 1973. Diagnosis of African swine fever by immunofluorescence. Trop. Anim. Health Prod. 5:181–186.

Letchworth, G.J., and Whyard, T.C. 1984. Characterization of African swine fever virus antigenic proteins by immunoprecipitation. Arch. Virol. 80:265–274.

McDaniel, H.A. 1981. African swine fever. In A.D. Leman, R.D. Glock, W.L. Mengeling, R.H.C. Penny, E. Scholl, and B. Straw, eds., Diseases of Swine, 5th ed. Iowa State University Press, Ames. Pp. 237–245.

McKercher, P.D., Hess, W.R., and Hamdy, F. 1978. Residual viruses in pork products. Appl. Environ. Microbiol. 35:142–145.

Malmquist, W.A. 1963. Serologic and immunologic studies with African swine fever virus. Am. J. Vet. Res. 24:450–459.

Malmquist, W.A., and Hay, D. 1960. Hemadsorption and cytopathic effect produced by African swine fever virus in swine bone marrow and buffy coat cultures. Am. J. Vet. Res. 21:104–108.

Maurer, F.D., Griesemer, R.A., and Jones, T.C. 1958. The pathology of African swine fever—A comparison with hog cholera. Am. J. Vet. Res. 19:517–539.

Montgomery, R.E. 1921. On a form of swine fever occurring in British East Africa (Kenya colony). J. Comp. Pathol. 34:159–191.

Moulton, J.E., Pan, I.C., Hess, W.R., DeBoer, C.J., and Tessler, J. 1975. Pathologic features of chronic pneumonia in pigs with experimentally induced African swine fever. Am. J. Vet. Res. 36:27–32.

Pan, I.C., Moulton, J.E., and Hess, W.R. 1975. Immunofluorescent studies on chronic pneumonia in swine with experimentally induced African swine fever. Am. J. Vet. Res. 36:379–386.

Pan, I.C., Shimizu, M., and Hess, W.R. 1978. African swine fever: Microplaque assay by an immunoperoxidase method. Am. J. Vet. Res. 39:491–497.

Pan, I.C., Trautman, R., DeBoer, C.J., and Hess, W.R. 1974. African swine fever: Hypergammaglobulinemia and the iodine agglutination test. Am. J. Vet. Res. 35:629–631.

Ribeiro, J.M., Azevedo, J.A.R., Teixeira, M.J.O., Forte, M.C.B., Ribeiro, A.M.R., Noronha, F.O., Pereira, C.G., and Vigario, J.D. 1958. Peste porcine provoquée par une souche différente (souche L) de la souche classique. Bull. Off. Int. Epizoot. 50:516–534.

Schlafer, D.H., and Mebus, C.A. 1984. Abortion in sows experimentally infected with African swine fever virus: Clinical features. Am. J. Vet. Res. 45:1353–1360.

Shimizu, M., Pan, I.C., and Hess, W.R. 1977. Cellular immunity demonstrated in pigs infected with African swine fever virus. Am. J. Vet. Res. 38:27–31.

Tabarés, E., Marcotegui, M.A., Fernández, M., and Sánchez-Botija, C. 1980. Proteins specified by African swine fever virus. I. Analysis of viral structural proteins and antigenic properties. Arch. Virol. 66:107–117.

Tabarés, E,. Martinez, J., Ruiz Gonzalvo, F., and Sánchez-Botija, C. 1980. Proteins specified by African swine fever virus. II. Analysis of proteins in infected cells and antigenic properties. Arch. Virol. 66:119–132.

Viñuela, E. 1985. African swine fever virus. Curr. Top. Microbiol. Immunol. 116:151–170.

Wardley, R.C., and Wilkinson, P.J. 1977. The association of African swine fever virus with blood components of infected pigs. Arch. Virol. 55:327–334.

Wardley, R.C., and Wilkinson, P.J. 1978. The growth of virulent African swine fever virus in pig monocytes and macrophages. J. Gen. Virol. 38:183–186.

Wardley, R.C., Abu Elzein, E.M., Crowther, J.R., and Wilkinson, P.J. 1979. A solid-phase enzyme-linked immunosorbent assay for the detection of African swine fever virus antigen and antibody. J. Hyg. 83:363–369.

45 The Poxviridae

The family Poxviridae contains two subfamilies: (1) Chordopoxvirinae, which comprises six genera that include all the animal poxviruses, and (2) Entomopoxvirinae, which includes all the insect poxviruses. This chapter covers the genera of animal poxviruses: *Avipoxvirus*, *Orthopoxvirus*, *Suipoxvirus*, *Capripoxvirus*, *Leporipoxvirus*, and *Parapoxvirus*. The diseases caused by members of the Poxviridae are listed in Table 45.1. The taxonomy of this family is based largely on three criteria: (1) similar morphology, (2) a group-specific nucleoprotein antigen shared by all poxviruses of vertebrates, and (3) other antigens shared by members of each genus (Matthews 1982, Moss 1985, Takahashi et al. 1959, Woodroofe and Fenner 1962).

The genus *Orthopoxvirus* includes the viruses of cowpox, vaccinia, variola, alastrim, ectromelia (mousepox), rabbitpox, monkeypox, buffalopox, camelpox, catpox, elephantpox, and horsepox. Fowlpox, pigeonpox, turkeypox, canarypox, quailpox, lovebirdpox, sparrowpox, juncopox, and starlingpox pathogens constitute the genus *Avipoxvirus*. The genus *Capripoxvirus* contains sheeppox, goatpox, and lumpy skin disease viruses. Myxoma viruses and rabbit, hare, and squirrel fibroma viruses are in the genus *Leporipoxvirus*. The genus *Suipoxvirus* includes swinepox virus. Contagious pustular dermatitis of sheep (orf), bovine papular stomatitis, sealionpox virus, and pseudocowpox (milker's nodules) are diseases caused by viruses of the genus *Parapoxvirus*. New poxviruses have been isolated from elephants, domestic and exotic cats, raccoons, and gerbils. Many of these isolates resemble cowpox virus, and it is uncertain whether these isolates are cowpox virus that has infected other species, or

different viruses closely related to cowpox virus. Interestingly, no poxviruses have been isolated from the dog. The taxonomic position of molluscum contagiosum virus of humans, tanapox virus, and Yaba monkey virus within the Poxviridae is unclear.

Formerly, poxviruses were classified on the basis of morphology and the animal species showing disease. The so-called true poxviruses (*Orthopoxvirus* and *Avipoxvirus*) and pseudopoxviruses (*Parapoxvirus*) were readily distinguished by morphology. (See sections on *Orthopoxvirus* and *Parapoxvirus* for data on size and morphology of particles.) The true poxviruses are slightly larger and less ovoid than the pseudopoxviruses. There is a pronounced difference in the arrangement of the threadlike structures; the true poxviruses display an irregular whorled (mulberrylike) appearance, while the pseudopoxviruses have a characteristic, highly regular crisscross pattern created by threadlike structures wound around the virion.

The serologic relationships of poxviruses are determined by the use of infected cell extracts (Joklik 1968). In these preparations up to 20 antigens can form precipitin lines with antiviral serum for orthopoxviruses (Appleyard et al. 1962, Rodriguez-Burgos et al. 1966) and for leporipoxviruses (Fenner 1965). One of these antigens is probably responsible for production of neutralizing antibody (Appleyard et al. 1964). It is generally assumed that these antigens are structural protein components. Viruses of the genus *Leporipoxvirus* are not neutralized by vaccinia antiserum, and none of the major antigens is shared by these two groups. The avianpox viruses are not related to other true poxvirus groups, but fowlpox virus produces experimental infection in some mammals, such as cattle, cats, and horses (see p. 563). Many poxviruses form a hemagglutinin. Alkaline digestion of all poxviruses yields a fraction called the NP antigen, which is shared by all poxviruses.

The brick-shaped or ovoid particles are 170 to 250 by 300 to 450 nm. Virions have a complex structure with an external coat surrounding a double membrane with filamentous subunits in irregular arrangement and an internal body (core) consisting of a double membrane with cylindrical subunits and containing the DNA. The buoyant density in cesium chloride is 1.1–1.33 g/ml, and the sedimentation coefficient is 5,000. The poxviruses contain large numbers of enzymes, including the key enzyme RNA polymerase (Moss 1985). Some poxviruses are ether-resistant. Members can recombine genetically, and all exhibit nongenetic reactivation.

Poxviruses replicate in the cytoplasm of cells, principally in epithelial types. The various stages of poxvirus replication have been reviewed by Moss (1985). The in-

Table 45.1. Diseases of domestic animals caused by viruses in the Poxviridae family

Common name of virus	Natural hosts	Type of disease produced
Genus *Avipoxvirus*		
Fowlpox virus	Chickens, turkeys, pheasants, canaries	Pox lesions appear on comb, wattles, nostrils and eyes; pustules dry into epithelial crusts. Affected animals may become lethargic and die
Pigeonpox virus	Pigeons	Lesions of mouth region. Occasionally eyes are affected, causing blindness
Turkeypox virus	Turkeys	Disease similar to fowlpox
Genus *Orthopoxvirus*		
Cowpox virus	Cattle, humans, cats, elephants, exotic felids, anteaters	Mild. Affecting teats and udder forming vesicles followed by crusting
Vaccinia virus	Cattle, humans	Mild. Affecting teats and udder forming vesicles followed by crusting
Catpox virus	Domestic and exotic felids	Chronic dermatological condition or an acute, sometimes fatal respiratory disease
Buffalopox virus	Cattle, buffalo	No significant information available
Rabbitpox virus	Rabbits	Acute generalized disease of domesticated rabbits. Wild animals appear immune. High mortality rate in domesticated rabbits
Camelpox virus	Camels	Acute, highly infectious disease similar to variola in humans
Horsepox virus	Horses, humans	Multiple lesions of lips and gums, tongue and cheeks. Pustules form. Fever may develop. There may be mortality among young animals
Genus *Suipoxvirus*		
Swinepox virus	Swine	Acute infectious disease that affects swine only. Pox lesions found primarily on abdomen and inside thighs and legs
Genus *Capripoxvirus*		
Sheeppox virus	Sheep	Acute disease—mortality 5% to 50% of infected animals Lesions occur on mucous membranes in pharynx and trachea. Hemorrhage and inflammation of digestive and respiratory tracts
Goatpox virus	Goats	Lesions occur on hairless regions. Similar to sheeppox, but not as severe
Lumpy skin disease virus	Cattle, buffalo	Nodules in the skin, pathological changes in mucous membranes and viscera
Genus *Leporipoxvirus*		
Myxoma virus	Rabbits, hares	Acute, generalized, highly fatal disease characterized by tumorlike masses having rubbery, gelatinous consistency
Shope fibroma virus	Rabbits	Fibrous tumor of cottontail rabbit located in subcutaneous tissue

Table 45.1—*continued*

Common name of virus	Natural hosts	Type of disease produced
Genus *Parapoxvirus*		
Contagious pustular dermatitis virus (orf virus)	Sheep, goats, humans	Formation of vesicles on lips and areas of nose and eyes—later forming pustules and scabs. Fatalities occur in sheep and goats from complications
Bovine papular stomatitis virus	Cattle	Mild. Causes proliferative lesions or craterlike ulcers of stoma
Pseudocowpox virus (milker's nodules virus)	Cattle, humans	Mild. Resembles lesions of cowpox

fected cells contain cytoplasmic inclusion bodies that harbor the virus particles, sometimes called elementary bodies.

The poxviruses contain 5 to 7.5 percent linear double-stranded DNA with a molecular mass of 85 to 240×10^6 daltons. Extensive research, with electron microscopy, restriction endonucleases, recombinant DNA technology, and rapid sequencing methods, has elucidated the basic structure of the genomes of poxviruses, especially vaccinia virus. The discovery of a mutant vaccinia virus with a smaller genome into which foreign genes could be inserted led to great interest in using recombinant poxvirus genomes as recombinant vaccines for viruses, bacteria, protozoa, and various parasites in both human and veterinary medicine (Mackett et al. 1982, Panicali and Paoletti 1982, Panicali et al. 1981). The genome that codes for the polypeptide antigen responsible for stimulating protective immunity against that pathogen is inserted into the genome of a vaccinia virus. When this recombinant hybrid vaccinia virus is injected into an animal, immunity to both the poxvirus and the pathogen in question is generated. Hybrid viruses that contain as many as 25,000 base pairs of foreign DNA may be constructed (Mackett et al. 1982, Moss 1985, Panicali and Paoletti 1982, Smith and Moss 1983).

Animal poxvirus diseases characterized by the formation of pustules on the skin, with or without general manifestations of illness, occur in all species of domestic animals except dogs.

In humans there are nine different poxviruses that produce disease (Fenner 1985). The most serious of these diseases is called *variola*, or *smallpox*, a disease which has been eradicated from the world by vaccination of humans with the closely related vaccinia virus vaccine. Humans can also be infected with monkeypox, cowpox, and vaccinia viruses, and by orf virus and paravaccinia virus in the genus *Parapoxvirus*.

The pox diseases of humans, sheep, goats, and fowl are severe and often fatal. Some researchers believe that all of our pox diseases came originally from one or more basic strains, which have changed over time as they adapted to different hosts. The disease in birds may be proliferative and tumorlike rather than pustular. It is seldom possible to establish an infection in a mammal with a bird pox, or vice versa. There are many types of bird poxes, but these are related immunologically, and many of them can readily be adapted to new bird hosts. The true pox diseases of mammals show immunological relationships, and in many instances they may be adapted to new mammalian hosts.

Pox in fowl, turkeys, pheasants, pigeons, canaries, and many wild birds is seen from time to time in the United States. Immunization of domestic fowl has reduced the incidence and importance of this disease.

Excellent review articles of pox disease have been written by Joklik (1966, 1968), Fenner (1985), Moss (1985), and Tripathy et al. (1981).

REFERENCES

Appleyard, G., Westwood, J.C., and Zwartouw, H.T. 1962. The toxic effect of rabbitpox virus in tissue culture. Virology 18:159–169.

Appleyard, G., Zwartouw, H.T., and Westwood, J.C. 1964. A protective antigen from the pox-viruses. I. Reaction with neutralizing antibody. Br. J. Exp. Pathol. 45:150–161.

Fenner, F. 1965. Viruses of the myxoma-fibroma subgroup of the poxviruses. II. Comparison of soluble antigens by gel diffusion tests, and a general discussion of the subgroup. Aust. J. Exp. Biol. Med. Sci. 43:143–156.

Fenner, F. 1985. Poxviruses. In B.N. Fields, D.M. Knipe, R.M. Chanock, J.L. Melnick, B. Roizman, and R.E. Shope, eds., Virology. Raven Press, New York. Pp. 661–684.

Joklik, W.K. 1966. The poxviruses. Bact. Proc. 30:33–66.

Joklik, W.K. 1968. The poxviruses. Ann. Rev. Microbiol. 22:359–390.

Mackett, M., Smith, G.L., and Moss, B. 1982. Vaccinia virus: A selectable eukaryotic cloning and expression vector. Proc. Natl. Acad. Sci. USA 79:7415–7419.

Matthews, R.E.F. 1982. Classification and nomenclature of viruses. Intervirology 17:42–46.

Moss, B. 1985. Replication of poxviruses. In B.N. Fields, D.M. Knipe, R.M. Chanock, J.L. Melnick, B. Roizman, and R.E. Shope, eds., Virology. Raven Press, New York. Pp. 685–703.

Panicali, D., and Paoletti, E. 1982. Construction of poxviruses as cloning vectors: Insertion of the thymidine kinase gene from herpes simplex virus into the DNA of infectious vaccinia virus. Proc. Natl. Acad. Sci. USA 79:4927–4931.

Panicali, D., Davis, S.W., Mercer, S.R., and Paoletti, E. 1981. Two major DNA variants present in serially propagated stocks of the WR strain of vaccinia virus. J. Virol. 37:1000–1010.

Rodriguez-Burgos, A., Chordi, A., Diaz, R., Torms, J. 1966. Immunoelectrophoretic analysis of vaccinia virus. Virology 30:569–572.

Smith, G.L., and Moss, B. 1983. Infectious poxvirus vectors have capacity for at least 25,000 base pairs of foreign DNA. Gene 25:21–28.

Takahashi, M., Kameyama, S., Kato, S., and Kamahora, J. 1959. The immunological relationship of the poxvirus group. Biken J. 2:27–29.

Tripathy, D.N., Hanson, L.E., and Crandell, R.A. 1981. Poxviruses of veterinary importance: Diagnosis of infections. In E. Kurstak and C. Kurstak, eds., Comparative Diagnosis of Viral Diseases, vol. 3. Academic Press, New York. Pp. 267–346.

Woodroofe, G.M., and Fenner, F. 1962. Serological relationships within the poxvirus group: An antigen common to all members of the group. Virology 16:334–341.

The Genus *Avipoxvirus*

Avianpox

SYNONYMS: Avian diphtheria, canarypox, chickenpox, contagious epithelioma, fowlpox, pigeonpox, quailpox, sorehead, turkeypox

Poxvirus infections in birds appear as proliferative lesions on the unfeathered areas of the head and body, or as proliferative or diphtheritic lesions in the upper respiratory and oral mucosa.

Several viruses in the genus *Avipoxvirus* infect birds. These include the viruses of fowlpox, pigeonpox, quailpox, canarypox, turkeypox, parakeetpox, and psittacinepox, as well as a variety of isolates found in wild and game birds (Tripathy et al. 1981). The viruses differ somewhat in pathogenicity in different species, usually being more virulent for the species from which they were recovered than for other kinds of birds. For example, fowlpox attacks chickens primarily but also affects turkeys, pheasants and other wild birds, and canaries. Pigeonpox virus is only slightly pathogenic for chickens but can cause severe disease in pigeons and several other species of birds.

Although the avian poxviruses share common antigens, many of these viruses are not cross-protective for domestic fowl. Pigeonpox immunizes chickens against fowlpox and constitutes a good vaccine for this purpose. On the other hand, chickens, turkeys, and quail vaccinated with pigeonpox and fowlpox vaccines are not protected against quailpox (Winterfield and Reed 1985).

Character of the Disease. Pox in chickens is manifested by characteristic lesions on the head. They appear on the comb and wattles and around the corners of the mouth, the nostrils, and the eyes (Figure 45.1). In some cases the lesions involve the mucous membranes of the mouth, larynx, pharynx, esophagus, and trachea. These appear as raised, whitish nodules of varying size that tend to coalesce, then become yellow, caseous, and necrotic (Tripathy et al. 1981). The lesions may ulcerate and form what are commonly called cankers. This form of pox was considered to be a separate disease and was called *avian diphtheria* for many years. In such infections the infraorbital sinus frequently becomes greatly distended and thus distorts the facial features.

The skin lesions are small pustules that soon dry and become warty epithelial crusts that may become quite thick. Affected birds become ill, refuse to eat, become emaciated, and stop laying; many die. The lesions are confined to the featherless part of the head, as a rule, but occasionally they are found around the vent, and even on the feet. If the infection remains on the skin and does not involve the mucous membranes of the head, the effect on the bird is much less severe and recoveries are more common. In favorable cases the course of the disease is 3 or 4 weeks; with complications it may be much longer.

An epornitic of avian pox in canaries and house sparrows within a research aviary was characterized by proliferative lesions in the upper and lower respiratory tracts, including proliferative air sacculitis, proliferative bronchopneumonia, and proliferative rhinitis (Donnelly and Crane 1984).

Pigeonpox frequently causes considerable trouble in squab-raising plants. The squabs may become infected while still in the nest, but more often the disease appears in well-developed birds. Cankers are found in the mouth, and the corners of the mouth are covered with crusts. The eyelids may also be affected and the birds blinded. The legs and toes are sometimes involved. The death rate may be high.

Avian pox infections have been reported in a variety of species of wild and zoo birds, including Canada geese (Cox 1980), birds of prey (Halliwell 1979), green-winged teal (Morton and Dieterich 1979), terns (Jacobson et al. 1980), peacocks (Al Falluji et al. 1979), bobwhite quail (Davidson et al. 1980), Amazon parrots (Boosinger et al. 1982, Graham 1978, McDonald et al. 1981), cherrug falcon (Thiele et al. 1979), and various species of pheasant (Dobson 1937, Ensley et al. 1978). Avipoxviruses have been isolated from several species of wild birds in western Australia (Annuar et al. 1983).

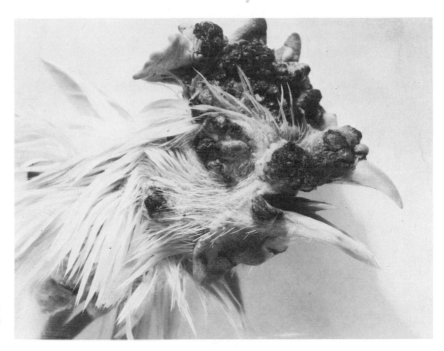

Figure 45.1. Fowlpox. Note the characteristic dry scabs on the comb and around the eye, nostrils, and corner of the mouth.

In cattle (Gillespie et al. 1984) and in cats (Scott et al. 1984) subcutaneous or intradermal inoculation of a vaccine strain of fowlpox virus produced well-defined, circumscribed, and localized lesions—typical fowlpox lesions—at the site of the injection (Figure 45.2) and stimulated the production of neutralizing antibodies. Fowlpox virus was recovered from the scabs taken from the cattle and cats at varying intervals after intradermal injection. Whether this recovery represented residual or replicating virus is unknown at present. In cattle subsequent repeated intradermal injection of virus into different sites at periods varying between 3 and 5 weeks continued to yield typical lesions at the injection sites, although after the second injection, the lesions were not as prominent. There was no transmission of virus from the infected cattle to control cattle with which they came in contact. Ponies inoculated intradermally with the same strain of virus did not show skin lesions at the injection sites, although neutralizing antibodies were demonstrated (Holmes et al. 1984). The viral titers of the stock virus could be assayed in heifers by the intradermal injection of a series of viral dilutions (Gillespie et al. 1984).

Properties of the Virus. Fowlpox virus has been studied in some detail, but the biochemical and biophysical properties of most of the other avian poxviruses have not been adequately characterized. Fowlpox virus is brick-shaped or rectangular, with dimensions of 258 by 354 nm (Tripathy et al. 1981). The virions contain linear double-stranded DNA of 200 to 240 $\times$ 10^6 molecular weight.

The Borrel (or elementary) have estimated dimensions

Figure 45.2. (*Top*) Inflammatory reaction in a cow 2 days after intradermal injection of 0.3 ml of fowlpox vaccine virus in three different sites. Each lesion was approximately 1 cm in diameter. Scabbing ensued 2 days later and the lesions persisted for about 13 days. (*Bottom*) Comparative reaction in the same cow 2 days after a second series of intradermal injections of the same stock virus in three different sites. The lesions persisted through day 9.

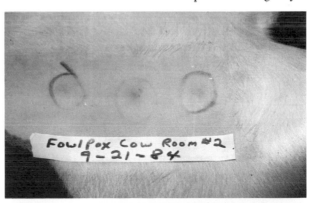

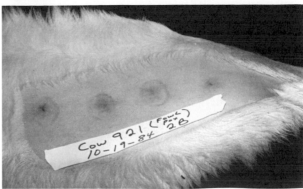

of 332 by 284 nm with a pepsin-resistant core (Woodruff and Goodpasture 1929 and 1930). They are located in the Bollinger body, a cytoplasmic inclusion body that consists of a matrix (Figure 45.3) which is dissolved by sodium lauryl sulfate but is quite resistant to enzymes. The matrix gives a positive Feulgen reaction after previous extraction of lipids. The developing elementary bodies initially are poorly defined but later acquire the characteristic poxvirus appearance of a dumbbell-like structure within an outer membrane. Virions are readily observed by electron microscopy.

Fowlpox virus is resistant to drying. In the dried crusts from epithelial lesions, virulence remains unimpaired for many months if the drying has been thorough. The disease tends to recur year after year on the same premises, but it is not known how the virus is preserved in the intervening periods. The virus is readily destroyed by alkalis and by most disinfectants. It is preserved for long periods by 50 percent glycerol and is inactivated by heating for 30 minutes at 50°C, or 8 minutes at 60°C. The virus is resistant to ether but sensitive to chloroform.

Neutralization tests can be performed with "pock" counting on chorioallantoic membranes. Precipitating antibodies can be revealed by gel diffusion, and complement-fixing antibodies by the complement-fixation test. The hemagglutination inhibition antibody can be used to measure virus and detect hemagglutination inhibition antibody.

Virus neutralization in cell culture is more reliable in differentiating avian poxviruses than the passive hemagglutination test, as cross-reactions were detected among avian poxviruses by the latter test.

Cultivation. Avian poxviruses can be isolated and grown in chick embryos and cell cultures (Goodpasture et al. 1932, Tripathy et al. 1973).

Epizootiology and Pathogenesis. Fowlpox is believed to be transmitted principally by direct inoculation from bird to bird through wounds incurred by fighting and by the birds' picking at one another. The disease may also be spread by the bites of mosquitoes (Kligler et al. 1929, Matheson et al. 1930) and possibly by other arthropods. Arthropod transmission is certainly not as important as direct contact in the spread of this disease within flocks, but it may be the usual way by which the infection is spread from one flock to another. Doyle and Minett (1927) placed susceptible birds in cages that had just been occupied by infected birds. Transmission did not occur except when the skin or mucous membranes of the susceptible birds had been scarified. Infection seems to depend, therefore, on breaks in the skin.

The incubation period is generally 4 to 10 days. Viral

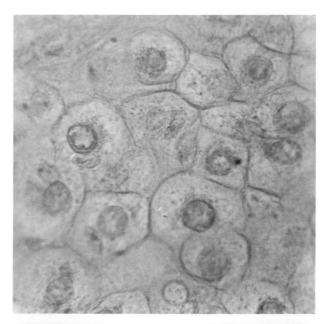

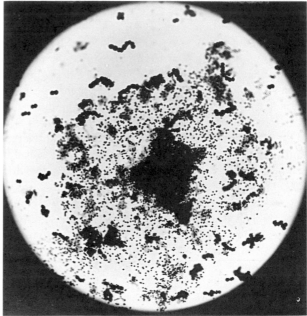

Figure 45.3. (*Top*) Fowlpox. Swollen epithelial cells in an early lesion show the Bollinger (inclusion) bodies. These bodies are spherical and prominent in the stained section. In several of the cells the nuclei are crowded against the cell wall. × 465. (*Bottom*) The Borrel, or elementary, bodies of fowlpox. These minute spherical bodies were obtained free of tissue debris by tryptic digestion of the Bollinger bodies contained in virus-infected cells. The bodies here are stained after admixture with *Streptococcus* sp. to indicate comparative sizes. × 350. (From E. W. Goodpasture, courtesy of *American Journal of Pathology*.)

replication occurs at the site of primary infection and produces a primary lesion that quickly progresses into papules within 1 or 2 days. Vesicles are present briefly, then the lesions become confluent within 4 or 5 days. Scabs are formed as desquamation occurs (Tripathy et al. 1981). Viral replication occurs in the cytoplasm, with characteristic intracytoplasmic inclusions observable by 36 to 48 hours.

The pathogenesis of infection in laying hens has been described in depth by Tripathy and Hanson (1978).

Immunity. Birds that have recovered from fowlpox are solidly immune thereafter. Both humoral and cellular immunity are involved in protection. There is a possibility of persistence of virus in the bird, which might also be a factor in long-term protection. In flocks in which the disease has occurred for some years, it is seen only in the young birds. This could be the result of carriers or persistence of the virus in the environment. In previously uninfected flocks, birds of all ages develop the disease.

Diagnosis. A clinical diagnosis of avianpox can usually be made based on signs and lesions and confirmed by microscopic examination of biopsy or necropsy lesions with the characteristic intracytoplasmic inclusion bodies, by virus isolation, and by electron microscopic identification of the characteristic brick-shaped virions in infected cells.

Treatment. There is no specific treatment for avianpox infections.

Prevention and Control. Pox infection in fowl can be prevented by immunization of the birds with the homologous strain of virus. Immunization of poultry flocks is encouraged only in regions where fowlpox or other avianpox is prevalent. Two types of fowlpox vaccines are available for immunizing chickens against fowlpox—vaccine virus propagated in chicken embryonating eggs or in susceptible cell cultures. A canarypox vaccine will protect chickens against canarypox (Hitchner 1981).

Vaccines are normally injected into the wing web. Fowlpox and pigeonpox vaccines given subcutaneously in one study depressed body weight gain (Springer and Truman 1981). Oral vaccination with the attenuated HP–1 cell culture strain in the 200th to 400th transfer is effective in 5-day-old chicks and is safer (Mayr and Danner 1976) than in older birds. A second vaccine dose should be given 3 to 4 weeks later. It is essential that the vaccine dose contain 10 $TCID_{50}$ of virus.

Fowlpox vaccines can be combined with Newcastle and/or Marek's virus vaccine, but inoculations usually are given parenterally.

The Disease in Humans. Fowlpox does not affect humans. The disease in humans known as *chickenpox* or *varicella* is caused by a herpesvirus and has no relationship with avianpox viruses, nor is it contracted from chickens or other fowl.

REFERENCES

Al Falluji, M.M., Tantawi, H.H., Al-Bana, A., and Al-Sheikhly, S. 1979. Pox infection among captive peacocks. J. Wildl. Dis. 15:597–600.

Annuar, B.O., Mackenzie, J.S., and Lalor, P.A. 1983. Isolation and characterization of avipoxviruses from wild birds in Western Australia. Arch. Virol. 76:217–229.

Boosinger, T.R., Winterfield, R.W., Feldman, D.S., and Dhillon, A.S. 1982. Psittacine pox virus: Virus isolation and identification, transmission, and cross-challenge studies in parrots and chickens. Avian Dis. 26:437–444.

Cox, W.R. 1980. Avian pox infection in a Canada goose (*Branta canadensis*). J. Wildl. Dis. 16:623–626.

Davidson, W.R., Kellogg, F.E., and Doster, G.L. 1980. An epornitic of avian pox in wild bobwhite quail. J. Wildl. Dis. 16:293–298.

Dobson, N. 1937. Pox in pheasants. J. Comp. Pathol. Therap. 50:401–404.

Donnelly, T.M., and Crane, L.A. 1984. An epornitic of avian pox in a research aviary. Avian Dis. 28:517–525.

Doyle, T.M., and Minett, F.C. 1927. Fowl pox. J. Comp. Pathol. Therap. 40:247–266.

Ensley, P.K., Anderson, M.P., Costello, M.L., Powell, H.C., and Cooper, R. 1978. Epornitic of avian pox in a zoo. J. Am. Vet. Med. Assoc. 173:1111–1114.

Gillespie, J.H., Schiff, E.I., Scott, F.W., Holmes, D.F., and Higgins, W.P. 1984. The response of heifer calves to a vaccine strain of fowlpox virus. Personal communication.

Goodpasture, E.W., Woodruff, A.M., and Buddingh, G.J. 1932. Vaccinal infection of the chorio-allantoic membrane of the chick embryo. Am. J. Pathol. 8:271–282.

Graham, C.L. 1978. Poxvirus infection in a spectacled Amazon parrot (*Amazona albifrons*). Avian Dis. 22:340–343.

Halliwell, W.H. 1979. Diseases of birds of prey. Vet. Clin. North Am. [Small Anim. Pract.] 9(3):541–568.

Hitchner, S.B. 1981. Canary pox vaccination with live embryo-attenuated virus. Avian Dis. 25:874–881.

Holmes, D.F., Gillespie, J.H., and Scott, F.W. 1984. The response of ponies to a vaccine strain of fowlpox virus. Personal communication.

Jacobson, E.R., Raphael, B.L., Nguyen, H.T., Greiner, E.C., and Gross, T. 1980. Avian pox infection, aspergillosis and renal trematodiasis in a royal tern. J. Wildl. Dis. 16:627–631.

Kligler, I.J., Muckenfuss, R.S., and Rivers, T.M. 1929. Transmission of fowl-pox by mosquitoes. J. Exp. Med. 49:649–660.

McDonald, S.E., Lowenstine, L.J., and Ardans, A.A. 1981. Avian pox in blue-fronted Amazon parrots. J. Am. Vet. Med. Assoc. 179:1218–1222.

Matheson, R., Burnett, E.L., and Brody, A.L. 1930. The transmission of fowl-pox by mosquitoes. Preliminary report. Poult. Sci. 10:211–223.

Mayr, A., and Danner, K. 1976. Oral immunization against pox. Studies on fowl pox as a model. Dev. Biol. Stand. 33:249–259.

Morton, J.K., and Dieterich, R.A. 1979. Avian pox infection in an American green-winged teal (*Anas crecca carolinensis*) in Alaska. J. Wildl. Dis. 15:451–453.

Scott, F.W., Geissinger, C., Gillespie, J.H., and Holmes, D.F. 1984. The response of cats to a vaccine strain of fowlpox virus. Personal communication.

Springer, W.T., and Truman, R.W. 1981. Effect of subcutaneous pox vaccination of young chicks on immune responses and weight gains. Poult. Sci. 60:1213–1220.

Thiele, J., Kiel, H., and Adolphs, H.D. 1979. Avian pox virus. An ultrastructural study on a cherrug falcon. Arch. Virol. 62:77–82.

Tripathy, D.N., and Hanson, L.E. 1978. Pathogenesis of fowlpox in laying hens. Avian Dis. 22:259–265.

Tripathy, D.N., Hanson, L.E., and Crandell, R.A. 1981. Poxviruses of veterinary importance: Diagnosis of infections. In E. Kurstak and C. Kurstak, eds., Comparative Diagnosis of Viral Diseases, vol. 3. Acaeds., Comparative Diagnosis of Viral Diseases, vol. 3. Academic Press, New York, Pp. 267–346.

Tripathy, D.N., Hanson, L.E., and Killinger, A.H. 1973. Studies on differentiation of avian pox viruses. Avian Dis. 17:325–333.

Winterfield, R.W., and Reed, W. 1985. Avian pox: Infection and immunity with quail, psittacine, fowl, and pigeon pox viruses. Poult. Sci. 64:65–70.

Woodruff, C.E., and Goodpasture, E.W. 1929. Infectivity of isolated inclusion bodies of fowl pox. Am. J. Pathol. 5:1–9.

Woodruff, C.E., and Goodpasture, E.W. 1930. Relation of virus of fowl-pox to specific cellular inclusions of the disease. Am. J. Pathol. 6:713–720.

The Genus *Orthopoxvirus*

For centuries, evidence indicates, true cowpox occurred frequently in both Europe and America and these outbreaks were often directly related to epidemics of smallpox (variola) in humans. Smallpox infection was also sometimes transmitted from milkers to the cows being milked, and the disease in these animals was called cowpox. There is evidence, too, that horsepox was often transmitted to cattle by the infected hands of milkers, the disease being indistinguishable from smallpox transmitted by humans and from cowpox transmitted by other cattle. Although smallpox, cowpox, and horsepox are regarded as distinct diseases, the differences in the causative viruses may result from adaptation to different hosts. These relationships were first recognized by Jenner (1798), who used the knowledge to immunize humans against deadly smallpox by vaccinating children and susceptible adults with vaccinia virus.

Bovine Vaccinia Mammillitis

SYNONYM: Vaccinia

There is no evidence that vaccinia as a disease entity in cattle now exists anywhere in the world because vaccinia virus vaccine is no longer used to immunize humans against smallpox. When vaccinia occurred in the past, it was an accidental infection caused by contact between cattle and humans recently vaccinated for smallpox (Boerner 1923, Gibbs 1984). The cattle became infected from vaccinia virus on the hands of the milkers. The disease often spread to many cows in the milking herd and from these cows to other people. In some cases nearly every unvaccinated person who had contact with the cows, or who used raw milk from them, became infected. These individuals developed typical vaccinia lesions on their hands, arms, faces, and other parts of their bodies.

A disease commonly called *cowpox* occurs in cattle, usually dairy cattle. The available evidence indicates that this condition is caused either by cowpox virus or pseudo-cowpox virus, agents separate and distinct from vaccinia virus. Investigators believe that cowpox does not exist in North America, although it does occur in cattle and other animals in western Europe (Baxby 1975, Gibbs 1984).

Character of the Disease. The mammillitis caused by vaccinia virus occurred as lesions on the teats and udders of cattle (Gibbs 1984, Kahrs 1981). The lesions resembled those shown in Figure 45.5. They appeared as small papules that gradually changed to pustules. A reddened areola appeared around each lesion. The pustule tended to develop a small pit, or umbilication. The lesions could be numerous, but generally they appeared in rather small numbers, mostly on the teats. The friction of the milking process generally caused the lesions to break and form raw areas that were very tender. When the pustules were not broken, they dried up and became covered with dry scabs that fell off in about 10 days, leaving an unscarred surface. Healing was greatly delayed by the friction of milking, and bacterial invasion of the udder often resulted in mastitis.

Properties of the Virus. Vaccinia virus has been studied extensively, and its properties and replication have been reviewed by Moss (1985). Extensive research into the genome of the native virus has led to the development of hybrid viruses through recombinant DNA technology. These hybrid viruses offer great hope for the development of new vaccines against infectious agents for which vaccines have not been available to protect humans and animals or for which available vaccines have not been effective. The accepted use of these hybrid vaccines would again put humans and cattle at risk of contracting vaccinia, although cases of disease would be rare.

Vaccinia virions, like other poxviruses, have a complex structure and lack icosahedral symmetry. The mature virions, known as elementary bodies, vary in size from 240 to 380 by 170 to 270 nm (Figure 45.4). A lipoprotein bilayer, called the outer membrane or envelope, is 9 to 12 nm thick. The virus contains a central biconcave core with two smaller lateral bodies beside it in the concavities. The core contains nucleoprotein. Negative staining subunits exist on the surface of the particle but within the outer membrane. Virions can be seen readily with a light microscopy.

The vaccinia genome contains 186,000 base pairs and consists of a single uninterrupted polynucleotide chain that is folded to form a linear duplex structure with hairpin loops at each end (Baroudy et al. 1982, Moss 1985).

More than 100 polypeptides, ranging in mass from 8,000 to 200,000 daltons, have been identified from the

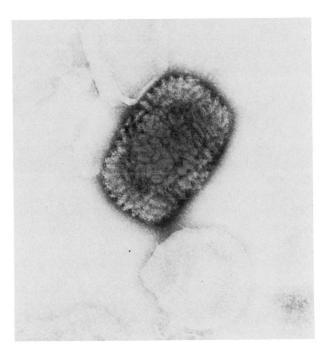

Figure 45.4. Virus of the variola-vaccinia-cowpox group, negatively stained. × 110,000. (Courtesy Viral Pathology and Viral Exanthems Branches, Centers for Disease Control.)

vaccinia virion (Essani and Dales 1979, Oie and Ichihashi 1981). Several polypeptides have been identified in the envelope, including a 58-kilodalton protein that constitutes the surface tubules and stimulates neutralizing antibodies and antibodies that inhibit cell fusion (Moss 1985). The hemagglutinin, one of seven glycosolated polypeptides located in the envelope, agglutinates the red cells of some fowl. The nucleoprotein antigen is involved in complement-fixation and precipitation reactions.

Vaccinia virus is quite stable and resistant. Suspensions of the virus are inactivated in 10 minutes at 60°C, but dried virus withstands temperatures of 100°C for 10 minutes. It is quite stable between pH 5 and 9. The virus is resistant to ether in the cold but is inactivated by chloroform. Oxidizing agents such as potassium permanganate or ethyl oxide readily inactivate the particle.

Cultivation. Vaccinia virus grows in primary cultures of chick embryo, rabbit kidney, rabbit testis, bovine embryo skin, and also in continuous cell lines such as HeLA and L-929. Cell destruction occurs early and includes the formation of giant cells. Plaques are formed in agar overlay systems. In embryonated eggs 7 to 13 days old the virus grows well on the chorioallantoic membrane and produces pocks, the formation of which may be used to titrate the virus. Embryo mortality varies from low to 100 percent, depending on the virus strain and the test conditions. Less sensitive routes of inoculation are the allantoic cavity and the yolk sac.

Epizootiology and Pathogenesis. In the past, outbreaks of bovine mammillitis caused by vaccinia virus have almost invariably been associated with the lesions of recently vaccinated humans who had direct contact with cattle. Once the outbreak started, the virus could be spread throughout the herd, usually by means of the milking process.

Immunity. After recovery from vaccinia, cattle are immune for a considerable time, perhaps for life. Second attacks have been reported, but these may have been infections of pseudopox virus. Experimentally, solid resistance is conveyed by one exposure.

Diagnosis. The mammillitis caused by vaccinia and cowpox is identical clinically. The two viruses are differentiated in the laboratory with some difficulty, and the results are based on the greater sensitivity of vaccinia virus on the chorioallantoic membrane of the hen's egg with the formation of pock lesions (Gibbs 1984, Gibbs et al. 1970). Other causes of mammillitis such as pseudocowpox virus, herpesvirus, and the pathogens of the various vesicular diseases must be differentiated from cowpox virus and vaccinia virus by electron microscopy. Laboratory confirmation of the diagnosis can be made by isolation of virus from lesions.

Prevention and Control. When the disease appeared in a milking herd in the past, affected animals were segregated from the others as far as practicable. They were milked last, and the milkers scrubbed their hands thoroughly with soap and water after milking them and before handling others animals.

The Disease in Humans. Humans who became infected with vaccinia virus through milking or handling vaccinia-infected cattle developed vaccinia lesions on their hands. Each lesion consisted of a papule that quickly became a pustule. It was reddened about its periphery; and, although it itched, it was not particularly painful. The characteristic umbilication appeared in most of the pustules. If not rubbed or scratched, the lesion became dehydrated after a few days; a scab formed and subsequently fell off after 10 to 14 days. The lesions usually were not numerous.

REFERENCES

Baroudy, B.M., Vankatesan, S., and Moss, B. 1982. Incompletely base-paired flip-flop terminal loops link the two DNA strands of the vaccinia virus genome into one uninterrupted polynucleotide chain. Cell 28:315–324.

Baxby, D. 1975. Identification and inter-relationships of the variola/vaccinia subgroup of poxviruses. Prog. Med. Virol. 19:215–228.

Boerner, F. 1923. An outbreak of cowpox introduced by vaccination, involving a herd of cattle and a family. J. Am. Vet. Med. Assoc. 64:93–97.

Essani, K., and Dales, S. 1979. Biogenesis of vaccinia: Evidence for more than 100 polypeptides in the virion. Virology 95:385–394.

Gibbs, E.P.J. 1984. Viral diseases of the skin of the bovine teat and udder. Vet. Clin. North Am. [Large Anim. Pract.] 6(1):187–202.

Gibbs, E.P.J., Johnson, R.H., and Osborne, A.D. 1970. Differential diagnosis of viral skin infection of the bovine teat. Vet. Rec. 87:602–609.

Jenner, E. 1798. An inquiry into the causes and effects of variolae vaccinae, a disease discovered in some of the western counties of England, particularly Gloucestershire, and known by the name of cowpox. London, Sampson Low. (Reprinted in Camac, L.N.B. 1959. Classics of Medicine and Surgery. Dover, New York. Pp. 213–240.)

Kahrs, R.F. 1981. Viral diseases of cattle: Poxvirus infections of the teats. Iowa State University Press, Ames. Pp. 189–196.

Moss, B. 1985. Replication of poxviruses. In B.N. Fields, D.M. Knipe, R.M. Chanock, J.L. Melnick, B. Roizman, and R.E. Shope, eds., Virology. Raven Press, New York. Pp. 685–703.

Oie, M., and Ichihashi, Y. 1981. Characterization of vaccinia polypeptides. Virology 113:263–276.

Cowpox

Cowpox virus produces a mammillitis in cattle indistinguishable from vaccinia, yet there is general agreement that the disease is distinct from vaccinia and pseudocowpox. Cowpox is only rarely recorded in cattle, and then only in western Europe (Gibbs 1984, Gibbs et al. 1973). It is believed that cowpox virus does not exist in the United States.

The antigenic properties of this virus are close to, but distinct from, vaccinia as determined by of complement-fixation, agar-gel diffusion, and antibody-absorption tests (Andrewes 1964). In general, the features of cowpox virus such as biochemical and biophysical properties, hemagglutination red cell spectrum, morphology, and cultivation in tissue culture and eggs, are similar to those of vaccinia.

In cattle the virus affects the skin, particularly the teats and udders (Figure 45.5). The papules develop into vesicles, followed by crusting, which may persist for weeks.

The epidemiology of cowpox is not known for certain. It is believed that a rodent host, in which the infection is subclinical, serves as a reservoir for the virus (Baxby 1977).

In western Europe cowpox virus or a closely related virus has been reported in several animal species other than cattle, including elephants, anteaters, domestic cats, and exotic felids (Baxby et al. 1982, Gaskell et al. 1983, Marennikova et al. 1977, Martland et al. 1983).

Lesions in humans resemble those of primary vaccination with vaccinia virus and may be found on the hands, arms, face, and eyes of milkers (Andrewes 1964). The disease may be severe.

REFERENCES

Andrewes, C. 1964. Viruses of Vertebrates. Williams & Wilkins, Baltimore.

Baxby, D. 1977. Poxvirus hosts and reservoirs. Arch. Virol. 55:169–179.

Baxby, D., Ashton, D.G., Jones, D.M., and Thomsett, L.R. 1982. An outbreak of cowpox in captive cheetahs: Virological and epidemiological studies. J. Hyg. 89:365–372.

Gaskell, R.M., Gaskell, C.J., Evans, R.J., Dennis, P.E., Bennett, A.M., Udall, N.D., Voyle, C., and Hill, T.J. 1983. Natural and experimental pox virus infection in the domestic cat. Vet. Rec. 112:164–170.

Gibbs, E.P.J. 1984. Viral diseases of the skin of the bovine teat and udder. Vet. Clin. North Am. [Large Anim. Pract.] 6(1):187–202.

Gibbs, E.P.J., Johnson, R.H., and Collings, D.F. 1973. Cowpox in a dairy herd in the United Kingdom. Vet. Rec. 92:56–64.

Marennikova, S.S., Maltseva, N.N., Korneeva, V.I., and Garanina, N.M. 1977. Outbreak of pox disease among Carnivora (Felidae) and Edentata. J. Infect. Dis. 135:358–366.

Martland, M.F., Fowler, S., Poulton, G.J., and Baxby, D. 1983. Pox virus infection of a domestic cat. Vet. Rec. 112:171–172.

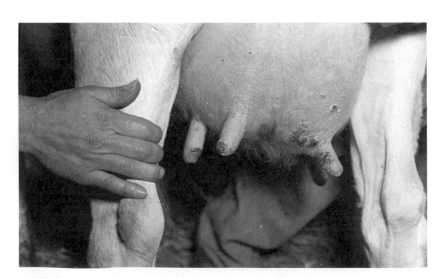

Figure 45.5. Cowpox. Note the well-advanced lesions on the teats and udder. (Courtesy Robert Graham.)

Catpox

SYNONYMS: "Cowpox," feline pox, orthopoxvirus infection, pox disease

Catpox virus causes a chronic dermatological and/or an acute, sometimes fatal, respiratory disease in domestic and exotic felids. Outbreaks have occurred in zoological parks.

Character of the Disease. Catpox has been reported from several countries of Europe, including the United Kingdom, Austria, and the Soviet Union. Morbidity is low in domestic cats; cases reported to date have involved only individual cats, or at most a few animals (Gaskell et al. 1983; Martland et al. 1983, 1985; Thomsett et al. 1978). In zoo outbreaks in the United Kingdom and the Soviet Union the morbidity was high, most cats within a holding area became infected (Baxby et al. 1982, Marennikova et al. 1977). Mortality from the dermal form of catpox is low, and most cats recover within a few weeks. During the outbreaks in British and Soviet zoos pneumonia and exudative pleuritis were common, and the mortality from this respiratory form of the disease was much higher. Most of these cases have occurred in the fall or winter, but the low number of reported cases makes it difficult to establish a definite seasonal incidence. There does not appear to be any specific age incidence, with cases reported in 12 week old kittens as well as in mature cats. There is no abnormal sex distribution of cases, and the only special population distribution has been in zoological parks and in rural free-roaming cats presumably in contact with an as yet unidentified virus carrier, probably a small mammal.

Clinical disease in the cat occurs in two forms, dermal and respiratory. The dermal form occurs as a general rash, a single skin lesion, or multiple skin lesions over the entire body. Localized crusty and slightly proliferative skin lesions 2 to 3 mm in diameter appear initially at the site of inoculation or scarification. Lesions may appear first on the paws, head, or lips, or around the edges of the conjunctiva; within a few days they often spread over much of the body. Cats may show severe edema of the distal limbs, head, and neck. Temperature usually remains normal, and appetite may be normal to severely depressed. The skin lesions were reported by Gaskell and co-workers (1983) to be circular, 3 to 6 mm in diameter, and to be one of three types. The first type appeared as "flat, glistening, red, hairless areas." Type 2 lesions were thick scabs that covered "shallow, crater-like ulcers filled with white pus," while type 3 lesions consisted of thick scabs over "smooth to granular red areas." Other clinical signs or concurrent problems noted include abscesses, sloughing of the metacarpal pad, ulcerated lick granuloma of the lip, and transient neurological signs. Pruritus may be slight in some cats, but in others it is severe with self-inflicted exacerbation of lesions. A mild conjunctivitis may occur. The usual respiratory form of the disease involves pneumonia, conjunctivitis, and exudative pleuritis. The clinical signs are characterized by anorexia, fever, dyspnea, lethargy, paroxysmal coughing, cyanosis, and openmouth breathing. The course for the respiratory form runs 3 to 8 days, and mortality is very high.

Properties of the Virus. Catpox virus is an orthopoxvirus of the Poxviridae family. It is closely related to, and perhaps identical to, the cowpox virus (Baxby et al. 1979). Variola (or smallpox), vaccinia, cowpox, horsepox, and elephantpox viruses are all closely related. These are large viruses—240 to 380 by 170 to 270 nm. The virions, which often appear brick-shaped on electron microscopic examination, have an outer membrane and a multitude of cross-hatched tubular structures. Orthopoxviruses are quite stable and resistant, and can survive in dried scabs from lesions for extended periods. They are resistant to many disinfectants that inactivate most enveloped viruses but can be inactivated by certain oxidizing agents such as potassium permanganate or ethyl oxide, and probably sodium hypochlorite.

Poxviruses replicate in the cytoplasm of cells, principally epithelial cells. Large eosinophilic intracytoplasmic inclusion bodies are evident in cells undergoing poxvirus replication.

Epizootiology and Pathogenesis. In addition to the domestic cat, catpox has been seen in the lion, puma, Far Eastern cat (*Felis bengalensis*), ocelot, cheetah, black panther, and jaguar (Baxby et al. 1982, Marennikova et al. 1977). In all likelihood, all members of the Felidae are susceptible to this virus. In addition the giant anteater is susceptible, and a very similar virus has been isolated from elephants.

The exact method of poxvirus transmission and infection in the domestic cat is not known. Virus is present in skin lesions, lungs, pleural exudate, and occasionally in liver, kidney, and spleen; and virus can persist for several weeks in some tissues. Presumably the initial infection in cats results from the ingestion of tissues of an infected rodent, followed by direct contact spread to other susceptible cats. In the Moscow zoo outbreak (Marennikova et al. 1977), the source of virus was shown to be ingestion of poxvirus infected white rats that were fed to the exotic cats. These rats had experienced severe dermal and respiratory disease with 50 percent mortality. An indistinguishable poxvirus has also been isolated from other rodents such as the big gerbil and the yellow suslik. In experimental rodents virus persisted in urine for at least 3 weeks, and in kidney tissue for 5 weeks.

Poxvirus infects the epithelial cells of the skin, mucosa, or respiratory tract. Viral replication results in cell lysis, tissue necrosis, edema, and inflammatory exudate. The host's immune response gradually reduces the quantity of virus in the lesions and allows the tissues to heal, provided the cat does not die from severe respiratory involvement before antibodies appear. The dermal form of catpox is characterized by focal necrotizing and pustular skin lesions, which are described in the section "Character of the Disease." Skin lesions may also take the form of a generalized skin rash and lesions may involve the mucosa of the hard palate, tongue, lips, and esophagus. In the pulmonary form, fibrinonecrotic bronchopneumonia and serofibrinous pleuritis often are found. The laryngeal, tracheal, and bronchial mucosa may be hyperemic with petechiae, and a vesicular rash is seen in some cases in these areas. Foamy fluid and fibrinous pellicles have been observed in the trachea. The bronchi and bronchioli may be filled with foamy, hemorrhagic fluid and fibrin. Peribronchial tissues may be edematous. Lobes of the lung often are bluish red and firm. Large quantities of yellow, serous fluid may be present in the pleural cavity.

Histopathological findings of skin lesions are characterized by necrosis, edema, and hemorrhage, with swollen epithelial cells that contain large, oval, eosinophilic intracytoplasmic inclusions. These inclusions are "type A" and are typical of those seen in several other poxvirus infections. Electron microscopy examination of biopsy specimens from skin lesions reveals electron-dense intracytoplasmic inclusion bodies that contain large virus particles with typical orthopoxvirus morphology. In the lung of animals with the respiratory form, foci of lysis are present, with fibrin and inflammatory cells in the lumina of bronchi, bronchioli, alveolar ducts, and alveoli. The walls of the alveolar ducts and the alveoli may be thickened, and peribronchiolar infiltration with fibrin may occur. The pleura are edematous and contain disintegrating leukocytes and fibrin.

Diagnosis. A clinical diagnosis of poxvirus infection can be made on the basis of history and clinical signs, but confirmation requires appropriate laboratory tests.

The causal virus can be isolated from samples of scabs or skin biopsy specimens. Virus has also been isolated from tonsils, thoracic fluid, lungs, regional lymph nodes, thymus, spleen, liver, and kidney. Isolation is made in feline cell cultures, embryonated eggs, or by inoculation of laboratory animals such as the rabbit, mouse, or rat. Direct immunofluorescence studies of tissues stained with a specific antipoxvirus conjugate can also be utilized.

Specific poxvirus antibodies in serum samples are indicative of previous poxvirus infection. Seroconversion as determined by a rise in antibody titers between paired serum samples confirms the diagnosis. Virus neutralization or hemagglutination inhibition tests can be used to identify antibodies. Biopsy specimens from skin lesions can be submitted for histopathological examination or for the direct identification of poxvirus by electron microscopy (Martland et al. 1985).

Treatment. Treatment for catpox virus infection is symptomatic and supportive. Most cases have been treated with broad-spectrum antibiotics, supplemented by fluids and other symptomatic treatment as indicated. One significant word of caution—treatment with corticosteroids or oral progestogen may transform a localized, relatively mild disease into a generalized, more severe disease that may even be fatal.

Prevention and Control. There is no vaccine available for catpox. Attempts to vaccinate cheetahs with vaccinia virus vaccine have failed. Control of outbreaks involves prompt diagnosis and isolation of infected cats, elimination of the source of virus (infected rodents or contaminated food), if possible, and disinfection of animal living quarters, food dishes, and water pans. Convalescent cats may shed virus for several weeks, and poxviruses are particularly stable in dried crusts from skin lesions. Caution should be exercised in how soon after an outbreak new or susceptible cats are reintroduced to infected areas or placed in contact with cats recovered from poxvirus infections.

The Disease in Humans. As with several other orthopoxviruses of animals, catpox virus can infect humans and produce localized skin lesions. There is one reported case of an animal caretaker infected during an outbreak of catpox in a zoological park (Marennikova et al. 1977). This person developed a localized rash that became generalized, with subsequent papules and pox lesions. A second case of transmission, this time from a domestic cat to its owner, has been reported (Willemse and Egberink 1985). Caution should be exercised in handling cats infected with poxvirus.

REFERENCES

Baxby, D., Ashton, D.G., Jones, D.M., and Thomsett, L.R. 1982. An outbreak of cowpox in captive cheetahs: Virological and epidemiological studies. J. Hyg. 89:365–372.

Baxby, D., Shackleton, W.B., Wheeler, J., and Turner, A. 1979. Comparison of cowpox-like viruses isolated from European zoos. Arch. Virol. 61:337–340.

Gaskell, R.M., Gaskell, C.J., Evans, R.J., Dennis, P.E., Bennett, A.M., Udall, N.D., Voyle, C., and Hill, T.J. 1983. Natural and experimental pox virus infection in the domestic cat. Vet. Rec. 112:164–170.

Marennikova, S.S., Maltseva, N.N., Korneeva, V.I., and Garanina, N.M. 1977. Outbreak of pox disease among Carnivora (Felidae) and Edentata. J. Infect. Dis. 135:358–366.

Martland, M.F., Fowler, S., Poulton, G.J., and Baxby, D. 1983. Pox virus infection of a domestic cat. Vet. Rec. 112:171–172.

Martland, M.F., Poulton, G.J., and Done, R.A. 1985. Three cases of cowpox infection of domestic cats. Vet. Rec. 117:231–233.

Thomsett, L.R., Baxby, D., and Denham, E.M.H. 1978. Cowpox in the domestic cat. Vet. Rec. 103:567.

Willemse, A., and Egberink, H.F. 1985. Transmission of cowpox virus infection from domestic cat to man. Lancet 1:1515

Horsepox

SYNONYMS: Contagious pustular stomatitis, "grease," "grease-heel," viral papular dermatitis

Horsepox is a rare dermatological viral disease of horses characterized by poxlike lesions in and around the mouth or on the legs. The disease has not been reported from the United States, and it seems to be much less common in Europe than it was a half-century ago (DeJong 1917, Tripathy et al. 1981, Zwick 1924). The horsepox pathogen is similar to vaccinia virus and cowpox virus.

Character of the Disease. The disease in horses takes two forms. The less important is an infection of the pastern region, apparently spread by the hands of horseshoers and hostlers. This condition is known as *grease* or *grease heel*. It is characterized by papular eruptions on the flexor surface of the joints in the lower leg. The papules change to vesicles, then to pustules, which finally dry up and form crusts. The legs become somewhat painful, but there is no general reaction as a rule.

The second, more important form is manifested by multiple lesions on the inside of the lips and the opposing surfaces of the gums, on the frenum of the tongue, and on the inside of the cheeks. The lesions begin as papules, change to vesicles, and then become pustules. The animal may have fever, and young horses may become sick and occasionally die. Food is refused, saliva drools from the corners of the mouth, and the animal likes to dip its mouth in water. At first a few lesions appear, but new crops occur and finally nearly all the mucous membranes of the mouth are involved. In some horses the lesions are found also in the nasal passages. Virus removed from lesions of horses will infect cattle, and that from cattle will infect horses.

Two poxviruses antigenically similar to vaccinia were isolated from horses with natural infections in Kenya (Kaminjolo et al. 1974). Although horsepox has not been reported in the United States, viral papular stomatitis in horses has been reported in Australia, New Zealand, and the United States (Bone 1972). The relationship of the two diseases is not clear.

Immunity. Recovery from horsepox leaves substantial immunity. Because lesions on the skin are less severe than those on the mucosa of the mouth, some European authors have suggested that intradermal vaccination produces good results. The cow and horse diseases reciprocally immunize against each other, and both will infect persons who have not been vaccinated against smallpox.

REFERENCES

Bone, J.F. 1972. Viral papular dermatitis. In E.J. Catcott and J.F. Smithcors, eds., Equine Medicine and Surgery. American Veterinary Publications, Wheaton, Ill. P. 77.

DeJong, D.A. 1917. The relationship between contagious pustular stomatitis of the horse, equine variola (horse-pox of Jenner), and vaccinia (cow-pox of Jenner). J. Comp. Pathol. Therap. 30:242–262.

Kaminjolo, J.S., Jr., Nyaga, P.N., and Gicho, J.N. 1974. Isolation, cultivation, and characterization of a poxvirus from some horses in Kenya. Zentralbl. Veterinärmed. [B] 21:592–601.

Tripathy, D.N., Hanson, L.E., and Crandell, R.A. 1981. Poxviruses of veterinary importance: Diagnosis of infections. In E. Kurstak and C. Kurstak, eds., Comparative Diagnosis of Viral Diseases, vol. 3. Academic Press, New York. Pp. 267–346.

Zwick, W. 1924. Über die Beziehungen der Stomatitis Pustulosacontagiosa des Pferdes zu den Pocken der Haustiere und des Menschen. Berl. Tierärztl. Wochenschr. 40:757–761.

Camelpox

Camelpox virus, an orthopoxvirus, causes a highly infectious and generalized disease in camels that spreads readily to susceptible contact animals. Camelpox is an important disease in northern and eastern Africa and the Middle East (Lane et al. 1981). The virus is closely related immunologically to variola (smallpox) virus; camels inoculated with variola virus are protected from camelpox upon subsequent inoculation with virulent camelpox virus (Baxby 1972, Baxby et al., 1975). Isolates from camels in Egypt, Iran, and the Soviet Union are closely related to vaccinia virus, but to varying degrees (Marennikova et al. 1974, Tantawi et al. 1978).

REFERENCES

Baxby, D. 1972. Smallpox-like virus from camels in Iran. Lancet 2:1063.

Baxby, D., Ramyar, H., Hessami, M., and Ghaboosi, B. 1975. Response of camels to intradermal inoculation with smallpox and camelpox viruses. Infect. Immun. 11:617–621.

Lane, J.M., Steele, J.H., and Beran, G.W. 1981. Pox and parapoxvirus infections. In J.H. Steele and G.W. Beran, eds., Handbook Series in Zoonoses, vol. 2: Viral Zoonoses. CRC Press, Boca Raton, Fla. Pp. 365–385.

Marennikova, S.S., Shinkman, L.S., Shelukhina, E.M., and Maltseva, N.N. 1974. Isolation of camel pox virus and investigation of its properties. Acta Virol. 18:423–428.

Tantawi, H.H., El-Dahaby, H., and Fahmy, L.S. 1978. Comparative studies on poxvirus strains isolated from camels. Acta Virol. 22:451–457.

The Genus *Suipoxvirus*

Swinepox

Swinepox is a relatively mild skin infection of swine. It has been reported in Europe, Japan, and the United States and can be common in the swine-raising areas of these countries. It has been studied by McNutt et al. (1929), Schwarte and Biester (1941), and Shope (1940) in the United States and has been reviewed by Kasza (1981). In the United States it is not generally considered very important; however, some veterinarians believe that its importance is underestimated.

So far as is known, all cases of swinepox in the United States are caused by a virus that is unrelated to the poxviruses of other animals, including vaccinia, with which there has been confusion. Swine are susceptible to both vaccinia virus and swinepox virus.

Character of the Disease. Swinepox affects principally young animals, with suckling pigs especially susceptible. McNutt and associates (1929) reported that the lesions are usually found on the lower part of the abdomen and inside the thighs and front legs (Figure 45.6), but in the outbreak in Iowa described by Schwarte and Biester (1941) the lesions were located on the backs and sides. As a rule, they do not appear on the head or on the lower parts of the legs. The lesions consist of red papules that appear 4 to 5 days after virus is placed on the scarified skin. A slight fever and mild general reaction occur at this time. The papules rapidly develop into raised, hard elevations, which may be from 1 to 3 cm in diameter. Hard crusts form on these areas, then drop off in a few days, and the whole process is completed in 12 to 14 days. Vesicles and pustules do not ordinarily appear in field cases, but typical lesions that pass through the papule, vesicle, and pustule stages are observed on the abdomen of artificially inoculated pigs.

Properties of the Virus. The swinepox virus is the sole member of the *Suipoxvirus* genus of the Chordopoxvirinae subfamily (Mathews 1982, Moss 1985). The virions are ovoid or prismatic in shape, measure 300 to 350 nm × 200 to 250 nm × 100 nm (Kasza 1981, Reczko 1959), and are composed of cores, lateral bodies, surface proteins, and membranes or envelopes (Kasza 1981).

Cultivation. The swinepox virus produces a cytopathic effect in porcine kidney, testes, embryonic lung, and embryonic brain cultures (Kazka et al. 1960). Minute plaques are observed in an agar overlay system. Attempts to cultivate the swinepox virus in embryonated hens' eggs, horses, calves, sheep, dogs, cats, fowl, rabbits, rats, mice, and humans have failed. In contrast, vaccinia has a wide experimental host spectrum.

Epizootiology and Pathogenesis. Swinepox virus may be transmitted directly from one animal to another by contact. However, the virus often is transmitted mechanically by the hog louse, *Hematopinus suis*; this parasite can provide the necessary skin injury to allow the virus to enter the skin and establish infection. Because the hog louse is found on the lower parts of the animal, on the belly, in the axilla, and on the inside of the thighs, pox lesions usually are found in these locations. In a large herd studied by Schwarte and Biester (1941), in which the pigs were free of lice, the lesions were found mainly on the back and sides. This pattern suggested that flies or other insects might be the transmitting agents, an idea supported by the fact that the disease disappeared as soon as cold weather killed the insects.

Once a herd of swine is infected with the swinepox virus, the virus will usually persist in that herd indefinitely. Because of the limited mortality and lack of eco-

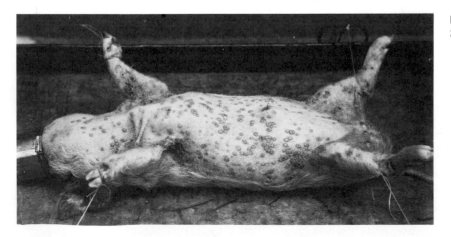

Figure 45.6. Swinepox. (Courtesy R. E. Shope.)

nomic importance, little attention is usually paid to this infection (Kasza 1981). The virus is resistant to inactivation when contained in the dried crusts that drop from the skin lesions, thus enabling it to persist on an infected farm.

Teppema and DeBoer (1975) and Kim et al. (1977) found the following ultrastructural changes in swinepox-infected cells: (1) intranuclear inclusions consisting of very fine filaments, (2) fibrillar structures with cross striations in the nuclear inclusions, and (3) similar striated fibrillar structures in or just adjacent to Cowdry's B type inclusions in the cytoplasm. These observations correlate well with descriptions of in vivo infection. Vacuoles in nuclei of stratum spinosum cells are observed with swinepox virus infection in pigs, but not in swinepox caused by vaccinia virus, the only other known cause of pox in swine.

Microscopically the earliest lesions appear on day 3 before the clinical lesions. The epidermis is thickened due to hydropic degeneration and epithelial hyperplasia. As the lesion progresses, cytoplasmic inclusions and nuclear vacuoles appear. There is an infiltration of inflammatory cells followed by formation of small vesicles, which coalesce (Kasza 1981). With the pustular stage of the lesions, there is a necrosis of the basilar layer with extensive infiltration of neutrophils. As the lesions begin to heal, crusts form and usually remain attached for up to 21 days. The regional lymph nodes may be edematous, hyperemic, and hyperplastic (Kasza 1981).

Immunity. Pigs that have recovered from the disease appear to be solidly immune for life. Vaccination is not generally practiced, the disease not being important enough for that.

Diagnosis. Swinepox usually can be diagnosed and differentiated from other skin diseases of swine because of its mild nature and characteristic lesions. The clinical diagnosis can be confirmed by histopathological examination of a skin lesion biopsy specimen, with observation of the typical intracytoplasmic inclusions and vacuolization of the epithelial nuclei (Kasza 1981), and/or by the virus neutralization test on paired serums. Swinepox virus in the skin lesions of naturally infected pigs can be rapidly identified by the electron microscopic method of negative staining (Garg and Meyer 1973).

The differences between vaccinia and swinepox virus were elucidated by DeBoer (1975) with challenge infections of convalescent pigs and with the agar-gel diffusion precipitin test and immunoelectrophoresis.

Treatment. There is no specific treatment for swinepox.

Prevention and Control. The best control measures are good sanitation practices and the elimination of lice and other external parasites. Because the virus can persist for extended periods in crusts that drop off lesions, disinfection of the environment, where possible, reduces the chance of new pigs becoming infected. New pigs should be purchased only from herds with no history of pox infection and should be examined for pox lesions before introduction into a herd.

The Disease in Humans. Swinepox virus does not infect humans. However, vaccinia virus can infect swine, and this virus can be transmitted to humans.

REFERENCES

DeBoer, G.F. 1975. Swinepox. Virus isolation, experimental infections and the differentiation from vaccinia virus infections. Arch. Virol. 49:141–150.

Garg, S.K., and Meyer, R.C. 1973. Studies on swinepox virus: Fluorescence and light microscopy of infected cell cultures. Res. Vet. Sci. 14:216–219.

Kasza, L. 1981. Swine pox. In A.D. Leman et al., eds., Diseases of Swine, 5th ed. Iowa State University Press, Ames. Pp. 254–260.

Kazka, L., Bohl, E.H., and Jones, D.O. 1960. Isolation and cultivation of swine pox virus in primary cell cultures of swine origin. Am. J. Vet. Res. 21:269–273.

Kim, U.H., Mukhajonpan, V., Nii, S., and Kato, S. 1977. Ultrastructural study of cell cultures infected with swinepox and orf viruses. Biken J. 20:57–67.

McNutt, S.H., Murray, C., and Purwin, P. 1929. Swine pox. J. Am. Vet. Med. Assoc. 74:752–761.

Mathews, R.E.F. 1982. Classification and nomenclature of viruses. Intervirology. 17:42–46.

Moss, B. 1985. Replication of poxviruses. In B.N. Fields, D.M. Knipe, R.M. Chanock, J.L. Melnick, B. Roizman, and R.E. Shope, eds., Virology. Raven Press, New York. Pp. 685–703.

Reczko, E. 1959. Elektronenmikroskopische Untersuchung der mitoriginären Schweinepocken infizierten Bauchhaut des Ferkels. Arch. Gesam. Virusforsch. 9:193–213.

Schwarte, L.H., and Biester, H.E. 1941. Pox in swine. Am. J. Vet. Res. 2.136–140.

Shope, R.E. 1940. Swine pox. J. Bact. 39:39.

Teppema, J.S., and DeBoer, G.F. 1975. Ultrastructural aspects of experimental swinepox with special reference to inclusion bodies. Arch. Virol. 49:151–163.

The Genus *Capripoxvirus*

Sheeppox

SYNONYM: *Clavelie*

Of all the animal poxes, sheeppox is the most damaging. In the past it has caused great losses in Europe, but it has now been controlled or eliminated from much of that area. It continues to exist in southern and eastern Europe, in the Middle East, in the Indian subcontinent, and in North Africa. It does not exist in the Western Hemisphere. Sheeppox has been reviewed by Davies (1981), Singh et al. (1979), and Tripathy et al. (1981).

Character of the Disease. The clinical disease caused by sheeppox virus has been discussed in several reports (Davies 1981, Lofstedt 1983, Robinson 1983, Singh et al.

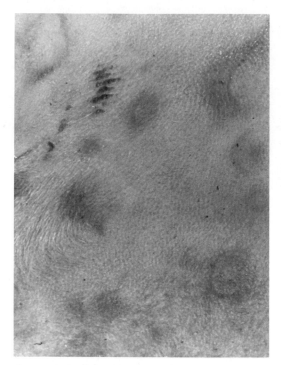 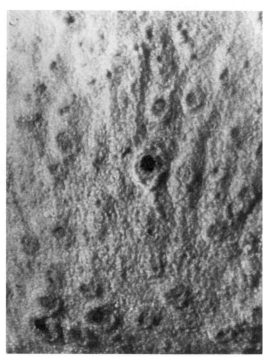

Figure 45.7 (*left*). Sheeppox. Rounded skin lesions in different stges of development. Early lesions are reddened plaques, and older lesions are raised and dark with irregular surfaces. (Courtesy D. A. Gregg, Plum Island Animal Disease Center, U.S. Dept. of Agriculture.)

Figure 45.8 (*right*). Sheeppox. Old skin lesions characterized by dried necrotic centers with raised edges. (Courtesy D. A. Gregg, Plum Island Animal Disease Center, U.S. Dept. of Agriculture.)

1979, Tripathy et al. 1981). Sheep of any age may be affected, but the disease is especially severe in young animals. Rhinitis, conjunctivitis, and fever are observed first in sheep that tend to stand with arched backs, are anorectic, and have poor coats. A generalized pox eruption occurs on the skin (Figures 45.7 and 45.8) within 1 or 2 days, and similar lesions often occur on the mucous membrane of the pharynx and trachea, sometimes even in the abomasum. Hemorrhagic inflammation of the respiratory passages (Figure 45.9) and of the digestive tract occurs. Caseous nodules and areas of catarrhal pneumonia occur in the lungs. Mortality varies from about 5 percent to higher than 50 percent.

Properties of the Virus. Sheeppox virus is classified in the genus *Capripoxvirus* along with goatpox virus and lumpy skin disease virus (Davies 1976, 1981).

The morphology of sheeppox virus is similar to that of the orthopoxviruses but distinct from that of the parapoxviruses (Abdussalam and Cosslett 1957, Davies 1981). The virus is more elongated than other poxviruses and measures 115 to 194 nm (Abdussalam and Cosslett 1957).

It is inactivated in 15 minutes by 2 percent phenol. Unlike most other poxviruses, the capripoxviruses are relatively sensitive to ether (Plowright and Ferris 1958).

Sheeppox virus is very resistant to inactivation in normal environmental conditions, especially when contained within scabs discharged from lesions.

All strains are serologically identical, and goatpox virus, which protects against sheeppox, is clearly related antigenically (Sharma and Dhands 1971, Subba Rao and Malik 1979).

Cultivation. A cytopathic effect is produced in the cultures of skin, kidney, and testis of sheep, goats, and calves with no change in virulence for sheep after serial passage (Plowright and Ferris 1958). An attenuated virus resulted after transfer in sheep embryo cultures (Aygun 1955). The inoculation of strain Perego induced only a local reaction and a temperature rise without generalization after it had undergone serial passage in lamb testes (Mateva and Stoichev 1975). The virus apparently can be adapted to embryonated hens' eggs with no apparent change in virulence for sheep (Sabban 1957).

Epizootiology and Pathogenesis. The epizootiology of sheeppox has been discussed by Belwal et al. (1982) and by Davies (1976). Plowright et al. (1959) discussed the pathogenesis of the infection in the skin of sheep, and Murray et al. (1973) reported on the histopathological and ultrastructural changes during experimental infection.

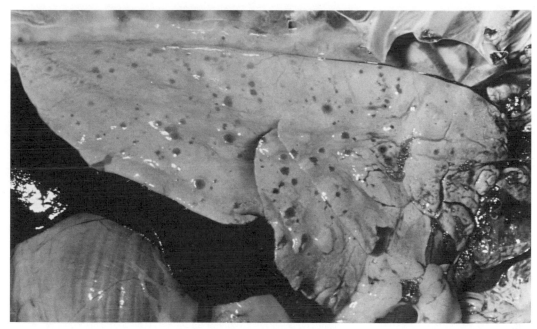

Figure 45.9. Sheeppox lesions in the lungs of an experimental sheep. Some lesions are firm, whitish nodules; others are reddened foci with dark red centers. (Courtesy D. A. Gregg, Plum Island Animal Disease Center, U.S. Dept. of Agriculture.)

Prevention and Control. Vaccination is essential in areas where the disease is enzootic. In Egypt a mild sheep strain from Iran is used to immunize sheep (Sabban 1955). In Turkey a tissue-cultured attenuated vaccine is used with success (Aygun 1955). A formaldehyde inactivated virus vaccine in Mongolia has proved effective (Solyom et al. 1982).

The Disease in Humans. There is no evidence that goatpox virus causes diesase in humans.

REFERENCES

Abdussalam, M., and Cosslett, V.E. 1957. Contagious pustular dermatitis virus. I. Studies on morphology. J. Comp. Pathol. Therap. 67:145–156.

Aygun, S.T. 1955. The propagation of variola ovina virus in sheep embryonic tissue cultures and its usefulness as a vaccine against this disease. Arch. Exp. Vet. Med. 9:415–441.

Belwal, L.M., Nivsarkar, A.E., Mathur, P.B., and Singh, R.N. 1982. Epidemiology of sheep pox. Trop. Anim. Health Prod. 14:229–233.

Davies, F.G. 1976. Characteristics of a virus causing a pox disease of sheep and goats in Kenya, with observations on the epidemiology and control. J. Hyg. 76:163–171.

Davies, F.G. 1981. Sheep and goat pox. In E.P.J. Gibbs, ed., Virus Diseases of Food Animals, vol. 2. Academic Press, London. Pp. 733–749.

Lofstedt, J. 1983. Dermatologic diseases of sheep. Vet. Clin. North Am. [Large Anim. Pract.] 5:427–448.

Mateva, V., and Stoichev, S. 1975. Adaptirane i kultivirane virusa nasharkata po ovtsete shtam Perego v tukanni kulturi i pretsenka naimmunogennite mu kachestva. Vet. Med. Nauki 12(10):18–23.

Murray, M., Martin, W.B., and Koylu, A. 1973. Experimental sheep

pox. A histological and ultrastructural study. Res. Vet. Sci. 15:201–208.

Plowright, W., and Ferris, R.D. 1958. The growth and cytopathogenicity of sheep-pox virus in tissue cultures. Br. J. Exp. Pathol. 39:424–435.

Plowright, W., MacLeod, W.G., and Ferris, R.D. 1959. The pathogenesis of sheep pox in the skin of sheep. J. Comp. Pathol. 69:400–413.

Robinson, R.A. 1983. Sheep and goat zoonoses. Vet. Clin. North Am. [Large Anim. Pract.] 5:711–717.

Sabban, M.S. 1955. Sheep pox and its control in Egypt using a desiccated live virus vaccine. Am. J. Vet. Res. 16:209–213.

Sabban, M.S. 1957. The cultivation of sheep pox virus on the chorioallantoic membrane of the developing chicken embryo. Am. J. Vet. Res. 18:618–624.

Sharma, N.S., and Dhands, M.R. 1971. Studies on the interrelationship between sheep and goat pox viruses. Indian J. Anim. Sci. 41:267–272.

Singh, I.P., Pandey, R., and Srivastava, R.N. 1979. Sheep pox—A review. Vet. Bul. 49:145–154.

Solyom, F., Perenlei, L., and Roith, J. 1982. Sheep-pox vaccine prepared from formaldehyde inactivated virus adsorbed to aluminum hydroxide gel. Acta Microbiol. Acad. Sci. Hung. 29:69–75.

Subba Rao, M.V., and Malik, B.S. 1979. Cross-neutralization tests on sheep pox, goat pox and contagious pustular dermatitis viruses. Acta Virol. 23:165–167.

Tripathy, D.N., Hanson, L.E., and Crandall, R.A. 1981. Poxviruses of veterinary importance: Diagnosis of infection. In E. Kurstak and C. Kurstak, eds., Comparative Diagnosis of Viral Diseases, vol. 3. Academic Press, New York. Pp. 267–346.

Goatpox

Like sheeppox, goatpox is a severe pox disease, especially of young animals. Goatpox virus causes gener-

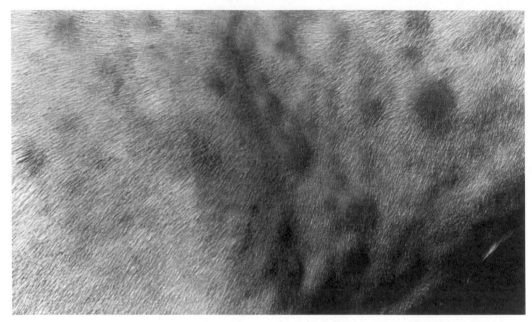

Figure 45.10. Goatpox lesions in different stages of development on the neck of a goat. (Courtesy D. A. Gregg, Plum Island Animal Disease Center, U.S. Dept. of Agriculture.)

alized skin pocks, fever, and upper respiratory infections. The course and type of disease produced in goats is similar to that produced in sheep with sheeppox virus (Tripathy et al. 1981).

The disease is prevalent in North Africa, the Middle East, and India and can occur in some European countries and Far Eastern countries (Davies 1981, Mohamed et al. 1982, Rafyi and Ramyar 1959, Tantawi et al. 1979, Tripathy et al. 1981). It also occurs in the Scandinavian countries and Australia, and there is a report of a similar virus in goats in the United States (Renshaw and Dodd 1978).

The virus causes generalized pocks on mucous membranes and skin after an incubation period of about 2 weeks. Goats have fever and lacrimal and nasal discharges; skin eruptions appear 1 to 2 days later. Lesions start out as papules, become umbilicated, then crust over to form scabs. They heal in 3 to 4 weeks, but scars are left at the lesion sites (Tripathy et al. 1981). Typical lesions are shown in Figures 45.10 and 45.11. Although strains of goatpox virus are generally host-specific, isolates from Kenya have also infected sheep (Tripathy et al. 1981).

The virus can be propagated in a number of cell cultures as well as embryonated eggs and produces a cytopathic effect and cytoplasmic inclusion bodies in many of these cultures (Tantawi and Al Fulliji 1979, Tantawi et al. 1979).

Both inactivated and attenuated vaccines have been used in endemic areas to protect goats (Kitching 1983). It is reported that goatpox immunizes against contagious ecthyma of sheep and sheeppox (Rafyi and Ramyar 1959); the reverse is not true. It also protects against lumpy skin disease of cattle (Capstick et al. 1959). Scubba Rao and Malik (1979) reported on the virus neutralization between sheeppox and goatpox viruses.

Human infection with goatpox virus can result when persons handle infected goats. Intensely pruritic lesions appear on the arms and hands, healing in 10 to 15 days (Tripathy et al. 1981).

REFERENCES

Capstick, P.B., Brydie, J., Coakley, W., and Burdin, M.L. 1959. Protection of cattle against the virus of lumpy skin disease. Vet. Rec. 71:422–423.

Davies, F.G. 1981. Sheep and goat pox. In E.P.J. Gibbs, ed., Virus Diseases of Food Animals, vol. 2. Academic Press, London. Pp. 733–749.

Kitching, P. 1983. Progress towards sheep and goat pox vaccines. Vaccine 1:4–9.

Mohamed, K.A., Hago, B.E., Taylor, W.P., Nayil, A.A., and Abu-Samra, M.T. 1982. Goat pox in the Sudan. Trop. Anim. Health Prod. 14:104–108.

Rafyi, A., and Ramyar, H. 1959. Goat pox in Iran. J. Comp. Pathol. Therap. 69:141–147.

Renshaw, H.W., and Dodd, A.G. 1978. Serological and cross immunity studies with contagious ecthyma and goat pox viruses isolated from the western United States. Arch. Virol. 56:201–210.

Scubba Rao, M.V., and Malik, B.S. 1979. Cross-neutralization tests on sheep pox, goat pox and contagious pustular dermatitis viruses. Acta Virol. 23:165–167.

Tantawi, H.H., and Al Fulluji, M.M. 1979. Laboratory characteristics of four strains of goatpox virus. Acta Virol. 23:455–460.

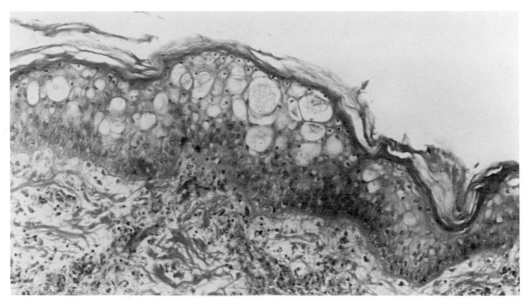

Figure 45.11. Micrograph of a section from an early skin lesion of goatpox. In the epidermis cells have undergone hydropic degeneration, and there are microvesicles. In the dermis there is histiocytic hyperplasia and necrosis. Hemotoxylin and eosin stain. × 57. (Courtesy C. A. Mebus, Plum Island Animal Disease Center, U.S. Dept. of Agriculture.)

Tantawi, H.H., Shony, M.O., and Hassan, F.K. 1979. Isolation and identification of the Sersenk strain of goat pox virus in Iraq. Trop. Anim. Health Prod. 11:208–210.

Tripathy, D.N., Hanson, L.E., and Crandell, R.A. 1981. Poxviruses of veterinary importance: Diagnosis of infections. In E. Kurstak and C. Kurstak, eds., Comparative Diagnosis of Viral Diseases, vol 3. Academic Press, New York. Pp. 267–346.

Lumpy Skin Disease

SYNONYMS: Exanthema nodularis bovis, *knopvelsiekte*, lumpy disease, pseudourticaria; abbreviation, LSD

Lumpy skin disease is an acute, subacute, chronic, or inapparent infection of cattle characterized by fever, development of nodular cutaneous lesions undergoing necrosis, generalized lymphadenitis, and edema of the ventral parts of the body and limbs (Tripathy et al. 1981). First observed in Zambia (then known as Northern Rhodesia) and Madagascar in 1929, it was recognized as infectious in 1943 to 1945, when it rapidly spread through southern and eastern Africa, affecting some 8 million cattle in one of the largest epizootics ever recorded (Davies 1981, Thomas and Mare 1945). The disease may occur in buffalo as well as cattle, and giraffes and impalas develop generalized, fatal disease after experimental inoculation with virus (Young et al. 1968).

Lumpy skin disease has been reviewed by Davies (1981), Tripathy et al. (1981), and Weiss (1968).

Character of the Disease. The clinical signs of LSD have been described by several investigators (Ayre-Smith 1960, Davies 1981, Haig 1957, Thomas and Mare 1945, von Backstromm 1945). In cattle fever develops, accompanied by multiple nodules in the skin, pathological changes in the mucous membranes and viscera, and adenitis. Skin lesions have a predilection for the head, neck, limbs, perineum, the genitalia, and udder. Morbidity and mortality may each vary from 1 percent to more than 50 percent in individual outbreaks.

Cytoplasmic inclusions are found in epithelial cells and histiocytes (Figure 45.12).

Properties of the Virus. Lumpy skin disease virus belongs to the *Capripoxvirus* genus within the family Poxviridae. Figure 45.13 shows its structure and size. The Neethling pox strain of LSD virus is closely related to the other capripoxviruses, African sheeppox virus and goatpox virus (Tripathy et al. 1981). Other isolates of LSD virus from various countries in Africa have been shown to be serologically identical to the Neethling strain of virus (Davies 1982).

Studies of isolates from LSD lesions resulted in identification of three viruses: an orphan herpes virus; the Allerton herpes virus, which is related to (but not identical to) bovine herpes mammillitis virus; and the Neethling group of poxviruses that were eventually shown to be the cause of LSD (Davies 1981).

Cultivation. LSD virus multiplies in the chick embryo and chorioallantoic membrane, producing pocks on the membrane. After adaptation the virus produces spindle

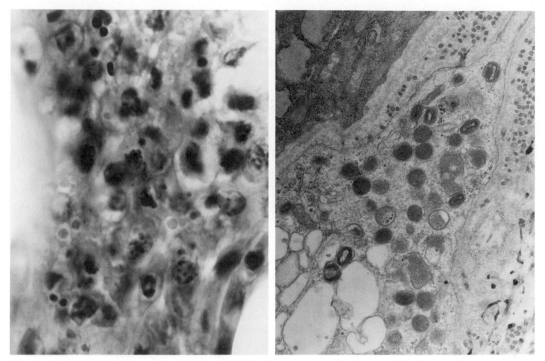

Figure 45.12 (*left*). Micrograph of nasal epithelium from a steer with lumpy skin disease. There are several eosinophilic cytoplasmic inclusion bodies in the epidermis. Hematoxylin and eosin stain. × 300. (Courtesy C. A. Mebus, Plum Island Animal Disease Center, U.S. Dept. of Agriculture.)

Figure 45.13 (*right*). Lumpy skin disease skin lesions and virus particles. × 16,000. (Courtesy S. S. Breese, Plum Island Animal Disease Center, U.S. Dept. of Agriculture.)

cells within 24 to 48 hours in cell cultures of embryonic calf and lamb kidney and of calf and lamb testis.

Epizootiology and Pathogenesis. The virus is believed to be transmitted by various biting insects (Davies 1981). The disease is more prevalent in rainy seasons and in low wetlands.

A survey of wildlife in Africa for serum-neutralizing antibodies indicated that only a few species and only an occasional animal had low levels of neutralizing antibodies against LSD virus, indicating that wildlife do not play an important role in the spread of LSD (Hedger and Hamblin 1983). Another study, however, indicates that the African buffalo (*Syncerus caffer*) may be involved in the maintenance cycle of LSD virus in enzootic areas (Davies 1982).

A study of the pathological changes in LSD lesions was conducted by Prozesky and Barnard (1982). The lesions are granulomatous reactions within the dermis and hypodermis. Vasculitis and lymphangitis with thrombosis and infarction results in necrosis and edema of the skin.

Prevention and Control. Restricting the movement of cattle from diseased to free areas has not always proved effective (Davies 1981, Haig 1957). The Isiolo or Kedong strains of sheeppox have been used to protect cattle against Neethling virus (Capstick and Coakley 1961), and an attenuated strain of the Neethling virus has been used effectively as a vaccine (Davies 1981).

Because this disease can have serious economic consequences, cattle from southern Africa should not be exported to other parts of the world until physical examinations and a study of their histories ensure that they are not infected.

The Disease in Humans. There is no evidence that the virus causes disease in humans.

REFERENCES

Ayre-Smith, R.A. 1960. The symptoms and clinical diagnosis of lumpy-skin diseases. Vet. Rec. 72:469–472.

Capstick, P.B., and Coakley, W. 1961. Protection of cattle against lumpyskin disease. I. Trials with a vaccine against Neethling type infection. Res. Vet. Sci. 2:362–368.

Davies, F.G. 1981. Lumpyskin disease. In E.P.J. Gibbs, ed., Virus Diseases of Food Animals, vol. 2. Academic Press, London. Pp. 751–764.

Davies, F.G. 1982. Observations on the epidemiology of lumpy skin disease in Kenya. J. Hyg. 88:95–102.

Haig, D. 1957. Lumpyskin disease. Bull. Epiz. Dis. Afr. 5:421–430.

Hedger, R.S., and Hamblin, C. 1983. Neutralising antibodies to lumpy skin disease virus in African wildlife. Comp. Immunol. Microbiol. Infect. Dis. 6:209–213.

Prozesky, L., and Barnard, B.J. 1982. A study of the pathology of lumpy skin disease in cattle. Onderstepoort J. Vet. Res. 49:167–175.

Thomas, A.D., and Mare, C.V.E. 1945. Knopvelsiekte. J. S. Afr. Vet. Med. Assoc. 16:36–43.

Tripathy, D.N., Hanson, L.E., and Crandell, R.A. 1981. Poxviruses of veterinary importance: Diagnosis of infections. In E. Kurstak and C. Kurstak, eds., Comparative Diagnosis of Viral Diseases, vol. 3. Academic Press, New York. Pp. 267–346.

von Backstromm, U. 1945. Ngamiland cattle disease: Preliminary report on a new disease, the aetiological agent being probably of an infectious nature. J. S. Afr. Vet. Med. Assoc. 16:29–35.

Weiss, K.E. 1968. Lumpyskin disease. Virol. Monogr. 3:111–131.

Young, E., Basson, P.A., and Weiss, K.E. 1968. Experimental infection of the giraffe, impala and the Cape buffalo with lumpyskin disease virus. Onderstepoort J. Vet. Res. 37:79–88.

The Genus *Leporipoxvirus*

Infectious Myxomatosis of Rabbits

A highly contagious and almost always fatal disease of domesticated rabbits, infectious myoxmatosis was first recognized in South America and later in Mexico, England, Western Europe, and the United States (California). It often destroys whole rabbitries. In 1976 an epizootic in western Oregon involved 26 rabbitries with mortality ranging from 20 to 50 percent (Patton and Holmes 1977).

It was first described by Sanarelli (1898), working in Montevideo, Uruguay, who ascribed the disease to a virus, since he could not see or cultivate any organisms in the lesions. It is interesting to note that Sanarelli's paper appeared in the same year as that of Loeffler and Frosch, who determined the causative agent of foot-and-mouth disease of cattle to be a virus (see Chapter 47). The myxoma virus takes its place, historically, as the second animal disease virus to be recognized.

Myxomatosis affects ordinary domestic rabbits, Angora rabbits, Belgian hares, and Flemish giants; but the wild rabbit of Brazil, the common cottontail, and the jackrabbit of the United States arc almost wholly resistant. The virus does not affect any animal species other than certain rabbits, and humans are also resistant.

Character of the Disease. The disease begins with inflammation of the eyes. The eyelids swell, and a copious discharge from the conjunctival mucous membranes appears. At first the discharge is serous, but shortly it becomes purulent. Within 24 to 48 hours the eyes cannot be opened because of the swelling. A nasal discharge also appears, and swellings involving the skin of the face and ears are noted. Similar swellings may then appear on other parts of the body. The genital openings become inflamed and discharge a purulent cxudate. Finally the tumorous masses may involve nearly the whole body (Figure 45.14); the affected animal almost invariably dies 7 to 15 days after the first signs are noted.

The tumorlike masses consist of tissue with a rubbery,

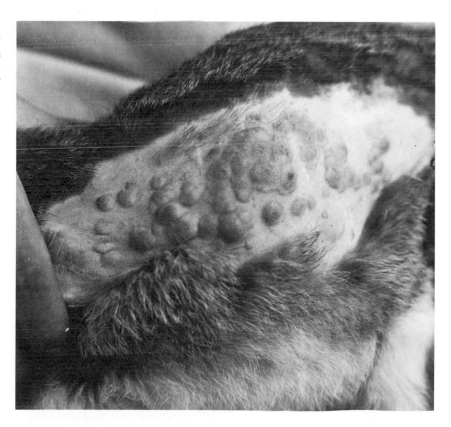

Figure 45.14. Myxomatosis in a rabbit. Multiple primary tumors were induced by virus on the freshly shaved skin. (From Rivers, 1926–1927, courtesy of *Proceedings of the Society for Experimental Biology and Medicine.*)

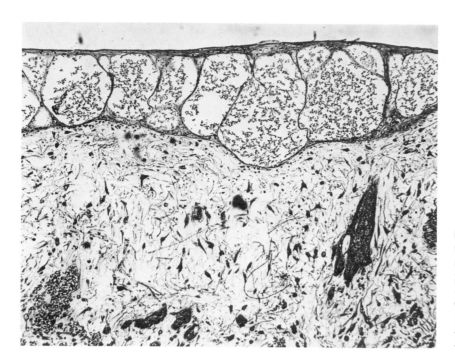

Figure 45.15. Myxomatosis. The virus attacks epidermal cells as well as those of the subcutaneous tissue. In the lower part of the photograph the myxomatous tissue is seen. In the upper part is a series of vesicles—the end result of infection of epithelial cells. × 100. (From Rivers, 1926–1927, courtesy of *Proceedings of the Society for Experimental Biology and Medicine.*)

gelatinous consistency. Usually the lungs, liver, and kidneys appear normal, but the spleen is always swollen and the lymph nodes are enlarged and hemorrhagic. Although the external genitalia are inflamed, the testicles, uterus, and ovaries are generally free of lesions. The testicular swelling mentioned by many authors is usually caused by changes in the scrotum rather than in the testicle.

Sections of the myxomata show tissue characteristic of that type of tumor, that is, large stellate cells embedded in a homogeneous, gelatinous substance that is largely if not wholly mucin (Figure 45.15). In addition, however, there is inflammation manifested by engorgement and hemorrhages and by collections of neutrophilic leukocytes. Rivers (1926–1927) was the first to call attention to another characteristic feature of these virus tumors, that is, a peculiar type of degeneration of the epithelial coverings. The epithelial cells are greatly swollen and vacuolated, and acidophilic bodies rapidly develop in their cytoplasm (Figure 45.16). These bodies contain blue-staining coccoid elements. The whole structure resembles the Bollinger bodies of fowlpox.

Rivers and Ward (1937) obtained suspensions of these elementary bodies, which they regarded as the virus, in a relatively pure form. Not only are such suspensions highly pathogenic, but the bodies are specifically agglutinated by the serum of recovered or immunized animals.

Properties of the Virus. Myxoma virus is indistinguishable from vaccinia virus by electron microscopy (Farrant and Fenner 1953). It is classified in the genus *Leporipoxvirus*. The cytoplasmic inclusion bodies, which presumably contain virus are Feulgen-positive. It is a reasonably stable virus in glycerol and when frozen or dried. The virus is heat inactivated by heat in 25 minutes at 55°C. The agent survives many months in the skins of affected rabbits that are maintained at ordinary temperatures (Jacotot et al. 1955). Unlike most other poxviruses, myxoma virus is ether-sensitive, but like them it is resistant to sodium deoxycholate (Andrewes and Horstmann 1949).

The viral antigen produces complement-fixing, precipitating, and neutralizing antibodies. The virus is closely related to the rabbit fibroma virus (Shope 1932).

Cultivation. Hoffstadt and Pilcher (1938) reported cultivation of myxoma virus on the chorioallantoic membrane of the developing chick embryo. The virus produces a cytopathic effect and grows in cell cultures from cottontail rabbits, squirrels, young rats, hamsters, guinea pigs, and certain human tissues (Andrewes 1964). Plaques develop on cell monolayers.

Epizootiology and Pathogenesis. Myxomatosis spreads readily by contact or close cohabitation of domesticated rabbits. The incubation period is about 5 days. The rabbit flea (*Spilopsyllus cuniculi*) also is a transmitting agent, but unless rabbit populations are very dense, flea transmission fails to produce epizootics.

Because this disease is not pathogenic for humans or any other animal species, investigators trying to reduce the unwanted rabbit population in Australia suggested it as a means of control. The wild Australian rabbit is a

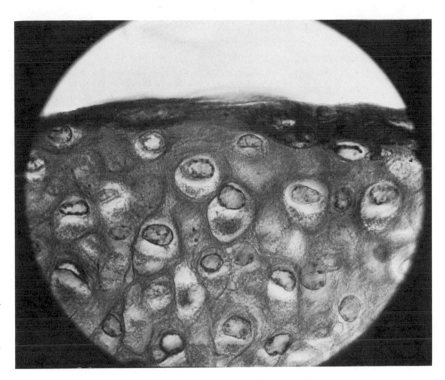

Figure 45.16. Myxomatosis. Epidermis of a tumor shows cytoplasmic inclusion bodies. × 850. (From Rivers, 1926–1927, courtesy of *Proceedings of the Society for Experimental Biology and Medicine.*)

descendant of European rabbits imported many years ago. Because there are no natural enemies of rabbits in Australia, they have thrived remarkably well; it is estimated that their numbers were 1 to 3 billion in 1950. They ate huge amounts of vegetation that could more profitably be used for feeding sheep and other animals. In 1950 myxoma-infected rabbits were released in seven locations in Australia in the hope that the disease would spread from these centers in the form of a great epizootic. In six centers the attempt was a failure. In the seventh, the Murray River Valley, many rabbits perished from the disease, and it was here that the importance of mosquito vectors was first appreciated. Hundreds of thousands of acres of land in this valley were cleared of rabbits. The following season, which was hot and dry, mosquitoes were not numerous and the disease did not flourish. However, in other areas with more moisture and many mosquitoes, the disease spread rapidly. In later years the kill has been lower, and there is evidence of some host-parasite adjustment.

In 1952 a French physician who had retired to his country estate released some infected rabbits in an attempt to destroy the rabbits that plagued his gardens. Not only did he destroy his own rabbits, but within 18 months the disease had spread through most of France, Belgium, Germany, and Holland; it had even crossed the English Channel into Great Britain. All attempts to stop the disease failed. Only fibroma virus vaccine saved some of the domesticated species. With time, resistant strains of rabbits have developed (Ross and Sanders 1984).

For papers dealing with the epizootiology of myxomatosis in wild rabbits, see Bull et al. (1954), Mead-Briggs and Vaughan (1975), Myers et al. (1954), Ritchie et al. (1954), Shepherd and Edmonds (1977), and Thompson (1954).

Immunity. Among experimental rabbits the mortality from myxoma infection is so nearly 100 percent that only a few survivors have been available for studies on immunity. These have shown, however, a high grade of resistance to reinfection.

In Australia the initial mortality from the induced outbreaks was estimated to be 99.5 percent. It was found, however, in some regions that mortality was not so high in successive seasons; hence a considerable number of survivors were available for study. According to Fenner et al. (1953), these showed serum antibodies that persisted at least 18 months. Inoculation of such rabbits with virulent myxoma virus produced a small lesion in some cases and no lesions at all in others. Fenner and Marshall (1954) showed that the young of immune mothers were passively protected, at least in part. In contrast, Sobey and Conolly (1975) reported that offspring with maternal antibody to myxoma virus that were exposed to fleas contaminated with myxoma virus and/or had contact with infected rabbits from birth died or became infected before 8 weeks of age. When compared with adult control animals the offspring with maternal antibodies showed no advantage in survival time or recovery rate.

Shope (1938) discovered that the virus of the Shope

fibroma, a benign tumor, immunized rabbits to the virus of myxomatosis. When first reported, this interesting observation was thought to have little practical value. Since 1953, however, it has been useful as a means of protecting breeding stocks in Europe. Ritchie et al. (1954) reported that in England the method gives about 90 percent serviceable immunity, and that few problems have resulted from its use. On very young rabbits, large tumors may be produced, but on older stock, immunity often is obtained without the production of tumors.

The Disease in Humans. There is no evidence that myxoma virus causes disease in humans.

REFERENCES

Andrewes, C. 1964. Viruses of Vertebrates. Williams & Wilkins, Baltimore.

Andrewes, C.H., and Horstmann, D.M. 1949. The susceptibility of viruses to ethyl ether. J. Gen. Microbiol. 3:290–297.

Bull, L.B., Ratcliffe, F.N., and Edgar, G. 1954. Myxomatosis: Its use in the control of rabbit populations in Australia. Vet. Rec. 66:61–62.

Farrant, J.L., and Fenner, F. 1953. A comparison of the morphology of vaccinia and myxoma viruses. Aust. J. Exp. Biol. Med. Sci. 31:121–125.

Fenner, F., and Marshall, I.D. 1954. Passive immunity in myxomatosis of the European rabbit (Oryctolagus cuniculus): The protection conferred on kittens born by immune does. J. Hyg. 52:321–336.

Fenner, F., Marshall, I.D., and Woodroofe, G.M. 1953. Studies in the epidemiology of infectious myxomatosis of rabbits. I. Recovery of Australian wild rabbits (Oryctolagus cuniculus) from myxomatosis under field conditions. J. Hyg. 51:225–244.

Hoffstadt, R.E., and Pilcher, K.S. 1938. A further study of the cultivation of virus Myxomatosum on the chorio-allantoic membrane of the chick embryo. J. Bact. 36:286.

Jacotot, H., Vallee, A., and Virat, B. 1955. Sur la conservation et la destruction dans les peaux du virus de la myxomatose des lapins. Ann. Inst. Pasteur 89:290–298.

Mead-Briggs, A.R., and Vaughan, J.A. 1975. The differential transmissibility of myxoma virus strains of differing virulence grades by the rabbit flea Spilopsyllus cuniculi (Dale). J. Hyg. 75:237–247.

Myers, K., Marshall, I.D., and Fenner, F. 1954. Studies in the epidemiology of infectious myxomatosis of rabbits. III. Observations on two succeeding epizootics in Australian wild rabbits on the riverine plain of south-eastern Australia, 1951–1953. J. Hyg. 52:337–360.

Patton, N.M., and Holmes, H.T. 1977. Myxomatosis in domestic rabbits in Oregon. J. Am. Vet. Med. Assoc. 171:560–562.

Ritchie, J.N., Hudson, J.R., and Thompson, H.V. 1954. Myxomatosis. Vet. Rec. 66:796–804.

Rivers, T.M. 1926–1927. Changes observed in epidermal cells covering myxomatous masses induced by virus Myxomatosum (Sanarelli). Proc. Soc. Exp. Biol. Med. 24:435–437.

Rivers, T.M., and Ward, S.M. 1937. Infectious myxomatosis of rabbits. Preparation of elementary bodies and studies of serologically active materials associated with the disease. J. Exp. Med. 66:1–14.

Ross, J., and Sanders, M.F. 1984. The development of genetic resistance to myxomatosis in wild rabbits in Britain. J. Hyg. 92:255–261.

Sanarelli, G. 1898. Das Myxomatogene Virus. Beitrag zur Studium der Krankheitserreger aus Berhalb des Sichtbaren. Zentralbl. Bakteriol. I. Abt. 23:865–874.

Shepherd, R.C., and Edmonds, J.W. 1977. Myxomatosis: The transmission of a highly virulent strain of myxoma virus by the European rabbit flea Spilopsyllus cuniculi (Dale) in the Mallee region of Victoria. J. Hyg. 79:405–409.

Shope, R.E. 1932. A filtrable virus causing a tumor-like condition in rabbits and its relationship to virus Myxomatosum. J. Exp. Med. 56:803–822.

Shope, R.E. 1938. Protection of rabbits against naturally acquired infectious myxomatosis by previous infection with fibroma virus. Proc. Soc. Exp. Biol. Med. 38:86–89.

Sobey, W.R., and Conolly, D. 1975. Myxomatosis: Passive immunity in the offspring of immune rabbits (Oryctolagus cuniculus) infested with fleas (Spilopsyllus cuniculi Dale) and exposed to myxoma virus. J. Hyg. 74:43–55.

Thompson, H.V. 1954. Myxomatosis of rabbits. Agriculture 60:503–508.

Shope Fibroma of Rabbits

SYNONYMS: Fibromatosis, rabbit fibroma

Shope (1932a, 1932b) described a type of fibrous tumor of the cottontail rabbit which proved to be transmissible to other cottontail rabbits and to the domestic species by the injection of cellular suspension and of Berkefeld filtrates. Although of interest on its own account, Shope fibroma virus has attracted much attention because of its relationship to the virus of myxomatosis.

Character of the Disease. In naturally infected rabbits the tumors occur subcutaneously. There may be one or several in the same animal. They are firm, spherical masses that can be moved about under the skin because they are only loosely attached (Figure 45.17). Sections show that the masses are made up of spindle-shaped, connective tissue cells, without evidence of inflammation or necrotic reaction (Figure 45.18).

Properties of the Virus. Shope fibroma virus is classified in the *Leporipoxvirus* genus of the family Poxviridae. This virus resembles vaccinia and myxoma viruses as determined by electron microscope studies, and it is similar to squirrel and hare fibroma viruses (Tripathy et al. 1981). In thin sections its size is estimated at 200 to

Figure 45.17. The Shope fibroma. This tumor on the shaved skin of the abdomen of a rabbit was produced by experimental inoculation 11 days previously. (Courtesy R. E. Shope.)

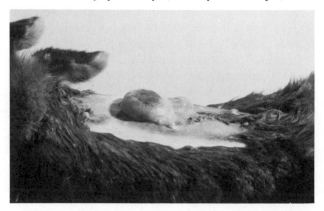

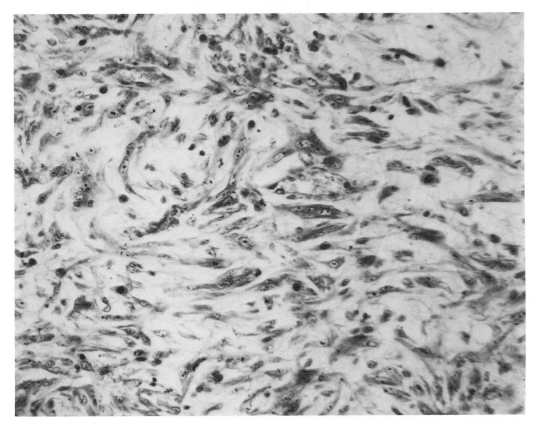

Figure 45.18. Shope fibroma. Section of a testicular tumor produced by experimental inoculation of a rabbit. × 330. (Courtesy R. E. Shope.)

240 nm. It is ether-sensitive and quite stable in glycerol and at low temperatures.

Rabbit fibroma virus is closely related immunologically to myxoma virus. Presumably there are minor antigenic differences as determined by the complement-fixation and agar-gel diffusion tests. Interference is reported by virus III, Semliki forest virus, and Murray Valley encephalitis virus.

Phosphonoacetic acid (PAA) has an inhibitory effect on this virus. A complete suppression of induced tumors was observed when 10 mg of PAA was inoculated into the lesion site for 5 days if treatment was begun 24 hours after virus inoculation (Friedman-Kien et al. 1976).

One strain of rabbit fibroma virus, after 18 passages in domestic rabbits, suddenly mutated and thereafter failed to produce tumors but instead caused inflammation at the injection sites. This change was detected by Andrewes (1936) in England, to whom Shope had sent the material. Shope (1936c) was able to confirm Andrewes' findings. Passage through a series of cottontail rabbits restored part of the virus' tumor-producing power. Other strains, however, have not changed. The altered strain continued to immunize against the tumor-producing strains.

Cultivation. The OA strain multiplies in the chorio-allantoic membrane of embryonated hens' eggs without producing lesions. The agent produces a cytopathic effect and propagates in cell cultures of tissues from the domestic rabbit, cottontail rabbit, guinea pig, rat, and humans (Chaproniere and Andrewes 1957). Foci appear on rabbit kidney monolayers (Padgett et al. 1962).

Epizootiology and Pathogenesis. The mode of natural transmission is not known. Virus is not spread from animal to animal by simple contact. Hyde and Gardner (1939) found that it was not transmitted from mother to young either through the placenta or through the milk. Experimentally the disease has been produced only by inoculation. In view of what is now known about the transmission of myxoma, it seems fairly safe to assume that natural transmission occurs by means of biting insects (Dalmat 1959).

Filtrates of tumor tissue, when injected into the testicles, regularly cause of similar tumors. Subcutaneous and intramuscular inoculations frequently, but not always, succeed. Intraperitoneal and intracerebral inoculations fail.

Inoculation transmits the tumors equally well in domestic and cottontail rabbits, but the behavior of the tumors in these species differs. In the cottontail rabbit, growth is slow and continues over many months. In the domestic rabbit, growth is rapid, but after about 10 days of active proliferation further growth does not occur and retrogression begins.

The virus in rabbit fibromatosis is found only in the tumors. It has not been demonstrated in the blood, viscera, or any of the secretions or excretions. In susceptible animals it stimulates a proliferation of the connective tissue at the point where it is deposited. The virus content of the cottontail tumors remains high for a long period (77 days at least), whereas in domestic rabbit tumors it is highest about 7 to 9 days after inoculation and disappears as retrogression occurs (Shope 1932b). Guinea pigs, rats, mice, and chickens proved refractory to inoculation. So far as is known, no animal other than rabbits can be infected with this virus.

Immunity. Shope (1932b) showed that domestic rabbits in which tumors had formed and retrogressed could not be reinfected with the same virus. To his surprise he found that such rabbits also had a high degree of resistance to the virus of myxomatosis. Whereas myxoma virus is almost always fatal to normal rabbits, it destroyed only 1 of a group of 15 fibroma-recovered animals. These animals then proved to be highly immune to myxoma virus as well as to fibroma virus. One rabbit that recovered from myxoma without having previously been affected with fibroma proved to be resistant to fibroma as well as myxoma (Shope 1938).

Thinking that fibroma might be the natural reaction of cottontail rabbits to the virus of myxomatosis, Shope (1936a) attempted to pass the myxoma virus serially through these animals. Only minimal reactions were induced, and these had the character of neither fibroma nor myxoma.

The unexpected finding of the immunological relationship between fibromatosis and myxomatosis suggested that the benign fibroma was caused by an attenuated strain of the malignant myxoma; however, Shope (1936b) expressed the opinion that such was not the case—that the viruses were qualitatively different.

The Disease in Humans. Shope fibroma does not occur in humans.

REFERENCES

Andrewes, C.H. 1936. A change in rabbit fibroma virus suggesting mutation. J. Exp. Med. 63:157–172.

Chaproniere, D.M., and Andrewes, C.H. 1957. Cultivation of rabbit myxoma and fibroma viruses in tissues of nonsusceptible hosts. Virology 4:351–365.

Dalmat, H.T. 1959. Arthropod transmission of rabbit fibromatosis (Shope). J. Hyg. 57:1–30.

Friedman-Kien, A.E., Fondak, A.A., and Klein, R.J. 1976. Phosphonoacetic acid treatment of Shope fibroma and vaccinia virus skin infections in rabbits. J. Invest. Dermatol. 66:99–102.

Hyde, R.R., and Gardner, R.E. 1939. Transmission experiments with fibroma (Shope) and myxoma (Sanarelli) viruses. Am. J. Hyg. 30:57–63.

Padgett, B.L., Moore, M.S., and Walker, D.L. 1962. Plaque assays for myxoma and fibroma viruses and differentiation of the viruses by plaque form. Virology 17:462–469.

Shope, R.E. 1932a. A transmissible tumor-like condition in rabbits. J. Exp. Med. 56:793–802.

Shope, R.E. 1932b. A filtrable virus causing a tumor-like condition in rabbits and its relationship to virus *Myxomatosum*. J. Exp. Med. 56:803–822.

Shope, R.E. 1936a. Infectious fibroma of rabbits. III. The serial transmission of virus *Myxomatosum* in cottontail rabbits, and cross-immunity tests with the fibroma virus. J. Exp. Med. 63:33–41.

Shope, R.E. 1936b. Infectious fibroma of rabbits. IV. The infection with virus *Myxomatosum* of rabbits recovered from fibroma. J. Exp. Med. 63:43–57.

Shope, R.E. 1936c. A change in rabbit fibroma virus suggesting mutation. II. Behavior of the variant virus in cottontail rabbits. J. Exp. Med. 63:173–178.

Shope, R.E. 1938. Protection of rabbits against naturally acquired infectious myxomatosis by previous infection with fibroma virus. Proc. Soc. Exp. Biol. Med. 38:86–89.

Tripathy, D.N., Hanson, L.E., and Crandell, R.A. 1981. Poxviruses of veterinary importance: Diagnosis of infections. In E. Kurstak and C. Kurstak, eds., Comparative Diagnosis of Viral Diseases, vol. 3. Academic Press., New York. Pp. 267–346.

The Genus *Parapoxvirus*

Pseudocowpox

SYNONYMS: Milker's nodules, paravaccinia; abbreviations, MN, PCP

Pseudocowpox is the most common poxlike lesion on the teats and udders of cattle. The causative parapovirus also produces milker's nodules (MN) on the hands and arms of people that have contact with infected cattle. Reviews have been written by Cheville and Shey (1967), Gibbs (1984), Gibbs et al. (1970), Hunt (1984), and Kahrs (1981).

Character of the Disease. Pseudocowpox clinically resembles cowpox and vaccinia, with lesions confined to the teats and udders of milking cows. Early lesions are accompanied by local pain, edema, and erythema (Cheville and Shey 1967, Gibbs et al. 1970). The lesions progress from papules to vesicles to raw areas that heal under a dry scab. The lesions expand centrifugally, and the center may become umbilicated or depressed.

The disease is very annoying because of the soreness of the teats, which makes the cows difficult to milk. The disease spreads to most of the cows that are milked, apparently on the hands of the milkers or through contamination of the milking machines. Dry cows, nonmilking heifers, and bulls rarely become involved. Mastitis sometimes results, apparently from secondary bacterial infections.

Healing usually occurs after several weeks and the disease disappears, although one herd outbreak lasted for 18 months, forcing the farmer to sell his cattle (Kahrs 1981). Antiseptic ointments facilitate healing and make milking less painful.

Properties of the Virus. Pseudocowpox was shown to be caused by a poxvirus that is classified in the *Parapoxvirus* genus of the family Poxviridae (Friedman-Kien et al. 1963, Rossi et al. 1977, Tripathy et al. 1981). The dimensions of the virus are approximately 220 to 300 nm by 140 to 170 nm. It has a spiral structure, as does the pathogen for contagious pustular dermatitis of sheep and bovine papular stomatitis.

No cross-immunity has been demonstrated between this virus and cowpox or vaccinia, but the virus is related antigenically to orf and bovine papular stomatitis viruses (Papadopoulos et al. 1968, Tripathy et al. 1981). Analysis of the genomes of several parapoxviruses, including pseudocowpox virus, indicates considerable genetic heterogeneity both between virus groups within the parapoxvirus genus and between strains of the same virus (Gassmann et al. 1985).

The genome of the MN virus codes for at least 40 polypeptides, 10 of which appear to be surface polypeptides (Thomas et al. 1980). The major polypeptide composing the threadlike tubules on the surface of the parapoxviruses appears to be approximately 42 to 45 kilodaltons.

Cultivation. The virus produces a cytopathic effect in bovine kidney cell cultures (Friedman-Kien et al. 1963). After cultivation in bovine kidney cell culture, it grew in human embryonic fibroblasts but not in rabbit and rhesus monkey kidney cultures. The infection has not been successfully transmitted to rabbits, mice, guinea pigs, or chick embryos.

Epizootiology and Pathogenesis. Transmission is by the hands of milkers, by nursing calves, or by milking machines. Infection usually occurs in cold weather, which facilitates breaks in the epithelial tissue of the teat or udder. The incubation period is about 1 week. Lactating dairy cows are the natural hosts.

Gibbs and Osborne (1974) studied the natural occurrence of pseudocowpox in dairy herds. Lesions occurred in cattle throughout the year, and most cases first appeared 1 to 2 weeks after calving. Lesions frequently recurred every 6 months in individual cows. Thirteen percent of cows going to slaughter were infected.

The replication of MN virus was studied in vitro by Thomas et al. (1980). Replication occurs within the cytoplasm of the infected cell and requires 30 to 36 hours to complete the replicative cycle. Host nuclear DNA synthesis is inhibited in the process.

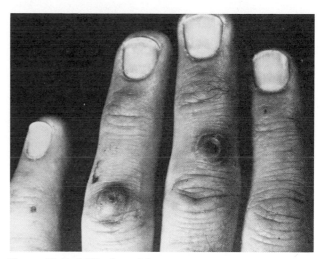

Figure 45.19. Milker's nodules.

Immunity. It has been suggested that the immunity may be transient in cattle, yet precipitating antibodies can be detected for at least 4 months after infection (Papadopoulos et al. 1968).

The Disease in Humans. In humans milker's nodules are hemispherical cherry red papules (Figure 45.19) that appear on the hands and sometimes on other parts of the body (Becker 1940). The papules appear 5 to 7 days after exposure. They gradually enlarge into firm, bluish red, smooth, hemispherical masses varying in size up to 2 cm in diameter. They are relatively painless but frequently itch. When fully developed they often show a dimple on the tip, but they do not break down with pus formation. They are highly vascular. The tense, grayish skin covering them remains intact. The granulation tissue that makes up the mass of the nodule is gradually absorbed. As this occurs, the lesions slowly flatten and finally, after 4 to 6 weeks, they disappear. Sometimes there is slight swelling of the axillary nodes, but otherwise there is no evidence of any generalization of the disease.

REFERENCES

Becker, F.T. 1940. Milker's nodules. J.A.M.A. 115:2140–2144.
Cheville, N.F., and Shey, D.J. 1967. Pseudocowpox in dairy cattle. J. Am. Vet. Med. Assoc. 150:855–861.
Friedman-Kien, A.E., Rowe, W.P., and Banfield, W.G. 1963. Milker's nodules: Isolation of a poxvirus from a human case. Science 140:1335–1336.
Gassmann, U., Wyler, R., and Wittek, R. 1985. Analysis of parapoxvirus genomes. Arch. Virol. 83:17–31.
Gibbs, E.P.J. 1984. Viral diseases of the skin of the bovine teat and udder. Vet. Clin. North Am. [Large Anim. Pract.] 6(1):187–202.
Gibbs, E.P.J., and Osborne, A.D. 1974. Observations on the epidemiology of pseudocowpox in south-west England and south Wales. Br. Vet. J. 130:150–159.

Gibbs, E.P.J., Johnson, R.H., and Osborne, A.D. 1970. Differential diagnosis of viral skin infection of the bovine teat. Vet. Rec. 87:602–609.

Hunt, E. 1984. Infectious skin diseases of cattle. Vet. Clin. North Am. [Large Anim. Pract.] 6(1):155–174.

Kahrs, R.F. 1981. Viral Diseases of Cattle. Iowa State University Press, Ames.

Papadopoulos, O.A., Dawson, P.S., Huck, R.A., and Stuart, P. 1968. Agar gel diffusion studies of paravaccinia viruses. J. Comp. Pathol. 78:219–225.

Rossi, C.R., Kiesel, G.K., and Jong, M.H. 1977. A paravaccinia virus isolated from cattle. Cornell Vet. 67:72–78.

Thomas, V., Flores, L., and Holowczak, J.A. 1980. Biochemical and electron microscopic studies of the replication and composition of milker's node virus. J. Virol. 34:244–255.

Tripathy, D.N., Hanson, L.E., and Crandell, R.A. 1981. Poxviruses of veterinary importance: Diagnosis of infection. In E. Kurstak and C. Kurstak, eds., Comparative Diagnosis of Viral Diseases, vol. 3. Academic Press, New York. Pp. 267–346.

Bovine Papular Stomatitis

SYNONYM: Stomatitis papulosa;
abbreviation, BPS

Bovine papular stomatitis is a common but mild or subclinical disease of young cattle characterized by proliferative lesions on the dental pad, buccal mucosa, on the margins of the lips, and on the muzzle. Reviews and descriptions of BPS have been presented by Crandell (1978), Griesemer and Cole (1960, 1961a, 1961b), Kahrs (1981), Nagington et al. (1967), and Tripathy et al. (1981).

Character of the Disease. Because BPS is usually a subclinical infection, clinical signs of disease typically are not detected. When lesions are present, the main problem is one of accurate diagnosis when concurrent infection or disease is present. The clinician must differentiate these lesions from those produced by the various vesicular diseases.

The lesions in the mouth and muzzle are usually raised and not depressed or ulcerated, although on occasion some lesions may degenerate into erosions. The lesions begin as raised hyperemic areas which then progress rather rapidly into roughened plaquelike lesions with irregular margins. Lesions may heal in a few weeks without scar formation, or they may persist for several months (Griesemer and Cole 1960).

Occasionally, BPS virus can cause teat lesions (Gibbs 1984), esophageal ulcers or lesions in the posterior oral cavity (Crandell and Gosser 1974), hyperkeratosis, or the so-called rat tail syndrome (necrotic dermatitis of the tail) in feedlot cattle (Brown et al. 1976, Irwin et al. 1976).

This disease of cattle may be the same as erosive stomatitis, stomatitis papulosa, ulcerative stomatitis, or pseudoaphthous stomatitis. It occurs in North America, Af-

rica, and Europe. Rossi et al. (1977) reported the isolation of a parapoxvirus from a calf with oral lesions and respiratory disease, but they were unable to produce signs of illness or elicit antibody production in experimental calves.

Properties of the Virus. BPS virus belongs to the *Parapoxvirus* genus of the family Poxviridae. The virus is similar to contagious pustular dermatitis virus of sheep and pseudocowpox virus of cattle. The reported size of the virus varies from 125 to 150 nm in diameter to 207 by 215 nm and the particles are poxlike structures with single or double membranes (Holscher et al. 1973, Pritchard et al. 1958, Reczko 1957).

Cultivation. BPS virus can be cultivated in cultures of calf testis, bovine kidney, and bovine turbinate cells with the production of cytopathic effects including cytolysis, stranding, and horseshoe-shaped intracytoplasmic inclusions (Crandell and Conroy 1974, Rossi et al. 1977).

Epizootiology and Pathogenesis. Transmission of BPS virus probably occurs by a variety of means. Nursing and bucket-fed calves probably acquire the virus from infected dams or from contaminated feeding utensils (Kahrs 1981). Direct contact or contaminated feed and water areas probably result in transmission in older young stock and adult cattle.

Immunity. Recovered animals are believed to be immune. In endemic herds infection usually occurs only in young cattle.

Diagnosis. Diagnosis is based on the presence of raised papular lesions or flat, irregular-edged brown lesions on the oral mucous membranes and muzzle in young cattle without other clinical signs, or with clinical signs of other diseases (Kahrs 1981). The diagnosis can be confirmed by demonstration of characteristic intracytoplasmic poxlike inclusions in a lesion biopsy specimen or by demonstration of the virus by electron microscopic examination of the biopsy sample. Virus can be isolated in cell culture or embryonated eggs. The main challenge in diagnosing BPS is to differentiate this benign infection from other more important diseases that may produce lesions in the mouth.

Treatment. The benign nature of the infection does not require treatment.

Prevention and Control. No prevention or control measures are necessary in most cases. Adequate disinfection of feeding utensils and milking machines will reduce the spread of virus within a herd.

The Disease in Humans. On occasion BPS virus may produce a benign, self-limiting local infection in humans. Therefore, precautions should be taken when handling and examining infected cattle.

REFERENCES

Brown, L.N., Irwin, L.R., and Bucerra, V.M. 1976. "Rat-tail syndrome" of feedlot cattle and bovine papular stomatitis virus infection. Proc. Am. Assoc. Vet. Lab. Diag. 19:405–410.

Crandell, R.A. 1978. Bovine papular stomatitis: Its occurrence in beef cattle. Univ. Ill. Agric. Exp. Sta. Bull. 20:14–15.

Crandell, R.A., and Conroy, J.D. 1974. The isolation and characterization of a strain of papular stomatitis virus. Proc. Am. Assoc. Vet. Lab. Diag. 17:223–234.

Crandell, R.A., and Gosser, H.A. 1974. Ulcerative esophagitis associated with a poxvirus infection in a calf. J. Am. Vet. Med. Assoc. 165:282–283.

Gibbs, E.P.J. 1984. Viral diseases of the skin of the bovine teat and udder. Vet. Clin. North Am. [Large Anim. Pract.] 6(1):187–202.

Griesemer, R.A., and Cole, C.R. 1960. Bovine papular stomatitis. I. Recognition in the U. S. J. Am. Vet. Med. Assoc. 137:404–410.

Griesemer, R.A., and Cole, C.R. 1961a. Bovine papular stomatitis. II. The experimentally produced disease. Am. J. Vet. Res. 22:473–481.

Griesemer, R.A., and Cole, C.R. 1961b. Bovine papular stomatitis. III. Histopathology. Am. J. Vet. Res. 22:482–486.

Holscher, M.A., Powell, H.S., Heath, J.E., and Bundza, A. 1973. Bovine papular stomatitis—Ultrastructural studies. Proc. U.S. Anim. Health Assoc. 77:638–643.

Irwin, M.R., Brown, L.N., Deyhle, C.E., and Bechtol, D.T. 1976. Association of bovine papular stomatitis with "rat-tail" syndrome in feedlot cattle. Southwest Vet. 20:120–124.

Kahrs, R.F. 1981. Viral Diseases of Cattle. Iowa State University Press, Ames.

Nagington, J.E., Lauder, M., and Smith, J.S. 1967. Bovine papular stomatitis, pseudocowpox, and milker's nodules. Vet. Rec. 81:306–313.

Pritchard, W.R., Clafin, R.M., Gustafson, D.P., and Ristic, M. 1958. An infectious ulcerative stomatitis of cattle. J. Am. Vet. Med. Assoc. 132:273–278

Reczko, E. 1957. Electronenmikroskopische Untersuchungen am Virus der Stomatitis Papulosa. Zentralbl. Bakt., I Abt. Orig. 169:425–453.

Rossi, C.R., Kiesel, G.K., and Jong, M.H. 1977. A paravaccinia virus isolated from cattle. Cornell Vet. 67.72–80.

Tripathy, D.N., Hanson, L.E., and Crandell, R.A. 1981. Poxviruses of veterinary importance: Diagnosis of infection. In E. Kurstak and C. Kurstak, eds., Comparative Diagnosis of Viral Diseases, vol. 3. Academic Press, New York. Pp. 267–346.

Contagious Pustular Dermatitis (Orf)

SYNONYMS: Contagious ecthyma of sheep, contagious pustular stomatitis, infectious labia dermatitis, orf, "scabby mouth," sore mouth; abbreviation, CPD

Contagious pustular dermatitis, a common acute viral disease of sheep and goats and occasionally other animals, is characterized by vesiculopapular eruptions or lesions on the lips, gums, and nose which progress into pustules and thick crusts. Infection sometimes occurs in humans who handle infected sheep and goats. The disease is frequent on the western ranges during the spring and summer, and it occurs occasionally in the farm flocks of the eastern United States. It has been reported in many sheep-raising countries and is thought to occur worldwide.

CPD apparently was first described by Walley (1890), who called it "contagious dermatitis" or "orf." An excel-

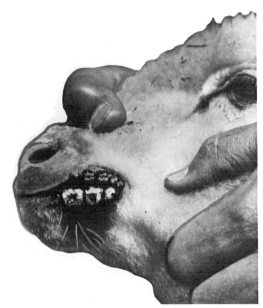

Figure 45.20. Contagious pustular dermatitis (sore mouth) in sheep. (Courtesy Jen-Sal Laboratories, Inc.)

lent review was presented by Robinson and Balassu (1981).

Character of the Disease. The virus of CPD is highly epitheliotropic. Lesions are usually restricted to the lips and nostrils, but on occasion can be seen on the skin, mucocutaneous junction, or mucous membranes of other parts of the body such as the inside of the thigh, the axilla, around the eyes, on the coronet of the feet, vulva, udder, palate, gums, and on the tongue (Aynaud 1923, Glover 1928, Howarth 1929, Robinson and Balassu 1981, Sharma and Bhatia 1959, Valder et al. 1979).

The disease is characterized by the formation of papules and vesicles that rapidly change to pustules, and finally by the appearance of heavy scabs (Figure 45.20). With their thickened, stiff, sensitive lips, affected lambs or kids can neither suckle nor graze, and rapid emaciation occurs. Healing usually is complete in about 1 month, by which time the scabs have fallen off and left the lips smooth and without scars.

In areas where the disease has been well established, it is seen principally in the lambs and kids because older animals are immune as a result of vaccination or having suffered the disease earlier in life. Ewes with suckling, infected lambs commonly develop lesions on their udders.

Fatalities are usually not numerous except when complications occur. In the more southerly states deaths commonly result from invasion of the lesions by the larvae of the flesh or screwworm fly (*Cochliomyia hominivorax*). Then losses in larvae-infested young lambs and kids fre-

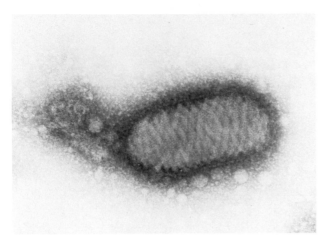

Figure 45.21. Contagious pustular dermatitis virus of sheep, a parapoxvirus. × 142,500. (Courtesy Viral Pathology and Viral Exanthems Branches, Centers for Disease Control.)

quently are great. The disease in older animals is usually less severe, and these animals are better able to resist the damage from the fly larvae. Where there are no screwworms, the only serious complication, according to Marsh and Tunnicliff (1937), is invasion of the lesions by the bacillus *Fusobacterium necrophorum*.

Unusually severe outbreaks of CPD have been reported in the United Kingdom, where the acute form of the disease, with severe involvement of the heart, lungs, and gastrointestinal tract, resulted in a mortality of 18 percent (Darbyshire 1961), and in Germany, where severe involvement of the feet, mouth, and esophagus resulted in high mortality, especially in young lambs (Valder et al. 1979).

Properties of the Virus. CPD virus is a member of the genus *Parapoxvirus* of the family Poxviridae. Its morphology is identical to that of bovine papular stomatitis virus (Robinson and Balassu 1981). Electron microscopy reveals an agent approximately 160 by 260 nm, with rounded ends and dense subpolar regions (Abdussalam and Coslett 1957, Kluge et al. 1972, Nagington and Horne 1962, Nagington et al. 1964, Yeh and Soltani 1974) (Figure 45.21). Virions appear on electron microscopy in one of two forms, either the type 1, or M (mulberry), form, which appears as the characteristic "ball of wool," or the type 2 form (C, or clear, form) (Nagington and Horne 1962, Nagington et al. 1964, Robinson and Balassu 1981).

It is an ether- and chloroform-resistant double-stranded DNA virus. The DNA of orf viruses and other parapoxviruses has been examined by restriction enzyme analysis (Gassmann et al. 1985, Raffii and Burger 1985, Robinson et al. 1982), and considerable heterogeneity was detected.

The virus is quite thermostable. Boughton and Hardy (1935) determined that the virus was destroyed by being heated to 58° to 60°C for half an hour, but its infectivity was not destroyed completely by the same exposure at 55°C.

Of the greatest practical importance is the resistance of this virus to natural conditions. It can remain viable for very long periods in the dried scabs that fall when the lesions heal. Premises have been known to harbor infection for more than a year after all animals have been removed. Boughton and Hardy (1935) showed that such scabs usually lost all virulence when placed in the sun for 30 to 60 days during the hot summer in western Texas, but if placed in the shade they retained their virulence for years. Scabs placed outside in the fall of the year were still virulent in the spring. Powdered, dry scabs retained virulence for at least 32 months when kept in the refrigerator but lost all infectivity in 54 to 120 days when stored in the dark at an average temperature of 83°F.

There has been confusion in the past between this disease and sheeppox and goatpox. There is no cross-immunization between orf and sheeppox; however, goatpox, which is a much milder disease, appears to give some protection against later exposure to orf.

Cultivation. The virus can be cultivated in a variety of cell cultures (Greig 1957, Schmidt and Hardy 1932). Mice, rabbits, guinea pigs, hamsters, and chick embryos are refractory to inoculation.

Epizootiology and Pathogenesis. Outbreaks of CPD are usually initiated by virus that persists in the soil or on equipment or feed and watering troughs from one season to the next. Transmission of virus within an outbreak is by direct contact with infected animals, or by contact with contaminated soil, equipment, or feed and water troughs. Rapid spread, severe disease, and high morbidity in an Australian herd were attributed to the concentration of sheep around a palatable scrub, *Templetonia retusa*, which caused extensive trauma to mucous membranes during grazing (Gardiner et al. 1967).

CPD is most often seen in domestic sheep, but it also can occur in goats and in wild animals such as the Rocky Mountain bighorn sheep (*Ovis canadensis*), mountain goats, Dall sheep (*Ovis dalli*), musk-oxen (*Ovibos moschatus*), and reindeer (Connell 1954; Dieterich et al. 1981; Falk 1978, Kummeneje and Krogsrud 1978, 1979; Lance et al. 1981; Robinson and Balassu 1981; Samuel et al. 1975; Smith et al. 1982; Zarnke et al. 1983). Experimental infection has been documented in the mule deer (*Odocoileus hemionus*), white-tailed deer (*Odocoileus virginianus*), pronghorn antelope (*Antilocapra americana*), and wapiti (*Cervus elaphus nelsoni*) with mild clinical disease (Lance et al. 1983), and in the moose

(*Alces alces*) and caribou (*Rangifer tarandus*) without clinical disease (Zarnke et al. 1983).

An outbreak of "contagious ecthyma" in camels in Mongolia was caused by a parapoxvirus similar to CPD virus of sheep and goats, but the CPD virus vaccines did not appear to protect camels against the camel strain of virus (Dashtseren et al. 1984).

Immunity. Animals that recover from the disease are immune for as long as 28 months, and perhaps much longer. Range animals that have been vaccinated have traditionally been considered immune for life. Schmidt and Hardy (1932) found that lambs and kids that had recovered from this disease were immune thereafter. Yet there are reports of outbreaks of CPD in flocks of vaccinated sheep (Beck and Taylor 1974, Buddle et al. 1984b, Hardy 1964, Peddie 1950).

Immune serums agglutinate elementary bodies, precipitate soluble antigen, and fix complement (Abdussalam and Coslett 1957). The virus shows a small amount of cross-reaction with vaccinia and ectromelia, as demonstrated by the complement-fixation and gel-diffusion tests, and contagious pustular dermatitis antiserums showed some neutralization of ectromelia virus (Trueblood and Chow 1963). Goatpox immunizes against CPD but the converse is not true (Bennett et al. 1944). Strains of CPD virus may not be serologically identical (Greig 1957) as there is heterogeneity among CPD virus isolates (Buddle et al. 1984a, Horgan and Haseeb 1947, Robinson et al. 1982, Wittek et al. 1980).

Diagnosis. The disease is recognized by its characteristic epithelial lesions with ballooning cells that lead to degeneration, vesicle formation, and possible granulomatous formation. Cytoplasmic inclusion bodies are found. Diagnosis is confirmed by the isolation and identification of the virus or by electron microscopy of negatively stained suspensions from lesions (Harkness et al. 1977).

There are some similarities to bluetongue in the initial stages of the disease (Gardiner et al. 1967) and also to skin forms of anthrax.

Prevention and Control. Where this disease is prevalent, it is wise to vaccinate all lambs or kids each spring before the pasture season begins because it tends to recur regularly each year on pastures that are once infected. Range animals can also be infected during shipment to fattening areas. Available vaccines are either live virus vaccines prepared from dried scabs of lesions or preparations from cell culture–grown attenuated live-virus (Mayr et al. 1981). With the live virus vaccine, animals are vaccinated intradermally on a woolless or hairless area of the skin such as inside the thigh. The skin is scarified and a drop of reconstituted vaccine is brushed into the area. A papule, pustule, and, finally, a scab appear at the vaccination site. The attenuated cell culture vaccine is administered parenterally. Buddle et al. (1984b) reported that the cell culture–propagated vaccines were less effective than those propagated in sheep.

Immune ewes transfer passive immunity to their lambs through the colostrum, which interferes with vaccination if it is present in sufficient titers (Jan et al. 1978). Vaccine failures, apparently from the heterogeneity of the strains of virus (Beck and Taylor 1974, Buddle et al. 1984b, Hardy 1964, Peddie 1950), have been reported.

The vaccines are infectious for humans, so special care must be exercised in handling the vaccine and recently vaccinated animals.

The Disease in Humans. Contagious pustular dermatitis in humans is often referred to as *orf,* and the virus is referred to as the *orf virus* (Robinson and Balassu 1981). Transmission often occurs with apparent ease from infected sheep to humans. Orf is an occupational disease of sheepherders, sheep shearers, slaughterhouse workers, and veterinarians, all of whom are apt to develop lesions on the hands, arms, or face. Transmission between individuals has been reported (Lang 1961).

Robinson and Petersen (1983) did a survey of the incidence of orf in workers in the meat industry. In 18 slaughterhouses handling lambs and sheep, there were 231 clinical cases of orf reported in 1 year. This was 1.4 percent of the total workers, with the employees with the highest incidence of disease being those who handled wool and pelts. Eighteen of these cases were reinfections.

There have been many reports on the nature of the disease in humans (Blackmore et al. 1948, Fastier 1957, Freeman et al. 1984, Hunter 1964, Leavell et al. 1968, Moore et al. 1983, Newsom and Cross 1934, Purdy 1955, Rucker 1977, Sanchez et al. 1985). The lesions begin in abrasions, as a rule. They consist of rather large vesicles that may be multiple in structure. The surrounding skin becomes reddened and moderately swollen. The individual may have fever, axillary lymph nodes may be swollen, and the local lesion is moderately painful. Secondary infection usually occurs, and healing is often rather slow (Marsh and Tunnicliff 1937).

REFERENCES

Abdussalam, M., and Cosslet, V.E. 1957. Contagious pustular dermatitis virus. I. Studies on morphology. J. Comp. Pathol. Therap. 67:145–156.

Aynaud, M. 1923. La stomatite pustuleuse contagieuse des ovins (chancre du mouton). Ann. Inst. Pasteur 37:498–527.

Beck, C.C., and Taylor, W.B. 1974. Orf: It's awful. Vet. Med./Small Anim. Clin. 69:1413–1417.

Bennett, S.C.J., Horgan, E.S., and Haseeb, M.A. 1944. The pox diseases of sheep and goats. J. Comp. Pathol. Therap. 54:131–160.

Blackmore, F., Abdussalam, M., and Goldsmith, W.N. 1948. A case of orf (contagious pustular dermatitis): Identification of the virus. Br. J. Dermatol. 60:404–409.

Boughton, I.B., and Hardy, W.T. 1935. Immunization of sheep and goats against soremouth (contagious ecthyma). Texas Agric. Exp. Sta. Bull. 504.

Buddle, B.M., Dellers, R.W., and Schurig, G.G. 1984a. Heterogeneity of contagious ecthyma virus isolates. Am. J. Vet. Res. 45:75–79.

Buddle, B.M., Dellers, R.W., and Schurig, G.G. 1984b. Contagious ecthyma virus vaccination failures. Am. J. Vet. Res. 45:263–266.

Connell, R. 1954. Contagious ecthyma in Rocky Mountain bighorn sheep. Can. J. Comp. Med. 18:59–60.

Darbyshire, J.H. 1961. A fatal ulcerative mucosal condition of sheep associated with the virus of contagious pustular dermatitis. Br. Vet. J. 117:97–105.

Dashtseren, T., Solovyev, B.V., Varejka, F., and Khokhoo, A. 1984. Camel contagious ecthyma (pustular dermatitis). Acta Virol. 28:122–127.

Dieterich, R.A., Spencer, G.R., Burger, D., Gallina, A.M., and Vanderschalie, J. 1981. Contagious ecthyma in Alaskan musk-oxen and Dall sheep. J. Am. Vet. Med. Assoc. 179:1140–1143.

Falk, E.S. 1978. Parapoxvirus infections of reindeer and musk ox associated with unusual human infections. Br. J. Dermatol. 99:647–654.

Fastier, L.B. 1957. Human infections with the virus of ovine contagious pustular dermatitis (scabby mouth). N.Z. Med. J. 56:121–123.

Freeman, G., Bron, A.J., and Juel-Jensen, B. 1984. Ocular infection with orf virus. Am. J. Ophthalmol. 97:601–604.

Gardiner, M.R., Craig, J., and Nairn, M.E. 1967. An unusual outbreak of contagious ecthyma (scabby mouth) in sheep. Aust. Vet. J. 43:163–165.

Gassmann, U., Wyler, R., and Wittek, R. 1985. Analysis of parapoxvirus genomes. Arch. Virol. 83:17–31.

Glover, R.E. 1928. Contagious pustular dermatitis of the sheep. J. Comp. Pathol. Therap. 41:318–340.

Greig, A.S. 1957. Contagious ecthyma of sheep. II. In vitro cultivation of the virus. Can. J. Comp. Pathol. Vet. Sci. 21:304–308.

Hardy, W.T. 1964. Contagious ecthyma in sheep and goats. Proc. U.S. Livestock Sanit. Assoc. 67:293–299.

Harkness, J.W., Scott, A.C., and Hebert, C.N. 1977. Electron microscopy in the rapid diagnosis of orf. Br. Vet. J. 133:81–87.

Horgan, E.S., and Haseeb, M.A. 1947. The immunological relationships of strains contagious pustular dermatitis virus. J. Comp. Pathol. Therap. 57:1–7.

Howarth, J.A. 1929. Infectious pustular dermatitis of sheep and goats. J. Am. Vet. Med. Assoc. 75:741–760.

Hunter, W.R. 1964. The cutaneous lesions of human orf. Br. J. Surg. 51:831–833.

Jan, C. le, L'Haridon, R., Madelaine, M.F., Cornu, C., and Asso, J. 1978. Transfer of antibodies against the CPD virus through colostrum and milk. Ann. Rech. Vét. 9:343–346.

Kluge, J.P., Cheville, N.F., and Perry, T.M. 1972. Ultrastructural studies of contagious ecthyma in sheep. Am. J. Vet. Res. 33:1191–1200.

Kummeneje, K., and Krogsrud, J. 1978. Contagious ecthyma (orf) in the musk ox (Ovibos moschatos). Acta Vet. Scand. 19:461–462.

Kummeneje, K., and Krogsrud, J. 1979. Contagious ecthyma (orf) in reindeer (Rangifer tarandus). Vet. Rec. 105:60–61.

Lance, W.R., Adrian, W., and Widhalm, B. 1981. An epizootic of contagious ecthyma in Rocky Mountain bighorn sheep in Colorado. J. Wildl. Dis. 17:601–603.

Lance, W.R., Hibler, C.P., and DeMartini, J. 1983. Experimental contagious ecthyma in mule deer, white-tailed deer, pronghorn and wapiti. J. Wildl. Dis. 19:165–169.

Lang, H.A. 1961. Human orf. Br. Med. J. 11:1566.

Leavell, U.W., McNamara, M.J., Muelling, R., Talbert, W.M., Rucker, R.C., and Dalton, A.J. 1968. Orf: Report of 19 human cases with clinical and pathological observations. J. Am. Med. Assoc. 204:657–664.

Marsh, H., and Tunnicliff, E.A. 1937. Stomatitis in young lambs involving Actinomyces necrophorus and the virus of contagious ecthyma. J. Am. Vet. Med. Assoc. 91:600–605.

Mayr, A., Herlyn, M., Mahnel, H., Danco, A., Zach, A., and Bostedt, H. 1981. Control of ecthyma contagiosum (pustular dermatitis) of sheep with a new parenteral cell culture vaccine. Zentralbl. Veterinärmed. [B] 28:535–552.

Moore, D.M., MacKenzie, W.F., Doepel, F., and Hansen, T.N. 1983. Contagious ecthyma in lambs and laboratory personnel. Lab. Anim. Sci. 33:473–475.

Nagington, J., and Horne, R.W. 1962. Morphological studies of orf and vaccinia viruses. Virology 16:248–260.

Nagington, J., Newton, A.A., and Horne, R.W. 1964. The structure of orf virus. Virology 23:461–472.

Newsom, I.E., and Cross, F. 1934. Sore mouth in sheep transmissible to man. J. Am. Vet. Med. Assoc. 84:799–802.

Peddie, J.J.G. 1950. Vaccination of sheep against scabby mouth. N.Z. J. Agric. 81:19.

Purdy, M.J. 1955. Orf. N.Z. Med. J. 54:572–575.

Raffii, F., and Burger, D. 1985. Comparison of contagious ecthyma virus genomes by restriction endonucleases. Arch. Virol. 84:283–289.

Robinson, A.J., and Petersen, G.V. 1983. Orf virus infection of workers in the meat industry. N.Z. Med. J. 96:81–85.

Robinson, A.J., Ellis, G., and Balassu, T. 1982. The genome of orf virus: Restriction endonuclease analysis of viral DNA isolated from lesions of orf in sheep. Arch. Virol. 71:43–55.

Rucker, R.C. 1977. Clinical picture of orf in northern California. Cutis 20:109–111.

Samuel, W.M., Chalmers, G.A., Stelfox, J.G., Loewen, A., and Thomsen, J.J. 1975. Contagious ecthyma in bighorn sheep and mountain goats in western Canada. J. Wildl. Dis. 11:26–31.

Sanchez, R.L., Hebert, A., Lucia, H., and Swedo, J. 1985. Orf. A case report with histologic, electron microscopic, and immunoperoxidase studies. Arch. Pathol. Lab. Med. 109:166–170.

Schmidt, H., and Hardy, W.T. 1932. Soremouth (contagious ecthyma) in sheep and goats. Texas Agric. Exp. Sta. Bull. 457.

Sharma, R.M., and Bhatia, H.M. 1959. Contagious pustular dermatitis in goats. Indian J. Vet. Sci. 28:205–210.

Smith, T.C., Heimer, W.E., and Foreyt, W.J. 1982. Contagious ecthyma in an adult Dall sheep (Ovis dalli) in Alaska. J. Wildl. Dis. 18:111–112.

Trueblood, M.S., and Chow, T.L. 1963. Characterization of the agents of ulcerative dermatosis and contagious ecthyma. Am. J. Vet. Res. 24:47–51.

Valder, W.A., Straub, O.C., Thiel, W., Wachendörfer, G., and Zettl, K. 1979. Ecthyma Contagiosum des Schafes—Wandel des klinischen Bildes. Tierärztl. Umsch. 34:828–836.

Walley, T. 1890. Contagious dermatitis: "Orf" in sheep. J. Comp. Pathol. Therap. 3:357–360.

Wittek, R., Herlyn, M., Schumperli, D., Bachmann, P.A., Mayr, A., and Wyler, R. 1980. Genetic and antigenic heterogeneity of different parapoxvirus strains. Intervirology 13:33–41.

Yeh, H.P., and Soltani, K. 1974. Ultrastructural studies in human orf. Arch. Dermatol. 109:390–392.

Zarnke, R.L., Dieterich, R.A., Neiland, K.A., and Ranglack, G. 1983. Serologic and experimental investigations of contagious ecthyma in in Alaska. J. Wildl. Dis. 19:170–174.

46 The Herpesviridae

The family Herpesviridae contains many viruses responsible for important human and animal diseases. It is divided into three subfamilies on the basis of shared biological properties (Matthews 1982, Roizman and Batterson 1985).

The subfamily Alphaherpesvirinae contains herpesviruses characterized by a variable host range, short replicative cycle with rapid cytolysis of infected cells, and latent infections, primarily in nerve ganglia. Two genera *Simplexvirus* and *Poikilovirus,* are recognized in this subfamily.

The Betaherpesvirinae subfamily comprises viruses characterized by a long replicative cycle, a slow progression of infection in cultures and hosts, frequent formation of cytomegalic cells, and the formation of latent infections in secretory glands, lymphoreticular cells, kidneys, and other tissues. This subfamily contains two genera, *Cytomegalovirus* and *Muromegalovirus.*

The subfamily Gammaherpesvirinae includes viruses characterized by a restricted host range, a predilection for T or B lymphocytes with occasional infection of epithelial fibroblastic cells, and latent infections of lymphoid tissues. Three genera, *Lymphocryptovirus, Thetalymphocryptovirus,* and *Rhadinovirus,* are recognized in this subfamily.

The physical, chemical, and replicative properties of herpesviruses have been reviewed by Roizman and Batterson (1985). Herpesviruses are medium-sized enveloped viruses. The herpesvirion is composed of four structural elements: (1) the central core containing the nucleic acid, (2) the icosahedral capsid surrounding the core, (3) an asymmetrical coat or layer surrounding the capsid called the tegument, and (4) an outer envelope surrounding the tegument and capsid. The morphologic features of a typical herpesvirus are depicted in Figure 46.1.

The core of the herpesvirus contains linear, double-stranded DNA in the form of a torus. The molecular mass of the nucleic acid varies from 54 to 92×10^6 daltons, which constitutes approximately 7 percent of the particle mass.

The capsids have diameters of 100 to 150 nm. They contain 162 hollow capsomeres, which are about 9 nm across and 12.5 nm deep, with central cavities of about 4 nm in diameter which run part way down the long axis of the capsomere.

The tegument has no distinctive features and frequently is distributed asymmetrically between the capsid and the envelope. The envelope or outer covering has a trilaminar structure derived from altered cell membranes. The surface is covered with short (8-nm) protrusions, or peplomers. The lipid content of the envelope makes the herpesvirus particles quite labile, and they generally are inactivated rapidly by environmental, physical, and chemical agents such as lipid solvents and detergents.

The number of individual proteins in various herpesviruses has been reported to be from 15 to 35. At least four glycoproteins are located on the surface, and the capsid contains at least six polypeptides.

Replication of herpesviruses in susceptible cells occurs within 12 or more hours for the rapidly cytolytic viruses, such as pseudorabies virus, to more than 70 hours for the slowly replicative viruses, such as cytomegaloviruses (Roizman and Batterson 1985). The virions attach to the cell at specific receptor sites and penetrate the capsid when a viral surface protein has been activated by the attachment. This process results in fusion of the viral envelope and plasma membrane of the cell, and the removal of the envelope to give the de-enveloped capsid, which is transported to the nucleus where the DNA is released.

Transcription and replication of the viral DNA occurs in the nucleus of the infected cell, and the capsids are formed in the nucleus. The viral DNA is transcribed by host RNA polymerase II, and protein synthesis and processing (cleavage, phosphorylation, sulfation, glycosylation) occur in the cytoplasm. The proteins are then transported back to the nucleus, where they are assembled into the capsids. The new viral DNA is inserted or packaged into the preformed capsids, and the nucleocapsids attach to patches or aggregations of viral membrane proteins on the inner lamella of the nuclear membrane. The nucleocapsids then bud through the nuclear membrane as they acquire their envelopes. The mature virions emerge through the cytoplasm and are released from the cell.

Intranuclear eosinophilic inclusion bodies are formed

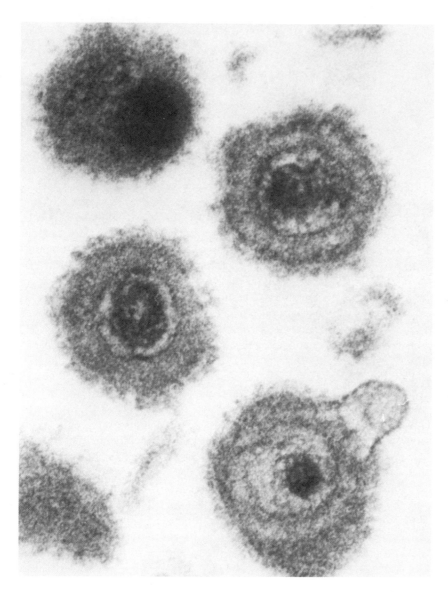

Figure 46.1. Thin section of herpes simplex virus particles. Lead citrate. × 192,000. (From Volk, 1978, courtesy of J. B. Lippincott Co., B. Roizman, and W. Volk.)

in infected cells. Most herpesviruses have an affinity for epithelial tissue and tend to produce latent infections. In cell culture and on embryonating chicken membranes they produce focal cytopathic effects in the form of plaques or pocks. Some members of the group are strongly cell-associated and require special procedures to release the virus into the tissue-culture medium in appreciable titers; others readily release virus into the medium. These viruses are rather poor interferon producers.

Diseases of domestic animals caused by viruses in the Herpesviridae family are listed in Table 46.1. All species of domestic animals can be infected with one or more herpesviruses. Many herpesviruses are species-specific in their infectivity range, whereas others affect a broad range of species. The character of the diseases caused by herpesviruses varies from acute inflammations to tumors. Subclinical infections from some herpesviruses may be common.

REFERENCES

Matthews, R.E.F. 1982. Classification and nomenclature of viruses. Fourth report of the International Committee on Taxonomy of Viruses. Intervirology 17:1–199.

Roizman, B., and Batterson, W. 1985. Herpesviruses and their replication. In B.N. Fields, D.M. Knipe, R.M. Chanock, J.L. Melnick, B. Roizman, and R.E. Shope, eds., Virology. Raven Press, New York. Pp. 497–526.

Volk, W., ed. 1978. Essentials of Medical Microbiology. Lippincott, Philadelphia.

Table 46.1. Diseases of domestic animals caused by viruses in the Herpesviridae family

Common name of virus	Natural hosts	Type of disease produced
Subfamily Alphaherpesvirinae		
Infectious bovine rhinotracheitis–infectious pustular vulvovaginitis virus (bovine herpesvirus 1)	Cattle	*Respiratory tract form:* Fever, depression, upper and lower catarrhal respiratory signs, and conjunctivitis. Average mortality is 10 percent
		Reproductive tract form: Fever, depression, inflammatory pustular lesions in vulva and vagina of cows and on prepuce and penis of bulls. Negligible mortality
		Encephalitis form: Usually in calves, with high mortality. Morbidity is usually low
Bovine mammillitis virus (bovine herpesvirus 2)	Cattle	Ulcerative lesions appear on teats and udder. Slow healing with formation of scabs
Equine rhinopneumonitis virus (subtypes 1 and 2)	Horses	Subtype 2 causes respiratory signs and leukopenia. Subtype 1 causes abortions in mares and occasionally produces paralysis.
Equine coital exanthema virus (equine herpesvirus 3)	Horses	Vesicular or pustular lesions occur in vulva or on penis
Pseudorabies virus	Cattle, sheep, goats, swine, dogs, cats, rats	Acute disease in all animals except adult swine. Severe pruritis (except swine), paralysis, cardiac and respiratory distress, convulsions. Mortality high in most species
Canine herpesvirus	Dogs	May cause fatal hemorrhagic disease in infant puppies. Mild signs in older dogs
Feline viral rhinotracheitis virus (feline herpesvirus 1)	Cats	Serious disease in kittens. Fever and depression. Signs largely referable to respiratory tract and eye. Pregnant females may abort. Mortality may be appreciable in young cats
Avian infectious laryngotracheitis virus	Chickens	Acute, highly contagious respiratory disease. Severe respiratory distress results from caseous plugs in trachea that cause death. Mortality can be significant; morbidity is high
Pigeon herpesvirus	Pigeons	Clinical signs of coryza are observed with lesions most prominent in larynx or pharynx
Duck plague virus	Ducks, geese (rarely)	Acute fatal disease involving the respiratory, enteric, and nervous systems of ducks
Subfamily Bethaherpesvirinae		
Feline urolithiasis virus (feline herpesvirus 2)	Cats	Experimental disease—virus causes urolithiasis often resulting in uremia and death unless appropriate treatment is applied
Subfamily Gammaherpesvirinae		
Malignant catarrhal fever virus	Cattle, wildebeest, sheep	Natural disease only in cattle. Wildebeest (in Africa) and sheep

Table 46.1.—*continued*

Common name of virus	Natural hosts	Type of disease produced
		have inapparent infection, but serve as carriers. African strains of virus readily produce disease; converse is true with U.S. isolates. It is a sporadic disease with a short febrile period, inflammation of mucous membranes of mouth, nose, and eyes, nervous signs, and a high death rate
Marek's disease virus	Chickens, turkeys, pheasants, quail (principal avian hosts)	Acute fulminating type of oncogenic disease in young chicks that spreads rapidly with a high mortality as a rule. Virus causes various forms of tumors—neurolymphomatosis, ocular lymphomatosis, and visceral lymphomatosis. Arterial sclerosis

The Subfamily Alphaherpesvirinae

Infectious Bovine Rhinotracheitis

SYNONYMNS: Bovine coital exanthema, infectious bovine necrotic rhinotracheitis, infectious pustular vulvovaginitis, necrotic rhinitis, "red nose" disease; abbreviations, IBR, IPV

Bovine herpesvirus 1 (BHV-1), also known as IBR virus and IPV virus, causes disease in cattle, goats, and pigs. The respiratory form, which usually occurs in the cold months of the years, was first recognized in beef cattle in Colorado feedlots (Madin et al. 1956). It was then seen in California and other western states. In the eastern part of the United States the virus first manifested itself in cases of infectious pustular vulvovaginitis (Gillespie et al. 1959). On occasion the major disease manifestation of this virus in a herd is meningoencephalitis in neonatal and young calves (French 1962) or a viremic disease in this age group, with lesions in the upper portion of the digestive tract and in the parenchymatous organs (Baker et al. 1960); keratoconjunctivitis (Abinanti and Plumer 1961); dermal infections; or abortions in cows (Chow et al. 1964, McKercher and Wada 1964). BHV-1 has also been isolated from vesicular lesions of the bovine udder (Guy et al. 1984). Some outbreaks cause marked economic loss.

BHV-1 has a worldwide distribution. All forms of the bovine disease now are recognized in the United States, Australia, many European countries, New Zealand, and Japan. The disease has assumed great importance in Europe and the United States. More than one form may be observed in a herd outbreak. In the United States the incidence of antibody in cattle ranges from 10 to 35 percent.

In goats the virus reputedly causes respiratory disease (Mohanty et al. 1972) and has been isolated from two stillborn pig fetuses (Derbyshire and Caplan 1976). Infections in various wildlife and zoological species have been recorded (Stauber et al. 1980, Zarnke and Yuill 1981).

Gibbs and Rweyemamu (1977) have written excellent review articles on the bovine herpesviruses. The literature on BHV-1 has expanded markedly since the last edition of this textbook (1981), but no recent review article has been written.

Character of the Disease. The respiratory form (IBR) may occur as a mild, unrecognized infection, or it may be very severe. The acute disease involves the entire respiratory tract with lesser damage to the alimentary canal. It begins with high fever (104.5° to 107.5°F), great depression, inappetence, and abundant mucopurulent nasal discharge (Figure 46.2). The nasal mucous membranes become very congested, and shallow ulcers appear. Necrosis of the wings of the nostrils and of the muzzle occurs. The highly inflamed tissues gave rise to the name "red nose." Dyspnea and mouth breathing result from closure of the nares by inflammatory exudate. Conjunctivitis and lacrimation may be seen, but necrosis of the lacrimal tissues does not occur. The breath usually becomes fetid because of the necrosis of the nasal mucosae. The respiratory rate usually is accelerated, and a deep bronchial cough is frequent. Blood-stained diarrhea sometimes occurs. Abortions may be associated with this disease form.

Infectious pustular vulvovaginitis (IPV) occurs in heifers, dairy cows, and bulls (Kendrick et al. 1958) (Fig-

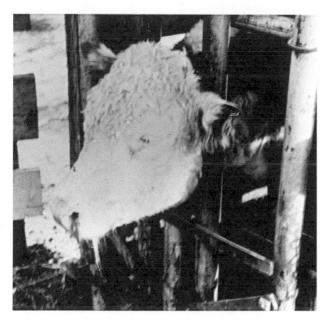

Figure 46.2. Respiratory form of infectious bovine rhinotracheitis with characteristic hemorrhagic exudate from the nose.

ure 46.3). The degree of reaction varies greatly in an infected herd. The fact that disease sometimes spreads rapidly through a herd suggests transmission by aerosal route or by individuals handling the herd. The disease usually begins with fever, and severely affected cows show considerable anxiety and pain, with frequent urination. The vulva swells, and a sticky exudate may appear on the vulval hair. The infection usually persists for 10 to 14 days in a herd. Bulls may have lesions on the penis and prepuce similar to those observed in the vulva of cows, and these may persist for 2 weeks or even longer if complications arise. Severe complications may result in temporary or perhaps permanent impairment of a bull's ability to mate. In general there is disagreement on the extent to which infected bulls may be a significant factor in infertility. Certainly every effort should be made to keep a stud free of IPV.

In the naturally transmitted disease the incubation period is from 4 to 6 days. Intratracheal inoculation or nasal or vulvovaginal instillation can shorten this period to 18 to 72 hours (Gillespie et al. 1957). The course of the disease varies widely, depending on the severity of the infection. Milder forms may be noticed. Some animals may die of the respiratory or brain form within a few hours after they are first noticed to be sick; most will be ill for only a few days.

Mortality varies widely, depending on the virulence of the virus, age and condition of cattle, form of the disease, and management conditions. In severe outbreaks in west-

ern feedlots 75 percent or more of the animals can show respiratory signs, with an average mortality of 10 percent. In a susceptible group of calves mortality from the meningoencephalitic form reached 50 percent. Calves that showed nervous signs seldom survived.

Properties of the Virus. Tousimis et al. (1958) studied the virus by electron microscopy and determined that the BHV-1 particles produced in bovine kidney cell cultures had a diameter of 145 to 156 nm. In tissue fluids the diameter was determined to be 136 ± 10 nm. Griffin et al. (1958) found this virus to be stable when suspended in culture mediums at pH 7.0. The original titer was maintained for 30 days at 4°C. Only one log of infectivity was lost after 5 days at 22°C. Equal parts of virus suspension and alcohol, acetone, or chloroform caused prompt inactivation. After exposure to 20 percent ethyl ether for 16 hours at 4°C, most field isolates were resistant (Crandall et al. 1975).

The density of BHV-1 in the potassium tartrate gradient is 1.22 g/ml. Armstrong et al. (1961) first suggested this was a DNA virus. The DNA of BHV-1 has an average molecular mass of 84×10^6 daltons (Scal et al. 1985).

Through the use of various biochemical procedures and of panels of monoclonal antibodies investigators are determining the number of polypeptides in the virion and, more important, the glycoproteins that are involved in the

Figure 46.3. Vulva of a heifer inoculated 48 hours previously with infectious pustular vulvovaginitis virus (BHV 1). The typical round pustules, some of which are in rows, are present on a reddened mucosa. Near the dorsal commissure the closely spaced pustules have coalesced to form a large, plaquelike lesion. (From Kendrick et al., 1958, courtesy of *Cornell Veterinarian.*)

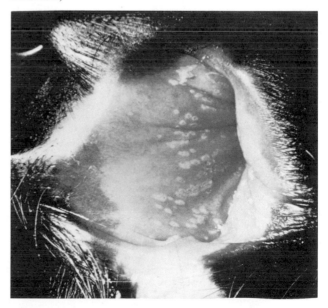

production of immunity. BHV-1 has been shown to have 33 polypeptides (Chang et al. 1986). Ten glycoproteins (Chang et al. 1986, Marshall et al. 1986) with molecular masses ranging from 45 kilodaltons (kDa) to 180 kDa (Marshall et al. 1986) and 1 nonglycosylated 107-kDa protein (Chang et al. 1986, Marshall et al. 1986) were located on the viral surface. Immunoprecipitations with monoclonal antibodies showed that three sets of coprecipitating glycoproteins—180 kDa/97 kDa, 150 kDa/77 kDa, and 130 kDa/74 kDa/55 kDa—were the major neutralizing antibody components of the BHV-1 envelope but that 130 kDa/74 kDa/55 kDa required complement for neutralization (Marshall et al. 1986). Four unique glycoproteins or glycoprotein complexes were recognized by a panel of monoclonal antibodies to the viral envelope of BHV-1 (Collins et al. 1985, Van Drunen Littel–van den Hurk and Babiuk 1985). In another study only few minor differences were noted among 14 viral isolates in regard to intracellular content of 19 proteins with molecular masses of 14 kDa to 145 kDa; a monoclonal antibody to the Cooper strain neutralized all other 13 strains immunoprecipitating the major 90-kDa glycoprotein (Trepanier et al. 1986). Another monoclonal antibody with a high hemagglutination titer inhibited the hemagglutination of the other 13 isolates and also reacted against the 90-kDa glycoprotein by immunoprecipitation. Lawrence et al. (1986) ascertained the map location of the gene for the 130,000-dalton glycoprotein of BHV-1. Experiments by Kit and Qavi (1983) strongly suggest that wild BHV-1 induces virus-specific thymidine kinase (TK) activity. Lui and Manning (1986) identified the TK gene of BHV-1 and elucidated its function in *Escherichia coli*. The various strains of IBR virus are antigenically homogeneous, although slight differences between strains have been demonstrated by neutralization tests in tissue culture (York et al. 1957).

Carmichael and Barnes (1961) showed some relationship of the virus to that of equine rhinopneumonitis with complement-fixation and gel diffusion tests. IBR, Marek's, and Burkitt's lymphoma viruses share a common antigen, as shown by agar-gel diffusion and indirect fluorescent antibody tests. BHV-1 and caprine herpesvirus 1 also have a common antigen (Berrios and McKercher 1975); but, on the basis of DNA restriction endonuclease patterns of caprine herpesviruses, it should be designated as the prototype virus of bovine herpesvirus 6 (Engels et al. 1983). As measured by liquid reassociation kinetics the homology between the genomes of BHV-1 and pseudorabies viruses was approximately 8 percent (Bush and Pritchett 1985). A probing of viral western immunoblots with rabbit hyperimmune sera showed a number of viral specific cross-reactive proteins between BHV-1 and pseudorabies virus (Bush and Pritchett 1986).

Differences between the genomes of several viral isolates of BHV-1 from the different forms of the disease were detected with DNA restriction enzyme analyses, but nucleic acid hybridization studies of viral DNAs indicated at least a 95 percent genetic homology (Seal et al. 1985).

In a recent study (Theodoridis 1985) indicated the BHV-4 strains may be the same as BHV-1 that has undergone certain biological changes, illustrating a pheomenon that he thought was a characteristic of herpesviruses.

Studies with a number of BHV-1 isolates representing various forms of the disease for molecular and antigenic characteristic implied that two antigenic variants exist and that most isolates of nonpurulent meningoencephalitis are a hitherto unrecognized antigenic variant (Metzler et al. 1985, 1986).

Cultivation. BHV-1 was first isolated by Madin et al. (1956). Several groups of workers also reported successful cultivation of the virus in bovine embryo tissue-culture cells and in bovine kidney cells (Gillespie et al. 1968, Studdert et al. 1964). The agent of IBR always exhibits a strong cytopathic effect for practically all cells in which it is cultivated within 24 to 48 hours. It also grows and produces a cytopathic effect in pig, dog, sheep, goat, horse, and WI-38 human diploid kidney cells. Intranuclear inclusion bodies are produced in these cells and can be demonstrated by fixation with Bouin's solution and hematoxylin and eosin stain (Cheatham and Crandell 1957). Plaques can be produced in bovine kidney monolayers and in many other cell cultures (York 1968).

Persistent infection can be established in hamster embryo cell cultures by inoculation of infective virus particles at approximately half the number of cells in culture. The persistence of virus is indicated by a minimal degree of cytopathic effect with a low level of released virus (Michalski and Hsiung 1976). Hamster embryo cells showed malignant transformation following BHV-1 inoculation.

BHV-1 grows to high titer, produces intranuclear inclusion bodies (Chetham and Crandell 1957), and prevents ciliary activity in nasal and tracheal organ cultures (Shroyer and Easterday 1968).

Epizootiology and Pathogenesis. Cattle are susceptible to BHV-1. The disease is readily transmitted by infected cattle, and certain individuals can remain carriers of the virus weeks after acute infection (Studdert et al. 1964). All forms of the disease are transmitted by contact, especially under crowded conditions, and the venereal form can also be transmitted by coitus. The virus has been isolated from semen.

Stress may cause cattle vaccinated with attenuated vaccines to BHV-1 to excrete virus (Sheffy and Rodman 1973), but whether the excreted virus regains virulence for cattle has not been established. Vaccinated and recovered cattle may contribute to perpetuation of the disease.

Young goats infected experimentally developed fever and mild respiratory disease (McKercher 1959, Wafula et al. 1985). Rabbits inoculated intradermally or intratesticularly developed local lesions (Armstrong et al. 1961), but serial passage of virus was unsuccessful. Newborn rabbits given the LA strain of BHV-1 developed severe, sometimes fatal, generalized infection with focal and diffuse necrosis of the liver and adrenal glands (Kelly 1977). Rabbits experimentally infected with BHV-1 produced diverse manifestations comparable to those seen in cattle (Lupton, Barnes, and Reed 1980). Pigs experimentally inoculated with BHV-1 developed mild clinical signs and specific neutralizing antibodies (Neill et al. 1984). Experimental infection of neonatal skunks (*Mephitis mephitis*) with BHV-1 caused fatal viremic disease comparable to the syndrome in neonatal calves (Lupton, Jorgenson, and Reed 1980). BHV-1 established long-term persistent infection in intracerebrally inoculated athymic nude mice, and in vitro inoculation of outbred mouse spleen macrophages (Gerder et al. 1981). The transformed macrophages induced fibrosarcomas and cystic tumors in athymic nude mice.

The pathogenesis of the various forms of the disease in cattle caused by BHV-1 has been a subject of great interest. Viremia occurs with the dissemination of the virus throughout the body, yet systemic disease is seldom seen, except in neonates and aborted fetuses from susceptible cows. Encephalitis is believed to gain access to the brain from the oropharynx by way of the cranial nerves. Persistent infection that commonly occurs in cattle can be activated experimentally by synthetic and natural steroids, resulting in the release of virus in excretions such as semen (Davies and Carmichael 1973, Shetty and Davies 1972) and occasionally in recrudescence of disease (Davies and Duncan 1974).

Recrudescence of disease caused by dexamethasone and other steroids became a subject of great interest to investigators and practitioners because it raised four concerns: (1) the health of the recovered animal under subsequent stress, (2) the use of attenuated virus vaccines, (3) the transmission of the disease, and (4) the location of the virus in the recovered animal. Not all of these questions can be answered now, but there are some answers. In a single trial six latently infected calves shed virus after corticosteroid administration but failed to transmit BHV-1 during 4 weeks of contact with susceptible calves (Homan and Easterday 1983). BHV-1 DNA was demonstrated intranuclearly in trigeminal ganglion neurons by in situ hybridization and by immunofluorescence during recrudescence in the six latently infected calves. Because isolation of virus from excretions depends on the route of inoculation, BHV-1 initially given intranasally can be isolated from nasal excretions, but not from the vagina, 30 days after dexamethasone treatment. The reverse is true for heifers initially infected vaginally (Rossi et al. 1982). BHV-1 DNA could be demonstrated only in sacral ganglia during latency after intravaginal infection with a strain isolated from a cow with IPV (Ackermann and Wyler 1984). Bullocks recovered from BHV-1, when given *Dictyocaulus viviparus* larvae 5 months later, developed typical clinical signs and lesions of IBR, and virus was recovered (Msolla et al. 1983).

Concurrent infection with BHV-1 and bacteria such as *Pasteurella multocida* and *P. haemolytica* can cause more severe disease (Forman et al. 1982, Jericho and Carter 1985, Newman et al. 1982, Yates et al. 1983). Evidence suggests that stress such as physical exhaustion may cause physiological alterations that modulate cellular immunity and viral replication (Bilecha and Minocha 1983). When infection with bovine virus diarrhea virus precedes BHV-1 infection by 7 days the respiratory disease is more severe; this finding suggests that bovine virus diarrhea virus may impair the clearance of BHV-1 from the lungs (Potgieter et al. 1984).

The exposure of recently hatched bovine embryos to four different strains of BHV-1 caused embryonic infection and death and viral replication (Bowen et al. 1985). In contrast the exposure of 6- to 8-day-old bovine embryo transfers with intact zona pellucida to BHV-1 had no effect on the embryos, and there was no evidence of viral penetration through the intact zona pellucida (Gillespie et al. 1988, Hare 1985, Singh et al. 1982).

The characteristic lesions in cattle are the highly inflamed mucous membranes of the respiratory tract, with shallow erosions covered with a glairy, fetid, mucopurulent exudate. These lesions may be found also in the pharynx, larynx, trachea, and larger bronchi. There may be patchy, purulent pneumonia. Ulceration and inflammation of the abomasal mucosa are frequent, and catarrhal enteritis may involve both small and large intestines. Abscesses may form in the lungs and liver in animals with chronic cases. Renal infarction is seen in many animals that die of the disease. Reactivation of virus by dexamethasone treatment causes trigeminal ganglionitis consisting of many proliferated microglia and inflammatory cells (Narita et al. 1981). In calves this disease may manifest as meningoencephalitis. This should not be surprising because the pathogen is a herpesvirus, and other herpesviruses produce encephalitis in the young.

This versatile virus also has an affinity for mucous membranes and causes keratoconjunctivitis, usually without ulceration of the cornea (Abinanti and Plumer, 1961). Under certain circumstances field virus or attenuated virus vaccine produces abortions, usually in first-calf

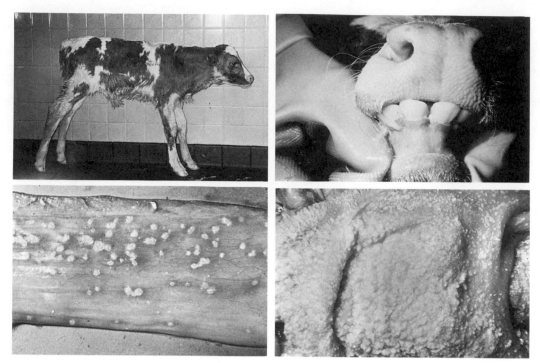

Figure 46.4. Acute infectious bovine rhinotracheitis–infectious pustular vulvovaginitis in infant calves. Calf in typical posture, with excessive salivation and pain (*top left*). Pustular lesions on gum, by margin of teeth (*top right*). Necrotic foci, distal portion of esophagus (*bottom left*). Diffuse necrosis in the rumen (*bottom right*). (From Baker et al., 1960, courtesy of *Cornell Veterinarian.*)

heifers in any stage of gestation (McKercher and Wada 1964). Abortions occur sometimes with no signs of illness in the dam.

Baker et al. (1960) produced a rather interesting form of the disease in experimental calves only a few days old by feeding, by intravenous injection, and by placing them in contact with infected calves (Figure 46.4). The characteristic pustular lesions, intranuclear inclusion bodies, and necrosis were found in the oral cavity, esophagus, and forestomachs. Necrotic foci were observed in the liver, lungs, and kidneys. Calves that survived the acute infection developed a chronic cough with ensuing pneumonia, but virus could no longer be isolated at this stage. Van Kruinigen and Bartholomew (1964) isolated BHV-1 from a natural case in a calf in contact with older animals suffering from the respiratory form of the disease. Postmortem examination revealed focal necrosis of the liver, necrosis of the suprapharyngeal lymph node, and necrosis of the rumen mucosa. In the epithelial cells of the respiratory tract inclusion bodies appear quite early in the course of the disease and disappear before it is fully developed.

In the vulva and vagina circumscribed, reddened areas become pustules that appear over the lymphatic follicles (Kendrick et al. 1958); many pustules coalesce, and a purulent exudate appears. Incomplete healing in some

cows results in a condition known as granular vulvovaginitis. Histologically there is a predominance of neutrophils and necrosis with a diffuse infiltration of lymphocytes in the connective tissue. Intranuclear bodies appear in the epithelial cells Figure 46.5).

The brain lesions in cases of meningoencephalitis are quite similar to changes described by French (1962). Intranuclear viral inclusions occur in the astrocytes and neurons. Perivascular edema and cuffing are common in the cerebrum. There are diffuse areas of degeneration of the cerebral cortex with vacuolation around the neurons. The superficial cortical lamina of the cerebrum may show rarefaction necrosis.

Aborted fetuses have some focal necrosis in the liver and spleen, and sometimes skin edema, but these findings are not consistent or severe enough to be pathognomonic (York 1968). Despite the widespread necrosis that occurs in the tissues of most aborted fetuses, there is little inflammation. Intranuclear inclusions may be seen in affected cells (Gibbs and Rweyemamu 1977).

If there is hematogenous spread of BHV-1 in heifers bred 7 or 14 days after infection, they develop mild oophoritis characterized by foci of necrosis and mononuclear cell accumulations in the corpus luteum (Miller and Van der Maaten 1986). Most heifers including those

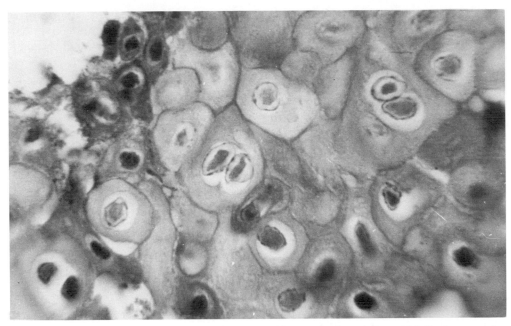

Figure 46.5. Inclusion bodies in the vulvar epithelium 48 hours after inoculation with infectious pustular vulvovaginitis virus (BHV-1). Two of the inclusion-bearing cells contain double nuclei. Schleifstein's Negri body stain. × 900. (From Kendrick et al., 1958, courtesy of *Cornell Veterinarian*.)

given virus 21 and 28 days after breeding, also had a few necrotic follicles in at least one ovary. Virus was isolated from a few of the affected tissues. Heifers inoculated 14 days after breeding were not pregnant at necropsy; but there was histological evidence that the cycle was longer than normal, suggesting early embryonic death. When the virus was administered by aerosol transmission to four heifers, no lesions or virus were found in the ovaries (Van der Maaten and Miller 1985).

Immunity. The immune response of cattle to BHV-1 can be attributed to antibody and cell-mediated components (Gibbs and Rweyemamu 1977, Wilkie 1982). Cattle that recover from natural disease are relatively resistant to challenge by any strain of BHV-1 regardless of the tissue from which it is isolated (Gillespie et al. 1959) and despite the latency of virus in local nerves (Castrucci et al. 1984). The duration of immunity is long term, although recrudescence and viral shedding usually occur after four or five treatments with corticosteroids on consecutive days.

Cattle immunized with attenuated or virulent virus are immune to challenge 3 to 4 weeks later with virulent virus instilled intranasally or intravaginally. A few transient lesions in the vulva and vagina have been observed after intravaginal instillation of a massive dose of virulent virus, but no fever results (Kendrick et al. 1958). The presence of neutralizing antibody has been correlated with protection against clinical signs of illness. An animal with

measurable neutralizing antibody against 100 tissue-cultured infective doses ($TCID_{50}$) is immune. Titers occasionally reach 1:256, with the average ranging between 1:8 and 1:64. Higher titers can be achieved by adding complement (Rossi and Kiesel 1974). The constant serum-varying virus neutralization test (House and Baker 1971) is reasonably sensitive in the detection of antibody. Neutralizing antibody can be detected on or about 7 days after infection, and the primary immune response is characterized by IgM and IgG antibodies in serum by day 7. Maximum IgG titer occurred after 35 days in nonpregnant heifers and after 14 days in pregnant heifers, with slow declines thereafter. Maximum IgM titers occurred at day 14 in open and pregnant heifers and declined rapidly thereafter (Guy and Potgieter 1985). Secondary responses to viral re-exposure involved IgG_2 as well as IgG_1 appearance and the reappearance of IgM. The latent virus state in all likelihood accounts for persisting neutralizing antibody in most animals, but re-exposure to virus resulting in reinfection without disease manifestations cannot be entirely dismissed.

Maternal neutralizing antibodies are readily detected in serum of calves from immune dams. The serum titers of dams are low and sometimes persist until the calf is 4 months old. Maternal antibody can interfere with production of active immunity and must be considered in a herd vaccination program.

In the past the role of antibody in the protection against

herpesviruses was questioned because these viruses spread from cell to cell by intracellular bridges (Christian and Ludovici 1971). Serum antibodies mediate virus neutralization and destroy virus-infected cells by two immune mechanisms (1) antibody and complement-mediated lysis and (2) antibody-dependent cell-mediated cytotoxicity (Van Drunen Littel–van den Hurk and Babiuk 1986). The role of secretory antibody in protecting the superficial epithelial tissues involved in some forms of the disease has not been defined. Babiuk and his group have studied extensively the mechanism of cell-mediated immunity associated with BHV-1 (Bielefeldt Ohmann and Babiuk 1985, 1986; Forman and Babiuk 1982; Grewal and Babiuk 1980; Rouse and Babiuk 1975; Rouse et al. 1980). To show the role of cell-mediated immunity and its synergistic role with *Pasteurella* organisms in cattle pneumonia, Rouse and Babiuk (1975) developed a viral plaque inhibition assay test that showed that blood lymphocytes from immune animals prevented viral plaque formation in cell monolayers infected with BHV-1. The reaction is specific and involves suppression of viral replication rather than the destruction of virus or virus-infected cells. A lymphokine produced by cooperation of macrophages and T-cell lymphocytes from immune animals is involved in the process. This phenomenon has been described as "immune interferon," not to be confused with interferon, which differs both in its mode of origin and in its biochemical and biophysical characteristics. The ability of bovine alveolar macrophages to participate in antibody-dependent cell toxicity is dramatically reduced within 2 hours after GHV-1 infection before morphologic cellular changes are apparent. Polymorphonuclear neutrophils in the presence of complement are also involved in cell-mediated immunity. Defective neutrophil and alveolar macrophage functions (McGuire and Babiuk 1984) as well as a lack of helper cell activity and development of suppressor cells by BHV-1 help to explain the interaction between the virus and *Pasteurella* organisms in the production and degree of pulmonary infection.

Interferon production to BHV-1 has been demonstrated in cattle (MacLachlan and Rosenquist 1982, Rosenquist and Loan 1969). Interferon produced by an interferon inducer administered 3 hours before infection reduced the severity of disease in calves, compared with untreated animals (Theil et al. 1971). Fasting enhanced the ability of calves to produce interferon; it was not produced in response to increased BHV-1 replication (d'Offay and Rosenquist 1986).

The levels of interferon in serum and the toxicity of *E. coli*–derived bovine alpha-1 interferon in dairy calves after intranasal, intramuscular, subcutaneous, and intravenous administration interferon (10^6 U/kg of body weight) were reported by Gillespie et al. (1986). The highest serum levels (10,000 U/ml) in the vesicular stomatitis viral assay system were obtained after intravenous administration, occurred within 30 minutes of one dose, and rapidly declined thereafter to insignificant levels by 24 hours. Levels after intramuscular and subcutaneous adminstration were five to ten times lower, with a plateau of 1,000–2,000 U/ml between 2 and 8 hours after one dose and a decline to insignificant levels by 24 hours. Serum interferon was not detected after intranasal dosing or in the control group given physiological buffered saline intramuscularly. A transitory, moderate fever, but no other clinical adverse effects, occurred after the first intramuscular dose, but not after subsequent doses at 1-day intervals for 5 days. No clinical signs were noted after intravenous, subcutaneous, or intranasal dosing or in the control calves. After intravenous, subcutaneous, and intramuscular administration, leukopenia, neutropenia, and lymphocytopenia were observed; these were most prominent within the first 24 hours after the initial dose.

In vitro protective effect of *E. coli*–derived bovine alpha-1 interferon against various strains of BHV-1 was of a low order (Babiuk et al. 1985, Gillespie et al. 1985). This same interferon product did not prevent respiratory disease when administered intranasally to experimental cattle slightly before or at the time of aerosol exposure to BHV-1, but ameliorated the resulting disease when compared to the controls with lesser signs of illness and a delayed incubation period (Babiuk et al. 1985; F.W. Scott, J.H. Gillespie, and C. Geissinger, 1987, unpublished data). There is some evidence that human leukocyte A interferon produces a comparable effect in experimental calves exposed to BHV-1 by the respiratory route (Roney et al. 1985).

Diagnosis. Quite frequently diagnosis can be rendered on the basis of the history and character of the disease. Confirmation of the field diagnosis may necessitate isolation of the virus.

Specimens for virus isolation should be collected from body systems displaying the signs and pathological lesions. Because calcium alginate wool swabs inactivate BHV-1, cotton or polyester swabs should be used (Hanson and Schipper 1976). Virus is readily isolated from specimens taken during the febrile stage of the infection by immunofluorescence and immunoperoxidase tests, by enzyme-linked immunosorbent assay (ELISA) and in cell culture (Edwards et al. 1983). Virus also has been isolated from the thoracic cavity fluid of aborted fetuses and from cotyledons, but not often.

BHV-1 is readily isolated on bovine kidney cells in tissue culture. It may also be recovered on swine tissue-cultured kidney cells (Cabasso et al. 1957, Schwarz et al.

1957). Many cell lines are susceptible; the most commonly used one is the bovine turbinate cell line. The virus can be identified tentatively by its rapid and characteristic cytolytic effects, and also by neutralization and fluorescent antibody tests with tissue culture cells as indicators.

Many other serologic tests are used to detect antibody: ELISA, passive hemagglutination (Kirby et al. 1974), complement fixation, agar-gel diffusion, and the direct and indirect fluorescent antibody. Most recent studies involve the improvement of micro and macro ELISAs as a rapid method of viral antigen detection and also for detection of antibody (Beccaria et al. 1982; Collins, Bulla, et al. 1985; Collins, Butcher, and Riegel 1985; Collins, Butcher, Teramoto, and Winston 1985; Darcel and Kozub 1984, Florent and de Marneffe 1986; Herbert et al. 1985). The ELISA is a more sensitive method for detecting antibody than the serum neutralization test.

DNA restriction endonuclease analyses patterns of field isolates could serve as a method for investigating epizootics of BHV-1 (Whetstone et al. 1986).

Cutaneous rections to BHV-1 occur in cattle (Darcell and Dorwood 1975). The accuracy and usefulness of this skin test as a simple diagnostic tool under field conditions have not been evaluated.

Prevention and Control. Numerous types of vaccines have been proposed for the prevention and control of BHV-1 disease in cattle. An attenuated vaccine modified by serial passage in cell culture was effective but not without some question about its safety and transmission (Sheffy and Rodman 1973). Inactivated virus vaccines circumvent the problem of safety and latency, but the duration of immunity is difficult to evaluate since antibodies are not always detectable. Yet field evidence suggests that inactivated virus vaccines are useful if periodic booster immunizations are given annually (Soulebot et al. 1982, Sweat 1983). If inactivated virus vaccine does not provide adequate protection against field exposure to BHV-1, mild disease may ensue with resulting viral latency (Frerichs et al. 1982).

More recently temperature-sensitive vaccines have been prepared through selection of temperature-sensitive mutant clones (Pastoret et al. 1980, Rossi and Kiesel 1982), but dexamethasone treatment produced latency and viral shedding.

There seems to be greater promise in using subunit vaccine that incorporates one or more of the envelope glycoproteins that induce high serum-neutralizing antibody titers without the production of latency in the cattle. These subunit vaccines are safe and provide protection upon challenge with virulent virus (Lupton and Reed 1980, Van Drunen Littel–van den Hurk and Babiuk 1985). There is evidence that thymidine kinase–negative

BHV-1 mutant is safe and efficacious (Kit et al. 1985, 1986). Experimentally vaccinated cattle did not show signs of illness, developed neutralizing antibodies, and resisted challenge with virulent virus. The TK-1 mutant could be isolated from the respective tracts after intranasal or intravaginal administration of vaccine and again, after five treatments with dexamethansone, from the tract into which the vaccine was originally introduced.

In one large field trial preimmunization with vaccine given at the farm failed to significantly reduce the overall treatment rate in calves entering feedlots (Martin et al. 1983), but then perhaps BHV-1 was not the only pathogen involved in the respiratory syndrome.

Vaccination of sheep with a multiple vaccine including BHV-1 is a questionable practice (Lehmkuhl and Cutlip 1985).

For a herd health program including BHV-1 immunization, see the report of the panel for the American Veterinary Medical Association Symposium on Immunity to the Bovine Respiratory Disease Complex (Gillespie et al. 1968).

The Disease in Humans. BHV-1 is not pathogenic for humans.

REFERENCES

Abinanti, F.K., and Plumer, G.J. 1961. The isolation of infectious bovine rhinotracheitis virus from cattle affected with conjunctivitis— Observations on experimental infection. Am. J. Vet. Res. 22:13–17.

Ackermann, M., and Wyler, R. 1984. The DNA of an IPV strain of bovid herpesvirus 1 in sacral ganglia during latency after intravaginal infection. Vet. Microbiol. 9:53–63.

Armstrong, J.A., Pereira, H.G., and Andrews, C.H. 1961. Observations on the virus of infectious bovine rhinotracheitis, and its affinity with the herpesvirus group. Virology 14:276–285.

Babiuk, L.A., Bielefeldt Ohmann, H., Gifford, G., Czarniek, C.W., Scialli, V.T., and Hamilton, E.D. 1985. Effect of bovine alpha 1 interferon on bovine herpesvirus type 1–induced respiratory disease. J. Gen. Virol. 66:2383–2394.

Baker, J.A., McEntee, K., and Gillespie, J.H. 1960. Effects of infectious bovine rhinotracheitis–infectious pustular vulvovaginitis (IBR-IPV) virus on newborn calves. Cornell Vet. 50:156–170.

Beccaria, E., Ferrari, A., Nachtmann, C., Boniolo, A., Bovis, M., Zannino, M., and Petruzzelli, E. 1982. Rapid detection of antibodies to infectious bovine rhinotracheitis by 'macro' and 'micro' ELISA. Dev. Biol. Stand. 52:141–146.

Berrios, P.E., and McKercher, D.G. 1975. Characterization of a caprine herpesvirus. Am. J. Vet. Res. 36:1755–1762.

Bielefeldt Ohmann, H., and Babiuk, L.A. 1985. Viral-bacterial pneumonia in calves: Effect of bovine herpes virus-1 on immunologic functions. J. Infect. Dis. 151:937–947.

Bielefeldt Ohmann, H., and Babiuk, L.A. 1986. Alteration of alveolar macrophage functions after aerosol infection with bovine herpesvirus type 1. Infect. Immun. 51:344–347.

Bilecha, F., and Minocha, H.C. 1983. Suppressed lymphocyte blastogenic responses and enhanced in vitro growth of infectious bovine rhinotracheitis virus in stressed feeder calves. Am. J. Vet. Res. 44:2145–2148.

Bowen, R.A., Elsden, R.P., and Seidel, G.E., Jr. 1985. Infection of early bovine embryos with bovine herpesvirus-1. Am. J. Vet. Res. 46:1095–1097.

Bush, C.E., and Pritchett, R.F. 1985. A comparison of the genomes of bovine herpesvirus type 1 and pseudorabies virus. J. Gen. Virol. 66:1811–1817.

Bush, C.E., and Pritchett, R.F. 1986. Immunologic comparison of the proteins of pseudorabies (Aujeszky's disease) virus and bovine herpesvirus-1. Am. J. Vet. Res. 47:1708–1712.

Cabasso, V.J., Brown, R.G., and Cox, H.R. 1957. Infectious bovine rhinotracheitis (IBR). I. Propagation of virus in cancer cells of human origin (HeLa). Proc. Soc. Exp. Biol. Med. 95:471–476.

Carmichael, L.E., and Barnes, F.D. 1961. The relationship of infectious bovine rhinotracheitis virus to equine rhinopneumonitis virus. Proc. U.S. Livestock Sanit. Assoc. 65:384–388.

Castrucci, G., Frigeri, F., Ranucci, S., Ferrari, M., Cilli, V., Pedini, B., Nettleton, P., Caleffi, F., Aldrovandi, V., and Herring, A.J. 1984. Comparative studies of strains of infectious bovine rhinotracheitis virus isolated from latently infected calves. Comp. Immunol. Microbiol. Infect. Dis. 7:1–10.

Chang, L.W., Zee, Y.C., Pritchett, R.F., and Ardans, A.A. 1986. Neutralizing monoclonal antibodies directed to infectious bovine rhinotracheitis virus. Arch. Virol. 88:203–215.

Cheatham, W.J., and Crandell, R.A. 1957. Occurrence of intranuclear inclusions in tissue cultures infected with virus of infectious bovine rhinotracheitis. Proc. Soc. Exp. Biol. Med. 96:536–538.

Chow, T.L., Mollelo, J.A., and Owen, N.V. 1964. Abortion experimentally induced in cattle by infectious bovine rhinotracheitis virus. J. Am. Vet. Med. Assoc. 144:1005–1007.

Christian, R.T., and Ludovici, P.P. 1971. Cell-to-cell transmission of herpes simplex virus in primary human amnion cells (36061). Proc. Soc. Exp. Biol. Med. 138:1109–1115.

Collins, J.K., Bulla, G.A., Riegel, C.A., and Butcher, A.C. 1985. A single dilution enzyme-linked immunosorbent assay for the quantitative detection of antibodies to bovine herpesvirus type 1. Vet. Mircrobiol. 10:133–147.

Collins, J.K., Butcher, A.C., and Riegel, C.A. 1985. Immune response to bovine herpes herpesvirus type 1 infections: Virus-specific antibodies in sera from infected animals. J. Clin. Microbiol. 21:546–552.

Collins, J.K., Butcher, A.C., Teramoto, Y.A., and Winston, S. 1985. Rapid detection of bovine herpesvirus type 1 antigens in nasal swab specimens with an antigen capture enzyme-linked immunosorbent assay. J. Clin. Microbiol. 21:375–380.

Crandell, R.A., Melloh, A.J., and Sorlie, P. 1975. Sensitivity of infectious bovine rhinotracheitis virus to ether. J. Clin. Microbiol. 2:465–468.

Darcel, C. le A., and Dorwood, W.J. 1975. Recovery of infectious bovine rhinotracheitis virus following corticosteroid treatment of vaccinated animals. Can. Vet. J. 16:87–88.

Darcel, C.L., and Kozeib, S.C. 1984. The effect on kaolin adsorption of serum on the virus neutralization and enzyme-linked immunosorbent assays of antibody to bovine herpesvirus 1. J. Biol. Stand. 12:87–92.

Davies, D.H., and Carmichael, L.E. 1973. Role of cell-mediated immunity in the recovery of cattle from primary and recurrent infections with infectious bovine rhinotracheitis virus. Infect. Immun. 8:510–518.

Davies, D.H., and Duncan, J.R. 1974. The pathogenesis of recurrent infections with infectious bovine rhinotracheitis virus induced in calves by treatment with corticosteroids. Cornell Vet. 64:340–366.

Derbyshire, J.B., and Caplan, B.A. 1976. The isolation and characterization of a strain of infectious bovine rhinotracheitis virus from still birth in swine. Can. J. Comp. Med. 40:252–256.

d'Offay, J.M., and Rosenquist, B.D. 1986. Interferon production and replication of infectious bovine rhinotracheitis virus in fasted calves. J. Interferon Res. 6:79–84.

Edwards, S., Chasey, D., and White, H. 1983. Experimental infectious bovine rhinotracheitis: Comparison of four antigen detection methods. Res. Vet. Sci. 34:42–45.

Engels, M., Gelderblom, H. Darai, G., and Ludwig, H. 1983. Goat herpesviruses: Biological and physiochemical properties. J. Gen. Virol. 64:2237–2247.

Florent, G., and de Marneffe, C. 1986. Enzyme linked immunosorbent assay used to monitor serum antibodies to bovine respiratory disease viruses. Vet. Microbiol. 11:309–317.

Forman, A.J., and Babiuk, L.A. 1982. Effect of infectious bovine rhinotracheitis virus infection on bovine alveolar macrophage function. Infect. Immun. 35:1041–1047.

Forman, A.J., Babiuk, L.A., Baldwin, F., and Friend, S.C. 1982. Effect of infectious bovine rhinotracheitis virus infection of calves on cell populations recovered by lung lavage. Am. J. Vet. Res. 43:1174–1179.

French, E.L. 1962. Relationship between infectious bovine rhinotracheitis (IBR) virus and a virus isolated from calves with encephalitis. Aust. Vet. Sci. 38:555–556.

Frerichs, G.N., Woods, S.B., Lucas, M.H., and Sands, J.J. 1982. Safety and efficacy of live and inactivated infectious bovine rhinotracheitis vaccines. Vet. Rec. 111:116–122.

Gerder, L., Lee, K.J., Dawson, M.S., Engle, R., Maliniak, R.M., and Lang, C.M. 1981. Induction of persistent infection in mice and oncogenic transformation of mouse macrophages with infectious bovine rhinotracheitis virus. Am. J. Vet. Res. 42:300–307.

Gibbs, E.P.J., and Rweyemamu, M.M. 1977. Bovine herpesvirus. I. Bovine herpesvirus 1. II. Bovine herpesvirus 2 and 3. Vet. Bull. 47:317–343, 411–425.

Gillespie, J.H., Foote, R.H., Schlafer, D.H., Quick, S., Dougherty, E., Schiff, E., and Allen, S. 1988. In press.

Gillespie, J.H., Jensen, R., McKercher, D., Peacock, G., Briston, R., Casselberry, N.H., Collier, J.R., Fox, F.H., Heijl, J., Mackey, D.R., Oberst, F., Pope, E.A., Jones, L.M., Freeman, A., and Bieber, L. 1968. Report of the panel for the Symposium on Immuity to the Bovine Respiratory Disease Complex. J. Am. Vet. Med. Assoc. 152:713–719.

Gillespie, J.H., Lee, K.M., and Baker, J.A. 1957. Infectious bovine rhinotracheitis. Am. J. Vet. Res. 18:530–535.

Gillespie, J.H., McEntee, K., Kendrick, J.W., and Wagner, W.C. 1959. Comparison of infectious pustular vulvovaginitis virus with infectious bovine rhinotracheitis virus. Cornell Vet. 49:288–297.

Gillespie, J.H., Robson, D.S., Scott, F.W., and Schiff, E.I. 1985. In vitro protective effect of bacteria-derived bovine alpha interferon Il against selected bovine viruses. J. Clin. Microbiol. 22:912–914.

Gillespie, J.H., Scott, F.W., Geissinger, C.M., Czarniecki, C.W., and Scialli, V.T. 1986. Levels of interferon in blood serum and toxicity studies of bacteria-derived bovine alpha-1 interferon in dairy calves. J. Clin. Microbiol. 24:240–244.

Grewal, A.S., and Babiuk, L.A. 1980. Complement-dependent, polymorphonuclear neutrophil-mediated cytotoxicity of herpesvirus-infected cells: Possible mechanism(s) of cytotoxicity. Immunology 40:151–161.

Griffin, T.P., Howells, W.V., R.A., Crandell, and F.D. Maurer. 1958. Stability of the virus of infectious bovine rhinotracheitis. Am. J. Vet. Res. 19:990–992.

Guy, J.S., and Potgieter, L.N. 1985. Bovine herpesvirus-1 infection of cattle: Kinetics of antibody formation after intranasal exposure and abortion induced by the virus. Am. J. Vet. Res. 46:893–898.

Guy, J.S., Potgieter, L.N., McCracken, M., and Martin, W. 1984. Isolation of bovine herpesvirus-1 from vesicular lesions of the bovine udder. Am. J. Vet. Res. 45:783–785.

Hanson, B.R., and Schipper, I.A. 1976. Effects of swab materials on infectious bovine rhinotracheitis virus. Am. J. Vet. Res. 37:707–708.

Hare, W.S.D. 1985. Diseases transmissible by semen and embryo transfer techniques. Technical Series no. 4. Office International Epizooties, Paris. Pp. 1–117.

Herbert, C.N,. Edwards, S., Bushnell, S., Jones, P.C., and Perry, C.T. 1985. Establishment of a statistical base for use of ELISA in diagnostic serology for infectious bovine rhinotracheitis. J. Biol. Stand. 13:243–253.

Homan, E.J., and Easterday, B.C. 1983. Experimental latent and recrudescent bovine herpesvirus-1 infections in calves. Am. J. Vet. Res. 44:309–313.

House, J.A., and Baker, J.A. 1971. Bovine herpesvirus IBR-IPV. The antibody virus neutralization reaction. Cornell Vet. 61:320–335.

Jericho, K.W., and Carter, G.R. 1985. Pneumonia in calves produced with aerosols of *Pasteurella multocida* alone and in combination with bovine herpesvirus 1. Can. J. Comp. Med. 49:138–144.

Kelly, D.F. 1977. Experimental infection of rabbits with the virus of infectious bovine rhinotracheitis. Br. J. Exp. Pathol. 58:168–176.

Kendrick, J.W., Gillespie, J.H., and McEntee, K. 1958. Infectious pustular vulvovaginitis of cattle. Cornell Vet. 48:458–495.

Kirby, F.D., Martin, H.T., and Ostler, D.C. 1974. An indirect hemagglutination test for the detection and assay of antibody to infectious bovine rhinotracheitis virus. Vet. Rec. 94:361–362.

Kit, S., and Qavi, H. 1983. Thymidine kinase (TK) induction after infection of TK-deficient rabbit cell mutants with bovine herpesvirus type 1 (BHV-1): Isolation of TK-BHV-1 mutants. Virology 130:381–389.

Kit, S., Kit, M., and McConnell, S. 1986. Intramuscular and intravaginal vaccination of pregnant cows with thymidine kinase-negative, temperature-resistant infectious bovine rhinotracheitis virus (bovine herpesvirus 1). Vaccine 4:55–61.

Kit, S., Qavi, H., Gaines, J.D., Billingsley, P., and McConnell, S. 1985. Thymidine kinase-negative bovine herpesvirus type 1 mutant is stable and highly attenuated in calves. Arch. Virol. 86:63–83.

Lawrence, W.C., D'urso, R.C., Kundel, C.A., Whitbeck, J.C., and Bello, L.J. 1986. Map location of the gene for a 130,000-dalton glycoprotein of bovine herpesvirus 1. J. Virol. 60:405–414.

Lehmkuhl, H.D., and Cutlip, R.C. 1985. Protection from parainfluenza-3 virus and persistence of infectious bovine rhinotracheitis virus in sheep vaccinated with a modified live IBR-PI-3 vaccine. Can. J. Comp. Med. 49:58–62.

Lui, K.Y., and Manning, J.S. 1986. Identification of the thymidine kinase gene of infectious bovine rhinotracheitis virus and its function in *Escherichia coli* hosts. Gene 44:279–285.

Lupton, H.W., and Reed, D.E. 1980. Evaluation of experimental subunit vaccines for infectious bovine rhinotracheitis. Am. J. Vet. Res. 41:383–390.

Lupton, H.W., Barnes, H.J., and Reed, D.E. 1980. Evaluation of the rabbit as a laboratory model for infectious bovine rhinotracheitis virus infection. Cornell Vet. 70:77–95.

Lupton, H.W., Jorgenson, R.D., and Reed, D.E. 1980. Experimental infection of neonatal striped skunks (*Mephitis mephitis*) with infectious bovine rhinotracheitis virus. J. Wildl. Dis. 16:117–123.

McGuire, R.L., and Babiuk, L.A. 1984. Evidence for defective neutrophil function in lungs of calves exposed to infectious bovine rhinotracheitis virus. Vet. Immunol. Immunopathol. 5:259–271.

McKercher, D.G. 1959. Infectious bovine rhinotracheitis. Adv. Vet. Sci. 5:299–328.

McKercher, D.G., and Wada, E.M. 1964. The virus of infectious bovine rhinotracheitis as a cause of abortion in cattle. J. Am. Vet. Med. Assoc. 144:136–142.

MacLachlan, N.J., and Rosenquist, B.D. 1982. Duration of protection of calves against rhinovirus challenge exposure by infectious bovine rhinotracheitis virus-induced interferon in nasal secretions. Am. J. Vet. Res. 43:289–293.

Madin, S.H., York, C.J., and McKercher, D.G. 1956. Isolation of the infectious bovine rhinotracheitis virus. Science 124:721–722.

Marshall, R.L., Rodriguez, L.L., and Letchworth, G.J. 1986. Characterization of envelope proteins of infectious bovine rhinotracheitis virus (bovine herpesvirus 1) by biochemical and immunological methods. J. Virol. 57:745–753.

Martin, W., Willson, P., Curtis, R., Allen, B., and Acres, S. 1983. A field trial, of preshipment vaccination, with intranasal infectious bovine rhinotracheitis–parainfluenza-3 vaccines. Can. J. Comp. Med. 47:245–249.

Metzler, A.E., Matile, H., Gassmann, L.L., Engels, M., and Wyler, R. 1985. European isolates of bovine herpesvirus 1: A comparison of restriction endonuclease sites, polypeptides, and reactivity with monoclonal antibodies. Arch. Virol. 85:57–69.

Metzler, A.E., Schudel, A.A., and Engels, M. 1986. Bovine herpesvirus 1: Molecular and antigenic characteristics of variant viruses isolated from calves with neurological disease. Arch. Virol. 87:205–217.

Michalski, F.J., and Hsiung, G.D. 1976. Persistent infection with bovine herpesvirus-1 (infectious bovine rhinotracheitis virus) in cultured hamster cells. In Vitro 12:682–686.

Miller, J.M., and Van der Maaten, M.J. 1986. Experimentally induced infectious bovine rhinotracheitis virus infection during early pregnancy: Effect on the bovine corpus luteum and conceptus. Am. J. Vet. Res. 47:223–228.

Mohanty, S.B., Lillio, M.G., Corselius, N.P., and Beck, J.D. 1972. Natural infection with infectious bovine rhinotracheitis virus in goats. J. Am. Vet. Med. Assoc. 160:879–880.

Msolla, P.M., Allan, E.M., Selman, I.E., and Wiseman, A. 1983. Reactivation and shedding of bovine herpesvirus 1 following *Dictyocaulus viviparus* infection. J. Comp. Pathol. 93:271–274.

Narita, M., Inui, S., Nanba, K., and Shimizu, Y. 1981. Recrudescence of infectious bovine rhinotracheitis virus and associated neural changes in calves treated with dexamethasone. Am. J. Vet. Res. 42:1192–1197.

Neill, J.D., Kelling, C.L., and Rhodes, M.B. 1984. Specificity of pseudorabies virus serotests. Am. J. Vet. Res. 45:2675–2676.

Newman, P.R., Corstvet, R.E., and Panciera, R.J. 1982. Distribution of *Pasteurella haemolytica* and *Pasturella multocida* in the bovine lung following vaccination and challenge exposure as an indicator of lung resistance. Am. J. Vet. Res. 43:417–422.

Pastoret, P.P., Babiuk, L.A., Misra, V., and Griebel, P. 1980. Reactivation of temperature-sensitive infectious bovine rhinotracheitis vaccine virus with dexamethasone. Infect. Immun. 29:483–488.

Potgieter, L.N., McCracken, M.D., Hopkins, F.M., and Walker, R.D. 1984. Effect of bovine viral diarrhea virus infection on the distribution of infectious bovine rhinotracheitis virus in calves. Am. J. Vet. Res. 45:687–690.

Roney, C.S., Rossi, C.R., Smith, P.C., Lauerman, L.C., Spano, J.S., Hanrahan, L.A., and William, J.C. 1985. Effect of human leukocyte A interferon on prevention of infectious bovine rhinotracheitis virus infection of cattle. Am. J. Vet. Res. 46.1251–1255.

Rosenquist, B.D., and Loan, R.W. 1969. Interferon induction in the bovine species by infectious bovine rhinotracheitis virus. Am. J. Vet. Res. 30:1305–1312.

Rossi, C.K., and Kiesel, G.K. 1974. Complement-requiring neutralizing antibodies in cattle to infectious bovine rhinotracheitis virus. Arch. Gesam. Virusforsch. 45:328–334.

Rossi, C.R., and Kiesel, G.K. 1982. Effect of infectious bovine rhinotracheitis virus immunization on viral shedding in challenge-exposed calves treated with dexamethasone. Am. J. Vet. Res. 43:1576–1579.

Rossi, C.R., Kiesel, G.K., and Rumph, P.F. 1982. Association between route of inoculation with infectious bovine rhinotracheitis virus and site of recrudescence after dexamethasone treatment. Am. J. Vet. Res. 43:1440–1442.

Rouse, B.T., and Babiuk, L.A. 1975. Host defense mechanisms against infectious bovine rhinotracheitis virus. II. Inhibition of viral plaque formation by immune peripheral blood lymphocytes. Cell Immunol. 17:43–56.

Rouse, B.T., Babiuk, L.A., and Henson, P.M. 1980. Neutrophils in antiviral immunity: Inhibition of virus replication by a mediator produced by bovine neutrophils. J. Infect. Dis. 141:223–232.

Schwarz, A.J.F., York, C.J., Zirbel, L.W., and Esteala, L.A. 1957. Modification of infectious bovine rhinotracheitis (IBR) virus in tissue culture and development of a vaccine. Proc. Soc. Exp. Biol. Med. 96:453–458.

Seal, B.S., St. Jeor, S.C., and Taylor, R.E. 1985. Restriction endonuclease analysis of bovine herpesvirus 1 DNA and nucleic acid homology between isolates. J. Gen. Virol. 66:2787–2792.

Sheffy, B.E., and Davies, D.H. 1972. Reaction of a bovine herpesvirus after corticosteroid treatment. Proc. Soc. Exp. Biol. Med. 140:974–976.

Sheffy, B.E., and Rodman, S. 1973. Activation of latent infectious bovine rhinotracheitis infection. J. Am. Vet. Med. Assoc. 163:850–851.

Shroyer, E.L., and Easterday, B.C. 1968. Growth of infectious bovine rhinotracheitis virus in organ cultures. Am. J. Vet. Res. 29:1355–1362.

Singh, E.L., Thomas, F.C., Englesome, M.D., Papp-Ved, G., and Hare, W.C.D. 1982. Embryo transfer as a means of controlling the transmission of viral infections. II. The in vitro exposure of pre-implantation embryos to infectious bovine rhinotracheitis virus. Theriogenology 18:13–140.

Soulebot, J.P., Guillemin, F., Brun, A., Dubourget, P., Espinasse, J., and Terre, J. 1982. Infectious bovine rhinotracheitis: Study on the experimentally induced disease and its prevention using an inactivated, adjuvanted vaccine. Dev. Biol. Stand. 52:463–483.

Stauber, E.H., Autenrieth, R., Markham, O.D., and Whitbeck, V. 1980. A seroepidemiologic survey of three pronghorn (*Antilocapra americana*) populations in southeastern Idaho, 1975–1977. J. Wildl. Dis. 16:109–115.

Studdert, M.J., Wada, E.M., Kortum, W.M., and Goverman, F.A. 1964. Bovine infectious pustular vulvovaginitis in the western United States. J. Am. Vet. Med. Assoc. 144:615–619.

Sweat, R.L. 1983. Persistence of antibodies and anamnestic response in calves vaccinated with inactivated infectious bovine rhinotracheitis virus and parainfluenza-3 virus vaccines. J. Am. Vet. Med. Assoc. 182:809–811.

Theil, K.W., Mohanty, S.B., Hetrick, F.M. 1971. Intracellular localization and sequential development of infectious bovine rhinotracheitis viral antigens. Am. J. Vet. Res. 32:1955–1962.

Theodoridis, A. 1985. Studies on bovine herpesviruses. I. Isolation and characterization of viruses isolated from the genital tract of cattle. Onderstepoort J. Vet. Res. 52:239–254.

Tousimis, A.J., Howells, W.V., Griffin, T.P., Porter, R.P., Cheatham, W.J., and Mauer, F.D. 1958. Biophysical characterization of infectious bovine rhinotracheitis virus. Proc. Sci. Exp. Biol. Med. 99:614–617.

Trepanier, P., Minocha, H.C., Bastien, Y., Nadon, F., Seguin, C., Lussier, G., and Trudel, M. 1986. Bovine herpesvirus 1: Strain comparison of polypeptides and identification of a neutralization epitope on the 90-kilodalton hemagglutinin. J. Virol. 60:302–306.

Van der Maaten, M.J., and Miller, J.M. 1985. Ovarian lesions in heifers exposed to infectious bovine rhinotracheitis virus by non-genital routes on the day after breeding. Vet. Microbiol. 10:155–163.

Van Drunen Littel–van den Hurk, S., and Babiuk, L.A. 1985. Antigenic and immunogenic characteristics of bovine herpesivrus type-1 glycoproteins GVP 3/9 and GVP 6/11a/16, purified by immunoadsorbent chromatography. Virology 144:204–215.

Van Drunen Littel–van den Hurk, S., and Babiuk, L.A. 1986a. Polypeptide specificity of the antibody response after primary and recurrent infection with bovine herpesvirus 1. J. Clin. Microbiol. 23:274–282.

Van Drunen Littel–van den Hurk, S., and Babiuk, L.A. 1986b. Synthesis and processing of bovine herpesvirus 1 glycoproteins. J. Virol. 59:401–410.

Van Kruiningen, H.J., and Bartholomew, R.C. 1964. Infectious bovine rhinotracheitis diagnosed by lesions in a calf. J. Am. Vet. Med. Assoc. 144:1008–1012.

Wafula, J.S., Mushi, E.Z., and Wamwayi, H. 1985. Reaction of goats to infection with infectious bovine rhinotracheitis virus. Res. Vet. Sci. 39:84–86.

Whetstone, C.A., Wheeler, J.G., and Reed, D.E. 1986. Investigation of possible vaccine-induced epizootics of infectious bovine rhinotracheitis, using restriction endonuclease analysis of viral DNA. Am. J. Vet. Res. 47:1789–1795.

Wilkie, B.N. 1982. Respiratory tract immune response to microbial pathogens. J. Am. Vet. Med. Assoc. 181:1074–1079.

Yates, W.D., Jericho, K.W., and Doige, C.E. 1983. Effect of bacterial

dose on pneumonia induced by aerosol exposure of calves to bovine herpesvirus-1 and *Pasteurella haemolytica*. Am. J. Vet. Res. 44:238–243.

York, C.J. 1968. Infectious bovine rhinotracheitis. J. Am. Vet. Med. Assoc. 152:758–760.

York, C.J., Schwartz, A.J.F., and Estella, L.A. 1957. Isolation and identification of infectious bovine rhinotracheitis virus in tissue culture. Proc. Soc. Exp. Biol. 94:740–744.

Zarnke, R.L., and Yuill, T.M. 1981. Serologic survey for selected microbial agents in mammals from Alberta, 1976. J. Wildl. Dis. 17:453–461.

Bovine Ulcerative Mammillitis

The Allerton virus strain was first isolated in 1957 from animals with lumpy skin disease in South Africa by Alexander et al. (1957). It now is known that the Allerton strain does not cause lumpy skin disease; a poxvirus does. In Ruanda-Urundi, Huygelen (1960) isolated, from cattle with extensive erosion of the teats, a virus similar to the Allerton strain. Martin et al. (1966) reported that bovine ulcerative mammillitis is caused by a herpesvirus, which they called bovine mammillitis virus (BMV), also known as bovine herpesvirus 2 (BHV-2). This disease exists in England (Rweyemamu et al. 1968), the United States (Weaver et al. 1972), and Scotland (Martin et al. 1966) and more recently has appeared in eastern and southern Africa and also in Australia. Allerton virus and BMV are indistinguishable antigenically and in physical properties. Neutralizing antibody has been demonstrated in buffalo, giraffes, and other wild animals in eastern Africa (Plowright and Jessett 1971). Excellent review articles have been written by Gibbs and Rweyemamu (1977), Cilli and Castrucci (1976), and Gibbs (1984).

Character of the Disease. The effect of bovine ulcerative mammillitis on a milking herd depends on whether the herd has been exposed to the disease before. In primary herd infections morbidity is high and affects all ages of milking cows; there is no mortality. In previously exposed herds the disease is limited principally to first-calf heifers. A retrospective study in a large herd of bulls revealed a natural spread of infection (Letchworth, Carmichael, and Lein 1982). A serologic study showed that BHV-2 infection occurs continually in 20 species of African wildlife, principally bovids (Hamblin and Hedger 1982).

The incubation period is 3 to 7 days. Ulcerative lesions appear on the teats and less frequently on the udders of affected milking cows. The infection usually causes gross swelling of the teat wall. Within 48 hours the skin over the affected areas becomes soft and sloughed, revealing an irregularly shaped, painful, deeply ulcerated area that heals slowly with formation of brown scabs within 5 or 6 days after skin lesions are observed (Figure 46.6). The

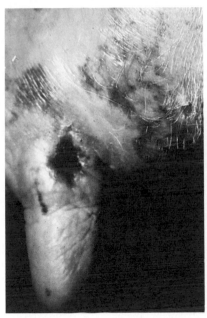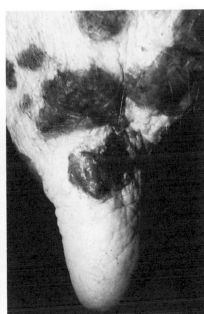

Figure 46.6. Early lesions caused by bovine mammillitis virus (*left*) and later scabby lesions of same teat (*right*). (Courtesy W. B. Martin.)

scabs begin shedding by day 14. Lymphadenitis occurs. Mastitis follows in approximately 22 percent of diseased animals.

Properties of the Virus. BHV-2 is a member of the herpes group and has all the biochemical and biophysical features of herpesviruses. Iodophors at concentrations used in dairy disinfectants inactivate the virus, but hypochlorite solutions are less effective.

Close antigenic relationships exist between strains of BHV-2 despite some variation in temperature lability (Castrucci et al. 1972) in a buffalo strain (Castrucci et al. 1975). Early work showed no relationship between this virus and other members of the Herpesviridae, including herpes simplex. Neutralization, complement-fixation, immunofluorescence, immunodiffusion, and mouse protection tests showed that herpes simplex and BHV-2 share at least one common antigen, most likely located in the envelope (Sterz et al. 1974). In an extension of these studies an antiserum produced to the oligomeric form of glycoprotein B (gB) induced by herpes simplex virus type 1 (HSV-1) gave a single common precipitin line in agar-gel diffusion with BHV-2, HSV-1, HSV-2, and equine herpes virus type 1 (EHV-1). The antiserum also neutralized HSV-1, HSV-2, and BHV-2, but not EHV-1. Absorption of the antiserum with excess BHV-2 and HSV-2 antigens resulted in an HSV-1–specific neutralizing antiserum. In immunoprecipitation tests two proteins, gB and pgB, were precipitated from cells infected with HSV-1 and HSV-2 and at least three from cells infected with BHV-2 and EHV-1. Infected cells labeled with ^{125}I and appropriate separation of the peptides of each virus

showed that the resulting profiles were almost identical. This finding suggests considerable structural conservation of the peptide backbone of the antigenically related glycoproteins of these four herpesvirus (Snowden et al. 1985). In cells infected with BHV-2 at least 12 acid-soluble peptides were extracted and separated by 5DS-PAGE (Halliburton and Freeman 1985).

Cultivation. The virus replicates in a wide variety of cell cultures, although primary cultures of bovine kidney tissue develop large syncytia, which appear as early as 8 hours or as late as 8 days after inoculation. Soon after syncytial formation, cell destruction is complete. Numerous large inclusions of Cowdry type A are present in the nuclei. The virus also replicates in baby hamster kidney cells, and the Allerton strain is known to multiply in lamb testes. The BHM-TVA strain produces uniform plaques in bovine cell cultures under carboxymethyl cellulose overlay.

Epizootiology and Pathogenesis. BMV is transmitted mechanically by means of milkers or by biting flies (Martin et al. 1966, Rweyemamu et al. 1968). Insects such as *Musca fasciata* may transmit the Allerton strain (Andrewes 1967).

BHV-2 (Allerton) produces skin nodules when inoculated into suckling mice and transient lesions when given intradermally to rabbits. It will also cause lesions in sheep and goats (Andrewes 1967, Westbury 1981). When the Allerton strain is inoculated intradermally into susceptible cattle, fever ensues and skin nodules erupt over the entire body. The nodules become necrotic, and lymphadenitis is another feature of the experimental disease.

Day-old rats, mice, and Chinese hamsters are susceptible to BHV-1, which causes stunting, with or without skin lesions, and high mortality; but older animals are resistant (Rweyemamu et al. 1968). In rabbits and guinea pigs, which are of lower susceptibility, no difference in age susceptibility was observed.

Local tissue temperature seems to be a critical factor in the pathogenesis of BHV-2. The reduced BHV-2 replication at elevated temperatures (39° to 40°C) contrasts with excellent titers in cell cultures maintained at 30° to 37°C (Letchworth et al. 1982). This phenomenon may account for the observed restriction of BHV-2 skin lesions to the udder and teats of cattle and restriction of disease outbreaks to months when the temperature is lower (Letchworth and Carmichael 1984).

Recent evidence suggests that latent infection of cattle (Castrucci et al. 1983), sheep, and goats (Westbury 1981) occurs after exposure to BHV-2; and virus is expressed after treatment with dexamethasone. In earlier studies, cattle unknowingly were exposed to BHV-1; and latency to BHV-2 was not achieved after inoculation, as dexamethasone treatment activated the BHV-1 but not BHV-2 (Castrucci et al. 1980, Letchworth and Carmichael 1982).

Histological changes (Martin et al. 1969) in the epidermis on the first day of the clinical reaction are severe inflammation accompanied by syncytia and inclusion body formation (Figure 46.7). Inflammation rapidly becomes more intense in the next few days, and great numbers of polymorphonuclear and other leukocytes appear in the epidermis and dermis. Syncytial masses containing many nuclei occur in the lesions during the first few days as well as intranuclear inclusion bodies, which vary somewhat in appearance depending on the age of the lesion.

More mast cells appear in the dermis during the reaction. Virus particles are found in sections examined with the electron microscope, and particles occur within the nucleus with single limiting membranes either packed in crystalline array (Figure 46.8) or dispersed irregularly. Particles in the cytoplasm usually have two limiting membranes, with the second one acquired at the nuclear membrane (Figure 46.9). Teat skin is not particularly susceptible to infection, but skin damage does permit viral entry.

Immunity. Neutralizing antibodies are found in the serums of recovered cattle. Complete protection results after recovery from natural or experimental BHV-1 disease. The duration of protection is unknown, but it does persist for at least 8 months (Rweyemamu and Johnson 1969). Maximal neutralizing antibody titers are achieved 3 weeks after experimental inoculation, but titers do not

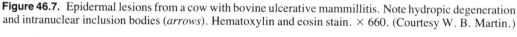

Figure 46.7. Epidermal lesions from a cow with bovine ulcerative mammillitis. Note hydropic degeneration and intranuclear inclusion bodies (*arrows*). Hematoxylin and eosin stain. × 660. (Courtesy W. B. Martin.)

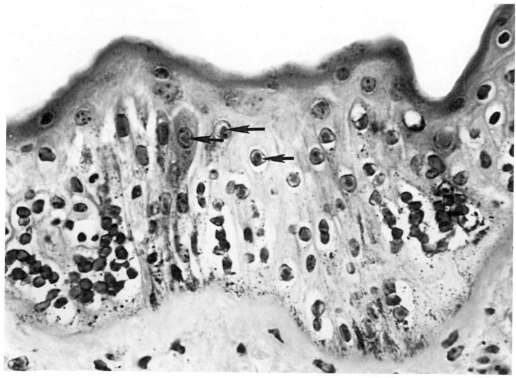

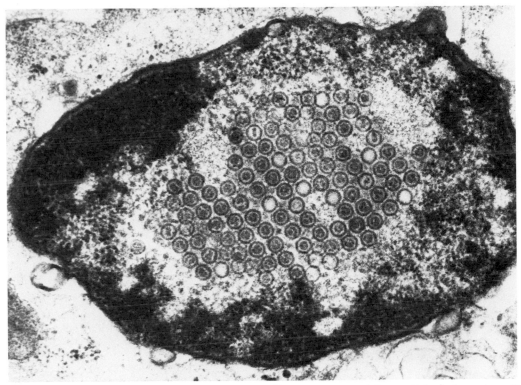

Figure 46.8. Bovine ulcerative mammillitis. Paracrystalline arrangement of virus particles in the nucleus. × 41,800. (Courtesy W. B. Martin.)

persist (Martin et al. 1969). In contrast, following recovery from natural disease, antibody titers persist for at least 2 years (Rweyemamu et al. 1969)

Diagnosis. In bovine ulcerative mammillitis the lesions are infective from the first to the tenth day. High infectivity titers of lesions and of exuding fluid are present during the first 4 days. With this material, virus readily produces a cytopathic effect in cell cultures (section on cultivation). Use of paired serums with a cell-culture system demonstrates a rising neutralizing antibody titer.

Paravaccinia, a common cause of teat lesions, can be differentiated from BMV by examination of biopsy material before scabbing occurs (Rweyemamu et al. 1968). Paravaccinia causes epithelial hyperplasia, intracellular edema of cells of the stratum spinosum, and cytoplasmic inclusions in the vesicular epithelial cells—this is in marked contrast to lesions caused by BMV.

Prevention and Control. In a study of various experimental vaccine preparations with BHV-1 the most practical virus vaccine was found to be an unaltered virus strain (TV) administered intramuscularly (Rweyemamu and Johnson 1969). This vaccine was safe for use in pregnant animals, and there was no evidence of excretion to susceptible contact animals. Protection lasted for at least 8 months. Animals inoculated with unaltered virus vaccine

should be monitored closely, since virus latency has been demonstrated in cattle, sheep, and goats.

The Disease in Humans. There is no evidence that Allerton virus or BMV strains cause disease in humans.

REFERENCES

Alexander, R.A., Plowright, W., and Haig, D.A. 1957. Cytopathogenic agents associated with lumpy skin disease of cattle. Bull. Epizoot. Dis. Afr. 5:489–492.

Andrewes, C., and Pereira, J.G. 1967. Viruses of Vertebrates, 2d ed. Williams & Wilkins, Baltimore.

Castrucci, G., Cilli, V., Frigeri, F., Ferrari, M., Ranucci, S., and Ramphichini, L. 1983. Reactivation of bovid herpesvirus 1 and 2 and parainfluenza 3 virus in calves latently infected. Comp. Immunol. Microbiol. Infect. Dis. 6:193–199.

Castrucci, G., Frigeri, F., Cilli, V., Tesei, B., Arush, A.M., Fedini, B., Ranucci, S., and Rampichini, L. 1980. Attempts to reactivate bovid herpesvirus-2 in experimentally infected calves. Am. J. Vet. Res. 41:1890–1893.

Castrucci, G., Martin, W.B., Pendini, B., Cilli, V., and Ranucci, S. 1975. A comparison in calves of the antigenicity of three strains of bovid herpesvirus 2. Res. Vet. Sci. 18:208–215.

Castrucci, G., Pendini, B., Cilli, V., and Arancia, G. 1972. Characterization of a viral agent resembling bovine herpes mammillitis virus. Vet. Rec. 90:325–335.

Cilli, V., and Castrucci, G. 1976. Infection of cattle with bovid herpesvirus 2. Folia Vet. Lat. 6:1–44.

Gibbs, E.P.J. 1984. Viral diseases of the skin of the bovine teat and udder. Vet. Clin. North Am. [Large Anim. Pract.] 6:187–202.

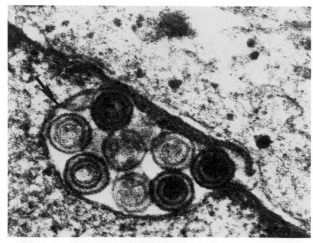

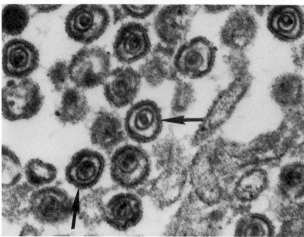

Figure 46.9. Bovine ulcerative mammillitis. Several enveloped virus particles within a vacuole formed by the nuclear membrane about to leave the nucleus (*top*). Extracellular virus particles (*bottom*). × 60,500. (Courtesy W. B. Martin.)

Gibbs, E.P.J., and Rweyemamu, M.M. 1977. Bovine herpesvirus. I. Bovine herpesvirus 1. II. Bovine herpesvirus 2 and 3. Vet. Bull. 47:411–425.

Halliburton, I.W., and Freeman, M.J. 1985. A comparison of the acid-soluble polypeptides of five herpesviruses. J. Gen. Virol. 66:2243–2248.

Hamblin, G., and Hedger, R.S. 1982. Prevalence of neutralizing antibodies to bovid herpesvirus 2 in African wildlife. J. Wildl. Dis. 18:429–436.

Huygelen, C. 1960. Allerton virus, a cytopathogenic agent associated with lumpy skin disease. I. Propagation in tissue cultures of bovine and ovine testis cells. Zentralbl. Veterinärmed. 7:664–670.

Letchworth, G.J., and Carmichael, L.E. 1982. Bovid herpesvirus 2 latency: Failure to recover virus from central sensory nerve ganglia. Can. J. Comp. Med. 46:76–79.

Letchworth, G.J., and Carmichael, L.E. 1984. Local tissue temperature: A critical factor in the pathogenesis of bovid herpesvirus 2. Infect. Immun. 43:1072–1079.

Letchworth, G.J., Carmichael, L.E., and Greisen, H.A. 1982. Sensitivity of bovid herpesvirus 2 replication to temperatures found in the natural host. Arch. Virol. 73:273–286.

Letchworth, G.J., Carmichael, L.E., and Lein, D.H. 1982. Bovid herpesvirus 2: Natural spread among breeding bulls. Cornell Vet. 72:200–210.

Martin, W.B., James, Z.H., Lauder, I.M., Murray, M., and Piru, H.M. 1969. Pathogenesis of bovine mammillitis virus infection in cattle. Am. J. Vet. Res. 30:2151–2166.

Martin, W.B., Martin, B., Hay, D., and Lauder, I.M. 1966. Bovine ulcerative mammillitis caused by a herpesvirus. Vet. Rec. 78:494–497.

Plowright, W., and Jessett, D.M., 1971. Investigations of Allerton type herpes virus infection in East African game animals and cattle. J. Hyg. 69:209–222.

Rweyemamu, M.M., and Johnson, R.H. 1969. The development of a vaccine for bovine herpes mammillitis. Res. Vet. Sci. 10:419–427.

Rweyemamu, M.M., Johnson, R.H., and Laurilord, R.E. 1969. Serological findings in bovine herpes mammillitis. Br. Vet. J. 125:317–325.

Rweyemamu, M.M., Johnson, R.H., and McCrea, M.R. 1968. Bovine herpes mammillitis virus. III. Observations on experimental infection. Br. Vet. J. 124:317–324.

Snowden, B.W., Kinchington, P.R., Powell, K. L., and Halliburton, I.W. 1985. Antigenic and biochemical analysis of gB of herpes simplex virus type 1 and type 2 and of cross-reacting glycoproteins induced by bovine mammillitis virus and equine herpesvirus type 1. J. Gen. Virol. 66:231–247.

Sterz, H., Ludwig, H., and Rott, R. 1974. Immunological and genetic relationship between herpes simplex virus and bovine herpes mammillitis virus. Intervirology 2:1–13.

Weaver, L.D., Dellers, R.W., and Dardin, A.H. 1972. Bovine herpes mammillitis in New York. J. Am. Vet. Med. Assoc. 160:1643–1644.

Westbury, H.A. 1981. Infection of sheep and goats with bovid herpesvirus 2. Res. Vet. Sci. 31:353–357.

Equine Herpesviruses

At present three equine herpesvirus serotypes are recognized. Equine herpesvirus 1 (EHV-1) is primarily a respiratory tract pathogen that is now classified EHV-1, subtype 2 (Patel et al. 1982, Turtinen et al. 1981). Another serotype causes abortions and nervous manifestations in pregnant mares; it is classified as EHV-1, subtype 1, by Patel et al. (1982) and by Turtinen et al. (1981) or simply as EHV-1 by Studdert et al. (1981). Equine herpesvirus 2 (EHV-2) is often isolated from the respiratory tract and other sites in normal horses and in those displaying a variety of diseases. Blakeslee et al. (1975) provided some evidence that it may cause pharyngitis in young foals. In general, the pathogenicity of this cytomegalovirus (EHV-2) is undetermined, so it is given little consideration here, except where it may be involved with the other two equine herpesvirus serotypes. Equine herpesvirus 3 (EHV-3) causes coital exanthema in the horse. Diseases caused by equine herpesvirus 1 and 3 are described below. Subtype designations of EHV-1 will be used to distinguish between the strains that cause respiratory disease and those that cause abortions or nervous manifestations or both.

REFERENCES

Blakeslee, J.R., Olsen, R.G., McAllister, E.S., Fassbender, J., and Dennis, R. 1975. Evidence of respiratory tract infection induced by equine herpesvirus, type 2, in the horse. Can. J. Microbiol. 21:1940–1946.

Patel, J.R., Edington, N., and Mumford, J.A. 1982. Variation in cellular tropism between isolates of equine herpesvirus-1 in foals. Arch. Virol. 74:41–51.

Studdert, M.J., Simpson, T., and Roizman, B. 1981. Differentiation of respiratory and abortogenic isolates of equine herpesvirus 1 by restriction endonucleases. Science 214:562–564.

Turtinen, L.W., Allen, G.P., Darlington, R.W., and Bryans, J.T. 1981. Serologic and molecular comparisons of several equine herpesvirus type 1 strains. Am. J. Vet. Res. 42:2099–2104.

Equine Rhinopneumonitis

SYNONYM: Equine virus abortion

Dimock and Edwards (1932) reported a form of epizootic abortion in mares in Kentucky which was shown to be due to a virus. Manninger and Csontos (1941) first called attention to similarities between the viruses of equine influenza and equine virus abortion. Doll and Kintner (1954) in the United States made a comparative study of several strains of equine abortion virus with two strains of virus isolated from horses suffering from respiratory infection that had been regarded as influenza. These strains proved to be identical, but different from influenza viruses. Because EHV-1 is essentially a respiratory tract pathogen and causes abortions secondarily, Doll et al. (1957) proposed that the disease that it causes be called equine rhinopneumonitis. Nervous manifestations occasionally appear in pregnant mares. The abortions and nervous manifestations usually are caused by EHV-1, subcaused by EHV-1, subtype 1, and the respiratory disease by EHV-1, subtype 2 (or EHV-4).

Natural disease occurs only in horses. It has been found in many areas of the United States, in Australia, and in many European countries and is viewed as an important disease in horses, especially on breeding farms. Most yearlings in Australia have neutralizing antibodies to both subtypes (Sabine et al. 1983).

Character of the Disease. The disease appears in two different forms—the first in weanlings, the second in pregnant mares—and occurs primarily in breeding establishments, where it is a serious economic disease.

The weanling disease is manifested by mild fever accompanied by rhinitis or nasal catarrh, which appears in the fall months. Although the disease is so mild as to cause little concern, Doll et al. (1957) showed that it is accompanied by the development of antibodies for the virus of equine rhinopneumonitis. Each September, before the rhinitis appeared, all foals were free of antibodies for this virus; but in each successive month while the disease was under way the number of animals positive for the antibodies increased until 80 to 100 percent were positive by December. Doll et al. (1957) also showed the etiological relationship between this respiratory virus and strains of virus obtained from aborting mares by inoculating sucklings and weanling horses. The animals that were inoculated both intravenously and intranasally with virus in fetal tissue developed fever, mild leukopenia, mild mucopurulent nasal discharge, and specific antibodies. There was no cough and no pulmonary or conjunctival involvement. The fever appears within 2 to 3 days, generally is diphasic, and persists for 8 to 10 days. Mortality in sucklings and weanlings is negligible. The disease, originally described in mares, was characterized by abortions and occasionally by nervous signs (Dimock et al. 1947). Abortions occurred in mares with few or no premonitory signs any time after the sixth month of gestation. After the virus was expelled, the genital tract returned to normal rather quickly. Lesions could be found only in the fetus. In aborting mares without nervous signs, no lesions have been recognized in the dam, but there are characteristic lesions in the fetus. Foals infected very late in pregnancy and born alive generally died within 36 hours. It is believed that abortions in natural outbreaks occur 3 to 4 weeks after a mare is infected. In the abortion disease, mortality in the mares is low, but losses of foals may be high. The disease strikes from 10 to 90 percent of the pregnant mares living on the same premises. When the infection appears late in the foaling season after many of the mares have foaled, the incidence of abortion is much lower. Some investigators reported that numerous cases of meningoencephalitis in European and U.S. pregnant mares often were preceded by respiratory signs (Charlton et al. 1976, Dinter and Klingeborn 1976, Jeffcoat and Rossdale 1976). EHV-1, subtype 1, also causes ataxia in stallions, geldings, and foals (Crowhurst et al. 1981, Greenwood and Simson 1980).

Properties of the Virus. EHV-1 is a DNA virus that produces intranuclear inclusion bodies (Figure 46.10). The genome has a molecular weight of 100×10^6. Parti-

Figure 46.10. Characteristic intranuclear inclusions of equine rhinopneumonitis virus (EHV-1) in the epithelium of a bronchus. × 930. (From Randall and Doll, 1956, courtesy of *Cornell Veterinarian.*)

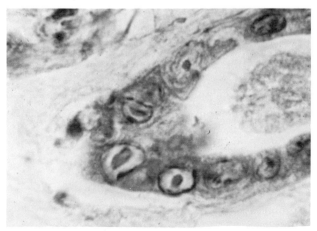

cles have been described in the nuclei of affected hepatic cells of hamsters. The virus bodies are 92 nm in diameter in and outside of the cytoplasm (Tajima et al. 1961). Particles in the nuclei may be in a crystalline array. EHV-1 morphology is similar to that of herpes simplex virus, the prototype virus for this subfamily.

Homology studies demonstrate that types 1 and 3 exhibit little genetic homology (Allen et al. 1977, Staczek et al. 1983), but closely related sequences may be conserved among the genomes of EHV-1, EHV-2, and EHV-3 (Staczek et al. 1983). Various biochemical techniques demonstrated 20 to 30 percent homology between the two subtypes of EHV-1 (Allen and Turtinen 1982). The restriction endonuclease DNA fingerprints of 20 low-passage, epidemiologically unrelated isolates of EHV-1, subtype 2, showed considerable heterogeneity in certain fragments assigned to restricted positions on the kilobase (Kb) genome (Studdert et al. 1986). Eleven envelope glycoproteins have been identified in three different EHV-1 strains (Caughman et al. 1985, Robinson et al. 1985, Turtinen and Allen 1982) and provided evidence for immediate early/early/late regulation of viral gene expression.

Antigenic studies of equine herpesvirus 1, 2, and 3 were undertaken with various serologic methods including neutralization, immunodiffusion, complement-fixation, and direct and indirect fluorescent antibody tests (Gutekunst et al. 1978). These studies indicated that each type contains specific antigenic components. EHV-1 and EHV-3 share a common antigen that is not shared with EHV-2. Cross-neutralization was not detected in reciprocal tests among the three types. Carmichael and Barnes (1961) showed that equine herpesvirus 1 and infectious bovine rhinotracheitis virus share common complement-fixing and precipitating antigens. Complement-fixing antibodies decline more rapidly than other types of antibody, but this is a consistent finding with most viral infections.

Virus survives for more than 457 days at −18°C. The agent is labile in saline suspensions, and it is inactivated by 0.35 percent formalin. Its density is 1.18 g/ml in cesium chloride.

Horse red blood cells are agglutinated by tissues of affected horses between 4° and 37°C (McCollum et al. 1956). The hemagglutinin is not neutralized by convalescent horse serums but is inhibited by hyperimmune serum from horses given infected hamster tissue.

Infection of permissive hamster embryo cells with virus preparations enriched with defective interfering particles of EHV-1 resulted in persistent infection and oncogenic transformation (Robinson et al. 1980). Baumann et al. (1986) mapped the DNA of EHV-1 defective interfering particles.

Cultivation. Strains of equine herpesvirus 1 from the respiratory tract and also from tissues of aborted horse fetuses were adapted to hens' eggs by alternation between the hamster virus and the fertile egg (Doll et al. 1953).

EHV-1 produces a cytopathic effect in cell cultures of fetal horse kidney, lamb kidney, and rabbit kidney (Plummer and Waterson 1964), with the production of intranuclear inclusion bodies of varying types depending on the virus isolate (Erasmus 1969, Randall 1957). With equine herpesvirus 1 the cytopathic effect is rapid and complete. It also produces a cytopathic effect in a number of other cell culture types (Doll and Kintner 1954). Plaque-assay methods, using monolayers of Earle's L cells (Randall and Lawson 1962) and horse kidney cells (Shimizu et al. 1963), are available for EHV-1.

EHV-1 causes extensive loss of the epithelial layer in equine tracheal and nasal turbinate organ cultures, and the classic stages of herpesvirus morphogeneses were seen in thin sections by electron microscopy (O'Neill et al. 1984).

It is possible to differentiate in vitro field strains of virus from a strain adapted to the NL-111 rabbit kidney cells (Holmes et al. 1979). The rabbit-adapted virus produces large, circular plaques, 2 to 3 mm in diameter, in NL-111 rabbit kidney cells, whereas field isolates produce small, irregular plaques. This phenomenon provides a mechanism for studying the epidemiology of the disease in areas where horses are vaccinated with rabbit-attenuated virus vaccine.

Epizootiology and Pathogenesis. The respiratory disease is undoubtedly transmitted by droplets from infected horses after outbreaks have started. The source of the virus that initiates outbreaks is unknown. Aborted fetuses contain much virus, and aborting mares often bring infections to new premises. There is no evidence, however, that virus is carried by an aborting mare very long after abortion occurs. It is known, though, that herpesviruses in general often persist for long periods after recovery. It is possible that dogs, foxes, and carrier birds may carry infection, from ingested fragments of aborted fetuses, from one farm to another. In mares with nervous manifestations in natural and experimental cases the disease is characterized by ataxia or paresis lasting up to several weeks. Little and Thorsen (1976) mention 12 naturally infected horses with disseminating necrotizing myeloencephalitis. Necrotic arteriolitis, nonsuppurative necrotizing myeloencephalitis, and gasserian ganglioneuritis were present in a paraparetic horse. In experimental trials with EHV-1 a neurological syndrome was produced in all mares between 3 and 9 months' gestation 6 to 8 days after inoculation (Jackson et al. 1977). Vascular changes and concomitant degeneration were present in the central nervous system of mares with neurological disease. Doll

(1953) developed a technique of inoculating fetuses in utero directly through the abdominal wall; this produced abortions in 100 percent of cases, regardless of whether the mare was immune to the virus.

The studies of Bruner et al. (1949), Dimock et al. (1942), and Kress (1946) indicate that the virus causes pregnant guinea pigs to abort. When virus material was injected into the guinea pig fetuses on the 35th day of gestation, the fetuses were aborted 7 to 9 days later. The injection of virus-free material into the fetuses of control animals did not cause abortions, and at birth the baby guinea pigs appeared entirely normal (Bruner et al. 1949).

Doll et al. (1953) succeeded in adapting this virus to suckling hamsters, after Anderson and Goodpasture (1942) had pointed the way by reporting the finding of intranuclear inclusions resembling those of viral abortion in suckling hamsters. Later Doll and associates succeeded in cultivating a number of strains of the abortion virus and the respiratory virus, which until then was considered to be different in suckling hamsters. All of these strains of EHV-1 produced identical lesions in the hamsters and resulted in their deaths (Doll et al. 1954). Typical acidophilic intranuclear inclusion bodies were found in the livers of all inoculated individuals; horse tissues fixed complement with hamster antibodies, and hamster tissues fixed complement with horse antibodies. The virus also has a tropism for the trophoblast cells of the syncytiotrophoblast zone of the placenta (Burek et al. 1975).

The pathogenesis of 11 isolates of subtype 1 was studied in suckling mice after intracerebral inoculation. The five less pathogenic isolates were restricted predominantly to the olfactory lobes, while the more pathogenic isolates were detected in neurons as well as the blood, the bronchial and renal epithelium, and the lymphoid cells in the spleen (Patel and Edington 1983).

Subtype-1 isolates of EHV-1 from a quadriplegic horse and from an aborted fetus were compared with each other and with a subtype-2 respiratory isolate (Patel et al. 1982). All three isolates were detected in the epithelium and macrophages of the respiratory tract. Both the paresis and fetal subtype-1 isolate replicated in the epithelium of the ileum, and this finding correlated with the recovery of virus from feces in vivo. The paresis subtype-1 isolate also had a predilection for vascular endothelial cells, particularly in the nasal mucosa, but also in the lung, central nervous system, adrenal, and thyroid. Of the nine foals inoculated with the paresis isolate, two developed hind limb dysfunction, four developed diarrhea, and one of these four died of intussusception.

In a series with 21 pregnant mares 19 became infected, as evidenced by clinical signs or viremia or both, but only one mare aborted. The viremias were leukocyte-associated and appeared as nonproductive latent infections of these cells (Gleeson and Coggins 1980).

More recently Edington et al. (1986) provided some excellent information on the pathogenesis of a subtype-1 isolate from a case of equine paresis. In two mares examined 4 days after inoculation immunofluorescence showed endothelial cell infection together with thromboses in the rete arteriosum of the nasal mucosa and also in the spinal cord of one mare. Circulating platelet counts in six other mares fell as early as 2 days after inoculation and remained depressed for 7 days. Circulating immune complexes started to appear 2 days after inoculation, reached maximum levels after 10 days, but were undetectable after 28 days. Three of these mares developed varying degrees of incoordination 8 and 9 days after inoculation. In the two incoordinate mares that were killed on the ninth and tenth postinoculation day the hemorrhages in the spinal cord and brain were associated with extensive endothelial cell fluorescence and thrombus formation. Clinical paresis coincided with an increase in circulating complement-fixing and neutralizing antibodies, which in all six mares were higher against the subtype-1 isolate than against subtype 2. In five yearlings infected with a subtype-2 isolate of EHV-1 platelet counts remained normal, and immune complexes, viremia, or incoordination were not detected.

Following experimental infection of eight ponies with EHV-1, subtype 1, animals showed clinical signs and serologic conversion. Virus was isolated from the nasal swabs and leukocytes. Immediately after recovery and 3 months later, virus was isolated from six of the eight ponies after immunosuppression with dexamethasone and prednisolone treatment, showing that EHV-1 remained latent in most recovered animals (Edington et al. 1985).

Studdert et al. (1984) showed the value of molecular epidemiology in establishing the subtypes of EHV-1 and its use in pathogenesis studies. In some sequential infection studies in horses with equine herpesviruses 1, 2, and 3, EHV-2 failed to produce a disease in foals (Wilks and Studdert 1976). The inoculation of EHV-3 into the genital tract of the same test horses resulted in lesions typical of equine coital exanthema. Intranasal inoculation of EHV-1 produced definite respiratory signs and lesions, but the disease was milder than expected in two of the three foals. Thus the investigators hypothesized that recent prior infection with EHV-2 and/or EHV-3 might give partial protection against EHV-1.

The most consistent lesions of aborted fetuses are multiple focal areas of necrosis in the liver. Many fetuses also exhibit petechiae in the heart muscle and in the capsules of the spleen and liver. Edema of the lungs with excessive fluid in the chest cavity is also characteristic. Considered diagnostic of this disease are the inclusion bodies, which in most cases are readily found in the liver and various other organs.

Immunity. Exposure of susceptible horses and ponies to EHV-1 subtypes elicits serum-neutralizing antibodies and cellular immune responses. A similar response occurs after a single injection of inactivated subtype-1 or subtype-2 virus vaccine (Fitzpatrick and Studdert 1984). Serum-neutralizing antibody responses were subtype-specific but were cross-reactive after exposure to other subtypes of EHV-1. Exposure to both subtypes provides better protection in foals that either subtype alone.

In infected ponies complement levels were depressed during the first 2 weeks, declined as early as the second day, and decreased to 35 percent of preinfection levels by the tenth day. Higher neutralizing antibody titers can be achieved by adding complement.

Engles et al. (1986), found that the Piber isolate of subtype 1 should protect horses against abortions but immunity against the paretic form was less certain. Protection against the respiratory disease form is unlikely with subtype 1.

Viral abortions are seldom, if ever, observed in the same mare in two successive seasons, although some have been known to have aborted a fetus several years after the first abortion. This phenomenon would indicate the presence of an immune mechanism that gives a somewhat transitory resistance, or possible chance infection with a highly virulent strain.

A serum-neutralizing titer of 10^2 or greater (against 50 to 100 $TCID_{50}$ of virus in a cell-culture system) in a mare prevents reinfection by intranasal challenge (Bryans 1969, Bryans and Prickett 1969). Horses with lower titers or no measurable neutralizing antibody may develop mild signs of respiratory illness. Cell-mediated immunity also plays a significant role in herpesvirus infections such as rhinopneumonitis. The response can be measured by the lymphocyte transformation test or by the in vitro cytotoxicity test (Wilks and Coggins 1976). It is believed that cytotoxic antibodies or peripheral blood leukocytes could play an important role in restricting virus spread after infection (Wilks 1977). Thus it appears that neutralizing antibody, cytotoxic antibody, and leukocytes all play a role in protection against EHV-1.

Diagnosis. Clinical diagnosis is usually not difficult. Autopsy of the aborted fetus generally will establish a precise diagnosis. In animals with respiratory disease the lungs are usually edematous, hemorrhages occur on the pericardium, and the liver lesions are most characteristic. The finding of the characteristic inclusion bodies is diagnostic. These bodies, described by Westerfield and Dimock in 1946, are acidophilic, intranuclear, and usually numerous in the liver cells. Often from 50 to 80 percent of

the liver cells are necrotic and contain these bodies. They may be found also in the epithelium lining the air passages and the bile ducts and in endothelial cells of the spleen, lymph nodes, and thymus. Virus typing may be indicated in certain instances.

Various serologic tests, such as serum neutralization, immunofluorescence, complement-fixation, and ELISA, can be used to detect antibody. The latter test can also be used to detect antigen (Dutta et al. 1983). Rapid typing of EHV-1 subtypes was done with monoclonal antibodies in enzyme immunofiltration of 50 epizootiologically unrelated field isolates (Yeargan et al. 1985). Restriction endonuclease characterization of the DNA is very useful in epidemiological studies and diagnosis (Allen et al. 1985, Studdert et al. 1981).

Prevention and Control. Because EHV-1 disease is highly contagious, isolation of infected animals is recommended. Indiscriminate movement of infected foals or mares following an outbreak may spread the disease. After an abortion the stall of the aborting animal should be thoroughly disinfected, particularly if other pregnant mares are kept in the same stable.

As a prophylactic measure mares have been vaccinated with inactivated virus vaccine (Bruner et al. 1948, 1949; Kress 1946), with hamster-adapted live virus vaccine (Doll et al. 1953), with attenuated vaccine produced in Vero cells (Purdy et al. 1977), and with attenuated virus vaccine produced in tissue-cultured equine cells (NL-EQ_4) (Gerber et al. 1977). Each product has its advantages and disadvantages; none is completely satisfactory. Only two products now are available. Because the hamster-adapted live virus vaccine may cause mild disease in many weanlings, it should be given to all horses on a farm late in June and again in October. This procedure has reduced the number of abortions. The attenuated virus vaccine produced in NL-EQ_4 equine cells does not cause any signs of illness, and after two injections the vaccine elicits neutralizing antibodies and a cell-mediated immune response. Although it is generally believed that this vaccine affords some protection, abortions still occur in some vaccinated mares.

Since 1979 the efficacy of inactivated virus vaccines has been the subject of considerable research and field evaluation (Bryans 1980, Bryans and Allen 1982, Campbell et al. 1982, Mumford and Bates 1984). A chemically inactivated EHV-1 with added adjuvant was used to immunize pregnant thoroughbred mares during a 5-year test. The incidence of EHV-1 abortions was 1.6/1,000 in vaccinated mares, compared with 6.8/1,000 in the remainder of the study population (Bryans and Allen 1982). A subtype-2 inactivated vaccine provided no protection to pregnant mares, with abortions occurring

but vaccinated yearlings and 2-year-old ponies had less severe respiratory disease than the controls in an experimental trial (Burrows et al. 1984). In another experimental trial three doses of an inactivated subtype-1 virus vaccine protected yearling ponies, whereas two doses gave incomplete protection (Mumford and Bates 1984). To provide more complete protection a vaccine containing both subtypes of EHV-1 may be desirable.

A single dose of bovine herpesvirus 1247 strain was inoculated subcutaneously in five pregnant pony mares (Crandell et al. 1980). No adverse clinical signs were observed, and virus was not recovered from nasal swabs taken during the 2-week period after vaccination. One mare had a dead foal, but pathological and virological examinations were negative for EHV-1. No field studies with this vaccine have been reported.

If equine cytomegaloviruses are found in the United States as a cause of respiratory disease and abortion, the control program for EHV-1 will require considerable modification (Bryans 1964).

The Disease in Humans. EHV-1 infection has not been reported in humans, although references to an obscure disease of a human fetus in which there were intranuclear inclusion bodies appear in the literature (Bryans 1964).

REFERENCES

Allen, G.P., and Turtinen, L.W. 1982. Assessment of the base sequence homology between the two subtypes of equine herpesvirus 1. J. Virol. 44:249–255.

Allen, G.P., Callaghan, D.J., and Randall, C.C. 1977. Genetic relatedness of equine herpesvirus types 1 and 3. J. Virol. 24:761–767.

Allen, G.P., Turtinen, L.W., Bryans, J.T., and McCollum. 1985. Molecular epizootiologic studies of equine herpesvirus-1 infections by restriction endonuclease finger printing of viral DNA. Am. J. Vet. Res. 44:263–268.

Anderson, K., and Goodpasture, E.W. 1942. Infection of newborn Syrian hamsters with the virus of mare abortion (Dimock and Edwards). Am. J. Pathol. 18:555–561.

Baumann, R.P., Staczek, J., and O'Callaghan, D.J. 1986. Cloning and fine mapping the DNA of equine herpesvirus type one defective interfering particles. Virology 153:188–200.

Bruner, D.W., Doll, E.R., and Hull, F.E. 1949. Studies on virus abortion. Blood-Horse 58:31.

Bruner, D.W., Edwards, P.R., and Hull, F.E. 1948. Equine virus abortion vaccine. Blood-Horse 53:666.

Bryans, J.T. 1964. Viral respiratory disease of horses. In Proceedings of the Annual Meeting of the American Veterinary Medical Association. Pp. 112–121.

Bryans, J.T. 1969. On immunity to disease caused by equine herpesvirus 1. J. Am. Vet. Med. Assoc. 155:294–300.

Bryans, J.T. 1980. Serologic responses of pregnant thoroughbred mares to vaccination with an inactivated equine herpesvirus 1 vaccine. Am. J. Vet. Res. 41:1743–1746.

Bryans, J.T., and Allen, G.P. 1982. Application of a chemically inactivated, adjuvanted vaccine to control abortigenic infection of mares by equine herpesvirus 1. Dev. Biol. Stand. 52:493–498.

Bryans, J.T., and Prickett, M.E. 1969. A consideration of the pathogenesis of abortigenic disease caused by equine herpesvirus 1. In J.T. Bryans and H. Gerber, eds., Proceedings of the 2d International Conference on Equine Infectious Disease. Karger, Basel. Pp. 34–40.

Burek, J.D., Roas, R.P., and Narayan, O. 1975. Virus induced abortion: Studies of equine herpesvirus 1 (abortion virus) in hamsters. Lab. Invest. 33:400–406.

Burrows, R., Goodridge, D., and Denyer, M.S. 1984. Trials of an inactivated equid herpesvirus 1 vaccine: Challenge with a subtype 1 virus. Vet. Rec. 114:369–374.

Campbell, T.M., Studdert, M.J., and Blackney, M.H. 1982. Immunogenicity of equine herpesvirus 1 (EHV-1) and equine rhinovirus type 1 (ERhV1) following inactivation by betapropiolactone (BPL) and ultraviolet (UV) light. Vet. Microbiol. 7:535–544.

Carmichael, L.E., and Barnes, F.D. 1961. The relationship of infectious bovine rhinotracheitis virus to equine rhinopneumonitis virus. Proc. U.S. Livestock Sanit. Assoc. 65:384–388.

Caughman, G.B., Staczek, J., and O'Callahan, D.J. 1985. Equine herpesvirus type 1 infected cell polypeptides: Evidence for immediate early/early/late regulation of viral gene expression. Virology 145:49–61.

Charlton, K.M., Mitchell, D., Girard, A., and Corner, A.H. 1976. Meningoencephalomyelitis in horses associated with equine herpesvirus 1 infection. Vet. Pathol. 13:59–68.

Crandell, R.A., Mock, R.E., and Lock, T.F. 1980. Vaccination of pregnant ponies against equine rhinopneumonitis. Am. J. Vet. Res. 41:994–996.

Crowhurst, F.A., Dickinson, G., and Burrows, R. 1981. An outbreak of paresis in mares and geldings associated with equid herpesvirus 1. Vet. Rec. 109:527–528.

Dimock, W.W., and Edwards, P.R. 1932. Infections of foetuses and foals. Ky. Agric. Exp. Sta. Bull. 333:291–339.

Dimock, W.W., Edwards, P.R., and Bruner, D.W. 1942. Equine virus abortion. Ky. Agric. Exp. Sta. Bull. 426:20.

Dimock, W.W., Edwards, P.R., and Bruner, D.W. 1947. Infections observed in equine fetuses and foals. Cornell Vet. 37:89–99.

Dinter, Z., and Klingeborn, B. 1976. Serological study of an outbreak of pareses due to equid herpesvirus 1 (EHV-1). Vet. Rec. 99:10–12.

Doll, E.R. 1953. Intrauterine and intrafetal inoculations with equine abortion virus in pregnant mares. Cornell Vet. 43:112–121.

Doll, E.R., and Kinter, J.H. 1954. A comparative study of the equine abortion and equine influenza viruses. Cornell Vet. 44:355–367.

Doll, E.R., Bryans, J.T., McCollum, W.H., and Crowe, M.E.W. 1957. Isolation of a filterable agent causing arteritis of horses and abortion in mares. Its differentiation from equine abortion (influenza) virus. Cornell Vet. 47:3–31.

Doll, E.R., Richards, M.G., and Wallace, M.E. 1953. Adaptation of the equine abortion virus to suckling Syrian hamsters. Cornell Vet. 43:551–558.

Doll, E.R., Richards, M.G., and Wallace, M.E. 1954. Cultivation of the equine influenza virus in suckling Syrian hamsters. Its similarity to the equine abortion virus. Cornell Vet. 44:133–138.

Dutta, S.K., Talbot, N.C., and Myrup, A.C. 1983. Detection of equine herpesvirus-1 antigen and the specific antibody by enzyme-linked immunosorbent assay. Am. J. Vet. Res. 44:1930–1934.

Edington, N., Bridges, D.G., and Huckle, A. 1985. Experimental reactivation of equid herpesvirus 1 (EHV 1) following the administration of corticosteroids. Equine Vet. J. 17:369–372.

Edington, N., Bridges, C.G., and Patel, J.R. 1986. Endothelial cell infection and thrombosis in paralysis caused by equid herpesvirus-1: Equine stroke. Arch. Virol. 90:111–124.

Engles, M., Nowotny, N., Metzler, A.F., Wyler, R., and Burki, F. 1986. Genomic and antigenic comparison of an equine herpesvirus 1 (EHV 1) isolate from the 1983 Lippizan abortion storm with EHV 1 reference strains. Microbiologica 9:221–234.

Erasmus, B.J. 1969. Equine cytomegaloviruses. In J.T. Bryans and H. Gerber, eds., Proceedings of the 2d International Conference on Equine Infectious Disease. Karger, Basel. Pp. 46–55.

Fitzpatrick, D.R., and Studdert, M.J. 1984. Immunologic relationships between equine herpesvirus type 1 (equine abortion virus) and type 4 (equine rhinopneumonitis virus). Am. J. Vet. Res. 45:1947–1952.

Gerber, J.D., Marron, A.E., Bass, E.P., and Beckenhauer, W.H. 1977. Effect of age and pregnancy on the antibody and cell-mediated immune responses of horses to equine herpesvirus 1. Can. J. Comp. Med. 41:471–478.

Gleeson, L.J., and Coggins, L. 1980. Response of pregnant mares to equine herpesvirus 1 (EHV 1). Cornell Vet. 70:391–400.

Greenwood, R.E., and Simson, A.R. 1980. Clinical report of a paralytic syndrome affecting stallions, mares, and foals on a thoroughbred stud farm. Equine Vet. J. 12:113–117.

Gutekunst, D.E., Malmquist, W.A., and Becvar, C.S. 1978. Antigenic relatedness of equine herpesvirus types 1 and 3. Arch. Virol. 56:33–45.

Holmes, D.F., Kemen, M.J., and Joubert, J. 1979. Differentiation of field strains and a vaccine strain of equine herpesvirus 1, using plaque characteristics. Am. J. Vet. Res. 40:305–306.

Jackson, T.A., Osburn, B.I., Cordy, D.R., and Kendrick, J.W. 1977. Equine herpesvirus 1, infection of horses: Studies on the experimentally induced neurologic disease. Am. J. Vet. Res. 38:709–719.

Jeffcoat, L.B., and Rossdale, P.D. 1976. Practical aspects of equine virus abortion in United Kingdom. Vet. Rec. 98:153–155.

Kress, F. 1946. Versuche zur Bekampfung des Virus bedingten Abortus beim Pferde mit Organvakzine. Wien. Tierärztl. Monatsschr. 33:121–126.

Little, P.B., and Thorsen, J. 1976. Disseminated necrotizing myeloencephalitis: A herpes-associated neurological disease of horses. Vet. Pathol. 13:161–171.

McCollum, W.H., Doll, E.R., and Bryans, J.T. 1956. Agglutination of horse erythrocytes by tissue extracts from hamsters infected with equine abortion virus. Am. J. Vet. Res. 17:267–270.

Manninger, R., and Csontos, J. 1941. Virusabortus der Stuten. D.T.W. 49:105–108.

Mumford, J.A., and Bates, J. 1984. Trials of an inactivated equid herpesvirus 1 vaccine: Challenge with a subtype 2 virus. Vet. Rec. 114:369–374.

O'Neill, F.D., Issel, C.J., and Henk, W.G. 1984. Electron microscopy of equine respiratory viruses in organ cultures of equine fetal respiratory tract epithelium. Am. J. Vet. Res. 45:1953–1960.

Patel, J.R., and Edington, N. 1983. The pathogenicity in mice of respiratory, abortion and paresis isolates of equine herpesvirus-1. Vet. Microbiol. 8:301–305.

Patel, J.R., Edington, N., and Mumford, J.A. 1982. Variation in cellular tropism between isolates of equine herpesvirus-1 in foals. Arch. Virol. 74:41–51.

Plummer, G., and Waterson, A.P. 1964. Quoted by Christopher Andrewes, ed., in Viruses of Vertebrates. Bailliere, Tindall & Cox, London.

Purdy, C.W., Ford, S.J., and Grant, W.Z. 1977. Equine rhinopneumonitis virus (herpesvirus type 1): Attenuation in stable monkey cell line. Am. J. Vet. Res. 38:1211–1215.

Randall, C.C. 1957. Adaptation of equine abortion virus to HeLa cells. Proc. Soc. Exp. Biol., 95:508–510.

Randall, C.C., and Doll, E.R., 1956. Further observation of the in vitro susceptibility of adult horse tissue to equine abortion virus. Cornell Vet. 46:64–67.

Randall, C.C., and Lawson, L.A. 1962. Adaptation of equine abortion virus to Earle's L cells in serum-free medium with plaque formation. Proc. Soc. Exp. Biol. 110:487–489.

Robinson, R.A., Vance, R.B., and O'Callaghan, D.J. 1985. Oncogenic transformation by equine herpesviruses. II. Coestablishment of persistent infection and oncogenic transformation of hamster embryo cells by equine herpesvirus type 1 preparations enriched for defective interfering particles. J. Virol. 36:204–219.

Sabine, M., Feilen, C., Herbert, L., Jones, R.F., Lomas, S.W., Love, D.N., and Wild, J. 1983. Equine herpesvirus abortion in Australia, 1977 to 1982. Equine Vet. J. 15:366–370.

Shimizu, T., Ishizaki, R., and Matumoto, M. 1963. A plaque assay for equine rhinopneumonitis virus on monolayer culture of horse kidney cells. Jpn. J. Exp. Med. 33:85–93.

Staczek, J., Atherton, S.S., and O'Callaghan, D.J. 1983. Genetic relatedness of the genomes of equine herpesvirus types 1, 2, and 3. J. Virol. 48:855–858.

Studdert, M.J., Fitzpatrick, D.R., Browning, G.F., Cullinane, A.A., and Whalley, J.M. 1986. Equine herpesvirus genomes: Heterogeneity of naturally occurring type 4 isolates and of a type 1 isolate after heterologous cell passage. Arch. Virol. 91:375–381.

Studdert, M.J., Fitzpatrick, D.R., Horner, G.W., Westbury, H.A., and Gleeson, L.J. 1984. Molecular epidemiology and pathogenesis of some equine herpesvirus type 1 (equine abortion virus) and type 4 (equine rhinopneumonitis virus) isolates. Aust. Vet. J. 61:345–348.

Studdert, M.J., Simpson, T., and Roizman, B. 1981. Differentiation of respiratory and abortigenic isolates of equine herpesvirus 1 by restriction endonucleases. Science 214:562–564.

Tajima, M., Shimizu, T., and Ishizaki, R. 1961. Electron microscopy of equine abortion virus. Am. J. Vet. Res. 22:250–265.

Turtinen, L.W., and Allen, G.P. 1982. Identification of the envelope surface glycoproteins of equine herpesvirus type 1. J. Gen. Virol. 63:481–485.

Turtinen, L.W., Allen, G.P., Darlington, R.W., and Bryans, J.T. 1981. Serologic and molecular comparisons of several equine herpesvirus type 1 strains. Am. J. Vet. Res. 42:2099–2104.

Westerfield, C., and Dimock, W.W. 1946. The pathology of equine virus abortion. J. Am. Vet. Med. Assoc. 109:101–111.

Wilks, C.R. 1977. In vitro cytotoxicity of serum and peripheral blood leukocytes for equine herpesvirus type 1–infected target cells. Am. J. Vet. Res. 38:117–121.

Wilks, C.R., and Coggins, L. 1976. Immunity to equine herpesvirus type 1 (rhinopneumonitis): In vitro lymphocyte response. Am. J. Vet. Res. 37:486–492.

Wilks, C.R., and Studdert, M.J. 1976. Equine herpesvirus. 6. Sequential infection of horses with types 1, 2, and 3. Aust. Vet. J. 52:199–203.

Yeargan, M.R., Allen, G.P., and Bryans, J.T. 1985. Rapid subtyping of equine herpesvirus 1 with monoclonal antibodies. J. Clin. Microbiol. 21:694–697.

Equine Coital Exanthema

SYNONYMS: Equine herpesvirus 3 (EHV-3) disease, equine venereal vulvitis or balanitis

Equine coital exanthema is spread by coitus, although it may occasionally produce skin lesions through contact with an affected horse (Crandell and Davis 1985). Infection usually occurs during breeding activities. The signs of illness and lesions are similar to those of pustular vulvovaginitis in cattle. Early lesions appear vesicular or pustular and occur in the vulva and perineum in mares and on the penile mucosa of stallions (Girard et al. 1968). Lesions may also occur on teats of the mare and the muzzle and lips of the nursing foal (Crandell and Davis 1985). Later, uncomplicated lesions appear circular and pocklike, and as healing progresses affected areas are depigmented. In the absence of secondary bacterial infection, healing is complete in 10 to 14 days. No effects on fertility are apparent, but affected stallions are reluctant to cover mares until healing is complete. The incubation period is 6 to 8 days. There is evidence that virus persists in both the stallion and mare from one breeding season to another (Burrows 1977).

The inoculation of the virus into the amniotic cavity of a pregnant mare (6 to 7 months' gestation) resulted in abortion 11 days later (Gleeson et al. 1976). Although this is an interesting experimental finding, the virus has not been reported to cause abortions in the field.

Girard et al. (1968) first isolated, from two stud outbreaks, a herpesvirus that differed immunologically and culturally from EHV-1. EHV-3, the causative pathogen, replicates only in cultured cells of equine origin and is known to infect only horses. The virus produces a cytopathic effect in cell culture, but it is slower than EHV-1, and the virus appears to be cell associated.

EHV-3 DNA exists in two isomeric forms and has a molecular structure similar to that of the EHV-1 genome (Jacob et al. 1985, Sullivan et al. 1984). Experiments with several laboratory and wild strains of EHV-3 showed them to be temperature sensitive at 39°C in equine dermal cells; a function required for the egress of nucleocapsids from the nucleus is absent at 39°C. This characterization influences the pathogenicity of the disease (Jacob 1986).

Complement-fixing antibodies disappear within 60 days, whereas neutralizing antibodies persist for at least 1 year. This fact provides a useful guide for determining recent infections and the temporal incidence of infection in groups of mares.

REFERENCES

Burrows, R. 1977. Herpesvirus infections of animals—A brief review. J. Antimicrob. Rev. 3(Suppl. A):9–14.
Crandell, R.A., and Davis, E.R. 1985. Isolation of equine coital exanthema virus (equine herpesvirus 3) from the nostril of a foal. J. Am. Vet. Med. Assoc. 187:503–504.
Girard, L.J., Greig, A.S., and Mitchell, D. 1968. A virus associated with vulvitis and balanitis in the horse—A preliminary report. Can. J. Comp. Med. 32:603–604.
Gleeson, L.J., Sullivan, N.D., and Studdert, M.J. 1976. Equine herpesviruses. Type 3 as an abortigenic agent. Aust. Vet. J. 52:349–354.
Jacob, R.J. 1986. Molecular pathogenesis of equine coital exanthema: Temperature-sensitive function(s) in cells infected with equine herpesviruses. Vet. Microbiol. 11:221–237.
Jacob, R.J., Price, R., and Allen, G.P. 1985. Molecular pathogenesis of equine coital exanthema: Restriction endonuclease digestions of EHV-3 DNA and indications of a unique Xba I cleavage site. Intervirology 23:172–180.
Sullivan, D.C., Atherton, S.S., Staczek, J., and O'Callaghan, D.J. 1984. Structure of the genome of equine herpesvirus type 3. Virology 132:352–367.

Pseudorabies

SYNONYMS: Aujeszky's disease, *Herpesvirus suis* disease, infectious bulbar paralysis, mad itch; abbreviation, PR

Pseudorabies was shown to be caused by a virus by Aujeszky (1902) in Hungary. It occurs in most European countries and in South America and has been diagnosed in North America in swine, cattle, and dogs (Eidson et al. 1953, McNutt 1943, Morrill and Graham 1941, Ray 1943, Shahan et al. 1947, Shope 1931).

The disease is usually transmitted from infected pigs to other hosts, although swine and dogs may become infected from contact with carcasses of rats, raccoons, swine, and other infected animals. Shope was the first to show that the disease was prevalent in swine in the midwestern United States and that cases in cattle stemmed from the swine reservoir. By inoculation the disease can be produced in nearly all warm-blooded animals, including birds. The rabbit is especially susceptible to inoculation.

Character of the Disease. This disease occurs naturally in swine, cattle, sheep, goats, dogs, cats, chickens, mink, rats, and raccoons. Cases have been diagnosed clinically in horses, but in the absence of laboratory confirmation there is some doubt about the susceptibility of the species. In all but adult swine it is a highly fatal disease.

The disease in swine. Pruritus does not occur in swine. In adult animals the signs may be vague and mild; and recovery, usually in 4 to 8 days, is the rule rather than the exception. There may be some fever and mental depression. Some animals vomit. In some sows respiratory signs signal the onset of the disease (Gustafson et al. 1968), and it may be limited to the respiratory tract. At this time the temperature is elevated, and the sows stop eating on the third day after exposure. Constipation and depression may be accompanied by vomiting during the next 2 days. If sows are pregnant, about 50 percent will abort and the remainder will farrow. Some fetuses will be macerated; others will be normal. A significant increase in mummified fetuses occurs about 1 month after outbreaks of PR in sows (Morrison and Jov 1985). A higher percentage of abortions occurs in the first month of pregnancy. Late pregnancies may go as long as 17 days beyond the expected date of delivery. In suckling and recently weaned pigs losses may be severe. According to Hirt (1935), McNutt (1943), and Ray (1943) losses in pigs younger than 15 days are frequently 100 percent. Such animals usually become prostrate within an hour or so after the first signs are observed and die in 12 to 24 hours. McNutt noted that losses are directly proportional to the ages of the animals, varying from none in mature animals to 100 percent in the very young.

The disease in cattle. The name *mad itch* has been applied to the disease in cattle. Intense pruritus of some portion of the skin is the principal manifestation and generally appears on one of the flanks or the hind legs, but it may be on any part of the body. If the part is accessible, the animal begins licking it incessantly until it becomes reddened and abraded. If the victim can reach a wall, post, or fence, it wll rub the part until the skin is broken and torn. The itching is so intense as to cause the animal to become frenzied. As the disease progresses, the medulla becomes involved, and this leads to paralysis of the pharynx, salivation, forced respiration, and cardiac irregularities. The animal remains conscious until death approaches. There may be grinding of the teeth, bellowing, mania, and convulsions. Death usually occurs within 48 hours and sometimes much sooner. Occasional victims die within several hours after signs are first observed and without showing the pruritic signs.

The disease in dogs and cats. Cases in dogs and cats seem to be common in some European countries; thus Galloway (1938) reported that Marek, in Budapest, had seen 118 cats and 29 dogs with the disease between 1902 and 1908. It is being recognized more frequently now, but some dogs and cats die so suddenly with or without typical signs that the diagnosis can be easily missed (Hawkins and Olson 1985). In about 18 percent of cases the animals are driven into a frenzy because of the intolerable itching and do great damage to themselves by biting and tearing at the affected parts. Bulbar paralysis is generally manifested early; paralysis of the jaws and of the pharynx appears; plaintive cries and howls are emitted; and saliva drools from the mouth. The appearance may simulate rabies; but, in contrast to the furious form of rabies, the affected animals show no tendency to attack other animals or humans. As in cattle, consciousness is maintained until the end. At no stage is there any fever. In some dogs fatal arrhythmias may result from myocardial lesions (Olson and Miller 1986).

The disease in goats. The disease is largely referable to the nervous system with extreme signs including restlessness, screaming, profuse sweating, and, in the terminal stage, spasms and paralysis. Death usually occurs in 24 to 48 hours. Pruritus often is not associated with the disease in these animals. Pseudorabies in goats is associated with close proximity to virus-carrier pigs.

Properties of the Virus. Shope (1931) reported that pseudorabies virus (PRV) stored in 50 percent glycerol survives for 154 days with little loss of titer at refrigerator temperature. Virus survives on hay for 30 days in summer and 46 days in winter. It is stable between a pH of 4 and 9. One-half percent sodium hydroxide rapidly inactivates it, but 3 percent phenol is considerably less effective. Lyophilized virus survives 2 years; at low temperatures virus in tissue remains viable many years. Ultraviolet light and drying on glass inactivates the virus (Davies and Beran 1981).

Various investigators have used various biochemical and immunological procedures to characterize and identify the major glycoproteins associated with immunity and also the production of neutralizing antibodies (Ben-porat et al. 1986, Hampl et al. 1984, Sun and Gustafson 1982). Originally Ben-porat and Kaplan (1970) described four major glycoproteins. Several additional minor glycoproteins have since been identified in the viral envelopes and also several nonglycosylated proteins (Hampl et al. 1984). Three of the four major glycoproteins are linked covalently by disulfide bridges and share extensive homology. Of the monoclonal antibodies used, only those reactive with the major 98-kilodalton glycoprotein (gIII) inhibit virus adsorption and neutralize viral infectivity in the absence of complement. In an extension of these studies Ben-porat and co-workers (Ben-porat, DeMarchi, Lomniczi, and Kaplan 1986) further assessed the role of glycoproteins of PRV in eliciting neutralizing antibodies during infection of swine. A larger part of the neutralizing activity of pooled convalescent swine serums is directed against glycoprotein gIII; no activity was directed against glycoprotein gI. Antigenic variation between strains of PRV from different geographic areas is readily detectable but less common in strains from same area. No antigenic drift in glycoprotein gII was observed; but gIII and, to some extent, gI showed a high degree of antigenic drift. In other studies Sun and Gustafson (1982) described four immunologically distinct antigens designated Ag1, Ag2, Ag3, and Ag4. Antigenic similarities in the virion and cellular membrane glycoproteins were found in cells infected with PRV.

The PRV gene encoding for glycoprotein gIII is not essential for viral replication (Robbins et al. 1986). Viral functions are necessary for the recombination of the genome in infected cells (Ihara and Ben-porat 1985).

The avirulent Bartha strain lacked genes in the short unique region of the genome coding for several translationally competent mRNAs and in thymidine kinase activity that is responsible, at least in part, for its lack of virulence (Lomniczi et al. 1984).

PR, varicella zoster, and herpes simplex viruses all have a cluster of homologous glycoprotein genes in the small unique components of their genomes, and the organization of these genes is conserved (Petrovskis et al. 1986). There are also a number of cross-reactive proteins between BHV-1 and PRV (Bush and Pritchett 1986).

Some strains of PRV produce lesions only in the central nervous systems of pigs; others cause rhinitis, pneumonia, and encephalitis (Ben-porat and Kaplan 1962).

Cultivation. Traub (1933) was the first to report success in cultivating PRV. He obtained replication in minced testicular tissue of rabbits and guinea pigs and also in minced chick embryo medium. Mesrobeanu (1938) obtained growth in chick embryos, and his work was quickly confirmed by several workers. The virus may

served on continued passage at high multiplicity of most DIPs of other viruses are not observed for DIPs of PRV. The defective genomes are enriched for an origin of replication but probably also for sequences necessary for efficient cleavage encapsidation. The nondefective genomes in this population of DIPs are modified and acquired the ability to compete with the defective genomes for cleavage encapsidation (Wu et al. 1986).

Epizootiology and Pathogenesis. The principal natural reservoir of PRV is swine. Symptomless animals harbor and transmit the virus. The brown rat may be important in disease transmission from farm to farm. Infected fresh or frozen meat or offal from swine and cattle consumed by dogs and cats is the usual route of exposure for these species. Other animal species contract the disease from one of these hosts, most often from swine, but are not involved in its transmission. The discovery of the reservoir in swine was made by Shope (1935a). European workers assumed that the virus escaped from swine in the saliva and urine, but Shope showed that these fluids were not infectious and that the virus escaped only by way of the nasal excretions. Beginning about the 6th day after inoculation, when there is a concomitant temperature rise, and continuing for several days thereafter, virus is demonstrable in the scanty nasal discharge. Rabbits are easily infected by rubbing a slightly scarified skin surface on the snouts of the pigs during this time.

Shope (1934, 1935a) also showed that the ordinary brown rat, which often frequents corn cribs and animal houses, readily develops pseudorabies by ingestion. Cassells and Lamont (1942) and Lamont and Gordon (1950) described cases in Ireland in dogs (rat terriers) that, it was believed, contracted the infection from killing rats on pig farms.

In the United States mad itch of cattle occurs most often in midwestern feedlots, where range-raised beef cattle are fattened for market. Swine are commonly allowed to run with such cattle to salvage feed wasted by the cattle, and apparently these infected pigs introduce the virus through minor bite wounds on the legs of the cattle.

In coitus, virus may be transmitted from the boar to the sow and vice versa (Akkermans 1963). That such transmission occurs was confirmed by the isolation of virus from the prepuce and vagina of infected swine. It is not known whether the virus is secreted with the sperm.

In England 7 out of 11 outbreaks of PR in Yorkshire could have resulted from air-borne virus (Gloster et al. 1984). Investigators have found antibodies to PRV in the serum of raccoons, and Kirkpatrick et al. (1980) showed that infected raccoons could transmit the disease to swine but not to each other. Infected swine can also transmit the disease to contact raccoons. The raccoon may serve as a

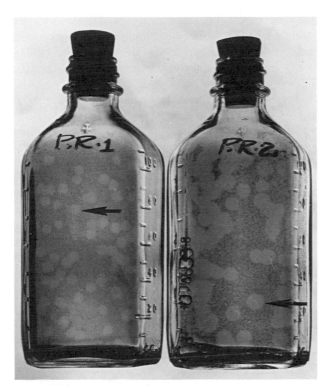

Figure 46.11. Comparison of plaque size (*arrows*) and count of pseudorabies virus on porcine kidney (*PR1*) and rabbit kidney (*PR2*) monolayers 9 days after virus seeding. (Courtesy K. V. Singh, *Cornell Veterinarian.*)

easily be passed in series in egg embryos after it has once been adapted. Bang (1942) called attention to the fact that the lesions which appear as whitish plaques on the chorioallantoic membrane after about 4 days' incubation are quickly followed by viral invasion of all parts of the central nervous system. Many strains produce hemorrhagic destruction of the nervous system, which leads to protrusion of the cranium of the embryo.

Tokumaru (1957) cultivated the virus in monkey kidney cells after it had first been adapted to eggs. Two cytopathogenic varieties were found; one produced typical cytopathic effects, the other a cell-rounding type of degeneration previously described for certain other viruses. The virus also grows in cultures of chick, rabbit, guinea pig, and dog tissues. It causes a cytopathic effect, and plaques are produced in agar overlays of pig kidney, rabbit kidney, and chick embryo cell cultures. The less virulent strains may produce larger plaques (Figure 46.11). Intranuclear inclusion bodies are found in infected cultures and eggs.

Serial passage of PRV at high multiplicity yields defective interfering particles (DIPs), but the sharp cyclical increases and decreases in titer of infectious virus ob-

short-term reservoir for PRV but is unlikely to be a long-term subclinical carrier (Wright and Thawley 1980).

Porcine embryo transfers are an excellent way to conserve valuable genetic material from swine herds with pseudorabies, because virus does not penetrate the zona pellucida (Bolin et al. 1983). When embryos from seropositive sows were transferred to seronegative sows, neither the recipients nor their progeny seroconverted (James et al. 1983). In vitro studies showed that PRV could not penetrate the zone pellucida of 8-day-old bovine embryos (Gillespie et al. 1988).

Numerous genomically different PRV strains are currently present in the United States. The combination of restriction endonuclease analysis and DNA hybridization offers useful epidemiological information about the various strains (Pirtle et al. 1984).

Latency of pseudorabies in swine has been studied by many scientists. It is possible to establish latent infection in piglets. During acute stages of disease the virus can be isolated readily by swabbing the oropharyngeal region, where replication is initiated, for 10 days. Months after the initial infection virus can be isolated from the tonsils, cervical lymph nodes, nasal mucosa, and Gasserian ganglia (Sabo 1985, Sabo and Rajcani 1976). PRV antigen was seen by immunofluorescence only in explants from Gasserian ganglia, where it was localized in the neurons and satellite cells. For 13 months after infection the stable PRV genome persisted both qualitatively and quantitatively in different areas of both the peripheral and central nervous system (Rhiza et al. 1986). The stress of farrowing may cause virus shedding in the nasal secretions for a few days (Davies and Beran 1980). Piglets with maternal antibodies may become latently infected, and virus shedding recurs after administration of large doses of corticosteroids (van Oirschot and Gielkens 1984a).

McFarlane et al. (1986) reported on DNA hybridization to detect PRV DNA in swine tissues; the procedure provides a useful tool for the study of latency and pathogenesis.

McNutt (1943) studied pseudorabies produced by inoculation in swine. When virus was injected into the muscles of one leg, a characteristic reaction, which varied according to the size and age of the animal, appeared. Pigs that weighed from 30 to 40 pounds usually became ill after an incubation period of 5 to 7 days and died about 2 days later. Larger pigs usually developed paralysis of the inoculated leg. Some of these died, others remained permanently paralyzed, and others recovered. The paralyzed pigs usually had good appetites, were active, had normal temperatures, and were not noticeably excitable. Virus was not found in the blood or in the visceral organs of most of these animals. It was found regularly, however, in the nerve trunks of the affected legs, and frequently in the spinal cord and brain. Pigs weighing more than 80 pounds seldom showed any appreciable signs, but virus could be recovered from their nervous systems and was discharged in their nasal secretions.

There is good evidence that natural infection in swine occurs by the naso-oropharyngeal route. Gustafson (1970) found that intranasal exposure to the virus resulted in a syndrome seen in natural infections as opposed to exposure via intramuscular, intratracheal, or intragastric routes. The primary sites of viral replication were the upper respiratory passages and tonsillar tissue. Virus was isolated from olfactory epithelium and tonsils after 18 hours and at 6- to 12-hour intervals thereafter for at least 5 days. Similarly, virus was isolated from the medulla and pons at 24 hours, suggesting transmission from the nasal and oral cavities in the epineural lymph of the fifth and ninth cranial nerves. Virus was not found in the blood during this period.

PRV infection can be established by preputial inoculation and may cause decreased spermatogenesis and consequent infertility of young, mature boars (Hall et al. 1984).

The pathogenesis of PRV in domestic cats after oral administration of an Iowa isolate was studied by Hagemoser et al. (1980). Several cats were studied at 1-day intervals, and tissues were examined to determine the initial sites of viral penetration and replication and the pathways traveled from the mouth to the central nervous system. Lesions were similar in the tonsils, along the pathways of the sensory branches of the ninth and tenth cranial nerves, in the nucleus tractus solitarii and the tractus solitarius, and in the area postrema in the medulla. Lesions were found less often in the ganglia and nuclei of the fifth cranial nerve, indicating a lesser role for the passage of virus via this nerve. Nervous lesions consisted of multifocal to diffuse microgliosis, mononuclear perivascular cuffing, and mononuclear inflammatory cell infiltration with a variable number of neutrophils occasionally forming microabscesses. Virus isolations correlated well with microscopic lesions. Virions were observed within the nucleus of the neurons in the medulla. Pruritus was consistently absent. Virus was isolated consistently from oral and nasal excretions for the first 2 or 3 days after inoculation but not after the third day.

The signs of naturally occurring cases can be produced experimentally by inoculating animals with the virus. Edematous tissue from a bovine lesion injected subcutaneously into rabbits results in typical mad itch signs, which begin after an incubation period of about 2 days. The animal first licks the point of inoculation, then becomes more frenzied, biting and tearing the skin of this area. This behavior lasts for 4 to 6 hours, after which the animal is exhausted. It then lies on its side, shows clonic spasms and labored respiration, and dies. Material from cattle does not infect guinea pigs or mice when inoculated subcutaneously, but, curiously, virus that has been passed through a rabbit brain causes mad itch signs in these animals (Shope 1933). Hurst (1934) studied the distribution of PRV in the rabbit. After parental inoculation the virus reaches the central nervous system by passage through the peripheral nerves. After intracerebral inoculation, virus passes centripetally from the nervous system to the lungs. After intravenous inoculation, the virus rapidly disappears from the blood and forms multiple infective foci in the organs, from which it passes through the nerves to the brain. When virus is injected subcutaneously into an area without nerves, signs are delayed because the virus must then pass through the blood to establish visceral foci from which the central nervous system is infected secondarily. Virus injected intracerebrally is uniformally fatal to guinea pigs, rats, and mice. Pruritus of the skin does not occur in such cases. After an incubation period of 24 to 48 hours, signs of excitement appear, and blindness eventually occurs. The animals frequently salivate and grind their teeth; they run about their cages wildly and injure themselves by running into the walls. Death follows after a short period of coma. Ferrets are also susceptible to the virus, which causes nonsuppurative meningoencephalitis as well as visceral lesions (Ahsima et al. 1976).

The gross lesions are not extensive in natural disease. In animals with pruritus the skin and underlying tissues at the point of infection usually are lacerated, torn, and covered with bloody exudate. The subcutaneous tissue of this region usually is very swollen. The lungs often are congested and edematous, and there may be fluid in the pericardial sac and hemorrhages on the epicardium. The other organs usually are normal. In adult swine, gross lesions generally are absent, but subcutaneous edema and sometimes necrosis may be found in some animals.

Infiltrations and necrosis of nerve elements can be seen microscopically. These lesions begin where the virus was introduced and proceed centripetally along the nerve trunks. Animals often die before the virus has reached the brain or even the anterior part of the spinal cord. This fact should be remembered when tissues are selected for laboratory diagnosis.

Immunity. Shope (1935b) showed that swine that have recovered from the disease have neutralizing antibodies in their serums. Using the neutralization test, he proved that the European and the American diseases cross-immunized perfectly and that the virus strains could be considered identical (Shope 1932). Shahan et al. (1947) showed that, after recovery from the disease, swine are immune to inoculation even by the intracerebral route.

PRV antibodies in experimentally infected swine were detected by indirect hemagglutination and serum-neutralizing antibody tests (Hoffer et al. 1980). Specific antibody titers were observed by the former method 5 days after inoculation but not until a few days later by the latter test. IgM was the predominant immunoglobulin class in serums after 5 and 7 days, as determined by sulfhydryl reductions. The virus-neutralization test lacked sensitivity to early Ig levels, while the indirect hemagglutination was highly sensitive. Competitive enzyme assay can differentiate serum antibodies of vaccinated pigs from those of animals infected with wild virus (van Oirschot et al. 1986). Pigs vaccinated with the Bartha, BVK, or NIA-4 strains did not produce antibody to the epitope of gI, whereas all wild viruses induced this antibody, which persisted for at least 15 weeks.

Colostral antibodies, which have a half-life of 8.5 days, protect against virulent virus but do not prevent the piglets from excreting virus (McFerran 1975), and latency develops.

The first cell-mediated immunity reaction of lymphocytes occurs 4 days after infection, whereas neutralizing antibodies can be detected 3 days later and reach optimal titer at day 14 (Wittman et al. 1976). Lymphocytes from the lymph nodes and spleen cause the most marked reaction, blood and thymus lymphocytes react less frequently, and those from bone marrow show no response during the test period from day 7 to 35. Reinfection causes little increase in neutralizing antibody titer. The sensitivity of the test can be enhanced by the addition of fresh guinea pig complement. Complement-fixing antibodies cannot be detected until 14 days after infection.

Diagnosis. In animals other than swine the clinical signs are quite characteristic and at least suggestive of the diagnosis. The clinician must be aware that pruritus is not observed in all animals, particularly in dogs, goats, and cats.

A definite diagnosis can be made in at least three ways: (1) isolation of the virus in rabbits or cell culture; (2) demonstration of a rising antibody titer with paired serums, using various serologic tests; or (3) a skin test in swine.

Edematous fluid from a lesion or tissues from the nerve trunk of the region, the spinal cord, and portions of the brain are appropriate tissues for isolating virus. Virus can be detected in rabbits as easily by subcutaneous as by intracerebral inoculation. The subcutaneous method has two advantages: intercurrent infections are not so apt to kill the rabbits and the characteristic pruritus aids recognition of the virus. For final recognition of the virus, virus-neutralization tests with known antiserum against the newly recovered virus may be conducted.

In rabbits acidophilic intranuclear inclusion bodies of the Cowdry A type are usually found in the spinal ganglia, in the posterior horn of the spinal cord, in the glial cells, and in a variety of cells in the local lesions, according to Hurst (1934). Such inclusions are found irregularly in cattle and have not been observed in swine. They have little diagnostic importance. There are no cytoplasmic inclusions in any species. Selected cell cultures described in the section on cultivation can be used for virus isolation.

Many serologic procedures, such as microtiter and macrotiter neutralization, microimmunodiffusion (Gutekunst et al. 1978), indirect radioimmunoassay, complement fixation, ELISA, single dilution indirect solid-phase radioimmunoassay, dot-enzyme immunoassay, indirect enzyme immunoassay, counterimmunoelectrophoresis, and indirect fluorescent antibody tests (Wirahadiredja and Rondhuis 1976), can be used to demonstrate rising serum antibody titers. Some tests, such as ELISA (Banks and Cartwright 1983), ELISA disc (Banks 1985), and single-dilution indirect solid-phase radio immunoassay (Wang and Hahn 1986), are more rapid, sensitive, and economical. The microimmunodiffusion test (MIDT), developed and evaluated for its sensitivity in revealing antibodies in swine serums (Gutekunst et al. 1978), appears to be as sensitive as the microtiter neutralization test. It also can be used to test serums that are cytotoxic, markedly hemolyzed, or too contaminated with bacteria to undergo the neutralization test. The MIDT is accurate, rapid, economical, and sensitive. In contrast, the indirect fluorescent antibody technique is not as sensitive as the microneutralization test for the detection of antibodies (Wirahadiredja and Rondhuis 1976).

A skin test is a promising diagnostic aid (Scherba et al. 1983, Smith and Mengeling 1977). The reaction, induced by subcutaneous injection in the lower eyelid, is easily evaluated. A positive response was detected as early as 7 days after exposure, reached near maximal levels by 28 days, and persisted for at least 90 days. Because control animals did not react, it appears the test is specific.

Pseudorabies virus in tissues can be detected with the immunofluorescent antibody test, but it is less sensitive than isolation of the virus in cell culture or in rabbits (Biancifiori et al. 1977). In cell-culture systems the plaque method is more indicative of the presence of virus in meat and meat products than is the cytopathic effect observed in cell monolayers (Kunev 1977). Virus can also be detected in animal tissues and in cell culture by immunoperoxidase labeling (Afshar and Dulac 1986, Allan et al. 1985).

Prevention and Control. Four types of vaccine have been fabricated for the protection of swine against PR: (1) attenuated virus vaccines such as the Bartha K vaccine strain, (2) inactivated virus vaccines, (3) thymidine kinase–deficient vaccines, and (4) subunit vaccines. As of 1987 the first three types have been approved for use by the U.S. Department of Agriculture.

When the Bartha K attenuated vaccine grown in Vero cells is inoculated intramuscularly into pigs, it causes no signs of illness or virus excretion (McFerran and Dow 1975). A single inoculation gives good protection. After intranasal administration there is minimal excretion of virus but a greater degree of protection. The lack of virulence of the Bartha vaccine strain may be related to its limited release of virus from some target cells (Ben-porat, DeMarchi, Pendrys, et al. 1986). After intranasal administration there is an absence of viral latency, but it does not prevent latency in swine exposed later to virulent virus (van Oirschot and Gielkens 1984b). Under field conditions the vaccine is effective in swine, even in a contaminated environment (Elsinghorst et al. 1976). The use of the Bartha vaccine in dogs is contraindicated because it causes adverse reactions.

Inactivated virus vaccines are not commonly used. Although they are safe, they fail to provide the same degree of protection as most attenuated virus vaccines (van Oirschot and DeLeeuw 1985).

A subunit vaccine against PRV was prepared by treating pelleted virions and infected cells with nonionic detergent Nonidet P-40 and emulsifying the extracted proteins with incomplete Freund's adjuvant. Two doses given intramuscularly 3 weeks apart to swine produced neutralizing antibodies, and the animals resisted intranasal challenge with virulent virus 30 days after the second administration. No virus was shed after challenge (Maes and Schultz 1983). This vaccine looks promising, but no further studies have been published.

Other forms of attenuated virus vaccines are the thymidine kinase–negative deletion mutants of PRV described by Kit et al. (1985) and McGregor et al. (1985). These mutants protect pigs, and latency does not develop after intranasal instillation. After challenge with virulent virus there is a secondary antibody response. One group of researchers could not isolate virus from the tonsils or trigeminal ganglia after challenge with virulent virus given 11 days after vaccination (Kit et al. 1985). A second group did recover virulent challenge virus from ganglia of a few pigs, but not from most animals, indicating that colonization of challenge virus was considerably reduced by vaccination (McGregor et al. 1985).

Swine vaccinated with attenuated PR virus vaccines showed breed differences in the serum-neutralizing antibody response (Rothschild et al. 1984). How this correlates with protection was not determined. Maternal antibody can interfere with the response of an inactivated and an attenuated virus vaccine after intranasal and parenteral adminstration (Vannier 1985, van Oirschot and DeLeeuw 1985). The efficacy of parenteral as well as intranasal vaccination decreases with the increasing levels of maternal antibody at the time of vaccination.

It has been postulated that a properly controlled and monitored vaccination, culling, and management program may eradicate pseudorabies from breeding herds (McCracken et al. 1984). The control of wildlife and segregation of infected swine from cattle are recommended.

The Disease in Humans. The danger to humans from pseudorabies is apparently slight, although several human cases have been diagnosed in Europe; investigators claim to have isolated virus from some of these patients. Usually the patient has come in contact with tissues of infected animals and has become contaminated through a skin wound. No fatalities have been reported, but severe pruritus has been noted in some patients.

REFERENCES

Afshar, A., and Dulac, G.C. 1986. Immunoperoixdase plaque staining for the detection of pseudorabies virus. Can. J. Vet. Res. 50:118–119.

Ahsima, K., Gorham, J.R., and Henson, J.B. 1976. Pathologic changes in ferrets exposed to pseudorabies virus. Am. J. Vet. Res. 37:591–596.

Akkermans, J.P.W. 1963. Aujeszky's disease in swine varies in severity. J. Am. Vet. Med. Assoc. 143:860.

Allan, G.M., McNulty, M.S., Todd, D., and McFerran, J.B. 1985. The rapid detection of Aujeszky's disease virus in pigs by direct immunoperoxidase labelling. Vet. Microbiol. 10:481–486.

Aujeszky, A. 1902. Über eine neue Infektionskrankheit bei Haustieren. Zentralbl. Bakteriol. I. Abt. Orig. 32:353–357.

Bang, F.B. 1942. Experimental infection of the chick embryo with the virus of pseudorabies. J. Exp. Med. 76:263–270.

Banks, M. 1985. Detection of antibodies to Aujeszky's disease virus in whole blood by Elisadisc. J. Virol. Methods. 12:41–45.

Banks, M., and Cartwright, S. 1983. Comparison and evaluation of four serological tests for detection of antibodies to Aujeszky's disease virus. Vet. Rec. 113:38–41.

Ben-porat, T., and Kaplan, A.S. 1962. The chemical composition of herpes simplex and pseudorabies viruses. Virology 16:261–266.

Ben-porat, T., and Kaplan, A.S. 1970. Synthesis of proteins in cells infected with herpesvirus. Virology 41:265–273.

Ben-porat, T., DeMarchi, J.M., Lomniczi, B., and Kaplan, A.S. 1986. Role of glycoproteins of pseudorabies virus in eliciting neutralizing antibodies. Virology 154:325–334.

Ben-porat, T., DeMarchi, J., Pendrys, J., Veach, R.A., and Kaplan, A.S. 1986. Proteins specified by the short unique region of the genome of pseudorabies virus play a role in the release of virions from certain cells. J. Virol. 57:191–196.

Biancifiori, F., Gilletti, L., Frescura, T., and Morozzi, A. 1977. Presence of Aujeszky's disease virus in organs and material from experimentally infected dogs. Folia Vet. Lat. 7:174–178.

Bolin, S.R., Turek, J.J., Runnels, L.J., and Gustafson, D.P. 1983. Pseudorabies virus, porcine parvovirus, and porcine enterovirus interactions with the zona pellucida of the porcine embryo. Am. J. Vet. Res. 44:1036–1039.

Bush, C.E., and Pritchett, R.F. 1986. Immunologic comparison of the proteins of pseudorabies (Aujeszky's disease) virus and bovine herpesvirus-1. Am. J. Vet. Res. 47:1708–1712.

Cassells, R.W., and Lamont, H.G. 1942. Aujeszky's disease in dogs. Vet. Rec. 54:21.

Davies, E.B., and Beran, G.W. 1980. Spontaneous shedding of pseudorabies virus from a clinically recovered postparturient sow. J. Am. Vet. Med. Assoc. 176:1345–1347.

Davies, E.B., and Beran, G.W. 1981. Influence of environmental factors upon the survival of Aujeszky's disease virus. Res. Vet. Sci. 31:32–36.

DeLeeuw, P.W., and van Oirschot, J.T. 1985. Vaccines against Aujeszky's disease: Evaluation of their efficacy under standardized laboratory conditions. Vet. Q. 7:191–197.

Eidson, M.E., Kissling, R.E., and Tierkel, E.S. 1953. Pseudorabies virus infections in dogs. J. Am. Vet. Med. Assoc. 123:34–37.

Elsinghorst, A.H., van der Linden, M.J., van Lieshout, J.A., and Schröder, P. 1976. Ziekte van aujeszky in de praktijk en de enting tegen de ziekte. Tijdschr. Diergeneeskd. 101:912–917.

Galloway, I.A. 1938. Aujeszky's disease. Common synonyms: "pseudo-rabies," "infectious bulbar paralysis," "mad itch." Vet. Rec. 50:745–762.

Gillespie, J.H., Foote, R.H., Schlafer, D.H., Quick, S., Dougherty, E., Schiff, E., and Allen, S. 1988. Bovine embryo transfers: Viral persistence of seven viruses on six- to eight-day-old bovine embryos after in vitro exposure. In press.

Gloster, J., Donaldson, A.I., and Hough, M.N. 1984. Analysis of a series of outbreaks of Aujeszky's disease in Yorkshire in 1981–82: The possibility of airborne disease spread. Vet. Rec. 114:234–239.

Gustafson, D.P. 1970. In H.W. Dunne, ed., Diseases of Swine, 3d ed. Iowa State University Press, Ames. Pp. 337–355.

Gustafson, D.P., Claflin, R.M., and Saunders, J.R. 1968. Immunology: Mechanisms of viral pathogenesis. Fed. Proc. 27:425.

Gutekunst, D.E., Pirtle, E.C., and Mengeling, W.L. 1978. Development evaluation of a microimmunodiffusion test for detection of antibodies to pseudorabies virus in swine serum. Am. J. Vet. Res. 39:207–210.

Hagemoser, W.A., Kluge, J.P., and Hill, H.T. 1980. Studies on the pathogenesis of pseudorabies in domestic cats following oral inoculation. Can. J. Comp. Med. 44:192–202.

Hall, L.B., Jr., Kluge, J.P., Evans, L.E., and Hill, H.T. 1984. The effect of pseudorabies (Aujeszky's) virus infection on young mature boars and boar fertility. Can. J. Comp. Med. 48:192–197.

Hampl, H., Ben-porat, T., Ehrlicher, L., Habermehl, K.O., and Kaplan, A.S. 1984. Characterization of the envelope proteins of pseudorabies virus. J. Virol. 52:583–590.

Hawkins, B.A., and Olson, G.R. 1985. Clinical signs of pseudorabies in the dog and cat: A review of 40 cases. Iowa State Univ. Vet. 47:116–119.

Hirt, G. 1935. Beiträge zur Aujeszkyschen Krankheit der Savgerkel. Arch. Wiss. Prakt. Tierheilk. 70:86–94.

Hoffer, K., Gustafson, D.P., and Kanitz, C.L. 1980. Detection of pseudorabies virus antibodies: Time of appearance by two serotests. Am. J. Vet. Res. 41:1317–1318.

Hurst, E.W. 1934. The histology of equine encephalomyelitis. J. Exp. Med. 59:529–542.

Ihara, S., and Ben-porat, T. 1985. The expression of viral functions is necessary for recombination of a herpes-virus (pseudorabies). Virology 147:237–240.

James, J.E., James, D.M., Martin, P.A., Reed, D.E., and Davis, D.L. 1983. Embryo transfer for conserving valuable genetic material from swine herds with pseudorabies. J. Am. Vet. Med. Assoc. 183:525–528.

Kirkpatrick, C.M., Kanitz, C.L., and McCrocklin, S.M. 1980. Possible role of wild mammals in transmission of pseudorabies to swine. J. Wildl. Dis. 16:601–614.

Kit, S., Kit, M., and Pirtle, E.C. 1985. Attenuated properties of thymidine kinase–negative deletion mutant of pseudorabies virus. Am. J. Vet. Res. 46:1359–1367.

Kunev, Z.H. 1977. Izpolzvane na plakoviya metod za izolirane na virusa na bolesti na Aueski. [Use of the plaque method to isolate Aujeszky's disease virus from meat, viscera and meat products.] Vet. Med. Nauki 14:79–83.

Lamont, H.G., and Gordon, W.A.M. 1950. Aujeszky's disease—A sporadic case in a fox terrier bitch. Vet. Rec. 62:596.

Lomniczi, B., Watanabe, S., Ben-porat, T., and Kaplan, A.S. 1984. Genetic basis of the neurovirulence of pseudorabies virus. J. Virol. 52:198–205.

McCracken, R.M., McFerran, J.B., McParland, P.J., and McKillop, E.R. 1984. Vaccination against Aujeszky's disease: Field experiences. Vet. Rec. 115:348–352.

McFarlane, R.G., Thawley, D.G., and Solorzano, R.F. 1986. Detection of latent pseudorabies virus in porcine tissue, using a DNA hybridization dot-blot assay. Am. J. Vet. Res. 47:2329–2336.

McFerran, J.B. 1975. Studies on immunity to Aujeszky's disease (pseudorabies) virus infection in pigs. Dev. Biol. Stand. 28:563–570.

McFerran, J.B., and Dow, C. 1975. Studies on immunisation of pigs with the Bartha strain of Aujeszky's disease virus. Res. Vet. Sci. 19:17–22.

McGregor, S., Easterday, B.C., Kaplan, A.S., and Ben-porat, T. 1985. Vaccination of swine with thymidine kinase–deficient mutants of pseudorabies virus. Am. J. Vet. Res. 46:1494–1497.

McNutt, S.H. 1943. Some infectious diseases involving the nervous system of swine. North Am. Vet. 24:409–417.

Maes, R.K., and Shutz, J.C. 1983. Evaluation in swine of a subunit vaccine against pseudorabies. Am. J. Vet. Res. 44:123–125.

Mesrobeanu, I. 1938. Culture du virus de la maladie d'Aujeszky dans la membrane chorioallantoi dienne du poulet. C.R. Soc. Biol. Paris 127:1183–1185.

Morrill, C.C., and Graham, R. 1941. An outbreak of bovine pseudorabies, or "mad itch." Am. J. Vet. Res. 2:35–40.

Morrison, R.B., and Jov, H.S. 1985. Prenatal and preweaning deaths caused by pseudorabies virus and porcine parvovirus in a swine herd. J. Am. Vet. Med. Assoc. 187:481–483.

Olson, G.R., and Miller, L.D. 1986. Studies on the pathogenesis of heart lesions in dogs infected with pseudorabies virus. Can. J. Vet. Res. 50:245–250.

Petrovskis, E.A., Timmins, J.G., and Post, L.E. 1986. Use of lambda gt11 to isolate genes for two pseudorabies virus glycoproteins with homology to herpes simplex virus and varicella-zoster virus glycoproteins. J. Virol. 60:185–193.

Pirtle, E.C., Wathen, M.W., Paul, P.S., Mengeling, W.L., and Sacks, J.M. 1984. Evaluation of field isolates of pseudorabies (Aujeszky's disease) virus as determined by restriction endonuclease analysis and hybridization. Am. J. Vet. Res. 45:1906–1912.

Ray, J.D. 1943. Pseudorabies (Aujeszky's disease) in suckling pigs in the United States. Vet. Med. 38:178–179.

Rhiza, H.J., Mettenleiter, T.C., Ohlinger, V., and Wittmann, G. 1986. Herpesvirus (pseudorabies virus) latency in swine: Occurrence and physical state of viral DNA in neural tissues. Virology 155:600–613.

Robbins, A.K., Whealy, M.E., Watson, R.J., and Enquist, L.W. 1986. Pseudorabies virus gene encoding glycoprotein gIII is not essential for growth in tissue culture. J. Virol. 59:635–645.

Rothschild, M.F., Hill, H.T., Christian, L.L., and Warner, C.M. 1984. Genetic differences in serum-neutralization titers of pigs after vaccination with pseudorabies modified live-virus vaccine. Am. J. Vet. Res. 45:1216–1218.

Sabo, A. 1985. Analysis of reactivation of latent pseudorabies virus infection in tonsils and gasserian ganglia of pigs. Acta Virol. 29:393–402.

Sabo, A., and Rajcani, J. 1976. Latent pseudorabies virus infection in pigs. Acta Virol. 20:208–214.

Scherba, G., Turek, J.J., and Gustafson, D.P. 1983. Pseudorabies virus nucleocapsid antigen for skin testing in swine. J. Clin. Microbiol. 17:539–544.

Shahan, M.S., Knudson, R.L., Seibold, H.R., and Dale, C.N. 1947. Aujeszky's disease (pseudorabies). A review with notes on two strains of the virus. North Am. Vet. 28:440–449, 511–521.

Shope, R.E. 1931. An experimental study of "mad itch" with especial reference to its relationship to pseudorabies. J. Exp. Med. 54:233–248.

Shope, R.E. 1932. Identity of the viruses causing "mad itch" and pseudorabies. Proc. Soc. Exp. Biol. Med. 30:308–309.

Shope, R.E. 1933. Modification of the pathogenicity of pseudo-rabies virus by animal passage. J. Exp. Med. 57:925–931.

Shope, R.E. 1934. Pseudorabies as a contagious disease of swine. Science 80:102–103.

Shope, R.E. 1935a. Experiments on the epidemiology of pseudo-rabies. I. Modes of transmission of the disease in swine and their possible role in its spread to cattle. J. Exp. Med. 62:85–99.

Shope, R.E. 1935b. Experiments on the epidemiology of pseudo-rabies. II. Prevalence of the disease among middle western swine and the possible role of rats in herd-to-herd infections. J. Exp. Med. 62:101–117.

Smith, P.C., and Mengeling, W.L. 1977. A skin test for pseudorabies virus infection (Aujeszky's disease) in swine. Can. J. Comp. Med. 41:364–368.

Sun, I.L., and Gustafson, D.P. 1982. Identification of immunologically distinct antigens in pseudorabies virus. J. Hyg. Epidemiol. Microbiol. Immunol. 26:285–290.

Tokumaru, T. 1957. Pseudorabies virus in tissue culture: Differentiation of two distinct strains of virus by cytopathogenic pattern induced. Proc. Soc. Exp. Biol. Med. 96:55–60.

Traub, E. 1933. Cultivation of pseudorabies virus. J. Exp. Med. 58:663–681.

Vannier, P. 1985. Experimental infection of fattening pigs with pseudorabies (Aujeszky's disease) virus: Efficacy of attenuated live—and inactivated—virus vaccines in pigs with or without passive immunity. Am. J. Vet. Res. 46:1498–1502.

van Oirschot, J.T.,and DeLeeuw, P.W. 1985. Intranasal vaccination of pigs against Aujeszky's disease. 4. Comparison with one or two doses of an inactivated vaccine in pigs with moderate maternal antibody titers. Vet. Microbiol. 10:401–408.

van Oirschot, J.T., and Gielkens, A.L. 1984a. In vivo and in vitro reactivation of latent pseudorabies virus in pigs born to vaccinated sows. Am. J. Vet. Res. 45:567–571.

van Oirschot, J.T., and Gielkens, A.L. 1984b. Intranasal vaccination of pigs against pseudorabies: Absence of vaccinal virus latency and failure to prevent latency of virulent virus. Am. J. Vet. Res. 45:2099–2103.

van Oirschot, J.T., Rziha, H.J., Moonen, P.J., Pol, J.M., and van Zaane, D. 1986. Differentiation of serum antibodies from pigs vaccinated or infected with Aujeszky's disease virus by a competitive enzyme immunoassay. J. Gen. Virol. 67:1179–1182.

Wang, F.I., and Hahn, E.C. 1986. Single-dilution indirect solid-phase radioimmunoassay for the detection of antipseudorabies immunoglobulin G in swine sera. Am. J. Vet. Res. 47:1495–1500.

Wirahadiredja, R.M.S., and Rondhuis, P.R. 1976. A comparative study of the neutralisation test and the indirect flourescent antibody technique for the detection of antibodies to the virus of Aujeszky in pig sera. Tijdschr. Diergeneeskd. 101:1125–1128.

Wittman, G., Bartenback, G., and Jakubik, J. 1976. Cell-mediated immunity in Aujeszky disease virus infected pigs. I. Lymphocyte stimulation. Arch. Virol. 50:215–222.

Wright, J.C., and Thawley, D.G. 1980. Role of the raccoon in the transmission of pseudorabies: A field and laboratory investigation. Am. J. Vet. Res. 41:581–583.

Wu, C.A., Harper, L., and Ben-porat, T. 1986. Molecular basis for interference of defective interfering particles of pseudorabies virus with replication of standard virus. J. Virol. 59:308–317.

Canine Herpesvirus Infection

A fatal septicemic disease of infant puppies caused by a herpeslike virus was described by Carmichael et al. (1965). A virus with characteristics of herpesviruses also was recovered by Stewart (1965) from young puppies that died of a hemorrhagic disease.

So far as is known, only dogs are susceptible. The disease has been observed in the United States, Great Britain, and Europe. Serologic studies indicate that the virus is widespread in the eastern and southeastern United States.

Character of the Disease. Severe disease has been recognized only in puppies less than 1 month old; fatal illness occurs in those less than 2 weeks old. The illness in infant puppies appears between the 5th and 14th day after birth; the principal signs are a soft, odorless, yellowish green stool; anorexia; labored breathing; abdominal pain; and crying.

The incubation period varies between 3 and 8 days in puppies inoculated intranasally or intraperitoneally. The route of inoculation and virus does not appear to be related to the time of onset or to the severity of illness.

The course of the disease is short in puppies; most animals die within 24 to 48 hours after the onset of clinical manifestations. Virus has been isolated from the nasopharynx of inoculated dogs for periods up to 21 days.

The disease in older dogs is confined largely to the reproductive system. Usually there are no external clinical signs associated with the genital infection in female dogs; the vaginal lesions consist of multiple lymphoid nodules in the mucosa interspersed with petechial and submucosal hemorrhages. Male dogs have a serous preputial discharge 3 to 7 days after exposure. Occasionally, the infection spreads to the conjunctiva; and, like the genital disease, it is self-limiting and regresses in 4 to 5 days (Hill and Mare 1974).

Pathological changes in fatal cases are characteristic. Lesions in inoculated and naturally infected puppies consist of disseminated focal necrosis and hemorrhages, and can be found in virtually all of the organs. Especially noteworthy changes occur in the kidneys, where subcapsular hemorrhages appear as bright red spots on the gray background of necrotic cortical tissue. The lungs are diffusely pneumonic. Focal necrosis and hemorrhages also are common in the liver, intestinal tract, and adrenal glands. Spleens characteristically are enlarged. Meningoencephalitic lesions are frequently found and virus isolated from them, even though other clinical signs are lacking (Huxsoll and Hemelt 1970, Percy 1970).

In pathogenetic studies of the dog, Carmichael (1970) suggested that virus enters the body by oral or nasal routes, with oral, nasal, and vaginal excretions the source of infection for susceptible dogs. Virus replicates primarily in the tonsils, nasal turbinate, mucosa, and pharynx and is transported in the blood, where it is associated with the leukocytes. Secondary viral replication takes place in blood vessels; reticuloendothelial cells of spleen, liver, and lymph nodes; parenchyma of liver, lungs, kidneys, spleen, and adrenal glands; lamina propria of intestinal tract; meninges; and brain.

Canine herpesvirus–induced retinal dysplasia and associated ocular anomalies were produced in newborn beagle puppies (Albert et al. 1976). In these studies histological fluorescent antibody and virus isolation procedures were applied to determine the pathogenesis of the eye disease.

Body temperature and its regulation are important pathogenetic factors in infant pups (Carmichael 1970, Huxsoll and Hemelt 1970). By maintaining puppies that were inoculated with virus at 1 day of age in an environment that increased their body temperature from 101° to 103.1°F, Carmichael (1970) was able to prolong survival, and viral growth was diminished. This phenomenon does not entirely explain the age resistance associated with canine herpesvirus (CHV) infection in the opinion of these authors.

The role of CHV in tracheobronchitis needs to be clarified (Percy 1970), although it is unlikely that it is involved in the etiology of this disease (Gillespie et al. 1970).

Properties of the Virus. Virus particles in thin sections of dog kidney cells have an average diameter of 142 nm. The particles contain a DNA core surrounded by two membranes. The protein coat is composed of 162 subunits, a characteristic shared by other herpesviruses. The virus is inactivated by chloroform and ether, and is destroyed in less than 4 minutes at 56°C. Infectivity is reduced by 50 percent after 5 hours at 37°C. Virus titers are maintained for months at -70°C in virus stocks that contain 10 percent serum. Infectivity is lost below pH 4.5 after 30 minutes. Hemagglutination has not been demonstrated with erythrocytes from a variety of species. The virus is not related serologically to infectious canine hepatitis, canine distemper, infectious bovine rhinotracheitis, equine rhinopneumonitis, avian laryngotracheitis, or herpes simplex viruses.

Cultivation. CHV grows readily in dog kidney cell cultures. Characteristic cytopathic effects—focal areas of rounded and degenerating cells which detach from the glass of the culture tube—occur in susceptible cell cultures, beginning 12 to 16 hours after inoculation. Cells occasionally have faintly acidophilic intranuclear changes, which consist of dissolution of chromatin and the formation of basophilic nucleoprotein bodies that are often most numerous adjacent to the nuclear membrane.

A plaque reduction test was developed by Binn et al. (1970) for comparing antigenic relationships of various strains of CHV, and no significant antigenic differences were noted in the comparison of four United States isolates.

Immunity. Puppies from inoculated pregnant females with antibody titers at the time of inoculation did not develop illness. In contrast, susceptible pregnant females that were inoculated intravaginally with virus gave birth to puppies, all of which died within 2 weeks. Virus was recovered from the dead puppies. Females whose puppies died naturally of the disease have been observed to give birth 1 year later to normal puppies. Neutralizing antibodies develop in older dogs inoculated with the virus; however, the duration of immunity is not known. The need for a vaccine does not seem great, and none is available at present (Carmichael 1970).

Epizootiology. The natural mode of transmission is by inhalation or ingestion or by vaginal contact. Infections occurred in puppies whose mothers were inoculated intravaginally 2 weeks before whelping. This phenomenon has also been observed in a naturally infected litter. Transmission by droplet infection has been observed between older inoculated dogs placed in close contact with uninoculated animals.

The problem of latency and carrier animals in CHV infection has not received much attention, as it is not considered an important disease of dogs. One report states that virus was isolated from the anterior vagina of a bitch 18 days after whelping a litter of herpesvirus-infected puppies (Love and Huxtable 1976).

Diagnosis. The uncomplicated disease in older dogs is so mild that it probably goes unnoticed; however, the disease-producing potential of this virus has not been fully explored. Pathological changes in affected puppies are characteristic. Necrotic and hemorrhagic lesions in the liver, lungs, and kidneys of dead puppies suggest a tentative diagnosis of CHV infection. Focal renal hemorrhages have not been reported in dogs infected with canine hepatitis or distemper viruses. Microscopic examination reveals characteristic intranuclear inclusions in cells in necrotic areas which must be differentiated from canine hepatitis inclusions. Virus is isolated readily from tissues of dead puppies in dog kidney cell cultures.

The neutralization or complement-fixation tests can be used to demonstrate antibody (Huxsoll and Hemelt 1970); but complement-fixing antibodies are not present in serums of all convalescent dogs, and they often disappear within 1 to 2 months after exposure. Neutralizing antibody titers are produced in low titer and generally persist longer than complement-fixing antibody. Neutralizing titers can be increased two- to eightfold by the addition of four units of guinea pig complement (C^1).

The Disease in Humans. There is no evidence that CHV is pathogenic for humans.

REFERENCES

Albert, D.M., Lahav, M., Carmichael, L.E., and Percy, D.H. 1976. Canine herpes induced retinal dysplasia and associated ocular anomolies. Invest. Ophthalmol. 15:267–268.

Binn, L.N., Koughan, W.P., Lazar, E. 1970. A simple plaque procedure for comparing antigenic relationships of canine herpesvirus. J.A.M.A. 156:1724–1725.

Carmichael, L.E. 1970. Herpesvirus canis: Aspects of pathogenesis and immune response. J. Am. Vet. Med. Assoc. 156:1714–1721.

Carmichael, L.E., Squire, R.A., and Krook, L. 1965. Clinical and pathologic features of a fatal viral disease of newborn pups. Am. J. Vet. Res. 26:803–814.

Gillespie, J.H., Carmichael, L.E., Gourlay, J.A., Dinsmore, J.R., Abbott, G.W., Binn, L.N., Cabasso, V., Fox, F.H., Gorham, J.R., Ott, R.L., Peacock, G.V., Sharpless, G.R., Decker, W.M., and Freeman, A. 1970. Introduction to the symposium on immunity to selected canine infectious diseases. J. Am. Vet. Med. Assoc. 156:1669–1671.

Hill, H., and Mare, C.J. 1974. Genital disease in dogs caused by canine herpesvirus. Am. J. Vet. Res. 35:669–672.

Huxsoll, D.L., and Hemmelt, I.E. 1970. Clinical observations of canine herpesvirus. J. Am. Vet. Med. Assoc. 156:1706–1713.

Love, D.N., and Huxtable, C.R.R. 1976. Naturally-occurring neonatal canine herpesvirus infection. Vet. Rec. 99:501–503.

Percy, D.H. 1970. Comments on canine herpesvirus: Pathogenesis and immune response. J. Am. Vet. Med. Assoc. 156:1721–1724.

Stewart, S.E., David-Ferreira, J., Lovelace, E., Landon, J., Stock, N. 1965. Herpes-like virus isolated from neonatal and fetal dogs. Science 148:1341–1343.

Feline Viral Rhinotracheitis

Feline viral rhinotracheitis (FVR) occurs in both the Eastern and Western hemispheres, principally as a respiratory infection. It is a very important and common disease of the domestic cat, and the causative virus—feline herpesvirus 1 (FHV-1), also known as FVR virus—is one of a number of viruses involved in respiratory disease of cats. An excellent short review of this disease is given by Crandell (1973).

The virus, which possesses the properties of the genus *Herpesvirus*, was first isolated by Crandell and Maurer (1958) from young kittens with respiratory disease. The first European isolation was made by Burki (1963).

Character of the Disease. The respiratory disease varies markedly, from an inapparent condition to severe respiratory involvement terminating in death. The disease principally affects the upper respiratory tract and is characterized by sudden onset; transient fever; neutrophilic leukocytosis; paroxysmal sneezing and coughing; nasal, turbinate (Figure 46.12), and conjunctival exudate; difficult breathing; and anorexia and weight loss (Bodle 1976). It may cause generalized disease in susceptible kittens and abortions in pregnant queens. A similar respiratory disease is seen in germ-free cats, suggesting that the severity of FVR does not depend on the secondary activity of respiratory microbes (Hoover and Griesemer 1971).

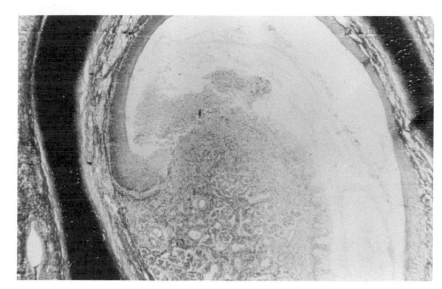

Figure 46.12. Feline herpesvirus 1 infection. Ulcerated area with cellular reaction in the turbinate. Hematoxylin and eosin stain. × 3.5. (From Walton and Gillespie, 1970a, courtesy of *Cornell Veterinarian.*)

Properties of the Virus. The nuclear virus particles have an average diameter of 148 nm and consist of a central, dense core surrounded by a clear zone bounded by an outer membrane (Crandell 1973). Cytoplasmic particles vary in size from 128 to 167 nm in diameter, whereas extracellular particles are 164 nm in diameter. The enveloped particle of cubic symmetry has 162 capsomeres (Figure 46.13). It is a DNA virus that is pH-labile and sensitive to ether and chloroform (Bartholomew and Gillespie 1968, Crandell 1973).

The virus is highly species-specific, having been isolated only from the domestic cat and other members of the cat family.

Hemagglutinating and hemadsorbing properties of the virus have been demonstrated with feline red blood cells (Gillespie et al. 1971). A hemagglutination test has been developed to detect feline herpes antibodies.

Investigators in the United States and Europe have compared many strains of feline herpesvirus and have concluded that only one serotype of feline respiratory herpesvirus is known to exist. Neutralization tests show no serologic relationship between FHV-1 and feline panleukopenia, infectious bovine rhinotracheitis, pseudorabies, certain feline calicivirus strains, and herpes simplex viruses. Complement-fixation tests show no antigenic relationship between FHV-1 and certain feline calicivirus strains (Crandell et al. 1961) or the human adenovirus group.

A biochemical study of FHV-1 revealed 23 viral proteins and 6 glycoproteins in the whole virus particle. Treatment with Tween 80 diethylether removed the major glycoproteins (Fargeaud et al. 1984). Immunoprecipitates of purified virions and Nonidet P-40 extracts contain three major glycoproteins with the same estimated molecular masses as those found by direct analysis—105 kilodaltons, 68 kilodaltons, and 60 kilodaltons (Maes et al. 1984). The physical structure of the genome of FHV-1 is similar to the genome of other alpha herpesviruses (Rota, Maes, and Ruyechan 1986).

Figure 46.13. Feline herpesvirus 1 particle, stained with phosphotungstic acid, showing capsomeres and other structures characteristic of the genus. × 200,500. (Courtesy J. Strandberg, D. Kahn, and P. Bartholomew.)

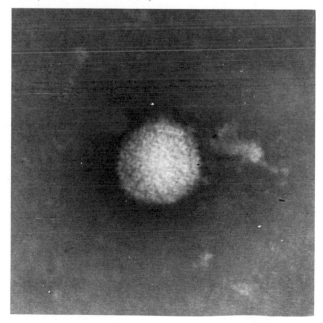

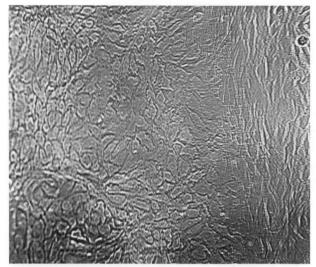

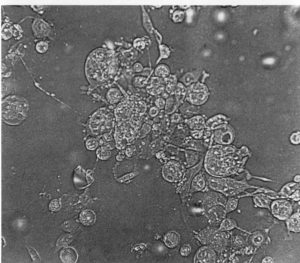

Figure 46.14. Feline herpesvirus 1 in feline kidney cell culture. Uninoculated monolayer (*top*) and inoculated culture showing characterisic cytopathic effect of a herpesvirus (*bottom*). × 100. (From Walton and Gillespie, 1970a, courtesy of *Cornell Veterinarian.*)

Cultivation. The virus replicates and produces a cytopathic effect in cell cultures of feline origin (Crandell 1973) (Figure 46.14). Although tests in cell cultures have not been exhaustive, cytopathology of FHV-1 is limited to cultures of feline origin (Lee et al. 1969).

The characteristic feature of its cytopathic effect is the formation of intranuclear inclusion bodies (Figure 46.15). Multinucleated giant cells or syncytia also are formed in cell cultures. Macroscopic plaques in cultures under agar are readily produced by many strains. Some cell lines show differences in plaque size (Tham and Studdert 1986). The appearance of the cytopathic effect is dose-dependent, but as a rule it is observed within 24 to 72

hours and reaches a maximum titer of 10^4 to 10^6 TCID$_{50}$ per 0.1 ml.

Epizootiology and Pathogenesis. All evidence suggests that the infection is transmitted by cats to cats, presumably by the respiratory route. Cats that recover from the disease may become carriers with virus localized principally in the pharyngeal region (Walton and Gillespie 1970a). The vast majority of cats are virus carriers, and approximately half shed virus spontaneously with or without stress (Gaskell and Povey 1977). Carriers are probably the most significant source of virus and account largely for the spread of virus, but intimate contact is required. Aerosol transmission is unlikely, but there is limited information on this point (Gaskell and Povey 1982). Because latency of FHV-1 in nerves has been demonstrated, this herpesvirus characteristic was anticipated (Ellis 1982, Gaskell et al. 1985).

FHV-1 has been isolated five times from dogs (Rota, Maes, and Evermann 1986). The significance of this finding in terms of disease and transmission is still not apparent.

In experimental studies pathogen-free queens given FHV-1 intravenously in the late stages of gestation (seventh or eighth week) had stillborn fetuses (Johnson 1964). Other animal herpesviruses produce a similar effect under natural conditions, and stillbirths have also been observed in natural FHV-1 infections in cats. Intracerebral inoculation of feline herpesvirus causes fatal encephalitis (Hoover and Griesemer 1971), thus we can anticipate occasional natural cases, especially in neonatal kittens.

Eosinophilic intranuclear inclusion bodies are associated with extensive nasal epithelial necrosis and focal epithelial necrosis in the conjunctiva, tonsils, epiglottis, larynx, trachea, and, rarely, in bronchi or bronchioles (Hoover and Griesemer 1971). Laryngotracheal lesions usually are mild, and pulmonary lesions are rare, with confinement to the bronchi and bronchioles. In natural cases pneumonia may occur as a result of secondary bacterial infection. In separate experimental studies in conventional cats (Walton and Gillespie 1970b) and in germ-free cats (Hoover and Griesemer 1971), lingual ulceration was not observed, but it was seen in feline calicivirus (picornavirus) infection (Kahn and Gillespie 1970) and more recently in a natural case of FVR (Shields and Gaskin 1977). Apparently the tongue lesions may occur in a cat with natural FVR. Intranuclear inclusion bodies were found in the lingual lesions and the multifocal liver lesions of the cat. Naturally occurring dendritic keratitis has been observed in conjunction with FVR in neonatal, juvenile, and adult domestic cats (Bodle 1976).

In addition to resorption of turbinate bone in conventional cats (Crandell 1973), Hoover and Griesemer (1971)

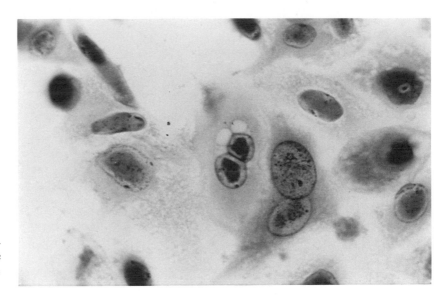

Figure 46.15. Typical Cowdry type A intranuclear inclusion bodies caused by feline herpesvirus 1. May-Grünwald-Giemsa stain. × 380.

observed severe osteolytic lesions simulating overt necrosis of bone in the turbinates of some germ-free cats with FHV-1 infection.

Immunity. An evaluation of the literature suggests that cats in the convalescent stage are completely immune, even though some may lack neutralizing antibody at 21 days; a partial but significant immunity still exists after 5 months.

In experimental studies Walton and Gillespie (1970b) confirmed that the initial antibody response after intranasal infection produced little or no neutralizing antibody (Bartholomew and Gillespie 1968, Crandell 1973). In addition, the kitten challenged by aerosol route at 21 days did not respond clinically or excrete virus, but serum-neutralizing antibody titers increased significantly (Bartholomew and Gillespie 1968, Walton and Gillespie 1970b). When challenged by the aerosol route at 150 days, the serum titers of the kittens as a group were significantly lower, and the animals showed only mild signs of illness; some kittens excreted virus for up to 6 days (Walton and Gillespie 1970b). Johnson and Thomas (1966) associated resistance to infection in older cats with and without detectable antibody levels. A transient antibody response was observed by Povey and Johnson (1967) in recovered cats, with the development of febrile reaction only upon challenge with virulent virus. They also reported a relatively persistent antibody response in cats that were resistant to challenge. Seroconversion does occur after exposure to intranasal vaccine virus or to parenteral inoculation with inactivated virus vaccine.

To provide some information on recovery mechanisms from feline viral tracheitis, Wardley et al. (1976) performed studies in cell cultures. They found that virus-infected cells could be destroyed in three ways: antibody-mediated and complement-mediated lysis, direct lymphocyte cytotoxicity, and antibody-dependent, cell-mediated cytotoxicity. Antibody-complement lysis and antibody-dependent, cell-mediated cytotoxicity occurred 6 hours after infection when intracellular infections virus spread takes place, while direct cytotoxicity occurred at 8 hours, just prior to extracellular viral spread.

Diagnosis. To clinically distinguish FVR from other feline respiratory conditions with other causes is difficult, if not impossible. Diagnosis requires isolation of FHV-1. The virus can be successfully isolated during the acute febrile stage of disease with sterile swabs applied to the pharynx, nasal passages, and conjunctiva, in that order. The material obtained is inoculated into cell cultures of feline origin, and with positive material a cytopathic effect is seen. The virus in a tissue-culture system can be quickly identified by a knowledge of its properties, as described earlier, and by fluorescent antibody test. The latter test can also be applied with good results (Bistner et al. 1971) directly to smear preparations of the conjunctiva and to other infected tissues as well.

Prevention and Control. FVR infection in a cattery causes great problems. When susceptible kittens are introduced into a group that has carriers, the disease remains endemic. Because depopulation is often impossible, the disease persists as one of the two major respiratory problems.

Attenuated and inactivated virus vaccines for FHV-1 are now available. The attenuated vaccine, singly or in combination with feline calicivirus, appears to be safe and reasonably efficacious (Bittle and Rubic 1975, Chappuis et al. 1982, Orr et al. 1980, Scott 1977, Yagami et al.

1985). Intranasal inoculation of attenuated virus vaccine presumably does not cause the carrier status. FHV-1 and feline calicivirus may also be combined with inactivated feline panleukopenia virus. Other inactivated combined vaccines have also been developed (Bush et al. 1981, Chappius et al. 1982).

A feline interferon and two recombinant human leukocyte interferons caused some reduction in viral activity in a feline lung monolayer culture (Fulton and Burge 1985). No studies have been made of interferon's effects on the experimental disease in cats.

A study of the virucidal effects of commercial disinfectants on feline viruses found 22 products were effective against FHV-1 (Scott 1980).

The Disease in Humans. There is no evidence that FHV-1 causes disease in humans.

REFERENCES

Bartholomew, P.T., and Gillespie, J.H. 1968. Feline viruses. I. Characterization of four isolates and their effect on young kittens. Cornell Vet. 58:248–265.

Bistner, S.I., Carlson, J.H., Shively, J.N., and Scott, F.W. 1971. Ocular manifestations of feline herpesvirus infection. J. Am. Vet. Med. Assoc. 159:1223–1237.

Bittle, J.L., and Rubic, W.J. 1975. Immunogenic and protective effects of the F-2 strain of feline viral rhinotracheitis virus. Am. J. Vet. Res. 36:89–91.

Bodle, J.E. 1976. Feline herpes virus infection. Surv. Ophthalmol. 21:209–215.

Burki, F. 1963. Viren des Respirationsapparates bei Katzen. 17th World Veterinary Congress, Hannover. Pp. 559–564.

Bush, M., Povey, R.C., and Koones, H. 1981. Antibody response to an inactivated vaccine for rhinotracheitis, caliciviral disease, and panleukopenia in nondomestic felids. J. Am. Vet. Med. Assoc. 179 1203–1205.

Chappuis, G., Benoit-Jeanin, C., and Fargeaud, D. 1982. Feline rhinotracheitis: A purified inactive vaccine and an experimental model. Dev. Biol. 52:485–491.

Crandell, R.A. 1973. Feline viral rhinotracheitis (FVR). Adv. Vet. Sci. Comp. Med. 17:201–224.

Crandell, R.A., and Maurer, F.D. 1958. Isolation of a feline virus associated with intranuclear inclusion bodies. Proc. Soc. Exp. Biol. Med. 97:487–490.

Crandell, R.A., Rehkemper, J.A., Niemann, W.H., Gamway, J.R., and Maurer, F.D. 1961. Experimental feline viral rhinotracheitis. J. Am. Vet. Med. Assoc. 138:191–196.

Ellis, T.M. 1982. Feline viral rhinotracheitis virus: Explant and cocultivation studies on tissues collected from persistently infected cats. Res. Vet. Sci. 33:270–274.

Fargeaud, D., Jeanin, C.B., Kato, F., and Chappius, G. 1984. Biochemical study of the feline herpesvirus 1. Identification of glycoproteins by affinity. Arch. Virol. 80:69–82.

Fulton, R.W., and Burge, L.J. 1985. Susceptibility of feline herpesvirus 1 and feline calicivirus to feline interferon and recombinant human leukocyte interferons. Antimicrob. Agents Chemother. 28:698–699.

Gaskell, R.M., and Povey, R.C. 1977. Experimental induction of feline viral rhinotracheitis and virus re-excretion in FVR-recovered cats. Vet. Rec. 100:128–133.

Gaskell, R.M., and Povey, R.C. 1982. Transmission of feline viral rhinotracheitis. Vet. Rec. 111:359–362.

Gaskell, R.M., Dennis, P.E., Goddard, L.E., Cocker, F.M., and

Willis, J.M. 1985. Isolation of field herpesvirus I from the trigeminal ganglia of latently infected cats. J. Gen. Virol. 66:391–394.

Gillespie, J.H., Judkins, A.B., and Scott, F.W. 1971. Feline viruses. XII. Hemagglutination and hemadsorption tests for feline herpesvirus. Cornell Vet. 61:159–171.

Hoover, E.A., and Griesemer, R.A. 1971. Comments: Pathogenicity of feline viral rhinotracheitis virus and effect on germfree cats, growing bone, and the gravid uterus. J. Am. Vet. Med. Assoc. 158:929–931.

Johnson, R.H., and Thomas, R.G. 1966. Feline viral rhinotracheitis in Britain. Vet. Rec. 79:188–190.

Johnson, R.T. 1964. The pathogenesis of herpes virus encephalitis. II. A cellular basis for the development of resistance with age. J. Exp. Med. 120:359–374.

Kahn, D.E., and Gillespie, J.H. 1970. Feline viruses. X. Characterization of a newly-isolated picornavirus causing interstitial pneumonia and ulcerative stomatitis in the domestic cat. Cornell Vet. 60:669–683.

Lee, K.M., Kniazeff, A.J., Fabricant, C.G., and Gillespie, J.H. 1969. Utilization of various cell culture systems for propagation of certain feline viruses and canine herpesvirus. Cornell Vet. 59:539–547.

Maes, R.K., Fritsch, S.L., Herr, L.L., and Rota, P.A. 1984. Immunogenic proteins of feline rhinotracheitis virus. J. Virol. 51:259–262.

Orr, C.M., Gaskell, C.J., and Gaskell, R.M. 1980. Interaction of an intranasal combined feline viral rhinotracheitis, feline calicivirus vaccine and the FVR carrier state. Vet. Rec. 106:164–166.

Povey, R.C., and Johnson, R.H. 1967. Further observations on feline viral rhinotracheitis. Vet. Rec. 81:686–689.

Rota, P.A., Maes, R.K., and Evermann, J.F. 1986. Biochemical and antigenic characterization of feline herpesvirus-1–like isolates from dogs. Arch. Virol. 89:57–68.

Rota, P.A., Maes, R.K., and Ruyechan, W.T. 1986. Physical characterization of the genomes of feline herpesvirus-1. Virology 154:168–179.

Scott, F.W. 1977. Evaluation of a feline viral rhinotracheitis–feline calicivirus disease vaccine. Am. J. Vet. Res. 38:229–234.

Scott, F.W. 1980. Virucidal disinfectants and feline viruses. Am. J. Vet. Res. 41:410–414.

Shields, R.P., and Gaskin, J.M. 1977. Fatal generalized feline viral rhinotracheitis in a young adult cat. J. Am. Vet. Med. Assoc. 170:439–441.

Tham, K.M., and Studdert, M.J. 1986. Variable sensitivity of a feline embryo cell line and of three kitten kidney cell cultures to feline herpes- and caliciviruses. Vet. Microbiol. 11:173–176.

Walton, T.E., and Gillespie, J.H. 1970a. Feline viruses. VI. Survey of the incidence of feline pathogenic agents in normal and clinically-ill cats. Cornell Vet. 60:215–232.

Walton, T.E., and Gillespie, J.H. 1970b. Feline viruses. VII. Immunity to the feline herpes virus in kittens inoculated experimentally by the aerosol method. Cornell Vet. 60:232–239.

Wardley, R.C., Rouse, B.T., and Babiuk, L.A. 1976. Observations on recovery mechanisms from feline viral rhinotracheitis. Can. J. Comp. Med. 40:257–264.

Yagami, K., Furukawa, T., Fukui, M., and Hamada, H. 1985. Evaluation of tricombinant vaccine for feline herpesvirus, calicivirus and panleukopenia virus infections in Japanese native cats. Jikken Dobutsu 34:287–294.

Avian Infectious Laryngotracheitis

Until the late 1940s a variety of diseases of the respiratory tract of birds were grouped together under the name *roup*. These have since been differentiated into nutritional, bacterial, parasitic, and viral disorders. Infectious laryngotracheitis (ILT) was shown by Beach (1930) to be a specific viral disease. First recognized in the United States, ILT is now known to exist in nearly all parts of the world where poultry are kept. It affects chickens, occasionally pheasants and ducks, and perhaps Japanese quail.

Character of the Disease. Infectious laryngotracheitis affects chickens of all ages. It is highly contagious and, when it enters a susceptible flock, does not stop until practically every bird has been infected. Infection occurs through the respiratory tract and the conjunctival sac (Hitchner et al. 1977). There is no viremia. The incubation period is short, less than 48 hours as a rule. The course of the disease is acute, some birds dying within 24 hours after the disease is first detected, others being ill for as long as 5 or 6 days. Birds that do not die during the first 5 days of signs practically always recover, and recovery generally is rapid. Although no single bird will show evidence of disease for as long as a week, the disease may require 3 or 4 weeks to run through a flock. An important fact is that a considerable number of recovered birds continue to harbor the virus, and such birds usually are sources for new infections when transferred to new flocks, or when new, susceptible birds are added, perhaps a season or more later (Gibbs 1953).

The signs depend on the age of the birds and the season of the year. Young birds during the warm months usually are less severely affected, and mortality is lower than in older birds during cold weather. Affected birds show respiratory distress in varying degree. In severe cases the chickens extend their necks, open their mouths, and inhale in a gasping manner (Figure 46.16). Gurgling and rattling sounds, sometimes best described as whistling, are often heard. These sounds are due to partial obstruction of the air passages by exudate. Not all birds show marked respiratory distress, since the exudate sometimes is in the nasal passages or nasal sinuses. In mature birds in heavy production mortality may be as high as 70 percent. Death appears to be due largely to suffocation.

Properties of the Virus. Beach (1930) found that infectious laryngotracheitis virus (ILTV) could be filtered readily through Berkefeld V filters, but not always. Evidence suggests that the particle is similar in size and structure to those of other herpesviruses (Cruickshank et al. 1963). The virus is present only in the air passages and is infective by this route. Subcutaneous, intramuscular, and intraperitoneal injections are harmless, but experimental infections may be rarely induced by intravenous inoculation.

The virus is moderately resistant. After diseased and carrier birds are removed, premises do not retain effective quantities of virus for long. Beaudette and Hudson (1939) reported that egg-propagated virus, when dried and kept in a refrigerator, retained its potency and immunizing properties for 421 days. It is inactivated by a concentration of 3 percent Iosan (iodoform preparation) and 2 per-

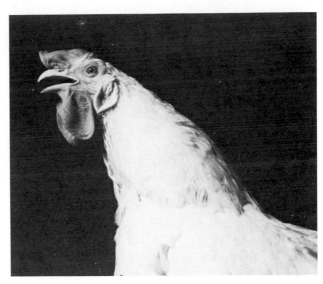

Figure 46.16. Chicken with infectious laryngotracheitis showing the characteristic gasping type of respiration. (Courtesy E. L. Brunett.)

cent Bradofen (quaternary ammonium preparation) after 45 minutes of exposure.

There is a single immunogenic type of ILTV. Strains examined by indirect immunofluorescence showed no intratypic differences; but the use of restriction endonucleases showed some differences between the strains, which may indicate the presence of submolar fragments (Kotiw et al. 1982).

Restricted DNA fragments were successfully cloned into *Escherichia coli* HB-101 cells and could be used for pathotyping ILTV strains and their differences from other avian viruses (Kotiw et al. 1986).

Cultivation. ILTV was cultivated on the chorioallantoic membrane of developing chick embryos by Burnet (1934), by Brandly (1936), and by many others. The virus produces whitish plaques on the membrane. Although two kinds of plaques have been described, the viruses appear to be identical immunologically. Diluted viruses, according to Burnet (1936), can be roughly assayed for virulence by counting the number of plaques produced per volume of virus.

Viral replication occurs in avian leukocyte cultures; cytopathic effect is characterized by multinucleated giant cells (Chang et al. 1977). Calnek et al. (1986) showed that chicken macrophage cultures were as susceptible as chicken kidney cells to infection by some strains, but replication of most virus strains in macrophages was markedly restricted. The authors suggested that both the cell genotype and viral genotype influence replication.

Epizootiology and Pathogenesis. The disease is transmitted naturally through droplet infection. Isolates of the virus with relatively low chicken embryo mortality have low or no pathogenicity for chickens, whereas isolates causing high chicken embryo mortality are markedly pathogenic (Izuchi and Hasegawa 1982).

The lesions, which are confined to the larynx, trachea, and bronchi, are reddened, petechiated, and covered with a slimy exudate containing streaks of bright red blood. Sometimes the exudate is caseous, and plugs of such material may completely block the trachea. Histological changes in the trachea include ciliary disruption, luminal debris, and epithelial sloughing (Bayer et al. 1977).

Seifried (1931) described inclusion bodies in the nuclei of epithelial cells of tracheal lesions. Burnet (1934) found similar bodies in the ectodermal cell lesions of the membranes of infected eggs.

Specific-pathogen–free 4-week-old chicks were infected intranasally with virulent ILTV strain CSW-1. High titers of virus were present in nasal washings 2 to 4 days after inoculation but declined rapidly and were not detectable by day 7 (Bagust et al. 1986). Virus was not isolated from blood leukocytes or lymphoid organs but was present in the trigeminal ganglia or brain of some chicks. However, it was not present in these tissues of five chicks examined 8 days after inoculation. Neutralizing antibodies were detected in the nasal washings 7 to 8 days after inoculation, but interferon was not detectable in serum or tracheal exudates within 14 days.

Immunity. Birds that recover from this disease are immune for the remainder of their lives. Cell-mediated immunity plays a significant role in this protection. Many of these birds are virus carriers; hence, when the disease has once occurred in a flock, annual recurrences must be expected in young stock unless they are artificially immunized. In small flocks it is often simpler and less expensive to dispose of all old stock.

The transfer of parental immunity is marginal and is unlikely to inhibit the response to primary vaccination (Hayles, Hamilton, and Newby 1976).

Diagnosis. Ordinarily once disease is well under way in a flock, a diagnosis can easily be made on the basis of signs and lesions. In individual birds it may not be so simple. If the question is important enough to warrant the trouble, the answer can be obtained by swabbing the larynx of one or two susceptible birds with tracheal exudate from the supposedly infected birds. The susceptible birds should develop signs between 2 and 5 days later if the disease is laryngotracheitis. If immunized birds are included in the test, they should prove resistant while the others sicken.

Direct electron microscopy of lysed tracheal cells and the agar-gel diffusion test are sometimes used to establish a quick diagnosis (Van Kammer and Spradbrow 1976).

Prevention and Control. Beaudette and Hudson (1933) developed a method of actively immunizing birds which has proved to be quite successful. Full immunity results about 9 days after cloacal administration of egg-propagated virus. This approach was not without risk and was used only in flocks with a history of the disease (Beaudette 1939).

Shibley et al. (1963) described the preparation and standardization of strain 146 for use as a conjunctivally administered vaccine, which causes conjunctivitis but no permanent tissue damage. Neutralizing antibodies were still present 372 days after vaccination.

Most investigators now recommend that broiler flocks be immunized as early as 4 weeks of age with commercial vaccine administered in the drinking water (Hayles, Newby, et al. 1976; Seimenis and Menasse 1976). The success of this method depends on introduction of the vaccine virus into the nasal passages while the birds drink (Robertson and Egerton 1981). In a study of a commercial vaccine administered in the drinking water success was correlated with the virus titer of the vaccine (Hilbink et al. 1981). The attenuated vaccine was safe, no contact infection occurred, and vaccinated birds were not carriers of the virus. Most producers now use commercial vaccine to prevent and control the disease.

The Disease in Humans. Infectious laryngotracheitis of poultry does not affect any mammals, including humans, so far as is known.

REFERENCES

Bagust, T.J., Calneck, B.W., and Fahey, K.J. 1986. Gallid-1 herpesvirus infection in the chicken. 3. Reinvestigation of the pathogenesis of infectious laryngotracheitis in acute and early post-acute respiratory disease. Avian Dis. 30:179–190.

Bayer, R.C., Bryan, R.A., Chawan, C.B., and Rittenburg, J.H. 1977. Comparison of tracheal histopathology and scanning electron microscopy of infectious laryngotracheitis. Poultry Sci. 56:964–968.

Beach, J.R. 1930. The virus of laryngotracheitis of fowls. Science 72:633–634.

Beaudette, F.R. 1939. Laryngotracheitis. Vet. Med. 34:743–747.

Beaudette, F.R., and Hudson, C.B. 1933. Experiments on immunization against laryngotracheitis in fowls. J. Am. Vet. Med. Assoc. 82:460–467.

Beaudette,F.R., and Hudson, C.B. 1939. The viability and immunizing value of egg-propagated laryngotracheitis virus. J. Am. Vet. Med. Assoc. 75:333–339.

Brandly, C.A. 1936. Studies on the egg-propagated viruses of infectious laryngotracheitis and fowl-pox. J. Am. Vet. Med. Assoc. 88:587–599.

Burnet, F.M. 1934. The propagation of the virus of infectious laryngotracheitis on the chorio-allantoic membrane of the developing egg. Br. J. Exp. Pathol. 15:52–55.

Burnet, F.M. 1936. Immunological studies with the virus of infectious laryngotracheitis of fowls using the developing egg technique. J. Exp. Med. 63:685–701.

Calnek, B.W., Fahey, K.J., and Bagust, T.J. 1986. In vitro infection studies with infectious larynogotracheitis virus. Avian Dis. 30:327–336.

Chang, P.W., Sculco, F., and Yates, V.J. 1977. An in vivo and in vitro study of infectious laryngotracheitis virus in chicken leukocytes. Avian Dis. 21:492–500.

Cruickshank, J.G., Berry, D.M., and Hay, B. 1963. The fine structure of infectious laryngotracheitis virus. Virology 20:376–378.

Gibbs, C.S. 1933. Filtrable virus carriers. J. Infect. Dis. 53:169–174.

Hayles, L.B., Hamilton, D., and Newby, W.C. 1976. Transfer of parental immunity to infectious laryngotracheitis in chicks. Can. J. Comp. Med. 40:218–219.

Hayles, L.B., Newby, W.C., Gasperdone, H., and Gilchrist, E.W. 1976. Immunization of broiler chickens with a commercial water. Can. J. Comp. Med. 40:129–134.

Hilbink, F., Smit, T., and Yadin, H. 1981. Drinking water vaccination against infectious laryngotracheitis. Can. J. Comp. Med. 45:120–123.

Hitchner, S.B., Fabricant, J., and Bagust, T.J. 1977. A fluorescent-antibody study of the pathogenesis of infectious laryngotracheitis. Avian Dis. 21:185–194.

Izuchi, T., and Hasegawa, A. 1982. Pathogenicity of infectious laryngotracheitis virus as measured by chicken embryo inoculation. Avian Dis. 26:18–25.

Kotiw, M., Sheppard, M., May, J.T., and Wilks, C.R. 1986. Differentiation between virulent and avirulent strains of infectious laryngotracheitis virus by DNA:DNA hybridization using a cloned DNA marker. Vet. Microbiol. 11:319–330.

Kotiw, M., Wilks, C.R., and May, J.T. 1982. Differentiation of infectious laryngotracheitis virus strains using restriction endonucleases. Avian Dis. 26:718–731.

Robertson, G.M., and Egerton, J.R. 1981. Replication of infectious larynogotracheitis virus in chickens following vaccination. Aust. Vet. J. 57:119–123.

Seifried, O. 1931. Histopathology of infectious laryngotracheitis in chickens. J. Exp. Med. 54:817–826.

Seimenis, A., and Menasse, I. 1976. Studies on vaccination against infectious laryngotracheitis by the drinking water. Dev. Biol. Stand. 33:328–331.

Shibley, G.P., Luginbuhl, R.E., and Helmboldt, C.F. 1963. A study of infectious laryngotracheitis virus. II. The duration and degree of immunity induced by conjunctival vaccination. Avian Dis. 7:184–192.

Van Kammer, A., and Spradbrow, P.D. 1976. Rapid diagnosis of some avian virus diseases. Avian Dis. 20:748–751.

Herpesvirus Infection in Pigeons

Cornwell and Wright (1970) isolated a herpesvirus from racing pigeons with a disease resembling ornithosis. Diphtheric foci were present in the pharynx or larynx of several birds; intranuclear inclusions were found in one of them. The herpesvirus produced pocks on the chorioallantoic membrane of the embryonated hen's egg and foci of necrosis in the embryonic liver. Vindevogel et al. (1975) isolated a herpesvirus from pigeons with clinical signs of coryza. Its characteristics were comparable to the virus isolated by Cornwell and Wright. Vindevogel's virus produces cytopathic effect in monolayer cultures in 24 hours and causes disease in experimental pigeons.

Two strains were pathogenic for young pigeons, but not for chicks (Cornwell et al. 1970). Intraperitoneal inoculation of these strains caused pancreatitis, peritonitis, and, in some birds, hepatic necrosis. Eosinophilic intranuclear inclusions and specific viral antigen were seen in pancreatic acinar and in hepatitic parenchymal cells. Intra-

nuclear inclusion bodies also were observed in the necrotic foci in the laryngeal epithelium after pigeons were given virus by the intralaryngeal route.

REFERENCES

Cornwell, H.J.C., and Wright, N.G. 1970. Herpesvirus infection of pigeons. I. Pathology and virus isolation. J. Comp. Pathol. 80:221–228.

Cornwell, H.J.C., Wright, N.G., and McCusker, H.B. 1970. Herpesvirus infection of pigeons. II. Experimental infection of pigeons and chicks. J. Comp. Pathol. 80:229–232.

Vindevogel, H., Pastoret, P.P., Burtonboy, G., Gouffaux, M., and Duchatel, J.P. 1975. Isolement d'un virus herpes dans un élevage de pigeons de carrière. Ann. Rech. Vét. 6:431–436.

Duck Plague

SYNONYM: Duck virus enteritis

Duck plague is an acute, highly fatal, viremic disease of ducks and geese caused by a herpesvirus. It has occurred in the Netherlands, Belgium, India, England, Japan, France, China, the United States, and Canada. The incidence in commercial duck flocks is about 10 percent (Mason et al. 1983).

An article describing the disease was written by Jansen (1968), who did much of the original work on the disease. Leibovitz and Hwang (1968) described the 1967 outbreak on Long Island, New York.

Character of the Disease. Naturally and experimentally infected ducks show similar signs of illness—listlessness; ruffled, dull feathers; wet areas around the eyes, which later become mucoid (Figure 46.17); nasal discharge and labored breathing; inappetence; watery diarrhea; and nervous manifestations. Not all of these signs may be present, and ducks frequently show temporary improvement before death occurs in 1 to 3 days. Mortality usually is high, and disease often lasts about 3 weeks on a farm.

Properties of the Virus. Duck plague virus is a member of the *Herpesvirus* genus (Figure 46.18). There is only one serotype and one immunogenic type, as complete cross-immunity has been demonstrated with various isolates by immunity tests in ducks and by neutralization tests in embryonated duck eggs.

Attempts to demonstrate a hemagglutinin have failed (Jansen 1968). The virus is quite stable at $-20°$ C and in the lyophilized state. Cloned duck hepatitis B virus DNA is infectious in Pekin ducks (Sprengel et al. 1984). The cell-associated antigen recognized by the antiserum elicited to viral DNA synthesis complexes (immature cores) appears to cross-react with a 35,000-dalton polypeptide fraction associated with the immature cores (Halpern et al. 1984).

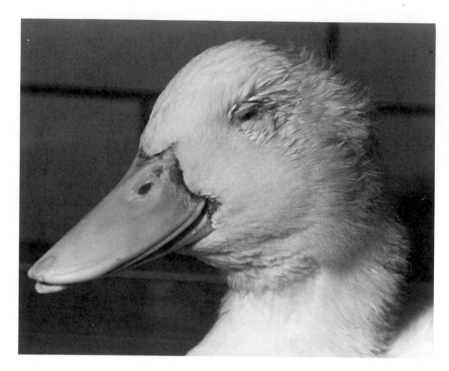

Figure 46.17. Duck with ocular discharge. (Courtesy D. A. Gregg, Plum Island Animal Disease Center, U.S. Dept. of Agriculture.)

Figure 46.18. Duck plague herpesvirus in duck embryo cells. × 17,100. (Courtesy S. S. Breese, Plum Island Animal Disease Center, U.S. Dept. of Agriculture.)

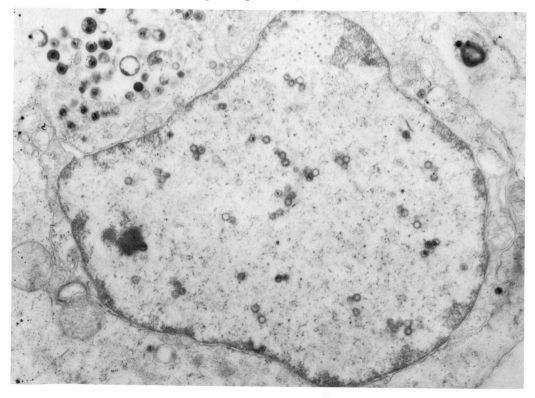

Cultivation. The virus can be cultivated readily by inoculation on the chorioallantoic membrane of 12-day-old embryonated duck eggs. The embryos die in 4 days and show extensive hemorrhage (Jansen 1968). Direct cultivation of the virus in the embryonated hens' eggs is not possible. Duck embryo–adapted virus can be established in the hen's embryo. Repeated passage in the latter host produces a virus that is attenuated for ducks (Jansen 1968). Cultivation of the virus in cell culture has been reported by Kunst (1967). Kocan (1976) compared duck embryo fibroblast cultures from seven species and found that Muscovy duck and wood duck cells gave the best virus yield and plaque quality.

Epizootiology and Pathogenesis. Under natural conditions duck plague is spread by contact because excretions from infected ducks contain virus. Free access to ponds, moats, and pools undoubtedly facilitates spread. The reproductive state and exercise are two factors that act in concert to stimulate the shedding of virus in oral secretions (Burgess and Yuill 1983). In wild waterfowl and Pekin ducks vertical transmission may be the main means of virus perpetuation from generation to generation (Burgess and Yuill 1981, O'Connell et al. 1983, Urban et al. 1985). Pathogenetic studies of this disease were undertaken by Proctor (1975, 1976) using light, electron, and fluorescent microscopy, which highlighted the necrosis that occurs in many types of cells in the body—lymphocytes, macrophages, fibrocytes, and epithelial cells. Subsequent studies showed that the viral replication starts in the liver and spreads to the pancreas, kidneys, and the spleen (Tagawa et al. 1985). The virus is tropic for exocrine cells (Halpern et al. 1985), and viral antigen has also been demonstrated in exocrine cells of the adrenal gland.

At necropsy the most striking lesions are multiple hemorrhages throughout the body, usually most pronounced in heart, serous membranes, and esophageal mucosa. Marked congestion occurs in the ovary that is in production. If the disease becomes subacute, diphtheric membranes may appear on the mucosa of the esophagus and cloaca and may extend to the salpinx and rectum. In many birds there is peritonitis, and the liver may be friable.

Immunity. The chick embryo–adapted strain of duck plague virus that is avirulent for ducks produces an effective immunity in the duck. It rapidly produces protection as a result of interference. Ducks given this vaccine were immune to challenge 12 to 14 months later, although most had no demonstrable neutralizing antibody (Jansen 1968). Dardiri (1975) found that a marked anamnestic serologic response resulted from challenge with virulent virus in ducks given chicken embryo–attenuated virus vaccine. There is evidence of parental antibody interference (Newcomb 1968). Superinfection in ducks persistently infected with duck plague may kill some birds despite the presence of low levels of neutralizing antibody (Burgess and Yuill 1982).

Diagnosis. The virus can be isolated in cell culture or in 12-day-old embryonated duck eggs. Immunofluorescence and immunoperoxidase tests can be used for detecting antigen in tissues. The reverse passive hemagglutination test is a rapid, simple procedure that is sufficiently sensitive for detection of virus in tissues of dying ducks (Deng et al. 1984).

The serum-neutralization test can be used for detection of antibody. The disease can be identified by serum neutralization with ducklings as the host system (Hanson and Willis 1976).

Prevention and Control. Because free-flying birds are involved, control other than by a vaccination program is exceedingly difficult. Apathogenic strains have been used as vaccines to protect ducks against virulent virus challenge by intramuscular inoculation or contact exposure (Lam and Lin 1986, Lin et al. 1984).

The Disease in Humans. Duck plague has not been reported in humans.

REFERENCES

Burgess, E.C., and Yuill, T.M. 1981. Vertical transmission of duck plague virus (DPV) by apparently healthy DPV carrier waterfowl. Avian Dis. 25:795–800.
Burgess, E.C., and Yuill, T.M. 1982. Superinfection in ducks persistently infected with duck plague virus. Avian Dis. 26:40–46.
Burgess, E.C., and Yuill, T.M. 1983. The influence of seven environmental and physiological factors on duck plague virus shedding by carrier mallards. J. Wildl. Dis. 19:77–81.
Dardiri, A.H. 1975. Duck viral enteritis (duck plague) characteristics and immune response of the host. Am. J. Vet. Res. 36:535–538.
Deng, M.Y., Burgess, E.C., and Yuill, T.M. 1984. Detection of duck plague virus by reverse passive hemagglutination test. Avian Dis. 28:616–628.
Halpern, M.S., Egan, J., McMahon, S.B., and Ewert, D.L. 1985. Duck hepatitis B virus is tropic for exocrine cells of the pancreas. Virology 146:157–161.
Halpern, M.S., England, J.M., Flores, L., Egan, J., Newbold, J., and Mason, W.S. 1984. Individual cells in tissues of DHBV infected ducks express antigens crossreactive with those on virus surface antigen particles and immature viral cores. Virology 137:408–413.
Hanson, J.A., and Willis, N.G. 1976. An outbreak of duck virus enteritis (duck plague) in Alberta. J. Wildl. Dis. 12:258–262.
Jansen, J. 1968. Duck plague. J. Am. Vet. Med. Assoc. 152:1009–1016.
Kocan, R.M. 1976. Duck plague virus in Muscovy duck fibroblast cells. Avian Dis. 21:574–580.
Kunst, H. 1967. Isolation of duck plague virus in tissue cultures. Tijdschr. Diergeneeskd. 92:713–714.
Lam, K.M., and Lin, W.Q. 1986. Antibody-mediated resistance against duck enteritis virus infection. Can. J. Vet. Res. 50:380–383.
Leibovitz, L., and Hwang, J. 1968. Duck plague on the American continent. Avian Dis. 12:361–378.
Lin, W.Q., Lam, K.M., and Clark, W.E. 1984. Active and passive immunization of ducks against duck viral enteritis. Avian Dis. 28:968–973.

Mason, W.S., Halpern, M.S., England, J.M., Seal, G., Egan, J., Coates, L., Aldrich, C., and Summers, J. 1983. Experimental transmission of duck hepatitis B virus. Virology 131:375–384.

Newcomb, S.S. 1968. Duck virus enteritis (duck plague) epidemiology and the related investigations. J. Am. Vet. Med. Assoc. 152:1349.

O'Connell, A.P., Urban, M.K., and London, W.T. 1983. Naturally occurring infection of Pekin duck embryos by duck hepatitis B virus. Proc. Natl. Acad. Sci. USA 80:1703–1706.

Proctor, S.J. 1975. Pathogenesis of digestive tract lesions in duck plague. Vet. Pathol. 12:349–361.

Proctor, S.J. 1976. Pathogenesis of duck plague in the bursa of Fabricius, thymus, and spleen. Am. J. Vet. Res. 37:427–431.

Sprengel, R., Kuhn, C., Manso, C., and Will, H. 1984. Cloned duck hepatitis B virus DNA is infectious in Pekin ducks. J. Virol. 52:932–937.

Tagawa, M., Omata, M., Yokosuka, O., Uchiumi, K., Imazek, F., and Okuda, K. 1985. Early events in duck hepatitis B virus infection. Sequential appearance of viral deoxyribonucleic acid in the liver, pancreas, kidney, and spleen. Gastroenterology 89:1224–1229.

Urban, M.K., O'Connell, A.P., and London, W.T. 1985. Sequence of events in natural infection of Pekin duck embryos with duck hepatitis B virus. J. Virol. 55:16–22.

The Subfamily Betaherpesvirinae

Herpesvirus-Induced Feline Urolithiasis

SYNONYMS: Feline herpesvirus 2 infection, feline urological syndrome; abbreviation, FUS

Feline urolithiasis, or feline urological syndrome, is an acute and recurring disease of male cats primarily characterized by bloody urine, hemorrhagic cystitis, straining to urinate, and complete tract blockage by urinary crystals.

Three viruses have been isolated from cats with natural cases: a feline calicivirus, a feline syncytium-forming virus, and a feline herpesvirus (Fabricant and Gillespie 1974). The herpesvirus may play a significant role in the urolithiasis syndrome of domestic cats. An excellent review was written by Fabricant (1979), and this section contains much of the information in that review.

Character of the Disease. FUS in domestic cats has a wide geographic distribution, including the United States and Europe. A case has been described in a cheetah (Weber et al. 1984). The disease occurs more frequently in the cold months, and although it is assumed to afflict cats fed dry food, cats on a variety of diets contract the disease. It can be an acute disease. The stones or sandy particles found most frequently have been identified as triple ammonium magnesium phosphates (struvite). Blockage results in retention of urine and uremia. Death may ensue as a result of a ruptured bladder or azotemia. In cats that recover the condition often recurs.

The etiology of FUS is complex, and many factors, including diet, metabolic disorders, anatomical and physiological reasons, and infection, have been suggested as important causes (Fabricant 1979, Finco et al. 1985,

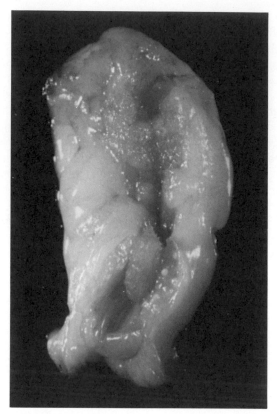

Figure 46.19. Section of urethral plugs from an experimental specific-pathogen–free cat inoculated with feline herpesvirus 2 (cell-associated). (From Fabricant, 1979, courtesy of *Comparative Immunology, Microbiology and Infectious Diseases*.)

Lewis and Morris 1984a, Osborne et al. 1984). Some or all of these factors may play either primary or secondary roles. Rich (1969) eliminated struvite crystals, pH, and bacterial infection as primary causes of the syndrome. After reproducing the disease in conventionally reared male cats with multiple inoculations of filtered urine from obstructed cats, he suspected a possible viral etiology. This led to a series of experiments, first in conventionally reared cats and later in specific-pathogen–free cats. He concluded that feline herpesvirus 2 (FHV-2) alone can produce FUS in all of its manifestations (Figure 46.19), but clinical signs developed earlier with more urinary tract complications when experimental specific-pathogen–free cats were inoculated with a feline calicivirus and FHV-2 (Fabricant 1977, 1979; Rich et al. 1971). The significance of the syncytium-forming feline virus as a complicating factor in the disease has not been established yet (Fabricant 1979).

Properties of the Virus. The feline herpesvirus (FHV-2) associated with this disease has all the physical, chemical, and biological properties of a herpesvirus (Fabricant and Gillespie 1974). The average diameter of the virus particles is 115 nm, as determined by electron microscopy.

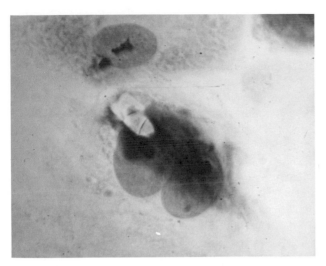

Figure 46.20. Intracellular phosphatelike crystals formed in a cell infected with feline herpesvirus 2 (cell-associated). May-Grünwald-Giemsa stain. × 58. (From Fabricant, 1979, courtesy of *Comparative Immunology, Microbiology and Infectious Diseases.*)

The virus is inactivated by ether and chloroform. The nucleic acid has been identified as DNA. This feline herpesvirus is neutralized by its homologous antiserum. At dilutions of 1.2, antiserums of various animal herpesviruses, including feline viral rhinotracheitis virus (feline herpesvirus 1) and herpes simplex, failed to neutralize FHV-2.

Cultivation. FHV-2 is strongly cell associated, and viral titers in infected cell cultures prepared by disrupting the supernatant and residual cells with ultrasound vary from TCID$_{50}$ $10^{1.8}$ to $10^{5.8}$ per 0.1 ml. The cytopathic changes in the Crandell feline kidney cell and in autogenous heart, bladder, and kidney cell cultures include condensation and reticulation of the nuclear chromatin, often with bizarre nucleolar changes and enlarged and transformed cells. Intranuclear inclusion bodies are seen, but differ from those produced by feline herpesvirus 1. Infected cell sheets remain attached to culture flask surfaces for months without a change of medium, whereas cell sheets of uninoculated cultures detach from the surface in 4 to 8 weeks. This virus has also induced several types of chemical crystals intracellularly (Figure 46.20) and extracellularly, as well as the formation of "tissue culture calculi," a unique finding (Fabricant et al. 1971). Cholesterol has been identified as one of the crystals in cell culture (Fabricant et al. 1973).

FHV-2 is extremely difficult to isolate in cell cultures, and therefore isolation attempts from clinical cases usually will be unsuccessful.

Epizootiology. The virus can be readily transmitted from an infected cat to a susceptible cat. The exact mechanism is unknown, although it is speculated that cats shed the virus in the urine, producing infective aerosols when they urinate (Fabricant 1979).

Immunity. We still do not know if FHV-2 can protect cats against urolithiasis. There is strong evidence that natural virus persists in cats, and under certain conditions it can be triggered by another feline virus or some other factor. Obviously studies are required to determine the immune mechanism and how it might be manipulated to the advantage of the cat. It is clear that neutralizing antibodies are produced, but in low titer. The role of cell-mediated immunity is entirely unknown, but it is reasonable to expect that its mechanism is similar to that of other herpesviruses.

Diagnosis. The diagnosis of the disease in males is simple, as the signs of illness are typical. The incidence of the infection in females is common, but the anatomical differences in the two sexes are responsible for the difference in incidence of urinary blockage, the severe form of the disease. The long, narrow urethra in males is the important factor accounting for blockage by calculi.

Prevention and Control. Herpes-induced feline urolithiasis presents a difficult problem to veterinarians. It is a common and serious disease that defies control as long as cats are allowed to have contact with other cats. In catteries, where close contact is constant, it is a particular problem. There is also evidence that the virus can persist in the ovaries. Horizontal transmission occurs as well, and field evidence strongly suggests that carrier queens can readily transmit the virus to their nursing progeny.

Once cats contract urolithiasis, they are at greater risk of repeated attacks. Such cats should be placed on diets with low magnesium and ash content. Special diets and feed additives to lower the pH of the urine will help to prevent uroliths from forming in the urine (Lewis and Morris 1984b, Taton et al. 1984).

The Disease in Humans. There is no evidence that FHV-2 causes disease in humans.

REFERENCES

Fabricant, C.G. 1977. Herpesvirus-induced urolithiasis in specific pathogen–free male cats. Am. J. Vet. Res. 38:1837–1842.
Fabricant, C.G. 1979. Herpesvirus induced urolithiasis—A review. Comp. Immun. Microbiol. Infect. Dis. 1:121–134.
Fabricant, C.G., and Gillespie, J.H. 1974. Identification and characterization of a second feline herpesvirus. Infect. Immun. 9:460–466.
Fabricant, C.G., Gillespie, J.H., and Krook, L. 1971. Intracellular and extracellular mineral crystal formation induced by viral infection of cell cultures. Infect. Immun. 3:416–419.
Fabricant, C.G., Krook, L., and Gillespie, J.H. 1973. Virus-induced cholesterol crystals. Science 181:566–567.
Finco, D.R., Barsanti, J.A., and Crowell, W.A. 1985. Characterization

of magnesium-induced urinary disease in the cat and comparison with feline urologic syndrome. Am. J. Vet. Res. 46:391–400.

Lewis, L.D., and Morris, M.L., Jr., 1984a. Diet as a causative factor of feline urolithiasis. Vet. Clin. North Am. [Small Anim. Pract.] 14(3):513–527.

Lewis, L.D., and Morris, M.L., Jr. 1984b. Treatment and prevention of feline struvite urolithiasis. Vet. Clin. North Am. [Small Anim. Pract.] 14(3):649–660.

Osborne, C.A., Clinton, C.W., Brunkow, H.C., Frost, A.P., and Johnston, G.R. 1984. Epidemiology of naturally occurring feline uroliths and urethral plugs. Vet. Clin. North Am. [Small Anim. Pract.] 14(3):481–489.

Rich, L.J. 1969. Influence of diets and urine pH on struvite and their relationship to urethral obstruction. Ph.D. dissertation, Cornell University, Ithaca, N.Y. Pp. 51–79.

Taton, G.F., Hamar, D.W., and Lewis, L.D. 1984. Urinary acidification in the prevention and treatment of feline struvite urolithiasis. J. Am. Vet. Med. Assoc. 184:437–443.

Weber, W.J., Raphael, B.L., and Boothe, H.W., Jr. 1984. Struvite uroliths in cheetah. J. Am. Vet. Med. Assoc. 185:1389–1390.

The Subfamily Gammaherpesvirinae

Malignant Catarrhal Fever

SYNONYMS: Bovine epitheliosis, bovine malignant catarrh, malignant head catarrh of cattle, *snotsiekte* (South Africa); abbreviation, MCF

Malignant catarrhal fever is a pansystemic herpesvirus disease of cattle and other ruminants characterized by a severe erosive rhinitis, keratoconjunctivitis and panophthalmia, encephalitis, erosive stomatitis and gastroenteritis, and an extremely high death rate. MCF usually occurs as a sporadic disease with low morbidity, but occasionally explosive outbreaks may occur (Blood et al. 1983, Kahrs 1981).

MCF occurs as one of two diseases: (1) American, European, or "sheep-associated," MCF; or (2) African, or "wildebeest-associated," MCF. While these diseases are similar enough to be considered as one disease or clinical pathological entity (Pierson et al. 1979, Plowright 1984), it appears that two viruses, or at least different strains of the same virus, are responsible for these two types of MCF. African MCF can be destructive in exotic ruminants in wild animal parks, zoological gardens, and deer farms (Castro et al. 1982; Hatkin 1980; Heuschele 1982, 1983; Heuschele et al. 1985; Ramsay et al. 1982; Westbury and Denholm 1982; Zimmer et al. 1981).

MCF has been reviewed by several authors, including Blood et al. (1983), Heuschele (1982), Kahrs (1981), Mare (1977), Mushi and Rurangirwa (1981), and Plowright (1968, 1984).

Character of the Disease. MCF is primarily a disease of cattle, but outbreaks also occur in wild animal parks among captive ruminants, farm deer (Heuschele 1982,

1983; Heuschele et al. 1985; Westbury and Denholm 1982; Whitenack et al. 1981), American bison (Ruth et al. 1977, Todd and Storz 1983), and buffalo (Hoffman et al. 1984). Sheep and African wildebeests can also be infected, but the signs in these species are vague or absent. African antelope of the subfamily Alcelaphinae (wildebeest, hartebeest, and topi) can carry MCF virus without signs of illness and thus serve as the source of outbreaks in cattle (Heuschele et al. 1985; Mushi et al. 1980; Plowright 1965a, 1965b; Plowright et al. 1960). Outbreaks of American MCF in cattle usually are associated with sheep contact. Stenius (1952), who made an extensive study of the disease in Finland, supported the hypothesis that sheep often serve as the reservoir of infection for cattle. It is clear, however, that natural disease also occurs in cattle that have had no contact with sheep.

In North America the disease is generally seen in late autumn and early spring, although Blood et al. (1983) found a seasonal incidence from late winter to summer. Most cases occur in any one herd during a single season. On some farms the disease appears regularly, season after season, causing severe losses over a period of years. Marshall et al. (1919–1920) described one outbreak in a large herd which began in the fall and continued until spring. A total of 31 animals died. The disease has been reported in most of the countries of Europe and Central Africa, in South Africa, and in North America.

The incubation period of African MCF in natural infections varies from 3 to 8 weeks; in experimental infections it may be shorter (Blood et al. 1961, 1983; Kalunda, Dardiri, and Lee 1981). In experimental infections, American MCF had a longer incubation period (mean, 32 days; range, 18 to 73 days) compared with African MCF (mean, 13 days; range, 7 to 28 days) (Pierson et al. 1979).

Several forms of MCF have been described based on the clinical disease produced and the organs involved: the peracute form, the alimentary tract form, the common head-and-eye form and the mild form (Blood et al. 1983). These forms are merely gradations of disease, and an individual strain of virus can produce all of them.

The course of the disease varies greatly. Some of the peracute cases may result in death in 24 hours or less (Pierson et al. 1973). In the head-and-eye form, the one most readily diagnosed, and therefore reported most often, the course varies from 5 to 14 days, but a few cases may last much longer. A comparison of the American-European and African types of MCF revealed that American-European MCF has a short course (mean, 4 days) with African MCF having a longer course (mean, 12 days) (Pierson et al. 1979). Mortality is always high. Goss et al. (1947) reported 16 deaths in 18 sporadic cases. Others report even higher cases.

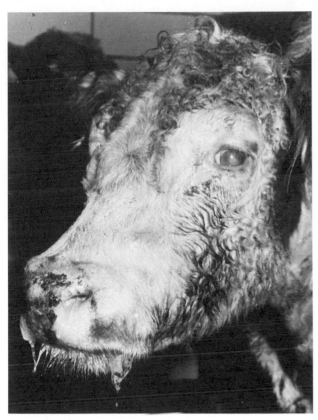

Figure 46.21. Head of a steer infected with an African isolate of malignant catarrhal fever virus. Some characteristic signs are corneal opacity, necrotic skin and exudate on the muzzle, and slobbering. (Courtesy D. A. Gregg, Plum Island Animal Disease Center, U.S. Dept. of Agriculture.)

The clinical disease of MCF has been described by several authors (Blood et al. 1983; Kahrs 1981; Kalunda, Dardiri, and Lee 1981; Marshall et al. 1919–1920; Pierson et al. 1973, 1979; Plowright 1968). The onset is usually sudden. The natural disease begins with fever and severe depression. Inflammation of the mucous membranes of the mouth, nasal passages, and eyes appears early (Figure 46.21). Generally there is panophthalmitis with photophobia, lacrimation, infection of the sclera, corneal opacity that begins at the limbus and progresses centrally, and even ulceration. There are erosions on the soft palate and tongue with blunting and loss of some conical buccal papillae (Figures 46.22 and 46.23). The nasal mucosa becomes deep red, edematous, and covered with a fibrinopurulent exudate.

Blood et al. (1983, p. 752) gave a vivid description of the clinical disease in cattle:

In the "head and eye" form there is a sudden onset of extreme dejection, anorexia, agalactia, high fever

(41–41.5°C, 106–107°F), rapid pulse rate (100–120/min), a profuse mucopurulent nasal discharge, severe dyspnea with stertor due to obstruction of the nasal cavities with exudate, ocular discharge, with variable degrees of edema of the eyelids, blepharospasm, and congestion of scleral vessels. Superficial necrosis is evident in the anterior nasal mucosa and on the buccal mucosa. . . . Discrete local areas of necrosis appear on the hard palate, gums and gingivae. The mouth is painful at this time and the animal moves its jaws carefully, painfully and with a smacking sound. The mucosa as a whole is fragile and splits easily. The mouth and tongue are slippery and the mouth is hard to open. The erosive mucosal lesions may be localized or diffuse. They may occur on the hard palate, the dorsum of the tongue, the gums below the incisors, the commissures of the mouth, or inside the lips. The cheek papillae inside the mouth are hemorrhagic, especially at the tips which are later eroded. At this stage there is excessive salivation with saliva, which is ropey and bubbly, hanging from the lips. The skin of the muzzle is extensively involved commencing with discrete patches of necrosis at the nostrils which soon coalesce causing the entire muzzle to be covered by tenacious scabs. Similar lesions may occur at the skin-horn junction of the feet especially at the back of the pastern. The skin of the teats, vulva and scrotum in acute cases may slough off entirely on touching or become covered with dry, tenacious scabs. Nervous signs, particularly weakness in one leg, incoordination, a demented appearance and muscle tremor may develop very early, and with nystagmus are common in the late stages. Head-pushing, paralysis and convulsions may occur in the final stages.

In cattle with the peracute form of MCF, characteristic signs and lesions of the head-and-eye form do not develop, since the disease lasts only for 1 to 3 days. The alimentary form of MCF is similar to the head-and-eye form except that eye involvement is less severe (conjunctivitis and not panophthalmitis) and there is severe diarrhea.

In three epizootics of MCF in American bison 6.9 percent of 333 animals were affected with mortality of 100 percent (Ruth et al. 1977). Clinical signs most consistently observed were "depression, separation from the herd, serous nasal and ocular discharge, conjunctivitis, gray cornea, diarrhea (occasionally with blood), and apparent muscular weakness."

Properties of the Virus. African MCF virus is a highly cell-associated virus classified in the Gammaherpesvirinae subfamily of the Herpesviridae family. It is called bovid herpesvirus 3 (Kahrs 1981, Ludwig 1984) and alcelaphine herpesvirus 1 (Heuschele 1983, Heuschele et al. 1985). It was first isolated from wildebeest and identified as a herpesvirus by Plowright et al. (1960).

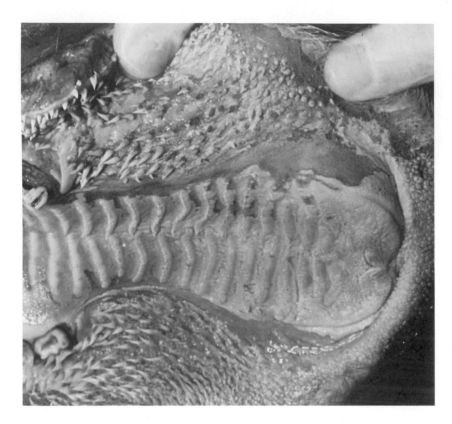

Figure 46.22. Palate and buccal mucosa from a steer infected with an African isolate of malignant catarrhal fever virus. There are erosions on the head and soft palate, with blunting and loss of some conical buccal papillae. (Courtesy D. A. Gregg, Plum Island Animal Disease Center, U.S. Dept. of Agriculture.)

The morphology of African MCF virions observed by electron microscopy is consistent with that of other herpesviruses (Castro and Daley 1982, Castro et al. 1984). The virions appear as icosahedral, enveloped particles 98 to 194 nm in diameter; develop in the nucleus of the cell; mature in the cytoplasm of the cell; and acquire one or more envelopes as they pass through the nuclear and plasma membranes. Virions are closely associated with the endoplasmic reticulum. (Figure 46.24).

The cause of American MCF is unclear. Various viruses have been isolated from cattle with MCF, but their role in the production of the disease is uncertain (Storz et

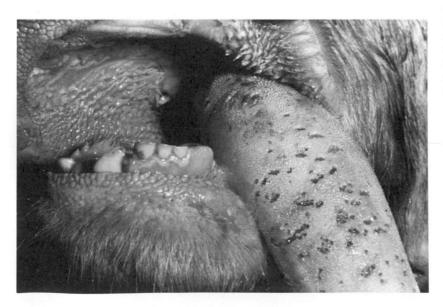

Figure 46.23. Multiple erosions on the tongue of a steer infected with an African isolate of malignant catarrhal fever virus. (Courtesy D. A. Gregg, Plum Island Animal Disease Center, U.S. Dept. of Agriculture.)

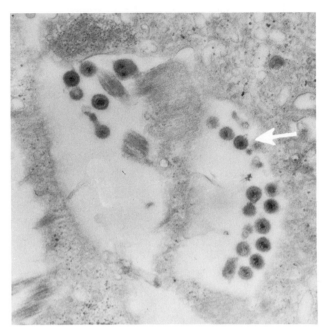

Figure 46.24. Electron micrograph showing malignant catarrhal fever virus particles (*arrow*) of an African strain inoculated into a bovine thyroid cell culture 8 days previously. × 24,900. (Courtesy S. S. Breese, Plum Island Animal Disease Center, U.S. Dept. of Agriculture.)

al. 1976). Most investigators believe the American form is caused by a herpesvirus similar to the African virus. There is evidence of a close antigenic association between the American or sheep-associated strain of virus and the African strain. Sheep in Australia, Britain, Austria, and Kenya, and cattle with non-wildebeest-associated MCF had high antibody titers to African MCF virus (Rossiter 1980, 1983). A rabbit cell line has been established which apparently is infected with the sheep-associated agent obtained from an affected deer, but the agent has not been identified (Buxton and Reid 1980; Buxton et al. 1984, 1985; Reid et al. 1984). Rabbits and sheep can be infected with this agent. These investigators propose that the virus infects a particular subpopulation of T lymphocytes, which in turn sets up a profound immunological perturbation involving T-lymphocytes hyperplasia and deregulation of cytotoxic natural killer cells with tissue necrosis as the final result.

Cultivation. Plowright et al. (1960) reported that African MCF virus can be grown in thyroid or adrenal gland cultures by inoculation of viable tissue suspensions or leukocytes from acutely or latently infected animals. Cowdry type A inclusion bodies and syncytia are produced. After several cell-culture transfers, the virus can be transferred to calf kidney cultures. The adapted virus also grows in cultures of sheep thyroid, calf testis or adrenal gland, and in wildebeest and rabbit kidney.

The American-European MCF virus has not been isolated or propagated in vitro. However, it appears that a cell culture of rabbit T lymphocytes contains the infectious agent of sheep-associated MCF (Reid et al. 1984).

Epizootiology and Pathogenesis. In most cases, transmission occurs only after contact with wildebeest or other antelope in the African form, and after contact with sheep in the American and European form. Transmission occurred when cattle were placed in direct contact with wildebeests in the early stage of infection (Plowright 1965b). Ocular and nasal secretions of young wildebeest often contain MCF virus, but saliva and urine do not (Mushi et al. 1980). Transmission usually does not occur naturally between cattle (Kahrs 1981, Mushi and Rurangirwa 1981, Plowright 1984). Attempts to transmit the disease from diseased cattle to contact cattle usually fail despite virus in excretions of diseased animals, but both the African form and the American and European form can readily be transmitted with whole blood of infected cattle injected into other cattle (Blood et al. 1961; Kalunda, Dardiri, and Lee 1981; Piercy 1952a, 1952b, Pierson et al. 1979; Plowright 1953). A survey of African wildlife that contain neutralizing antibodies for African MCF virus has been reported by Hamblin and Hedger (1984).

Stenius (1952) inoculated a number of sheep with tissues from diseased cattle and a number of cattle with tissues from the infected sheep. In sheep, an inapparent disease resulted; however, characteristic lesions of virus encephalitis were present. In cattle, mild lesions of catarrhal fever were produced with materials derived from the infected sheep.

MCF infection was readily reproduced in U.S. cattle with the African virus (Kalunda, Dardiri, and Lee 1981). Of 53 cattle inoculated with virus, 47 showed the head-and-eye form (of these, 28 died), 3 had mild signs, and 3 had inapparent infection. Plowright (1953), employing one of Piercy's strains, reported that in rabbits there was fever followed by mild leukocytosis in nine instances, mild leukopenia in three, and no blood change in two. In all cases there was an increase in the nongranular cells during the reaction. Using his African strain, Kalunda (1975) and co-workers Ferris et al. (1981) infected guinea pigs, rabbits, and hamsters, all of which had abnormal discharges, became paralyzed, and died.

The experimental disease in the wildebeest was studied by Plowright (1965a, 1965b). A viremic state persisted in one wildebeest calf for 31 weeks and in another for 8 weeks. Neither calf showed signs of illness. Bovine calves in contact with the first wildebeest calf during the early weeks of infection (2 to 12) developed typical malignant head catarrh. In conjunction with these studies virus was isolated from 7 percent of 282 blood samples from wildebeests in northern Tanganyika (Mettam 1923). Some calves were probably infected in utero, as they were viremic during the first week of life. Transplacental infection was confirmed, as virus was isolated from a fetal spleen.

The lesions of MCF have been described by several investigators (Goss et al. 1947, Liggitt and DeMartini 1980, Stenius 1952, Whiteley et al. 1985, Zimmer et al. 1981). The dark, swollen, glassy membranes of the turbinates and nasal sinuses are covered with shreds of fibrin and a dirty, purulent secretion. Shallow ulcers generally are found on these surfaces. Similar lesions are found in the larynx, trachea, and the larger bronchi; and there may be areas of bronchopneumonia in the anterior lung lobes. The lymph nodes of the head are generally swollen. The mucous membrane of the abomasum often is inflamed, edematous, and sometimes eroded; and there may be similar lesions in the small intestine.

The meninges of the brain often are congested and may show hemorrhages, but the brain itself usually appears normal. Histologically, however, there are lesions of nonpurulent encephalitis of the virus type, associated in some cases with acidophilic inclusion bodies. Some early workers reported finding inclusion bodies in the nerve cells of cattle dying from this disease. Stenius (1952) found, in all 50 animals examined, acidophilic inclusions in degenerated motor neurons, especially in the vagoglossopharyngeal nucleus, and more sparsely in other areas in the medulla oblongata and elsewhere in the brain. The ultrastructural changes in MCF lesions have been described by Castro et al. (1985).

The epidemology of MCF has been reviewed by Mushi and Rurangirwa (1981).

Immunity. The rare bovine that recovers from MCF probably is immune for life (Plowright 1984). Neutralizing, complement-fixing, and precipitating antibodies are formed in these cattle; but there is little, if any, correlation between antibody titer and protection (Plowright 1984, Rossiter 1983, Rossiter and Jessett 1980). In a controlled field trial, vaccinated cattle showed no evidence of protection against natural challenge by exposure to wildebeest herds (Plowright et al. 1975). In all likelihood, cell-mediated immunity plays a key role in resistance to this disease.

Immunity to the American form of MCF has been impossible to evaluate because few animals survive the disease, and the precise etiology still has not been ascertained.

Diagnosis. The clinical diagnosis of MCF is relatively easy when history, signs, and lesions are properly con-

sidered (Kahrs 1981). However, the clinical signs may be similar to those of a composite of diseases that have been labeled "the mucosal diseases." The sporadic character of malignant catarrhal fever and the presence of eye lesions in most cases are evidence of encephalitic changes that tend to differentiate MCF from other, similar diseases characterized by mouth, nasal, and intestinal lesions.

The African form of the disease can be confirmed by special procedures that isolate the virus from buffy coat cells or explant cultures of thyroids. Serologic assays for MCF antibodies can help to confirm the presence of MCF virus in a single animal or within a herd.

The American and European form of MCF is difficult to confirm by laboratory assays. Virus has not been isolated from this form of the disease. There appears to be cross-reactivity with the African strain, so serologic assays may be of some help.

Prevention and Control. The sporadic nature of the disease would make control measures difficult, even if effective methods were known. In enzootic herds where multiple cases are occurring on the same premises cattle should be separated completely from possible chronic carriers of virus, such as sheep (or wildebeest in Africa). Effective vaccines are not available.

The Disease in Humans. No evidence has been found that humans are susceptible to MCF virus.

REFERENCES

Blood, D.C., Radostits, O.M., and Henderson, J.A. 1983. Bovine malignant catarrh. In Veterinary Medicine, 6th ed. Bailliere Tindall, London. Pp. 750–754.

Blood, D.C., Rowsell, H.C., and Savan, M. 1961. An outbreak of bovine malignant catarrh in a dairy herd. II. Transmission experiments. Can. Vet. J. 2:319–325.

Buxton, D., and Reid, H.W. 1980. Transmission of malignant catarrhal fever to rabbits. Vet. Rec. 106:243–245.

Buxton, D., Reid, H.W., Finlayson, J., and Pow, I. 1984. Pathogenesis of "sheep-associated" malignant catarrhal fever in rabbits. Res. Vet. Sci. 36:205–211.

Buxton, D., Reid, H.W., Finlayson, J., Pow, I., and Berrie, E. 1985. Transmission of a malignant catarrhal fever–like syndrome to sheep; Preliminary experiments. Res. Vet. Sci. 38:22–29.

Castro, A.E., and Daley, G.G. 1982. Electron microscopic study of the African strain of malignant catarrhal fever virus in bovine cell cultures. Am. J. Vet. Res. 43:576–582.

Castro, A.E., Daley, G.G., Zimmer, M.A., Whitenack, D.L., and Jensen, J. 1982. Malignant catarrhal fever in an Indian gaur and greater kudu: Experimental transmission, isolation, and identification of a herpesvirus. Am. J. Vet. Res. 43:5–11.

Castro, A.E., Heuschele, W.P., Schramke, M.L., and Dotson, J.F. 1985. Ultrastructure of cellular changes in the replication of the alcelaphine herpesvirus-1 of malignant catarrhal fever. Am. J. Vet. Res. 46:1231–1237.

Castro, A.E., Ramsay, E.C., Dotson, J.F., Schramke, M.L., Kocan, A.A., and Whitenack, D.L. 1984. Characteristics of the herpesvirus of malignant catarrhal fever isolated from captive wildebeest calves. Am. J. Vet. Res. 45:409–415.

Goss, L.W., Cole, G.R., and Kissling, R.E. 1947. The pathology of malignant catarrhal fever (bovine epitheliosis) with special reference to cytoplasmic inclusion. Am. J. Pathol. 23:837–841.

Hamblin, C., and Hedger, R.S. 1984. Neutralizing antibodies to wildebeest-derived malignant catarrhal fever virus in African wildlife. Comp. Immunol. Microbiol. Infect. Dis. 7:195–199.

Hatkin, J. 1980. Endemic malignant catarrhal fever at the San Diego wild animal park. J. Wildl. Dis. 16:439–443.

Heuschele, W.P. 1982. Malignant catarrhal fever in wild ruminants—A review and current status report. Proc. U.S. Anim. Health Assoc. 86:552–570.

Heuschele, W.P. 1983. Diagnosis of malignant catarrhal fever due to alcelaphine herpesvirus-1. In Proceedings of the 3d International Symposium on Veterinary Laboratory Diagnosis. Pp. 707–713.

Heuschele, W.P., Nielsen, N.O., Oosterhuis, J.E., and Castro, A.E. 1985. Dexamethazone-induced recrudescence of malignant catarrhal fever and associated lymphosarcoma and granulomatous disease in a Formosan sika deer (Cervus nippon taiouanus). Am. J. Vet. Res. 46:1578–1583.

Hoffmann, D., Soeripto, S., Sobironingsih, S., Campbell, R.S., and Clarke, B.C. 1984. The clinico-pathology of a malignant catarrhal fever syndrome in the Indonesian swamp buffalo (Bubalus bubalis). Aust. Vet. J. 61:108–112.

Kahrs, R.F. 1981. Malignant catarrhal fever. In R.F. Kahrs, ed., Viral Diseases of Cattle. Iowa State University Press, Ames. Pp. 157–163.

Kalunda, M. 1975. African malignant catarrhal fever virus: Its biologic properties and the response of American cattle. Ph.D. dissertation, Cornell University, Ithaca, N.Y.

Kalunda, M., Dardiri, A.H., and Lee, K.M. 1981. Malignant catarrhal fever. I. Response of American cattle to malignant catarrhal virus isolated in Kenya. Can. J. Comp. Med. 45:70–76.

Kalunda, M., Ferris, D.H., Dardiri, A.H., and Lee, K.M. 1981. Malignant catarrhal fever. III. Experimental infection of sheep, domestic rabbits and laboratory animals with malignant catarrhal fever virus. Can. J. Comp. Med. 45:310–314.

Liggitt, H.D., and DeMartini, J.C. 1980. The pathomorphology of malignant catarrhal fever. I. Generalized lymphoid vasculitis. II. Multisystemic epithelial lesions. Vet. Pathol. 17:58–72, 73–83.

Ludwig, H. 1984. Herpesviruses of Bovidae: The characterization, grouping and role of different types, including latent viruses. In G. Wittman, R. Gaskell, and H. Rziha, eds., Latent Herpes Virus Infections in Veterinary Medicine. Martinus Nijhoff, Boston. Pp. 171–189.

Mare, C.J. 1977. Malignant catarrhal fever: An emerging disease of cattle in the USA. Proc. U.S. Anim. Health Assoc. 81:151–157.

Marshall, C.J., Munce, T.E., Barnes, M.F., and Boerner, F. 1919–1920. Malignant catarrhal fever. J. Am. Vet. Med. Assoc. 56:570–580.

Mushi, E.Z., and Rurangirwa, F.R. 1981. Epidemiology of bovine malignant catarrhal fevers, a review. Vet. Res. Commun. 5:127–142.

Mushi, E.Z., Karstad, L., and Jessett, D.M. 1980. Isolation of bovine malignant catarrhal fever virus from ocular and nasal secretions of wildebeest calves. Res. Vet. Sci. 29:168–171.

Piercy, S.E. 1952a. Studies in bovine malignant catarrh I. Experimental infection in cattle. Br. Vet. J. 108:35–46.

Piercy, S.E. 1952b. Experimental infection of cattle (continued). I. Infectivity of materials other than lymph gland. II. Rates of inoculation. Br. Vet. J. 108:214–220.

Pierson, R.E., Hamdy, R.M., Dardiri, A.H., Ferris, D.H., and Schloer, G.M. 1979. Comparison of African and American forms of malignant catarrhal fever: Transmission and clinical signs. Am. J. Vet. Res. 40:1091–1095.

Pierson, R.E., Thake, D., McChesney, A.E., and Storz, J. 1973. An epizootic of malignant catarrhal fever in feedlot cattle. J. Am. Vet. Med. Assoc. 163:349–350.

Plowright, W. 1953. The blood leukocytes in infectious malignant catarrh of the ox and rabbit. J. Comp. Pathol. Therap. 63:618–634.

Plowright, W. 1965a. Malignant catarrhal fever in East Africa I. Behavior of the virus in free-living populations of blue wildebeest. Res. Vet. Sci. 6:56–68.

Plowright, W. 1965b. Malignant catarrhal fever in East Africa II. Obser-

vations on wildebeest calves at the laboratory and contact transmission of the infection to cattle. Res. Vet. Sci. 6:69–83.

Plowright, W. 1968. Malignant catarrhal fever. J. Am. Vet. Med. Assoc. 152:795–806.

Plowright, W. 1984. Malignant catarrhal fever virus: A lymphotropic herpesvirus of ruminants. In G. Wittman, R. Gaskell, and H. Rhiza, eds., Latent Herpes Virus Infections in Veterinary Medicine. Martinus Nijhoff, Boston. Pp. 279–305.

Plowright, W., Ferris, R.D., and Scott, G.R. 1960. Blue wildebeest and the aetiological agent of bovine malignant catarrhal fever. Nature 188:1167–1169.

Plowright, W.K., Herniman, A.J., Jessett, D.M., Kalunda, M., and Rampton, C.S. 1975. Immunisation of cattle against the herpesvirus of malignant catarrhal fever: Failure of inactivated culture vaccines with adjuvant. Res. Vet. Sci. 19:159–166.

Ramsay, E.R., Castro, A.E., and Baumeister, B.M. 1982. Investigations of malignant catarrhal fever in ruminants at the Oklahoma City Zoo. Proc. U.S. Anim. Health Assoc. 86:571–582.

Reid, H.W., Buxton, D., Berrie, E., Pow, I., and Finlayson, J. 1984. Malignant catarrhal fever. Vet. Rec. 114:581–583.

Rossiter, P.B. 1980. A comparison of immunofluorescence and immunoperoxidase techniques for use in the study of malignant catarrhal fever. Bull. Anim. Health Prod. Afr. 28:109–114.

Rossiter, P.B. 1983. Antibodies to malignant catarrhal fever virus in cattle with non-wildebeest–associated malignant catarrhal fever. J. Comp. Pathol. 93:93–97.

Rossiter, P.B., and Jessett, D.M. 1980. A complement fixation test for antigens of and antibodies to malignant catarrhal fever virus. Res. Vet. Sci. 28:228–233.

Ruth, G.R., Reed, D.E., Daley, C.A., Vorhies, M.W., Wohlgemuth, K., and Shave, H. 1977. Malignant catarrhal fever in bison. J. Am. Vet. Med. Assoc. 171:913–917.

Stenius, P. 1952. Bovine malignant catarrh: A statistical, histopathological and experimental study. Institute of Pathology, Veterinary College, Helsinki.

Storz, J., Okuna, N., McChesney, A.E., and Pierson, R.E. 1976. Virologic studies on cattle with naturally occurring and experimentally induced malignant catarrhal fever. Am. J. Vet. Res 37:875–878.

Todd, W.J., and Storz, J. 1983. Morphogenesis of a cytomegalovirus from an American bison affected with malignant catarrhal fever. J. Gen. Virol. 64:1025–1030.

Westbury, H.A., and Denholm, L.J. 1982. Malignant catarrhal fever in farmed Rusa deer (Cervus timorensis). 2. Animal transmission and virological studies. Aust. Vet. J. 58:88–92.

Whiteley, H.E., Young, S., Liggitt, H.D., and DeMartini, J.C. 1985. Ocular lesions of bovine malignant catarrhal fever. Vet. Pathol. 22:219–225.

Whitenack, D.L., Castro, A.E., and Kocan, A.A. 1981. Experimental malignant catarrhal fever (African form) in white-tailed deer. J. Wildl. Dis. 17:443–451.

Zimmer, M.A., McCoy, C.P., and Jensen, J.M. 1981. Comparative pathology of the African form of malignant catarrhal fever in captive Indian gaur and domestic cattle. J. Am. Vet. Med. Assoc. 179:1130–1135.

Marek's Disease

SYNONYMS: Avian leukosis, fisheye, gray eye, iritis, neural leukosis, neuritis, neurolymphomatosis, polyneuritis, range paralysis, skin leukosis, uveitis; abbreviation, MD

Most so-called avian leukosis cases (Marek's disease) are caused by an avian herpesvirus, a member of the subfamily Gammaherpesvirinae. The chicken is the primary host for the virus, but it also is found in turkeys, pheasants, and possibly quail. Similar lesions are observed in the pigeon, duck, goose, canary, budgerigar, and swan (Wight, 1963). The economic loss in chickens as a result of Marek's disease is extremely high, and it is a major disease of chicken flocks throughout the world. It is an acute fulminating type of oncogenic disease in young chicks which spreads quite rapidly.

There is now rather good proof that two virus groups are involved in the production of the various forms of the avian leukosis complex (Biggs 1961). One group of isolates termed *lymphoid leukosis virus,* a retrovirus, produces visceral lymphomatosis, erythroblastosis, myeloblastosis, and possibly osteopetrosis (Walter et al. 1963). In 1962 it was proposed that the nephroblastoma produced by the BAI strain A be considered an additional tumor in this group (Walter et al. 1962). The herpesvirus strains of the Marek group cause neurolymphomatosis, ocular lymphomatosis, and, to a lesser degree, a form of visceral lymphomatosis. All the various forms included in the complex have been reproduced by experimental inoculation of filtrates.

Our knowledge of the etiology of MD has progressed from the point of complete ignorance to virtual control of this oncogenic disease by vaccination, which saves the poultry industry millions of dollars each year. MD is the first oncogenic disease to be controlled by vaccination. It also is an important model for studying viral and host factors that influence the outcome of infection by an oncogenic herpesvirus.

Excellent review articles have been written by Calnek (1980) and by Payne (1985a).

Character of the Disease. Marek's disease consists of inflammatory and neoplastic lesions. It affects primarily the nervous system, but visceral organs and other tissues may also be involved. The disease is seen most often in young birds about the time they are turned out on the range, but it sometimes occurs in birds as young as 3 or 4 weeks old and sometimes in those more than a year old. The disease is manifested by a flaccid or spastic paralysis of a leg, wing, or, less commonly, the neck. Sometimes both legs or wings are affected, but more commonly the disease is unilateral. The affected wing droops and may brush the ground as the bird walks. Affected legs usually are stretched forward or backward; and, when the disease has progressed far, the bird is unable to stand or walk. When the neck is affected, the head is depressed or there may be twisting (torticollis). The location and intensity of the paralysis vary widely in different birds in the same flock.

The Marek group of viruses is probably responsible for

ocular lymphomatosis, manifested by a diffuse bluish gray fading of the iris of one or both eyes. Depigmentation sometimes occurs in a spotty fashion and sometimes in the form of annular fading. The pupils frequently become irregular in outline.

Visceral lymphoid tumors commonly involve the gonad, liver, lung, and skin. All degrees of severity are seen. The disease may occur in older birds, but the most acute forms may be observed in birds as young as 6 to 8 weeks old. Morbidity and mortality may exceed 50 percent of the flock.

Properties of the Virus. The molecular biology and properties of the virus were thoroughly reviewed by Calnek (1980) and Schat (1985). The herpesvirus of Marek's disease belongs to the cytomegalovirus group of cell-associated herpesviruses. All field isolates appear to be antigenically identical, as they cross-react in agar-gel precipitin and fluorescent antibody tests (Chubb and Churchill 1968, Purchase 1969); however, some are altered somewhat after cell-culture passage (Churchill, Chubb, and Baxendale 1969). A herpesvirus isolated from turkeys is antigenically similar to Marek's disease virus and is nonpathogenic for chickens and turkeys (Witter et al. 1970).

The DNA virus particles are 85 to 100 nm in diameter, and the capsid has 162 hollow cylindrical capsomeres. The particles from feather follicles have a similar morphology but a loose irregular envelope up to 400 nm in diameter (Figure 46.25). The extracted DNA has a high guanine-cytosine content.

Because Marek's disease virus is highly cell-associated, whole cells must be used as inoculum from all of the infected bird's tissues except the feather follicles, from which the completed enveloped virus particles are excreted (Calnek and Hitchner 1969). Preservation of virus-containing cells requires the following storage conditions: the addition of dimethyl sulfoxide, slow freezing, and holding at $-196°C$. Virus preparations from feather follicles remain infectious after lyophilization and maintenance at room temperature.

Antibody can be demonstrated in serums of recovered birds by agar-gel precipitin (Chubb and Churchill 1968), indirect fluorescent antibody (Purchase 1969), or passive hemagglutination tests (Edison and Schmittle 1969). In the precipitin test up to six lines may form; the major line is called the precipitin line (Purchase 1969). This test is most widely used for the detection of antibody to Marek's disease. The indirect fluorescent antibody test is used to distinguish between Marek's disease virus and the herpesvirus of turkeys.

Cultivation. Marek's disease virus produces cytopathic effect plaques in duck embryo fibroblasts. In chick

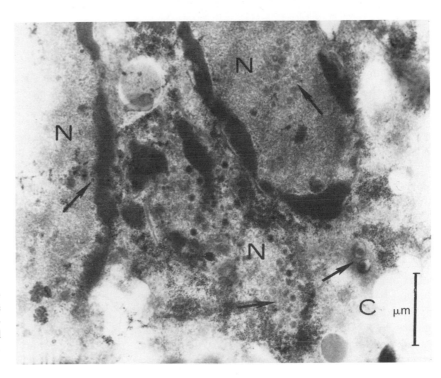

Figure 46.25. Marek's disease. In the nucleus (*N*) naked, incomplete virions are found; but in the cytoplasm (*C*) of the infected feather follicle, numerous enveloped particles are observed. (Courtesy B. Calnek.)

kidney cell cultures the virus produces rounded, highly retractile cells or syncytia, or both (Figure 46.26) (Churchill and Biggs 1967, Solomon et al. 1968). The cell plaques appear in 6 to 14 days and consist of rounded and fusiform cells and polykaryocytes containing Cowdry type A intranuclear inclusion bodies. Naked and occasionally enveloped virus particles are seen in the nucleus of the infected cells and occasionally in the cytoplasm.

The virus produces pocks on the chorioallantoic membrane route. The yolk sac route is preferred.

Epizootiology and Pathogenesis. Most birds have antibody to Marek's disease by maturity. Infection persists in birds for long periods of time, possibly for life. Congenital (vertical) infection probably does not occur, so embryos and young chicks are virus-free and susceptible. Consequently disease transmission occurs after maternal

Figure 46.26. Cytopathic effect (*C*) caused by Marek's virus in chicken kidney cell culture, unstained. × 240. (From Calnek and Madin, 1969, courtesy of *American Journal of Veterinary Research.*)

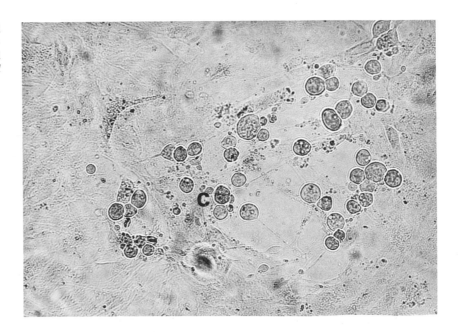

immunity subsides (by 3 weeks of age) by exposure to infected chickens or an environment with persisting virus in excreta, litter, and poultry house dust.

The pathogenesis of this disease is reasonably well known (Calnek 1980, 1985; Payne 1981). Inhalation is the usual means of viral entry. It is speculated that virus is transmitted by macrophages to lymphoid tissues. Viral replication can be found in the spleen, thymus, and bursa of Fabricius within 3 days. The early infection is characterized by inflammatory, necrotic, and cytolytic (of lymphocytes) pathological changes. During the 5 to 7 days after inoculation a marked change in the infection occurs; there is a switch from cytolytic to latent infection. The latter involves primarily Ia-bearing (activated) T cells, but some B cells also are latently infected. When viral activity wanes in the lymphoid organs during the second week of infection, a variety of other tissues, notably those of epithelial origin, become infected by latently infected peripheral blood lymphocytes. Focal necrosis and intranuclear inclusion bodies may be seen in many organs, including the kidney, pancreas, and adrenal gland. In general, infection of the epithelial cells is the productive-restrictive type. The feather follicle epithelium deserves special attention because it is the only tissue in which fully infectious virus particles are released more than 2 weeks after infection, and it is the mechanism by which the disease is transmitted to susceptible birds (Calnek et al. 1970, Edison and Schmittle 1969). The ultimate event is the development of gross tumors in a variety of tissues described below. The neoplastic element of lymphomas is transformed thymus-derived T lymphoblast.

Fabricant et al. (1978) observed grossly occlusive atherosclerosis in a significant number (24 percent) of chickens during a 7-month period after a strain of relatively low oncogenicity was inoculated into newly hatched, specific-pathogen–free chicks. The lesion type and distribution resembled those seen in human chronic arteriosclerosis. The mechanism of induction is not understood, but the investigators suggested that oncogenic transformation of arterial smooth muscle cells, or a response to direct insult by the virus or to indirect insult by immune complexes, should be considered.

The gross lesions of Marek's disease consist of grayish white swellings of the principal nerve trunks in the region involved. When the leg is involved, the swelling generally is found in the sciatic nerve on the inside of the thigh. By comparing the size of the nerve trunks on the two sides of the bird, one can detect even small tumors, but generally the growths are sufficiently great to be readily observed. Histological examination of the swollen nerve trunks shows extensive infiltration of the small round cells, which generally cannot be distinguished from lymphocytes but sometimes appear like mononuclear cells or histiocytes. The lesion may be edematous, and there may be myelin degeneration of the nerve sheaths, but degeneration of the neuroaxons is not conspicuous. Histologically infiltrations of lymphocytic or mononuclear cells are found in the iris, and often there are similar infiltrations in the optic nerve. This form of the disease usually occurs in flocks affected with neurolymphomatosis, but the eye condition generally appears later in life. Many pathologists consider it a latent form of neurolymphomatosis.

For more detailed information about pathology of Marek's disease, see the review by Payne (1985b).

Immunity. Schat (1987) reviewed in depth the immunity to Marek's disease. Although there is no effective immunity to infection, resistance of chickens to tumor formation may be affected by the genetic line of the birds (Cole 1968, Crittenden 1968), age at infection (Sevoian and Chamberlain 1963), antibody status of the dam (Chubb and Churchill, 1969), and exposure to avirulent viruses (Churchill, Payne, and Chubb 1969; Rispens et al. 1969; Witter et al. 1970). The resistance of chickens to tumor formation can be evaluated by intra-abdominal challenge with virulent virus or by exposure to infected chickens. For a test to be valid, known susceptible controls must be challenged in a similar manner at the same time. A satisfactory challenge response is achieved in 6 to 20 weeks, depending on the virulence of the challenge virus, age of the chicken, and the susceptibility of the chicken line (Nazerian and Witter 1970).

Passive immunity conferred by the dam may persist for 3 weeks after hatch. It will delay the onset and reduce the incidence of disease in 1-day-old birds challenged by a natural route. It has little effect when birds are challenged intra-abdominally (Chubb and Churchill 1969).

The indirect-hemagglutination antibody titer of chickens infected with Marek's disease virus suggests a direct relationship with the chicken's ability to survive the disease (Edison and Schmittle 1969).

Diagnosis. Detection of gross or microscopic lesions or both in nerves or viscera, demonstration of specific antigen in feather follicles by immunofluorescence test, virus isolation in cell culture, or demonstration of a rising antibody titer in paired serum samples are all suitable methods of diagnosis.

Virus isolation can be made in cell culture with infected cells or with virus from feathered follicles, but it is 10- to 1,000-fold less sensitive than chicken inoculation (Witter et al. 1969). Direct cultivation of cells in culture from test chickens is more sensitive than inoculation of cell suspensions on monolayers of susceptible cell cultures.

If the passive hemagglutination test is used, a positive

serum has a titer of 1:16 or greater (Edison and Schmittle 1969). The agar-gel test is most widely used for detection of antibody and also for distinguishing between virulent and attenuated tissue cultured strains.

Prevention and Control. Present knowledge makes it possible to develop a flock that is free of Marek's disease virus. Such flocks can be kept free of the infection by strict isolation, constant surveillance, and frequent monitoring for virus and antibody.

Three types of commercial vaccines now available are extremely effective. These are (1) attenuated oncogenic MD virus, (2) a natural pathogenic turkey herpesvirus antigenically related to MD virus and (3) a natural pathogenic or nononcogenic MD virus. More information about the vaccines and their use is presented by Witter (1985). All vaccines are given subcutaneously. The significant immune responses are probably T-cell–mediated, since an immunosuppressive drug, Cy, interferes with vaccination response only during the transient period when the drug suppresses T-cell activities. The immune responses appear to be aimed at both viral and tumor antigens.

The Disease in Humans. Marek's disease is not known to occur in humans.

REFERENCES

Biggs, P.M. 1961. A discussion on the classification of the avian leucosis complex and fowl paralysis. Br. Vet. J. 117:326–334.

Calnek, B. 1980. Marek's disease virus and lymphoma. In F. Rapp, ed., Oncogenic Herpesvirus. CRC Press, West Palm Beach, Fla.

Calnek, B.W. 1985. Pathogenesis of Marek's disease—A review. In B.W. Calnek and J.L. Spencer, eds., Proceedings of the International Symposium on Marek's Disease. American Association of Avian Pathologists, Kennett Square, Pa. Pp. 374–390.

Calnek, B.W., and Hitchner, S.B. 1969. Localization of viral antigen in chickens infected with Marek's disease herpesvirus. J. Natl. Cancer Inst. 43:935–949.

Calnek, B.W., and Madin, S.H. 1969. Characteristics of in vitro infection of chicken kidney cell cultures with a herpesvirus from Marek's disease. Am. J. Vet. Res. 30:1389–1402.

Calnek, B.W., Aldinger, H.K., and Kahn, D.E. 1970. Feather follicle epithelium: A source of enveloped and infectious cell-free herpesvirus from Marek's disease. Avian Dis. 14:219–233.

Chubb, R.C., and Churchill, A.E. 1968. Precipitating antibodies associated with Marek's disease. Vet. Rec. 83:4–7.

Chubb, R.C., and Churchill, A.E. 1969. Effect of maternal antibody on Marek's disease. Vet. Rec. 85:303–304.

Churchill, A.E., and Biggs, P.M. 1967. Agent of Marek's disease in tissue culture. Nature 215:528–530.

Churchill, A.E., Chubb, R.C., and Baxendale, W. 1969. The attenuation with loss of oncogenicity, of the herpes-type virus of Marek's disease (strain HPRS-16) on passage in cell culture. J. Gen. Virol. 4:557–564.

Churchill, A.E., Payne, L.N., and Chubb, R.C. 1969. Immunization against Marek's disease using a live attenuated virus. Nature 221:744–747.

Cole, R.K. 1968. Studies on genetic resistance to Marek's disease. Avian Dis. 12:9–28.

Crittenden, L.B. 1968. Avian tumor viruses: Prospects for control. World Poult. Sci. J. 24:18–36.

Edison, C.S., and Schmittle, S.C. 1969. Studies on acute Marek's disease. XII. Detection of antibodies with a tannic acid indirect hemagglutination test. Avian Dis. 13:744–782.

Fabricant, C.G., Fabricant, J., Litrenta, M.M., and Minick, C.R. 1978. Virus-induced atherosclerosis. J. Exp. Med. 148:335–340.

Nazerian, K., and Witter, R.L. 1970. Cell-free transmission and in vivo replication of Marek's disease virus. J. Virol. 5:388–397.

Payne, L.N. 1981. Biology of Marek's disease virus and the herpesvirus of turkeys. In B. Roizinav, ed., The Herpesvirus. Plenum Press, New York. Pp. 347–431.

Payne, L.N. 1985a. Marek's disease: Scientific basis and methods of control. In L.N. Payne, ed., Developments in Veterinary Virology. Martinus Nijhoff, Boston. Pp. 1–349.

Payne, L.N. 1985b. Pathology. In L.N. Payne, ed., Marek's Disease. Martinus Nijhoff, Boston. Pp. 1–34.

Purchase, H.G. 1969. Immunofluorescence in the study of Marek's disease. I. Detection of antigen in cell culture and an antigenic comparison of eight isolates. J. Virol. 3:557–565.

Rispens, B.H., Van Vloten, J., Maas, H.J.L. 1969. Some virological and serological observations on Marek's disease: A preliminary report. Br. Vet. J. 125:445–453.

Schat, K.A. 1985. Molecular biology of the virus. In L.N. Payne, ed., Marek's disease. Martinus Nijhoff, Boston. Pp. 113–150.

Schat, K.A. 1987. Immunity in Marek's disease and other tumors. In A. Torvanen and P. Torvanen, eds., Basis and Practice of Avian Immunology. CRC Press, Boca Raton, Fla.

Sevoian, M., and Chamberlain, D.M. 1963. Avian lymphomatosis. III. Incidence and manifestations in experimentally infected chickens of various ages. Avian Dis. 7:97–102.

Solomon, J.J., Witter, R.L., Nazerian, K., and Burmester, B.R. 1968. Studies on the etiology of Marek's disease. I. Propagation of the agent in cell culture (32649). Proc. Soc. Exp. Biol. Med. 127:173–177.

Walter, W.G., Burmester, B.R., and Cunningham, C.H. 1962. Studies on the transmission and pathology of a viral-induced avian nephroblastoma (embryonal nephroma). Avian Dis. 6:455–477.

Walter, W.G., Burmester, B.R., and Fontes, A.K. 1963. Variation in the occurrence of erythroblastosis and osteopetrosis induced by virus from individual chickens infected with avian leukosis strain RPL12. Avian Dis. 7:79–89.

Wight, P.A.L. 1963. Lymphoid leucosis and fowl paralysis in the quail. Vet. Rec. 75:685–687.

Witter, R.L. 1985. Principles of vaccination. In L.N. Payne, ed., Marek's Disease. Martinus Nijhoff, Boston. Pp. 203–250.

Witter, R.L., Nazerian, K., Purchase, H.G., and Burgoyne, G.H. 1970. Isolation from turkeys of a cell-associated herpesvirus antigenically related to Marek's disease virus. Am. J. Vet. Res. 31:525–538.

Witter, R.L., Solomon, J.J., and Burgoyne, G.H. 1969. Cell culture techniques for primary isolation of Marek's disease–associated herpesvirus. Avian Dis. 13:101–118.

The nucleic acid core of the RNA group of viruses is ribonucleic acid. There are 11 families recognized by the International Committee on Taxonomy of Viruses in the RNA group: Picornaviridae, Reoviridae, Togaviridae, Orthomyxoviridae, Paramyxoviridae, Rhabdoviridae, Retroviridae, Bunyaviridae, Arenaviridae, Caliciviridae, and Coronaviridae.

47 The Picornaviridae

The viruses in the Picornaviridae family are classified in four genera: *Rhinovirus, Enterovirus, Aphthovirus,* and *Cardiovirus.* There are no known pathogens of domestic animals in the genus *Cardiovirus.* Viruses in this rather large family have a primary affinity for superficial tissues and cause many important animal virus diseases, particularly foot-and-mouth disease (FMD) (Table 47.1). Most viruses in these four genera have been well studied and share certain biochemical and biophysical characteristics. All the families except Reoviridae contain single-stranded RNA. Viruses in the Reoviridae family have double-stranded RNA. All are nonenveloped isometric particles of small size that are ether-resistant and are synthesized in the cytoplasm of cells.

The Genus *Aphthovirus*

The seven virus types that cause foot-and-mouth disease (FMD) are the only members of the genus *Aphthovirus.* FMD is considered by many to be the most important animal disease in the world. It markedly affects world trade. Countries that are free of the disease limit trade to selected processed foods and to importation of livestock only after rigorous and costly laboratory tests for virus and/or antibody. For this reason, FMD is called a political as well as an economic disease.

Foot-and-Mouth Disease

SYNONYMS: Aphthous fever, epizootic aphthae, infectious aphthous stomatitis, *aftosa* (Italian and Spanish), *fievre aphtheuse* (French), *Maul- und Klauenseuch* (German); abbreviation, FMD

Foot-and-mouth disease occurs in many cattle-raising regions of the world. It has never gained a firm foothold in Australia, New Zealand, Japan, the British Isles, and North America, regions that have long used drastic means to prevent its establishment. The disease is exceedingly contagious. On at least nine occasions it has broken out in the United States, but all of these outbreaks were successfully stamped out without excessive cost. At the time of this writing, March 1988, there have been no outbreaks in the United States since 1929. The disease has been of great interest to animal disease control authorities in the United States because of the outbreak that occurred in Mexico between 1946 and 1954. In 1951–1952 a small outbreak in western Canada, very close to the international border, also caused considerable concern in the United States.

FMD affects cloven-footed animals, especially cattle and swine as well as sheep and goats and there have been outbreaks in wild ruminants, particularly deer and antelope. Naturally infected hedgehogs have been found in England. An outbreak has been reported in Indian elephants (Pyakural et al. 1976). Human cases occasionally

Table 47.1. Diseases of domestic animals caused by viruses in the Picornaviridae family

Common name of virus	Natural hosts	Type of disease produced
Genus *Aphthovirus*		
Foot-and-mouth disease virus, 7 types, innumerable subtypes	Cattle, swine, sheep, goats, deer, hedgehogs, elephants, rarely humans	The most important political and economic disease of animals in the world. In cattle is characterized by depression, fever, and the appearance of vesicles first on the mucous membranes of the oral cavity, then in the interdigital skin, and occasionally on the teats and udder. High morbidity with low mortality; death results from cardiac muscle necrosis. The disease is similar in other natural hosts, except that in swine lameness is the most conspicuous sign. It is important to differentiate FMD from vesicular exanthema of swine, vesicular stomatitis, and swine vesicular disease
Genus *Rhinovirus*		
Bovine rhinovirus types 1 and 2	Cattle	Acute disease in cattle with fever, depression, coughing, nasal discharge, and dyspnea. As a rule it is a mild, inapparent disease, and some strains do not produce disease; morbidity is high in affected herds
Equine rhinovirus types 1 and 2; perhaps a third one	Horses	Infected stables have a high morbidity, negligible mortality. Signs referable to upper respiratory tract
Genus *Enterovirus*		
Teschen disease virus (porcine enterovirus type 1)	Swine	The disease may be acute or chronic, also inapparent. Initial signs are fever, lassitude, and inappetence, followed by nervous signs. No gross lesions except possible myocardial alterations. Microscopic lesions are typical of a diffuse encephalomyelitis
Porcine enterovirus types 2–8	Swine	Some types produce disease; others do not. Most pathogenic strains cause polioencephalomyelitis; others cause abortions, stillbirths, mummification, and infertility (porcine SMEDI groups). One strain causes pneumonitis
Swine vesicular disease virus (porcine enterovirus type 9)	Swine	This enterovirus causes signs and lesions in pigs similar to FMD. Swine vesicular disease is important in its own right but must be differentiated from FMD
Bovine enterovirus types 1–7	Cattle	These viruses have been isolated from normal cattle and from cattle with disease. Except for one report, these viruses fail to produce disease in experimental calves
Avian encephalomyelitis virus	Chicks and pheasants	The disease manifestations occur only in very young birds which show incoordination, ataxia, and rapid tremors of head and neck. The losses may be as high as 50 percent in a given hatch with an average of 10 percent. Characteristic microscopic lesions are found in the central nervous system

Table 47.1.—*continued*

Common name of virus	Natural hosts	Type of disease produced
Duck hepatitis virus, 2 types	Ducks	The virus causes disease in young duck-lings. Both viral types cause altera-tions in parenchymatous organs. The major changes are in the liver, which is enlarged with petechial and ecchy-motic hemorrhages; there is also focal necrosis of liver cells, high morbidity, and high mortality
Turkey hepatitis virus	Turkeys	Probable enterovirus. Highly contagious disease with high mortality in poults under 2 weeks of age. Principal lesions are in the liver
Human enterovirus	Dogs	ECHO virus type 6 may cause enteric disease in dogs
Equine enterovirus	Horses	Significance as a pathogen undetermined

occur, but these are rare and entail minor localized skin lesions. Carnivorous animals are resistant, and solipeds are completely resistant.

Character of the Disease. FMD is the most feared dis-ease of cattle in the world. From time to time, it has spread over the entire continent of Europe in great panzootics that usually run a year or two and then seem to disappear. The disease never completely disappears, however, for in-fected centers always remain somewhere, from which it again spreads when a new, highly susceptible animal pop-ulation becomes established. The disease causes its great-est losses in cattle and may be serious in swine, but in sheep and goats it usually is not very important.

The importance of FMD lies not so much in its killing power, for mortality usually is not great, but in morbidity losses—the loss of milk and of flesh, and long periods in which affected animals are not productive.

FMD spreads most rapidly during the summer months because of the greater traffic in animals then. The disease would now be especially difficult to control in the United States because of the highly developed transportation sys-tem and the practice of shipping animals long distances—from range to feedlots, from feedlots to slaughtering cen-ters, from farms to marketing centers, and back to other farms.

In cattle the disease is characterized by depression, fever, and the appearance of vesicles filled with clear fluid in certain mucous membranes and portions of the skin. The essential pathological change in the tongue is necrosis of epithelial cells in the stratum spinosum, intracellular

edema, and granulocytic infiltration (Seibold 1963). Cir-cumscribed, slightly elevated, blanched areas termed "initial lesions" develop in the lingual mucosa. Separa-tion of the mucosa from the underlying tissue causes much of this initial lesion to develop into vesicles (Figures 47.1 and 47.2) When some initial lesions fail to separate from the underlying tissue, the desiccating, necrotic mucosa becomes discolored without vesicle formation. Failure to vesiculate in the interdigital skin is the exception, but the initial lesion is similar to the lingual process.

The vesicles appear principally on the mucous mem-branes of the mouth (tongue, cheeks, dental pad, and gums); on the skin of the muzzle, the interdigital space, and around the tops of the claws, and on the teats and occasionally the surface of the udder. More rarely they may be seen around the base of the horns and in the pharynx, larynx, trachea, esophagus, and wall of the rumen, especially around the esophageal groove.

Within 24 to 48 hours after multiplying in the epi-thelium, which is first invaded, the virus escapes into the blood, which carries it to all organs and tissues. This often results in the appearance of secondary vesicles in epi-thelium remote from the point of entry of the virus. The virus does not multiply in the blood, but presumably does so in certain organs. It produces degenerative changes in the muscular tissues, particularly those of the heart. Yellow-whitish streaks, foci of parenchymatous degener-ation, and sometimes necrosis (Figure 47.3) are the man-ifestations of this damage. Severe damage of this type is seen most often in young calves, and this accounts for the

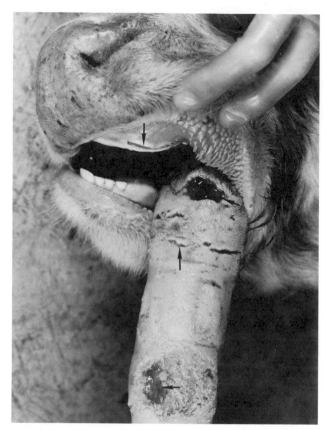

Figure 47.1. Ruptured vesicles (*arrows*) of the tongue epithelium in a steer infected with foot-and-mouth disease virus. Note ruptured vesicle (*arrow*) on dental pad. (Courtesy J. Callis and staff, U.S. Dept. of Agriculture.)

greater mortality in young stock than in adult animals. In some outbreaks, the heart damage is great and mortality of adults as well as young stock may be much higher than usual. This is said to be the malignant form of FMD. In these outbreaks many of the deaths occur early in the course of the infection and are attributed to the specific action of the virus.

Affected cattle become lame as a result of the foot lesions (Figure 47.4), and they champ their jaws and drool because of the mouth soreness (Figure 47.5). They lie down as much as possible, move with great reluctance, and do not eat. As a result, they lose flesh rapidly and milk secretion diminishes greatly. The vesicles in the mouth rupture a few hours after forming, leaving large flaps of whitish, detached epithelium under which are raw, bleeding surfaces. Many times a large part of the tongue is denuded. Secondary bacterial infections of the denuded areas between the claws usually occur, and these result in deep necrosis of tissue and suppurations that frequently undermine the claws, causing them to become loosened from the soft tissues and eventually cast off. The mouth

lesions usually heal quite promptly so that the soreness disappears within a week, but the foot lesions often require much longer to heal.

Much of the damage in most FMD outbreaks is caused by bacterial complications, such as the foot infections described above. These often require slaughter of the animal. In the few cases in which vesicles develop in the upper respiratory tract, pneumonia may occur. A common and serious complication in dairy cattle is udder infection (Figure 47.6). Early in the course of the disease, the udder swells acutely, and the milk becomes thick and viscid, assuming the appearance of colostrum. Whether this is a result of viral action is not clear, but many European workers have so regarded it. In any case streptococcic, staphylococcic, and other bacterial infections resulting in mastitis often develop.

Figure 47.2. Micrograph of part of a vesicular lesion of foot-and-mouth disease on the muzzle of a cow. The cells in the stratum spinosum are rounded and separated from each other (spongiosis), and there is a mild leukocytic infiltrate. Hematoxylin and eosin stain. × 58. (Courtesy C. A. Mebus, Plum Island Animal Disease Center, U.S. Dept. of Agriculture.)

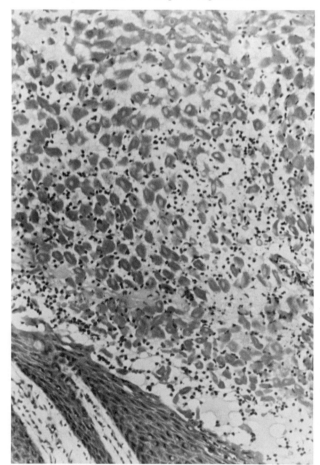

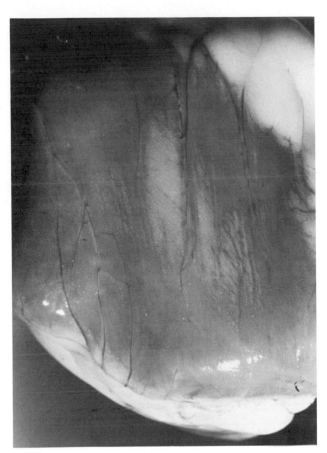

Figure 47.3. Foot-and-mouth disease. The longitudinal yellow-whitish streaks are areas of myocardial necrosis. (Courtesy D. A. Gregg, Plum Island Disease Center, U.S. Dept. of Agriculture.)

In swine lameness is usually the most conspicuous sign and the first noticed. The animals have little appetite, have fever, and move with great reluctance. The lesions in the mouth, between the claws (Figure 47.7), and in the heart muscle are much like those seen in cattle. Large vesicles usually develop in the snout (Figure 47.8).

In sheep and goats lameness is also usually the most conspicuous sign. As a general rule, these animals are not severely affected by FMD. There are exceptions, however. There have been outbreaks in Europe in which sheep and goats were more severely affected than cattle.

The incubation period in FMD is very short. Inoculated animals develop local lesions at the point of inoculation in less than 24 hours, and generalized lesions elsewhere and fever in less than 48 hours. When cattle and swine are exposed naturally, the incubation period is usually no longer than 4 days and may be shorter than 48 hours.

Animals without complications from pyogenic bacteria usually recover completely within 2 to 3 weeks, although milk production may be depressed much longer and their original body weight may not have been re-established at that time. Complications are common, however, and may cause trouble for many weeks or months.

In most outbreaks of FMD the mortality is not high. It seldom averages more than 3 percent and often is less than 1 percent. Occasionally it may be much higher, even as high as 50 percent (McFadyean 1926). The death rate among young stock is higher than that among adults, and somewhat greater in young pigs than in calves. It is usually very low in sheep and goats.

FMD can be readily produced in naturally susceptible species by parental inoculation. Also cattle are easily infected by rubbing virus-containing material on the mucous membrane of the mouth. When cattle are used to detect virus in suspected materials, the most sensitive procedure is to inoculate intradermally into the dorsum of the tongue. After inoculation vesicles appear within 10 to 12 hours at the point of injection, and fever and viremia occur within 20 to 24 hours. Secondary vesiculation generally appears in the interdigital space within 2 to 4 days following this method of inoculation. In cattle infected with the virus of foot-and-mouth disease (FMDV), three types of lesions may be observed. The first type is a vesicle developed mainly from the lysis of swollen, spherical cells and the release of intracellular fluid. The second type is formed mainly by the accumulation of intercellular edema. The third type is characterized by the absence of a vesicle due to seepage and loss of edema fluid and desiccation of the lesion.

In earlier times, research on FMD was greatly hampered because infections could not be produced in small laboratory animals. Swine and cattle, which are very expensive, had to be used. Another difficulty was that the great contagiousness of the disease necessitated elaborate equipment and housing facilities to prevent infection from escaping and spreading uncontrolled to all susceptible stock in large animal quarters. The discovery by Waldmann and Pape (1921) that guinea pigs could be infected with FMDV by a special technique was an advance of great importance. These animals can be used to detect virus in animal tissues and in materials that have been in contact with infected animals. Furthermore, the disease in guinea pigs is not naturally transmissible, and thus the problem of keeping susceptible animals on the premises for experimental work was immediately solved.

Very young and very old guinea pigs are not satisfactory for work with this virus. Half-grown animals weighing about 350 g are best. The virus is inoculated intradermally into the footpads of the hind feet either with a fine hypodermic needle or by scarification. A primary vesicle usually appears at the point of inoculation within 24 hours, occasionally longer. When the primary vesicle ap-

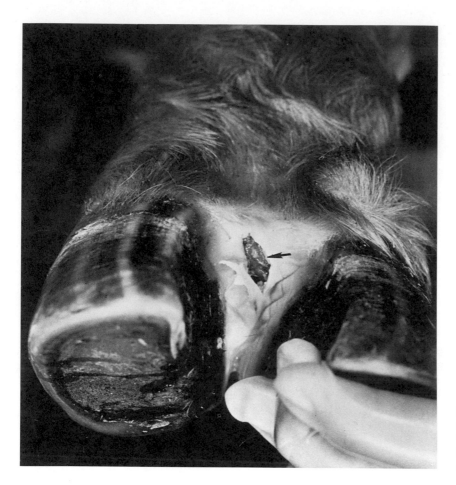

Figure 47.4. Ruptured vesicles (*arrow*) in the interdigital region of a steer infected with foot-and-mouth disease virus. (Courtesy J. J. Callis and staff, U.S. Dept. of Agriculture.)

pears, virus can be detected in the blood. Within 18 to 36 hours, secondary vesicles appear in the mouth, and the virus disappears from the blood. Complete repair of the lesions requires several weeks. Only an occasional animal dies of the disease. There is no evidence that the virus multiplies elsewhere than at the site of the lesions. Intralingual injection has been reported to be more sensitive than footpad inoculation (Hyde and Graves 1963). It is not known why the disease in this animal is not naturally transmissible.

Skinner (1951) showed that unweaned white mice are very sensitive to FMDV and that these animals constitute the best laboratory species for detecting small amounts of virus in suspected materials. Those from 7 to 10 days old prove most suitable. The mice are inoculated intraperitoneally. A spastic paralysis of the hind legs generally appears after several days, but some mice die before exhibiting this sign. Those that die or are destroyed after several days show a marked degeneration of the musculature of the hindquarters and often of the lumbar and intercostal regions. Half or more of all animals exhibit myocardial degeneration.

It was shown by Skinner and confirmed by others that unweaned mice were 10 to 100 times more sensitive to FMDV than were guinea pigs (by footpad inoculation) and always fully as susceptible, and occasionally more so, than cattle inoculated intralingually. The placenta is an active site of infection for FMDV in pregnant mice, but fetuses are relatively resistant to infection (Andersen and Campbell 1976). Other animals such as armadillos, cats, dogs, hamsters, wildebeests, wild and white rats, deer, and rabbits have been infected artificially.

Various investigators have successfully cultivated the virus in birds and chick embryos. Gillespie (1954) infected day-old chicks with tissue-cultured adapted FMDV types A, O, and C and 6-week-old birds with type A virus. Degenerative gizzard muscle lesions developed in most chicks and heart lesions in a small percentage. With some cattle strains Skinner (1954) infected day-old chicks and observed lingual lesions; injection of FMDV into the tongue or footpads resulted in characteristic lesions in bantams, ducks, geese, guinea fowl, and turkeys.

Traub and Schneider (1948) adapted guinea pig virus to the hen's egg, but this virus was no longer pathogenic or

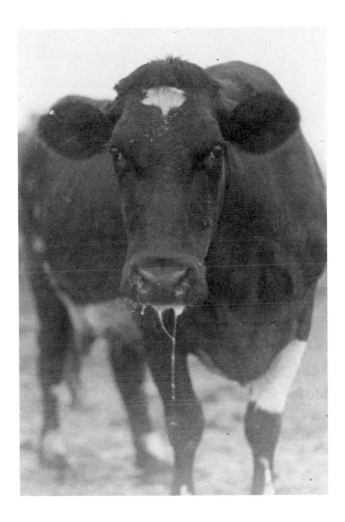

Figure 47.5. Cow with foot-and-mouth disease showing the characteristic drooling of saliva. Affected animals do not eat because of the soreness of their mouths. They champ their jaws, making a smacking sound. (Courtesy L. M. Hurt)

immunogenic for cattle. Skinner (1954) succeeded in passing several cattle strains for many generations in chick embryos by intravenous injection. Gillespie (1955) did likewise with chick-adapted type C virus by inoculating the chorioallantoic membrane and he noted some attenuation for cattle with the 25th egg transfer. Embryos, which usually died in 2 to 6 days, showed edema and hemorrhages in the skin, liver and kidneys; serous or blood-tinged fluid in the body cavity and pericardial sac; and, occasionally, enlarged white areas in the heart muscle. The greatest concentration of virus was in the heart muscle.

Properties of the Virus. The French workers Vallee and Carre (1922) discovered two different types of FMDV. Waldmann and Trautwein (1926) confirmed the

French findings and added a third viral type. The original French types are now designated A (*Allemand*—French for "German") and O (for the Oise Valley, from which the virus came). The German type is known as C. Thus we have three types, O, A, and C, which are known as the European types. Several years ago three new types were found in South Africa. These are designated SAT 1, SAT 2, and SAT 3. The English FMD laboratories reported on a seventh type found in widely separated parts of Asia, which they designated Asiatic type 1.

In addition to the seven basic FDMV types, at least 70 subtypes were recognized before subtyping was discontinued at the World Reference Laboratory in England. Some of these have been designated by subscripts such as A_5 and O_1. Some field subtypes are sufficiently different

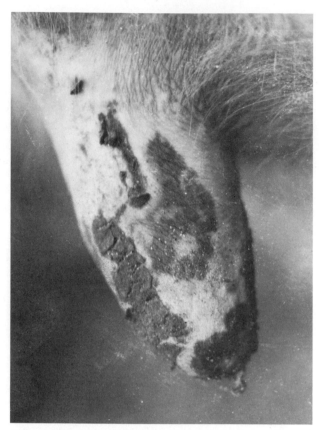

Figure 47.6. Lesions on the teat of a cow with foot-and-mouth disease. Beginning as papules that change to vesicles, the latter rupture, leaving raw surfaces that become infected with bacteria. Mastitis often develops as a result of infection that extends into the teat canal. The surface lesions finally heal under scabs, as depicted here. (Courtesy L. M. Hurt.)

immunologically from the parent strains to make successful immunization dependent upon the use of specific variant vaccines.

The virus of FMD appears to be unusually variable. In later stages of outbreaks in Europe new types or variants appeared which seemed to be derived from the original one rather than from being introduced from outside. Ramon (1952) suggested that such variations may arise as a result of vaccines that imperfectly immunize animals, thus setting up within them the means for forcing variations in the field strains. In a series of papers a group of investigators (Lake et al. 1975, McCahon et al. 1977, MacKenzie and Slade 1975) presented the evidence for recombination between immunological types of FMDV and developed genetic recombination maps.

Animals that have recovered from FMD caused by one viral type generally are sufficiently resistant to that type to withstand additional exposure for 1 year. Such animals

may, however, be immediately infected with one of the other types.

The differentiation of viral types is a laboratory procedure. It may be done with guinea pigs, unweaned mice, complement-fixation or biochemical procedures. In the animal tests one must have high-titer immune serum of a known type. The unknown virus is mixed in appropriate dilutions with the known antiserums, and the mixtures are injected into the animals. The virus is typed to correspond to the type of antiserum that proves to be able to neutralize it. The complement-fixation test for virus typing has been highly developed and in competent hands is highly reliable in differentiating between FMD and other vesicular diseases and slightly less efficient in differentiating among the FMDV types. The technique has been extensively studied by Brooksby (1952b) in England. Complement-fixation typing results are confirmed by cross-neutralizations between virus strains and strain-specific antisera. Other serologic tests such as the indirect complement-fixation (Sakaki et al. 1977, Tekerlekov and Mitev 1976) and hemagglutination-inhibition (Booth et al. 1975) tests have been found comparable to the serum-neutralization test in specificity and sensitivity for detecting virus antibody. The typing of FMDV also may be done by fluorescent-antibody (Sugimura and Eissner 1976) and radioimmunoassay (Crowther 1976) techniques. Progress is also being made in using cloned FMDV cDNA hybridization probes to detect FMDV RNA sequences in infected cells (De La Torre et al. 1985).

In their excellent review articles on FMD Shahan (1962) and Bachrach (1968, 1977) covered the biochemical and biophysical properties of FMDV. The virus is resistant to alcohol, ether, chloroform, and other fat solvents. Glycerol has a preservative effect, especially when mixed with a buffer solution, which prevents the development of acidity. Infected lymph and tissues may be stored for long periods in such a solution without loss of virulence, especially if the solution is kept cold.

In early investigations two complement-fixing antigens were demonstrated in infected guinea pig and bovine vesicular fluids with two different sedimentation coefficients (S rates). The infectious virion (particle) has an S rate of 140S and a diameter of 23 ± 2 nm (Figure 47.9); and the smaller particle, without infectivity, has an S rate of 12S and a diameter of 7 to 8 nm. This smaller particle is composed of three of the four capsid proteins of the virus and is more stable to heat, acids, and enzymes than the infective particle.

Additional virus-specific antigens have been identified in infected tissues. Graves et al. (1968) described empty

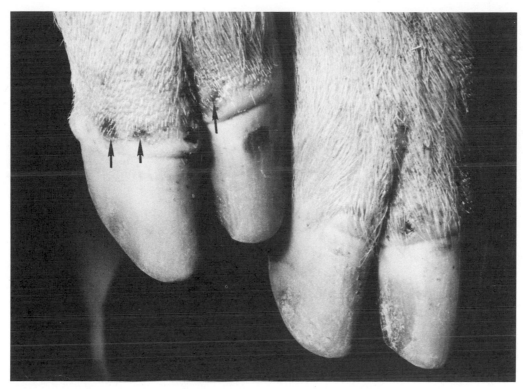

Figure 47.7. Ruptured vesicles (*arrows*) on the coronary band of the feet of a pig infected with foot-and-mouth disease virus. (Courtesy J. Callis and staff, U.S. Dept. of Agriculture.)

Figure 47.8. A large unruptured vesicle on the snout of a pig with foot-and-mouth disease. (Courtesy D. A. Gregg, Plum Island Animal Disease Center, U.S. Dept. of Agriculture.)

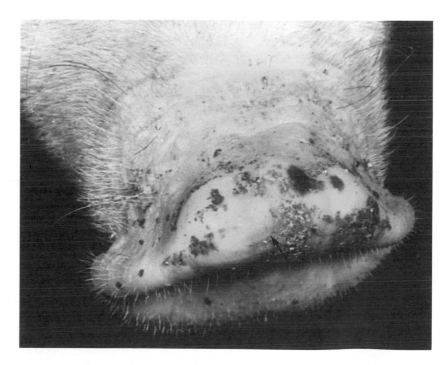

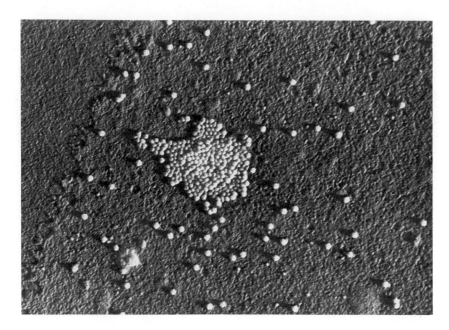

Figure 47.9. Foot-and-mouth disease virus, 23 ± 2 nm. (From Bachrach and Breese, 1958, courtesy of *Proceedings of the Society for Experimental Biology and Medicine.*)

viral capsids with an S rate of 75S, and Cowan and Graves (1966) reported a virus-infection–associated (VIA) antigen with an S rate less than 4.5S. Empty capsids are precipitated by antibody to virions as well as by antibody to 12S viral subunit. The VIA antigen is probably an enzymatically inactive form of FMDV-specific RNA polymerase, because its antibody inhibits polymerase activity. The VIA-RNA polymerase antigen is formed before virions and only when virus replicates in cells of animals, indicating its translation from noncapsid cistrons of the viral genome. Consequently, animals vaccinated with inactivated virus do not produce VIA antigen or its antibody. The test for VIA antibody is a powerful tool in determining whether an animal has ever replicated virus. Thus it is useful in epidemiological studies, in safety evaluation of inactivated-virus vaccine preparations, and in detection of infection in an animal population in eradication programs. All VIA antigens are immunologically identical regardless of viral type. VIA antigen as well as 12S protein subunits interfere with typing FMDV. The adverse effect of these two antigens in this test can be minimized by the use of a short high-temperature test at 37°C for 30 to 90 minutes at high dilutions of antiserum.

All four antigens of the FMD system are active in complement fixation and agar-gel precipitation tests. Only antibodies to 140S virion are known to be type-specific. Only the 140S and 75S antigens appear to produce neutralizing antibody and immunity. As little as 160 nanograms of purified 140S antigen is required to produce measurable neutralizing antibody in guinea pigs (Morgan et al. 1969). Antigenic potencies of 75S naturally occur-

ring empty capsids are quite high; however, a direct comparison of the activities of the 75S and 140S antigens to induce protective immunity was not reported (Rowlands et al. 1975).

The agar-gel diffusion test coupled with acridine orange staining differentiates the 140S RNA-containing virions from the other RNA-free 75S, 12S, and VIA antigens, because only the 140S antigen–acridine orange complex fluoresces under ultraviolet light. In contrast, the fluorescent antibody (FA) is probably antibody to VIA antigen, because FA labeling is not type-specific and occurs only with antiserum from animals in which virus replicates. Direct and indirect FA tests detect FMD infection.

Many strains of FMDV have been characterized by their resistance to thermal inactivation (Bachrach et al. 1960). There is an initial rapid first-order inactivation of tissue-cultured virus followed by tailing, which suggests the presence of a small, heat-resistant population of virus. The heating of virus yields infectious RNA in absence of RNase. The thermal stability of the FMDV is largely determined by the nature of its protein capsid.

The spherical infectious particle is readily inactivated by heat, but its stripped RNA core remains infectious after boiling for 5 minutes. Extensive practical experience has shown that the ability to transmit the disease usually is removed from milk by ordinary pasteurization, but not always. Experiments, however, have shown that a minute fraction of active virus remains in fluids subjected to temperatures above those for pasteurization for periods as long as 7 hours (Bachrach et al. 1957). Virus survived in the milk of acutely infected cows after high-temperature, short-time pasteurization at 72°C for 15 to 17 seconds (Hyde et al. 1975) and survived in the pasteurized milk after evaporation at 65°C to 50 percent of the original volume. FMDV survived in the cream after it was heated at 93°C for 25 minutes (Blackwell and Hyde 1976). Other dairy products remain infective depending on the process.

Viral resistance to drying varies according to the way it is done. If the virus is contained in albuminous material, is dried quickly and completely, and is kept dried, it will persist for very long periods. Virus in epithelial fragments appears to be more resistant than when free in fluids. Schoening (1927) found that virus dried on hay and on soil particles remained viable for about a month, and Trautwein (1926) found epithelial fragments still infective after exposure to winter weather for more than 2 months. Gailiunas and Cottral (1967) found that virus persisted in bovine skin for varying periods of time after treatment by one of four conventional methods for preservation of hides. The shortest period for virus inactivation was 21 days, and the longest was 352 days. FMDV may survive even longer under field conditions. The virus types isolated from hides stored under experimental conditions were virulent and occasionally highly pathogenic for cattle. Cattle hides imported into the United States from countries with FMD are obviously a potential hazard, although this practice has continued since 1930 and no outbreak has occurred.

The resistance of FMDV to drying and its persistence in infected tissues are matters of great importance, since they have a distinct bearing on possible new outbreaks in distant regions due to accidental transfer of the virus. There is no evidence, for example, that any of the last half-dozen outbreaks of this disease in the United States resulted from importing infected animals. At least two outbreaks originated with imported meat scraps that found their way into garbage and then into native swine (Mohler 1926, Mohler 1929), and at least one with vaccine virus imported from a foreign country (Mohler and Rosenau 1909). The origins of several other outbreaks were never discovered, but they may well have begun with virus dried on straw packing materials or on other objects.

FMDV is very sensitive to acidity. At pH 6.5 there is a 10-fold loss every 14 hours at 4°C, and at pH 6 and pH 5 inactivation rises to 90 percent per minute and second, respectively. It is quite stable at 4°C at pH 7 to 7.5 and only slightly less stable at pH 8 to 9. In the absence of RNase, purified FMDV RNA is more stable at pH 4 than crude virus preparations, because RNase in crude virus inactivates the RNA released from virions by acidification (Bachrach 1960).

Phenol and hexylresorcinol release single-stranded infectious RNA from FMDV by stripping off the protein coat. The RNA has an S rate of 37S. RNA extracted from crude virus still contains some RNase to cause slow inactivation, so storage at −196°C or in 70 percent ethanol at −20°C is required to retard inactivation. The FMDV protein is recovered from the phenol phase in pure form by precipitation with methanol and resuspension in phenol, formic acid, or 0.1 percent sodium dodecyl sulfate (Bachrach and Vande Woude 1968).

RNA-containing viruses such as that of FMD, are inactivated by ultraviolet light through changes in their uracil components. FMDV retains its antigenicity and ability to attach to cells after ultraviolet treatment and has a maximum rate of inactivation at 265 nm.

The FMD virion has a molecular mass of approximately 7.3×10^6 daltons and contains 69 percent protein and 31 percent RNA (Bachrach et al. 1964). There are 32 capsomeres, which form a symmetrical icosahedral (20 sides) capsid for the RNA core. During replication in tissue culture cytoplasmic crystalline arrays of complete virus (Figure 47.10) and empty capsids may be observed. Its RNA base composition is G.24:A.26:C.28:U.22. Its isodensity is cesium chloride is 1.43 g/ml.

Figure 47.10. Cytoplasmic crystalline array of foot-and-mouth disease virus particles (*V*) in a bovine kidney tissue-culture cell. × 36,000. (Courtesy S. Breese, U.S. Dept. of Agriculture.)

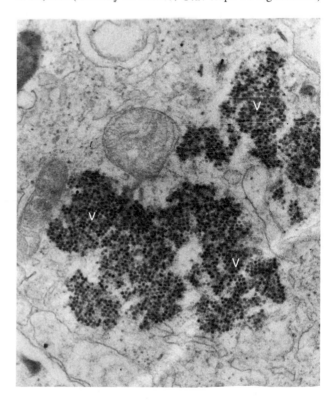

FMDV contains four major peptides: VP_1, VP_2, VP_3, and VP_4. (Publications by Bachrach and collaborators before 1983 [approximately] referred to the protective protein [24 kDa] immunogen as VP_3 because of its position in SDS–8M urea polyacrylamide gel electrophoresis. Subsequently, and in this chapter as well, it has been called VP_1 to conform to the *convention* for the numbering of loci on picornavirus genomes.) The N-terminal amino acids for representative strains of FMDV types A, O, and C were glycine in VP_3, aspartic acid in VP_2, and theonine in VP_1 (Matheka and Bachrach 1975). The complete amino acid sequences of the capsid and noncapsid proteins of FMDV type A_{12} have been determined by sequencing cloned DNA derived from viral RNA (Robertson et al. 1985).

FMDV induces the production of interferon in cell culture (Dinter and Philipson 1962). It has been suggested that FMDV with low virulence, or with many defective particles, is a better inducer of interferon than highly virulent strains. Synthetic polyribonucleotide duplexes that induce interferon interfere with FMDV replication in tissue-culture cells. Bogel (1967) found a thermostable inhibitor of FMDV in normal pig serum which is probably a beta-macroglobulin and not interferon. Andersen (1977) extended the studies with normal swine serums and concluded that the cross-reactions result from IgM or a similar macroglobulin. Using plaque reduction and radio-immunodiffusion tests, Andersen (1975) examined serums from normal cattle and found high levels of cross-reactions with one or two FMDV types per serum tested. The increases of cross-reactions after shipping suggest that an infective agent may be responsible (Andersen 1978b). A bovine enterovirus (E76T) isolated from a bull in the United States produced serologic cross-reactions to FMD SAT 1 virus but not to the other antigenic types of FMDV (Andersen 1978a).

Cultivation. The virus can be propagated in embryonated hens' eggs or in tissue cultures.

In embryonated hens' eggs. Reference has already been made to the studies in adapting a number of FMDV strains to chick embryos. More recently other investigators have used chick-adapted strains for successful transfer in hens' eggs. Some of these studies, egg-adapted and chick-adapted strains have undergone a marked loss of pathogenicity for certain breeds of cattle.

In tissue cultures. Frenkel (1947, 1951) developed a method by which the virus of FMD can be propagated in bovine epithelial tissue suspended in a solution of peptone, glucose, and salt with small amounts of Baker's solution (Parker 1938). The epithelial tissue is obtained at slaughterhouses from the tongues of freshly killed cattle. After inoculation with virus, the stainless steel fermenters are held at 37°C, and a stream of sterile air bubbled through the medium. The fermenters are harvested after 24 hours' incubation, when the virus titer is usually 10^5 to 10^6. The Frenkel method is one of best for the commercial production of vaccine.

Propagation of FMDV in monolayer cultures of bovine and porcine kidney cells was first reported by Bachrach et al. (1955) and by Sellers (1955). Other cell cultures that have been used include those of embryonic bovine skin and muscle, embryonic heart and lung, lamb kidney, fetal rabbit kidney, and murine mammary carcinomatous tissue. The stable line of baby hamster kidney cells (BHK-21) is now commonly used in monolayers and in suspension cultures for research and vaccine virus production, since it is highly susceptible to FMDV. Suspended BHK-21 cell cultures for production of viral vaccine antigen have a number of obvious advantages over BHK-21 cells grown on surfaces, but they have some disadvantages as well. Virus titers from BHK-21 cells grown in suspension are so much lower than those from BHK-21 cells on surfaces that suspension virus must be concentrated during vaccine formulation. Moreover, FMDV from BHK-21 cells grown either way diverge rapidly in antigenic specificity and plaque size (toward small plaque) from the field virus inoculum.

With the plaque method or the production of a cytopathic effect, certain cell cultures can be used to assay for virus. The sensitivity and precision of plaque assays for FMDV depend on the virus-strain cell-substrate system, and on environmental factors (Bachrach 1968). The MVPK–1 cell line derived from fetal pig kidneys is as susceptible as bovine kidney cell cultures to all seven FMDV types in a plaque assay system (Swaney 1976).

Epizootiology. Most of the virus in affected animals is concentrated in the epithelial lesions, but during the early febrile period all tissues and organs and all secretions and excretions contain virus. The disease spreads very rapidly to all susceptible animals on infected farms, probably through infected saliva.

Cottral et al. (1968) demonstrated FMDV in semen before clinical signs appeared and for 10 days after inoculation, and showed that the disease could be transmitted by artificial insemination. This fact should be borne in mind when artificial breeding is considered. No insect vector has been identified as important in the spread of FMD. However, there are a few reports that ticks transmit the disease to cattle. FMD can occur in any season and often seems to be related to the movement of livestock.

Within a comparatively short time after an outbreak on a farm has subsided, or after all infected animals have been removed, the virus generally disappears. Residual virus may remain in dark, damp areas for a long time, however; hence it is necessary to clean and thoroughly disinfect infected premises before they are restocked with susceptible stock. It is also wise to allow the premises to remain unstocked for a considerable time after disinfection.

The U.S. Department of Agriculture permits gradual restocking of premises 30 days after disinfection (Bureau of Animal Industry 1943). A few yearling calves or hogs are first introduced. These are carefully inspected every other day for 10 days, and then twice weekly until the end of the second month. Additional stock may be introduced at this time, but the herd is kept under quarantine and surveillance for a third month. If at the end of 90 days after disinfection there is no evidence of FMD on the premises or on any farms in the immediate neighborhood, the farm is released from quarantine.

It has long been recognized that FMDV can be shipped to distant parts of the world in infected meat. England has had much experience with this source of infection because it had to import most of its fresh meat from countries where the disease is enzootic.

The last two outbreaks of FMD in the United States occurred in California in 1924 and 1929. They began in swine fed on ships' garbage that contained scraps of meat from infected areas of the Orient and South America. As a result of this experience, ships coming from countries where this disease occurs are no longer allowed to land garbage in any U.S. ports.

Stockman and Minett (1927) studied the survival of FMDV in carcasses of animals slaughtered while suffering from this disease. They showed that the acidity that develops in muscular tissue after the onset of rigor mortis rapidly destroys any virus. Usually virus cannot be demonstrated after a few days, even when the meat is refrigerated normally. Virus in visceral organs, however, and in the marrow of the long bones is not subject to the action of tissue acids; and virus was often found in such refrigerated materials after 40 days or more.

Under a provision of the Hawley-Smoot Tariff Act of 1930, the U.S. Secretary of Agriculture is required to place an embargo on fresh meat, fresh hides, and fresh offal from countries where FMD is known to exist. This legislation excludes meat from such countries which has been canned, dried, or otherwise processed in a way that destroys the virus. The enforcement of this provision is largely responsible for the United States' freedom from the disease since 1929 despite a marked increase of international plane and ship traffic. The control officials of the U.S. Department of Agriculture should be congratulated for a job well done despite enormous political pressures to relax their vigilance.

There has been much speculation about the possible role of wild birds in the spread of FMD. Since birds are not naturally susceptible to this virus, they would have to be mechanical carriers if they carried it at all. Many species of birds associate closely with farm livestock, and it seems reasonable to believe that they might have some role in spreading the disease, particularly since no practical quarantine measures have been devised to control their movements. More recently, winds have been incriminated in the spread of FMD. The initial pattern of outbreaks in England in 1967–1968 suggested that spread was air-borne. The movement of trucks containing infected milk also contributed to disease spread. Most animals that recover from FMD are not contagious for other animals within a very short time after complete clinical recovery from the disease. The fact that many outbreaks of FMD have occurred in isolated areas, where it has been difficult to explain the origin of the infection, has caused many to believe that recovered animals may continue to harbor virus long after all signs of the disease have vanished, and that such animals often are the cause of new outbreaks. Most attempts to demonstrate virus in recovered animals have failed, but van Bekkum et al. (1959) found virus in the saliva of cattle several months after their recovery, the virus being capable of infecting unweaned mice and other cattle upon inoculation (Figure 47.11). The disease did not pass naturally to susceptible contact cattle. These studies have been confirmed by many other investigators. Burrows (1968) reported on the persistence of FMDV in the tonsils, pharynx, and dorsal surface of the soft palate of sheep for 1 to 5 months. Cattle become carriers after infection with attenuated or virulent virus, and the virus recovered from carriers is more virulent for pigs than for cattle (Sutmoller et al. 1968). In a field study, 1-year-old calves from cows immunized with rabbit-attenuated virus became carriers; most lacked demonstrable antibody. Carrier virus in esophageal-pharyngeal fluid may be partially masked by antibodies or other inhibitors because fluorocarbon treatment increases the infectivity of the test fluid by 10- to 100-fold. It has also been demonstrated that cattle immunized with inactivated-virus vaccine may become carriers after exposure to virulent test virus without showing clinical signs of illness. Cattle may be carriers for at least 15 months. Animal handlers exposed to infected cattle can inhale the virus and carry it in their throats and nasal passages for at least 28 hours (Sellers et al. 1970).

Many unsuccessful attempts to transmit FMDV from carrier to contact cattle under experimental conditions suggest the existence of unknown factors accountable for successful transmission. Carrier cattle undoubtedly contribute to changes in virulence and antigenicity of FMDV, and probably account for the emergence of new viral sub-

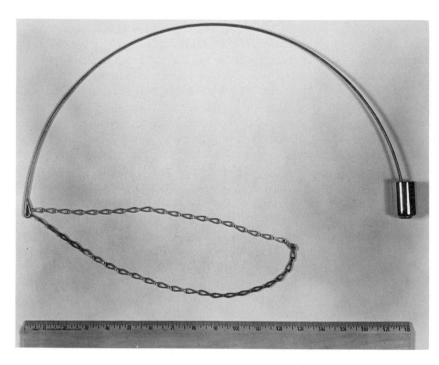

Figure 47.11. Cup probang used to collect saliva and mucus samples for foot-and-mouth disease virus isolation from the bovine posterior pharynx and esophagus. (Courtesy J. J. Callis and staff, U.S. Dept. of Agriculture.)

types where the disease is enzootic and vaccination is practiced. New variants often are available for selection, since the mutation rate of some strains is 1:10,000 (Pringle 1964).

Immunity. Cattle that have recovered from FMD generally have enough immunity to protect them from the same type of virus for a year or more, but the resistance is not lifelong. Natural immunity in cattle and swine is negligible, although some individuals have greater resistance than others. Little is known about duration of immunity in swine, except that it is shorter than in cattle. Even less is known about such other animals as sheep and goats (Cunliffe and Graves 1970).

Antibodies that develop in immunized or convalescent animals are of two types—early and late (Brown and Graves 1959). The early antibody is present 7 days after inoculation but persists for 30 days only. It is a 19S or IgM, which adsorbs strongly to DEAE-cellulose and is sensitive to 2 M mercaptoethanol. This antibody neutralizes and precipitates homotypic and heterotypic FMD virus but has little or no complement-fixation activity. The late antibody appears in 10 to 14 days and may persist for several months. It is a low-molecular-weight 7S IgG, which adsorbs weakly to DEAE-cellulose and is resistant to 2 M mercaptoethanol. The 7S antibody has neutralizing, precipitating and complement-fixing activities that are type-specific.

Immunity in animals, particularly cattle, can be evaluated qualitatively and quantitatively. Various qualitative techniques, such as contact exposure, "cloth infection,"

intranasal or intrapharyngeal instillation, and arbitrary dose of virus on the tongue, are employed. Intralingual titration of virus, and tongue, intramuscular, or subcutaneous inoculations of a standardized dose of virus may produce more quantifiable data; but contact exposure is more representative of field exposure. The correlation between pig protection and neutralizing antibody titer depends on the strain of virus, so the use of antibody titer alone for evaluating protection is unreliable (Bauer et al. 1975).

Graves (1963) reported that the transfer of neutralizing antibody to calves born of dams vaccinated against FMD was by colostrum only. Immunoelectrophoresis showed that calves were born with no gamma globulin in the serum, but that it was present 2 hours after the ingestion of colostrum. Transfer of antibody could be blocked by prior feeding of skim milk or immune bovine serum. A passively immune calf did not respond to vaccination until the serum antibody reached low levels, whereas calves of the same age from nonimmune mothers could be vaccinated, as evidenced by the production of neutralizing antibody. Piglets derive their maternal immunity through the colostrum.

Passive immunity. Susceptible animals can be protected against some of the damages of FMD by injection with immune serum just before, or simultaneously with the exposure to virus. The protection is short-lived—only 1 or 2 weeks—and often it is not sufficient to prevent infection and is seldom used.

Inactivated vaccines. Schmidt and Hansen (1935) and

Schmidt (1936) reported on the use of adjuvants with inactivated FMDV to enhance immunizing power. Waldmann and Kobe (1938) reported the successful use of this vaccine in the field. This type of vaccine is now known as the Schmidt-Waldmann vaccine. Although it has been used very successfully in many European countries, it has not been as successful in Latin America. A Schmidt-Waldmann type of vaccine was used to control the Mexican outbreak. Inactivated vaccines of tissue-culture origin are also frequently used now.

Production of Schmidt-Waldmann vaccine differs somewhat from one laboratory to another, but the principles are the same. Virus is obtained by inoculating susceptible cattle with diluted virus. The inoculum is injected in many places over the surface of the tongue, the virus being deposited in the deeper layer of the tongue epithelium. In about 18 hours large confluent vesicles, loosening practically all of the epithelium of the dorsal surface of the tongue, should appear. If the vesicles have reached a satisfactory stage of development, the animals are slaughtered. The tongues are now carefully removed and saved for the harvest of virus. The processed virus suspension is mixed in about 1.5 percent concentration in a colloidal suspension of aluminum hydroxide particles that absorb the smaller virus particles. Formalin is added to a concentration of 0.1 percent, and the suspension is held at 26°C for 24 hours. This constitutes the vaccine. After being appropriately tested for both innocuousness and immunizing ability, it is ready to be bottled for field use. The finished vaccine has the opalescent appearance of the aluminum hydroxide colloidal suspension. The material must be kept cold, but it is spoiled by freezing and by heat. It is injected subcutaneously in a dose of 30 ml.

Immunity develops after 7 to 10 days, but does not reach its peak until 21 days. European workers consider that a serviceable degree of immunity lasts for 1 year in cattle. In Latin America, where management practices are different, cattle must be vaccinated three times per year for maximum protection. In 1963, van Bekkum et al. stated that the serum titers of Dutch dairy cattle given two or more annual vaccinations remained high for at least 2 years.

The method devised by Frenkel (1947) of Holland for cultivating the virus of FMD has been described in an earlier section. Frenkel and his co-workers were successful in adapting their methods to mass production of high-titer virus. From this virus, vaccine is made by the same procedures used for making the Schmidt-Waldmann vaccine (Bachrach 1968, Frenkel 1951). Henderson (1953) checked several vaccines made in this way and found them fully as good and perhaps better in some instances than those made from cattle tongues.

Other inactivated virus vaccines have utilized FMDV produced in calf kidney cell cultures in Roux flasks and later in large roller bottles (Ubertini et al. 1963). Cell production is limited by the difficulty of processing kidneys and the relatively low cell density reached in the monolayers. The stable baby hamster kidney (BHK) cell line is an improvement, as its cell population in roller bottles is eight times greater than primary bovine kidney monolayers, and it can also be grown in 30- to 100-liter submerged cultures with automatic control of temperature and pH (Capstick et al. 1962). Vaccines prepared with BHK cells can—by restricting the virus passage number and concentrating the virus harvest—be made as potent as other inactivated vaccines. Also, they lack other latent kidney viruses, such as bovine virus diarrhea virus and bovine adenoviruses, and are apparently free of tumorigenicity.

Brown et al. (1963) reported that vaccines prepared by the inactivation of virus with acetylethylenimine were as potent as the corresponding formalin vaccines. With the addition of an oil adjuvant, vaccines become more efficient than the standard formalin—aluminum hydroxide gel vaccines because the duration of immunity is lengthened in cattle and pigs. McKercher and Graves (1976) wrote a review on the status of oil adjuvants in FMD vaccines. Binary ethylenimine can be used as the inactivant instead of acetylethylenimine with comparable results and considerable reduction of the potential danger in handling pure ethylenimine and other aziridines (Bahnemann 1975).

In summary, tissue-cultured FMDV inactivated by acetylethylenimine or binary ethylenimine and emulsified with adjuvant provides a satisfactory vaccine.

Modified live-virus vaccines. The adaptation of FMDV to unweaned mice by Skinner (1951) and to chick embryos and day-old chicks by Skinner (1954) and by Gillespie (1954, 1955), to other small animals (Shahan 1962), and to tissue cultures led to the development of modified live-virus vaccines. Virulent virus was transferred through one or more of these hosts until the virulence for cattle was markedly reduced. Attenuation for one host, however, does not imply reduction of virulence for another host, or even avirulence for the same host under stressful conditions. There is also an indication that, in a combined modified live-virus vaccine, two serotypes may interfere with each other to some degree, although this is not true in all instances, since it is possible for certain subtypes within serotypes to cross-protect (Palacios 1967). Although modified live-virus vaccines undoubtedly conferred longer-lasting immunity than inactivated vaccines and showed some promise under field conditions in certain areas of the world, many problems arose, such as disease in young cattle, potential activation of other infectious latent agents, and post-vaccinal teat lesions leading to mastitis. At present (1987), only Venezuela uses modified live virus vaccine in cattle.

Experimental subunit vaccines. The outermost capsid protein VP_1 (24 kilodaltons) of the FMD virus plays a major role in immunity (Bachrach et al. 1975). This capsid protein isolated from type A_{12} virions and emulsified with incomplete Freund's adjuvant was inoculated, in 100 mg doses, into swine on days 1, 28, and 60. It induced protection by day 82 against exposure to infected swine. However, the serums from prechallenged swine vaccinated with VP_1, contained virus-precipitating and virus-neutralizing antibodies but recognized fewer viral antigenic determinants than antiviral serums. In addition, a 13-kDa peptide (amino acid residues 55-179) excised from VP_1 with cyanogen bromide elicited neutralizing antibodies in guinea pigs (Bachrach et al. 1979) and protective immunity in swine and cattle (Bachrach et al. 1982). Kaaden et al. (1977) have studied the immunogenic capacity of VP_1, cleaved from FMDV type 0_1 in guinea pigs with similar results. Isolated VP_2 and VP_3 are not involved in immune (protective) mechanisms. The detection of fewer antigenic determinants on type A_{12} VP_1 compared with virions (Bachrach et al. 1975) is in accord with the mapping of neutralization epitopes on VP_1 and virions using monoclonal antibodies generated against virions, VP_1 and the 13-kDa fragment (Robertson et al. 1983, Baxt et al. 1984, Grubman and Morgan 1986). Of five epitopes detected, three are on both virions and VP_1, whereas two appear to be conformational epitopes present only in intact virions.

Advances with subunit vaccines for the prevention of FMD in cattle and pigs have been made using bio-synthesized and organically-synthesized VP_1-specific peptides and proteins. A 44-kDa fusion protein cloned and expressed in *Escherichia coli* (having amino acid residues 7-211 of type A_{12} VP_1) in Freund's incomplete adjuvant induces protective immunity in swine and cattle (Kleid et al. 1981). This achievement was described by the U.S. Secretary of Agriculture as being *the first production through gene splicing of an effective vaccine against any disease in animals or humans.* The animals resisted challenge 1.5 months following the first of two vaccinations. With a similarly cloned 26-kDa fusion protein vaccine having residues 1–211 of VP_1 cattle vaccinated on day zero and again at 3.5 or 7.5 months were resistant to challenge at 7 and 10.5 months respectively (McKercher et al. 1985). Results similar to those with the type A_{12} 44-kDa fusion protein have been obtained with VP_1-specific fusion proteins for current field viruses A_{24}, A_{27}, A_{79}, and C_3 but not for type O viruses. In type O viruses two intrachain-linked regions of VP_1 may compromise a dom-

inant immunogenic epitope, as evidenced by the induction of protective immunity in cattle using a 40-residue synthetic peptide *Cys cys 200–213 pro pro ser 141–158 pro cys Gly* in Freund's complete adjuvant (Di Marchi et al. 1986). The foundations are thus in place for artificially produced VP_1-specific protein subunit vaccines for current FMD A, O, and C field types and for production of a completely safe trivalent vaccine that is needed in Europe and South America. For example, 44 percent of the outbreaks in Europe from 1969 to 1981 have been linked to the production of virus used in FMD vaccines (Bachrach 1982).

Diagnosis. In countries like the United States where FMD does not exist, it is of the utmost importance that cases caused by imported virus be quickly recognized. The stamping-out method is not as costly if the disease has not spread far from the initial site. This is why the U.S. Department of Agriculture provides a course in foreign animal disease diagnosis annually or sometimes twice annually at its Plum Island Animal Disease Center in New York State.

Veterinarians and others should always suspect this disease when a number of animals of susceptible species develop stomatitis or lameness at about the same time. In these cases the mouths of a number of animals should be examined for the characteristic vesicles or the denuded areas that follow rupture of the vesicles. The feet should be examined for similar lesions. The epithelial coverings of unruptured vesicles of tongue and feet are the best source of virus (Scott et al. 1966). Three other diseases of farm livestock present with mouth vesicles and sometimes foot lesions that are indistinguishable from those of FMD. These are swine vesicular disease (SVD), vesicular stomatitis (VS), and vesicular exanthema (VE). Differentiation of these diseases from FMD must be done by laboratory experts. Although the tests are relatively simple, it should be strongly emphasized that the importance of an accurate, early diagnosis is so great that those who have had no experience with them should not ordinarily attempt them. *When a disease that resembles FMD is seen in any part of the United States, it should be reported promptly to the chief disease control officer of the state, who will quickly assign experts to the diagnostic problem.*

Differential diagnosis of these four vesicular viruses by laboratory experts is achieved on the basis of history, clinical signs, and laboratory in vitro and in vivo tests. Disease in horses presents no difficulty, for horses are naturally susceptible only to vesicular stomatitis virus. When disease occurs in cattle, the question to be decided is whether it is FMD or VS; in swine it may be any of the four diseases.

Both field and laboratory methods are used to reach a

Table 47.2. Results of inoculating animals with the viruses of foot-and-mouth disease, vesicular stomatitis, and vesicular exanthema

	FMD	VS	VE
Horse (intradermal-lingual)	−	+	−*
Cow (intradermal-lingual)	+	+	−
Cow (intramuscular)	+	−	−
Guinea pig (intradermal-footpad)	+	+	−

*Small local lesions often produced; no generalization.

decision. If a suitably equipped laboratory is available, not only can these viruses be quickly differentiated from each other by the complement-fixation test but also the viral types can be determined (Brooksby 1952a, Camargo 1955, Camargo et al. 1950). In experienced hands the tests are not only much more rapid than the field or inoculation tests but also more accurate and more sensitive.

The field methods for differentiating FMD, VS, and VE viruses depend on animal inoculation (Table 47.2). The procedures, as recommended by Traum (1936), are as follows:

1. Inoculate at least two cows with fresh vesicular fluid. One should be injected intravenously or intramuscularly; the other should be injected in the mucosa of the tongue, lips, or dental pad, or the fluid may be rubbed into scarified areas. If the virus is FMDV, both animals should develop the disease. If it is VSV, the animal injected intravenously or intramuscularly will fail to develop the disease; the other should do so. If it is VEV, both animals will fail to develop the disease.

2. Inoculation of swine is useless because the animals usually will develop disease when any of the four viruses is present.

3. Inoculation of horses is very helpful in differentiating between FMD and VS. The horse is susceptible to the virus of VS but is entirely resistant to that of FMD. The virus of VE is mildly pathogenic for horses. Some animals develop small vesicles near the point of inoculation, others do not. Horses should be injected in the mucous membrane of the dorsum of the tongue, or the virus may be introduced through scarification at this site.

4. Guinea pigs are helpful in differentiating between the virus of VE and of FMD and VS, since VE does not cause infections when introduced through the foot-pad, whereas FMD and VS viruses quite regularly produce vesicular lesions.

Nardelli et al. (1968) described a vesicular viral disease (swine vesicular disease, SVD) in Italian pigs which is clinically indistinguishable from FMD, VE, and VS. The Italian virus is classified as an enterovirus, as it has all the characteristics of that genus. By careful study of its properties one can distinguish it from the other vesicular disease viruses of the pig. An approach for differentiation between SVD and FMD is provided by Buckley et al. (1975). The complement-fixation test can be used, but its sensitivity is limited, so epithelial diagnostic specimens should also be inoculated into tube cultures of primary bovine thyroid cells and into 8-oz bottles of the $IBRS_2$ line of pig kidney cells. FMDV generally grows and causes a cytopathic effect in both types of cell cultures, whereas SVD can be detected only in the porcine cells.

Prevention and Control. The control of FMD is made difficult by four factors: (1) multiplicity of animal hosts, (2) the high contagiousness, (3) multiplicity and variability of viral antigenicity, and (4) short-lived immunity following infection or vaccination and the carrier state in cattle and sheep.

In general two methods of control are used.

Slaughter. This method has been successful in the United States and in other countries (such as Britain and Ireland) that are sufficiently isolated geographically to make it economically feasible (Figure 47.12). It has been used less often and with less success on the European mainland.

When this procedure is chosen, drastic quarantine measures must be established immediately and enough quarantine officers placed on duty to enforce them. Not only the affected farms but also those within a radius of several miles are included in the quarantine. On all farms in the area cattle are confined to their stables or corrals, swine are restricted to buildings or small pens, sheep are restrained, and even dogs and cats are confined to the premises. It is just as important that people be confined and allowed to move from one place to another only by special permission, and then only after thorough disinfection if they are thought to have been in contact with infectious materials. Affected animals and all other susceptible stock that may have been in contact with them, whether or not they show any evidence of the disease, are slaughtered as quickly as possible and buried on the premises. The infected premises are then thoroughly cleaned and disinfected with a strong alkali solution. The U.S. Department of Agriculture uses a disinfectant made of 5 lb of hydrated or water-slacked (*not* air-slacked) lime, 1 lb of concentrated lye or caustic soda, and 10 gallons of hot water to disinfect floors, stanchions, walls, fences, and any other objects that may have been contaminated with virus. If lime is not available, lye or soda is used alone at the rate of 2 lb to each 10 gallons of water. The solution should be applied with a power spray, and all objects should be well soaked. A 4 percent solution of formaldehyde is suitable for harness, blankets, ropes, and finished surfaces that

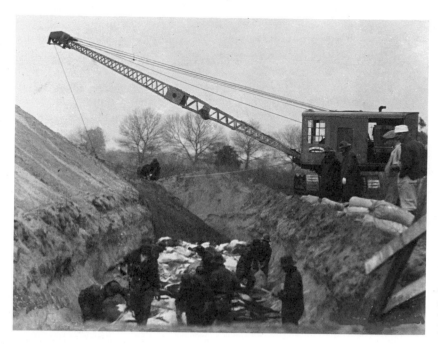

Figure 47.12. Burial of a herd of cattle infected with foot-and-mouth disease. Outbreaks of this disease in the United States are stamped out by the drastic method of slaughter and burial on the premises of all infected and all exposed animals. Trenches are dug; and the cattle are driven into them, slaughtered there, and the hides of the carcasses slashed and covered with a layer of quicklime. All carcasses are then covered with a thick layer of soil. (Courtesy L. M. Hurt.)

would be damaged by alkali. Dwellings, milkhouses, and other tight buildings may be fumigated with formaldehyde gas.

Persons whose work requires them to come in contact with infected animals must wear rubber clothing—hats, coats, pants, boots, and gloves. These may be disinfected with a 2 percent lye solution or with one of the cresylic acid disinfectants. The lye is caustic and will burn the skin if it is permitted to remain on it. Immediate washing with water usually prevents this, or the lye may be neutralized with vinegar. The alkali solutions may be stored in containers made of wood, earthenware, or any of the common metals except aluminum. Infected haystacks can be made safe by removing the surface layers and spraying the remainder with a 4 percent solution of formalin. Old straw, dried manure, and old structures of small value should be burned. Manure piles may be burned, if sufficiently dry, or the material may be thinly spread on fields to which cattle will not have access and plowed underground. All procedures must be done thoroughly.

In the United States the owners of destroyed animals are indemnified from government funds to facilitate the control of FMD. They may also be indemnified for losses of feed, hay, or any other materials destroyed in the course of the cleaning and disinfecting.

All susceptible livestock on farms in the vicinity of infected premises are frequently and thoroughly inspected for evidence of the disease. Stations receiving milk from the quarantined area are inspected to see that they have suitable sterilizing equipment, properly used, to insure

that any milk containers returned to farms are free of virus.

Quarantine and vaccination. This method of FMD control has never been used in the United States, and it is unlikely that it ever will be unless the disease is so widespread that the slaughter method would be impracticable. It has been used successfully in some of the countries of continental Europe, and it appears to have contributed to the success of the campaign that ended a very long and extensive outbreak in Mexico. Since the 1967–1968 epizootic, when close to half a million infected or exposed cattle, sheep, goats and pigs had to be destroyed, Britain has maintained stocks of vaccine for possible immediate use in conjunction with slaughter in future outbreaks. A similar preparedness policy has been adopted in the United States.

The method consists of rigid quarantine of infected premises and immediate use of inactivated vaccine in all susceptible animals within a several mile radius of the center of infection. These measures should be implemented as quickly as the virus type has been determined and vaccine can be procured. When large areas become involved, as in Mexico, all susceptible animals in the entire infected area should be vaccinated.

When vaccines are used, the importance of strict quarantine measures should not be ignored. So far as possible the movement of livestock and of people in contact with livestock should be restricted. Feeding of uncooked garbage to swine in such regions should be prohibited, and unpasteurized milk should not be fed to calves. In

1951–1952 an exceptionally virulent and widespread outbreak of FMD occurred in Europe. Efforts to control this outbreak by vaccination were not very successful, as the disease spread faster than animals could be vaccinated. Also, a number of variant viral types, against which the current vaccines were not potent, appeared. According to Ramon (1952), too little attention was paid to sanitation and quarantine—the old accepted methods—since these measures were no longer considered necessary when the cattle had been vaccinated.

The Disease in Humans. Human beings are only slightly susceptible to the virus of FMD. There have been no recognized cases of human infection in any of the more recent outbreaks of the disease in the United States, and none in the last one in Mexico, although countless people have had close contact with active virus. Many of the early reports of FMD in humans must be discounted because of lack of unequivocal evidence that the conditions described were caused by this virus.

There are some clear-cut records of the disease in humans, however. Gins (1924) described the case of a worker in one of the vaccine laboratories who cut his hand on a broken flask that had contained vesicular fluid. FMDV was identified in the fluid of vesicles that developed, along with other symptoms, in the individual. There are other authentic cases on record, but the number is less than fifty. The susceptibility of humans to FMDV has been reviewed by Betts (1952), who concludes that "the number of credible cases in relation to the number of persons exposed is infinitesimal."

The symptoms in humans are fever, vomiting, a sense of heat and dryness in the mouth, and small vesicles on the lips, tongue, and cheeks. Lesions on the hands have also been described. The course of the disease is short, and there are no records of serious complications or deaths.

FMD in humans may be confused with a vesicular exanthema of the hand, foot, and mouth caused by certain serotypes of Coxsackie virus group A, a subgroup of the genus *Enterovirus*.

REFERENCES

Andersen, A.A. 1975. Cross-reactions of normal bovine serums to foot-and-mouth disease virus in plaque-reduction neutralization and radial immunodiffusion. Am. J. Vet. Res. 36:979–983.

Andersen, A.A. 1977. Occurrence of cross reactions to foot-and-mouth disease virus in normal swine sera. Am. J. Vet. Res. 38:1757–1759.

Andersen, A.A. 1978. Cross reaction between bovine enterovirus and South African Territories. I. Foot-and-mouth disease virus. Am. J. Vet. Res. 39:59–63.

Andersen, A.A. 1978. Cross reactions of normal bovine sera with foot-and-mouth disease virus: Incidence, duration, and effect of shipping stress. Am. J. Vet. Res. 39:603–606.

Andersen, A.A., and Campbell, C.H. 1976. Experimental placental transfer of foot-and-mouth disease virus in mice. Am. J. Vet. Res. 37:585–589.

Bachrach, H.L. 1960. Ribonucleic acid of foot-and-mouth disease virus: Its preparation, stability and plating efficiency on bovine-kidney cultures. Virology 12:259–271.

Bachrach, H.L. 1968. Foot-and-mouth disease. Ann. Rev. Microbiol. 22:201–244.

Bachrach, H.L. 1977. Foot-and-mouth disease virus: Properties, molecular biology and immunogenicity. Beltsville Symposia in Agricultural Research. I. Virology in Agriculture. Allanheld, Osmun & Co., Montclair, N.J. Pp. 3–32.

Bachrach, H.L. 1978. Foot-and-mouth disease: World-wide impact and control measures. In E. Kurstak and K. Maramorosch, eds., Virus and Environment. Academic Press, New York. Pp. 229–310.

Bachrach, H.L. 1982. Recombinant DNA technology for the preparation of subunit vaccines. J. Am. Vet. Med. Assoc. 181:992–999.

Bachrach, H.L., and Breese, S.S., Jr. 1958. Purification and electron-microscopy of foot-and-mouth disease virus. Proc. Soc. Exp. Biol. Med. 97:659–665.

Bachrach, H.L., and Vande Woude, G.F. 1968. Amino acid composition and C-terminal sequence of foot-and-mouth disease virus protein. Virology 34:282–289.

Bachrach, H.L., Breese, S.S., Jr., Callis, J.J., Hess, W.R., and Patty, R.E. 1957. Inactivation of foot-and-mouth disease virus by pH and temperature changes and by formaldehyde. Proc. Soc. Exp. Biol. Med. 95:147–152.

Bachrach, H.L., Hess, W.R., and Callis, J.J. 1955. Foot-and-mouth disease virus: Its growth and cytopathogenicity in tissue culture. Science 122:1269–1270.

Bachrach, H.L., Moore, D.M., McKercher, P.D., and Polatnick, J. 1975. Immune and antibody responses to an isolated capsid protein of foot-and-mouth disease virus. J. Immunol. 115:1636–1641.

Bachrach, H.L., Morgan, D.O., McKercher, P.D., Moore, D.M., and Robertson, D.H. 1982. Immunogenicity and structure of fragments derived from foot-and-mouth disease virus capsid protein VP₃ and of virions having intact and cleaved VP₃. Vet. Microbiol. 7:85–96.

Bachrach, H.L., Morgan, D.O., and Moore, D.M. 1979. Foot-and-mouth disease virus immunogenic capsid protein VP_T: N-terminal sequences and immunogenic peptides obtained by CNBr and tryptic cleavages. Intervirology 12:65–72.

Bachrach, H.L., Patty, R.E., and Pledger, R.A. 1960. Thermal-resistant populations of foot-and-mouth disease virus. Proc. Soc. Exp. Biol. Med. 103:540–542.

Bachrach, H.L., Trautman, R., and Breese, S.S., Jr. 1964. Chemical and physical properties of virtually pure foot-and-mouth disease virus. Am. J. Vet. Res. 25:333–342.

Bahnemann, H.G. 1975. Binary ethylenimine as an inactivant for foot-and-mouth disease virus and its application for vaccine production. Arch. Virol. 47:47–56.

Bauer, K., Lorenz, R.J., and Wittmann, G. 1975. Studies on the relationship between immunity and the level of neutralizing antibodies in pigs vaccinated against foot-and-mouth disease. Arch. Virol. 49:349–357.

Baxt, B., Morgan, D.O., Robertson, B.H., and Timpone, C.A. 1984. Epitopes of foot-and-mouth disease outer capsid protein VP₁ involved in neutralization and cell attachment. J. Virol. 51:298–305.

Betts, A.O. 1952. The susceptibility of man to the virus of foot-and-mouth disease. Vet. Rec. 64:640–641.

Blackwell, J.H., and Hyde, J.L. 1976. Effect of heat on foot-and-mouth disease virus (FMDV) in the components of milk from FMDV-infected cows. J. Hyg. 77:77–83.

Bogel, K. 1967. A thermostable inhibitor in pig serum against foot and mouth disease virus. II. Resistance to treatments which destroy, precipitate or adsorb inhibitors. Zentralbl. Veterinärmed. [B] 14:79–92.

Booth, J.C., Pay, T.W.F., Hedger, R.S., and Barnett, I.T. 1975. The use of the haemagglutination-inhibition test for detecting antibodies to type SAT 2 foot-and-mouth disease viruses in cattle sera. J. Hyg. 74:115–122.

Brooksby, J.B. 1952a. Vesicular stomatitis and foot-and-mouth disease: Analysis of mixed infection in cattle. J. Hyg. 50:394–404.

Brooksby, J.B. 1952b. The technique of complement-fixation in foot-

and-mouth disease research. Agr. Res. Council (Gt. Brit.), Rpt. Series no. 12. H.M. Stationery Office, London.

Brown. F, and Graves, J.H. 1959. Changes in specificity and electrophoretic mobility of the precipitating antibodies present in serum of cattle recovering from foot-and-mouth disease. Nature 183:1688–1689.

Brown, F., Hyslop, N. St. G., Crick, J., and Morrow, A.W. 1963. The use of acetyleneimine in the production of inactivated foot-and-mouth disease vaccines. J. Hyg. 61:337–344.

Buckley, L.S., Osborne, R.W., Periera, H.G. 1975. Laboratory diagnosis of foot-and-mouth disease and swine vesicular disease. Bull. Off. Int. Epiz. 83:123–129.

Burrows, R. 1968. The persistence of foot-and-mouth disease virus in sheep. J. Hyg. 66:633–640.

Camargo, N.F. 1955. A contribution to the study of vesicular stomatitis in Mexico. Proc. U.S. Livestock Sanit. Assoc. 58:379–389.

Camargo, N.F., Eichhorn, E.A., Levine, J.M., and Giron, A.T. 1950. A complement-fixation technique as applied to the study of foot-and-mouth disease and vesicular stomatitis. J. Am. Vet. Med. Assoc. 117:107–108.

Capstick, P.B., Telling, R.C., Chapman, W.G., and Stewart, D.L. 1962. Growth of a cloned strain of hamster kidney cells in suspended cultures and their susceptibility to the virus of foot-and-mouth disease. Nature 195:1163–1164.

Cottral, G.E., Gailiunas, P., and Cox, B.F. 1968. Foot-and-mouth disease virus in semen of bulls and in transmission by artificial insemination. Arch. Gesam. Virusforsch. 23:362–377.

Cowan, K.M., and Graves, J.H. 1966. A third antigenic component associated with foot-and-mouth disease infection. Virology 30:528–540.

Crowther, J.R. 1976. Examination of differences between foot-and-mouth disease virus strains using a radioimmunoassay technique. Dev. Biol. Stand. 35:185–193.

Cunliffe, H.R., and Graves, J.H. 1970. Immunologic response of lambs to emulsified foot-and-mouth disease vaccine. Arch. Gesam. Virusforsch. 32:261–268.

De La Torre, J.C., Davila, M., Sobrine, F., Ortin, J., and Domingo, E. 1985. Establishment of cell lines persistently infected with foot-and-mouth disease virus. Virology 145:24–35.

Di Marchi, R., Brooke, G., Gale, C., Cracknell, V., Doel, T., and Mowat, N. 1986. Protection of cattle against foot-and-mouth disease with a synthetic peptide. Science 232:639–641.

Dinter, Z., and Philipson, L. 1962. An interferon produced by foot and mouth disease virus (FMDV) in calf kidney cells. Proc. Soc. Exp. Biol. Med. 109:893–897.

Frenkel, H.S. 1947. La culture du virus de la fièvre aphteuse sur l'epithelium de la langue des bovides. Bull. Off. Int. Epiz. 28:155–162.

Frenkel, H.S. 1951. Research on foot-and-mouth disease. III. The cultivation of the virus on a practical scale in explanations of bovine tongue epithelium. Am. J. Vet. Res. 12:187–190.

Gailiunas, P., and Cottral, G.E. 1967. Survival of foot-and-mouth disease virus in bovine hides. Am. J. Vet. Res. 28:1047–1053.

Gillespie, J.H. 1954. The propagation and effects of type A foot-and-mouth virus in the day-old chick. Cornell Vet. 44:425–433.

Gillespie, J.H. 1955. Propagation of type C foot-and-mouth-disease virus in eggs and effects of the egg-cultivated virus on cattle. Cornell Vet. 45:170–179.

Gins, H.A. 1924. Foot-and-mouth disease. Klin. Wochenschr. 3:1135.

Graves, J.H. 1963. Transfer of neutralizing antibody by colostrum to calves born of foot-and-mouth disease vaccinated dams. J. Immunol. 91:251–256.

Graves, J.H., Cowan, K.M., and Trautman, R. 1968. Immunochemical studies of foot-and-mouth disease. II. Characterization of RNA-free viruslike particles. Virology 34:269–274.

Grubman, M.J., and Morgan, D.O. 1986. Antigenic comparison of foot-and-mouth disease virus serotypes with monoclonal antibodies. Virus Res. 6:33–43.

Henderson, W.A. 1953. Foot-and-mouth disease. In Proceedings of the 15th International Veterinary Congress, Stockholm. P. 191.

Hyde, J.L., and Graves, J.H. 1963. The comparative titration of foot-and-mouth disease virus inoculated into the tongue and foot pads of guinea pigs. Am. J. Vet. Res. 24:642–643.

Hyde, J.L., Blackwell, J.H., and Callis, J.J. 1975. Effect of pasteurization and evaporation on foot-and-mouth disease virus in whole milk from infected cows. Can. J. Comp. Med. 39:305–309.

Kaaden, O.R., Adam, K.H., and Strohmaier, K. 1977. Induction of neutralizing antibodies and immunity in vaccinated guinea pigs by cyanogen bromide peptides of VP$_3$ of foot-and-mouth disease virus. J. Gen. Virol. 34:397–400.

Kleid, D.G., Yansura, D., Small, B., Dowbenko, D., Moore, D.M., Grubman, M.J., McKercher, P.D., Morgan, D.O., Robertson, B.H., and Bachrach, H.L. 1981. Cloned viral protein vaccine for foot-and-mouth disease: Responses in cattle and swine. Science 214:1125–1129.

Lake, J.R., Priston, A.J., and Slade, W.R. 1975. A genetic recombination map of foot-and-mouth disease virus. J. Gen. Virol. 27:355–367.

McCahon, D., Slade, W.R., Priston, R.A., et al. 1977. An extended genetic recombination map for foot-and-mouth disease virus. J. Gen. Virol. 35:555–565.

McFadyean, J. 1926. Foot-and-mouth disease. Vet. Rec. 6:358–359.

MacKenzie, J.S., and Slade, W.R. 1975. Evidence for recombination between two different immunological types of foot-and-mouth disease virus. Aust. J. Exp. Biol. Med. Sci. 53:251–256.

McKercher, P.D., and Graves, J.H. 1976. A review of the current status of oil adjuvants in foot-and-mouth disease vaccines. Dev. Biol. Stand. 35:107–112.

McKercher, P.D., Moore, D.M., Morgan, D.O., Robertson, B.H., Callis, J.J., Kleid, D.G., Shire, S.J., Yansura, D.G., Dowbenko, D., and Small, B. 1985. Dose response evaluation of genetically engineered foot-and-mouth disease virus polypeptide immunogen in cattle. Am. J. Vet. Res. 46:587–590.

Matheka, H.D., and Bachrach, H.L. 1975. N-terminal amino acid sequences in the major capsid proteins of foot-and-mouth disease virus types A, O, and C. J. Virol. 16:1248–1253.

Mohler, J.R. 1926. Foot-and-mouth disease with special reference to outbreaks in California, 1924 and Texas, 1924 and 1925. U.S. Department of Agriculture Circ. 400.

Mohler, J.R. 1929. Foot-and-mouth disease barriers. Rpt. Chief, Bur. Anim. Indus., U.S. Department of Agriculture.

Mohler, J.R., and Rosenau, M. 1909. The origin of the 1908 outbreak of foot-and-mouth disease in the United States. U.S. Department of Agriculture Circ. 147.

Morgan, D.O., Bachrach, H.L., and McKercher, P.D. 1969. Immunogenicity of nanogram to milligram quantities of inactivated foot-and-mouth disease virus. Appl. Microbiol. 17:441–445.

Nardelli, L., Lodetti, E., Gualandi, G.L., Burrows, R., Goodridge, D., Brown, F., and Cartwright, B. 1968. A foot-and-mouth disease syndrome in pigs caused by an enterovirus. Nature 219:1275–1276.

Palacios, C.A. 1967. Studies on live foot-and-mouth disease vaccines. In Rpt. Manufacturers Res. Group Standing Tech. Comm., European Comm. Control FMD, Rome. Paper 8. P. 86.

Parker, R.C. 1938. Methods of Tissue Culture. Paul B. Hoeber, New York.

Pringle, C.R. 1964. Genetic aspects of the thermal inactivation properties of foot-and-mouth disease virus strains. Bull. Off. Int. Epiz. 61:619–628.

Pyakural, S., Singh, U., and Singh, N.B. 1976. An outbreak of foot-and-mouth disease in Indian elephants (*Elephas maximus*). Vet. Rec. 99:28–29.

Ramon, G. 1952. II. Travaux originaux. Foot-and-mouth disease. Epidemiologic, virologic and immunologic considerations. Lessons drawn from a large epizootic. Bull. Off. Int. Epiz. 37:625–661.

Robertson, B.H., Grubman, M.J., Weddell, G.N., Moore, D.M., Welsh, J.D., Fischer, T., Dowbenko, D.J., Yansura, D.G., Small, B., and Kleid, D.G. 1985. Nucleotide and amino acid sequence coding for polypeptides of foot-and-mouth disease virus type A$_{12}$. J. Virol. 54:651–660.

Robertson, B.H., Morgan, D.O., and Moore, D.M. 1983. Location of neutralizing epitopes defined by monoclonal antibodies generated against the outer capsid polypeptide VP_1, of foot-and-mouth disease virus A_{12}. Virus Res. 1:489–500.

Rowlands, D.J., Sangar, D.V., and Brown, F. 1975. A comparative chemical and serological study of the full and empty particles of foot-and-mouth disease virus. J. Gen. Virol. 26:227–238.

Sakaki, K., Suphavilai, P., and Toxuda, G. 1977. Antibody estimation by indirect complement fixation test for foot-and-mouth disease in cattle. Natl. Inst. Anim. Health Q. 17:45–53.

Schmidt, S. 1936. Immunization of guinea pigs against foot-and-mouth disease by three types of virus suspended in aluminum hydroxide. Z. Hyg. 88:91–103.

Schmidt, S., and Hansen, A. 1935. Immunisation contre la fièvre aphteuse au moyen de virus aphteux. Comp. Rend. Soc. Biol. (Paris) 121:1244–1246.

Schoening, H.W. 1927. Recent research on foot-and-mouth disease with special reference to the work of the American Commission. J. Bacteriol.13:21–23.

Scott, F.W., Cottral, G.E., and Gailiunas, P. 1966. Persistence of foot-and-mouth disease virus in external lesions and saliva of experimentally infected cattle. Am. J. Vet. Res. 27:1531–1536.

Seibold, H.R. 1963. A revised concept of the lingual lesions in cattle with foot-and-mouth disease. Am. J. Vet. Res. 24:1123–1130.

Sellers, R.F. 1955. Growth and titration of the viruses of foot-and-mouth disease and vesicular stomatitis in kidney monolayer tissue cultures. Nature 176:547–549.

Sellers, R.F., Donaldson, A.I., and Herniman, K.A.J. 1970. Inhalation, persistence and dispersal of foot-and-mouth disease by man. J. Hyg. 68:565–573.

Shahan, M.S. 1962. The virus of foot-and-mouth disease. N.Y. Acad. Sci. 101:444–454.

Skinner, H.H. 1951. Propagation of strains of foot-and-mouth disease virus in unweaned white mice. Proc. R. Soc. Med. 44:1041–1044.

Skinner, H.H. 1954. Infection of chickens and chick embryos with the viruses of foot-and-mouth disease and of vesicular stomatitis. (Correspondence.) Nature 174:1052–1053.

Stockman, S., Minett, F.C., Davies, G.O., and Watt, W. 1927. Favorable conditions for the survival of virus of foot-and-mouth disease. In Second Progress Report of the Foot-and-Mouth Disease Research Commission, H.M. Stationery Office, London. Pp. 39–40.

Sugimura, T., and Eissner, G. 1976. Typing foot-and-mouth disease virus by fluorescent antibody technique. Natl. Inst. Anim. Health Q. 16:152–159.

Sutmoller, P., McVicar, J.W., and Cottral, G.E. 1968. The epizootiological importance of foot-and-mouth disease carriers. I. Experimentally produced foot-and-mouth disease carriers in susceptible and immune cattle. Arch. Gesam. Virusforsch. 23:227–235.

Swaney, L.M. 1976. Susceptibility of a new fetal pig kidney cell line (MVPK–1) to foot-and-mouth disease virus. Am. J. Vet. Res. 37:1319–1322.

Tekerlekov, P., and Mitev, G. 1976. Izpolzvano na indirektnata reaktsiia za svurzvane na komplementa pri prouchvane na shapnite virusi. Vet. Med. Nauki 13:35–41.

Traub, E., and Schneider, B. 1948. Cultivation of the virus of foot-and-mouth disease in incubated hen eggs. Z. Naturforsch. 3B:178–187.

Traum, J. 1936. Vesicular exanthema of swine. J. Am. Vet. Med. Assoc. 88:316–334.

Trautwein, K. 1926. Versuche zur Tenazität des Maul- und Klauenseuche Virus in der Aussenwelt. Arch. Tierheilk. 54:273–279.

Ubertini, B., Nardelli, L., Prato, A., Panina, G., and Santero, G. 1963. Large scale cultivation of foot-and-mouth disease virus on calf kidney cell monolayers in rolling bottles. Zentralbl. Veterinärmed. [B] 10:93–101.

U.S. Department of Agriculture, Bureau of Animal Industry. 1943. Instruction for employees engaged in eradicating foot and mouth disease. Washington, D.C.

Vallee, H.P., and Carre, H. 1922. Sur la contagiosité de la fièvre aphteuse. Note de MM. H. Valle. Comp. Rend. Acad. Sci. 175:292–294.

Van Bekkum, J.G., Fish, R.C., and Dale, C.N. 1963. Immunogenic studies in Dutch cattle vaccinated with foot-and-mouth vaccines under field conditions. I. Neutralizing antibody responses to O and A types. Am. J. Vet. Res. 24:77–82.

Van Bekkum, J.G., Frenkel, H.S., Frederiks, H.H.J., and Frenkel, S. 1959. Observations on the carrier state of cattle exposed to foot-and-mouth disease virus. Tijdschr. Diergeneeskd. 84:1159–1164.

Waldmann, O., and Kobe, K. 1938. Die aktive Immunisierung des Rindes gegen Maul- und Klauenseuche. Berl. Tierärztl. Wochenschr. 22:317–320.

Waldmann, O., and Pape, J. 1921. Experimentelle Untersuchungen über Maul- und Klauenseuche. Berl. Tierärztl. Wochenschr. 37:349–354.

Waldmann, O., and Trautwein, K. 1926. Experimentelle Untersuchungen über die Pluralität des Maul- und Klauenseuchevirus. Berl. Tierärztl. Wochenschr. 42:569.

The Genus *Rhinovirus*

The type species for the genus *Rhinovirus* is *Rhinovirus* h-1A of humans. Other members in the genus are numerous human rhinoviruses (more than 100), equine rhinoviruses, and two bovine rhinoviruses. The particles contain 30 percent of single-stranded RNA with a molecular mass of 2.4 to 2.8 × 10^6 daltons. Isometric nonenveloped particles are 20 to 30 nm in diameter, probably with icosahedral symmetry. Thirty-two capsomeres seem to form a symmetrical capsid for the RNA core. Ether-resistant particles are labile at pH 3, and some viruses are stabilized by magnesium chloride. They have a sedimentation rate of 140 to 150S and a buoyant density in cesium chloride of 1.38 to 1.43 g/ml. The viruses multiply in the cytoplasm and normally reside in respiratory and ancillary structures.

Bovine Rhinovirus Infection

Bovine rhinovirus is one of a number of viruses isolated from the respiratory tract of cattle; it was first described by Bogel and Bohm (1962). Its significance as a pathogen of economic importance is still unclear, but fragmentary evidence suggests that it is a widespread infection in cattle (Bogel 1968). Limited serologic surveys have always found rather high percentages of antibodies to rhinovirus in test cattle populations (Bogel 1968, Mohanty 1968). The virus appears to be highly specific for cattle, with a strict affinity for mucous membranes of the respiratory tract, principally the nasal mucosa.

Character of the Disease. Field experience with respiratory disease caused by bovine rhinovirus is limited. It is rarely isolated from bovine respiratory outbreaks, but this failure may be due in part to the difficulties associated with isolating the virus.

In natural and experimental cases the disease is usually characterized by a serous nasal discharge that is seen 2 to 4 days after exposure (Bogel 1968). Other signs of illness may be a rise in temperature, depression, coughing, anorexia, hyperpnea, and dyspnea (Mohanty et al. 1969). A pneumonic condition may occur in some experimental calves without other signs of illness (Mohanty et al. 1969, Wizigmann and Schiefer 1966). In their experiments Mohanty et al. (1969) observed pneumonia in calves inoculated intratracheally but not in calves exposed to their isolate by the intranasal route. Mayr et al. (1965) failed to produce disease in calves with their isolate of bovine rhinovirus. Thus, virulence of a strain may play an important role in the production of disease, but a great deal more needs to be learned about host susceptibility and immunity. The principal pathological changes occur in the nasal passages.

Apparently morbidity in affected herds is high, but mortality is negligible. The infection has been reported in West Germany (Bogel 1968), Great Britain (Ide and Darbyshire 1969), the United States (Bogel 1968, Mohanty et al. 1969), and Africa (Eisa 1980).

Properties of the Virus. Bovine rhinovirus is an RNA virus less than 30 nm in diameter. It is resistant to lipid solvents such as chloroform, ether, and sodium dodecyl sulfate. It is inactivated at pH 4 to 5.

The original isolates of bovine rhinovirus were serologically related or identical (Bogel 1968, Ide and Darbyshire 1969). A second type is now known to exist. In comparative studies with 11 human rhinovirus serotypes, no serologic relationship was found. More than 100 rhinovirus serotypes have been described in humans, so it will not be surprising if additional serotypes are subsequently described in cattle.

Researchers' attempts to demonstrate a viral hemagglutinin utilizing red blood cells from various species failed (Ide and Darbyshire 1969).

Cultivation. Bovine rhinovirus replicates in primary cultures and low passaged Madin-Darby (MD) bovine kidney-cell cultures (Bogel 1968). Cytopathic effects are observed in monolayer cultures maintained at 33°C 1 to 3 days after inoculation. Rotation of MD cell cultures did not increase viral titers but enhanced cytopathogenicity (Lupton et al. 1980). At 33°C viral replication leads to more marked cytopathic changes and a higher infectivity yield than at 37°C. At 33°C viral titers usually are approximately 10^5 $TCID_{50}$, and disruption of cells produces higher virus yields. Viral plaques are visible in this cell-culture system 4 days after inoculation.

Bovine rhinovirus failed to produce a cytopathic effect in cell cultures of other bovine tissues and kidney cells from other species. Clinical signs were not observed when mice of varying ages were inoculated by various routes.

No alterations were observed in guinea pigs or in embryonated hens' eggs injected with bovine rhinovirus.

The virus is quite stable at −60°C for long periods. It is readily inactivated by heat.

Epizootiology. Virus can be isolated from the nasal exudate of cattle only for a few days after inoculation. It is obvious that our knowledge of the transmission and maintenance of this virus in cattle is extremely limited. Somehow the virus is maintained in nature and commonly transmitted to cattle, as the morbidity in this host is high.

Immunity. Cattle with low titers of serum-neutralizing antibodies can be infected with challenge virus of the same serotype, and maternal immunity in calves is never complete (Bogel 1968). These experimental observations suggest that cattle may be reinfected with the same serotype if the titer drops to a low level.

In cattle with no serum-neutralizing antibody, active immunity is accompanied by the production of serum-neutralizing titers that range from 1:2 to 1:100 against 100 $TCID_{50}$ of rhinovirus. The mean antibody titer seems to increase with age, possibly as a result of reinfection with some serotype (Bogel 1968).

Calves given a vaccine strain of infectious bovine rhinotracheitis virus intranasally had interferon levels in the nasal excretions within 1 day and these levels persisted for 5 to 10 days (MacLachlan and Rosenquist 1982). The interferon provided protection at day 2 and day 6, when the calves were given bovine rhinovirus. Although some rhinovirus shedding occurred (but less than in the controls), the antibody titers of nasal secretions more closely correlated with protective immunity to rhinovirus infection than with serum antibody titer.

There is no evidence that recovered cattle are carriers of the virus, although exhaustive studies have not been done. Virus carriers have been detected in other animal species recovered from Picornaviridae infections.

Diagnosis. Clinically, differentiating rhinovirus infection from other respiratory pathogens of cattle is difficult, if not impossible. A rising serum-neutralizing titer with paired serums is a sound basis for a positive diagnosis. Isolation of the virus in tissue culture is rather difficult but is the only method available at present. Characteristics of rhinovirus include resistance to chloroform, sensitivity to acid media (pH 4 to 5), optimum growth at 33°C, and a lack of demonstrable pathogenicity for embryonated hens' eggs or small laboratory animals.

Prevention and Control. Until we have further information regarding the economic importance of this disease there is no need for a vaccine.

The Disease in Humans. There is no evidence that bovine rhinovirus causes disease in humans.

REFERENCES

Bogel, K. 1968. Bovine rhinoviruses. J. Am. Vet. Med. Assoc. 152: 780–783.

Bogel, K., and Bohm, H. 1962. Ein Rhinovirus des Rindes. Zentralbl. Bakteriol. 187:2–14.

Esia, M., 1980. Isolation of a rhinovirus of bovine origin in Sudan. Vet. Rec. 106:225–227.

Ide, P.R., and Darbyshire, J.H., 1969. Rhinoviruses of bovine origin. Br. Vet. J. 125:7–8.

Lupton, H.W., Smith, M.H., and Frey, M.L., 1980. Identification and characterization of a bovine rhinovirus isolated from Iowa cattle with acute respiratory disease. Am. J. Vet. Res. 41:1029–1034.

MacLachlan, N.J., and Rosenquist, B.D., 1982. Duration of protection of calves after rhinovirus challenge exposure by infectious bovine rhinotracheitis virus-induced interferon in nasal secretions. Am. J. Vet. Res. 43:289–293.

Mayr, A., Wizigmann, G., Wizigmann, I., et al. 1965. Untersuchungen über infektiose Kalbererkrankungen während der Neugeborenenphase. Zentralbl. Veterinärmed. [B] 12:1–12.

Mohanty, S.B. 1968. Comments on bovine rhinoviruses. J. Am. Vet. Med. Assoc. 152:784–785.

Mohanty, S.B., Lillie, M.G., Albert, T.F., and Sass, B. 1969. Experimental exposure of calves to a bovine rhinovirus. Am. J. Vet. Res.30:1105–1111.

Wizigmann, G., and Schiefer, B. 1966. Isolierung von Rhinoviren bei Kalbern und Untersuchungen über die Bedeutung dieser Viren für die Entstehung von Kalbererkrankungen. Zentralbl. Veterinärmed. [B] 13:37–50.

Equine Rhinovirus Infection

Equine rhinovirus infection occurs in North America, South America, Europe, and Africa. Holmes et al. (1978) provided information about the incidence of the disease in selected United States horse populations. In most instances the infection is inapparent, but the virus may cause mild to severe upper respiratory disease. Plummer (1962, 1963) first characterized the virus and disease in horses. Until recently all subsequent isolates from horses were serologically related to Plummer's first isolate except one isolated and described in Canada (Ditchfield and MacPherson 1965) but no longer available for confirmation of a second type. Newman et al. (1977) isolated and described the properties of a second serotype recovered from sick horses in a Swiss army remount station (Hofer et al. 1972). Steck et al. (1978) reported a probable third serotype.

Character of the Disease. The incubation period is 3 to 7 days. The signs of illness in natural outbreaks include fever, anorexia, and a copious nasal discharge (Ditchfield and MacPherson 1965). The discharge is initially serous but later mucopurulent. There may be a mild cough and marked pharyngitis. Lymphadenitis and abscesses of the submaxillary lymph nodes sometimes result from secondary bacterial infection, usually with *Streptococcus equi* or *zooepidemicus*, and this prolongs the disease beyond a few days. Infected stables have a high morbidity but a negligible mortality. Virus is recovered from nasopharyngeal swabs taken from horses with high antibody levels (Burrows 1969, Plummer and Kerry 1962).

Plummer and Kerry (1962) described the clinical signs and virological findings of experimental infection in horses. The clinical signs were similar to those observed in natural disease. Most susceptible horses developed viremia that lasted 4 to 5 days and terminated with the appearance of serum-neutralizing antibodies. At necropsy virus was recovered from the pharyngeal tissues of horses but not from the intestinal tract. On the basis of virus recovery from the feces of live horses it was estimated that virus persisted for at least 1 month in the pharyngeal tissues.

Equine rhinovirus differs from human and bovine rhinoviruses in its pathogenicity for other animal species (Plummer 1963). Virus was isolated from blood of humans, monkeys, and rabbits for a few days after virus instillation and from the upper respiratory tract and associated lymph nodes of the laboratory animals for as long as 10 days after infection. Virus also was isolated from the urine and kidneys of some laboratory animals. Neutralizing antibody appeared in the serum of all species about 7 days after exposure.

Unsuccessful attempts to infect mice, hamsters, chickens, and embryonated hens' eggs have been reported (Burrows 1969). A Canadian strain also failed to produce infection in the guinea pig (Burrows 1969).

Properties of the Virus. The physicochemical properties are similar to those of bovine rhinovirus (Burrows 1969). Its particle diameter is 25 to 30 nm with an RNA genome. It is reasonably heat-stable, with little loss of infectivity over several days at 37°C, and with no appreciable loss of titer of two virus strains maintained at 50°C for 1 hour (Wilson et al. 1965). The virus is not stabilized against inactivation at 50°C with 1 M magnesium chloride.

There are two serologically distinct equine rhinoviruses—perhaps three (Hofer et al. 1972). Types 1 and 2 have slightly different sedimentation coefficients and buoyant densities (Hofer et al. 1972). A limited number of base composition analyses also showed differences between the two virus RNAs. The polypeptide profile of each serotype in polyacrylamide gels was similar to those of other picornaviruses, but the two serotypes could be readily differentiated from each other. No hemagglutinin has been demonstrated for these viruses.

Cultivation. The equine rhinovirus strains differ from human and bovine rhinoviruses since they will grow in cultures prepared from several animal species (Burrows 1969). A cytopathic effect is produced by equine rhinovirus in primary kidney cultures prepared from the horse, monkey, rabbit, dog, and hamster, in diploid cells of equine origin, and in stable cell lines such as HeLa and HEP 2 from humans, LLC-MK$_2$ from monkeys, and RK–13 from rabbit. Field isolations have been made in several of these cell culture types. The cytopathic changes in cell culture are typical of rhinoviruses, and plaques are present under suitable cultural conditions. A temperature of 33° C and the special requirement of low bicarbonate for human and bovine rhinoviruses are not essential for optimum growth with known strains of equine rhinovirus. Equine rhinovirus 1 replicates in organ cultures derived from nasal turbinate epithelium (O'Neill and Issel 1984)).

Epizootiology. Rhinovirus infections of horses are spread mainly by direct or indirect contact with nasal excretions from infected horses and by aerosol inhalation over limited distances (Burrows 1969). Horses can carry the virus for at least 1 month after infection, so carrier horses as well as those in the acute stage of infection with or without signs of illness are good sources of virus for perpetuating the disease on a premises. The virus is also quite stable and conceivably can survive on inanimate objects for a long time.

Immunity. Our knowledge of immunity to equine rhinovirus is rather limited, and some of our present ideas are based on our general knowledge of immunity to other rhinovirus infections in animals and humans.

The serologic test presently used is the serum-neutralization procedure (Ditchfield 1969). Neutralizing antibody to equine rhinovirus is detected 7 to 14 days after infection, and some horses develop maximum serum titers ($<$log 10^3) that presumably persist for long periods. The persisting titers are based on field observations, so reinfection cannot be excluded as the factor accounting for persisting antibody. The relationship of antibody level and protection against disease is not known for equine rhinovirus infection. There probably is an established relationship for rhinovirus infectons of other species since a low level of antibody ($>$log 10$^{0.5}$) does not protect against infection, whereas higher levels do. There is indirect evidence that maternal neutralizing antibody protects, as 22 foals less than 6 months old had no antibody (Ditchfield and MacPherson 1965). It is assumed these foals were protected against this common infection without the development of an active immunity and by 5 to 6 months of age lost their maternal antibody. This speculation was confirmed in a study of 5-month-old foals from immune mares that had no antibody (Burrows 1969). In contrast, a high percentage of Thoroughbreds in training had antibody (Plummer and Kerry 1962). Other small serologic surveys have demonstrated that the infection is highly contagious and common in horses.

Diagnosis. Isolation of the virus from the blood or the nasal excretions during the acute stage of disease can be readily made in a tissue-culture system. Virus can also be isolated from the pharynx of some horses for as long as 30 days after onset of infection. The virus has the characteristics of a typical rhinovirus: it is a small RNA virus with resistance to lipid solvents, susceptibility to pH 4 to 5, lack of demonstrable pathogenicity in embryonated hens' eggs, and typical Picornaviridae cytopathic effect in cell culture.

The demonstration of a rising serum titer with paired serums is another excellent means of diagnosis. Immune electron microscopy is another good, and more rapid means of diagnosis.

Prevention and Control. Present knowledge suggests that a suitable vaccine to protect horses against this disease could be developed (Burrows 1969). An inactivated equine vaccine produced primary immune responses in mice, rabbits, and probably in horses (Campbell et al. 1982). If a number of serotypes are subsequently found, vaccine production may not be feasible. This is the problem in humans, where numerous serotypes are known to exist. Because IgG is absorbed efficiently from both serum and colostrum, the use of reconstituted lyophilized serum as a prophylactic measure of conferring passive immunity to a newborn foal has been suggested (Burton et al. 1981).

The Disease in Humans. Plummer's studies (1962, 1963) suggest that humans can acquire infection without symptoms from contact with diseased horses, but he found no evidence of transmission from person to person or from laboratory animal to laboratory animal.

REFERENCES

Burrows, R. 1969. The general virology of the herpesvirus group. In J.T. Bryans and H. Gerber, eds., Equine Infectious Diseases , vol. 2. S. Karger, New York. Pp. 1–12.

Burton, S.C., Hintz, H.F., Kemen, M.J., and Holmes, R.F. 1981. Lyophilized hyperimmune equine serum as a source of antibodies for neonatal foals. Am. J. Vet. Res. 42:308–310.

Campbell, T.M., Studdert, M.J., and Blackney, M.H. 1982. Immunogenicity of equine herpesvirus type 1 (EHV$_1$) and equine rhinovirus type 1 (ERhV$_1$) following inactivation with betapropiolactone (BPL) and ultraviolet (UV) light. Vet. Microbiol. 7:535–544.

Ditchfield, W.J. 1969. Rhinoviruses and parainfluenza viruses of horses. J. Am. Vet. Med. Assoc. 155:384–387.

Ditchfield, W.J., and MacPherson, L.W. 1965. The properties and classification of two new rhinoviruses recovered from horses in Toronto, Canada. Cornell Vet. 55:181–189.

Hofer, B., Steck, F., Gerber, H., Lohrer, J., Nicolet, J., and Paccaud, M.F. 1972. An investigation of the etiology of viral respiratory disease in a remount depot. In J.T. Bryans and H. Gerber, eds., Equine Infectious Diseases, vol. 3. S. Karger, New York.

Holmes, D., Kemen, M., and Coggins, L. 1978. Equine rhinovirus infection—Serologic evidence of infection in selected United States horse populations. In J.T. Bryans and H. Gerber, eds., Equine Infectious Diseases, vol. 4. Veterinary Publications, Princeton, N.J. Pp. 315—319.

Newman, J.F., Rowlands, D.J., Brown, F., et al. 1977. Physicochemical characterization of two serologically unrelated equine rhinoviruses. Intervirology 8:145–154.

O'Neill, F.D., and Issel, C.J. 1984. Growth kinetics of equine respiratory tract viruses in cell and organ cultures. Am. J. Vet. Res. 45:1961–1966.

Plummer, G. 1962. An equine respiratory virus with enterovirus properties. Nature 195:519–520.

Plummer, G. 1963. An equine respiratory enterovirus. Some biological and physical properties. Arch. Gesam. Virusforsch. 12:694–700.

Plummer, G., and Kerry, J.B. 1962. Studies on an equine respiratory virus. Vet. Rec. 74:967–970.

Steck, F., Hofer, B., Schaeren, B., Nicolet, J., and Gerber, H. 1978. Equine Rhinoviruses: New serotypes. In J.T. Bryans and H. Gerber, eds., Equine Infectious Diseases, vol. 4. Veterinary Publications, Princeton, N.J. Pp. 321–328.

Wilson, J.C., Bryans, J.T., Doll, E.R., and Tudor, L. 1965. Isolation of a newly identified equine respiratory virus. Cornell Vet. 55:425–431.

The Genus *Enterovirus*

The type species of the genus *Enterovirus* is *Enterovirus* polio 1. Other members of the genus are at least 63 human enteroviruses including polioviruses, Coxsackie viruses, human hepatitis A virus, and echoviruses; seven bovine enteroviruses; 11 porcine enteroviruses including Teschen virus; one swine vesicular disease enterovirus; simian enteroviruses; Nodamura virus; murine encephalomyelitis virus; encephalomyocarditis virus, avian encephalomyelitis virus, and acute bee paralysis virus.

The particles contain 20 to 30 percent single-stranded RNA with an appropriate molecular mass of 2.5×10^6 daltons. Nonenveloped isometric particles with icosahedral symmetry are 20 to 30 nm in diameter. The particles have a sedimentation rate of 150 to 160S and a buoyant density in cesium chloride of 1.34–1.35 g/ml. Naturally occurring protein shells have a sedimentation rate of 80S. The particles are naked (no envelope) and inactivated at 50° to 60°C after 30 minutes. The virions are acid-stable at pH 3 and are resistant to ether and other lipid solvents. The virus is synthesized in the cytoplasm and resides principally in the intestinal tract. Replication involves functional protein formation by posttranslational cleavage or an unpunctuated precursor.

Porcine Enteroviruses

Porcine enteroviruses are cytopathogenic agents isolated in cell cultures from the feces, alimentary tract, and the nasopharynges of pigs. The prototype porcine enterovirus is the virus of Teschen disease, porcine enterovirus type 1.

The physicochemical characteristics of porcine enteroviruses are typical of the genus *Enterovirus*. The viruses replicate principally in the alimentary tract but can also be recovered from the brains of colostrum-deprived pigs that develop nervous manifestations as a result of experimental infection. All porcine enteroviruses grow well on primary porcine kidney cells. Most isolates replicate well on the PK 15 stable kidney cell line, but isolation is more difficult to achieve in this line than in primary cultures. The viruses produce two different types of cytopathic effect, and most strains cause plaque formation. The viruses are host-specific, as attempts to adapt them to other hosts have failed except for those of Moscovici et al. (1959), who reported pathogenicity for the hen's embryonated egg. Knowles and Buckley obtained similar findings with the virus of swine vesicular disease.

There are 11 porcine enterovirus serotypes, and some are pathogenic for the natural host. Most pathogenic strains produce polioencephalomyelitis, although others called SMEDI (stillbirth, mummification, embryonic death, infertility) viruses are principally implicated with reproductive disorders. One strain of porcine enterovirus reputedly causes severe pneumonia when instilled into the nostril (Meyer et al. 1966), and other strains produce mild pneumonitis by the same route (Betts 1970). Pericarditis and myocarditis have been observed in experimentally infected germ-free pigs that also developed encephalomyelitis (Long et al. 1966). Swine vesicular disease enterovirus causes vesicular disease, and, as previously stated, porcine enterovirus type 1 causes Teschen disease.

Serologic surveys have shown that porcine enteroviruses are distributed world wide and the infection rate among pig populations is high. It is extremely difficult to prevent the spread of these agents, and it is rare indeed to find a pig herd, even specific-pathogen–free herds, without antibodies to one or more of the porcine enteroviruses. The antibody response of the pig to enteroviruses varies, but in general, higher neutralizing-antibody titers are produced by the pathogens. In some inapparent cases of Teschen disease only low titers of neutralizing antibody are produced and precipitating antibodies are absent (Mayr and Wittmann 1959). Perhaps these infections were limited to the gastrointestinal tract, and high titers occurred in cases in which viremia was part of the infectious process.

Porcine embryo transfers were exposed to two different strains of pig enteroviruses. As observed by electron microscopy, virus particles entered the pores of the zona pellucida and were associated with sperm at or near the outer surface. There was no evidence of a productive viral infection of the blastomeres of the embryos (Bolin et al. 1983).

These viruses are not known to cause disease in humans or in animals other than the pig.

REFERENCES

Betts, A.L. 1970. Porcine enteroviruses. In H.W. Dunne, ed., Diseases of Swine, 2d ed. Iowa State University Press, Ames.

Bolin, S.R., Turek, J.J., Runnells, L.J., and Gustafson, D.P. 1983. Pseudo-rabies virus, porcine parvovirus, and porcine enterovirus interactions with the zona pellucida of the porcine embryo. Am. J. Vet. Res. 44:1036–1039.

Knowles, N.J., and Buckley, L.S. 1980. Differentiation of porcine enterovirus serotypes by complement fixation. Res. Vet. Sci. 29:113–115.

Long, J.F., Koestner, A., and Kasza, L. 1966. Pericarditis and myocarditis in germfree and pathogen-free pigs experimentally infected with a porcine polioencephalomyelitis virus. Lab. Invest. 15:1128.

Mayr, A., and Wittmann, G. 1959. Antikörperuntersuchungen bei Schweinen nach Flitterung mit dem Virus der ansteckenden Schweinelähmung. Z. Immunoforsch. 117:45–52.

Meyer, R.C., Woods, G.T., and Simon, J. 1966. Pneumonitis in an enterovirus infection in swine. J. Comp. Pathol. 76:397–405.

Moscovivi, C., Ginevri, A., and Mazzaracchio, V. 1959. Isolation of a cytopathogenic agent from swine with enteritis. Am. J. Vet. Res. 20:625–626.

Teschen Disease

SYNONYMS: Infectious porcine encephalomyelitis, porcine poliomyelitis, Talfan disease

Teschen disease, a virus-induced encephalomyelitis of swine, has caused serious losses in Czechoslovakia, southeastern Germany, Hungary, Yugoslavia, and Poland. It has also been reported in Switzerland, France, Sweden, Denmark, Great Britain, and Madagascar. In England it was known as Talfan disease before it was identified as a milder form of Teschen disease. This disease has not been recognized in Asia. Mild strains of the causative virus are present in Canada (Richards and Savan 1960), the United States (Koestner et al. 1962), and Australia. A condition described by Thordal-Christensen (1959) in Denmark as benign enzootic paresis of swine may be a mild form of Teschen disease.

The disease, named for a town in Czechoslovakia where it was first recognized, was first accurately described in 1929. So far as is known, natural infection with this virus occurs only in swine.

Character of the Disease. The incubation period averages about 14 days, though it may be considerably longer or shorter. Sometimes the disease is sporadic, affecting only a few individuals; at other times it may affect nearly the whole herd. The disease may be acute or chronic, and there is an inapparent form. The prodromal signs are fever, lassitude, and inappetence. These may be followed by a variety of nervous signs—irritability, convulsions, prostration, stiffness, and then paralysis of the legs, particularly of the hind legs. Opisthotonos is frequent. Often the animals lie on their sides and make running motions with their forelegs. Sometimes they squeal when dis-

turbed. Mortality averages about 70 percent, varying from 50 to 90. Animals that recover from the acute stages frequently have residual paralysis. If such animals are carefully nursed, they may live a long time, but affected muscles may atrophy. Animals that live more than 1 week often develop pneumonia and succumb.

There are no gross lesions, with the possible exception of myocardial lesions. The microscopic lesions are confined to the central nervous system and are typical of diffuse encephalomyelitis. Cytoplasmic masses occur in nerve cells. With minor exceptions the lesions are confined to the gray matter. Horstmann et al. (1951), although demonstrating that the cord lesions resemble those of human poliomyelitis, thought that the diffuseness of the lesions, and especially their great concentration in the cerebrum, made them very different from those of the human disease.

Properties of the Virus. The virus particles of Teschen virus strain are approximately 20 to 25 nm in diameter (Horstmann 1952). The viral antigen has been demonstrated in the cytoplasm and to a lesser degree at the periphery of the nucleus (Mussgay 1958). Cold phenol has been used to extract the infectious RNA, and its physicochemical properties were described by Tsybanov et al. (1982).

It has a wide range of pH stability, shows ether resistance, and survives well at 6°C or lower. A temperature of 60°C for 20 minutes or 0.15 percent formalin inactivates the virus. The International Committee on Taxonomy of Viruses has designated the Teschen virus strain as the prototype virus for porcine enterovirus type 1. The Talfan strain is a representative of type 2. The neutralization test in pig kidney cell cultures and the gel diffusion test demonstrate antibodies.

Cultivation. Fortner (1941) was able to grow the virus in chick embryos. Horstmann (1952) obtained survival in tissue cultures for 17 days but was unable to prove that replication had occurred. Mayr and Schwobel (1956) successfully cultivated the virus in swine kidney cell tissue cultures. After some passages the virus grew well, produced cytopathic effects, and retained its virulence for swine. It also produced plaques on monolayers.

Epizootiology. The disease apparently is transmitted by direct contact. Experimentally it can be transmitted by feeding and by intranasal instillation. Fortner (1941), however, was not able to demonstrate virus in the nasal secretions. The virus is usually a harmless inhabitant of the intestinal tract. Seldom does the disease spread rapidly in a herd. Fortner obtained infection by pen contact in only 3 out of 29 trials.

It was suggested that the disease might be due to the virus of hog cholera, but Diernhofer (1940) found that animals immune to hog cholera can be infected with the Teschen virus and that animals that have recovered from the latter can be infected with hog cholera. It seems clear that the Teschen virus is not related to any other disease-producing agent.

The virus has been inoculated by various workers into mice, rats, guinea pigs, sheep, cattle, and monkeys, generally intracerebrally, with negative results.

Immunity. Animals that have recovered from Teschen disease are solidly immune thereafter, at least for a few months.

Infected piglets immunosuppressed with cyclophosphamide to impair normal recovery mechanisms provided evidence that humoral immune response plays an important role in immunity to Talfan virus (Derbyshire 1983).

Prevention and Control. Several attempts have been made to make a brain-virus vaccine. Fortner (1941) had only indifferent success with a formalin-treated vaccine. Single injections failed completely. Better but still unsatisfactory results were obtained with two injections.

Rapid passage in pig kidney cultures attenuates the virulence of the virus for piglets. This attenuated virus vaccine or formalin-inactivated vaccine made from cultured virus gave 80 to 86 percent protection (Mayr and Correns 1959).

Trials with inactivated and attenuated virus vaccines have been reported to protect pigs against porcine enterovirus serotype 2 (T–80 strain) (Hazlett and Derbyshire 1977a, 1977b).

If virulent strains of Teschen disease virus are not known to exist in a country or territory, there is every justification to guard against introduction of vaccines.

Fortner (1941) found that the blood serum of recovered pigs had little effect in protecting against virus exposure.

The Disease in Humans. There is no evidence that Teschen or Talfan virus serotypes cause disease in humans.

REFERENCES

Derbyshire, J.B. 1983. The effect of immunosuppression with cyclophosphamide on an experimental porcine enterovirus infection in piglets. Can. J. Comp. Med. 47:235–237.

Diernhofer, K. 1940. Die ansteckende Schweinelähmung. Deut. Tierärztl. Wochenschr. 48:213–217.

Fortner, J. 1941. Experimentelle Untersuchungen über die ansteckende Schweinelähme. Deut. Tierärztl. Wochenschr. 49:43–44.

Hazlett, D.T., and Derbyshire, J.B. 1977a. The protective effect of two porcine enterovirus vaccines in swine. Can. J. Comp. Med. 41:264–273.

Hazlett, D.T. and Derbyshire, J.B. 1977b. Characterization of the local and systemic virus neutralizing activity in swine vaccinated with a porcine enterovirus. Can. J. Comp. Med. 41:257–263.

Horstmann, D.M. 1952. Experiments with Teschen disease (virus encephalomyelitis of swine). J. Immunol. 69:379–394.

Horstmann, D.M., Manuelidis, E., and Sprinz, H. 1951. Neuropathology of Teschen disease (virus encephalomyelitis of swine). Proc. Soc. Exp. Biol. Med. 77:8–13.

Koestner, A., Long, J.F., and Kasza, L. 1962. Occurrence of viral polio encephalomyelitis in suckling pigs in Ohio. J. Am. Vet. Med. Assoc. 140:811–814.

Mayr, A., and Correns, H. 1959. Experimentelle Untersuchungen über Lebend- und Totimpfstoffe aus einem modifizierten Gewebekulturstamm des Teschenvirus (Poliomyelitis suum). Zentralbl. Veterinärmed. 6:416–428.

Mayr, A., and Schwobel, W. 1956. Züchtung des Virus der ansteckenden Schweinelähmung (Teschener Krankheit) in der Gewebekultur. Monatsh. Tierheilk. 8:49–51.

Mussgay, M. 1958. Der Nachweis von Teschenvirus-Antigen in Gewebekulturzellen mit Hilfe von fluoreszierenden Antikörpern. Zentralbl. Bakt., I Abt. Orig. 171:231–247.

Richards, W.P.C., and Savan, M. 1960. Viral encephalomyelitis of pigs: A preliminary report on the transmissibility and pathology of a disease observed in Ontario. Cornell Vet. 50:132–155.

Thordal-Christensen, A. 1959. A study of benign enzootic paresis of pigs in Denmark. On Commission to Carl Fr. Mortensen, Ltd., Copenhagen. From the Medical Clinic and Department of Special Pathology and Therapeutics, Royal Veterinary and Agricultural College, Nordlundes Bogtrykkeri, Copenhagen, Denmark. Pp. 13–190.

Tsybanov, S.Zh., Sergeev, V.A., and Balysheva, 1982. Physicochemical properties of virion RNA of Teschen disease virus. Vofer Virusol. 80:3.

Porcine SMEDI Enterovirus Infection

Dunne et al. (1965) reported on two serologically distinct groups of swine enteroviruses that are associated with stillbirth, mummification, embryonic death, and infertility in swine. These groups were designated as SMEDI A and SMEDI B. Subsequently SMEDI group C was described, and these viruses fall into porcine enterovirus serotype 1 (Huang et al. 1980). During a 6-year period of porcine abortions viruses were shown to be involved in 22 percent of cases. Enteroviruses (10.9 percent) were most commonly isolated, followed by parvoviruses (4.9 percent), reoviruses (4.4 percent), pseudorabies virus (1 percent), and adenoviruses (0.8 percent) (Kirkbride and McAdaragh 1978).

Character of the Disease. The problem herds from which enteroviruses were isolated had similar disease syndromes and epizootiological pictures (Dunne et al. 1965). The most consistent observation was a decrease or absence of living pigs at birth and the passage of 1 to 12 mummified fetuses of varying sizes. Many pigs alive at birth died a few hours later. The number of live pigs farrowed by infected sows was less than half the average number of unaffected sows. Some infected sows that were bred returned to heat but never farrowed. Repeat breedings were more frequent. At no time during the course of infection did sows show signs of illness. No other diseases were observed in these herds, and certain ones such as brucellosis and leptospirosis were eliminated on the basis of serologic testing. Both Yorkshire and Berkshire breeds were involved. In one herd two serologic types of SMEDI viruses were isolated in kidney cells from fetal or newborn pigs.

At necropsy the gross lesions in experimental and field stillborn pigs were limited to mild edema, particularly of the spiral colon, hydrothorax, and hydropericardium. Preliminary histological findings in a few stillborn pigs included cellular infiltration, edema, and hemorrhage. The lesions were in most, but not all of the stillborn pigs examined. Encephalitic lesions were seen in a number of the animals.

In England, swine herds affected with similar reproductive disorders were studied by Cartwright and Huck (Cartwright and Huck 1967). Fifteen enteroviruses were isolated; and five were placed in the SMEDI A group, three in the SMEDI B group, two in the SMEDI C group, and one in the T80 group of porcine enteroviruses. A parvovirus also was isolated from many of their test materials. Steck and Addy in Switzerland isolated 30 enteroviruses from 47 aborted fetuses. Their isolates fell into two serologic groups with some cross-reaction with SMEDI B and SMEDI C groups.

Properties of the Virus. In the tissue culture neutralization test the SMEDI group A and B viruses were compared with many other viruses of swine. The SMEDI group A appeared somewhat related to a group of swine enteroviruses not yet fully classified but designated as group II. The SMEDI group B showed some relationship to edema disease virus and the virus of Ontario (Canada) polioencephalitis of swine. There was no relationship of either group with Ontario (Canada) hemagglutinating, Teschen (Talfan), hog cholera, or transmissible gastroenteritis viruses.

Hemagglutination and hemadsorption trials were negative.

Cultivation. The SMEDI viruses were isolated from infected fetuses, still alive or dead for only a short time, in kidney cell cultures from healthy fetuses or newborn pigs. Virus could not be isolated from a mummified fetus (Links et al. 1986). The viruses produced a cytopathic effect in these cultures.

Immunity. After infection, sows develop a significant neutralizing antibody titer. The importance of these antibodies in terms of protection or duration of immunity have not been ascertained.

Prevention and Control. No control measures can be suggested because the means of transmission of this disease are not definitely known.

The Disease in Humans. There is no evidence that porcine SMEDI enterovirus disease occurs in humans.

REFERENCES

Cartwright, S.F., and Huck, R.A. 1967. Viruses isolated in association with herd infertility, abortions and stillbirths in pigs. Vet. Rec. 81:196–197.
Dunne, H.W., Gobble, J.L., Hokanson, J.F., et al. 1965. Porcine reproductive failure associated with a newly identified "SMEDI" group of picorna viruses. Am. J. Vet. Res. 26:1284–1297.
Huang, J., Gentry, R.F., and Zarkower, A. 1980. Experimental infection of pregnant sows with porcine enteroviruses. Am. J. Vet. Res. 41:469–473.
Kirkbride, C.A., and McAdaragh, J.P. 1978. Infectious agents associated with fetal and early neonatal death and abortion in swine. J. Am. Vet. Med. Assoc. 172:480–483.
Links, I.J., Whittington, R.J., Kennedy, D.J., Grewal, A., and Sharrock, A.J. 1986. An association between encephalomyocarditis virus and reproductive failure in pigs. Aust. Vet. J. 63:150–152.
Steck, F., and Addy, P. 1968. Personal communication.

Swine Vesicular Disease

In 1966 swine vesicular disease (SVD) appeared on two farms in large numbers of pigs; the disease was indistinguishable from other porcine vesicular diseases including foot-and-mouth disease, vesicular stomatitis, and vesicular exanthema (Nardelli et al. 1968). The disease was disseminated rapidly to many countries in Europe, including Great Britain, as well as to Japan and Taiwan. At present there is no evidence of the disease in Great Britain (Hendrie et al. 1977). It has not been observed in pigs from the United States. This virus has been designated porcine enterovirus type 9, and it has a close serologic relationship to Coxsackie virus B5 of humans (Brown et al. 1973, Graves 1973).

Terpstra (1975) has written a comprehensive review of SVD.

Character of the Disease. The clinical signs include fever and vesicular lesions on the coronary band and bulbs of the heel and in the interdigital spaces. Vesicles are found also on the snout and on the skin overlying the metacarpals and metatarsals of some animals. Vesicles rupture after 2 to 3 days, and healing is rapid in most animals without secondary bacterial infection. The clinical disease is indistinguishable from other swine vesicular diseases. Pigs can be infected by a number of pathways, and the skin is probably the most frequent route of infection (Mann and Hutchings 1980).

Reports of natural and experimental infections with SVD indicate that some pigs show no clinical signs but develop significant levels of neutralizing antibody (Nardelli et al. 1968). Morbidity in natural outbreaks has ranged from 25 to 65 percent. In experimental pigs in contact with clinically affected donors morbidity usually has been 100 percent, with animals showing moderate to severe lesions. Under experimental conditions sows showed slight clinical signs, and lesions were not obvious on casual examination (Burrows et al. 1977).

In a pathogenetic study (Lai et al. 1979) contact pigs developed vesicular lesions by day 2. Lesions first appeared on the coronary band and then on the dewclaw, tongue, snout, lips, and bulbs of the heels. The onset of viremia coincided with the appearance of fever and the vesicles. Virus was isolated from the nasal discharge, esophageal-pharyngeal fluid, and feces as early as postinoculation day 1. Greater amounts of virus were isolated from samples collected during the first week of infection, and lesser amounts from samples collected during the second week. The appearance and the distribution of specific fluorescence in various tissues indicated that, during the development of swine vesicular disease virus (SVDV) infection, the epithelial tissues were initially involved, followed by generalized infection of lymph tissues, and, subsequently, primary viremia. Seroconversion was detectable as early as postinoculation day 4.

Mild, nonsuppurative meningoencephalomyelitis throughout the central nervous system was observed in both inoculated and contact-exposed pigs. The olfactory bulbs were most severely and most frequently affected, particularly in contact pigs. The most severe brain lesions were found in pigs 3 to 4 days after the onset of viremia; contact pigs showed more severe brain lesions than inoculated pigs. Microscopic changes were also found in the coronary band, snout, tongue, and heart.

The injection of the tongue dermis of a donkey, two cattle, rabbits, and chickens with infective vesicular epithelium failed to induce frank disease. Injection of the footpads of guinea pigs or of the abdominal skin of hamsters failed to elicit inflammation. Large doses of tissue-cultured virus given intracerebrally or intraperitoneally to day-old mice produced nervous signs 4 to 5 days after inoculation and death in 5 to 10 days. Virus was distributed in the brain, spinal cord, and muscular tissues. No signs of illness were produced in 7-day-old mice with the same inoculum by the same routes.

Properties of the Virus. This porcine virus has all the characteristics of an enterovirus. It is stable at pH 5, and it is stabilized by 1 M magnesium chloride at 50°C. Its buoyant density in cesium chloride is 1.34 g/ml. The virion is resistant to ether. The sedimentation rate is 150S in sucrose gradients. Viewed with the electron microscope it is roughly spherical, 30 to 32 nm in diameter.

SVDV and Coxsackie virus B5 were shown to be related but not identical by serologic and molecular analysis. Both viruses contain single-stranded RNA and four major polypeptides referred to as VP_1, VP_2, VP_3, and VP_4. Four M rads of gamma irradiation inactivates SVDV in liquid animal feces (Thomas et al. 1982).

The SVDV isolates from the Italian outbreak in 1966 and in Hong Kong in 1971 were different from those from England, Italy, and Austria in 1972–1973 as determined by polyacrylamide-gel electrophoresis. By comparison, there was less antigenic drift between SVDV isolates than in the 1952 and 1973 Coxsackie B5 isolates from humans, and the isolates were intermediate between the Coxsackie B5 isolates of 1952 and 1953 (Harris et al. 1977). Although Coxsackie virus B5 will not cause vesiculation in experimental pigs, it does produce micropathological lesions in the brain and spinal cord (Monlux et al. 1975).

Various serologic tests—complement-fixation, fluorescent antibody, immunodiffusion, and neutralizing-antibody procedures—are used to evaluate the properties of the virus and immunity.

Cultivation. The virus produces a cytopathic effect in primary and secondary pig kidney monolayer cultures and in cultures of pig kidney cell lines PR 15 and IBRS 2. No effect was observed in primary calf kidney or in thyroid monolayer cultures or in first-passage baby hamster kidney cell-line cultures. The sequential appearance of SVD viral antigens and virus (in pig kidney cell line MVPK) was studied by immunofluorescence and electron microscopy (Lai et al. 1979). The replication cycle was approximately 3 to 4 hours. Viral antigens were demonstrable in the cytoplasm 2 hours after inoculation. After 3 hours, a few virus particles were seen by electron microscopy in the cytoplasm. Morphological changes of cells, margination, and condensation of nuclear chromatin occurred at the same time. A compact mass of fluorescence was seen when cells showed cytopathic effect at 5.5 hours. Cytoplasmic crystalline arrays of virus were first detected at 7 hours.

Epizootiology. The disease appeared on two farms at the same time in the 1966 outbreak in Italy. Both farms had received pigs for fattening from the same source. All introduced pigs were afflicted, and approximately 25 percent of the resident pigs in the same pens showed signs of illness. No new cases were seen after 3 weeks. Subclinical infection undoubtedly occurs in the field. Virus was isolated from the feces of healthy pigs on several farms in Japan during a nonepizootic period (Kodama et al. 1980). Carrier pigs may also serve as a means for transmitting the virus, especially if they are stressed.

Immunity. The duration of immunity to SVDV is unknown. Neutralizing antibodies are formed in the pig after exposure. Their relationship to protection is not known, but it is reasonable to assume that there is a correlation.

Diagnosis. The appearance of vesicular disease in pigs

requires the immediate attention of a state or federal control official, especially in countries where other diseases such as foot-and-mouth disease, vesicular exanthema, or vesicular stomatitis do not occur. Differential diagnosis can be made only in a laboratory with competent personnel and appropriate reagents. These procedures were discussed in the section on diagnosis of foot-and-mouth disease.

Prevention and Control. There are no reports in the literature on the development and use of a vaccine against SVD. Great Britain and Ireland control disease by requiring that garbage be cooked and, when an outbreak occurs, by immediately imposing a strict quarantine and slaughter policy.

The Disease in Humans. The close relationship of Coxsackie virus B5 and SVDV suggests that these viruses could cause disease in both hosts, humans and pigs. Several individuals in a laboratory working with SVDV became ill with symptoms that occur in Coxsackie virus infections, and high levels of antibody to SVD were found in their serums (Brown et al. 1976). Coxsackie virus B5 produces an inapparent infection in pigs.

REFERENCES

Brown, F., Goodridge, D., and Burrows, R. 1976. Infection of man by swine vesicular disease virus. J. Comp. Pathol. 86:409–414.

Brown, F., Talbot, P., and Burrows, R. 1973. Antigenic differences between isolates of swine vesicular disease virus and their relationship to Coxsackie B5 virus. Nature 245:315–316.

Burrows, R., Mann, J.A., Goodridge, D., et al. 1977. Swine vesicular disease—Studies in pregnant sows. Zentralbl. Veterinärmed. [B] 24:177–182.

Graves, J.H. 1973. Serological relationship of swine vesicular disease virus and Coxsackie B5 virus. Nature 245:314–315.

Harris, T.J.R., Doel, T.R., and Brown, F. 1977. Molecular aspects of the antigenic variation of swine vesicular disease and Coxsackie B5 virus. J. Gen. Virol. 35:299–315.

Hendrie, E.W., Watson, J., Hedger, R.S., Rowe, L.W., and Garland, Y.J. 1977. Swine vesicular disease: Continuing serological surveys of pigs presented for slaughter in the United Kingdom. Vet. Rec. 100:363–365.

Kodama, M., Ogawa, T., Saito, T., Tokuda, G., and Sasahara, J. 1980. Swine vesicular disease viruses isolated from healthy pigs in nonepizootic period. I. Isolation and identification. Natl. Inst. Anim. Health Q. 20:1–10.

Lai, S.S., Breese, S.S., Moore, D.M., and Gillespie, J.H. 1981. Comparison of proliferation and cytopathogenicity of swine vesicular virus and coxsackievirus B5. Chung-Hua Min Kuo Wei Sheng Wu Chi Mien I Hsueh Tsa Chih 14:167–172.

Lai, S.S., McKercher, P.D., Moore, D.M., and Gillespie, J.H. 1979. Pathogenesis of swine vesicular disease in pigs. Am. J. Vet. Res. 40:463–468.

Mann, J.A., and Hutchings, G.H. 1980. Swine vesicular disease: Pathways of infection. J. Hyg. 84:355–365.

Monlux, V.S., McKercher, P.D., and Graves, J.H. 1975. Brain and spinal cord lesions in pigs inoculated with swine vesicular disease (UKG strain) virus and coxsackievirus B5. Am. J. Vet. Res. 36:1745–1749.

Nardelli, L., Lodetti, E., Gualandi, G.L., et al. 1968. A foot and mouth disease syndrome in pigs caused by an enterovirus. Nature 219:1275–1276.

Terpstra, C. 1975. Vesiculaire varkensziekte, een overzicht. Tijdschr. Diergeneeskd. 100:555–561.

Thomas, F.C., Ouwerkerk, T., and McKercher, P. 1982. Inactivation by gamma irradiation of animal viruses in simulated laboratory effluent. Appl. Environ. Microbiol. 43:1051–1056.

Bovine Enteroviruses

Bovine enteroviruses have been isolated from normal cattle and from cattle showing signs of illness. More than 60 isolates in various parts of the world have failed to produce disease in experimental cattle, although Van Der Matten and Packer (1967) claim that some of their strains caused diarrhea. Andersen and Scott (1976) did a serologic comparison of the French WE–42 enterovirus isolate with bovine winter dysentery and found that the WD–42 isolate failed to produce signs of illness. Serologic studies of paired acute and convalescent serum samples from 10 New York state herds naturally infected with winter dysentery essentially showed no relationship of winter dysentery occurring in New York state to WD–42 isolate.

At present, bovine enterovirus types 1 through 7 are recognized by the International Committee on Taxonomy of Viruses. La Placa has divided bovine enteroviruses into two major groups based on the hemagglutination of rhesus monkey red blood cells and sensitivity to hydroxybenzyl-benzimidole (HBB). Knowles and Barnett (1985), using criteria to differentiate other human and animal picornavirus serotypes, proposed that BEV types 1, 4, 5, and 6 be placed in a single serotype and that types 2, 3, and 7 be placed in a second serotype. There were some variants in both serotypes and these should be designated as subtypes.

The bovine enteroviruses have the same physicochemical properties as other members of the genus *Enterovirus*. One type was shown to have four major proteins termed VP_1, VP_2, VP_3, and VP_4 (Carthew 1976). Bovine enteroviruses are present in feces and produce a characteristic enterovirus cytopathic effect in cell cultures of embryonic bovine or lamb kidney, calf testicle, human kidney, rhesus monkey kidney and testes, rabbit kidney, established bovine kidney, and diploid embryonic bovine trachea (Moll and Davis 1959). Embryonic bovine kidney or calf testicle cell cultures are recommended for initial isolations.

Neutralizing antibody can be produced in various laboratory animals. The rooster and goat are preferred to produce hyperimmune antiserums. Rabbits should be avoided because their serums contain a naturally occurring inhibiting substance. Nonspecific inhibitors to bovine enteroviruses have been found in serum, allantoic, and amniotic fluids of bovine fetuses (Rossi et al. 1976). Cross-reactions to foot-and-mouth disease virus have been observed in normal swine serums in plaque-reduction neutralization and mouse protection tests (Andersen 1977).

Bovine enteroviruses can be inactivated in liquid cattle manure by anaerobic digestion heat treatment at 70°C for 30 minutes, by 1.0 M rads of gamma irradiation in ensilage, or by composting for 30 days (Monteith et al. 1986).

REFERENCES

Andersen, A.A. 1977. Occurrence of cross reactions to foot-and-mouth disease virus in normal swine sera. Am. J. Vet. Res. 38:1757–1759.
Andersen, A.A., and Scott, F.W. 1976. Serological comparison of French WD–42 enterovirus isolate with bovine winter dysentery in New York State. Cornell Vet. 66:232–239.
Carthew, P. 1976. The surface nature of proteins of a bovine enterovirus, before and after neutralization. J. Gen. Virol. 32:17–23.
Knowles, N.J., and Barnett, I.T. 1985. A serological classification of bovine enteroviruses. Arch. Virol. 83:141–155.
La Placa, M. 1964. The basis of a classification of bovine enteroviruses. Arch. Gesam. Virusforsch. 17:98.
Moll, T., and Davis, A.D. 1959. Isolation and characterization of cytopathogenic enteroviruses from cattle with respiratory disease. Am. J. Vet. Res. 20:27–32.
Monteith, H.D., Shannon, E.E., and Derbyshire, J.B. 1986. The inactivation of a bovine enterovirus and a bovine parvovirus in cattle manure by anaerobic digestion, heat treatment, gamma irradiation, ensilage, and composting. J. Hyg. 97:175–184.
Rossi, C.R., Kiesel, G.K., and Hubbert, W.T. 1976. Immunoglobulin concentrations and bovine enterovirus inhibitors in fetal bovine fluids. Cornell Vet. 66:381–386.
Van Der Matten, M.J. and Packer, R.A. 1967. Isolation and characterization of bovine enteric viruses. Am. J. Vet. Res. 28:677–684.

Avian Encephalomyelitis
SYNONYM: Epidemic tremor of chicks

Avian encephalomyelitis, an enterovirus disease, was first described by Jones (1932) in Massachusetts. In a more complete description of the disease and the virus that causes it, Jones (1934) called the disease *epidemic tremor* because of the peculiar vibration of the head and neck that characterizes many cases. Because this sign is not so frequently seen as others that indicate damage of the nervous system, Van Roekel et al. (1938) proposed that it be named *infectious avian encephalomyelitis*. The word *infectious* is now generally dropped from the name.

Character of the Disease. For some years avian encephalomyelitis was believed to be confined to the northeastern part of the United States. In later years, according to Feibel et al. (1952), it was also reported from other parts of the United States and from Canada, Great Britain, Sweden, South Africa, Korea, and Australia. The disease has a seasonal prevalence in the United States, where it is seen more frequently in winter and spring than in summer.

The disease has been recognized only in very young chickens and pheasants. It generally appears when the chicks are 2 to 3 weeks old, but it may appear earlier or later. Van Roekel and associates observed signs in chicks as they were removed from the incubator within 24 to 48 hours after they had been hatched. Other researchers have reported cases that appeared as late as 42 days after birds hatched.

Chicks infected by intracerebral inoculation rarely show signs in less than 9 or 10 days. There are no precise data on the incubation period in natural infections; however, it probably is 2 weeks or more.

The first sign noted is ataxia, or incoordination of the leg muscles. The signs become more obvious as the disease progresses, and finally the bird may lose all control of its legs and be unable to stand. Before this stage is reached, the bird is reluctant to move and may walk on its shanks. The characteristic vibration of the head and neck muscles usually appears well after the ataxic signs. This tremor is periodic, continuing for varying lengths of time. Finally the victim is unable to feed, becomes somnolent, and dies. In many cases the course of the disease is very rapid and somnolence appears within 24 hours after the first signs are noted.

The course of the disease varies greatly. Many birds become incapacitated so that they cannot reach food and hence die of starvation; others are killed by being trampled by other birds. If separated and given individual care, many severely affected birds live for a long time, and some even recover.

The losses may be very high, more than 50 percent in some cases. The average mortality is about 10 percent.

There are no gross lesions. Microscopically, the islands of lymphatic tissue, which, in birds, are scattered throughout the organs, show marked hyperplasia. The most characteristic lesions, however, are found in the central nervous system. Exceptionally large masses of lymphocytes and monocytes surround all the blood vessels. Extensive neuronal degeneration occurs, especially in the anterior horn of the cord, in the medulla, and in the pons. No specific inclusion bodies have been identified in this disease.

Avian encephalomyelitis is not known to occur naturally in species other than chickens and pheasants; however, ducklings, turkey poults, and young pigeons may be infected by inoculation. All mammals are refractory. Workers have found that the most certain way of reproducing the disease is by intracerebral injection. Miyamae (1983) used immunofluorescence to show the presence of the virus in the proventriculae, duodeneum, jejunum, and cecum of all infected chicks within 24 hours. After viremia occurred, infection spread rapidly to the pancreas, followed by the liver, kidney, and spleen. Subsequently, the virus spread to the central nervous system. Injection of virus peripherally—intravenously, intraperitoneally, or intramuscularly—induces signs in only a small proportion of those inoculated. Chicks from hatching time to 3 weeks of age are most susceptible to inoculation, but Van Roekel (1938) and others produced the disease in birds up to 3 months old and Feibel et al. (1952) has infected birds more than 6 months old by intraperitoneal injection.

Properties of the Virus. Virus is regularly present in the nervous system of infected birds. Virus suspensions regularly pass V and N Berkefeld filters and Seitz disks. Olitsky and Bauer (1939) showed by filtration through Gradocol membranes that the virus particle is about 20 to 30 nm in diameter. The virus is readily preserved for long periods by rapid freeze-drying, and it has retained viability for at least 80 days when suspended in 50 percent neutral glycerol. The use of polyethylene glycol and fluorocarbon can create a 50-fold increase of avian encephalomyelitis virus over the original homogenate (Matsumoto and Murphy 1977). Olitsky (1939) found no relationship between the virus of avian encephalomyelitis and that of equine encephalomyelitis. The chick virus proved innocuous for mice, guinea pigs, and monkeys, which are susceptible to the equine virus; furthermore, there were no cross-immunological reactions between the two viruses.

Cultivation. Jungherr et al. (1956) successfully propagated the virus in embryonated eggs by inoculation into the orb of the eye. Wills and Moulthrop (1956) succeeded by inoculating into the yolk sac and into the allantoic cavity. Kligler and Olitsky (1940) failed with chick embryos but succeeded in obtaining growth in a medium of minced chick embryos suspended in a mixture of rabbit serum and Tyrode's solution. Neutralizing antibodies are demonstrable by the use of the cytopathic effect produced in monolayers of chick fibroblast cultures (Hwang et al. 1959) and in monkey kidney cell cultures.

Monolayer cell cultures consisting of epithelioid cells from pancreatic tissue of 10- to 13-day-old chicks provided a substrate for the propagation of an embryo-adapted strain of the virus (Kodama et al. 1975).

Epizootiology. Convincing information exists which shows that horizontal and vertical transmission of the disease takes place. The disease is transmitted from infected chickens of various ages to susceptible birds or by placing susceptible birds in quarters that previously housed infected chickens (Calnek et al. 1960). Virus has been recovered from the feces of normal chicks. Vertical transmission, which occurs by means of infected eggs from carrier birds, produces clinical infection in the progeny (Calnek et al. 1960). Virus is transmitted when egg-infected chicks are placed with susceptible contact chicks following exposure within the incubator during hatching (Van Roekel et al. 1938) or in batteries following hatching with an incubation period of 11 to 16 days following contact (Calnek et al. 1960). Because the disease usually occurs during winter, it is unlikely that insect vectors play a role in its transmission.

Immunity. Schaaf and Lamoreux (1955) observed that, after a flock had suffered from an outbreak of this disease, generally there was very little further trouble from it; apparently the flock had been immunized. Following this observation they injected virus into the birds of the breeding flock when they were 16 to 20 weeks old. Birds at this age react very mildly to the virus, but they become solidly immune thereafter and apparently do not lay infected eggs when they come into production. Schaaf and Lamoreux claim to have eliminated the disease from a flock by following this procedure. Chicks that have recovered from this disease are resistant to reinoculation, and neutralizing antibodies can be demonstrated in them. Serum-antibody titers demonstrated by enzyme-linked immunosorbent assay have been correlated with protection of hens and their embryonated eggs. Embryos from hens with titers of 400 or greater were protected against virus challenge (Garrett et al. 1985).

Other procedures such as the fluorescent antibody (Miyamae 1977), immunodiffusion (Ikeda 1977), and neutralization tests are available for virus and antibody assay.

Diagnosis. Clinical diagnosis of avian encephalomyelitis in young chicks is not difficult. In doubtful cases other chicks can be inoculated intracerebrally with brain tissue. This procedure is not always successful because the virus content of brain tissue of diseased chicks sometimes is below the infectivity level. Blood vessel cuffing, gliosis, and neuronal degeneration point toward viral encephalitis but do not necessarily indicate the disease. Combining the infectivity of the virus in chicken embryo brain cell cultures with the sensitivity of the indirect fluorescent antibody test is a more sensitive method for virus detection than embryo inoculation assay (Berger 1982). The demonstration of rising antibody titer with paired serums is also useful.

Prevention and Control. A simple test based on the failure of embryos from immune hens to support the growth of virus can be used to select resistant-breeder flocks and to avoid disease in their progeny (Taylor and Schelling, 1960). It is possible to produce an immune breeder flock with live and inactivated vaccines used under the appropriate circumstances (Calnek et al. 1961).

In the United States birds approximately 2 to 4 months old are vaccinated with the embryo-propagated strain

1143 placed in the drinking water. The virus produces no clinical signs of illness in birds of this age and protects against infection with natural virus. Other vaccine strains available for use in some other countries include the NSW-1 (Westbury and Sinkovic 1976), Philips-Duphar (Folkers et al. 1976), and chicken pancreas cell culture (Miyamae 1978).

The Disease in Humans. Avian encephalomyelitis is not known to occur in humans.

REFERENCES

Berger, R.G. 1982. An in vitro assay for quantifying the virus of avian encephalomyelitis. Avian Dis. 26:534–541.

Calnek, B.W., Luginbuhl, R.E., McKercher, P.D., and Van Roekel, H. 1961. Committee report on a tentative program for the control of avian encephalomyelitis. Avian Dis. 5:456–460.

Calnek, B.W., Taylor, P.J., and Sevoian, M. 1960. Studies on avian encephalomyelitis. IV. Epizootiology. Avian Dis. 4:325–347.

Fiebel, F., Helmboldt, C.F., Jungherr, E.L., and Carson, J.R. 1952. Avian encephalomyelitis—Prevalence, pathogenicity of the virus, and breed susceptibility. Am. J. Vet. Res. 13:260–266.

Folkers, C., Jaspers, D., Stumpel, M.E., et al. 1976. Vaccination against avian encephalomyelitis with special reference to the spray method. Dev. Biol. Stand. 33:364–369.

Garrett, J.K., Davis, R.B., and Ragland, W.L. 1985. Correlation of serum antibody titer for avian encephalomyelitis virus (AEV) in hens with the resistance of progeny embryos to EAV. Avian Dis. 29:878–880.

Hwang, J., Luginbuhl, R.E., and Jungherr, E.L. 1959. Synthesis, cytopathogenicity, and modification of avian encephalomyelitis virus (AEV) in chick kidney cell culture. Proc. Soc. Exp. Biol. Med. 102:429–431.

Ikeda, S. 1977. Immunodiffusion test in avian encephalomyelitis. II. Detection of precipitating antibody in infected chickens in comparison with neutralizing antibody. Natl. Inst. Anim. Health Q. 17:88–94.

Jones, E.E. 1934. Epidemic tremor, an encephalomyelitis affecting young chickens. J. Exp. Med. 59:781–798.

Jones, S.S. 1932. An encephalomyelitis virus in the chicken. Science 76:331–332.

Jungherr, E., Sumner, F., and Luginbuhl, R.E. 1956. Pathology of egg-adapted avian encephalomyelitis. Science 124:80–81.

Kligler, I.J., and Olitsky, P.K. 1940. Experiments on cultivation of virus of infectious avian encephalomyelitis. Proc. Soc. Exp. Biol. Med. 43:680–683.

Kodama, H., Sato, G., and Miura, S. 1975. Avian encephalomyelitis virus in chicken pancreatic cell cultures. Avian Dis. 19:556–565.

Matsumoto, M., and Murphy, M.L. 1977. Use of polyethylene glycol and fluorocarbon for the purification of avian encephalomyelitis virus. Avian Dis. 21:300–309.

Miyamae, T. 1977. Immunofluorescent study on egg-adapted avian encephalomyelitis virus infection in chickens. Am. J. Vet. Res. 38:2009–2012.

Miyamae, T. 1978. Pancreas-passaged avian encephalomyelitis virus and its immunogenicity. Am. J. Vet. Res. 39:503–504.

Miyamae, T. 1983. Invasion of avian encephalomyelitis virus from the gastrointestinal tract to the central nervous system in young chickens. Am. J. Vet. Res. 44:508–510.

Olitsky, P.K. 1939. Experimental studies on the virus of infectious avian encephalomyelitis. J. Exp. Med. 70:565–582.

Olitsky, P.K., and Bauer, J.H. 1939. Ultrafiltration of the virus of infectious avian encephalomyelitis. Proc. Soc. Exp. Biol. Med. 42:634–636.

Schaaf, K., and Lamoreux, W.F. 1955. Control of avian encephalomyelitis by vaccination. Am. J. Vet. Res. 16:627–633.

Taylor, J.R.E., and Schelling, E.P. 1960. The distribution of avian encephalomyelitis in North America as indicated by an immunity test. Avian Dis. 4:122–133.

Van Roekel, H., Bullis, K.L., and Clarke, M.K. 1938. Preliminary report on infectious encephalomyelitis. J. Am. Vet. Med. Assoc. 93:372–375.

Westbury, H.A., and Sinkovic, B. 1976. The immunisation of chickens against infectious avian encephalomyelitis. Aust. Vet. J. 52:374–377.

Wills, F.K., and Moulthrop, I.M. 1956. Propagation of avian encephalomyelitis virus in the chick embryo. Southwest Vet. 10.39–42.

Viral Hepatitis of Ducklings

First recognized and described by Levine and Fabricant (1950), viral hepatitis of ducklings had not been seen previously by experienced observers on Long Island, where ducklings had been raised commercially for many years. Dougherty (1953) reported finding the disease in Massachusetts and in the western part of New York State. Hanson and Alberts (1956) reported an outbreak in Illinois. Asplin and McLauchlan (1954) reported the disease in England. Virus isolated from English birds was neutralized by antiserum obtained from New York. The disease was recognized in Canada in 1957 and the virus isolated (MacPherson and Avery 1957). It has since been recognized in Michigan and also in various other countries of the world.

This virus affects only young ducklings. There are no signs in adult birds, although they often harbor infection. Young chicks and turkey poults in close association with infected ducks have not developed the disease. The most recent review of viral hepatitis of ducklings was written by Fabricant and Levine (1984).

Until recently, there were three distinct serotypes that were considered to be enteroviruses. Serotype 2 is now known to be an astrovirus (Gough 1986) that causes the same type of disease as serotypes 1 and 3. A naturally occurring infection of ducklings caused by a hepatitis B virus also has been described (Robinson 1980).

Character of the Disease. In the earlier outbreaks of viral hepatitis of ducklings, losses occurred only among ducklings between 2 and 3 weeks old, but later losses were incurred on many farms in birds as young as 3 days. The disease is acute, with a short incubation period of about 2 to 3 days. In most instances signs were not observed longer than 1 hour before death. The affected birds lagged behind the remainder of the hatch; they quickly became somnolent, fell on their sides, and died after a brief struggle. Nearly all deaths in a particular hatch occurred within 4 days, the peak of the death rate usually occurring on the second day. Mortality varies from flock to flock, and from hatch to hatch in the same flock. Sometimes it is as high as 85 to 95 percent of large hatches. In other cases it may be as low as 35 percent.

The principal lesions of serotype 1 are found in the liver, which is usually enlarged and contains petechiae and ecchymotic hemorrhages. Mottling of the parenchyma is commonly seen, and focal necrosis of liver cells occurs, although not as often. The spleen and kidneys often are swollen. The microscopic changes (Fabricant et al. 1957) consist of necrosis of the parenchymal cells and proliferation of bile duct epithelium. These changes are accompanied by hemorrhages and varying degrees of inflammation. In ducklings that do not die, liver parenchyma regenerates.

Toth (1969) reported the isolation of an agent from liver suspensions from ducks under 2 weeks old that died of hepatitis despite parenteral immunity to duck hepatitis virus (DVH). This agent caused hepatic disease in susceptible and immune ducks. The clinical signs and lesions were similar. Toth's agent is an enterovirus that is serologically different from the classical duck hepatitis virus (Haider and Calnek 1979). These investigators recommended that Toth's virus be designated type 3 DHV, whereas the classic virus is called type 1 DHV. The duck hepatitis astrovirus produces hepatitis with features comparable to those of classic DHV. In contrast, duck hepatitis B virus usually produces an inapparent infection, but its real significance as a pathogen is still undetermined.

Properties of the Virus. The agent is classified as an enterovirus. Electron micrographs showed it to be spherical and quite small, 20 to 30 nm. It is an RNA virus and is ether-resistant. Its thermostability at various temperatures was reported by Hwang (1975). It resists 0.1 percent formalin held for 8 hours at 37°C.

Attempts to demonstrate hemagglutinins have failed. Two lines of precipitate have been demonstrated in the gel-diffusion test. Sueltenfuss and Pollard (1963) described a technique for the cytochemical assay of interferon produced by duck hepatitis virus.

Cultivation. The virus can be propagated in developing chick embryos and kills most of them in 4 days without observable lesions. Embryos that die after the fourth day show characteristic stunting of growth; severe edema; greenish discoloration of the embryo liver, egg fluids, and yolk sac; and necrotic foci of the liver (Levine and Fabricant 1950).

In cultures of chick embryo tissues the virus replicates without producing a cytopathic effect (Pollard and Starr 1959).

Epizootiology. The means of transmission is not entirely clear. The high incidence of the disease in infected flocks indicates a high rate of transmissibility; yet there have been many instances in which hatches with high

mortality have been kept in the same buildings, and sometimes in the same rooms, with other hatches in which the disease has failed to develop. Transmissibility through eggs has not been proved, and there is considerable evidence that this does not occur. Hatches, and parts of hatches, that have been removed to other premises directly from incubators have failed to develop the disease, whereas the remainder, kept on the premises, have exhibited high mortality. Present evidence indicates that the disease spreads during brooding by contacts other than through droppings.

Immunity. Ducks recovering from the natural disease or from inoculation with egg-propagated virus are resistant to reinoculation, and their serums contain neutralizing antibodies for the virus. Virus-neutralizing activity was revealed in both IgM and IgG classes of serums of actively immunized ducks (Toth and Norcross 1981).

Diagnosis. The diagnosis is based on clinical signs and is made by inoculation of chick embryos with organ suspensions, blood, or brain material.

Prevention and Control. Artificial immunization of ducklings has been attempted. Active immunization with vaccines made from allantoic fluid and embryo livers inactivated with formalin and from living virus of egg origin did not give satisfactory results. The failure apparently was due to the fact that the disease usually struck before the animals had had time to produce protective antibody levels. Much better results were obtained with antiserum from ducks that had recovered from the disease. This serum, secured at the slaughterhouse when the birds were dressed for market, was administered intramuscularly in 0.5-ml doses, protected most ducklings aged three to eleven days from the disease. In eight trials the treated ducklings showed mortality rates varying from 0 to 19 percent, whereas control ducklings, raised in the same pens, had mortality percentages varying from 26 to 80. This procedure has been used with success on many thousands of ducklings in the concentrated duck-raising area of eastern Long Island, New York.

Asplin (1956) reported success in actively immunizing breeder ducks with virulent virus. He also reported the success of a vaccine from an attenuated strain of virus that had been modified by growth in chick embryos. Ducklings were vaccinated with a needle dipped in virus and thrust through one of the foot webs (Asplin 1958).

Hanson and Tripathy (1976) have successfully immunized 350,000 ducklings from susceptible and immune breeders by placing an attenuated live duck hepatitis virus in the drinking water. This procedure, if successful, would be ideal, as it circumvents handling the birds.

The type 3 DHV (Toth 1969) is now included in the immunization program against viral hepatitis of ducks on

Long Island and has reduced the number of immunization problems there.

An attenuated virus vaccine produced with duck hepatitis astrovirus is safe and efficacious (Gough 1986). It should further reduce field problems with duck hepatitis.

The Disease in Humans. There is no evidence to connect duck hepatitis enteroviruses with illness in humans. Comparisons of enteroviruses of duck hepatitis with those of viral hepatitis of dogs and humans show no serologic relationships (Fabricant et al. 1957). There is no evidence that the duck hepatitis astrovirus or the duck hepatitis B virus causes disease in humans.

REFERENCES

Asplin, F.D. 1956. The production of ducklings resistant to virus hepatitis. Vet. Rec. 68:412–413.

Asplin, F.D. 1958. An attenuated strain of duck hepatitis virus. Vet. Rec. 70:1226–1230.

Asplin, F.D., and McLauchlan, J.D. 1954. Duck virus hepatitis. Vet. Rec. 66:456–458.

Dougherty, F. III. 1953. Ill. Proc. Am. Vet. Med. Assoc. P. 359.

Fabricant, J., and Levine, P.R. 1984. Duck hepatitis virus. In M.S. Hofstad, ed., Diseases of Poultry, 8th ed. Iowa State University Press, Ames. Pp. 535–542.

Fabricant, J., Rickard, C.G., and Levine, P.P. 1957. The pathology of duck virus hepatitis. Avian Dis. 1:256–275.

Gough, R.E. 1986. Duck hepatitis type 2 associated with an astrovirus. In J.B. McFerran and M.S. McNulty, eds., Acute Virus Diseases of Poultry. Martinus Nyhoff, Dordrecht, Netherlands. Pp. 321–328.

Haider, S.A., and Calnek, B.W. 1979. In vitro isolation, propagation, and characterization of duck hepatitis virus type III. Avian Dis. 23:715–729.

Hanson, L.E., and Alberts, J.O. 1956. Virus hepatitis in ducklings. J Am. Vet. Med. Assoc. 128:37–38.

Hanson, L.E., and Tripathy, D.N. 1976. Oral immunization of ducklings with attenuated duck hepatitis virus. Dev. Biol. Stand. 33:357–363.

Hwang, J. 1975. Thermostability of duck hepatitis virus. Am. J. Vet. Res. 36:1683–1684.

Levine, P.P., and Fabricant, J. 1950. A hitherto undescribed virus disease of ducks in North America. Cornell Vet. 40:71–86.

MacPherson, L.W., and Avery, R.J. 1957. Duck virus hepatitis in Canada. Can. J. Comp. Med. 21:26–31.

Pollard, M., and Starr, T.J. 1959. Propagation of duck hepatitis virus in tissue culture. Proc. Soc. Exp. Biol. Med. 101:521–524.

Robinson, W.S. 1980. Genetic variation among hepatitis B and related viruses. Ann. N.Y. Acad. Sci. 354:371–378.

Sueltenfuss, E.A., and Pollard, M. 1963. Cytochemical assay of interferon produced by duck hepatitis virus. Science 139:595–596.

Toth, T.E. 1969. Studies of an agent causing mortality among ducklings immune to duck virus hepatitis. Avian Dis. 13:834–846.

Toth, T.E., and Norcross, N.L. 1981. Humoral immune response of the duck to duck hepatitis virus: Neutralizing antibody vs. virus precipitating antibodies. Avian Dis. 25:17–28.

Viral Hepatitis of Turkeys

Two groups of workers in the eastern United States (Mongeau et al. 1959, Snoeyenbos et al. 1959) independently and almost simultaneously described a hitherto unknown viral hepatitis of turkey poults. Both successfully propagated the virus in the yolk sacs of embryonating eggs and produced disease in day-old poults by inoculation into the unabsorbed yolk sacs.

The virus is classified provisionally as an enterovirus. Baby chicks inoculated with the virus show little or no disease.

The disease is very contagious and produces high death rates in poults less than 2 weeks old. Investigations by Tzianabos and Snoeyenbos (1965) revealed that turkeys recovered from infection developed resistance to reinfection, although no serum-neutralizing antibodies were detected in the serums of these birds or in the serums of chickens, turkeys, or rabbits repeatedly inoculated with this virus. An antigen common to turkey and duck hepatitis viruses was demonstrated by agar-gel diffusion, but other characteristics of the two viruses were found to be dissimilar. Attempts to infect ducklings, quail, and pheasants proved unsuccessful.

REFERENCES

Mongeau, J.D., Truscott, R.B., Ferguson, A.E., and Connell, M.C. 1959. Virus hepatitis in turkeys. Avian Dis. 3:388–396.

Snoeyenbos, G.H., Basch, H.I., and Sevoian, M. 1959. An infectious agent producing hepatitis in turkeys. Avian Dis. 3:377–388.

Tzianabos, T. and Snoeyenbos, G.H. 1965. Clinical, immunological, and serological observations on turkey virus hepatitis. Avian Dis. 9:578–591.

Human Enteroviruses in Dogs

The human enteroviruses—ECHO virus type 6, Coxsackie viruses B1, B2, and B3—have been isolated from nasopharyngeal and rectal specimens of beagle dogs with no signs of illness (Lundgren et al. 1968, Pindak and Clapper 1964). Low neutralizing antibody titers against Coxsackie viruses B1 and B5 were present in some of the serums collected from these dogs. No titers were demonstrated for Coxsackie virus B1 or ECHO virus type 6. There was no correlation between virus isolation and serum titers.

Feeding ECHO virus 6 to dogs produced signs of enteric disease (Pindak and Clapper 1966). Although virus was recovered from fecal samples of five of the six dogs, antibody was not demonstrated.

Neutralizing antibody to poliovirus types 1 and 3, Coxsackie virus A9 and B2, and ECHO virus types 6, 7, 8, 9, and 12 has been found in dog serums. Replication of these viruses and production of canine disease have not been ascertained.

REFERENCES

Lundgren, D.L., Clapper, W.E., and Sanchez, A. 1968. Isolation of human enteroviruses from beagle dogs. Proc. Soc. Exp. Biol. Med. 128:463–466.

Pindak, F.F., and Clapper, W.E. 1964. Isolation of enteric cytopathogenic human orphan virus type 6 from dogs. Am. J. Vet. Res. 25:52–54.

Pindak, F.F., and Clapper, W.E. 1966. Experimental infection of beagles with echo virus type 6. Texas Rep. Biol. Med. 24:466–472.

Equine Enterovirus

An equine enterovirus was isolated from the liver and spleen of an aborted foal (Bohm 1964). An RNA virus, it measures less than 28 nm in diameter. It is resistant to ether, chloroform, and trypsin and is relatively stable to cations at normal temperatures and over a wide pH range. Its significance as a pathogen is yet to be ascertained.

REFERENCE

Bohm, H.O., 1964. Über die Isolierung und Charakterisierung eines Picornavirus vom Pferd. Zentralbl. Veterinärmed. [B] 11:240–250.

48   The Caliciviridae

The family Caliciviridae contains a single proposed genus, *Calicivirus*, which includes vesicular exanthema of swine virus, San Miguel sea lion virus and other marine or pinniped viruses, feline calicivirus, and several recently identified caliciviruses including canine, bovine, avian, nonhuman primate, and human caliciviruses (Barlough et al. 1986, Schaffer 1979, Schaffer et al. 1980, Studdert 1978)

Originally caliciviruses were classified as picornaviruses, then as a separate genus, *Calicivirus*, within the Picornaviridae family. The caliciviruses do resemble picornaviruses in many respects. Viruses in both families are small, nonenveloped agents that contain a positive single-strand of nonsegmented RNA. Yet there are some clear differences; the caliciviruses are larger, with a diameter of 35 to 40 nm compared with 24 to 30 nm for picornaviruses. Their capsid is composed of a single major polypeptide instead of four polypeptides for the picornaviruses, and their morphology is unique with 32 cup-shaped depressions arranged in icosahedral symmetry. The term *calicivirus* is derived from *calyx* ("chalice"), which describes the cup-shaped depressions on the capsid (Bachrach and Hess 1973, Burroughs and Brown 1974, Schaffer et al. 1980).

The type species for the family Caliciviridae is vesicular exanthema of swine virus serotype A. Its single-stranded RNA has a molecular mass of approximately 2×10^6 daltons, and its buoyant density in cesium chloride is 1.36–1.39 g/ml. The virus particles are unstable at pH 3 and have variable stability at pH 5. Excellent review articles on the caliciviruses have been written by Barlough et al. (1986), Schaffer (1979), Smith (1981), and Studdert (1978).

REFERENCES

Bachrach, H.L., and Hess, W.R. 1973. Animal picornaviruses with a single major species of capsid protein. Biochem. Biophys. Res. Commun. 55:141–149.

Barlough, J.E., Berry, E.S., Skilling, D.E., and Smith, A.W. 1986. The marine calicivirus story. Compend. Cont. Ed. Pract. Vet. 8:F5–F14, F75–F83.

Burroughs, J.N., and Brown, F. 1974. Physico-chemical evidence for reclassification of the caliciviruses. J. Gen. Microbiol. 22:281–286.

Schaffer, F.L. 1979. Caliciviruses. In H. Fraenkel-Conrat, and R.R. Wagner, eds., Comprehensive Virology, vol. 14. Plenum Press, New York. Pp. 249–283.

Schaffer, F.L., Bachrach, H.L., Brown, F., Gillespie, J.H., Burroughs, J.N., Madin, S.H., Madeley, C.R., Povey, R.C., Scott, F., Smith, A.W., and Studdert, M.J. 1980. Caliciviridae. Intervirology. 14:1–6.

Smith, A.W. 1981. Marine reservoirs for caliciviruses. In J.H. Steele, ed., CRC Handbook Series in Zoonoses, vol. 2, sect. B. CRC Press, Boca Raton, Fla, Pp. 182–190.

Studdert, M.J. 1978. Caliciviruses: Brief review. Arch. Virol. 58:157–191.

Vesicular Exanthema of Swine

Vesicular exanthema of swine (VES) is an acute viral disease caused by serotypes of VES virus and is characterized by the formation of vesicles in the mouth, on the lips, snout, and feet. It has been recognized only in the continental United States, Hawaii, and Iceland, where it undoubtedly was carried in American pork. The disease was officially "eradicated" in the United States in 1959.

In the spring of 1932 an outbreak of what was regarded as foot-and-mouth disease (FMD) appeared in a number of swine herds in southern California. Thirty-seven infected herds eventually were identified, and more than 18,000 hogs were slaughtered and buried in an effort to eradicate the disease. It reappeared the following year, but on a much smaller scale, and was again handled as if it were FMD. Investigations conducted during these outbreaks led to the conclusion that the disease was not FMD but a hitherto unknown virus-induced malady. The disease was first differentiated from FMD by Traum (1936), who proposed the name by which it is now known.

VES continued to appear in California year after year and less effort was made to control it once it was recognized not to be FMD. In 1952, 20 years after it had first been seen, the disease suddenly spread eastward across the United States. Within a few months outbreaks had been reported in 42 states and the District of Columbia. Vigorous control measures were then initiated, and the disease was "eradicated" by 1959.

In 1972 a calicivirus was isolated from California sea lions during an outbreak of premature parturition on San

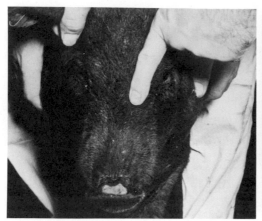 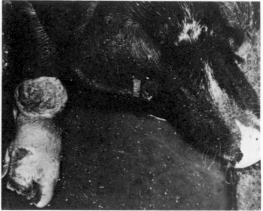

Figure 48.1. Vesicular exanthema, showing ruptured vesicles on the snout (*left*) and on the forelimb (*right*). These lesions cannot be distinguished from those of foot-and-mouth disease. (Courtesy L. M. Hurt.)

Miguel Island, California. This virus, called the San Miguel sea lion virus (SMSV), produced a disease clinically indistinguishable from VES (Smith and Akers 1976) when it was injected into swine. The close morphological and physicochemical resemblance between the two viruses reinforced the conclusion that for all practical purposes, SMSV and VESV were variants of a single calicivirus type. Madin (1973) and Smith and Akers (1976) postulated that VESV may have arisen from a marine source. A graphic description of the scenario of this isolation and the establishment of the similarity of SMSV and VESV has been presented by Smith (1981).

Antibodies to a number of VESV serotypes also have been demonstrated in marine and feral mammals (Smith and Latham 1978). Studies by Gelberg and co-workers (Gelberg and Lewis 1982; Gelberg, Dieterich, and Lewis 1982; Gelberg, Mebus, and Lewis 1982) demonstrated the similarity of disease in both swine and sea mammals inoculated with either VESV or SMSV.

Accumulating evidence suggests that caliciviruses are present in many ocean reservoirs in the Pacific and that these viruses occasionally infect terrestrial mammals. It also appears that this transmission from marine to domestic livestock is continuing today (Barlough et al. 1986). Current evidence suggests that SMSV infections occur in both terrestrial and marine mammals inhabiting the California coastal zones. Frozen meat from seal carcasses fed to minks on ranches in Utah has been shown to contain SMSV (Sawyer et al. 1978). Thus, domestic species in the United States occasionally may be exposed to SMSV.

Although marine mammals are a source of SMSV, the primary reservoir is thought to be one or more submammalian marine species common to the southern California coastline. SMSV has been isolated on several occasions

from the opaleye fish (*Girella nigricans*) (Barlough et al. 1986, Smith et al. 1980). Such a primary reservoir presumably is the source of new SMSV serotypes infecting marine mammals and may have been the original source of the VESV serotypes that infected swine through raw garbage containing fish scraps and/or marine mammal remains.

Neutralizing antibodies to some VESV types were found in California sea lions, in certain species of whales, in feral swine, and in one donkey along the coast of southern California (Smith and Latham 1978). These findings clearly show that certain marine and terrestrial mammals are susceptible to infection with either or both viruses.

Character of the Disease. Several reports describe the clinical disease produced by VESV (Crawford 1936; Madin 1981a, 1981b; Madin and Traum 1953; Mott et al. 1954; Smith and Akers 1976; Traum 1936; Watson 1981; White 1940). In VES, as in FMD, vesicles of varying size occur on the snout, lips, tongue, footpads, and skin between the claws, around the coronary bands and dew claws, and on the teats of nursing sows (Figure 48.1). As in FMD, these vesicles rupture easily leaving raw surfaces with ragged margins to which whitish flaps of partially detached epithelium often adhere. About 12 hours before the lesions appear a febrile period occurs in most animals. Failure of the animals to come for feed when called is frequently the first sign noted. It is then noticed that the animals are lame. Lameness is generally more severe in heavier animals than lighter ones. The foot soreness causes most animals to lie down, and they protest by squealing when they are forced to rise to their feet and walk. Sometimes animals will walk knuckled over on their fetlocks or knees to remove weight from their feet. During this time there is rapid weight loss, which has been estimated to be the equivalent of 1 month's feeding in growing pigs. All experienced observers agree that the lesions of VES cannot be distinguished from those of FMD by gross inspection.

The incubation period usually is about 48 hours, although sometimes it may be as short as 18 hours; in a few instances it has been very much longer. The course of the primary disease is relatively short. The mouth lesions heal quickly, but the foot lesions may cause lameness for several weeks because of secondary bacterial infections. The presence of the disease in an infected herd may last for several weeks to months, because the virus does not spread as rapidly as FMDV. Some animals may escape infection even though they are susceptible.

Mortality among adult animals is low, but heavy losses often occur among suckling pigs. The baby pigs are believed to die of suffocation from vesicles that form in their nostrils or from starvation because of lactation failure in the sows.

Properties of the Virus. Crawford (1936) was the first to demonstrate a plurality of VES viruses. He identified four serologic types, which he designated A, B, C, and D. Unfortunately the strains with which he worked have been lost, so they cannot be compared with present-day strains. Madin and Traum (1953) proposed that three types found in southern California be named A, B, and C, and to these Bankowski et al. (1954) added a fourth, D. At least 9 more types were identified in California, making a total of 13. As in FMD, all of these types are immunologically distinct from one another. Slight differences in pathogenicity for swine have been recognized among the several types. Multiple viral types have been found only in California.

Resistance is similar to that of FMDV. VESV is inactivated in 60 minutes at 62°C, or in 30 minutes at 64°C. The virus survives 6 weeks at room temperature and for 2 years in the refrigerator in 50 percent glycerol. It is susceptible to 2 percent sodium hydroxide, 0.1 percent sodium hypochlorite, and 2 percent citric acid (Madin 1981a). The virus is not disrupted by mild detergents. Thermal inactivation is accelerated by high concentrations of magnesium ions.

Precipitin reactions indicate antigenic relationships among caliciviruses, which are reflected in the similar base compositions of the RNAs. Homology studies show that VESV is closely related to SMSV but is not related to feline calicivirus (Burroughs et al. 1978). Tryptic peptide maps of the single major polypeptide composing the capsid of each virus also show that SMSV and VESV are more closely related to each other than either is to feline calicivirus.

Cultivation. The viruses grow with considerable ease in kidney, skin, or embryonic tissue cultures from swine, horses, dogs, and cats and produce a cytopathic effect (Madin 1981a, 1981b). On monolayers of pig kidney cultures plaques of two sizes occur; the larger ones are more virulent (McClain et al. 1958).

Epizootiology and Pathogenesis. The disease may be produced readily in swine by inoculation with virus-containing materials or by feeding organs or tissues containing virus. All attempts to infect cattle, calves, sheep, goats, rabbits, rats, mice, hedgehogs, and chick embryos have failed.

In horses intradermal lingual injection gives variable results. Certain strains produce vesiculation at the points of injection; others do not. Crawford (1936) found that two strains with which he worked regularly produced such lesions in horses and two others did not. Because those that succeeded were of a different serologic type than those that failed, he believed that the difference was a type characteristic, but this hypothesis has not been confirmed. It may be only a question of relative virulence without reference to serologic grouping.

Unlike the viruses of FMD and vesicular stomatitis, the virus of VES does not ordinarily infect guinea pigs.

Bankowski and Wood (1953) reported occasional successes in infecting dogs by intradermal lingual injection. The lesions produced at the inoculation site were mild and characterized by eroded epithelium and blanching. Often the animals showed some fever. Virus was recovered on one occasion from the spleen of a dog 16 hours after inoculation; it was not recovered from several others that did not become febrile. Dogs were successfully infected with strains belonging to the three types of virus then known.

Madin and Traum (1953) successfully infected hamsters with VESV. With one strain they succeeded in making six serial passages by intradermal inoculation of the skin of the abdomen. The strain then lost its ability to cause further infections. Another strain proved to be regularly pathogenic for hamsters. Secondary lesions were never found. The development of local lesions was definitely associated with a fever curve.

Nearly all of the past outbreaks of VES have occurred in herds of swine that were fed raw garbage. White (1940) reported that in the 1939–1940 outbreak in California, only 8 of the 123 herds involved had not been fed raw garbage, and four of these had some contact with herds that had been fed garbage. It has long been recognized that new herd infections are initiated in one of two ways: by the introduction of infected animals into the herd, or by the feeding of uncooked garbage that originated off the premises. Garbage-fed swine undoubtedly become infected from pork scraps and trimmings from carcasses that contained virus at the time of slaughter. Meat-inspection authorities try to prevent the use of such meat, but it often cannot be detected and the meat enters trade channels.

Because SMSV and VESV infections occur in marine and terrestrial mammals, it is clear that hosts other than domestic swine and their by-products are involved in the ecology of these viruses.

Mott et al. (1953) found it difficult to infect susceptible pigs placed in uncleaned pens that had previously contained infected animals. These findings agree with field experience that the disease is not so easily transmitted as FMD.

Immunity. Swine inoculated with any of the types of VESV develop, within 3 weeks, a solid immunity to that viral type which lasts for at least 6 months and perhaps much longer. Animals recovering from infection with one type may, however, almost immediately develop the disease again as a result of infection with one of the other types of virus. Madin and Traum (1953) made a formalin-killed vaccine adsorbed to an aluminum gel, by essentially the same technique as that used for the Schmidt-Waldmann vaccine for FMD, and found that it created solid immunity. No attempt has been made to make such a vaccine for field use.

Diagnosis. With VES, the diagnostic matter of greatest importance is the determination that the disease outbreak is not FMD. In California, during the many years when little was done to control VESV, those feeding garbage to swine were required to keep a few young calves in the same pens with the swine as a precaution. When a vesicular disease struck a herd, authorities felt safe in assuming the disease to be VES rather than FMD if the calves remained free of infection. It is still important to establish the range of species susceptibility to a new vesicular viral disease outbreak.

Laboratory diagnosis must be obtained as soon as possible when an outbreak of vesicular disease occurs in a herd of domestic animals. This is easy to do with today's rapid diagnostic procedures utilizing isolation of virus in cell culture and serologic procedures. Wilder (1980) discussed the diagnosis of swine caliciviruses with indirect immunofluorescence. Plaque-reduction neutralization tests (or other reliable serologic tests) with known antiserums are important to establish the identity of the viral isolate (Madin 1981a).

The differentiation of FMD, VES, and vesicular stomatitis is discussed in the section on FMD in Chapter 47.

Prevention and Control. Because this disease does not have the high infectivity level of FMD, it is not as difficult to control. For 20 years the disease was confined to a single state, and little effort was made to control it once it was determined not to be FMD. When it was thought to be FMD, two attempts were made to eradicate it by the drastic methods employed for FMD. On both occasions all herds in which the disease was recognized were slaughtered and buried, and yet the disease reappeared in other herds the following year. At that time investigators assumed that refrigerated pork was responsible for reinfection in the area. Now we recognize that another source may have been virus in meat from infected marine or feral animals.

Experience has shown that VES is more readily controlled than FMD. The methods used since 1952 in the United States are described below.

Quarantine of infected herds. Animals from infected herds should not be slaughtered until at least 2 weeks after all evidence of active disease in the herd has disappeared. Even this time period may not always be sufficient. A better procedure is to allow animals from recently infected swine herds or meat from marine and feral mammals to go to only those processing plants where all meat is cooked or otherwise processed by methods that destroy the virus.

Enactment and enforcement of garbage-cooking laws. Legislation is undoubtedly the most effective and practical single procedure. If such laws were universally enforced, they would quickly eliminate VES from domestic swine. They would also remove part of the danger of infection with FMDV and would greatly reduce the trichinosis hazard to humans. The U.S. government has assisted by banning the interstate shipment of pork from pigs fed uncooked garbage at any time in their lives unless it has been processed in such a way as to destroy any virus it might contain.

The Disease in Humans. There is no evidence that VESV infects humans. However, the recent infection of a research worker with one of the serotypes of SMSV indicates that the potential may exist.

REFERENCES

Bachrach, H.L., and Hess, W.R. 1973. Animal picornaviruses with a single major species of capsid protein. Biochem. Biophys. Res. Commun. 55:141–149.

Bankowski, R.A., and Wood, M. 1953. Experimental vesicular exanthema in the dog. J. Am. Vet. Med. Assoc. 123:115–118.

Bankowski, R.A., Keith, H.B., Stuart, E.E., and Kummer, B.A. 1954. Recovery of the fourth immunological type of vesicular exanthema virus in California. J. Am. Vet. Med. Assoc. 125:383–384.

Barlough, J.E., Berry, E.S., Skilling, D.E., and Smith, A.W. 1986. The marine calicivirus story. Compend. Cont. Ed. Pract. Vet. 8:F5–F14, F75–F83.

Burroughs, N., Doel, T., and Brown, F. 1978. Relationship of San Miguel sea lion virus to other members of the calicivirus group. Intervirology 10:51–59.

Crawford, A.B. 1936. Experimental vesicular exanthema of swine. In Proceedings of the 40th Annual Meeting of the U.S. Livestock Sanitary Association. Pp. 380–395.

Gelberg, H.B., and Lewis, R.M. 1982. The pathogenesis of vesicular exanthema of swine virus and San Miguel sea lion virus in swine. Vet. Pathol. 19:424–443.

Gelberg, H.B., Dieterich, R.A., and Lewis, R.M. 1982. Vesicular exanthema of swine and San Miguel sea lion virus: Experimental and field studies in otarid seals, feeding trials in swine. Vet. Pathol. 19:413–23.

Gelberg, H.B., Mebus, C.A., and Lewis, R.M. 1982. Experimental vesicular exanthema of swine virus and San Miguel sea lion virus infection in phocid seals. Vet. Pathol. 19:406–412.

McClain, M.E., Hackett, A.J., and Madin, S.H. 1958. Plaque morphology and pathogenicity of vesicular exanthema virus. Science 127:1391–1392.

Madin, S.H. 1973. Pigs, sea lions and vesicular exanthema. In M. Pollard, ed., Second International Conference on Foot and Mouth Disease. Academic Press, New York. Pp. 78.

Madin, S.H. 1981a. Vesicular exanthema. In A.D. Leman, R.D. Glock, W.L. Mengeling, R.H.C. Penny, E. Scholl, and B. Straw, eds., Diseases of Swine, 5th ed. Iowa State University Press, Ames. Pp. 302–309.

Madin, S.H., 1981b. Vesicular exanthema of swine. In E.P.J. Gibbs, ed., Virus Diseases of Food Animals, vol. 2. Academic Press, New York. Pp. 383–397.

Madin, S.H., and Traum, J. 1953. Experimental studies with vesicular exanthema of swine. Vet. Med. 48:395–400.

Mott, L.O., Patterson, W.C., Songer, J.R., and Hopkins, S.R. 1954. Experimental infections with vesicular exanthema. In Proceedings of the 57th Annual Meeting of the U.S. Livestock Sanitary Association. Pp. 334–363.

Sawyer, J.C., Madin, S.H., and Skilling, D.E. 1978. Isolation of San Miguel sea lion virus from samples of an animal food product produced from northern fur seal (Callorhinus ursinus) carcasses. Am. J. Vet. Res. 39:137–139.

Schaffer, F.L. 1979. Caliciviruses. In H. Fraenkel-Conrat and R.R. Wagner, eds., Comprehensive Virology, vol 14. Plenum Press, New York. Pp. 249–283.

Schaffer, F.L., Bachrach, H.L., Brown, F., Burroughs, J.N., Gillespie, J.H., Madin, S.H., Madeley, C.R., Povey, R.C., Scott, F., Smith, A.W., and Studdert, M.J. 1980. Caliciviridae. Intervirology 14:1–6

Smith, A.W. 1981. Marine reservoirs for caliciviruses. In J.H. Steele, ed., CRC Handbook Series in Zoonoses. vol. 2, Sect. B. CRC Press, Boca Raton, Fla. Pp. 182–190.

Smith, A.W., and Akers, T.G. 1976. Vesicular exanthema of swine. J. Am. Vet. Med. Assoc. 169:700–703.

Smith, A.W., and Latham, A.B. 1978. Prevalence of vesicular exanthema of swine antibodies among feral mammals associated with the southern California coastal zones. Am. J. Vet. Res. 39:291–296.

Smith, A.W., Skilling, D.E., Dardiri, A.H., and Latham, A.B. 1980. Calicivirus pathogenic for swine: A new serotype isolated from opaleye Girella nigricans, an ocean fish. Science 209:940–941.

Studdert, M.J. 1978. Caliciviruses. Brief review. Arch. Virol. 58:157–191.

Traum, J. 1936. Vesicular exanthema of swine. J. Am. Vet. Med. Assoc. 88:316–334.

Watson, W.A. 1981. Vesicular diseases: Recent advances and concepts of control. Can. Vet. J. 22:311–320.

White, B.B. 1940. Vesicular exanthema of swine. J. Am. Vet. Med. Assoc. 97:230–232.

Wilder, F.W. 1980. Detection of swine caliciviruses by indirect immunofluorescence. Can. J. Comp. Med. 44:87–92.

San Miguel Sea Lion Virus Infection

SYNONYM: Marine calicivirus infection; abbreviation, SMSV infection

Marine caliciviruses, including the San Miguel sea lion viruses (SMSVs), are a group of at least 16 virus serotypes that infect a variety of pinnipeds and other marine life as well as terrestrial mammals. This group of caliciviruses perhaps will be best remembered as the first viruses from marine animals shown to be infectious for terrestrial animals (Smith et al. 1973). The SMSVs are closely related to VESV in every respect—biochemically, biophysically, and biologically.

The 14 known serotypes of SMSV (Smith 1981) can produce disease similar to VES in domestic pigs (Barlough et al. 1986, Breese and Dardiri 1977; Gelberg and Lewis 1982; Gelberg, Dieterich, and Lewis 1982; Gelberg, Mebus, and Lewis 1982). They have been associated with vesicular lesions on the flippers of pinnipeds and with abortions and neonatal deaths in pinniped pups.

SMSV has been isolated from California sea lions, northern fur seals, elephant seals, walrus, opaleye fish, and a liver fluke of sea lions (Barlough et al. 1986, Schaffer 1979, Sawyer et al. 1978; Smith 1981, Smith et al. 1981, Smith, Ritter, et al. 1983; Smith, Skilling, and Ridgway 1983). Neutralizing antibody to the virus has been found in Steller sea lions, northern elephant seals, and California gray whales. SMSV serum-neutralizing antibodies have also been in feral swine, sheep, and foxes inhabiting the Channel Islands of California. SMSV–4 has been isolated from swine in California (Smith 1981).

The host range for the marine caliciviruses, once thought to be narrow, is now known to be quite extensive. For example, SMSV-5, isolated from a northern fur seal, will infect several species including fish, mink, nonhuman primates, cattle, pigs, and humans (Barlough et al. 1986, Smith et al. 1977).

A research scientist at Oregon State University working with an SMSV isolated from a northern fur seal became infected and developed temporary deep vesicles on the hands and feet. The lesions lasted for a little more than a week and regressed without complications. This appears to be the first documented case of human infection caused by one of the animal caliciviruses. Other strains could potentially infect humans, and cause serious disease.

REFERENCES

Barlough, J.E., Berry, E.S., Skilling, D.E., and Smith, A.W. 1986. The marine calicivirus story. Compend. Cont. Ed. Pract. Vet. 8:F5–F14, F75–F83.

Breese, S.S., and Dardiri, A.H. 1977. Electron microscope observations on a virus transmissible from pinnipeds to swine. J. Gen. Virol. 36:221–225.

Gelberg, H.B., and Lewis, R.M. 1982. The pathogenesis of vesicular exanthema of swine virus and San Miguel sea lion virus in swine. Vet. Pathol. 19:424–443.

Gelberg, H.B., Dieterich, R.A., and Lewis, R.M. 1982. Vesicular exanthema of swine and San Miguel sea lion virus: Experimental and field studies in otarid seals, feeding trials in swine. Vet. Pathol. 19:413–23.

Gelberg, H.B., Mebus, C.A., and Lewis, R.M. 1982. Experimental vesicular exanthema of swine virus and San Miguel sea lion virus infection in phocid seals. Vet. Pathol. 19:406–412.

Sawyer, J.C., Madin, S.H., and Skilling, D.E. 1978. Isolation of San Miguel sea lion virus from samples of an animal food product produced from northern fur seal (*Callorhinus ursinus*) carcasses. Am. J. Vet. Res. 39:137–139.

Schaffer, F.L. 1979. Caliciviruses. In H. Fraenkel-Conrat and R.R. Wagner, eds., Comprehensive Virology, vol. 14. Plenum Press, New York. Pp. 249–283.

Smith, A.W. 1981. Marine reservoirs for caliciviruses. In J.H. Steele, ed., CRC Handbook Series in Zoonoses, vol. 2, Sect. B. CRC Press, Boca Raton, Fla. Pp. 182–190.

Smith, A.W., Akers, T.G., Madin, S.H., and Vedros, N.A. 1973. San Miguel sea lion virus isolation, preliminary characterization and relationship to vesicular exanthema of swine virus. Nature 244:108–110.

Smith, A.W., Prato, C.M., and Skilling, D.E. 1977. Characterization of two new serotypes of San Miguel sea lion virus. Intervirology 8:30–36.

Smith, A.W., Ritter, D.G., Ray, G.C., Skilling, D.E., and Wartzok, D. 1983. New calicivirus isolates from feces of walrus (*Odobenus rosmarus*). J. Wild. Dis. 19:86–89.

Smith, A.W., Skilling, D.E., and Latham, A.B. 1981. Isolation and identification of five new serotypes of calicivirus from marine mammals. Am. J. Vet. Res. 42:693–694.

Smith, A.W., Skilling, D.E., and Ridgway, S. 1983. Calicivirus-induced vesicular disease in cetaceans and probable interspecies transmission. J. Am. Vet. Med. Assoc. 183:1223–1225.

Feline Calicivirus Infection

SYNONYM: Feline picornavirus infection; abbreviation, FCV infection

An acute, highly contagious viral disease of cats, feline calicivirus infection is characterized by upper respiratory disease, pneumonia, ulcerative stomatitis, and, occasionally, enteritis or arthritis. The causative agent, feline calicivirus (FCV), was originally called "feline picornavirus." The first isolation of the virus was reported by Fastier (1957). Reviews have been written by Gaskell and Wardley (1978), Gillespie and Scott (1973), Kahn and Hoover (1976b), Ott (1983), Povey (1976, 1985), Schaffer (1979), Scott (1986), and Studdert (1978).

Character of the Disease. Several different types of disease, including: upper respiratory infection, pneumonia, ulceration, enteritis, acute arthritis, and plasmacytic-lymphocytic stomatitis, are produced by the FCVs.

The clinical signs vary greatly depending on the strain of virus, the age of the cat, and any coexisting infections. Severity may vary from subclinical or mild disease of one to a few days' duration to severe, fatal pneumonia. Fever is a consistent finding in all FCV infections. It is usually diphasic with the initial asymptomatic spike occurring 1 or 2 days after exposure, followed by a period of normal temperature for a day or two; the main febrile response occurs simultaneously with the clinical signs. Sick cats exhibit varying degrees of general signs of illness, including anorexia, depression, and rough coat. In the upper respiratory form of FCV infection, there is mild ocular and nasal discharge for one to a few days (Figure 48.2). The discharge usually remains serous, or it may become mucoid or mucopurulent, but it rarely progresses to the severe, purulent discharge with crust formation that is so common with feline viral rhinotracheitis (FVR). The mild nasal involvement does not result in the paroxysmal sneezing associated with FVR-1. The conjunctiva may be

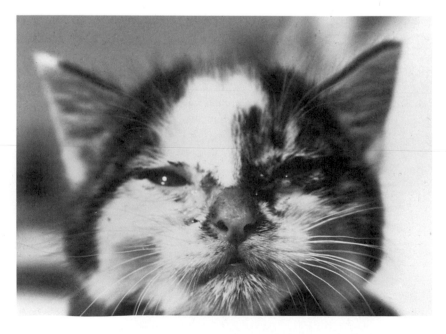

Figure 48.2. Upper respiratory infection caused by feline calicivirus strain 255. Note the serous ocular discharge with wetting and staining of the hair. (Courtesy D. E. Kahn.)

mildly hyperemic, with some swelling. Ulcerative keratitis has not been observed.

Many, if not all, strains of FCV will produce some degree of pneumonia. In most cases this is transient and does not result in any outward signs of illness attributable to the lung involvement. Other strains, however, may consistently produce extensive interstitial pneumonia and up to 30 mortality. FCV is the most common cause of interstitial pneumonia in young cats. In the initial stages of pneumonia outward clinical signs are usually difficult to detect. There is little inflammation in the trachea, bronchi, or bronchioli, and therefore rales are not prominent. Cats may mask the lung involvement for the first 1 or 2 days of illness, then suddenly exhibit severe respiratory distress. The deep, forced respirations enable the clinician to diagnose pneumonia in a febrile cat. Radiographs of the thorax in a suspect case will reveal a generalized increased interstitial pattern in the lungs.

The ulcerative form of FCV infection is common and may occur alone or in combination with one or more of the other forms of the disease. Excessive salivation may be seen. Ulcers may occur on the tongue, the hard palate, at the angle of the jaws, on the tip of the nose, and, rarely, on the skin or around the claws. The most characteristic lesions occur on the dorsum of the tongue either as discrete, circular, shallow ulcers 2 to 5 mm in diameter (Figure 48.3) or as a large horseshoe-shaped necrotic ulcer on the anterior dorsal surface of the tongue (Figure 48.4). These ulcers begin as transient vesicular eruptions which quickly rupture and release clear or serum-colored fluid. They last for 7 to 10 days and heal without complications. The ulcers or, more correctly, necrotic areas that occur on the hard palate are small (1 to 2 mm) are brownish red, and are not erosions like those on the tongue. The ulcers at the angles of the jaws tend to be similar in appearance to those of the hard palate. Rarely, there may be ulcerative erosions at the angles of the jaws and along the lips. The ulceration on the tip of the nose is superficial and results in a raw-appearing nose. This lesion may progress to form crusts. Its location on the tip of the nose, not in and around the nares, differentiates FCV from FVR-1. Ulcerations rarely occur on the feet, especially around the claws, to produce the condition known as *paw-and-mouth disease* (Cooper and Sabine 1972).

Certain strains of FCV may produce acute arthritis as part of the *limping kitten syndrome* (Pedersen et al. 1983). In addition to fever, anorexia, depression, and oral ulcerations, cats affected with this syndrome exhibit acute swelling and pain of the joints of the distal limbs. Affected cats are reluctant to move, and they cry out in pain if these joints are manipulated. Although this form of FCV infection usually occurs in young kittens, one outbreak of acute

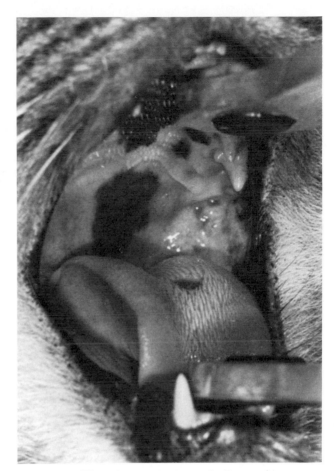

Figure 48.3. Ulceration of the tongue of a 5-year-old domestic shorthair cat caused by feline calicivirus infection. Note the round ulcer on the dorsum of the tongue.

arthritis and fever in adult cats investigated by Scott (unpublished data) resulted in more than 25 percent mortality.

FCV has been isolated from the feces and intestines of experimentally infected kittens, and clinical enteritis has been associated with natural infections of FCV. An outbreak of persistent, chronic enteritis within a cattery appeared to be caused by a stud cat persistently infected with FCV (F. Scott, unpublished data). Little is known about the noncultivatable enteric calicivirus of cats, but what little information is available points to this virus being distinct and unrelated to the respiratory and ulcerative caliciviruses (Y. Hoshino and F. Scott, unpublished data). Nothing is known about the disease-producing capabilities of the enteric caliciviruses.

Properties of the Virus. Feline caliciviruses were originally called picornaviruses, then classified in the *Calicivirus* genus of the family Picornaviridae, and finally moved to the Caliciviridae family. There has not been a picornavirus identified in the cat, so that all of the

tongue, tonsils, and pneumocytes of the alveoli of the lung. Replication appears to involve the synthesis of subgenomic RNAs, which in turn are translated into the main coat protein. Infected cells frequently have perinuclear arrays of calicivirus virions (Figure 48.6). These cells quickly round up, then release the virions by cytolysis. In cell culture, the growth curve or replicative cycle of FCV may produce progeny virus as early as 3 hours after infection, with maximum viral titers by 8 hours (Studdert 1978). This growth curve is slower in vivo.

Following the initial isolation of FCV, a number of reports of isolations and characterization of various strains were published (Bürki 1966, Crandell 1967, Crandell et al. 1960, Gillespie et al. 1971, Kahn and Gillespie 1970, Peterson and Studdert 1970). It was originally believed that there were multiple serotypes of FCV, similar to the situation with human rhinoviruses. After extensive

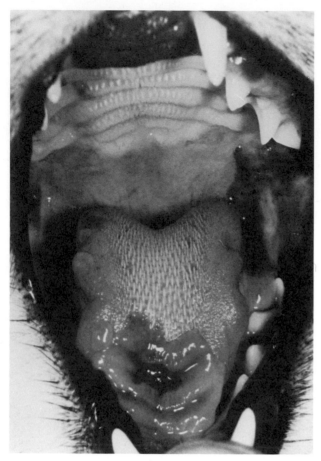

Figure 48.4. Ulcerations of the tongue of a kitten 8 days after exposure to feline calicivirus strain 255. Note the vesicle on the margin of the tongue (*left*) and the large ulcer on the tip of the tongue.

original reports of "feline picornavirus" were in fact describing feline calicivirus.

The caliciviruses are unique among viruses in that they contain only one major polypeptide with a molecular mass of approximately 65,000 to 70,000 daltons (P65 or P70) (Black and Brown 1977, Studdert 1978).

FCV is nonenveloped and therefore resistant to lipotrophic solvents and disinfectants (Scott 1980). The virions, 35 to 40 nm in diameter, appear as spheres or polyhedrons on electron micrographs (Figure 48.5)(Almeida et al. 1968, Peterson and Studdert 1970, Studdert 1978, Zwillenberg and Bürki 1966). Caliciviruses are moderately resistant to environmental conditions and can survive for several days on contaminated objects. They are susceptible to acids (pH 3) and have variable stability at pH 5.

Feline caliciviruses replicate in the cytoplasm of epithelial cells of the upper respiratory tract, conjunctiva,

Figure 48.5. Feline calicivirus crystals. × 69,000. (*Inset*) A single virion of strain KCD showing thin and rodlike capsomeres. Negative strain. × 230,000. (Courtesy J. Strandberg, D. Kahn, and P. Bartholomew.)

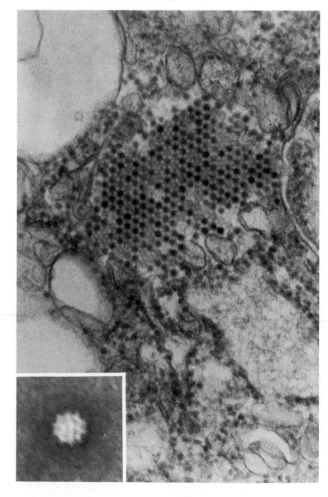

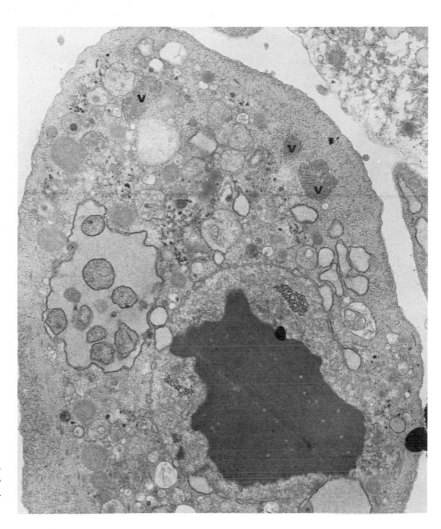

Figure 48.6. Feline calicivirus. Note crystalline arrays of virus particles (v) in the cytoplasm. × 12,560. (Courtesy J. Strandberg, D. Kahn, and P. Bartholomew.)

research, however, it was concluded that there was a single major antigenic type with multiple subtypes that have varying degrees of antigenic cross-reactivity (Bürki et al. 1976, Gillespie and Scott 1973, Kalunda et al. 1975, Povey 1974, Povey and Ingersoll 1975). FCV isolates from clinical cases of limping kitten syndrome appear to be of different serotypes (Pedersen et al. 1983). In addition, calicviruslike particles have been observed by electron microscopy in fecal samples of cats with enteritis. These enteric caliciviruses have not been grown in cell cultures, and nothing is known about possible antigenic relationships with other FCVs. However, they appear to resemble noncultivatable caliciviruses identified in the feces of several other species of animals with clinical enteritis.

Epizootiology and Pathogenesis. FCV is a very common pathogen of cats worldwide. The incidence of clinical disease, the prevalence of virus-neutralizing antibodies in healthy cats, and the percentage of healthy cats shedding FCV vary considerably from population to population. Up to 40 percent of clinical respiratory disease in cats may be due to FCV, and 20 percent of healthy cats may be shedding FCV.

The morbidity of FCV infection is nearly 100 percent when an outbreak occurs in a susceptible population. With most strains of the virus mortality is usually quite low, but it can reach 30 percent with some more pathogenic strains, especially those that cause severe pneumonia.

FCV infection can be seen year round, but the highest incidence occurs when large numbers of susceptible, unvaccinated kittens expand the cat population in a given area. It is most often seen in kittens 2 to 6 months old but can occur in cats of any age. There is no sex predilection. As with FVR-1, FCV is more common where many cats are housed and can be especially troublesome on farms, in adoption shelters, and in commercial breeding catteries.

The domestic cat is the primary host for FCV. The virus has also been isolated from cheetahs in zoological parks

(Sabine and Hyne 1970, Scott 1986), and probably all felids are susceptible. There is no known susceptibility to FCV in species other than felids, although there is some similarity between FCV and other caliciviruses that infect swine and pinnipeds.

FCV is transmitted primarily by direct contact of acutely infected cats, but the virus is maintained in the cat population between outbreaks by persistently infected carrier cats. Carrier queens infect their kittens when they are between 3 and 9 weeks old; the resulting disease can be subclinical, mild, or severe (August 1984, Johnson and Povey 1984, Scott 1986).

In the acute disease large quantities of virus are shed in the secretions of the mouth and nose, and occasionally in the feces as well. It was originally speculated that aerosol transmission played a major role, but controlled studies showed that this route was minimal in the epidemiology of FCV outbreaks (Wardley and Povey 1977a). Contaminated objects such as feed and water dishes, as well as the hands, feet, and clothing of people, can spread the virus to susceptible cats. Serum-neutralizing antibodies appear in the serum by day 6 or 7 after infection, and the viral titers in the lung and other tissues, except the tonsil, decrease to negative by day 10 to 14 after infection (Kahn and Gillespie, 1971). Tonsils retain high viral titers in some cats for many months (Wardley and Povey 1977b, 1977c). Low titers of virus were isolated from tissues of the respiratory tract, oral cavity, and regional lymph nodes of recovered cats by Wardley and Povey (1977b, 1977c). Although virus persists in tonsils and possibly other tissues for long periods of time, the humoral immune response of cats eliminates any clinical signs or chronic lesions in cats recovered from FCV infection.

The incubation period for FCV infection is extremely short. Fever may occur on day 1, with the main febrile response and clinical signs generally first being observed on day 3 after exposure. The incubation period in natural exposure varies with the dose of virus exposure and the virulence of the infecting strain. The course of the disease is generally 5 to 7 days, although some strains of FCV may produce only a transient disease with clinical signs evident for only 1 or 2 days. Complicated, prolonged cases of FCV infection usually do not occur as they do with FVR or chlamydiosis.

Local infection with FCV occurs in the oropharyngeal epithelium tissue and possibly the epithelium of the upper respiratory tract and the conjunctiva. After rapid replication and release from these infected cells, the virus spreads quickly to other epithelial cells. Some strains may spread down the respiratory tract directly or through the bloodstream to involve the alveolar pneumocytes of the lung. Necrosis of the alveolar pneumocytes may occur as early as 12 hours after infection (Langloss et al. 1978). Viral titers reach a peak of 5 to 6 logs of virus per gram of tissue in lungs and tonsils 1 day after aerosol exposure to virulent FCV strain 255 (Kahn and Gillespie 1971). Lower titers of virus occur in the trachea, third eyelid, and pharyngeal lymph nodes. Although viremia may occur, it is not a major factor in the pathogenesis of FCV infection.

Necrosis and cytolysis of infected cells result in microscopic and macroscopic lesions of the mouth and lungs. Enteric shed of virus may occur, and enteritis or acute arthritis may be seen rarely.

Gross pathological findings. Cats that die of FCV infection succumb because of the interstitial pneumonia. These cats generally die suddenly, with no observable lesions. If the disease course was more prolonged, dehydration and loss of body fat may have occurred. There may be mild discharges from the eyes and nose, and ulcerations often are present on the tongue, hard palate, nose, or lips. Joints of the distal limbs may be swollen. On rare occasions, ulcerations may be evident on the skin, especially around the claws.

The lungs of cats with fatal FCV cases have consolidated areas that may vary from diffuse to patchy. Often an entire lobe or several lobes will be involved (Figure 48.7). Early lesions tend to be focal and bright red, but as the disease progresses the lesions appear more diffuse and red-gray to purple (Holzinger and Kahn 1970, Hoover and Kahn 1975, Studdert 1978).

Concurrent infections with other respiratory pathogens are common, and the pathological changes due to these agents, especially feline herpesvirus 1, may be present.

Histopathological findings. The histopathological lesions of significance in FCV infection involve the alveolar pneumonia. Lesions are usually restricted to the alveoli, alveolar ducts, and the terminal bronchioli. In early lesions (2 to 4 days after exposure), there is edema, hemorrhage, leukocyte infiltration, and necrosis of the pneumocytes composing the alveolar walls. As the disease progresses, exudation decreases; but hyperplasia, hypertrophy, and exfoliation of the pneumocytes are evident. Cellular infiltration (lymphocytes, plasma cells, and macrophages) of the interstitial areas thicken the alveolar septa (Holzinger and Kahn 1970, Hoover and Kahn 1975, Studdert 1978).

Microscopic changes associated with the ulcerations of lingual and mucosal epithelium include epithelial necrosis and polymorphonuclear leukocyte infiltration (Hoover and Kahn 1975). Tonsillar crypt epithelium may have necrosis and inflammatory cell infiltration.

Inclusion bodies are not produced in cells infected with FCV.

Immunity. Cats recovered from FCV infection have

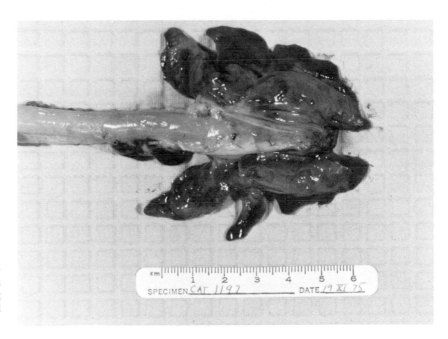

Figure 48.7. Lungs of a kitten with pneumonia caused by feline calicivirus strain 255. One or several entire lobes of the lung may be involved, with consolidation and hepatization present.

good immunity that will protect against subsequent clinical disease, although immune cats may still become infected and shed virus for a time. Queens immune to FCV transfer high levels of maternally derived immunity to their kittens (Johnson and Povey 1983).

Diagnosis. Feline respiratory disease is easily diagnosed by clinical signs, but the exact agent involved is often very difficult to identify without laboratory confirmation. The diagnosis of viral respiratory disease is often sufficient, since treatment and management are similar in most cases regardless of the cause.

In many cases a presumptive diagnosis of FCV infection can be made in many cases based on history and clinical signs, especially if these include ulceration of the tongue. If the clinical syndrome includes severe pneumonia or acute upper respiratory disease without much sneezing, a tentative diagnosis of FCV is warranted.

A diagnosis of FCV can be confirmed by virus isolation or by demonstration of seroconversion to FCV. Virus is best isolated on swabs from the oropharynx or, in animals with fatal cases, from the lung. FCV is easily isolated in most all feline cell cultures. Although antibody titers to FCV are not high following the first exposure, they are usually sufficient to allow identification of the specific virus. Paired serum samples should be taken at least 2 weeks apart and submitted together for antibody titer assay.

For virus isolation, samples should be placed in a transport medium and quickly submitted to the laboratory. Although the caliciviruses are not as susceptible to inactivation by environmental conditions as the her-

pesviruses, precautions should still be taken to prevent inactivation during transport.

Because most cats recovered from FCV will carry and shed the virus from the oropharynx for long periods, the mere isolation of FCV is not absolute proof that this virus is the cause of the disease in question. However, the isolation of FCV in acute respiratory disease with a clinical picture consistent with FCV usually is sufficient to justify a definitive diagnosis. One should always be aware of potential concurrent infection with other agents, especially FHV-1. Unless special precautions are taken, FCV, but not FHV-1, will be isolated from a sample containing both viruses, because FCV replicates faster and thus masks the herpesvirus cytopathology.

Clinicopathological findings with FCV infection are generally of little significance. The initial viral infection may produce transient lymphopenia the day after infection, but the leukocyte counts are normal by the time clinical signs appear (Kahn and Gillespie 1971).

Treatment. The treatment of cats infected with FCV entails supportive and good nursing care, broad-spectrum antibiotics for secondary bacterial infections, and specific therapy to relieve the respiratory distress from the interstitial pneumonia. There are no antiviral compounds effective against FCV.

Most cats with upper respiratory infection due to FCV respond satisfactorily without treatment. Secondary complications or concurrent infection may necessitate therapy. The eyes and nose may have to be cleaned several times a day, and the application of antibiotic ophthalmic ointment may be indicated. The ulcerations of the tongue and mouth do not require specific therapy. They heal in a few days without complications. Of course bland foods and perhaps forced feeding may be indicated during this period.

Viral pneumonia and possible secondary bacterial pneumonia should receive prompt and careful attention. While there is no specific antiviral drug effective against the FCV, supportive therapy, especially oxygen, can make the difference between death and survival. One should remember that the primary lesion in FCV pneumonia involves the alveolar pneumocytes; thus the air-exchange tissues are directly affected (Langloss et al. 1978). Barring complications, alveolar lesions heal 7 to 10 days after exposure with minimal permanent lesions. The role of the clinician is to provide supportive care through this critical period until natural healing occurs.

Antibiotics such as ampicillin, chloramphenicol, or gentamicin, which are effective against respiratory bacteria, should be given until the pneumonia has resolved. Chloramphenicol should not be administered for more than 7 days to avoid toxic complications.

Intestinal involvement with respiratory FCV generally is of minimal concern and usually does not require specific therapy. If it does, supportive therapy for viral enteritis should be sufficient.

Prevention and Control. Although FCV infection can be acute and highly contagious, vaccination and disinfection are often effective in its control.

Vaccination. Inactivated and attenuated or modified live-virus vaccines of cell culture origin are available for immunization of cats against FCV by parenteral administration (August 1984; Bittle and Rubic 1976; Bittle et al. 1982; Bush et al. 1981; Gaskell et al. 1982; Kahn and Hoover 1976; Kahn et al. 1975; Povey 1979; Povey and Wilson 1978; Scott 1977, 1986). In addition, modified live-virus vaccines for administration by nasal and ocular drops are available (Davis and Beckenhauer 1976, Wilson 1978). An experimental subunit vaccine, which is antigenically similar to the whole virus, has been studied (Komolafe and Jarrett 1985).

A parenteral vaccine given in two doses at least 3 weeks apart or a single dose of intranasal modified live-virus vaccine produces significant protection for at least 1 year. Cats should be revaccinated annually with a single dose of vaccine.

FCV vaccines are available in combination with FHV-1, as a triple vaccine with feline parvovirus and FHV-1, or in a variety of combinations with feline pneumonitis and rabies agents. These vaccines produce significant protection and should be part of the routine immunization program. Immunized cats, while protected against systemic and severe respiratory disease, are not protected completely against local viral replication. Exposed immunized cats develop localized viral infection and shed virus for a short time; they generally do not develop clinical illness. A rapid anamnestic immune response occurs in these exposed cats.

Intranasal FVR-FCV vaccines may produce mild sneezing and slight ocular and nasal discharge 4 to 7 days after vaccination, and owners should be warned to expect this reaction.

Most vaccination programs start when kittens are about 8 weeks old, with a second dose of vaccine 3 to 4 weeks later. In some catteries it is necessary to begin vaccinations in kittens as young as 4 weeks old, with repeated doses every 3 to 4 weeks until the kittens are 12 weeks old.

Two new serotypes of FCV have been identified from kittens with acute arthritis (Pedersen et al. 1983). Two vaccine strains of FCV (F-9 and M-8) did not protect cats against these serotypes.

Exotic cats should be routinely immunized with either modified live-virus or inactivated parenteral vaccines. Until tested further, the intranasal vaccines should not be used in these species. Age at vaccination and other recommendations for FCV immunization are similar to those for domestic cats.

Disinfection. FCV is more resistant to environmental conditions and disinfectants than is FHV-1, but it is more labile than feline parvovirus. The caliciviruses are susceptible to sodium hypochlorite (household bleach) and the substituted phenolic compounds but are resistant to quaternary ammonium, chlorhexidine, and many of the iodine-containing disinfectants (Scott 1980). The routine use of bleach at a concentration of 1:20 to 1:32 is highly effective in removing FCV from a contaminated environment and should be routine procedure for control of FCV.

The Disease in Humans. There are no known public health dangers posed by FCV.

REFERENCES

Almeida, J.D., Waterson, A.P., Prydie, J., and Fletcher, E.W.L. 1968. The structure of a feline picornavirus and its relevance to cubic viruses in general. Arch. Gesam. Virusforsch. 25:105–114.

August, J.R. 1984. Feline viral respiratory disease. The carrier state, vaccination, and control. Vet. Clin. North Am. [Small Anim. Pract.]. 14:1159–1171.

Bittle, J.L., and Rubic, W.J. 1976. Immunization against feline calicivirus infection. Am. J. Vet. Res. 37:275–278.

Bittle, J.L., Grant, W.A., and Scott, F.W. 1982. Canine and feline immunization guidelines—1982. J. Am. Vet. Med. Assoc. 181:332–335.

Black, D.N., and Brown, F. 1977. Proteins induced by infection with caliciviruses. J. Gen. Virol. 38:75–82

Bürki, F. 1965. Picornaviruses of cats. Arch. Gesam. Virusforsch. 15:690–696.

Bürki, F., Starustka, B., and Ruttner, O. 1976. Attempts to serologically classify feline caliciviruses on a national and an international basis. Infect. Immun. 14:876–881.

Bush, M., Povey, R.C., and Koonse, H. 1981. Antibody response to an inactivated vaccine for rhinotracheitis, caliciviral disease, and panleukopenia in nondomestic felids. J. Am. Vet. Med. Assoc. 179:1203–1205.

Cooper, L.M., and Sabine, M. 1972. Paw and mouth disease in a cat. Aust. Vet. J. 48:644.

Crandell, R.A. 1967. A description of eight feline picornaviruses and an attempt to classify them. Proc. Soc. Exp. Biol. Med. 126:240–245.

Crandell, R.A., Niemann, W.H., Ganaway, J.R., and Maurer, F.D. 1960. Isolation of cytopathic agents from the nasopharyngeal region of the domestic cat. Virology 10:283–285.

Davis, E.V., and Beckenhauer, W.H. 1976. Studies on the safety and efficacy of an intranasal feline rhinotracheitis-calicivirus vaccine. Vet. Med./Small Anim. Clin. 71:1405–1410.

Fastier, L.B. 1957. A new feline virus isolated in tissue culture. Am. J. Vet. Res. 18:382–389.

Gaskell, R.M., and Wardley, R.C. 1978. Feline viral respiratory disease: A review with particular reference to its epizootiology and control. J. Small Anim. Pract. 19:1–16.

Gaskell, C.J., Gaskell, R.M., Dennis, P.E., and Wooldridge, M.J. 1982. Efficacy of an inactivated feline calicivirus (FCV) vaccine against challenge with United Kingdom field strains and its interaction with the FCV carrier state. Res. Vet. Sci. 32:23–26.

Gillespie, J.H., and Scott, F.W. 1973. Feline viral infections. Adv. Vet. Sci. Comp. Med. 17:163–200.

Gillespie, J.H., Judkins, A.B., and Kahn, D.E. 1971. Feline viruses. XIII. The use of the immunofluorescent test for the detection of feline picornaviruses. Cornell Vet. 61:172–179.

Holzinger, E.A., and Kahn, D.E. 1970. Pathologic features of picornavirus infections in cats. Am. J. Vet. Res. 31:1623–1630.

Hoover, E.A., and Kahn, D.E. 1975. Experimentally induced feline calicivirus infections: Clinical signs and lesions. J. Am. Vet. Med. Assoc. 166:463–468.

Johnson, R.P., and Povey, R.C. 1983. Transfer and decline of maternal antibody to feline calicivirus. Can. Vet. J. 24:6–9.

Johnson, R.P., and Povey, R.C. 1984. Feline calicivirus infection in kittens borne by cats persistently infected with the virus. Res. Vet. Sci. 37:114–119.

Kahn, D.E., and Gillespie, J.H. 1970. Feline viruses. X. Characterization of a newly-isolated picornavirus causing interstitial pneumonia and ulcerative stomatitis in the domestic cat. Cornell Vet. 60:669–683.

Kahn, D.E., and Gillespie, J.H. 1971. Feline viruses: Pathogenesis of picornavirus infection in the cat. Am. J. Vet. Res. 32:521–531.

Kahn, D.E., and Hoover, E.A. 1976a. Feline caliciviral disease: Experimental immunoprophylaxis. Am. J. Vet. Res. 37:279–283.

Kahn, D.E., and Hoover, E.A. 1976b. Infectious respiratory diseases of cats. Vet. Clin. North. Am. 6:399–413.

Kahn D.E., Hoover, E.A., and Bittle, J.L. 1975. Induction of immunity to feline caliciviral disease. Infect. Immun. 11:1003–1009.

Kalunda, M., Lee, K.M., Holmes, D.F., and Gillespie, J.H. 1975. Serologic classification of feline caliciviruses by plaque-reduction neutralization and immunodiffusion. Am. J. Vet. Res. 36:353–356.

Komolafe, O.O., and Jarrett, O. 1985. Feline calicivirus subunit vaccine—A prototype. Antiviral Res. 5:241–248.

Langloss, J.M., Hoover, E.A., and Kahn, D.E. 1978. Ultrastructural morphogenesis of acute viral pneumonia produced by feline calicivirus. Am. J. Vet. Res. 39:1577–1583.

Ott, R.L. 1983. Systemic viral diseases. In P.W. Pratt, ed., Feline Medicine, 1st ed. American Veterinary Publications, Santa Barbara, Calif. Pp. 85–139.

Pedersen, N.C., Laliberte, L., and Ekman, S. 1983. A transient febrile "limping" syndrome of kittens caused by two different strains of feline calicivirus. Feline Pract. 13:26–35.

Peterson, J.E., and Studdert, M.J. 1970. Feline picornavirus. Arch. Gesam. Virusforsch. 32:249–260.

Povey, R.C. 1974. Serological relationships among feline caliciviruses. Infect. Immun. 10:1307–1314.

Povey, R.C. 1976. Feline respiratory infections—A clinical review. Can. Vet. J. 17:93–100.

Povey, R.C. 1979. The efficacy of two commercial feline rhinotracheitis-calicivirus-panleukopenia vaccines. Can. Vet. J. 20:253–260.

Povey, R.C. 1985. Infectious Diseases of Cats. A Clinical Handbook. Centaur Press, Guelph, Ontario.

Povey, R.C., and Ingersoll, J. 1975. Cross protection among feline caliciviruses. Infect. Immun. 11:877–885.

Povey, R.C., and Wilson, M.R. 1978. A comparison of inactivated feline viral rhinotracheitis and feline caliciviral disease vaccines with live-modified viral vaccines. Feline Pract. 8:35–42.

Sabine, M., and Hyne, R.H.J. 1970. Isolation of feline picornavirus from cheetahs with conjunctivitis and glossitis. Vet. Rec. 87:794–796.

Schaffer, F.L. 1979. Caliciviruses. In H. Fraenkel-Conrat and R.R. Wagner, eds. Comprehensive Virology, vol. 14. Plenum Press, New York. Pp. 249–283.

Scott, F.W. 1977. Evaluation of a feline viral rhinotracheitis-feline calicivirus disease vaccine. Am. J. Vet. Res. 38:229–234.

Scott, F.W. 1980. Virucidal disinfectants and feline viruses. Am. J. Vet. Res. 41:410–414.

Scott, F.W. 1986. Feline respiratory viral diseases. In F.W. Scott, ed., Infectious Diseases. Contemporary Issues in Small Animal Practice, vol. 3. Churchill Livingstone, New York. Pp. 155–175.

Studdert, M.J. 1978. Caliciviruses. Arch. Virol. 58:157–191.

Wardley, R.C. 1976. Feline calicivirus carrier state. A study of the host/virus relationship. Arch. Virol. 52:243–249.

Wardley, R.C., and Povey, R.C. 1977a. Aerosol transmission of feline caliciviruses. An assessment of its epidemiological importance. Br. Vet. J. 133:504–508.

Wardley, R.C., and Povey, R.C. 1977b. The clinical disease and patterns of excretion associated with three different strains of feline caliciviruses. Res. Vet. Sci. 23:7–14.

Wardley, R.C., and Povey, R.C. 1977c. The pathology and sites of persistence associated with three different strains of feline calicivirus. Res. Vet. Sci. 23:15–19.

Wilson, J.H.G. 1978. Intranasal vaccination against upper respiratory tract disease (URD) in the cat. II. Results of field studies under enzootic conditions in the Netherlands with a combined vaccine containing live attenuated calici- and herpesvirus. Comp. Immunol. Microbiol. Infect. Dis. 1:43–48.

Zwillenberg, L.O., and Bürki, F. 1966. On the capsid structure of some small feline and bovine RNA viruses. Arch. Gesam. Virusforsch. 19:373–384.

Canine Calicivirus Infection

Evermann et al. (1981) first isolated a calicivirus from a dog with glossitis. Two of three dogs from a household had multiple small ulcers and vesicles over the dorsal surface of the tongue, and additional ulcers were present on the gingiva above the upper incisors. The course of the disease was about 4 weeks, and the dogs did not stop eating and did not have fever.

The canine glossitis isolate characterized by Evermann et al. (1981, 1983) was found to be very similar antigenically to feline calicivirus. Electron microscopy revealed that this virus had the morphology of caliciviruses.

Caliciviruses were isolated from seven dogs and a captured coyote with enteritis (Evermann et al. 1985). A high fatality rate occurred in pups 4 to 16 weeks of age; but because these dogs were also infected with other bacterial and viral pathogens, the exact pathogenicity of these isolates for dogs was not determined. These enteric isolates were similar to feline calicivirus.

Schaffer et al. (1985) reported another calicivirus isolate from the feces of a dog with diarrhea. Its morphology and physicochemical properties showed it to be a calicivirus. Antigenically this isolate differed from several known caliciviruses from other species. Serologic studies indicated that many dogs in one area had been infected with it.

Foxes have been shown to have antibodies against certain caliciviruses (Prato et al. 1977).

The Disease in Humans. An outbreak of gastroenteritis occurred in a retirement home 24 hours after the proprietor's dog became ill (Humphrey et al. 1984). A calicivirus was isolated from one of the residents, and this isolate appeared to be capable of infecting dogs.

REFERENCES

Evermann, J.F., Bryan, G.M., and McKeirnan, A.J. 1981. Isolation of a calicivirus from a case of canine glossitis. Canine Pract. 8:36–39.
Evermann, J.F., McKeirnan, A.J., Smith, A.W., Skilling, D.E., and Ott, R.L. 1985. Isolation and identification of caliciviruses from dogs with enteric infections. Am. J. Vet. Res. 46:218–220.
Evermann, J.F., Smith, A.W., Skilling, D.E., and McKeirnan, A.J. 1983. Ultrastructure of newly recognized caliciviruses of the dog and mink. Arch. Virol. 76:257–261.
Humphrey, T.J., Cruickshank, J.G., and Cubitt, W.D. 1984. An outbreak of calicivirus associated gastroenteritis in an elderly persons home. A possible zoonosis? J. Hyg. 93:293–299.
Prato, C.M., Akers, T.G., and Smith, A.W. 1977. Calicivirus antibodies in wild fox populations. J. Wildl. Dis. 13:448–450.
Schaffer, F.L., Soergel, M.E., Black, J.W., Skilling, D.E., Smith, A.W., and Cubitt, W.D. 1985. Characterization of a new calicivirus isolated from feces of a dog. Arch. Virol. 84:181–195.

Bovine Calicivirus Infection

SYNONYMS: Newbury agent infection,
Tillamook calicivirus infection

A bovine calicivirus was isolated from calves in an Oregon herd that had persistent respiratory disease (Smith et al. 1983). This isolate, the Tillamook calicivirus (TCV), has been shown to produce small skin lesions in calves inoculated with it and mild vesicular exanthema in swine. Antibody titers to this virus were present in 4 percent of serum samples from California sea lions and Steller sea lions sampled from the Bering Sea to southern California (Barlough et al. 1987).

Oregon cattle have been shown to contain neutralizing antibodies to SMSV-5 and SMSV-13 (Barlough et al. 1987, Berry et al. 1987). It appears that cattle occasionally are susceptible to infection with the marine caliciviruses.

Two serotypes of bovine calicivirus (Newbury agent SRV-1 and SRV-2) isolated from calves with diarrhea. In the initial isolation, astrovirus particles were found in fecal samples (Woode and Bridger 1978). Experimental infection of the villous cells of the anterior small intestine resulted in exfoliation of degenerate enterocytes and stunted villi (Hall et al. 1984). Cross-protection tests in gnotobiotic calves showed that these two serotypes were antigenically distinct, and infection of gnotobiotic calves with one virus did not protect them against infection with the other serotype (Bridger et al. 1984).

REFERENCES

Barlough, J.E., Berry, E.S., Smith, A.W., and Skilling, D.E. 1987. Prevalence and distribution of serum neutralizing antibodies to Tillamook (bovine) calicivirus in selected populations of marine mammals. J. Wildl. Dis. 23:45–51.
Berry, E.S., Barlough, J.E., Skilling, D.E., Smith, A.W., Gage, L., Dierauf, L. and Vedros, N.A. 1987. Calicivirus isolation from an outbreak of vesicular disease among California pinnipeds, and experimental production of vesicular exanthema in pigs. Am. J. Vet. Res. Submitted.
Bridger, J.C., Hall, G.A., and Brown, J.F. 1984. Characterization of a calici-like virus (Newbury agent) found in association with astrovirus in bovine diarrhea. Infect. Immun. 43:133–138.
Hall, G.A., Bridger, J.C., Brooker, B.E., Parsons, K.R., and Ormerod, E. 1984. Lesions of gnotobiotic calves experimentally infected with a calicivirus-like (Newbury) agent. Vet. Pathol. 21:208–215.
Smith, A.W., Mattson, D.E., Skilling, D.E., and Schmitz, J.A. 1983. Isolation and partial characterization of a calicivirus from calves. Am. J. Vet. Res. 44:851–855.
Woode, G.N., and Bridger, J.C. 1978. Isolation of small viruses resembling astroviruses and caliciviruses from acute enteritis of calves. J. Med. Microbiol. 11:441–452.

Other Calicivirus Infections

A caliciviruslike agent has been isolated from gut homogenate of stunted broiler chicks and partially characterized (Cubitt and Barrett 1985). Its morphology and biophysical properties are similar to those of feline calicivirus. Caliciviruses have been identified in mink (Evermann et al. 1983), in four species of nonhuman primates (Smith et al. 1983, 1985), and in reptiles and amphibians (Smith et al. 1986).

REFERENCES

Cubitt, W.D., and Barrett, A.D. 1985. Propagation and preliminary characterization of a chicken candidate calicivirus. J. Gen. Virol. 66:1431–1438.

Evermann, J.F., Smith, A.W., Skilling, D.E., and McKeirnan, A.J. 1983. Ultrastructure of newly recognized caliciviruses of the dog and mink. Arch. Virol. 76:257–261.

Smith, A.W., Anderson, M.P., Skilling, D.E., Barlough, J.E., and Ensley, P.K. 1986. First isolation of calicivirus from reptiles and amphibians. Am. J. Vet. Res. 47:1718–1721.

Smith, A.W., Skilling, D.E., and Benirschke, K. 1985. Calicivirus isolation from three species of primates: An incidental finding. Am. J. Vet. Res. 46:2197–2199.

Smith, A.W., Skilling, D.E., Ensley, P.K., Benirschke, K., and Lester, T.L. 1983. Calicivirus isolation and persistence in a pygmy chimpanzee (*Pan paniscus*). Science 221:79–81.

49   The Reoviridae

The family Reoviridae consists of three genera now recognized by the International Committee on Taxonomy of Viruses: *Reovirus, Rotovirus,* and *Orbivirus.* Infectious bursal disease virus of chickens and infectious pancreatic necrosis virus of salmonids are included in this family even though they do not fit into any of the three genera because they have no envelope and contain marked differences in RNA segmentation. Reoviridae infections are extremely common in birds and mammals (Table 49.1). Consequently, antibodies to these pathogens can be readily detected in most domestic animals. A review article on orbivirus and reovirus infections of mammals and birds was published by Stanley in 1981.

The Genus *Reovirus*

Viruses in the genus *Reovirus* are characterized by double-stranded RNA. The total molecular mass is about 15 $\times$ 10^6 daltons. The particle's capsid is isometric with icosahedral symmetry, usually naked; but a pseudo-membrane, probably of host origin, is seen. The capsid diameter is 75 nm. Most viruses in this genus have two-layer capsids (Fenner 1976). The buoyant density in cesium chloride is 1.36 g/ml. The particle resists treatment with lipid solvents. Synthesis and maturation occur in the host cell's cytoplasm, with the formation of inclusion bodies that sometimes contain particles in crystalline arrays.

Some characteristics of reoviruses that help to distinguish them from other mammalian viruses are (1) their distinctive cytopathic effects, including intracytoplasmic inclusion bodies, in cell cultures from a variety of animal species, (2) a common complement-fixing antigen, and (3) their ability to agglutinate human group O and bovine erythrocytes, but not chick or guinea pig erythrocytes.

The type species for this genus is *Reovirus* h-1 (human type), one of three mammalian serotypes. Members of the genus, morphologically and serologically indistinguishable from each other, occur commonly in various animal species. The natural occurrence of these three serotypes in different species suggests transmission from one animal species to another in nature; this phenomenon, however, has not been proved.

At present the economic importance of reoviral disease in domestic mammals is still largely undetermined. Most infections are mild or inapparent (Fenner 1976). Avian reoviruses, however, are important pathogens in chickens, turkeys, and ducks and cause significant economic losses. In his review article Rosen (1968) discusses five avian reovirus serotypes that are officially recognized by the International Committee on Taxonomy of Viruses.

REFERENCES

Fenner, F. 1976. Classification and nomenclature of viruses. Second report of the International Committee on Taxonomy of Viruses. Intervirology 7:34.

Rosen, L. 1968. Reoviruses. In S. Gard, C. Hallauer, and K.F. Meyer, eds., Virology Monographs, vol. 1. Springer-Verlag, New York. Pp. 73–107.

Stanley, N.F. 1981. Reoviridae: Orbivirus and reovirus infections of mammals and birds. In E. Kurstak and C. Kurstak, eds., Comparative Diagnosis of Viral Diseases, vol. 4, pt. B. Academic Press, New York. Pp. 67–104.

Bovine Reovirus Infection

Bovine reoviruses are widespread in nature, and their incidence in cattle is common. Their importance as pathogens in the respiratory syndrome is still undetermined, however. Reovirus serotypes 1, 2, and 3 have been recovered from the feces of naturally infected cattle (Rosen and Abinanti 1960).

Character of the Disease. Present evidence strongly suggests that bovine reoviruses cause an inapparent infection in nature (Lamont 1968, Rosen and Abinanti 1960), although Trainor et al. (1966) reported mild respiratory disease in calves with the Lang strain of reovirus 1 of human origin.

In a study of colostrum-deprived calves infected with reovirus 1 strains of human and bovine origin, no clinical signs of illness were produced, yet macroscopic and microscopic lesions of interstitial pneumonia were seen 4 and 7 days after a regimen of combined intranasal and intratracheal routes of inoculation (Lamont 1966, 1968). Nonspecific lymphadenitis of the retropharyngeal, bron-

Table 49.1. Diseases of domestic animals caused by viruses in the Reoviridae family

Common name of virus	Natural hosts	Type of disease produced
Genus *Reovirus*		
Reovirus serotypes 1–3	Cattle	Usually inapparent disease; possibly mild respiratory disease on occasion
Reovirus serotypes 1 and 2	Dogs	Mild or inapparent upper respiratory infection
Reovirus serotypes 1 and 3	Cats	Mild upper respiratory infection when it occasionally occurs
Reovirus serotypes 1, 2, 3	Horses	Coughing, nasal and ocular discharge
At least 5 avian reovirus serotypes recognized	Birds	Cloacal pasting; infectious tenosynovitis (4 serotypes recognized)
Genus *Rotavirus*		
Bovine rotavirus—1? serotype	Cattle	Acute gastroenteritis of neonatal calves
Porcine rotavirus—2 serotypes	Pigs	Acute gastroenteritis of piglets
Equine rotavirus—3 serotypes	Horses	Acute gastroenteritis of neonatal foals and young horses
Ovine rotavirus—1 serotype	Sheep	Acute gastroenteritis of neonatal lambs
Human rotavirus—4 scrotypes	Humans	Acute gastroenteritis of infants and occasionally adults
Feline rotavirus—1 serotype	Cats	Diarrhea in cats (experimental)
Canine rotavirus—1 serotype	Dogs	Acute gastroenteritis of puppies
Chicken rotavirus—1 serotype	Chickens	
Turkey rotavirus—1 serotype	Turkeys	
Genus *Orbivirus*		
African horsesickness virus, serotypes 1–9	Horses; less severe disease in donkeys and mules	Acute form—pulmonary signs. Chronic form—hydropericardium and edema of head, neck, and shoulder regions
Bluetongue virus, serotypes 1–24 (5 in USA)	Sheep, cattle, goats, and wild ruminants	Acute form—usually in feeder lambs—characterized by edema erosions in oral cavity, respiratory signs, and stiffness. Abortions in ewes, occasionally other signs. Less serious consequences in cattle as a rule, but disease manifestations are similar

Table 49.1. —*continued*

Common name of virus	Natural hosts	Type of disease produced
Epizootic hemorrhagic disease (EHD) virus, serotypes 1–3; Ibaraki virus may be the third serotype of EHD virus	Deer (*Odocoileus virginianus*), cattle	Acute disease—high morbidity with high mortality in confined deer. Severe shock, edema, and hemorrhages are characteristic
Unspecified genera		
Infectious bursal disease virus, serotypes 1 and 2	Young chickens	Highly contagious disease. Enteric disease with bursa of Fabricius as the target organ. Principal lesions in lymphoid structures
Infectious pancreatic necrosis virus, serotypes 1–3	Salmonids	Acute disease—high morbidity; mortality usually high in young fish. Disease manifested by catarrhal enteritis and pancreatic necrosis

*In many cases animals in all species have mixed enteric infections and accompanying pneumonia associated with rotavirus disease.

chial, mediastinal, and mesenteric lymph nodes and some congestion and degenerative changes in the liver were also seen. Virus in low titers was recovered for 4 days from nasal swabs and for 7 days from rectal swabs. In a virus distribution study, suspensions of respiratory tissues had higher titers than other body tissues (Lamont 1968).

Trainor et al. (1966) suggested that a strain of *Pasteurella multocida* did not enhance reovirus infection in calves; however, *Pasteurella haemolytica* did enhance reovirus 1 infection in day-old calves deprived of colostrum (Lamont 1968).

Properties of the Virus. Properties of the three reovirus serotypes recovered from cattle are indistinguishable from the same serotypes isolated from other species.

Cultivation. Bovine reoviruses 1, 2, and 3 have been propagated in bovine kidney cell cultures (Rosen and Abinanti 1960, Rosen et al. 1963) and also in pig kidney, monkey kidney, and mouse fibroblast (L strain) cell cultures (Lamont 1968). The three bovine serotypes cause a cytopathic effect in these cell cultures, but the bovine kidney cell cultures seem to be more resistant to pathological change (Lamont 1968).

Epizootiology. Bovine reoviruses can be detected in the feces of naturally and experimentally infected cattle for as long as a month, although the organisms usually disappear in a shorter period of time (Moscovici et al. 1961, Rosen and Abinanti 1960, Rosen et al. 1963). Virus also is discharged from the nasal passages and the conjunctiva, probably for a comparable period of time. Through contact with these infectious sources, susceptible cattle may become infected. Although it has not been proved, cattle possibly may become infected with the three reovirus serotypes common to many animal species.

Immunity. Maternally acquired immunity does not appear to protect calves from infection under natural conditions (Rosen et al. 1963) and perhaps under experimental conditions as well (Lamont 1968).

The degree and duration of protection of cattle after active infection is unknown, but neutralizing antibodies are formed and presumably persist for a while.

Diagnosis. As potential respiratory pathogens, reoviruses must be distinguished from numerous other microbial respiratory pathogens of cattle. This is difficult, if not impossible, unless one resorts to virus isolation or serology.

The only practical means for virus isolation and identification is tissue culture. The neutralization or hemagglutination-inhibition (HI) test can be used for demonstrating a rising serum titer with paired serums. An HI test with a rise in titer of four-fold or greater between the acute and convalescent samples is considered positive (Lamont 1968).

The Disease in Humans. Although not proved, it is conceivable that the bovine reoviruses may infect humans.

REFERENCES

Lamont, P.H. 1966. Some bovine respiratory viruses. Proc. R. Soc. Med. 59:50–51.
Lamont, P.H. 1968. Reoviruses. J. Am. Vet. Med. Assoc. 152:807–813.
Moscovici, C., LaPlaca, M., Maisel, J., and Kempe, C.H. 1961. Studies of bovine enteroviruses. Am. J. Vet. Res. 22:852–863.
Rosen, L., and Abinanti, F.R. 1960. Natural and experimental infection of cattle with human types of reoviruses. Am. J. Hyg. 71:250–257.
Rosen, L., Abinanti, F.R., and Hovis, J.F. 1963. Further observations of the natural infection of cattle with reoviruses. Am. J. Hyg. 77:38.
Trainor, P.D., Mohanty, S.B., and Hetrick, F.M. 1966. Experimental

infection of calves with reovirus type 1. Am. J. Epidemiol. 83:217–223.

Canine Reovirus Infection

Reovirus serotype 1 isolated from dogs with respiratory signs of illness has produced interstitial pneumonia in naturally and experimentally infected dogs (Lou and Venner 1963). Inoculation of this isolate into dogs free of germs (gnotobiotic) and specific pathogens failed to produce signs of illness or pathological changes, but it did cause infection as shown by the fact that virus was isolated and seroconversion occurred (Holzinger and Griesimer 1966). Massie and Shaw (1966) recovered reovirus 1 from 4 of 133 dogs, and one of these isolates produced signs of illness referable to the respiratory and enteric tracts in 4 experimentally infected puppies. Further studies in conventional and pathogen-free dogs are essential to determine the factors responsible for the pathogenicity of reovirus 1.

Reovirus serotype 2 was isolated from the throat and feces of an immature dog with upper respiratory disease (Binn et al. 1977), but viral pathogenicity in experimental dogs was not reported. The affected pup had an increase in antibody titer to reovirus 2 and 3, providing evidence for possible heterotypic responses in dogs to reovirus infection. A serologic survey of dogs in Japan showed that young puppies have antibodies to the three types of reovirus (Murakami et al. 1979).

REFERENCES

Binn, L.N., Marchwicki, R.H., Kennan, K.P., Strano, A.J., and Engler, W. 1977. Recovery of reovirus type 2 from an immature dog with respiratory tract disease. Am. J. Vet. Res. 38:927–929.
Holzinger, E.A., and Griesimer, R.A. 1966. Effects of reovirus, type 1, on germfree and disease-free dogs. Am. J. Epidemiol. 84:426–430.
Lou, T.Y., and Wenner, H.A. 1963. Natural and experimental infection of dogs with reovirus, type 1: Pathogenicity of the strain for other animals. Am. J. Hyg. 77:293–304.
Massie, E.L., and Shaw, E.D. 1966. Reovirus type 1 in laboratory dogs. Am. J. Vet. Res. 27:783–785.
Murakami, T., Anzai, T., Ogawa, T., Fukazawa, Y., Ono, K., and Hirano, N. 1979. A survey of reovirus antibodies in dogs in Morioka. J. Fac. Agric. 14:337–441.

Feline Reovirus Infection

Scott et al. (1970) isolated reovirus type 3 from a cat suspected of having died of feline infectious panleukopenia. Cell cultures inoculated with a suspension of intestinal tract from this cat produced intracytoplasmic inclusion bodies that were later attributed to reovirus 3. Three subsequent isolations of reovirus 3 from cats have been reported. Hong (1970) also produced three isolations of reovirus from feline neoplasm cell cultures, and all were typed as reovirus 1 as determined by the hemagglutination test.

Character of the Disease. The experimental disease produced by feline reovirus 3 is mild (Scott 1968, Scott et al. 1970). It is characterized by conjunctivitis, photophobia, gingivitis, serous lacrimation, and depression. Most cats that come in contact with reovirus 3 have similar signs of illness 4 to 19 days after exposure, and signs persisted from 1 to 29 days. Virus is isolated from the pharynx, eye, and rectum of the experimentally infected cats, with 6 to 10 days being the optimal period for isolation. Cytoplasmic reovirus 1 inclusion bodies are found in the bronchiolar epithelium of severely stressed neonatal experimental kittens (Hong 1970).

Properties of the Virus. Feline reovirus 3 particles in negatively stained preparations have a diameter of 75 nm and exhibit prominent hollow-cored capsomeres (Scott et al. 1970) (Figure 49.1). The hexagonal particle has icosahedral symmetry and is composed of 92 capsomeres. With acridine staining, infected cell cultures have green-staining inclusion masses, and the borders of the

Figure 49.1. Feline reovirus particles (75 nm in diameter). Prominent capsomeres with hollow cores are evident in a negatively stained preparation. (From Scott et al., 1970, courtesy of *American Journal of Veterinary Research.*)

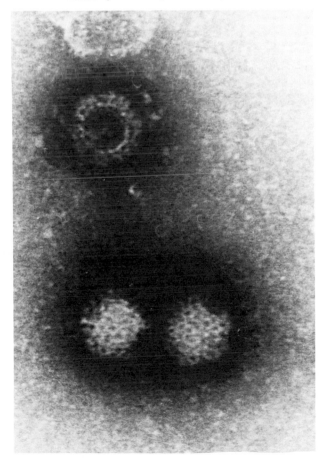

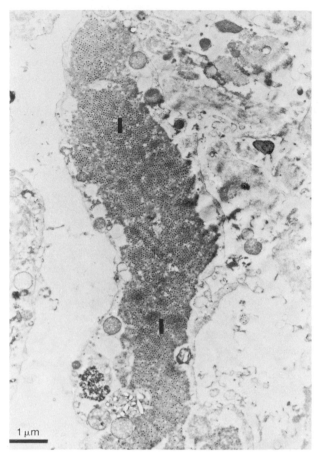

Figure 49.2.   Single cytoplasmic inclusion (*I*) of feline reovirus particles in a closely packed paracrystalline array. (From Scott et al., 1970, courtesy of *American Journal of Veterinary Research.*)

cytoplasm fluoresce reddish orange. Virus particles in infected cell cultures examined by electron microscopy are either arranged in closely packed, highly ordered paracrystalline arrays or spread through osmophilic reticular masses (Figure 49.2). A few cells contain masses of virus particles in membrane-bound cytoplasmic vesicles within their cytoplasms.

The virus is quite thermostabile, as it is not destroyed after heating for 30 minutes at 56°C.

Cultivation.   Reovirus 3 is propagated in primary cultures of feline kidney cells and of bovine fetal kidney cells (Scott et al. 1970). Feline kidney cell cultures give a titer of approximately 10^6 TCID$_{50}$/ml, whereas the titer is about 1 log less in the bovine kidney cultures. The virus produces a typical cytopathic effect in unstained cultures. In May-Grünwald-Giemsa-stained preparations large, irregularly shaped, blue-staining, intracytoplasmic inclusions begin to appear on the third or fourth day after inoculation (Figure 49.3).

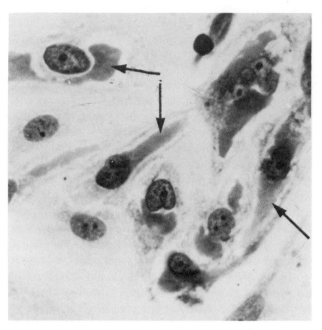

Figure 49.3.   Large cytoplasmic inclusion bodies (*arrows*) in a 4-day-old feline kidney cell culture. May-Grünwald-Giemsa stain. × 650. (From Scott et al., 1970, courtesy of *American Journal of Veterinary Research.*)

Epizootiology.   Reovirus is readily transmitted from infected cats to susceptible cats maintained in the same room. This is the only known means of transmission. The incidence of the disease is not known, although it probably is widespread (Scott 1971). The virus has been isolated from cats in California and New York, and neutralizing antibodies are present in a significant percentage of cats in the Ithaca, New York, area (50 percent for reovirus 3, 71 percent for reovirus 1).

Immunity.   Little is known about immunity to feline reoviruses. Neutralizing antibodies to the homotypic virus are produced in cats. The high incidence of neutralizing antibody in a small feline population suggests that it is a common disease and that most cats are immune. Obviously, considerably more research must be done.

It is not practical to develop a vaccine against feline reoviruses until more is known about the immunity to these viruses and their pathological effects and pathogenicity.

Diagnosis.   Reovirus infection in the cat can be confused with other feline respiratory diseases. The importance of the reoviruses as feline pathogens is still undetermined. Scott (1971) made the following observations that help to differentiate reovirus infection from other respiratory diseases. The clinical disease is mild and usually of short duration. The signs of illness are restricted primarily to the eyes; a nasal discharge usually is associated with other respiratory infections. Fever, leukopenia or leukocytosis, and anorexia generally are not observed.

Certain rules must be observed in attempts to isolate feline reoviruses from feline tissues in cell culture. Because the cytopathic effect in unstained cell cultures may not be visualized for up to 10 days, cultures must be retained for this period of time. Although not proved, it may be necessary to make blind passages before declaring a test sample negative. At present cell-culture appears to be the method of choice for virus isolation.

Serologic methods such as the neutralization or the hemagglutination test can be used to demonstrate a rising titer with paired serums from active cases.

The Diseases in Humans. The natural occurrence of reovirus 1 and 3 in cats and humans suggests the possible transmission between these species and others that harbor these viruses. Such transmission has not been demonstrated, but it is almost inconceivable that it does not occur on occasion (Rosen 1968).

REFERENCES

Hong, C. 1970. Studies on a strain of reovirus type 1 isolated from a feline leukemia cell culture. Ph.D. dissertation, Cornell University, Ithaca, N.Y.
Rosen, L. 1968. Reoviruses. In S. Gard, C. Hallauer, and K.F. Meyer, eds., Virology Monographs, vol. 1. Springer-Verlag, New York. Pp. 1:73–107.
Scott, F.W. 1968. Feline panleukopenia. Ph.D. dissertation, Cornell University, Ithaca, N.Y.
Scott, F.W. 1971. Feline reovirus. J. Am. Vet Med Assoc. 158:944–945.
Scott, F.W., Kahn, D.E., and Gillespie, J.H. 1970. Feline viruses: Isolation, characterization, and pathogenicity of a feline reovirus. Am. J. Vet. Res. 31:11–20.

Equine Reovirus Infection

Antibodies to reovirus serotypes 1, 2, and 3 have been found in horses with respiratory disease and also in healthy horses from West Germany, the Netherlands, England, and Belgium. The incidence in 415 individual and 184 paired serum samples was 23 percent to serotype 1, 7 percent to serotype 2, and 50 percent to serotype 3 (Thein and Mayr 1974). Subsequent serologic surveys in the United States (Conner, Kita, et al. 1984), Chile (Reinhardt et al. 1983), and Canada (Sturm et al. 1980) reported the occurrence of antibodies to the three reovirus types. The incidence for the three types varied markedly in each country.

In a respiratory outbreak among horses in an Arabian stud, both reovirus types 1 and 3 were isolated. The horses coughed and had an ocular discharge but no fever. Experimental horses inoculated with reovirus types 1 and 3

showed typical signs of illness, and specificity was confirmed virologically and serologically. Further studies with these two isolates confirmed that they produce an upper respiratory infection and conjunctivitis in experimental horses, but the disease is much less severe (Conner, Gillespie, et al. 1984). The horses were maintained in isolation units and were not under stress, perhaps accounting for the less severe disease. All horses except one seroconverted.

Reovirus type 3 was isolated from the feces of a foal with diarrhea (Conner, Kita, et al. 1984). Attempts to produce enteric disease in neonatal or older foals with this isolate failed (Conner, Gillespie, et al. 1984), but this strain did produce mild upper respiratory disease and conjunctivitis in experimental horses and ponies. There was little or no protection against subsequent inoculation with the homologous reovirus type 3 strain. The characteristics of this enteric isolate were typical of reovirus (Conner, Kita, et al. 1984).

Equine reoviruses are respiratory pathogens of minor significance in horses under ordinary circumstances.

REFERENCES

Conner, M., Gillespie, J., Schiff, E., Holmes, D., Frey, M., and Quick, S. 1984. Experimental infection of horses and ponies by oral and nasal routes with New York State reovirus type 3 and Germany reovirus types 1 and 3 equine isolates. Zentralbl. Veterinärmed. [B] 31:707–717.
Conner, M., Kita, A., Quick, S., Schiff, E., Joubert, J., and Gillespie, J.H. 1984. Isolation and characteristics of an equine reovirus type 3 and an antibody prevalence survey to reoviruses in horses located in New York State. Vet. Microbiol. 9:15–25.
Reinhardt, G., Polette, M., and Yevenes, J.R. 1983. Serological study on equine reoviruses on two regions of southern Chile. Zentralbl. Veterinärmed. [B] 30:195–202.
Sturm, R.T., Lang, G.H., and Mitchell, W.R. 1980. Prevalence of reovirus 1, 2, and 3 antibodies in Ontario racehorses. Can. Vet. J. 21:206–209.
Thein, P., and Mayr, A. 1974. Studies on significance of reovirus infections for respiratory diseases in horses. (In German.) Zentralbl. Veterinärmed. [B] 21:219–233.

Avian Reovirus Infection

Most chicken reoviruses have been recovered from feces or from rectal swabs, but on two occasions reoviruses were isolated from the trachea (Kawamura et al. 1965). Reoviruses were isolated from the intestinal tracts of turkeys with bluecomb disease in widely separated geographic areas of the United States and Canada (Deshmukh et al. 1968). A reovirus (strain WVU-2937) is responsible for viral arthritis in chickens. At present five avian reovirus serotypes are recognized. Many isolates have been made, but much more study is required to establish the precise number of avian reovirus serotypes.

Three reovirus serotypes related to the human reovirus serotypes 1, 2, and 3, as demonstrated by hemagglutination-inhibition, complement-fixation, serum-neutralization, and agar-gel diffusion tests, were isolated from chicks with severe cloacal pasting (Deshmukh and Pomeroy 1969a). No clinical signs were seen in chickens inoculated orally or intravenously with three chicken serotypes isolated by Kawamura (1968). Attempts to reproduce cloacal pasting in chicks maintained in isolation with two reovirus isolates from chicks with cloacal chick disease were successful but inconsistent. The chicks in which cloacal pasting developed were depressed and lost weight. In contrast, cloacal pasting failed to develop in germ-free chicks. Day-old turkey poults also failed to show signs or lesions after virus inoculation with these cloacal isolates (Deshmukh and Pomeroy 1969b, Deshmukh et al. 1969).

The properties of avian reoviruses generally are consistent with reoviruses isolated from other species (Kawamura et al. 1965). A major difference is the lack of hemagglutinins that are characteristic of mammalian reoviruses. Avian reoviruses produce pocks on the chorioallantoic membrane of embryonated chicken eggs. The 7-day-old embryos die when inoculated by the chorioallantoic membrane, yolk sac, and chorioallantoic cavity routes. These findings were extended by Deshmukh and Pomeroy (1969a), who observed embryo stunting and necrosis of the liver with two of their strains. Two reovirus strains associated with chick cloacal disease produced a syncytial type of cytopathic effect in whole chicken embryo primary cell culture, although the virus titer was not high (Deshmukh and Pomeroy 1969b). Plaques also are produced in this type of culture. A similar cytopathic affect was observed in chicken embryo kidney cell cultures but not seen in cultures of bovine fetal kidney, liver, endocardial, or corneal cells.

There have been reports that isolates of avian reovirus cause viral arthritis (infectious tenosynovitis) in chickens (Menendez et al. 1975, Olson and Sahu 1975, Sahu and Olson 1975, Van DerHeide and Kalbac 1975). The disease is characterized by tenosynovitis with a generalized infection that largely subsides in 2 weeks but may persist in the tendons, oviduct, and intestinal tract for up to 30 days. Isolation in chick kidney cell culture is more reliable than fluorescent antibody tests for detection of the virus that causes the arthritis (Menendez et al. 1975). Virus is found in embryos of eggs 8 to 12 days after inoculation of hens (Van DerHeide and Kalbac 1975) but not in chicks hatched from eggs laid 12 to 35 days after inoculation of the breeders (Menendez et al. 1975). Maternal antibodies protect progeny for at least 3 weeks after oral administration of virus, but subcutaneous injection overrides maternal immunity (Van DerHeide et al. 1976). Viral isolates that can experimentally produce viral arthritis have a common agar-gel precipitin line (Sahu and Olson, 1975). On the basis of the plaque reduction test in primary chicken kidney cells, the viruses in the group were classified into four major serotypes (Sahu and Olson 1975).

In summary, five avian reovirus serotypes have been incriminated in the production of disease. Selected strains are shown to cause one or more of the following disorders: (1) tenosynovitis (viral arthritis) with a generalized infection in chicks; (2) osteopetrosis, principally in broilers; (3) maladsorption syndrome (characterized by stunting and leg weakness) in chicks; (4) enteronephritis in turkeys; (5) generalized infection (characterized by necrotic foci in liver spleen and kidney) in Muscovy ducks; (6) chick enteritis; and (7) chick embryo death. Protective antibodies are formed as a result of natural disease or vaccination with commercial vaccine; however, the vaccine strain apparently does not protect against all reoviral pathogens isolated from field outbreaks of diseases.

REFERENCES

Deshmukh, D.R., and Pomeroy, B.S. 1969a. Avian reoviruses. I. Isolation and serological characterization. II. Physiochemical characterization and classification. Avian Dis. 13:239–243.

Deshmukh, D.R., and Pomeroy, B.S. 1969b. Avian reoviruses. III. Infectivity and egg transmission. Avian Dis. 13:427–439.

Deshmukh, D.R., Larson, C.T. and Pomeroy, B.S. 1968. Characterization of viruses isolated from turkeys with bluecomb disease. J. Am. Vet. Med. Assoc. 152:1346.

Deshmukh, D.R., Sayed, H.I., and Pomeroy, B.S. 1969. Avian reoviruses. IV. Relationship to human reoviruses. Avian Dis. 13:16–22.

Kawamura, H. 1968. Quoted by L. Rosen in S. Gard, C. Hallauer, and K.F. Meyer, eds., Virology Monographs, vol. 1. Springer-Verlag, New York. Pp. 73–107.

Kawamura, H., Shimizu, F., Maeda, T., and Tsubahara, H. 1965. Avian adenovirus: Its properties and serological classification. Natl. Inst. Anim. Health Q. 5:115.

Menendez, N.A., Calnek, B.W., and Cowan, B.S. 1975. Localization of avian reovirus (FPO isolant) in tissues of mature chickens. Avian Dis. 19:112.

Olson, N.O., and Sahu, S.P. 1975. Avian viral arthritis: Antigenic types and immune response. Am. J. Vet. Res. 36:545–547.

Sahu, S.P., and Olson N.O. 1975. Comparison of the characteristics of avian reoviruses isolated from the digestive and respiratory tract, with viruses isolated from the synovia. Am. J. Vet. Res. 36:847–850.

Van DerHeide, L., and Kalbac, M. 1975. Infectious tenosynovitis (viral arthritis): Characterization of a Connecticut viral isolant as a reovirus and evidence of viral egg transmission by reovirus-infected broiler breeders. Avian Dis. 19:683–688.

Van DerHeide, L., Kalbac, M. and Hall, W.C. 1976. Infectious tenosynovitis (viral arthritis): Influences of maternal antibodies on the development of tenosynovitis lesions after experimental infection by day-old chickens with tenosynovitis virus. Avian Dis. 20:641–648.

The Genus *Rotavirus*

A wide range of mammals, including calves, piglets, lambs, foals, rabbits, deer, pronghorn antelope, monkeys, cats, dogs and humans, are infected with rotaviruses (Baldwin 1983, Carmichael and Pollock 1979, Eugster and Sidwa 1979, Flewett and Woode 1978). Frequently, diarrheal animal feces that contain rotavirus also contain other viruses.

The resemblance of rotaviruses to reoviruses was recognized soon after rotaviruses were first identified (Banfield et al. 1968, Derbyshire and Woode 1978). Bovine rotavirus (Fernelius et al. 1972) and porcine rotavirus (Lecce et al. 1976) were initially described as reoviruslike agents. As more information on basic rotavirus properties was gained, it became clear that these organisms were sufficiently different to justify their classification in a separate genus. The name *Rotavirus* was recommended because the virion resembles a small wheel with short spikes and a narrow rim.

Rotaviruses are not related antigenically to the members of the other two genera in the family. The virions, 65nm in diameter with a double-capsid shell, share a common antigen in the inner capsid, demonstrable by complement fixation, immunofluorescence, immunodiffusion, and immune electron microscopy (Flewett and Woode 1978). Rotaviruses from various animal species can be distinguished by a virus-neutralization test. Investigators testing a number of isolates found no cross-neutralization between the bovine and ovine rotaviruses (Snodgrass et al. 1976) or among human, porcine, murine, and bovine strains (Thouless et al. 1977). In the latter comparative studies, some viruses showed a degree of cross-neutralization, which was restricted to high concentrations of antibody; homologous titers were eight- to ten-fold higher than heterologous titers. Some degree of specificity can be shown for the outer capsid layer, but this does not correlate entirely with neutralization specificity (Schoub et al. 1977; Woode, Bridger, Jones, et al. 1976). The serologic specificity of neutralization is associated with infectivity and thus with outer capsid polypeptides (Schoub et al. 1977, Thouless et al. 1977), and it can be correlated with certain RNA virion segments of varying electrophoretic mobility and with the glycosylated polypeptides (Rodger et al. 1977) of the outer capsid for which the RNA may code.

Present evidence suggests there are 7 immunogenic serotypes of rotaviruses which infect domestic animals and humans. A discussion of these can be found in the section titled "Properties of the Virus."

The importance of rotaviruses in the etiology of diarrheal disease in young animals worldwide has been well established. Further, transmission of human, bovine, porcine, and equine strains to calves, monkeys, and pigs has been confirmed. Not all strains are transferable among mammalian species, and virulence depends on the host in which the strain is experimentally cultured (Woode 1976). Biological differences among strains may be reflected in serologic differences, but these must await more extensive study of many rotavirus strains from various susceptible hosts.

The importance of rotaviruses as a natural cause of diarrhea in other domestic animals such as dogs, cats, and goats awaits further investigation.

The natural history of rotavirus diseases in humans, domestic animals, and others is so similar that, in general, infections from organisms in this genus can be treated as a single entity. Exceptions or differences among the species will be presented. In general, the format used by Woode and Crouch (1978) will be followed for rotavirus diseases of cattle, pigs, sheep, horses, and dogs. The literature on diseases in cattle, humans, sheep, and pigs is particualarly voluminous; for the reader interested in more detailed information, rotavirus infections in these four species are covered in three excellent review articles (Estes et al. 1983, Flewett and Woode 1978, Kurstak et al. 1981).

Viruses that resemble rotaviruses in physical and chemical characteristics and in tropism for enterocytes, but which are antigenically distinct, have recently been reported in swine and chickens. Bohl et al. (1982) have suggested that these antigenically distinct organisms be called pararotaviruses. They may eventually constitute a separate subgroup within the *Rotavirus* genus. The pararotavirus pathogens can be distinguished from the Rotavirus group in all animal species only by immunological means and not by electron microscopy. The signs of illness are indistinguishable from rotavirus infection.

Character of the Disease. Rotaviruses have been isolated from feces of neonatal calves, foals, pigs, dogs, and lambs with diarrhea. The disease is sometimes severe and fatal in such young animals. Infections occur at all ages; even adult cattle (Woode and Bridger 1975) and horses (Conner and Darlington 1980) are sometimes afflicted.

As a rule rotavirus infection is a sudden and rapidly spreading epizootic in domestic animals. A high percentage of a population may be affected by disease. Many horses have subclinical infection. The incubation period of the disease is 18 to 96 hours and is followed by depression, diarrhea, and sometimes a fever. The disease in calves, pigs, lambs, and foals usually becomes apparent some time between 3 days and 15 weeks after birth.

In all species rotavirus infects the epithelial cells of the

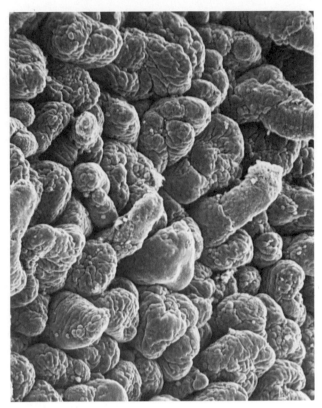

Figure 49.4. Scanning electron micrograph of lower ileum, from a gnotobiotic calf infected with bovine rotavirus. Shortened villi are covered by irregular-sized epithelial cells. Tips of several villi are denuded. × 100. (Courtesy C. A. Mebus, Plum Island Animal Disease Center, U.S. Dept. of Agriculture).

absorptive portion of the villus, and not crypt cells. Desquamation of infected cells is followed by shortening of the villi and proliferation of the crypt cells (Figure 49.4). The epithelial cells in gnotobiotic lambs given human rotavirus contain cytoplasmic vesicles, and rotavirus is observed in these and subepithelial phagocytic cells.

In calves on a total milk diet, feces are usually brilliant yellow to white, not always putrid, and similar to those of classic milk scours. In other calves, feces may be watery and brown, gray, or light green with fresh blood and mucus. The color appears to depend on the diet. If diarrhea is prolonged, dehydration becomes apparent and the calf may die within 4 to 7 days. Severely ill calves usually recover after administration of glucose and saline mixtures instead of milk. Continued feeding of milk is harmful and probably accounts for the severe epizootics in calves maintained in a cow-calf operation. Inclement weather complicates an outbreak, as many calves contract severe pneumonia after the onset of diarrhea and die 2 to 3 weeks later.

In pigs there is marked weight loss associated with severe diarrhea. Vomiting and other signs of illness often precede the diarrhea. Milk should be withdrawn from the diet of suckling or newly weaned pigs and replaced with glucose and saline feedings. A drop of 10 to 20 degrees in ambient temperature increases mortality.

Dual infection in gnotobiotic pigs given porcine rotavirus and transmissible gastroenteritis (TGE) virus produced a more severe disease (Woode and Crouch 1978). Another set of animal experiments showed that rotavirus infection did not interfere with the virulence of the TGE virus.

In lambs the signs of illness are similar to those described for foals, calves, and piglets. Viral replication takes place in the enterocytes of the small intestine throughout its length in fatal cases and may extend into the large intestine. The pathogenesis is similar to transmissible gastroenteritis in pigs. Diarrhea causes a disordered sodium transport system with a net extracellular fluid-to-lumen flux of sodium ions. Because villous tip cells are rich in thymidine kinase rather than sucrase, they have an immature enzyme profile similar to that in crypt cells (Middleton 1978). This finding explains the accelerated migration of secretory crypts to the villi normally lined by mature enterocyte cells. The failure of enterocytes to differentiate fully as they migrate up villi appears to be a major cause of electrolyte transport defect.

In foals the illness usually begins within the first week after birth. There is profuse diarrhea with a characteristic fetid odor. The animal rapidly becomes dehydrated, and, unless fluids are given soon after disease onset, the foal may die. With proper and immediate therapy, however, death is rare. The disease usually spreads quickly to all susceptible foals and horses on the premises unless strict quarantine procedure are instituted. In young horses the disease is milder, as a rule. Most horses have antibodies (Conner and Darlington 1980).

In laboratory research on rotavirus infection the most satisfactory results are obtained with gnotobiotic animals, particularly pigs, cattle, dogs, cats, and sheep. To quantitate the effects of diarrhea caused by rotavirus disease in pigs, one group of researchers used daily weight record. Mortality in experimental pigs varied between 0 and 100 percent according to age, with some individual variation within litters (Woode, Bridger, Hall, et al. 1976). Experimentally infected pigs, calves, and lambs have a shorter period of illness than naturally infected animals. Bacteria such as pathogenic *E. coli* presumably enhance the severity of the disease.

In another study with experimental animals foal, human, or lamb rotaviruses fed to gnotobiotic pigs did not cause disease, but infection occurred and the viruses were excreted in quantities similar to those observed in pigs given virulent porcine rotavirus (Woode, Bridger, Jones, et al. 1976). Another strain of human rotavirus fed to pigs and calves produces diarrhea in the experimental animals (Mebus et al. 1976)

It has been demonstrated that equine rotavirus isolates produce diarrhea in experimentally neonatal ponies (Conner 1985, Kanitz 1976). Electron microscopy and Rotazyme tests (enzyme-linked immunosorbent assay [ELISA]) revealed virus in the feces of foals maintained in isolation units with their dams. The foals produced serum-neutralizing antibodies and transferred the virus to the mares as a silent infection that resulted in their seroconversion (Conner et al. 1983). Two separate serotypes of cell-cultured adapted strains of equine rotavirus each produced diarrhea in the majority of neonatal ponies given virus by mouth. These two serotypes cross-reacted in protection experiments in neonates (Higgins 1986).

In dogs rotaviruses have been implicated as a cause of diarrhea (Carmichael and Pollock 1979, Eugster and Sidwa 1979), although this sign is usually associated with parvovirus disease. In an experimental trial conducted by England and Poston (1980) puppies given a field isolate failed to show signs of illness, and virus was not shed in the feces. In gnotobiotic puppies a canine isolate given orally produced diarrhea and dehydration in 20 to 24 hours; examination with electron microscopy revealed that virus was present in the feces between 12 and 154 hours (Johnson, Fulton, et al. 1983). Lesions referable to the gastrointestinal tract characterized rotavirus infection in other susceptible species (e.g., cats) (Johnson, Snider, et al. 1983).

Conventional laboratory cats given a feline isolate of rotavirus failed to show signs of illness, although virus was shed in the feces. In gnotobiotic cats intestinal lesions were evident 30 to 36 hours after oral administration of a feline rotavirus. The lesions were typical of rotavirus infection (Baldwin 1983). Feline rotavirus is probably an etiological factor in diarrhea in the neonatal cat.

Properties of the Virus. Electron microscopy studies of the double-stranded RNA of the Nebraska strain of bovine rotavirus showed that the organism has four size classes of RNA in contrast to the well-described three classes of double-stranded RNA reoviruses. The RNA migration pattern for the Nebraska strain is stable, whereas there are three different RNA migration patterns in electrophoresis among human rotaviruses. These differences do not necessarily imply antigenic difference.

Rotaviruses have a distinctive outer capsid (Figure 49.5) more clearly defined than the reoviruses (Figure 49.1) and different from that of the orbiviruses, which is amorphous (Figure 49.16). In other physical and chemical characteristics rotaviruses closely parallel other genera in the family except that they have 5 to 10 structural polypeptides, whereas reoviruses and orbiviruses have 7.

At present, seven serotypes are recognized on the basis

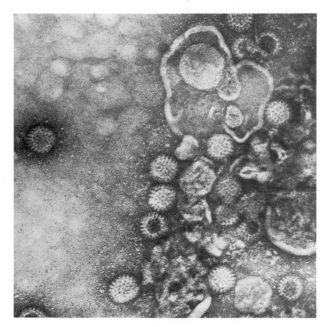

Figure 49.5. Bovine rotavirus particles in a fecal preparation. Note the sharply defined outer capsid membrane—a characteristic of rotaviruses. × 95,000. (Courtesy Alfonso Torres-Medina.)

of a ≥ 20-fold or greater difference between the titers of homologous and heterologous reciprocal neutralizing antibodies in mammals and birds (Hoshina et al. 1984). Only one serotype is found in cats. Serotypes 1 and 2 are found in humans. Serotype 3 is recognized in humans, monkeys, dogs, and horses. Serotype 4 occurs in humans and pigs. Porcine and equine rotavirus strains constitute serotype 5; bovine virus, serotype 6; and chicken and a turkey rotavirus are members of serotype 7. A third equine serotype (strain EID_4) has been identified by cross-neutralization tests (Conner 1985, Higgins 1986). Its relation to rotavirus serotypes 1, 2, 4, 6, and 7 is still to be determined, but it is clearly different from serotypes 3 and 5. Other serotypes will probably be demonstrated in future studies.

Cultivation. There was no serious interest in the propagation of rotaviruses in cell culture until bovine rotavirus (Nebraska strain) was recognized as a cause of neonatal calf diarrhea and was adapted to cell-culture passage in fetal bovine kidney cells. With the production of plaques the cytopathic effect of this virus was readily recognizable (Mebus et al. 1971). Despite this successful propagation, the adaptation of rotaviruses of various species met with little or no success until the pancreatic enzymes, trypsin and alpha-chymotrypsin, were found to be important determinants in the replication and adaptation of porcine rotaviruses in porcine kidney cell cultures (Theil et al. 1978). Specifically, trypsin (15 μg/ml) and alpha-chymotrypsin (15 μg/ml) were added to sonicated virus-

Table 49.2. Attempted propagation of equine rotavirus isolates in MA-104 cell cultures

Foal number	Electron microscopy		ELISA*–cell cultures† (Rotazyme)	
	Fecal sample	TC† virus	Visual reading	Spectrophotometer
1	+	+	+ + + +	1.89
2	+	−	+ + +	1.33
3	+	+	+ + +	1.12
4	+	+	+ + + +	1.96
5	+	+	+ + +	1.82
6	+	+	+ + + +	1.97
7	+	+	+ + + +	1.91
8	+	+	±	0.47
9	+	+	+ + + +	1.75
10	+	−	+ + + +	1.68
11	+	+	+ + + +	1.87
12	+	−	±	0.20
13	+	+	+ + + +	1.86
14	+	+	+ + +	1.26
15	+	+	+ + + +	1.91
16	+	−	+ + + +	1.61
17	+	+	+ +	0.50
18	+	−	+ + + +	1.67
19	+	+	+ +	0.63
20	+	−	+ + +	0.44
21	+	−	+ + +	1.99
22	+	+	+ + +	1.17
23	+	+	+ + + +	2.55
24	+	+	+ + +	1.11

*Virus positive control values; + + + and 0.67 negative control values; − and 0.08.
†Either fifth or seventh tissue-culture (TC) passage; + = cytopathic effect.
From Gillespie et al., 1984, courtesy of *Veterinary Microbiology*.

laden culture fluid, and this mixture was inoculated on washed monolayers of either primary or cell-line (MDPK–15) pig kidney cells. After an hour of incubation the inoculum was removed, and the monolayers were washed once to remove the residual enzymes and then maintained with serum-free medium. After 18 to 24 hours, more than 90 percent of cells contained virus, as demonstrated by fluorescent antibody procedure. This modified procedure with pancreatic enzymes made possible repeated transfers in cell cultures at 24-hour intervals. Certain influenza viruses (Lazarowitz and Choppin 1975) and paramyxoviruses (Nagai and Klenk 1977) require proteolytic cleavage of envelope glycoproteins to activate their infectivity. The pancreatic enzymes act similarly on proteins or glycoproteins in the rotavirus capsid. When replication of rotaviruses in cell cultures is unsatisfactory, the use of pancreatic enzymes or lactase, found in microvilli, as possible receptors for rotaviruses may facilitate or enhance viral reproduction.

Bovine rotavirus (Lincoln strain) formed distinct plaques in monolayers of MA-104 cells, an established rhesus monkey kidney cell line, when diethylaminoethyl dextran (100 μg/ml) and trypsin (2 μg/ml) were added (Matsuno et al. 1977). In this system discrete plaques 2 to 3 mm in diameter were formed with viral plaque titers reaching 1.5×10^7 after 3 to 4 days of incubation at 37°C; the plaques were inhibited by homologous antiserum.

Twenty-four field isolates of equine rotavirus, as determined by electron microscopy, were studied for their replication and the production of cytopathic effect in MA-104 cell cultures (Table 49.2) (Gillespie et al. 1984). Of this group, 21 isolates were cultured through the seventh passage and 3 isolates through the fifth passage. Most of the isolates produced a cytopathic effect 2 to 6 days after transfer (Figure 49.6). In some instances they were sufficiently adapted to produce with regularity a cytopathic effect at a sufficiently high dilution to provide a useful procedure for virus assay. Rotavirus particles were observed by electron microscopy in 17 of the 24 cultures, and ELISA revealed virus in 22 of 24 cultures. Successful adaptation of a high percentage of equine rotavirus field isolates depended on the availability of the

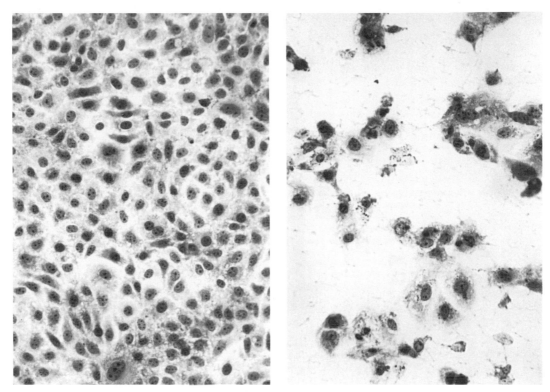

Figure 49.6. (*Left*) Uninfected MA-104 cell culture. × 141. (*Right*) Cytopathic effect in MA-104 cells infected with equine rotavirus. × 282. May-Grünwald-Giemsa stain. (From Gillespie et al., 1984, courtesy of *Veterinary Microbiology*.)

right batch of commercial trypsin to provide the appropriate virus cleavage during viral pretreatment and its use in cell culture without being toxic to the cells. An equine rotavirus produced plaques in MA-104 cells (Figure 49.7). Tissue-cultured adapted equine rotavirus strains attained titers of ±10^6 $TCID_{50}$/ml based on a cytopathic effect in MA-104 cell culture (Gillespie et al. 1984).

Epizootiology. The duration of immunity is not known, nor is the length of the virus persists in the feces after illness (Conner 1985, Conner et al. 1983, Higgins 1986). The effectiveness of cell-mediated immunity in individuals apparently influences its persistence. Because immunity may be only partial and temporary, adults can become diseased from infected neonates. As the incidence of the disease is extremely high and a host may be reinfected, the disease probably is perpetuated through viral persistence within an animal species. Interspecies infection may be an important factor in disease transmission, since three rotavirus serotypes occur in more than one animal species, including humans. It is well documented that rotaviruses of one species can provide another means for transmission and viral existence in nature.

Immunity. Resistance to rotavirus disease appears to be mediated by local immunity at the epithelial surface of the small intestine (Snodgrass and Wells 1976a). Unfortunately, in calves the passive protection afforded by the

Figure 49.7. Plaque assay test utilizing virus dilutions of 10^{-2}, 10^{-3}, and 10^{-4} of tissue-cultured equine rotavirus strain EID_1 that produces small plaques, >10^5 plaque-forming units/ml. (From Gillespie et al., 1984, courtesy of *Veterinary Microbiology*.).

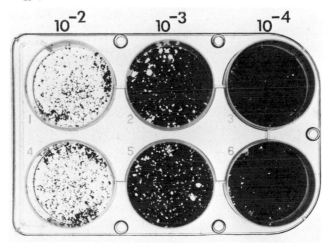

colostrum has limited value. Some dams have low levels of protective antibody in the colostrum; in other immune dams the antibody in the colostrum rapidly declines tenfold 24 to 48 hours after birth. A similar situation occurs with pigs. Breastfed children in Bangladesh, however, had virtually no rotavirus diarrhea. Using the ELISA blocking test, Yolken et al. (1978) found a high level of antibody was found in breast milk, and the amount fell to lower but detectable levels for 1 year after birth. Totterdell et al. (1980) found that factors other than the rotavirus antibodies in expressed human milk are important in preventing rotavirus infection in newborns. These factors have not been identified in the milk of domestic animals. There obviously is a difference in hosts. Calves are protected when fed colostrum with rotavirus antibody of high content, but it must be given continually in the face of constant viral exposure. The same is true of lambs infected with lamb or human rotavirus and fed daily with sheep colostrum or human gamma globulin (Snodgrass and Wells 1976b, Snodgrass et al. 1977).

There is no direct correlation between rotavirus antibody in serum and protection in domestic animals, yet the antibody classes and subclasses in serum, and particularly in body fluids, are relevant to rotavirus immunity. After rotavirus infection ensues, IgM appears early in the course of the disease and persists during the disease syndrome. IgG usually is correlated with history of exposure. Secretory IgA antibody probably plays as important a role in protection as it does in the case of transmissible gastroenteritis in pigs (Bohl et al. 1972, 1982; Hess and Bachmann 1981). Natural or experimental infection by the oral route produces higher IgA levels in the colostrum and milk than in the serum and affords greater protection than parenteral injection of virus. IgG was shown to be protective in calves when antibody was present in high concentrations in the colostrum and milk (Snodgrass et al. 1980). Cell-mediated immunity also may have a significant role in protection against intestinal infections, but its mechanism is unclear except that proper T-cell function is essential (Welliver and Ogra 1978).

Rotaviruses isolated from the various species do not show optimal cross neutralization activity. Despite this fact there may be some degree of cross-protection between some species. In one study calves were inoculated with foal rotaviruses and then exposed to a bovine strain. The foal rotaviruses did not induce neutralizing antibodies to the bovine strain, but 30 percent of the calves were protected against a virulent bovine rotavirus. Similar results were observed in pigs after inoculation with bovine or foal rotavirus. A bovine strain inoculated into calf fetuses induced resistance to diarrheal disease caused by

the human type 2 virus as well as the homologous bovine virus (Wyatt et al. 1979).

Diagnosis. For routine diagnosis of rotavirus infection there are various techniques such as tissue culture, ELISA, immunocytochemical unlabeled soluble enzyme peroxidase-antiperoxidase method (Graham and Estes 1979), immunofluorescence test, electron microscopy, cross-electrophoresis, or complement fixation (Flewett 1978). Specificity of rotaviruses of the various animal species can be determined by a cross neutralization test in cell culture, which is the only method of differentiating the rotaviruses and pararotaviruses.

When new diarrheal epizootics or valuable neonatal animals are involved, fecal specimens should be prepared and examined by electron microscopy for organisms other than rotavirus (Flewett 1978). Many times, one or more other potentially viral pathogens, such as coronavirus, adenovirus, and/or parvovirus, may be detected. If mixed viral infections are found, this knowledge is useful in determining appropriate control, treatment, and preventive measures.

Prevention and Control. Neonatal diarrheal disease caused by rotaviruses is extremely serious, often fatal, unless treatment is initiated within hours after onset. It must be reemphasized that protection against intestinal disease is mediated by a system that operates largely in the intestinal tract. As a consequence, colostrum initially is extremely important in the control of this disease. The mother's colostrum and milk must contain reasonably high levels of antibody to the rotavirus involved, and the infant must be fed every day during the crucial period of susceptibility. Snodgrass et al. (1976) used various regimens in lambs, such as daily feeding of colostrum with high antibody content throughout the period of greatest risk, thus providing clinical protection while reducing the degree of viral multiplication and permitting development of active immunity. Serum or serum products with high antibody titer could replace colostrum but they are not commercially available. Vaccination of ewes before conception may also be a logical approach because it increases the antibody levels in colostrum and milk.

Active immunization of the newborn is another approach to providing protection. At present, there is only one licensed vaccine for rotavirus disease in the United States—the bovine attenuated tissue-cultured vaccine given to day-old calves (Mebus et al. 1973). There is some question about its efficacy (Acres and Radostits 1976), as no significant differences were observed in the incidence or severity of rotavirus-associated diarrhea between calves given a placebo (76) and vaccinated calves (74) in two endemically infected herds (Leeuw et al.

1980). Mebus et al. (1973) also found that a combined attenuated vaccine containing rotavirus and coronavirus provides some protection against diarrheal disease. Because more than one immunogenic serotype has been described for other species, the present bovine vaccine virus may not protect against all field rotavirus strains, and some failures may result.

The Disease in Humans. Rotavirus infection in infants is a common and serious malady. Two different serotypes (perhaps three) that do not provide cross-protection exist in humans. Because human rotavirus produces disease in newborn monkeys, calves, and pigs, it would not be surprising to find that animal rotaviruses cause infection in humans.

REFERENCES

Acres, S.D., and Radostits, O.M. 1976. The efficacy of a modified live reo-like virus vaccine and an *E. coli* bacterin for prevention of acute undifferentiated neonatal diarrhea of beef calves. Can. Vet. J. 17:197–212.

Baldwin, C.A. 1983. Feline rotavirus. M.S. thesis, Cornell University, Ithaca, N.Y.

Banfield, W.G., Kasnic, G., and Blackwell, J.H. 1968. Further observations on the virus of epizootic diarrhea of infant mice. An electron microscopic study. Virology 36:411–421.

Bohl, E.H., Gupta, R.K.P., Olquin, M.V.F., and Saif, L.J. 1972. Antibody responses in serum, colostrum, and milk of swine after infection or vaccination with transmissible gastroenteritis virus. Infect. Immun. 6:289–301.

Bohl, E.H., Saif, L.T., Thiel, K.W., Agnes, A.G., and Cross, R.F. 1982. Porcine pararotavirus detection, differentiation from rotavirus and pathogenesis in gnotobiotic pigs. J. Clin. Microbiol. 15:312–319.

Carmichael, L.E., and Pollock, R.V. 1979. Viral diseases of puppies. Gaines Progress. Pp. 1–6.

Conner, M.E. 1985. Studies of equine reovirus and rotavirus. Ph.D. dissertation, Cornell University, Ithaca, N.Y.

Conner, M.E., and Darlington, R.W. 1980. Rotavirus infection in foals. Am. J. Vet. Res. 41:1699–1703.

Conner, M.E., Gillespie, J.H., Schiff, E.I., and Frey, M.S. 1983. Detection of rotavirus in horses with and without diarrhea by electron microscopy. Cornell Vet. 73:280–287.

Derbyshire, J.B., and Woode, G.N. 1978. Classification of rotaviruses: Report form the World Health Organization/Food and Agriculture Organization Comparative Virology Program. J. Am. Vet. Med. Assoc. 173:519–521.

England, J.J., and Poston, R.P. 1980. Electron microscopic identification and subsequent isolation of a rotavirus from a dog with fatal neonatal diarrhea. Am. J. Vet. Res. 41:782–783.

Estes, M.K., Palmer, E.L., and Obijeski, J.F. 1983. Rotaviruses: A review. Curr. Top. Microbiol. Immunol. 105:123–184.

Eugster, A.K., and Sidwa, T. 1979. Rotaviruses in diarrheic feces of a dog. Vet. Med./Small Anim. Clin. 74:817–819.

Fernelius, A.L., Ritchie, A.E., Classick, L.G., Norman, J.O., and Mebus, C.A. 1972. Cell culture adaptation and propagation of a reovirus-like agent in calf diarrhea from a field outbreak in Nebraska. Arch. Gesam. Virusforsch. 37:114–130.

Flewett, T.H. 1978. Electron microscopy in the diagnosis of infectious diarrhea. J. Am. Vet. Med. Assoc. 173:538–543.

Flewett, T.H., and Woode, G.M. 1978. The rotaviruses. Brief review. Arch. Virol. 57:1–23.

Gillespie, J.H., Kalica, A., Conner, M., Schiff, E., Barr, M., Holmes, D., and Frey, M. 1984. The isolation, propagation, and characterization of tissue-cultured equine rotaviruses. Vet. Microbiol. 9:1–14.

Graham, D.Y., and Estes, M.K. 1979. Comparison of methods for immunocytochemical detection of rotavirus infections. Infect. Immun. 26:686–689.

Hess, R.G., and Bachman, P.A. 1981. Distribution of antibodies to rotavirus in serum and lacteal secretions of naturally infected swine and their suckling pigs. Am. J. Vet. Res. 42:1149–1152.

Higgins, W. 1986. Field and laboratory studies of equine viral pathogens. Ph.D, dissertation, Cornell University, Ithaca, N.Y.

Hoshina, Y., Wyatt, R.G., Greenberg, H.B., Flores, J., and Kapikian, A. 1984. Serotypic similarity and diversity of rotaviruses of mammalian and avian origin as studied by plaque-reduction neutralization. J. Infect. Dis. 149:694–702.

Johnson, C.A., Fulton, R.W., Henk, W.G., and Snider, T.G. 1983. Inoculation of neonatal gnotobiotic dogs with a canine rotavirus. Am. J. Vet. Res. 44:1682–1686.

Johnson, C.A., Snider, T.G., Fulton, R.W., and Cho, D. 1983. Gross and light microscopic lesions in neonatal gnotobiotic dogs inoculated with a canine rotavirus. Am. J. Vet. Res. 44:1687–1693.

Kanitz, C. 1976. Identification of an equine rotavirus as a cause of neonatal foal diarrhea. Annu. Proc. Am. Assoc. Equine Pract. 22:155–163.

Kurstak, E., Kurstak, C., van den Hurk, J., and Morrisset, M. 1981. Animal rotaviruses. In E. Kurstak and C. Kurstak, eds., Comparative Diagnosis of Viral Diseases, vol. 4, pt. B. Academic Press, New York. Pp. 105–148.

Lazarowitz, S.G., and Choppin, P.W., 1975. Enhancement of the infectivity of influenza A + B viruses by proteolytic cleavage of the hemagglutinin polypeptide. Virology 68:440–454.

Lecce, J.G., King, M.W., and Mock, R. 1976. Reovirus-like agent associated with fatal diarrhea in neonatal pigs. Infect. Immun. 14:816–825.

Leeuw, P.W., Ellens, D.J., Talmon, F.P., Zimmer, G., and Kommery, R. 1980. Rotavirus infections in calves: Efficacy of oral vaccination in endemically infected herds. Res. Vet. Sci. 29:142–147.

Matsuno, S., Inouye, S., and Konu, R. 1977. Plaque assay of neonatal calf diarrhea virus and the neutralizing antibody in human sera. J. Clin. Microbiol. 5:1–4.

Mebus, C.A., Kono, M., Underdahl, N.R., and Twiehaus, M.J., 1971. Cell culture propagation of neonatal calf diarrhea (scours) virus. Can. Vet. J. 12:69–72.

Mebus, C.A., White, R.G., Bass, E.P., and Twiehaus, M.J., 1973. Immunity to neonatal calf diarrhea virus. J. Am. Vet. Med. Assoc. 163:880–883.

Mebus, C.A., Wyatt, R.G., Sharpee, R.L., Sereno, M.M., Kalica, A.R., Kapikian, A.Z., and Twiehaus, M.J. 1976. Diarrhea in gnotobiotic calves caused by the reovirus-like agent of human infantile gastroenteritis. Infect. Immun. 14:471–474.

Middleton, P.J. 1978. Pathogenesis of rotaviral infection. J. Am. Vet. Med. Assoc. 173:544–545.

Nagai, Y., and Klenk, H.D. 1977. Activation of precursors to both glycoproteins of Newcastle disease virus by proteolytic cleavage. Virology 77:125–134.

Rodger, S.M., Schnagl, R.D., and Holmes, I.H. 1977. Further biochemical characterization, including the detection of surface glycoproteins, of human, calf, and simian rotaviruses. J. Virol. 24:91–98.

Schoub, B.D., Lecatsas, G., and Prozesky, O.W., 1977. Antigenic relationship between human and simian rotaviruses. J. Med. Microbiol. 10:1–6.

Snodgrass, D.R., and Wells, P.W. 1976a. The immunoprophylaxis of rotavirus infection in lambs. J. Am. Vet. Med. Assoc. 173:565.

Snodgrass, D.R., and Wells, P.W. 1976b. Rotavirus infection in lambs: Studies on passive protection. Arch. Virol. 52:201–205.

Snodgrass, D.R., Herring, J.A., and Gray, E.W. 1976. Experimental rotavirus infection in lambs. J. Comp. Pathol. 86:637–642.

Snodgrass, D.R., Madeley, D.R., Wells, P.W., and Angus, K.W.

1977. Human rotavirus in lambs: Infection and passive protection. Infect. Immun. 16:268–270.

Snodgrass, D.R., Fahey, K.J., Wells, P.W., Campbell, I., and White-law, A. 1980. Passive immunity in calf rotavirus infections: Maternal vaccination increases and prolongs immunoglobulin G₁ antibody secretion in milk. Infect. Immun. 28:344–349.

Theil, K.W., Bohl, E.H., and Saif, L.J. 1978. Techniques for rotaviral propagation. J. Am. Vet. Med. Assoc. 173:548–551.

Thouless, M.E., Bryden, A.S., Flewett, T.H., Woode, G.N., Bridges, J.C., Snodgrass, D.R., and Herring, J.A. 1977. Serological relationships between rotaviruses from different species as studied by complement fixation and neutralization. Arch. Virol. 53:287–294.

Totterdell, B.M., Chrystie, I.L., and Banatvala, J.E. 1980. Cord blood and breast milk antibodies in neonatal rotavirus infection. Br. Med. J. 280:828–830.

Welliver, R.C., and Ogra, P.L. 1978. Importance of local immunity in enteric infection. J. Am. Vet. Med. Assoc. 173:560–564.

Woode, G.N. 1976. Acute diarrhea in childhood. Ciba Found. Symp. 42:251.

Woode, G.N., and Bridger, J.C. 1975. Viral enteritis of calves. Vet. Rec. 96:85–88.

Woode, G.N., and Crouch, C.F. 1978. Naturally occurring and experimentally induced rotaviral infections of domestic and laboratory animals. J. Am. Vet. Med. Assoc. 173:520–526.

Woode, G.N., Bridger, J., Hall, G.A., Jones, J.M., and Jackson, G. 1976. The isolation of reovirus-like agents (rotaviruses) from acute gastroenteritis of piglets. J. Med. Microbiol. 9:203–209.

Woode, G.N., Bridger, J.C., Jones, J.M., Flewett, T.H., Bryden, A.S., Davis, H.A., and White, G.B.B. 1976. Morphological and antigenic relationships between viruses (rotaviruses) from acute gastroenteritis of children, calves, piglets, mice, and foals. Infect. Immun. 14:804–810.

Wyatt, R.G., Mebus, C.A., Yolken, R.H., Kalica, A.R., James, H.P. Jr., Kapikian, A.Z., and Chanock, R.M. 1979. Rotaviral immunity in gnotobiotic calves: Heterologous resistance to human virus induced by bovine virus. Science 203:548–550.

Yolken, R.H., Barbour, B.A., Wyatt, R.G., and Kapikian, A.Z., 1978. Immune response to rotaviral infection—Measurement of enzyme immunoassay. J. Am. Vet. Med. Assoc. 173:552–554.

The Genus *Orbivirus*

The genus *Orbivirus* contains some important pathogens, including those that cause African horsesickness, bluetongue in sheep and cattle, epizootic hemorrhagic disease in deer, and Colorado tick fever in human. Morphologically the particles of infectious bursal disease (IBD) virus of chickens, infectious pancreatitis necrosis (IPN) virus of salmonid fish, and bluetongue virus are similar, but serologically they are not related. At present the chicken and trout viruses are tentatively assigned to the genus *Birnavirus*. Many orbiviruses have been found in wild birds but do not have any known significance in domestic animals.

The outer capsid of members in the genus is indistinct. The inner capsid has icosahedral symmetry (T-3 plus complex secondary symmetry). The particles, 60 to 80 nm in diameter, are partially resistant to ether; most are sensitive to acid pH (except IBD and IPN viruses, which are very resistant to acid pH). Member viruses contain double-stranded RNA, but there may be significant differences in the number of segments in the strands of the viruses now placed in this genus.

African Horsesickness

SYNONYMS: Equine plaque, *pestis equorum*; abbreviation, AHS

African horsesickness, an acute or subacute infectious disease of solipeds, occurs principally in southern and central Africa and along the Nile Valley in Egypt, although it has raged through the Middle East and parts of Asia since 1944 when cases were diagnosed in Palestine, Syria, Lebanon, and Transjordan. The disease occurs in warm, humid regions, particularly during unusually wet seasons. It is found mostly in relatively flat coastal plains, but it also occurs in valleys at considerably high altitudes. It is definitely a seasonal disease, occurring mostly in the late summer and disappearing quickly after frosts come. The disease remains a threat to Europe and the Soviet Union. It is unknown in the Western Hemisphere. With modern transport, however, no country is safe from infection as the vector can survive plane trips.

Horses are most susceptible and constitute the greatest number of fatalities. Mules are considerably more resistant than horses. Donkeys in most parts of Africa are quite resistant, but Alexander (1948) found donkeys in the Near East to be fairly susceptible. Outbreaks have been reported in zebras, but generally this species is highly resistant. There have been a few reports of sickness and death in dogs, the disease usually being attributed to ingestion of infected horse meat. In the locales from which these reports were made, dogs are not often infected by insects. Angora goats are known to be susceptible. Elephants and zebras are possible reservoirs for virus (Davies and Otieno 1977).

Character of the Disease. Some cases are very mild, recovery occurring in 3 to 5 days. There is fever (105°F or higher), inappetence, redness of the conjunctivae, and labored breathing. The highly acute form that accounts for most deaths is the pulmonary type in which there is severe lung edema and the victims literally drown in their own fluids. Coughing, severe dyspnea, fever, and copious foamy discharge from the nostrils are the principal signs of this form of the disease. A somewhat more chronic form is characterized by heart lesions and edema of the head and neck tissues. Many of these animals recover. A combination of both disease forms is most commonly observed in field cases.

The incubation period generally is about 7 to 9 days in the experimental disease, but occasionally it is much

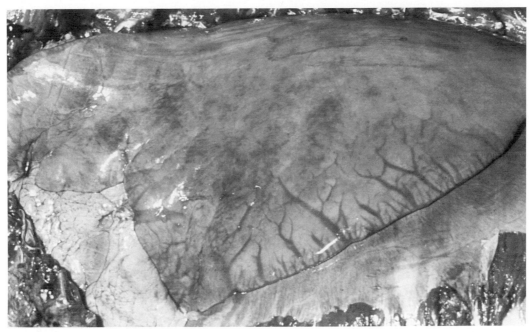

Figure 49.8. African horsesickness. The lung is distended, and there is severe pulmonary edema, which is manifested by the greatly widened interlobular septa and rounded edge. (Courtesy D. A. Gregg, Plum Island Animal Disease Center, U.S. Dept. of Agriculture.)

shorter or longer. No new cases of the natural disease have been noted later than 9 days after the first severe frost.

In the severe forms of the disease the course is rarely longer than 5 days, since the animal generally dies within that time period. In the milder forms the course may be several weeks. Mortality varies considerably. In some outbreaks in which the agent is highly virulent the death rate may be as high as 90 to 95 percent. In others it may be as low as 25 percent.

The lesions depend on the severity of the disease. In the acute type the thorax generally contains several liters of fluid, and the lungs are distended with fluid (Figure 49.8). The interlobular tissue generally is separated from the alveolar portions by a yellowish infiltrate. Upon sectioning the lungs do not collapse; the surface is wet, and fluid runs out of the cut surface. The pericardial sac may contain some fluid, and subendocardial hemorrhages generally are present. There is usually some fluid in the abdominal cavity, the liver is swollen, and the intestines are reddened.

In the more chronic form, characterized by edema of the head, neck, and sometimes the shoulder region, hydropericardium generally is found, and there is hydropic degeneration of the myocardium, but the lungs and pleural cavity show only moderate edema.

Histologically, the abundance of fibrin and inflammatory cells in the edematous lung suggests that the primary lesion is an exudative pneumonia (Newsholme 1983). Lymphoid depletion and necrosis in germinal centers is present. Ultrastructural evidence of vascular injury is not apparent in edematous tissues. Virus particles or virus-associated structures are not observed in the tissues by electron microscopy.

Horses can readily be infected by parenteral injection of small amounts of blood, tissue emulsions, and bronchial secretions. The urine is infective only occasionally. The disease is transmitted irregularly by feeding, and only with large amounts of material.

In addition to naturally susceptible animals, the disease can be transmitted by inoculation to goats, ferrets, rats, guinea pigs, and mice.

Properties of the Virus. African horsesickness was first shown to be caused by a virus in 1900. Polson and Madsen (1954) suggested that there are two different-sized particles, 50.8 nm and 31.2 nm in diameter. According to Breese et al. (1969) the spherical particle has an average diameter of 49 nm in negative-stained preparations and about 71 nm with an inner-core diameter of 36 nm in thin sections. The core of African horsesickness virus (AHSV) contains RNA (Ozawa 1967) that is double-stranded. The particle has 92 capsomeres. Virus particles are shown in Figure 49.9.

The virus is stable between a pH of 6 and 10, and it survives for years in the cold in an oxalate-phenolglycerol

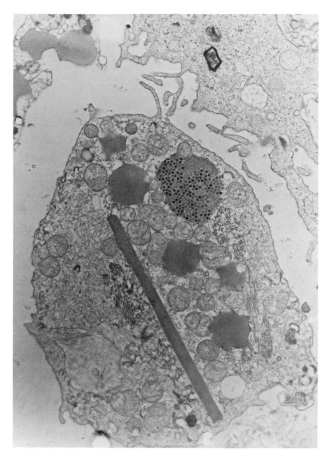

Figure 49.9. African horsesickness virus type 9 in green monkey kidney cells, 48 hours after inoculation. × 15,000. (Courtesy S. S. Breese, Plum Island Animal Disease Center, U.S. Dept. of Agriculture.)

mixture (Alexander 1935). It is resistant to ether and sodium deoxycholate but readily inactivated by a 1:1,000 dilution of formalin in 48 hours. The virus is relatively resistant to heat. The neurotropic virus is destroyed at 60°C within 15 minutes, but infective virus in tissue-culture medium persists after heating at 50°C for 3 hours or at 37°C for 37 days. At 4°C, the cultured virus retains its infectivity for a long time. The best method of storage is to freeze-dry the virus with lactone and peptone or to maintain virus suspensions or infected tissues at −70°C. Inactivated virus prepared with 0.4 percent or lower concentrations of betapropiolactone were immunogenic in guinea pigs (Parker 1975).

There are nine immunological virus types as determined by cross-neutralization tests in mice (Howell 1962). Each virus strain possesses a common complement-fixing antigen, which has a diameter of 12 nm (Polson and Madsen 1954). The virus in mouse brain tissue also hemagglutinates horse erythrocytes at pH 6.4 at 37°C for 2 hours (Pavri 1961).

Cultivation. Various cell lines such as Vero, MS (monkey kidney), baby hamster kidney (BHK), and primary cultures of BHK support replication of AHSV (Ozawa and Hazrati 1964). Not all virus serotypes produce a cytopathic effect on first passage of field specimens, but on subsequent passages characteristic cytopathic effect may be produced in 48 to 96 hours. The onset of cytopathic effect occurs soonest in the MS cell line—within 24 hours after infection in some strains (Ozawa 1967). Plaques are produced in Vero and MS cell cultures (Ozawa 1967).

Infected cell cultures have multiple inclusion bodies near the nucleus, and these bodies show immunofluorescence (Ozawa 1967). AHSV propagated in suckling mouse brains may be readily adapted to adult mice and chick embryos.

Epizootiology. Horsesickness is not directly transmissible from animal to animal. Affected animals stabled with susceptible horses do not cause outbreaks of the disease. Outbreaks usually occur in warm, damp weather, on swampy, low-lying farms, and only in horses that are pastured at night. These facts indicate that night-flying insects are the probable vectors. Certain species of *Culicoides* (midges), including *C. variipennis*, have been shown to harbor AHSV and to be capable of transmitting the infection by bite (Du Toit 1944). These insects feed at night and are believed to be the main and perhaps the only vector of the disease. Multiplication and persistence of the virus in *Aedes* mosquitoes has been demonstrated experimentally (Ozawa et al. 1966). Mules, asses, elephants, zebras, and dogs, none of which are as susceptible to the disease as horses, have been suggested as possible reservoirs of virus.

The virus may be spread by the wind.

Immunity. Animals that have recovered from horsesickness are not always permanently immune to the disease. Cases have been reported of animals having the disease a second time. Reinfection occurs because there are at least nine types of virus and immunization against one type does not fully protect against all others. Usually second attacks of the disease are mild. Immune mares convey a passive immunity to their foals, which are usually protected until they are 6 months old.

An immune serum provides passive protection from the disease for a limited time. This serum is made by hyperimmunizing recovered horses by transfusing them directly with blood from horses in the febrile stage of horsesickness. To obtain a lasting immunity, veterinarians used to give horses simultaneous injections of large doses of immune serum and small doses of virus. Fever developed in about 85 percent of these horses, in which case another dose of immune serum was given. A considerable number always contracted severe disease, and a mortality of about 4 percent was expected. This method has been abandoned in favor of vaccines.

Du Toit et al. (1933) developed a vaccine for horsesickness made from formalinized spleen pulp emulsion. Four doses were given, the first having been treated with formalin in a concentration of 1:1,000, the second in 1:2,000, the third in 1:3,000, and the fourth in 1:4,000. The results were generally satisfactory, but the immunity was not permanent.

Alexander and Du Toit (1934), Alexander (1936), and Alexander et al. (1936) reported successful immunization of horses with live vaccine made by modifying the virulence of AHSV by intracerebral passage through mice. As the virus became adapted as a neurotropic strain for mice, its virulence for mice increased, but that for horses decreased. After it had gone through more than 100 passages in mice, the virulence became fixed and the virus could no longer produce disease in horses. Because of the several immunological types, it was necessary to make fixed virus from each type. The field vaccine is manufactured from a mixture of nine viral types, because a polyvalent vaccine made from nine selected virus strains usually protects against all the types found in South Africa. A single dose containing 100 mouse-infecting doses of each type is enough to afford protection.

The mouse brain vaccines have now displaced all others for protecting horses against this disease. The immunity conferred may not be permanent, however, so exposed animals should be vaccinated annually before the horsesickness season.

Diagnosis. When AHS first appears in a country that has been free of the disease, the condition is frequently diagnosed as equine infectious arteritis, equine infectious anemia, trypanosomiasis, or anthrax because these diseases induce similar clinical signs and postmortem findings. Consequently a field diagnosis should be confirmed by virus isolation and identification or by serologic means, using paired serums.

Suckling mice are most commonly used for virus isolation from infectious blood or tissues. They are inoculated intracerebrally with 0.03 ml of each preparation. The incubation period varies from 4 to 20 days, and mortality may reach 100 percent in the first passage. Serial passages of brain virus shorten the incubation period, and suckling mice die within 2 to 7 days after inoculation. Tissue-cultured cells also may be used for field isolations, but these cells are not as susceptible as suckling mice or horses.

The demonstration of a rising titer utilizing paired serums is ample proof that the disease is AHS. Complement-fixation, agar-gel diffusion, and immunofluores-cence tests are disease-specific, as all nine serotypes share a common antigenic component. There are at least two precipitating antigenic components common to the nine serotypes.

Viral typing is usually done by the serum-neutralization test, but the hemagglutination test also may be used. The neutralization tests are performed in mice (Alexander 1935) or in tissue culture. Some cross-neutralization occurs among some of the nine serotypes, with the greatest level occurring between types 6 and 9.

Prevention and Control. Vaccination is the best means of control in infected regions (see "Immunity"), but nonvaccinated animals can be protected by stabling them at night in insectproof buildings.

The Disease in Humans. AHSV has not been reported to cause disease in humans.

REFERENCES

Alexander, R.A. 1935. Studies on the neurotropic virus of horse-sickness. I. Neurotropic fixation. II. Some physical and chemical properties. III. The intracerebral protection test and its application to the study of immunity. IV. The pathogenesis in horses. Onderstepoort J. Vet. Sci. Anim. Indus. 4:291–388.

Alexander, R.A. 1936. Studies on the neurotropic virus of horsesickness. V. The antigenic response of horses to simultaneous trivalent immunization. Onderstepoort J. Vet. Sci. Anim. Indus. 7:11–16.

Alexander, R.A. 1948. The 1944 epizootic of horsesickness in the Middle East. Onderstepoort J. Vet. Sci. Anim. Indus. 23:77–92.

Alexander, R.A., and Du Toit, P.J. 1934. The immunization of horses and mules against horsesickness by means of the neurotropic virus of mice and guinea-pigs. Onderstepoort J. Vet. Sci. Anim. Indus. 2:375–391.

Alexander, R.A., Neitz, W.O., and Du Toit, P.J. 1936. Horsesickness: Immunization of horses and mules in the field during the season 1934–1935 with a description of the technique of preparation of poly valent mouse neurotropic vaccine. Onderstepoort J. Vet. Sci. Anim. Indus. 7:17–30.

Breese, S.S., Ozawa, Y., and Dardiri, A.H. 1969. Electron microscopic characterization of African horsesickness virus. J. Am. Vet. Med. Assoc. 155:391–400.

Davies, F.G., and Otieno, S. 1977. Elephants and zebras as possible reservoir hosts for African horse sickness virus. Vet. Rec. 100:291–292.

Du Toit, R.M. 1944. The transmission of blue-tongue and horse sickness by Culicoides. Onderstepoort J. Vet. Sci. Anim. Indus. 19:7–16.

Du Toit, P.J., Alexander, R.A., and Neitz, W.O. 1933. The immunization of horses against horse sickness by the use of formalized viruses. Part II. Onderstepoort J. Vet. Sci. Anim. Indus. 1:25–50.

Howell, P.G. 1962. Bluetongue—Recent advances in research. Onderstepoort J. Vet. Res. 29:139.

Newsholme, S.J. 1983. A morphological study of the lesions of African horsesickness. Onderstepoort J. Vet. Res. 50:7–24.

Ozawa, Y. 1967. Studies on the virus in two different cell line cultures. Arch. Gesam. Virusforsch. 21:155–160.

Ozawa, Y., and Hazrati, A. 1964. Growth of African horsesickness virus in monkey kidney cell culture. Am. J. Vet. Res. 25:505–511.

Ozawa, Y., Shad-Del, F., Nakata, G., and Navai, S. 1966. Transmission of African horse-sickness by a species of mosquito. In Proceedings of the 1st International Conference on Equine Infectious Diseases, Stressa, Italy. S. Karger, Basel. P. 196.

Parker, J. 1975. Inactivation of African horse-sickness virus by betapropiolactone and by pH. Arch. Virol. 47:357–365.

Pavri, K.M. 1961. Hemagglutination and hemagglutination inhibition with African horse-sickness virus. Nature 189:249.

Polson, A., and Madsen, T. 1954. Particle size distribution of African horsesickness virus. Biochim. Biophys. Acta 14:366–373.

Bluetongue

SYNONYMS: Catarrhal fever of sheep, range stiffness in lambs, sore muzzle of sheep

Bluetongue is an infectious viral disease of ruminants transmitted by the insect vector *Culicoides variipennis*. In sheep the disease is characterized by fever, emaciation, oral lesions, lameness, and a substantial death rate, primarily in lambs.

Although the heaviest losses are in sheep, the disease also occurs in cattle and in goats. Cattle have sometimes been the suspected source of infection for sheep. In certain areas of South Africa, the disease has developed in sheep brought into areas where no sheep or cattle had existed previously; hence it is highly probable that other natural hosts for this virus—such as goats, wild ruminants, and, possibly, certain wild rodents—transmitted the disease. In 1966 Howell reported that at least 18 immunological serotypes existed worldwide; as of 1986 24 have been recognized. Using the neutralization test, Luedke and Hochim (1968) recognized at least six antigenic types in 1967 in the United States. In 1986 five serotypes were recognized in the United States: 2, 10, 11, 13, 17.

Bluetongue was first reported in South Africa in 1905 and has been a serious problem there ever since. A clinical diagnosis of bluetongue in sheep was made in California by McGowan (1952), and the following year the virus was isolated by McKercher et al. (1953). These authors sent a strain of their virus to South Africa, where it was compared immunologically with South African strains and the identification confirmed. Soon afterward a disease in Texas which had been described by Hardy and Price (1952) under the name *sore muzzle* was identified as bluetongue. According to Price (1954) laboratory diagnosis of bluetongue in sheep has been made not only in California and Texas but also in Arizona and Colorado. Since then it has been identified in Kansas, Missouri, Nebraska, New Mexico, Oklahoma, Oregon, Florida, Louisiana, Utah, and other states. In 1977–1978 a U.S. survey of serums collected from brucellosis laboratories showed a prevalence of bluetongue virus antibody of from 0 to 79 percent in the samples from various states, with a national prevalence of 18.2 percent. The prevalence was generally low in the northern states and high in the southwestern states. The wide distribution of the disease reveals that it was not recently introduced. Apparently it has existed unrecog-

nized for many years on sheep ranges in the western United States.

Bluetongue virus now exists in many other countries including Mexico, Cyprus, Israel, Greece, Japan (serotypes 1, 12, 20), the Soviet Union, Turkey, India, and Australia (types 1, 20, 21). Virus has been recovered from insects and antibodies have been detected in cattle in Australia, but no evidence of disease has been found in sheep or cattle. Canada once had the infection in cattle but antibodies have not been found in cattle there since the mid-1970s.

The disease is seen only in midsummer and early fall and is especially prevalent in wet seasons, although seroconversion occurs in some animals during the dry season. The disease disappears abruptly with the onset of frosts.

More detailed information on bluetongue can be found in two useful sources: U.S. Department of Agriculture (1979) and Verwoerd et al. (1979).

Character of the Disease. In sheep with bluetongue the principal losses are in feeder lambs, but losses in older animals do occur. There is an early temperature rise (to 105°F or higher) that lasts only a short time. The victims are greatly depressed, do not feed, and lose weight rapidly. Edema of the lips, tongue, throat, and brisket develops in many animals. The buccal mucosa sometimes becomes flushed or even cyanotic. Erosions usually appear on the dental pad, tongue, gums, margins of the lips, and corners of the mouth. The lips bleed easily. Frequently there is a thick, tenacious nasal discharge that dries and crusts on the muzzle. There may be an eye discharge, and edema of the lungs and pneumonia (Figure 49.10) sometimes occur. Occasionally there is diarrhea, especially in young animals. Other lesions include edema and hemorrhages in the musculature, hemorrhages in many of the serous membranes of the rumen, abomasum,

Figure 49.10. Acute, bilateral inhalation pneumonia in a sheep that died of bluetongue. (Courtesy T. Walton, Arthropod-Borne Animal Diseases Branch, U.S. Dept. of Agriculture.)

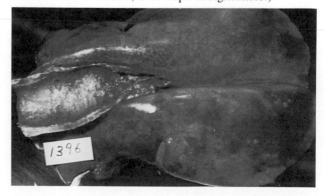

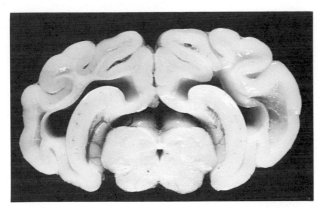

Figure 49.11. Subcortical cavitation (hydranencephaly) in the brain of a lamb infected with bluetongue virus in utero. (Courtesy D. Cordy.)

and intestines. Frequently, hyperemic areas of the skin develop into localized dermatitis. Leukopenia is found in the early stages of the disease. Later there may be leukocytosis and anemia. Abortions may occur in pregnant ewes. Hydranencephaly (Figures 49.11 and 49.12) and other congenital deformities may occur in infected fetuses.

A characteristic sign is stiffness or lameness due to muscular changes and, in many animals, to laminitis. The feet often have a reddish or purplish line or zone in the skin of the coronet (Figure 49.13), and the hemorrhages frequently extend into the horny tissue. Following recovery, a definite ridge, which persists for many months, can be seen in the horn of the hoof.

The virulence of the causative agent varies widely, and there may be differences in susceptibility in different breeds of sheep. Very young lambs suckling immune ewes are protected by colostral antibodies. Price (1954) believes that the syndrome that has long been known in Texas under the name *range stiffness in lambs* is a mild form of bluetongue contracted by lambs before they have wholly lost their colostral immunity. In most outbreaks many older animals have only very mild attacks, manifested principally by a short febrile period.

Mortality varies widely. In Africa, where the virus obviously is much more virulent than in the United States, it is said to range from 2 to 30 percent. In California mortality has been considerably less. In highly susceptible virgin cattle or sheep mortality is usually higher.

Studies in sheep indicate that the incubation period in bluetongue is relatively short—from 3 to 10 days. Death seldom occurs before 8 to 10 days following the appearance of the first signs. In many animals the course is much shorter, the mild signs having disappeared after several days. Severely affected animals, if they survive, are apt to have a prolonged period of convalescence.

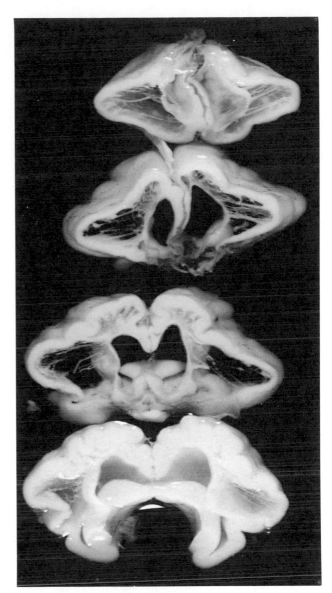

Figure 49.12. Severe hydranencephaly in a lamb following in utero infection with bluetongue virus. Secondary hydrocephalus *ex vacus* also is present. (Courtesy D. Cordy, *Journal of Neuropathology and Experimental Neurology*.)

The disease in cattle is similar to that in sheep except that cattle generally suffer only mild infections and have a low mortality rate (Bekker et al. 1934, Luedke et al. 1970). In Africa infections have been diagnosed only by inoculating sheep. Sometimes there may be frank signs and well-developed lesions. Mouth lesions, crusts and excoriations on the muzzle, nasal discharge, laminitis, which is often severe, and acute, patchy dermatitis involving the flanks, groin, perineum, udder, and teats are characteristic. Necrosis of the skin in the interdigital spaces is often seen. In utero transmission occurs in cattle

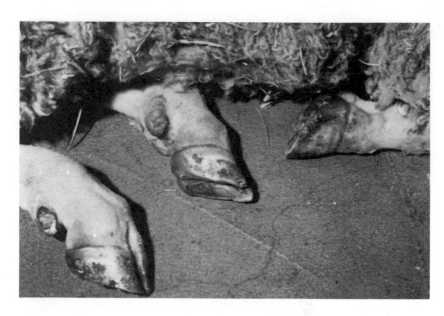

Figure 49.13. Coronitis in a sheep with bluetongue. (Courtesy T. Walton, Anthropod-Borne Animal Diseases Branch, U.S. Dept. of Agriculture.)

and can result in abortion, hydranencephaly, congenital deformity, and immunologically tolerant calves (Figure 49.14) (Hourrigan and Klingsporn 1975). The virus can produce pathological changes in the reproductive tract of bulls, such as focal degeneration of the seminiferous tu-

bules and hemorrhage and hyperemia in the colliculus seminalis. Some recovered animals may be carriers of the virus (Luedke et al. 1970).

Bluetongue can be produced in sheep experimentally by inoculation of blood or tissues, which yields a disease

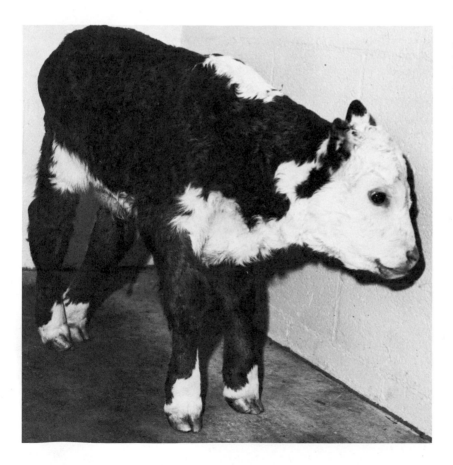

Figure 49.14. Newborn dwarf calf with congenital deformities of the rear legs born to a dam with bluetongue. (Courtesy T. Walton, Arthropod-Borne Animal Diseases Branch, U.S. Dept. of Agriculture.)

similar to the one observed in nature. The mutton breeds are more susceptible than the wool breeds, and native African sheep are resistant to the disease.

Goats are susceptible to virus, but there is no evidence of clinical signs either experimentally or during natural outbreaks. The experimental infection in cattle also is inapparent.

Disease has been produced experimentally in the blesbok and white-tailed deer. Naturally occurring cases have been observed in a bighorn sheep and a captive deer herd. Based on a serologic survey for bluetongue virus in wild ruminants of North America (Trainer and Jochim 1969), elk, antelope, big horn sheep, Barbary sheep, moose, and three species of deer should be susceptible to the virus. Experimental bluetongue in white-tailed deer usually terminates in death (Vosdingh et al. 1968). The lesions and signs of illness are similar to those of epizootic hemorrhagic disease. In fatal cases of bluetongue the lesions are subendocardial hemorrhages, hemorrhages in the tongue, and enteritis in the small and large intestine. The predominant histological changes are extensive thrombosis with hemorrhages, degenerative changes, and necrosis in affected tissues and organs. Bluetongue virus is readily recovered from the blood and a variety of tissues. Neutralizing antibodies are detected in all convalescent serums.

Cabasso et al. (1955) have successfully propagated this virus in suckling hamsters, and Van den Ende and co-workers (1954) successfully transmitted it in series in mice by intracerebral inoculation.

Properties of the Virus. The bluetongue virus is a sphere 60 to 80 nm in diameter (Figures 49.15 and 49.16). It appears to consist of 32 capsomeres rather than the 92 accepted for reoviruses. Knudsen et al. (1982) analyzed the viral genome using polyacrylamide-gel electrophoresis and found that it comprises 10 segments of double-stranded RNA. Estimates of the molecular mass of the segments showed that the U.S. bluetongue serotypes were similar, but each virus serotype had a distinct double stranded RNA profile. There is a difference of opinion regarding the presence of a true envelope—it apparently depends on the degree of purification. The virus has a hemagglutinin.

Bluetongue virus is somewhat resistant to ether, chloroform, and deoxycholate. It is sensitive to trypsin and has a narrow zone of pH stability—between 6 and 8. It is extraordinarily resistant to influences that quickly destroy most other viruses; for example, it will withstand a considerable amount of putrefaction and has been recovered unchanged by filtering highly decomposed blood. Neitz (1944) isolated virulent virus from infective blood that had been preserved more than 25 years at room

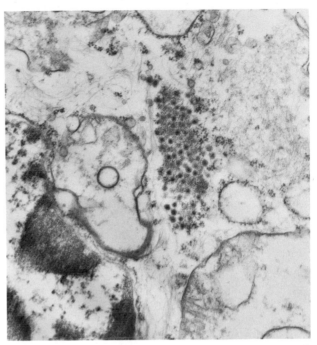

Figure 49.15. A cluster of bluetongue virions in pig kidney cell culture 24 hours after inoculation. × 29,000. (Courtesy S. S. Breese, Plum Island Animal Disease Center, U.S. Dept. of Agriculture.)

Figure 49.16. A single bluetongue virus particle. × 662,000. (Courtesy T. Walton, Arthropod-Borne Animal Diseases Branch, U.S. Dept. of Agriculture.)

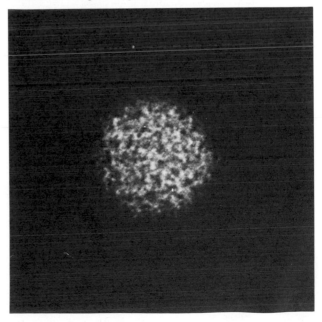

temperature in a glycerol-oxalate-phenol mixture. Air-dried virus keeps unusually well, and freeze-dried organisms remain viable for many months. McCrory et al. (1959) found the virus comparatively resistant to several common disinfectants, such as sodium hydroxide, sodium carbonate, and ethyl alcohol. The most effective chemical disinfectant tried was Wescodyne, a proprietary preparation.

In Africa 19 different antigenic strains of bluetongue virus have been recognized. Serotypes 2, 10, 11, 13, and 17 are known to exist in the United States. In recent years new serotypes have been isolated in Australia, where intensive research is in progress, but none have been associated with disease in livestock. Three serotypes (1, 12, 20) exist in Japan.

A group-specific precipitating antigen (V7) that has a molecular mass of 39,000 daltons can be readily purified by chromatofocusing. So far all the bluetongue virus (BTV) serotypes have been shown to possess this protein (Hubschle and Yang 1983). The other major polypeptide of the BTV core is P3 and these two polypeptides are surrounded by an outer capsid layer composed primarily of two polypeptides, P2 and P5 (Huismans and Erasmus 1981). P2 is the main determinant of serotype specificity, and P2-precipitating antibodies in the serum correlate with neutralizing antibody titers (Appleton and Letchworth 1983, Huismans and Erasmus 1981). Antibodies directed against a single epitope on BTV-17 can prevent bluetongue (Letchworth and Appleton 1983).

Temperature-sensitive mutants of BTV have been isolated and classified in genetic recombination groups (Shipham and DeLaRey 1976). The frequency of recombination varied both within and among groups. The period of incubation required for maximum recombination was 48 hours at 28°C.

Both genetic drift and genetic recombination were demonstrated in BTV-11 isolates over a 12-year period in the United States. Reassortant BTV from mixed, dual, wild-type viral infections were obtained with BTV-10 and BTV-11 (Sugiyama et al. 1982).

The virus has a close affinity for erythrocytes. When virus is isolated from the blood, washed erythrocytes, rather than cell cultures, should be used and injected into susceptible lambs.

Cultivation. Alexander (1947) in South Africa showed that BTV could be propagated readily in chick embryos, providing the temperature did not exceed 33.5°C. This is considerably below the optimum temperature for development of the embryo. Serial passage in egg embryos rapidly reduces the virulence of the virus. The yolk sac or intravascular route of inoculation is satisfactory, but the latter method is more sensitive and more time-consuming (Luedke et al. 1970).

Haig et al. (1956) demonstrated that egg-adapted strains of virus could be cultivated on monolayers of sheep kidney cells and that cytopathogenic activity was exhibited. This activity could be neutralized with homologous antiserum. Cytolytic phenomena were not seen with virulent, unmodified virus on the same cells. Two adapted strains produced a cytopathogenic effect in bovine kidney cells. Since the original studies, it has been demonstrated that the virus propagates in various primary and established cell lines, including the baby hamster kidney cell line. Using egg-adapted strains of virus, Howell et al. (1967) produced plaques in a mouse fibroblast cell line under agarose. Jochim and Jones (1976) used a plaque assay system in plastic panels with baby hamster cells grown under an overlay of gum tragacanth. Plaques also are formed by virus in Vero cells (Figure 49.17). Bovine macrophage cultures and organ cultures of tracheal rings were susceptible to bovine BTV strains (Rossi and Kiesel 1977), and with few exceptions viruses cytopathogenic for bovine embryonic lung cultures also were cytopathogenic for bovine macrophages. Although the viruses were initially cytopathogenic in macrophages, cytopathogenicity was lost on repeated passages, despite replication.

Figure 49.17. Plaque formation by bluetongue virus in African green monkey cells (Vero). Stained with neutral red in a Noble agar overlay. (Courtesy T. Walton, Arthropod-Borne Animal Diseases Branch, U.S. Dept. of Agriculture.)

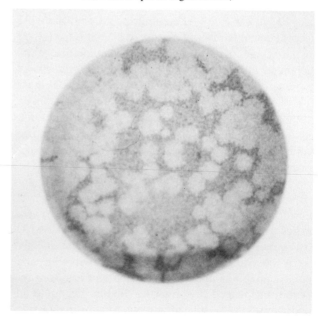

Epizootiology. Bluetongue is not transmissible by simple contact. It has long been known that an insect vector must be involved. Mosquitoes were suspected but largely acquitted by experimental work. Du Toit (1944) showed that gnats (*Culicoides*) were natural transmitters. In the United States, Price and Hardy (1954) found the virus in *C. variipennis*, which happened to be the most common gnat in the infected regions of Texas. *C. pallidipennis* often is involved in transmission. Any other natural insect carriers of this disease have not yet been identified.

Because of the need for a vector, the disease occurs only in warm weather, generally in midsummer or later when the insect population has built up to maximum numbers, and it is generally worse in wet seasons. In California it occurs in animals on irrigated pastures, where conditions for insect development are ideal.

The carrier status of cattle after infection and the susceptibility of domestic and wild ruminants, and possibly of rodents, must be considered in the ecology of the disease. The suggestion that the virus may be recovered from the semen of immunologically incompetent bulls indicates another potential mechanism for the transmission of the virus (Luedke, Jones, et al. 1977). Abnormalities have been observed in spermatozoa and BTV isolated from the semen of two known BTV carrier bulls and two of four BTV seropositive field bulls. (Foster et al. 1980). Others (Howard 1983, Parsonson et al. 1981) have found that approximately 25 percent of the bulls experimentally infected with BTV had virus in the semen during the limited test periods. Another group has suggested that transplacental infection of bluetongue in sheep may be another overwintering mechanism for the virus in certain areas of the world (Gibbs et al. 1979).

At present there is no evidence that 7- to 9-day-old bovine embryos transferred to recipient heifers can transmit BTV to the heifers (Bowen et al. 1982, Singh et al. 1982).

Immunity. Sheep that have recovered from an attack of bluetongue are solidly resistant for months to infection by the same viral strain. If more than one type of virus exists in the same locality, second infections may occur within a short time, but such infections do not happen often, since some different viral types partially immunize against each other. Because there is a plurality of viral serotypes and variability in susceptibility of sheep breeds, no clear pattern of the duration and degree of immunity has been ascertained. Active immunity in sheep produced by virulent virus is associated with the formation of neutralizing and complement-fixing antibodies. Neutralizing antibodies at a high level persist for more than 2 years. In contrast, complement-fixing antibodies are detectable for

6 to 8 weeks after infection but are barely detectable after 1 year.

Oellerman et al. (1976) described a modified hemolytic plaque technique for detection of bluetongue antibody–forming cells. Primary IgM response in mice to sheep red blood cells or virus occurred after 4 days but declined rapidly to less than 5 percent by day 9. IgG response was detected from day 6 onward and dominated the response.

Calves that are infected in utero may become latently infected, and virus can be isolated from washed erythrocyte samples for more than 1 year, and in one instance 5 years, after challenge with bluetongue virus. The latently infected calves are either immunologically competent or incompetent in producing virus antibodies (Luedke, Jochim, et al. 1977). Immunologically tolerant cattle can become competent after repeated exposures from bites of virus-infected *C. variipennis*. These results suggest a means by which the virus survives the winter (Luedke, Jones, et al. 1977).

Diagnosis. In regions where the disease commonly occurs, the diagnosis is usually based on the clinical signs. Bluetongue resembles, but must be differentiated from, such diseases as foot-and-mouth disease, mycotic stomatitis, infectious bovine rhinotracheitis, bovine virus diarrhea–mucosal disease, rinderpest, Ibaraki disease, and vesicular stomatitis. Ibaraki disease virus and bluetongue virus are similar in morphology, but neutralization tests, complement-fixation tests, and ferritin tagging have indicated antigenic differences (Campbell et al. 1975). In newly infected regions confirmation of bluetongue should be obtained by transmission experiments, serologic tests, or serum-protection tests.

Virus can be isolated from blood, semen, or tissues by inoculation of susceptible sheep, embryonated hens' eggs (Luedke 1969), susceptible cell cultures (Howell 1963, 1966), and suckling mice and hamsters (Howell 1963). The system of choice at present for field isolations is the inoculation of the embryonated hens' eggs and Vero cells. If blood is used, quantitation of virus depends on ultrasonic disruption of blood samples. Glycerol-oxalate-phenol preservative mixture is an excellent stabilizer for the virus and enhances its isolation.

Six separate serologic tests can be used to aid the diagnosis of bluetongue. They are the serum-neutralization test done in cell culture, micro agar-gel diffusion test (Jochim and Chow 1969), fluorescent antibody direct and indirect tests (Livingston and Moore 1962), complement-fixation test (Luedke et al. 1970), ELISA, and modified complement-fixation test. The serum-neutralization test has been used most widely in diagnosis and virus typing and is based on inhibition of cytopathic effects in a cell culture by specific antibody. Because agar-gel diffusion is simple, sensitive, and economical, it is the in vitro test of choice for studying group-specific antigens. The direct flourescent antibody test can be used for detecting antigen in bovine labial mucosa and chicken embryonic membranes. Plaque neutralization is the most sensitive serological test for detecting reactors.

Prevention and Control. In South Africa a vaccine was used for many years which had been produced by inoculating virus serially in sheep, without intervention of the natural vector. Attenuation was obtained in this way, and a serviceable vaccine developed. A better, more uniform vaccine was developed by Alexander et al. (1947). Their vaccine was a strain of BTV attenuated by serial passage through chick embryos until it no longer produced signs of illness in sheep. Generally several types of strains must be combined in a single vaccine to protect against the multiple types found in the field. McKercher and co-workers (1957) introduced a modified virus vaccine for use in the United States. American strains also were attenuated by serial passage in embryonated hens' eggs. A freeze-dried product was successfully tested in the laboratory and field. This vaccine produces only nominal reactions when injected into sheep, it does not regain virulence by sheep passage, and it immunizes solidly against massive challenges with virulent virus. When stored under proper refrigeration, the vaccine deteriorates very slowly.

Luedke and Jochim (1968) reported a variation in the clinical and immunological response of sheep to vaccination. An egg vaccine produced fairly good serum-neutralizing antibody indices, but a tissue-cultured vaccine produced little or no antibody response in a 21-day exposure period. A poor correlation also was apparent between the clinical response of sheep after challenge and their serum-neutralizating antibody indices. There also was evidence of immunological nonspecificity for one of the serotypes.

Pregnant ewes and cows should not be vaccinated with attenuated virus vaccines.

A bluetongue virus grown in baby hamster kidney cells and inactivated with 0.2 percent beta propiolactone produced neutralizing antibodies that reached a high level that persisted for at least 1 year (Parker et al. 1975). After revaccination a secondary response was elicited. Similar results were obtained with a bivalent inactivated virus vaccine.

Ordinary isolation measures will not stop the spread of bluetongue in regions infested with *Culicoides*. Control must be aimed at reducing the gnat population, moving lambs out of the gnat-infested regions, using repellent sprays on lambs to discourage gnat bites, keeping lambs indoors from late afternoon until well into the next day, or immunizing lambs shortly after they are weaned and before the gnat season begins. South African workers claim that gnats, unlike mosquitoes, seldom enter buildings (even though unscreened) at night unless they are attracted by lights.

Immunization is the most practical scheme, but ewes must not be vaccinated during early pregnancy (particularly 4 to 8 weeks gestation) because vaccine virus can produce stillborn, spastic, "dummy" or "crazy," putrefied, and deformed lambs (Schultz and Delay 1955). Sheep should be vaccinated after shearing, as wool fiber breaks in severely reacting sheep (Howell 1963). Maternal immunity protection persists for 3 to 6 months, and this fact must be considered in any immunization program.

There is some evidence for a sheep-breed difference in the immune response to a binary ethylenimine-inactivated BTV vaccine (Berry et al. 1982). Serologic conversion of Hampshire and Suffolk lambs was poor at 43 percent as compared with 84 percent in Columbia and Finn lambs.

The Disease in Humans. There is no evidence that BTV causes disease in humans.

REFERENCES

Alexander, R.A. 1947. The propagation of blue-tongue virus in the developing chick embryo with particular reference to the temperature of incubation. Onderstepoort J. Vet. Sci. Anim. Indus. 22:7–26.

Alexander, R.A., Haig, D.A., and Adelaar, T.F. 1947. The attenuation of bluetongue virus by serial passage through fertile eggs. Onderstepoort J. Vet. Sci. Anim. Indus. 21:231–241.

Appleton, J.A., and Letchworth, G.J. 1983. Monoclonal antibody analysis of serotype restricted and unrestricted bluetongue viral antigenic determinants. Virology 124:286–299.

Bekker, J.G., DeKock, G.W., and Quinlan, J.B. 1934. The occurrence and identification of bluetongue in cattle—The so-called pseudo-foot and mouth disease in South Africa. Onderstepoort J. Vet. Sci. Anim. Indus. 2:393–507.

Berry, L.J., Osburn, B.I., Scott, J.L., Farver, T., Heron, B., and Patton, W. 1982. Inactivated bluetongue virus vaccine in lambs: Differential serological responses related to breed. Vet. Res. Commun. 5:289–293.

Bowen, R.A., Howard, T.H., and Pickett, B.W., 1982. Interaction of bluetongue virus with preimplantation embryos from mice and cattle. Am. J. Vet. Res. 43:1907–1911.

Cabasso, V.J., Roberts, G.I., Douglas, J.M., Zorzi, R., Stebbins, M.R., and Cox, H.R., 1955. Bluetongue. I. Propagation of bluetongue virus of sheep in suckling hamsters. Proc. Soc. Exp. Biol. Med. 88:678–681.

Campbell, C.H., Breese, S.S., and McKercher, P.D. 1975. Antigenic and morphologic comparisons of Ibaraki and bluetongue viruses. Can. J. Microbiol. 21:2098–2102.

Du Toit, R. 1944. Transmission of horse-sickness and bluetongue in South Africa. Onderstepoort J. Vet. Sci. Anim. Indus. 19:7.

Els, H.J., and Verwoerd, D.W. 1969. Morphology of bluetongue virus. Virology 38:213–219.

Foster, N.M., Alders, M.A., Luedke, A.J., and Walton, T.E. 1980. Abnormalities and virus-like particles in spermatozoa from bulls latently infected with bluetongue virus. Am. J. Vet. Res. 41:1045–1048.

Gibbs, E.P., Lawman, M.J., and Herniman, K.A. 1979. Preliminary observations on transplacental infection of blue tongue virus in sheep—A possible overwintering mechanism. Res. Vet. Sci. 27:118–120.

Haig, D.A., McKercher, D.G., and Alexander, R.A. 1956. The cytopathogenic action of bluetongue virus on tissue cultures and its application to the detection of antibodies in the serum of sheep. Onderstepoort J. Vet. Sci. Anim. Indus. 27:171–177.

Hardy, W.T., and Price, D.A. 1952. Soremuzzle of sheep. J. Am. Vet. Med. Assoc. 120:23–25.

Hourrigan, J.L., and Klingsporn, A.L. 1975. Bluetongue: The disease in cattle. Aust. Vet. J. 51:170–174.

Howard, T.H. 1983. The pathogenesis of bluetongue in the bull. Diss. Abstr. Int. B. Sci. Eng. 43:,7, 2130–2131.

Howell, P.G., 1966. Some aspects of the epizootiology of bluetongue. Bull. Off. Int. Epiz. 66:341–352.

Howell, P.G., Verwoerd, D.W., and Oellermann, R.A. 1967. Plaque formation by bluetongue virus. Onderstepoort J. Vet. Res. 34:317–332.

Hubschle, O.J., and Yang, C. 1983. Purification of the group-specific antigen of bluetongue virus by chromatofocusing. J. Virol. Methods 6:171–178.

Huismans, H., and Erasmus, B.J.1981. Identification of the serotype-specific and group-specific antigens of blue tongue. Onderstepoort J. Vet. Res. 48:51–58.

Jochim, M.M. and Chow, T.L.,1969. Immunodiffusion of bluetongue virus. Am. J. Vet. Res. 30:33–41.

Jochim, M.M., and Jones, S.C., 1976. Plaque neutralization of blue-tongue virus and epizootic hemorrhagic disease virus in BHK_{21} cells. Am. J. Vet. Res. 37:1345–1347.

Knudson, D.L., Butterfield, W.K., Shope, R.E., Walton, T.E., and Campbell, C.H., 1982. Electrophoretic comparison of the genomes of North American blue tongue viruses, one Australian blue tongue virus, and three related orbiviruses. Vet. Microbiol. 7:285–293.

Letchworth, G.J., and Appleton, J.A., 1983. Passive protection of mice and sheep against bluetongue virus by a neutralizing monoclonal antibody. Infect. Immun. 39:208–212.

Livingston, C.W., and Moore, R.W. 1962. Cytochemical changes of bluetongue virus in tissue culture. Am. J. Vet. Res. 23:701–710.

Luedke, A.J. 1969. Bluetongue in sheep: Viral assay and viremia. Am. J. Vet. Res. 30:499–509.

Luedke, A.J., and Jochim, M.M., 1968. Bluetongue virus in sheep. Intensification of the clinical response by previrus oral administration. Am. J. Vet. Res. 29:841.

Luedke, A.J., Jochim, M.M., Bowne, J.G.,and Jones, R.H. 1970. Observations on latent bluetongue virus infection in cattle. J. Am. Vet. Med. Assoc. 156:1871–1879.

Luedke, A.J., Jochim, M.M., and Jones, R.H., 1977. Bluetongue in cattle: Effects of *Culicoides variipennis* transmitted bluetongue virus on pregnant heifers and their calves. Am. J. Vet. Res. 38:1697.

Luedke, A.J., Jones, R.H., and Walton, T.E., 1977. Overwintering mechanism for bluetongue virus: Biological recovery of latent virus from a bovine by bites of *Culicoides variipennis*. Am. J. Trop. Med. Hyg. 26:313–325.

McCrory, B.R., Foster, N.M., and Bay, R.C. 1959. Virucidal effect of some chemical agents on bluetongue virus. Am. J. Vet. Res. 20:665–669.

McGowan, B. 1952. An epidemic resembling sore-muzzle or blue-tongue in California sheep. Cornell Vet. 42:213–216.

McKercher, D.G., McGowan, B., Cabasso, V.J., Roberts, G.I., and Saito, J.K. 1957. Studies on bluetongue. III. The development of a modified live vaccine employing American strains of bluetongue virus. Am. J. Vet. Res. 18:310–316.

McKercher, D.G., McGowan, B., Howarth, J.A., and Saito, J.K. 1953. A preliminary report on the isolation and identification of the bluetongue virus from sheep in California. J. Am. Vet. Med. Assoc. 122:300–301.

Neitz, W.O. 1944. The susceptibility of the springbuck (*Antidorcas marcupialis*) to heartwater. Onderstepoort J. Vet. Sci. Anim. Indus. 20:93.

Oellerman, R.A., Carter, P., and Marx, M.J. 1976. Modified hemolytic plaque technique for the detection of bluetongue virus antibody-forming cells. Infect. Immun. 13:1321–1324.

Parker, J., Herniman, K.A.J., Gibbs, E.P.J., and Sellers, R.F. 1975. An experimental inactivated vaccine against bluetongue. Vet. Rec. 96:284–287.

Parsonson, I.M., Della-Porta, A.J., McPhee, D.A., Cybinski, D.H., Squire, K.R., Standfast, H.A., and Aren, M.F. 1981. Isolation of bluetongue virus serotype 20 from the semen of an experimentally-infected bull (correspondence). Aust. Vet. J. 57:252–253.

Price, D.A. 1954. The problem of bluetongue control in range sheep. Proc. U.S. Livestock Sanit. Assoc. 58:256–259.

Price, D.A., and Hardy, W.T. 1954. Isolation of the bluetongue virus from Texas sheep—*Culicoides* shown to be a vector. J. Am. Vet. Med. Assoc. 124:255–258.

Rossi, C.R., and Kiesel, G.K. 1977. Susceptibility of bovine macrophage and tracheal ring cultures to bovine viruses. Am. J. Vet. Res. 38:1705–1708.

Schultz, G., and DeLay, P.D. 1955. Losses in newborn lambs associated with bluetongue vaccination of pregnant ewes. J. Am. Vet. Med. Assoc. 127:224–226.

Shipham, S.O., and DeLaRey, M. 1976. The isolation and preliminary genetic classification of temperature-sensitive mutants of bluetongue virus. Onderstepoort J. Vet. Res. 43:189–192.

Singh, E.L., Eaglesome, M.D., Thomas, F.C., Papp-Vid, G., and Hare, W.C.D. 1982. Embryo transfer as a means of controlling the transmission of viral infections. I. The in vitro exposure of preimplantation bovine embryos to akabane, bluetongue, and bovine viral diarrhea viruses. Theriogenology 17.437–444.

Sugiyama, K., Bishop, D.H., and Roy, P. 1982. Analysis of the genomes of blue tongue viruses recovered from different states of the United States and at different times (1953–1975). Am. J. Epidemol. 115:332–347.

Trainer, D.O., and Jochim, M.M. 1969. Serologic evidence of blue-tongue in wild ruminants of North America. Am. J. Vet. Res. 30.2007–2011.

U.S. Department of Agriculture. 1979. Bluetongue bibliography, July, 1979. Animal and Plant Health Inspection Services, Hyattsville, Md.

Van den Ende, M., Linder, A., and Kaschula, V.R. 1954. Experiments with the Cyprus strain of bluetongue virus: Multiplication in the central nervous system of mice and complement-fixation. J. Hyg. 52:155.

Verwoerd, D.W., Huismans, H., and Erasmus, B.J. 1979. Orbiviruses. In H. Fraenkel-Conrat and R.R. Wagner, eds., Comprehensive Virology, vol. 14. Plenum, New York. Pp. 285–345.

Vosdingh, R.A., Trainer, D.O., and Easterday, B.C. 1968. Experimental bluetongue disease in white-tailed deer. Can. J. Comp. Med. Vet. Sci. 32:382–387.

Epizootic Hemorrhagic Disease

SYNONYM: Ibaraki disease of cattle; abbreviation, EHD

Epizootic hemorrhagic disease occurs in the Virginia white-tailed deer (*Odocoileus virginianus*) and is caused by a virus classified as an orbivirus. Shope et al. (1960) first described the natural disease. It is characterized by an incubation period of 6 to 8 days, severe shock, and multiple hemorrhages, and associated edema in various tissues and serous sacs, coma, and death. Prothrombin deficiency may cause the hemorrhages (Karstad et al. 1961). Other epizootics have occurred in the United States (Fosberg et al. 1977, Roughton 1975). The clinical signs and lesions were consistent with the original description of the disease. In one instance the infection rate among captive and free-ranging park deer in Mammoth Cave National Park (Kentucky) was high (±90 percent) with a high mortality (62 percent) in captive deer and with negligible mortality in free-ranging deer. The highest mortality occurred in fawns and adults, the lowest in yearlings.

Mule deer and other species of deer are not susceptible to the virus. The biting gnat *Culicoides variipennis* is responsible for transmitting the disease. Infection does not occur from direct contact. Intracerebral inoculation of suckling mice causes 100 percent mortality, and after four transfers in this host the virus produces an inapparent infection in deer (Mettler et al. 1962).

The Washington strain of EHD virus (EHDV) replicates in fetal deer cells derived from an entire fetus. The cytopathic effect is characterized by focal development of rounded and clumped cells (Fosberg et al. 1977). The staining of infected cells with acridine orange indicates double-stranded nucleic acid in the cytoplasm. The New Jersey strain produces a cytopathic effect in HeLa cells (Mettler et al. 1962). A similar effect is produced by the South Dakota strain in embryonic deer kidney cells (Pirtle and Layton 1961).

Purified EHDV contains 10 double-stranded RNA segments and a double-layered protein capsid with four major and four minor polypeptides. The virus differs from bluetongue virus, the orbivirus prototype, by having an additional minor polypeptide component that, together with P2 and P5, compromise the outer capsid layer. The extra polypeptide gives the virus more stability than bluetongue virus. Two noncapsid polypeptides, P5A and P6A, are present in addition to the light capsid polypeptides (Huismans et al. 1979).

A plaque-neutralization test demonstrated the existence of two serotypes of EHDV (EHD-Alberta and EHD-New Jersey) (Barber and Jochim 1975). Antibodies to both serotypes and to bluetongue virus have been found in cattle in the United States. These results emphasize the need to consider both diseases in cattle when either agent is suspected as the clinical signs and lesions can be similar.

Ibaraki virus, a virus closely related to EHVD, causes a disease similar to bluetongue in cattle in Japan. Antibodies to Ibaraki virus are common in cattle in all regions of the United States except the northeastern states (Anderson and Campbell 1979). There is no antigenic relation between bluetongue virus and Ibaraki virus, but Ibaraki virus and the two EHDV serotypes are related antigenically, as shown by agar-gel diffusion and immunofluorescent antibody tests for group antigens (Campbell et al. 1978). Yet a common complement-fixing antigen is shared by the EHDV serotypes and the bluetongue virus serotypes (Moore and Lee 1972). The EHD, Ibaraki, and bluetongue viruses have all been placed in a single serologic group, but it is clear that considerably more comparative study must be done. Results of plaque-neutralization tests indicate that Ibaraki virus may be a third serotype of EHDV. Its significance as a pathogen in U.S. cattle is unknown, but, judging from its effects in Japanese cattle and its wide distribution in the United States, one can anticipate problems similar to those seen with bluetongue in sheep.

REFERENCES

Anderson, A.B., and Campbell, C.H. 1979. Personal communication.

Barber, T.L., and Jochim. M.M. 1975. Production of high titering antibody in rabbits for identification of bluetongue viral antigen by the indirect fluorescent antibody technique. Proceedings of the 18th Annual Meeting of the Association of Veterinary Laboratory Diagnosticians, Portland, Oregon. P. 149.

Campbell, C.H., Barber, T.L., and Jochim, M.M. 1978. Antigenic relationship of Ibaraki, bluetongue, and epizootic hemorrhagic disease viruses. Vet. Microbiol. 3:15–22.

Fosberg, S.A., Stauber, and Renshaw, H.W. 1977. Isolation and characterization of epizootic hemorrhagic disease virus from white-tailed deer (*Odocoileus virginianus*) in eastern Washington. Am. J. Vet. Res. 38:361–364.

Huismans, H., Bremer, C.W., and Barber, T.L. 1979. The nucleic acid and proteins of epizootic hemorrhagic disease virus. Onderstepoort J. Vet. Res. 46:95–104.

Karstad, L., Winter, A., and Trainer, D.O. 1961. Pathology of epizootic hemorrhagic disease of deer. Am. J. Vet. Res. 22:227–235.

Mettler, N.E., MacNamara, L.G., and Shope, R.E. 1962. The propagation of the virus of epizootic hemorrhagic disease of deer in newborn mice and HeLa cells. J. Exp. Med. 116:665–678.

Moore, D.L., and Lee, V.H. 1972. Antigenic relationship between the virus of epizootic haemorrhagic disease of deer and bluetongue virus. Brief report. Arch. Gesam. Virusforsch. 37:282.

Pirtle, E.C., and Layton, J.M. 1961. Epizootic hemorrhagic disease in white tailed deer—Characteristics of the South Dakota strain of virus. Am. J. Vet. Res. 22:104–108.

Roughton, R.D. 1975. An outbreak of a hemorrhagic disease in white-tailed deer in Kentucky. J. Wildl. Dis. 11:177–186.

Shope, R.E., MacNamara, L.G., and Mangold, R. 1960. A virus-induced epizootic hemorrhagic disease of the Virginia white-tailed deer (*Odocoileus virginianus*). J. Exp. Med. 111:155–170.

Other Viruses Assigned to the Reoviridae Family

Infectious bursal disease (IBD) virus and infectious pancreatitis necrosis (IPN) virus have a morphology similar to that of the orbiviruses, yet they are not related serologically to them. For this reason, the IBD and IPN viruses are tentatively assigned to the proposed genus *Birnavirus*. Members of this proposed group have a genome consisting of two segments of double-stranded RNA. The viruses are assembled in the cytoplasm. The particles are isometric with a diameter of 61 nm; tubular and smaller virus particles are also observed. The virus is a single-shelled capsid composed of 132 interconnected morphologic units with dextrosymmetry (T-13).

Infectious Bursal Disease

SYNONYMS: Avian nephrosis, Gumboro disease; abbreviation, IBD

Infectious bursal disease of chickens was described as a specific entity by Cosgrove (1962) and is also termed *avian nephrosis*. As it was first observed in the neighborhood of Gumboro, Delaware, in the United States, *Gumboro disease* became another name for the condition. Winterfield and Hitchner (1962) confirmed the original observations of Cosgrove and successfully propagated the virus in chicken embryos. The disease is prevalent in the United States and in other parts of the world in concentrated poultry-producing areas. Two viral serotypes have been described (Jackwood et al. 1982).

Character of the Disease. According to Mandelli et al. (1967), the natural disease occurs in chickens only, and white leghorns react more severely than the heavy breeds. The disease is principally limited to young chickens, with the greatest incidence in chicks 3 to 6 weeks old. The initial outbreak is usually the most severe; subsequent outbreaks in succeeding broods often are unnoticed.

The incubation period is short, as clinical signs are detected in 2 to 3 days. The birds display ruffled feathers and appear droopy. Other signs include soiled vent feathers, whitish or watery diarrhea, anorexia, depression, trembling, severe prostration, and, finally, death. In affected flocks morbidity approaches 100 percent, and mortality varies from negligible to 30 percent. Proudfoot (1975) observed that groups of birds fed the highest protein starter diet (24 percent protein) had a significantly higher mortality and a larger number of stunted birds.

Birds that die are dehydrated, with discoloration of pectoral muscles that also may show hemorrhages. There is increased mucus in the intestine, and the kidneys are enlarged from accumulated urates. Fluorescence has been observed in the renal glomeruli of infected chickens indicating that gamma globulins, probably in the form of immune complexes, lodge in the glomeruli (Ley et al. 1979). The bursa of Fabricius is the target structure for the IBD virus (IBDV). Initially, the bursa is edematous, hyperemic, and cream-colored with prominent longitudinal striations; by the time of death it is atrophied and gray. It often shows necrotic foci and may have hemorrhages on the serosal surface (Mandelli et al. 1967). The spleen may be enlarged, with small gray foci on the surface. On occasion, hemorrhages are seen in the mucosa at the junction of the proventriculus and gizzard. The condition is regarded as an infectious lymphocidal disease, with the principal histological lesions appearing in the lymphoid structures such as the bursa of Fabricius, spleen, thymus, and cecal tonsil (Helmboldt and Garner 1964). In neonates the virus produces aplastic anemia, liver necrosis, and hemorrhage.

In young chicks with mixed infections of IBD and other pathogens such as infectious bronchitis virus, Newcastle disease virus, or *Eimeria tenella* (coccidial agent), the disease is more severe and a higher mortality ensues. Aflatoxicosis is more severe in young broilers infected with IBDV. IBDV infection also enhances the production of lesions by *Aspergillus fumigatus*. Because IBD damages the chicken's immune mechanism, administration of certain attenuated virus vaccines to a flock suffering from IBD will exacerbate the morbidity.

Natural infection with serotype 2 occurs in turkeys but with no clinical evidence of disease (Jackwood et al. 1982). Experimentally, poults given IBDV do not show signs of illness but produce precipitating and neutralizing antibodies. Six-week-old ducklings inoculated intraperitoneally with IBDV contract mild disease without mortality (Christopher 1982).

A strain of IBDV has been isolated from the mosquito *Aedes vexans*, and designated 743 virus. This strain is comparable to other IBDV strains except it is nonpathogenic for fowls (Howie and Thorzen 1981).

Properties of the Virus. IBDV is resistant to ether and chloroform and also to pH 2. It is quite resistant to heat, being viable after 5 hours at 56°C. The virus is unaffected by immersion for 1 hour at 30°C in 0.5 percent phenol or 0.125 percent merthiolate solutions. There is a marked reduction in titer when exposed to 0.15 percent formalin for 6 hours. Chloramine in 0.5 percent concentration destroys the virus in 10 minutes.

Electron microscopy studies show that the virus particle is 58 to 65 nm in diameter (Cheville 1967, Mandelli et al. 1967). In immune electron microscopy studies negatively stained preparations reveal morphologic similarities to both the bluetongue virus group and the infectious pancreatic necrosis virus of salmonids. Small particles found in such preparations are a degradation product of the large particle (Harkness et al. 1975).

Cultivation. Isolation and serial propagation of the virus in 10-day-old embryonated hens' eggs is not difficult if eggs are obtained from a flock free of the disease. Infected chorioallantoic membranes of embryos are used as the source of virus for passage, and the virus is inoculated into the chorioallantoic membrane (Hitchner 1971).

Embryo adaptation of the virus by serial passage can increase virus titers in amniotic-allantoic fluid (Winterfield 1969). Embryo mortality occurs between the third and seventh days after inoculation (Hitchner 1971). The dead embryos show edematous distention of the abdomen, cutaneous congestion and petechial hemorrhages on toe joints and in the cerebrum, occasional necrosis and hemorrhages in the liver, a pale, "parboiled" appearance of the heart, congestion and necrosis of the kidneys, congestion of the lungs, and a pale spleen, sometimes with necrotic foci. The chorioallantoic membrane may have hemorrhagic areas, but the bursa of Fabricius does not undergo marked change.

Landgraf et al. (1967) reported on the propagation of the virus in monolayer cultures of chick embryo fibroblast. Petek and Mandelli (1968) observed cytopathic changes in chick embryo kidney cell cultures.

A variant strain was established that produces smaller plaques than the parent Cu-1 virus. It does not produce overt disease in fowls and causes only minor lesions in the bursa of Fabricius. Infection with the variant strain confers solid protective immunity against virulent virus (Cursiefen et al. 1979).

Epizootiology. The disease is highly contagious and spreads readily. The virus is resistant to heat, acids, and many chemicals, so it can remain viable on infected premises for at least 122 days after removal of the infected birds (Benton et al. 1967).

Carrier birds are unknown, but it is suspected that they exist. The lesser mealworm, *Alphitobius diaperinus*, taken from an infected premises 8 weeks after an outbreak, was infectious in susceptible chickens. Conceivably, insects may play a role in disease transmission.

Immunity Antibodies are transferred from immune hens to their progeny through the yolk sac of the egg. These chicks with maternal antibodies are protected for at least 4 to 5 weeks after hatching.

In one study, 4-week-old susceptible birds had an excellent neutralizing antibody response to chicken embryo–adapted virus with a mean titer of $10^{3.5}$ (Winterfield 1969). In contrast, 3-day-old chicks had titers between $10^{1.5}$ to $10^{2.0}$. Hitchner (1971) observed excellent titers in 12-week-old birds that were about $10^{3.8}$ after 27 weeks. Adult birds usually did not respond as well to virus. The delayed and poor response is probably caused by the absence of an active bursa of Fabricius. Chicks inoculated orally with IBDV 1 day after hatching showed a 50 percent incidence of immunodeficiency but little mortality. The antibody response to IBDV and subsequent inoculations with vaccine viruses was suppressed. Serum IgG concentration was decreased, whereas IgM occurred exclusively in its 7S monomeric form. The same IBDV inoculated into 3-week-old chicks resulted in 50 percent mortality but little immunodeficiency (Ivanyi and Morris 1976). Paradoxically serum IgG concentration was elevated in comparison with normal birds. It appears that bursal but not peripheral B cells are targets of IBDV and that the immunodeficiency results from impaired peripheral seeding of B cells in infected day-old chicks. More specifically, the surface IgM-bearing B lymphocytes probably are the target cells for infection.

Diagnosis. In acute outbreaks in susceptible flocks the high morbidity, the rapidity of onset and recovery from clinical signs (5 to 7 days) in 3- to 6-week-old chicks, and the spiked mortality curve should make the diagnostician consider IBD. Pathological confirmation can be obtained by examining the bursa of Fabricius and other sites for lesions typical of this disease. Virus particles in smear preparations of infected bursa can be readily detected.

Counterimmunoelectrophoresis is used to detect IBD precipitating antibodies in chicken serum (Berg 1982). The test is sensitive, simple, reproducible, and provides results in 45 minutes. It is comparable in sensitivity to the agar-gel diffusion test.

The virus can be readily isolated in embryonated hens' egg and identified by the use of a known positive antiserum against the isolate in the neutralization test. Paired serums are rarely used to demonstrate a rising neutralizing antibody serum titer because the history, signs of illness, and gross pathological changes, particularly of the bursa, usually are sufficient to render a correct diagnosis.

Prevention and Control. Infection is often controlled naturally because chicks exposed at an early age develop an active immunity without showing signs of illness. The resulting infection without disease may result from the natural resistance of young chicks or from maternal antibodies. Administration of an attenuated virus vaccine (Vielitz and Landgraf 1976) is recommended when management practices do not control the disease and to prevent Newcastle disease, infectious bronchitis, infectious laryngotracheitis, Marek's disease, and possibly other diseases as well. Oral administration of attenuated virus vaccines is effective in 15-week-old birds, but not in birds 23 weeks and older. Chickens of all ages respond to intramuscular inoculation (Yadin et al. 1980). Many inactivated and attenuated virus vaccines provide serviceable immunity against IBD.

The Disease in Humans. IBD has not been reported in humans.

REFERENCES

Benton, W.J., Cover, M.S., and Rosenberger, J.K. 1967. Studies on the transmission of the infectious bursal agent (IBA) of chickens. Avian Dis. 11:430–438.

Berg, N.W. 1982. Rapid detection of infectious bursa disease antibodies by counter-immuno-electrophoresis. Avian Pathol. 11:611–614.

Cheville, N.F. 1967. Studies on the pathogenesis of Gumboro disease in the bursa of Fabricius, spleen, and thymus of the chicken. Am. J. Pathol. 51:527–551.

Christopher, K.H. 1982. Experimental infection of chick infectious bursal disease virus to ducklings. Vet. Archiv. 52:189–195.

Cosgrove, A.S. 1962. Effects of a new nitrofuran feed additive on production efficiency in chickens. Avian Dis. 6:385.

Cursiefen, D., Kaufer, I., and Becht, H. 1979. Loss of virulence in a small plaque mutant of the infectious bursal disease virus. Arch. Virol. 59:39–46.

Harkness, J.W., Alexander, D.J., Pattison, M., and Scott, A.C. 1975. Infectious bursal disease agent: Morphology by negative stain electron microscopy. Arch. Virol. 48:63–73.

Helmboldt, C.F., and Garner, E. 1964. Experimentally induced Gumboro disease (IBA). Avian Dis. 8:561–575.

Hitchner, S.F. 1971. Personal communication.

Howie, R.I., and Thorzen, J. 1981. Identification of a strain of infectious bursal disease virus isolated from mosquitoes. Can. J. Comp. Med. 45:315–320.

Ivanyi, J., and Morris, R. 1976. Immunodeficiency in the chicken. IV. An immunological study of infectious bursal disease. Clin. Exp. Immunol. 23:154–165.

Jackwood, D.J., Saif, Y.M., and Hughes, J.H. 1982. Characteristics and serologic studies of two serotypes of infectious bursal disease virus in turkeys. Avian Dis. 26:871–878.

Landgraf, H., Vielitz, E., and Kirsch, R. 1967. Occurrence of an infectious disease affecting the bursa of Fabricius (Gumboro disease). D.T.W. 74:6–10.

Ley, D.H., Yamamoto, R., and Beckford, A.A. 1979. Immune-complex involvement in the pathogenesis of infectious bursal disease in chickens. Avian Dis. 23:219–224.

Mandelli, G., Rinaldi, A., Cerioli, A., and Cervio, G. 1967. Ultramicroscopic features of the bursa of Fabricius in natural and experimental Gumboro disease of chickens. Atti Soc. Itali. Sci. Vet. 21:1.

Muller, H., and Becht, H. 1982. Biosynthesis of virus-specific proteins in cells infected with infectious bursal disease virus and their significance as structural elements for infectious virus and incomplete particles. J. Virol. 44:384–392.

Petek, M., and Mandelli, G. 1968. Biological properties of a reovirus isolated in outbreak of Gumboro disease. Atti Soc. Ital. Sci. Vet. 22:875–879.

Proudfoot, F.G. 1975. The effect of diet on the severity of losses from infectious bursal disease (Gumboro) in a commercial broiler genotype. Poultry Sci. 54:294–296.

Vielitz, E., and Landgraf, H. 1976. Comparative tests on safety and potency of IBA vaccines. Dev. Biol. Stand. 33:332–339.

Winterfield, R.W. 1969. Immunity response to the infectious bursal agent. Avian Dis. 13:548–557.

Winterfield, R.W., and Hitchner, S.B. 1962. Etiology of an infectious nephritis–Nephrosis syndrome of chickens. Am. J. Vet. Res. 23:1273–1279.

Yadin, H., Hoekstra, J., Oei, H.L., and Van Roozelaar, D.J. 1980. Investigations on live virus vaccines against infectious bursal disease. Vet. Q. 2:48–57.

Infectious Pancreatic Necrosis

Infectious pancreatic necrosis (IPN) is an acute, highly contagious viral disease of salmonid fishes, often causing high mortality and significant economic loss in salmonid hatcheries throughout the world. The disease, apparently first recognized in Canadian hatcheries in 1941, was described as catarrhal enteritis resulting from excess mucus in the stomach and intestines of diseased fish. It subsequently was reported in the United States, where it was described as infectious pancreatic necrosis on the basis of histopathological findings. Five years later Wolf et al. (1960) demonstrated the viral etiology of IPN, using brook trout explants and susceptible brook trout fry and thus making the causative agent of IPN the first virus to be isolated from fish. The indiscriminant movement of salmonid fish and eggs worldwide has resulted in the spread of IPN throughout Europe and Japan.

IPN typically causes clinical signs and mortality in very young trout. Outbreaks usually occur shortly after fry have begun feeding and may result in mortality ranging from less than 10 percent to more than 90 percent, depending on the viral strain and fish population involved. Fish surviving an acute infection often become persistent carriers and may shed virus in the feces and seminal or ovarian fluids, thus allowing for horizontal and vertical transmission of IPN. Species reported to be susceptible to infection with IPN virus (IPNV) include brook trout (*Salvelinus fontinalis*), rainbow trout (*Salmo gairdneri*), cutthroat trout (*Salmo clarkii*), and brown trout (*Salmo trutta*). Atlantic salmon (*Salmo salar*) also become infected following exposure to IPN (Swanson and Gillespie 1979).

Utilizing virus isolation, histopathology, and immunofluorescence, Swanson et al. (1982) studied the pathogenesis of IPN by sequential sampling of brook trout after intraperitoneal injection of IPNV. Virus entering the peritoneal cavity within 2 days interacted with the pancreatic exocrine cells. Replication in these cells resulted in the production of IPNV-specific antigen, necrosis of infected cells, and spread of infective virus to adjacent tissue. Areas of viral replication were at first multifocal but tended to merge as they grew. Eventually most of the acinar tissue became involved, and only small pockets of normal acinar cells remained. Twelve-week-old brook trout survived with only a small amount of functional exocrine pancreas, and limited viral replication continued in this tissue for weeks. Extensive viral replication appeared to take place only in the pancreas, although viral antigen and slight pathological changes were found in the renal interstitium and livers of some fish.

Classification of IPNV has been somewhat controversial, but Underwood et al. (1977) noted its resemblance to the infectious bursal disease virus based on RNA segmentation and a similar polypeptide composition hence their tentative inclusion in the proposed genus *Birnavirus*. Studies indicate that IPNV is an unenveloped icosahedral virus approximately 60 nm in diameter and contains two species of double-stranded RNA in its genome (Dobos et al. 1977, MacDonald and Yamamoto 1977, Underwood et al. 1977). Dobos and Robert (1983) have published a brief review of the molecular biology of IPNV. There are three serotypes, as determined by neutralization kinetics in the presence of excess antibody (MacDonald and Gower 1981). Although IPNV does share certain characteristics with the Reoviridae, differences in capsid structure and nucleic acid may warrant its exclusion from this family in the future.

The virus is easily propagated in many of the piscine cell lines and produces cytopathic effect in 2 to 3 days at 20°C.

IPN is usually diagnosed by the isolation of virus from tissues of fish with active cases and subsequent identification using specific antiserum in the serum-neutralization method. High titers of virus are present in tissues from moribund fish, and diagnosis is rarely difficult during acute outbreaks. The indirect immunofluorescence test (Swanson et al. 1982), indirect immunoperoxidase technique (Nicholson and Henchal 1978), and ELISA (Dixon and Hill 1983) also have been recommended for the rapid diagnosis of IPN. Cleator and Burney (1980) have described a hemagglutination test that may be useful.

Diagnosis in apparently healthy carriers remains one of the most perplexing problems associated with IPN. Adult carriers seem to excrete virus only intermittently and are often too valuable to sacrifice in the numbers necessary to sample a population. Such nondestructive methods as examining feces, peritoneal washes, and seminal and ovarian fluids have been employed with varying degrees of success. Serologic testing of adult fish has proved inadequate because carriers tend to be poor antibody producers.

Owing to the absence of vaccines or chemotherapeutic treatments, the control of IPN currently is limited to preventive measures and the propagation of virus-free salmonid stocks. Measures employed by hatcheries to eradicate IPN vary, but slaughter of all infected stock and disinfection of the water supply are the only certain means of avoiding recurring epidemics. An attenuated vaccine (currently experimental) that could be administered at a very early age in the feed shows considerable promise. Some progress has been made in the attenuation of certain IPNV strains (Dorson 1977, Wolf 1966), but the safety and effectiveness of these have not been tested in the field. With the recognition of three serotypes among IPNV isolates, an additional concern is the degree of protection any vaccine would afford following exposure to heterologous strains.

REFERENCES

Cleator, G.M., and Burney, L.A. 1980. The hemagglutinating properties of infectious pancreatic necrosis virus. Arch. Virol. 63:81–85.

Dixon, P.F., and Hill, B.J. 1983. Rapid detection of infectious pancreatic necrosis virus (IPNV) by the enzyme-linked immunosorbent assay (ELISA). J. Gen. Virol. 64:321–330.

Dobos, P., and Roberts, T.E. 1983. The molecular biology of infectious pancreatic necrosis virus: A review. Can. J. Microbiol. 29:377–384.

Dobos, P., Hallett, R., Kells, D.T., Sorensen, O., and Rowe, D.. 1977. Biophysical studies of infectious pancreatic necrosis virus. J. Virol. 22:150–159.

Dorson, M. 1977. Vaccination trials of rainbow trout fry against infectious pancreatic necrosis. Bull. Off. Int. Epiz. 87:405.

MacDonald, R.D., and Gower, D.A. 1981. Genomic and phenotypic divergence among three serotypes of aquatic birnaviruses (infectious pancreatic necrosis virus). Virology 114:187–195.

MacDonald, R.D., and Yamamoto, T. 1977. Quantitative analysis of defective interfering particles in infectious pancreatic necrosis virus preparations. J. Gen. Virol. 35:235.

Nicholson, B.L., and Henchal, E.A. 1978. Rapid identification of infectious pancreatic necrosis virus in infected cell cultures by immunoperoxidase techniques. J. Wildl. Dis. 14:465–469.

Swanson, R.N., and Gillespie, J.H. 1979. Pathogenesis of infectious pancreatic necrosis in Atlantic salmon (Salmo salar). J. Fish Res. Board Can. 36:587–591.

Swanson, R.N., Carlisle, J.C., and Gillespie, J.H. 1982. Pathogenesis of infectious pancreatic necrosis virus infection in brook trout Salvelinus fontinales (Mitchill), following intraperitoneal injection. J. Fish Dis. 5:449–460.

Underwood, B.O., Smale, C.J., and Brown, F. 1977. Relationship of a virus from Tellina tenuis to infectious pancreatic necrosis virus. J. Gen. Virol. 36:93.

Wolf, K. 1966. The fish viruses. Adv. Virus Res. 12:35–101.

Wolf, K., Snieszko, S.F., Dunbar, C.E., and Pyle, E. 1960. Virus nature of infectious pancreatic necrosis in trout. Proc. Soc. Exp. Biol. Med. 104:105–108.

50 The Togaviridae

At present, four genera are included in the Togaviridae. The genus *Pestivirus* consists of hog cholera virus (also known as swine fever virus), bovine virus diarrhea virus (also known as bovine virus diarrhea–mucosal disease virus, see p. 741), lactic dehydrogenase virus, border disease virus, and possibly simian hemorrhagic fever virus. The genus *Rubivirus* includes rubella virus (of humans) and possibly equine arteritis virus. The genus *Alphavirus* includes former members of the arbovirus A group, and the genus *Flavivirus* formerly was called the arbovirus B group. A study group has recommended to the Vertebrate Virus Subcommittee of the International Committee on Taxonomy of Viruses that the flaviviruses be placed in a new family, the Flaviviridae, consisting of one genus, *Flavivirus*. The same group recommended that an additional genus, *Arterivirus*, be added to the Togaviridae family (Westaway et al. 1985).

There are more than 200 recognized arboviruses, and an appreciable number belong to the Togaviridae family. Most replicate in arthropod as well as vertebrate hosts. Because many arboviruses now are better characterized, it is possible to place them in specific genera in various families. Important diseases of domestic animals caused by members of the Togaviridae are listed in Table 50.1.

REFERENCE

Westaway, E.G., Brinton, M.A., Gaidamovich, S.Y., Horzinek, M.C., Igarashi, J.S., Kääriäinen, L., Lvov, D.K., Porterfield, J.S. Russell, P.K., and Trent, D.W. 1985. Flaviviridae. Intervirology 24:183–192.

The Genus *Pestivirus*

Hog cholera, bovine virus diarrhea, and border disease of lambs are the only diseases caused by viruses in the genus *Pestivirus* which are covered in this book. Hog cholera, bovine virus diarrhea, and border disease viruses are closely related to each other biophysically, biochemically, and biologically.

Hog Cholera
SYNONYM: Swine fever (Europe);
abbreviation, HC

Classical hog cholera is an acute, highly contagious disease of swine characterized by degeneration in the walls of the smaller blood vessels, which results in multiple hemorrhages, necrosis, and infarctions in the internal organs. Affected animals are prone to suffer from the effects of bacterial agents that frequently accompany the virus, but these secondary agents are not necessary for production of the disease. The sole cause of the disease is a virus.

Hog cholera was first recognized as a disease entity by Salmon and Smith in 1885, but it was erroneously believed to be caused by the bacterium they called *Bacillus cholerae-suis*, now known as *Salmonella choleraesuis*. The error was corrected when other researchers in 1903 proved that the disease was caused by a virus and that the "hog cholera bacillus" played a secondary role.

Hog cholera appeared in England in 1862 and on the European continent in 1887. In the United States the disease seems to have been first seen in Ohio in 1883; from there it spread to all parts of the United States through the shipment of stock. Its greatest prevalence was in the north central states, the so-called Corn Belt, where the swine population is greatest. The disease now has been eradicated from hogs in the United States, Canada, Hungary, Denmark, Finland, Norway, Sweden, Switzerland, the United Kingdom, Ireland, and possibly Luxembourg. Where hog cholera still exists, it is a tremendously destructive disease that causes large losses despite fairly satisfactory immunization procedures. Outbreaks have been recorded in nearly all European countries as well as in Africa, Taiwan, and Australia (Lee 1981).

Several publications provide a comprehensive review of the literature and add to our present knowledge on hog cholera (Commission of the European Communities 1977; Harkness 1985; Liess 1981, 1987; U.S. Department of Agriculture 1981).

Character of the Disease. Present knowledge suggests that hog cholera virus (HCV) produces natural disease only in domestic and wild pigs. The disease is first manifested by fever (104°F or higher), although often the first

Table 50.1. Diseases of domestic animals caused by viruses in the Togaviridae family

Viral disease	Natural hosts	Characteristics of disease produced
Genus *Pestivirus*		
Hog cholera (swine fever)	Swine	Acute, highly contagious disease with variable mortality depending on virus strain and herd susceptibility. Fever, depression, and degeneration of small blood vessels resulting in multiple hemorrhages, necrosis, and infarction.
Bovine virus diarrhea–mucosal disease	Cattle, swine, sheep, deer, and goats	Principally a disease in cattle of all ages. High morbidity, low disease occurrence and mortality as a rule. Fever, leukopenia, depression, excessive salivation caused by erosions in oral cavity, nasal discharge, and abortions in pregnant cows.
Border disease of lambs	Lambs	A mucosal disease caused by a virus antigenically similar to BVD virus.
Genus *Rubivirus*		
Equine arteritis	Horses	Acute, contagious disease characterized by fever, stiffness of gait, edema of limbs and around eyes, and abortions precipitated by lesions in the small arteries.
Genus *Alphavirus*		
Western and eastern equine encephalomyelitis	Horses, humans, wild and domesticated birds, invertebrate hosts (mosquitoes and chicken mites)	WEE and EEE affect horses of all ages. EEE causes greater mortality than WEE in horses. Epizootics occur during mosquito season. Fever and depression may be followed by signs referable to CNS if the virus invades that system, with death usually resulting 1 to 2 days after nervous signs begin. Can cause encephalitis in humans and pheasants.
Venezuelan equine encephalomyelitis	Horses, humans, many mammals, reptiles, mosquitoes	Signs of illness in horses similar to WEE and EEE. Can cause encephalitis in humans.

sign noticed is loss of appetite. In a fully susceptible herd the disease generally begins in a few animals, then gradually spreads to others until practically all are sick. The affected animals appear dull and drowsy; they crowd together in corners, under haystacks, or in any other protected place as if chilled. Vomiting is common, a mucopurulent discharge from the eyes frequently is seen, and many animals suffer from diarrhea. Sometimes the diarrheal attacks alternate with periods of constipation. In white-skinned animals a livid coloring of the skin frequently appears, especially on the abdomen and the inside of the thighs and flanks. Cutaneous hemorrhages may also appear in these areas. If the course of the disease is prolonged beyond 1 week, as it often is, bacterial complications usually occur, principally in the form of pneumonia and ulcerative enteritis.

Nervous signs—for instance, grinding of the teeth, local paralyses, locomotor disturbances, and, occasionally, lethargy and convulsions—occur quite commonly. These are manifestations of encephalomyelitis that occurs in a large percentage of all cases. Seifried (1931) found brain and cord changes in 33 of 39 animals. although most did not manifest unusual nervous signs. Macroscopically, hemorrhages are often found in the meninges and in the brain parenchyma. Microscopically, besides the hemorrhages, the usual evidence of encephalomyelitis is found—i.e., perivascular "cuffing" with lymphocytes, mononuclear cells, and a few plasma and eosinophilic

Table 50.1.—*continued*

Viral disease	Natural hosts	Characteristics of disease produced
Genus *Flavivirus*		
St. Louis encephalitis	Horses, wild and domesticated birds, humans, insects	Encephalitis in humans. Inapparent infections in horses and birds.
Japanese encephalitis	Horses, pigs, cattle, humans, wild birds, mosquitoes	Causes encephalitis in humans; domesticated animals may occasionally have disease in mild form, with occasional deaths in cattle, swine, and horses. Stillbirths and abortions occur in pregnant sows.
California encephalitis	Foals, suckling pigs, hares, humans, mosquitoes	In humans it causes an influenzalike disease with some individuals developing meningoencephalitis and atypical pneumonia. Antibodies found in foals, hares, and suckling pigs, but no disease.
Louping ill	Primarily sheep, also horses, deer, humans, ticks, cattle, piglets, dogs	Generalized infection in lambs that may involve CNS. Mortality negligible unless CNS signs occur; then death usually ensues. Horse disease similar to disease in sheep. The disease in humans is initially a febrile disease of short duration that may be followed by CNS disease.
Central European tick-borne fever	Cows, sheep, goats, humans, ticks	Diphasic disease in humans—influenzalike signs followed by CNS involvement. Virus may cause infection in cattle, sheep, and goats and be present in the milk.
Murray Valley encephalitis	Horses, feral pigs, birds, humans, insects	Infection but no disease in horses. Principally a disease of humans; birds and mosquitoes play a role in its ecology.
Wesselsbron disease	Sheep, cattle, humans, mosquitoes, dogs	Causes epizootics in sheep with abortions accompanied by death of newborn lambs and pregnant ewes. Abortions in cattle. In humans causes fever and muscular pains.
Israel meningoencephalitis	Turkeys	Progressive paralysis associated with a nonpurulent meningoencephalitis.
Powassan disease	Goats, humans	Antibodies to this virus found in a small percentage of goats in New York State. It causes disease in humans.

cells (Figure 50.1). The glial cells proliferate both diffusely and in the form of compact nodes. There is nerve cell degeneration and some neuronophagia. Changes of this type are found in some pigs very early in the disease, before recognizable signs appear. They represent a true virus-induced reaction.

Inclusion bodies have been recognized in hog cholera. Boynton et al. (1942) believed that certain bodies that they saw in the nuclei of epithelial cells of the gallbladder of pigs with cholera were of this type. Intranuclear inclusion bodies were observed in reticuloendothelial cells of various organs from more than half of the pigs given three different strains of virulent virus, but inclusion bodies were not found in pigs injected with various strains of modified HCV (Urman et al. 1962).

There is a precipitous fall in the number of circulating leukocytes in the blood—severe leukopenia (Dhennin et al. 1976, Kamijo et al. 1977). Within 48 hours after inoculation of HCV, the leukocytes, which vary between 14,000 and 24,000/μl in normal pigs, decrease to less

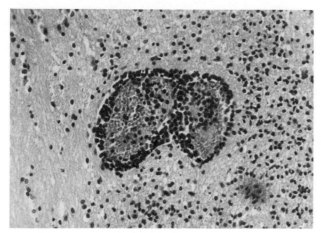

Figure 50.1. Lesions of encephalitis, which commonly occur in hog cholera. Perivascular cuffing and infiltrations of round cells into the nerve tissue are shown. Hematoxylin and eosin stain. × 210. (Courtesy S. H. McNutt.)

than 4,000 and sometimes no leukocytes can be found. So far as is known, no other common disease of pigs involves this reaction. Late in hog cholera, when secondary bacterial action plays a prominent part in the disease picture, leukopenia is replaced by leukocytosis.

Animals that die within 1 week after first showing signs usually exhibit lesions that are purely of virus origin. The pure viral disease is best seen in inoculated animals kept under good hygienic conditions. When these animals die at the height of the temperature reaction, generally on the fifth or sixth day, many have practically no gross lesions. If lesions are found, they consist only of petechial hemorrhages in the kidney cortex and in the mucosa of the urinary bladder, larynx, and trachea. Sometimes they are found also on some of the serous membranes. Larger hemorrhages often are found in the intestinal mucosa, lungs, spleen, and especially the cortex of many of the lymph nodes (Figure 50.2). These hemorrhages are caused by the rupture of capillaries that have undergone retrogressive changes as the result of virus action. The endothelial linings of the vessels commonly show swelling and proliferation, and many lymphatic channels are plugged with such desquamated cells. Many small vessels degenerate into hyaline tubes, which readily rupture and allow blood to leak into the lymph channels.

In animals with cases that run a longer course, fibrinous pneumonia, often with necrotic foci in the consolidated portions, and fibrinopurulent enteritis with ulceration are commonly found. In these animals "button" ulcers of the mucosa may appear, especially in the region of the ileocecal valve. Because of the deposition of concentric layers of fibrin over the mucosal perforations, raised, buttonlike deposits are formed—hence the name. These lesions may

be associated with the activities of the "hog cholera bacillus" (*Salmonella choleraesuis*) and the necrosis bacillus (*Fusobacterium necrophorum*). The latter lives saprophytically in the alimentary canal of most swine and causes damage only when the intestinal mucosa is altered by the presence of another pathogenic agent such as *S. choleraesuis*.

Infections of pregnant sows cause small litters, fetal deaths, premature births, stillbirths, cerebellar ataxic piglets, runting, and tremors (Hermanns et al. 1981). Immune pregnant sows as well as susceptible dams can give birth to piglets with congenital disease (Carbrey 1965, Young et al. 1955). Some piglets that survive are immunotolerant and unthrifty and remain virus carriers. Immunotolerant piglets have a disease totally different from classic hog cholera (Dunne and Clark 1968).

Following inoculation with virulent virus, pigs remain apparently well for at least 3 days. Field exposures to much smaller quantities of virus by natural routes may prolong this incubation period to 6 or 7 days. Most swine die within 7 to 10 days from the time signs first appear. Sometimes individuals live longer, in which case pneumonia and enteric complications are apt to appear. The mortality in some natural outbreaks is close to 100 percent. Since the introduction of attenuated virus vaccines, many outbreaks of HC with low mortality have occurred. Some veterinarians suggest that these outbreaks represent strains of attenuated virus which have increased in virulence by transfer in nature.

In experimental studies only swine show clinical signs of illness with HCV. The virus has been adapted to rabbits, and after several passages, the only sign of illness is a slight rise in body temperature (Baker 1947). Growth of virus has been demonstrated by serial transfer in cattle, goats, sheep, and peccaries. Significant antibody production was detected in peccaries, calves, goats, sheep, and deer after inoculation with HCV. The inoculated animals failed to transmit the virus by contact to penmates of the same species, and calves failed to transmit the infection to susceptible cohabiting pigs (Loan and Storm 1968). Antibody production was not detected in wild mice, cottontail rabbits, sparrows, wild rats, raccoons, or pigeons after HC virus inoculation (Loan and Storm 1968).

In experimental studies in pigs, the virus is introduced into the body either by the respiratory system or the upper digestive tract (Dunne et al. 1959). According to Lin et al. (1969) the tonsil is a prime target because the greatest concentration of virus is found there. Infectious virus is present in the bloodstream 24 hours after respiratory or tonsillar exposure. Leukocytes of the peripheral blood are infected and capable of viral replication. Regional lymph nodes are the first tissues to show edema and hemorrhage.

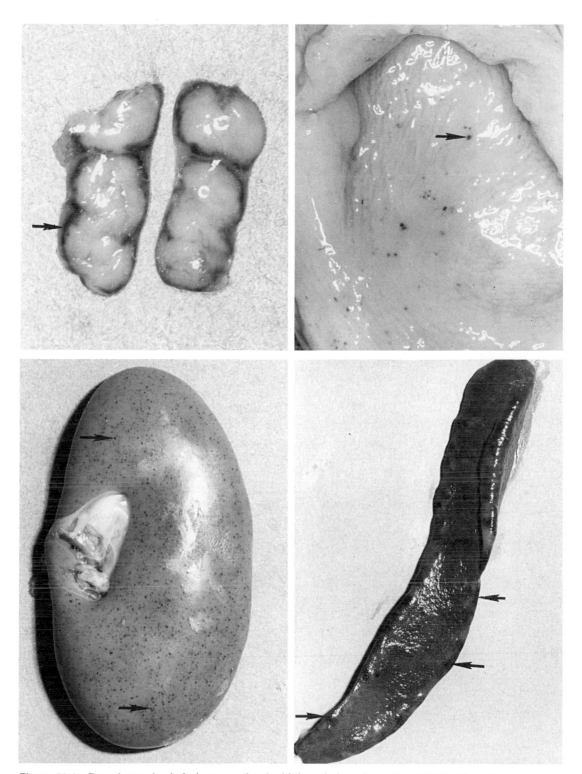

Figure 50.2. Gross hemorrhagic lesions associated with hog cholera virus. (*Top left*) Peripheral hemorrhage in cervical lymph node. (*Top right*) Submucosal hemorrhages in urinary bladder. (*Botton left*) Subcapsular petechiation of kidney. The white areas are photographic artifacts. (*Bottom right*) Hemorrhagic areas along margin of the spleen. (Courtesy D. Gustafson.)

After intravenous inoculation of HCV, infective virus can not be demonstrated at 0.5, 5, 8, and 13 hours after injection, but blood samples at 16 and 18 hours contain infective virus (Dunne et al. 1959). Apparently many reticuloendothelial cells become infected. Many internal organs contain virus, but not until 48 hours after infection.

Properties of the Virus. The particle size of HCV is 38 to 50 nm (Dunne 1970, Enzmann and Rehberg 1977). Small particles ranging from 3 to 23 nm have been observed in many tissue-cultured HCV preparations (Dunne 1970). In some instances they are parvoviruses. A ring of light particle projections 6 to 8 nm long, observed at the particle surface, probably represents the soluble antigen of HCV (Ritchie and Fernelius 1967). This RNA virus is spherical with an envelope (Dinter, 1963). The molecular mass of the viral RNA is about 4×10^6 daltons in polyacrylamide–agarose-gel electrophoresis (Enzmann and Weiland 1978). The virus is sensitive to ether and chloroform. In a sucrose density gradient the particles are seen as a visible band at a density of 1.13 to 1.14 g/ml. (Coggins 1964). The HC virus has at least three polypeptides as resolved by polyacrylamide-gel electrophoresis after disruption of the virus with sodium dodecyl sulfate (Enzmann and Rehberg 1977, Enzmann and Weiland 1978). The molecular masses of the structural proteins are 55,000 daltons (gp 55), 46,000 daltons (gp 46), and 36,000 (p 36).

A relatively stable virus, it can survive temperatures of 50°C for 3 days, 37°C for 7 to 15 days, and −70°C for many years without appreciable loss of infectivity. After an initial drop upon lyophilization it remains viable at 6°C for years. The greatest pH stability of the virus in defibrinated blood occurs at levels of 5 to 5.5. Dimethyl sulfoxide helps to stabilize the virus (Tessler et al. 1975). Hydrolytic enzymes such as trypsin and phospholipase C reduce viral infectivity, suggesting that it is dependent on the integrity of membrane phospholipids (Laude 1977). The virus also is inactivated by Roccal, cresol, sodium hypochloride, sodium-*o*-phenylphenate, and betapropiolactone.

The agglutinin of *Ricinus communis* has been used to develop simple concentration and purification procedures for HCV. The lectin both precipitates and binds the virus in affinity chromatography (Neukirch et al. 1981).

Kamijo et al. (1977) divided strains of HCV into two groups, H and B, based on the difference in the neutralization capacity. Group H consists of strains reacting poorly in the neutralization test and causing acute illness in experimental pigs. Group B consists of strains reacting well with bovine virus diarrhea antiserum and producing a chronic illness in pigs. The investigators found that pigs immunized with bovine diarrhea virus resisted challenge with a group B virus, but succumbed to challenge with a group H virus. This finding indicates a significant biological difference in HCV strains, yet the attenuated hog cholera virus vaccines clearly protect pigs against challenge with virulent strains (group H).

A number of serologic methods to study HC antigen and antibody have been described. A conglutination-complement-absorption test for the detection of HC antibody was described by Millian and Englehard (1961). A hemagglutination test used to measure HCV and antibody was based on the linkage of formalinized erythrocytes through diazo bonds with eitherHCV or HC antibody (Segre 1962). The agar-gel method of Ouchterlony is used to demonstrate a specific antigen-antibody precipitation. The neutralization test in pig kidney cultured cells is possible since the isolation of a cytopathogenic strain of HCV by Gillespie and co-workers (1960). An indirect neutralization test called the END method was developed by Japanese workers (Kumagai et al. 1961); its cytopathogenicity is based on the exaltation effect of Newcastle virus on HCV in a cell-culture system. More recently, a simple and rapid microtiter procedure for the END method has been described for determining HC antibody titers (Lai et al. 1980). A complement-fixation test was used to demonstrate that HCV and bovine virus diarrhea virus (BVDV) share a soluble antigen (Gutekunst and Malmquist 1964). An enzyme-labeled antibody microtiter technique for rapidly detecting hog cholera antibodies was developed by Saunders (1977). Because it measures the same antibody as the complement-fixation test, cross-reactions with antiserums to HCV and BVDV occur. A peroxidase-linked antibody assay based on the use of microplates with fixed viral antigen has been developed (Jensen 1981). Use of this test with the complement-fixation test permits some differentiation between HC and BVD antibodies.

Cultivation. Virus multiplies in embryonated hens' eggs only when freshly minced testicular tissue is placed on the chorioallantoic membrane (TenBroeck 1941).

HCV was first grown in cell culture by Hecke in Maitland plasma cell type cultures (Dunne 1970). He also cultivated the virus in suspended porcine spleen tissue. In general, HCV strains grow most successfully in primary or stable cell cultures derived from swine leukocytes, bone marrow, lymph node, lung, kidney, testicle, and spleen. In most instances no cytopathic effect is observed following inoculation with HCV. A slight cytopathology in spleen cultures was reported by Gustafson and Pomerat (1957). Gillespie et al. (1960) described a PAV-1 strain that produces marked cytopathology in primary swine kidney cells and also grows in swine testicular cells. Subsequent studies by a Munich group (Bachmann et al.

1967) with this PAV-1 cytopathogenic strain have shown that it contains no adenovirus, BVDV, or mycoplasma (Bodon 1965, Horzinek and Uberschar 1966). The Munich group also reported that their virus preparations of PAV-1 had particles of two sizes, 39 to 40 nm and 14 to 16 nm, which both banded in cesium chloride fractions between 1.14 and 1.20 g/ml. The larger ones are believed to be the principal HCV particles since the smaller particles were not found in the Ames or strain A preparations. The exact nature of the smaller particle or its relation to the larger HCV particle, if any, has not been ascertained (Bachmann et al. 1967). Whether the larger particles of the PAV-1 strain have unique cytopathogenic properties or whether the presence of both particles are required for the cytopathic effect in cell culture remains to be determined.

Direct plaque formation with representative strains of HCV was observed in several pig kidney cell lines under agar overlay (Laude 1978b). The infected cells appear as hazy plaques under indirect light and as white plaques after neutral red staining.

The production of cytopathogenesis by the exalted effect of Newcastle virus on HCV was described by Kumagai et al. in 1961. Any strain of virus can be detected in tissue culture by the use of fluorescent antibody technique (Mengeling et al. 1963, Solorzano 1962). Reverse plaque formation, based on viral interference with vesicular stomatitis virus, is a simple and rapid procedure to assay for HCV in cell culture (Fukusho et al 1976, Laude 1978a).

HCV usually persists in cell cultures without a cytopathic effect. It is known to survive and multiply in leukocyte cultures for more than 2 months (Dunne 1970) and has persisted in subcultural leukocytes for more than 471 days (Loan and Gustafson 1961).

An end-point dilution–fluorescent antibody technique has been used to clone HCV (Kreese et al. 1982). The derived virus clone yielded a homogenous population of HCV that retained the characteristics of the parent strain.

Epizootiology. Hog cholera is transmitted principally by direct contact with sick animals and directly or indirectly with fresh secretions and excretions. How the virus passes from farm to farm is not known precisely in every case. Birds have been suspected of carrying virus on their bodies, and undoubtedly virus may be carried on the shoes and clothing of people and the feet of animals if they travel directly from infected premises. The disease may be transmitted to new locations by careless handling of blood, virus used for immunization, or bottles that have contained such virus.

Probably one of the most common ways by which hog cholera infects isolated swine herds is through the feeding of kitchen scraps or garbage. In 1915 many pigs were slaughtered for food while in the early stages of the disease when their tissues contained a great deal of virus, it was shown that HCV persisted for considerable periods in fresh pork and even in pickled and smoked hams from these animals. Trimmings from infected meat, thrown into garbage, can readily start outbreaks. These findings have been amply confirmed by Doyle (1933) in England. Claxton (1954) point out that most English outbreaks were initiated in this way. Between 1944 and 1949 England imported very little pork, and during this time the incidence of hog cholera fell far below the usual level. In studies by McKercher et al. (1978) in the United States, virus was not recovered from partly cooked hams and from dried pepperoni sausages after the required curing period.

Dunne et al. (1959) showed that HCV, incorporated into double gelatin capsules and passed into the stomach, did not produce infection in test pigs. Infection was readily instigated through the tonsils and also through the respiratory tract when precautions were taken to avoid tonsillar infection.

Mosquitoes trapped during an epizootic of hog cholera contained virus (Stewart et al. 1975). Pigs inoculated with positive pools of mosquitoes developed chronic hog cholera with persistent viremia. Experimental studies demonstrated that *Aedes aegypti* and *Culex tarsalis* may mechanically transmit the virus to susceptible pigs.

As the virus does not persist on the premises after swine have been removed, it was a mystery for a long time how outbreaks of cholera began, since it is largely a seasonal disease. Most sows are bred to farrow in the spring and fall of each year and most cholera outbreaks occur in those seasons. A highly significant report by Baker and Sheffy (1960) provides the most reasonable and logical explanation for the persistence of virus between outbreaks. They showed that some piglets given low-passage attenuated rabbit HCV were stunted and unthrifty. The virus reverted to virulence in the piglets and persisted in the bloodstream in high concentrations until death 2 to 3 months later. Carbrey et al. (1980) confirmed these findings by studies of 135 HC field isolates. Persistent viremic infections may also occur as a result of vertical transmission in utero (see reviews by Harkness [1985] and Liess [1987]). The infected pigs may live for as long as 152 days.

In summary, the persistently infected pig clearly is potentially very important in the transmission of natural disease. The success or failure of a regional or countrywide hog cholera eradication program seems to hinge on this single factor—elimination of the infected pig (and herd).

Immunity. Animals that recover from an attack of hog

cholera have long-lasting and durable immunity. It is generally accepted that a single immunological type of virus exists. Dale et al. (1951) described a variant strain that required larger doses of antiserums, which was produced against standard virus for protection against the variant strain, than the normal homotypic virus strain. An encephalitic strain described by Dunne et al. (1952) was only partially neutralized by commercial HC antiserum.

In preliminary tests with the PAV-1 cytopathogenic strain of HCV, neutralizing antibody titers were correlated with resistance to hog cholera infection, suggesting that resistance is related to the presence of circulating antibody or to its rapid production (Coggins 1962). The neutralization test is accurate and specific. The presence of antibody appears to indicate resistance to hog cholera. The test has also been used to assess the efficacy of vaccines. Immune serums to other strains of HCV neutralize the PAV-1 cytopathogenic strain. The neutralization test has been used to study maternal and active immunity and the relation of HCV to BVDV (Coggins 1964).

The newborn pig obtains most, if not all, of its antibody from the colostrum of its immune dam. Colostral antibody is lost from the young pig at a constant rate. Antibody half-life is 13 days, and pigs that have maternal antibody titers of 1:1,000 or above still have some antibody at age 4 months and therefore resist virulent HCV. Pigs with sufficient antibody to resist virulent virus become solidly immune following challenge (Coggins 1962).

Colostral or serum antibody may interfere with the development of immunity following vaccination (Dunne 1970). Coggins (1964) showed that the interference is not an all-or-none phenomenon. Interference depends on the amount of antibody in the host and the amount of virus in the vaccine. Tissue-cultured vaccine containing 10,000 immunizing doses of virus overcomes maternal immunity at antibody levels of 1:1,000 or above. It was found that high levels of antibody depressed the antibody response to vaccine and such animals consistently developed lower titers. The amount of viable virus thus appears to be the most important single factor in overcoming maternal antibody interference. Two other groups of scientists (Lai et al. 1978, Launais et al. 1978) showed that the HC maternal antibody titers decline sufficiently in piglets 30 to 35 days old of age to permit successful vaccination.

Diagnosis. Prompt diagnosis of hog cholera is extremely important because delays often mean the loss of entire herds when many animals might have been saved by prompt use of antiserum. If the diagnosis is in doubt, it is best to treat a disease as hog cholera rather than delay prophylaxis for a day or two until the nature of the disease becomes clearer. It is a case of risking the cost of unnecessary serum treatment against that of losing many animals.

The fluorescent antibody method is preferred in diagnostic laboratories for the detection of HCV. Direct examination of tissues from infected pigs makes diagnosis possible with a few hours. It appears that the field strain of HCV grows in tissue culture without producing a cytopathic effect, but viral activity can be detected by the fluorescent antibody technique, a powerful tool for the diagnosis and eradication of hog cholera. Solorzano et al. (1966), using the PK-15 cell line for virus propagation and the flourescent antibody test for identification of viral replication, tested specimens from 462 animals with suspected hog cholera. By this procedure, 146 (32 percent) were positive; 169 (37 percent) were positive when brain lesions were used as diagnostic criteria. The two methods agreed in 82 percent of cases and disagreed in 18 percent. With fluorescent antibody testing, 32 animals (7 percent) that had no brain lesions were found to have HCV, and the presence of virus in 53 animals (11 percent) with brain lesions could not be confirmed. The investigators concluded that the fluorescent antibody method is superior to conventional methods for hog cholera diagnosis.

A two-step technique for the isolation of HC virus, consisting of an initial culture on buffy coat cultures and subinoculation to PK-15 cell line, is a more efficient and sensitive procedure for isolating virus from field cases, but it is not infallible (Kresse et al. 1975). Pig inoculation with field test specimens is still the most sensitive method for isolation of HCV.

Testing acute and convalescent serum samples for antibody and then detecting a significant rise between the paired serums is another method that can be profitably used to diagnose hog cholera. The serum-neutralization test is commonly used for this purpose (Gillespie et al. 1960).

The differential diagnosis of hog cholera and acute erysipelas infection often presents serious difficulties even to experienced veterinarians. In erysipelas infections it is not uncommon for several animals to die suddenly with few or no premonitory signs. This does not happen with cholera. In both infections the sick animals have high temperatures, but more animals are apt to develop signs at about the same time in erysipelas than in cholera. In both cases the sick animals lie on their bedding, refuse food, and are reluctant to move; but, whereas in cholera they are mentally depressed and sleepy, they are mentally alert in erysipelas. The joint swellings that appear in many cases of erysipelas are absent in cholera. Vomiting occurs in both diseases. The characteristic "diamond skin" lesions of erysipelas appear most often in the chronic rather than the acute form of the disease, but they are sometimes seen in acute cases and may be helpful in diagnosis. In some cases of acute erysipelas infection, edema of the lungs develops, and this causes the animals to pant and show evidence of shortness of breath. This is not seen in cholera.

Autopsy findings often are not very helpful in the more acute cases of erysipelas and cholera because these diseases may cause only minimal lesions. Blood cell counts show leukopenia in cholera and leukocytosis in erysipelas. The organism of erysipelas can usually be isolated from the spleen of affected animals, thus confirming the field diagnosis.

The introduction of African swine fever into a country where hog cholera exists poses very serious problems in diagnosis. It is impossible to differentiate these two important diseases in swine except by laboratory tests performed by competent personnel who are familiar with test procedures for both diseases.

Prevention. Several methods have been developed for the prophylactic immunization of swine against cholera. Passive immunity is obtained with a hyperimmune antiserum made in swine. Active immunity may be conferred with simultaneous injection of antiserum and active virus, with vaccines containing only inactivated virus, or with vaccines containing living, attenuated virus. The use of BVDV as a means of protecting pigs against hog cholera has been proposed by Atkinson et al. (1962). Another group (Kamijo et al. 1977) showed that BVDV protects pigs against certain biotypes of HCV but not others.

Leebken et al. (1967) used the fluorescent antibody test to differentiate the effects of virulent, attenuated, and inactivated HCV strains on tonsillar tissue in young swine. Bright cytoplasmic fluorescence was diffusely distributed throughout the epithelial and lymphoid tissues in tonsils of pigs given virulent HCV. After injection of attenuated HC vaccines bright fluorescence was observed, primarily in plaquelike areas in the tonsillar crypt epithelium. In pigs given either of two inactivated virus vaccines, fluorescence was granular and limited to the tonsillar germinal centers.

Passive immunity. The value of antiviral serum was first reported in 1908 by a group of workers with the U.S. Department of Agriculture. The serum was prepared in pigs. As a prophylactic agent it is very effective, immunity being established immediately. As a curative agent its usefulness is limited because most animals showing definite signs will die in spite of serum treatment. The principal use for serum alone is at the beginning of outbreaks to protect animals that have not yet contracted the infection. It is effective, but the immunity is short-lived.

Table 50.2. Minimum dose of hog cholera antiserum required to induce passive immunity in pigs

Pig weight	Minimum dose (ml)
Suckling pigs	20
20 to 40 pounds	30
40 to 90 pounds	35
90 to 120 pounds	45
120 to 150 pounds	55
150 to 180 pounds	65
180 pounds and over	75

Doses of antiserum for hog cholera must be gauged by the weight of the animal (Table 50.2). It is important that doses not be underestimated, particularly when serum is used simultaneously with virus. It is far better to give too much serum than too little.

After pasteurization of anti–hog cholera serum became a requirement, a type of serum shock occurring immediately after its injection was noticed. Serum shock occurs in only a few animals. The signs vary from animal to animal, but usually consist of rapid respiration and prostration, and sometimes vomiting and convulsions. These signs are seen more often in young animals than in older ones. Deaths are rare; consequently, the reactions are not considered serious enough to cause hesitancy in the use of serum. The shock-provoking agent can be isolated from heated serum by ammonium sulfate in concentrations great enough to precipitate the euglobulin. Some evidence indicates that there is a relation between serum shock and anemia in young pigs (Ritchie and Fernelius 1967). For a discussion of this problem, see Mathews and Buthala (1958).

Active immunity. The simultaneous injection of antiserum and virus was the first method used in the United States to protect pigs against hog cholera. This method sometimes caused a reaction in pigs and occasionally caused death, but the survivors were solidly immune. When serum breaks occur, they indicate a failure of the antiserum to protect against the virus administered. Serum breaks always occur within a few days. Virus breaks are significant when cholera develops several weeks or months following the simultaneous treatment. These failures occur when the virus is not sufficiently potent or when pigs fail to react properly to virus. Such animals are only passively immunized and become susceptible 2 to 3 weeks later.

Crystal violet vaccine was once a commonly used inactivated-virus agent, but neutralizing antibody titers following one injection of crystal violet vaccine were low or undetectable (Coggins 1962). A second injection improved its effectiveness.

The use of BVDV of cattle for protection against hog cholera has been recommended (Atkinson et al. 1962). Vaccination with strain NY-1 of BVDV protects against some HCV strains, but not all. This protection is based on the secondary response because immunization with strain NY-1 produces BVDV antibody but no HC antibody. Upon challenge with virulent HVC, pigs usually produce HC antibody quickly, and this antibody may render clinical protection. Its potential use as an immunizing agent has certain advantages: it is not pathogenic for pigs; it is safer than attenuated HCV vaccine because HCV is not involved; and with no HC antibodies produced, the presence of HC antibody in a pig population means that the animals have been naturally exposed to HCV. Studies by Kamijo et al. (1977) suggest that BVD vaccine might be used successfully where the chronic form of hog cholera predomina.es.

The first attenuated HCV vaccines were modified by passage in rabbits (Atkinson et al. 1962). Certain attenuated vaccines were given simultaneously with HC antiserum. Serum use depended on the degree of virus attenuation by rabbit passage or by tissue-culture passage (Gillespie et al. 1961). More recently there has been great interest in a lapinized HCV vaccine strain developed by Taiwanese investigators (Lin and Lee 1981). This high-passage vaccine strain—it underwent over 800 passages in rabbits—caused no clinical signs, viremia, leukopenia, virus excretion, or contact infection. Its use in Taiwan reduced the rate of hog cholera from 0.8 to 0.02 percent in a relatively short time. This product is now being evaluated and used in some European countries.

Tissue-cultured vaccines cost less to produce and are reputed to contain more virus with higher antigenicity. The use of the cytopathogenic strain or the fluorescent antibody technique for the detection of noncytopathic vaccine strains makes production control and virus assay much simpler. There is evidence that most rabbit vaccines spread to susceptible pigs. Apparently tissue-cultured vaccines also spread.

The immunity derived from these attenuated vaccines lasts a long time. Parenteral or intranasal vaccination provides a good systemic and local immune response (Corthier and Aynaud 1977). Maternal immunity may suppress primary antibody response depending, on the serum antibody concentration in the piglets. The inhibition of antibody production is either partial or complete, but a primary response of the immune system does occur, as evidenced by the clinical signs and the type of immune response following challenge with virulent virus (Corthier 1976). It may be necessary to revaccinate breeder stock.

Rabbit vaccine virus should not be given to pregnant sows because the virus produces a variety of fetal abnormalities, with fetal death and partial reabsorption sometimes occurring (Sautter et al. 1953). Low-passage rabbit virus should not be used in young pigs because stunting and death may occur (Baker and Sheffy 1960). The use of tissue cultured virus vaccines in pregnant sows should also be avoided.

Control. HCV is spread through fresh pork, the trimmings of which often find their way back to swine in garbage. When cholera appears in herds of swine of marketable size, farmers frequently rush their stock to market. In federally inspected slaughtering establishments efforts are made to prevent the slaughter of swine obviously ill from cholera, but frequently such animals are not detected in the short time they are held in the yards. This means that many hogs that harbor active virus are slaughtered and contaminated pork enters the market. Abbatoirs that are not under federal control probably distribute more virus through infected pork than those where some, but insufficient, control is exercised.

Laws requiring the cooking of all garbage fed to swine have long been in effect in many European countries, the United States, and Canada. These were enacted in most cases to reduce foot-and-mouth disease transmission, but they also serve, of course, to reduce the hazards of other diseases, including hog cholera.

Pigs that recover from hog cholera or piglets infected in utero may be carriers of the virus. Some vaccine strains also may persist in immunized pigs. As a consequence, pigs on any premises that have been exposed to live virus constitute a potential source of infection for other susceptible pigs. At present, swine are the only known source of virus, but the natural history of this disease has not been completely studied. Other virus reservoirs may exist.

Hog cholera has been eliminated in various European countries, the United States, and Canada. Eradication procedures are extremely expensive, but officials believe the benefits outweigh the costs. To effect a successful program requires the unqualified support of control officials, veterinarians, and the swine industry officials. As of 1988, the United States has been free of disease for 10 years, 20 years after the start of a federal eradication program. The tremendous effort and continued vigilance on the part of individuals in the Department of Agriculture and others clearly have led to a major victory for all concerned, with the swine industry and the general public the major benefactors. This freedom from disease also strongly supports the hypothesis that eliminating hog cholera virus from the swine population effectively eradicates the disease in an area or country.

Relation of HCV to BVDV. Using the agar-gel diffusion test, Darbyshire (1960) showed that the two viruses were related. The precipitation reaction was specific, and antibody could be absorbed with heterologous antigen as well as with homologous antigen. In neutralization tests their respective antibodies did not cross-neutralize (Sheffy et al. 1961). Each virus is capable of stimulating a primary response for the other, and an accelerated antibody to the heterologous virus appears in 5 to 7 days. In the case of hog cholera, this secondary response confers protection to pigs against virulent HCV but apparently not against all strains (Sheffy et al. 1962). Resistance was not clearly demonstrated in calves because they had only a mild clinical infection when given BVDV, making challenge evaluation difficult. Nevertheless, an anamnestic type of antibody response has been found in these animals (Sheffy et al. 1962). HCV and BVDV each multiply in rabbits without producing disease. In these animals heterotypic neutralizing antibody responses are seen, regardless of the virus injected (Coggins and Seo 1963).

Knowledge of the physical, chemical, and morphologic features of both viruses show that similarities exist. They interfere with each other in tissue-culture systems. There is cross-staining when immunofluorescence is employed. Furthermore, heterologous reactions indicate a common soluble antigen (Mengeling et al. 1963). This antigen has been used in a complement-fixation test to further characterize their relation (Gutekunst and Malmquist 1964). Hyperimmune antiserums contain detectable levels of the heterotypic neutralizing antibody.

The Disease in Humans. There is no evidence that HCV causes infection in humans.

REFERENCES

Atkinson, G.F., Baker, J.A., Campbell, C., Coggins, L., Nelson, D., Robson, D., Sheffy, B.E., Sippel, W.,and Nelson, S. 1962. Bovine virus diarrhea (BVD) vaccine for protection of pigs against hog cholera. Proc. U.S. Livestock Sanit. Assoc. 66:326–338.

Bachmann, P.A., Sheffy, B.E., and Siegl, G. 1967. Viruses contributing to the cytopathic effect of hog cholera strain PAV-1. Arch. Gesam. Virusforsch. 22:467–471.

Baker, J.A. 1947. Attenuation of hog-cholera virus by serial passage in rabbits. J. Am. Vet. Med. Assoc. 111:503–505.

Baker, J.A., and Sheffy, B.E. 1960. A persistent hog cholera viremia in young pigs. Proc. Soc. Exp. Biol. Med. 105:675–678.

Bodon, L. 1965. Contamination of various hog cholera virus strains with adenoviruses or virus diarrhoea virus. Preliminary report. Acta Vet. Acad. Sci. Hung. 15:471–472.

Boynton, W.H., Woods, G.M., Wood, F.W., and Castleberry, N.H. 1942. Immunological studies with hog cholera tissue vaccine. J. Am. Vet. Med. Assoc. 101:523.

Carbrey, E.A. 1965. The role of immune tolerance in transmission of hog cholera. J. Am. Vet. Med Assoc. 146:233–237.

Carbrey, E.A., Stewart, W.C., Kresse, J.I., and Snyder, M.L. 1980. Persistent hog cholera infection detected during virulence typing of 135 field isolates. Am. J. Vet. Res. 41:946–949.

Claxton, B.A. 1954. Progress in the control of swine fever [in Great Britain]. Agriculture (Lond.) 60:473–478.

Coggins, L. 1962. Hog cholera and virus diarrhea maternal antibodies in swine. Ph.D. dissertation, Cornell University, Ithaca, N.Y.

Coggins, L. 1964. Study of hog cholera colostral antibody and its effect on active hog cholera immunization. Am. J. Vet. Res. 25:613–617.

Coggins, L., and Seo, S. 1963. Serological comparison with rabbit antisera of hog cholera virus and bovine virus diarrhea virus. Proc. Soc. Exp. Biol. Med. 114:778.

Commission of the European Communities. 1977. Agricultural research seminar on hog cholera/classical swine fever and African swine fever. Hanover, Sept. 6–11, 1976. Luxembourg, Directorate-General XIII. P. 804.

Corthier, G. 1976. Swine fever: Influence of passive immunity on pig immune response following vaccination with a live virus vaccine. (Thiverval strain). Ann. Rech. Vét. 7:361.

Corthier, G., and Aynaud, J.M. 1977. Comparison of the immune response in serum and bucco pharyngeal secretions following immunization by different routes with a live hog cholera virus vaccine (Thiverval strain). Ann. Rech. Vét. 8:159–165.

Dale, C.N., Schoening, H.W., Cole, C.G, Henley, R.R., and Zinober, M.R. 1951. Variations (variants) of hog cholera virus. J. Am. Vet. Med. Assoc. 118:279–285.

Darbyshire, J.H. 1960. A serological relationship between swine fever and mucosal disease of cattle. Vet. Res. 72:331.

Dhennin, L., Larenaudie, B., and Remond, M. 1976. Etude d'un nouveau vaccin inactif contre la peste porcine classique. Acad. Sci. D (Paris) 283:1457.

Dinter, Z. 1963. Relationship between bovine virus diarrhoea virus and hog cholera virus. Zentralbl. Bakteriol. 188:475–486.

Doyle T.M. 1933. Transmission of tuberculosis by contact from infected to healthy guinea-pigs, with reference to some recent work on B.C.G. vaccine. J. Comp. Pathol. Therap. 46:25–34.

Dunne, H.W. 1970. Hog cholera. In Diseases of Swine, 3d ed. Iowa State University Press, Ames. Pp. 177–239.

Dunne, H.W., and Clark, C.D. 1968. Embryonic and neonatal death in pigs of gilts vaccinated with live-virus hog cholera vaccine. Am. J. Vet. Res. 29:787.

Dunne, H.W., Hokanson, J.F., and Luedke, A.J. 1959. The pathogenesis of hog cholera. I. Route of entrance of the virus into the animal body. Am. J. Vet. Res. 20:615–618.

Dunne, H.W., Smith, E.M., Runnells, R.A., Stafseth, H.J., and Thorp, F. 1952. A study of an encephalitic strain of hog cholera virus. Am. J. Vet. Res. 13:277–289.

Enzmann, P.J., and Rehberg, H. 1977. The structural components of hog cholera virus. Z. Naturschrift 32:456–458.

Enzmann, P.J., and Weiland, F. 1978. Structural similarities of hog cholera virus with togaviruses. Arch. Virol. 57:339–348.

Fukusho, A. N., Ogawa, H., Yamamoto, M., Sawada, T., and Sazawa, H. 1976. Reverse plaque formation by hog cholera virus of the GPE-strain inducing heterologous interference. Infect. Immun. 14:332–336.

Gillespie, J.H., Sheffy, B.E., and Baker, J.A. 1960. Propagation of hog cholera virus in tissue culture. Proc. Soc. Exp. Biol. Med. 105:679–681.

Gillespie, J.H., Sheffy, B.E., Coggins, L., Madin, S.H., and Baker, J.A. 1961. Propagation and attenuation of hog cholera virus in tissue culture. Proc. U.S. Livestock Sanit. Assoc. 65:57–63.

Gustafson, D.P., and Pomerat, C.M. 1957. Cytopathogenic effects of hog cholera virus on embryonic swine tissues in vitro. Am. J. Vet. Res. 18:473–480.

Gutekunst, D.E., and Malmquist, W.A. 1964. Complement-fixing and neutralizing antibody response to bovine viral diarrhea and hog cholera antigens. Can. J. Comp. Med. Vet. Sci. 28:19–23.

Harkness, J.W. 1985. Classical swine fever and its diagnosis: A current view. Vet. Rec. 116:288–293.

Hermanns, W., Trautwein, G., Meyer, H., and Liess, B. 1981. Experimental transplacental transmission of hog cholera virus in pigs. V. Immunopathological findings in newborn pigs. Zentralbl. Veterinärmed. [B] 28:669–683.

Horzinek, M., and Uberschar, S. 1966. Characterization of a porcine adenovirus in connection with studies on swine fever virus. Arch. Gesam. Virusforsch. 18:406–421.

Jensen, M.H. 1981. Detection of antibodies against hog cholera virus and bovine viral diarrhea virus in porcine serum. A comparative examination using CF, PLA, and NPLA assays. Acta Vet. Scand. 22:85–98.

Kamijo, Y., Ohkuma, S., Shimizu, M., and Shimizu, Y. 1977. Effect of dexamethasone on the multiplication of attenuated strains of hog cholera virus in pigs. Natl. Inst. Anim. Health Q. (Tokyo) 17:133.

Kresse, J.I., Stewart, W.C., Carbrey, E.A., and Snyder, M.L. 1975. Swine buffy coat culture: An aid to the laboratory diagnosis of hog cholera. Am. J. Vet. Res. 36:141–144.

Kresse, J.I., Stewart, W.C., Cabrey, E.A, and Snyder, M.L. 1982. End-point dilution–fluorescent antibody technique for cloning hog cholera virus. Am. J. Vet. Res. 43:497–498.

Kumagai, T., Shimizu, T., Ikeda, S., and Matumato, M. 1961. A new in vitro method (END) for detection and measurement of hog cholera virus and its antibody by means of effect of HC virus on Newcastle disease virus in swine tissue culture. I. Establishment of standard procedure. J. Immunol. 87:245–256.

Lai, S.S., Chen, C.S., Huang, T.H., Ho, W.C., Wang, J.T., and Wu, F.M. 1980. Immune response of pigs with different levels of colostral antibody to inoculation with LPC—Chinese strain of hog cholera vaccine. J. Chin. Soc. Vet. Sci. 6:77–81.

Lai, S.S., Ho, W.C., Huang, T.S., Wan, S.K., and Lin, T.C. 1978. A simple and rapid microtiter procedure for END method to determine hog cholera antibody titers. J. Chin. Soc. Vet. Sci. 4:109–111.

Laude, H. 1977. Hog cholera virus. I. Sensitivity to hydrolytic enzymes. II. Isoelectric focusing. Ann. Rech. Vét. 8:59–65.

Laude, H. 1978a. Swine fever virus: Interference with vesicular stomatitis virus and titration by the reverse plaque formation method. Arch. Virol. 56:273–277.

Laude, H. 1978b. A direct plaque assay for hog cholera virus. J. Gen. Virol. 40:225–228.

Launais, M., Aynaud, J.M., and Corthier, G. 1978. Hog cholera virus: Active immunization of piglets with the thiverval strain in the presence and absence of colostral passive immunity. Vet. Microbiol. 3:31–43.

Lee, R.C.T. 1981. Animal health and economics with special reference to hog cholera control in Taiwan, ROC. Bull. Off. Int. Epiz. 93:929–946.

Liess, B. 1981. Hog cholera. In E.P.J. Gibbs, ed., Virus Diseases of Food Animals, vol. 2. Academic Press, London. Pp.627–650.

Liess, B. 1987. Pathogenesis and epidemiology of hog cholera. Ann. Rech. Vét. 18:139–145.

Lin, T.C., Kang, B.J., Shimizu, Y., Kumagai, T., and Sasahara, J. 1969. Evaluation of the fluorescent antibody cell culture test for detection and titration of hog cholera virus. Natl. Inst. Anim. Health Q. (Tokyo) 9:10–19.

Lin, T.T.C., and Lee, R.C.T. 1981. An overall report on the development of a highly safe and potent lapinized hog cholera virus strain for hog cholera control in Taiwan. Natl. Sci. Council 7:44.

Loan, R.W., and Gustafson, D.P. 1961. Cultivation of hog cholera virus in subculturable swine buffy coat cells. Am. J. Vet. Res. 22:741–745.

Loan, R.W., and Storm, M.M. 1968. Propagation and transmission of hog cholera virus in nonporcine hosts. Am. J. Vet. Res. 29:807–811.

McKercher, P.D., Hess, W.R., and Hamdy, F. 1978. Residual viruses in pork products. Appl. Environ. Microbiol. 35:142–145.

Martin, W.W. 1978. Hog cholera eradicated (in U.S.)—A case history. Agric. Res. 26:8–12.

Mathews, J., and Buthala, D.A. 1958. Toxicity of heated swine serum. Am. J. Vet. Res. 19:32–36.

Mengeling, W.L., Pirtle, E.C., and Torrey, J.P. 1963. Identification of hog cholera viral antigen by immunofluorescence. Applications as a diagnostic and assay method. Can. J. Comp. Med. Vet. Sci. 27:249–252.

Millian, S.J., and Englehard, W.E. 1961. Application of the conglutina-tion complement absorption test to detect hog cholera antibodies. I. The technique. Am. J. Vet. Res. 22:396–400.

Neukirch, M., Moennig, V., and Liess, B. 1981. A simple procedure for the concentration and purification of hog cholera virus (HCV) using the lectin of *Ricinus communis*. Arch. Virol. 69:287–290.

Ritchie, A.R., and Fernelius, A.L. 1967. Electron microscopy of hog cholera virus and its antigen-antibody complex. Vet. Rec. 69:417–418.

Saunders, G.C. 1977. Development and evaluation of an enzyme-labeled antibody test for the rapid detection of hog cholera antibodies. Am. J. Vet. Res. 38:21–25.

Sautter, J.H., Young, G.A., Luedke, A.J., and Kitchell, R.L. 1953. The experimental production of malformations and other abnormalities in fetal pigs by means of attenuated hog cholera virus. In Proceedings of the 90th Annual Meeting of the American Veterinary Medical Association. Pp. 146–150.

Segre, D. 1962. Detection of hog cholera virus by a hemagglutination test. Am. J. Vet. Res. 95:748–751.

Seifried, O. 1931. Histological studies on hog cholera. I. Lesions in the central nervous system. J. Exp. Med. 53:277.

Sheffy, B.E., Coggins, L., and Baker, J.A. 1961. Protection of pigs against hog cholera with virus diarrhea virus of cattle. Proc. U.S. Livestock Sanit. Assoc. 65:347–358.

Sheffy, B.E., Coggins, L., and Baker, J.A. 1962. Relationship between hog cholera virus and virus diarrhea virus of cattle. Proc. Soc. Exp. Biol. Med. 109:349–352.

Solorzano, R.F. 1962. Ph.D disseration, Penn. State University.

Solorzano, R.F., Thigpen, J.E., Bedell, D.M., and Schwartz, W.L. 1966. The diagnosis of hog cholera by a fluorescent antibody test. J. Am. Vet. Med. Assoc. 149:31–34.

Stewart, W.C., Carbrey, B.A., Jenny, E.W., Kresse, J.I., Snyder, M.L., and Wessman, S.J. 1975. Transmission of hog cholera virus by mosquitoes. Am. J. Vet. Res. 36:611–614.

Teebken, D.L., Aiken, J.M., and Twiehaus, M.J. 1967. Differentiation of virulent, attenuated, and inactivated hog cholera viruses by fluorescent-antibody technique. J. Am. Vet. Med. Assoc. 150:53–61.

TenBroeck, C. 1941. Cultivation of the hog cholera virus. J. Exp. Med. 74:427–432.

Tessler, J., Stewart, W.C., and Kresse, J.I. 1975. Stabilization of hog cholera virus by dimethyl sulfoxide. Can. J. Comp. Med. 39:472–473.

U.S. Department of Agriculture. 1981. Hog cholera bibliography, July, 1981. Emergency Programs Foreign Animal Disease Data Bank. Hyattsville, Md. 209 pp. 3,156 references.

Urman, H.K., Underdahl, N.R., Aiken, J.M., Stair, E.L., and Young, G.A. 1962. Intranuclear inclusion bodies associated with hog cholera. J. Am. Vet. Med. Assoc. 141:571–581.

Young, G.A., Kitchell, R.L., Luedke, A.J., and Sautter, J.H. 1955. The effect of viral and other infections of the dam on fetal development in swine. I. Modified live hog cholera viruses—immunological, virological, and gross pathological studies. J. Am. Vet. Med. Assoc. 126:155–171.

Bovine Virus Diarrhea–Mucosal Disease

SYNONYMS: Mucosal disease, virus diarrhea of cattle; abbreviations, VD, BVD, BVD-MD

Olafson et al. (1946) described a disease of dairy cattle that had a striking resemblance to rinderpest, except that it was much milder. Olafson and Rickard (1947) had no difficulty in transmitting the disease with defibrinated blood, spleen tissue, or other organ tissue by parenteral injection, and the disease proved highly contagious under natural conditions. Pritchard et al. (1956) described a similar disease in dairy and beef cattle. It was thought that there were some immunological differences and also some clinical variations between the New York and the Indiana diseases, and for a time they were identified as virus diarrhea–New York and virus diarrhea–Indiana. The original Indiana strain had been lost, but Gillespie and Baker (1959), using cross-protection tests in disease-free cattle, compared another Indiana strain and two New York strains and found no differences among them.

Cytopathogenic strains of virus isolated from clinical cases of mucosal disease first described by Ramsey and Chivers (1953) are immunologically related to many available cytopathogenic and noncytopathogenic strains of VD virus (Gillespie et al. 1960, 1961, 1962). As these two entities are now considered clinical variations of the same viral disease, the Ad Hoc Committee on Terminology for the American Veterinary Medical Association Symposium (1971) named it bovine virus diarrhea–mucosal disease. An awkward name, perhaps, but it clearly indicates that the two diseases have a common cause. For simplicity we use the name *bovine virus diarrhea* (BVD) in this chapter. The diseases have been reviewed recently (Baker 1987, Brownlie et al. 1987, Duffell and Harkness 1985).

Bovine virus diarrhea has been diagnosed in cattle worldwide. Virtually all reported clinical cases of this disease involve cattle. BVD occurs as a natural infection, usually without signs of illness, in domestic swine in the United States (Carbrey et al. 1976, Stewart et al. 1971).

Virus strain NY-1 was isolated by Baker et al. (1954) from a New York herd; it was the original type strain until the cytopathogenic strain Oregon (C24V) was isolated by Gillespie et al. (1960). The availability of strain Oregon for comparative serological and virological studies has enabled various investigators throughout the world to evaluate clinical entities that resemble BVD (Gillespie et al. 1961, Knaizeff et al. 1961).

Serologic surveys have been conducted in various parts of the United States and abroad. In a New York State survey 53 percent of cows selected at random within 500 herds (two cows per herd) distributed through 53 counties had antibodies (Kahrs et al. 1964). Serum samples from cattle in 22 Florida counties showed that 65 percent of beef cattle and 61 percent of dairy cattle were positive for BVD antibodies (Knaizeff 1962). In another survey of states where 100 or more cattle serums were tested, 59 percent in Illinois, 69 percent in Iowa, and 73 percent in Nebraska were positive (Newberne et al. 1961). Incidence studies in Europe yielded similar results.

Neutralizing antibodies have been demonstrated in serums of white-tailed deer from New York State (Kahrs et al. 1964). A disease of white-tailed deer and mule deer with lesions similar to BVD infection of cattle has been described in North Dakota by Richards et al. (1956). Antibodies to BVD are found in pronghorns (Barrett and Chalmers 1975) and caribou located in Canada. Various deer species in European countries have antibodies to bovine virus diarrhea virus (BVDV).

Neutralizing antibodies to BVDV have been demonstrated in sheep and goats (Taylor et al. 1977). The virus causes a mild or inapparent infection in both species (Gratzek 1961, Rossi and Kiesel 1977). A condition in lambs called border disease, characterized by hairiness of the birth coat and poor viability, is caused by a virus that is antigenically related to BVD and HC viruses (Plant et al. 1973).

Character of the Disease. BVD occurs most frequently in late winter and in spring. It affects cattle of all ages, but young stock are more likely to show signs of illness, possibly because of the higher susceptibility rate of younger animals. A recent paper provides an excellent description of the clinical syndromes associated with BVD (Perdrizet et al. 1987).

The high incidence of antibodies in cattle suggests that most cattle experience a mild or inapparent infection. When the disease occurs in a herd, it may be a mild or a severe acute infection; occasionally it is chronic. As a herd disease, it varies from one with a high morbidity and low mortality to one with a high morbidity and high mortality. Since 1975 the disease in dairy cattle has become more severe and has caused considerable economic loss.

Severely affected cattle have a diphasic temperature reaction and leukopenia. Other signs of illness include depression, anorexia, dehydration, reduced milk supply, mucoid and sometimes blood-tinged diarrhea, bluish discoloration of the muzzle, cessation of rumination, conjunctivitis, congestion and ulcerations in the mucous membrane of the oral cavity, a dry, hard, nonproductive cough, excessive salivation, nonpurulent vaginitis, infertility, and abortions in pregnant cows. Field observations of abortions and the isolation of noncytopathogenic BVDV from two aborted fetuses confirmed the diagnosis in two New York State dairy herds (Gillespie et al. 1967). Nervous signs caused by hydrocephalus in neonatal calves have been observed. Lameness, probably caused by laminitis, occurs in some animals. Occasionally there is a mucoid nasal discharge that leads veterinarians to confuse BVD with infectious bovine rhinotracheitis, parainfluenza 3 infection, or some other respiratory illness. BVDV is just one of many bovine viruses involved in

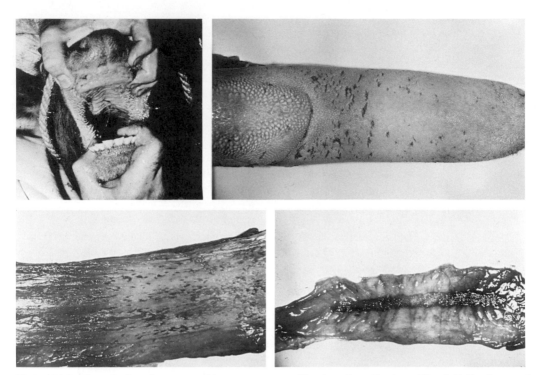

Figure 50.3. Gross lesions in a cow with a severe case of bovine virus diarrhea. (*Top left*) Erosions and hemorrhages of gums. (*Top right*) Erosions on dorsal surface of the tongue. (*Bottom left*) Erosions and necrosis in esophagus. (*Bottom right*) Hemorrhage and necrosis of Peyer's patches of intestinal tract. (Courtesy K. McEntee.)

neonatal respiratory diseases. Often, mixed viral and bacterial infections occur, to the detriment of the host.

The gross lesions associated with natural cases were first described by Olafson and co-workers (1946). Subsequent investigators mentioned other pathological changes (Carlson et al. 1957, Pritchard et al. 1954, Ramsey and Chivers 1953). The eyes are sunken and the carcasses gaunt and dehydrated. Erosions are found on the dental pad, palate, and lateral tongue surface, around the incisors, and on the inside of the cheeks. Occasionally erosions are seen on the muzzle and at the entrance of the nostrils, and the nasal mucosa is reddened. Ulceration of the pharynx and larynx or diffuse necrosis of the mucous membranes in these regions occurs in some animals with fatal cases. Secondary pneumonia is rarely observed. Characteristic lesions were irregular, shallow, punched-out erosions of varying sizes and shapes arranged in linear fashion in the mucous membranes of the esophagus. Some of the ulcers coalesce, and sometimes the necrotic material remains intact. An occasional calf does not have oral ulcers.

The forestomachs sometimes show small necrotic areas areas and a few ulcers. The small intestine may have a diffusely, reddened mucosa. The cecum often shows petechiae and small ulcers. Hemorrhages are sometimes seen in the subcutaneous tissue, in the epicardium, and in the vaginal mucosa. Hemorrhage, edema, necrosis, and ulceration of the pyloric portion of the abomasum are observed. Similar changes are occasionally noted in the small intestine, with marked lesions in Peyer's patches (Figure 50.3). Other significant lesions are atrophic changes in lymphatic tissues and degenerative alterations in the kidney, skin, and adrenals. Erosions or ulcerations develop in interdigital regions of some cattle, and extensive necrosis sometimes follows. The lymph nodes often appear normal, but in some animals they are greatly enlarged and edematous.

Various investigators (Carlson et al. 1957, Ramsey and Chivers 1953, Trapp 1960, Whiteman 1960) have reported on the microscopic changes associated with the natural and the experimental disease. The most striking changes occur in the digestive system. Probably the first change in that portion lined by stratified squamous epithelium is the vacuolation of the cytoplasm in cells, particularly those in the stratum germinativum and stratum spinosum. The intercellular bridges are destroyed, and the nuclei become pyknotic. With cellular destruction, lesions develop and coalesce, forming erosions. In the early lesions there is marked hyperemia with minimal infiltration of mononuclear cells. Some old lesions have deep ulcerations and marked inflammation because bacteria have invaded the denuded epithelium.

Ulcers involving the fundus of the abomasum are formed by localized necrosis, erosion of the epithelium, and damage to the lamina propria. Accompanying changes are edema of the lamina propria and submucosa with moderate leukocytic infiltration and hemorrhage. Edema, hemorrhage, erosions, and ulcerations sometimes occur in the pyloric mucosa. Occasionally, the lesions indicate necrotic abomasitis.

In cattle with severe cases marked changes occur in the intestinal tract. The crypts of the intestinal glands are filled with mucus, necrotic cells, and a varying number of leukocytes. Edema is evident in some animals. The glandular epithelium is destroyed, especially in animals with acute cases. In the submucosal lymphatic tissue, necrosis sometimes initiates changes that lead to erosion. Depletion of lymphocytes in Peyer's patches may be prominent. Ulcers are especially evident over Peyer's patches. Similar changes can be found in the colonic mucosa. Severe typhlitis, colitis, and proctitis, varying from a catarrhal to necrotic inflammation, are often found.

The thymus is smaller than normal and occasionally contains grayish white foci. There is loss of differentiation between the medulla and cortex and widespread depletion of thymocytes. Lymphocytes are replaced by large mononuclear cells in the tonsils.

Subepicardial and subendocardial hemorrhages are observed. Vessel changes occur only in the media of the arterioles located in the submucosa of the digestive tract, where severe changes occur, especially in the germinal centers. The subcapsular sinus may be extended and filled with leukocytes. Neutrophils occasionally infiltrate the cortex and the medulla. Similar histological changes occur in the spleen and hemal nodes.

In studies of experimental disease susceptible cattle are infected by mouth and by parenteral injection. The incubation period is 2 to 3 days. The first temperature response usually lasts for 1 to 2 days; the second response starts 2 to 3 days later and persists 2 to 3 days with temperatures ranging from 104° to 107°F. Leukopenia occurs and may be followed by leukocytosis. Diarrhea seldom is noted, and reddening and ulceration of the gums sometimes occurs (Baker et al. 1954).

Using a noncytopathogenic strain (Studdert) of BVDV isolated from an aborted fetus (Gillespie et al., 1967), Ward et al. (1969) inoculated 11 pregnant dairy cows intravenously at varying stages of gestation ranging from 150 to 217 days. The fetus that was 150 days old showed ataxia, blindness, and buccal lesions at birth. Two other calves had buccal lesions at birth, and the 8 other calves were normal. All 11 calves, including 4 from whom blood

samples were collected before they began suckling, had BVD antibodies at birth. The antibody levels persisted for 6 months without decline, and 6 of these calves showed no signs of illness after being given virulent virus at that time. This evidence was substantial proof that the bovine fetus produces active antibody against BVDV as early as the fifth month of embryonic development. Subsequent experiments by Scott et al. (1970, 1973) extended these studies. These investigators gave the same Studdert strain intravenously to susceptible cows that were 3 to 5 months pregnant. Infection in the cows was followed by fetal death, fetal mummification, abortion, or birth at term of calves with cerebellar or ocular defects. Kahrs et al. (1970) made similar observations of natural disease in a dairy herd; BVDV was isolated from one aborted fetus, and rising serum neutralizing antibody titers were demonstrated in some cows. These results proved BVDV causes abortions and congenital defects in cattle. In studies of pathogenesis in the bovine fetus, acute ocular lesions occurred in fetuses taken 17 to 21 days from susceptible pregnant cows given BVDV at approximately 150 days' gestation (Brown et al. 1975). The acute lesions were characterized by mild to moderate retinitis. After 28 days the acute lesions had begun to resolve, and in newborn animals focal to total retinal atrophy was seen.

In an experiment, 15 susceptible pregnant Jersey heifers were inoculated intramuscularly with a pool of 10 cytopathogenic strains of BVDV isolated from cattle in Great Britain and grown in primary calf testes tissue cultures (Done et al. 1980). Because the heifers had been pregnant for 100 days, the virus pool had the usual effects—inapparent infection in the heifers but serious consequences in the fetuses. Of the 10 liveborn fetuses 2 produced neutralizing antibodies, and noncytopathogenic—not cytopathogenic—virus was isolated from the remaining neonates. In most instances noncytopathic virus is isolated from infected aborted fetuses in natural disease.

Nine susceptible bulls were inoculated parenterally and orally with 100 tissue-cultured doses of BVDV (Whitmore et al. 1978). Semen samples were collected throughout the 14 days after inoculation, and virus was detected in 4 of 96 semen samples and in the testes of 1 of 6 bulls slaughtered 60 to 90 days later. The virus did not affect the semen quality or cause lesions in the reproductive tract. Although BVDV may be shed in semen after inoculation, the probability of this occurring is low.

Sheep and goats are susceptible to experimental inoculation with BVDV. An English strain produced a rise in temperature between the fifth and eighth day after inoculation (Huck 1957). Lack of appetite and diarrhea also were noted in the sheep. Ward (1971) inoculated pregnant sheep and reported congenital anomalies and antibody response in the fetuses. Other investigators had similar results (Barlow et al. 1980, Barrett and Chalmers 1975, Vantsis et al. 1979)

Strain NY-1 has been maintained in rabbits for more than 100 transfers and strain Indiana for more than 20 transfers without producing signs of illness in this species.

In experimental pigs BVDV replicates, and specific antibodies are formed. No signs of illness occur.

The virus fails to elicit a response in white mice.

Properties of the Virus. BVDV is an RNA, helical, enveloped virus. Neither 5-iodo-deoxyuridine nor 5-bromo-deoxyuridine inhibits the Oregon strain (Hermodsson and Dinter 1962). Inactivation occurs after treatment with chloroform and ether (Gillespie et al. 1963, Hermodsson and Dinter 1962). The sedimentation coefficient of the virus particle is 80 to 90S. In a sucrose density gradient its buoyant density is 1.13 to 1.14 g/ml. Gratzek (1961) reported a 10-fold loss of virus in 24 hours at 26°C or 37°C. The virus is readily maintained in a lyophilized or frozen state ($-60°$ to $-70°$C) for many years.

Electron photomicrographs of strain Oregon shadowed with chromium reveal somewhat spherical particles 35 to 55 nm in diameter (Knaizeff 1962). Ultrathin sections of virus pellets also reveal spherical particles approximately 40 nm in diameter (Hermodsson and Dinter 1962). In other studies Richie and Fernelius (1969) observed by electron microscopy three major size classes of particulate entities of negatively stained (phosphotungstic acid) crude and partially purified preparations of one noncytopathogenic and two cytopathogenic (including strain Oregon) BVDV strains cultured in embryonic bovine kidney cells: (1) 15- to 20-nm virus-specific precursor particles considered to represent a ribosomelike soluble antigen; although quite similar in size to the 15- to 16-nm unknown particlelike entities associated with the PAV-1 strain of HCV, these BVD particles were different in appearance; (2) 30- to 35-nm particles, a heterogenous population of three types of particulate entities; and (3) 80- to 100-nm pleomorphic membrane-bound particles. The two larger components had infectious particles, and the surface of the largest unit generally was smooth with rare prominent projections.

Immune complexes are formed between BVDV structural polypeptides and bovine anti-BVDV hyperimmune serums as well as porcine anti-HCV hyperimmune serums, by precipitation and by affinity chromatography on protein A-Sepharose tested for antigens by SDS-PAGE (sodium dodecyl sulfate–polyacrylamide electrophoresis) procedure. Analyses showed differences in the reactivity of the two species of antibodies. In contrast to the BVD antibodies, the HC antibodies failed to react with p 34.

When the glycoproteins gp 57 and gp 44 of the viral envelope were compared, the HC antibodies revealed a more intense reaction with gp 44, whereas the BVD antibodies reacted more intensely with gp 57 (Matthaeus 1981).

Most strains of BVDV but not all, are closely related serologically, and cross-protection tests in cattle further confirm this close relation (Castrucci et al. 1975). The virus produces neutralizing, precipitating, and complement-fixing antibodies. No hemagglutination has been associated with the BVDV particle.

Greiser-Wilke et al. (1986) and Donis et al. (1987) have produced monoclonal antibodies to BVDV. The availability of these antibodies should help to elucidate the antigenic characteristics of noncytopathogenic and cytopathogenic strains of BVDV.

Cultivation. Isolates of BVDV are either cytopathogenic or noncytopathogenic in various cell-culture systems. Strain NY-1 multiplies in embryonic bovine skin-muscle cells or embryonic bovine kidney cells without cytopathic changes (Lee and Gillespie 1957). Similar results in embryonic bovine kidney cells were obtained with strain Indiana 46 and the Saunders strain (Coggins et al. 1961). Noncytopathic virus is most conveniently demonstrated in tissue culture by the interference phenomenon (Gillespie et al. 1962) (Figure 50.4), by the exaltation effect produced by the addition of Newcastle disease virus (Inaba et al. 1963), or by the immunofluorescence test (Gutekunst and Malmquist 1963).

Noice and Schipper (1959) and Underdahl et al. (1957) isolated virus from mucosal disease cases which showed some minor alterations in cell culture. Gillespie et al. (1960) isolated a cytopathogenic strain, designated strain Oregon of BVDV, from the spleen of a calf supplied by investigators at Oregon State University (Figure 50.5). This strain produced experimental infection in calves and high titers of cytopathogenic virus in cell cultures, and the cell-adapted virus was neutralized by the homologous antiserum as well as antiserums produced in calves inoculated with the NY-1 strain, Indiana strain, and others. These same investigators, and others, soon isolated many cytopathogenic strains from field cases.

Some viruses produce a cytopathic effect more quickly than others and completely destroy the cell sheet. Various strains produce plaques, and the plaque-formation method can be used for more accurate viral titration (Gillespie et al. 1962). Throughout the growth cycle, the fluid phase of the culture has a greater concentration than the cells, and this suggests that the completely infective particle is formed in the cytoplasm (Gillespie et al. 1963). Other monolayer cell cultures of bovine origin that support viral replication include fetal lung (Goldsmit and Barzilai

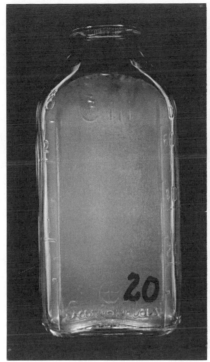
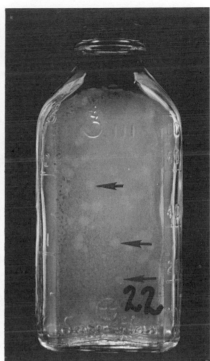

Figure 50.4. Interference test for bovine virus diarrhea virus. (*Left*) Culture inoculated first with noncytopathogenic virus followed by 50 plaque-forming units (PFU) of cytopathogenic virus 3 days later. No plaques are visible, as interference with viral replication occurred. (*Right*) Plaques (*arrows*) are clearly visible because this control culture was inoculated with only 50 PFU of cytopathogenic virus.

1975), fetal endometrium (Soto-Belloso et al. 1976), and blood macrophages (Rossi and Kiesel 1977). The virus also replicates in bovine tracheal-ring organ cultures and readily destroys ciliary activity (Rossi and Kiesel 1977). All investigative groups except one (Carbrey et al. 1976) have failed to propagate BVD virus in embryonated hens' eggs.

Endogenous bovine virus contaminants, including BVDV, occur in commercially supplied fetal bovine serum. Noncytopathogenic virus constitutes the gravest problem because it can go undetected but it can interfere with virus assay of cytopathogenic strains. Fetal calf serum also may contain BVD antibody and interferon or noncytopathogenic BVDV that can affect viral or antibody assay procedures.

Epizootiology. Because BVD is a viremic disease, it is assumed that body excretions (e.g., feces) contain infective virus during the acute stage of infection. Blood and splenic tissue also contain virus during this stage. Despite the presence of serum-neutralizing antibodies, BVDV was isolated from buffy coat of cattle given virus 3 weeks earlier (Gutekunst and Malmquist 1963). Infection can be produced with virus given orally or injected parenterally. There is excellent field evidence that the infection can be carried readily from one herd to another by mechanical means.

Natural BVD infection probably occurs in sheep and goats, and they may play a role in transmission of the virus to cattle. It is also a natural infection in swine, so transmission to other susceptible animals is possible. Neutralizing antibodies have been found in a small percentage of New York white-tailed deer (Kahrs et al. 1964). A disease resembling BVD has been described in white-tailed and mule deer in North Dakota (Richards et al 1956). One or more of these wildlife hosts may play a significant role in the ecology of this disease.

The virus may persist in the blood of recovered or chronically ill cattle, which may be a potential source of infection to other susceptible livestock

Immunity. The immune mechanism to BVDV has not been clearly defined because of viral immunosuppressive effects and the existence of several biotypes, but certain facts suggest that the virus produces a long and durable immunity in most cattle under natural conditions. These animals usually undergo an inapparent infection with no obvious long-term consequences.

Most field isolates of noncytopathogenic and cytopathogenic BVDV protect against themselves and each other. For example, the MD England LS strain protected cattle that were challenged with virulent virus at 13 and 22 months following inoculation (Huck 1957). Cattle immunized with strain Indiana 46, strain NY-1, or strain Oregon were resistant to homologous virulent virus for at least 12 to 16 months (Gillespie and Baker 1959, Prit-

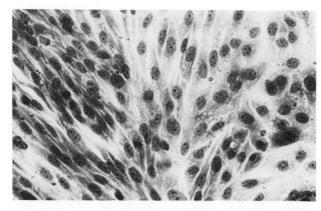

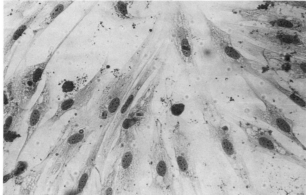

Figure 50.5. (*Top*) Uninoculated 8-day-old tissue culture of embryonic bovine kidney cell. Hematoxylin and eosin (H and E) stain. (*Bottom*) Eight-day-old culture of strain Oregon of bovine virus diarrhea virus on embryonic bovine kidney cells. Note cytopathic effect. H and E stain. × 100. (From Gillespie et al., 1960, courtesy of *Cornell Veterinarian*.)

chard 1963). Calves that were infected with virus in utero had an active immunity at 6 months of age and were resistant to challenge (Ward et al. 1969). Cattle immunized with strain Oregon, strain Indiana, and strain NY-1 were protected against themselves and each other. Apparently some antigen field variants are sufficiently different from strain Oregon virus vaccine so that protection does not ensue (Steck et al. 1980). Among 209 seronegative animals successfully immunized in a field trial, 4 produced good antibody titers to strain Oregon but nevertheless died from disease caused by the antigenic variant, against which neutralizing antibodies were lacking. Further study is needed to evaluate the antigenic variations of BVDV and their significance in the protection of cattle; such evaluation will require monoclonal antibody studies, viral amino acid sequencing, and identifying viral glycoproteins involved in protection (Donis and Dubovi 1987a, 1987b, 1987c, 1987d).

Robson et al. (1960) showed that no serum neutralizing

antibodies are detectable 1 week after inoculation with BVDV, but titers at 2 weeks range from 80 to 280 and at 4 weeks between 210 and 2,500. High concentrations of IgG are present in the serum and follicular fluid (Whitmore and Archbald 1977). IgG, IgM, and IgA concentrations are low in uterine and vaginal secretions. Steck et al. (1980) reported that the serum levels of IgG, IgM, and IgA in diseased cattle were normal, whereas those of IgA_2 were reduced and 24 of 25 diseased cattle lacked neutralizing antibody to BVDV.

Interferon can be produced by BVDV in heifers and fetuses from the middle of the second trimester to birth (Rinaldo et al. 1976).

Serum-neutralizing antibody resulting from an active immunity is a good indication of protection in cattle. The relation between this test and immunity to challenge with virulent virus in a sequential experiment showed that the neutralization test is at least 95 percent accurate and thus is an acceptable substitute for direct challenge (Robson et al. 1960). To assure reasonable accuracy, the test was standardized by the use of 100 $TCID_{50}$ of cytopathogenic virus against serial threefold dilutions of test serum (Gillespie et al. 1960). The serum titer varies according to the amount of virus in the test, with an increase of 1 log of virus causing a decrease of 0.44 log of serum titer (Coggins 1962). The neutralization test is quite accurate, varying as little as 0.26 log within tests and 0.41 log between tests.

Calves given BVDV form complement-fixing antibodies before serum-neutralizing antibodies, and the former remain at high levels for at least 15 weeks (Gutekunst and Malmquist 1963).

Maternal immunity studies were performed by Brar et al. (1978), Kahrs et al. (1967), and Malmquist (1968). Antibody titers persist for 6 to 9 months in calves whose dams are immune. The half-life of maternal antibody to BVDV is 21 days. Before calves lose their maternal antibody entirely, they respond to virus with the production of an active immunity. Production of an active immunity may not occur if the antibody titer derived from the dam is sufficiently high.

Unfortunately, more and more cattle are encountering field strains of BVDV that have a marked effect on the reticuloendothelial system. As a result the animals contract a chronic, debilitating disease with persisting virus in the blood stream and no antibody. These animals rarely recover from the marked pathological lesions and usually die in a few weeks after the onset of illness.

A unique situation occurs in neonatal and young cattle. Presumably some fetuses infected with BVDV in utero develop immunological tolerance and have persisting noncytopathogenic virus in the bloodstream. Upon subsequent exposure to some virulent strains, field or experimental, these animals develop mucosal disease and usually die (Bolin et al. 1985, Brownlie et al. 1984, Roeder and Drew 1984).

Diagnosis. The diagnosis is based generally on clinical signs and more specifically on lesions. This disease can be readily confused clinically with malignant catarrhal fever or rinderpest in some instances, and on occasion with bovine respiratory infections.

As far as we know, all noncytopathogenic and cytopathogenic field isolates replicate in cell-culture systems, including embryonic bovine cultures of kidney, spleen, testicle, and trachea. Virus has been isolated from the blood, urine, and nasal or ocular discharges of animals with acute cases. At necropsy, spleen, bone marrow, or mesenteric lymph nodes are good sources for virus. If cytopathic changes are not observed after three passages in cell culture, noncytopathogenic strains can be identified by the immunofluorescence test, by the END method, or by the cellular resistance test.

A rising titer with paired serums in the serum-neutralizing or complement-fixation test constitutes a good basis for diagnosis, but, in practice, the serum-neutralization test is preferred. Because serologic variants do occur, one strain may not reveal antibody to a heterologous virus if the antibody titer is low. This problem can be largely circumvented by the addition of complement to the neutralization test system (Haralambiev 1975).

Prevention. No alteration in virulence in calves was noted with strain NY-1 after 100 transfers in embryonic bovine kidney cells (J.H. Gillespie, unpublished data). In contrast, strain Oregon showed attenuation for calves by the 32d passage in this same cell system and did not spread to a limited number of contact calves (Coggins et al. 1961). Laboratory and field tests of strain Oregon by other workers confirmed these observations and supported its use in the field (York et al. 1960). This vaccine strain is commercially produced and probably creates long-lasting immunity. Another virus vaccine that is attenuated by passage in a continuous porcine cell line has been described for vaccination of cattle (Phillips et al. 1975). It is reputed to be safe and efficacious without spread to contact animals.

The immunization of calves against BVD with an ethanol saponin vaccine caused neutralizing antibodies to form in high titers (Zwetkow et al. 1975); the vaccinated calves resisted challenge with virulent BVD virus. The duration of immunity to this inactivated virus vaccine is unknown.

Bacteria-derived bovine alpha interferon I1 (BoIFN-α_{I1}) caused a marked inhibitory effect in cell culture against the Singer and NADL strains of BVDV (Gillespie et al. 1985). In dairy cattle protection tests bacteria-derived BoIFN-α_{I1}, given at doses of 10,000 U/kg of body weight, delayed the onset of illness and reduced its severity under experimental conditions. The interferon, given intramuscularly, caused a slight rise in temperature for 12 to 24 hours and mild leukopenia for a few days after administration (Gillespie et al. 1986).

At an American Veterinary Medical Association Symposium on Bovine Diseases in 1967 a panel included BVD vaccination in its recommendations for herd health programs. A herd health program for beef cattle should include the following vaccination regimen. As a preconditioning program for calves, BVD modified-live virus of tissue-culture origin singly or in combination with *Leptospira pomona* bacterin should be given to 5-month-old calves. Calves that arrive at feedlots without preconditioning should not be given BVD vaccine unless the feedlot has had problems with BVD, and then only 48 hours or more after arrival, depending on recovery from the stress of shipping. In the self-contained dairy herd calves should be inoculated with BVD vaccine at 6 to 8 months of age only if the disease is prevalent in the area. Additions to the open herd should be isolated for 30 days and immunized with BVD vaccine if the disease is common in the herd.

The panel recognized that BVD modified living vaccines are quite effective and relatively safe for most cattle under field conditions (Bovine Respiratory Disease Symposium, 1971). Reports following field use indicate that in some cattle this vaccine may be a predisposing factor, or possibly the primary cause of, severe reactions. Such adverse reactions, which usually involve low morbidity and high mortality, may result from the combination of stress and/or infectious agents and of the vaccine. BVDV has an immunosuppressive effect, and the combined factors may tip the balance with frank disease ensuing after vaccination. In consideration of these reactions, attenuated BVD vaccine is recommended only when previous or anticipated disease problems are of sufficient magnitude to warrant the risk involved. It should be recognized that detectable levels of BVD antibody of maternal origin may persist in a small percentage of calves up to 9 months of age.

BVDV causes abortions and congenital anomalies, so the use of vaccine in pregnant cows is ill-advised.

Inactivated virus vaccine shows promise and ultimately should replace attenuated virus vaccine.

Control. The economic importance of this disease has been reasonably well established, particularly in feedlot operations. Regular use of the attenuated virus vaccine is not advised despite the high incidence of infection in cattle unless severe disease appears in a given area or herd. There is a clear need for a vaccine that is safe and efficacious and protects against all field viruses (Liess et al. 1983, Steck et al. 1980).

The Disease in Humans. There is no evidence to suggest that humans are infected with BVDV.

REFERENCES

Baker, J.A., York, C.J., Gillespie, J.H., and Mitchell, G.B. 1954. Virus diarrhea in cattle. Am. J. Vet. Res. 15:525–531.

Baker, J.C. 1987. Bovine viral diarrhea virus: A review. J. Am. Vet. Med. Assoc. 190:1449–1458.

Barlow, R.M., Rennie, J.C., and Gardiner, A.C. 1980. Infection of pregnant sheep with the NADL strain of bovine virus diarrhea virus and their subsequent challenge with border disease. J. Comp. Pathol. 90:67–72.

Barrett, M.W., and Chalmers, G.A. 1975. A serologic survey of pronghorns in Alberta and Saskatchewan. J. Wildl. Dis. 11:157–163.

Bolin, S.R., McClurkin, A.W., Cutlip, R.C., and Coria, M.F. 1985. Severe clinical disease induced in cattle persistently infected with noncytopathic bovine viral diarrhea virus by superinfection with cytopathic bovine viral diarrhea virus. Am. J. Vet. Res. 46:573–576.

Bovine Respiratory Disease Symposium. 1971. Panel report. J. Am. Vet. Med. Assoc. 152:940.

Brar, J.S., Johnson, D.W., Muscoplat, C.C., Shope, R.E., and Meiske, J.C. 1978. Maternal immunity to infectious bovine rhinotracheitis and bovine viral diarrhea viruses: Duration and effect of vaccination in young calves. Am. J. Vet. Res. 39:241–244.

Brown, T.T., Bistner, S.I., DeLahunta, A., Scott, F.W., and McEntee, K. 1975. Pathogenetic studies of infection of the bovine fetus with bovine viral diarrhea virus. II. Ocular lesions. Vet. Pathol. 12:394–404.

Brownlie, J., Clarke, M.C., and Howard, C.J. 1984. Experimental production of fatal mucosal disease in cattle. Vet. Rec. 114:535–536.

Brownlie, J., Clarke, M.C., Howard, C.J., and Pocock, D.H. 1987. Pathogenesis and epidemiology of bovine virus diarrhoea virus infection of cattle. Ann. Rech. Vét. 18:157–166.

Carbrey, E.A., Stewart, W.C., Kresse, J.I., and Snyder, M.L. 1976. Bovine viral diarrhea infection in pigs and its differentiation from infection with hog cholera strains of low virulence. J. Am. Vet. Med. Assoc. 169:1217–1229.

Carlson, R.G., Pritchard, W.R., and Doyle, L.P. 1957. The pathology of virus diarrhea of cattle in Indiana. Am. J. Vet. Res. 18:560–568.

Castrucci, G., Avellini, G., Cilli, V., Pedini, B., McKercher, D.G., and Valente, C. 1975. A study of immunologic relationships among serologically heterologous strains of bovine viral diarrhea virus by cross immunity test. Cornell Vet. 65:65–72.

Coggins, L. 1962. Hog cholera and virus diarrhea maternal antibodies in swine. Ph.D. dissertation, Cornell University, Ithaca, N.Y.

Coggins, L., Gillespie, J.H., Robson, D.S., Thompson, J.D., Wagner, W.C., and Baker, J.A. 1961. Attenuation of virus diarrhea virus (strain Oregon C24V) for vaccine purposes. Cornell Vet. 51:540–545.

Done, J.T., Terlecki, S., Richardson, C., Harkness, J.W., Sands, J.J., Patterson, D.S., Sweasey, D., Shaw, I.G., Winkler, C.E., and Dhiffell, S.J. 1980. Bovine virus diarrhoea–mucosal disease: Pathogenicity for the fetal calf following maternal infection. Vet. Rec. 106:473–479.

Donis, R.O., and Dubovi, E.J. 1987a. Molecular specificity of the antibody responses of cattle naturally and experimentally infected with cytopathic and noncytopathic bovine viral diarrhea virus biotypes. Am. J. Vet. Res. 48:1549–1554.

Donis, R.O., and Dubovi, E.J. 1987b. Differences in virus-induced polypeptides in cells infected by cytopathic and noncytopathic biotypes of bovine virus diarrhea–mucosal disease virus. Virology 158:168–173.

Donis, R.O., and Dubovi, E.J. 1987c. Characterization of bovine viral diarrhoea–mucosal disease virus-specific proteins in bovine cells. J. Gen. Virol. 68:1597–1605.

Donis, R.O., and Dubovi, E.J. 1987d. Glycoproteins of bovine viral diarrhoea–mucosal disease virus in infected bovine cells. J. Gen. Virol. 68:1607–1616.

Donis, R.O., Corapi, W., and Dubovi, E.J. 1987. Neutralizing monoclonal antibodies to bovine viral diarrhoea virus bind to the 56K and 58K glycoprotein. J. Gen. Virol. In press.

Duffell, S.J., and Harkness, J.W. 1985. Bovine virus diarrhoea-mucosal disease infection in cattle. Vet. Rec. 117:240–245.

Gillespie, J.H., and Baker, J.A. 1959. Studies on virus diarrhea. Cornell Vet. 49:439–443.

Gillespie, J.H., Baker, J.A., and McEntee, K. 1960. A cytopathogenic strain of virus diarrhea virus. Cornell Vet. 40:73–79.

Gillespie, J.H., Bartholomew, P.T., Thompson, R.G., and McEntee, K. 1967. The isolation of noncytopathic virus diarrhea virus from two aborted bovine fetuses. Cornell Vet. 57:564–571.

Gillespie, J.H., Coggins, L., Thompson, J., and Baker, J.A. 1961. Comparison by neutralization tests of strains of virus isolated from virus diarrhea and mucosal disease. Cornell Vet. 51:155–159.

Gillespie, J.H., Madin, S.H., and Darby, N.B. 1962. Cellular resistance in tissue culture, induced by noncytopathogenic strains, to a cytopathogenic strain of virus diarrhea virus of cattle. Proc. Soc. Exp. Biol. Med. 110:248–250.

Gillespie, J.H., Madin, S.H., and Darby, N.B. 1963. Studies on virus diarrhea virus of cattle, with special reference to its growth in tissue culture and its ether susceptibility. Cornell Vet. 53:276–282.

Gillespie, J.H., Robson, D.S., Scott, F.W., and Schiff, E.I. 1985. In vitro protective effect of bacteria-derived bovine alpha interferon I1 against selected bovine viruses. J. Clin. Microbiol. 22:912–914.

Gillespie, J.H, Scott, F., Geissinger, D., and Schiff, E. 1986. The prophylactic effects of E. coli–derived bovine interferon alpha₁1 on bovine virus diarrhoea in calves after intramuscular administration. J. Vet. Med. 771–776.

Goldsmit, L., and Barzilai, E. 1975. Propagation of bovine viral diarrhea viruses in bovine fetal lung cell cultures. Am. J. Vet. Res. 36:407–411.

Gratzek, J.B. 1961. Characteristics of two bovine viral diarrhea agents. Ph.D. dissertation, University of Wisconsin.

Greiser-Wilke, J., Peters, W., Moennig, V., and Leiss, B. 1986. Characterization of various strains of bovine viral diarrhea virus by means of monoclonal antibodies. Personal communication.

Gutekunst, D.E., and Malmquist, W.A. 1963. Separation of a soluble antigen and infectious particles of bovine viral diarrhea viruse and their relationship to hog cholera. Can. J. Comp. Med. 28:19–20.

Haralambiev, H. 1975. Immunologic relationships between two strains of mucosal disease/viral diarrhea virus. Arch. Exp. Veterinärmed. 29:777–780.

Hermodsson, S., and Dinter, Z. 1962. Properties of bovine virus diarrhoea virus. Nature 194:893–894.

Huck, R.A. 1957. A mucosal disease of cattle. Vet. Rec. 69:1207–1215.

Inaba, Y., Omori, T., and Kumagai, T. 1963. Detection and measurement of non-cytopathogenic strains of virus diarrhea of cattle by the END method. Arch. Gesam. Virusforsch. 13:245.

Kahrs, R., Atkinson, G., Baker, J.A., Carmichael, L., Coggins, L., Gillespie, J., Langer, P., Marshall, V., Robson, D., and Sheffy, B. 1964. Serological studies on the incidences of bovine virus diarrhea, infectious bovine rhinotracheitis, bovine myxovirus parainfluenza–3, and *Leptospira pomona* in New York State. Cornell Vet. 54:360–369.

Kahrs, R.F., Robson, D.S., and Baker, J.A. 1967. Epidemiological considerations for the control of bovine virus diarrhea. In Proceedings of the 70th Annual Meeting of the U.S. Livestock Sanitation Association. Pp. 145–153.

Kahrs, R.F., Scott, F.W., and de Lahunta, A. 1970. Bovine viral diarrhea–mucosal disease, abortion, and congenital cerebellar hypoplasia in a dairy herd. J. Am. Vet. Med. Assoc. 156:1443.

Knaizeff, A.J. 1962. Personal communication to W.R. Pritchard, Davis, Calif.

Knaizeff, A.J., Huck, R.A., Jarrett, W.F.H., Pritchard, W.R., Ramsey, F.K, Schipper, I.A., Stoeber, M., and Liess, B. 1961. Antigenic relationship of some bovine viral diarrhoea–mucosal disease viruses from the United States, Great Britain, and West Germany. Vet. Rec. 73:768–769.

Lee, K.M., and Gillespie, J.H. 1957. Propagation of virus diarrhea virus of cattle in tissue culture. Am. J. Vet. Res. 18:952–953.

Liess, B., Frey, H.R., Orban, S., and Hafer, S.M. 1983. Bovine virus diarrhoea (BVD)–mucosal disease: Persistente BVD-feldvirus Infektionen der serologisch selektierten Rindern. D.T.W. 90:261–266.

Malmquist, W.A. 1968. Bovine viral diarrhea–mucosal disease: Etiology, pathogenesis, and applied immunity. J. Am. Vet. Med. Assoc. 152:763–768.

Matthaeus, W. 1981. Differences in reaction behavior of structural polypeptides of viral diarrhoea virus (BVDV) with antisera against BVDV and hog cholera virus (HCV). Zentralbl. Veterinärmed. [B] 28:126–132.

Newberne, J.W., Robinson, V.B., and Alter, M.L. 1961. Incidence of infectious bovine rhinotracheitis and bovine virus diarrhea. Vet. Med. 56:395–398.

Noice, F., and Schipper, I.A. 1959. Isolation of mucosal disease virus by tissue cultures in mixture 199, Morgan, Morten and Parker. Proc. Soc. Exp. Biol. Med. 100:84–87.

Olafson, P., and Rickard, C.G. 1947. Further observations on the virus diarrhea (new transmissible disease) of cattle. Cornell Vet. 37:104–106.

Olafson, P., MacCallum, A.D., and Fox, F.H. 1946. An apparently new transmissible disease of cattle. Cornell Vet. 36:205–213.

Perdrizet, J.A., Rebhun, W.C., Dubovi, E.J., and Donis, R.A. 1987. Bovine virus diarrhea—Clinical syndromes in dairy herds. Cornell Vet. 77:46–74.

Phillips, R.M., Heuschele, W.P., and Todd, J.D. 1975. Evaluation of a bovine viral diarrhea vaccine produced in a porcine kidney cell line. Am. J. Vet. Res. 36:135–140.

Plant, J.W., Littlejohn, I.R., Gardiner, A.C., Vantsis, J.T., and Huck, R.A. 1973. Immunological relationship between border disease, mucosal diseases and swine fever. Vet. Rec. 92:455.

Pritchard, W.R. 1963. The bovine viral diarrhea–mucosal disease complex. Adv. Vet. Sci. 8:1–47.

Pritchard, W.R., Taylor, D.B., Moses, H.E., and Doyle, L.P. 1954. A virus diarrhea in cattle. Proj. no. 724. Detailed Annual Report, Dept. of Veterinary Science, Indiana Agriculture Experiment Station.

Pritchard, W.R., Taylor, D.B., Moses, H.E., and Doyle, L.P. 1956. A transmissible disease affecting the mucosae of cattle. J. Am. Vet. Med. Assoc. 128:1–5.

Ramsey, F.K., and Chivers, W.H. 1953. Mucosal disease of cattle. North Am. Vet. 34:629–633.

Richards, S.H., Schipper, I.A., Eveleth, D.F., and Shumard, R.F. 1956. Mucosal disease of deer. Vet. Med. 51:538–542.

Richie, A.E., and Fernelius, A.L. 1969. Characterization of bovine viral diarrhea viruses. V. Morphology of characteristic particles studied by electron microscopy. Arch. Gesam. Virusforsch. 28:369–389.

Rinaldo, C.R., Isackson, D.W., Overall, J.C., Glasgow, L.A., Brown, T.T, Bistner, S.I., Gillespie, J.H., and Scott, F.W. 1976. Fetal and adult bovine interferon production during bovine viral diarrhoea virus infection. Infect. Immun. 14:660–666.

Robson, D.S., Gillespie, J.H., and Baker, J.A. 1960. The neutraliza-

tion test as an indication of immunity to virus diarrhea. Cornell Vet. 50:503–509.

Roeder, P.L., and Drew, T.W. 1984. Mucosal disease of cattle: A late sequel to fetal infection. Vet. Rec. 114:309–313.

Rossi, C.R., and Kiesel, G.K. 1977. Bovine peripheral blood monocyte cultures: Growth characteristics and cellular receptors for immunoglobulin G and complement. Am. J. Vet. Res. 38:1705–1709.

Scott, F.W., Kahrs, R.F., DeLahunta, A., Brown, T.T., McEntee, K., and Gillespie, J.H. 1973. Virus induced congenital anomalies of the bovine fetus. Cerebellar degeneration (hypoplasia), ocular lesions and fetal mummification following experimental infection with bovine viral diarrheal–mucosal disease virus. Cornell Vet. 63:536–560.

Scott, F.W., Kahrs, R.F., and Parsonson, I.M. 1970. A mummified bovine fetus following experimental bovine viral diarrhea–mucosal disease in a pregnant cow. J. Am. Vet. Med. Assoc. 156:867.

Soto-Belloso, E.R., Archbald, L.F., and Zemjanis, R. 1976. Development of a cell culture line of bovine fetal endometrial cells. Am. J. Vet. Res. 37:1103–1105.

Steck, F., Lazary, S., Fey, H., Wandeler, A., Huggler, C., Opplinger, G., Baumberger, H., Kaderli, R., and Martig, J. 1980. Immune responsiveness in cattle fatally affected by bovine virus diarrhea–mucosal disease. Zentralbl. Veterinärmed. [B] 27:429–445.

Stewart, W.C., Carbrey, E.A., Jenny, E.W., Brown, C.L., and Kresse, J.I. 1971. Bovine viral diarrhoea infection in pigs. Program, 108th Annual Meeting, American Veterinary Medical Association. P. 163.

Taylor, W.P., Okeke, A.N., and Shidali, N.N. 1977. Prevalence of bovine virus diarrhoea and infectious bovine rhinotracheitis antibodies in Nigerian sheep and goats. Trop. Anim. Health Prod. 9:171–175.

Terlecki, S., Richardson, C., Done, J.T., Harkness, J.W., Sands, J.J., Shaw, I.G., Winkler, C.E., Duffell, S.J., Patterson, D.S., and Sweazey, D. 1980. Pathogenicity for the sheep foetus of Bourne virus diarrhoea–mucosal disease virus of Bourne origin. Br. Vet. J. 136:602–611.

Trapp, A.L. 1960. Pathology of the blood-vascular and lymphatic systems of cattle affected with mucosal disease. Ph.D. dissertation, Iowa State University, Ames.

Underdahl, N.R., Grace, O.P., and Hoerlein, A.B. 1957. Cultivation in tissue-culture of cytopathogenic agent from bovine mucosal disease. Proc. Soc. Exp. Biol. Med. 94:795–797.

Vantsis, J.T., Linklater, K.A., Rennie, J.C., and Barlow, R.M. 1979. Experimental challenge infection of ewes following a field outbreak of border disease. J. Comp. Pathol. 89:331–339.

Ward, G.M. 1971. Bovine viral diarrhea–mucosal disease implicated in a calf with cerebellar hypoplasia and ocular disease. A case report. Cornell Vet. 61:179–181.

Ward, G.M., Roberts, S.J., McEntee, K., and Gillespie, J.H. 1969. A study of experimentally induced bovine viral diarrhea–mucosal disease in pregnant cows and their progeny. Cornell Vet. 59:525–538.

Whiteman, C.E. 1960. Histopathology of the adrenal cortex and adenohypophysis in cattle with mucosal disease. Ph.D. dissertation, Iowa State University, Ames.

Whitmore, H.L., and Archbald, L.F. 1977. Demonstration and quantitation of immunoglobulins in bovine serum, follicular fluid, and uterine and vaginal secretions with reference to bovine viral diarrhea and infectious bovine rhinotracheitis. Am. J. Vet. Res. 38:455–457.

Whitmore, H.L., Gustafsson, B.K., Havareshti, P., Duchateau, P.U., and Mather, E.C. 1978. Inoculation of bulls with bovine virus diarrhea virus: Excretion of virus in semen and effects on semen quality. Theriogenology 9:153–163.

York, C.J., Rosner, S.F., and McLean, G.J. 1960. Evaluation of vaccines for virus diarrhea of cattle. Proc. U.S. Livestock Sanit. Assoc. 64:339–343.

Zwetkow, P., Boyadgiev, S., and Haralambiev, H. 1975. Investigation on the immunogenity of concentrated ethanol saponin vaccine against mucosal disease–bovine viral diarrhea. Arch. Exp. Vet. 29:759–761.

Border Disease of Lambs

SYNONYM: "Hairy shaker" disease

Border disease is a neonatal condition of lambs characterized by excessive hairiness of the birth coat, poor growth, and nervous abnormalities ("hairy shaker" lambs). The disease occurs in many flocks in Australia, Canada, Europe, the United States, New Zealand, the British Isles, and a number of other countries and causes considerable economic loss. As a result considerable research is now in progress. Excellent review articles have been prepared (Barlow et al. 1982, Nettleton 1987).

The disease in lambs often occurs in flocks with abortions that may take place during any stage of gestation. Acute focal necrotizing placentitis develops about 10 days after maternal infection (Barlow and Gardiner, 1969).

The disease can be induced experimentally with crude suspensions of brain, spinal cord, and spleen tissue from affected lambs which are injected intraperitoneally or subcutaneously into pregnant ewes sometime between the 7th and 85th day of gestation (Gard et al. 1976). The virus persists in the blood of lambs that survive and are immunologically tolerant. Susceptible sheep in contact with hairy lambs become infected with a mucosal disease virus. Experimentally infected ewes develop antibodies and are immune to subsequent challenges during pregnancy.

All present evidence suggests that border disease is caused by a virus that shares virtually all of the characteristics of BVDV and some of HCV (Acland et al. 1972). Sheep that recover from natural or experimental border disease contain precipitating and neutralizing antibodies to the other two viruses. Pregnant cattle inoculated early in gestation with tissues from affected lambs with border disease virus frequently abort and develop antibodies to BVDV. Similarly, pregnant ewes inoculated with certain BVDV strains abort or bear mummified or malformed fetuses (Barlow et al. 1980, Terlecki et al. 1980, Vantsis et al. 1979). It appears that the outcome of infection with these viruses depends on the genetic make-up and immune status of the dam, the strain of infecting virus, and the gestational age of fetus at infection (Barlow et al. 1980). The border disease virus replicates in cell culture, producing a cytopathic effect, and is considered similar, if not identical, to BVDV (Harkness et al. 1977). All of these facts point to a close antigenic relation between border disease virus, BVDV, and HCV, particularly between the first two.

Inactivated and live virus experimental vaccines have been tested in sheep. The vaccines were given by various routes, and two doses were more effective than one (Vantsis et al. 1980). These vaccines have not been approved for use in the United States. Therefore, border disease is currently controlled most effectively by eliminating infected lambs from the flock.

REFERENCES

Acland, H.M., Gard, G.P., and Plant, J.W. 1972. Infection of sheep with a mucosal disease virus. Aust. Vet. J. 48:70.

Barlow, R.M. and Gardiner, A.C. 1969. Experiments in border disease. I. Transmission, pathology and some serological aspects of the experimental disease. J. Comp. Pathol. 79:397–405.

Barlow, R.M., Patterson, D.S.P., Gardiner, A.C., Harkness, J.W., Orr, M.B., Richardson, C., Sweazey, D., Vantsis, J.T., and White, E.G. 1982. Border disease of sheep: A virus-induced teratogenic disorder. Fortschr. Veterinärmed. 36:90

Barlow, R.M., Rennie, J.C., and Gardiner, A.C. 1980. Infection of pregnant sheep with the NADL strain of bovine virus diarrhea virus and their subsequent challenge with border disease II B pool. J. Comp. Pathol. 90:67–72.

Gard, G.P., Acland, H.M., and Plant, J.W. 1976. A mucosal disease virus as a cause of abortion, hairy birth coat and unthriftiness in sheep. II. Observations on lambs surviving for longer than seven days. Aust. Vet. J. 52:64–68.

Harkness, J.W., King, A.A., Terlecki, S., and Sands, J.J. 1977. Border disease of sheep: Isolation of the virus in tissue culture and experimental reproduction of the disease. Vet. Rec. 100:71–72.

Nettleton, P.F. 1987. Pathogenesis and epidemiology of border disease. Ann. Rech. Vét. 18:147–155.

Terlecki, S., Richardson, C., Done, J.T., Harkness, W., Sands, J.J., Shaw, T.G., Winkler, C.E., Duffell, S.T., Patterson, D.S., and Sweazey, D. 1980. Pathogenicity for the sheep foetus of bovine virus diarrhoea–mucosal disease virus of bovine origin. Br. Vet. J. 136:602–611.

Vantsis, J.T., Linklater, K.A., Rennie, J.C., and Barlow, R.M. 1979. Experimental challenge infection of ewes following a field outbreak of border disease. J. Comp. Pathol. 89:331–339.

The Genus *Rubivirus*

Equine Arteritis

SYNONYMS: Epizootic cellulitis-pinkeye syndrome, *rotlaufseuche;* abbreviation, EA

Equine arteritis may be the same disease described by German scientists as *rotlaufseuche* and by English writers as epizootic cellulitis-pinkeye syndrome or typhoid fever. In 1953 the virus was isolated from outbreaks in Ohio (USA) which were characterized by illness in horses and abortions in mares (Doll et al. 1957). Since then, virus has been isolated from other epizootics in the United States. In Europe equine arteritis virus (EAV) was first isolated in Switzerland and later in Vienna, Austria (Burki 1969). There is serologic evidence of the disease in India (Burki 1969). Evidence of the infection in horses has been reported in France, Italy, Poland, and other European countries as well as Morocco and other African countries. In

1984 a number of severe clinical outbreaks occurred in Kentucky (Timoney et al. 1987, Traub-Dorgatz et al. 1985).

In the past this disease has been confused with equine influenza and equine rhinopneumonitis. The horse is the only susceptible animal, and the principal natural infections have been observed only on breeding farms (Bryans 1964).

Character of the Disease. The horses have fever, leukopenia, mild anemia, stiffness of gait, edema of the limbs, and swelling around the eyes. The disease spreads rapidly to susceptible horses on the premises. Pregnant mares abort—the essential feature of the disease in one natural outbreak. Stallions may also contract the disease. It usually occurs on breeding farms, and fatalities rarely result nor is there residual damage.

Inoculation of the virus into pregnant mares or young horses caused death in almost 50 percent of the animals in one experimental study (Doll et al. 1957). The mares aborted. These findings suggest that EAV conceivably can cause mortality under unfavorable circumstances.

The incubation period is 3 to 5 days (Doll et al. 1957). Fever is a constant sign; the other signs depend on the site and amount of damage to the arteries. Other signs in animals with fatal cases include pronounced conjunctivitis, palpebral edema and edema of the nictitating membrane, and excessive lacrimation. The nasal membrane becomes congested, and a serous nasal discharge is noted. Pulmonary dyspnea is frequent, and there is marked depression and muscular weakness. Mild or severe colic may be accompanied by watery diarrhea. There is edema of the limbs. On occasions keratitis, hypopyon, icterus, edema of the abdomen, and marked loss of weight are observed. Panleukopenia characterized by lymphopenia occurs.

The basic lesions involve small arteries about 0.5 mm in diameter, the smallest vessels that have well-developed muscular coats (Jones et al. 1957). The arterioles (less than 0.3 mm in diameter) and the large muscular and elastic arteries are free of specific lesions. Veins and lymphatics are often distended with blood or lymph, respectively, but are neither inflamed nor necrotic. The specific lesions in small arteries are distributed randomly in vessels throughout the body. Arterial lesions are found in every organ, but more conspicuously in the cecum, colon, spleen, lymph nodes, and adrenal capsule.

The microscopic lesion starts with necrosis of muscle cells in the arterial media. Edema and a few leukocytes then appear in the adventitia. The arterial media becomes edematous and infiltrated by lymphocytes, some with karyorrhectic or pyknotic nuclei. Initially, these changes may be limited to one microscopic segment of the artery viewed in cross-section. As the lesion progresses, most of the arterial media is involved and replaced by edema and

leukocytes. At this stage the artery is tortuous, and the intact endothelium becomes surrounded by leukocytes and edema, which replaces the media and adventitia. The lumen usually is empty and contains a few erythrocytes. In the large intestine and spleen, frank thrombosis and infarction occur. Consequently, the effects of these arterial changes are most often edema and hemorrhage. The mechanism of death is not definitely known, but the probable changes in electrolytes in cell and tissue fluids might be important (Jones et al. 1957).

The gross lesions are explained entirely on the basis of their distribution in small arteries (Jones et al. 1957). Edema and petechiae are conspicuous in adult animals and fetuses. Fetuses are particularly edematous, but no distinct microscopic lesion is found in the arteries. Edema is found in the subcutis of the legs and abdomen, near the injection site, and in the adjacent fascia. Edema and petechia are also found in the omental, mesenteric, and perirenal fat, the subpleural and interlobular septa of the lungs, the intra-abdominal lymph nodes, the broad ligament, and the adrenal cortex. Similar hemorrhages and edema are evident along the course of the ileocecocolic and anterior mesenteric arteries. The intestines, especially the cecum and colon, are severely involved, with sharply demarcated segments 1 to 2 m long. The entire wall is edematous and the mucosa markedly hemorrhagic. These lesions are related to typical changes in submucosal arteries, with thrombosis in most vessels. Sharply demarcated, often elevated hemorrhagic infarcts are seen in the spleen, particularly in younger horses.

Properties of the Virus. The incorporation of 5-iodo-2-deoxyuridine in tissue cultures does not inhibit the replication of virus, indirect evidence that EAV is an RNA virus (Burki 1969). EAV is readily inactivated by lipid solvents and by sodium deoxycholate. It survives 20, but not 30, minutes at 56°C (McCollum et al. 1961) and is quite stable at low temperatures. It is resistant to trypsin. In sucrose gradients its density is 1.18 to 1.20 g/ml (Maess et al. 1969).

By filtration the particle size is estimated to be from 50 to 100 nm (Burki 1969). Maess et al. (1966) concentrated and purified virus by ultracentrifugation and again by zonal centrifugation in sucrose gradients. This preparation was treated with uranyl acetate and phosphotungstic acid. The negatively stained particles observed with the electron microscope were spherical and had an average diameter of 60 ± 13 nm. The inner core of the virion had an average diameter of 35 ± 9 nm. Breese and McCollum (1969) found that in the cytoplasm of infected tissue-cultured cells, virus particles in the cytoplasmic vacuoles were 43 ± 2 nm, with a core diameter of 35 ± 2 nm. These particles were observed 18 hours after inoculation but not after 12 hours. The virus particles were found in increasing concentration and in increasing numbers of cells at 24, 30, 34, and 43 hours postinfection.

In an attempt to demonstrate an antigenic relation between lactic dehydrogenase and EAV (both non-arthropod-borne togaviridae), Berlo et al. (1983) showed that no relation existed at the level of envelope proteins or nucleocapsid proteins. They found that VP, the nucleocapsid protein of EAV, binds directly to staphylococcal protein A.

The virion apparently lacks a hemagglutinin but does contain a complement fixing antigen component. Only one immunogenic type of virus is known to exist, and it produces neutralizing antibodies. The prototype virus is the Bucyrus strain (Doll et al. 1957).

Cultivation. Attempts to propagate EAV in embryonated hens' eggs and in laboratory animals have failed (Doll et al. 1957). The virus produces a cytopathic effect in cultures of horse kidney cells and becomes attenuated so it can be used for immunization (McCollum et al. 1961). It also grows in hamster kidney cells (Wilson et al. 1962) and in rabbit kidney cells (McCollum et al. 1962) and produces plaques in overlay cultures. Thus far, only cells of equine origin show a cytopathic effect when inoculated with material from infected horses. Adapted strains replicate in tissue cultures from other species. In cell culture the Bucyrus strain usually yields 10^6 $TCID_{50}$/ml. EAV replication in RK-13 cells is enhanced by pretreatment of cells with 6-azauridine (Tozzini 1976). Sonified tissue-culture preparations are a good source of complement-fixing antigen (Burki 1969).

Epizootiology. The virus is spread in the air and is contracted by inhalation (Bryans 1964). It remains viable in nasal secretions for 8 to 10 days. The tissues and fluids of infected aborted fetuses also contain virus. Semen can contain virus and can be a vehicle of transmission to mares (Timoney et al. 1987).

Immunity. Horses that recover from infection or immunization with a modified live virus have solid immunity. Vaccinated horses are immune to virulent virus challenge for at least a year and presumably for many years (McCollum 1969). Antibodies against EAV can be demonstrated by the complement-fixation and neutralization tests. Complement enhances viral binding to antibody in the neutralization test.

McCollum (1976) reported that neonatal foals from immune dams with colostrum developed serum-neutralizing antibody titers equivalent to the dams' titers soon after suckling. The titers persisted in the foals for 2 to 6 months. When given virulent virus intranasally at 6 days of age, the foals showed no signs of illness or had a very mild clinical reaction. These foals had no neutralizing antibodies at 6 months and either died or contracted severe disease when given virulent virus intranasally. Maternal immunity did not provide full protection to some neonatal foals but clearly interfered with the production of active immunity. This point should be taken into account in any vaccination program for horses.

Diagnosis. Equine arteritis occurs sporadically, and in the typical outbreak mortality does not occur, although abortions occur in 50 to 60 percent of pregnant mares. Aborted fetuses often are autolyzed, in contrast with fresh aborted fetuses usually associated with rhinopneumonitis virus infection.

For diagnosis by virus isolation, samples can be taken from the nostrils, blood, or conjunctival sac. The nasal or conjunctival exudate is placed in Hank's balanced salt solution with antibiotics and 1 percent bovine albumin. These specimens can be stored at $-20°C$ for weeks. At necropsy, many different organ tissues can be used for virus isolation. Virus isolation attempts are made in primary cell cultures of horse origin or by horse inoculation. The demonstration of a rising antibody titer by the use of the complement-fixation or the neutralization test is another suitable means for making a diagnosis.

Prevention and Control. According to the Panel of the American Veterinary Medical Association Symposium on Immunity to Selected Equine Diseases (1969), equine arteritis can be prevented and controlled by good management practices and vaccination. The panel recommended that the attenuated HK-131 RK-111 Bucyrus virus vaccine be licensed when justified by supplementary data received by the Veterinary Biologics Division, U.S. Department of Agriculture, from potential commercial producers (Equine Disease Symposium, 1969). The vaccine now is licensed. The panel also recommended continued research on an inactivated virus vaccine.

To create the vaccine, researchers modified the Bucyrus strain by transferring it 131 times in primary cell cultures of horse kidney, followed by 111 transfers in primary cell cultures in rabbit kidney. The vaccine strain has undergone further passage in equine dermal cells (NBL-6), a continuous diploid cell line, and is used as vaccine virus between the 16th and 25th passage in this line (Harry and McCollum 1981). This vaccine virus causes either no reaction or slight fever and leukopenia. As little as 200 $TCID_{50}$ injected intramuscularly protects horses against challenge with virulent virus but vaccine administered intranasally does not immunize effectively. The vaccine protects pregnant mares without causing any ill effects on their fetuses. Serial passage of the vaccine virus does not restore its virulence, and the virus does not spread to susceptible horses maintained in direct contact with vaccinated horses. The use of the vaccine to control the disease in the stallion has been described by Timoney et al. (1987).

The Disease in Humans. Equine arteritis is not known to occur in humans.

REFERENCES

Berlo, M.F., Zeegers, J.J.W., Horzenek, M.C., van der Zeijst, B.A.M. 1983. Antigenic comparison of equine arteritis virus (EAV) and lactic dehydrogenase (LDV). Binding of staphylococca protein A to the nucleocapsid protein of EAV. Zentrabl. Veterinärmed. [B] 1983:297–304.

Breese, S.S., and McCollum, W.H. 1969. Electron microscopic characterization of equine arteritis virus. In J.T. Bryans and H. Gerber, eds., Proceedings of the 2d International Conference on Equine Infectious Disease. S. Karger, Basel. Pp. 133–139.

Bryans, J.T. 1964. Viral respiratory disease of horses. In Proceedings of the 101st Meeting of the American Veterinary Medical Association. Pp. 112–121.

Burki, F. 1969. III. Equine viral arteritis. In J.T. Bryans and H. Gerber, eds., Proceedings or the 2d International Conference on Infectious Disease. S. Karger, Basel. Pp.125–129.

Doll, E.R., Bryans, J.T., McCollum, W.H., and Crowe, M.E.W. 1957. Isolation of a filterable agent causing arteritis of horses and abortion of mares. Its differentiation from equine abortion (influenza) virus. Cornell Vet. 47:3–41.

Equine Disease Symposium. 1969. Panel report. J. Am. Vet. Med. Assoc. 155:237.

Harry, T.O., and McCollum, W.H. 1981. The stability of viability and immunizing potency of lyophilized, modified equine arteritis live virus and vaccine. Bull. Anim. Health Prod. Africa 29:177–185.

Jones, T.C., Doll, E.R., and Bryans, J.T. 1957. The lesions of equine arteritis. Cornell Vet. 47:3–68.

McCollum, W.H. 1969. Development of a modified virus strain and vaccine for equine viral arteritis. J. Am. Vet. Med. Assoc. 155:318–322.

McCollum, W.H. 1976. Studies of passive immunity in foals to equine viral arteritis. Vet. Microbiol. 1:45–54.

McCollum, W.H., Doll, E.R., Wilson, J.C., and Cheatham, J. 1962. Isolation and propagation of equine arteritis virus in monolayer cell cultures of rabbit kidney. Cornell Vet. 52:454–458.

McCollum, W.H., Doll, E.R., Wilson, J.C., and Johnson, C.B. 1961. Plaque formation by equine rhino-pneumonitis virus on monolayer cell cultures of equine, ovine, and porcine kidneys. Am. J. Vet. Res. 22:731–735.

Maess, J., Reczko, E., and Bohm, H.O. 1969. An investigation of the morphology of equine arteritis virus. In J.T. Bryans and H. Gerber, eds., Proceedings of the 2d International Conference on Equine Infectious Disease. S. Karger, Basel. Pp. 130–132.

Timoney, P.J., McCollum, W.H., Roberts, A.W., and McDonald, M.J. 1987. Status of equine viral arteritis in Kentucky, 1985. J. Am. Vet. Med. Assoc. 191:36–39.

Tozzini, F. 1976. In vitro sensitivity of myxomatosis virus to 6-azauridine. Boll. Ist. Sieroter. Milan 55:279.

Traub-Dorgatz, J.L., Falston, S.L., Collins, J.K., Bennett, D.G., and Timoney, P.J. 1985. Equine viral arteritis. Compend. Cont. Ed. Pract. Vet. 7:S490–S496.

Wilson, J.C., Doll, E.R., McCollum, W.H., and Cheatham, J. 1962. Propagation of equine arteritis virus previously adapted to cell cultures of equine kidney in monolayer cultures of hamster kidney. Cornell Vet. 52:200–205.

The Genus *Alphavirus*

The type species for the genus *Alphavirus* is *Alphavirus sindbis*. Some members in the group are Aura virus, Chikungunya virus, eastern equine encephalomyelitis virus, Getah virus, Mayaro virus, Middleburgh virus, Mucambo virus, Ndumu virus, O'Nyong-nyong virus, Pixuna virus, Ross River virus, Semliki forest virus, Una virus, Venezuelan equine encephalomyelitis virus, western equine encephalomyelitis virus, and Whataroa virus.

These viruses contain 4 to 6 percent single-stranded RNA with a molecular mass of approximately 3×10^6 daltons. They are spherical, enveloped particles, with a diameter between 25 and 70 nm. They contain lipid and are sensitive to ether. The buoyant density in cesium chloride is 1.25 g/ml. Trypsin does not destroy the infectivity of the particle. Hemagglutination is not inhibited by phospholipids and occurs over a narrower range of temperature and pH than that of flaviviruses. Alphaviruses are less inhibited by bile salts than flaviviruses. The virion replicates in the cytoplasm, and maturation occurs by budding. All members of the genus *Alphavirus* show cross-reactions in the hemagglutination inhibition test, but not with members of the genus *Flavivirus*. All members replicate in arthropod vectors, including the mosquito.

Three viruses in this genus are pertinent to a discussion of infectious diseases of domestic animals—eastern equine encephalomyelitis (EEE) virus, western equine encephalomyelitis (WEE) virus, and Venezuelan equine encephalomyelitis (VEE) virus.

Hayes and Wallis (1977) have written a review article on the ecology of WEE in the eastern United States. A comprehensive bibliography on VEE has been prepared by the U.S. Department of Agriculture (1980).

Western and Eastern Equine Encephalomyelitis

It appears certain that an enzootic encephalomyelitis of horses of viral origin has occurred in the United States for many years. In the late summer and early fall of 1912 many horses were lost in Kansas, Nebraska, Colorado, Oklahoma, and Missouri from what was most certainly viral encephalitis, although it was not recognized as such at the time. The outbreak and the characteristic lesions were described by Udall (1913). An estimated 35,000 horses died of the disease from midsummer until October, when the heavy frosts put an end to the outbreak. In later years small outbreaks of the malady have appeared in many western states. Natural infections occur in pheasants, and some die of it.

In July 1930 encephalomyelitis appeared among horses in the San Joaquin Valley in California. The outbreak continued through August, reached its peak in September, and disappeared with the advent of cool weather in November. It was studied by Meyer et al. (1931), who estimated that 3,000 horses and mules, representing about half the total recognized cases, perished. These workers isolated and studied the virus of the disease. The following year the disease recurred in the same area and appeared for the first time in several neighboring states. It reappeared each successive summer, and spread over a larger and larger area. In 1937 the disease was recognized in every state west of the Mississippi River and in several east of it. The peak incidence occurred in 1938, when 184,000 horses were estimated by the U.S. Bureau of Animal Industry to have died of encephalomyelitis. By this time every state west of the Appalachian Mountains had cases.

In 1933 an isolated focus of the disease appeared along the coastal plains of Delaware, Maryland, Virginia, and southern New Jersey; at least 1,000 horses died of the disease that year. The signs of illness were much like those exhibited by horses in the western parts of the country, but the mortality was much higher, approximating 90 percent. It was generally believed at first that the disease was identical to that which prevailed west of the Appalachian Mountains, but TenBroeck and Merrill (1933) pointed out that the virus was immunologically different because animals immunized against the virus of the eastern disease were not protected against the virus of the western disease and vice versa. These results were quickly confirmed by others, and it was generally accepted that there were two types of the disease: the *western type* and *eastern type*. Both types produce encephalomyelitis in horses; the signs of illness and pathological changes are practically identical. The principal differences are that the eastern type is much more virulent in horses, most experimental animals, and humans, and that there is little or no cross-immunity between the two types.

Randall and Eichhorn (1941) recognized a small outbreak near Brownsville, Texas, as caused by eastern-type virus. More recently the eastern-type virus has been found in Michigan, Wisconsin, Missouri, and other midwestern states. Large and severe outbreaks have occurred in Louisiana.

The virus of western equine encephalomyelitis has caused outbreaks in horses and humans in all states west of the Appalachian Mountains, and outbreaks have also been recognized in western Canada. The western-type virus was not recognized on the Eastern Seaboard until 1954, when it was isolated from sparrows in New Jersey by Holden (1955) and later from chukars in Florida. Late in 1955 the North Carolina State Board of Health reported finding virus of this type in a number of mosquitoes trapped in that state. WEE is a rare disease in horses or humans along the Eastern Seaboard.

The U.S. Department of Agriculture has collected sta-

Table 50.3. Annual cases of equine encephalomyelitis in U.S. horses, 1971–1985

Year	WEE	EEE	VEE	Cases submitted
1971	4	76	139	—
1972	446	30	0	965
1973	111	206	0	738
1974	312	27	0	730
1975	703	59	0	1172
1976	38	7	0	444
1977	617	4	0	1140
1978	17	4	0	353
1979	73	7	0	314
1980	27	44	0	397
1981	328	42	0	805
1982	27	47	0	519
1983	77	17	0	426
1984	9	11	0	274
1985	7	9	0	296
Total	2,796	590	139	8,573

Note: Cases confirmed by testing at the National Veterinary Services Laboratories of the Animal and Plant Health Inspection Service, U.S. Department of Agriculture.

Courtesy K. R. Hook, Ames, Iowa.

tistics on the yearly occurrence of equine encephalomyelitis. Although these figures are not complete, they do indicate the importance of this disease in the United States. The latest figures are given in Table 50.3, and the map in Figure 50.6 provides information about its distribution.

An encephalomyelitis of horses occurs in Brazil. According to Carneiro and Cunha (1943) the virus is closely related, if not identical, to the eastern type of North America. Livesay (1949) and Mace et al. (1949) reported the eastern type virus in native Philippine monkeys (*Macacus philippinensis*) suffering from a disease that resembled poliomyelitis. This disease has not been recognized in Philippine horses, but Mace and co-workers found neutralizing antibodies for eastern type virus in 26 of a series of 86 horses.

Equine encephalomyelitis occurs in Argentina. According to Meyer et al. (1934), the Argentine virus is very closely related, or perhaps identical, to the western-type virus of North America.

Character of the Diseases. In the United States and Canada both WEE and EEE are distinctly seasonal. In all but the most southerly parts of the United States they occur from June to November; in the warmer states sporadic cases may be seen during the winter months. As a rule, disease is sporadic during the summer, assumes epizootic proportions during August and September, and di-

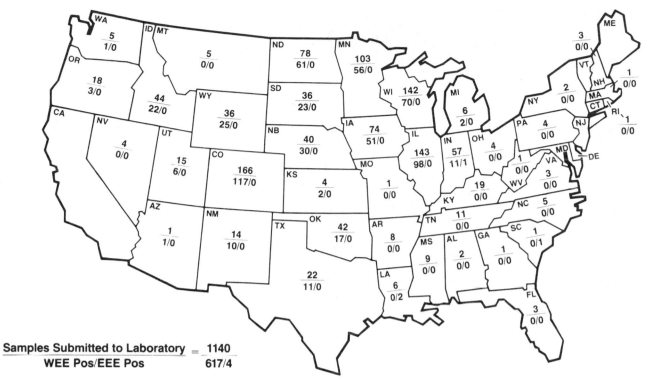

Figure 50.6. Equine encephalomyelitis serology (calendar year 1977). (Courtesy R. P. Jones, Animal and Plant Health Inspection Service, U.S. Dept. of Agriculture.)

minishes in intensity afterward In most of the country all outbreaks cease by the middle of November, because the mosquito population has been killed by frosts.

Horses of all ages may succumb, but younger animals appear somewhat more susceptible than older ones. It is unusual for more than 20 percent of the horses in any one place to become affected, and considerable periods often elapse between cases on the same farm.

The incubation period is from 1 to 3 weeks. In this respect the American forms of encephalomyelitis differ markedly from the German Borna disease, in which incubation is 4 to 7 weeks or more.

It is known from observations of experimental animals that fever is the first manifestation of the infection. The depression that occurs at this time may be so mild as to be unnoticed. At this stage there is viremia—an opportunity for bloodsucking insects to obtain virus. Invasion of the nervous system does not occur in all animals. If it does not, the animal does not appear ill, but will possess neutralizing antibodies in its blood serum for some time thereafter. When the nervous system is involved, the signs are, in general, those of deranged consciousness. Fever has disappeared by this time, and the blood is no longer infective. In the early stages of neural involvement, the victim may be restless or mildly excited. The animal may walk in

circles, crash through fences, or walk aimlessly into obstacles of any kind. It may shy at low doorsills and jump high in clearing them. It refuses food and water. Later a sleepy attitude develops, and the horse stands with head lowered resting it on the manger or on a fence (Figure 50.7). The animal can be aroused, but it quickly relapses into the sleep posture when not prodded into activity. It may sit on its hindquarters, stand with its front legs crossed, or assume other unusual and unnatural postures. Evidence of paralysis of portions of the body may become evident: the lower lip often becomes pendulous, the tongue may protrude, or there is difficulty in walking because the horse lacks full control of its hind legs. Finally, the paralysis may become general; the animal lies on the ground and is unable to rise. Death usually occurs within a day or two after the nervous signs begin. Horses that recover frequently show permanent cerebral damage, manifested by loss of ability to react to normal stimuli. Such animals are often called "dummies" by horsemen.

The course of the disease varies widely. In some cases animals die within a few hours of the time that the first signs are noted. At the height of outbreaks most deaths occur within 2 to 4 days. Animals that survive the effects of the virus may contract terminal pneumonia and die from this after a week or more. Others may recover com-

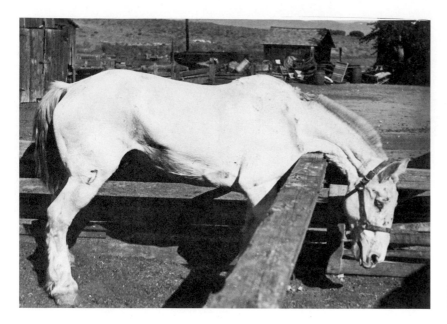

Figure 50.7. Equine encephalomyelitis. (Courtesy Edward Records.)

pletely or show various paralytic effects for many weeks or permanently.

The eastern-type virus is considerably more virulent for horses than the western-type. With the former, mortality generally exceeds 90 percent; with the latter, it may be as high as 50 percent, but averages from 20 to 30 percent.

There are no characteristic gross lesions in animals that die of this disease. Hurst (1934), who studied the histology of the lesions in the central nervous system, says that the gray matter is affected to a greater extent than the white and that the lesions are most marked in the cerebral cortex, thalamus, and hypothalamic regions, with the brain stem and spinal cord as a rule being less involved. The lesions consist of degeneration of the nerve cells, perivascular cuffing with mononuclear and polymorphonuclear cells in varying proportion, polymorphonuclear leukocyte infiltrations into the gray matter, and proliferation of glial cells (Figure 50.8). The lesions produced by the western-type virus are, as a rule, less than those caused by the eastern type.

Meyer et al. (1931) found that guinea pigs were highly susceptible to intracerebral inoculation with virus of equine origin and that these animals were the most suitable for diagnostic work. Death occurs in 4 to 6 days as a rule and is preceded by a fever followed by muscular tremors, flabbiness of the abdominal muscles, salivation, and trotting movements after the animal becomes prostrate. Rabbits are much less susceptible. Fever occurs and virus exists in the blood, but signs are very mild or absent, and the animals generally recover. White mice are very susceptible. They may be infected by inoculation intra-

cerebrally or through the undamaged nasal mucosa. According to Medearis and Kebrick (1958) suckling mice are even more susceptible to this virus than chicken embryos and constitute the most sensitive means of virus detection. Calves can be infected by intracerebral inoculation; they begin to display marked nervous signs approximately 5 days after injection. By the 14th day recovery usually is complete, according to Giltner and Shaham (1933). These authors found that sheep, dogs, and cats were refractory to inoculation. The common ground squirrel of the western states, *Citellus richardsoni,* may readily be infected by intracranial inoculation.

Karstad and Hanson (1959) showed that swine were highly susceptible to infection with the virus of eastern encephalomyelitis, either naturally or by inoculation. No signs were exhibited by the infected animals, but high antibody titers quickly developed. Inasmuch as they were unable to demonstrate viremia in swine, they concluded that this species probably has little or nothing to do with the natural propagation of this virus.

The eastern-type virus generally produces fatal infections when inoculated into pheasants, quail, pigeons, blackbirds, cardinals, cedar waxwings, sparrows, juncos, thrushes, young chickens, ducklings, chukar partridges, and turkey poults. Adult domesticated fowl (including turkeys) and some wild birds are resistant to infection. Ordinarily these birds do not show recognizable signs, but high-titer viremias generally appear for a day or two, followed by high antibody titers.

The subcutaneous inoculation of Texas tortoises (*Gopherus berlandieri*) with WEE virus results in pro-

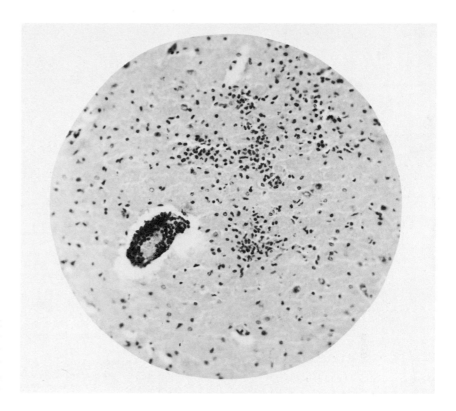

Figure 50.8. Brain tissue of a guinea pig inoculated with western-type equine encephalomyelitis virus. Note cellular infiltrations of both gray and white matter and perivascular cuffing. Hematoxylin and eosin stain. × 180. (Courtesy S. H. McNutt.)

longed viremia of up to 105 days' duration (Bowen 1977). The nature of the viremia is markedly affected by environmental temperature.

Properties of the Viruses. Strains of EEE virus are isometric, enveloped, and range from 50 to 70 nm in diameter (Figures 50.9 and 50.10). The capsids have ico-

sahedral symmetry. The virus replicates in vertebrate and arthropod hosts. Its RNA central core is infectious. Its specific gravity is 1.13, and the particle is inactivated in 10 minutes at 60°C. The virus withstands freezing and thawing and is readily maintained at low temperatures. Ether and deoxycholate inactivate the agent; formalin, but

Figure 50.9. Eastern equine encephalomyelitis virus in a mosquito salivary gland. The nucleocapsids are labeled *B* to differentiate them from the ribosomes (*arrows*) in the cytoplasmic matrix. Distention of the reticulum appears to be a consequence of accumulation of enveloped virus. Stained with phosphotungstic acid. × 74,300. (Courtesy S. G. Whitfield, F. A. Murphy, and W. D. Sudia, Centers for Disease Control.)

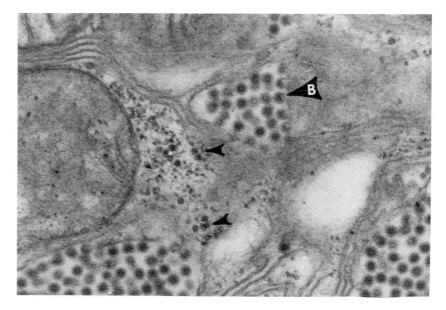

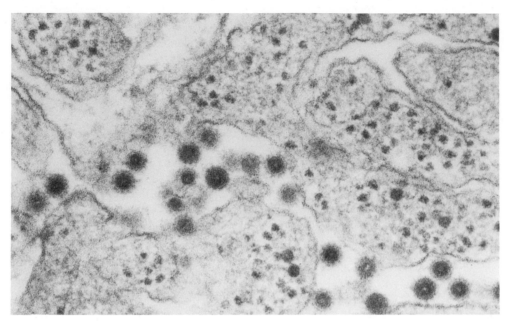

Figure 50.10. Higher magnification (than Figure 50.9) of eastern equine encephalomyelitis virus, which has infected a mouse brain cell. The nucleocapsids are clearly distinguishable from the ribosomes. The electron micrograph shows typical extracellular EEE virus particles with dense centers and enveloped surfaces with projections. Stained with phosphotungstic acid. × 90,000. (Courtesy F. A. Murphy and S. G. Whitfield, Centers for Disease Control.)

not phenol, destroys it. The virus disappears rapidly from tissues after death probably because of the acidity. A hemagglutinin has been demonstrated, and a hemolysin also exists. Complement-fixation and neutralization tests in mice inoculated intracerebrally and plaque-inhibition tests in tissue culture show the virus to be distinct from other arboviruses. Hemagglutination-inhibition tests demonstrate some antigenic components common to other alphaviruses. Some slight antigenic variations are demonstrated among strains of EEE virus coming from different areas. Interference, probably through the production of interferon, occurs between this virus and certain other arboviruses, myxoviruses, and picornaviruses.

WEE virus is essentially the same size as EEE and shares most of its physical and chemical characteristics. It has been estimated that 100 infectious particles are released from an infected cell, but only a few at a time. WEE is more closely related to sindbis virus than other alphaviruses, as shown by the plaque-inhibition test. This similarity has been confirmed by the hemagglutination-inhibition test, which also shows some crossing with other alphaviruses. WEE virus also produces interferon in appreciable amounts so that it is commonly used to study this nonspecific protein substance, which is produced in tissue culture by many viruses.

The molecular basis for the antigenic differences between WEE virus and a serologically related alphavirus

designated Highlands J (HJ), from the eastern United States, was examined. The structural proteins of WEE virus had molecular weights of 55×10^3 (E1), 47×10^3 (E2) and 33×10^3 for the nucleocapsid. The E1 glycoprotein had an isoelectric point (pI) of 6.4 and induced hemagglutination-inhibiting antibody specific for WEE virus. The E2 glycoprotein of WEE virus had a pI of 8.4 and induced antibody that was virus-specific by neutralization but that cross-reacted with HJ virus in the radioimmunoprecipitation test. Envelope glycoproteins of HJ virus isolates had molecular weights of 58×10^3 (E1) and 49×10^3 (E2), respectively. The E1 glycoprotein from HJ virus had a pI of 9.1 and induced antibodies that were reactive at equal titer with both WEE and HJ viruses by radioimmunoprecipitation. Two-dimensional gel electrophoresis of RNase T1 oligonucleotides of WEE virus and HJ virus genome RNase T1 oligonucleotides showed that the primary structures of the RNase of these two alphaviruses were distant. The fingerprints of the oligonucleotides from 16 WEE viruses from western and central North America, Mexico, and South America were similar to each other and easily distinguished from those of the 8 HJ viruses isolated in the eastern United States from Massachusetts to Louisiana (Trent and Grant 1980).

Cultivation. Higbie and Howitt (1935) reported successful cultivation of both eastern and western types of equine encephalomyelitis virus in chick embryos. Minute amounts of brain virus placed on the chorioallantoic membrane resulted in deaths of the embryos in 15 to 24 hours, the embryonic tissues being saturated with virus of a very high titer. The sensitivity of chick embryos to the virus of this disease is very great; less than 0.1 minimum lethal dose (MLD) for the guinea pig is frequently sufficient to infect. Both viruses produce a cytopathic effect in hamster kidney cell cultures (Kissling 1957). They also grow in cell cultures from many other species. Plaques are produced on monolayers of chick embryo cells. A color test in tissue culture depending on a change of pH has been used as means to titrate WEE virus.

A germ-free method to cultivate *Aedes aegypti* and *Aedes triseriatus* mosquitoes permits primary tissue cell cultures to be prepared from minced larvae of both species (Johnson 1969). The Louisiana strain of EEE grew in larval tissue cultures of both mosquitoes. There was some evidence of a virus-inactivating substance in the cultures of both species.

Epizootiology. Vawter and Records (1933) showed that horses could be readily infected by intranasal instillation of WEE virus, and that transmission in this way probably occurs at times. The epizootiology of the disease indicates, however, that this is not the usual way. Transmission by bloodsucking insects, particularly by mosquitoes, had previously been suspected, but Kelser (1933) was the first to show that mosquitoes could be infected and could convey the disease from animal to animal. In his work he used yellow fever mosquitoes (*Aedes aegypti*), which, 6 to 8 days after they had fed on infected guinea pigs, infected other guinea pigs and a horse. In the following year Merrill et al. (1934) showed that the ordinary salt-marsh mosquito (*Aedes sollicitans*) was capable of transmitting both the eastern and western types of virus. Another salt-marsh mosquito (*Aedes cantator*) proved capable of transmitting the eastern type of virus but not the western. *Anopheles quadrimaculatus* and *Culex pipiens* were incapable of transmitting either type. Madsen and Knowlton (1935) showed that local species of *Aedes* mosquitoes in Utah, *Aedes dorsalis* and *Aedes nigromaculis*, can transmit western-type virus. Other investigators have shown that *Aedes albopictus*, *Aedes taeniorhynchus*, and *Aedes vexans* can also transmit western-type virus. Merrill and TenBroeck (1935) proved that the virus multiplies in affected *Aedes aegypti*.

In the summer of 1941 Hammon et al. detected naturally infected wild mosquitoes and demonstrated western-type virus in one lot of *Culex tarsalis*) caught in the Yakima Valley in Washington during an outbreak of WEE in horses. This species of mosquitoes, widely distributed west of the Mississippi River, feeds on humans, horses, mules, cattle, and various birds. A number of other species of mosquitoes have been found naturally infected with western-type virus. Hammon et al. (1945) proved that *Culiseta inornata* and *Culex tarsalis* in the Yakima Valley could transmit the virus. The first isolation of eastern-type virus from naturally infected mosquitoes was reported by Howitt et al. (1949). The species was *Mansonia perturbans*, and the mosquitoes were captured in Georgia. The same workers (1948) found naturally infected chicken mites (*Dermanyssus gallinae*) and chicken lice (*Menapon pallidum* and *Eomenacanthus stramineus*) in Tennessee. The virus isolated was the eastern type. Neutralizing antibodies for this virus were found in one cow and a few chickens in the locality where the strain originated.

Although both types of equine encephalomyelitis virus can be transmitted by a considerable number of species of mosquitoes, the western type is transmitted to both birds and mammals principally by *Culex tarsalis*, and the principal vector of the eastern type to birds but not to mammals is the freshwater swamp mosquito *Culiseta melanura*. It is not yet clear whether there is a principal transmitter of the eastern-type virus from the bird reservoir to horses and humans, but it cannot be *C. melanura*, since this species attacks only swamp-inhabiting birds (Chamberlain 1958).

Kitselman and Grundman (1940) demonstrated the western-type virus in a large bloodsucking insect known as the assassin bug (*Triatoma sanguisuga*) captured in a pasture in Kansas. Since this insect is common in many parts of the west and feeds on horses, it is possible that it sometimes plays a part in virus transmission.

Smith et al. (1944) reported the recovery of western type virus from the chicken mite (*Dermanyssus gallinae*). These mites may be of some importance in conveying the disease since they feed on horses stabled near chicken houses. Furthermore, it is possible that chicken mites may harbor virus from one season to the next, as has been found to be true of the virus that St. Louis encephalitis.

Syverton and Berry (1937) showed that the spotted fever tick, *Dermacentor andersoni*, was a vector for WEE virus. Adult and nymphal stages of this tick were allowed to feed on normal guinea pigs and ground squirrels; the disease was transmitted to these animals. Continuity of the virus through all stages, including the eggs, was demonstrated. Virus remained in these ticks for 130 days, long enough to suggest that this might be one way by which the virus was preserved from one season to the next.

The work of many investigators makes it clear that this disease is transmitted primarily by mosquitoes of various kinds. Transmission by direct contact and by other arthropods undoubtedly occurs, but this is of slight importance in the total picture. There is experimental proof that mosquitoes may transmit the disease from infected horses to others by mosquitoes, but many workers believe that the virus reservoir in horses is much less important than that in various wild and domesticated birds. The presence of virus in hibernating *Culex tarsalis* in all months except December and the experimental overwintering of virus in garter snakes appears to be important in setting the stage for epidemics in horses and humans. Moreover, WEE is readily transmitted from snakes by infected *Culex tarsalis* (Gebhardt et al. 1966).

The overwintering of WEE and EEE viruses has been studied by many investigators interested in their epidemiology. Main (1979) suggested that hibernating colonial bats in southern New England in the United States may provide such a mechanism. Natural infections with EEE occur in the genera *Myotis* and *Eptesicus* in the area, but WEE virus was not isolated. After monthly observations of viruses and their bird and insect hosts in 1974 and 1975 it was suggested that *Oeciacus vicarius* (cliff swallow bug), with its overwintering capability and its relation to susceptible nestling birds in the spring, supports the endemic persistence of WEE-related alphavirus in Colorado (Hayes et al. 1977).

Immunity. Immunity to WEE and EEE persists for years after natural infection or after vaccination with attenuated virus vaccines. Foals of dams exposed to WEE are temporarily protected by colostral antibody. There is a suggestion that active immunity is produced by inactivated virus despite colostral antibodies in the foal.

In one study, vaccines prepared from the envelope component of WEE and EEE viruses stimulated the production of humoral antibodies in mice with varying degrees of homologous protection upon challenge (Pedersen 1976).

Diagnosis. Although the clinical signs are characteristic, they are not always diagnostic, especially in isolated cases. Several cases thought to be equine encephalomyelitis have turned out to be dumb rabies.

For a specific diagnosis, the virus usually must be isolated. This is best done by intracerebral injection of animals, preferably guinea pigs, or of embryonated eggs. Fresh brain tissue should be used for inoculation. The virus is not always isolated, even when other indications make it clear that viral encephalitis is present, for the organism often disappears from the tissues very quickly after the victim dies. For laboratory confirmation it is best to destroy the animal when it is obvious that it is not going to survive, rather than to let it die naturally. The brain should be removed promptly, cooled quickly, and delivered to the laboratory as soon as possible.

If the virus is isolated, it often is desirable to determine whether it is of the eastern or western type. This is most readily accomplished by inoculating several guinea pigs that have been previously immunized with eastern-type vaccine and several more that have received the western-type vaccine. Since there is relatively little cross-immunization between these virus types, the homologous animals should survive and the heterologous should die. Another approach is to incubate the unknown virus in antiserums specific for each viral type, then inject the mixtures into a susceptible laboratory animal or a susceptible tissue culture to establish which of the two specific antiserums causes virus neutralization.

Microscopic lesions in the brain are characteristic of viral encephalitis. In diagnostic work it is well to fix material for sectioning in case virus isolation fails. The histological changes never prove the precise type of virus involved but can strongly indicate this disease.

Meyer et al. (1931) were unable to find inclusion bodies in this disease and made a point of this fact in differentiating it from Borna disease in Germany. During the Kansas horse plague of 1912 a number of workers, including Joest, sought unsuccessfully to demonstrate inclusion bodies similar to the Joest bodies of Borna disease. Hurst (1934), on the other hand, described acidophilic intranuclear bodies in some of the degenerated neurons.

A relatively new diagnostic procedure for the identification of western, eastern, and Venezuelan equine encephalomyelitis may replace the use of laboratory animals and also provide results more quickly (Levitt et al. 1975). Virus is precipitated with fluorescein-conjugated gamma globulin followed by cellulose acetate electrophoresis. Clinical specimens are inoculated into primary duck embryo cell cultures, and within 24 hours there is sufficient virus for detection by microprecipitation.

If brain tissue from horses with clinical encephalomyelitis can be obtained within 24 hours after onset of signs of illness, examination of frozen sections or impression smears by the indirect fluorescent antibody test will give positive results for EEE. The most intense fluorescence is in the thalamus and the pons (Monath et al. 1981). It also has been suggested that high hemagglutination, complement-fixation, and/or serum-neutralizing antibody titer in a single serum sample obtained from a horse during the acute phase of WEE can be used as a presumptive diagnosis (Calisher et al., 1983).

Prevention and Control. Annual vaccination of horses with inactivated virus vaccine gives highly satisfactory results. The vaccine currently licensed in the United States is made from infected tissue-culture fluids (Gutekunst et al. 1966). Formerly other inactivated virus or attenuated virus vaccines were recommended for use in horses. The inactivated chick embryo vaccine virus was quite effective, but complications sometime arose when it was given subcutaneously rather than intradermally. A malady characterized by icterus, constipation, nervous signs, and often death usually occurred 30 days after vaccination (Kissling et al. 1954).

The immunity induced by inactivated virus vaccine is excellent and persists during an epizootic season. Annual vaccination usually is practiced in areas where encephalomyelitis is expected. Foals vaccinated during the first 8 months of life should be vaccinated again at 1 year of age.

At one time an encephalomyelitis antiserum was available, but apparently its manufacture has been discontinued in the United States. Large doses of this serum will protect horses for a short time against homologous viruses. After signs of neural involvement have appeared, antiserums have little or no value.

Given that the transmitting agents are a number of species of mosquitoes, another means of reducing the incidence of the disease is to implement antimosquito measures.

The Diseases in Humans. Meyer (1932) reported three cases of encephalitis in persons who had associated with horses suffering from western-type encephalomyelitis. One proved fatal. Virus was not isolated from any of these people. The first human cases proved to be caused by the equine encephalomyelitis virus were described by Fothergill and coworkers (1938). Shortly afterward Wesselhoeft et al. (1938) reported 40 cases—mostly in children—occurred in eastern Massachusetts during the height of an outbreak in horses. Eastern-type virus was isolated in nine cases. There were no multiple cases in families, and no afflicted person had had any contact with horses. The season had been very wet, however, and mosquitoes were common.

The onset of EEE in humans was sudden and was characterized by high fever, convulsions, vomiting, and drowsiness, which rapidly progressed to coma. Nearly all patients died. The high death rate distinguishes this illness from other forms of human viral encephalitis, which ordinarily have a much lower mortality.

Howitt (1938) reported the first proved case of equine encephalomyelitis virus infection in humans caused by WEE virus—in a 20-month-old infant who died after an illness of 5 days. The most extensive outbreak of human encephalitis ever recorded was reported by Leake (1941) and occurred in the north central part of the United States. Nearly 3,000 human cases were recognized. In general, the cases were mild; however, 195 deaths occurred. During the same period Jackson (1943) reported numerous human cases in Manitoba, Canada, just north of the epidemic area in the United States. Most of these were in infants less than a year old or in elderly persons. Cox et al.

(1941) isolated WEE from eight individuals with fatal cases, and virus neutralization with serums of recovered cases left no doubt that the equine virus was the cause of the outbreak. The disease in horses at the time of the human outbreak was not nearly so prevalent as it had been in several previous years when human cases were not recognized. It was a rather damp summer, however, and mosquitoes were unusually numerous. An interesting feature of this outbreak was that more than twice as many males as females were afflicted, which means, presumably, that men working in the harvest fields were more exposed to mosquitoes than were women.

In 1939 a number of laboratories began manufacturing a vaccine from virus propagated in chick embryos to protect horses. Soon afterward several fatal infections occurred in these laboratory workers. Manufacturers then began to immunize workers with a somewhat refined form of the vaccine used on horses (Beard et al. 1939). This protective measure has proved effective and has not caused unusual discomfort or resulted in undesirable sequelae. The vaccine is still recommended for persons exposed to unusual danger of infection. Workers exposed to both western and eastern types of virus should be given a mixture of both types of vaccine.

In the epidemic area in Manitoba in the summer of 1941, Jackson (1943) reported the vaccination of more than 3,000 adults with chick-embryo vaccine. There were no untoward results, although more than half the people suffered mild reactions.

REFERENCES

Beard, J.W., Beard, D., and Finkelstein, H. 1939. Human vaccination against equine encephalomyelitis virus with formalized chick embryo vaccine. Science 90:215–216.

Bowen, G.S. 1977. Prolonged western equine encephalitis viremia in the Texas tortoise (*Gopherus berlandieri*). Am. J. Trop. Med. Hyg. 26:171–175.

Calisher, C.H., Emerson, J.K., Muth, D.J., Lazuick, J.S., and Monath, T.P. 1983. Serodiagnosis of western equine encephalitis virus infections: Relationships of antibody titer and test to observed onset of clinical illness. J. Am. Vet. Med. Assoc. 183:438–440.

Carneiro, V., and Cunha, R. 1943. Equine encephalomyelitis in Brazil. Arch. Inst. Biol. (São Paulo) 14:157–194.

Chamberlain, R.W. 1958. Vector relationships of the arthropod-borne encephalitides in North America. Ann. N.Y. Acad. Sci. 70:312–319.

Cox, H.R., Jellison, W.L., and Hughes, L.E. 1941. Isolation of western equine encephalomyelitis virus from a naturally infected prairie chicken. Public Health Rep. 56:1905–1906.

Fothergill, L.D., Dingle, J.H., Farber, S., and Connerley, M. 1938. Human encephalitis caused by virus of the eastern variety of equine encephalomyelitis. N. Engl. J. Med. 219:411.

Gebhardt, L.P., Stanton, G.J., and St. Jeor, S. 1966. Transmission of WEE virus to snakes by infected *Culex tarsalis* mosquitoes. Proc. Soc. Exp. Biol. Med. 123:233–235.

Giltner, L.T., and Shaham, M.S. 1933. Transmission of infectious equine encephalomyelitis in mammals and birds. Science 78:63–64.

Gutekunst, D.E., Martin, M.J., and Langer, P.H. 1966. Immunization against equine encephalomyelitis with a new tissue culture origin vaccine. Vet. Med. 61:348–351.

Hammon, W.McD., Reeves, W.C., Benner, S.R., and Brookman, B. 1945. Human encephalitis in the Yakima Valley, Washington, 1942. With forty-nine virus isolations (western equine and St. Louis types) from mosquitoes. J.A.M.A. 128:1133.

Hammon, W.McD., Reeves, W.C., Brookman, B., Izumi, E.M., and Gjullin, C.M. 1941. Isolation of viruses of western equine and St. Louis encephalitis from Culex tarsalis mosquitoes. Science 84:328–330.

Hayes, C.G., and Wallis, R.C. 1977. An ecology of western equine encephalomyelitis in the eastern United States. Adv. Virus Res. 21:37–83.

Hayes, R.O., Francy, D.B., Lazuick, J.S., Smith, and Gibbs, E.P.J. 1977. Role of the cliff swallow bug (Oeciacus vicarius) in the natural cycle of a western equine encephalitis–related alphavirus. J. Med. Entomol. 14:257–262.

Higbie, E., and Howitt, B. 1935. The behavior of the virus of equine encephalomyelitis on the chorioallantoic membrane of the developing chick. J. Bacteriol. 29:399–406.

Holden, P. 1955. Recovery of western equine encephalomyelitis virus from naturally infected English sparrows of New Jersey, 1953. Proc. Soc. Exp. Biol. Med. 88:490–492.

Howitt, B.F. 1938. The Moscow 2 strain of equine encephalitic virus as compared with other strains of equine encephalitic virus. J. Infect. Dis. 63:269–286.

Howitt, B.F., Dodge, H.R., Bishop, L.K., and Gorrie, R.H. 1948. Virus of eastern equine encephalomyelitis isolated from chicken mites (Dermanyssus gallinae) and chicken lice (Comenacanthus stramineus). Proc. Soc. Exp. Biol. Med. 68:622–625.

Howitt, B.F., Dodge, H.R., and Gorrie, R.H. 1949. Recovery of the virus of eastern equine encephalomyelitis from mosquitoes (Mansonia perturbans) collected in Georgia. Science 110:141–142.

Hurst, E.W. 1934. The histology of equine encephalomyelitis. J. Exp. Med. 59:529–542.

Jackson, F.W., 1943. Encephalitis (western equine) in Manitoba, 1941. Am. J. Public Health 33:833–838.

Johnson, J.W. 1969. Growth of Venezuelan equine encephalitis virus in tissue cultures of minced Aedes aegypti pupae. Am. J. Trop. Med. Hyg. 18:103–114.

Karstad, L., and Hanson, R.P. 1959. Natural and experimental infections in swine with the virus of eastern equine encephalitis. J. Infect. Dis. 105:293–296.

Kelser, R.A. 1933. Mosquitoes as vectors of the virus of equine encephalomyelitis. J. Am. Vet. Med. Assoc. 82:767–771.

Kissling, R.E. 1957. Growth of several arthropod-borne viruses in tissue cultures. Proc. Soc. Exp. Biol. Med. 96:290–294.

Kissling, R.E., Chamberlain, R.W., Sikes, R.K., and Eidson, M.E. 1954. Studies on the North American arthropod-borne encephalitides. III. Eastern equine encephalitis in wild birds. Am. J. Hyg. 60:251–265.

Kitselman, C.H., and Grundman, A.W. 1940. Equine encephalomyelitis virus isolated from naturally infected Tratoma sanguisuga Le Conte. Kans. Agric. Exp. Sta. Tech. Bull. 50. P. 15.

Leake, J.P. 1941. Epidemic of infectious encephalitis. Public Health Rep. 56:1902–1905.

Levitt, N.H., Miller, H.V., Pederson, D.E., and Eddy, G.A. 1975. A microprecipitation test for rapid detection and identification of Venezuelan, eastern and western equine encephalitis viruses. Am. J. Trop. Med. Hyg. 24:127–130.

Livesay, H.R. 1949. Isolation of eastern equine encephalomyelitis virus from naturally infected monkey (Macacus philippinensis). J. Infect. Dis. 84:306–309.

Mace, D.L., Ott, R.L., and Cortez, F.S. 1949. Evidence of the presence of equine encephalomyelitis virus in Philippine animals. Bull. U.S. Army Dept. 9:504–507.

Madsen, D.E., and Knowlton, G.F. 1935. Mosquito transmission of equine encephalomyelitis (Aedes). J. Am. Vet. Med. Assoc. 86:662–666.

Main, A.J. 1979. Virologic and serologic survey for eastern equine

encephalomyelitis and certain other viruses in colonial bats of New England. J. Wildl. Dis. 15:455–466.

Medearis, D.N., and Kebrick, S. 1958. An evaluation of various tissues in culture for isolation of eastern equine encephalitis virus. Proc. Soc. Exp. Biol. 97:152–158.

Merrill, M.H., and TenBroeck, C. 1935. The transmission of equine encephalomyelitis virus by Aedes aegypti. J. Exp. Med. 62:687–695.

Merrill, M.H., Lacaillade, D.W., Jr., and TenBroeck, C. 1934. Mosquito transmission of equine encephalomyelitis. Science 80:251–252.

Meyer, K.F. 1932. Summary of recent studies on equine encephalomyelitis. Ann. Intern. Med. 6:645–654.

Meyer, K.F., Haring, C.M., and Howitt, B. 1931. Newer knowledge of neurotropic virus infections of horse. J. Am. Vet. Med. Assoc. 79:376–389.

Meyer, K.F., Wood, F., Haring, C.M., and Howitt, B. 1934. Susceptibility of non-immune hyperimmunized horses and goats to eastern, western and Argentine virus of equine encephalomyelitis. Proc. Soc. Exp. Biol. Med. 32:56–58.

Monath, T.P., McLean, R.G., Croop, C.B., Parkam, G.L., Lazuick, G.L., and Calisher, C.H. 1981. Diagnosis of eastern equine encephalomyelitis by immunofluorescent staining of brain tissue. Am. J. Vet. Res. 42:1418–1421.

Pedersen, C.E., Jr. 1976. Preparation and testing of vaccines prepared from envelopes of Venezuelan, eastern and western equine encephalomyelitis virus. J. Clin. Microbiol. 3:113–118.

Randall, R., and Eichorn, E.A. 1941. Westward spread of eastern type equine encephalomyelitis virus. Science 93:595.

Smith, M.G., Blattner, R.J., and Heys, F.M. 1944. The isolation of the St. Louis encephalitis virus from chicken mites (Dermanyssus gallinae) in nature. Science 100:362–363.

Syverton, J.T., and Berry, G.P. 1937. The tick as a vector for the virus disease, equine encephalomyelitis. J. Bacteriol. 33:60

TenBroeck, C., and Merrill, M.H. 1933. A serological difference between eastern and western equine encephalomyelitis virus. Proc. Soc. Biol. Med. 31:217–220.

Trent, D.W., and Grant, J.A. 1980. A comparison of New World alphaviruses in the western equine encephalomyelitis complex by immunochemical and oligonucleotide fingerprint techniques. J. Gen. Virol. 47:261–282.

Udall, D.H. 1913. A report on the outbreak of "cerebro-spinal meningitis" (encephalitis) in horses in Kansas and Nebraska in 1912. Cornell Vet. 3:17–43.

U.S. Department of Agriculture. 1980. Venezuelan equine encephalomyelitis bibliography. Veterinary Services, Animal and Plant Health Inspection Service, U.S. Dept. of Agriculture, Hyattsville, Md. 94 pp.

Vawter, L.R., and Records, E. 1933. Respiratory infection in equine encephalomyelitis. Science 78:41–42.

Wesselhoeft, C., Smith, E.C., and Branch, C.F. 1938. Human encephalitis: 8 fatal cases with 4 due to virus of equine encephalomyelitis. J.A.M.A. 111:1735–1741.

Venezuelan Equine Encephalomyelitis

Venequelan equine encephalomyelitis is a member of the genus *Alphavirus* and is often abbreviated VEE virus or VE virus. It was first isolated from a disease outbreak in horses in Venezuela. Beck and Wyckoff (1938) compared the virus with WEE and EEE viruses and found that all three shared many physical, biochemical, and biological characteristics but that VEE virus was immunologically distinct from WEE and EEE viruses.

In 1943 an explosive outbreak of equine encephalomyelitis appeared on Trinidad, off the coast of Venezuela. Gilyard (1944) isolated the virus, which proved to be of the Venezuelan type, and vaccine made from this type of virus brought the outbreak under control. The virus was obtained from the local mosquito *Mansonia titillans,* but other species were not excluded as vectors. A U.S. Navy seaman stationed on the island died of encephalitis about 6 weeks before the animal outbreak. Venezuelan type of virus was isolated from his brain. This is the first reported case of human infection with VEE virus. Later experience showed that this type of virus is highly infectious in humans.

From 1962 through 1964 a severe epidemic of VEE subtype 1B in Venezuela and Colombia caused innumerable cases in horses and 30,000 cases in humans, with 300 deaths. From 1960 through 1964 VEE antibodies were found in Seminole Indians in Florida, and virus later was isolated from rodents, mosquitoes, and three humans. This strain causes a mild disease in horses, but it produces immunity.

In 1968 VEE subtype 1B appeared in Central America, where it spread rapidly and caused severe disease in horses and humans. This subtype then appeared in Mexico in 1970 and by midsummer of 1971 was diagnosed in Texas in both horses and humans. The disease moved northward into the United States despite an effort to control the disease in Central America and Mexico by the use of a modified VEE vaccine (developed for humans) in horses and a mosquito-spraying program. In certain localities these efforts were begun too late or were hampered by logistical problems. The disease moved very fast, causing considerable havoc in the U.S. horse population and marked concern in public health department.

Because of its multiple-host distribution (among mammals, reptiles, and insects) elimination of this disease from a given area is extremely difficult. Consequently, it usually must be controlled by vaccination and by spraying of mosquitoes.

Character of the Disease. The signs of illness in horses are similar to those of WEE and EEE. Fever is accompanied by viremia for approximately 5 days. Marked diarrhea and neurological manifestations usually occur on the fifth or sixth day, and horses with fatal cases usually die 1 to 2 days later. Not all fatally ill horses have nervous manifestations. Survivors have detectable antibodies within the first 2 weeks after the onset of illness.

The gross and microscopic lesions (Figures 50.11 and 50.12) are typical of viral encephalitis with no distinguishing features that separate them of WEE, EEE, and most other encephalitides.

Properties and Cultivation of the Virus. In general, properties of the VEE virus are similar to those of the WEE and EEE viruses (Figure 50.13). There is evidence

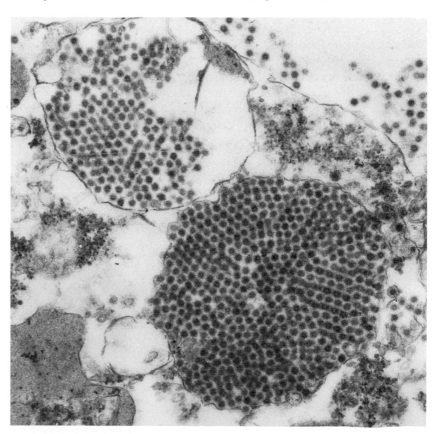

Figure 50.11. Accumulation of enveloped particles of Venezuelan equine encephalomyelitis virus in an area where brain cells are completely disrupted. Apparently virus particles that bud into vacuoles are trapped there upon disruption of the host cell. Stained with phosphotungstic acid (negative stain). × 44,500. (Courtesy F. A. Murphy and A. K. Harrison, Centers for Disease Control.)

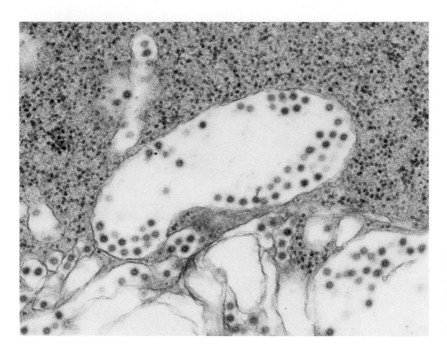

Figure 50.12. Mononuclear inflammatory cell (monocyte-macrophage) containing numerous mature Venezuelan equine encephalomyelitis virus particles within vacuoles. Stained with phosphotungstic acid (negative stain). × 38,000. (Courtesy F. A. Murphy and A. K. Harrison, Centers for Disease Control.)

that VEE virus is not inactivated by treatment with formalin, as are EEE and WEE viruses (Kubes 1944, Young and Johnson 1969). Safety tests indicated there was no residual VEE virus, but the use of the inactivated vaccine did not prevent clinical disease. This problem led to the development of an attenuated virus vaccine for humans.

One hundred fifty-eight strains of VEE virus were typed antigenically and classified epidemiologically as either epizootic or enzootic (Martin et al. 1982). Only antigenic variant group IABC strains could be classified epidemiologically as epizootic. In vitro, these strains were characterized by the formation of small plaques in Vero cells and a relatively narrow pH range for optimum

hemagglutinin-antibody reactivity. Experimental studies in horses confirmed that only IABC strains have epizootic potential. It was concluded that plaque size in Vero cell monolayers would be useful for detecting equine virulent strains. Indirect evidence suggested that small plaques resulted from sensitivity to an anionic substance in the agar overlay medium.

VEE virus has essentially the same mammalian host range and tissue-culture cell range as WEE and EEE viruses, so comparable methods are used for its cultivation and assay.

Epizootiology. The culicine mosquitoes *Aedes taeniorhynchus* and *Masonia titillans* and tabanid flies are

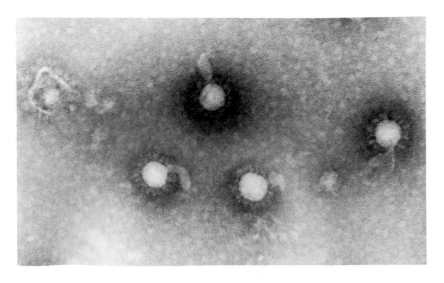

Figure 50.13. Negative stain of Venezuelan equine encephalomyelitis virus revealing spherical particles with surface projections ranging from precise, postlike structures to a halo of massed filamentous material. × 158,500. (Courtesy F. A. Murphy and A. K. Harrison, Centers for Disease Control.)

known field vectors of VEE, and there may be others. Experimental transmission with *Aedes triseriatus* has been proved in horses. *Mansonia indubitans, M. perturbans*, and *Psorophora ferox* are susceptible to laboratory infection with VEE virus. The genus *Aedes* is abundant in the United States; *M. perturbans* and *P. ferox* are common in southeastern United States; *M. indubitans* and *M. titillans* occur in Florida. Tabanid flies are found throughout the United States.

Many birds, including migratory birds, are susceptible to VEE. Birds generally have lower virus levels than certain mammals (such as rodents); this finding suggests that the natural cycle more likely occurs in mammals and insects than birds.

Direct contact transmission occurs between horses, presumably by the respiratory route. VEE virus is found in oral, nasal, and ocular excretions and in the milk and urine of infected animals.

In a pregnant mare near term virus may be transmitted transplacentally to the fetus (Justines et al. 1980). Virus can be recovered from fetal blood and organs but not from maternal blood.

The disease coincides with mosquito activity, so it is a warm-season malady in colder climates.

Immunity. Infection with VEE virus produces solid, long-lasting immunity. The protection appears to be a function of the neutralizing antibody's specificity, avidity, and ability to bind to virion antigenic determinants close to the critical neutralization site (Mathews and Roehrig 1982). The biological functions of hemagglutination and virus neutralization are primarily associated with only one antigenic epitope on the glycoprotein of the TC-83 vaccine strain (Roehrig et al. 1982).

Diagnosis. In horses the disease is identified as one of the viral encephalitides by the typical neurological signs; fatal cases can occur without neurological signs, however.

A specific diagnosis can be made only by laboratory procedure, either by the isolation of the virus from central nervous tissue, blood, or nasopharyngeal washings or by the demonstration of a rising serum-neutralization or complement-fixing antibody titer. Serologic confirmation is difficult or impossible, since animals often die before a convalescent serum sample can be obtained. Because the virus is hazardous to humans, few laboratories are willing to attempt viral isolation unless they have special facilities and vaccinated personnel. Erickson and Mare (1975) recommended a combined tissue-culture and fluorescent antibody system to isolate and identify VEE virus. A similar system, described in the diagnosis section for WEE and EEE, also works for VEE (Levitt et al. 1975).

Certain other diseases can be confused with VEE. Toxic encephalitis causes similar nervous manifestations but occurs commonly in the fall and winter from eating moldy corn or fodder. Purpura head swellings are similar in appearance, but VEE fails to cause respiratory distress or hemorrhages common to purpura. Rabies may be confused with VEE, but the history often aids in differentiating the two diseases. African horse sickness virus (AHSV) produces head swellings but it is very difficult to differentiate from the encephalitides, including VEE, because AHSV has many immunological types. Botulism can be differentiated from VEE chiefly by its nonseasonal nature and history.

Prevention and Control. Vector control should be considered first, but to be effective it must be complete. If vaccination of horses is permitted by state and local officials, it should be a part of the control program.

An attenuated virus vaccine produced by U.S. Army scientists (Berge et al. 1961, McKinney et al. 1963) for use in humans was used to control the 1969 Central American epizootic in horses (Spertzel and McKinney 1970). The horses at the periphery of the epizootic were vaccinated to create an artificial barrier to limit the spread of VEE. Horses within the epizootic area were also vaccinated. Within 7 to 10 days after vaccination, even on ranches where the disease was rampant, all equine cases subsided. Vaccination completely protected horses in affected areas and prevented the spread of VEE into Guatemala by an immune barrier of vaccinated horses, 50 km wide, established on the Pacific coastal plain. In 1970 this virulent strain somehow breached the immune barrier and became established in Costa Rica and then Mexico. It reached the United States in 1971; yet no epizootic occurred in 1970 or 1971 in either Guatemala or Nicaragua, evidence that strongly supports the view that attenuated virus vaccine gives lasting protection against the disease. Vaccination of pregnant mares does not appear to affect the developing fetus, but it should be avoided if possible.

Primary chicken-embryo cell cultures were evaluated as an alternate cell-culture system for the production of attenuated VEE (TC-83 strain) vaccine (Cole et al. 1976). The virus remained biologically stable through 10 serial passages.

There is no evidence that vaccination against EEE or WEE provides protection against VEE. Claims that multiple doses or the combination of EEE and WEE vaccines will provide protection probably are not correct, so it is advisable to use VEE vaccine to protect horses. Because some horses may not produce detectable vaccine-induced VEE antibody (Calisher et al. 1973, Moore et al. 1977), revaccination is recommended in high-risk areas.

Suspected cases should be reported immediately to the proper agencies so early typing of the virus as well as immediate quarantine can be initiated. Acutely ill animals should be isolated in stalls that are mosquito-proof, if possible.

The Disease in Humans. Naturally occurring epidemics of VEE in humans have been reported in Colombia, Panama, Venezuela, Mexico, and the state of Texas in the United States. Serologic evidence indicates that the infection has occurred in Brazil and in the state of Florida.

Numerous infections in laboratory workers attest to the marked susceptibility of humans to this agent. Further evidence is the production of disease in humans with inactivated virus vaccines that have been proved safe in animals. The isolation of VEE virus from the upper respiratory tract of an infected laboratory worker has important epidemiological implications. There is strong field evidence that the disease can be transmitted from person to person.

REFERENCES

Beck, C.E., and Wyckoff, R.W.G. 1938. The antigenic stability of western equine encephalomyelitis virus. Science 88:264.

Berge, T.O., Banks, I.S., and Tigertt, W.D. 1961. Attenuation of Venezuelan equine encephalomyelitis virus by in vitro cultivation in guinea-pig heart cells. Am. J. Hyg. 73:209–218.

Calisher, C.H., Sasso, D.R., and Sather, G.E. 1973. Possible evidence for interference with Venezuelan equine encephalitis virus vaccination of equines by pre-existing antibody to eastern or western equine encephalitis virus or both. Appl. Microbiol. 26:485–488.

Cole, F.E., Pederson, C.E., Robinson, D.M., and Eddy, G.A. 1976. Improved method of production of attenuated Venezuelan equine encephalomyelitis (TC-83) strain vaccine. J. Clin. Microbiol. 3:460–462.

Erickson, G.A., and Mare, C.J. 1975. Rapid diagnosis of Venezuelan equine encephalomyelitis by fluorescence microscopy. Am. J. Vet. Res. 36:167–170.

Gilyard, R.T. 1944. Mosquito transmission of Venezuelan virus equine encephalomyelitis in Trinidad. U.S. Army Med. Dept. 75:96–107.

Justines, G., Sucre, H. and Alvarez, O. 1980. Transplacental transmission of Venezuelan equine encephalitis virus in horses. Am. J. Trop. Med. Hyg. 29:653–656.

Kubes, V. 1944. Venezuelan-type equine encephalomyelitis virus in Trinidad. Science 99:41–42.

Levitt, N.H., Miller, H.V., Pederson, C.E., and Eddy, G.A. 1975. A microprecipitation test for rapid detection and identification of Venezuelan, eastern and western equine encephalomyelitis viruses. Am. J. Trop. Med. Hyg. 24:127–130.

McKinney, R.W., Berge, T.O., Sawyer, W.D., Tigertt, W.D., and Crozier, D. 1963. Use of an attenuated strain of Venezuelan equine encephalomyelitis virus for immunization in man. Am. J. Trop. Med. Hyg. 12:597–603.

Martin, D.H., Dietz, W.H., Alvaerz, O., Jr., and Johnson, K.M. 1982. Epidemiological significance of Venezuelan equine encephalomyelitis virus in vitro markers. Am. J. Trop. Med. Hyg. 31:561–568.

Mathews, J.H., and Roehrig, J.T. 1982. Determination of the protective epitopes on the glycoproteins of Venezuelan equine encephalomyelitis virus by passive transfer of monoclonal antibodies. J. Immunol. 129:2763–2767.

Moore, R.M., Jr., Moulthrop, J.I., Sather, G.E., Holmes, C.L., and Parker, R.L. 1977. Venezuelan equine encephalitis vaccination sur-

vey in Arizona and New Mexico, 1972. Public Health Rep. 92:357–360.

Roehrig, J.T., Day, J.W., and Kinney, R.M. 1982. Antigenic analysis of the surface glycoproteins of a Venezuelan equine encephalomyelitis virus (TC-83) using monoclonal antibodies. Virology 118:269–282.

Spertzel, R.O., and McKinney, R.W. 1970. V.E.E. A disease on the move. In Proceedings of the 74th Annual Meeting of the U.S. Animal Health Association. Pp. 268–275.

Young, N.A., and Johnson, K.M. 1969. Antigenic variants of Venezuelan equine encephalitis virus: Their geographic distribution and epidemiologic significance. Am. J. Epidemiol. 89:286–307.

The Genus *Flavivirus*

The genus *Flavivirus* includes a number of causative organisms for arthropod-borne viral encephalitides of humans in which domestic animals are involved. The viral encephalitides described in this section include St. Louis encephalitis, Japanese encephalitis, California encephalitis, louping ill of sheep, central European tick-borne fever, Murray Valley encephalitis, Wesselsbron disease, Israel turkey meningoencephalitis, and Powassan disease.

The type species for the genus is *Flavivirus febricis*, otherwise known as yellow fever virus. A typical member of the group contains approximately 7 to 8 percent of single stranded RNA. Its molecular mass is 3×10^6 daltons. Spherical enveloped particles, measuring $\pm$ 40 nm in diameter (Figure 50.14), have a buoyant density in cesium chloride of 1.25 g/ml. The particles contain lipid and a hemagglutinin; they are sensitive to ether and trypsin. The virions multiply in the cytoplasm and mature by budding. Not all viruses in this genus replicate in arthropods, but all are serologically related.

St. Louis Encephalitis

A warm-weather viral disease that occurs sporadically in the central and western United States, St. Louis encephalitis was first identified during a rather large outbreak in and around St. Louis, Missouri (USA), in the summer of 1933—hence its name. It occurs in the late summer and early fall. A number of species of mosquitoes, including many of those that transmit western equine encephalomyelitis, are known to be transmitting agents, and it is believed that they ordinarily convey the disease to humans. Hammon and Reeves (1945) isolated this virus from eight pools of *Culex tarsalis* captured in the Yakima Valley in Washington State during 1941, 1942, and 1944, and from other species elsewhere. They found that chickens were easily infected with this virus, and viremia of 2 to 3 days' duration followed. The infected birds showed no clinical signs. Neutralizing anti-

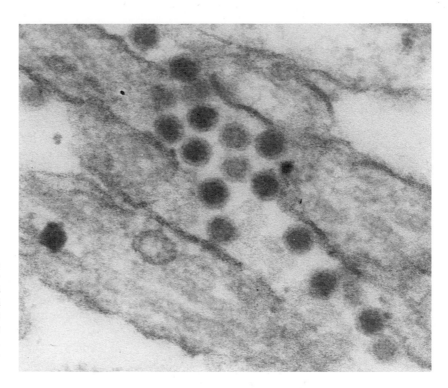

Figure 50.14. St. Louis encephalitis virus, a flavivirus, free in extracellular space. Virions consist of an electron-dense core or a closely bound lucid halo or envelope, 38 nm in diameter. Stained with phosphotungstic acid (negative stain). × 226,000. (Courtesy F. A. Murphy, A. K. Harrison, G. W. Gary, Jr., S. G. Whitfield, and F. T. Forester, Centers for Disease Control.)

bodies were found in many chickens in areas where the disease was occurring in humans. Smith et al. (1948) showed that certain mosquitoes could easily be infected by being fed virus-containing materials and that these insects could transmit the infection to chickens and hamsters for several weeks thereafter, viremia but no encephalitis was produced. They also demonstrated that the chicken mite (*Dermanyssus gallinae*) could be infected with the virus, which could then be transmitted through the eggs from generation to generation. Infection in these mites could continue indefinitely, providing the mechanism by which virus is maintained from one season to the next. The virus can also be maintained in *Culex pipiens* in temperate zones during the winter months—constituting another means for natural dissemination and persistence (Bailey et al. 1978).

In an epidemiological study of the 1962 epidemic of St. Louis encephalitis in four Florida counties, 222 laboratory-confirmed cases occurred in humans, with 43 deaths (Bond et al. 1965). The virus was recovered from four humans and from 42 mosquito pools of which 40 were *Culex nigripalpus*. All fatal cases occurred in persons more than 45 years old, and the death rate was unusually high in persons more than 65 years old. Widespread viral activity in nature was demonstrated by mosquito collections and serologic findings in wild or domestic birds in these four counties.

Whenever this disease appears in humans, neutralizing antibodies, hemagglutinating antibodies, and inhibiting antibodies can be found in horses and some other vertebrates. Lord et al. (1974) found antibodies in urban-dwelling wild birds (immature house sparrows). Because the appearance of antibodies in birds often precedes the disease in humans, monitoring may provide a clue for an impending epidemic, which can then be averted by intensifying mosquito control.

Hammon et al. (1942) inoculated horses with virus freshly isolated from mosquitoes. No signs were produced, but viremia occurred in some animals and high antibody titers in all. There is no evidence that horses ever suffer from a clinically recognizable disease as a result of infection with this agent or that they play any significant role in the propagation of the disease in humans. The virus has also been isolated from the brain of a California gray fox, *Urocyon cinereoargenteus* (Emmons and Lennette 1967), and from the Mexican free-tailed bat, *Tadarida b. mexicana*, during an outbreak in Texas in 1964 (Sulkin et al. 1966).

Trent et al. (1976) described a micro solid-phase radioimmunoassay test (SPRIAT) for antibodies reactive with nonstructural viral protein that is as specific and sensitive as the plaque-reduction neutralization test. The test, performed with wells precoated with purified St. Louis encephalitis viral antigen, can be completed in a day and can be adapted for use in testing a large number of serum samples.

REFERENCES

Bailey, C.L., Eldridge, B.F., Hayes, D.E., Watts, D.M., Tammarrello, R.F., and Dalrymple, J.M. 1978. Isolation of St. Louis encephalitis virus from overwintering *Culex pipiens* mosquitoes. Science 199:1346–1349.

Bond, J.O., Quick, D.T., Witte, J.J., and Oard, L. 1965. The 1962 epidemic of St. Louis encephalitis is Florida. I. Epidemiologic observations. Am. J. Epidemiol. 681:392–404.

Emmons, R.W., and Lennette, E.H. 1967. Isolation of St. Louis encephalitis virus from a naturally-infected gray fox, *Urocyon cinereoargenteus.* Proc. Soc. Exp. Biol. Med. 125:443–447.

Hammon, W.McD., and Reeves, W.C. 1945. Recent advances in the epidemiology of the arthropod-borne virus encephalitides including certain exotic types. Am. J. Public Health 35:994–1004.

Hammon, W.McD., Carle, B.N., and Izumi, E.M. 1942. Infection of horses with St. Louis encephalitis virus, experimental and natural. Proc. Soc. Exp. Biol. Med. 49:335–340.

Lord, R.D., Calisher, C.H., Chappell, W.A., Metzger, W.R., and Rischer, G.W. 1974. Urban St. Louis encephalitis surveillance through wild birds. Am. J. Epidemiol. 99:360–363.

Smith, M.G., Blattner, R.J., Heys, F.M., and Miller, A. 1948. Experiments on the role of the chicken mite, *Dermanyssus gallinae,* and the mosquito in the epidemiology of St. Louis encephalitis. J. Exp. Med. 87:119–138.

Sulkin, S.E., Sims, R.A., and Allen, R. 1966. Isolation of St. Louis encephalitis virus from bats (*Tadarida b. mexicana*) in Texas. Science 152:223–225.

Trent, D.W., Harvey, C.L., and Qureshi Lestourgeon, A. 1976. Solid-phase radioimmunoassay for antibodies to flavivirus structural and nonstructural proteins. Infect. Immun. 13:1325–1333.

Japanese Encephalitis

A virus-induced encephalitis (Japanese encephalitis) occurs in humans in Japan, Korea, Manchuria, Malaya, China, Indochina, and Sumatra; the causative organism has been classified as a member of the B group of arboviruses, now known as the flaviviruses. A disorder called Australian X disease is probably an identical infection. Large outbreaks with high mortality have occurred from time to time. A milder form evidently exists, since many people in the Orient carry neutralizing antibodies for the virus. It is reported, for example, that more than 90 percent of all Koreans exhibit such antibodies. The attention of western workers was first directed to this infection when American military personnel contracted the disease in infected regions during World War II. The disease was also found in Guam in 1948.

The disease is mosquito-borne. Hammon et al. (1949) confirmed earlier Japanese findings that *Culex tritaeniorhynchus* and a local variety of *Culex pipiens* could transmit the virus; they captured virus-carrying mosquitoes of the first species in the wild, where the disease was endemic. In Japan and neighboring regions the disease occurs only during the summer. In Guam and other tropical regions the disease may occur year round.

Hodes et al. (1946), Sabin (1947), and Hammon (1948), working at different times on Okinawa, showed

that most of the horses, pigs, and cattle carried neutralizing antibodies. They all agreed that chickens rarely had such antibodies; apparently these birds do not play the role that they do in disseminating western equine encephalomyelitis virus and the St. Louis encephalitis virus. Hammon et al. (1951) found that finches and redwinged blackbirds circulated more virus following inoculation than did chickens and concluded that some wild birds may be important in the propagation of this disease. In Sarawak, it appears that the pig acts as a maintenance host of Japanese encephalitis in a cycle involving *Culex gelidus* mosquitoes and, toward the end of the year, in a cycle involving *C. tritaeniorhynchus* (Simpson et al. 1976). More than 50 percent of fresh-water turtles (*Trionyx sinesis* Wiegman) from China have hemagglutination-inhibiting and/or virus-neutralizing antibodies, and there are no obvious differences in positive results between spring-summer and autumn-winter seasons (Shortridge et al. 1975).

Various surveys in the endemic areas showing the high incidence of horses, cattle, and swine with high antibody titers indicate that the infection must occur frequently in a mild form. Infections in pregnant sows may cause stillbirths and constitute a significant loss in herds in the Orient. Experimental infection in boars causes reproductive disorders. Patterson et al. (1952) described deaths of a number of race horses in Malaya, and Japanese authors have described fatal cases in cattle and swine. When intracerebrally inoculated with virus, all test animals of these three species die.

Two attenuated virus vaccines for protection of domestice animals against Japanese encephalitis have been developed in cell-culture systems (Fujisaki et al. 1975, Halle and Zebovitz 1977). Both are reputed to be safe and efficacious in test animals. Fujisaki et al. (1975) performed extensive experiments in piglets and pregnant sows with excellent results, so it is presumed that the S strain is safe for use in swine. Vaccination of gilts before mating, using the M strain of vaccine virus developed by Halle and Zebovitz (1977), markedly reduced stillbirths at a large breeding farm on Taiwan (Hsu et al. 1972).

REFERENCES

Fujisaki, Y., Sugimori, T., Morimoto, T., and Miura, Y. 1975. Development of an attenuated strain for Japanese encephalitis live virus vaccine for porcine use. Natl. Inst. Anim. Health Q. (Tokyo) 15:15–23.

Halle, S., and Zebovitz, E. 1977. A spontaneous temperature sensitive mutant of Japanese encephalitis virus: Preliminary characterization. Arch. Virol. 54:165–176.

Hammon, W.McD. 1948. Japanese B encephalitis. Proc. Fourth Int. Congr. Trop. Dis. Malaria 1:568–575.

Hammon, W.McD., Reeves, W.C., and Sather, G.E. 1951. Japanese B encephalitis virus in the blood of experimentally inoculated birds. Epidemiologic implications. Am. J. Hyg. 53:249—261.

Hammon, W.McD., Tigertt, W.D., Sather, G., and Schenker, H. 1949. Isolation of Japanese B encephalitis virus from naturally infected *Culex tritaeniorhynchus* collected in Japan. Am. J. Hyg. 50:51–56.

Hodes, H.L., Thomas, L., and Peck, J.L. 1946. Complement fixing and neutralizing antibodies against Japanese B virus in the sera of Okinawan horses. Science 103:357–359.

Hsu, S.T., Chang, L.C., Lin, S.Y., Chuang, H., Ma, L., Inoue, W.Y., and Okuno, L.O. 1972. The effect of vaccination with a live attenuated strain of Japanese encephalitis virus on stillbirths in swine in Taiwan. Bull. WHO 46:465–471.

Patterson, P.Y., Ley, H.L., Jr., Wisseman, D.L., Jr., Pond, W.L., Smadel, J.E., Dierchs, F.H., Hetherington, H.D.G., Sneath, P.H.A., Witherington, D.H., and Lancaster, W.E. 1952. Japanese encephalitis in Malaya. I. Isolation of virus and serological evidence of human and equine infections. Am. J. Hyg. 56:320–333.

Sabin, A.B. 1947. Epidemic encephalitis in military personnel: Isolation of Japanese B virus on Okinawa in 1945, serologic diagnosis, clinical manifastation, epidemiological aspects and use of mouse brain vaccine. J.A.M.A. 133:281–293.

Shortridge, K.F., Oya, A., Kobayashi, M., and Yip, L. 1975. Arbovirus infections in reptiles: Studies on the presence of Japanese encephalitis virus antibody in the plasma of the turtle, *Trionyx sinesis*. Southeast Asian J. Trop. Med. Public Health 6 :161–169.

Simpson, D.I., Smith, C.E., Marshall, T.F., et al. 1976. Arbovirus infections in Sarawak: The role of the domestic pig. Trans. R. Soc. Trop. Med. Hyg. 70:66–72.

California Encephalitis

California encephalitis is caused by a group of closely related flaviviruses. Hammon et al. (1952) were the first to describe one of these viruses, which they isolated from mosquitoes (*Aedes dorsalis* and *Culex tarsalis*) in Kern County, California (USA). Encephalitis, sometimes fatal, developed in mice, cotton rats, and hamsters following inoculation, especially when the inoculum was introduced intracerebrally. The signs and lesions in the experimental animals were indistinguishable from those induced by equine encephalomyelitis and St. Louis viruses. Guinea pigs, rabbits, ground squirrels, a calf, and a monkey showed serologic responses, but no signs after injection of the virus. Squirrel and rabbit reactions were of particular interest, since both species developed viremias that could infect mosquito vectors. Chickens proved to be wholly refractory.

Both species of mosquitoes that harbor this virus in nature can readily be infected by feeding, and they maintain the virus for at least 7 to 8 days. In one instance artificially infected *A. dorsalis* transmitted the infection to a rabbit. More recently a virus of this group was isolated from the mosquito *Culex inornata*.

In the north central United States, California encephalitis is caused by the La Crosse strain of virus, and transovarian transmission of the virus in *Aedes triseriatus* is the mechanism for its survival during the winter (Watts et al. 1974). Venereal transmission of La Crosse virus strain from male to female *A. triseriatus* has been shown by

experimental studies (Thompson and Beaty 1978). Human cases of encephalitis have been associated with virus isolated from various stages of *A. triseriatus* captured from tree holes close to the patients' homes (Balfour et al. 1974, Watts et al. 1974).

The Tahyna virus is a member of the California group of flaviviruses and occurs in practically all European countries (Bardos 1976). Antibodies to the virus have been found in foals, suckling pigs, and hares. In humans it causes an influenzalike disease; some patients have meningoencephalitis and atypical pneumonia. A human case of nonfatal encephalitis was suspected to have been caused by this virus because neutralizing antibodies were demonstrated after recovery. Wenner and co-workers (1951) believed the evidence indicated that this virus has a natural reservoir in the wild and perhaps also in domestic mammals; the infection is propagated by mosquitoes. Cross-neutralization tests indicated a close relation with a virus that caused an outbreak of human encephalitis in Barnes County, North Dakota, in the summer of 1949.

A member placed in this group which was antigenically different form the prototype BFS-283 strain for the group was isolated form a pool of 23 *Aedes cinerus* mosquitoes in New York State (Whitney et al. 1969).

Other viral isolates are closely related to the original California isolate. In addition to the five previously recognized viruses in the group, two of which were from the United States, there now appear to be at least eight antigenically related viruses in the United States (Hammon and Sather 1966). The complement-fixation test for these eight viruses in the California group had only twofold reciprocal differences with the closely related La Crosse and snowshoe hare viruses (Sprance and Shope 1977).

REFERENCES

Balfour, H.H., Jr., Edelman, D.K., Cook. F.E., Barton, W.I., Buzicky, A.W., Siem, R.A., and Bauer H. 1974. Isolates of California encephalitis (La Crosse) virus from field collected eggs and larvae of *Aedes triseriatus*: Identification of the overwintering site of California encephalitis. J. Infect. Dis. 131:712–715.

Bardos, V. 1976. Zur Ökologie und medizinischen Bedeutung des Tahyna-virus. Münch. Med. Wochenschr. 118:1617–1620.

Hammon, W.McD., and Sather, G. 1966. History and recent reappearance of viruses in the California encephalitis group. Am. J. Trop. Med. Hyg. 15:199–204.

Hammon, W.McD., Reeves, W.C., and Sather, G. 1952. California encephalitis virus, a newly described agent. II. Isolations and attempts to identify and characterize the agent. J. Immunol. 69:493–510.

Sprancem H.E., and Shope, R.E. 1977. Single inoculation immune hamster sera for typing California group arboviruses by the complement-fixation test. Am. J. Trop. Med. Hyg. 26:544–546.

Thompson, W.H., and Beaty, B.J. 1978. Venereal transmission of La Crosse virus from male to female *Aedes triseriatus*. Am. J. Trop. Med. Hyg. 27:187–196.

Watts, D.M., Thompson, W.H., Yuill, T.M., DeFoliart, G.R., and

Hanson, R.P. 1974. Overwintering of La Crosse virus in *Aedes triseriatus*. Am. J. Trop. Med. Hyg. 23:694–700.

Wenner, H.A., Kamtsuka, P., Krammer, M.C., Cockburn, T.A., and Price, E.R. 1951. Encephalitis in the Missouri River Basin. II. Studies on a focal outbreak of encephalitis in North Dakota. Public Health Rep. 66:1075–1085.

Whitney, E., Jamnback, H., Means, R.G., Roz, A.P., and Rayner, G.A. 1969. California encephalitis virus complex from *Aedes cinerus*. Am. J. Trop. Med. Hyg. 18:123–131.

Louping III

SYNONYM: Infectious encephalomyelitis of sheep

Louping ill has occurred in the highland sheep of Scotland and the northern part of England for more than a century. It also exists in Ireland. Although similar to spring-summer encephalitis, which afflicts humans in Czechoslovakia and the Soviet Union, it is not the same disease. It is not known to occur in the Western Hemisphere. The disease gets its name from the peculiar leaping gait of the ataxic animals. Poole et al. (1930) showed that it is inoculable by intracerebral injection. Greig et al. (1931) proved, the following year, that the causative agent was a filterable virus.

The disease is primarily one of sheep, but it occasionally affects cattle pastured on the same lands with infected sheep. An outbreak in piglets has been described in Scotland. The piglets had been fed raw meat from lambs that presumably had louping ill. Most animals had nervous signs and died of severe meningoencephalomyelitis; virus was isolated from the brain (Bannatyne et al. 1980). Timoney et al. (1976) described an outbreak in a group of free-ranging horses in Ireland. Antibodies to the virus have been found in wild red deer in Scotland, which may therfore serve as a tangential host (Adam et al. 1977). A case has been described in a dog that partially recovered from severe nervous manifestations. Human infection also occurs.

Character of the Disease. Under conditions of natural exposure, the incubation time in sheep is from 6 to 18 days. The earliest signs are dullness and high temperature, which may be 107°F or more. At this stage virus is present in the blood. The temperature generally falls after a day or so, and the animal appears better; but improvement is only temporary for a second temperature rise usually occurs about the fifth day. At this time the nervous system may become involved. If it does not, the animal recovers rapidly and thereafter is immune. Nervous signs begin with muscular incoordination, tremors, cerebellar ataxia, and progress to paralysis. A high percentage of animals that do not die usually are permanently damaged. In very acute cases death may occur within a day or two of the time the first signs are observed. In chronic cases

paralysis may exist for months. The disease resembles human poliomyelitis in that it is always begins as a generalized infection, which may or may not be followed by an invasion of the central nervous system.

If only generalized or viremic changes occur, without nervous system involvement, the death rate is practically nil. In the highly infected areas of the British Isles sheep more than 1 year old seldom develop the disease; they are immune as a result of unrecognized infections. This disease is seen mostly in young lambs.

The disease in horses is characteristic of louping ill disease in sheep. Timoney et al. (1976) described three horses that displayed signs of central nervous system disturbance; two died after 2 and 12 days of illness, respectively. Virus was isolated from the brain and cervical spinal cord. Serum samples from the infected horses contained hemagglutinating, complement-fixing, precipitating, and neutralizing antibodies to louping ill virus.

The microscopic lesions of fatally ill animals are typical viral encephalomyelitis and meningitis. Degeneration of neurons, particularly the Purkinje cells of the cerebellum, is characteristic. There are no typical gross lesions.

By intracerebral inoculation of brain virus the disease can be produced in sheep, cattle, swine, mice, hamsters, and monkeys. Rabbits and guinea pigs do not appear to be susceptible. According to Galloway and Perdrau (1935) monkeys and mice can be readily infected by instilling virus in their nostrils. The incubation period in these cases varied from 13 to 22 days, averaging 17 days. Hurst (1931) found characteristic cytoplasmic inclusion bodies in the brains of mice, but he could not find them in other species. Edward (1947b) produced encephalitis in 44 percent of susceptible lambs by inoculating virus subcutaneously. Injection of sterile starch solution intracerebrally 3 days after inoculation of the virus increased the number of cases of encephalitis to nearly 100 percent.

Four red deer and one roe deer had no signs of illness after subcutaneous inoculation with the SB-526 strain of louping ill virus. All of the deer had viremia and produced antibodies (Reid et al. 1982).

Experimental studies in a group of ponies confirmed that the horse was susceptible to louping ill virus (Timoney 1980). Most of the ponies had viremia of sufficient concentration for 2 to 3 days to potentially infect nymphs of the castor bean tick *Ixodes ricinus*.

Properties of the Virus. The virus has properties characteristic of other flaviviruses. Infectious RNA has been extracted from the particles, which are spherical. The virus hemagglutinates red blood cells in roosters. Crossing occurs with the other flaviviruses in hemagglutination-inhibition tests, but not to the same degree as with other members of the genus. The agent is well preserved by freezing and by glycerol, but deteriorates rapidly in saline or broth, especially in dilute and somewhat acid suspensions.

A complement-fixation test is available, but complement-fixing antibodies are transient, so the test has limited value in diagnosis and research (Williams 1968).

Cultivation. Rivers and Ward (1933) were successful in obtaining artificial cultures of the virus on minced chick embryo medium. The virus also grows in cultures of pig kidney. Edward (1947a) grew it in embryonated eggs by inoculating either the yolk sac or the embryo.

Epizootiology Experiments have shown that monkeys and humans can contract infection by inhaling infective droplets. Infection may occur similarly in sheep, but most transmissions occur via bloodsucking arthropods. McLeod and Gordon (1932) showed that in the louping ill districts of the British Isles the principal transmitter was the castor bean tick, *Ixodes ricinus*. The larval tick, feeding on infected sheep, conveys the infection to new hosts when it nexts feed as a nymph; or if the tick becomes infected as a nymph, it conveys the disease to a new host as an adult. The disease is prevalent in the early summer, subsides during midsummer, and reappears in early fall. These periods correspond to the seasons of tick activity in the area.

Further epizootiological studies of this disease on the Scottish heather moorland showed that the maintenance of louping ill virus depends on sheep, with the red grouse occasionally acting as the amplifier host (Reid 1978).

Immunity. Recovery from natural or artificial infections always results in solid, enduring immunity. Suckling lambs whose dams are immune are protected by colostral antibody (Reid and Boyce 1976). A vaccine developed by Gordon (1936) and consisting of formalinized nerve tissue provides effective protection for young lambs.

Diagnosis. Diagnosis from the clinical signs may be difficult unless the animals are in a louping ill district. Virus may be most readily demonstrated by inoculating mice intracerebrally with nerve tissue. Serologic tests may be necessary to make a definitive diagnosis in many cases.

Prevention and Control. Louping ill may be controlled in two ways: (1) by immunizing all newborn lambs with nerve tissue vaccine shortly after weaning and (2) by dipping flocks to remove all castor bean ticks.

In a study by Shaw and Reid (1981) two injections of commercially available vaccine were required to provoke an adequate antibody response, and maximal titers were achieved when 2 to 8 weeks elapsed between injections.

After challenge, viremia could not be detected in animals with titers of 20 or greater. Vaccinated sheep with titers less than 20 had viremia without any signs of illness, signifying adequate protection had been conferred.

Toxoplasma gondii infection in sheep will suppress the immunizing effect of a single injection of virus vaccine but not that of two injections.

The Disease in Humans. Although louping ill has occurred for many years, human infections were not recognized until recently. The first cases, described by Rivers and Schwenther (1934), occurred in three laboratory workers engaged in research on the disease in the Rockefeller Institute in New York City in 1933. The illness was of an influenzal nature. Virus was not recovered from these patients, but neutralizing antibodies appeared in their serums shortly after recovery.

Several cases have been recognized in the British Isles. One described by Brewis et al. (1949) is typical. A young shepherd whose flock was affected by the disease was the victim. His disease was diphasic. An initial febrile illness of short duration was followed by apparent recovery. About 1 week later, he became delirious and was comatose for 36 hours. The virus was isolated by the inoculation of mice, intracerebrally and intramuscularly, with cerebrospinal fluid; neutralizing antibodies later appeared in the patient's blood. He recovered almost completely except for some mild symptoms of ataxia.

REFERENCES

Adam, K.M.G., Beasley, S.J., and Blewett, D.A. 1977. The occurrence of antibody to *Babesia* and to the virus of louping-ill in deer in Scotland. Res. Vet. Sci. 23:133–138.

Bannatyne, C.C., Wilson, R.L., Reid, H.W., Buxton, D., and Pow, I. 1980. Louping-ill virus infection of pigs. Vet. Rec. 106:13.

Brewis, E.G., Neubauer, C., and Hurst, E.W. 1949. Another case of louping-ill in man. Isolation of the virus. Lancet 256:689–691.

Edward, D.G. 1947a. Culture of louping-ill virus in the embryonated egg. Br. J. Exp. Pathol. 28:237–247.

Edward, D.G. 1947b. Methods of investigating immunization against louping-ill. Br. J. Exp. Pathol. 28:368–376.

Galloway, I.A., and Perdrau, J.R. 1935. Louping-ill in monkeys. Infection by the nose. J. Hyg. 35:339–346.

Gordon, W.S. 1936. Comparative aspects of louping-ill in sheep and poliomyelitis of man. Vet. J. 92:84–92.

Greig, J.R., Brownlee, A., Wilson, D.R., and Gordon, W.S. 1931. The nature of louping ill. Vet. Rec. 11:325–333.

Hurst, E.W. 1931. The transmission of louping-ill to the mouse and the monkey: Histology of the experimental disease. J. Comp. Pathol. Ther. 44:231–245.

McLeod, J., and Gordon, W.S. 1932. Studies in louping ill (an encephalomyelitis of sheep). II. Transmission by the sheep tick, *Ixodes ricinus*. J. Comp. Pathol. Ther. 45:240–256.

Pool, W.A., Brownlee, A., and Wilson, D.R. 1930. The aetiology of "louping-ill." J. Comp. Pathol. Ther. 43:253–290.

Reid, H.W. 1978. The epidemiology of louping-ill. Tick-borne diseases and their vectors. In J.K.H. Wilde, ed., Proceedings of the International Conference of the Centre for Tropical Veterinary Medicine, Edinburgh. Pp. 501–507.

Reid, H.W., and Boyce, J.B. 1976. The effect of colostrum derived antibody on louping-ill virus infection in lambs. J. Hyg. 77:349–354.

Reid, H.W., Buxton, D., Pow, I., and Finlayson, J. 1982. Experimental louping-ill virus infection in two species of British deer. Vet. Rec. 111:61.

Rivers, T.M., and Schwenther, F.F. 1934. Louping ill in man. J. Exp. Med. 59:669–685.

Rivers, T.M., and Ward, S.M. 1933. Cultivation of louping ill virus. Proc. Soc. Exp. Biol. Med. 30:1300–1301.

Shaw, B., and Reid, W.H. 1981. Immune responses of sheep to louping ill virus vaccines. Vet. Rec. 109:529–531.

Timoney, P.J. 1980. Susceptibility of the horse to experimental inoculation with louping-ill virus. J. Comp. Pathol. 90:73–86.

Timoney, P.J., Donnelly, W.J.C., Clements, L.O., and Fenlon, M. 1976. Encephalitis caused by louping ill virus in a group of horses in Ireland. Equine Vet. J. 8:113–117.

Williams, H.E. 1968. Complement-fixation test for louping ill in sheep. Am. J. Vet. Res. 29:1619–1624.

Central European Tick-Borne Fever

SYNONYMS: Diphasic milk fever, Russian spring-summer encephalitis (western form)

Central European tick-borne fever, a member of the tick-borne encephalitis complex, is a diphasic disease in humans. The initial phase is influenzalike, and the second stage, after an afebrile period of 4 to 10 days, is characterized by meningitis or meningoencephalitis. Virus may be present in the milk of infected goats may infect humans. Experimentally, virus may localize in the mammary glands of infected goats, cows, and sheep and may be present in the urine. The vector is the tick *Ixodes ricinus*, probably the most important reservoir of infection for humans. An attenuated virus vaccine is being tested for immunization of cattle, sheep, and goats (Blaskovic 1962).

REFERENCE

Blaskovic, D. 1962. Studies on tick-borne encephalitis. Bull. WHO 36(Suppl. 1).

Murray Valley Encephalitis

SYNONYM: Australian X disease; abbreviation, MVE

Murray Valley encephalitis is caused by a flavivirus with the usual characteristics of the genus. In humans the disease resembles Japanese encephalitis and occurs in certain areas of Australia and Papua. Horses may be infected, but do not contract encephalitis (Anderson 1954, Gard et al. 1977). The hemagglutination-inhibition test showed—they produce antibodies to MVE virus—antibody in 58 percent of feral pigs in New South Wales (Gard et al. 1976). Liehne et al. (1976) found antibodies to MVE virus in humans, birds, and cattle in the Ord River area in Australia. The important vector is *Culex annulirostris* (McLean 1953), but certain members of *Aedes* may also serve as vectors (Kay et al. 1979, Lehmann et al. 1976).

Like all flaviviruses, the virus replicates in various cell-culture systems, such as Vero cells, and also in embryonated hens' eggs. For isolation of field virus, the hen's egg seems more sensitive (Lehmann et al. 1976). For information about the proteins of MVE virus, the reader is referred to the article by Westway (1975). Clinical cases of MVE in humans can be diagnosed by the detection of MVE immunoglobulin M (Wiemers and Stallman 1975).

A survey of antibody in domestic fowls may suggest widespread activity in a given area and warn health authorities to reduce the mosquito population immediately before the first encephalitis case occurs in a human (Doherty et al. 1976).

REFERENCES

Anderson, S.G. 1954. Murray Valley encephalitis and Australian X disease. J. Hyg. 52:447–468.

Doherty, R.L., Carley, J.G., Kay, B.H., Filippich, C., and Marks, E.N. 1976. Murray Valley encephalitis virus infection in mosquitoes and domestic fowls in Queensland. Aust. J. Exp. Biol. Med. Sci. 54:237–243.

Gard, G.P., Giles, J.R., Dwyer-Gray, R.J., and Woodroofe, G.M. 1976. Serological evidence of inter-epidemic infection of feral pigs in New South Wales with Murray Valley encephalitis virus. Aust. J. Exp. Biol. Med. Sci. 54:297–302.

Gard, G.P., Marshall, I.D., Walker, K.H., Acland, H.M., and Sarem, W.D. 1977. Association of Australian arboviruses with nervous diseases in horses. Aust. Vet. J. 53:61–66.

Kay, B., Carley, J.G., Fanning, I.D., and Filippich, C. 1979. Quantitative studies of the vector competence of *Aedes aegyptae*, *Culex annulirostris*, and other mosquitoes (Distoera: Culicidae) with Murray Valley encephalitis and other Queensland viruses. J. Med. Entomol. 16:59–66.

Lehmann, N.I., Gust, I.D., and Doherty, R. 1976. Isolation of Murray Valley encephalitis virus from the brains of three patients with encephalitis. Med. J. Aust. 2:450–454.

Liehne, C.G., Stanley, N.F., Alpers, M.P., Paul, S., Liehne, P.F.S., and Chan, K.H. 1976. Ord River arboviruses—Serological epidemiology [man, cattle, birds]. Aust. J. Exp. Biol. Med. Sci. 54:505–512.

McLean, D.M. 1953. Transmission of Murray Valley encephalitis virus by mosquitoes. Aust. J. Exp. Biol. Med. Sci. 31:481–490.

Westway, E.G. 1975. The proteins of Murray Valley encephalitis virus. J. Gen. Virol. 27:283–292.

Wiemers, M.A., and Stallman, N.D. 1975. Immunoglobin M in Murray Valley encephalitis. Pathology 7:187–191.

Wesselsbron Disease

Wesslsbron disease occurs in South Africa, Rhodesia, and Mozambique. The causative virus, a member of the genus *Flavivirus*, may infect humans producing fever and muscular pains. It is known to cause epizootics in sheep, with abortions and death of newborn lambs and pregnant ewes as characteristic features. Jaundice and hemorrhages may appear, and meningoencephalitis may occur in fetuses. The virus also causes abortion in cattle and congenital porencephaly and cerebellar hypoplasia in calves (Coetzer et al. 1979). A fatal case was described in a dog with nervous signs. The virus has a diameter of 30 nm (Weiss et al. 1956), grows in the chick embryo after yolk sac inoculation, and propagates in cultures of lamb kidney. The mosquitoes *Aedes caballus* and *A. circumluteolus* (Kokernot et al. 1960) are primarily responsible for virus transmission.

REFERENCES

Coetzer, J.A., Theodoridis, A., Herr, S., and Kritzinger, L. 1979. Wesselsbron disease: A cause of congenital porencephaly and cerebellar hypoplasia in calves. Onderstepoort J. Vet. Res. 46:165–169.
Kokernot, R.H., Smithburn, K.C., Paterson, H.E., and DeMeillon, B. 1960. Further isolations of Wesselsbron virus from mosquitoes. S. Afr. J. Med. Sci. 34:871–874.
Weiss, K.A., Haig, D.A., and Alexander, R.A. 1956. Wesselsbron virus—A virus not previously described, associated with abortion in domestic animals. Onderstepoort J. Vet. Res. 27:183–195.

Israel Turkey Meningoencephalitis

Komarov and Kalmar (1960) described a disease of turkeys in the Shomron area of Israel. It was characterized by a progressive paralysis associated with nonpurulent meningoencephalitis. The agent was a filterable virus, cultivable in embryonated hens' eggs, and it produced plaques on chick embryo cell-culture monolayers. Turkeys and mice were susceptible to the virus, whereas chickens, ducks, pigeons, hamsters, and guinea pigs were resistant. Turkeys that recovered were resistant to infection. In 1961 Porterfield showed that this virus belongs to the genus *Flavivirus*.

Following serial passages of the virus in chicken eggs, modification of its virulence for turkeys and mice results, without loss of antigenicity. Mice immune to the turkey virus are susceptible to representative members of the alphaviruses and the flaviviruses.

Preliminary studies suggest that a species of mosquito may be involved in transmission of the disease.

REFERENCES

Komarov, A., and Kalmar, E. 1960. A hitherto undescribed disease—Turkey meningo-encephalitis. Vet. Rec. 72:257–261.
Porterfield, J.S. 1961. Israel turkey meningo-encephalitis virus. Vet. Rec. 73:392–394.

Powassan Disease

A member of the genus *Flavivirus*, Powassan disease virus occasionally causes encephalitis in humans. In a serum survey of 499 goats in New York State, 9 animals had neutralizing antibodies to the virus (Woodall and Roz 1977). The goats with positive serums came from widely scattered areas in the state, including counties where human cases were confirmed. A lactating goat with a 74-day-old kid was inoculated with mouse virulent virus and developed infection without disease. Its nursing progeny became infected but also failed to show clinical signs of illness.

REFERENCE

Woodall, J.P., and A. Roz. 1977. Experimental milk-borne transmission of Powassan virus in the goat. Am. J. Trop. Med. Hyg. 26:190–192.

Spontaneous Viral Diseases of the Nervous System in Experimental Animals

No attempt is made here to describe in any detail the spontaneous encephalitides that occur in animals commonly used for the isolation and study of viruses that infect humans and animals. It is sufficient merely to mention that such viruses exist and that they may affect an investigator's experimental results.

Viruses causing spontaneous encephalitis have been found in rabbits, guinea pigs, and mice and occur occasionally in all species. These viruses often are latent or masked and become evident only when inoculations containing foreign material irritate the nerve tissue. Having been activated in this way, such viruses may then be passed readily from animal to animal in series. Traub (1936) demonstrated that the virus of lymphocytic choriomeningitis may sometimes occur spontaneously in colonies of white mice. The herpes simplex virus of humans has been found to occur spontaneously in rabbit colonies.

In studies of neurotropic viruses two or more viruses sometimes exist in the same material, or a virus may become contaminated with another that occurred spontaneously in some animal through which the original material was passed. While studying the etiology of St. Louis encephalitis in humans, Armstrong and Lillie (1934) first encountered the virus now known to cause lymphocytic choriomeningitis. In another instance Dalldorf et al. (1938) produced a nervous disease in monkeys by injecting them with distemper virus. This surprising discovery was explained later when Dalldorf (1939) found that the distemper virus had been contaminated with the lymphatic virus choriomeningitis, which caused the signs of illness.

REFERENCES

Armstrong, C., and Lillie, R.D. 1934. Experimental lymphocytic choriomeningitis of monkeys and mice produced by virus encountered in studies of 1933 St. Louis encephalitis epidemic. U.S. Public Health Rep. 49:1019–1027.

Dalldorf, G. 1939. The simultaneous occurrence of the viruses of canine distemper and lymphocytic choriomeningitis. A correction of "canine distemper in the rhesus monkey." J. Exp. Med. 70:19–27.

Dalldorf, G., Douglass, M., and Robinson, H.E. 1938. Canine distemper in the rhesus monkey (*Macaca mulatta*). J. Exp. Med. 67:323–332.

Traub, E. 1936. An epidemic in a mouse colony due to the virus of acute lymphocytic choriomeningitis. J. Exp. Med. 63:533–546.

51 The Orthomyxoviridae

Members of the family Orthomyxoviridae contain 1 percent of single-stranded RNA. The molecular mass is approximately 4×10^6 daltons. The helical capsid is 6 to 9 nm in diameter and is composed of eight separate pieces. The enveloped particle, 80 to 120 nm in diameter, is spherical or elongated with numerous hollow and cylindrical spheres about 9 nm long and 1.5 to 2 nm wide (Figure 51.1). The virion contains lipid, carbohydrate, and neuraminidase, and is ether-sensitive, heat-sensitive, and acid-labile. Hemagglutination occurs at neuraminidase sensitive receptors. Replication is inhibited by dactinomycin. Nucleocapsids form in the nucleus, and maturation takes place by budding at the cell surface.

Genetic recombination is common, since the RNA genome contains eight segments and antigenic variation frequently occurs (Figure 51.2). There are three discrete antigenic types (A, B, and C) distinguished by the specificity of the ribonucleoprotein (or soluble) antigen. Antigenic crossing does occur among subtypes of the three types. The hemagglutinin subunits are likely composed of two different hemagglutinins in the viral envelope of influenza A viruses and constitute the main component of the spikes. They carry the specific receptors for the mucins and also the subtype- and strain-specific antigens commonly called "V" antigens. Antibodies are formed to these antigens and are demonstrated by serum neutralization, hemagglutination, and complement-fixation tests against homologous antigen.

The neuraminidase subunits are most likely located between the spikes of the envelope, a double membrane 6 to 7 nm thick. On the basis of neuraminidase (NASE) thermostability, sensitivity to pH treatment, and specific enzymatic activity (NASE activity per hemagglutinin unit) influenza viruses are placed in two major groups—hemagglutinins and neuraminidases—according to a nomenclature revised by the World Health Organization (WHO). Neuraminidases represent the enzymatic activity of the virus and contain antigens that differ from the hemagglutinins. Antibodies to the enzyme inhibit neuraminidase activity but not viral infectivity, although they do delay or even prevent liberation of infectious particles from cells.

Classification of the orthomyxoviruses is based on shared antigens. As mentioned previously, there are three discrete types—A, B, and C—each of which includes one or more subtypes. Each subtype may comprise several strains. The type species for the genus *Orthomyxovirus* is *Orthomyxovirus* h-A (human influenza A) virus. Other types and representative subtypes are as follows:

Type A
  Human influenza viruses
    A/PR8/34
    Al/Cam/46
    A2/Singapore/1/57
  Equine influenza viruses
    A/Equi-1/Praha/56
    A/Equi-2/Miami/63
  Porcine influenza viruses
    A/SW/Iowa/31
    A/SW/Wis/61
    A/SW/Wis/68
  Avian influenza viruses
    fowl plague/27
    A/Duck/Czech/56
    A/Duck/Eng/56
    A/Chick/Scot/59
    A/Turkey/Can/63
    A/Turkey/Ontario/7732/66
    A/Quail/Italy/1117/65

Type B
  Human influenza viruses
    B/Lee/40
    B/Johannesburg/59
    B/Taiwan/62

Type C
  Human influenza virus
    C/Taylor/1233/47

The RNA genome is coated with basic proteins that carry the type-specific antigen mentioned earlier. This antigen can be detected with the complement-fixation or the flocculation test. As a rule, antibodies against this antigen are developed only after infection. Consequently

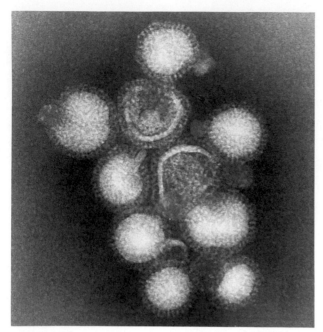

Figure 51.1. Negatively stained particles of influenza virus A2/Hong Kong/1/68 from chick embryo chorioallantoic fluid. The pleomorphism is typical. All influenza virus strains are 80 to 120 nm in diameter and have prominent surface projections, or spikes, covering a membranous envelope. × 142,000. (Courtesy F. Murphy.)

they are not produced in animals given inactivated or disrupted viruses unless a special procedure is used (Zavadova et al. 1967).

The principal diseases in domestic animals caused by members of the genus include equine influenza, swine influenza, and avian influenza (fowl plague), which occurs in chickens, turkeys, and ducks. In mammals the disease syndrome is largely confined to the respiratory tract from which virus can be isolated in high titer. Virus is also found in the bronchial lymph nodes but in low titer.

When an antigenic change is gradual, it is called a *drift*; a sudden major change in either or both antigens is called a *shift*. A drift is usually attributed to the selection of preexisting mutants by pressure from increasing immunity in a population. The cause of an antigenic shift is less clear, but it may occur from mammalian or avian reservoirs or by genetic strains (Dowdle and Schild 1976).

The orthomyxoviruses are stable at −70°C and can remain in the lyophilized state for years. Most are inactivated by temperatures of 56°C for 30 minutes, but some require a longer period. Phenol, ether, and formalin inactivate the virus.

Excellent review articles of orthomyxoviruses are available (Andrewes and Pereira 1967, Chanock and Coates 1964, Easterday et al. 1981, Kaplan and Webster 1977).

REFERENCES

Andrewes, C., and Pereira, H.G. 1967. Viruses of Vertebrates, 2d ed. Bailliere, Tindall & Cassell, London.
Chanock, R.M., and Coates, H.V. 1964. Myxoviruses—A comparative description. In Robert P. Hanson, ed., Newcastle Disease Virus: An Evolving Pathogen. University of Wisconsin Press, Madison. Pp. 279–298.
Dowdle, W.R., and Schild, G.C. 1976. Influenza: Its antigenic variation and ecology. Bull. Pan Am. Health Org. 10:193–195.
Easterday, B.C., Byrans, J.T., Campbell, C.H., and Butterfield, W.K. 1981. Influenza (I), swine influenza (II), equine influenza (III), influenza of domestic fowl (IV), influenza virus infections of wild birds. In J.H. Steel and G.W. Beran, eds., CRC Handbook Series in Zoonosis, vol. 2. Section B: Viral Zoonosis. CRC Press, Boca Raton, Fl. Pp. 225–246.
Kaplan, M.M., and Webster, R.G. 1977. The epidemiology of influenza. Sci. Am. 237(6):88–106.
Zavadova, H., Kutinova, L., and Vonka, V. 1967. Preparation of antisera against the S antigen of influenza A virus by immunization of guinea pigs with internal S antigen. Arch. Gesam. Virusforsch. 20:421–429.

Figure 51.2. An unusually large particle of influenza virus A2/Aichi/2/68 with three ribonucleoprotein (RNP) capsid coils (*arrows*). The RNP helix consists of a varying number of turns of a 9-nm diameter strand, which replicates as eight separate pieces of RNA and thus makes genetic recombination (and antigenic variation) common. Negatively stained. × 138,750. (Courtesy F. Murphy.)

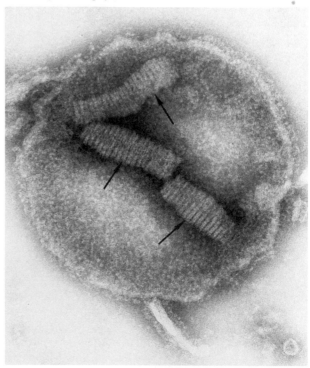

Equine Influenza

SYNONYMS: Epizootic cellulitis of horses,
   pinkeye, shipping fever, stable
   pneumonia

The disease known as equine influenza resembles influenzas in swine and humans. The virus is also included with the influenza A viruses and is a member of the *Orthomyxovirus* genus. Two immunological types are known to exist; they have been designated A/Equi-1/Praha/56 (H7N7) and A/Equi-2/Miami/63 (H3N8) (Bryans 1964).

The disease spreads rapidly among susceptible horses. It affects animals of all ages but occurs mostly in young animals that have been moved into new surroundings, particularly those that come in contact with older animals. In the past it has given much trouble in sales stables, in dealers' herds, and in army remount stations (Dale and Dollahite 1939). In centers where fresh "green" horses arrive from time to time, the new, highly susceptible stock serves to keep the disease alive and virulent. Under such conditions the death rate may be very high, but usually does not exceed 5 percent. Like human influenza, this disease has a history of great panzootics on various continents in which nearly every horse was a victim. The last one of this kind in the United States occurred in the winter of 1872–1873. At that time traffic in many large cities was nearly stopped because of the lack of horses well enough to do their normal work of drawing horsecars, drays, and delivery wagons.

Like human influenza, equine influenza formerly occurred every year in a milder, less contagious form, and few horses escaped the disease. As the horse population decreased, equine influenza became less common. With increasing numbers of horses its importance and incidence has again increased, particularly in Thoroughbred and Standardbred populations, as evidenced by many reports from all continents in recent years.

At present only members of the equine family are known to be susceptible to equine subtypes A_1 and A_2.

Character of the Disease. The disease is highly contagious; practically every young horse and many of the older ones become infected when the disease appears on the premises. The period of incubation varies from 1 to 3 days, with extremes of 0.5 and 7 days. Its course varies greatly depending on whether complications occur. Animals with uncomplicated cases may be essentially well again within 1 week. Mortality usually is low, and the chief economic loss stems from the victim's inability to work or train for 1 to 3 weeks, occasionally longer (Doll et al. 1957).

The disease affects horses, ponies, asses, and mules. The onset is sudden and is manifested by a high temperature—103° to 106°F—which lasts about 3 days. A/Equi-2 virus causes higher temperatures than A/Equi-1 virus (Gerber 1969). At the same time there is inappetence and great mental depression. The animal stands with head down and with ears depressed, taking little interest in its surroundings. Coughing is the most common sign of illness.

Photophobia and lacrimation are usually exhibited, and often the congested conjunctivae protrude from between the closed eyelids because of the infiltration of the tissues. A mucopurulent discharge from the eyes appears, the corneas often become clouded, and occasionally the function of one or both eyes is lost. Nasal catarrh is usually present, and the lymph nodes of the head may become swollen. Pneumonia occasionally occurs, in which case the victim often dies, usually from secondary bacterial infection.

In some horses edematous swellings appear on the ventral parts of the trunk especially in the legs, where the tendon sheaths often are inflamed. This form of the disease has been called *epizootic cellulitis*. Mild icterus is not infrequent. Catarrhal and even hemorrhagic enteritis occur in some animals, and kidney damage is not uncommon. Leukopenia appears in the early stages of the disease.

In the classic accounts of equine influenza, abortions in mares are mentioned, but they do not appear to have happened frequently. In all likelihood equine influenza was a misdiagnosis, and the respiratory disease associated with abortions was equine rhinopneumonitis.

The principal lesions in animals with fatal cases of equine influenza occur in the lungs, where there may be extensive edema or bronchopneumonia with pleurisy. The thorax is usually filled with fluid. Gelatinous infiltrations around the larynx and in the legs are common. Usually the lymph nodes are swollen.

In experimental horses influenza virus is recoverable for 5 days after intranasal instillation (Bryans 1964). Edema of the throat and the intermandibular lymph nodes occurs in some animals. A thick, purulent nasal discharge usually follows the acute stage and is associated with secondary bacterial infection.

Blaskovic (1969) reported that horses given equine influenza virus A/Equi-2 by the intranasal route had an elevated temperature 2 to 3 days later, followed by coughing and other signs of illness referable to the lower respiratory tract 2 or 3 days after the onset of fever. A contact horse also caught the disease. During the first 5 days after inoculation virus was readily recovered from the nasal mucosa of all animals, including the contact horse. Other horses given the same virus intramuscularly did not show signs of illness.

The virus has been adapted to produce pneumonia in mice after intranasal instillation, and encephalitis results after intracerebral inoculation of suckling mice. It causes inapparent infection in ferrets.

Properties of the Virus. All equine cases are caused by type A virus, which has the main characteristics described for the type species of the genus, human influenza A virus (Paccaud 1969).

Equine influenza viruses are divided into the two subtypes according to hemagglutination-inhibition test results. Variants showing slight antigenic differences are distinguished in A/Equi-2, but in the winter of 1978–1979 there was sufficient drift of equine influenza A_2 virus isolated from an enzootic in Holland to warrant consideration of its incorporation in future vaccines (Van Oirschot et al. 1981). No antigenic relation has been demonstrated between the hemagglutinin and neuraminidase antigens of these two subtypes with antiserums produced in laboratory animals. However, horses recovering from A/Equi-2 infections may have antibody rises to A/Equi-1 strains, to certain human A2 strains, and to the infecting virus—findings that suggest the existence of shared minor antigens.

Certain antigenic relations have been observed among the equine viruses, strains of avian influenza A and strains of human origin. Both the hemagglutinin and neuraminidase antigens of A/Equi-1 are antigenically related to those of fowl plague/27 and A/Turkey/Can/63 viruses. A/Equi-1 has a hemagglutinin that is antigenically related to the hemagglutinin of fowl plague virus strain Rostock and a neuraminidase that cross-reacts with the enzyme of avian virus N (A/Chick/Germany/49) (Rott et al. 1975). A/Equi-2 viruses show some crossing with avian virus N and A/Quail/Italy/1117/65. A/Equi-2 shows some cross-reaction with the human A2/Hong Kong/1/68 hemagglutinin antigens.

Like other influenza viruses (Tumova and Fiserova-Sovinova 1959), both equine subtypes hemagglutinate erythrocytes of a wide range of species; the highest titers are attained with pigeon cell suspensions (Paccaud 1969).

The properties of equine virus neuramidases, such as pH sensitivity, thermostability, and specific activities, are attributed directly to the properties of the subunits, such as glycoprotein entities, rather than to some association with hemagglutinin (Lipkind et al. 1977).

Cultivation. Andrewes and Worthington (1959) cultivated the A/Equi-1 virus in fertile eggs and in cell cultures of bovine kidney, chick embryo kidney and fibroblasts, and rhesus monkey and human embryo kidney. Equine viruses usually are isolated and propagated in embryonated hens' eggs. A/Equi-2 is usually isolated without difficulty, but A/Equi-1 is rather difficult to isolate.

In general, isolation of virus in cell cultures is more difficult than isolation in embryonated eggs. A/Equi-2 viruses are isolated in primary cultures of monkey kidney cells, but other primary kidney cell cultures of bovine, equine, and human origin are not satisfactory for this purpose (Paccaud 1969). The equine influenza viruses have been cultivated in the Madin-Darby canine kidney cell line (Nath and Minocha 1977). Certain strains can be adapted to replicate in chick and bovine cell cultures.

Epizootiology. The respiratory form of equine influenza presumably results from droplet infection. Numerous reports have appeared on the transmission of this disease by stallions used for breeding purposes months after having recovered from influenza. Several reports of virus in the semen of such animals for periods varying from 1 to 6 years are in the literature (Gaffky 1912). Schofield (1937) in Canada observed two outbreaks apparently initiated by breeding stallions that had had the disease some months previously. Examination of the semen of one of these animals 6 months later failed to show the virus. A/Equi-2 virus has been isolated from a single dead foal.

The pattern and incidence of infectious disease among horses are influenced by the immune status of the population, its concentration of antibody, and the antigenic characteristics of the virus. Although natural resistance to influenza does not seem to be an important factor, it may account for a certain number of horses that show no signs of illness during epizootics (Gerber 1969). Higgins et al. (1986) studied the epidemiology of equine influenza A_2 outbreaks during 1983 and 1984 at five racetracks in the northeastern United States. Virus was isolated from four outbreaks and serologically diagnosed in six. Only horses not vaccinated within 6 months before the outbreak became ill. Clinically normal horses showed no serologic conversion.

When the disease occurs in a susceptible population, it is explosive and the rapid aerosol spread is due principally to the strong and frequent cough. The short incubation period and the high concentration of virus in the respiratory tract also account for its rapid transmission from horse to horse.

Immunity. Infected animals generally produce antibodies to the three major components of the virus particle. The horse given inactivated or disrupted virus produces antibodies against the main envelope antigens, hemagglutinins and neuraminidase. Complement-fixing antibodies against type-specific S antigen may be detected as early as 4 to 6 days after illness has begun, reach their peak at 12 to 20 days, and usually are not detectable after 8 to 12 weeks. Complement-fixing antibodies against strain-specific V antigen, serum-neutralizing antibodies, and hemagglutination-inhibiting antibodies develop later than S-specific complement-fixing antibodies but reach their peak at 15 to 20 days and decline until the third month. The hemagglutination-inhibiting and serum-neutralization antibodies level off at this time then remain constant for years. The V-specific complement-fixing antibody is no longer detectable, as a rule, at the sixth month.

It is generally agreed that antibody on the respiratory mucosa surface confers protection against this pneumotropic infection. The mucosal titer is a good index for determining the level of protection. Although the mucosal titer does not always parallel the serum titer, the serum titer is an approximate measure of resistance in humans, and the same is likely to be true for equine influenza (Beveridge 1969) in both vaccinated and unvaccinated individuals. Older horses that have had the disease earlier in life usually escape infection later. In past enzootics this immunity was frequently not adequate to protect horses completely. Information on the duration of immunity is based on field observations; natural infection reportedly produces rather solid immunity that persists for 1 year (Gerber 1969).

Maternal immunity plays a role in protecting neonates and young foals. In one study antibody and IgG levels in foals that had nursed were equivalent to those in the dam's serum. The half-life of maternally acquired serum antibody in foals was found to be 28 days for A/Equi-1 virus and 29.1 days for A/Equi-2 virus. Antibody and IgG levels in colostrum were two to eight times higher than those in the mare's serum (Higgins et al. 1987).

Diagnosis. Equine influenza is generally diagnosed on clinical evidence. When the disease is epizootic, the signs of illness are generally sufficient to make a diagnosis, given that it is a highly contagious disease. When brood mares abort as a result of this infection, they are sick when the abortions occur.

Positive diagnosis can be assured only by isolation of the virus or by demonstration of a rising hemagglutination or of a neutralizing antibody titer with paired serums. In an initial outbreak the virus must be isolated for typing. This information is essential for an effective vaccination program in an area and also for a correct diagnosis. If a new type of virus is involved, serologic tests alone will not give a satisfactory answer.

Prevention and Control. Inactivated and attenuated virus vaccines have been used to immunize horses against influenza.

At least two types of inactivated virus vaccine are available (Bryans 1966, Peterman et al. 1969). According to Burki et al. (1975) inactivated vaccines must contain both serotype A/Equi-1 and A/Equi-2 and an adjuvant. Two doses are required for basic immunization. In young horses the doses should be spaced 3 months apart, but 2 weeks apart in older horses with unknown immunity. Until horses are 2 years old, they should be revaccinated twice yearly, preferably in January and July. An annual booster dose should be given to older horses every January. This schedule will not interfere with vaccination for rhinopneumonitis, which is prevalent in the fall. A vaccine was produced in France that combined A/Equi-1 virus, A/Equi-2 virus, and the tetanus bacterium as a product inactivated with aluminum hydroxide adjuvant. This vaccine was given together with rabies vaccine; a second dose was administered 28 days later and satisfactory antibody titers were produced (Brun et al. 1980). The duration of immunity to inactivated equine influenza virus vaccine is controversial, but most investigators believe it affords protection for a few months. In some recent outbreaks at racetracks strong evidence suggested that horses vaccinated within 6 months of the start of the outbreak were protected against disease (Higgins et al. 1986).

Attenuation of equine virus is achieved by serial passage in the chick embryo chorioallantois in the presence of normal horse serum (Bondreault et al. 1976). Colts immunized by the intranasal route were completely protected, whereas one-third of those immunized orally shed small quantities of virus after challenge.

Live temperature-sensitive equine influenza virus vaccines currently are under investigation. Clones with desirable genetic characteristics for vaccine strains are obtained by mating wild equine A_1 or A_2 influenza viruses with human or avian influenza A viruses. Preliminary tests in ponies given selected clones by the intranasal route are very encouraging because the vaccines appear to be safe and efficacous (Nath and Minocha 1977). Attenuated virus vaccines should give a longer-lasting immunity than inactivated virus vaccines.

The successful incorporation of the hemagglutination gene of A/PR8/34 (human influenza virus) into vaccinia virus and the excellent serologic response of domestic animals, including horses, to the hemagglutination gene provides another potential avenue for a better influenza vaccine for horses (Holmes et al. 1988).

During outbreaks, isolation and quarantine measures are advised in addition to vaccination.

The Disease in Humans. There is a minor antigenic relation between A/Equi-2 and A2/Hong Kong (human) strains, but there is no evidence that the A/Equi-2 produces infection in humans; nor does the reverse occur (McQueen et al. 1969).

REFERENCES

Andrewes, C.H., and Worthington, G. 1959. Some new or little known respiratory viruses. Bull. WHO 20:435–443.

Beveridge, W.I.B. 1969. Opening discussion of influenza papers. In J.T. Bryans and H. Gerber, eds., Proceedings of the 2d International Conference on Equine Infectious Disease. S. Karger, Basel. Pp. 119–124.

Blaskovic, D. 1969. Experimental infection of horses with equine influenza virus. In J.T. Bryans and H. Gerber, eds., Proceedings of the 2d

International Conference on Equine Infectious Disease. S. Karger, Basel. Pp. 111–117.

Bondreault, A., Boulay, G., and Marois, P. 1976. Immunization of man and animals against influenza by oral and intranasal routes. Dev. Biol. Stand. 33:171–177.

Brun, A., Duret, C., Devaux, B., and Calmels, D. 1980. Simple, simultaneous, or combined vaccination of horses against equine influenza, rabies, and tetanus. Comp. Immunol. Microbiol. Infect. Dis. 3:93–99.

Bryans, J.T. 1964. Viral respiratory disease of horses. In Proceedings of the American Veterinary Medical Association. Pp. 112–121.

Bryans, J.T., Doll, E.R., Wilson, J.C., and McCollum, W.H. 1966. Immunization for equine influenza. J. Am. Vet. Med. Assoc. 148:413–417.

Burki, F., Sibalin, M., and Jaksch, W. 1975. Ein neuer Impfplan gegen Pferdeninfluenza. [A new immunization schedule against equine influenza.] Zentralbl. Veterinärmed. [B] 22:3–17.

Dale, C.N., and Dollahite, J.W. 1939. Experimental transmission of equine influenza. J. Am. Vet. Med. Assoc. 95:534–535.

Doll, E.R., Bryans, J.T., McCollum, W.H., and Crowe, M.E.W. 1957. Isolation of a filterable agent causing arteritis of horses and abortion by mares. Its differentiation from equine abortion (influenza) virus. Cornell Vet. 47:3–41.

Gaffky. 1912. Anatomische miskroskopische und kulturelle Untersuchungen. Infektionsversuche an kleinen Versuchstieren. Z. Vetkde. 24:209–223.

Gerber, H. 1969. Clinical features, sequelae and epidemiology of equine influenza. In J.T. Bryans and H. Gerber, eds., Proceedings of the 2d International Conference on Equine Infectious Disease. S. Karger, Basel. Pp. 63–80.

Higgins, W.P., Gillespie, J.H., Holmes, D.F., and Robson, D.S. 1986. Surveys of equine influenza outbreaks during 1983 and 1984. Equine Vet. Sci. 6:15–19.

Higgins, W.A., Gillespie, J.H., and Robson, D.S. 1987. Studies of maternally acquired antibodies in the foal to equine influenza A_1 and A_2 and equine rhinopneumonitis. Equine Vet. Sci. 7:207–210.

Holmes, D.F., Lamb, L.M., Gillespie, J.H., Scott, F.W., Perkus, M., and Paoletti, E. 1988. Preliminary studies of the response of horses to vaccinia virus and vaccinia virus expressing foreign genes. In Proceedings of the 5th International Conference on Equine Infectious Diseases, Lexington, Ky. In press.

Lipkind, M.A., Tsvethova, I.V., and Muraviyor, V.N. 1977. Animal influenza virus neuraminidase: Studies on dependence of some of its properties on its association with hemagglutinin. Dev. Biol. Stand. 39:447–452.

McQueen, J.L., Kaye, H.S., Coleman, M.T., and Dowdle, W.R. 1969. Immunology of equine influenza. Equine Dis. Suppl., J. Am. Vet. Med. Assoc. 155:265–271.

Nath, D.M., and Minocha, H.C. 1977. Replication of swine and equine influenza viruses in canine kidney cells. Am. J. Vet. Res. 38:1059–1061.

Paccaud, M.F. 1969. The virology of equine influenza. In J.T. Bryans and H. Gerber, eds., Proceedings of the 2d International Conference on Equine Infectious Disease. Pp. 81–93.

Peterman, H.G., Fayet, M.T., Fontaine, M., and Fontaine, M.P. 1969. Vaccination against equine influenza. In J.T. Bryans and H. Gerber, eds., Proceedings of the 2d International Conference on Equine Infectious Disease. S. Karger, Basel. Pp. 105–110.

Rott, R., Becht, H., and Orlich, L. 1975. Antigenic relationship between surface antigens of avian and equine influenza viruses. Med. Microbiol. Immunol. 161:253–261.

Schofield, F.W. 1937. A report of 2 outbreaks of equine influenza due to virus carriers (stallions). Report of the Ontario Veterinary College. P. 15.

Tumova, B., and Fiserova-Sovinova, O. 1959. Properties of influenza viruses A/ASIA/57 and A-EQUI/PRAHA/56. I. Agglutination of red blood cells. Bull. WHO 20:445–454.

Van Oirschot, J.T., Masurel, N., Huffels, A.D., and Anker, W.J. 1981. Equine influenza in the Netherlands during the winter of 1978–79: Antigenic drift of A-equi 2 virus. Vet. Q. 3:80–84.

Swine Influenza

SYNONYM: Hog "flu"

Swine influenza is an acute disease of the respiratory organs which occurs in the colder months of the year. The onset is sudden, and practically all animals in an affected herd show signs almost simultaneously. The signs are similar to those of epidemic influenza in humans, and the virus of swine influenza is closely related to that of human influenza.

The disease was first recognized as an entity in the midwestern United States in the fall of 1918, when a pandemic of human influenza was under way. The similarity of the diseases in humans and pigs was recognized by Dorset et al. (1922). When the causative agents of the two diseases were better understood, the hypothesis that swine may have become infected from humans, thus giving rise to a new disease in the species, became much more plausible than before. The swine virus is more closely related to type A human virus than the three human virus types (A, B, C) are to each other. The fact that many adult humans carry antibodies that neutralize the virus of swine influenza has been regarded by some as evidence that these persons have been infected at some time with the same type of virus that exists in pigs. This idea was supported by the isolation of a strain of swine influenza virus from a soldier who died of influenza at Fort Dix, New Jersey, in the United States, in 1976. This same strain, Hsw 1/Nsw 1, was isolated from five other soldiers, but at the same time A/Victoria/3/75 also was infecting service personnel. Serologic investigations showed that approximately 500 persons at Fort Dix produced antibodies to the swine strain. Fortunately, this strain did not spread further. There have been other recent incidents on farms in which the swine strain has infected humans, but they were self-limiting. Naturally, public health officials are concerned about swine strains because the possibility always exists that any strain may have an unusual capacity for dissemination and for virulence in humans and may create a pandemic comparable to the 1918 episode. Another cause for concern is the isolation, from pigs in Hong Kong in 1977, of A2 Hong Kong/1/68 (H3N2) influenza virus, which had not been isolated from humans for several years, and the simultaneous occurrence of A/Victoria/3/75 (Shortridge et al. 1977).

Character of the Disease. Swine and, to a lesser degree, humans appear to be naturally susceptible to the virus of swine influenza. In the United States the disease occurs primarily in the midwestern and north central states, but there is serologic evidence for its existence in every state. The virus has also been isolated in England, France, the Netherlands, Argentina, China, Russia, Poland, Kenya, Italy, Germany, and Czechoslovakia. Periodically serious epidemics are reported in many countries, including the United States. The disease usually occurs in the fall and early winter months, rarely during the warm months (Kaplan and Webster 1977).

The disease usually appears suddenly in swine herds, and whole groups commonly show signs of illness almost simultaneously. The development of the disease in many animals at almost the same time has commonly been attributed to an extreme degree of contagiousness.

Preliminary signs are fever, anorexia, extreme weakness, and prostration. The animals crowd together, lying down, and are moved only with difficulty. When moved or handled they exhibit evidence of muscular stiffness and pain. In some cases lung edema and bronchopneumonia develop, and these animals usually die. At the height of the disease animals exhibit a jerky type of respiration, caused by spasms of the diaphragm, which is commonly known as *thumps*. Bronchitis is indicated by coughing. When the animals are initially in good condition and are kept during the course of the disease in a dry, fairly warm place, well bedded with straw, the principal losses usually are in growth retardation and weight loss.

The period of incubation is very short—from a few hours to several days. In animals with uncomplicated cases the disease runs a course varying from 2 to 6 days; recovery occurs almost as suddenly as the disease begins. If pneumonia develops, the course is longer. As a rule the mortality rate does not exceed 4 percent if the animals are given good care. In some instances it has been as high as 10 percent.

Animals killed at the height of the disease exhibit no significant lesions outside the thoracic cavity. The lung lesions are characteristic. They are limited, as a rule, to the medius, cardiac, and azygos lobes. These portions are collapsed, deep purplish red and do not crepitate. They are not pneumonic. This condition is an atelectasis caused by a thick, mucilaginous exudate in the bronchioles and bronchi of the parts (Shope 1931a). The remainder of the lungs is usually pale because of the interstitial emphysema. The cervical, bronchial, and mediastinal lymph nodes are swollen and filled with fluid. When pneumonia occurs, the consolidated portions are the same as the atelectatic areas in animals with milder cases. The nonpneumonic lung portions in these animals are congested and edematous. The spleen often is moderately enlarged. There is hyperemia of the mucosa of the stomach in most animals. The other abdominal organs generally are normal.

Viral pneumonia of pigs presents lesions that can easily be confused with those of influenzal pneumonia.

Andrewes et al. (1934) demonstrated that the virus of swine influenza was pathogenic for mice when introduced by a special technique into the nasal passages. The virus also causes pneumonia in ferrets and lambs and a respiratory disease in squirrel monkeys. Mouse passage virus retains its virulence for swine indefinitely (Shope 1935).

The experimental disease can be induced by the concurrent action of two agents, the swine influenza and the bacterium *Haemophilus (suis) parasuis*. The virus alone, administered to normal pigs in an area where swine influenza does not exist, produces a very mild, almost inapparent, disease, which surely would be overlooked on the farm. *H. suis*, on the other hand, is virtually nonpathogenic for swine. When both agents are given simultaneously, however, typical influenza results. The virulence of *H. parasuis* may decline with repeated passage in mice, however, in which case new cultures are needed to supply the bacterial factors necessary to produce a more severe form of the swine influenza. In natural outbreaks *H. parasuis* is not always isolated. Scott (1941) reported the isolation of *Pasteurella multocida* and influenza virus, and others (Nakamura and Easterday 1970, Urman et al. 1958) reported the isolation of influenza virus only.

In experimental trials with pregnant sows there was evidence of transplacental transmission of swine influenza virus in 1 of 10 piglets born to sows that were exposed 10, 24, and 39 days before parturition (Wallace and Elm 1979). In other experiments porcine fetuses between 51 and 57 days old were inoculated intra-allantoically with swine influenza virus and examined 3, 7, 13, 28, and 58 days later (Brown et al. 1980). At 3 and 7 days severe epithelial necrosis was seen in most bronchial buds and moderate epithelial necrosis was observed in more fully differentiated major bronchi. The disorders resulted in pulmonary hypoplasia. Vertical transmission in natural disease has not been reported.

Properties of the Virus. Shope (1931b) isolated the virus and at the same time determined that *H. suis* was regularly present (Lewis and Shope, 1931). This virus was type A.

It shares a common ribonucleoprotein (S) antigen with the human, equine, and avian members of the type A influenza viruses (Easterday 1970). Among the swine influenza virus strains, insufficient antigenic differences have been observed to justify designation of subtypes. Instead, three antigenic groupings have been made on the basis of hemagglutination and strain-specific complement-fixing reactions (Easterday 1970). The representative strains of the three groups are A/SW/Iowa/31 (the original Shope isolate), A/SW/Wis/61, and A/SW/Wis/68. Accumulated evidence suggests that swine influenza virus is or is closely related to the virus that caused the 1918 pandemic of human influenza. An antigen relation between swine influenza virus and the A/Chick/Scot/59 virus of chickens has also been described (Tumova and Pereira 1968). Using polyacrylamide-gel electrophoresis, Palese and Ritchey (1977) succeeded in establishing a complete genetic map for influenza A viruses. On a farm, two isolates from pigs and one isolate from a human had identical RNA patterns that differed from other recently identified swine isolates. This finding suggested that swine virus is transmitted to humans and that swine viruses may occasionally infect humans without causing pandemics. It also is interesting that the Hong Kong strain isolated from swine has caused disease in dogs and in cattle in the Soviet Union.

By use of the hemagglutination test, 11 influenza A swine strains were divided into three antigenic subgroups (DeJong and DeRonde-Verloop 1977). Neuraminidases are placed into two subgroups—N1 or N2—yet there is considerable heterogeneity within subgroup N1.

Cultivation. In affected pigs the virus is found in nasal secretions, in the tracheal and bronchial exudates, in the lungs, and in the lymph nodes draining the lungs. It is not ordinarily found in the blood, spleen, liver, kidneys, mesentric lymph nodes,and brain (Orcutt and Shope 1935).

Kobe and Fertig (1938) and Scott (1940) reported the successful cultivation of swine influenza virus on the chorioallantoic membrane of the developing chick. Scott reported that his cultures as far as the 50th generation were virulent for mice and swine, but that the 85th and later generations had lost their virulence. Intra-allantoic or intra-amniotic routes of inoculation into 10- to 12-day-old embryonated hens' eggs are the most commonly employed methods for cultivation of the virus. The virus is not lethal for the embryo, but it is readily detected by its hemagglutinating property. Strain A/SW/Wis/68 had higher hemagglutination and egg infectivity titers when the embryonated eggs were incubated at 33°C (Pirtle and Ritchie 1975).

Various cell-culture monolayer systems involving primary or stable cell cultures have been used for propagation and assay (Easterday 1970). Depending on the culture system, the virus is recognized by plaque production or by hemadsorption of red cells. The virus also propagates in organ cultures of fetal pig trachea, lung, or nasal epithelial tissue (Nakamura and Easterday 1970).

The immunofluorescence test has been used extensively in the study of influenza viruses, including swine influenza virus (Nakamura and Easterday 1970).

Epizootiology. Swine influenza appears each autumn in the midwestern United States. The epizootics coincide with the onset of autumn rains and marked fluctuating temperatures. The disease appears simultaneously on many farms, suggesting that the virus is widely seeded before the outbreak and then provoked by climatic conditions and management procedures. It appears that all pigs become ill at the same time on individual farms, but more observant owners often report that one or a few pigs are ill 2 to 5 days before the diffuse herd disease appears.

It has been shown that pigs free of parasites can be infected and can transmit infection to contact pigs kept with them for at least 3 months thereafter (Shope 1939, 1941). Nakamura and Easterday (1970) extended these findings in a study of the natural history of the disease.

Domestic fowl may play a role in disseminating swine influenza virus to other susceptible hosts. In Hong Kong, an influenza virus was isolated from a duck that had Hsw 1 antigens related to strain Hsw 1/Nsw 1 of swine influenza virus (Butterfield et al. 1978). Two outbreaks of influenza occurred in two turkey breeder flocks raised in consecutive years on an Ohio farm that also produced swine. The antibody detected indicated the virus causing the disease in turkeys had the Hsw 1 hemagglutinin of swine influenza virus (Mohan et al. 1981).

A study of 12 influenza viruses, antigenically related to Hσ, Hl, and Hsw 1 subgroup, which were isolated from cloacal samples from feral ducks in Canada suggested that these birds serve as a substantial reservoir of antigenically diverse influenza viruses. These viruses were closely related to Hsw 1/Nsw 1 isolates from humans and swine (Hinshaw et al. 1978).

Immunity. Various serologic methods, including the complement-fixation, hemagglutination-inhibition, serum-neutralization, and hemadsorption-inhibition tests, have been used in swine influenza immunity studies.

Present evidence supports the belief that swine recovered from influenza are resistant to subsequent infection. A subsequent respiratory outbreak of respiratory illness in a herd in a given season is caused by another pathogen. There is no unanimity of opinion on this point, however. According to Scott (1940), experimental pigs with neutralizing antibody are not necessarily immune to challenge by the intranasal route with virus and *H. parasuis* combined. Pigs exposed to aerosols of virus 83 days after earlier intranasal and aerosol exposure all had hemagglutinin-inhibition titers of 80 or above at the time of challenge and resisted that challenge. Increasing evidence suggests that local antibody is very important in influenzal immunity, as local and systematic cell-mediated responses were detected by in vitro transformation tests during the second week after intranasal inoculation (Charley 1977). Local and serum-neutralizing antibodies also appeared.

Maternal immunity plays a role in the epidemiology of the disease. Piglets from immune sows are protected as long as 13 to 18 weeks, depending on the serum-titer level of the dam. In addition to providing protection, colostral antibody often inhibits propagation of the virus in the host and development of active immunity. Infection of piglets with low titers led to immunological priming (Renshaw 1975). A second exposure to virus produced a secondary response that resulted in mild clinical disease of shorter duration than in piglets in which antibody completely blocked viral replication.

Diagnosis. Swine influenza should be suspected in any herd with respiratory disease in the fall or early winter. A clinical diagnosis is presumptive because influenza does not always follow the typical pattern and because other respiratory diseases are similar (Easterday 1972).

Definitive diagnosis requires virus isolation or the demonstration of a rising titer with paired serum samples. In the past, mice or ferrets were inoculated intranasally, but today the generally accepted method is chorioallantoic or amniotic inoculation of the 10- to 12-day-old embryonated hen's egg. Nasal exudate and lung tissue from a febrile pig usually contains virus. Proper treatment to eliminate bacteria and molds from test material is desirable to enhance virus isolation. After 72 to 96 hours of incubation the chorioallantoic and amniotic fluids are tested for hemagglutinating activity. If positive, the isolate is tested against influenza antiserums for specificity.

The hemagglutination-inhibition test is used most frequently in diagnosis when serology is applied. Paired serums are used. The first serum sample is taken during the acute phase of illness, and the second one is obtained 2 to 3 weeks later. A rising titer constitutes a positive result. The serologist must be aware of possible nonspecific inhibitors of hemagglutination and the methods by which the serums can be treated to remove them (Nakamura and Easterday 1967).

Prevention and Control. Experimental vaccines including a subunit vaccine, have been produced with swine influenza virus, but none has proved effective enough to be manufactured commercially. Although the economic aspects of the disease are not known, there appears to be a need for a safe, efficacious vaccine that probably would be more effective if administered by the respiratory route. Techniques are available for producing strains in the laboratory by recombinations that are safe and immunogenic (Easterday 1972), so it should be only a matter of time before a satisfactory vaccine is available to immunize pigs.

Careful nursing of sick animals, with provision of comfortable and draft-free quarters with clean, dry, and dust-free bedding is important. Fresh, clean water and a good source of feed are essential. The animals should not be disturbed or moved during the disease course. Antibiotics and sulfonamides are useful to control secondary bacterial infections in herds.

Much research has been done on potential antiviral substances that would effectively control influenza A viruses. All strains of influenza A continue to be sensitive to amantadine-hydrochloride, but until the 1980s this drug had not been used in outbreaks of swine influenza. 5-Iododeoxyuridine showed antiviral activity in swine with influenza, but toxicity also was observed (Steffenhagen et al. 1976).

The Disease in Humans. Since the mid-1970s swine influenza virus has infected humans. Antibodies in the serum of elderly persons suggests that they were infected with a swine influenza virus many years ago or with a human influenza virus that shared a common antigen(s) with the early swine strain. Pigs with influenza A viruses have transmitted the infection to humans, but fortunately, no pandemics have been associated with these episodes (Kaplan and Webster 1977).

REFERENCES

Andrewes, C.H., Laidlaw, P.P., and Smith, W. 1934. The susceptibility of mice to the viruses of human and swine influenza. Lancet 227:859–862.

Brown, T.T., Mengeling, W.L., Paul, P.S., and Pirtle, E.C. 1980. Porcine fetuses with pulmonary hypoplasia resulting from experimental swine influenza virus infection. Vet. Pathol. 17:455–468.

Butterfield, W.K., Campbell, C.H., Webster, R.G., and Shortridge, K.F. 1978. Identification of a swine influenza virus (Hsw_1N_1) isolated from a duck in Hong Kong. J. Infect. Dis. 138:686–689.

Charley, B. 1977. Local immunity in the pig respiratory tract. I. Cellular and humoral immune responses following swine influenza infection. Ann. Microbiol. 128B.95–107.

DeJong, J.C., and DeRonde-Verloop, F.M. 1977. Antigenic subgroups of influenza A (HSW1 N1) virus differentiated by hemagglutination inhibition. Dev. Biol. Stand. 39:453–455.

Dorset, M., McBryde, C.N., and Niles, W.B. 1922. Remarks on "hog flu." J. Am. Vet. Med. Assoc. 62:162–171.

Easterday, B.C. 1970. Swine influenza. In H.W. Dunne, ed., Diseases of Swine, 3d ed. Iowa State University Press, Ames. Chap. 5, p. 127.

Easterday, B.C. 1972. Immunologic considerations in swine influenza. Swine Disease Suppl. J. Am. Vet. Med. Assoc. 160:645–648.

Hinshaw, V.S., Webster, R.G., Bean, W.J., Downie, J., and Sinne, D.A. 1983. Swine influenza like viruses in turkeys: Potential source of virus for humans. Science 220:206–208.

Hinshaw, V.S., Webster, R.G., and Turner, B. 1978. Novel influenza A viruses isolated from Canadian feral ducks: Including strains antigenically related to swine influenza (Hsw1N1) viruses. J. Gen. Virol. 41:115–127.

Kaplan, M.M., and Webster, R.G. 1977. The epidemiology of influenza. Sci. Am. 237:88–106.

Kobe, V.K., and Fertig, H. 1938. Die Züchtung des Ferkelgrippe und swine influenza Virus. Zentralbl. Bakteriol. I Abt. Orig. 141:1–14.

Lewis, P.A., and Shope, R.E. 1931. Swine influenza. II. A hemophilic bacillus from the respiratory tract of infected swine. J. Exp. Med. 54:361–371.

Mohan, R., Saif, Y.M., Erickson, G.A., Gustafson, G.A., and Easterday, B.C. 1981. Serologic and epidemiologic evidence of infection in turkeys with an agent related to the swine influenza virus. Avian Dis. 25:11–16.

Nakamura, R.M., and Easterday, B.C. 1967. Serological studies of influenza in animals. Bull. WHO 37:559–567.

Nakamura, R.M., and Easterday, B.C. 1970. Studies of swine influenza. III. Propagation of swine influenza virus in explants of respiratory tract tissues from fetal pigs. Cornell Vet. 60:27–35.

Orcutt, M.L., and Shope, R.E. 1935. The distribution of swine influenza virus in swine. J. Exp. Med. 62:823–826.

Palese, P., and Ritchey, M.B. 1977. Polyacrylamide gel electrophoresis of the RNAs of new influenza virus strains: An epidemiological tool. Dev. Biol. Stand. 39:411–415.

Pirtle, E.C., and Ritchie, A.E. 1975. Morphologic heterogeneity of a strain of swine influenza virus (A/swine/Wisconsin/1/68, Hsw 1/Nsw 1) propagated at different temperatures. Am. J. Vet. Res. 36:1783–1787.

Renshaw, H.W. 1975. Influence of antibody-mediated immune suppression on clinical, viral and immune responses to swine influenza infection. Am. J. Vet. Res. 36:5–13.

Scott, J.P. 1940. Swine influenza. J. Bacteriol. 40:327.

Scott, J.P. 1941. Swine influenza associated with hog cholera. Vet. Extension Q., Univ. Pa. 82:3–12.

Shope, R.E. 1931a. Swine influenza. I. Experimental transmission and pathology. J. Exp. Med. 54:349–360.

Shope, R.E. 1931b. Swine influenza. III. Filtration experiments and etiology. J. Exp. Med. 54:373–385.

Shope, R.E. 1935. The infection of mice with swine influenza virus. J. Exp. Med. 62:571–572.

Shope, R.E. 1939. An intermediate host for the swine influenza virus. Science 89:441–442.

Shope, R.E. 1941. The swine lungworm as a reservoir and intermediate host for swine influenza virus. II. The transmission of swine influenza virus by the swine lungworm. J. Exp. Med. 74:49–68.

Shortridge, K.F., Webster, R.G., Butterfield, W.K., and Campbell, C.H. 1977. Persistence of Hong Kong influenza virus variants in pigs. Science 196:1454–1455.

Steffenhagen, K.A., Easterday, B.C., and Galasso, G.J. 1976. Evaluation of 6-azauridine and 5-iododeoxyuridine in the treatment of experimental viral infections. J. Infect. Dis. 133:603–612.

Tumova, B., and Pereira, H.G. 1968. Antigenic relationship between influenza A viruses of human and animal origin. Bull. WHO 38:415–420.

Urman, H.K., Underdahl, N.R. and Young, G.A. 1958. Comparative histopathology of experimental swine influenza and virus pneumonia of pigs in disease-free, antibody-devoid pigs. Am. J. Vet. Res. 19:913–917.

Wallace, G.D., and Elm, J.L., Jr. 1979. Transplacental transmission and neonatal infection with swine influenza virus (Hsw1N1) in swine. Am. J. Vet. Res. 40:1169–1172.

Avian Influenza

SYNONYMS: Fowl pest, fowl plague

Avian influenza is typically an acute, highly fatal disease of chickens, turkeys, pheasants, and certain wild birds. Ducks, geese, and other waterfowl are less susceptible but do contract the disease at times. Natural infection among pigeons is uncommon. In 1978–1979 an avian influenza A virus caused primary pneumonia and death in harbor seals on the Cape Cod peninsula in the United States (Wilson 1980). There is evidence that avian influenza viruses can naturally infect other mammals (Lu et al. 1982). Artificial infection of ducks, geese, and pigeons by the injection of large amounts of virus from naturally infected chickens often fails. The signs of illness and lesions of avian influenza are similar to those of fowl cholera.

Avian influenza has been known since about 1880, when it was recognized in Italy as a separate disease. Early in the twentieth century it spread throughout the greater part of Europe. The virus was brought into the United States illegally in 1923 by a laboratory worker. In the fall of 1924 the virus escaped from the laboratory into the New York poultry market, where it was estimated to have killed more than 500,000 birds (Mohler 1925). From this market it spread to many eastern poultry farms, probably on the contaminated crates of dealers, causing large losses. The disease was stamped out within 1 year by rigid quarantine methods. After the 1924–1925 outbreak, avian influenza was diagnosed again in the United States by Beaudette and co-workers (1934). The second outbreak was small, involving a few flocks in New Jersey. As with the earlier, larger outbreak, the disease was brought under control by strict quarantine measures. No birds were vaccinated. In Canada (Lang et al. 1965) and later in the United States (Olesuik et al. 1967, Smithies et al. 1969) an influenza was reported as an acute respiratory disease in turkeys, with high morbidity and low mortality (Smithies et al. 1969). In 1978 to 1981 the disease occurred more frequently in turkeys than in chickens and caused considerable economic loss in North America and Europe. The disease in chickens occurred in laying flocks in 1976, with a substantial mortality and severe drop in egg production (Johnson and Maxfield, 1976). Between 1964 and 1981 the disease was reported in turkeys in 14 U.S. states, in chickens in two states, and in other avian species in two states (Pomeroy 1981).

Since the mid-1970s molecular virologists have used the avian influenza virus strains to study the genetics, biochemistry, and replication of influenzal viruses because convenient and accurate in vitro and in vivo systems exist to elucidate these areas of interest. As a consequence the literature on avian influenza virus is voluminous, but it is outside the realm of this book to cover in depth these areas of molecular virology.

A comprehensive review of avian influenza was presented during the First International Symposium on Avian Influenza, sponsored by the U.S. Animal Health Organization and the United States Department of Agriculture (Bankowski 1981).

Character of the Disease. The nature of the disease has been characterized best in chickens and turkeys.

The disease in chickens. The period of incubation is rather short—3 to 5 days as a rule. Inoculated birds may show signs within 24 to 36 hours. A high temperature rapidly develops (110° to 112°F), the appetite is lost, and the birds rapidly become lethargic. The comb and wattle commonly have whitish, necrotic areas of skin (Figure 51.3). A mucoid nasal discharge appears, and often edema of the head and neck develops. The hock may be swollen and discolored because of subcutaneous hemor-

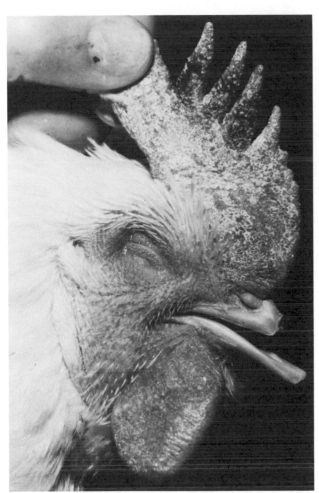

Figure 51.3. A chicken with avian influenza. The comb and wattles have whitish, necrotic areas of skin. (Courtesy D. A. Gregg, Plum Island Animal Disease Center, U.S. Dept. of Agriculture.)

rhage and edema (Figure 51.4). The course of the disease often is very rapid, death usually occurring within a few hours after the appearance of the first signs. The temperature commonly falls to subnormal shortly before death. Mortality sometimes is close to 100 percent.

Chickens with acute cases generally have few lesions. They consist of petechial hemorrhages on the heart, the fatty tissue around the gizzard, the serosa of the body cavity, and the mucous membranes of the proventriculus. In some animals a serofibrinous exudate appears in the pericardial sac. The principal organs may show petechiae and cloudy swelling. The nervous system appears normal, but microscopic examination shows a diffuse encephalitis with cuffing of the blood vessels, degeneration of nerve cells, and necrotic foci around which there is proliferation of glia cells. The spleen shows necrotic lymphoid nodules (Figure 51.5).

The disease in turkeys. The first outbreaks in Canada appeared as acute respiratory disease and caused a severe production problem for turkey farms (Lang et al. 1965). The viral isolate from the outbreaks was designated A/Turkey/Can/63 (Wilmot) and was found to be related to the influenza A group of viruses. In transmission experiments the virus regularly produced sinusitis in turkey poults less than 4 weeks old but was not pathogenic for older turkeys and chickens of any age. In contrast, a later isolate designated A/Turkey/Ontario/7732/66 was highly pathogenic for turkeys and chickens (Lang et al. 1968).

A Massachusetts isolate produced an air sac disease characterized by depression and acute death in some semimature turkeys (Olesuik et al., 1967). The antigenic relation of the isolate to the Canadian Wilmot virus was demonstrated by the hemagglutinin-inhibition test.

The Wisconsin isolate is a type A influenza virus that produces an acute respiratory disease in turkeys (Smithies et al. 1969). The disease, with high morbidity and low mortality, was seen in 9 breeding flocks in northwestern

Figure 51.4. The hock of a chicken with avian influenza. The hock is discolored, swollen, and hemorrhagic. (Courtesy D. A. Gregg, Plum Island Animal Disease Center, U.S. Dept. of Agriculture.)

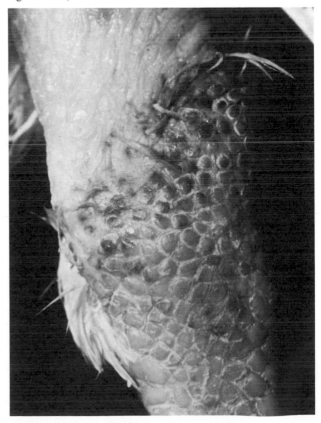

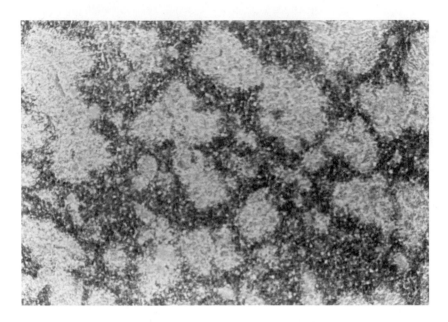

Figure 51.5. Micrograph of a spleen from a chicken infected with avian influenza virus. The light areas are necrotic lymphoid nodules. Hematoxylin and eosin stain. (Courtesy C. A. Mebus, Plum Island Animal Center, U.S. Dept. of Agriculture.)

Wisconsin, and serologic evidence was demonstrated in 11 turkey flocks.

In Minnesota during a two-year study (1980–1981) eight influenza virus subtypes were involved in turkey outbreaks; seven of these subtypes also were detected in sentinel mallard ducks and/or other avian species (Halvorson et al. 1983).

Properties of the Virus. Various tests—such as complement fixation, enzyme-linked immunosorbent assay, counterimmunoelectrophoresis, electron microscopy, indirect hemagglutination, hemagglutination, and serum neutralization tests—are common for the study of avian influenza viruses. These viruses are members of the *Orthomyxovirus* type A group, and they exhibit a wide range of antigenic variation. Of 108 possible antigenic combinations of avian influenza A virus, 47 have been recorded among the Hong Kong isolates during a 5-year period of testing the cloacal and tracheal swabs of fowl at a Hong Kong poultry dressing plant (Shortridge 1981). Ten different hemagglutinin variant types have been recognized. Variant types 1 and 5 are pathogenic, but they must be present in the cleaved form, indicating that the hemagglutinin alone is not responsible for pathogenicity—it is a sum of the total genome. Apparently there is no correlation between the antigenic subtype and the virulence of avian influenza viruses (Allan et al. 1975). Rott et al. (1974) provided conclusive evidence that the neuraminidase of influenza viruses plays a significant role in protection.

The virus particles are spherical, 80 to 100 nm in diameter (Figure 51.6). Associated filaments average 80 nm in diameter and are up to 8 nm in length (Dawson and

Elford 1949). By electron microscopy Waterson et al. (1961) showed that the avian viruses resembles human influenza A viruses.

The ribonucleoprotein is a continuous strand, 6 nm in diameter, which is formed in the nucleus of infected cells (Almeida and Brand 1975); the hemagglutinin is developed in the cytoplasm (Breitenfeld and Schafer 1957). Hemagglutination of red blood cells from fowl, rhesus monkeys, horses, and cattle has been demonstrated.

The avian viruses have a complement-fixing antigen common to the influenza A virus group. They also share hemagglutinins and neuraminidases with other species.

Cultivation. The viruses multiply readily in embryonated hens' eggs. A cytopathic effect is produced in cell cultures of various fowl and mammalian tissues. Attenuation of virus for fowl is reported after transfers in chick, pigeon, and human cell cultures (Hallauer and Kronauer 1959).

Noninfectious virus particles produced by an avian influenza virus in infected Ehrlich ascitic carcinoma cells have the same morphology, size, and sedimentation rate as standard virions. Apparently the particles are very fragile. In isopyknic fractionation they are detected in two forms. Particles with a density of 1.23 g/ml. retain their hemagglutinating but not their neuraminidase activity. Those with a density of 1.27 g/ml lack both hemagglutinating and neuraminidase activity (Gitelman et al. 1976).

The virus has been known to grow in mouse peritoneal macrophages in vitro, and Lindenmann et al. (1978) did some experiments to show that macrophages and resistance of mice are two facets of the same phenomenon.

Epizootiology. Migratory birds are probably responsi-

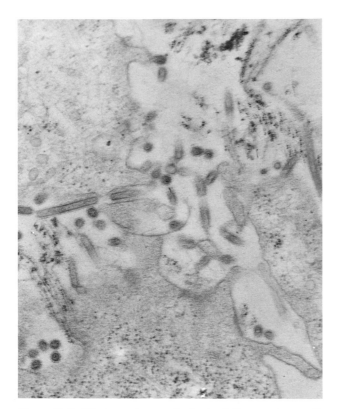

Figure 51.6. Electron micrograph of avian influenza virus particles in infected cells of a chick embryo cell culture. Negatively stained, × 38,400. (Courtesy S. S. Breese, Plum Island Animal Disease Center, U.S. Dept. of Agriculture.)

ble for the spread of avian influenza viruses throughout the world (Kaplan and Webster 1977). These birds can harbor the virus without showing signs of illness. Further, it has been shown that the virus can replicate in the intestinal tract of feral ducks, which then shed virus in high concentrations into water where it remains viable for days or weeks depending on water temperature (Webster et al. 1977). As a consequence, there is a real possibility that influenza viruses are transmitted between wild birds and domestic birds and eventually to mammals, including humans, which helps to explain the epidemiology of the influenza viruses. Various investigators, including Fukumi et al. (1977), have reported that some species of migrating ducks, such as pintail, mallard, widgeon, and falcated teal, possess antibodies in their serums against hemagglutinin antigens of human or avian influenza viruses.

Kaplan and Webster (1977) concluded that, from an evolutionary point of view, the family of influenza viruses originated in the bird kingdom, an animal group some 100 million years old, and that birds can now be infected with most of the influenza viruses without becoming diseased.

Avian influenza viruses can infect mammals, so they also may contribute to the antigenic pool from which new pandemic strains may originate (Hinshaw et al. 1981)

Hinshaw et al. (1983) reported that a laboratory worker developed respiratory signs of illness after working with strain H1N1 of turkey influenza. Virus was recovered from the patient, and seroconversion resulted. This suggests that turkeys as well as swine are involved in the maintenance of influenza viruses and that they can transmit them to humans.

Immunity. Recovered birds are solidly immune for several months at least. The serum of recovered birds gives considerable immunity to susceptible fowls, but because the immunity is short-lived and only a small amount of serum can be obtained from immune birds, the method has no practical value.

Avian influenza viruses replicate in a variety of mammals and birds, yet hemagglutination inhibition tests on serum from these animals have only low levels of hemagglutinin-inhibiting antibody. In reality there is a good antibody response; the failure to detect hemagglutinin-inhibiting antibodies to avian viruses with intact virions was overcome by using hemagglutinin subunits as antigen (Lu et al. 1982).

Diagnosis. The enzyme-linked immunosorbent assay (ELISA) for antibodies is an excellent diagnostic test whose sensitivity is 100 times greater than the complement-fixation or hemagglutination-inhibition test (Leinikki and Passila 1977), but the latter is the usual test of choice for diagnosis and research. Occasionally the serum neutralization is employed to confirm the results of the hemagglutination-inhibition test. The isolation of virus also provides a positive approach in the diagnosis of the disease. The embryonated hen's egg is the most sensitive substrate for this purpose, although cell-culture can be employed as well.

Prevention and Control. As mentioned earlier, the outbreaks of avian influenza in the United States during the 1920s and 1930s were controlled by rigid quarantine methods. These included controls for shipping birds and for cleaning and disinfecting poultry crates, egg crates, and other objects that might carry virus from infected flocks. The birds were not vaccinated.

To eliminate the disease in its present form from Canada and the United States would require formidable costs and effort. Naturally, U.S. government control officials are concerned with the potential danger that avian influenza viruses pose to commercial poultry flocks. When epizootics occur in chickens or turkeys or both, stringent quarantine and slaughter measures are put into effect through collaboration between state and federal governments.

There is an extensive European literature on vaccines for avian influenza. Attempts have been made to produce vaccines from blood and from tissues. Treatment with heat, phenol, glycerol, ether, and formaldehyde weakens and finally destroys the virus. Moses et al. (1948) obtained a high degree of immunity, which persisted for 18 to 21 weeks, following vaccination with whole-egg adjuvant vaccines (inactivated virus) and with living variant virus. Daubney et al. (1949), in experiments designed to improve the quality of the inactivated avian influenza vaccines, noted that serial passage of one strain of influenza virus through pigeon embryos resulted in a mutant that was completely nonpathogenic for chickens, turkeys, and young pigeons but which induced solid immunity against virulent avian influenza virus. A cold variant, which is an attenuated virus derived by genetic recombination at 25°C in embryonating eggs, provides protection against virulent virus (Merritt and Maassab 1977). There may be some reservation about its use as a vaccine because virus can be recovered from lung and turbinate (Rott et al. 1976). Through recombination of avian influenza virus with other influenza A viruses nonpathogenic for fowl, it is possible to produce a number of antigenic hybrids that are nonpathogenic for chickens. These results have led to the conclusion that the surface components do not by themselves determine the pathogenicity of influenza A viruses.

Vaccines could be used during outbreaks, but the constant drift and shift of influenza viruses pose a special problem, and the stockpiling of appropriate antigens for this purpose is not technically feasible at present (1986).

The Disease in Humans. Epidemiological studies suggest that avian influenza viruses could conceivably infect humans because avian and human strains may share common hemagglutinins. A human case of keratoconjunctivitis that was caused by an avian influenza virus (HAV/1/NEQ/1) occurred as the result of a laboratory accident. A turkey isolate of avian influenza virus produced respiratory signs and a fever in another laboratory worker. The ease by which antigen hybrids of influenza viruses can be produced in vivo supports the hypothesis that new influenza viruses can arise in nature from birds and mammals and cause disease in humans (Webster and Campbell 1972).

REFERENCES

Allan, W.H., Alexander, D.J., Pomeroy, B.S., and Parsons, G. 1977. Use of virulence index test for avian influenza viruses. Avian Dis. 21:359–363.

Almeida, J.D., and Brand, C.M. 1975. A morphological study of the internal component of influenza virus. J. Gen. Virol. 27:313–318.

Bankowski, R.A. 1981. In Proceedings of the 1st International Symposium on Avian Influenza. Beltsville, Md. April 22–24, 1981. P. 215. (Available from Carter Compos., 3408 W. Leigh St., Richmond, VA, 23230, U.S.A.)

Beaudette, F.R., Hudson, C.B., and Saxe, A.H. 1934. An outbreak of fowl plague in New Jersey in 1929. J. Agric. Res. 49:83–92.

Breitenfeld, P.M., and Schafer, W. 1957. The formation of fowl plague virus antigens in infected cells as studied with fluorescent antibodies. Virology 4:328–345.

Daubney, R., Mansi, W., and Zaharan, G. 1949. Vaccination against fowl plague. J. Comp. Pathol. Therap. 59:1–18.

Dawson, I.M., and Elford, W.J. 1949. The investigation of influenza and related viruses in the electron microscope, by a new technique. J. Gen. Microbiol. 3:298–311.

Fukumi, H., Nerome, K., Nakayama, M., and Ishida, M. 1977. Serological and virological investigations for orthomyxovirus in birds in South-east Asian area. Dev. Biol. Stand. 39:475–482.

Gitelman, A.K., Martynenko, V.B., Molibog, E.V., and Vorkunova, J.B. 1976. Abortivnaia infektsiia virusa grippa v kletkakh astsitnogo raka Erlikha. Dal' neishu izuchenie svoistv astsitnogo virusa. Vopr. Virusol. 6:713–721.

Hallauer, C., and Kronauer, G. 1959. Further studies on cultivation and variants of the classical fowl plague virus in human tissue explants. (In German.) Arch. Gesam. Virusforsch. 9:232–250.

Halvorson, D., Karunakaran, D., Senne, D., Kelleher, C. Bailey, C., Abraham, A., Hinshaw, V., and Newman, J. 1983. Epizootiology of avian influenza—Simultaneous monitoring of sentinel ducks and turkeys in Minnesota. Avian Dis. 27:77–85.

Hinshaw, V.S., Webster, R.G., Easterday, B.C., and Bean, W.B., Jr. 1981. Replication of avian influenza viruses in mammals. Infect. Immun. 34:354–361.

Johnson, D.C., and Maxfield, B.G. 1976. An occurrence of avian influenza virus infection in laying chickens. Avian Dis. 20:422–424.

Kaplan, M.M., and Webster, R.G. 1977. The epidemiology of influenza. Sci. Am. 237:88–106.

Lang, G., Ferguson, A.E., Connell, M.C., and Wills, C.G. 1965. Isolation of unidentified hemagglutinating virus from the respiratory tract of turkeys. Avian Dis. 9:495–504.

Lang, G., Narayan, O., Rouse, B.T., Ferguson, A.E., and Connell, M.C. 1968. A new influenza A virus infection in turkeys. II. A highly pathogenic variant, A/Turkey/Ontario 7732/66. Can. Vet. J. 9:151–160.

Leinikki, P.O., and Passila, S. 1977. Quantitative, semiautomated, enzyme-linked immunosorbent assay for viral antibodies. J. Infect. Dis. 136 (Suppl.):294–299.

Lindenmann, J., Deuel, E., Fanconi, S., and Haller, O. 1978. Inborn resistance of mice to myxoviruses: macrophages express phenotype in vitro. J. Exp. Med. 147:531–540.

Lu, B.L., Webster, R.G., and Hinshaw, V.S. 1982. Failure to detect hemagglutination-inhibiting antibodies with intact avian influenza virions. Infect. Immun. 38:530–535.

Merritt, S.N., and Maassab, H.F. 1977. Characteristics of a live avian influenza virus. Health Lab. Sci. 14:122–125.

Mohler, J.R. 1925. Dangerous microbial immigrants. J. Am. Vet. Med. Assoc. 67:764–772.

Moses, H.E., Brandly, C.A., Jones, E.E., and Jungherr, E.L. 1948. Immunization of chickens against fowl plague. Am. J. Vet. Res. 9:399–420.

Olesuik, O.M., Snoeyenbos, G.H., and Roberts, D.H. 1967. An influenza A virus isolated from turkeys. Avian Dis. 11:203–208.

Pomeroy, B.S. 1981. Avian influenza in the United States (1964–1981). In Proceedings of the 1st International Symposium on Avian Influenza. Beltsville, Md., April 22–24, 1981. Pp. 13–17. (Available from Carter Compos., 3408 W. Leigh St., Richmond, VA, 23230, U.S.A.)

Rott, R., Becht, H., and Orlich, M. 1974. The significance of influenza virus neuraminidase in immunity. J. Gen. Virol. 22:35–41.

Rott, R., Orlich, M., and Scholtissek, C. 1976. Attenuation of pathogenicity of fowl plague virus by recombination with other influenza A viruses nonpathogenic for fowl: Nonexclusive dependence of pathogenicity on hemagglutinin and neuraminidase of the virus. J. Virol. 19:54–60.

Shortridge, K.F. 1981. Epidemiology of avian influenza and sources of infection in domestic species. In Proceedings of the 1st International Symposium on Avian Influenza. Beltsville, Md, April 22–24, 1981. (Available from Carter Compos., 3408 W. Leigh St., Richmond, VA, 23230, U.S.A.)

Smithies, L.K., Radloff, D.B., Friedell, R.W., Albright, G.W., Misner, V.E., and Easterday, B.C. 1969. Two different type A influenza virus infections in turkeys in Wisconsin. I. 1965–1966 outbreak. Avian Dis. 13:603–606.

Waterson, A.P., Rott, R., and Schafer, W. 1961. The structure of fowl plague virus and virus N. Z. Naturforsch. 16B:154–156.

Webster, R.G., and Campbell, C.H. 1972. An inhibition test for identifying the neuraminidase antigen on influenza viruses. Avian Dis. 16:1057–1066.

Webster, R.G., Hinshaw, V.S., Bean, W.J., Jr., Turner, B., and Shortridge, K.F. 1977. Influenza viruses from avian and porcine sources and their possible role in the origin of human pandemic strains. Dev. Biol. Stand. 39:461–468.

Wilson, M. 1980. Fowl plague in North American seals. Anim. Dis. Rep., U.K., no. 3. Pp. 3–4.

52 The Paramyxoviridae

The family Paramyxoviridae contains several viruses that produce significant diseases in both animals and humans. Members of this family are medium to large, enveloped, pleomorphic viruses containing a helical nucleocapsid with one negative nonsegmented strand of RNA. There are three genera: *Morbillivirus*, *Paramyxovirus*, and *Pneumovirus*. A triad of important viruses—canine distemper virus, rinderpest virus, and measles virus—in addition to peste des petits ruminants virus, constitute the genus *Morbillivirus*. The genus *Paramyxovirus* includes a number of pathogens including Newcastle disease virus, four serotypes of parainfluenza viruses (including bovine parainfluenza virus and canine parainfluenza virus), several serotypes of avain paramyxoviruses, and mumps virus. The respiratory syncytial viruses of humans and cattle along with pneumonia virus of mice are included in the genus *Pneumovirus*.

Important pathogens of domestic animals within the Paramyxoviridae family with salient features of the clinical diseases produced are listed in Table 52.1. Reviews have been written by Appel et al. (1981), Bishop and Compans (1984), Chanock and McIntosh (1985), Choppin and Compans (1975), Frank (1981), Kelen and McLeod (1977), Kingsbury (1985), and White and Fenner (1986).

The spherical, enveloped pleomorphic particles range in diameter from 100 to 300 nm and have characteristic glycoprotein projections, or "spikes." The helical nucleocapsid is approximately 18 nm in diameter and 1 μm long. The particles are ether-sensitive but antigenically stable.

Viruses in this family contain a single molecule of single-stranded, nonsegmented RNA of negative polarity and molecular weight of 5 to 8×10^6. A complete set of six or more viral genes is present in each genome. The negative-strand genome is complementary to viral mRNA, and thus it must be transcribed by an RNA polymerase to give the positive-strand mRNA. The nucleocapsids develop in the cytoplasm. Genetic reassortment does not occur as it does in the orthomyxoviruses.

In the prototype paramyxovirus (Sendai virus), at least three proteins are present in the nucleocapsid, protein L (largest), a polymerase-associated protein (P), and a nucleocapsid structural protein (NP). Three proteins are present in the envelope. One of these is the hemagglutinin-neuraminidase (HN) glycoprotein, which contains both neuraminidase and hemagglutinating activity, and is involved in the virus-cell attachment. Several viruses in the family—including measles virus, other morbilliviruses, respiratory syncytial virus, and other pneumoviruses—do not contain neuraminidase. A second glycoprotein, the fusion (F) protein, is involved in the fusion of infected cells to give the syncytia so common in paramyxovirus-infected cells. The third protein is the membrane (M) protein, which is nonglycosylated. At least one nonstructural protein (C) may be present (Kingsbury 1985, White and Fenner 1986).

Paramyxoviruses enter the cell by attachment of the envelope to the cell membrane, then fusion of the viral envelope with the cellular membrane. Thus these viruses enter the cell directly without the internalization through endosomes which occurs with many other viruses (Kingsbury 1985). The virus replicates in the cytoplasm.

REFERENCES

Appel, M.J.G., Gibbs, E.P.J., Martin, S.J., Ter Meulen, V., Rima, B.K., Stephenson, J.R., and Taylor, W.P. 1981. Morbillivirus diseases of animals and man. In E. Kurstak and C. Kurstak, eds., Comparative Diagnosis of Viral Diseases. vol. 4. Academic Press, New York. Pp. 187–233.

Bishop, D.H.L., and Compans, R.W., eds. 1984. Non-Segmented Negative Strand Viruses: Paramyxoviruses and Rhabdoviruses. Academic Press, New York.

Chanock, R.M., and McIntosh, K. 1985. Parainfluenza viruses. In B.N. Fields, D.M. Knipe, R.M. Chanock, J.L. Melnick, B. Roizman, and R.E. Shope, eds., Virology. Raven Press, New York. Pp. 1241–1253.

Choppin, P.W., and Compans, R.W. 1975. Reproduction of paramyxoviruses. In H. Fraenkel-Conrat and R.R. Wagner, eds., Comprehensive Virology, vol. 4. Plenum, New York. Pp. 95–178.

Frank, G.H. 1981. Paramyxovirus and pneumovirus diseases of animals and birds: Comparative aspects and diagnosis. In E. Kurstak and C. Kurstak, eds., Comparative Diagnosis of Viral Diseases, vol. 4. Academic Press, New York. Pp. 187–233.

Kelen, A.E., and McLeod, D.A. 1977. Paramyxoviruses: Comparative diagnosis of parainfluenza, mumps, measles, and respiratory syncytial virus infections. In E. Kurstak and C. Kurstak, eds., Comparative Diagnosis of Viral Diseases. vol. 1. Academic Press, New York. Pp. 503–607.

Table 52.1. Diseases of domestic animals caused by viruses in the Paramyxoviridae family

Common name of virus	Natural hosts	Type of disease produced
Genus *Morbillivirus*		
Canine distemper virus	Dogs, other canines, ferrets, and mink	Highly contagious disease of young dogs manifested by diphasic temperature curve, acute rhinitis, followed by bronchitis and catarrhal pneumonia, severe gastroenteritis and, occasionally, nervous signs. Morbidity high; mortality varies, largely dependent on development of nervous manifestations
Rinderpest virus	Cattle, water buffalo, sheep, and perhaps goats	A very important disease in cattle and water buffalo which occurs in Asia and Africa. It is an acute febrile disease with lesions largely confined to the digestive tract with ulceration and hemorrhages in the pharynx and larynx and throughout the rest of the tract including Peyer's patches. The respiratory tract shows reddening and often petechiation and a patchy peumonia. In a susceptible population it is explosive with a high morbidity and mortality
Peste des petits ruminants virus	Sheep, goats	Rinderpestlike disease
Genus *Paramyxovirus*		
Newcastle disease virus (avian paramyxovirus 1)	Chickens, turkeys, guinea fowl, ducks, geese, pheasants, and many wild avian species	The intensity of the disease varies markedly depending on the virulence of the viral strain involved. The disease usually begins with respiratory signs followed by diarrhea and then nervous signs, particularly by involving younger chickens. The disease spreads rapidly with a high morbidity and a variable mortality
Parainfluenza 3 virus	Cattle	One agent involved in shipping fever syndrome of cattle. Acute respiratory signs and distress accompanied by fever, inappetence, and depression. Morbidity and mortality likely to be high. Stress and concurrent infections contribute to the severity of the disease
Canine parainfluenza virus	Dogs	In outbreaks the disease is severe and probably involves other pathogens as well. There is a sudden onset, copious nasal discharge, fever, and coughing resembling a disease called kennel cough
Parainfluenza 3 virus	Sheep	Respiratory disease comparable to parainfluenza 3 infections in cattle. Viral strains in sheep comparable but not identical to bovine and human PI-3 viruses
Parainfluenza 3 virus	Horses	Rather obscure disease. Respiratory signs observed in diseased foals or yearlings. The infection may be common in horses

Table 52.1.—*continued*

Common name of virus	Natural hosts	Type of disease produced
Sendai virus (para-influenza 1 virus)	Swine, humans	In swine, reputedly causes broncho-pneumonia in young pigs and abortions in sows in Japan
Avian paramyxoviruses (PMV-2 to PMV-9)	Chickens, turkeys, ducks, geese, caged birds, wild birds	Cause respiratory illness, fatal illness in caged birds
Mumps virus	Cats, dogs, humans	Present evidence suggests that cats and dogs are susceptible to mumps and it occasionally can produce clinical disease
Genus *Pneumovirus* Bovine respiratory syncytial viruses	Cattle, sheep, goats	Certain viral isolates produce respiratory disease characterized by pyrexia, rhinitis, and pneumonia. The human respiratory syncytial virus causes disease in experimental calves; it is not known if BRSV causes disease in humans

Kingsbury, D.W. 1985. Orthomyxo- and paramyxoviruses and their replication. In B.N. Fields, D.M. Knipe, R.M. Chanock, J.L. Melnick, B. Roizman, R.E. Shope, eds., Virology. Raven Press, New York. Pp. 1157–1178.

White, D.O., and Fenner, F.J., eds. 1986. Paramyxoviruses. In Medical Virology, 3d ed. Academic Press, Orlando, Fla. Pp. 521–539.

The Genus *Morbillivirus*

Canine Distemper

SYNONYM: Carré's disease; abbreviation, CD

Canine distemper is a worldwide, highly contagious disease of young dogs. It is manifested first by a diphasic fever curve and acute rhinitis, and later by bronchitis and catarrhal pneumonia, severe gastroenteritis, and nervous signs. The initiating agent is a virus, first described by Carré (1905), but many of the pathological changes in naturally occurring cases are due to bacterial complications. Carré's studies were not generally accepted until the classical reports of Laidlaw and Dunkin (Dunkin and Laidlaw 1926a, 1926b; Laidlaw and Dunkin 1926, 1928a, 1928b). Investigators in England (MacIntyre et al. 1948) described a disease in dogs which they termed *hard pad disease*. This is simply one of the many manifestations that canine distemper virus (CDV) produces.

There are many review articles about canine distemper (Appel and Gillespie 1972, Appel et al. 1981, Gillespie 1962, Gorham 1960, Greene 1984).

Character of the Disease. Over the years CD has caused the death or permanent disability of more young dogs than any other disease. It occurs in all members of the Canidae family (wolves, foxes, jackals, coyotes, dingoes), all members of the Mustelidae family (ferrets, mink, skunks, badgers, martins, otters, stoats, weasels), and members of the Procyonidae family (lesser pandas, kinkajous, coatis, raccoons). Ferrets are exceedingly susceptible to distemper virus and almost always die of the disease. For this reason they are used frequently as experimental animals. Feline panleukopenia, a viral disease of cats, is sometimes called distemper, but this disease is caused by the feline parvovirus. Neither any of the other domesticated animals or humans are susceptible to CDV, although inapparent experimental infection has been produced in the domestic cat (Appel et al. 1974). Fatal CD in a Bengal tiger has been described (Blythe et al. 1983).

CD is well controlled in many parts of the world by vaccination. However, in areas with unvaccinated populations, CD occurs wherever dogs are raised. It is a disease of young, unvaccinated dogs which is especially common in cities, pet stores, shelters, dog colonies, or other places where there are many contacts with other dogs. Puppies born of immune mothers acquire a passive immunity through the colostral milk which protects them until that immunity is lost. Unless the young dog is raised in relative isolation from other dogs, it is likely to develop the disease at this time. Farm dogs, which often live in relative isolation, may escape distemper entirely or perhaps have it when they are old. Old dogs are not immune to distemper because of age, but only because they have had previous contacts with the virus.

The onset of the disease is usually manifested by a serous discharge from the eyes and nose, lassitude, inappetence, and fever, which may reach 105°F or higher. The lachrymal discharge may become purulent within 24 hours. The initial temperature rise lasts about 2 days and is followed by a period of 2 or 3 days in which the temperature may be nearly or quite normal. During this time the animal may appear to feel better and may eat its food. This period is followed by a secondary temperature rise that may last for several weeks. Again the dog obviously feels bad, has no appetite, and usually vomits. Pneumonia frequently develops, and in many victims severe diarrhea appears. The feces are watery, mixed with mucus, fetid, and often bloody. Under these conditions the dog loses weight rapidly. The death rate is high; hence the prognosis should be guarded.

Along with the initial temperature rise a few young dogs suffer a skin eruption. This consists of pustules, which occur on the abdomen, the inside of the thighs, and elsewhere. They are secondary bacterial infections usually caused by *Staphylococcus intermedius*. As the animal recovers, these lesions dry up and disappear.

Neurological manifestations may occur. On occasion catarrhal signs are not severe, and the nervous signs predominate. If dogs develop an effective level of neutralizing antibodies by the 10th day after infection, neurological signs usually do not develop and the dogs recover without complications. If, however, neutralizing antibodies are not produced by the 10th day, the dogs usually develop neurological disease and most eventually die (Appel et al. 1981). Dogs with nervous manifestations have a syndrome characterized by several or all of the following signs: depression, myalgia, myoclonus, incoordination, circling, epileptiform convulsions, and coma. In general when dogs show convulsions, death results. In some cases chorea and paralysis may remain after other signs subside. Encephalitis in old dogs also may be another form of CD (Adams et al. 1975, Lincoln et al. 1973).

In the early febrile stage of the disease, leukopenia occurs; but later, if bacterial infection is not controlled by treatment, marked leukocytosis appears. Immunosuppresion caused by the virus may play a major role in the outcome of the disease.

Dunkin and Laidlaw (1926b) showed that the uncomplicated viral infections in dogs maintained in isolation produced severe signs in many cases, but with a relatively low death rate. The high mortality usually seen in this disease is due, in most cases, to complications of bacterial infections to which the animal is predisposed by the action of the virus, and the result of viral action on the central nervous system.

Another viral disease, infectious canine hepatitis, may be confused with distemper, or both diseases may occur in a dog simultaneously. There is no interference between the viruses of these two diseases, according to Gillespie et al. (1952). In experiments dogs infected with both viruses develop a more severe type of illness than that seen in others receiving only one virus. Both viruses are recovered from the blood of such dogs, and the typical inclusion bodies of both viruses are found in their tissues.

The disease in ferrets. Ferrets are exceedingly susceptible to the virus of CD (Dunkin and Laidlaw 1926a). Natural outbreaks of the disease often occur, and the mortality is very nearly 100 percent. The virus is readily transmitted through the air by infectious droplets.

The incubation period in ferrets is about 10 days as a rule but may occasionally be 1 or 2 days shorter. A serous discharge from the eyes and the nose indicates the onset of the disease. This discharge quickly becomes purulent, and the eyelids become swollen and pasted together. The chin becomes reddened, and small vesicles form around the mouth where the hair meets the naked skin of the lips. The feet swell, the footpads become red, and sometimes the skin of the abdomen also reddens. On the third day the vesicles on the chin become pustules, and the animal, refusing all food, remains curled up in the cage. It becomes weaker and generally dies on the fifth or sixth day. Occasionally an animal lives longer and develops pneumonia or nervous signs, but ultimately it almost always dies. Heath (1940) described a neurotropic strain of CDV. After a few passages in ferrets in which typical signs were produced, the signs changed suddenly and nervous manifestations predominated in ferrets inoculated thereafter. The incubation period became longer (about 16 days). Some animals died suddenly without manifesting any signs. Others exhibited intermittent convulsions and died 2 to 4 days after the first spasms were seen.

The disease in raccoons. Raccoons and other members of the Procyonidae family are susceptible to CDV (Appel and Gillespie 1972, Potgieter and Patton 1984). It is the most common cause of neurological disease in raccoons in the northeastern United States.

The disease in hamsters. Cabasso et al. (1955) reported success in adapting a chick embryo–adapted strain of CD virus to suckling hamsters. The infected animals died 4 to 7 days following inoculation.

The disease in suckling mice. CD was first adapted to suckling mice by Morse et al. (1953). Intracerebral inoculation of chick embryo–adapted strains into suckling mice produced nervous manifestations and death.

The disease in nonhuman primates. Encephalomyeli-

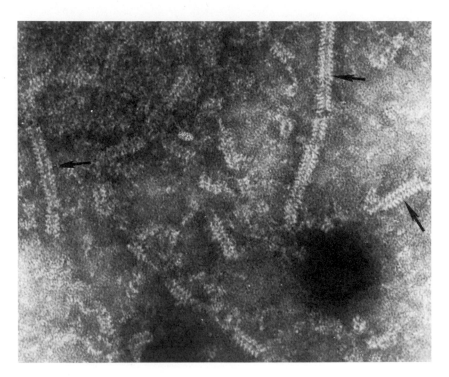

Figure 52.1. Helical cores (*arrows*) of canine distemper virus. × 225,000. (Courtesy J. Almeida.)

tis was induced by a neurovirulent strain of CDV (Yamanouchi et al. 1970). Intracerebral inoculation produced histological lesions in monkeys comparable to those described in the dog.

Properties of the Virus. CDV, an ether-sensitve RNA virus, has physical and biochemical properties consistent with those of other morbilliviruses within the Paramyxoviridae family. Ultrafiltration experiments by Palm and Black (1961) revealed a particle size between 115 and 160 nm in diameter. Subsequent electron micrographs of Cruickshank et al. (1962) showed that most particles range between 150 and 300 nm and that the central core contains helices 15 to 17 nm in diameter (Figure 52.1). Filamentous forms of virus are described.

Many studies have been done to identify the proteins and glycoproteins in CDV particles (Campbell et al. 1980, Hall et al. 1980, Orvell 1980, Orvell and Norrby 1980, Rima et al. 1983, Sato et al. 1981), and these reports have been reviewed and summarized by Appel et al. (1981). The H glycoprotein has a molecular mass of 76 to 80 kilodaltons, whereas the fusion glycoprotein (F) is 59 to 62 kilodaltons in size. There also are an M protein lining the inner membrane of the virus and at least two nucleocapsid proteins.

Several published reports have identified the gene sequences for CDV and several have compared the sequences of CDV, peste des petits ruminants virus, rinderpest virus, and measles virus (Barrett and Mahy 1984; Barrett et al. 1985; Rozenblatt, Eizenberg, Ben-Levy, et al. 1985; Rozenblatt, Eizenberg, England, and Bellini 1985). Plasmid DNA containing a virus-specific insert, representing more than 98 percent of the genes derived from the P protein in RNA of CDV showed significant cross-hybridization with all the other morbilliviruses.

The mRNAs produced by the CDV genome have been characterized (Barrett and Underwood 1985, Hirayama et al. 1985, Russell et al. 1985). When analyzed on denaturing agarose-formaldehyde gels, the major RNA components from all viruses in the genus *Mobillivirus* were identical, except for CDV; in CDV one of the virus-specific mRNAs (mRNA$_5$), which probably codes for the viral hemagglutinin, was smaller than the corresponding mRNA induced by the other viruses.

CDV remains viable for years at −70°C. Lyophilization provides a convenient method to preserve it in the laboratory and for commercial use. Either lyophilized virulent or attenuated virus can be maintained at approximately 6°C for years with little or no loss of titer, provided the moisture content is low.

Various chemical compounds, including 0.75 percent formalin, can inactivate CDV (Celiker and Gillespie 1954). Hydroxylamine inactivates it under certain conditions, and beta propriolactone in a final concentration of 0.1 percent inactivates it within 2 hours at 37°C.

The plate and microscope slide procedures of the Ouchterlony agar-gel diffusion test have been used to study CDV. Soluble antigens distinct from the infective particle precipitate specific antibody. Antigen can be de-

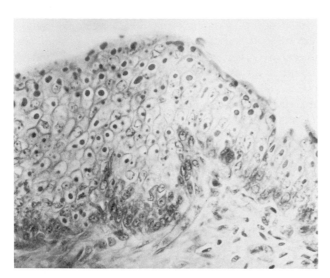

Figure 52.2. Canine distemper virus inclusion bodies in the urinary bladder of a raccoon. The bodies are located in the epithelial cells. They are not always as numerous. × 600.

rived from tissue fragments of mesenteric lymph node or spleen of infected animals or from supernatant fluid of infective tissue-culture fluids.

The immunofluorescence test has been used effectively in pathogenesis studies of the dog because viral antigen is readily demonstrated in tissue cells (Appel and Gillespie 1972). It has been located in inclusion bodies of infected tissues from dogs (Moulton and Brown 1954) and also from raccoons (Figure 52.2). Yamanouchi et al. (1970) claimed V (envelope) and S (soluble) antigens are formed in cytoplasm because intranuclear fluorescence in tissue-cultured cells appeared only after 48 to 72 hours, and a single growth cycle is approximately 18 hours. Complete virus on cell surfaces fluoresced, indicating activity

against V antigen. Activity against S antigen was not observed.

The virus of CD, like that of measles, is sensitive to light in fluid suspension and during replication. Calf serum or glutathione reduces the inactivation rate. Certain components of tissue-culture media enhanced light sensitivity, but their presence was not essential for light inactivation. It has been suggested that a substance derived from the host cell which is incorporated into the viral overcoat serves to make CDV light-sensitive (Appel and Gillespie 1972).

Neutralizing antibodies are formed and can be demonstrated in various systems such as embryonated hens' eggs, suckling hamsters, suckling mice, ferrets, dogs, and various tissue-culture systems. The chick-embryo system has been used to study viral antigenicity.

Various serologic and protection tests in animals have proved that the viruses of measles, canine distemper, and rinderpest of cattle share some common antigenic material. There is some similarity in the lesions that they produce in their respective susceptible hosts and in certain tissue-culture systems.

Cultivation. CDV can be grown on the chorioallantoic membrane of embryonated chicks (Cabasso and Cox 1949). Dedie and Klapotke (1951) successfully cultivated the virus in tissue culture. Rockborn (1958) propagated the virus in dog kidney monolayer cultures, and it produced syncytia, intranuclear and cytoplasmic inclusion bodies, and stellate cells. In chick embryo cell cultures, egg-adapted virus produced cellular granulation and fragmentation without the syncytia (Karzon and Bussell 1959). Isolation of virulent CDV in tissue culture is difficult, although it has been done in various cell systems. Dog lung macrophages give good results (Figure 52.3).

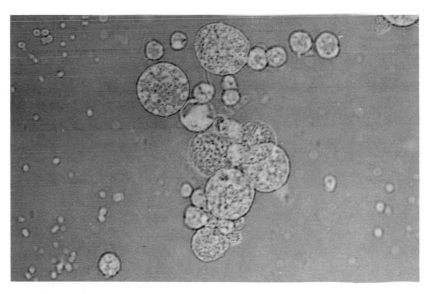

Figure 52.3. The effects of Snyder Hill strain of canine distemper virus in dog macrophage culture. × 360. (Courtesy M. Appel.)

Once adapted to embryonating eggs or tissue culture, the virus can be propagated in a large number of primary and stable cell cultures derived from canine, mustelid, avian, bovine, simian, and human tissues (Appel and Gillespie 1972). Karzon and Bussell (1959) used the plaque overlay method to quantitate virus or antibody.

Epizootiology and Pathogenesis. Distemper virus is transmitted principally by droplet infection, virus being present in abundance in the serous excretions that run from the eyes and nose during the early febrile stage of the disease. Dunkin and Laidlaw found that it was impossible to keep susceptible dogs in the same room with infected dogs without the former becoming infected, no matter what precautions were taken. In their experimental work they set up individual kennels 100 to 150 feet apart and depended on air dilution to prevent the passage of virus from one to another. This experiment generally succeeded, but there were some instances when they believed that infected droplets had bridged these gaps. Urine and feces contain virus and can transmit the disease. Kennels, runs, and other places inhabited by dogs generally harbor virus. Arthropod carriers of this virus have not been found. There is a suggestion that transplacental transmission of CDV may occur (Krakowka, Hoover, et al. 1977).

Dunkin and Laidlaw (1926b) found the incubation period to be remarkably constant. In most dogs fever appeared on the fourth day after exposure. Rarely it occurred on the third day, occasionally on the fifth, and rarely on the sixth.

The course of the disease varies greatly, depending on the character and severity of the secondary complications. In uncomplicated cases dogs may show very mild signs, which may not be recognized, or they may suffer a febrile illness that may last 2 weeks or longer. When complicated with catarrhal pneumonia and enteritis, the course may be much longer. Nervous signs may be evident for many weeks after recovery from all other signs.

The death rate varies widely, depending on the breed, and age of the dog and the kind of nursing care and treatment given. It probably averages about 20 percent.

Distemper virus has an affinity for lymphatic and epithelial cells. The viral antigen first appears in the bronchial lymph nodes and tonsils 24 hours after exposure, as determined by immunofluorescence. It appears in the mononuclear cells of the blood by the second or third day, followed by widespread dissemination by the ninth day. This accounts for the widespread appearance of lesions in the dog. In the skin vesicular and pustular dermatitis occur. These changes are confined to the malpighian layer of the epidermis, but congestion of the dermis usually occurs and lymphocytic infiltration may occur. Proliferation of the keratin layer of the footpad epidermis results in a

hardened pad—a condition that British investigators have termed *hard pad disease*. The urinary tract epithelium may show vascular congestion with cytoplasmic and intranuclear inclusion bodies, these occur particularly in the bladder and renal pelvis. The reproductive organs may also show lesions, and mild interstitial epididymitis and orchitis are common. Few lesions are observed in the stomach and intestine; however, cytoplasmic acidophilic inclusion bodies may be found in the epithelial lining. Intranuclear acidophilic inclusions also may be seen occasionally in these cells. Excessive mucus is often seen in the large intestine. Catarrhal or purulent bronchopneumonia, where bronchi and alveoli are filled with exudate, was found more commonly before the introduction of sulfa drugs and antibiotics. In other cases mononuclear cells lining alveolar walls or partially filling the alveoli are the only evidence of involvement. Epithelioid cells with fused cytoplasm (giant cells) line the bronchioles and alveoli adjacent to the pleura, and the condition appears microscopically as giant-cell pneumonia. Inclusion bodies are found in giant cells, other mononuclear cells, and bronchiolar and bronchial epithelium. The spleen may be grossly enlarged, and congested necrosis of lymphoid cells in the splenic follicles may be observed microscopically. In uncomplicated cases the most significant change is a size reduction of the thymus gland, which may be gelatinous. Degenerative changes may occur in the adrenal glands, usually in the cortex.

Intraocular lesions associated with CD were described by Jubb et al. (1957). Leukocytes infiltrate the ciliary body. Exudative or degenerative changes are seen in retinal ganglion cells and proliferation in pigment epithelium. Edema causes focal retinal detachments. Ulcerative keratitis sometimes complicates purulent conjunctivitis.

Susceptible dogs exhibit the typical picture of acute distemper when inoculated with virus. Some viral strains develop neurotropic properties for dogs and cause a high percentage of cases in which nervous signs are prominent (Gillespie and Rickard 1956, Mansi 1951, Summers et al. 1984). In susceptible puppies 1 to 2 weeks old, the only signs of illness are hemorrhagic diarrhea, dehydration, and inappetence, usually terminating in death 2 weeks after the onset of illness (Gillespie et al. 1958). In studies with R252 strain, 85 percent of gnotobiotic dogs less than 1 week old died of acute encephalitis 2 to 5 weeks after infection. The percentage of mortality was considerably lower in older dogs. Physiological immaturity may account for the difference (Krakowka and Koestner 1976).

The distribution of CDV in the central nervous system of dogs with demyelinating encephalitis has been studied (Vandevelde and Kristensen 1977, Vandevelde et al.

1985). In the gray matter there was a good correlation between the presence and severity of lesions and the presence and amount of viral antigen. Large amounts of virus were found in the neurons and their processes. Most demyelinating lesions contained small amounts of viral antigen located mostly in the astrocytes, which presumably play an important part in this process.

Dogs with nervous manifestations may show perivascular cuffing, nonsuppurative leptomeningitis, and vacuoles in the white matter. Many Purkinje cells show degenerative changes. Numerous cells show pyknosis, whereas other cells appear swollen, with small, indistinct Nissl granules. Some Purkinje cells fade so that they are almost unrecognizable. Gliosis is seen in the cerebellum and is most marked in dogs that develop nervous manifestations a considerable time after onset of infection. Degenerated myelin is not demonstrable in the cerebellum of experimental dogs that are destroyed after displaying nervous signs 7 to 16 days after intracerebral inoculation with Snyder Hill strain (Gillespie and Rickard 1956). Demyelinization, accompanied by usual gitter cells and by intranuclear inclusion bodies in glial cells, is found in the cerebellums of dogs with nervous manifestations observed at the longer intervals. These data support the concept that demyelinization may be the response of a self-imposed antigen-antibody reaction. However, a direct viral effect on oligodendroglial cells that produce myelin has to be considered. By electron microscopy, crystallike structures similar to CDV nucleocapsids are seen in the cytoplasm of endothelial and adventitial cells of meningeal veins and arteries, in the endothelium of cortical and plexus capillaries, in mononuclear cells within the lumina of blood vessels, in histiocytes and macrophages within the arachnoid space, in reactive microglial cells, and in ependymal cells (Blinzinger and Deutschlander 1969).

Immunity. Dogs that recover from an infection with canine distemper virus usually are immune for life. CDV produces an antibody-mediated and a cell-mediated response, while measles virus causes only a cell-mediated response in dogs (Gerber and Marron 1976). Antibody titers vary inversely with the disease severity. Recovered dogs have the highest titers, whereas fatally infected dogs have little or no antibody activity. Dogs with chronic persistent infection form a third group with intermediate antibody levels. The inability to produce antibodies to envelope antigens may be a crucial factor in the establishment of a persistent infection. Although immunodepressive effects can be demonstrated in vitro, complete suppression of immune functions in the course of CDV infection in the dog does not occur (Krakowka, Cockerell, et al. 1975; Krakowa, Olsen, et al. 1975). A method for the rapid in vivo assessment of cell-mediated immunity in the dog is the intradermal mitogen test (Krakowka, Cockerell, and Koestner 1977).

The virus is so widespread that most dogs, except a few that lead sheltered lives, have been infected before they are a year old and are immune. Appel and Gillespie (1972) found that immunity persisted for at least 7 years in dogs retained in isolation. Occasionally older, previously vaccinated dogs that reside in an urban community develop clinical distemper. Immunity challenge in dogs is difficult to evaluate because contact exposure to diseased dogs is unreliable and parenteral inoculation does not result in frank disease in some susceptible dogs. A more reliable method is the intracerebral challenge with brain-adapted strains of CDV. Ferrets given egg-attenuated virus vaccine are immune for at least 5 years.

Neutralizing antibody has been used to evaluate the duration of immunity, and determining neutralizing antibody levels appears at present to be the only in vitro method for measuring immunity in dogs. A maternal antibody titer (passive immunity) of 1:100 or greater can be correlated with absolute protection against intracerebral or aerosol challenge with the Snyder Hill strain of CDV. Puppies with maternal titers of less than 1:20 are susceptible. On the other hand, dogs given inactivated distemper virus or measles virus had little or no measurable neutralizing CD antibody. When these dogs are challenged, no frank disease is produced and they react with an anamnestic antibody response. Consequently the amount of neutralizing antibody is only a relative index of protection in the dog.

At an American Veterinary Medical Association symposium on canine distemper (1966), the Committee on Standardized Methods and Test Procedures made recommendations for the standardization of the neutralization test. These recommendations were based on the statistical evaluation tests of Robson et al. (1959). Neutralization tests are performed in various tissue-culture systems, (embryonated hens' eggs, mice, ferrets, dogs, and suckling hamsters) with the properly adapted viral test strain used in each system.

Neutralizing antibodies first appear in the circulation 8 to 9 days after aerosol exposure to virulent virus; maximal titers are reached at 4 weeks and serum levels range from 1:300 to 1:3,000 when tested against approximately 10^2 EID_{50} (egg-infective dose$_{50}$) of virus. Titers to vaccine virus are slightly lower. The main fraction of CD-neutralizing antibody is found in the gamma globulin fraction of the serum. CD-neutralizing antibody is found in the cerebrospinal fluid of most dogs with demyelinating CD encephalitis. Most of these dogs also have a marked elevation of IgG and IgM in the cerebrospinal fluid.

Complement-fixing (CF) antibodies develop 3 to 4 weeks after initial infection but persist for only a few weeks thereafter. Consequently, this test is a means by which a recent initial infection can be diagnosed. Dogs given inactivated virus develop CF antibodies that rapidly disappear. Upon challenge with virulent virus a few months later, CF titers appear in 4 to 8 days and persist for at least 7 months at significant levels (Gillespie and Karzon 1960).

CD antibody produced with the Rockborn strain of CDV inhibits the hemagglutination of monkey erythrocytes by Tween 80 ether-treated measles virus. In contrast, CD antibody produced by the Snyder Hill strain of CDV failed; yet the serum-neutralization titers of both antiserums were similar.

Puppies born of immune mothers obtain effective immunity from the mother, but this is passive antibody and disappears within a few weeks. This passive neutralizing antibody is transferred in utero (3 percent) (Figure 52.4) and by combined placental and colostral antibody transfer equivalent to 77 percent of the mother's serum titer. The half-life of maternally transferred distemper antibody is 8.4 days (Gillespie et al. 1958) (Figure 52.5).

For many years it was believed that very young puppies could not produce distemper antibodies. These failures now can be attributed to maternal immunity interference or improper immunization. No effect of age on distemper antibody was discernible when the nomograph was used to determine this age (Figure 52.6). Titers produced in puppies of any age to egg-virus vaccine were identical

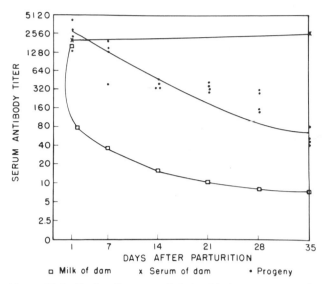

Figure 52.5. Canine distemper. Relationship between serum titer of the mother and her milk and the serum titer of her progeny during nursing. (From Gillespie et al., 1958, courtesy of *Cornell Veterinarian.*)

(Gillespie et al. 1958). Puppies that do no suckle their immune mothers and receive no colostrum can be vaccinated at 2 weeks of age because the amount of antibody transferred in utero is relatively small.

Diagnosis. The clinical diagnosis and laboratory confirmation of the diagnosis of CD has been reviewed by several workers, including Appel and Gillespie (1972), Appel et al. 1981, Dhein and Gorham (1986), Gorham (1960), Greene (1984), and Moise (1985). A clinical diagnosis of CD may be possible on the basis of clinical signs during an acute infection. Atypical infections, chronic infections, and neurological disease caused by CDV may make clinical diagnosis of CD difficult. With extensive vaccination against CD, less acute disease is seen by the clinician, and more cases are seen without pathognomonic signs (Appel and Gillespie 1972, Lauder et al. 1954).

Typical cytoplasmic or intranuclear inclusion bodies by histopathological techniques in affected tissues are presumptive evidence for a definite diagnosis. The possible persistence of inclusion bodies could conceivably lead to a false-positive diagnosis unless supported by serologic or virological evidence.

A positive diagnosis is assured by the isolation of CDV. Because distemper is a pantropic infection, virus can be readily isolated (by ferret or dog inoculation) from the blood, lymph nodes, spleen, lung, liver, and other visceral organs during the acute stage of infection. Virus has also been isolated from the brain of dogs with epileptiform convulsions long after it was impossible to isolate the

Figure 52.4. Canine distemper. Relationship between titer of mother and antibodies acquired by progeny through placental transfer. (From Gillespie et al., 1958, courtesy of *Cornell Veterinarian.*)

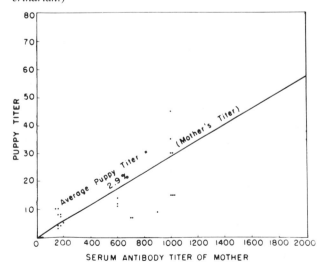

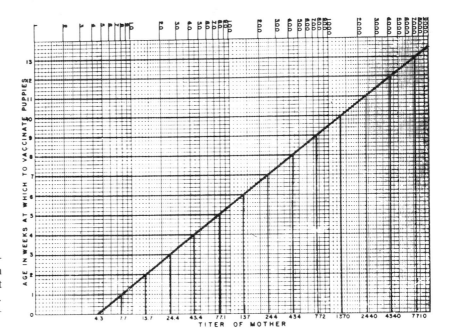

Figure 52.6. A nomograph for canine distemper showing the relationship between serum titer of mother and the age in weeks at which her progeny should be vaccinated. (From Baker et al., 1959, courtesy of *Cornell Veterinarian.*)

pathogen from the blood (Gillespie and Rickard 1956). No virus was isolated from the blood, urine, and brains of fully recovered dogs injected with virulent virus 30 days earlier.

The immunofluorescent antibody technique has been used to diagnose CD by demonstrating CDV antigen in cells from conjunctival or vaginal imprints, buffy coat preparations, central nervous system cells, or biopsy specimens from the footpads (Appel and Gillespie 1972, Appel et al. 1981, Cello et al. 1959). However, this method often results in negative tests if the samples are collected after neutralizing antibodies have appeared.

For many years susceptible dogs or ferrets were used for the primary isolation of CDV. The response in dogs can be slight, so the use of paired serum samples to demonstrate a rising antibody titer is essential in these instances.

Isolating virus from clinical cases of CD in cell culture systems is difficult, but several techniques enable primary isolation. Lung macrophage cultures from dogs are especially susceptible. The use of hens' eggs, suckling mice, and suckling hamsters for primary isolation is inadvisable because these hosts respond only to adapted strains.

The diagnosis of CD can also be confirmed by demonstrating seroconversion with neutralizing antibody tests, enzyme-linked immunosorbent assay (Noon et al. 1980), or various other assays.

The clinical diagnosis of CD has, in the past, been considered relatively simple. It is now quite certain that under this single designation several different diseases of dogs have been included. The enteric viruses have as-

sumed great importance, and to a lesser degree, infectious hepatitis has been important. A specific diagnosis of distemper, obviously, is not always simple because, as has already been pointed out, many animals show neither signs of illness nor lesions pathognomonic of the disease.

Relationship of CDV to Certain Other Viruses. Adams and Imagawa (1957) found that a strain of the virus of human measles was neutralized by the serum of ferrets that had been actively immunized against CDV. The serum of normal ferrets had no such effect. These neutralization studies were conducted in a tissue-culture system. In animal studies, ferrets that had been immunized with measles virus showed partial protection when challenged with CDV. Also, a mouse-adapted strain of CDV was completely neutralized by measles antiserum prepared in ferrets.

Cabasso et al. (1959) found that puppies vaccinated against CD developed high levels of homologous antibodies but failed to develop either neutralizing or complement-fixing antibodies for measles virus. Similarly chickens hyperimmunized against CDV, did not develop antibodies for measles, although their homologous titers were high.

Most dogs immunized with measles virus developed low distemper neutralizing antibody titers and excellent homotypic antibody titers. On challenge with a brain-adapted strain of CDV all dogs were protected, but the controls sickened and some died. Protection depended on a rapid secondary response of distemper antibody following the distemper challenge (Gillespie and Karzon 1960).

The relationship of measles virus (MV) and CDV in

animal species is variable (Appel and Gillespie 1972). Monkeys infected with MV react like humans and produce antibodies to both viruses. Infection of ferrets, rabbits, and guinea pigs with MV produces measles antibody titers but only low distemper neutralizing antibody titers in some of the animals, even after two infections with MV. Ferrets immunized with MV are partially protected against CDV challenge. When CDV is inoculated into various species, production of MV antibody is found less frequently, and protection against MV less effective.

In East Africa, Polding and Simpson (1957), noting that a group of dogs in constant intimate contact with cattle suffering from rinderpest remained free from CD, wondered if the apparent protection stemmed from exposure to rinderpest virus. They tested the hypothesis by injecting rinderpest virus into a group of CD-susceptible dogs and, after 25 days, inoculated these and a similar group of nontreated dogs with CDV. Those injected with rinderpest virus remained healthy; those that were not so treated developed distemper. Later Polding et al. (1959) inoculated cattle with CDV. No response was elicited, and all animals later proved susceptible to rinderpest when challenged with virus. Again a group of dogs given a single dose of rinderpest virus later proved refractory to CDV; but other dogs, given large doses of antirinderpest immune serum, received only slight protection against a subsequent inoculation with CDV.

For more information about CDV, MV, and rinderpest virus, see the monograph by Appel and Gillespie (1972) and the paper by Yamanouchi (1980).

Immunization. At the American Veterinary Medical Association symposia in 1966 and 1970 panels made recommendations for the immunization of dogs against CD. These recommendations, which are still valid, have led to a more standardized approach to the prevention and control of this most important disease. The panels' recommendations as well as a Special Report by the Council on Biologic and Therapeutic Agents (Bittle et al. 1982), are incorporated into this section.

Passive immunization of dogs. CD antiserum, if the antibody titer is sufficiently high, may protect susceptible dogs from the disease for a limited time. Formerly, the antiserum was used in some animal hospitals to protect young, unvaccinated dogs from infection during hospitalization or other period of imminent exposure to virus. Usually one 10-ml dose of antiserum was given for a few days' stay in the hospital or at a dog show. If the sojourn was prolonged, another dose was given on about the 10th day.

According to the American Veterinary Medical Association panels for the canine distemper symposiums (1966, 1970) there is evidence that the routine prophylac-tic use of agents that passively immunize pups against CD has less merit than multiple doses of attenuated live-virus vaccines. Because it may block active immunization, the use of antiserum or concentrated antiserum for short-term protection is discouraged. Small-animal clinicians now generally believe that this procedure has less merit than vaccination with modified live-virus vaccines, and antiserum for temporary protection against CDV is no longer used.

Antiserum or concentrated antiserum is of questionable value in the treatment of dogs with clinical signs of distemper.

Active immunization of dogs. Vaccination is the most effective means for the prevention of distemper. Over the years several types of vaccines have been used, including: (1) formalin-treated virus vaccines; (2) ferret-passaged modified vaccine; (3) modified hen's-egg virus vaccine; (4) a combination of distemper antiserum and virulent distemper virus; (5) modified cell-culture virus vaccines; (6) polyvalent virus vaccines containig various combinations for distemper, infectious canine hepatitis, canine adenovirus 2 infection, parainfluenza, parvovirus infection, and rabies; and (7) measles vaccine, either alone or in combination with CDV and parvovirus.

The modified live-virus distemper vaccines presently available usually do not cause illness, are efficacious, rarely spread to susceptible dogs, and give a relatively long immunity. The egg-adapted CD vaccines produced in chick fibroblasts or in the hen's egg are safer for use in dogs than some CD vaccine strains propagated in tissue-cultured canine cells. Immunity after vaccination can be assessed by determination of humoral antibody levels and also by the use of lymphocyte transformation to evaluate the cell-mediated immune response.

Neutralizing antibody titers in dogs receiving inactivated CD vaccines reach their maximum 30 days after the last injection, but titers seldom rise much above 1:100 and are no longer measurable 16 weeks after the first injection. Dogs are still sensitized to the distemper antigen 3 to 6 months later, and a secondary antibody response occurs which confers clinical protection when dogs are challenged with virulent virus (Gillespie 1965, Montali et al 1983). Efforts to develop an inactivated vaccine that will consistently produce high protective antibody titers have been less than encouraging. The combination of distemper antiserum and virulent distemper virus is no longer employed in the United States.

As distemper virus causes the greatest mortality in young dogs, protection is desirable at an early age. Interference with active immunity by maternal antibody complicates vaccination because the immune status of a pup varies. A solution to this problem might be vaccination of puppies between 6 and 10 weeks old with measles virus vaccines (Norrby and Appel 1980). However, protection against CD from measles vaccines is incomplete (Appel et al. 1984). Because maternal measles antibody interferes with an active immunity to that virus, maternally derived measles antibody as well as distemper antibody must also be considered in a distemper immunization program.

There has been much controversy in the past about the best age at which to immunize young animals. There are still differences of opinion, and it is not always possible to decide this precisely for an individual animal. When the mother is immune to CD, antibodies are stored in the colostral milk, and these convey a passive immunity to the puppies. The concentration of antibodies in the colostrum varies in different immune bitches, however, and this variation affects the length of time the sucklings will have sufficient antibodies to protect them against natural exposure. If active immunization is attempted while the young animals retain substantial antibody levels derived from their mothers, enduring immunity will not result, because the antigenic properties of the vaccines are wholly neutralized by the passively acquired antibody. On the other hand, if the mother is not immune to CD, there will be no antibody in her colostrum, and her puppies will at once be highly susceptible to the disease.

Depending on their level of colostral antibodies, young dogs, therefore, may contract CD at any age. Because immunization will fail if done too early and also if deferred too long, allowing natural infection to intervene, the selection of the best time for artificial immunization is difficult. Gillespie et al. (1958) and Baker et al. (1959) attempted to solve this problem by developing a nomograph that relates the serum antibody titer of the dam to the time after birth when, in most instances, the antibody titers of its offspring will have decreased to the point that artificial active immunization is effective (Figure 52.6). The system predicts when the antibody loss of the young makes them susceptible. The system is based on sound scientific facts and generally is quite effective, but it is more expensive than many dog owners will accept because it involves taking a blood sample from the dam before the offspring are born and determining its virus-neutralizing titer by laboratory tests.

Then, too, individuals often purchase a puppy whose mother's serum titer has not been determined. Under these circumstances approximately 82 percent of the puppies vaccinated at 9 weeks of age with egg or tissue-culture virus vaccine were successfully immunized (Gillespie et al. 1958). Revaccination at 15 weeks of age took care of the other 18 percent that failed to respond earlier because of maternal antibody interference. One-third of these vaccinated puppies had titers of less than 1:100 at 1 year of age (Robson et al. 1959). At 2 years of age another third had titers below this figure. A serum titer of 1:100 is the standard level for indicating immunity to CD, although some dogs with lower titers may be immune. Dogs should be vaccinated yearly with modified virus vaccine until a more sensitive test, which measures cellular immunity as well as neutralizing antibody, can be devised. In lieu of this procedure yearly blood tests can be performed. If the serum titer falls below 1:100, revaccination is indicated. More than 90 percent of vaccinated dogs will show a significant rise in titer above the 1:100 level—the absolute criterion that a dog will withstand challenge with virulent CDV.

Many clinicians now use a combination of attenuated MV and CDV for the first dose of vaccine between 6 and 10 weeks of age, then follow with a polyvalent vaccine containing attenuated CD, canine adenovirus, parainfluenza, and parvovirus viruses at 4-week-intervals until the puppy is at least 14 weeks old. The parvovirus component may need to be repeated when the puppy is 18 weeks old.

Recommended vaccination procedures. On the basis of available knowledge, the two American Veterinary Medical Association panels concerned with canine distemper immunization (AVMA 1966, 1970) offered the guidelines for CD immunization. These recommendations have been generally accepted by veterinarians in the United States, and their main features are described in previous sections.

Immunization of foxes, mink, and ferrets. CDV causes natural epizootics among foxes, mink, and ferrets raised in captivity; the losses are often great. The virus is the same one that infects dogs, and the disease can be easily transmitted from any of these species to any other species susceptible to CD. In foxes the heaviest losses occur in the fall when the animals are turned loose on the range.

Immunization of wild canids presents a serious problem. The inactivated vaccines have not produced consistent protection (Montali et al. 1983), and because some of the modified live-virus vaccines have not been attenuated sufficiently for the wild and exotic canids, they often produce clinical disease with the dog vaccines. Halbrooks et al. (1981) evaluated three commercial modified live-virus CD vaccines in gray foxes. A chicken tissue-culture vaccine appeared to be safe and effective, but two canine tissue-culture–propagated vaccines produced fatal CD in vaccinated foxes.

Green and Carlson (1945) showed that these losses could be greatly reduced by treating all animals with distemperoid, a ferret-passage virus, and West and Brandly (1949) had excellent success with formalin-inactivated vaccines made from virulent fox tissues (lungs, liver, spleen, kidneys, urinary bladder, and lymph nodes). A 20 percent suspension of these tissues was used, and a 5-ml dose was given subcutaneously or intramuscularly. Some of the vaccines that contained adjuvants (alumina gel and fatty agents) were somewhat more effective than those that did not contain them.

Distemper infection in foxes must be differentiated from fox encephalitis caused by infectious canine hepatitis virus; the two diseases may exist concurrently. Green and Carlson (1945) state that this can be done by inoculating ferrets, which are susceptible to distemper but resistant to the other virus. They also point out that a search for inclusion bodies is helpful. Typical intracytoplasmic inclusion bodies, resembling those seen in dogs, may be found in the epithelial cells of the air passages and urinary bladder in cases of distemper, whereas they are not found in these cells in encephalitis infection.

Laidlaw and Dunkin (1926), using a formalin-inactivated tissue vaccine, found it much easier to immunize ferrets than dogs. Pinkerton (1940) reported satisfactory results in immunizing mink with vaccine made from lung tissue of infected mink. At the beginning of an outbreak on a ranch, some of the first animals infected were used as a source of vaccine virus. The finely ground tissue was made into a 10 percent emulsion, which was treated with 0.3 percent formalin. Several injections were given of 2 to 4 ml at weekly intervals.

Certain attenuated vaccines can be used for immunizing ferrets (Shen et al. 1984) and mink. On many large mink farms, mink are routinely immunized by means of aerosol from a fine-particle nebulizer.

The Disease in Humans. So far as is known, the virus of CD is nonpathogenic for humans. Several investigators have suggested that CDV might be involved in multiple sclerosis of humans (Cook et al. 1978, 1979), but others questioned this association. Evidence now supports the lack of association between CD and multiple sclerosis (Appel et al. 1981). Krakowka et al. (1983) could not identify reactivity to unique canine distemper virus-virion polypeptides in serums or cerebrospinal fluid of multiple sclerosis patients.

REFERENCES

Adams, J.M., Brown, W.J., Snow, H.D., Lincoln, S.D., Sears, A.W., Jr., Barenfus, M., Holliday, T.A., Cremer, N.E., and Lennette, E.H. 1975. Old dog encephalitis and demyelinating disease in man. Vet. Pathol. 12:220–226.

Adams, J.M., and Imagawa, D.T. 1957. Immunological relationship between measles and distemper viruses. Proc. Soc. Exp. Biol. Med. 96:240–244.

American Veterinary Medical Association. 1966. Canine Distemper Symposium. J. Am. Vet. Med. Assoc. 149:599–718.

American Veterinary Medical Association. 1970. Canine Infectious Diseases Report. J. Am. Vet. Med. Assoc. 156:1655–1817.

Appel, M., and Gillespie, J.H. 1972. Canine distemper virus. Virol. Monogr. 11:1–96.

Appel, M.J.G., Gibbs, E.P.J., Martin, S.J., Ter Meulen, V., Rima, B.K., Stephenson, J.R., and Taylor, W.P. 1981. Morbillivirus diseases of animals and man. In E. Kurstak and C. Kurstak, eds., Comparative Diagnosis of Viral Diseases, vol. 4. Academic Press, New York. Pp. 187–233.

Appel, M., Sheffy, B.E., Percy, D.H., and Gaskin, J.M. 1974. Canine distemper virus in domesticated cats and pigs. Am. J. Vet. Res. 35:803–806.

Appel, M.J., Shek, W.R., Shesberadaran, H., and Norrby, E. 1984. Measles virus and inactivated canine distemper virus induce incomplete immunity to canine distemper. Arch. Virol. 82:73–82.

Baker, J.A., Robson, D.S., Gillespie, J.H., Burgher, J.A., and Doughty, M.F. 1959. A nomograph that predicts the age to vaccinate puppies against distemper. Cornell Vet. 49:158–167.

Barrett, T., and Mahy, B.W. 1984. Molecular cloning of the nucleoprotein gene of canine distemper virus. J. Gen. Virol. 65:549–557.

Barrett, T., and Underwood, B. 1985. Comparison of messenger RNAs induced in cells infected with each member of the morbillivirus group. Virology 145:195–199.

Barrett, T., Shrimpton, S.B., and Russell, S.E. 1985. Nucleotide sequence of the entire protein coding region of canine distemper virus polymerase-associated (P) protein mRNA. Virus Res. 3:367–372.

Bittle, J.L., Grant, W.A., and Scott, F.W. 1982. Canine and feline immunization guidelines—1982. J. Am. Vet. Med. Assoc. 181:332–335.

Blinzinger, K., and Deutschlander, N. 1969. Über eigentumliche-kristallgitterartige Strukturkomplexe in Gehrin von staupekranken Hunden. Verh. Dtsch. Ges. Pathol. 53:283–287.

Blythe, L.L., Schmitz, J.A., Roelke, M., and Skinner, S. 1983. Chronic encephalomyelitis caused by canine distemper virus in a Bengal tiger. J. Am. Vet. Med. Assoc. 183:1163–1167.

Cabasso, V., and Cox, H.R. 1949. Propagation of canine distemper virus on the chorio-allantoic membrane of embryonated hen eggs. Proc. Soc. Exp. Biol. Med. 71:246–250.

Cabasso, V.J., Douglas, J.M., Stebbins, M.R., and Cox, H.R. 1955. Propagation of canine distemper virus in suckling hamsters. Proc. Soc. Exp. Biol. Med. 88:199–202.

Cabasso, V.J., Kiser, K.H., and Stebbins, M.R. 1959. Distemper and measles viruses. I. Lack of immunogenic crossing in dogs and chickens. Proc. Soc. Exp. Biol. Med. 101:227–230.

Campbell, J.J., Cosby, S.L., Scott, J.K., Rima, B.K., Martin, S.J., and Appel, M. 1980. A comparison of measles and canine distemper virus polypeptides. J. Gen. Virol. 48:149–159.

Carré, H. 1905. On the disease of young dogs. C. R. Hebd. Seances Acad. Sci. 140:689–690, 1489–1491.

Celiker, A., and Gillespie, J.H. 1954. The effect of temperature, pH, and certain chemicals on egg cultivated distemper virus. Cornell Vet. 44:276–280.

Cello, R.M., Moulton, J.E., and McFarland, S. 1959. The occurrence of inclusion bodies in the circulating neutrophils of dogs with canine distemper. Cornell Vet. 49:127–146.

Cook, S.D., Dowling, P.C., and Russell, W.C. 1979. Neutralizing antibodies to canine distemper and measles virus in multiple sclerosis. J. Neurol. Sci. 41:61–70.

Cook, S.D., Natelson, B.H., Levin, B.E., Chavis, P.S., and Dowling, P.C. 1978. Further evidence of a possible association between house dogs and multiple sclerosis. Ann. Neurol. 3:141–143.

Cruickshank, J.G., Waterson, A.P., Kanarek, A.D., and Berry, D.M. 1962. The structure of canine distemper virus. Res. Vet. Sci. 3:485–486.

Dedie, K., and Klapotke, E. 1951. Die Züchtung des Virus der Hundestaupe im Gewebsexplantat. Arch. Exp. Vet. Med. 4:137–146.

Dhein, C.R., and Gorham, J.R. 1986. Canine respiratory infections. In F.W. Scott, ed., Infectious Diseases. Contemporary Issues in Small Animal Practice, vol. 3. Churchill Livingstone, New York. Pp. 177–205.

Dunkin, G.W., and Laidlaw, P.P. 1926a. Studies in dog distemper. I. Dog distemper in the ferret. J. Comp. Pathol. Therap. 39:201–212.

Dunkin, G.W., and Laidlaw, P.P. 1926b. Studies in dog distemper. II. Experimental distemper in the dog. J. Comp. Pathol. Therap. 39:213–221.

Gerber, J.D., and Marron, A.E. 1976. Cell-mediated immunity and age at vaccination associated with measles inoculation and protection of dogs against canine distemper. Am. J. Vet. Res. 37:133–138.

Gillespie, J.H. 1962. The virus of canine distemper. Ann. N.Y. Acad. Sci. 101:540–547.

Gillespie, J.H. 1965. A study of inactivated distemper virus in the dog. Cornell Vet. 55:3–8.

Gillespie, J.H., and Karzon, D.T. 1960. A study of the relationship between canine distemper and measles in the dog. Proc. Soc. Exp. Biol. Med. 105:547–551.

Gillespie, J.H., and Rickard, C.G. 1956. Encephalitis in dogs produced by distemper virus. Am. J. Vet. Res. 17:103–108.

Gillespie, J.H., Baker, J.A., Burgher, J., Robson, D., and Gilman, B. 1958. The immune response of dogs to distemper virus. Cornell Vet. 48:103–126.

Gillespie, J.H., Robinson, J.I., and Baker, J.A. 1952. Dual infection of dogs with distemper virus and virus of infectious canine hepatitis. Proc. Soc. Exp. Biol. Med. 81:461–463.

Gorham, J.R. 1960. Canine distemper. In C.A. Brandly and E.L. Jungherr, eds., Advances in Veterinary Sciences, vol. 6. Academic Press, New York. Pp. 287–351.

Green, R.G., and Carlson, W.E. 1945. The immunization of foxes and dogs to distemper with ferret-passage virus. J. Am. Vet. Med. Assoc. 107:131–142.

Greene, C.E. 1984. Canine distemper. In C.E. Greene, ed.,Clinical Microbiology and Infectious Diseases of the Dog and Cat. W.B. Saunders, Philadelphia. Pp. 386–405.

Halbrooks, R.D., Swango, L.J., Schnurrenberger, P.R., Mitchell, F.E., and Hill, E.P. 1981. Response of gray foxes to modified live-virus canine distemper vaccines. J. Am. Vet. Med. Assoc. 179:1170–1174.

Hall, W.W., Lamb, R.A., and Choppin, P.W. 1980. The polypeptides of canine distemper virus: Synthesis in infected cells and relatedness to the polypeptides of other morbilliviruses. Virology 100,433–449.

Heath, L.M. 1940. Distemper studies. A note on a distemper virus with neurotrophic tendency. Can. J. Comp. Med. 4:352–354.

Hirayama, N., Senda, M., Yamamoto, H., Yoshikawa, Y., and Yamanouchi, K. 1985. Isolation and characterization of canine distemper virus-specific RNA. Microbiol. Immunol. 29:47–54.

Jubb, K.V., Saunders, L.L., and Coates, H.V. 1957. The intraocular lesions of canine distemper. J. Comp. Pathol. Med. 67:21–28.

Karzon, D.T., and Bussell, R.H. 1959. Cytopathic effect of canine distemper virus in tissue culture. Science 130:1708–1709.

Krakowka, S., and Koestner, A. 1976. Age-related susceptibility to infection with canine distemper virus in gnotobiotic dogs. J. Infect. Dis. 134:629–632.

Krakowka, S., Cockerell, G., and Koestner, A. 1975. Effects of canine distemper virus infection on lymphoid function in vitro and in vivo. Infect. Immun. 11:1069–1078.

Krakowka, S., Cockerell, G., and Koestner, A. 1977. Intradermal mitogen response in dogs: Correlation with outcome of infection by canine distemper virus. Am. J. Vet. Res. 38:1539–1542.

Krakowka, S., Hoover, E.A., Koestner, A., and Ketring, K. 1977. Experimental and naturally occurring transplacental transmission of canine distemper virus. Am. J. Vet. Res. 38:919–922.

Krakowka, S., Miele, J.A., Mathes, L.E., and Metzler, A.E. 1983. Antibody responses to measles virus and canine distemper virus in multiple sclerosis. Ann. Neurol. 14:533–538.

Krakowka, S., Olsen, R., Confer, A., Koestner, A., and McCullough, B. 1975. Serologic response to canine distemper viral antigens in gnotobiotic dogs infected with canine distemper virus. J. Infect. Dis. 132:384–392.

Laidlaw, P.P., and Dunkin, G.W. 1926. Studies in dog distemper. III. The nature of the virus. J. Comp. Pathol. Therap. 39:222–230.

Laidlaw, P.P., and Dunkin, G.W. 1928a. Studies in dog distemper. IV. The immunization of ferrets against dog distemper. J. Comp. Pathol. Therap. 41:1–17.

Laidlaw, P.P., and Dunkin, G.W. 1928b. Studies in dog distemper. V. The immunization of dogs. J. Comp. Pathol. Therap. 41:209–227.

Lauder, I.M., Martin, W.B., Gordon, E.D., Lawson, D.D., Campbell, R.S.F., and Watrach, A.M. 1954. A survey of canine distemper. Vet. Rec. 66:607–611, 623–631.

Lincoln, S.D., Gorham, J.R., Davis, W.C., and Ott, R.L. 1973. Studies of old dog encephalitis: Electron microscopic and immunohistologic findings. Vet. Pathol. 10:124–129.

MacIntyre, A.B., Trevan, D.J., and Montgomerie, R.F. 1948. Observations on canine encephalitis. Vet. Rec. 60:635–644.

Mansi, W. 1951. The isolation of a neurotropic virus from a dog suffering from the so-called nervous distemper. Br. Vet. J. 107:214–229.

Moise, N.S. 1985. Viral respiratory diseases. Vet. Clin. North Am. [Small Anim. Pract.] 15:919–928.

Montali, R.J., Bartz, C.R., Teare, J.A., Allen, J.T., Appel, M.J., and Bush, M. 1983. Clinical trials with canine distemper vaccines in exotic carnivores. J. Am. Vet. Med. Assoc. 183:1163–1167.

Morse, H.G., Chow, T.L., and Brandly, C.A. 1953. Propagation of a strain of egg-adapted distemper virus in suckling mice. Proc. Soc. Exp. Biol. Med. 84:10–12.

Moulton, J.E., and Brown, C.H. 1954. Antigenicity of canine distemper inclusion bodies as demonstrated by fluorescent antibody technic. Proc. Soc. Exp. Biol. Med. 86:99–102.

Noon, K.F., Rogul, M., Binn, L.N., Keefe, T.J., Marchwicki, R.H., and Appel, M.J. 1980. Enzyme-linked immunosorbent assay for evaluation of antibody to canine distemper virus. Am. J. Vet. Res. 41:605–609.

Norrby, E., and Appel, M.J. 1980. Humoral immunity to canine distemper after immunization of dogs with inactivated and live measles virus. Arch. Virol. 66:169–177.

Orvell, C. 1980. Structural polypeptides of canine distemper virus. Arch. Virol. 66:193–206.

Orvell, C., and Norrby, E. 1980. Immunological relationships between homologous structural polypeptides of measles and canine distemper virus. J. Gen. Virol. 50:231–245.

Palm, C.R., and Black, F.L. 1961. A comparison of canine distemper and measles viruses. Proc. Soc. Exp. Biol. Med. 107:588–590.

Pinkerton, H. 1940. Immunological and histological studies on mink distemper. J. Am. Vet. Med. Assoc. 96:347–355.

Polding, J.B., and Simpson, R.M. 1957. A possible immunological relationship between canine distemper and rinderpest. Vet. Rec. 69:582–584.

Polding, J.B., Simpson, R.M., and Scott, G.R. 1959. Links between canine distemper and rinderpest. Vet. Rec. 71:643–645.

Potgieter, L.N., and Patton, C.S. 1984. Multifocal cerebellar cortical necrosis caused by canine distemper virus infection in a raccoon. J. Am. Vet. Med. Assoc. 185:1397–1399.

Rima, B.K., Roberts, M.W., and Martin, S.J. 1983. Comparison of morbillivirus proteins by limited proteolysis. Med. Microbiol. Immunol. (Berl.) 171:203–213.

Robson, D.S., Kenneson, R., Gillespie, J.H., and Benson, T.F. 1959. Statistical studies of distemper in dogs. Proc. 9th Gaines Vet. Sympos. 9:10–14.

Ruckborn, G. 1958. Canine distemper virus in tissue culture. Arch. Gesam. Virusforsch. 8:485–492.

Rozenblatt, S., Eizenberg, O., Ben-Levy, R., Lavie, V., and Bellini, W.J. 1985. Sequence homology within the morbilliviruses. J. Virol. 53:684–690.

Rozenblatt, S., Eizenberg, O., Englund, G., and Bellini, W.J. 1985. Cloning and characterization of DNA complementary to the canine distemper virus mRNA encoding matrix, phosphoprotein, and nucleocapsid protein. J. Virol. 53:691–694.

Russell, S.E., Clarke, D.K., Hoey, E.M., Rima, B.K., and Martin, S.J. 1985. cDNA cloning of the messenger RNAs of five genes of canine distemper virus. J. Gen. Virol. 66:433–441.

Sato, T.A., Hayami, M., and Yamanouchi, K. 1981. Analysis of structural proteins of measles, canine distemper, and rinderpest viruses. Jpn. J. Med. Sci. Biol. 34:355–364.

Shen, D.T., and Gorham, J.R. 1980. Survival of pathogenic distemper virus at 5C and 25C. Vet. Med./Small Anim. Clin. 75:69–72.

Shen, D.T., Gorham, J.R., Evermann, J.F., and McKeirnan, A.J. 1984. Comparison of subcutaneous and intramuscular administration of a live attenuated distemper virus vaccine in ferrets. Vet. Rec. 114:42–43.

Summers, B.A., Greisen, H.A., and Appel, M.J. 1984. Canine distemper encephalomyelitis: variation with virus strain. J. Comp. Pathol. 94:65–75.

Vandevelde, M., and Kristensen, B. 1977. Observations on the distribution of canine distemper virus in the central nervous system of dogs with demyelinating encephalitis. Acta Neuropathol. (Berl.). 40:233–236.

Vandevelde, M., Zurbriggen, A., Higgins, R.J., and Palmer D. 1985. Spread and distribution of viral antigen in nervous canine distemper. Acta Neuropathol. (Berl.) 67:211–218.

West, J.L., and Brandly, C.A. 1949. The production of immunity to distemper in foxes by means of vaccines. Cornell Vet. 39:292–301.

Yamanouchi, K. 1980. Comparative aspects of pathogenicity of measles, canine distemper, and rinderpest viruses. Jpn. J. Med. Sci. Biol. 33:41–66.

Yamanouchi, K., Kobune, F., Fukuda, A., et al. 1970. Comparative immunofluorescent studies on measles, canine distemper, and rinderpest viruses. Immunofluorescence of measles, distemper, and rinderpestviruses. Arch. Gesam. Virusforsch. 29:90–100.

Rinderpest

SYNONYMS: Cattle plague, oriental cattle plague; abbreviation, RP

Rinderpest is an acute, febrile disease of ruminants characterized by fever, necrotic stomatitis, gastroenteritis, and high mortality. Known and feared since antiquity, it is an ancient plague of cattle and buffalo in Asia (Scott 1981). The disease originated in Asia and spread into Europe and Africa over the centuries by the numerous military campaigns. It is currently restricted to parts of Africa and Asia. Excellent review articles have been prepared by Appel et al. (1981), Plowright (1968), and Scott (1964, 1981).

Character of the Disease. The disease affects principally cattle, hence its name. In the Orient, water buffalos are frequent victims. Sheep, yaks, goats, some wild ungulates, camels, pigs, and even warthogs are susceptible to infection; but the disease is seldom serious, although a few large outbreaks have been reported.

The virulence of rinderpest virus (RPV) varies greatly from time to time and from place to place. The susceptibility of animals differs widely also. European and American cattle, which have had no contacts with the disease for many years, are generally highly susceptible. In Asia, where the disease is enzootic, the native cattle are much more resistant, probably because the more susceptible strains of such cattle have gradually been changed through many years of exposure. Some breeds of cattle appear to be more susceptible than others. In India so-called hill cattle are usually much more susceptible than

plains cattle. In the same outbreak the mortality of the former may be high and that of the latter light or negligible. The carabao, or water buffalo, the common beast of burden in much of southern Asia, is susceptible to rinderpest, sometimes more so than native cattle (Naik 1946, Pfaff 1940).

When the resistance of the host is high and the virus comparatively mild, the signs may be so slight as to be overlooked. It is thought that such animals often are the means of importing the disease into new localities or countries. They acquire permanent resistance as a result of the experience. Young calves from immune mothers often suffer only slightly from rinderpest and acquire an immunity because of it.

Acute rinderpest is the most common form and the only one that is likely ever to be seen in European cattle or in those of the Western Hemisphere, where this disease does not exist and where susceptibility is high.

Rinderpest is usually quite explosive; large numbers of animals are likely to exhibit signs almost simultaneously after an incubation period of 3 to 8 days. High fever (104° to 108°F) is an early sign and is seen about the third day of the disease; later the temperature falls and usually becomes subnormal before death. Rumination is suspended; there is dullness, and the coat becomes rough. The buccal mucosa becomes very congested. Early in the disease there is often constipation. The victim strains in defecating, and the bowel discharges are dry, often coated with mucus and sometimes with blood. Later there is severe diarrhea, and the feces becomes quite fluid and very fetid. Frequently there is a profuse nasal discharge and lacrimation. The breath becomes offensive because of the many shallow erosions on the lips, dental pads, and gums. The abdomen becomes very tender, the animal moans, becomes dull, goes down, and is unable to rise; death usually occurs between the second and sixth day after the first signs are exhibited. Some of the more resistant breeds may linger for 2 or 3 weeks. In some outbreaks the virulence of the virus is low, and many animals may show a longer course than usual. Mortality varies, although it is almost always high. In European and American cattle mortality of 90 to 100 percent must always be expected. It is lower than this in regions where the disease is enzootic.

For many years it was thought that rinderpest could be transmitted only to cattle, water buffalo, and a few other species of ruminants. However, a few authentic oubreaks in sheep and goats have been recognized in Nigeria. White-tailed deer given a virulent strain succumbed to experimental infection after showing typical signs of rinderpest (Hamdy et al. 1975).

Properties of the Virus. RPV is a member of the *Morbillivirus* genus and shares antigenic properties with the

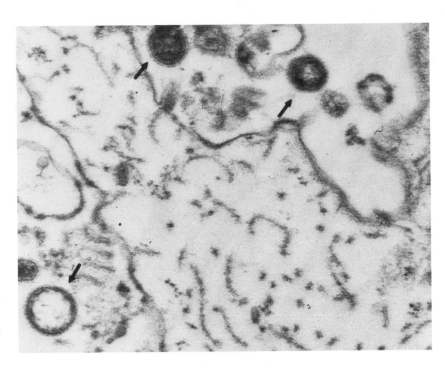

Figure 52.7. Rinderpest virus particles. Two mature particles (dark center) at top (*arrows*) and one immature particle (ghost particle) at bottom (*arrow*) in cell vacuoles. × 48,000. (Courtesy S. Breese, Plum Island Animal Disease Center, U.S. Dept. of Agriculture.)

other three members of this genus—canine distemper virus, measles virus, and peste des petits ruminants virus (Gibbs et al. 1979, Imagawa 1968, Polding and Simpson 1957, Sato et al. 1981).

The morphologic characteristics have been well described (Breese and de Boer 1963, Plowright 1962, Scott 1981, Tajima et al. 1971) (Figure 52.7). The particles are pleomorphic with an average diameter of 120 to 300 nm. Like other paramyxoviruses it has an internal helical component that is 17.5 nm in diameter with a periodicity of 5 to 6 nm, and this nucleocapsid is coiled like a ball of wool. There is an enclosing membrane, and the envelope bristles with minute filaments or projections.

The mRNAs involved in the replication of RPV and other morbilliviruses have considerable homology (Barrett and Underwood 1985).

RPV is quite stable after lyophilization and at very low temperatures (−70°C or less). High-passaged, tissue-cultured virus is relatively stable between pH 4 and 10, with the greatest stability between pH 7.2 and 7.9. Virulent strains are less stable under comparable conditions. The virus is stable in glycerol. Strong alkalis are the best disinfectants for its destruction. Certain chemicals, such as phenol, chinosol, formalin, and beta propiolactone, inactivate rinderpest-infected tissues without loss of antigenicity. Trypsin and 1 M hydroxylamine also inactivate the virus. A small fraction of tissue-cultured virus survives heating at 56°C for 50 to 60 minutes and at 60°C for 30 minutes.

Virus is inactivated rather quickly (in 1 or 2 days) in dried secretions, but in the presence of moisture it retains its activity somewhat longer. Boynton (1928) found that virus could never be detected by placing susceptible animals in corrals from which infected animals had been removed longer than 36 hours previously, even when water was present and parts of the area were shaded from the sun. He concluded that RPV does not survive long in pastures after affected animals are removed from them.

The virus contains antigens that produce neutralizing, complement-fixing and precipitating antibodies. Double diffusion in agar reveals a heat-stable and a heat-labile antigen. The viruses of measles, canine distemper, and rinderpest share a common antigen. RPV protects dogs against a challenge with virulent canine distemper virus. Interference with Rift Valley fever virus occurs, and attenuated rinderpest strains interfere with virulent ones. No hemagglutinin has been unequivocally demonstrated for RPV. Infected cell cultures do not cause hemadsorption of erythrocytes.

The peste des petits ruminants virus causes a rinderpestlike disease in goats and sheep in western Africa. It has all the characteristics of rinderpest virus (Hamdy et al. 1976) and originally was thought to be a biotype or strain of RPV, but now it is considered to be a separate virus in the genus (Gibbs et al. 1979, Hamdy et al. 1976).

Cultivation. Shope et al. (1946, 1946) succeeded in cultivating an African strain (the Kabete strain) on the chorioallantoic membranes of embryonated hens' eggs. They were not successful in adapting several other strains.

Kabete O strain of RPV multiplies and produces a

cytopathic effect in primary monolayer cultures of calf and lamb testes; bovine embryonic kidney cells; bovine skin-muscle tissue; pig, goat, sheep, and hamster kidneys; calf thyroid; and dog kidney (Plowright 1962). Virulent field strains selected from tissues of infected cattle regularly produce a cytopathic effect in primary calf kidney cultures (Plowright 1962). The cytopathogenic strains in calf kidney monolayers produce syncytia or multinucleated giant cells together with eosinophilic cytoplasmic and type B intranuclear inclusions. Strains of low virulence have a tendency to produce stellate cells that are large and sometimes multinucleated. There is more free virus in culture than cell-associated virus until the ninth day when the titers are comparable and drop rapidly (Plowright 1962).

Initially immunofluorescence antigen was not found in the nuclei except for a few granules in the later stages of infection. Using air-dried instead of acetone-fixed preparations, Liess (1966) showed fluorescent particles, often accompanied by perinuclear fluorescence, in the nucleus of infected cell cultures in as little as 8 hours. Cytoplasmic fluorescence was first noticed at 19 hours. It was concluded that the first synthesis of virus-specific materials probably occurred in the nucleus.

The Pendik strain of RPV in primary monolayers of bovine kidney cells produces plaques that become visible by 7 to 8 days and attain a diameter of 3 mm by day 12 and 5 mm by day 19 (McKercher 1963). Virus assay by plaque formation gives lower titers (approximately 2 $\log_{10}$ units) than 50 percent end points in monolayers. Plaque inhibition by specific immune serum is a usable system for virus identification.

Interferon produced in calf kidney cells by Sindbis virus suppresses the growth of a small amount of virulent RPV in the same cell type (Plowright 1968). It suppressed the yield of released virus more than the cell-associated virus replication for which there is no explanation.

Nakamura et al. (1938) adapted several strains to rabbits so the virus could be propagated in that species. In the early passages there are no signs except a slight temperature rise, which can easily be overlooked. After the virus has passed through several generations of rabbits, however, the animals show a sharp temperature rise during which they exhibit lassitude, inappetence, increased respiratory rate, and sometimes diarrhea. The febrile state lasts only about 36 to 48 hours, after which the signs subside and the animals again appear to be normal. Animals killed at the height of the temperature reaction often exhibit small necrotic areas in the intestinal mucosa, especially in the Peyer's patches. During this time there is a marked leukopenia. Further passage of the Nakamura III strain of lapinized RPV causes a very high mortality—

greater than 95 percent. It is a useful system to study rinderpest immunity.

Baker also adapted a strain of RPV to rabbits (Baker 1946) and guinea pigs (Baker et al. 1946). It also proliferates in mice, hamsters, dogs, ferrets, giant rats, and susliks (Plowright 1962)

Epizootiology and Pathogenesis. The disease is enzootic in parts of Asia and Africa. On many occasions, especially in times of war, it has spread from Asia to Europe where it has affected cattle principally (Hall 1962, Scott 1981). The results have often been devastating. During some of these epizootics a large portion of the entire cattle population perished. Only once has the disease appeared in the Western Hemisphere—in 1920 in Brazil—where it apparently had been imported in zebu cattle from India. This outbreak was quickly recognized and stamped out after fewer than 1,000 cattle had developed the disease; about 2,000 were slaughtered. Modern air travel has greatly increased the hazard of its bridging the oceans which have been our protectors in the past. Rinderpest could do great damage to the cattle population of North and South America should it ever gain a secure foothold, and veterinarians should constantly be on guard to detect it early.

Transmission. Rinderpest can be transmitted to susceptible animals by feed contaminated with infected blood, urine, feces, nasal discharges, and perspiration. Urine is believed to be especially important in the transmission of this disease. Some animals of the more resistant types may suffer from the disease and eliminate virulent infectious material while showing only mild signs themselves. When these animals are sent to market or shipped to distant points, they may introduce the disease into new localities. Because the virus is not particularly hardy, infected premises usually become free of infection within a relatively short time after diseased animals have been removed. There is little evidence that droplet infection plays any part in transmission, but infected meat may, since European pigs can acquire the disease by ingesting infected meat and can then spread the virus by contact to other pigs or to cattle or vice versa (Delay and Barber 1962, Scott et al. 1962). It has been suggested that the virus produces an exceedingly mild infection in pigs which may be overlooked and presumably the virus may persist in this host for as long as 36 days.

In cattle the disease is usually found in yearlings with no maternal immunity. It is of a mild type, especially in the resistant native breeds. Control is more difficult in Africa, where large populations of susceptible wildlife have the infection without any detectable mortality and morbidity.

Field experiments in Nigeria showed that RPV can be

spread, although irregularly, by close contact from cattle to sheep and goats and then to small ruminants; but spreading from sheep to cattle was not demonstrable and there was infrequent transfer from goats to cattle (Plowright 1968). Investigators have concluded that immunization of sheep and goats is not necessary once the disease has been eliminated from cattle. Obviously there is a slight element of risk, but the economic concerns warrant this risk in some countries.

The incubation period for naturally acquired rinderpest varies from 3 to 8 days. The virus enters through the respiratory mucosa or the pharyngeal area. Initial replication occurs in the tonsils or the pharyngeal and mandibular lymph nodes (Plowright 1964). Viremia occurs before fever is evident and terminates as neutralizing antibodies appear in the serum (Liess and Plowright 1964). During the acute disease virus is shed in ocular and nasal secretions (Mushi and Wafula 1984). Virus may persist for a few days in tissue, but there is no evidence that virus carriers exist (Scott 1981).

The gross and microscopic lesions of rinderpest are well described by Maurer et al. (1955). The principal ones are found in the digestive tract. Shallow ulcers are usually found in the mucosa of the mouth—in all parts except the dorsum of the tongue (Figures 52.8 and 52.9). These ulcers, which may also be found in the pharynx and esophagus, are shallow, have a "punched-out" appearance, and are filled with whitish caseous material. The mucosa of the abomasum is usually deeply congested. The livid membrane has areas of blood extravasation and dark purplish stripes. Ulceration of the pyloric orifice and folds is frequent. Sometimes the inflammatory exudate forms a false membrane that can easily be peeled off. The small intestine may exhibit similar lesions. The fluid con-

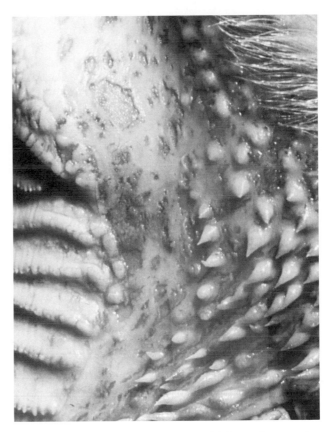

Figure 52.9. Rinderpest in a steer. Multiple erosions on the labial and buccal mucosa. (Courtesy D. A. Gregg, Plum Island Animal Disease Center, U.S. Dept. of Agriculture.)

Figure 52.8. Rinderpest in a steer. Multiple focal areas of necrosis on the mucosa of the lower lip. (Courtesy D. A. Gregg, Plum Island Animal Disease Center, U.S. Dept. of Agriculture.)

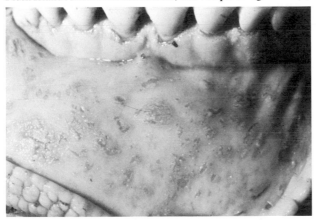

tent usually is fetid. Lesions in the large intestine include hemorrhages (Figure 52.10), and the rectum sometimes shows linear, bright red stripes—the so-called zebra striping. The Peyer's patches are usually ulcerated, and ulcers may be found on other parts of the mucosa.

The respiratory tract shows deep reddening of the upper passages and often petechiation. Patchy pneumonia, a purely secondary lesion, sometimes develops. If the animal lives more than a few days after becoming infected, there is marked dehydration of all tissues and extreme emaciation.

Plowright (1962) reported that lymphoid tissues also degenerate. Formation of syncytia with cytoplasmic inclusion bodies has been demonstrated in the stratum spinosum of stratified squamous epithelia of the buccal mucosa and upper alimentary tract and in lymphoid tissues (Figure 52.11 and 52.12) (Plowright 1962, Thiery 1956). Intranuclear inclusion bodies in vivo have been described by Thiery (1956).

Immunity. Animals surviving an attack of rinderpest from a living virus preparation are generally permanently

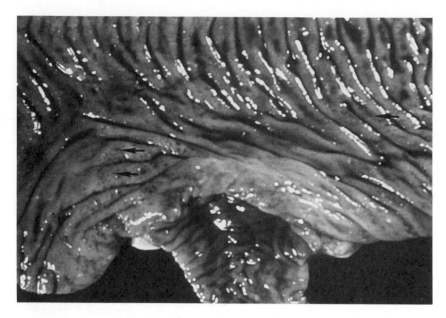

Figure 52.10. Rinderpest. Petechial and ecchymotic hemorrhage areas in the mucosal wall of the gastrointestinal tract. (Courtesy J. J. Callis and staff, Plum Island Animal Disease Center, U.S. Dept. of Agriculture.)

immune. Cattle vaccinated with a single dose of rinderpest cell-culture vaccine and isolated for 6 to 11 years were immune to challenge with RPV (Plowright 1984). These vaccinated cattle did not develop clinical signs, no viremia was detected, and they did not shed virus following virus challenge.

Immune animals have significant levels of neutralizing antibodies which are indicative of resistance. A small percentage of resistant animals may have no detectable circulating antibody. Vaccinated cattle develop both IgG and IgM antibodies, but not IgA antibodies (Sharma et al. 1985).

The hemagglutination-inhibition test, using measles virus hemagglutination, is applicable for detection of hemagglutination-inhibition antibodies, but its sensitivity is inferior to the neutralization test. Complement-fixing antibodies appear irregularly in the serums of recovered or vaccinated cattle, and they persist for only a short time; thus the test is suitable as a diagnostic method for individual herds but not for epidemiological surveys.

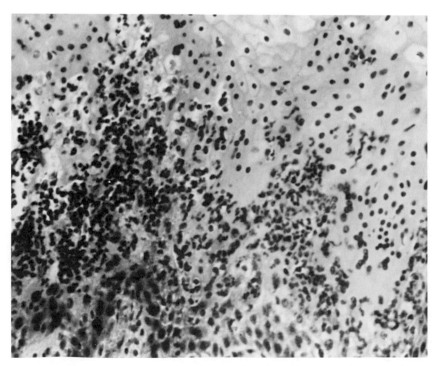

Figure 52.11. Rinderpest. The epithelial cells in the stratum spinosum of the buccal cavity of a steer are enlarged, and some have formed syncytia. Note the heavy infiltration of leukocytes in the epithelium on the left side. Hematoxylin and eosin stain. × 160. (Courtesy C. A. Mebus, Plum Island Animal Disease Center, U.S. Dept. of Agriculture.)

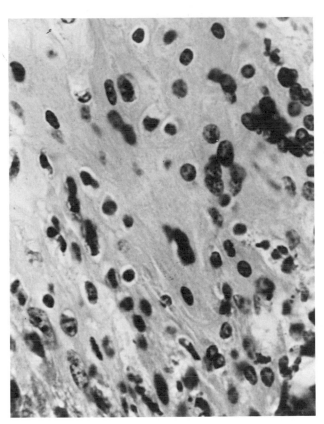

Figure 52.12. Rinderpest. The same pathological changes as in Figure 52.11, shown at a higher magnification (× 400). (Courtesy C. A. Mebus, Plum Island Animal Disease Center, U.S. Dept. of Agriculture.)

Antibody titers can be detected by the fluorescent antibody test, the immunoperoxidase test, or by the counterimmunoelectrophoresis test (Joshi et al. 1984, Rossiter and Mushi 1980). Enzyme-linked immunosorbent assay (ELISA) is a rapid and accurate test for antibody detection (Anderson et al. 1982, 1983).

Diagnosis. In areas where rinderpest is indigenous, the diagnosis usually presents few problems. It is based on the signs and lesions found at autopsy and also on the fact that the disease is highly contagious. In regions where the disease is not known, the diagnosis should be based on one or more of the following techniques: (1) the isolation of the virus from sick or dead animals; (2) detection of virus-specific antigens in the tissues; (3) demonstration of antibody production; (4) histological examination of tissues for virus-specific changes (Plowright 1968).

A tentative diagnosis is possible on the basis of gross examination and specific cytological changes, including the formation of syncytia and the presence of eosinophilic intracytoplasmic and perhaps intranuclear inclusion bodies as well (Plowright 1968). The best tissues for examination are lymphoid-epithelial, such as those from the tonsil, Peyer's patches, and lymph nodes, and also from lesions of the tongue, palate, and cheek papillae.

Studies in eastern Africa (Plowright and Ferris 1962) showed that naturally occurring strains can be readily recovered from the blood of infected cattle or wild animals in primary calf kidney cultures, making this a simple, rapid, and excellent aid in the diagnosis of rinderpest. The neutralization of the isolate with rinderpest antiserum confirms the isolation of RPV. The fluorescent antibody test also can be used for the detection of RPV.

Biopsies of lymph nodes of infected cattle can be performed and antigen can be tested for with the gel-diffusion agar technique (Brown and Scott 1960). A rapid complement-fixation test for the diagnosis of rinderpest by the use of tissue extracts of lymph node biopsy specimens from infected cattle gave excellent results (Stone and Moulton 1961). The testing of paired serum samples by the neutralization tests in cell cultures and in embryonated hens' eggs is also useful in its diagnosis.

A disease that closely resembles rinderpest, except that the mortality is much lower, is bovine virus diarrhea–mucosal disease (BVD-MD). Both BVD-MD and malignant catarrhal fever may have lesions that resemble those of rinderpest.

Prevention and Control. Methods for artificially immunizing animals both actively and passively are available. The earliest method was the injection of nasal and ocular secretions under the skin of the dewlap. Because this method often served to propagate the disease and the reactions usually were severe, it is no longer used. Robert Koch in 1897 introduced a great improvement when he showed that cattle could be successfully immunized with bile from animals killed on the fifth or sixth day of the disease. Normal bile is of no value. In 2 years more than 2 million cattle in South Africa were successfully immunized by this method. It has now been abandoned in favor of better vaccination procedures.

The methods used for artificially immunizing cattle against rinderpest today differ markedly in different parts of the world. Procedures that seem to be highly satisfactory in one area often prove too drastic or ineffective in others. Obviously the viral strains in different regions differ greatly in virulence, breeds of cattle differ greatly in susceptibility, and the efficacy of biologicals is sometimes questionable. For these reasons methods must be adapted to the particular areas and breeds involved.

Passive immunization. Serum from animals that have recovered from the disease possesses antibodies that are protective for susceptible animals. The value of such serum is greatly increased by hyperimmunization. Hyperimmune serum gives immediate protection, but resistance can be expected to last for only 10 days to 2 weeks. Immune serum has no value in treating the disease. Its principal use is to protect cattle against transient exposure, such as when they are driven or shipped through infected regions, and to stop the progress of the disease in recently infected herds.

Calves born of immune mothers obtain transient immunity through the colostral milk of their dams. Such animals resist infection. Active immunization of young calves from immune mothers is unsuccessful because maternal antibody interferes with active immunity.

Active immunization: Inactivated virus vaccines. A number of inactivated virus vaccines have been used with success. All are prepared by chemical treatment of tissue suspensions. They have the advantage of safety but the disadvantage of immunity that is only temporary. Generally they protect against ordinary exposure for up to 1 year. Because they did not give permanent immunity, these vaccines have been largely replaced by attenuated virus vaccines.

Active immunization: Host-adapted vaccines. These vaccines contain living virus that has been altered in virulence by serial passage through alien hosts. These vaccines cause mild, active infections that generally immunize cattle and carabao permanently, or at least for several years. The following is a list of host-adapted vaccines developed for rinderpest:

1. Caprinized (goat-adapted) vaccines. The goat-tissue vaccine has been used with success on many millions of cattle and carabao and appears to be most popular in southern Asia (Plaff 1938, Stirling 1932). In some highly susceptible breeds the vaccine may cause too much mortality. This could be offset in some cases by the administration of a small dose of antiserum with the vaccine.

2. Lapinized (rabbit-adapted) vaccines. Nakamura et al. (1938) attenuated the rinderpest virus by 100 passages in rabbits. The vaccine was made from the mesenteric lymph nodes of the infected rabbits. No preservatives were added. This virus keeps its viability for a short time only; hence it must be used promptly. It was employed extensively in China and Korea. Korean cattle are more susceptible to rinderpest than those of Manchuria, where the disease is enzootic. The vaccine alone served satisfactorily on the latter, but for the Korean cattle it was necessary to give a small dose of antiserum simultaneously. This vaccine is claimed to be less virulent than goat-adapted vaccine.

Cheng and Fischman (1948) vaccinated many cattle and carabao in China with a lapinized virus produced in the field with excellent results. When vaccine was needed, the vaccine strain was inoculated into rabbits. On the third or fourth day, when the temperature reaction was at its height, the rabbits were bled to death from the heart. The spleen and lymph nodes were pooled, finely ground, and diluted with the defibrinated blood in the proportion of 1:4. Next the mixture was diluted 1:100 with saline solutions. It was then ready for use and was always used within 8 hours of its preparation. Vaccine was also made by lyophilization of tissues; it kept satisfactorily for several months in the refrigerator.

3. Avianized (chick embryo–adapted) vaccines. Jenkins and Shope (1946) attenuated the Kabete strain of rinderpest virus by adapting it to develop in egg embryos. After 19 to 24 passages by yolksac inoculation the strain had lost enough virulence for cattle while retaining antigenicity to make it useful as an immunizing agent for cattle. After 50 to 60 passages the strain lost its immunizing properties. At the appropriate passage level, the strain solidly immunized calves against inoculation with fully virulent spleen virus. Vaccinated calves do not transmit the virus to susceptible animals, and thus this vaccine can be safely used in noninfected areas. Because the vaccine deteriorates rapidly, lyophilization must be employed and even then the vaccine must be stored and handled carefully. Hale and Walker (1946) described in detail large-scale production of the vaccine. Field tests in eastern Africa were satisfactory.

Brotherston (1951) propagated in rabbits the Nakamura lapinized strain of rinderpest virus in eastern Africa and used it successfully on many thousands of cattle of many different breeds. Most cattle show little reaction to the vaccine but are solidly immunized by it. Vaccinated cattle were tested by subcutaneous inoculation with virulent virus 8 to 15 months afterward and were found to be solidly immune. Natural exposure after 13 months likewise failed to break the immunity.

4. Tissue-cultured vaccines. After 70 or more passages in calf kidney monolayers the virulent Kabete O strain produced no detectable clinical reaction in eastern African cattle and was stable on serial cattle passage. The duration of immunity was probably at least 4 years, and the infective titer for cattle with this modified strain was comparable to the tissue-culture infectivity titer.

Cattle with East Coast fever have a diminished response, caused by massive lymphoid cell involvement, to rinderpest vaccination (Wagner et al. 1975).

In western Asia, India, and parts of Africa where rinderpest is indigenous, the disease is controlled principally by prophylactic vaccination. For this purpose the modified viruses seem to be the safest and most effective. In other parts of the world, including the Western Hemisphere, an embargo on the shipment of susceptible animals from infected areas has generally succeeded in excluding this disease. Because the virus is a rather delicate one which does not remain viable very long outside the body of infected animals, there appears to be relatively little danger of infection being imported into areas remote from enzootic regions by means of meat, hides, or other contaminated objects. The principal danger appears to be in the importation of live animals of the more resistant types that sometimes suffer from rather chronic, almost inapparent infections.

If the disease should manage to reach the United States, or any other country remote from the enzootic regions, it would undoubtedly be dealt with as foot-and-mouth disease has been handled in this country—by quarantine and slaughter. In countries free of the disease for long periods, or in those which have never been infected, rinderpest can be rapidly and completely eliminated by quarantine and vaccination (as in the Philippines in 1955), by movement restrictions and slaughter as (in Brazil and Australia), or by quarantine, slaughter, and antiserum as in Belgium (Plowright 1968).

The Disease in Humans. There is no evidence that RPV causes disease in humans.

REFERENCES

Anderson, J., Rowe, L.W., and Taylor, W.P. 1983. Use of an enzyme-linked immunosorbent assay for the detection of IgG antibodies to rinderpest virus in epidemiological surveys. Res. Vet. Sci. 34:77–81.

Anderson, J., Rowe, L.W., Taylor, W.P., and Crowther, J.R. 1982. An enzyme-linked immunosorbent assay for the detection of IgG, IgA, and IgM antibodies to rinderpest virus in experimentally infected cattle. Res. Vet. Sci. 32:242–247.

Appel, M.J.G., Gibbs, E.P.J., Martin, S.J., Ter Meulen, V., Rima, B.K., Stephenson, J.R., and Taylor, W.P. 1981. Morbillivirus diseases of animals and man. In E. Kurstak and C. Kurstak, eds, Comparative Diagnosis of Viral Diseases, vol. 4. Academic Press, New York. Pp. 187–233.

Baker, J.A. 1946. Rinderpest. Rinderpest infection in rabbits. Am. J. Vet. Res. 7:179–182.

Baker, J.A., Terrance, J., and Greig, A.S. 1946. Rinderpest. X. The response of guinea pigs to the virus of rinderpest. Am. J. Vet. Res. 7:189–192.

Barrett, T., and Underwood, B. 1985. Comparison of messenger RNAs induced in cells infected with each member of the morbillivirus group. Virology 145:195–199.

Boynton, W.H. 1928. Rinderpest, with special reference to its control by new method of prophylactic treatment. Philipp. J. Sci. 36:1–35.

Breese, S.S., Jr., and deBoer, C.J. 1963. Electron microscopy of rinderpest virus in bovine kidney tissue culture cells. Virology 19:340–348.

Brotherston, J.G. 1951. Lapinised rinderpest virus and a vaccine: Some observations in East Africa. I. Laboratory experiments. II. Field trials with lapinised vaccine. J. Comp. Pathol. 61:263–288, 289–306.

Brown, R.D., and Scott, G.R. 1960. Diagnosis of rinderpest by lymph node biopsy. Vet. Rec. 72:1055–1056.

Cheng, S.C., and Fischman, H.R. 1948. Lapinized rinderpest virus. In Food and Agricultural Organization Conference on Rinderpest, Nairobi, Kenya, no. 8, pp. 47–65.

Delay, P.O., and Barber, T.L. 1962. Transmission of rinderpest virus from experimentally infected cattle to pigs. Proc. U.S. Livestock Sanit. Assoc. 66:132–136.

Gibbs, E.P.J., Taylor, W.P., Lawman, M.J.P., and Bryant, J. 1979. Classification of peste des petits ruminants virus as the fourth member of the genus *Morbillivirus*. Intervirology 11:268–274.

Hale, M.W., and Walker, R.V.L. 1946. Rinderpest. XIII. The production of rinderpest vaccine from an attenuated strain of virus. Am. J. Vet. Res. 7:199–211.

Hall, S.A. 1962. The cattle plague of 1865. Med. Hist. 6:45–58.

Hamdy, F.M., Dardiri, A.H., Ferris, D.H., and Breese, S.S., Jr. 1975. Experimental infection of white-tailed deer with rinderpest virus. J. Wildl. Dis. 11:508–515.

Hamdy, F.M., Dardiri, A.H., Nduaka, O., Breese, S.S., and Ihemelandu, E.C. 1976. Etiology of the stomatitis pneumonenteritis complex in Nigerian dwarf goats. Can. J. Comp. Med. 40:276–284.

Imagawa, D.T. 1968. Relationship among measles, canine distemper, and rinderpest viruses. Prog. Med. Virol. 10:160–193.

Jenkins, D.L., and Shope, R.E. 1946. Rinderpest. VII. The attenuation of rinderpest virus for cattle by cultivation in embryonating eggs. Am. J. Vet. Res. 7:174–178.

Joshi, R.C., Sharma, B., Bandyopadhyay, S.K., and Bansal, R.P. 1984. Detection of rinderpest antibodies. Trop. Anim. Health Prod. 16:167–170.

Liess, B. 1966. Untersuchungen über das Virus der Rinderpest unter Verwendung von Zellkulturen. Arch. Exp. Vet. Med. 20:157–257.

Liess, B., and Plowright, W. 1964. Studies on the pathogenesis of rinderpest in experimental cattle. I. Correlation of clinical signs, viraemia and virus excretion by various routes. J. Hyg. 62:81–100.

McKercher, P.D. 1963. Plaque production by rinderpest virus in bovine kidney cultures: A preliminary report. Can. J. Comp. Med. 27:71–72.

Maurer, F.D., Jones, T.C., Easterday, B., and DeTray, D. 1955. The pathology of rinderpest. In Proceedings of the Annual Meeting of the American Veterinary Medical Association. Pp. 201–211.

Mushi, E.Z., and Wafula, J.S. 1984. The shedding of a virulent Kabete O strain of rinderpest virus by cattle. Vet. Res. Commun. 8:173–179.

Naik, R.N. 1946. Rinderpest and its control in the province of Bombay. Indian Vet. J. 23:203–216.

Nakamura, J., Wagatsuma, S., and Fukusko, K. 1938. On the experimental infection with rinderpest virus in the rabbit. I. Some fundamental experiments. J. Jpn. Soc. Vet. Sci. 17:185–204.

Pfaff, G. 1938. Immunization against rinderpest, with special reference to the use of dried goat spleen. Onderstepoort J. Vet. Sci. 11:263–330.

Pfaff, G. 1940. Rinderpest in buffaloes. The immunizing value of dried goat spleen vaccine. Onderstepoort J. Vet. Sci. 15:175–184.

Plowright, W. 1962. Rinderpest virus. Comp. Virol. N.Y. Acad. Sci. 101:548–563.

Plowright, W. 1964. Studies on the pathogenesis of rinderpest in experimental cattle. II. Proliferation of the virus in different tissues following intranasal infection. J. Hyg. 62:267–281.

Plowright, W. 1968. Rinderpest virus. Virol. Monogr. 3:27–110.

Plowright, W. 1984. The duration of immunity in cattle following inoculation of rinderpest cell culture vaccine. J. Hyg. 92:285–296.

Plowright, W., and Ferris, R.D. 1962. Studies with rinderpest virus in tissue culture. The use of attenuated culture virus as a vaccine for cattle. Res. Vet. Sci. 3:172–182.

Polding, J.B., and Simpson, R.M. 1957. A possible immunological relationship between canine distemper and rinderpest. Vet. Rec. 69:582–584.

Rossiter, P.B., and Mushi, E.Z. 1980. Rapid detection of rinderpest virus antigens by counter-immunoelectrophoresis. Trop. Anim. Health Prod. 12:209–216.

Sato, T.A., Hayami, M., and Yamanouchi, K. 1981. Analysis of structural proteins of measles, canine distemper, and rinderpest viruses. Jpn. J. Med. Sci. Biol. 34:355–364.

Scott, G.R. 1964. Rinderpest. Adv. Vet. Sci. 9:113–224.

Scott, G.R. 1981. Rinderpest and peste des petits ruminants. In E.P.J. Gibbs, ed., Virus Diseases of Food Animals, vol. 2. Academic Press, London. Pp. 401–432.

Scott, G.R., DeTray, D.E., and White, G. 1962. Rinderpest in pigs of European origin. Am. J. Vet. Res. 23:452–456.

Sharma, B., Bandyopadhyay, S.K., Joshi, R.C., and Bansal, R.P. 1985. Antibody response of cattle to rinderpest vaccine. Vet. Microbiol. 10:189–192.

Shope, R.E., Griffiths, H.J., and Jenkins, D.L. 1946. Rinderpest. I. The cultivation of rinderpest virus in the developing hen's egg. Am. J. Vet. Res. 7:135–141.

Shope, R.E., Maurer, F.D., Jenkins, D.L., Griffiths, H.J., and Baker, J.A. 1946. Rinderpest. IV. Infection of the embryos and the fluids of developing hens' eggs. Am. J. Vet. Res. 7:152–163.

Stirling, R.F. 1932. Some experiments in rinderpest vaccination: Active immunisation of Indian plains cattle by inoculation with goat-adapted virus alone in field conditions. Vet. J. 88:192–204.

Stone, S.S., and Moulton, W.M. 1961. A rapid serologic test for rinderpest. Am. J. Vet. Res. 22:18–22.

Tajima, M., Motohashi, T., Kishi, S., and Nakamura, J. 1971. A comparative electron microscopic study on the morphogenesis of canine distemper and rinderpest viruses. Jpn. J. Vet. Sci. 33:1–10.

Thiery, G. 1956. Hématologie, histopathologie et histochimie de la peste bovine. Intérêt de l'étude histochimique des inclusions cellulaires de la peste bovine pour la signification générale des inclusions dans les maladies à virus. Rev. Elev. Méd. Vét. Pays Trop. 9:117–140.

Wagner, G.G., Jessett, D.M., Brown, C.G.D., and Radley, D.E. 1975. Diminished antibody response to rinderpest vaccination in cattle undergoing experimental East Coast fever. Res. Vet. Sci. 19:209–211.

Peste des Petits Ruminants

SYNONYMS: Kata, stomatitis pneumoenteritis complex; abbreviations, PPR, SPC

Peste des petits ruminants is a rinderpestlike disease of goats, sheep, and other small ruminants such as deer which occurs in western Africa and certain other African countries (Scott 1981). It is caused by a morbillivirus similar to the other three morbilliviruses—canine distemper virus, measles virus, and rinderpest virus. PPR has been reviewed by Appel et al. (1981) and Scott (1981). PPR was first recognized and named by Gargadennec and Lalanne (1942) in the Ivory Coast of western Africa in sheep and goats that were experiencing a rinderpestlike disease. For many years the causative virus was considered to be a strain of rinderpest virus, but eventually it was shown that PPR virus (PPRV), although antigenically similar in some respects to rinderpest virus, was in fact a separate virus in the genus *Morbillivirus* (Gibbs et al. 1979, Hamdy et al. 1976).

Character of the Disease. The clinical disease produced by PPRV in sheep and goats mimics that of rinderpest, but the course is much more rapid. The incubation period is short (2 to 6 days), the onset of fever and signs is rapid, and lesions appear within hours of the onset of fever. Affected animals usually have ocular and nasal discharges, which start out serous but become mucopurulent with crust formation around the eyes and nostrils. Diarrhea frequently occurs within 2 or 3 days,

and affected animals may have secondary pasteurella pneumonia terminally. Mortality is high, death usually occurs within 1 week of the onset of signs. Pregnant animals may abort (Appel et al. 1981, Scott 1981).

Goats appear to be most susceptible to disease, but sheep are also susceptible. The white-tailed deer (*Odocoileus virginianus*) is fully susceptible to PPRV (Hamdy and Dardiri 1976). Cattle have subclinical infections, or at most mild clinical disease, with the development of active immunity.

Properties of the Virus. PPRV is very similar to rinderpest virus in physical and chemical properties (Durojaiye et al. 1985, Gibbs et al. 1979).

Epizootiology and Pathogenesis. PPR spreads rapidly by direct contact (Whitney et al. 1967), and indirect spread may also occur (Gargadannec and Lalanne 1942). Endemic areas are the tropical zones of western Africa and Chad; explosive outbreaks in isolated areas usually follow purchase or marketing of animals (Durtnell 1972, Scott 1981, Taylor 1979a, Whitney et al. 1967). Virus has been isolated in Sudan (El Hag Ali and Taylor 1984) and in Nigeria (Obi et al. 1983); and serologic evidence indicates that the virus is more widespread in some areas, such as Nigeria (Obi et al. 1984, Taylor 1979a). The pathological changes in goats dying of PPR include dehydration, mucopurulent ocular and nasal discharges with crusts, erosive stomatitis and pharyngitis, enteric lesions appearing as "zebra stripes" in the large intestine, and pneumonia (Scott 1981).

Immunity. Goats that have recovered from PPR are resistant to reinfection, but the duration of the resistance is not known (Scott 1981).

Diagnosis. The diagnosis of PPR is usually based on clinical signs and post mortem findings. If further confirmation is needed, virus can be isolated in cell culture, and immunofluorescence tests can be run on sections of infected tissues (Hamdy et al 1976, Scott 1981, Taylor and Abegunde 1979). Agar-gel precipitation tests and counterimmunoelectrophoresis tests can be run to detect PPR antigen (Obi and Patrick 1984). Antibodies against PPRV can be detected by a variety of tests, including microneutralization (Rossiter et al. 1985).

Prevention and Control. PPR can be prevented by immunization with rinderpest vaccine (Gibbs et al. 1979, Taylor 1979b), or by the simultaneous administration of PPR hyperimmune bovine serum and virulent PPRV (Adu and Joannis 1984). Methods such as quarantine and movement control would be quite difficult to implement in endemic areas (Appel et al. 1981). Hyperimmune serum has also been used to control PPR (Ihemelandu et al. 1985).

The Disease in Humans. There is no known susceptibility of humans to this virus.

REFERENCES

Adu, F.D., and Joannis, T.E. 1984. Serum-virus simultaneous method of immunisation against peste des petits ruminants. Trop. Anim. Health Prod. 16:119–122.

Appel, M.J.G., Gibbs, E.P.J., Martin, S.J., Ter Meulen, V., Rima, B.K., Stephenson, J.R., and Taylor, W.P. 1981. Morbillivirus diseases of animals and man. In E. Kurstak and C. Kurstak, eds., Comparative Diagnosis of Viral Diseases, vol. 4. Academic Press, New York. Pp. 187–233.

Durojaiye, O.A., Taylor, W.P., and Smale, C. 1985. The ultrastructure of peste des petits ruminants virus. Zentralbl. Veterinärmed. [B] 32:460–465.

Durtnell, R.E. 1972. A disease of Sokoto goats resembling "peste des petits ruminants." Trop. Anim. Health Prod. 4:162–164.

El Hag Ali, B., and Taylor, W.P. 1984. Isolation of peste des petits ruminants virus from the Sudan. Res. Vet. Sci. 36:1–4.

Gargadennec, L., and Lalanne, A. 1942. La peste des petits ruminants. Bull. Serv. Zootech. Epizoot. l'Afrique Occid. Fr. 5:16–21.

Gibbs, E.P.J., Taylor, W.P., Lawman, M.J.P., and Bryant, J. 1979. Classification of peste des petits ruminants virus as the fourth member of the genus *Morbillivirus*. Intervirology 11:268–274.

Hamdy, F.M., and Dardiri, A.H. 1976. Response of white-tailed deer to infection with peste des petits ruminants virus. J. Wildl. Dis. 12:516–522.

Hamdy, F.M., Dardiri, A.H., Nduaka, O., Breese, S.S., and Ihemelandu, E.C. 1976. Etiology of the stomatitis pneumoenteritis complex in Nigerian dwarf goats. Can. J. Comp. Med. 40:276–284.

Ihemelandu, E.C., Nduaka, O., and Ojukwu, E.M. 1985. Hyperimmune serum in the control of peste des petits ruminants. Trop. Anim. Health Prod. 17:83–88.

Obi, T.U., and Patrick, D. 1984. The detection of peste des petits ruminants (PPR) virus antigen by agar gel precipitation test and counterimmunoelectrophoresis. J. Hyg. 93:579–586.

Obi, T.U., Ojo, M.O., Durojaiye, O.A., Kasali, O.B., Akpavie, S., and Opasina, D.B. 1983. Peste des petits ruminants (PPR) in goats in Nigeria: Clinical, microbiological and pathological features. Zentralbl. Veterinärmed. [B] 30:751–761.

Obi, T.U., Rowe, L.W., and Taylor, W.P. 1984. Serological studies with peste des petits ruminants and rinderpest viruses in Nigeria. Trop. Anim. Health Prod. 16:115–118.

Rossiter, P.B., Jessett, D.M., and Taylor, W.P. 1985. Microneutralization systems for use with different strains of peste des petits ruminants virus and rinderpest virus. Trop. Anim. Health Prod. 17:75–81.

Scott, G.R. 1981. Rinderpest and peste des petits ruminants. In E.P.J. Gibbs, ed., Virus Diseases of Food Animals, vol. 2. Academic Press, London. Pp. 401–432.

Taylor, W.P. 1979a. Serological studies with the virus of peste des petits ruminants in Nigeria. Res. Vet. Sci. 26:236–242.

Taylor, W.P. 1979b. Protection of goats against peste des petits ruminants with attenuated rinderpest virus. Res. Vet. Sci. 26:321–324.

Taylor, W.P. and Abegunde, A. 1979. Isolation of peste des petits ruminants virus from Nigerian sheep and goats. Res. Vet. Sci. 26:94–96.

Whitney, J.C., Scott, G.R., and Hill, D.H. 1967. Preliminary observations on a stomatitis and enteritis of goats in southern Nigeria. Bull. Epizoot. Dis. Afr. 15:31–41.

The Genus *Paramyxovirus*

Newcastle Disease

SYNONYMS: Avian paramyxovirus, pneumoencephalitis, pseudo fowl pest, pseudoplague of fowls, Ranikhet disease; abbreviation, ND

Newcastle disease, an acute, highly contagious, viral disease of chickens, turkeys, and other birds, is characterized by respiratory disease, neurological disease, enteritis, hemorrhagic lesions, and often high mortality. Severity of outbreaks may vary from extremely destructive, with mortality up to 90 percent, to subclinical infections.

The disease was first encountered by Kraneveld (1926) in Djakarta, Indonesia. Its name was derived from an outbreak that occurred in a flock of chickens in Newcastle-on-Tyne, England (Doyle 1927). By the 1940s Newcastle disease had been recognized worldwide. Its identification in California marked the first recognition of the malady in the Western Hemisphere (Beach 1942, 1944). Although the virus frequently produces grave epizootics and high mortality among fowl in the Eastern Hemisphere, the percentages of losses in the Western Hemisphere vary considerably and depend on many factors.

Chickens, turkeys, guinea fowl, ducks, geese, pigeons, doves, pheasants, partridges, and many wild birds are susceptible to infection (Biancifiori and Fioroni 1983; Brandly et al. 1946; Brugh and Beard 1984; Lancaster 1966; Mackenzie et al. 1984; Vickers and Hanson 1982a, 1982b). The virus sometimes causes conjunctivitis in humans.

ND has been reviewed by several writers, including Beard and Hanson (1984), Brandly (1959), Frank (1981), Hanson (1978), Hanson and Brandly (1958), and Lancaster (1966, 1981).

Character of the Disease. Outbreaks of ND vary greatly in intensity. Five forms are recognized: viscerotropic velogenic, neurotropic velogenic, mesogenic, lentogenic, and asymptomatic (Alexander and Allan 1974, Beard and Hanson 1984, Frank 1981, Lancaster 1981). All five forms are caused by various strains of Newcastle disease virus (NDV).

Velogenic forms. The velogenic form may appear as the Doyle's form (Doyle 1927) caused by the strain of virus known as the *viscerotropic velogenic* Newcastle disease (VVND) virus (Hanson et al. 1973, McDaniel and Osborn 1973), or the Beach's form (Beach 1942), which is also called avian pneumoencephalitis and is caused by the *neurotropic velogenic* strain of virus. The onset of the velogenic form of disease is sudden and peracute deaths are common. Marked depression, dyspnea, and progressive prostration occur. Diarrhea and dehydration are frequently seen, and edema of the head may occur. The mortality of the velogenic form of disease in a susceptible flock may approach 100 percent.

Mesogenic form. Also known as Beaudette's form (Beaudette and Black 1946), the mesogenic form of ND is characterized by rapid spread of respiratory infection with dyspnea and cough, followed by the appearance of neurological signs. Mortality may approach 50 percent.

Lentogenic form. Also called Hitchner's form (Hitchner and Johnson 1948), the lentogenic form is character-

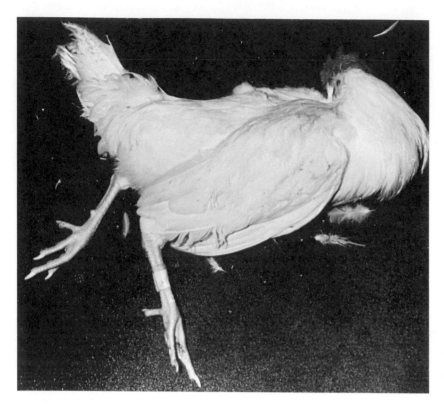

Figure 52.13. Torticollis in a chicken after inoculation with Texas GB strain of Newcastle disease virus. (Courtesy D. A. Gregg, Plum Island Animal Disease Center, U.S. Dept. of Agriculture.)

ized by mild respiratory signs without neurological signs and with negligible mortality.

Asymptomatic form. Several countries report the asymptomatic form, which has no clinical signs of illness.

Birds of all ages are susceptible to ND, but young ones are usually more severely affected than older ones. The disease usually begins with respiratory signs, often followed by diarrhea. The incubation period varies from 4 to 14 days, with an average of about 5 days.

The severity of the disease in a flock depends on the age and immunity status of birds, strain virulence, route of infection, and concurrent infections. In chicks from a few days to a few weeks old the velogenic form of the disease begins with respiratory signs often followed by profuse diarrhea. The infection spreads rapidly, and respiratory distress is evidenced by gasping, which may be accompanied by moist rales and crackling sounds. In many outbreaks nervous signs appear a few days after the onset of the respiratory syndrome. Very young chicks may show profound stupor. Birds often rest on their hocks with toes slightly flexed, head depressed, and eyes closed, or they appear to be unable to use one or both legs and remain in lateral recumbency. Others may show signs of ataxia, such as staggering, torticollis (Figure 52.13), opisthotonos, and posterior propulsion. Handling them often intensifies the nervous manifestations. The death rate usually is high, and those that survive often are worthless. In adult birds the signs are quite comparable to those in chicks, with a mortality of 90 to 100 percent. The mesogenic form causes less severe disease, and in laying flocks there is a sudden drop in egg production along with the appearance of grossly abnormal eggs. The eggs that are laid after the nonlaying period are frequently misshapen and usually have soft, imperfectly formed shells. Often the only change observed in a laying flock with the lentogenic form is a slight reduction in egg production, which may not return to former levels until 4 to 8 weeks after the birds recover.

In turkey poults the disease may be severe and may result in 50 percent mortality.

Properties of the Virus. NDV belongs to the *Paramyxovirus* genus and it has the same structural features as other members of this genus. It is a single-stranded RNA virus. There are at least nine distinct antigenic types of avian paramyxoviruses (PMV-1 to PMV-9); NDV is the prototype and is designated avian PMV-1/NDV (Alexander 1980, Beard and Hanson 1984). Research on NDV, including characterization of the nucleic acid, has been extensive (Collins et al. 1980, 1982; Hamaguchi et al. 1985; Kurilla et al. 1985). These avian paramyxoviruses share biochemical and biophysical properties with other paramyxoviruses (reviewed by Chanock and McIntosh 1985). Antigenically NDV is closely related to human parainfluenza virus type 1.

There is a high degree of cross-reactivity between avian

paramyxovirus type 1 isolated from racing pigeons and NDV (Alexander et al. 1984). However, these viruses could be differentiated on the basis of varying hemagglutination-inhibition titers.

NDV is destroyed by pasteurization and exposure to ultraviolet light. Pulp of infected organs dried in vacuo over phosphorus pentoxide and stored in the refrigerator remains virulent for years. Allantoic-amniotic fluid from infected embryonated eggs retains its virulence for several years if stored in the moist or lyophilized state at −70°C. Boyd and Hanson (1958) studied the survivability of the virus in soils at varying temperatures and humidities. In the presence of some moisture the virus proved to be surprisingly resistant. NDV is inactivated by formalin and by heating to 60°C for 30 minutes.

Cultivation. NDV is readily cultivated in embryonated chicken eggs. Bacteriologically sterile suspensions of virus-containing material are inoculated through the chorioallantoic membrane; the virus kills the embryo in about 2 to 6 days. In eggs with embryos dead on the third day or later, and occasionally in eggs with embryos dead on the second day, a small opaque area is found on the chorioallantois at the point of inoculation. Sometimes the membrane is edematous. The yolk sac vessels are congested, and the embryo is reddened, especially in the feet and legs. The skin around the head often shows hemorrhages, and the liver is usually congested.

NDV produces a cytopathic effect in a variety of cell cultures. In some cell lines the effect is only visible microscopically. Cytoplasmic inclusion bodies and multinucleated cells also occur in cultures. Occasionally well-defined intranuclear inclusion bodies are observed. Cell cultures may become chronically infected with or without virus release and frequently show no cytopathic effect. When interferon mediates persistent infections, the cells usually are resistant to other closely related viruses.

Epizootiology and Pathogenesis. NDV spreads readily by direct contact or by aerosol between infected and susceptible birds. Chicks may carry the virus from an infected hatchery, or from contact with diseased fowl while en route, to the poultry farm. Susceptible birds can contract the disease from infected excretions or organs of diseased fowl, from water contaminated by such fowl, and from infected feed bags and feed containers. Eggs laid by hens with acute infection may contain virus; after a flock has returned to full production, no virus is found in the eggs.

Transmission may also occur from chronically infected asymptomatic birds in the family Psittacidae (Lancaster 1981) and from wild pigeons that contaminate foodstuffs. In Great Britain in 1983 and 1984, 19 of 22 outbreaks of ND were caused directly or indirectly by avian paramyxovirus 1–infected pigeons infesting feed stores and thus contaminating feed (Alexander et al. 1985).

The virus generally enters the susceptible bird either by mouth or by aerosol transmission. Early replication occurs in the upper respiratory tract, and the virus can be readily isolated from the trachea. The tissues affected after the initial replication depend on the strain of NDV involved and the species of bird infected. The less virulent strains result only in intestinal infections, while the more virulent strains, such as the velogenic, produce severe, often fatal infections of the respiratory or nervous systems (Lancaster 1981).

The nature and extent of the lesions are governed by the pathogenicity of the disease. In mild cases the only changes may be cloudy air sac membranes, an enlarged spleen, and fluid or mucus in the trachea. In the velogenic form petechial hemorrhages, and sometimes erosions, may be present in the mucosa of proventriculus, cloaca (Figure 52.14), gizzard, and intestinal tract. The spleen may be enlarged and other organs congested. In the laying hen there often is an accumulation of fresh, watery yolk in the ovum and accompanying congestion of the ovarian blood vessels. When nervous signs are observed, microscopic lesions of mild encephalitis usually are found.

The pathogenesis of tracheal infections in chickens and turkeys has been studied in detail (Abdul-Aziz and Arp 1983a, 1983b; Lai and Ibrahim 1983).

Immunity. Fowl that recover from Newcastle disease are immune for years. The hemagglutination-inhibiting and serum-neutralizing antibodies are criteria of immunity, and they both persist for years. Some birds without antibody may withstand exposure to virulent virus; in them, cell-mediated mechanisms as well as humoral immunity probably are involved in protection.

In mammals the antibody activity in secretions is associated with secretory IgA. This association is also found in chickens, except that chicken IgA lacks the secretory component (Katz and Kohn 1976). After injection with NDV, there is an increase in total serum protein which parallels an increase in serum-neutralizing (SN), hemagglutination-inhibition (HI), and precipitating (P) antibodies. The SN, HI, and P antibodies are detected in both IgM and IgG immunoglobulins. Serum IgM appears during the first week after injection of virus, then diminishes, but rises again after secondary vaccination (Khare et al. 1976).

Mechanisms of host resistance to inactivated and mesogenic strains of NDV were studied in normal and immunodeficient birds (Perey and Dent 1975). Most normal birds resisted mesogenic NDV, but T cell–deficient birds were more susceptible, and agammaglobulinemic birds were extremely susceptible. There was no difference in the kinetics and levels of HI activity of plasma in control,

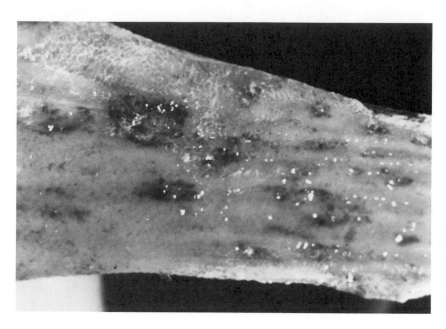

Figure 52.14. Cloaca of a chicken showing hemorrhagic areas and shallow erosions on mucosal surface after inoculation with a velogenic strain of Newcastle disease virus. (Courtesy D. A. Gregg, Plum Island Animal Disease Center, U.S. Dept. of Agriculture.)

irradiated, and T cell–deficient birds or between dying and surviving birds. Agammaglobulinemic chickens can be partially protected against a lethal challenge following immunization with lentogenic NDV or beta propiolactone–inactivated NDV mixed with complete Freund's adjuvant. Chickens immunized with a lentogenic strain of NDV 2 to 9 weeks before challenge with virulent virus remain normal, but virus can be found in the circulating leukocytes for as long as 10 days (Turner et al. 1976).

Diagnosis. Newcastle disease should be suspected when respiratory disease in chicks is associated with or followed by nervous or paralytic signs and when tracheal exudates and clouded air sacs are found on autopsy. Since the disease is primarily a respiratory infection, in the absence of nervous signs it is most likely to be confused with infectious bronchitis. Laryngotracheitis also exhibits respiratory signs, but gasping is more pronounced and respiration more rhythmical. Nervous signs appear in vitamin-deficiency diseases of chicks and in encephalomyelitis (epidemic tremor), but in these diseases no initial respiratory signs are seen. The fowl plague syndrome also simulates that of ND and must be considered in the differential diagnosis in countries where it exists.

Virus isolation and identification or serum-neutralization tests establish the identity of ND. Early in the course of the disease good sources of the virus are tracheal exudate, spleen, and brain. Within a few days after onset, surviving birds show positive serum-neutralization reactions.

Fabricant (1949) compared the results of HI and serum-neutralization SN tests in infected chickens and found that the HI test reached a positive level sooner than the SN test.

His studies indicated that the HI titer became positive from 2 days before to 5 days after (average, 2 days after) the first appearance of respiratory signs. This test has proved quite satisfactory for rapid diagnosis of ND.

Enzyme-linked immunosorbent assays (ELISAs) are also effective in the diagnosis of antibodies against NDV (Miers et al. 1983).

Prevention and Control. The prevention and control of ND in commercial flocks involves a combination of strict measures by control officials to prevent entrance into a country of virulent or exotic strains of NDV; vaccination programs; good husbandry techniques, including the prevention of contamination of feedstuffs; and, when necessary, government-controlled quarantine and slaughter programs (Walker et al. 1973).

Because ND is highly contagious and spreads readily through direct contact, in an outbreak removal of birds from the infected house may eliminate the infection. Frequently, though, the disease has spread so quickly that birds in other houses on the premises are exposed by the time it is diagnosed. Levine et al. (1950) concluded that birds recovered from ND do not harbor sufficient virus to infect susceptible birds 1 month after the flock recovers from respiratory signs.

Annual replacement of the laying flock at the end of the first laying year, with segregation of the replacement stock and the application of all sanitary precautions, has effectively controlled the disease on certain poultry farms.

Inactivated, inactivated oil-emulsion, and modified live-virus vaccines have been used with varying degrees of success to protect birds against NDV (Bankowski

1957; Beaudette et al. 1949; Brugh et al. 1983; Gale et al. 1965; Giambrone 1985; Hitchner 1950; Hitchner and Johnson 1948; Hofstad 1956; Ibrahim et al. 1980, 1983; Iyer and Dobson 1940; Komarov and Goldsmit 1947; Lancaster 1981; Shuaib et al. 1985; Stone 1985; Westbury et al. 1984; Winterfield et al. 1980). The production and use of vaccines have been reviewed by Allan et al. (1979). Vaccination programs that have controlled NDV in one country have failed in others (Lancaster 1981).

Interference with vaccination in young chicks by passive maternal antibody in the yolk sac, may affect vaccination programs. Chicks from flocks with high levels of antibodies in the yolk sac against NDV may be resistant to vaccination up to 3 weeks of age (Lancaster 1981).

Because of the large number of birds housed together and the usual requirement of multiple vaccinations per bird, individual vaccination is often impractical. Thus, vaccination of groups of birds by addition of modified live-virus vaccine in the drinking water or by aerosolization of vaccine virus is popular (Lancaster 1981).

Studies of the residual virulence of three vaccine strains of NDV indicated that strain V4 is less virulent for chickens than the B1 strain, which in turn is less virulent than the La Sota strain (Westbury et al. 1984).

Mineral oil–emulsion vaccines were shown to be superior to vaccines containing metabolizable lipid emulsion adjuvant (Brugh et al. 1983).

Birds infected with infectious bursal disease virus may have immunosuppression due to damage of the bursa of Fabricius and thus may have a decreased immune response to ND vaccines (Almassy and Kakuk 1976, Faragher et al. 1974, Lancaster 1981).

Infectious bronchitis (IB) virus interferes with NDV replication (Raggi et al. 1963), therefore the practice of combining IB and ND vaccines should be discouraged.

The Disease in Humans. NDV causes conjunctivitis in humans, and several reports of its isolation from patients with this condition have been published (Chang 1981, Freymann and Bang 1949, Ingalls and Mahoney 1949). Patients show acute unilateral or bilateral conjunctivitis. No systemic symptoms appear, and no ill effects are noted other than a mild conjunctival irritation that lasts about 3 to 7 days. In pathogenesis studies of ocular infection with NDV in rabbits and monkeys, conjunctivitis could be established in these species only when conjunctival epithelium was traumatized, whereas intact epithelium was resistant to infection (Charan et al. 1984).

Agglutinins against NDV-modified human group O erythrocytes and antibodies against NDV have been detected in serums from patients with various diseases (Powell et al. 1985). The incidence varied between 17 and 30 percent for such human diseases as multiple sclerosis, leprosy, systemic lupus erythematosus, and cancer. There is no indication that NDV is associated with any of these diseases.

REFERENCES

Abdul-Aziz, T.A., and Arp, L.H. 1983a. Pathology of the trachea in turkeys exposed by aerosol to lentogenic strains of Newcastle disease virus. Avian Dis. 27:1002–1011.

Abdul-Aziz, T.A., and Arp, L.H. 1983b. Progression of tracheal lesions in turkeys exposed by aerosol to LaSota strain of Newcastle disease virus. Avian Dis. 27:1131–1141.

Alexander, D.J. 1980. Avian paramyxoviruses. Vet. Bull. 50:737–752.

Alexander, D.J., and Allan, W.H. 1974. Newcastle disease virus pathotypes. Avian Pathol. 3:269–278.

Alexander, D.J., Russell, P.H., and Collins, M.S. 1984. Paramyxovirus type 1 infections of racing pigeons: Characterization of isolated viruses. Vet. Rec. 114:444–446.

Alexander, D.J., Wilson, G.W., Russell, P.H., Lister, S.A., and Parsons, G. 1985. Newcastle disease outbreaks in fowl in Great Britain during 1984. Vet. Rec. 117:429–434.

Allan, W.H., Lancaster, J.E., and Toth, B. 1979. Newcastle disease vaccines, their production and use. Animal Production and Health Series no. 10. Food and Agriculture Organization of the United Nations, Rome.

Almassy, K., and Kakuk, T. 1976. Immunosuppressive effect of a naturally acquired subclinical bursal agent infection on vaccination against Newcastle disease. Vet. Rec. 99:435–437.

Bankowski, R.A. 1957. A modified live Newcastle disease virus vaccine. Proc. Soc. Exp. Biol. Med. 96:114–118.

Beach, J.R. 1942. Avian pneumoencephalitis. In Proceedings of the 46th Annual Meeting of the U.S. Livestock Sanitary Association, Chicago. Pp. 203–223.

Beach, J.R. 1944. The neutralization in vitro of avian pneumoencephalitis virus by Newcastle disease immune serum. Science 100:361–362.

Beard, C.W., and Hanson, R.P. 1984. Newcastle disease. In M.S. Hofstad et al., eds., Diseases of Poultry, 8th ed. Iowa State University Press, Ames. Pp. 452–470.

Beaudette, F.R., and Black, J.J. 1946. Newcastle disease in New Jersey. In Proceedings of the 49th Annual Meeting U.S. Livestock Sanitary Association, Pp. 49–58.

Beaudette, F.R., Bivins, J.A., and Miller, B.R. 1949. Newcastle disease immunization with live virus. Cornell Vet. 39:302–334.

Biancifiori, F., and Fioroni, A. 1983. An occurrence of Newcastle disease in pigeons: Virological and serological studies on the isolates. Comp. Immunol. Microbiol. Infect. Dis. 6:247–252.

Boyd, R.J., and Hanson, R.P. 1958. Survival of Newcastle disease virus in nature. Avian Dis. 2:82–93.

Brandly, C.A. 1959. Newcastle disease. In H.E. Biester, and L.H. Schwarte, eds., Diseases of Poultry, 4th ed. Iowa State University Press, Ames. Pp. 464–503.

Brandly, C.A., Moses, H.E., Jones, E.E., and Jungherr, E.L. 1946. Epizootiology of Newcastle disease of poultry. Am. J. Vet. Res. 7:243–249.

Brugh, M., and Beard, C.W. 1984. Atypical disease produced in chickens by Newcastle disease virus isolated from exotic birds. Avian Dis. 28:482–488.

Brugh M., Stone, H.D., and Lupton, H.W. 1983. Comparison of inactivated Newcastle disease viral vaccines containing different emulsion adjuvants. Am. J. Vet. Res. 44:72–75.

Chang, P.W. 1981. Newcastle disease. In J.H. Steele, ed., CRC Handbook Series in Zoonoses, vol. 2. CRC Press, Boca Raton, Fla. Pp. 261–264.

Chanock, R.M., and McIntosh, K. 1985. Parainfluenza viruses. In B.N. Fields, D.M. Knipe, R.M. Chanock, J.L. Melnick, B. Roizman, and R.E. Shope, eds., Virology. Raven Press, New York. Pp. 1241–1253.

Charan, S., Mahajan, V.M., Rai, A., and Balaya, S. 1984. Ocular pathogenesis of Newcastle disease virus in rabbits and monkeys. J. Comp. Pathol. 94:159–163.

Collins, P.L., Hightower, L.E., and Ball, L.A. 1980. Transcriptional map for Newcastle disease virus. J. Virol. 35:682–693.

Collins, P.L., Wertz, G.W., Ball, L.A., and Hightower, L.E. 1982. Coding assignments of the five smaller mRNAs of Newcastle disease virus. J. Virol. 43:1024–1031.

Doyle, T.M. 1927. A hitherto unrecorded disease of fowls due to a filter-passing virus. J. Comp. Pathol. Therap. 40:144–169.

Fabricant, J. 1949. Studies on the diagnosis of Newcastle disease and infectious bronchitis of fowls. I. The hemagglutination-inhibition test for the diagnosis of Newcastle disease. Cornell Vet. 39:202–220.

Faragher, J.T., Allan, W.H., and Wyeth, P.J. 1974. Immunosuppressive effect of infectious bursal agent on vaccination against Newcastle disease. Vet. Rec. 95:385–388.

Frank, G.H. 1981. Paramyxovirus and pneumovirus diseases of animals and birds: Comparative aspects and diagnosis. In E. Kurstak and C. Kurstak, eds., Comparative Diagnosis of Viral Diseases. vol. 4. Academic Press, New York. Pp. 187–233.

Freymann, M.W., and Bang, F.B. 1949. Human conjunctivitis due to Newcastle virus in the U.S.A. Johns Hopkins Hosp. Bull. 84:409–413.

Gale, C., Gard, D.I., Ose, E.E., and Berkman, R.N. 1965. Evaluation of a tissue-culture Newcastle disease vaccine. Avian Dis. 9:348–358.

Giambrone, J.J. 1985. Laboratory evaluation of Newcastle disease vaccination programs for broiler chickens. Avian Dis. 29:479–487.

Hamaguchi, M., Nishikawa, K., Toyoda, T., Yoshida, T., Hanaichi, T., and Nagai, Y. 1985. Transcriptive complex of Newcastle disease virus. II. Structural and functional assembly associated with the cytoskeletal framework. Virology 147:295–308.

Hanson, R.P. 1978. Newcastle disease. In M.S. Hofstad, ed., Diseases of Poultry, 7th ed. Iowa State University Press, Ames. Pp. 513–538.

Hanson, R.P., and Brandly, C.A. 1958. Newcastle disease. Ann. N.Y. Acad. Sci. 70:585–597.

Hanson, R.P., Spalatin, J., and Jacobson, G.S. 1973. The viscerotropic pathotype of Newcastle disease virus. Avian Dis. 17:354–361.

Hitchner, S.B. 1950. Further observations on a virus of low virulence for immunizing fowls against Newcastle disease (avian pneumoencephalitis). Cornell Vet. 40:60–70.

Hitchner, S.B., and Johnson, E.P. 1948. A virus of low virulence for immunizing fowls against Newcastle disease (avian pneumoencephalitis). Vet. Med. 43:525–530.

Hofstad, M.S. 1956. Further studies on the evaluation of immunity in chickens vaccinated with formalin-inactivated Newcastle disease virus vaccine. Am. J. Vet. Res. 17:738–741.

Ibrahim, A.L., Chulan, U., and Babjee, A.M. 1980. The immune response of chickens vaccinated against Newcastle disease with live Newcastle disease V4 vaccine. Aust. Vet. J. 56:29–33.

Ibrahim, A.L., Lai, M.C., and Aini, I. 1983. Spray vaccination with an improved F Newcastle disease vaccine. A comparison of efficacy with the B1 and La Sota vaccines. Br. Vet. J. 139:213–219.

Ingalls, W.L., and Mahoney, A. 1949. Isolation of the virus of Newcastle disease from human beings. Am. J. Public Health 39:737–740.

Iyer, S.G., and Dobson, N. 1940. A successful method of immunization against Newcastle disease of fowls. Vet. Rec. 52:891–894.

Katz, D., and Kohn, A. 1976. Antibodies in blood secretions of chickens immunized parenterally and locally with killed Newcastle disease virus vaccine. Dev. Biol. Stand. 33:290–296.

Khare, M.L., Kumar, S., and Grun, J. 1976. Immunoglobulins of the chicken antibody to Newcastle disease virus. (Mukteswar and F strain). Poult. Sci. 55:152–159.

Komarov, A., and Goldsmit, L. 1947. The use of live viruses in Palestine for the vaccination of poultry against Newcastle disease. Cornell Vet. 37:368–372.

Kraneveld, F.C. 1926. A poultry disease in the Dutch East Indies. Ned. Ind. Bland. Diergeneesk. Dierenteelt 38:448–450.

Kurilla, M.G., Stone, H.O., and Keene, J.D. 1985. RNA sequence and transcriptional properties of the 3′ end of the Newcastle disease virus genome. Virology 145:203–212.

Lai, M.C., and Ibrahim, A.L. 1983. Scanning electron microscopy of tracheal epithelium of chickens infected with velogenic viscerotropic Newcastle disease virus. Avian Dis. 27:393–404.

Lancaster, J.E. 1966. Newcastle disease. A review of the literature published between 1926 and 1964. Monograph no. 3, Canada Dept. of Agriculture, Ottawa.

Lancaster, J.E. 1981. Newcastle disease. In E.P.J. Gibbs, ed., Virus Diseases of Food Animals, vol. 2. Academic Press, London. Pp. 433–465.

Levine, P.P., Fabricant, J., Gillespie, J.H., Angstrom, C.I., and Mitchell, G. 1950. The results of pen contact exposure of susceptible chickens to chickens recovered from Newcastle disease. Cornell Vet. 40:206–210.

McDaniel, H.A., and Osborn, J.S. 1973. Diagnosis of velogenic viscerotropic Newcastle disease. J. Am. Vet. Med. Assoc. 163:1075–1079.

Mackenzie, J.S., Edwards, E.C., Holmes, R.M., and Hinshaw, V.S. 1984. Isolation of ortho- and paramyxoviruses from wild birds in Western Australia, and the characterization of novel influenza A viruses. Aust. J. Exp. Biol. Med. Sci. 62:89–99.

Miers, L.A., Bankowski, R.A., and Zee, Y.C. 1983. Optimizing the enzyme-linked immunosorbent assay for evaluating immunity of chickens to Newcastle disease. Avian Dis. 27:1112–1125.

Perey, D.Y., and Dent, P.B. 1975. Host resistance mechanisms to Newcastle disease virus in immunodeficient chickens. Proc. Soc. Exp. Biol. Med. 148:365.

Powell, J.A., Kano, K., and Milgrom, F. 1985. Antibodies to Newcastle disease virus in various human diseases. Int. Arch. Allergy Appl. Immunol. 76:331–335.

Raggi, L.G., Lee, G.G., and Sohrab-Haghighat, V. 1963. Infectious bronchitis virus interference with growth of Newcastle disease virus. I. Study of interference in chicken embryos. Avian Dis. 7:106–122.

Shuaib, M.A., Spalatin, J., McMillan, B., and Hanson, R.P. 1985. Studies on the development of pelleted Newcastle disease virus (NDV) vaccine. Vaccine 3:385–388.

Stone, H.D. 1985. Determination of hemagglutination activity recovered from oil-emulsion Newcastle disease vaccines as a prediction of efficacy. Avian Dis. 29:721–728.

Turner, A.J., Spalatin, J., and Hanson, R.P. 1976. The occurrence of virus in leukocytes of vaccinated chickens following challenge with virulent Newcastle disease virus. Avian Dis. 20:375–381.

Vickers, M.L., and Hanson, R.P. 1982a. Characterization of isolates of Newcastle disease virus from migratory birds and turkeys. Avian Dis. 26:127–133.

Vickers, M.L., and Hanson, R.P. 1982b. Newcastle disease virus in waterfowl in Wisconsin. J. Wildl. Dis. 18:149–158.

Walker, J.W., Heron, B.R., and Mixson, M.A. 1973. Exotic Newcastle disease eradication program in the United States. Avian Dis. 17:486–503.

Westbury, H.A., Parsons, G., and Allan, W.H. 1984. Comparison of the residual virulence of Newcastle disease vaccine strains V4, Hitchner B1 and La Sota. Austr. Vet. J. 61:47–49.

Winterfield, R.W., Dhillon, A.S., and Alby, L.J. 1980. Vaccination of chickens against Newcastle disease with live and inactivated Newcastle disease virus. Poult. Sci. 59:240–246.

Parainfluenza 3 Virus Infection in Cattle

SYNONYMS: Hemorrhagic septicemia, shipping fever, shipping pneumonia, stockyard fever

Parainfluenza 3 (PI-3) virus is a common respiratory pathogen of cattle and sheep. Infection with PI-3 virus alone usually results in mild respiratory disease or subclinical infection with seroconversion. However, with stress or concurrent infection with other viruses (Stott et al. 1980) or certain bacteria, PI-3 virus infection of cattle plays an important role in the acute respiratory disease commonly termed shipping fever, shipping pneumonia, stockyard fever, or hemorrhagic septicemia. *Mycoplasma* and particularly *Pasteurella* species are frequently involved with PI-3 virus. Some animals with respiratory disease are infected both with PI-3 virus and with bovine virus diarrhea–mucosal disease virus, infectious bovine rhinotracheitis virus, enteroviruses, or a variety of opportunistic bacteria.

Shipping fever has been recognized for many years and has been the cause of heavy losses, especially in cattle shipped during the cold months. It formerly was believed to be caused only by organisms in the genus *Pasteurella*, particularly *P. haemolytica*. PI-3 virus was first isolated from cattle with shipping fever by Reisinger et al. (1959) who designated the isolate SF-4 virus. Shortly thereafter the virus was identified in cattle throughout the world.

PI-3 virus infections of cattle have been reviewed by Frank (1981), Frank and Marshall (1973), Gale (1970), Kahrs (1981), Reisinger (1962), Sinha and Abinanti (1962), and Woods (1968).

Character of the Disease. The first signs of illness occur in calves 24 to 30 hours after exposure and may include increased temperature, lacrimation, serous nasal discharge, depression, and dyspnea followed by coughing. In some animals the signs may be mild and easily missed. A calf can have marked pneumonia with meager clinical signs. More severe disease results when *P. multocida* is given intranasally 24 to 48 hours following exposure to PI-3 virus.

Colostrum-deprived calves have mild illness after intranasal inoculation of PI-3 virus (Woods et al. 1965). In utero injection of virus into pregnant cows produces pathological changes in the fetus (Sattar et al. 1967), but there is no evidence that the virus affects natural breeding efficiency (Call et al. 1978).

In adult cattle, shipping fever syndrome takes the form of fibrinous pneumonia, which conceivably could be caused by one or more viruses and *Pasteurella* species. The animals cough, have very high temperatures (107°F and higher), and soon exhibit signs of great respiratory obstruction. Often they stand with the forelegs wide apart and the neck extended far forward. Breathing, often through the mouth, may become stertorous. Foamy saliva frequently is blown on the floor and walls before the animal. Such animals usually die within a few hours after the severe respiratory obstruction begins, and within 3 or 4 days after the first signs of illness are observed.

In cattle with typical cases of shipping fever the lesions are located in the respiratory tract; all other sites are secondary. The lungs often fill the thorax and are covered with a white, fibrinous mass that can be peeled off the surface like coagulated egg albumin; the underlying surfaces are rough and congested. The lungs, especially the main lobes, may be solid and heavy. Cut sections show deep red lobules and grayish ones separated by interlobular tissue that has been greatly thickened by infiltration of coagulated exudate like that on the serous surface. Histological examination reveals broncheolitis, alveolitis, serocellular exudate in the lung, intracytoplasmic acidophilic inclusion bodies in nasal and bronchial epithelium, and alveolar macrophages, together with marked fluorescence with specific antibody (Woods 1968).

Properties of the Virus. The causative virus (bovine PI-3 virus) is one of four serotypes of parainfluenza viruses classified in the genus *Paramyxovirus*. The properties of all four of these viruses are quite similar.

The intact virus particles vary from 140 to 250 nm in diameter. An RNA virus, it is labile at pH 3 and in the presence of ether or chloroform. The virion hemagglutinates red blood cells from birds, cattle, swine, guinea pigs, and human beings. Guinea pig cells are most sensitive. Infected cell cultures show hemadsorption. The virus induces interferon in fetal bovine kidney cell cultures (Rosenquist and Loan 1967). The human, bovine, and sheep PI-3 viruses are closely related but not identical. The human and bovine strains were differentiated by neutralization, hemagglutination-inhibition, and complement fixation tests with guinea pig antiserum (Ketler et al. 1961). Strains differ in their neuraminidase activity. The whole virion and the peplomers are active as antigens in leukocyte migration inhibition, lymphocyte stimulation, and skin hypersensitivity tests (Hoglund et al. 1977).

Cultivation. The virus replicates in many types of cultured cells, including bovine, swine, equine, and rabbit kidneys, and also in cells from the chicken embryo. Multiplication in cell cultures usually produces syncytia and intracytoplasmic and intranuclear inclusion bodies. Plaques are produced in 3 to 5 days in agar overlay preparations. The virus also replicates in calf alveolar macrophages from the lung but to a higher titer at 32°C than at 37°C (Tsai 1977), and in bovine fetal tracheal mucosa and bovine fetal lung organ cultures, where it produces alterations (Kita et al. 1969) (Figures 52.15 and 52.16).

Epizootiology and Pathogenesis. Susceptible calves naturally exposed to clinically ill calves excreting virus become infected in 5 to 10 days. Virus can be isolated from the nasal excretions for 7 to 8 days after infection and from the lungs for 17 days and sometimes longer despite the presence of serum antibodies. Infected cattle probably are the prime source for the continuity of the bovine PI-3 virus in nature.

After aerosol exposure the incubation period may be as

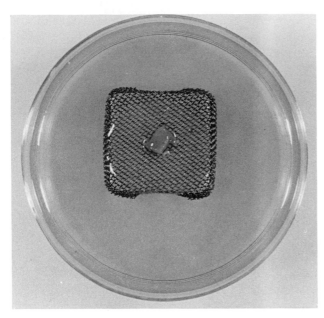

Figure 52.15. An organ culture of bovine fetal lung mounted on a wire grid and partially submerged in tissue-culture media. (From Kita et al., 1969, courtesy of *Cornell Veterinarian.*)

short as 2 days. This is followed by fever that may last 6 to 10 days (Frank and Marshall 1973, Kahrs 1981).

Pathogenicity studies of calves infected with PI-3 virus alone or in combination with *Pasteurella* sp. have been reported (Bryson et al. 1983, Carriere et al. 1983, Jericho et al. 1982, Tsai and Thomson 1975). The virus inhibits the clearance of *Pasteurella haemolytica* from the lungs of infected calves (Lopez et al. 1976), apparently by impairing the function of the alveolar macrophages (Liggitt et al. 1985). The cytotoxic cells in lung washings from calves are alveolar macrophages, and they destroy virus-infected calf kidney cells in culture and reduce the yields of virus. In infected bovine tracheal organ cultures, virus yield is initially reduced, but the macrophages become infected in 2 to 3 days and toxicity in the cultures decreases (Probert et al. 1977). Epithelial cells of the respiratory tract are the primary target cells for PI-3 virus, with more productive infection in the bronchoalveolar regions and the trachea. The replication of virus in the alveolar type 2 cells suggests that changes in surfactant production may occur during the peak of infection. Virus budding through the basement membrane of small bronchioles and particles in the interstitial regions imply that the basement membrane may be impaired (Tsai and Thomson 1975).

Figure 52.16. (*Left*) Uninoculated bovine fetal lung organ culture, 14 days. Note apparent cell viability with occasional large basophilic nucleoli and infrequency of pyknoses. Fixed in alcohol. Hematoxylin and eosin stain. × 1,100. (*Right*) Replicate culture, 13 days after inoculation with C3F-11 strain of bovine parainfluenza 3 virus. Note many intranuclear inclusion bodies (*arrows*), pyknosis, and karyorrhexis. Fixed in alcohol. H and E stain. × 1,100. (From Kita et al., 1969, courtesy of *Cornell Veterinarian.*)

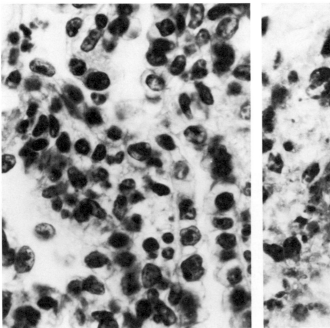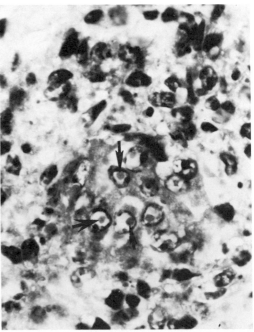

PI-3 virus has been isolated from humans, cattle, water buffalo, horses, and monkeys. Guinea pigs, hamsters, sheep, and swine are susceptible to experimental infection. PI-3 antibodies are found in humans, horses (Ditchfield et al. 1963), guinea pigs, swine, deer, and bighorn sheep. Their role in the transmission of the disease is unknown, but they may be involved in the ecology of the cattle disease, which occurs worldwide.

Immunity. The antibody level for bovine PI-3 virus increases before parturition and decreases to former levels during lactation. Antibodies are transferred to the calf in the colostrum and result in a blood level equal to or greater than that of the mother. Levels of this passive antibody decrease with age and are no longer detectable by weaning at 6 to 8 months of age. The antibody does not interfere with virus received by the aerosol route, but infection is less severe in calves given colostrum than in those deprived of it. The immunological response to virus in calves with colostrally acquired maternal immunity is less than in colostrum-deprived calves as the levels of serum and nasal secretion neutralizing antibody are lower (Marshall and Frank 1975).

Several reports have been published on immunity to PI-3 virus in calves (Burroughs et al. 1982, Fukumi 1975, Hoglund et al. 1977, Hussain and Mohanty 1984, Marshall 1981, Mukkur et al. 1975, Todd 1975, Woods et al. 1975, Zygraich et al. 1976). Active antibody develops in a calf when it comes in contact with PI-3 virus. After intranasal infection, IgA is found in the nasal secretions, and IgM and IgG immunoglobulins are demonstrable in the serum. Most investigators agree that the IgA antibodies, presumably synthesized locally, contribute heavily to the total antibody activity present in the secretions of the respiratory tract and to the protection provided to the animal. Reinfections with PI-3 virus are common and seem to depend more or less on circulating antibody levels. These antibody levels may determine whether an anamnestic response occurs, and, on occasion, mild clinical signs may also occur (Hamparian et al. 1961, Sweat 1983). It seems reasonable to assume that reinfections occur, as most adult beef and dairy cattle have demonstrable HI antibody.

Diagnosis. The virus can be readily isolated from respiratory tract exudates in tissue culture and identified by a combination of features: (1) production of syncytia and cytoplasmic and intranuclear inclusion bodies, (2) hemadsorption, (3) fluorescence by a specific conjugate, and (4) neutralization of the isolate by specific antiserum.

The demonstration of a rising titer in paired serums by a variety of antibody assays confirms a PI-3 infection (Assaf et al. 1983, Frank 1981, Kahrs 1981).

Certain clinical features may vary from those of other specific respiratory diseases of cattle, yet there is considerable overlap in the signs, making a positive diagnosis by this means often impossible (Bovine Respiratory Disease Symposium 1968).

Treatment. Clinical evidence indicates that animals with shipping fever sometimes may be successfully treated with various antibiotics if they are administered early in the course of the disease. Since these agents do not have any antiviral effect, their virtue lies only in their effect on the concurrent bacterial agents, especially *Pasteurella* species. For many years *Pasteurella* organisms were considered especially susceptible to antibiotics such as the penicillins and tetracyclines, but in recent years strains have developed which are resistant to most all antibiotics approved for use in food-producing animals.

Prevention and Control. The recommended procedures for the prevention and control of bovine PI-3 virus infection or disease in beef and dairy cattle have been outlined (Bovine Respiratory Disease Symposium 1968, Kahrs 1981). In brief, beef calves should be given PI-3 vaccine at 4 months of age. One month later another injection of virus vaccine should be administered. In open and closed dairy herds it is recommended that calves be vaccinated at 6 to 8 months of age with PI-3.

Studies by Woods et al. (1962) and Gale et al. (1963) show that two injections of inactivated virus vaccine are required to produce high HI titers. The vaccine produced by Gale et al. contained *Pasteurella* bacteria in addition to inactivated PI-3 virus. Some investigators have found that the vaccine does not always inhibit the disease in beef cattle, but the disease in the vaccinates is less severe and weight loss, if any, is minimal. Unvaccinated cattle lose considerable weight. Sweat (1983) evaluated the persistence of antibodies and anamnestic response in calves vaccinated with inactivated PI-3 vaccines.

Attenuated PI-3 virus vaccines, used singly and in combination with attenuated infectious bovine rhinotracheitis and bovine adenovirus 3, have been employed to immunize calves by the intranasal route. These vaccines are safe and efficacious. Several authors have compared the efficacy of PI-3 attenuated vaccines given by various routes (Burroughs et al. 1982; Martin et al. 1983; Mukkur et al. 1975; Todd 1975, 1976; Woods et al. 1975; Zygraich et al. 1976).

Transport of cattle, inclement weather, and the associated stresses have a marked influence on the severity of disease. Every effort should be made to make the cattle as comfortable as possible.

The Disease in Humans. There is no evidence that the bovine strains of PI-3 virus produce illness in humans, nor have human strains of PI-3 been proved to infect cattle.

REFERENCES

Assaf, R., Montpetit, C., and Marsolais, G. 1983. Serology of bovine parainfluenza virus type 3: Comparison of the enzyme linked immunosorbent assay and hemagglutination inhibition. Can. J. Comp. Med. 47:140–142.

Bovine Respiratory Disease Symposium. 1968. J. Am. Vet. Med. Assoc. 152(pt. 2):705–940.

Bryson, D.G., McNulty, M.S., McCracken, R.M., and Cush, P.F. 1983. Ultrastructural features of experimental parainfluenza type 3 virus pneumonia in calves. J. Comp. Pathol. 93:397–414.

Burroughs, A.L., Morrill, J.L., Bostwick, J.L., Ridley, R.K., Fryer, H.C. 1982. Immune responses of dairy cattle to parainfluenza-3 virus in intranasal infectious bovine rhinotracheitis–parainfluenza-3 virus vaccines. Can. J. Comp. Med. 46:264–266.

Call, J.W., Smart, R.A., Blake, J.T., Butcher, J.E., and Shupe, J.L. 1978. Parainfluenza-3 virus exposure of beef heifers prior to natural breeding. J. Am. Vet. Res. 39:527–528.

Carriere, P.D., Maxie, M.G., Wilkie, B.N., Savan, M., Valli, V.E., and Johnson, J.A. 1983. Exposure of calves to aerosols of parainfluenza-3 virus and *Pasteurella haemolytica*. Can. J. Comp. Med. 47:422–432.

Ditchfield, J., Zbitnew, A., MacPherson, L.W. 1963. Association of myxovirus para-influenzae 3 (RESS) with upper respiratory infecion of horses. Can. Vet. J. 4:175–180.

Frank, G.H. 1981. Paramyxovirus and pneumonvirus diseases of animals and birds: Comparative aspects and diagnosis. In E. Kurstak and C. Kurstak, eds., Comparative Diagnosis of Viral Diseases, vol. 4. Academic Press, New York. Pp. 187–233.

Frank, G.H., and Marshall, R.G. 1973. Parainfluenza-3 virus infection of cattle. J. Am. Vet. Med. Assoc. 163:858–860.

Fukumi, H. 1975. Meaning of circulating antibody titers in the infections of parainfluenza 3 virus and R.S. virus. Dev. Biol. Stand. 28:159–166.

Gale, C. 1970. Role of parainfluenza-3 in cattle. J. Dairy Sci. 53:621–625.

Gale, C., Hamdy, A.H., and Trapp, A.L. 1963. Studies on an experimental vaccine for prophylaxis of shipping fever. J. Am. Vet. Med. Assoc. 142:884–887.

Hamparian, V.V., Washko, F.V., Ketler, A., and Hilleman, M.R. 1961. Laboratory and field investigations of bovine myxovirus parainfluenza 3 virus and vaccine. III. Evaluation of an SF-4 (shipping fever) virus vaccine in cattle. J. Immunol. 87:139–146.

Hoglund, S., Moreno-Lopez, J., and Morein, B. 1977. Components of parainfluenza-3 virus, SLP-strain, reacting in assays of cell-mediated immunity in cattle. Arch. Virol. 53:323–333.

Hussain, A., and Mohanty, S.B. 1984. Antibody and complement-mediated cytotoxicity for bovine parainfluenza-3 virus-infected cells. Am. J. Vet. Res. 45:1219–1221.

Jericho, K.W., Darcel, C.L., and Langford, E.V. 1982. Respiratory disease in calves produced with aerosols of parainfluenza-3 virus and *Pasteurella haemolytica*. Can. J. Comp. Med. 46:293–301.

Kahrs, R.F. 1981. Parainfluenza-3. In R.F. Kahrs, ed., Viral Diseases of Cattle. Iowa State University Press, Ames. Pp. 171–181.

Ketler, A., Hamparian, V.V., and Hilleman, M.R. 1961. Laboratory field investigations of bovine myxovirus parainfluenza 3 virus and vaccine. I. Properties of the SF-4 (shipping fever) strain of virus. J. Immunol. 87:126–133.

Kita, J., Kenney, R.M., and Gillespie, J.H. 1969. The propagation and cytomorphological effects of bovine parainfluenza type 3 virus in organ cultures of bovine fetal tissues. Cornell Vet. 59:355–369.

Liggitt, D., Huston, L., Silflow, R., Evermann, J., and Trigo, E. 1985. Impaired function of bovine alveolar macrophages infected with parainfluenza-3 virus. Am. J. Vet. Res. 46:1740–1744.

Lopez, A., Thomson, R.G., and Savan, M. 1976. The pulmonary clearance of *Pasteurella hemolytica* in calves infected with bovine parainfluenza-3 virus. Can. J. Comp. Med. 40:385–391.

Marshall, R.G. 1981. Antibody response of calves after intranasal inoculation with parainfluenza-3 virus and resistance of inoculated calves to experimental homologous viral infection. Am. J. Vet. Res. 42:907–911.

Marshall, R.G., and Frank, G.H. 1975. Clinical and immunologic responses of calves with colostrally acquired maternal antibody against parainfluenza-3 virus to homologous viral infection. Am. J. Vet. Res. 36:1085–1089.

Martin, W., Wilson, P., Curtis, R., Allen B., and Acres, S. 1983. A field trial, of preshipment vaccination, with intranasal infectious bovine rhinotracheitis–parainfluenza-3 vaccines. Can. J. Comp. Med. 47:245–249.

Mukkur, T.K., Komar, R., and Sabina, L.R. 1975. Immunoglobulins and their relative neutralizing efficiency in cattle immunized with infectious bovine rhinotracheitis–parainfluenza-3 (IBR-PI-3) virus vaccine. Arch. Virol. 48:195–201.

Probert, M., Stott, E.J., and Thomas, L.H. 1977. Interactions between calf alveolar macrophages and parainfluenza-3 virus. Infect. Immun. 15:576–585.

Reisinger, R.C. 1962. Parainfluenza 3 virus in cattle. Ann. N.Y. Acad. Sci. 101:576–582.

Reisinger, R.C., Heddleston, K.L., and Manthei, C.A. 1959. A myxovirus (SF-4) associated with shipping fever of cattle. J. Am. Vet. Med. Assoc. 135:147–152.

Rosenquist, B.D., and Loan, R.W. 1967. Interferon production with strain SF-4 of parainfluenza-3 virus. Am. J. Vet. Res. 28:619–628.

Sattar, S.A., Bohl, E.H., Trapp, A.L., and Hamdy, A.H. 1967. In utero infection of bovine fetuses with myxovirus parainfluenza-3. Am. J. Vet. Res. 28:45–49.

Sinha, S.K., and Abinanti, F.R. 1962. Shipping fever of cattle. Adv. Vet. Sci. 7:225–271.

Stott, E.J., Thomas, L.H., Collins, A.P., Crouch, S., Jebbett, J., Smith, G.S., Luther, P.D., and Caswell, R. 1980. A survey of virus infections of the respiratory tract of cattle and their association with disease. J. Hyg. 85:257–270.

Sweat, R.L. 1983. Persistence of antibodies and anamnestic response in calves vaccinated with inactivated infectious bovine rhinotracheitis virus and parainfluenza-3 virus vaccines. J. Am. Vet. Med. Assoc. 182:809–811.

Todd, J.D. 1975. Immune response of cattle to intranasally or parenterally administered parainfluenza type 3 virus vaccines. Dev. Biol. Stand. 28:473–476.

Todd, J.D. 1976. Intranasal vaccination of cattle against IBR and PI3: Field and laboratory observations in dairy, beef, and neonatal calf populations. Dev. Biol. Stand. 33:391–395.

Tsai, K.S. 1977. Replication of parainfluenza type 3 virus in alveolar macrophages: Evidence of in vivo infection and of in vitro temperature sensitivity in virus maturation. Infect. Immun. 18:780–791.

Tsai, K.S., and Thomson, R.G. 1975. Bovine parainfluenza type 3 virus infection: Ultrastructural aspects of viral pathogenesis in the bovine respiratory tract. Infect. Immun. 11:783–803.

Woods, G.T. 1968. The natural history of bovine myxovirus parainfluenza-3. J. Am. Vet. Med. Assoc. 152:771–777.

Woods, G.T., Crandell, R.A., and Mansfield, M.E. 1975. A comparison of immunologic response to intranasal and intramuscular parainfluenza-3 live virus vaccines in beef calves challenged experimentally in the feedlot. Res. Commun. Chem. Pathol. Pharmacol. 11:117–128.

Woods, G.T., Mansfield, M.E., Sege, D., Holper, J.C., Brandly, C.A., and Barthel, C. 1962. The role of viruses in respiratory diseases of cattle. III. Respiratory disease in beef calves vaccinated before weaning with bovine myxovirus para-influenza 3 (SF-4) vaccine. Am. J. Vet. Res. 23:832–836.

Woods, G.T., Sibinovic, K., and Starkey, A.L. 1965. Exposure of colostrum-deprived calves to bovine myxovirus parainfluenza-3. Am. J. Vet. Res. 26:262–266.

Zygraich, N., Vascoboinic, E., and Huygelen, C. 1976. Immunity studies in calves vaccinated with a multivalent live respiratory vaccine composed of I.B.R., parainfluenza 3 and bovine adenovirus type 3. Dev. Biol. Stand. 33:379–383.

Canine Parainfluenza

SYNONYMS: Canine infectious tracheobronchitis, kennel cough; abbreviation, CPI

Canine parainfluenza is an acute viral respiratory disease of dogs characterized by sudden onset, nasal discharge, fever, and coughing. It often occurs as a co-infection with other viruses or bacteria, especially *Bordetella bronchiseptica* (Appel 1981, Appel and Bemis 1978, Wagener et al. 1984). It is an important component of the canine respiratory disease complex.

In 1967 a parainfluenza virus closely related to SV-5 parainfluenza virus of monkeys, a member of the parainfluenza 2 virus group, was implicated in an epizootic of respiratory disease in laboratory dogs (Binn et al. 1967). Two separate outbreaks occurred a year earlier in military dogs in the United States, and the isolates from the two outbreaks were identical (Binn et al. 1968, Crandell et al. 1968).

CPI and its causative virus (CPIV) have been reviewed by Appel (1981), Appel and Bemis (1978), and Frank (1981). Canine respiratory infections, including CPI, were reviewed by Dhein and Gorham (1986) and Thayer (1984).

Character of the Disease. The disease syndrome in field outbreaks is severe and probably involves other pathogens as well as CPIV (Appel and Percy 1970). The disease is characterized by sudden onset, nasal discharge, fever, and coughing in some dogs. CPIV can produce a disease that resembles kennel cough if *Mycoplasma* and certain bacterial organisms are also involved (Appel et al. 1970).

With their original isolate, Crandell et al. (1968) produced mild respiratory signs in dogs infected intranasally. The young dogs had tonsillitis and a slight nasal discharge but no fever. Others (Bittle and Emery 1970) observed similar signs in dogs exposed to Crandell's isolate by intranasal or intratracheal routes.

Properties of the Virus. CPIV is a negative-stranded, nonsegmented RNA virus classified in the *Paramyxovirus* genus of the family Paramyxoviridae. The canine virus is similar but distinct from SV-5 virus isolated from monkeys (Appel 1981, Binn et al. 1968, Crandell et al. 1968). Its hemagglutination and hemadsorbing properties are used in the study and diagnosis of the virus and the resulting disease.

Cultivation. CPIV replicates in a variety of cell cultures, including primary cultures of dog kidney, Madin-Darby canine kidney cell line, African green monkey kidney, rhesus monkey kidney, feline kidney, and human embryonic kidney. The virus produces multinucleated giant cells and eosinophilic inclusion bodies in the cytoplasm of cells.

Propagation of the virus in the amniotic cavity of the hen's embryonated egg was demonstrated by hemagglutination (Crandell et al. 1968). No embryonic deaths were observed. Both amniotic and allantoic fluids contained virus. The virus failed to replicate when inoculated into the allantoic cavity.

Epizootiology and Pathogenesis. The infection is readily transmitted from dogs in the acute stage to susceptible dogs. It is an important disease in places where dogs are introduced into a new environment, such as laboratories or military bases (Binn and Lazar 1970).

Virus cannot be recovered from the respiratory tract beyond 9 days after exposure. Natural infections in dogs seem to be limited to the respiratory tract. In the general canine population CPIV infection is quite widespread (Bittle and Emery 1970), and the virus has frequently been isolated from clinical outbreaks of kennel cough (Appel 1981).

The host range for CPIV is unclear but probably includes monkeys, humans, and dogs. Cats infected experimentally shed large quantities of virus for several days (Saona Black and Lee 1970).

In a pathogenetic study Appel and Percy (1970) inoculated dogs by various routes. Intramuscular and subcutaneous inoculation did not cause infection. In contrast, aerosol or contact exposure produced disease restricted to the respiratory tract. Virus inoculated into the urinary bladder directly resulted only in local viral replication and cystitis. With aerosol exposure to 10^4 TCID$_{50}$ of virus a slight rise in temperature was noted in most of the experimental dogs; it occurred 2 to 3 days after exposure and persisted for 1 to 2 days. A few dogs had a slight nasal discharge, and slightly less than half developed a slight nonproductive cough that could be forced by laryngeal palpation. The cough never persisted more than 1 week. At necropsy there were no lesions except for a few petechial hemorrhages in a few dogs examined 4 days after exposure. Microscopic inflammatory changes were evident in the upper and lower respiratory tract and in regional lymph nodes. Between the first and eighth day after exposure, virus was isolated from the oronasal specimens but not from the blood. The highest viral titers were found from respiratory specimens collected between the third and sixth days. Viral antigen, as demonstrated by the immunofluorescence test, is observed in the epithelial cells of nasal mucosa, trachea, bronchi, and bronchioli and in the peribronchial lymph nodes 1 to 6 days after exposure, with considerable reduction in fluorescence by the sixth day.

When *Mycoplasma* sp. and *Bordetella bronchiseptica*

were given intranasally after aerosol exposure to CPIV, the respiratory illness was more severe in all dogs; a dry cough persisted in some for several weeks. All dogs exposed to CPIV developed serum-neutralizing antibody, but levels declined thereafter with little or no antibody 3 to 4 months later (Appel et al. 1970).

Acute encephalitis and hydrocephalus caused by CPIV have been reported in dogs (Baumgartner et al. 1982a, 1982b; Evermann et al. 1980, 1981).

Immunity. Dogs infected with CPIV by the respiratory route are fully immune to challenge by this same route 3 weeks later. There are no signs of illness, and virus is not isolated from the respiratory tract. In contrast, dogs given virus parenterally develop good antibody titers but are not completely protected from an aerosol challenge (Appel and Percy 1970).

Neutralizing antibody may persist for at least 3 to 4 months (Appel et al. 1970). The serum-neutralization test is slightly more sensitive than the standard hemagglutination-inhibition test (Bittle and Emery 1970).

The level and frequency of neutralizing antibody in the dog population is such that maternal immunity does not play a significant role in protection or in immunization (Appel et al. 1970).

Diagnosis. To differentiate this viral disease from others in the dog at the clinical level is extremely difficult. Many other canine viruses produce comparable respiratory signs of illness.

Field strains from dogs grow quite readily and produce a cytopathic effect in cell cultures. A further distinguishing feature is the virus's hemadsorbing effect. Consequently tissue culture is an excellent method of virus isolation and identification. The use of paired serums in the hemagglutination-inhibition and serum-neutralization tests and the demonstration of a rising antibody titer are other means of diagnosis.

Treatment. Because bacterial infections often appear to be involved in canine respiratory disease associated with CPIV infection, antibiotics and sulfa compounds may aid in reducing the severity of the disease.

Prevention and Control. Prevention of CPI is primarily through vaccination with modified live-virus vaccines, either parenterally or intranasally. Emery et al. (1976) developed an attenuated-virus vaccine that may be given subcutaneously or intramuscularly. It is safe and provides sufficient immunity to protect dogs against an aerosol challenge with virulent virus. An anamnestic response occurs in vaccinated dogs after challenge exposure. The duration of immunity has not been ascertained.

Vaccines are available which combine the attenuated CPIV with an avirulent strain of *Bordetella bronchisep-* *tica* for intranasal administration (Appel 1981, Chladek et al. 1981, Glickman and Appel 1981, Kontor et al. 1981). These appear to be safe and to give rapid protection against clinical disease. Appel (1981) showed that if canine adenovirus 2 vaccine was included in this intranasal vaccine, the incidence of coughing in breeding kennels was reduced compared with kennels where dogs were vaccinated with only the bivalent vaccine or the *B. bronchiseptica* vaccine alone. This study supports the need for using all three antigens in respiratory vaccines for dogs.

Concentrations of ribavirin as low as 1 μg/ml showed some in vitro activity against CPIV but its effectiveness in a clinical situation has not been evaluated (Povey 1978).

The Disease in Humans. In studies of epizootiology in military dogs, handlers were not infected with CPIV (Crandell et al. 1968). The exact role if any of dogs in the epizootiology of parainfluenza virus infection in other species, including humans, is unknown. CPI is considered to be a model for lower respiratory infection in humans (Wagener et al. 1983).

REFERENCES

Appel, M.J. 1981. Canine infectious tracheobronchitis (kennel cough): A status report. Compend. Cont. Ed. Pract. Vet. 3:70–81.

Appel, M., and Bemis, D.A. 1978. The canine contagious respiratory disease complex (kennel cough). Cornell Vet. (Suppl.) 68:70–75.

Appel, M.J.G., and Percy, D.H. 1970. SV-5 like parainfluenza virus in dogs. J. Am. Vet. Med. Assoc. 156:1778–1781.

Appel, M.J.G., Pickerill, P.H., Menegus, M., Percy, D.H., Parsonson, I.M., and Sheffy, B.E. 1970. Current status of canine respiratory disease. In Gaines Veterinary Symposium, October 22, 1970. Pp. 15–23.

Baumgartner, W.K., Krakowka, S., Koestner, A., and Evermann, J. 1982a. Acute encephalitis and hydrocephalus in dogs caused by canine parainfluenza virus. Vet. Pathol. 19:79–92.

Baumgartner, W.K., Krakowka, S., Koestner, A., and Evermann, J. 1982b. Ultrastructural evaluation of the acute encephalitis and hydrocephalus in dogs caused by canine parainfluenza virus. Vet. Pathol. 19:305–314.

Binn, L.N., and Lazar, E.C. 1970. Comments on epizootiology of parainfluenza SV-5 in dogs. J. Am. Vet. Med. Assoc. 156:1774–1777.

Binn, L.N., Eddy, G.A., Lazar, E.C., Helms, J., and Murmane, T. 1967. Viruses recovered from laboratory dogs with respiratory disease. Proc. Soc. Exp. Biol. Med. 126:140–145.

Binn, L.N., Lazar, E.C., Rogul, M., Shepler, V.M., Swango, L.J., Claypoole, T., Hubbard, D.W., Asbill, S.G., and Alexander, A.D. 1968. Upper respiratory disease in military dogs: Bacterial, mycoplasma, and viral studies. Am. J. Vet. Res. 29:1809–1815.

Bittle, J.L., and Emery, J.B. 1970. The epizootiology of canine parainfluenza. J. Am. Vet. Med. Assoc. 156:1771–1773.

Chladek, D.W., Williams, J.M., Gerber, D.L., Harris, L.L., and Murdock, F.M. 1981. Canine parainfluenza–*Bordetella bronchiseptica* vaccine immunogenicity. Am. J. Vet. Res. 42:266–270.

Crandell, R.A., Brimlow, W.B., and Davison, V.E. 1968. Isolation of a parainfluenza virus from sentry dogs with upper respiratory disease. Am. J. Vet. Res. 29:2141–2147.

Dhein, C.R., and Gorham, J.R. 1986. Canine respiratory infections. In F.W. Scott, ed., Contemporary Issues in Small Animal Practice:

Infectious Diseases, vol. 3. Churchill Livingstone, New York. Pp. 177–205.

Emery, J.B., House, J.A., Bittle, J.L., and Spotts, A.M. 1976. A canine parainfluenza viral vaccine: Immunogenicity and safety. Am. J. Vet. Res. 37:1323–1327.

Evermann, J.F., Krakowka, S., McKeirnan, A.J., Baumgartner, W. 1981. Properties of an encephalitogenic canine parainfluenza virus. Arch. Virol. 68:165–172.

Evermann, J.F., Lincoln, J.D., McKiernan, A.J. 1980. Isolation of a paramyxovirus from the cerebrospinal fluid of a dog with posterior paresis. J. Am. Vet. Med. Assoc. 177:1132–1134.

Frank, G.H. 1981. Paramyxovirus and pneumovirus diseases of animals and birds: Comparative aspects and diagnosis. In E. Kurstak and C. Kurstak, eds., Comparative Diagnosis of Viral Diseases, vol. 4. Academic Press, New York. Pp. 187–233.

Glickman, L.T., and Appel, M.J. 1981. Intranasal vaccine trial for canine infectious tracheobronchitis (kennel cough). Lab. Anim. Sci. 31:397–399.

Kontor, E.J., Wegrzyn, R.J., and Goodnow, R.A. 1981. Canine infectious tracheobronchitis: Effects of an intranasal live canine para-influenza–Bordetella bronchiseptica vaccine on viral shedding and clinical tracheobronchitis (kennel cough). Am. J. Vet. Res. 42:1694–1698.

Povey, R.C. 1978. In vitro antiviral efficacy of ribavirin against feline calicivirus, feline viral rhinotracheitis virus, and canine parainfluenza virus. Am. J. Vet. Res. 39:175–177.

Saona Black, L., and Lee, K.M. 1970. Infection of dogs and cats with a canine parainfluenza virus and the application of a conglutinating-complement absorption test on cat scrums. Cornell Vet. 60:120–134.

Thayer, G.W. 1984. Canine infectious tracheobronchitis. In C.E. Greene, ed., Clinical Microbiology and Infectious Diseases of the Dog and Cat. W.B. Saunders, Philadelphia. Pp. 430–436.

Wagener, J.S., Minnich, L., Sobonya, R., Taussig, L.M., Ray, C.G., and Fulginiti, V. 1983. Parainfluenza type II infection in dogs. A model for viral lower respiratory tract infection in humans. Am. Rev. Respir. Dis. 127:771–775.

Wagener, J.S., Sobonya, R., Minnich, L., and Taussig, L.M. 1984. Role of canine parainfluenza virus and Bordetella bronchiseptica in kennel cough. Am. J. Vet. Res. 45:1862–1866.

Parainfluenza 3 Virus Infection in Sheep

Parainfluenza 3 virus of sheep origin produces acute respiratory disease in sheep comparable to that produced in cattle by bovine parainfluenza viruses. Sheep PI-3 virus was first isolated from the pneumonic lungs of five sheep in three flocks in Australia (St. George 1969). Mild pneumonia was produced in sheep when they were exposed to one of the isolates (CSL 6) under experimental conditions. The CSL 6 strain is closely related antigenically to bovine and human PI-3 viruses, but it is not identical to these viruses.

Exposure of 1-week-old colostrum-deprived lambs to a sheep isolate of PI-3 virus resulted in a biphasic febrile response, cough, rapid respiration, anorexia, and depression (Cutlip and Lehmkuhl 1982; Lehmkuhl and Cutlip 1982, 1983). The lungs of these lambs had multifocal areas of consolidation. Virus was detected by immunofluorescence and electron microscopy in small airways and alveolar epithelium. Microscopically the lung lesions were characterized by bronchiolitis and interstitial pneumonitis.

The incidence of antibody to PI-3 virus in various sheep populations were reported as 87 percent (Lehmkuhl et al. 1985), 74 percent (Brako et al. 1984), 50 to 56 percent (Adair et al. 1984), and 28 percent (Lamontagne et al. 1985). PI-3 virus antibodies in goat populations were also reported by Elazhary et al. (1984), Fulton et al. (1982), and Taylor et al. (1975).

The immunity of sheep to PI-3 virus was reviewed by Wells (1981), and Smith and his colleagues published a series of papers on the immune response of sheep to virulent, inactivated, and attenuated PI-3 virus (Smith 1975; Smith et al. 1975; Smith, Dawson, et al. 1976; Smith, Wells, et al. 1976; Wells et al. 1976). The nature of immunity is similar to that observed for PI-3 infection in cattle. The concentration of antibody in the respiratory tract and anamnestic response governed by cell mediation both play a significant role in protection against the subsequent respiratory disease. These investigators reported that immunity to challenge as assessed by viral shedding from the nose was conferred by attenuated virus administered intranasally or intramuscularly, by two doses of inactivated virus in Freund's complete adjuvant (FCA) given intramuscularly, and by intramuscular injection of inactivated virus in FCA followed by intranasal instillation of inactivated virus.

A subunit vaccine containing a mixture of the hemagglutinin and fusion glycoproteins of PI-3 virus stimulated protective immunity in sheep (Morein et al. 1983). A commercial bovine PI-3 vaccine produced some protection in challenged sheep, but it did not instill complete protection against infection and clinical disease (Lehmkuhl and Cutlip 1985). Clinical disease, however, was milder and virus was shed for a shorter period in vaccinated sheep.

REFERENCES

Adair, B.M., McFerran, J.B., McKillop, E.R., and McCullough, S.J. 1984. Survey for antibodies to respiratory viruses in groups of sheep in Northern Ireland. Vet. Rec. 115:403–406.

Brako, E.E., Fulton, R.W., Nicholson, S.S., and Amborski, G.F. 1984. Prevalence of bovine herpesvirus-1, bovine viral diarrhea, parainfluenza-3, goat respiratory syncytial, bovine leukemia, and bluetongue viral antibodies in sheep. Am. J. Vet. Res. 45:813–816.

Cutlip, R.C., and Lehmkuhl, H.D. 1982. Experimentally induced parainfluenza type 3 virus infection in young lambs: Pathologic response. Am. J. Vet. Res. 43:2101–2107.

Elazhary, M.A., Silim, A., and Dea, S. 1984. Prevalence of antibodies to bovine respiratory syncytial virus, bovine viral diarrhea virus, bovine herpesvirus-1, and bovine parainfluenza-3 virus in sheep and goats in Quebec. Am. J. Vet. Res. 45:1660–1662.

Fulton, R.W., Downing, M.M., and Hagstad, H.V. 1982. Prevalence of bovine herpesvirus-1, bovine viral diarrhea, parainfluenza-3, bovine adenovirus-3 and -7, and goat respiratory syncytial viral antibodies in goats. Am. J. Vet. Res. 43:1454–1457.

Lamontagne, L., Descôteaux, J.P., Roy, R. 1985. Epizootiological survey of parainfluenza-3, reovirus-3, respiratory syncytial and infectious bovine rhinotracheitis viral antibodies in sheep and goat flocks in Quebec. Can. J. Comp. Med. 49:424–428.

Lehmkuhl, H.D., and Cutlip, R.C. 1982. Characterization of parainfluenza type 3 virus isolated from the lung of a lamb with pneumonia. Am. J. Vet. Res. 43:626–628.

Lehmkuhl, H.D., and Cutlip, R.C. 1983. Experimental parainfluenza type 3 infection in young lambs: Clinical, microbiological, and serological response. Vet. Microbiol. 8:437–442.

Lehmkuhl, H.D., and Cutlip, R.C. 1985. Protection from parainfluenza-3 virus and persistence of infectious bovine rhinotracheitis virus in sheep vaccinated with a modified live IBR-PI-3 vaccine. 49:58–62.

Lehmkuhl, H.D., Cutlip, R.C., Bolin, S.R., and Brogden, K.A. 1985. Seroepidemiologic survey for antibodies to selected viruses in the respiratory tract of lambs. Am. J. Vet. Res. 46:2601–2604.

Morein, B., Sharp, M., Sundquist, B., and Simons, K. 1983. Protein subunit vaccines of parainfluenza type 3 virus: Immunogenic effect in lambs and mice. J. Gen. Virol. 64:1557–1569.

St. George, T.D. 1969. The isolation of myxovirus parainfluenza type 3 from sheep in Australia. Aust. Vet. J. 45:321–325.

Smith, W.D. 1975. The nasal secretion and serum antibody response of lambs following vaccination and aerosol challenge with parainfluenza 3 virus. Res. Vet. Sci. 19:56–62.

Smith, W.D., Dawson, A.M., Wells, P.W., and Burrells, C. 1976. Immunoglobulins in the serum and nasal secretions of lambs following vaccination and aerosol challenge with parainfluenza 3 virus. Res. Vet. Sci. 21:341–348.

Smith, W.D., Wells, P.W., Burrells, C., and Dawson, A.M. 1975. Immunoglobulins, antibodies and inhibitors of parainfluenza 3 virus in respiratory secretions of sheep. Arch. Virol. 49:329–337.

Smith, W.D., Wells, P.W., Burrells, C., and Dawson, A.M. 1976. Maternal immunoglobulins and parainfluenza 3 virus inhibitors in the nasal and lachrymal secretions and serum of newborn lambs. Clin. Exp. Immunol. 23:544–553.

Taylor, W.P., Momoh, M., Okeke, A.N.C., et al. 1975. Antibodies to parainfluenza-3 virus in cattle, sheep, and goats from Northern Nigeria. Vet. Rec. 97:183–184.

Wells, P.W. 1981. Immunity to parainfluenza type 3 virus and *Pasteurella haemolytica* in sheep. Adv. Exp. Med. Biol. 137:667–676.

Wells, P.W., Sharp, J.M., and Burrells, C., 1976. The assessment in sheep of an inactivated vaccine of parainfluenza 3 virus incorporating double stranded RNA (BRL 5907) as adjuvant. J. Hyg. 77:255–261.

Paramyxovirus Infection in Other Domestic Animals

Horses. Information about parainfluenza 3 virus in the horse is rather sparse. The virus was first isolated in 1961 from yearling Thoroughbred horses with acute upper respiratory disease (Ditchfield et al. 1963). A serologic survey of the horses on the affected premises showed that a large number of horses 2 years or older had hemagglutinating-inhibition (HI) antibodies to the equine PI-3 virus isolate. In a reciprocal HI test with HA-1 (human type) and SF-4 (bovine type) PI-3 strains the equine PI-3 strain (RE 55) gave virtually identical results with the HA-1 strain and similar, but not identical, results with the SF_4 strain.

In Illinois a PI-3 virus was isolated from four colts that had a disease diagnosed as strangles (Sibinovic et al. 1965). All the animals in their herd of 10 horses had a mucopurulent discharge and/or a history of recent respiratory disease. Significant serum HI titers were demonstrated in six of the colts.

Complement-fixing antibody apparently disappears about 4 months after infection. In contrast the HI and neutralizing antibody persisted for at least 1 year (Ditchfield 1969). Sibinovic et al. (1965) tested 130 horse serums from 14 counties in Illinois, and approximately half had high HI titers to equine PI-3 virus. Although Todd (1969) had negative test results for PI-3 neutralizing antibodies in his serologic survey, it is likely that PI-3 infection is common in horses. However, its significance in the horse as a pathogen capable of producing disease is yet to be ascertained.

Pigs. The hemagglutinating virus of Japan (HVP), also known as Sendai virus, is a PI-1 virus that infects mice and perhaps swine and humans. In swine Sendai virus reputedly causes bronchopneumonia in young pigs, although there is no serologic evidence in the swine population in Japan to support this contention. In pregnant sows inoculation of the virus early in pregnancy produces mummified fetuses and stillborn pigs (Shimuzu et al. 1954).

Greig et al. (1971) isolated a PI-3 virus from the brain of a pig. It crosses antigenically with PI-2 virus. Its pathogenicity for swine has not been ascertained.

Birds. At least nine serotypes of avian paramyxoviruses (PMV) have been identified (Alexander 1980, Clubb 1986, Gerlack 1984). Avian PMV-1 is Newcastle disease virus. The remaining eight serotypes (designated avian PMV-2 to PMV-9) have been isolated from a variety of domestic, pet, and wild birds.

PMV-2. A hemagglutinating agent designated Yucaipa virus was isolated from chickens with a mixed respiratory infection (Bankowski and Corstvet 1961). PMV-2 has been isolated on several occasions from normal chickens, turkeys, and caged birds, or from birds that had concurrent infections with other pathogens. This virus appears to be worldwide in distribution and is common in caged birds (Alexander 1980). PMV-2 is immunologically and serologically distinct from other known avian viruses and the paramyxoviruses of mammals. It causes a mild respiratory disease in chickens by the intratracheal route, but most reports indicate the virus is relatively nonpathogenic.

PMV-3. PMV-3 was first isolated by Lang in 1967 in Canada from turkeys with respiratory infections (Tumova et al. 1979). Similar isolates have been made from turkeys in the United States (Kelly 1985) and from caged birds of the psittacine and passerine species from several countries

(Ashton and Alexander 1980, Smit and Rondhuis 1976). This virus has been associated with either fatal respiratory disease or neurological disease in imported caged birds. It commonly infects turkeys in California (Kelly 1985).

PMV-4. Isolations of nonpathogenic PMV-4 have been made from ducks, geese, and other fowls in Hong Kong and from wild ducks in the United States and Czechoslovakia (Alexander 1980, Shortridge and Alexander 1978, Webster et al. 1976).

PMV-5. PMV-5 has been shown to be the cause of several outbreaks of fatal disease in caged budgerigars (*Melopsittacus undulatus*) in Japan and other countries (Nakayama et al. 1976, Nerome et al. 1978, Yoshida et al. 1977).

PMV-6. There have been several isolations of PMV-6 from healthy ducks in Hong Kong (Alexander 1980, Shortridge et al. 1980) and from sentinel ducks that were intermingled with wild ducks in the United States (Kelleher et al. 1985). There is no known disease associated with this serotype of PMV.

Several other avian paramyxoviruses have been isolated from various species of domestic and wild birds. Some of these isolates make up PMV-7 (Alexander 1980), whereas others are classified as PMV-8 and PMV-9 (Alexander et al. 1983). Undoubtedly additional serotypes of avian paramyxoviruses will be discovered.

REFERENCES

Alexander, D.J. 1980. Avian paramyxoviruses. Vet. Bull. 50:737–752.

Alexander, D.J., Hinshaw, V.S., Collins, M.S., and Yamane, N. 1983. Characterization of viruses which represent further distinct serotypes (PMV-8 and PMV-9) of avian paramyxoviruses. Arch. Virol. 78:29–36.

Ashton, W.L.G., and Alexander, D.J. 1980. A two-year survey on the control of the importation of captive birds into Great Britain. Vet. Rec. 106:80–83.

Bankowski, R.A., and Corstvet, R. 1961. Isolation of a hemagglutinating agent distinct from Newcastle disease from the respiratory tract of chickens. Avian Dis. 5:253–269.

Clubb, S.L. 1986. Viral and chlamydial diseases of pet birds. In F.W. Scott, ed., Contemporary Issues in Small Animal Practice: Infectious Diseases, vol. 3. Churchill Livingstone, New York. Pp. 225–244.

Ditchfield, W.J.B. 1969. Rhinovirus and parainfluenza viruses in horses. J. Am. Vet. Med. Assoc. 155:384–387.

Ditchfield, W.J.B., MacPherson, L.W., and Zbitnew, A. 1963. Association of myxovirus parainfluenza 3 (RE 55) with upper respiratory infection of horses. Can. Vet. J. 4:175–180.

Gerlack, H. 1984. Viral diseases in pet birds. Vet. Clin. North Am. [Small Anim. Pract.] 14:299–316.

Greig, A.S., Johnson, C.M., and Bouillant, A.M. 1971. Encephalomyelitis of swine caused by a hemagglutinating virus. VI. Morphology of the virus. Res. Vet. Sci. 12:305–307.

Kelleher, C.J., Halvorson, D.A., Newman, J.A., and Senne, D.A. 1985. Isolation of avian paramyxoviruses from sentinel ducks and turkeys in Minnesota. Avian Dis. 29:400–407.

Kelly, B.J. 1985. Paramyxovirus type 3 (PMV-3) in California turkeys: Serologic study of PMV-3 antibody with an enzyme-linked immunosorbent assay. Avian Dis. 29:364–372.

Nakayama, M., Nerome, K., Ishida, M., Fukumi, H., and Morita, A. 1976. Characterization of virus isolated from budgerigar. Med. Biol. 93:449–454.

Nerome, K., Nakayama, M., Ishida, M., Fukumi, H., and Morita, A. 1978. Isolation of a new avian paramyxovirus form budgerigar (*Melopsittacus undulatus*). J. Gen. Virol. 38:293–301.

Shimuzu, T., Kawakami, Y., Fukuhara, S., and Matomoto, M. 1954. Experimental stillbirth in pregnant swine infected with Japanese encephalitis virus. Jpn. J. Exp. Med. 24:363–375.

Shortridge, K.F., and Alexander, D.J. 1978. Incidence and preliminary characterization of a hitherto unreported, serologically distinct, avian paramyxovirus isolated in Hong Kong. Res. Vet. Sci. 25:128–130.

Shortridge, K.F., Alexander, D.J., and Collins, M.S. 1980. Isolation and properties of viruses from poultry in Hong Kong which represent a new (sixth) distinct group of avian paramyxoviruses. J. Gen. Virol. 49:255–262.

Sibinovic, K.H., Woods, G.T., Hardenbrook, H.J., and Marquis, G. 1965. Myxovirus parainfluenza-3 associated with an outbreak of strangles. Vet. Med. 60:600–604.

Smit, T., and Rondhuis, P.R. 1976. Studies on a virus isolated form the brain of a parakeet (*Neophema* sp.). Avian Pathol. 5:21–30.

Todd, J.D. 1969. Comments on rhinoviruses and parainfluenza viruses in horses. J. Am. Vet. Med. Assoc. 155:387–390.

Tumova, B., Robinson, J.H., and Easterday, B.C. 1979. A hitherto unreported paramyxovirus of turkeys. Res. Vet. Sci. 27:135–140.

Webster, R.G., Morita, M., Pridgen, C., and Tumova, B. 1976. Ortho- and paramyxoviruses from migrating feral ducks: Characterization of a new group of influenza A viruses. J. Gen. Virol. 32:217–225.

Yoshida, N., Miyamoto, T., Fukusho, K., Sekine, J., and Tajima, M. 1977. Properties of paramyxovirus isolated from budgerigars with an acute fatal disease. J. Jpn. Vet. Med. Assoc. 30:599–603.

Mumps Virus Infection in Cats and Dogs

Clinical observations suggest that both cats and dogs are susceptible to human mumps virus. A number of cases of parotitis have been seen in pet cats or dogs at the same time that members of the household were infected with mumps virus (Kirk 1970, Noice et al. 1959).

Mumps virus is classified in the genus *Paramyxovirus* of the family Paramyxoviridae. The only known natural host is humans. While natural transmission appears to occur from infected humans to dogs and cats, and experimental transmission has been produced in laboratory animals such as hamsters, suckling mice, guinea pigs, ferrets, and monkeys, animal-to-animal transmission of the virus, or transmission from animals to humans, has not been reported. An excellent review of mumps virus and mumps infection was published by (Wolinsky and Server 1985).

Mumps virus was isolated from the saliva of two dogs with swollen parotid glands (Noice et al. 1959). Both cases occurred during outbreaks of mumps in two households. These isolates produced cytopathic effect in HeLa cells, and the hemagglutinating properties of the virus were inhibited by human mumps antiserum. Stone (1969) reported that mumps virus may produce meningoencephalitis in the dog without involvement of the parotid gland. Morris et al. (1956) reported that 38 of 209 dog serum samples collected at random from a population fixed complement in the presence of mumps virus. In another study Cuadrado (1965) found that the serums of 20 dogs had hemagglutination-inhibition titers greater than 1:20 against mumps virus. Mumps virus given to dogs by the intraparotid route failed to produce signs of illness, and virus was not recoverable from the saliva, but dogs did develop mumps antibody. Binn (1970) suggested that observations on mumps virus should be viewed with caution, especially because SV-5 virus antigens are commonly noted in monkey kidney cell cultures and SV-5 antibodies are often seen in guinea pig serum used as a source of complement in the complement-fixation test (Hsuing et al. 1962).

Wollstein (1916, 1918) published two reports on the infectiousness of human mumps virus for the domestic cat. When bacteria-sterile saliva and blood from infected humans was inoculated into the parotid salivary gland and the testes of cats, orchitis and parotitis resulted. The experimental cats had a febrile response, leukocytosis, tenderness, and swelling of the injected glands and histological lesions similar to those seen in human mumps. Saliva from infected cats was infectious when inoculated into other cats, and virus could be recovered from infected parotid glands and regional lymph nodes of affected cats.

Scott et al. (1972) and Schultz and Scott (1973) showed that mumps virus replicated in feline kidney and feline lung cells in vitro. They also demonstrated that direct inoculation of virulent mumps virus into the parotid salivary gland and testes of an adult male cat resulted in parotitis and orchitis. Infection spread to the opposite gland, and virus was recovered from the parotid salivary gland 59 days after inoculation. Oral and intravenous inoculation of pregnant cats with mumps virus resulted in viral replication within the fetuses, indicating that virus had crossed the placenta.

Present evidence suggests that mumps virus infection does occur as a natural infection in dogs and cats. Its significance as a pathogen and its incidence in these hosts, as well as its importance in the transmission of this virus to humans, are yet to be ascertained.

REFERENCES

Binn, L.N. 1970. A review of viruses recovered from dogs. J. Am. Vet. Med. Assoc. 156:1672–1677.

Cuadrado, R.R. 1965. An epidemiological study on parainfluenza, DA and mumps virus infections in domestic animals in New England. Bull. WHO 33:803–808.

Hsuing, G.D., Isacson, P., and McCollum, R.W. 1962. Studies of a myxovirus isolated from human blood. I. Isolation and properties. J. Immunol. 88:284–290.

Kirk, R.W. 1970. Personal communication. College of Veterinary Medicine, Cornell University, Ithaca, N.Y.

Morris, J.A., Blount, R.E., and McCown, J.M. 1956. Natural occurrence in dog serum of antibodies against mumps virus. Cornell Vet. 46:525–531.

Noice, F., Bolin, F.M., and Eveleth, D.F. 1959. Incidence of viral parotitis in the domestic dog. J. Dis. Child. 98:350–352.

Schultz, R.D., and Scott, F.W. 1973. Experimental infection of mumps virus in cats (abstract). In Proceedings of the Annual Meeting of the American Society of Microbiologists. P. 227.

Scott, F.W., Schultz, R.D., and Gillespie, J.H. 1972. Unpublished findings.

Stone, A.B. 1969. Studies on mumps complement fixation titers in dogs. I. Complement fixation (c.f.) titers in normal dogs. II. Complement fixation (c.f.) titers in dogs with central nervous system (c.n.s.) damage. J. Small Anim. Pract. 10:555–557.

Wolinsky, J.S., and Server, A.C. 1985. Mumps virus. In B.N. Fields, D.M. Knipe, R.M. Chanock, J.L. Melnick, B. Roizman, and R.E. Shope, eds., Virology. Raven Press, New York. Pp. 1255–1284.

Wollstein, M. 1916. An experimental study of parotitis (mumps). J. Exp. Med. 23:353–374.

Wollstein, M. 1918. A further study of experimental parotitis. J. Exp. Med. 28:377–385.

The Genus *Pneumovirus*

Bovine Respiratory Syncytial Virus Infection

SYNONYMS: Atypical interstitial pneumonia, pulmonary adenomatosis, pulmonary emphysema; abbreviation, AIP

Bovine respiratory syncytial virus (BRSV) infection, an acute, highly contagious viral disease in cattle and sheep, is characterized by sudden onset of fever, nasal discharge, coughing, and signs of bronchial pneumonia or respiratory distress. Baker and Frey (1985), Frank (1981), Kahrs (1981), and Woods (1974) provided reviews of the virus and the clinical disease produced. The antigenically related human virus, the most important human virus causing lower respiratory tract disease, was reviewed extensively by McIntosh and Chanock (1985).

In studies on human respiratory syncytial virus (RSV), it was found that certain batches of bovine serum contained neutralizing antibodies against the human virus (Doggett et al. 1968). The first bovine RSV was isolated from an acute outbreak of respiratory disease in cattle in Switzerland (Paccaud and Jacquier 1970). BRSV was implicated in a large outbreak of respiratory disease in cattle in Japan (Inaba et al. 1970) and in calves in Great Britain (Jacobs and Edington 1971). The first isolations in the United States were reported in 1974 from Missouri and Iowa (Rosenquist 1974, Smith et al. 1974). Subsequently numerous isolations of BRSV have been made from several countries, and numerous investigations of the virus and the resulting clinical disease have been reported.

One must be aware of another bovine virus, bovine syncytial virus, which is unrelated to BRSV, does not produce disease (Scott et al. 1973), and is now classified in the genus *Spumavirus* of the Retroviridae family (see Chapter 54).

Character of the Disease. In cattle BRSV can cause an acute lower respiratory tract disease, varying in severity from relatively mild or even subclinical to severe. There are many descriptions of the natural and experimental clinical disease in cattle (Baker and Frey 1985; Bryson et al. 1983; Castleman, Torres-Medina, et al. 1985; Elazhary et al. 1980, 1982; Frank 1981; Gillette and Smith 1985; Harrison and Pursell 1985; Inaba et al. 1970, 1972; Jacobs and Edington 1975; Kahrs 1981; McNulty et al. 1983; Mohanty et al. 1975; Paccaud and Jacquier 1970; Pirie et al. 1981; Rosenquist 1974; Smith et al. 1975; Van Den Ingh et al. 1982; Verhoeff and van Niewstadt 1984; Verhoeff et al 1984; Woods 1974).

Affected cattle usually show fever, nasal discharge, respiratory distress, coughing, and, occasionally, lacrimation. As the disease progresses, signs may become more severe, with dyspnea, mouth breathing, excess salivation, and subcutaneous edema. Other signs reported include decreased milk production, diarrhea, abortion, and subcutaneous emphysema. Morbidity may be quite high, but mortality is usually low or negligible. The duration of the disease varies but usually is 1 to 2 weeks.

RSV is associated with respiratory disease in sheep (Al-Darraji et al. 1982, Berthiaume et al. 1973, Brako et al. 1984, Cutlip and Kehmkuhl 1979, Khristozova et al. 1985, LeaMaster et al. 1983). Sheep may be infected with bovine strains of virus or isolates that appear to be primarily sheep-adapted strains. Clinical disease is similar to that in the bovines. RSV has also been identified in goats with respiratory disease (Fulton et al. 1982, Smith et al. 1979).

Properties of the Virus. BRSV is classified in the *Pneumovirus* genus of the family Paramyxoviridae. It has physical and biochemical properties similar to those of human RSV (Frank 1981, McIntosh and Chanock 1985). The respiratory syncytial viruses differ antigenically from the pneumonia virus of mice, another pneumovirus.

The virions are pleomorphic, enveloped particles 150 to 300 nm in diameter with short, closely spaced projections on the surface of the bilayer membrane (McIntosh and Chanock 1985). The nucleocapsid contains a nonsegmented, negative-stranded RNA genome that codes for 10 separate proteins.

Cultivation. BRSV has been propagated in several bovine cell cultures by routine methods. The addition of 40 μg of diethylaminoethyl-dextran per milliliter of viral inoculum produces a cytopathic effect more rapidly (Rossi and Kiesel 1978). Trypsin, thrombin, and plasmin increase the cytopathology produced by human RSV (Dubovi et al. 1983).

Epizootiology and Pathogenesis. Transmission of infection between animals is probably by direct contact, by aerosol routes, or by feed and water contaminated by infected cattle. The incubation period is usually short (3 to 4 days) and followed by acute respiratory disease. The incidence of BRSV in cattle is not known, but serologic evidence indicates that the incidence is probably high. One outbreak in Japan involved more than 40,000 cattle (Inaba et al. 1970, 1972). Several studies in the United States found the incidence of antibody-positive cattle to be from 65 to 81 percent (Baker and Frey 1985, Potgieter and Aldridge 1977, Smith et al. 1975).

Cattle are believed to be the natural host for BRSV; under experimental conditions BRSV also infects sheep (Baker and Frey 1985). Respiratory syncytial viruses have been isolated from sheep (LeaMaster et al. 1983) and goats (Smith et al. 1979) but it is not known if sheep and goat respiratory syncytial viruses produce disease in cattle. Serum antibodies to RSV have been reported in cats (Pringle and Cross 1978, Richardson-Wyatt et al. 1981), dogs (Lundgren et al. 1969), sheep (Berthiaume et al. 1973, Brako et al. 1984, Elazhary et al. 1984, LeaMaster et al. 1983), goats (Elazhary et al. 1984, Fulton et al. 1982, Richardson-Wyatt et al. 1981), pigs (Woods 1974), and horses (Berthiaume et al. 1973).

During infection of the respiratory tract, BRSV causes bronchitis, bronchiolitis, interstitial pneumonia, multinucleation of alveolar and epithelial cells, and in the process destroys the ciliated respiratory epithelium (Baker and Frey 1985; Castleman, Chandler, and Slauson 1985; Castleman, Lay, et al. 1985). This destruction probably interferes with the clearance of bacteria from the respiratory tract, which in turn leads to secondary bacterial infections. Microscopic and ultrastructural studies of the pathogenesis of the respiratory infection in calves were reported by Bryson et al. (1983); Castleman, Chandler, and Slauson (1985); Castleman, Lay, et al. (1985); Thomas et al. (1984); and Van Den Ingh et al. (1982). Virus particles were present in epithelial cells of the trachea and bronchi from day 3 to day 7 after inoculation. Viral assembly and release of virions resulted in loss of cilia, swelling of mitochondria and endoplasmic reticulum, cell necrosis, and the formation of syncytial epithelial cells (Figure 52.17).

Immunity. Recovery from BRSV infection appears to confer partial immunity. Subsequent exposures to virus cause mild or inapparent disease. Cell-mediated immunity as well as humoral immunity is involved (Field and Smith 1984).

Diagnosis. BRSV infection cannot be diagnosed on the basis of clinical signs but must be identified by virus isolation, immunofluorescence (Thomas and Stott 1981),

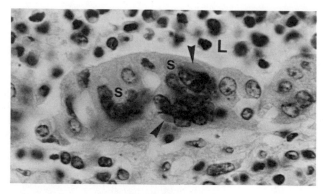

Figure 52.17. Histopathological specimen of the bronchiolar epithelium of a 4-month-old Holstein heifer with pneumonia caused by bovine respiratory syncytial virus. Two multinucleated syncytial epithelial cells are present (*S*), and one of these syncytial cells contains intracytoplasmic eosinophilic inclusions (*arrowheads*). The bronchiolar lumen (*L*) contains macrophages, neutrophils, and necrotic cellular debris. Hematoxylin and eosin stain. × 540. (From Castleman, Torres-Medina, et al., 1985, courtesy of *Cornell Veterinarian* and W. L. Castleman.)

demonstration of seroconversion in paired serum samples, or demonstration of typical lung lesions in animals that have undergone necropsy (Baker and Frey 1985). For virus isolation, samples must be taken early in the disease. Antibody assays can be made by indirect immunofluorescence neutralization, hemagglutination-inhibition, or enzyme-linked immuosorbent assay (Berthiaume et al. 1973, Elazhary et al. 1981, Gillette 1983, Martin 1983, Potgieter and Aldridge 1977, van Nieuwstadt and Verhoeff 1983, Westenbrink et al. 1985).

Prevention and Control. Inactivated and modified live-virus vaccines are available for immunization of cattle and appear to confer good immunity (Bohlender 1984, Kuchera et al. 1983, Stott et al. 1984, Verhoeff and van Nieuwstadt 1984b). Stress should be avoided during infection.

The Disease in Humans. BRSV is very similar to human RSV, but it has not been adequately established that the bovine agent infects humans.

REFERENCES

Al-Darraji, A.M., Cutlip, R.C., Lehmkuhl, H.D., and Graham, D.L. 1982. Experimental infection of lambs with bovine respiratory syncytial virus and *Pasteurella haemolytica:* Pathologic studies. Am. J. Vet. Res. 43:224–229.

Baker, J.C., and Frey, M.L. 1985. Bovine respiratory syncytial virus. Vet. Clin. North Am. [Food Anim. Pract.]. 1:259–275.

Berthiaume, L., Joncas, J., Boulay, G., and Pavilanis, V. 1973. Serological evidence of respiratory syncytial virus infections in sheep. Vet. Rec. 93:337–338.

Bohlender, R.E. 1984. Field trials of a bovine respiratory syncytial virus vaccine. Mod. Vet. Pract. 65:606–609.

Brako, E.E., Fulton, R.W., Nicholson, S.S., and Amborski, G.F. 1984. Prevalence of bovine herpesvirus-1, bovine viral diarrhea, parainfluenza-3, goat respiratory syncytial, bovine leukemia and bluetongue viral antibodies in sheep. Am. J. Vet. Res. 45:813–816.

Bryson, D.G., McNulty, M.S., Logan, E.F., and Cush, P.F. 1983. Respiratory syncytial virus pneumonia in young calves: Clinical and pathologic findings. Am. J. Vet. Res. 44:1648–1655.

Castleman, W.L., Chandler, S.K., and Slauson, D.O. 1985. Experimental bovine respiratory syncytial virus infection in conventional calves: Ultrastructural respiratory lesions. Am. J. Vet. Res. 46:554–560.

Castleman, W.L., Lay, J.C., Dubovi, E.J., and Slauson, D.O. 1985. Experimental bovine respiratory syncytial virus infection in conventional calves: Light microscopic lesions, microbiology, and studies on lavaged lung cells. Am. J. Vet. Res. 46:547–553.

Castleman, W.L., Torres-Medina, A., Hawkins, K.L., Dubovi, E.J., and Atz, J.M. 1985. Severe respiratory disease in dairy cattle in New York State associated with bovine respiratory syncytial virus infection. Cornell Vet. 75:473–483.

Cutlip, R.C., and Lehmkuhl, H.D. 1979. Lesions in lambs experimentally infected with bovine respiratory syncytial virus. Am. J. Vet. Res. 40:1479–1482.

Doggett, J.E., Taylor-Robinson, D., and Gallop, R.G.C. 1968. A study of an inhibitor in bovine serum activated against RS virus. Arch. Gesam. Virusforsch. 23:126–137.

Dubovi, E.J., Geratz, J.D., and Tidwell, R.R. 1983. Enhancement of respiratory syncytial virus-induced cytopathology by trypsin, thrombin, and plasmin. Infect. Immun. 40:351–358.

Elazhary, M.A., Galina, M., Roy, R.S., Fontaine, M., and Lamothe, P. 1980. Experimental infection of calves with bovine respiratory syncytial virus (Quebec strain). Can. J. Comp. Med. 44:390–395.

Elazhary, M.A.S.Y., Silim, A., and Dea, S. 1984. Prevalence of antibodies to bovine respiratory syncytial virus, bovine viral diarrhea virus, bovine herpesvirus-1, and bovine parainfluenza-3 virus in sheep and goats in Quebec. Am. J. Vet. Res. 45:1660–1662.

Elazhary, M.A., Silim, A., and Morin, M. 1982. A natural outbreak of bovine respiratory disease caused by bovine respiratory syncytial virus. Cornell Vet. 72:325–333.

Elazhary, M.A., Silim, A., and Roy, R.S. 1981. Interferon, fluorescent antibody, and neutralizing antibody responses in sera of calves inoculated with bovine respiratory syncytial virus. Am. J. Vet. Res. 42:1378–1382

Field, E.W., and Smith, M.H. 1984. Cell-mediated immune response in cattle to bovine respiratory syncytial virus. Am. J. Vet. Res. 45:1641–1643.

Frank, G.H. 1981. Paramyxovirus and pneumovirus diseases of animals and birds: Comparative aspects and diagnosis. In E. Kurstak and C. Kurstak, eds., Comparative Diagnosis of Viral Diseases, vol. 4. Academic Press, New York. Pp. 187–233.

Fulton, R.W., Downing, M.M., and Hagstad, H.V. 1982. Prevalence of bovine herpesvirus-1, bovine viral diarrhea, parainfluenza-3, bovine adenovirus-3 and -7, and goat respiratory syncytial viral antibodies in goats. Am. J. Vet. Res. 43:1454–1457.

Gillette, K.G. 1983. Enzyme-linked immunosorbent assay for serum antibody to bovine respiratory syncytial virus: Comparison with complement-fixation and neutralization test. Am. J. Vet. Res. 44:2251–2255.

Gillette, K.G., and Smith, P.C. 1985. Respiratory syncytial virus infection in transported calves. Am. J. Vet. Res. 46:2596–2600.

Harrison, L.R., and Pursell, A.R. 1985. An epizootic of respiratory syncytial virus infection in a dairy herd. J. Am. Vet. Med. Assoc. 187:716–720.

Inaba, Y., Tanaka, Y., Omori, T., and Matumoto, M. 1970. Isolation of bovine respiratory syncytial virus. Jpn. J. Exp. Med. 40:473–474.

Inaba, Y., Tanaka, Y., Sato, K., and Omori, T. 1972. Bovine respiratory syncytial virus: Studies on an outbreak in Japan, 1968–1969. Jpn. J. Microbiol. 16:373–383.

Jacobs, J.W., and Edington, N. 1971. Isolation of respiratory syncytial virus from cattle in Britain. Vet. Rec. 88:694.

Jacobs, J.W., and Edington, N. 1975. Experimental infection of calves with respiratory syncytial virus. Res. Vet. Sci. 18:299–306.

Kahrs, R.F. 1981. Respiratory syncytial virus. In R.F. Kahrs, ed., Viral Diseases of Cattle. Iowa State University Press, Ames. Pp. 215-220.

Khristozova, S., Tsvetkov, P., and Kharalambiev, Kh. E. 1985. Experimental infection of lambs with strains of the bovine respiratory syncytial virus. Vet. Med. Nauki 22:31–35.

Kucera, C.J., Feldner, T.J., and Wong, J.C.S. 1983. The testing of an experimental bovine respiratory syncytial virus vaccine. Vet. Med./Small Anim. Clin. 78:1599–1604.

LeaMaster, B.R., Evermann, J.F., Meuller, G.M., et al. 1983. Serologic and virologic studies on naturally occurring respiratory syncytial virus and *Haemophilus somnus* infections in sheep. Proc. Am. Assoc. Vet. Lab. Diag. 26:265–267.

Lundgren, D.L., Magnuson, M.G., and Clapper, W.E. 1969. A serological survey in dogs for antibody to human respiratory viruses. Lab. Anim. Care 19:352–359.

McIntosh, K., and Chanock, R.M. 1985. Respiratory syncytial virus. In B.N. Fields, D.M. Knipe, R.M. Chanock, J.L. Melnick, B. Roizman, and R.E. Shope, eds., Virology. Raven Press, New York. Pp. 1285–1304.

McNulty, M.S., Bryson, D.G., and Allan, G.M. 1983. Experimental respiratory syncytial virus pneumonia in young calves. Am. J. Vet. Res. 44:1656–1659.

Martin, H.T. 1983. Indirect haemagglutination test for the detection and assay of antibody to bovine respiratory syncytial virus. Vet. Rec. 113:290–293.

Mohanty, S.B., Ingling, A.L., and Lillie, M.G., 1975. Experimentally induced respiratory syncytial viral infection in calves. Am. J. Vet. Res. 36:417–419.

Paccaud, M.F., and Jacquier, C. 1970. A respiratory syncytial virus of bovine origin. Arch. Gesam. Virusforsch. 30:327–342.

Pirie, H.M., Petrie, L., Pringle, C.R., Allen, E.M., and Kennedy, G.J. 1981. Acute fatal pneumonia in calves due to respiratory syncytial virus. Vet. Rec. 108:411–416.

Potgieter, L.N.D., and Aldridge, P.L. 1977. Use of the indirect fluorescent antibody test in the detection of bovine respiratory virus antibodies in bovine serum. Am. J. Vet. Res. 38:1341–1343

Pringle, C.R., and Cross, A. 1978. Neutralization of respiratory syncytial virus by cat serum. Nature 276:501–502.

Richardson-Wyatt, L.S., Belshe, R.B., London, W.T., Sly, D.L. Camargo, F., and Chanock, R.M. 1981. Respiratory syncytial virus antibodies in nonhuman primates and domestic animals. Lab. Anim. Sci. 31:413–415.

Rosenquist, B.D. 1974. Isolation of respiratory syncytial virus from calves with acute respiratory disease. J. Infect. Dis. 130:177–182.

Rossi, C.R., and Kiesel, G.K. 1978. Bovine respiratory syncytial virus infection of bovine embryonic lung cultures: Enhancement of infectivity with diethylaminoethyl-dextran and virus-infected cells. Arch. Virol. 56:227–236.

Scott, F.W., Shively, J.N., Gaskin, J., and Gillespie, J.H. 1973. Bovine syncytial virus isolations. Arch. Gesam. Virusforsch. 43:43–52.

Smith, M.H., Frey, M.L., and Dierks, R.E. 1974. Isolation and characterization of a bovine respiratory syncytial virus. Vet. Rec. 94:599.

Smith, M.H., Frey, M.L., and Dierks, R.E. 1975. Isolation, characterization, and pathogenicity studies of a bovine respiratory syncytial virus. Arch. Virol. 47:237–247.

Smith, M.H., Lehmkuhl, H.D., and Phillips, S.M. 1979. Isolation and characterization of a respiratory syncytial virus from goats. Proc. Am. Assoc. Vet. Lab. Diag. 22:259–268.

Stott, E.J., Thomas, L.H., Taylor, G., Collins, A.P., Jebbett, J., and Crouch, S. 1984. A comparison of three vaccines against respiratory syncytial virus in calves. J. Hyg. 93:251–261.

Thomas, L.H., and Stott, E.J. 1981. Diagnosis of respiratory syncytial virus infection in the bovine respiratory tract by immunofluorescence. Vet. Rec. 108:432–435.

Thomas, L.H., Stott, E.J., Collins, A.P., Jebbett, J. 1984. Experimental pneumonia in gnotobiotic calves produced by respiratory syncytial virus. Br. J. Exp. Pathol. 65:19–28.

Van Den Ingh, T.S., Verhoeff, J., and van Nieuwstadt, A.P. 1982. Clinical and pathological observations on spontaneous bovine respiratory syncytial virus infections in calves. Res. Vet. Sci. 33:152–158.

van Nieuwstadt, A.P., and Verhoeff, J. 1983. Serology for diagnosis and epizootiological studies of bovine respiratory syncytial virus infections. Res. Vet. Sci. 35:153–159.

Verhoeff, J., and van Nieuwstadt, A.P. 1984a. BRS virus, PI3 virus and BHV1 infections of young stock on self-contained dairy farms: Epidemiological and clinical findings. Vet. Rec. 114:288–293.

Verhoeff, J., and van Nieuwstadt, A.P. 1984b. Prevention of bovine respiratory syncytial virus infection and clinical disease by vaccination. Vet. Rec. 115:488–492.

Verhoeff, J., Van der Ban, M., and van Nieuwstadt, A.P. 1984. Bovine respiratory syncytial virus infections in young dairy cattle: Clinical and haematological findings. Vet. Rec. 114:9–12.

Westenbrink, F., Brinkhof, J.M., Straver, P.J., Quak, J., and De Leeuw, P.W. 1985. Comparison of a newly developed enzyme-linked immunosorbent assay with complement fixation and neutralization tests for serology of bovine respiratory syncytial infections. Res. Vet. Sci. 38:334–340.

Woods, G.T. 1974. Bovine parvovirus 1, bovine syncytial virus and bovine respiratory syncytial virus and their infections. Adv. Vet. Sci. Comp. Med. 18:273–286.

53 The Rhabdoviridae

The rhabdoviruses are an important and widely distributed group of single-stranded RNA viruses that infect vertebrates, invertebrates, and plants (Bishop and Smith 1977, Brown et al. 1979, Emerson 1985, Winkler 1981). The enveloped virions have an elongated, cylindrical morphology (Greek *rhabdos,* "rod, stick"), which is either bullet-shaped or bacilliform in silhouette (Figure 53.1). The particles vary considerably in size, ranging from 130 to 380 nm in length and 60 to 95 nm in width. Surface projections (peplomers) approximately 5 to 10 nm long, which protrude through the unit-membrane envelope, contain a hemagglutinin and mediate viral penetration of host cells. The buoyant density of the particles is 1.17–1.19 g/ml in sucrose and 1.19–1.20 g/ml in cesium chloride. Infectivity is destroyed by lipid solvents, low pH, and heat.

The genomic RNA of rhabdoviruses is composed of a single linear molecule of single-stranded RNA (molecular weight 3.5 to 4.6×10^6), which is not infectious. Replication proceeds by the production of five monocistronic mRNAs via a virus-encoded RNA-dependent RNA polymerase. The five mRNAs are translated into the five major rhabdovirus proteins:

1. N (for nucleocapsid), which is the major structural protein and encapsidates the genomic RNA to form a ribonucleoprotein core
2. G (for glycoprotein), which forms the viral peplomers
3. M (for matrix), which is inserted between the envelope lipid and the ribonucleoprotein core (in some rhabdoviruses two M proteins are found)

4. L (for large), which has polymerase activity and is associated with the ribonucleoprotein core
5. NS (for nonstructural), which, like L, is associated with the ribonucleoprotein core and shows polymerase activity

Viral replication occurs in the cytoplasm of infected cells and may be accompanied by cytopathic changes. The site of virion maturation is variable, depending on the individual virus and on the host cell type. Some rhabdoviruses produce morphologically distinct defective-interfering particles (so-called T, or truncated, particles), which play a role in inhibiting replication of normal virus (Figure 53.2).

Certain members of the Rhabdoviridae have been assigned to two genera *(Lyssavirus* and *Vesiculovirus),* but the majority of viruses in this family remain unclassified (Table 53.1). An antigenic grouping of the rhabdoviruses into at least three major subgroups and four minor ones has been proposed (Tesh et al. 1983). Rhabdoviruses are widely distributed in nature, and many are transmitted, biologically or mechanically or both, by arthropod vectors. Member viruses have been associated with a variety of clinical manifestations in a number of host species. The important diseases of domestic animals caused by rhabdoviruses are listed in Table 53.2.

REFERENCES

Bishop, D.H.L., and Smith, M.S. 1977. Rhabdoviruses. In D.P. Nayak, ed., The Molecular Biology of Animal Viruses, vol. 1. Marcel Dekker, New York. Pp. 167–280.

Brown, F., Bishop, D.H.L., Crick, J., Francki, R.I.B., Holland, J.J., Hull, R. Johnson, K., Martelli, G., Murphy, F.A., Obijeski, J.F., Peters, D., Pringle, C.R., Reichmann, M.E., Schneider, L.G., Shope, R.E., Simpson, D.I.H., Summers, D.F., and Wagner, R. R. 1979. Rhabdoviridae. Intervirology 12:1–7.

Emerson, S.U. 1985. Rhabdoviruses. In B.N. Fields, ed., Virology. Raven Press, New York. Pp. 1119–1132.

Tesh, R.B., Travassos da Rosa, A.P.A., and Travassos da Rosa, J.S. 1983. Antigenic relationship among rhabdoviruses infecting terrestrial vertebrates. J. Gen. Virol. 64:169–176.

Winkler, W.G. 1981. The rhabdoviruses. In E. Kurstak and C. Kurstak, eds., Comparative Diagnosis of Viral Diseases, vol. 4, part B. Academic Press, New York. Pp. 529–550.

The Genus *Lyssavirus*

Rabies

SYNONYMS: Hydrophobia, *Tollwut, le rage, la rabia, derriengue*

Rabies has been known in Europe and Asia since the days of antiquity. The first mention of it may be in the law tablets of ancient Mesopotamia: "If a dog is vicious and the authorities have brought the fact to the knowledge of

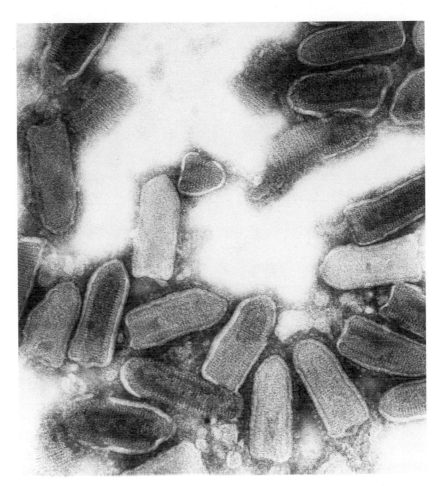

Figure 53.1. Vesicular stomatitis virus in negative stain preparation showing the characteristic bullet-shaped morphology. The envelope layer appears as a thickened line; the helically coiled nucleocapsid is seen as a series of cross-striations about 5 nm apart. × 94,300 (Courtesy F. A. Murphy and J. F. Obijeski, Centers for Disease Control.)

its owner, (if nevertheless) he does not keep it in, it bites a man and causes (his) death, then the owner of the dog shall pay two-thirds of a mina of silver. If it bites a slave and causes (its) death, he shall pay 15 shekels of silver" (Goetze 1955). Rabies was well known to the ancient Greeks, among them Democritus, Xenophon, and Aristotle, and in Roman times Celsus recognized the role of wild animals in transmitting the disease and wisely recommended treatment of bite wounds by excision and cauterization (Steele 1975).

Rabies occurs in all continents of the world except Australia and Antarctica. It is normally a disease of bats and carnivores, including the domestic dog and cat and many wild species. Cases of rabies in humans, however, continue to evoke a unique horror because of the unsettling nature of the clinical signs and the virtually universal lethality of the outcome once those signs are manifest.

A number of excellent reviews on different aspects of rabies are available (Baer 1975a, 1985; Beran and Crowley 1983; Clark and Prabhakar 1985; Dierks 1981; Kaplan and Koprowski 1980; Koprowski 1984; Kuwert and Scheiermann 1985; Martin and Sedmak 1983; Murphy 1977; Sedmak and Martin 1984; Sikes 1981).

Character of the Disease. The clinical signs of rabies are similar overall for the various species, but signs seen in individual cases can vary widely. Two principal forms or manifestations of the disease are generally recognized: (1) an excitatory, or "furious," form; and (2) a paralytic,

Table 53.1. Partial listing of rhabdoviruses isolated from vertebrates

Genus *Lyssavirus*
 Rabies virus
 Duvenhage virus
 Lagos bat virus
 Mokola virus

Genus *Vesiculovirus*
 Vesicular stomatitis virus, serotypes Indiana and New Jersey
 Chandipura virus
 Piry virus

Unclassified
 Ephemeral fever virus
 Viral hemorrhagic septicemia virus
 Infectious hematopoietic necrosis virus
 Red disease of pike virus
 Spring viremia of carp virus

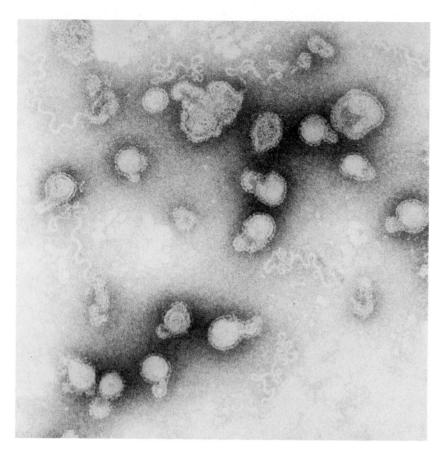

Figure 53.2. Defective-interfering (T, or truncated) particles of vesicular stomatitis virus. Negative stain. × 105,621. (Courtesy F. A. Murphy and J. F. Obijeski, Centers for Disease Control.)

or "dumb," form. In reality, most cases of rabies exhibit some manifestations of both forms. The paralytic form always represents the terminal stage; however, some animals die during convulsive seizures in the furious stage without exhibiting the final stage. Some show few or no signs of excitement, the clinical picture reflecting instead the effects of paresis or paralysis. Rarely, rabid animals die suddenly, without exhibiting any recognizable signs of illness. In the stage of excitation, many animals become aggressive and dangerous. They frequently snap at imaginary objects and may attempt to bite any animals or humans that approach. Within a short time these signs give way to those of the final stage, which usually lasts only for a day or two and terminates in death.

Table 53.2. Rhabdoviruses that cause diseases of importance in domestic animals

Virus	Natural hosts	Type of disease produced
Rabies virus, one serotype	Humans and most warm-blooded animals, especially dogs, cats, skunks, foxes, wolves, raccoons, mongooses, and bats	Variable incubation period, followed by excitatory and/or paralytic signs resulting from infection of the nervous system. Highly fatal once clinical signs are manifest. Worldwide distribution
Vesicular stomatitis virus, two serotypes	Horses, mules, cattle, swine	Vesicular disease, with lesions variably present in the mouth, on the feet, or on the teats. The lesions are indistinguishable from those of foot-and-mouth disease. Limited to the Western hemisphere
Ephemeral fever virus, one serotype?	Cattle, water buffalo	Acute febrile illness with respiratory signs and lameness. Course is usually short, with rapid recovery. Widespread in Africa, Asia, and Australia

An earlier prodromal stage is recognized in human rabies and may also be seen in some closely observed pet animals. In the prodrome, which usually lasts for 1 to 3 days, vague changes in temperament occur. Humans in this stage experience a feeling of unease, restlessness, and apprehension, accompanied frequently by a tingling sensation at the site of the bite wound. Dogs and cats that have been affectionate may shy away and shun company; more nervous animals may become unusually attentive, possibly manifesting a feeling of insecurity. The prodrome, however, when and if it occurs in animal species, may frequently pass unnoticed by human companions.

In dogs the furious stage lasts variably for 1 to 7 days and is manifested by restlessness, nervousness (often characterized by biting or snapping at insects, real or imaginary), and a developing viciousness. At first this behavior is more likely to be manifested toward strangers, but later the animal apparently does not recognize its owner and is as likely to injure him or her as others. Excitability, photophobia, and hyperesthesia may become apparent. If restrained, the dog will chew vigorously on metal chains or on the bars of the cage, often severely wounding itself. It frequently breaks its teeth, lacerates its mouth and tongue, and drools a ropy slobber tinged with blood. Sometimes heavy, rapid respiration through the mouth causes a frothing of the saliva. The dog seems oblivious to pain and discomfort. It often swallows pieces of wood, stones, straw, fecal material, or other foreign bodies. No real hydrophobia (aversion to water) appears to occur, as it does in humans. Frequently the dog utters strange cries and hoarse yowls (altered phonation) because of a partial paralysis of the laryngeal musculature. It usually shows little interest in food during this stage but may demonstrate spastic attempts to swallow. Sometimes the animal is unable to close its eyes, and the cornea becomes dry and dull. Pupillary dilation frequently produces a staring or far-away look (Figure 53.3). Convulsive seizures and muscular incoordination herald the onset of the final, paralytic stage of rabies.

The paralytic stage is much less spectacular than the aggressive or excitatory stage and may be difficult to diagnose. Paralysis usually appears first in the muscles of the head and neck, with the most characteristic signs being mandibular and pharyngeal paralysis. The dog cannot chew its food or swallow, or it does so only with great difficulty. A ropy saliva drools from the mouth. The owner often imagines that a bone or other foreign object has become lodged in the dog's throat. In trying to examine the animal's mouth for an object that is not there, the owner may be exposed to the rabies virus by scratching the hands or fingers on the dog's teeth or by merely

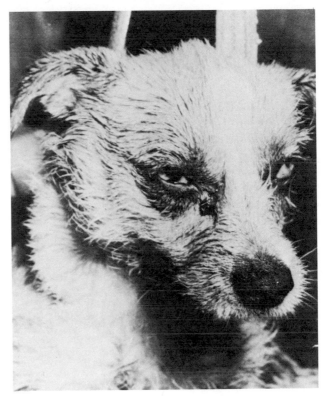

Figure 53.3. A dog with rabies showing the typical staring or far-away look. (From Tierkel, 1975b, courtesy of Academic Press and G. M. Baer.)

bathing already abraded hands in the copious, virus-laden saliva. The signs of localized paralysis are quickly succeeded by more generalized signs, with death following usually within 2 to 4 days of onset.

In cats rabies can assume the furious form with signs similar to those seen in dogs. Rabid cats are extremely dangerous animals for human attendants and owners because of their viciousness and quickness of action. The very few cases of vaccine-induced rabies in cats frequently have been paralytic in nature, however (Bellinger et al. 1983, Esh et al. 1982).

In horses clinical signs of rabies are extremely variable (Joyce and Russell 1981). The first manifestation may be rubbing and biting at the site of the bite wound. The horse often is alert and tense, holding its ears erect and moving them quickly back and forth as if listening to sounds from many directions. Genital excitement may be evident. The horse may try to break or bite through its halter rope or may attack the manger with such force that it breaks its teeth or even its mandible. It may paw the ground with its front feet and lash out with its rear limbs. The animal often refuses food but may swallow bits of straw, wood, manure, or other foreign objects. Hyperesthesia, ataxia, paralysis, fever, behavioral changes, and seizures all may be seen. The first signs of paralysis usually appear in the throat, manifested by an inability to swallow water. Saliva drools from the lips. Locomotor difficulties then appear, and finally the animal becomes recumbent. Death occurs in a few hours, sometimes following a series of violent convulsions.

In cattle signs of rabies are often particularly vague and confusing until late in the course of the disease. In the furious form the animals bawl, paw the earth, and, if provoked, may attack other animals or humans. The bellowing may be incessant and characterized by an altered pitch of the voice. More often the animals show no evidence of excitement. Salivation with drooling from the mouth is seen in many but not all cases, depending on whether pharyngeal paralysis develops. The eyes have a wide-open stare and frequently follow any moving object with a fixed look. Anorexia and an abrupt cessation of lactation are seen. Many animals strain more or less continuously for many hours in an apparent attempt to defecate or urinate. Usually air is aspirated into the rectum when the animal relaxes between straining periods. Another frequent sign is a knuckling over of the hind fetlock joints. The tail often becomes paralyzed. In bulls the penis may be protruded in a flaccid state. Conditions diagnosed as indigestion, milk fever, or esophageal foreign body may turn out to be rabies. Bovine paralytic rabies *(derriengue)* is particularly well recognized in the Latin American countries, where the offending vector frequently is the vampire bat (Baer 1975b, Dierks 1981).

In sheep and goats rabies does not often occur. Clinical signs can include restlessness, excitement, twitching of the lips, a wild and staring gaze, pruritus, pica, genital excitement, depression, and terminal paralysis.

In pigs rabies is considered rare but may be manifested by signs similar to those seen in sheep and goats.

The incubation period of rabies is extremely variable, ranging from a week to a year, depending on viral strain, host species, and dose and site of inoculation. In humans, it has long been recognized that bites in the region of the head and neck, particularly those that result in severe lacerations, are associated with a shorter incubation period and higher lethality than those received on other parts of the body. In humans the incubation period averages 3 to 6 weeks but may be as short as 15 days or as long as a year or more. A similar average incubation period is seen in the dog. The incubation period in cattle varies from 20 to 165 days, with an average of 1 to 2 months. The relatively short duration of the clinical illness is in contrast to the frequently lengthy incubation periods. In dogs and other carnivores, the course of the disease rarely exceeds 5 days, although a few may linger a day or two longer but rarely more than 9 to 10 days. The course of the disease in cattle is similar to that in carnivores.

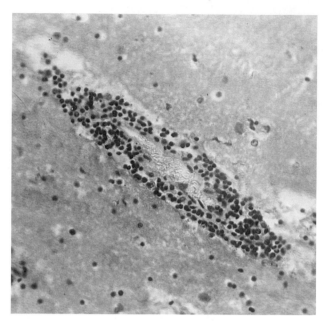

Figure 53.4. Perivascular cuffing produced by rabies virus in the brain of a rabbit. × 320. (Courtesy S. H. McNutt, University of Wisconsin, Madison.)

Rabies produces no pathognomonic gross pathological lesions. There may be some congestion of the meningeal vessels and mild cerebral edema. The brain tissue itself may appear unusually pink. The histological changes are notable primarily for their failure to reflect the severity of the clinical disease (Perl 1975). Perivascular cuffing is evident in the central nervous system (Figure 53.4), with vascular congestion, neuronophagia, and neuronal degeneration. There is a striking proliferation of the capsular cells surrounding ganglionic neurons. Negri bodies—cytoplasmic inclusions containing rabies viral antigen—may be found especially in the hippocampal ganglionic cells and the Purkinje cells of the cerebellum; they are considered diagnostic for rabies (Figure 53.5) (Lépine 1973, Tierkel 1973). They are present in only about 75 percent of confirmed cases, however. In the absence of Negri bodies, rabies encephalitis lesions cannot be distinguished from those produced by certain other viral encephalitides. The observed histological changes in general are not well correlated with the severity of the course of the disease, and a neurophysiological lesion sufficient to produce death of the host has yet to be identified.

Properties of the Virus. Rabies virus is a typical member of the Rhabdoviridae. It is heat-labile, ether-sensitive, and inactivated by many common detergents and disinfectants. Antigens of the rabies virus N protein are group-specific and have been detected by complement fixation, immunofluorescence, and agar-gel immunodiffusion. As

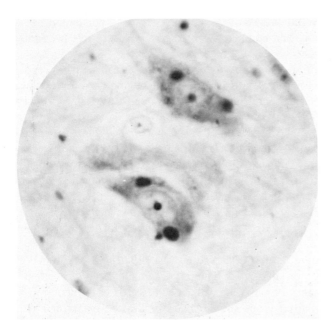

Figure 53.5. Negri bodies in the brain of a rabid dog. The clear vesicular nuclei containing sharply stained nucleoli occupy the center of each cell. The Negri bodies are located outside the nuclei in the cytoplasm. × 1,200. (Courtesy S. H. McNutt, University of Wisconsin, Madison.)

group-specific antigens, they show varying degrees of cross-reactivity with N protein antigens of other lyssaviruses. Antigens of the rabies virus G protein (peplomer protein) are responsible for the induction of virus-neutralizing antibody. The G protein antigens are type-specific and thus are useful for the differentiation of individual rabies virus strains.

Strains of rabies virus are classified as either *street* or *fixed*. Street viruses are the wild type or feral strains. They are characterized by a variable incubation period, salivary shedding, and moderate to low infectious virus titer levels in the brain (Clark and Prabhakar 1985). Fixed viruses are strains that have been passaged in laboratory animals. They have a shorter (fixed), more predictable incubation period and do *not* infect the salivary glands but produce higher titer levels in the brain. Virtually all strains of rabies virus adapted to growth in cell culture are fixed, or passaged, strains (Wiktor and Clark 1975). Among these are the common animal vaccine strains, such as the Flury high egg passage and ERA strains (Sikes 1975).

It is now well recognized that important antigenic and pathogenetic differences exist in rabies virus strains isolated from dogs, foxes, bats, and certain other reservoir species, although all field viruses and laboratory strains are still generally considered to belong to a single serotype (Beran and Crowley 1983). In addition, several rabies-related but serotypically distinct rhabdoviruses causing

rabieslike illness in humans and animals have been identified in Africa (Beran and Crowley 1983, Dierks 1981, Shope 1975). These include Duvenhage, Lagos bat, and Mokola viruses, which are placed together with rabies virus in the genus *Lyssavirus* of the Rhabdoviridae (see Table 53.1).

Cultivation. Rabies virus can be adapted to growth in a variety of primary cell cultures, including those derived from dogs, pigs, monkeys, chickens, and bats (Wiktor and Clark 1975). Many common vaccine strains have been propagated in embryonated duck or chicken eggs. One of the most useful systems for propagating the virus employs the BHK-21 (baby hamster kidney) cell line (Sokol et al. 1968, Wiktor et al. 1969). Human diploid cell strains (WI-38, MRC-5) also are widely employed and are especially useful today for production of human rabies vaccines. Cultures of neuroblastoma cells from humans and mice also will support replication of rabies virus. The virus has also been grown in cell lines derived from vertebrate poikilotherms. Cells infected by rabies virus generally can be maintained in culture for prolonged periods in the absence of noticeable cytopathic effect. Even with a highly susceptible cell line such as BHK-21, relatively little cytopathic effect may be observed.

A number of laboratory animal species are also employed in diagnostics and/or research including mice, rats, guinea pigs, hamsters, rabbits, dogs, and monkeys.

Epizootiology and Pathogenesis. Rabies is considered to be a universal infection (Koprowski 1984). The virus infects most warm-blooded animals and occurs worldwide. It is transmitted most commonly by the bite of an infected animal, which introduces virus-laden saliva into the wound. Rarely, infections occur through contamination of existing wounds or abrasions. Humans have contracted the disease through scratch wounds while endeavoring to find a supposed obstruction in the throats of animals with rabies-induced pharyngeal paralysis. Rabies has been shown to be transmissible through inhalation of virus-contaminated aerosols (as in caves inhabited by bats) (Constantine 1967, Winkler 1968), and it may also be acquired in the laboratory (Tillotson et al. 1977, Winkler et al. 1972), but these are both very rare phenomena, occurring under unique conditions. Transmission following ingestion of the virus is also very rare. It does not appear that either ingestion or inhalation of rabies virus is of great epizootiological significance (Dierks 1981). Vertical transmission has also been reported (Howard 1981, Martell et al. 1973).

Rabies is primarily maintained in nature by wild and domestic carnivores and by certain other wildlife species. In the United States skunks play a major role in spreading the disease and are now the primary reservoir in that country (Baer 1985, Parker 1975). Raccoons are important in the transmission of rabies in the southeastern states and have recently begun to spread the disease to more northern areas of the Atlantic seaboard (Hubbard 1985, McLean 1975, Smith et al. 1984). Wild foxes are reservoir hosts in many parts of Europe and in North America as well (Bögel et al. 1976, Winkler 1975). Wolves are major vectors in some areas of the world, especially in Iran and the Soviet Union (Selimov et al. 1959). In the Caribbean and much of the Americas, bats are important reservoirs. In the Latin American countries, vampire bats are particularly notorious for transmission of paralytic rabies *(derriengue)* to domestic cattle (Baer 1975c, Dierks 1981). The mongoose is another effective reservoir host in certain parts of the world, such as South Africa and the Caribbean (Everard et al. 1974, 1981). The only rodent species of any importance in rabies epizootiology appears to be the woodchuck, in the mid-Atlantic and midwestern regions of the United States (Fishbein et al. 1986). Of the domestic species only the dog and cat are significant vectors of the virus. In most developing areas today, the dog remains the primary reservoir of the disease and the principal source of human exposure (Beran and Crowley 1983). All domestic species in areas where wildlife rabies is enzootic, however, should be considered at risk of contracting the disease and of transmitting it to humans.

Seasonal variations in the occurrence of clinical rabies have been observed in a number of populations of wild animals, including foxes, skunks, raccoons, and bats (Baer and Adams 1970, Bigler et al. 1973, Dierks 1981, Johnston and Beauregard 1969, Verts 1967, Wandeler et al. 1974). Seasonal cycles may relate to mating and nesting behaviors, the presence of young susceptible offspring, and dispersal of animals by migration. Three-year cycles of rabies epizootics in foxes have also been reported (Johnston and Beauregard 1969, Kauker and Zettl 1960).

Although rabies is considered to be fatal once clinical signs of the disease are manifest, a certain proportion of infected animals merely seroconverts in the absence of clinical disease (Sikes 1981, Winkler 1981). These animals and their offspring, together with uninfected cohabitants and other animals migrating in from areas of higher population density, may constitute the foundation for interepizootic buildup of a new susceptible population. Because of the variable (and frequently lengthy) incubation period, a number of animals in the new and growing population may be expected to harbor rabies virus. Once the population has expanded sufficiently, and the ratio of infected to susceptible animals has attained an optimal value, a new epizootic of the disease would be expected to occur. In this way rabies virus infections may be perpetuated through a series of interrelated epizootic-enzootic cycles, powered by changing shifts in population densities and numbers of infected and susceptible host animals.

Experimental evidence indicates that rabies virus replicates in myocytes at the site of inoculation before reaching the peripheral nerves (Charlton and Casey 1979, 1981; Murphy, Bauer, et al. 1973; Murphy, Harrison, et al. 1973). Amputation of tissue inoculated with rabies virus markedly reduces mortality, even when performed weeks after viral injection (Baer and Cleary 1972). Prolonged retention of virus in myocytes following inoculation thus may be one contributing factor to the variable length of the rabies incubation period. When the incubation period is short, the virus may invade the peripheral nervous system soon after inoculation, with limited replication in extraneural tissues (Charlton and Casey 1979, 1981). Following this variable and still largely enigmatic period of encampment within muscle cells, the virus crosses the neuromuscular junctions and advances into the peripheral nerves, perhaps by using the acetylcholine receptor complex as a cellular receptor (Burrage et al. 1985; Lentz et al. 1983, 1984; Spriggs 1985), and then is transported centripetally in the axoplasm between the axons and their myelin sheaths. Upon reaching the spinal ganglia of the infected nerves, virions replicate and move rapidly up the spinal cord to the brain (Johnson 1965; Murphy, Bauer, et al. 1973; Murphy, Harrison, et al. 1973; Schneider 1969a, 1969b; Schneider and Hamann 1969). Invasion of the central nervous system is followed by centrifugal spread (again via nerve axons) to a wide variety of tissues in the respiratory, gastrointestinal, and urogenital tracts (Murphy, Harrison, et al. 1973; Schnieder 1975). Of greatest epizootiological significance is excretion of rabies virus from the salivary glands (Figure 53.6) (Charlton et al. 1983, 1984; Dierks et al. 1969; Winkler et al. 1985). The amount of virus produced may be substantial—as high as six to seven logs in undiluted saliva (Parker and Wilsnack 1966). Salivary shedding of virus can begin as early as 1 to 2 weeks *before* the onset of clinical signs in a number of species, including the dog (Baer 1985, Fekadu et al. 1982, Parker and Wilsnack 1966, Sikes 1962). Asymptomatic bats may excrete virus over longer periods (Baer 1975c), and some dogs may continue to shed virus in the saliva for months after rare clinical recovery from the disease (Fekadu 1972, Fekadu et al. 1981, 1983). Depending on conditions of temperature and humidity and the percentage and number of infected bats, the air in caves heavily infested by certain bat species (e.g., the Mexican freetail) can actually become infectious for susceptible mammals (Baer 1975b, 1975c; Constantine 1967; Winkler 1968).

Immunity. The peplomer (G) protein of the rabies

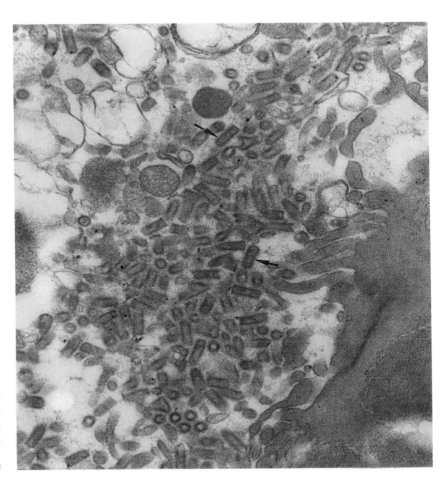

Figure 53.6. Rabies virus in the salivary gland of a rabid fox. Virions appear either in silhouette (bullet-shaped forms) or in cross-section (circular forms). Transmission electron microscopy. × 41,300. (Courtesy F. A. Murphy, Centers for Disease Control.)

virus particle is of greatest importance immunologically and is responsible for the induction of neutralizing antibody (Dietzschold et al. 1978, Wiktor et al. 1973). It may also play a role in determining the virulence of individual viral strains (Dietzschold et al. 1983, Seif et al. 1985). Immunization experiments using purified G protein or vaccinia-rabies G protein recombinants in mice and rabbits have demonstrated protection against rabies virus challenge (Atanasiu et al. 1976, Kieny et al. 1984, Wiktor et al. 1973, 1984). The presence of preformed neutralizing antibody in an individual animal usually (but not always) guarantees protection following challenge-exposure. Additional host factors that may also be involved in control of rabies virus infection include the production of interferon, action of cytotoxic T lymphocytes, and local effects resulting from pyrexia and the inflammatory process (Baer 1985, Bell 1975, Clark and Prabhakar 1985, Murphy 1977, Wiktor et al. 1968).

Many rabies vector species (dogs, skunks, raccoons, mongooses, vampire bats) are in actuality relatively resistant to rabies virus infection, as indicated in part by the presence of neutralizing antibodies in numerous healthy individuals from enzootic areas (Bigler et al. 1983, Doege and Northrop 1974, Everard et al. 1981, Lord et al. 1975, Tierkel 1959, 1975a, 1975b). It is generally assumed that most of these seropositive animals have experienced abortive infections, that is, they have contained the virus without developing fatal encephalitis (Bell 1975). Other vector species, such as foxes, are exquisitely sensitive to infection, as are certain dead-end hosts (cattle) (Dierks 1981, Tierkel 1959, Winkler 1975). Chronic infections, characterized by prolonged salivary shedding in asymptomatic animals or by an unusually prolonged incubation period, are generally considered to be extremely rare (Clark and Prabhakar 1985).

Diagnosis. The clinical signs of rabies, while considered to be characteristic for the disease, are not pathognomonic; a definitive diagnosis can be made only by laboratory examination. Considering the grave prognosis for recovery from rabies once clinical signs have appeared, an accurate diagnosis is imperative when attempting to determine whether exposure to a rabid animal has occurred.

Any wild or domestic mammal that has bitten a human

being and is showing clinical signs suggestive of rabies should be killed and the head submitted to a qualified laboratory for diagnostic tests. In addition, any bat or wild carnivore, regardless of symptoms manifested, which has bitten a human being should be destroyed immediately and its brain examined for the presence of rabies virus. This latter action is in consideration of the variable period of presymptomatic salivary shedding that is known to occur in a number of susceptible species. Any bat that has bitten a human being should be presumed rabid until confirmed negative for the disease by laboratory examination. *Any* healthy domestic animal that has bitten a human being should be confined for at least 10 days and observed for the development of clinical signs of rabies (ACIP 1984, NASPHV 1988, WHO 1984).

Unvaccinated domestic animals that have been bitten by or exposed to a rabid animal should be destroyed. If the owner is unwilling or unable to have this done, the unvaccinated animal should be placed in quarantine for 6 months and vaccinated for rabies 1 month before release. Vaccinated animals should be given a booster dose immediately after exposure to a rabid animal and observed by the owner for 90 days. If signs of rabies occur during this period, these animals should be killed and their brains examined. Livestock known to have been bitten by a rabid animal should be slaughtered or quarantined for 6 months for observation. If they are slaughtered within 7 days of being bitten, their meat may be consumed without fear of infection if liberal portions of the exposed region are discarded (NASPHV 1988, WHO 1984).

Currently three principal methods are available for the laboratory diagnosis of rabies.

Histopathology. Sections or smears of the hippocampus, cerebral cortex, and cerebellum are examined for signs of acute encephalitis and for the presence of Negri bodies (see Figure 53.5). Unfortunately, Negri bodies are not identified in all confirmed cases of rabies; however, this method is still used for the diagnosis of rabies in many parts of the world.

Immunofluorescence microscopy. Slides of brain tissue are examined for the presence of rabies virus antigen with fluorescein-tagged conjugates (Dean and Abelseth 1973, Kissling 1975). Immunofluorescence microscopy is more sensitive than histopathological examination because it can detect minute quantities of viral antigen earlier in the course of the disease. It is the most rapid and accurate method for the detection of rabies virus and is the current test of choice for the diagnosis of rabies. Immunofluorescence microscopy is being investigated also for antemortem detection of rabies virus antigen in biopsy specimens (Blenden 1981, Blenden et al. 1983, Wright 1983), although this procedure is definitely not

sensitive enough to replace other techniques (Fekadu and Shaddock 1984).

Mouse inoculation. In this method Swiss mice are inoculated intracerebrally with test suspensions and observed for the development of neurological signs (Koprowski 1973). Brains of affected mice are then examined for the presence of rabies virus antigen by immunofluorescence microscopy or for Negri bodies by histopathology. The mouse inoculation test is slightly less sensitive than immunofluorescence microscopy and has the added disadvantage of requiring several days for a positive diagnosis. The procedure today is frequently used to confirm positive results obtained by immunofluorescence microscopy or histopathology and to investigate further suspected cases in which results have proved negative by the other two methods.

Treatment. Because of the potential risk of exposing susceptible humans to rabies virus, treatment of domestic and wild animals following exposure to the virus, regardless of symptoms, must be strongly discouraged. Treatment of humans exposed to the virus, however, must be aggressively applied. Once clinical signs have appeared, recovery from rabies is exceedingly rare; only three human survivors have been documented (Hattwick et al. 1972, Porras et al. 1976, Tillotson et al. 1977).

Postexposure treatment for humans is essentially a three-pronged process (Baer 1985, Hattwick and Gregg 1975, Sikes 1981):

Local wound treatment. The importance of immediate and thorough flushing and cleansing of the wound with soap and water cannot be overemphasized (Dean 1975, Dean et al. 1963). Ethanol and/or a quaternary ammonium compound such as benzalkonium chloride should be applied following the soap and water scrub. In the case of deep puncture wounds, a catheter should be placed and the wound flushed at periodic intervals. Suturing of the wound is discouraged.

Rabies immune globulin (human origin). Administration of rabies immune globulin (including local infiltration of the wound site) along with vaccination is recommended and is considered to be the best specific postexposure treatment. Individuals who have been vaccinated (preimmunized) and who have adequate antibody titers should not be given immune globulin, however, because of its possible interference with the anamnestic response to human diploid cell rabies vaccine.

Human diploid cell vaccine. Five 1-ml doses of vaccine are given on days 0, 3, 7, 14, and 28 after exposure, following the administration of one dose of immune globulin. Preimmunized individuals with adequate antibody titers generally are given only two doses, on days 0 and 3. The presence of preformed antibody from previous immunizations is no guarantee of protection following exposure to rabies virus; *all preimmunized individuals regardless of rabies virus antibody titer should seek postexposure prophylaxis* (Kuwert and Scheiermann 1985). Preimmunized individuals with low or negative antibody titers should be considered unprotected and receive the full course of immunizations, including rabies immune globulin.

Prevention and Control. In the United States and most other countries of the world, effective rabies vaccines are available for prevention of rabies virus infection in domestic animals (Table 53.3) and humans. In the domestic species rabies vaccines are used primarily for preexposure prophylaxis; treatment after exposure is not advised. Mass immunization of dogs has been employed for many years to control the spread of rabies by creating an immunological barrier between wildlife reservoirs of the disease and human populations (Baer 1985, Steele 1975, Tierkel 1975b). Several nations, including Japan, England, Iceland, and the Scandinavian countries, have eradicated rabies by implementing control programs and strict quarantine regulations. Despite these successes, however, canine rabies remains a serious health hazard in many developing regions of the world (Beran and Crowley 1983, Tierkel 1975a, Turner 1976). In humans preexposure immunization is generally restricted to those individuals considered to be at high risk of exposure to rabies virus, for example, veterinarians, laboratory personnel, wildlife researchers, and animal control workers. At present, there are no rabies vaccines licensed for use in wild animals.

The first vaccine for rabies was developed in the 1880s by Pasteur, who successfully attenuated street virus by serial passage in rabbits (Steele 1975). Most present-day vaccines are produced in cell culture, embryonated eggs, or in suckling mouse brain, and are available as inactivated or modified live-virus preparations. It is generally recommended that vaccines with a 3-years' duration of immunity be administered to dogs and cats because their use constitutes the most effective method of increasing the proportion of immunized animals in comprehensive control programs (NASPHV 1988). Annual boosters are recommended, however, for horses and ruminants. Cats should never be immunized with modified live rabies virus vaccines not approved for use in the feline species because this may result in vaccine-induced rabies in a small proportion of vaccinated animals (Bellinger et al. 1983, Esh et al. 1982). Unless otherwise specified by the product label or package insert, all vaccines must be given intramuscularly at one site in the thigh (NASPHV 1988).

All dogs and cats should be vaccinated for rabies at 3 months of age and revaccinated as required by vaccine specifications (see Table 53.3). It is neither economically feasible nor medically justifiable to vaccinate all livestock; however, veterinary clinicians and owners of valuable animals may consider immunizing certain animals in areas where wildlife rabies is epizootic and where colonies of bats exist (NASPHV 1988). Wild animals in the United States *should not* be vaccinated for rabies, even with inactivated virus preparations, until vaccines approved for use in wildlife species are available.

Present regulations governing the importation of wild and domestic canines, felines, and other potential vectors of rabies are minimal for preventing the introduction of rabid animals into the United States (NASPHV 1988). All dogs and cats imported from countries with enzootic rabies should be vaccinated at least 30 days before entry. The requirements of the Centers for Disease Control (CDC) should be coordinated with interstate shipment requirements, and the health authority of the state of destination should be notified within 72 hours of any animal's being conditionally admitted into its area of jurisdiction. Failure to comply with these requirements should be reported promptly to the director of the CDC.

Accidental inoculation or other exposure of humans may occur while administering animal rabies virus vaccines. Available data indicate that such exposure to inactivated vaccines constitutes *no known* health hazard. Moreover, no cases of human rabies resulting from needle or other exposure to licensed modified live-virus rabies vaccines in the United States have been reported (NASPHV 1988).

Because rabies is transmitted almost exclusively through the bites of rabid animals, its control depends on the success achieved in controlling the activities of the reservoir species. In wild populations—skunks, foxes, raccoons, bats, mongooses—the disease can be eliminated only by destruction of the reservoir species or by greatly reducing its numbers. This is not ecologically, aesthetically, or logistically desirable. Some progress has been made in recent years in attempts to vaccinate certain wildlife species against rabies, most notably foxes, with various oral and parenteral virus preparations (commercial animal vaccines or virus sequestered in sausage baits, chicken heads, eggs, etc.) (Baer 1985, Baer et al. 1971, Debbie et al. 1972, Steck et al. 1982, Winkler and Baer 1976). Unfortunately, few other wildlife species appear to be immunized as readily as the fox. In urban settings immunization of dogs (and cats) remains the best deterrent to the spread of rabies to human populations (Beran and Crowley 1983).

The Disease in Humans. The signs and course of rabies in humans are similar to those seen in animals (Hattwick and Gregg 1975). Both excitatory and paralytic

Table 53.3. Compendium of animal rabies vaccines in the United States, 1988

Product name	Produced by	Marketed by	For use in*	Dose†	Recommended frequency of boosters‡
Modified live virus					
Endurall-R	Norden, license no. 189	Norden	Dogs	1 ml	Triennially
			Cats	1 ml	Annually
Neurogen-TC	Boehringer Ingelheim, license no. 124	Bio-Ceutic	Dogs	1 ml	Triennially
Inactivated					
Trimune	Fort Dodge, license no. 112	Fort Dodge	Dogs	1 ml	Triennially
			Cats	1 ml	Triennially
Annumune	Fort Dodge, license no. 112	Fort Dodge	Dogs	1 ml	Annually
			Cats	1 ml	Annually
Biorab-1	Schering, license no. 165-A	Biologics Corp.	Dogs	1 ml	Annually
			Cats	1 ml	Annually
Biorab-3	Schering, license no. 165-A	Biologics Corp.	Dogs	1 ml	Triennially
			Cats	1 ml	Annually
Rabmune 3	Schering, license no. 165-A	Beecham	Dogs	1 ml	Triennially
			Cats	1 ml	Annually
Dura-Rab 1	ImmunoVet, license no. 302-A	ImmunoVet and Vedco, Inc.	Dogs	1 ml	Annually
			Cats	1 ml	Annually
Dura-Rab 3	ImmunoVet, license no. 302-A	ImmunoVet & Vedco, Inc.	Dogs	1 ml	Triennially
			Cats	1 ml	Triennially
Rabcine	Beecham, license no. 225	Beecham	Dogs	1 ml	Annually
			Cats	1 ml	Annually
Rabcine 3	ImmunoVet, license no. 302-A	Beecham	Dogs	1 ml	Triennially
			Cats	1 ml	Triennially
Endurall-K	Norden, license no. 189	Norden	Dogs	1 ml	Annually
			Cats	1 ml	Annually
Rabguard-TC	Norden, license no. 189	Norden	Dogs	1 ml	Triennially
			Cats	1 ml	Triennially
			Cattle	1 ml	Annually
			Horses	1 ml	Annually
Cytorab	Coopers Animal Health Inc., license no. 107	Coopers	Dogs	1 ml	Annually
			Cats	1 ml	Annually
Trirab	Coopers Animal Health Inc., license no. 107	Coopers	Dogs	1 ml	Triennially
			Cats	1 ml	Annually
Rabvac 1	Fromm, license no. 195-A	Solvay Veterinary	Dogs	1 ml	Annually
			Cats	1 ml	Annually
Rabvac 3	Fromm, license no. 195-A	Solvay Veterinary	Dogs	1 ml	Triennially
			Cats	1 ml	Triennially
Imrab	Merieux, license no. 298	Pitman-Moore	Dogs	1 ml	Triennially
			Cats	1 ml	Triennially
			Sheep	1 ml	Triennially
			Cattle	2 ml	Annually
			Horses	2 ml	Annually
Imrab-1	Merieux, license no. 298	Pitman-Moore	Dogs	1 ml	Annually
			Cats	1 ml	Annually
Combination					
Eclipse 3 KP-R	Fromm, license no. 195-A	Solvay Veterinary	Cats	1 ml	Annually
Eclipse 4 KP-R	Fromm, license no. 195-A	Solvay Veterinary	Cats	1 ml	Annually

Table 53.3.—*continued*

Product name	Produced by	Marketed by	For use in*	Dose†	Recommended frequency of boosters‡
Cytorab RCP	Coopers Animal Health Inc., license no. 107	Coopers	Cats	1 ml	Annually
Fel-O-Vax PCT-R	Fort Dodge, license no. 112	Fort Dodge	Cats	1 ml	Triennially
Eclipse 4-R	Fromm, license no. 195-A	Solvay Veterinary	Cats	1 ml	Annually

*Refers only to domestic species of this group of animals.
†All vaccines must be administered intramuscularly at one site in the thigh unless otherwise specified by the label.
‡Primary immunization recommended at 3 months of age, with subsequent boosters as indicated.
Modified from a table supplied by M. K. Abelseth, N.Y. State Dept. of Health, on behalf of the National Association of State Public Health Veterinarians, Inc.

signs may be manifested. The incubation period, as in animals, is quite variable—from about 2 weeks to as long as a year—but averages between 3 and 6 weeks. The course of the disease is short—only a few days—and the mortality rate is essentially 100 percent once clinical signs have appeared. There are only three reports of individuals surviving documented clinical rabies (Hattwick et al. 1972, Porras et al. 1976, Tillotson et al. 1977). Mortality varies markedly according to the location of the bite (Hattwick and Gregg 1975; also see "Character of the Disease" above). The risk of rabies developing in the exposed individual varies with many factors but even in those with the most severe exposures does not reach 100 percent.

Preexposure prophylaxis is recommended only for individuals at high risk of exposure, but aggressive treatment after exposure is *essential* for all individuals known or suspected of having been exposed to a rabid animal. Human diploid cell vaccine is currently the recommended product for preexposure human rabies prophylaxis, whereas human diploid cell vaccine plus human rabies immune globulin is the preferred combination for postexposure treatment (ACIP 1984; Anderson, Sikes, et al. 1980, Anderson, Winkler, et al. 1980; Beran and Crowley 1983; Dreesen et al. 1982; Hafkin et al. 1978; Kuwert and Scheiermann 1985; WHO 1984).

Rabies is a classic zoonosis in that it is primarily a disease of animals that occasionally spills over into human beings, who are dead-end hosts. The vast majority of human deaths from rabies are attributable to dog bites, and the key to eradication of the disease from human populations is canine rabies control (Beran and Crowley 1983). In the developed nations of the world, control of rabies in dogs by immunization and quarantine procedures has resulted in a dramatic decline in the number of

human deaths from rabies, despite the persistence of wildlife reservoirs. In the last 10 years, significant advances in research have been made, particularly with regard to the improvement of human and animal vaccines. The gap between these new scientific developments and their implementation in the developing nations is appreciable, however; its closure represents one of the great challenges facing public health professionals today.

REFERENCES

ACIP (Immunization Practices Advisory Committee). 1984. Rabies prevention—United States, 1984. M.M.W.R. 33:393–402, 407–408.

Anderson, L.J., Baer, G.M., Smith, J.S., Winkler, W.G., and Holman, R.C. 1981. Rapid antibody response to human diploid rabies vaccine. Am. J. Epidemiol. 113:270–275.

Anderson, L.J., Sikes, R.K., Langkop, C.W., Mann, J.M., Smith, J.S., Winkler, W.G., and Deitch, M.W. 1980. Postexposure trial of a human diploid cell strain rabies vaccine. J. Infect. Dis. 142:133–138.

Anderson, L.J., Winkler, W.G., Hafkin, B., Keenlyside, R.A., D'Angelo, L.J., and Deitch, M.W. 1980. Clinical experience with a human diploid cell rabies vaccine. J.A.M.A. 244:781–784.

Atanasiu, P., Tsiang, H., Perrin, P., and Favre, S. 1976. Analyse du pouvoir immunogène et protecteur de la glycoprotéine extraite du virus rabique: Comparaison de préparations purifiées par des techniques différentes et résultats. Ann. Microbiol. (Inst. Pasteur) 127B:257–267.

Baer, G.M., ed. 1975a. The Natural History of Rabies, vols. 1 and 2. Academic Press, New York. 454 and 387 pp.

Baer, G.M. 1975b. Rabies in nonhematophagous bats. In G.M. Baer, ed., The Natural History of Rabies, vol. 2. Academic Press, New York. Pp. 79–97.

Baer, G.M. 1975c. Bovine paralytic rabies and rabies in the vampire bat. In G.M. Baer, ed., The Natural History of Rabies, vol. 2. Academic Press, New York. Pp. 155–175.

Baer, G.M. 1985. Rabies virus. In B.N. Fields, ed., Virology. Raven Press, New York. Pp. 1133–1156.

Baer, G.M., and Adams, D.B. 1970. Rabies in insectivorous bats in the United States, 1953–65. Public Health Rep. 85:637–645.

Baer, G.M., and Cleary, W.F. 1972. A model in mice for the pathogenesis and treatment of rabies. J. Infect. Dis. 125:520–527.

Baer, G.M., Abelseth, M.K., and Debbie, J.G. 1971. Oral vaccination of foxes against rabies. Am. J. Epidemiol. 93:487–490.

Bell, J.F. 1975. Latency and abortive rabies. In G.M. Baer, ed., The Natural History of Rabies, vol. 1. Academic Press, New York. Pp. 331–354.

Bellinger, D.A., Chang, J., Bunn, T.O., Pick, J.R., Murphy, M., and Rahija, R. 1983. Rabies induced in a cat by high-egg-passage Flury strain vaccine. J. Am. Vet. Med. Assoc. 183:997–998.

Beran, G.W., and Crowley, A.J. 1983. Toward worldwide rabies control. WHO Chron. 37:192–196.

Bigler, W.J., Hoff, G.L., Smith, J.S., McLean, R.G., Trevino, H. A., and Ingwersen, J. 1983. Persistence of rabies antibody in free-ranging raccoons. J. Infect. Dis. 148:610.

Bigler, W.J., McLean, R.G., and Trevino, H.A. 1973. Epizootiologic aspects of raccoon rabies in Florida. Am. J. Epidemiol. 98:326–335.

Blenden, D.C. 1981. Rabies in a litter of skunks predicted and diagnosed by skin biopsy. J. Am. Vet. Med. Assoc. 179:789–791.

Blenden, D.C., Bell, J.F., Tsao, A.T., and Umoh, J.U. 1983. Immunofluorescent examination of the skin of rabies-infected animals as a means of early detection of rabies virus antigen. J. Clin. Microbiol. 18:631–636.

Bögel, K., Moegle, H., Knorpp, F., Arata, A., Dietz, K., and Diethelm, P. 1976. Characteristics of the spread of a wildlife rabies epidemic in Europe. Bull. WHO 54:433–447.

Burrage, T.G., Tignor, G.H., and Smith, A.L. 1985. Rabies virus binding at neuromuscular junctions. Virus Res. 2:273–289.

Charlton, K.M., and Casey, G.A. 1979. Experimental rabies in skunks. Immunofluorescence light and electron microscopic studies. Lab. Invest. 41:36–44.

Charlton, K.M., and Casey, G.A. 1981. Experimental rabies in skunks: Persistence of virus in denervated muscle at the inoculation site. Can. J. Comp. Med. 45:357–362.

Charlton, K.M., Casey, G.A., and Campbell, J.B. 1983. Experimental rabies in skunks: Mechanisms of infection of the salivary glands. Can. J. Comp. Med. 47:363–369.

Charlton, K.M., Casey, G.A., and Webster, W.A. 1984. Rabies virus in the salivary glands and nasal mucosa of naturally infected skunks. Can. J. Comp. Med. 48:338–339.

Clark, H.F., and Prabhakar, B.S. 1985. Rabies. In R.G. Olsen, S. Krakowka, and J.R. Blakeslee, eds., Comparative Pathobiology of Viral Diseases, vol. 2. CRC Press, Boca Raton, Fla. Pp. 165–214.

Constantine, D.G. 1967. Rabies transmission by air in bat caves. U.S. Dept. of Health, Education, and Welfare, Public Health Service, publication no. 1617. U.S. Government Printing Office, Washington, D.C. 51 pp.

Dean, D.J. 1975. Local wound treatment. In G.M. Baer, ed., The Natural History of Rabies, vol. 2. Academic Press, New York. Pp. 305–317.

Dean, D.J., and Abelseth, M.K. 1973. The fluorescent antibody test. In M.M. Kaplan and H. Koprowski, eds., Laboratory Techniques in Rabies, 3d ed. World Health Organization, Geneva. Pp. 73–84.

Dean, D.J., Baer, G.M., and Thompson, W.R. 1963. Studies on the local treatment of rabies-infected wounds. Bull. WHO 28:477–486.

Debbie, J.G., Abelseth, M.K., and Baer, G.M. 1972. The use of commercially available vaccines for the oral vaccination of foxes against rabies. Am. J. Epidemiol. 96:231–235.

Dierks, R.E. 1981. Bovine rabies. In M. Ristic and I. McIntyre, eds., Diseases of Cattle in the Tropics. Martinus Nijhoff, The Hague. Pp. 107–121.

Dierks, R.E., Murphy, F.A., and Harrison, A.K. 1969. Extraneural rabies virus infection. Virus development in fox salivary gland. Am. J. Pathol. 54:251–273.

Dietzschold, B., Cox, J.H., Schneider, L.G., Wiktor, T.J., and Koprowski, H. 1978. Isolation and purification of a polymeric form of the glycoprotein of rabies virus. J. Gen. Virol. 40:131–139.

Dietzschold, B., Wunner, W.H., Wiktor, T.J., Lopes, A.D., Lafon, M., Smith, C.L., and Koprowski, H. 1983. Characterization of an antigenic determinant of the glycoprotein that correlates with pathogenicity of rabies virus. Proc. Natl. Acad. Sci USA 80:70–74.

Doege, T.C., and Northrop, R.L. 1974. Evidence for inapparent rabies infection. Lancet 2:826–829.

Dreesen, D.W., Sumner, J.W., Brown, J., and Kemp, D.T. 1982. Intradermal use of human diploid cell vaccine for preexposure rabies immunizations. J. Am. Vet. Med. Assoc. 181:1519–1523.

Esh, J.B., Cunningham, J.G., and Wiktor, T.J. 1982. Vaccine-induced rabies in four cats. J. Am. Vet. Med. Assoc. 180:1336–1339.

Everard, C.O.R., Baer, G.M., Alls, M.E., and Moore, S.A. 1981. Rabies serum neutralizing antibody in mongooses from Grenada. Trans. R. Soc. Trop. Med. Hyg. 75:654–666.

Everard, C.O.R., Baer, G.M., and James, A. 1974. Epidemiology of mongoose rabies in Grenada. J. Wildl. Dis. 10:190–196.

Fekadu, M. 1972. Atypical rabies in dogs in Ethiopia. Ethiop. Med. J. 10:79–86.

Fekadu, M., and Shaddock, J.H. 1984. Peripheral distribution of virus in dogs inoculated with two strains of rabies virus. Am. J. Vet. Res. 45:724–729.

Fekadu, M., Shaddock, J.H., and Baer, G.M. 1981. Intermittent excretion of rabies virus in the saliva of a dog two and six months after it had recovered from experimental rabies. Am. J. Trop. Med. Hyg. 30:1113–1115.

Fekadu, M., Shaddock, J.H., and Baer, G.M. 1982. Excretion of rabies virus in the saliva of dogs. J. Infect. Dis. 145:715–719.

Fekadu, M., Shaddock, J.H., Chandler, F.W., and Baer, G.M. 1983. Rabies virus in the tonsils of a carrier dog. Arch. Virol. 78:37–47.

Fishbein, D.B., Belotto, A.J., Pacer, R.E., Smith, J.S., Winkler, W.G., Jenkins, S.R., and Porter, K.M. 1986. Rabies in rodents and lagomorphs in the United States, 1971–1984: Increased cases in the woodchuck (Marmota monax) in mid-Atlantic states. J. Wildl. Dis. 22:151–155.

Goetze, A. 1955. The laws of Eshnunna. In J.B. Pritchard, ed., Ancient Near Eastern Texts Relating to the Old Testament, 2d ed. Princeton University Press, Princeton, N.J. Pp. 161–163.

Hafkin, B., Hattwick, H.A.W., Smith, J.S., Alls, M.E., Yager, P.A., Corey, L., Hoke, C.H., and Baer, G.M. 1978. A comparison of a WI-38 vaccine and duck embryo vaccine for preexposure rabies prophylaxis. Am. J. Epidemiol. 107:439–443.

Hattwick, M.A.W., and Gregg, M.B. 1975. The disease in man. In G.M. Baer, ed., The Natural History of Rabies, vol. 2. Academic Press, New York. Pp. 281–304.

Hattwick, M.A.W., Weis, T.T., Stechschulte, C.J., Baer, G.M., and Gregg, M.B. 1972. Recovery from rabies. A case report. Ann. Intern. Med. 76:931–942.

Howard, D.R. 1981. Transplacental transmission of rabies virus from a naturally infected skunk. Am. J. Vet. Res. 42:691–692.

Hubbard, D.R. 1985. A descriptive epidemiological study of raccoon rabies in a rural environment. J. Wildl. Dis. 21:105–110.

Johnson, R.T. 1965. Experimental rabies. Studies of cellular vulnerability and pathogenesis using fluorescent antibody staining. J. Neuropathol. Exp. Neurol. 24:662–674.

Johnston, D.H., and Beauregard, M. 1969. Rabies epidemiology in Ontario. Bull. Wildl. Dis. Assoc. 5:357–370.

Joyce, J.R., and Russell, L.H. 1981. Clinical signs of rabies in horses. Compend. Cont. Ed. Pract. Vet. 3:S56–S61.

Kaplan, M.M., and Koprowski, H. 1960. Rabies. Sci. Am. 242(1):120–134.

Kauker, E., and Zettl, K. 1960. Die Ökologie des Rotfuchses und ihre Beziehung zur Tollwut. D.T.W. 67:463–467.

Kieny, M.P., Lathe, R., Drillien, R., Spehner, D., Skory, S., Schmitt, D., Wiktor, T., Koprowski, H., and Lecocq, J.P. 1984. Expression of rabies virus glycoprotein from a recombinant vaccinia virus. Nature 312:163–166.

Kissling, R.E. 1975. The fluorescent antibody test in rabies. In G.M. Baer, ed., The Natural History of Rabies, vol. 1. Academic Press, New York. Pp. 401–416.

Koprowski, H. 1973. The mouse inoculation test. In M.M. Kaplan and H. Koprowski, eds., Laboratory Techniques in Rabies, 3d ed. World Health Organization, Geneva. Pp. 85–93.

Koprowski, H. 1984. Rabies. In A.L. Notkins and M.B.A. Oldstone, eds., Concepts in Viral Pathogenesis. Springer-Verlag, New York. Pp. 344–349.

Kuwert, E., and Scheiermann, N. 1985. Rabies: Post-exposure prophylaxis in man. Ann. Inst. Pasteur/Virol. 136E:425–445.

Lentz, T.L., Burrage, T.G., Smith, A.L., and Tignor, G.H. 1983. The acetylcholine receptor as a cellular receptor for rabies virus. Yale J. Biol. Med. 56:315–322.

Lentz, T.L., Wilson, P.T., Hawrot, E., and Speicher, D.W. 1984. Amino acid sequence similarity between rabies virus glycoprotein and snake venom curaremimetic neurotoxins. Science 226:847–848.

Lépine, P. 1973. Histopathological diagnosis. In M.M. Kaplan and H. Koprowski, eds., Laboratory Techniques in Rabies, 3d ed. World Health Organization, Geneva. Pp. 56–72.

Lord, R.D., Delpietro, H., Fuenzalida, E., Díaz, A.M.O., and Lazaro, L. 1975. Presence of rabies neutralizing antibodies in wild carnivores following an outbreak of bovine rabies. J. Wildl. Dis. 11:210–213. 11:210–213.

McLean, R.G. 1975. Raccoon rabies. In G.M. Baer, ed., The Natural History of Rabies, vol. 2. Academic Press, New York. Pp. 53–77.

Martell, M.A., Montes, F.C., and Alcocer, B.R. 1973. Transplacental transmission of bovine rabies after natural infection. J. Infect. Dis. 127:291–293.

Martin, M.L., and Sedmak, P.A. 1983. Rabies. I. Epidemiology, pathogenesis, and diagnosis. Compend. Cont. Ed. Pract. Vet. 5:521–528.

Murphy, F.A. 1977. Rabies pathogenesis. Arch. Virol. 54:279–297.

Murphy, F.A., Bauer, S.P., Harrison, A.K., and Winn, W.C. 1973. Comparative pathogenesis of rabies and rabies-like viruses. Viral infection and transit from inoculation site to the central nervous system. Lab. Invest. 28:361–376.

Murphy, F.A., Harrison, A.K., Winn, W.C., and Bauer, S.P. 1973. Comparative pathogenesis of rabies and rabies-like viruses. Infection of the central nervous system and centrifugal spread of virus to peripheral tissues. Lab. Invest. 29:1–16.

NASPHV (National Association of State Public Health Veterinarians). 1988. Compendium of animal rabies control, 1988. J. Am. Vet. Med. Assoc. 192:18–22.

Parker, R.L. 1975. Rabies in skunks. In G.M. Baer, ed., The Natural History of Rabies, vol. 2. Academic Press, New York. Pp. 41–51.

Parker, R.L., and Wilsnack, R.E. 1966. Pathogenesis of skunk rabies virus: Quantitation in skunks and foxes. Am. J. Vet. Res. 27:33–38.

Perl, D.P. 1975. The pathology of rabies in the central nervous system. In G.M. Baer, Ed., The Natural History of Rabies, vol. 1. Academic Press, New York. Pp. 235–272.

Porras, C., Barboza, J.J., Fuenzalida, E., Adaros, H.L., Díaz, A.M.O., and Furst, J. 1976. Recovery from rabies in man. Ann. Intern. Med. 85:44–48.

Schneider, L.G. 1969a. Die Pathogenese der Tollwut bei der Maus. I. Die Virusausbreitung vom Infektionsort zum Zentralnervensystem. Zentralbl. Bakteriol. Parasit. Infekt. Hyg. Abt. I. Orig. 211:281–308.

Schneider, L.G. 1969b. Die Pathogenese der Tollwut bei der Maus. II. Die Virusausbreitung innerhalb des ZNS. Zentralbl. Bakteriol. Parasit. Infekt. Hyg. Abt. I. Orig. 212:1–13.

Schneider, L.G. 1975. Spread of virus from the central nervous system. In G.M. Baer, ed., The Natural History of Rabies, vol. 1. Academic Press, New York. Pp. 273–301.

Schneider, L.G., and Hamann, I. 1969. Die Pathogenese der Tollwut bei der Maus. III. Die zentrifugale Virusausbreitung und die Virusgeneralisierung im Organismus. Zentralbl. Bakteriol. Parasit. Infekt. Hyg. Abt. I. Orig. 212:13–41.

Sedmak, P.A., and Martin, M.L. 1984. Rabies. II. Prophylaxis and control. Compend. Cont. Ed. Pract. Vet. 6:49–57.

Seif, I., Coulon, P., Rollin, P.E., and Flamand, A. 1985. Rabies virulence: Effect on pathogenicity and sequence characterization of rabies virus mutations affecting antigenic site III of the glycoprotein. J. Virol. 53:926–934.

Selimov, M., Boltucij, L., Semenova, E., Kobrinskij, G., and Zmusko, L. 1959. The use of antirabies gamma globulin in subjects severely bitten by rabid wolves or other animals. J. Hyg. Epidemiol. Microbiol. Immunol. (Praha) 3:168–180.

Shope, R. 1975. Rabies virus antigenic relationships. In G.M. Baer, ed., The Natural History of Rabies, vol. 1. Academic Press, New York. Pp. 141–152.

Sikes, R.K. 1962. Pathogenesis of rabies in wildlife. I. Comparative effect of varying doses of rabies virus inoculated into foxes and skunks. Am. J. Vet. Res. 23:1041–1047.

Sikes, R.K. 1975. Canine and feline vaccines—past and present. In G.M. Baer, ed., The Natural History of Rabies, vol. 2. Academic Press, New York. Pp. 177–187.

Sikes, R.K. 1981. Rabies. In J.W. Davis, L.H. Karstad, and D.O. Trainer, eds., Infectious Diseases of Wild Mammals, 2d ed. Iowa State University Press, Ames. Pp. 3–17.

Smith, J.S., Sumner, J.W., Roumillat, L.F., Baer, G.M., and Winkler, W.G. 1984. Antigenic characteristics of isolates associated with a new epizootic of raccoon rabies in the United States. J. Infect. Dis. 149:769–774.

Smith, W.B., Blenden, D.C., Fuh, T.H., and Hiler, L. 1972. Diagnosis of rabies by immunofluorescent staining of frozen sections of skin. J. Am. Vet. Med. Assoc. 161:1495–1501.

Sokol, F., Kuwert, E., Wiktor, T.J., Hummeler, K., and Koprowski, H. 1968. Purification of rabies virus grown in tissue culture. J. Virol. 2:836–849.

Spriggs, D.R. 1985. Rabies pathogenesis: Fast times at the neuromuscular junction. J. Infect. Dis. 152:1362–1363.

Steck, F., Wandeler, A., Bichsel, P., Capt, S., Häfliger, U., and Schneider, L. 1982. Oral immunization of foxes against rabies. Laboratory and field studies. Comp. Immunol. Microbiol. Infect. Dis. 5:165–171.

Steele, J.H. 1975. History of rabies. In G.M. Baer, ed., The Natural History of Rabies, vol. 1. Academic Press, New York. Pp. 1–29.

Tierkel, E.S. 1959. Rabies. Adv. Vet. Sci. 5:183–226.

Tierkel, E.S. 1973. Rapid microscopic examination for Negri bodies and preparation of specimens for biological test. In M.M. Kaplan and H. Koprowski, eds., Laboratory Techniques in Rabies, 3d ed. World Health Organization, Geneva. Pp. 41–55.

Tierkel, E.S. 1975a. Canine rabies. In G.M. Baer, ed., The Natural History of Rabies, vol. 2. Academic Press, New York. Pp. 123–137.

Tierkel, E.S. 1975b. Control of urban rabies. In G.M. Baer, ed., The Natural History of Rabies, vol. 2. Academic Press, New York. Pp. 189–201.

Tillotson, J.R., Axelrod, D., and Lyman, D.O. 1977. Follow-up on rabies—New York. M.M.W.R. 26:249–250.

Turner, G.S. 1976. A review of the world epidemiology of rabies. Trans. R. Soc. Trop. Med. Hyg. 70.175–178.

Verts, B.J. 1967. The Biology of the Striped Skunk. University of Illinois Press, Urbana. 218 pp.

Wandeler, A., Wachendörfer, G., Förster, U., Krekel, H., Schale, W., Müller, J., and Steck, F. 1974. Rabies in wild carnivores in central Europe. I. Epidemiological studies. Zentralbl. Vetinarmed. [B] 21:735–756.

WHO (World Health Organization). 1984. Seventh report of the expert committee on rabies. WHO Tech. Rep. Ser. No. 709.

Wiktor, T.J., and Clark, H.F. 1975. Growth of rabies virus in cell culture. In G.M. Baer, ed., The Natural History of Rabies, vol. 1. Academic Press, New York. Pp. 155–179.

Wiktor, T.J., György, E., Schlumberger, H.D., Sokol, F., and Koprowski, H. 1973. Antigenic properties of rabies virus components. J. Immunol. 110:269–276.

Wiktor, T.J., Kuwert, E., and Koprowski, H. 1968. Immune lysis of rabies virus-infected cells. J. Immunol. 101:1271–1282.

Wiktor, T.J., Macfarlan, R.I., Reagan, K.J., Dietzschold, B., Curtis, P.J., Wunner, W.H., Kieny, M.P., Lathe, R., Lecocq, J.P., Mackett, M., Moss, B., and Koprowski, H. 1984. Protection from rabies by a vaccinia virus recombinant containing the rabies virus glycoprotein gene. Proc. Natl. Acad. Sci. USA 81:7194–7198.

Wiktor, T.J., Sokol, F., Kuwert, E., and Koprowski, H. 1969. Immunogenicity of concentrated and purified rabies vaccine of tissue culture origin. Proc. Soc. Exp. Biol. Med. 131:799–805.

Winkler, W.G. 1968. Airborne rabies virus isolation. Bull. Wildl. Dis. Assoc. 4:37–40.

Winkler, W.G. 1975. Fox rabies. In G.M. Baer, The Natural History of Rabies, vol. 2. Academic Press, New York. Pp. 3–22.

Winkler, W.G. 1981. The rhabdoviruses. In E. Kurstak and C. Kurstak, eds., Comparative Diagnosis of Viral Diseases, vol. 4, part B. Academic Press, New York. Pp. 529–550.

Winkler, W.G., and Baer, G.M. 1976. Rabies immunization of red foxes *(Vulpes fulva)* with vaccine in sausage baits. Am. J. Epidemiol. 103:408–415.

Winkler, W.G., Baker, E.F., and Hopkins, C.C. 1972. An outbreak of non-bite transmitted rabies in a laboratory animal colony. Am. J. Epidemiol. 95:267–277.

Winkler, W.G., Shaddock, J.H., and Bowman, C. 1985. Rabies virus in salivary glands of raccoons *(Procyon lotor).* J. Wildl. Dis. 21:297–298.

Wright, B.G. 1983. Diagnosis of rabies in a living calf. Vet. Med./Small Anim. Clin. 78:237–238.

The Genus *Vesiculovirus*

Vesicular Stomatitis

SYNONYMS: Erosive stomatitis, stomatitis contagiosa of horses, aphthous stomatitis of cattle and swine, sore mouth, sore nose, red nose of pigs, *mal de tierra, seudoaftosa;* abbreviation, VS

Vesicular stomatitis is a disease recognized primarily in horses, cattle, and swine, characterized by fever and the development of vesicular and ulcerative lesions on the oral mucosa, coronary band, and teats (Blood et al. 1983; Hanson 1981; Knight and Messer 1983; Smith 1986a, 1986b; Watson 1981; Yuill 1981). Humans and certain wildlife species are also susceptible to infection. In cattle and swine the lesions of VS are indistinguishable from those of the more contagious foot-and-mouth disease (FMD).

VS is caused by a group of antigenically related viruses of the genus *Vesiculovirus.* The disease apparently is restricted to the Western hemisphere, where it occurs in certain key enzootic areas from which it periodically erupts in epizootic form. Despite decades of scientific inquiry, however, much of the natural history of VS—most important, the identification of reservoir species and mechanisms of virus transmission to domestic livestock—remains an enigma.

Character of the Disease. *In horses* the principal lesions are found in the mouth, especially on the lips and dorsum of the tongue. Most appear initially as blanched areas with little or no fluid accumulation, which then erode to form ulcerated lesions. Vesicles, when present, form early in the course of the disease and rupture rapidly. Excessive salivation is frequently the first clinical manifestation of illness, concomitant with or closely following a febrile reaction. The animals are often depressed and

anorectic but usually will accept water. They champ their jaws and grind their teeth, drooling a clear, ropy saliva from the mouth. Affected horses often rub their lips on the edges of mangers or other convenient objects. Lesions may involve the oropharynx and nasal turbinates, resulting in dysphagia, mild epistaxis, or respiratory difficulty. Lesions of the feet consist primarily of hyperemia and ulceration of the coronary band (coronitis), which in severe cases can lead to cracking of the hoof wall and persistent lameness. Secondary bacterial infection of these lesions is a serious complication. Lesions of the teats, commonly seen in dairy cattle with VS, are generally quite rare in horses.

In cattle mouth lesions are common, occurring primarily on the lips, dorsum of the tongue, dental pad, and buccal mucosa. In nonlactating animals the first clinical manifestation usually is hypersalivation. The animals drool, smack their lips, and produce a characteristic sucking noise. Vesicles form and rupture early in the course of the disease and may all have eroded by the time veterinary attention is sought. The cattle usually are anorectic and depressed. Coronitis and lameness are not as common as they are in horses and swine with VS. Teat lesions, on the other hand, are frequently observed. In lactating cows, teat lesions and a sudden drop in milk yield are often the first manifestations of the disease. The lesions in such cows may be severe and extensive and can lead to the development of mastitis.

In swine lesions develop on or behind the snout, on the oral mucosa, and on the feet. Lesions of the feet appear to be more common than oral lesions, and the first manifestation of VS in pigs frequently is lameness. Lesions on the teats are uncommon.

In general, the course of the disease in all species is fairly short, and mortality is negligible. After 3 or 4 days most animals begin to eat and regain lost weight. Barring complications of secondary bacterial infection, most lesions heal rapidly, with complete recovery in 2 to 3 weeks. Oral lesions tend to heal more quickly than foot and teat lesions. Damage to the coronary band and hoof wall may result in persistant lameness in severely affected animals. In some cows mastitis can lead to permanent loss of mammary gland function. The economic toll of VS among dairy cattle may be particularly great because of depressed milk yields, expense of mastitis treatment, and culling of severely affected cows (Buisch 1983, Corrêa 1964, Ellis and Kendall 1964, Heiny 1945, Jenney et al. 1984).

An important aspect of clinical VS in cattle and swine is the resemblance of the lesions, in form and distribution, to those of FMD, which is caused by a picornavirus. A swift and accurate diagnosis thus is critical in order to distinguish VS from this important and devastating livestock disease. In pigs VS must also be differentiated from swine vesicular disease (caused by a picornavirus) and vesicular exanthema (caused by a calicivirus).

Properties of the Virus. At present, two serotypes of VS virus (VSV) are recognized, Indiana and New Jersey. The Indiana serotype has been further divided into three subtypes: Indiana 1 (the original isolate from the United States), Indiana 2 (Cocal virus, from Trinidad, Brazil, and Argentina), and Indiana 3 (Alagoas virus, from Brazil) (Federer et al. 1967, Hanson 1981, Jonkers et al. 1964). Although the New Jersey virus has long been considered monotypic, there is evidence of considerable genetic diversity among different strains. Subdivision into two subtypes, Concan and Hazelhurst, has been proposed (Byrd et al. 1984, Reichmann et al. 1978). In general, the New Jersey serotype produces a more virulent disease and has been responsible for most of the epizootics recorded in the United States.

The causative agents are typical members of the Rhabdoviridae (see Figure 53.1). They are heat-labile, ether-sensitive, and inactivated by many common detergents and disinfectants. Antigens of the G protein (peplomer protein) are responsible for the induction of neutralizing antibody and are useful for the differentiation of VSV serotypes and subtypes (Gallione and Rose 1983, Kelley et al. 1972, Mackett et al. 1985, Wilks and House 1985, Wilks et al. 1984, Yilma et al. 1985).

Cultivation. The VSVs replicate in many mammalian and avian cell-culture systems, including Vero, BHK-21, mouse L, and primary chick embryo cells. Unlike rabies virus, development of cytopathic effect is common with these viruses. They have also been grown in cell cultures derived from fish, reptiles, amphibians, and insects. A number of laboratory animal species are also used, including mice, rabbits, and guinea pigs.

Epizootiology and Pathogenesis. VS is enzootic in the lowland forested tropical and subtropical regions of the Americas (Hanson 1981, Jonkers 1967, Sudia et al. 1967, Yuill 1981). Outbreaks of the disease occur at more frequent intervals in the tropics and less often as one travels north from the equator. In most areas VS has the seasonal prevalence of an arthropod-borne contagion, in the temperate zone appearing late in the warm season and disappearing with the onset of killing frosts, in the tropics appearing at the close of the rainy season and disappearing as the countryside dries out. A typical feature is the irregular or patchy distribution of affected farms in an epizootic area. Frequently, outbreaks originate in animals in pastures and then spread unevenly through the surrounding population, skipping certain pastures or entire farms in the affected area for no apparent reason. Premises that remain clean for the duration of an outbreak often are located immediately adjacent to farms that are severely affected. The disease has a tendency to recur in certain geographical areas, especially along riverbeds. In areas with repeated outbreaks, some farms or pastures are regularly involved, whereas others regularly escape. Affected areas in both temperate and tropical regions are often characterized by the presence of shade-giving trees, moist pastureland, and natural surface waters. Spread of the disease does not appear to follow routes of movement of either humans or animals, and transmission by direct contact, although known to occur, is usually of limited significance in the field. The extensive 1982–1983 epizootic (New Jersey serotype) in cattle and horses in the western United States defied some of these traditional patterns, however, by persisting over the winter months, during which time contact transmission and movement of infected cattle continued to spread the disease (Bridgewater 1983, Buisch 1983, Jenney et al. 1984). Recrudescence of infection also was noted in some affected and recovered cattle that developed fresh lesions after movement to a new location (Bridgewater 1983). Some observers have reported that VS appears almost simultaneously in several localities within an affected area, suggesting preseeding of pastureland with virus (Jonkers 1967). Others have reported more direct movement along river valleys or across individual states (Brandly et al. 1951, Buisch 1983, Heiny 1945). Still others indicate that the disease spreads outward in expanding circles from independent foci of infection (Lauerman 1967).

One outstanding feature of most VS epizootics is rapidity of spread. This observation, when taken together with the recognized seasonality of the disease and its apparent predilection for well-watered areas, has suggested the possibility of arthropod transmission from unidentified reservoir hosts. Seroepizootiological and virological studies have shown that the VSVs naturally infect a constellation of wild species, including rodents, raccoons, opossums, coyotes, bobcats, feral swine, deer, elk, bighorn sheep, antelope, porcupines, bats, monkeys, sloths, birds, and arthropods (Fletcher et al. 1985; Glazener et al. 1967; Jenney et al. 1970, 1980; Johnson et al. 1969; Karstad et al. 1956; Shelokov and Peralta 1967; Srihongse 1969; Stallknecht et al. 1985; Tesh et al. 1969, 1974; Trainer and Hanson 1969; Trainer et al. 1968; Webb 1983; Yuill 1981). Cattle, horses, mules, and pigs are the principal domestic species involved. To date, however, no vertebrate species, wild or domestic, in any of the enzootic areas has been shown to develop a viremia sufficiently intense for infection of bloodsucking vectors. Indeed, available data suggest that at least one of the VSVs (the classic Indiana serotype) probably does not totally conform to a conventional insect-vertebrate transmission cycle characteristic of so many of the mosquito-borne viruses.

In Panama, VSV-Indiana has been isolated repeatedly from phlebotomine sand flies (Shelokov and Peralta 1967, Tesh et al. 1969), and it now appears that these insects may serve both as biological vectors and as reservoir hosts of the virus in this region of the Americas. The virus has been shown to replicate within sand flies and can be passed to subsequent generations by transovarial transmission and to mammalian hosts by biting (Tesh and Chaniotis 1975, Tesh et al. 1971). Interestingly, virus transmission appears to preferentially involve creatures that inhabit the forest canopy, since arboreal species have been shown to have higher antibody prevalence rates than ground-living animals (Johnson et al. 1969, Srihongse 1969, Tesh et al. 1969). Experimental studies of VSV-Indiana infection in animals and humans, however, have confirmed that the viremia produced by this virus is ephemeral at best and unlikely to be of significance in transmission to hematophagous arthropods (Tesh et al. 1970). Considering also the very limited flight range of sand flies and their relatively short lifespans as adults, it has been proposed that transovarial transmission is the principal maintenance mechanism for the virus in nature and may actually be critical for its survival (Tesh and Chaniotis 1975). One negative note has been sounded, however, by the observed inefficiency of transovarial passage of the virus in the flies and by the absence to date of an attractive source of virus for replenishment of the transovarial cycle.

In the United States, a single isolation of VSV-Indiana has been made in New Mexico from a pool of *Aedes* mosquitoes (Sudia et al. 1967). Experimental studies have shown that the virus can replicate in and be transmitted by mosquitoes of this genus (Bergold et al. 1968, Liu and Zee 1976a, Mussgay and Suárez 1962), although acquisition of a "natural" infection by feeding on a viremic host (as opposed to intrathoracic injection of the virus) was largely unsuccessful (Liu and Zee 1976b). Mechanical transmission by mosquitoes, stable flies, and horseflies has also been demonstrated (Ferris et al. 1955). The epizootiological significance of these varied findings remains clouded, however, by repeated failures to regularly isolate VSVs from biting flies and mosquitoes in most enzootic and epizootic areas—failures that have tended to cast doubt on the notion that hematophagous arthropods are important vectors of the disease (Watson 1981).

In contrast to VSV-Indiana, arthropod vector transmission has not been demonstrated for VSV-New Jersey. This virus has, however, been isolated from mosquitoes in Guatemala (Clewley et al. 1977, Reichmann et al. 1978) and from blackflies (Simuliidae) in Colorado (Jenney et al. 1984, Schnitzlein and Reichmann 1985). Reservoir hosts remain unidentified, although many wild vertebrates show serologic evidence of infection.

Thus despite many decades of intense scientific investigation, much of the natural history of VS remains an enigma, and many basic questions remain unanswered. For instance, how important and widespread are arthropod vectors in transmission and maintenance of the VSVs? How do the viruses circulate in enzootic areas, and what are the important reservoir hosts? What factors govern periodic eruption of the disease in epizootic form, and how is it introduced into VS-free areas? What are the important methods of spread among domestic species? Why are certain premises repeatedly affected and others repeatedly spared? And what are the origins of the VSVs themselves?

Outbreaks of VS frequently are characterized by the development of lesions in affected animals at certain preferential body sites—that is, oral lesions are produced almost exclusively during some epizootics—whereas lesions of the feet or teats predominate during others (Hanson 1981, Jonkers 1967). This observation has raised the possibility that the virus enters through preexisting, nonspecific lesions common to certain body areas. Jonkers (1967) has suggested that the pasture is the basic epizootiological unit and that it is already preseeded with virus prior to an outbreak, either in or on the soil or vegetation. Johnson et al. (1969) have taken this idea one step further by hypothesizing that the VSVs are actually plant rhabdoviruses that become infectious for vertebrates only after ingestion by arthropods. These workers suggest that the plant form of the VSVs might contain an outer coat or shell that is removed following replication in insects, producing the familiar single-coated VSV particles. According to this theory, only this single-coated form would be infectious for vertebrates. Infected insects might then spread the viruses to other plants and also to animals that either eat the insects or are bitten by them. Preexisting wounds or abrasions on the mouth, feet, or teats might provide preferential areas for insect biting, or the virus might be liberated as insect-infested forage is chewed and enter through abrasions in the oral mucosa. Herds feeding on coarse roughage and hard-pelleted concentrates (which could produce multiple oral abrasions and allow for viral penetration) might be expected to show higher VS attack rates than herds feeding fine, leafy forage; this, indeed, has been shown to be the case (Hansen et al. 1985). Many plant rhabdoviruses are currently recognized and some are known to be infectious for arthropods, such as the sowthistle yellow vein virus, which is transmitted by aphids (Hackett et al. 1968, Richardson and Sylvester

1968, Sylvester and Richardson 1969). Recovery of the proposed double-shelled form of the VSVs from plants, however, has not yet been reported. Alternatively, VSVs might be insect viruses infectious for vertebrates (Gomez 1970), or simple plant parasites without requirements for arthropod intermediates.

VSV infection of the epithelium is characterized initially by changes in the stratum spinosum, followed by extension to the basal layer and stratum granulosum (Ribelin 1958). The viruses have a particular predilection for the prickle cells of the stratum spinosum (Chow and McNutt 1953, Chow et al. 1951). The cytopathic changes begin as a contraction of the cytoplasm, with an increasing prominence of the intercellular bridges and development of spongiosis. Transudates form in lacunae and coalesce to form vesicles. Cytoplasmic shrinkage progresses to nuclear pyknosis, with cellular debris floating freely in the vesicular fluid (Ribelin 1958). Infiltration of the area by polymorphonuclear leukocytes occurs, and the thin tissue overlying the vesicles breaks, leaving raw, eroded areas. Experimental data have tended to suggest that the lesions frequently are initiated in situ (i.e., by direct introduction of virus at the site of each lesion) rather than by viremic seeding (Hanson 1981). Like rabies virus, VSV apparently cannot penetrate intact skin but may enter through skin breaks or mucous membranes.

Immunity. On the basis of seroepizootiological studies, it is apparent that the great majority of VSV infections in domestic animals are subclinical. Usually only 10 to 15 percent of animals in a herd show clinical signs, although the incidence can be as high as 100 percent on severely affected premises. Serum-neutralizing antibody appears shortly after infection and persists at fluctuating levels (Geleta and Holbrook 1961, Sorensen et al. 1958). In individual cows this antibody may persist for many years (Sorensen et al. 1958). Immunity, however, is serotype-specific and relatively short-lived (6 months); animals can become reinfected with the same serotype and redevelop clinical illness despite the presence of significant levels of neutralizing antibody (Castañeda et al. 1964, Geleta and Holbrook 1961, Holbrook and Geleta 1962, Sorensen et al. 1958). In general, levels of complement-fixing antibody seem to be better correlated with immunity to reinfection (Geleta and Holbrook 1961, Holbrook and Geleta 1962). Protection against challenge is mediated by the G protein (peplomer protein) of the virion (Mackett et al. 1985, Yilma et al. 1985).

Diagnosis. Federal and state regulatory agencies should be notified *immediately* if a vesicular disease in livestock is suspected. Prompt and accurate diagnosis of VS is critical because the disease is clinicopathologically indistinguishable from the other three important viral vesicular

diseases—foot-and-mouth disease (FMD), swine vesicular disease, and vesicular exanthema. In a country where FMD does not occur, such as the United States, every outbreak of vesicular disease must be carefully scrutinized for the possible presence of FMD virus. A mistake in one direction might lead to disastrous consequences, and a mistake in the opposite direction to serious and expensive livestock restrictions.

A definitive diagnosis of VS can only be made in the laboratory. In the United States, testing for the diagnosis of the viral vesicular diseases can be performed at the Plum Island Animal Disease Center of the U.S. Department of Agriculture, located near Greenport, Long Island, New York. Specimens for identification of viral antigen or for virus isolation or for both should be collected from several affected animals and should include fresh vesicular fluid together with associated epithelial coverings, and/or tissue scraped from the margins of eroded lesions (when intact vesicles are absent). Serum samples should also be obtained. Samples should be promptly frozen and shipped to the laboratory on dry ice in tightly sealed Styrofoam containers.

Three principal laboratory methods are available for establishing a definitive diagnosis of VS: (1) demonstration of specific viral antigen by the tissue microtitration complement-fixation test (Snyder et al. 1982), which can be performed within hours of receipt of sample material; (2) virus isolation in cell cultures or laboratory animals; and (3) demonstration of a rise in complement-fixing antibody titer in paired (acute and convalescent) serum samples.

Treatment. There is no specific therapy for VS Affected animals should be removed from woodlot pastures and isolated from healthy susceptible animals, and water and a readily palatable feed provided. Insect control measures should be instituted, if possible. Severely affected horses should be given prophylactic antibiotic therapy and mouthwashes containing mild disinfectant solutions in order to control secondary bacterial infections (Knight and Messer 1983). Nasogastric tube feeding and intravenous fluid therapy may be required for anorectic patients. Lesions of the feet should be promptly and assiduously cared for in order to prevent loss of the hoof. General attention to hygiene will help to limit the spread of the disease, especially in dairy herds, where cow-to-cow transmission by human handlers and milking machines may be a problem (Hanson 1981, Yuill 1981).

Prevention and Control. Owing to the generally sporadic nature of the disease, severely restrictive control measures probably are not warranted for VS. Prudence dictates, however, that infected premises be quarantined and that infected animals not be transported to other areas until signs of the disease have subsided. A primary problem is our imperfect understanding of the epizootiology of the disease, which makes rational control procedures difficult to formulate.

Modified live and inactivated VS vaccines have been developed, primarily for use in dairy cattle, and have afforded some protection against the disease (Corrêa 1964; Lauerman and Hanson 1963a, 1963b; Lauerman et al. 1962). Conditional approval and licensure of two inactivated VS vaccines were granted in the United States during the 1982–1983 epizootic (Buisch 1983). More recent developments include testing of a subunit vaccine composed of the G protein (Yilma et al. 1985) and a vaccinia virus–VSV G protein recombinant vaccine (Mackett et al. 1985).

The Disease in Humans. VS is a recognized zoonosis and is manifested in humans by febrile influenzalike signs (Bridgewater 1983, Ellis and Kendall 1964, Hanson et al. 1950, Johnson et al. 1969, Shelokov and Peralta 1967). Sometimes vesicles are formed, especially in the mouth and on the lips. Most cases are subclinical, however. Antibody to the VSVs is regularly found in humans living in enzootic areas in both temperate and tropical America (Brody et al. 1967, Johnson et al. 1969, Shelokov and Peralta 1967). Serologic surveys indicate that the antibody prevalence can be as high as 50 percent of the population. Recognizable clinical signs, however, are rare. Most cases of VS occur in laboratory workers and researchers in contact with large quantities of virus derived from cell cultures (Bridgewater 1983).

REFERENCES

Bergold, G.H., Suárez, O.M., and Munz, K. 1968. Multiplication in and transmission by *Aedes aegypti* of vesicular stomatitis virus. J. Invertebr. Pathol. 11:406–428.

Blood, D.C., Radostits, O.M., and Henderson, J.A. 1983. Veterinary Medicine, 6th ed. Baillière Tindall, London. Pp. 743–744.

Brandly, C.A., Hanson, R.P., and Chow, T.L. 1951. Vesicular stomatitis with particular reference to the 1949 Wisconsin epizootic. Proc. Am. Vet. Med. Assoc. 88:61–67.

Bridgewater, D.R. 1983. Public health aspects of vesicular stomatitis in Colorado during the 1982–1983 epidemic. Proc. U.S. Anim. Health Assoc. 87:476–481.

Brody, J.A., Fischer, G.F., and Peralta, P.H. 1967. Vesicular stomatitis in Panama. Human serologic patterns in a cattle raising area. Am. J. Epidemiol. 86:158–161.

Buisch, W.W. 1983. Fiscal year 1982–1983 vesicular stomatitis outbreak. Proc. U.S. Anim. Health Assoc. 87:78–84.

Byrd, A.D., Kennedy-Morrow, J., Marks, M.D., and Lesnaw, J.A. 1984. Functional relationships within the New Jersey serotype of vesicular stomatitis virus: Genetic and physiological comparisons of the Hazelhurst and Concan subtypes. J. Gen. Virol. 65:1769–1779.

Castañeda, J., Lauerman, L.H., and Hanson, R.P. 1964. Evaluation of virus neutralization tests and association of indices to cattle resistance. Proc. U.S. Livestock Sanit. Assoc. 68:455–468.

Chow, T.L., and McNutt, S.H. 1953. Pathological changes of experimental vesicular stomatitis of swine. Am. J. Vet. Res. 14:420–424.

Chow, T.L., Hanson, R.P., and McNutt, S.H. 1951. The pathology of vesicular stomatitis in cattle. Proc. Am. Vet. Med. Assoc. 88:119–124.

Clewley, J.P., Bishop, D.H.L., Kang, C.Y., Coffin, J., Schnitzlein, W.M., Reichmann, M.E., and Shope, R.E. 1977. Oligonucleotide fingerprints of RNA species obtained from rhabdoviruses belonging to the vesicular stomatitis virus subgroup. J. Virol. 23:152–166.

Corrêa, W.M. 1964. Prophylaxis of vesicular stomatitis: A field trial in Guatemalan dairy cattle. Am. J. Vet. Res. 25:1300–1302.

Ellis, E.M., and Kendall, H.E. 1964. The public health and economic effects of vesicular stomatitis in a herd of dairy cattle. J. Am. Vet. Med. Assoc. 144:377–380.

Federer, K.E., Burrows, R., and Brooksby, J.B. 1967. Vesicular stomatitis virus—The relationship between some strains of the Indiana serotype. Res. Vet. Sci. 8:103–117.

Ferris, D.H., Hanson, R.P., Dicke, R.J., and Roberts, R.H. 1955. Experimental transmission of vesicular stomatitis virus by diptera. J. Infect. Dis. 96:184–192.

Fletcher, W.O., Stallknecht, D.E., and Jenney, E.W. 1985. Serologic surveillance for vesicular stomatitis virus on Ossabaw Island, Georgia. J. Wildl. Dis. 21:100–104.

Gallione, C.J., and Rose, J.K. 1983. Nucleotide sequence of a cDNA clone encoding the entire glycoprotein from the New Jersey serotype of vesicular stomatitis virus. J. Virol. 46:162–169.

Geleta, J.N., and Holbrook, A.A. 1961. Vesicular stomatitis—Patterns of complement-fixing and serum-neutralizing antibodies in serum of convalescent cattle and horses. Am. J. Vet. Res. 22:713–719.

Glazener, W.C., Cook, R.S., and Trainer, D.O. 1967. A serologic study of diseases in the Rio Grande turkey. J. Wildl. Mgmt. 31:34–39.

Gomez, G. 1970. Experimental infection of vegetation-associated insects with vesicular stomatitis. M.S. thesis, University of Wisconsin, Madison. 91 pp.

Hackett, A.J., Sylvester, E.S., Richardson, J., and Wood, P. 1968. Comparative electron micrographs of sowthistle yellow vein and vesicular stomatitis viruses. Virology 36:693–696.

Hansen, D.E., Thurmond, M.C., and Thorburn, M. 1985. Factors associated with the spread of clinical vesicular stomatitis in California dairy cattle. Am J. Vet. Res. 46:789–795.

Hanson, R.P. 1968. Discussion of the natural history of vesicular stomatitis. Am. J. Epidemiol. 87:264–266.

Hanson, R.P. 1981. Vesicular stomatitis. In E.P.J. Gibbs, ed., Virus Diseases of Food Animals, vol. 2. Academic Press, New York. Pp. 517–539.

Hanson, R.P., Rasmussen, A.F., Brandly, C.A., and Brown, J.W. 1950. Human infection with the virus of vesicular stomatitis. J. Lab. Clin. Med. 36:754–758.

Heiny, E. 1945. Vesicular stomatitis in cattle and horses in Colorado. North Am. Vet. 26:726–730.

Holbrook, A.A., and Geleta, J.N. 1962. Duration of immunity and serologic patterns in swine convalescing from vesicular stomatitis. J. Am. Vet. Med. Assoc. 141:1463–1464.

Jenney, E.W., Erickson, G.A., Buisch, W.W., Stewart, W.C., and Mixson, M.A. 1980. Surveillance for vesicular stomatitis in the United States 1972 through 1979. Proc. Am. Assoc. Vet. Lab. Diagn. 23:83–89.

Jenney, E.W., Erickson, G.A., and Snyder, M.L. 1984. Vesicular stomatitis outbreaks and surveillance in the United States January 1980 through May 1984. Proc. U.S. Anim. Health Assoc. 88:337–349.

Jenney, E.W., Hayes, F.A., and Brown, C.L. 1970. Survey for vesicular stomatitis virus neutralizing antibodies in serums of white-tailed deer *Odocoileus virginianus* of the southeastern United States. J. Wildl. Dis. 6:488–493.

Johnson, K.M., Tesh, R.B., and Peralta, P.H. 1969. Epidemiology of vesicular stomatitis virus: Some new data and a hypothesis for transmission of the Indiana serotype. J. Am. Vet. Med. Assoc. 155:2133–2140.

Jonkers, A.H. 1967. The epizootiology of the vesicular stomatitis virus: A reappraisal. Am. J. Epidemiol. 86:286–291.

Jonkers, A.H., Shope, R.E., Aitken, T.H.G., and Spence, L. 1964. Cocal virus, a new agent in Trinidad related to vesicular stomatitis virus, type Indiana. Am. J. Vet. Res. 25:236–241.

Karstad, L.H., Adams, E.V., Hanson, R.P., and Ferris, D.H. 1956. Evidence for the role of wildlife in epizootics of vesicular stomatitis. J. Am. Vet. Med. Assoc. 129:95–96.

Kelley, J.M., Emerson, S.U., and Wagner, R.R. 1972. The glycoprotein of vesicular stomatitis virus is the antigen that gives rise to and reacts with neutralizing antibody. J. Virol. 10:1231–1235.

Knight, A.P., and Messer, N.T. 1983. Vesicular stomatitis. Compend. Cont. Ed. Pract. Vet. 5:S517–S522.

Lauerman, L.H. 1967. Vesicular stomatitis in temperate and tropical America. Ph.D dissertation, University of Wisconsin, Madison. 193 pp.

Lauerman, L.H., and Hanson, R.P. 1963a. Field trial of live virus vaccination procedure for prevention of vesicular stomatitis in dairy cattle. III. Evaluation of emergency vaccination in Georgia. Proc. U.S. Livestock Sanit. Assoc. 67:473–482.

Lauerman, L.H., and Hanson, R.P. 1963b. Field trial of live virus vaccination procedure for prevention of vesicular stomatitis in dairy cattle. II. Second year evaluation in Panama. Proc. U.S. Livestock Sanit. Assoc. 67:483–490.

Lauerman, L.H., Kuns, M.L., and Hanson, R.P. 1962. Field trial of live virus vaccination procedure for prevention of vesicular stomatitis in dairy cattle. I. Preliminary immune response. Proc. U.S. Livestock Sanit. Assoc. 66:365–369.

Liu, I.K.M., and Zee, Y.C. 1976a. The pathogenesis of vesicular stomatitis virus, serotype Indiana, in *Aedes aegypti* mosquitoes. Am. J. Trop. Med. Hyg. 25:177–185.

Liu, I.K.M., and Zee, Y.C. 1976b. The pathogenesis of vesicular stomatitis virus, serotype Indiana, in *Aedes aegypti* mosquitoes, after imbibition of a viremic blood meal. Arch. Virol. 52:259–262.

Mackett, M., Yilma, T., Rose, J.K., and Moss, B. 1985. Vaccinia virus recombinants: Expression of VSV genes and protective immunization of mice and cattle. Science 227:433–435.

Mussgay, M., and Suárez, O. 1962. Multiplication of vesicular stomatitis virus in *Aedes aegypti* (L.) mosquitoes. Virology 17:202–204.

Reichmann, M.E., Schnitzlein, W.M., Bishop, D.H.L., Lazzrini, R.A., Beatrice, S.T., and Wagner, R.R. 1978. Classification of the New Jersey serotype of vesicular stomatitis virus into two subtypes. J. Virol. 25:446–449.

Ribelin, W.E. 1958. The cytopathogenesis of vesicular stomatitis virus infection in cattle. Am. J. Vet. Res. 19:66–73.

Richardson, J., and Sylvester, E.S. 1968. Further evidence of multiplication of sowthistle yellow vein virus in its aphid vector *Hyperomyzus lactucae*. Virology 35:347–355.

Schnitzlein, W.M., and Reichmann, M.E. 1985. Characterization of New Jersey vesicular stomatitis virus isolates from horses and black flies during the 1982 outbreak in Colorado. Virology 142:426–431.

Shelokov, A., and Peralta, P.H. 1967. Vesicular stomatitis virus, Indiana type: An arbovirus infection of tropical sandflies and humans? Am. J. Epidemiol. 86:149–157.

Smith, A.W. 1986a. Vesicular stomatitis virus in cattle. In J.L. Howard, ed., Current Veterinary Therapy: Food Animal Practice, 2d ed. W.B. Saunders, Philadelphia. Pp. 504–505.

Smith, A.W. 1986b. Vesicular stomatitis virus in swine. In J.L. Howard, ed., Current Veterinary Therapy: Food Animal Practice, 2d ed. W.B. Saunders, Philadelphia. P. 555.

Snyder, M.L., Jenney, E.W., Erickson, G.A., and Carbrey, E.A. 1982. The 1982 resurgence of vesicular stomatitis in the United States: A summary of laboratory diagnostic findings. Proc. Am. Assoc. Vet. Lab. Diag. 25:221–228.

Sorensen, D.K., Chow, T.L., Kowalczyk, T., Hanson, R.P., and Brandly, C.A. 1958. Persistence in cattle of serum-neutralizing antibodies of vesicular stomatitis virus. Am. J. Vet. Res. 19:74–77.

Srihongse, S. 1969. Vesicular stomatitis virus infections in Panamanian primates and other vertebrates. Am. J. Epidemiol. 90:69–76.

Stallknecht, D.E., Nettles, V.F., Erickson, G.A., and Jessup, D.A. 1986. Antibodies to vesicular stomatitis virus in populations of feral swine in the United States. J. Wildl. Dis. 22:320–325.

Stallknecht, D.E., Nettles, V.F., Fletcher, W.O., and Erickson, G.A. 1985. Enzootic vesicular stomatitis New Jersey type in an insular feral swine population. Am. J. Epidemiol. 122:876–883.

Sudia, W.D., Fields, B.N., and Calisher, C.H. 1967. The isolation of vesicular stomatitis virus (Indiana strain) and other viruses from mosquitoes in New Mexico, 1965. Am. J. Epidemiol. 86:598–602.

Sylvester, E.S., and Richardson, J. 1969. Additional evidence of multiplication of the sowthistle yellow vein virus in an aphid vector—Serial passage. Virology 37:26–31.

Tesh, R.B., and Chaniotis, B.N. 1975. Transovarial transmission of viruses by phlebotomine sandflies. Ann. N.Y. Acad. Sci. 266:125–134.

Tesh, R.B., Chaniotis, B.N., and Johnson, K.M. 1971. Vesicular stomatitis virus, Indiana serotype: Multiplication in and transmission by experimentally infected phlebotomine sandflies (*Lutzomyia trapidoi*). Am. J. Epidemiol. 93:491–495.

Tesh, R.B., Chaniotis, B.N., Peralta, P.H., and Johnson, K.M. 1969. Ecologic studies of vesicular stomatitis virus. I. Prevalence of infection among animals and humans living in an area of endemic VSV activity. Am. J. Epidemiol. 90:255–261.

Tesh, R.B., Chaniotis, B.N., Peralta, P.H., and Johnson, K.M. 1974. Ecology of viruses isolated from Panamanian phlebotomine sandflies. Am. J. Trop. Med. Hyg. 23:258–269.

Tesh, R.B., Peralta, P.H., and Johnson, K.M. 1970. Ecologic studies of vesicular stomatitis virus. II. Results of experimental infection in Panamanian wild animals. Am. J. Epidemiol. 91:216–224.

Trainer, D.O., and Hanson, R.P. 1969. Serologic evidence of arbovirus infections in wild ruminants. Am. J. Epidemiol. 90:354–358.

Trainer, D.O., Glazener, W.C., Hanson, R.P., and Nassif, B.D. 1968. Infectious disease exposure in a wild turkey population. Avian Dis. 12:208–214.

Watson, W.A. 1981. Vesicular diseases: Recent advances and concepts of control. Can. Vet. J. 22:311–320.

Webb, P. 1983. Centers for Disease Control report. In L.J. King, ed., Summary of Vesicular Stomatitis Meeting, January 11–12, 1983. U.S. Dept. of Agriculture, Animal and Plant Health Inspection Service, Washington, D.C. 56 pp.

Wilks, C.R., and House, J.A. 1985. The glycoproteins of seven vesiculoviruses are antigenically distinct. Arch. Virol. 86:335–340.

Wilks, C.R., Jenney, E.W., and House, J.A. 1984. Development of an immunoelectroosmophoresis test for the detection and typing of antibodies to vesicular stomatitis viruses. Can. J. Comp. Med. 48:179–183.

Yilma, T., Breeze, R.G., Ristow, S., Gorham, J.R., and Leib, S.R. 1985. Immune responses of cattle and mice to the G glycoprotein of vesicular stomatitis virus. Adv. Exp. Med. Biol. 185:101–115.

Yuill, T.M. 1981. Vesicular stomatitis. In J.H. Steele, ed., CRC Handbook Series in Zoonoses, section B, vol. 1. CRC Press, Boca Raton, Fla. Pp. 125–142.

Unclassified

Ephemeral Fever

SYNONYMS: Bovine epizootic fever, three-day sickness or stiff sickness, tongue fever of cattle, dengue fever of cattle, lazy man's disease; abbreviation, EF

Ephemeral fever is an acute disease of ruminants (cattle and domestic water buffalo) characterized by fever, depression, respiratory signs, stiffness, lameness, and sometimes paresis or paralysis (Combs 1978, Kahrs 1981, Martin 1981, St. George 1981, Spradbrow 1986). The term *ephemeral* aptly describes the most striking features of the disease, namely, its abrupt onset, short course, and rapid resolution. It occurs in Africa, Asia, and Australia. Sporadic cases occur in enzootic areas from which the disease periodically erupts in major epizootics. The mortality rate is low. Insect vectors have not been definitively identified but are believed to include biting midges and mosquitoes.

Character of the Disease.   The incubation period is generally 2 to 4 days in length but may be as long as a week. Clinical signs include anorexia, a fever that becomes biphasic, muscle fibrillations, and lameness, either constant or shifting, which may be spontaneous or induced by movement. A sudden and severe drop in milk production occurs in lactating cows. A characteristic feature of EF is the apparent presence of pain in the throat region, which may be accompanied by dysphagia and hypersalivation. In more severe cases, rales, oculonasal discharges, cessation of rumination, joint swelling, and subcutaneous emphysema may be seen. Affected animals stand stiffly, with the head hanging down and the back arched, and appear very depressed. They may go down in sternal or lateral recumbency with the head turned to one side. Pregnant animals do not abort, but a reduction in semen quality is seen in some bulls (Parsonson et al. 1981).

Clinical signs are much more severe in older and heavier cattle than in calves and are exacerbated by exercise. The onset of the disease is sudden, but clinical recovery may be equally rapid, sometimes occurring within hours. The usual disease course lasts from 1 to 3 days. Occasionally lameness persists for several weeks after other signs have vanished. The loss of milk production in lactating cows is one of the most serious economic effects of the disease; in some cases milk yield may be permanently depressed (Davis et al. 1984, Newton and Wheatley 1970), and mastitis is often a complicating sequela.

The hematological pattern in EF is characterized by a rapidly developing neutrophilia and a lymphopenia, both of which are associated with the onset of fever (Mackerras et al. 1941, St. George et al. 1984).

When mortality occurs it usually involves less than 1 percent of the affected animals and often is attributable to complications arising from prolonged recumbency. The most severely affected animals are paralyzed, possibly because of traumatic damage to the spinal cord (Hill and Schultz 1977). Some assume a sitting position and show a loss of reflexes, dysphagia, rumen atony, and rapid pulse. Fatal pulmonary emphysema has also been reported (Theodoridis and Coetzer 1979). Deaths may occur in remote areas where affected animals cannot reach water.

Sometimes death is attributable to inhalation pneumonia in animals with impaired swallowing reflexes. Fatalities are most common among fattened steers, high-producing dairy cows, and mature bulls.

The clinical disease course in water buffalo apparently is similar to that reported in cattle (Malviya and Prasad 1977, Mohan 1968).

Very few natural cases of EF have been studied post mortem; hence most information on the pathology of the disease has come from experimental work (Basson et al. 1970, Mackerras et al. 1940). Findings have included splenomegaly, renal engorgement, and a fibrinous exudate in the pericardial, pleural, and peritoneal cavities. A serofibrinous synovitis often is present, with accumulation of fluid and an accompanying periarthritis. The nasal mucosa may be severely inflamed. The lung and lymph nodes frequently are congested, and evidence of inhalation pneumonia may be present. The brain may show cerebral edema and hemorrhage. Focal necrosis of skeletal muscle has also been reported. Histological changes may include perivascular cuffing, endothelial hyperplasia, necrosis of arterial muscle walls, and vascular thrombosis. Edematous and pneumonic changes in the lung may be extensive. The peripheral lymph nodes are congested, with activation of germinal centers.

Properties of the Virus.   The causative virus is an unclassified member of the Rhabdoviridae (see Table 53.1) (Della-Porta and Brown 1979). It is heat-labile, ether-sensitive, and quite susceptible to changes in pH (Heuschele 1970). A certain degree of morphologic variability has been recognized in that some particles tend to be bullet-shaped, whereas others have a more conical appearance (Figure 53.7) (Della-Porta and Brown 1979, Holmes and Doherty 1970, Lecatsas et al. 1969, Murphy et al. 1972, van der Westhuizen 1967). Most strains isolated from cattle are antigenically similar, although variants have been reported (St. George et al. 1977). Antigenic differences have been reported also among strains isolated from mosquitoes in Australia (St. George et al. 1976). Also present in Australia are some newly characterized rhabdoviruses (Berrimah, Kimberley, and Adelaide River viruses) that show a distant antigenic similarity to EF virus; all have tentatively been placed together into a separate EF virus serogroup within the Rhabdoviridae (Cybinski and Zakrzewski 1983; Gard et al. 1983, 1984). A fifth proposed member virus (Fukuoka) has recently been reported from Japan (Kaneko et al. 1986).

Cultivation.   Primary isolations of the virus from cattle have frequently been made by intracerebral inoculation of suckling mice (Doherty et al. 1969; Inaba et al. 1968a, 1968b; Sasaki et al. 1968; Spradbrow and Francis 1969;

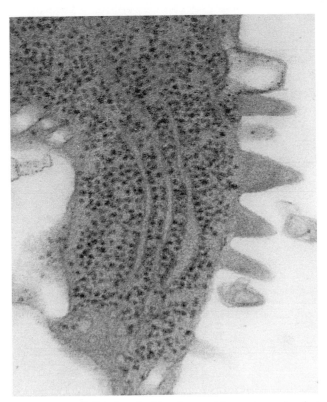

Figure 53.7. Cell infected with ephemeral fever virus, showing characteristic broad-based, cone-shaped virions. Transmission electron microscopy. × 123,750. (From Murphy et al., 1972, courtesy of *Archiv für die gesamte Virusforschung.*)

van der Westhuizen 1967). Further passage through mice at first attenuates the virus for cattle but then renders it nonimmunogenic, although this latter finding has been disputed (Della-Porta and Snowdon 1979). Isolating the virus from insects is more difficult (Davies and Walker 1974). Mouse-adapted strains and some field strains can be grown in cell-culture systems such as Vero and BHK-21 (St. George 1981, Snowdon 1970). Cytopathic effect usually is observed in these systems with well-adapted strains. Most successful primary isolations in cell culture of EF virus of bovine origin have been made from experimentally infected cattle rather than from natural cases (Snowdon 1970).

Epizootiology and Pathogenesis. EF is a disease of cattle and domestic water buffalo; other domestic species appear to be resistant. Its geographical range is considerable and extends through the tropical regions of Africa, Asia, and Australia, with spillover into subtropical and certain temperate latitudes. In Australia EF is the most economically important viral disease of cattle today (Vanselow et al. 1985). It has never been reported in the Americas and is absent from New Zealand and most tropical Pacific islands. In enzootic areas the occurrence of the disease is sporadic, except during periods of epizootic activity.

EF is not known to be transmitted from animal to animal by direct contact. Rather, there is a growing body of evidence that the virus is probably vectored by hematophagous arthropods. The occurrence of the disease generally is seasonal and correlated with rainy periods and the wet summer months. In Kenya an association with excessive rainfall has been noted (Davies et al. 1975). In Australia EF occurs primarily in summer and fall, and in the eastern half of the country it travels in a general north-south pattern that is aligned with the prevailing winds, suggesting spread by wind-borne insects (Murray 1970, Newton and Wheatley 1970, St. George et al. 1977, Seddon 1938). Isolations of the virus have been reported from *Culicoides* midges in Kenya (Davies and Walker 1974) and from mosquitoes in Australia (St. George et al. 1976), and experimental studies indicate that the virus will replicate in both insect types (St. George et al. 1977). Experimental transmission by insects to susceptible animals has not yet been reported, however. Other potential arthropod vectors have been identified, but isolations of virus from them have not been made (Mackerras et al. 1940, Murray 1975, Standfast and Dyce 1972).

Cattle are believed to be natural reservoirs of the disease, but the role (if any) of wildlife species as perpetuating or amplifying hosts remains poorly defined. Antibodies to the virus have been found in buffalo, waterbuck, wildebeest, and hartebeest in Africa (Davies et al. 1975) and in deer in Australia (St. George 1981). Clinical disease in these species has not been reported, even during major epizootics; however, these wild species and others are frequently found in close proximity to cattle herds in affected areas, and for this reason they must be considered potential reservoir hosts for livestock (Martin 1981).

The pathogenesis of the disease is incompletely understood. Following infection there is a brief period of viremia (about 5 days) that corresponds to the presence of clinical signs and during which virus is available to hematophagous arthropods. The virus is associated with the buffy coat fraction of the blood, but the site of replication in vivo is unknown. Occasionally virus is present in nasal discharges, but the infectivity is quite low. Some animals develop viremia in the absence of clinical disease. The basic lesion of EF is a serofibrinous polyserositis, presumably a result of vascular damage to the serosal surfaces of body cavities, including the joints (Basson et al. 1970, Spradbrow 1986). Effusion fluids are characterized by the presence of large numbers of neutrophils containing viral antigen (Young and Spradbrow 1980, 1985). This neutrophil influx, combined with evidence of increased permeability of small serosal vessels, suggests that EF may represent an acute, neutrophil-dependent, immune complex disease (Young and Spradbrow 1980).

Immunity. Information regarding immunity following natural infection is conflicting (Martin 1981; Spradbrow 1975, 1986; van der Westhuizen 1967). Most reports indicate that immunity is long-lasting, but some have suggested that it may be relatively brief. Experimental studies, however, have indicated that immunity may last for years (Mackerras et al. 1940, Snowdon 1970, Spradbrow 1975). Strain variation could play an important role in some of the observed discrepancies. Resistance to challenge appears to be correlated with the presence of serum-neutralizing antibodies, although this relationship has been questioned (Della-Porta and Snowdon 1979).

Diagnosis. EF frequently is diagnosed on the basis of clinical signs, especially during an epizootic. The very characteristic clinical course—abrupt onset, short duration, and rapid recovery—makes a presumptive field diagnosis quite probable. A definitive diagnosis, however, rests on the results of supportive laboratory tests.

The neutrophilia observed in field cases is a consistent finding, and unless it is present, the disease probably is not EF (St. George 1981). The most reliable specific procedure is detection of a rise in neutralizing antibody titer in paired (acute and convalescent) serum samples. Diagnosis is also possible by detection of specific viral antigen in leukocytes obtained from viremic animals; staining of blood smears with fluorescein-tagged conjugates is a useful way of accomplishing this. Primary isolation of EF virus from clinical cases generally is difficult and may require several passages in suckling mice or in cell cultures.

Treatment. No specific therapy exists for EF. Recovery from the disease usually is spontaneous, and treatment is purely supportive. Recumbent animals should be provided with drinking water and protected from the elements. Nonspecific therapy aimed at reducing fever and joint pain often includes aspirin or phenylbutazone. Antibiotics may be administered to guard against secondary bacterial pneumonia. Some recumbent cattle may respond to intravenous administration of calcium borogluconate. Oral feeding or medication is contraindicated in dysphagic animals because of the risk of inhalation pneumonia.

Prevention and Control. Vaccines of various types have been devised to protect cattle against EF. The rapid loss of virulence observed following passage in mice or cell cultures has prompted investigation of such mutant viruses for use as potential modified live-virus vaccines. Commercial vaccines are available in Japan and South Africa. In Japan, modified live-virus vaccination followed by inoculation with inactivated virus has met with success (Inaba et al. 1974). In Australia, modified live- and inactivated-virus vaccines have been tested, but none is yet available for widespread use (Della-Porta and Snowdon 1979, Spradbrow 1975, Tzipori and Spradbrow 1978, Tzipori et al. 1975, Vanselow et al. 1985). Control of EF by means other than vaccination (e.g., vector control) probably is not feasible.

The Disease in Humans. EF is not known to occur in humans.

REFERENCES

Basson, P.A., Pienaar, J.G., and van der Westhuizen, B. 1970. The pathology of ephemeral fever: A study of the experimental disease in cattle. J. S. Afr. Vet. Med. Assoc. 40:385–397.

Combs, G.P. 1978. Bovine ephemeral fever. Proc. U.S. Anim. Health Assoc. 82:29–35.

Cybinski, D.H., and Zakrzewski, H. 1983. The isolation and preliminary characterization of a rhabdovirus in Australia related to bovine ephemeral fever virus. Vet. Microbiol. 8:221–235.

Davies, F.G., and Walker, A.R. 1974. The isolation of ephemeral fever virus from cattle and *Culicoides* midges in Kenya. Vet. Rec. 95:63–64.

Davies, F.G., Shaw, T., and Ochieng, P. 1975. Observations on the epidemiology of ephemeral fever in Kenya. J. Hyg. (Cambridge) 75:231–235.

Davis, S.S., Gibson, D.S., and Clark, R. 1984. The effect of bovine ephemeral fever on milk production. Aust. Vet. J. 61:128–130.

Della-Porta, A.J., and Brown, F. 1979. The physico-chemical characterization of bovine ephemeral fever virus as a member of the family Rhabdoviridae. J. Gen. Virol. 44:99–112.

Della-Porta, A.J., and Snowdon, W.A. 1979. An experimental inactivated virus vaccine against bovine ephemeral fever. 1. Studies of the virus, and 2. Do neutralizing antibodies protect against infection? Vet. Microbiol. 4:183–208.

Doherty, R.L., Standfast, H.A., and Clark, I.A. 1969. Adaptation to mice of the causative virus of ephemeral fever of cattle from an epizootic in Queensland, 1968. Aust. J. Sci. 31:365–366.

Gard, G.P., Cybinski, D.H., and St. George, T.D. 1983. The isolation in Australia of a new virus related to bovine ephemeral fever virus. Aust. Vet. J. 60:89–90.

Gard, G.P., Cybinski, D.H., and Zakrzewski, H. 1984. The isolation of a fourth bovine ephemeral fever group virus. Aust. Vet. J. 61:332.

Heuschele, W.P. 1970. Bovine ephemeral fever. I. Characteristics of the causative virus. Arch. Gesam. Virusforsch. 30:195–202.

Hill, M.W.M., and Schultz, K. 1977. Ataxia and paralysis associated with bovine ephemeral fever infection. Aust. Vet. J. 53:217–221.

Holmes, I.H., and Doherty, R.L. 1970. Morphology and development of bovine ephemeral fever virus. J. Virol. 5:91–96.

Inaba, Y., Kurogi, H., Takahashi, A., Sato, K., Omori, T., Goto, Y., Hanaki, T., Yamamoto, M., Hishi, S., Kodama, K., Harada, K., and Matumoto, M. 1974. Vaccination of cattle against bovine ephemeral fever with live attenuated virus followed by killed virus. Arch. Gesam. Virusforsch. 44:121–132.

Inaba, Y., Tanaka, Y., Sato, K., Ito, H., Omori, T., and Matumoto, M. 1968a. Propagation in laboratory animals and cell cultures of a virus from cattle with bovine epizootic fever. Jpn. J. Microbiol. 12:253–255.

Inaba, Y., Tanaka, Y., Sato, K., Ito, H., Omori, T., and Matumoto, M. 1968b. Bovine epizootic fever. I. Propagation of the virus in suckling hamster, mouse and rat, and hamster kidney BHK21-W12 cell. Jpn. J. Microbiol. 12:457–469.

Kahrs, R.F. 1981. Virus Diseases of Cattle. Iowa State University Press, Ames. Pp. 251–254.

Kaneko, N., Inaba, Y., Akashi, H., Miura, Y., Shorthose, J., and

Kurashige, K. 1986. Isolation of a new bovine ephemeral fever group virus. Aust. Vet. J. 63:29.

Lecatsas, G., Theodoridis, A., and Erasmus, B.J. 1969. Electron microscopic studies on bovine ephemeral fever virus. Arch. Gesam. Virusforsch. 28:390–398.

Mackerras, I.M., Mackerras, M.J., and Burnet, F.M. 1940. Experimental studies of ephemeral fever in Australian cattle. Council for Scientific and Industrial Research, Australia, Bull. 136. 116 pp.

Malviya, H.K., and Prasad, J. 1977. Ephemeral fever—A clinical and epidemiological study in cross-bred cows and buffaloes. Ind. Vet. J. 54:440–444.

Martin, W.B. 1981. Ephemeral fever. In M. Ristic and I. McIntyre, eds., Diseases of Cattle in the Tropics. Martinus Nijhoff, The Hague. Pp. 181–187.

Mohan, R.N. 1968. Diseases and parasites of buffaloes. I. Viral, mycoplasmal and rickettsial diseases. Vet. Bull. (Weybridge) 38:567–576.

Murphy, F.A., Taylor, W.P., Mims, C.A., and Whitfield, S.G. 1972. Bovine ephemeral fever virus in cell culture and mice. Arch. Gesam. Virusforsch. 38:234–249.

Murray, M.D. 1970. The spread of ephemeral fever of cattle during the 1967–68 epizootic in Australia. Aust. Vet. J. 46:77–82.

Murray, M.D. 1975. Potential vectors of bluetongue in Australia. Aust. Vet. J. 51:216–220.

Newton, L.G., and Wheatley, C.H. 1970. The occurrence and spread of ephemeral fever of cattle in Queensland. Aust. Vet. J. 46:561–568.

Parsonson, I.M., Della-Porta, A.J., and Snowdon, W.A. 1981. Developmental disorders of the fetus in some arthropod-borne virus infections. Am. J. Trop. Med. Hyg. 30:660–673.

St. George, T.D. 1981. Ephemeral fever. In E.P.J. Gibbs, ed., Virus Diseases of Food Animals, vol. 2. Academic Press, New York. Pp. 541–564

St. George, T.D., Cybinski, D.H., Murphy, G.M., and Dimmock, C.K. 1984. Serological and biochemical factors in bovine ephemeral fever. Aust. J. Biol. Sci. 37:341–349.

St. George, T.D., Standfast, H.A., Christie, D.G., Knott, S.G., and Morgan, I.R. 1977. The epizootiology of bovine ephemeral fever in Australia and Papua-New Guinea. Aust. Vet. J. 53:17–28.

St. George, T.D., Standfast, H.A., and Dyce, A.L. 1976. The isolation of ephemeral fever virus from mosquitoes in Australia. Aust. Vet. J. 52:242.

Sasaki, N., Kodama, K., Iwamoto, I., Izumida, A., and Matsubara, T. 1968. Serial transmission in suckling mice of a virus from cattle with bovine epizootic fever. Jpn. J. Microbiol. 12:251–252.

Seddon, H.R. 1938. The spread of ephemeral fever (three-day sickness) in Australia in 1936–37. Aust. Vet. J. 14:90–101.

Snowdon, W.A. 1970. Bovine ephemeral fever: The reaction of cattle to different strains of ephemeral fever virus and the antigenic comparison of two strains of virus. Aust. Vet. J. 46:258–266.

Spradbrow, P.B. 1975. Attenuated vaccines against bovine ephemeral fever. Aust. Vet. J. 51:464–468.

Spradbrow, P.B. 1986. Bovine ephemeral fever. In J.L. Howard, ed., Current Veterinary Therapy: Food Animal Practice, 2d ed. W.B. Saunders, Philadelphia. Pp. 505–506.

Spradbrow, P.B., and Francis, J. 1969. Observations on bovine ephemeral fever and isolation of virus. Aust. Vet. J. 45:525–527.

Standfast, H.A., and Dyce, A.L. 1972. Potential vectors of arboviruses of cattle and buffalo in Australia. Aust. Vet. J. 48:224–227.

Theodoridis, A., and Coetzer, J.A.W. 1979. Subcutaneous and pulmonary emphysema as complications of bovine ephemeral fever. Onderstepoort J. Vet. Res. 46:125–127.

Tzipori, S., and Spradbrow, P.B. 1978. A cell culture vaccine against bovine ephemeral fever. Aust. Vet. J. 54:323–328.

Tzipori, S., Spradbrow, P.B., and Doyle, T. 1975. Laboratory and field studies with a bovine ephemeral fever vaccine. Aust. Vet. J. 51:244–250.

van der Westhuizen, B. 1967. Studies on bovine ephemeral fever. I. Isolation and preliminary characterization of a virus from natural and experimentally produced cases of bovine ephemeral fever. Onderstepoort J. Vet. Res. 34:29–40.

Vanselow, B.A., Abetz, I., and Trenfield, K. 1985. A bovine ephemeral fever vaccine incorporating adjuvant Quil A: A comparative study using adjuvants Quil A, aluminum hydroxide gel and dextran sulphate. Vet. Rec. 117:37–43.

Young, P.L., and Spradbrow, P.B. 1980. The role of neutrophils in bovine ephemeral fever virus infection of cattle. J. Infect. Dis. 142:50–55.

Young, P.L., and Spradbrow, P.B. 1985. Transmission of virus from serosal fluids and demonstration of antigen in neutrophils and mesothelial cells of cattle infected with bovine ephemeral fever virus. Vet. Microbiol. 10:199–207.

54 The Retroviridae

The retroviruses are an important and diverse group of single-stranded RNA viruses that are widely distributed among vertebrate species (Bishop 1978, Lowy 1985, Robinson 1982, Tronick and Aaronson 1984, Varmus 1982). Enveloped virions vary in size from 80 to 130 nm in diameter (mean 100 nm) and contain an inner electron-dense core, or *nucleoid*. The nucleoid is composed of ribonucleoprotein surrounded by an icosahedral protein capsid. The envelope surface is studded with regularly spaced glycoprotein projections (peplomers). The buoyant density in sucrose is 1.16–1.18 g/ml. The particles are sensitive to lipid solvents, detergents, and heat (56°C for 30 minutes).

The genome of retroviruses is capped, polyadenylated, and infectious. It is composed of two identical RNA subunits joined noncovalently near their 5′ termini. The genome is replicated in the host cell through a double-stranded DNA intermediate that is integrated into the chromosomal DNA. This reaction is catalyzed by a virus-encoded RNA-dependent DNA polymerase, *reverse transcriptase*. The integrated DNA intermediate, known as a *provirus* or *proviral DNA,* then divides whenever the host cell divides and can serve as a template for the production of new virus particles. Because a DNA version of their genetic material becomes a part of the total genetic information of the cells they infect, retroviruses are among the most intimate parasites known in nature. In most cases infected cells continue to grow and develop normally while synthesizing new virus particles, which are released by budding at the plasma membrane.

At least three distinct virus-encoded genes (protein coding domains) are required for the replication of retroviruses:

1. *gag* (for *g*roup-specific *a*ntigen), which encodes the viral core proteins
2. *pol* (for *pol*ymerase), which encodes the reverse transcriptase
3. *env* (for *env*elope), which encodes the viral envelope proteins

Some cancer-causing retroviruses contain in addition a viral-transforming gene, or *oncogene* (abbreviated v-*onc*), of which more than 20 types are currently recognized. Oncogenes appear to represent normal cellular genes that have been acquired by the virus by genetic recombination, subjected to minor alterations, and then placed under the control of viral regulatory elements. The cellular genes (so-called proto-oncogenes, abbreviated c-*onc*) are highly conserved in eukaryotic evolution; the ability of their virus-modified counterparts to produce abnormal cellular growth (neoplasia) suggests that c-*onc* genes are involved in regulation of very basic cellular processes of growth and differentiation.

At present, the family Retroviridae is divided into three subfamilies: oncogenic viruses (Oncovirinae); viruses inducing chronic degenerative diseases (Lentivirinae); and symbiotic viruses evoking little or no host cell response (Spumavirinae). The most important diseases of domestic animals caused by retroviruses are listed in Table 54.1.

REFERENCES

Bishop, J.M. 1978. Retroviruses. Annu. Rev. Biochem. 47:35–88.
Lowy, D.R. 1985. Transformation and oncogenesis: Retroviruses. In B. N. Fields, ed., Virology. Raven Press, New York. Pp. 235–263.
Robinson, H.L. 1982. Retroviruses and cancer. Rev. Infect. Dis. 4:1015–1025.
Tronick, S.R., and Aaronson, S.A. 1984. Unique interactions of retroviruses with eukaryotic cells. In A.L. Notkins and M.B.A. Oldstone, eds., Concepts in Viral Pathogenesis. Springer-Verlag, New York. Pp. 165–171.
Varmus, H.E. 1982. Form and function of retroviral proviruses. Science 216:812–820.

The Subfamily Oncovirinae

The Oncovirinae comprise the oncogenic retroviruses (RNA tumor viruses) and their nononcogenic relatives. Oncoviruses have been isolated from a wide variety of species, including humans. Many oncoviruses have proved oncogenic capabilities in their natural hosts as well as in other species under experimental conditions.

On the basis of morphology, the oncoviruses can be

Table 54.1. Retroviruses that cause diseases of importance in domestic animals

Virus	Natural host	Type of disease produced
Subfamily Oncovirinae		
Avian leukosis-sarcoma viruses	Chickens	Complex of neoplastic diseases, including lymphoid leukosis, erythroblastosis, myeloblastosis, myelocytomatosis, osteopetrosis, and others. Worldwide distribution
Feline leukemia-sarcoma viruses	Cats	Complex of neoplastic (lymphosarcoma, fibrosarcoma, myeloproliferative disorders) and non-neoplastic (anemia, thymic atrophy, immunosuppression, glomerulonephritis) diseases. Worldwide
Enzootic bovine leukosis virus	Cattle	Adult form of lymphosarcoma and persistent lymphocytosis. Worldwide
Subfamily Lentivirinae		
Maedi-visna virus	Sheep	Slow virus infection producing respiratory, neurologic, and/or arthritic signs. Worldwide
Caprine arthritis-encephalitis virus	Goats	Multisystemic disease producing neurological signs in kids and arthritic signs in adults. Worldwide
Equine infectious anemia virus	Horses	Diversity of signs and a variable course; anemia and hemorrhages are typically found. May appear in acute, subacute, or chronic form. Worldwide

divided into four groups, designated A, B, C, and D. The vast majority of oncoviruses are C-type viruses, that is, the particles are formed during budding at the plasma membrane. B-type oncoviruses, such as the mouse mammary tumor viruses, first form their nucleoids in the cytoplasm of the cell and then acquire an envelope during budding. D-type oncoviruses, such as the Mason-Pfizer monkey virus, form similarly to B-type viruses, but the mature (budded) virions are morphologically more similar to C-type particles. A-type particles (cisternaviruses) are found only intracellularly and are not infectious.

Some oncoviruses (acute transforming viruses) produce tumors within a very short time (days to weeks) after infection and in a high percentage of infected hosts. These viruses contain v-*onc* gene sequences that apparently mediate the rapid transformation of host cells. Examples of such v-*onc*+ viruses are the feline sarcoma viruses, simian sarcoma virus, and avian erythroblastosis virus. Other oncoviruses (chronic transforming viruses) cause cancers late after infection and in only a relatively low percentage of inoculated hosts. These viruses do not carry v-*onc* genes; instead, insertion of their proviral DNA into host cell chromosomes, in certain key locations, may activate potentially oncogenic c-*onc* sequences normally found in the cellular genome. Examples of v-*onc*− viruses are the feline leukemia virus, bovine leukemia virus, and human T-lymphotropic viruses I and II.

Avian Leukosis-Sarcoma Complex

The avian leukosis-sarcoma complex of neoplastic disease includes lymphoid leukosis, erythroblastosis, myeloblastosis, myelocytomatosis, osteopetrosis, and various other epithelial, endothelial, and connective tissue tumors (Essex and Worley 1981, Purchase and Payne 1984). These neoplasms are produced in chickens, and to a much lesser extent in other avian species, by a constellation of type C oncovirus strains, many of which have been studied intensively in the laboratory in an attempt to uncover the molecular mechanisms of oncogenesis. Avian leukosis-sarcoma viruses were first identified as agents of transmissible neoplastic disease over 70 years ago (Ellermann and Bang 1908, Rous 1911). The term *leukosis* is used to signify abnormal proliferation of primitive leukocyte precursor cells and is favored by most investigators over the older term, *leukemia,* which refers to the presence of neoplastic cells in the blood or bone marrow or both. There are many forms of disease in this complex in which such cells are found in the tissues but not in the bloodstream. The terms *pseudoleukemia* or *aleukemic leukemia* are sometimes used to differentiate these forms.

Character of the Major Diseases. The avian leukosis-sarcoma complex comprises several important disease entities, including the following:

Lymphoid leukosis. From the standpoint of the poultry producer, lymphoid leukosis (LL) is the most common and also the most important retroviral disease of chickens. Field outbreaks occur in birds over 3 months of age. Clinical signs of LL are generally nonspecific. Anorexia, emaciation, and weakness are commonly seen. The bird's comb may be pale and shriveled and sometimes cyanotic. Often there is abdominal enlargement reflecting growth of tumors in the liver, kidneys, and bursa. The clinical course of LL is rapid.

Erythroblastosis. As with LL, field cases of erythroblastosis usually occur in birds more than 3 months old. The earliest clinical signs are weakness, lethargy, and paleness or cyanosis of the comb. Diarrhea may develop, as may hemorrhages from the feather follicles. With severe anemia, the bird's comb may become light yellow. The course of the disease lasts from a few days to several months.

Myeloblastosis. Clinical signs are similar to those of erythroblastosis. The disease course is highly variable but is generally longer than that for erythroblastosis.

Myelocytomatosis. Most field cases are seen in immature birds. The clinical signs are similar to those of myeloblastosis. Additionally, skeletal growths resulting in abnormal protuberances occur on the head, thorax, and shanks. The disease course is usually lengthy.

Osteopetrosis. This disease is observed most commonly in birds 8 to 12 weeks old. The long bones of the limbs are affected, with a uniform or irregular thickening of the diaphyseal or metaphyseal regions producing characteristic bootlike shanks in severely diseased birds. Affected birds are stunted and pale and walk with difficulty.

Properties of the Viruses. The avian leukosis-sarcoma viruses that occur in chickens have been classified into five subgroups—A, B, C, D, and E—on the basis of their host range in chicken cells of differing genetic types, the host cell receptor interference patterns, and the viral envelope antigens identified by neutralization tests (Vogt 1970). Subgroups A and B are the most important in terms of field outbreaks. Subgroups C and D have been recovered much less frequently, whereas subgroup E viruses represent genetically inherited (endogenous) nononcogenic agents. Subgroup F and G viruses are found primarily in pheasants. Viruses within a subgroup cross-neutralize to varying extents, but with the exception of partial cross-neutralization between subgroups A and D, viruses belonging to different subgroups do not. There is evidence for antigenic variation within individual subgroups. Strains of viruses within subgroups are classified according to the predominant lesions they produce and the particular subgroup envelope they possess. The avian leukosis-sarcoma viruses cannot be distinguished on the basis of morphologic characteristics.

Acute transforming viruses, such as the Rous, Fujinami, and PRCII sarcoma viruses, avian erythroblastosis virus, and avian myeloblastosis virus, carry specific v-*onc* sequences that mediate oncogenic transformation of infected cells. Chronic transforming viruses, such as LL virus, are v-*onc*$^-$ but may be capable of activating c-*onc* sequences following proviral insertion. The exact mechanisms by which c-*onc* genes are activated and induce abnormal proliferation are still unknown.

Cultivation. In general, most avian leukosis viruses replicate in cultured chick embryo fibroblasts without producing a cytopathic effect or transformation. Cells infected with a leukosis virus, however, are resistant to superinfection with a sarcoma virus of the same subgroup. This property of *interference* has been exploited as a convenient assay procedure for leukosis viruses, the resistance-inducing factor (RIF) test (Hanafusa et al. 1964, Rubin 1960).

Certain avian sarcoma viruses, such as Rous virus, readily and quickly transform cells in culture. The morphology of the transformed cells and the shape of the neoplastic focus are characteristic of the infecting virus. Virus can be conveniently quantitated on the basis of focus-forming units per unit volume.

Epizootiology and Pathogenesis. The natural host for viruses of subgroups A through E is the chicken. Subgroup F and G viruses have been isolated from pheasants. Experimentally, however, some of the viruses show a broader host range. The Rous sarcoma virus, for example, can produce tumors in several species of birds. Some avian sarcoma viruses can produce tumors also in monkeys and other mammals (Kumanishi et al. 1973, Vogt 1965).

Leukosis viruses are transmitted horizontally in droppings and saliva and vertically through the egg. Although vertical transmission is much less common, it is nevertheless important as a means by which infections are maintained from one generation to the next (Robinson and Eisenman 1984). Most birds become infected through direct contact with congenitally infected chickens. Horizontal transmission is most efficient when chickens are in direct contact with infected birds or their excreta.

Lymphoid leukosis. The solid tumors of lymphoid leukosis are composed of large, primitive lymphoid cells that have been referred to as lymphoblasts, hemocytoblasts, and reticulolymphocytes. They are believed to be bursal in origin. Most tumor nodules are clonal, that is, they are derived from very small numbers of transformed cells. LL tumor cells have IgM rather than IgG or IgA on their surfaces because neoplastic transformation is accompanied by interference with the normal switch of B lymphocyte immunoglobulin production from IgM to IgG. Both of these events are believed to result from LL virus-induced activation of c-*onc* sequences in B cells.

Erythroblastosis. The primary cell involved in this disease is the erythroblast. Unlike in LL and myeloblastosis, the neoplastic cells in erythroblastosis remain entirely within the blood vascular system. Sinusoids and capillaries of the liver, spleen, and bone marrow become swollen and engorged with tumor cells. Eventually sinusoidal swelling results in pressure atrophy of the the surrounding parenchymal tissue. Varying degrees of anemia are frequently observed, and extramedullary hematopoiesis is common. The tumor arises from proviral DNA-mediated blockage of erythroblastic differentiation, resulting in the uncontrolled proliferation of precursor cells.

Myeloblastosis. This disease is characterized by a spectacular leukemia; as many as 2×10^6 myeloblasts per cubic millimeter of blood may be found. Parenchymatous organs are choked with intravascular and extravascular accumulations of myeloblasts and variable numbers of promyelocytes. Infiltration and proliferation are especially extensive around sinusoids and portal tracts in the hepatic parenchyma. The tumor arises in the bone marrow.

Myelocytomatosis. The tumors of this disease are composed of compact accumulations of nondescript myelocytes similar morphologically to those found in normal marrow. As the myelocytes proliferate, however, they overgrow the marrow cavity, expanding outward in discrete tuberclelike growths that extend through the periosteum. The disease is usually aleukemic.

Osteopetrosis. This disease consists essentially of an osteoblastic proliferation that is aleukemic but is usually accompanied by a secondary anemia. The periosteum is thickened by an increasing number of enlarged, basophilic osteoblasts.

Immunity. Chickens that are immunologically competent develop neutralizing antibodies after exposure to leukosis viruses. These antibodies are often of high titer and persist for the life of the bird (Rubin et al. 1962, Solomon et al. 1966). They are passed via the yolk to the chicks, providing temporary passive immunity that delays leukosis virus infection and reduces the occurrence of neoplasms (Burmester 1955, Witter et al. 1966). Cytotoxic lymphocytes and tumor-associated cell surface antigens are considered to be important factors in tumor regression and the elimination of neoplastic foci.

Genetic factors also are of importance in resistance to avian leukosis-sarcoma virus-induced tumors. Two levels of resistance are recognized: cellular resistance to viral infection and resistance to tumor development (Crittenden 1975; Pani 1976a, 1976b). Inheritance of cellular resistance to infection is of a simple Mendelian type, with susceptibility genes coding for subgroup-specific virus receptors on the cell surface. Resistant cells are believed to lack virus receptor sites. Genetic resistance to tumor development in the Rous sarcoma virus system is determined by a dominant gene that lies within the major histocompatibility complex (Collins et al. 1977). Resistance to LL tumor development is mediated by bursal cells (Purchase et al. 1977).

Diagnosis. Diagnosis of the individual neoplastic disease entities is made most commonly at necropsy. Identification of the causative retroviruses can be done in a number of ways, including direct isolation in cell culture. The RIF test is used for the assay of viruses that are not rapidly cytopathic (leukosis viruses) (Hanafusa et al. 1964, Rubin 1960). The complement-fixation test for avian leukosis viruses (COFAL) is used for detection of core antigens in cultures of infected cells (Sarma et al. 1964). Radioimmunoassay, immunofluorescence assay, and enzyme-linked immunosorbent assay are also available for core antigen detection. Phenotypic mixing is exploited in the nonproducer cell activation test (Rispens et al. 1970). The presence of adenosine triphosphatase (ATPase) on the surface of avian myeloblastosis virus can be used for quantitating virus in plasma or in supernatants of myeloblast cultures (Beaudreau and Becker 1958). Focus assays are commonly used to detect sarcoma virus–transformed cells in monolayers of susceptible chick cells (Temin and Rubin 1958).

Treatment. Tumors induced by avian leukosis-sarcoma viruses are not amenable to treatment. No practical therapeutic measures are available.

Prevention and Control. Pathogenic avian leukosis viruses can be eradicated and commercial breeder flocks free of infection can be established (Spencer et al. 1977) by rearing and maintaining in isolation chickens that are free of congenital infection. The embryos are obtained from hens selected for freedom from transovarial passage of virus.

Immunization procedures reported thus far are not suitable for commercial application. Attempts to produce attenuated virus strains for use in vaccines have been unsuccessful (Okazaki et al. 1982).

The Disease in Humans. Avian leukosis-sarcoma complex is not known to occur in humans.

REFERENCES

Beaudreau, G.S., and Becker, C. 1958. Virus of avian myeloblastosis. X. Photometric microdetermination of adenosinetriphosphatase activity. J. Natl. Cancer Inst. 20:339–349.

Burmester, B.R. 1955. Immunity to visceral lymphomatosis in chicks following injection of virus into dams. Proc. Soc. Exp. Biol. Med. 88:153–155.

Collins, W.M., Briles, W.E., Zsigray, R.M., Dunlop, W.R., Corbett, A.C., Clark, K.K., Marks, J.L., and McGrail, T.P. 1977. The *B* locus (MHC) in the chicken: Association with the fate of RSV-induced tumors. Immunogenetics 5:333–343.

Crittenden, L.B. 1975. Two levels of genetic resistance to lymphoid leukosis. Avian Dis. 19:281–292.

Ellermann, V., and Bang, O. 1908. Experimentelle Leukämie bei Hühnern. Zentralbl. Bakteriol. Parasiten. Infektion. I. Abt. Orig. 46:595–609.

Essex, M., and Worley, M. 1981. Naturally occurring retroviruses of animals and birds. In E. Kurstak and C. Kurstak, eds., Comparative Diagnosis of Viral Diseases, vol. 4, part B. Academic Press, New York. Pp. 553–597.

Hanafusa, H., Hanafusa, T., and Rubin, H. 1964. Analysis of the defectiveness of Rous sarcoma virus. I. Characterization of the helper virus. Virology 22:591–601.

Kumanishi, T., Ikuta, F., Nishida, K., Ueki, K., and Yamamoto, T. 1973. Brain tumors induced in adult monkeys by Schmidt-Ruppin strain of Rous sarcoma virus. Gann 64:641–643.

Okazaki, W., Purchase, H.G., and Crittenden, L.B. 1982. Pathogenicity of avian leukosis viruses. Avian Dis. 26:553–559.

Pani, P.K. 1976a. Further studies in genetic resistance of fowl to RSV(RAV O): Evidence for interaction between independently segregating tumour virus *b* and tumour virus *e* genes. J. Gen. Virol. 32:441–453.

Pani, P.K. 1976b. Genetics of resistance of fowl to infection by RNA tumour viruses. Proc. R. Soc. Med. 69:43–48.

Purchase, H.G., and Payne, L.N. 1984. Leukosis/sarcoma group. In M.S. Hofstad, H.J. Barnes, B.W. Calnek, W.M. Reid, and H.W. Yoder, eds., Diseases of Poultry, 8th ed. Iowa State University Press, Ames. Pp. 360–405.

Purchase, H.G., Gilmour, D.G., Romero, C.H., and Okazaki, W. 1977. Postinfection genetic resistance to avian lymphoid leukosis resides in B target cell. Nature 270:61–62.

Rispens, B.H., Long, P.A., Okazaki, W., and Burmester, B.R. 1970. The NP activation test for assay of avian leukosis/sarcoma viruses. Avian Dis. 14:738–751.

Robinson, H.L., and Eisenman, R.N. 1984. New findings on the congenital transmission of avian leukosis viruses. Science 225:417–419.

Rous, P. 1911. A sarcoma of the fowl transmissible by an agent separable from the tumor cells. J. Exp. Med. 13:397–411.

Rubin, H. 1960. A virus in chick embryos which induces resistance in vitro to infection with Rous sarcoma virus. Proc. Natl. Acad. Sci. USA 46:1105–1119.

Rubin, H., Fanshier, L., Cornelius, A., and Hughes, W.F. 1962. Tolerance and immunity in chickens after congenital and contact infection with an avian leukosis virus. Virology 17:143–156.

Sarma, P.S., Turner, H.C., and Huebner, R.J. 1964. An avian leucosis group-specific complement fixation reaction. Application for the detection and assay of non-cytopathogenic viruses. Virology 23:313–321.

Solomon, J.J., Burmester, B.R., and Fredrickson, T.N. 1966. Investigations of lymphoid leukosis infection in genetically similar chicken populations. Avian Dis. 10:477–484.

Spencer, J.L., Crittenden, L.B., Burmester, B.R., Okazaki, W., and Witter, R.L. 1977. Lymphoid leukosis: Interrelations among virus infections in hens, eggs, embryos, and chicks. Avian Dis. 21:331–345.

Temin, H.M., and Rubin, H. 1958. Characteristics of an assay for Rous sarcoma virus and Rous sarcoma cells in tissue culture. Virology 6:669–688.

Vogt, P.K. 1965. Avian tumor viruses. Adv. Virus Res. 11:293–385.

Vogt, P.K. 1970. Envelope classification of avian RNA tumor viruses. Bibl. Haematologica 36:153–167.

Witter, R.L., Calnek, B.W., and Levine, P.P. 1966. Influence of naturally occurring parenteral antibody on visceral lymphomatosis virus infection in chickens. Avian Dis. 10:43–56.

Feline Leukemia-Sarcoma Complex

In 1964 Jarrett and co-workers showed that a virus similar to those causing murine leukemia was present in feline lymphosarcoma (LSA) cells (Jarrett et al. 1964). This finding was soon confirmed by others (Kawakami et al. 1967, Rickard et al. 1967, Theilen et al. 1969). The virus, subsequently named feline leukemia virus (FeLV), is the causative agent of the most important fatal infectious disease complex in domestic cats (Barton 1986; Cotter 1984; Essex 1982; Gerstman 1985; Hardy 1981a, 1981b; Ott 1983; Pedersen and Madewell 1980). It is widespread in feline populations throughout the world.

Character of the Diseases. Cats persistently infected with FeLV are susceptible to diseases that are directly or indirectly caused by the virus. Those directly caused by FeLV include lymphoid malignancies, a number of myeloproliferative disorders, several types of anemia, the panleukopenialike and thymic atrophy syndromes, at least one form of kidney disease, certain reproductive disorders, and several other conditions. Diseases indirectly caused by FeLV include a myriad of conditions that develop secondary to FeLV-induced immunosuppression.

Lymphoid malignancies. LSA and its leukemic counterpart are the most common tumors of American domestic cats. Several forms of LSA have been identified, and their classification is based most commonly on their anatomical distribution. The tumors consist primarily of solid masses of proliferating lymphocytes and constitute the majority of the malignancies caused by FeLV.

The *alimentary form* of LSA is characterized by tumor cell infiltration of the gastrointestinal tract and other organs, including the intestinal lymph nodes, liver,

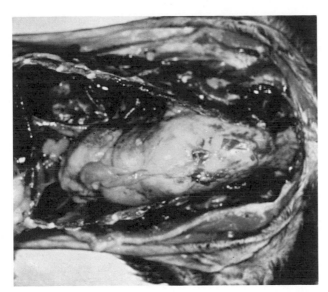

Figure 54.1. Experimental thymic lymphosarcoma in a neonatal kitten. (Courtesy C. Rickard, J. Post, and K. Lee, Cornell University.)

kidneys, and spleen. Common presenting signs include anorexia, weight loss, vomiting, diarrhea, bloody stool, and icterus. Occlusion of the bowel lumen by the proliferating tumor results in constipation or obstipation.

The *thymic,* or *mediastinal, form* is characterized by the presence of a large tumor mass (or masses) infiltrating the thymus gland and spreading to regional lymphoid tissue and sometimes to extrathoracic structures (Figure 54.1). Clinical signs reflect pressure effects of the mass and the severe intrathoracic fluid accumulation that frequently accompanies the tumor. Physical examination thus may reveal labored respiration, cyanosis, muffled heart sounds, coughing, difficulty in swallowing, and incompressibility of the chest wall.

The *multicentric form* is characterized by primary involvement of many lymphoid tissues of the body and additional involvement of other structures, such as the liver, bone marrow, kidneys, spleen, and lungs. Presenting signs are variable and depend on the precise anatomical distribution of the tumor, but they often include painless swelling of peripheral lymph nodes and enlargement of the spleen and liver and often of the mesenteric nodes.

Atypical forms of LSA also occur and consist usually of solitary or multiple tumor masses involving primary sites of origin in nonintestinal, nonlymphoid structures, including the kidneys, central nervous system, and eyes, and, rarely, the skin or bones. Presenting signs vary according to the location of the neoplasm.

Lymphocytic leukemia is characterized by the presence of circulating neoplastic lymphocytes in the blood and in the bone marrow. It may precede the development of LSA, or it may be associated secondarily with LSA. Presenting signs usually consist of nonspecific anorexia, weight loss, and depression. More specific signs that may be seen include anemia, fever, icterus, and enlargement of the liver, spleen, and lymph nodes.

Lymphoid tumors occur in cats of all ages, but certain age-related tendencies have been observed. Thus the thymic form of LSA and lymphocytic leukemia occur more commonly in younger cats, the multicentric form of LSA in middle-aged animals, and the alimentary form in middle-aged and older cats.

FeLV-negative lymphoid malignancies. During the course of investigations into the biology of FeLV, it has become apparent that 10 to 50 percent of lymphoid malignancies in cats are negative for FeLV-related material, such as virus particles, viral structural antigens, or proviral DNA (Francis, Cotter, et al. 1979; Hardy et al. 1969, 1980). Most of these FeLV-negative tumors are of the alimentary type and occur proportionally more often in older age groups than in younger ones. The cause of FeLV-negative LSAs is uncertain, but it is believed, for a number of reasons, that FeLV is ultimately responsible for their development.

Myeloproliferative disorders. Myeloproliferative disorders are a group of primary bone marrow disorders characterized by abnormal proliferation of one or more hematopoietic cell lines. Granulocytic (myelogenous) leukemia, erythroleukemia, erythremic myelosis, megakaryocytic leukemia, polycythemia rubra vera, and reticuloendotheliosis are all terms that have been applied to various forms of these disorders. Classification depends on the cell line(s) of origin. Clinicopathological differentiation among different forms is sometimes difficult, if not impossible, however, because more than one hematopoietic cell line may be involved, either sequentially or simultaneously. Presenting signs can include anorexia, depression, weight loss, relentless and progressive anemia, fever, icterus, peripheral lymphadenopathy, and enlargement of the liver and spleen secondary to massive infiltration by abnormally proliferating cells.

Nonregenerative anemia. Nonregenerative anemia (NRA) is probably one of the most common manifestations of FeLV infection. This type of anemia, also known as hypoplastic, aplastic, or depression anemia, is characterized by a severe reduction in the number of red cell precursors in the bone marrow, resulting in failure to produce an adequate number of circulating red cells. Sometimes a pancytopenia occurs in which red cell, white cell, and platelet precursors are all affected. NRA may occur alone or in conjunction with LSA or myeloproliferative disease, or it may precede the development of an FeLV-induced malignancy. Since many severely ill cats with NRA are destroyed, the true incidence of subsequent malignancy cannot be determined. Unfortunately, clinical signs usually are not detected until the anemia is well advanced. Common signs include anorexia, depression, weight loss, pallor of the mucous membranes, respiratory difficulty, and increased heart rate. Coinfection of such cats with *Haemobartonella felis* may contribute to the severity of the anemia.

Other anemias. In addition to NRA, other types of anemia may occur in cats in association with FeLV infection. These include (1) *leukoerythroblastic anemia,* characterized by the simultaneous presence of circulating nucleated red blood cells in numbers out of proportion to the severity of the anemia and of certain immature white cells (this type of anemia has been observed in some cases of LSA); (2) *megaloblastic anemia* (similar to the anemia of vitamin B_{12}-folate deficiency), sometimes seen in cats with myeloproliferative disorders; (3) *hemolytic anemia,* characterized by premature destruction of circulating erythrocytes by an immunological process; and (4) *anemia of chronic disease,* caused by the ineffective reutilization of iron for hemoglobin synthesis.

Panleukopenialike syndrome. A syndrome somewhat similar to panleukopenia has been observed in some FeLV-infected cats known to be properly immunized against panleukopenia. Presenting signs include anorexia, depression, dehydration, weight loss, fever, vomiting, diarrhea (which may be bloody), and a profound reduction in the number of circulating leukocytes. Anemia may also be present. Although affected cats may respond transiently to supportive therapy, the disease is progressive and usually fatal.

Thymic atrophy syndrome. Kittens born to persistently viremic queens often develop a syndrome of lethargy, anorexia, wasting, stunted growth, atrophy of the thymus and other lymphoid structures, and enhanced susceptibility to infection with other pathogens (fading kitten syndrome). The degree of thymic atrophy can be severe, amounting to virtual disappearance of the organ in some cases. Such kittens do not gain weight and often do not nurse vigorously. Many die from secondary bacterial or viral infections within the first few weeks of life. Those that survive are carriers of FeLV and thus are capable of transmitting the virus to other susceptible cats. The syndrome may also precede the development of an FeLV-induced malignancy.

Glomerulonephritis. Glomerulonephritis has been described in cats in association with LSA, lymphocytic leukemia, and granulocytic leukemia. In addition, glomerular disease in the absence of malignancy has been reported in FeLV-infected cats. In one study the leading cause of

death in an FeLV-infected household over 5 and a half years was glomerulonephritis (Francis et al. 1980). Other studies suggest that immune-complex disease, ranging from subclinical microscopic lesions to the nephrotic syndrome, may be caused by formation of antigen-antibody complexes that accumulate in renal glomeruli.

Reproductive disorders. Queens infected with FeLV may experience one or more reproductive disorders, including fetal resorption, abortion, infertility, endometritis, and birth of fading kittens. Abortions characteristically occur late in gestation and are more frequent in high-density multiple cat FeLV households than in solitary cat households or multiple cat households free of FeLV.

Miscellaneous disorders. Infection with FeLV has been associated with osteochondromatosis (aberrant growth of cartilage-capped bony protrusions from certain long bones) and persistent pupillary dilation (probably induced by paralysis of ciliary nerves in the eye).

Diseases secondary to immunosuppression. Secondary disease entities associated with FeLV-induced immunosuppression constitute one of the most important manifestations of FeLV infection. It has been estimated that nearly 50 percent of all cats with severe bacterial infections and infectious anemia and 75 percent of cats with toxoplasmosis have an underlying FeLV infection. In addition to these disorders, FeLV-induced immunosuppression has been associated with chronic gingivitis and stomatitis, poorly healing or recurrent abcesses, deep pyodermas, chronic respiratory infections, acute colitis, and feline infectious peritonitis. FeLV-induced immunosuppression probably also contributes to the development of FeLV-induced malignancies.

Multiple fibrosarcomas. The feline sarcoma virus (FeSV), a replication-defective mutant of FeLV, is the causative agent of certain fibrosarcomas in cats. Multiple fibrosarcomas arising in the skin of younger cats (generally less than 5 years of age) usually are associated with FeLV-FeSV infection, whereas solitary fibrosarcomas found in older cats usually are not. FeSV-induced malignancies occur only rarely in cats, however, and thus are of relatively minor clinical significance when compared with the array of problems associated with persistent FeLV infection.

Properties of the Virus. FeLV is a typical C-type oncovirus (Figure 54.2). A 27-kilodalton protein moiety, p27, is a structural component of the inner viral core and is the major FeLV group-specific antigen. It can be found in great abundance in the cytoplasm of infected leukocytes and platelets and in soluble form in the plasma and serum of viremic cats. This protein provides the major antigenic basis for currently available FeLV antigen detection tests.

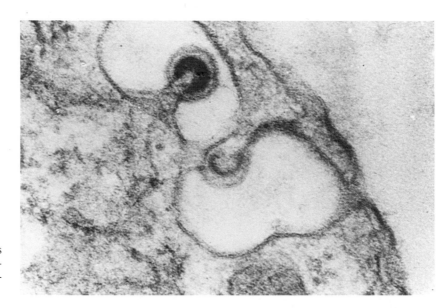

Figure 54.2. Budding feline leukemia virus particles characteristic of C-type oncoviruses. (Courtesy C. Rickard, Cornell University.)

A glycoprotein moiety, gp70, is the principal antigenic component of the viral peplomers, which are responsible for attachment of the virus to cells during infection. Neutralizing antibody directed against gp70 is an essential component of a successful immunological response to FeLV. A major cause of FeLV-induced immunosuppression appears to be a specific FeLV structural protein, p15(E), which, like gp70, is associated with the viral envelope. Both intact and disrupted (inactivated) virus particles retain immunosuppressive capabilities (Hebebrand et al. 1977, Mathes et al. 1979). All FeLV isolates are v-*onc*⁻.

The antigens of oncoviruses are classified according to the degree of cross-reactivity exhibited. Thus, interspecies-specific determinants cross-react among all mammalian C-type viruses, whereas species-specific determinants are shared by oncoviruses isolated from the same species (Figure 54.3). Type-specific determinants differentiate viral strains isolated within a species. At present, three subgroups or serotypes (A, B, and C) of FeLV are recognized (Sarma and Log 1973).

In common with many other enveloped viruses, FeLV is extremely labile once outside the cat and is rapidly inactivated by alcohol and most common household detergents and disinfectants. The infectivity of saliva left to dry at room temperature has been shown to decline to inconsequential levels within 3 or 4 hours (Francis, Essex, et al. 1979); however, the infectivity of FeLV that is suspended in liquid at room temperature may persist for several days or even longer at refrigerator temperature.

FeSV, a replication-defective mutant of FeLV, apparently arises within individual cats by a recombinational event in which a small piece of chromosomal DNA is incorporated into an FeLV provirus. The resulting FeSV is v-*onc*⁺ but unable to replicate without FeLV (helper virus) because a portion of its genetic information is lost during recombination. In nature, FeSV recombinational events apparently occur infrequently, and the recombinant viruses are probably not contagious per se (Hardy 1981b).

Figure 54.3. Demonstration of species and interspecies antigens of oncoviruses by agar-gel immunodiffusion. The broad interior line is the interspecies antigen-antibody complex, showing its presence in the murine leukemia virus (MuLV) and feline leukemia virus (FeLV). The lighter exterior line demonstrates species-specific antigens. (Courtesy F. Noronha, Cornell University.)

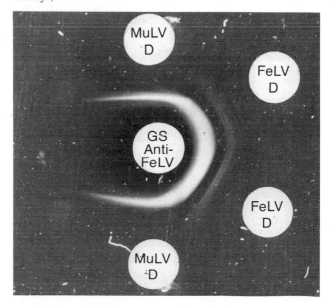

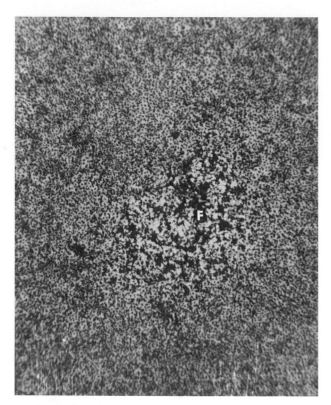

Figure 54.4. A single focus (F) of transformed cells in the Crandell feline kidney cell line induced by the murine sarcoma–feline leukemia hybrid virus of Fischinger and O'Connor. May-Grünwald-Giemsa stain. × 26. (Courtesy K. Lee, Cornell University.)

Cultivation. FeLV replicates in feline cell cultures in the absence of cytopathic effect. Some antigenic types (such as subgroup B) also replicate in canine, porcine, and human cell culttures. FeSV grows in a variety of cell cultures in the presence of helper FeLV, forming foci of transformed cells (Figure 54.4).

Epizootiology and Pathogenesis. In nature FeLV-FeSV infections appear to be restricted to members of the cat family, including domestic breeds and certain exotic cats—sand cats, European wild cats, jungle cats, and possibly leopards.

After infection of lymphoid tissues surrounding the site of initial viral penetration, a low grade (transient) viremia involving small numbers of mononuclear cells occurs within 2 weeks of exposure (Rojko et al. 1979). In this way the virus is transported to other regions of the body, especially to systemic lymphoid tissue, the intestine, and bone marrow. These areas contain populations of rapidly dividing cells, where FeLV replication can be enhanced. Infection of leukocyte and platelet precursors in the bone marrow and the subsequent release of infected cells into the circulation result in a second, more profound viremia

(persistent viremia). In those cats that resist widespread infection and replication of FeLV, containment of the virus occurs in the early lymphoid stage of infection, after transient viremia. In those cats destined to become persistently viremic, infection proceeds to extensive involvement of the bone marrow, pharynx, esophagus, stomach, bladdcr, rcspiratory tract, and salivary glands.

All persistently viremic cats are excretors of infectious FeLV and probably remain so for the rest of their lives (Hardy 1981a). They thus serve as reservoirs of infection for healthy, uninfected, susceptible cats with which they come into contact. During the initial transient viremia, even in animals destined to resist widespread infection, infectious FeLV may be shed from the oropharynx (Jarrett 1983; Jarrett, Golder, and Stewart 1982). In all cases excretion of FeLV occurs primarily by way of salivary secretions, although virus may also be present in respiratory secretions, milk, feces, and urine (Hardy 1981a, Hardy et al. 1973). Thus, the social grooming habits of cats, biting, sneezing, and the urban practice of sharing litter boxes and feeding bowls probably represent the major modes of spread of FeLV among pet cats. In addition, in utero transfer of virus across the placenta and its excretion in colostrum also are known to occur, so that kittens may become infected either through a carrier queen or by close contact with other infected cats (Hardy et al. 1976; Jarrett, Golder, and Weijer 1982). Prolonged close contact (days to weeks) between cats is probably required for effective transmission of FeLV. The time period between initial exposure to an infective dose of FeLV and the development of either persistent viremia or immunity is quite variable and may be dependent in part upon the route of virus transmission (Grant et al. 1980).

Immunity. The presence of virus-neutralizing antibody directed against peplomer gp70 is an indication of past exposure to FeLV. Most persistently viremic cats produce little or no neutralizing antibody. In addition, most cats in the general feline population do not have levels of neutralizing antibody that are considered protective against infection, probably because they have not been exposed to a sufficient FeLV dose. On the other hand, about 40 to 50 percent of healthy cats in FeLV-infected multiple cat households have protective neutralizing antibody titers. These cats are generally believed to be resistant to subsequent FeLV infection, and most will not become persistently viremic. The significance of the immunological response to the core protein, p27, is at present uncertain, because antibodies directed against it are not protective, preventing neither viremia nor FeLV-related disease (Essex et al. 1976).

A certain percentage of cats exposed to FeLV develop antibody against the feline oncornavirus–associated cell membrane antigen (FOCMA), a tumor-specific antigen found on the surface of FeLV-infected cells that have undergone malignant transformation (Essex and Grant 1979, Essex et al. 1976, Hardy 1981a). This antigen appears to be structurally similar to the gp70 of FeLV subgroup C (Snyder et al. 1983). Antibody titers to FOCMA tend to be higher in cats that have resisted generalized FeLV infection and in persistently viremic but healthy cats and lower (often undetectable) in cats with FeLV-induced neoplasia. In general, the higher the FOCMA antibody titer, the greater the probability that a cat is protected against the oncogenic effects of FeLV (Hardy 1981a). FOCMA antibody does not protect against the development of persistent viremia, however.

The problem of latency. The persistence of the integrated provirus in infected cells and their descendants is an important aspect of the replication cycle of retroviruses (Hughes 1983). Cells so infected frequently persist in the face of an active immunological response, a phenomenon well recognized in equine infectious anemia, maedi-visna, and enzootic bovine leukosis. Evidence continues to accumulate that many cats that mount an effective immune response following FeLV infection nevertheless harbor persistent infections in bone marrow cells. Recent studies have shown that many recovered cats develop a persistent infection of myelomonocytic precursor cells in the bone marrow and of certain nodal T lymphocytes (Madewell and Jarrett 1983, Pedersen et al. 1984, Rojko et al. 1982). Thus FeLV-negative cats are not necessarily free of FeLV. Cats latently infected with FeLV are not viremic and, thus, do not shed infectious FeLV into their environment. Administration of corticosteroids, however, can reactivate latent infections, with reemergence of FeLV into the bloodstream (and reversion to FeLV-positive status) (Pedersen et al. 1984, Post et al. 1980, Rojko et al. 1982). Most latent infections appear to dissipate within a relatively short period of time (less than a year), perhaps because the infected cells differentiate to extinction or are scavenged by immunological processes (Barton 1986, Pedersen et al. 1984).

Diagnosis. Two serodiagnostic procedures are commercially available for determining the FeLV status of an animal.

Detection of viral antigens. The FeLV p27 core protein provides the major antigenic basis for both the immunofluorescence assay (IFA) and the enzyme-linked immunosorbent assay (ELISA). A positive IFA for FeLV implies that a cat is excreting FeLV and is a potential health hazard to uninfected cats, especially kittens and cats on immunosuppressive drugs. Approximately 97 percent of cats with a positive IFA remain positive for life (Hardy 1981a). A negative IFA indicates that no detect-

able infected blood cells are present (leukocytes, platelets). A positive ELISA signifies the presence of circulating FeLV p27 in the blood fraction (serum, plasma, or whole blood) tested. Most but not all cats that test positive by ELISA are actively excreting FeLV. A negative ELISA indicates that no detectable p27 is present, but, as with IFA, it does not exclude the possibility of viral incubation and is not an indication of immunity to FeLV. It is thus important that positive FeLV tests be repeated within 2 to 3 months in order to determine whether the viremia is transient or persistent.

In the last several years, comparative studies have identified some cats that remain positive by ELISA but negative by IFA or by virus isolation for many months (Hirsch et al. 1982; Jarrett, Golder, and Weijer 1982; Lutz et al. 1980, 1983). As many as 30 percent of cats with positive reactions to ELISA may be negative according to one or both of the other methods (Jarrett, Golder, and Weijer 1982). Tests performed 1 to 10 months after initial testing have shown that the FeLV status of most of these cats remains unchanged. Published studies indicate that these cats, unlike their persistently viremic counterparts, do not give birth to infected kittens and do not appear to excrete FeLV (Jarrett 1983; Jarrett, Golder, and Weijer 1982). Long-term studies are in progress to determine whether these cats are still at risk of developing one or more of the FeLV-related diseases.

Detection of neutralizing antibodies. Cats with protective levels of neutralizing antibody have resisted generalized FeLV infection and in most cases are protected against subsequent development of persistent viremia. However, because a DNA copy of the FeLV genome stably integrates into the host cell chromosomal DNA during viral infection and replication, latent FeLV proviral infection resulting in malignant transformation at some time in the future cannot be excluded in cats with neutralizing antibody. The presence of this antibody indicates previous exposure to FeLV.

Treatment. Several treatments are available for certain FeLV-induced diseases:

Lymphoid malignancies. Chemotherapy, surgery, and radiation therapy are currently available for treatment of lymphoid malignancies. In general, lymphoid malignancies are quite responsive to radiation, but their widespread anatomical distribution usually dictates other methods of treatment. Consequently, chemotherapy has become the treatment of choice for these tumors. Lymphoid malignancies that respond best to treatment include the thymic and multicentric forms of LSA; those that respond least to treatment include the alimentary form of LSA and lymphocytic leukemia.

Myeloproliferative disorders. The profound anemia

that often accompanies these disorders is the overriding concern of the veterinarian when determining treatment. Thus the most important initial therapeutic procedure is the transfusion of fresh whole blood from healthy FeLV-negative cats. Chemotherapeutic regimens consist of many of the same drugs used in treating lymphoid malignancies. The results of therapy of myeloprolifcrative disorders, however, have been generally disappointing.

Nonregenerative anemia. Administration of fresh whole blood to cats with NRA is imperative when erythrocyte counts fall below acceptable levels. NRA is generally a relentless, progressive condition, however, and repeated transfusions are frequently required. The prognosis, as with all FeLV-related diseases, is poor.

Prevention and Control. Elimination of FeLV from an infected household can be achieved by implementation of an FeLV test-and-removal program using IFA (Hardy 1981a). This program has been highly effective in removing infectious FeLV from multiple cat households. In a survey of 45 households from which 159 FeLV-positive cats were removed, 561 of 564 (99.5 percent) FeLV-negative cats remained negative upon subsequent retesting (Hardy et al. 1976). Infected multiple cat households in which FeLV test and removal has not been implemented have experienced infection rates over 40 times higher than those in households in which the program has been successfully introduced.

Research into development of an effective vaccine for the prevention of FeLV infection has progressed slowly. Despite an increase in knowledge of the biological behavior of FeLV and of the pathogenesis of infection, development of a safe, protective vaccine has been elusive. Several strategies for immunization have been investigated, including both inactivated and live virus vaccines, tumor cell vaccines, and an envelope protein vaccine. Most recently developed is the soluble tumor cell antigen vaccine (STAV), which contains neither tumor cells nor FeLV but is composed only of immunogenically important antigens that are naturally released from lymphoid tumor cells grown in culture (Lewis et al. 1981, Sharpee et al. 1986, Wolff et al. 1979). Studies have shown that adult cats as well as kittens vaccinated with STAV produce protective neutralizing and FOCMA antibody and that most are protected against the development of lymphoid malignancies. In addition, although STAV contains the p15(E) protein, its immunosuppressive action is apparently not exerted in vaccinated animals. The STAV is commercially available and has been the subject of some controversy (Olsen and Sharpee 1986, Ott 1986, Pedersen 1986, Pedersen et al. 1985, Sharpee et al. 1986). It is hoped that questions regarding efficacy of the vaccine will be resolved over the next several years.

The Disease in Humans. The public health significance of FeLV, particularly the question of oncogenic potential for human beings, is still largely unsettled. Surveys designed to determine the prevalence of circulating FeLV in human serum have produced conflicting results over the years (Hardy 1981a), but most recent surveys have failed to find evidence of FeLV infection of human beings, including those with lymphoid (and other) malignancies. However, most cats with FeLV-induced malignancies have little or no circulating neutralizing antibodies, and a variable number of such cases are FeLV-negative. Until a more complete understanding of the public health implications of FeLV can be obtained, it is considered prudent to restrict human exposure to persistently viremic cats as much as possible. It must be emphasized, however, that there is no conclusive evidence to date that any human illness (including cancer) has ever been caused by a feline retrovirus.

REFERENCES

Barton, C.L. 1986. The feline leukemia virus: Pathogenesis of disease. In F.W. Scott, ed., Contemporary Issues in Small Animal Practice, vol. 3: Infectious Diseases. Churchill Livingstone, New York. Pp. 109–128.

Cotter, S.M. 1984. Feline viral neoplasia. In C.E. Greene, ed., Clinical Microbiology and Infectious Diseases of the Dog and Cat. W.B. Saunders, Philadelphia. Pp. 490–513.

Essex, M.E. 1982. Feline leukemia: A naturally occurring cancer of infectious origin. Epidemiol. Rev. 4:189–203.

Essex, M., and Grant, C.K. 1979. Tumor immunology in domestic animals. Adv. Vet. Sci. Comp. Med. 23:183–228.

Essex, M., Sliski, A., Hardy, W.D., and Cotter, S.M. 1976. Immune response to leukemia virus and tumor-associated antigens in cats. Cancer Res. 36:640–645.

Francis, D.P., Cotter, S.M., Hardy, W.D., and Essex, M. 1979. Comparison of virus-positive and virus-negative cases of feline leukemia and lymphoma. Cancer Res. 39:3866–3870.

Francis, D.P., Essex, M., and Gayzagian, D. 1979. Feline leukemia virus: Survival under home and laboratory conditions. J. Clin. Microbiol. 9:154–156.

Francis, D.P., Essex, M., Jakowski, R.M., Cotter, S.M., Lerer, T.J., and Hardy, W.D. 1980. Increased risk for lymphoma and glomerulonephritis in a closed population of cats exposed to feline leukemia virus. Am. J. Epidemiol. 111:337–346.

Gerstman, B.B. 1985. The epizootiology of feline leukemia virus infection and its associated diseases. Compend. Cont. Ed. Pract. Vet. 7:766–776.

Grant, C.K., Essex, M., Gardner, M.B., and Hardy, W.D. 1980. Natural feline leukemia virus infection and the immune response of cats of different ages. Cancer Res. 40:823–829.

Hardy, W.D. 1981a. The feline leukemia virus. J. Am. Anim. Hosp. Assoc. 17:951–980.

Hardy, W.D. 1981b. The feline sarcoma viruses. J. Am. Anim. Hosp. Assoc. 17:981–997.

Hardy, W.D., Geering, G., Old, L.J., deHarven, E., Brodey, R.S., and McDonough, S. 1969. Feline leukemia virus: Occurrence of viral antigen in the tissues of cats with lymphosarcoma and other diseases. Science 166:1019–1021.

Hardy, W.D., Hess, P.W., MacEwen, E.G., McClelland, A.J., Zuckerman, E.E., Essex, M., Cotter, S.M., and Jarrett, O. 1976.

Biology of feline leukemia virus in the natural environment. Cancer Res. 36:582–588.

Hardy, W.D., McClelland, A.J., Zuckerman, E.E., Snyder, H.W., MacEwen, E.G., Francis, D., and Essex, M. 1980. Development of virus non-producer lymphosarcomas in pet cats exposed to FeLV. Nature 288:90–92.

Hardy, W.D., Old, L.J., Hess, P.W., Essex, M., and Cotter, S. 1973. Horizontal transmission of feline leukemia virus. Nature 244:266–269.

Hebebrand, L.C., Mathes, L.E., and Olsen, R.G. 1977. Inhibition of concanavalin A stimulation of feline lymphocytes by inactivated feline leukemia virus. Cancer Res. 37:4532–4533.

Hirsch, V.M., Searcy, G., and Bellamy, J.E.C. 1982. Comparison of ELISA and immunofluorescence assays for detection of feline leukemia virus antigens in blood of cats. J. Am. Anim. Hosp. Assoc. 18:933–938.

Hughes, S.H. 1983. Synthesis, integration, and transcription of the retroviral provirus. Curr. Top. Microbiol. Immunol. 103:23–49.

Jarrett, O. 1983. Recent advances in the epidemiology of feline leukaemia virus. Vet. Ann. 23:287–293.

Jarrett, O., Golder, M.C., and Stewart, M.F. 1982. Detection of transient and persistent feline leukaemia virus infections. Vet. Rec. 110:225–228.

Jarrett, O., Golder, M.C., and Weijer, K. 1982. A comparison of three methods of feline leukaemia virus diagnosis. Vet. Rec. 110:325–328.

Jarrett, W.F.H., Crawford, E.M., Martin, W.B., and Davie, F. 1964. A virus-like particle associated with leukaemia (lymphosarcoma). Nature 202:567–568.

Kawakami, T.G., Theilen, G.H., Dungworth, D.L., Munn, R.J., and Beall, S.G. 1967. "C"-type viral particles in plasma of cats with feline leukemia. Science 158:1049–1050.

Lewis, M.G., Mathes, L.E., and Olsen, R.G. 1981. Protection against feline leukemia by vaccination with a subunit vaccine. Infect. Immun. 34:888–894.

Lutz, H., Pedersen, N.C., Harris, C.W., Higgins, J., and Theilen, G.H. 1980. Detection of feline leukemia virus infection. Feline Pract. 10(4):13–23.

Lutz, H., Pedersen, N.C., and Theilen, G.H. 1983. Course of feline leukemia virus infection and its detection by enzyme-linked immunosorbent assay and monoclonal antibodies. Am. J. Vet. Res. 44:2054–2059.

Madewell, B.R., and Jarrett, O. 1983. Recovery of feline leukaemia virus from non-viraemic cats. Vet. Rec. 112:339–342.

Mathes, L.E., Olsen, R.G., Hebebrand, L.C., Hoover, E.A., Schaller, J.P., Adams, P.W., and Nichols, W.S. 1979. Immunosuppressive properties of a virion polypeptide, a 15,000-dalton protein, from feline leukemia virus. Cancer Res. 39:950–955.

Olsen, R.G., and Sharpee, R.L. 1986. FeLV vaccine commentary. Feline Pract. 16(1):4–8.

Ott, R.L. 1983. Feline leukemia virus infection. In P.W. Pratt, ed., Feline Medicine. American Veterinary Publications, Santa Barbara, Calif. Pp. 123–133.

Ott, R.L. 1986. FeLV vaccine commentary: Reply. Feline Pract. 16(1):9–11.

Pedersen, N.C. 1986. FeLV vaccine commentary: Reply. Feline Pract. 16(1):8–9.

Pedersen, N.C., and Madewell, B.R. 1980. Feline leukemia virus disease complex. In R.W. Kirk, ed., Current Veterinary Therapy, Vol. 7. W.B. Saunders, Philadelphia. Pp. 404–410.

Pedersen, N.C., Johnson, L., and Ott, R.L. 1985. Evaluation of a commercial feline leukemia virus vaccine for immunogenicity and efficacy. Feline Pract. 15(6):7–20.

Pedersen, N.C., Meric, S.M., Ho, E., Johnson, L., Plucker, S., and Theilen, G.H. 1984. The clinical significance of latent feline leukemia virus infection in cats. Feline Pract. 14(2):32–48.

Post, J.E., and Warren, L. 1980. Reactivation of latent feline leukemia virus. In W.D. Hardy, M. Essex, and A.J. McClelland, eds., Feline Leukemia Virus. Elsevier, New York. Pp. 151–155.

Rickard, C.G., Barr, L.M., Noronha, F., Dougherty, E., and Post, J.E.

1967. C-type virus particles in spontaneous lymphocytic leukemia in a cat. Cornell Vet. 57:302–307.

Rojko, J.L., Hoover, E.A., Mathes, L.E., Olsen, R.G., and Schaller, J.P. 1979. Pathogenesis of experimental feline leukemia virus infection. J. Natl. Cancer Inst. 63:759–768.

Rojko, J.L., Hoover, E.A., Quackenbush, S.L., and Olsen, R.G. 1982. Reactivation of latent feline leukemia virus infection. Nature 298:385–388.

Sarma, P.S., and Log, T. 1973. Subgroup classification of feline leukemia and sarcoma viruses by viral interference and neutralization tests. Virology 54:160–169.

Sharpee, R.L., Beckenhauer, W.H., Baumgartener, L.E., Haffer, K.N., and Olsen, R.G. 1986. Feline leukemia vaccine: Evaluation of safety and efficacy against persistent viremia and tumor development. Compend. Cont. Ed. Pract. Vet. 8:267–277.

Snyder, H.W., Singhal, M.C., Zuckerman, E.E., Jones, F.R., and Hardy, W.D. 1983. The feline oncornavirus-associated cell membrane antigen (FOCMA) is related to, but distinguishable from, FeLV-C gp70. Virology 131:315–327.

Theilen, G.H., Kawakami, T.G., Rush, J.D., and Munn, R.J. 1969. Replication of cat leukaemia virus in cell suspension cultures. Nature 222:589–590.

Wolff, L.H., Mathes, L.E., and Olsen, R.G. 1979. Recovery of soluble feline oncornavirus-associated cell membrane antigen from large volumes of tissue culture fluids. J. Immunol. Methods 26:151–156.

Enzootic Bovine Leukosis

Studies reported in the 1970s have led to the identification and characterization of a leukemogenic oncovirus of cattle. On the basis of transmission experiments and seroepizootiological studies of well-characterized herds, this virus, known as the bovine leukemia virus (BLV), is now recognized as the cause of two related, genetically determined abnormalities of cattle: (1) the adult form of lymphosarcoma (LSA), probably the most common malignant neoplasm of cattle, which affects primarily dairy cattle between 4 and 8 years of age; and (2) persistent lymphocytosis (PL), a benign lymphoproliferative condition often observed in clinically healthy cattle in herds with a high incidence of LSA. Although PL precedes the development of LSA in about 65 percent of cases, most cattle with PL do not develop LSA. The term *enzootic bovine leukosis* is generally used to describe both conditions. The identification of BLV (Miller et al. 1969) and the subsequent development of sensitive serologic assays have led to the recognition that BLV infections are widespread in cattle in many countries of the world.

A number of excellent reviews on different aspects of bovine leukosis are available (Evermann 1983, Ferrer 1979, Ferrer et al. 1979, Ghysdael et al. 1984, Kahrs 1981, Miller 1986, Straub 1981).

Character of the Disease. The adult form of LSA is seen in cattle more than 2 years old and most commonly in those between 4 and 8 years old. The location of tumors is unpredictable, but tissues commonly involved include the lymph nodes, abomasum, heart, kidneys, spleen, uterus, spinal cord, and retrobulbar lymphatics. Under field conditions cattle in affected herds can show enlarged and firm superficial lymph nodes, weight loss, decreased milk production, and emaciation. Chronic bloating occurs in some because of enlargement of thoracic nodes. Abomasal tumors can lead to ulcers that are detected by the presence of dark blood in the feces. Lameness and paralysis often occur because of pressure on the spinal cord or peripheral nerves from the disseminated masses. Sometimes an eyeball may protrude (exophthalmos) because of tumor formation in the retrobulbar tissue. Uterine and pelvic lymph node tumors may cause infertility and can often be detected by palpation. Hematological examination may show as many as several hundred thousand lymphocytes per cubic millimeter of blood. An elevated cell count in the milk is sometimes detected by the California mastitis test.

PL is characterized by an elevated lymphocyte count (above 7,500 cells/mm³ of blood) in at least two samples collected not less than 3 months apart. Most of these lymphocytes carry B-cell surface markers. Animals with PL frequently do not show any clinical signs. PL tends to aggregate along familial lines and precedes the development of LSA in about 65 percent of cases. PL is a distinct entity and is *not* a subclinical form of LSA.

Properties of the Virus. BLV has all the characteristics of a typical C-type oncovirus and is v-*onc*⁻. In LSA the tumor cell populations show a consistent proviral integration pattern for all cells of the same tumor (Kettmann et al. 1980), although different tumors show different individual patterns, indicating that multiple integration sites for tumor induction probably exist. Experimental results, however, have thus far failed to demonstrate a preferential integration site for the BLV provirus. This clonality of the integration site in individual tumors is in sharp contrast to the polyclonality (different sites in different cells) of integration seen in PL (Kettmann et al. 1980).

In both LSA and PL, BLV proviral information appears to be repressed at the transcriptional level (Baliga and Ferrer 1977, Driscoll and Olson 1977, Kettmann et al. 1982). When isolated from the host and maintained in short-term cell culture, however, BLV-infected lymphocytes will produce viral mRNA, proteins, and intact virus particles (Balifa and Ferrer 1977, Miller et al. 1969, Stock and Ferrer 1972). With only a single exception, BLV viremia has not been reported (Kawakami et al. 1970).

Cultivation. BLV replicates in monolayers of bovine embryonic spleen and fetal ovine kidney cells, in bat lung cells, and in human diploid embryonic lung cells, with the formation of syncytia. Pretreatment of cells with DEAE-dextran greatly increases the sensitivity of the system.

Epizootiology and Pathogenesis. Cattle are the primary natural host for BLV. Sheep also develop LSA, and

under some circumstances it appears to occur preferentially in certain flocks. A retrovirus has been found in some cases, and there appears to be a very close relationship between the ovine agent and BLV (Rohde et al. 1978). BLV will infect and produce LSA in sheep under experimental conditions, so that it seems probable that the ovine agent is indeed BLV or a minor variant of it. In contrast to BLV infection of cattle, however, horizontal transmission of virus does not occur among sheep, PL is not seen, and the LSA produced is, interestingly, a T-cell neoplasm.

Although vertical transmission of BLV has been demonstrated, horizontal (contact) transmission is the major mode of spread among cattle. Transmission appears to require prolonged close contact between animals, and it is believed that most infections are the result of inoculation with infected blood cells, that is, transfer by hematophagous arthropods, by blood-contaminated needles, syringes, and surgical instruments, or by blood contamination from traumatic injuries. All current evidence suggests that BLV transmission is strictly cell-associated (lymphocytes); BLV-infected cattle do not produce significant amounts of cell-free virus in tissues, secretions, or excretions, although the virus has been detected in the semen of bulls. BLV-infected lymphocytes are frequently present in milk and colostrum of infected cows, but transmission to nursing calves seems to be a rare event, possibly because of the simultaneous presence of neutralizing antibody. Prenatal transmission, which apparently occurs via the placenta after the third month of gestation, usually involves less than 10 to 20 percent of calves from infected dams.

Data indicate that most BLV-infected cattle in dairy herds acquire infection by direct contact after the age of 18 months (Ferrer 1979). This is most likely because calves in these herds are protected during the first months of life by maternal antibody and are usually kept separate from other infected adults until sexual maturity. The relatively slow rate at which BLV infections spread among susceptible cattle suggests that the virus is not highly contagious.

In the United States the prevalence of BLV infections ranges from 10 to 50 percent in different parts of the country. On the basis of seroepizootiological data, it appears that at least 20 percent of adult dairy cattle in the United States are infected with BLV. The frequency of enzootic bovine leukosis and of BLV infection is considerably higher in dairy cattle than in beef cattle, probably because dairy herds contain a larger proportion of older animals and are kept under more confined conditions (Ferrer 1979). In most cases BLV infections are clinically inapparent; about 65 percent of infected cattle are asymptomatic, chronic carriers of the virus (Ferrer et al. 1979). The frequency of LSA among BLV-infected cattle is probably no greater than 5 percent, and the frequency of PL is probably less than 30 percent.

Host genetic factors strongly influence the development of both LSA and PL. It has been demonstrated that LSA and PL tend to aggregate in different herds as well as in different families within the same herd (Abt et al. 1970, Croshaw et al. 1963, Ferrer et al. 1979). It thus appears that the genetic factors determining susceptibility to LSA and PL are independent but frequently coincidental.

The mechanism of tumorigenesis utilized by BLV has not been elucidated. The virus is known to be v-onc⁻ and may require a multistep process for efficient tumor induction (Ghysdael et al. 1984). The process apparently does *not* involve either continuous expression of BLV genetic information or activation of c-onc sequences adjacent to the site of provirus integration.

Immunity. Calves nursing BLV-infected cows are protected for the duration of suckling by maternal antibody. Mechanisms of immunity in older cattle are less clear; in general, the presence of antibody in older animals is correlated with persistent BLV infection, forming the basis for the detection of infected individuals within a herd.

Diagnosis. A definitive diagnosis of LSA requires histopathological examination of the neoplastic tissue; PL is diagnosed by hematological parameters and the absence of clinical signs. Demonstration of BLV infection is provided by detection of BLV antibody, because circulating viral antigen is usually not present. The most widely used assay for antibody is the agar-gel immunodiffusion (AGID) test, which in most cases is designed to detect a BLV envelope glycoprotein antigen. BLV infections can be detected by AGID within 1 to 3 months after exposure. Colostral antibody interferes with testing, however, so that detection of active infection in calves is more difficult. The test is technically uncomplicated but has a relatively high false-negative rate (about 28 percent) (Gupta and Ferrer 1978), although this latter finding has been questioned (Miller et al. 1981). A technically more elaborate procedure is the radioimmunoassay (RIA), which detects the major BLV internal core antigen (Levy et al. 1977). It has been stated that BLV infection can be excluded on the basis of two negative RIA results on samples collected at 3-month intervals, provided that no exposure to BLV-infected cattle has occurred during the intervening period (Ferrer 1979).

Treatment. There is no treatment for enzootic bovine leukosis. BLV infection is persistent by its very nature and cannot be eliminated by any method currently available.

Prevention and Control. Control of BLV infection is based on identification and removal of BLV-infected cattle (BLV antibody-positive animals). Because the virus is transmitted primarily by contact, control measures must be instituted at the herd level unless isolation facilities are available. Countries of the European Economic Community have declared enzootic bovine leukosis to be a notifiable disease, and some have instituted programs to reduce its spread. A few countries in which moderate to high rates of infection existed have successfully eradicated BLV.

Eradication and control programs rely on serologic testing of cattle—testing that is now almost universally incorporated into international trade regulations. The success of such programs depends on the sensitivity of the method used for diagnosis of infection. For this reason, some have advocated use of the RIA as a standard for the detection of chronic virus carriers (Ferrer 1982). Eradication is accomplished by repeated serologic testing of cattle more than 6 months old, with prompt removal of infected animals. A testing interval of 3 months has been recommended. Insect control measures also should be instituted where feasible, and care should be taken to prevent transfer of blood from infected animals, particularly during procedures such as vaccination, collection of blood samples, dehorning, castration, and ear tagging.

Preliminary experiments suggest that vaccination against BLV is feasible (Miller and Van der Maaten 1978, Miller et al. 1983, Onuma et al. 1984, Theilen et al. 1982). Vaccination using whole virus would have the relative disadvantage of producing seropositive animals and making them ineligible for export certification. Use of a purified BLV envelope protein vaccine would obviate such a situation by seroconverting cattle to only the envelope protein itself (Onuma et al. 1984). Another approach has involved vaccination with live cells derived from a sporadic case of bovine leukosis (Theilen et al. 1982).

The Disease in Humans. To date, there is no evidence of a risk to human health associated with BLV.

REFERENCES

Abt, D.A., Marshak, R.R., Kulp, H.W., and Pollack, R.J. 1970. Studies on the relationship between lymphocytosis and bovine leukosis. Bibl. Haematologica 36:527–536.

Baliga, V., and Ferrer, J.F. 1977. Expression of the bovine leukemia virus and its internal antigen in blood lymphocytes. Proc. Soc. Exp. Biol. Med. 156:388–391.

Croshaw, J.E., Abt, D.A., Marshak, R.R., Hare, W.C.D., Switzer, J., Ipsen, J., and Dutcher, R.M. 1963. Pedigree studies in bovine lymphosarcoma. Ann. N.Y. Acad. Sci. 108:1193–1202.

Driscoll, D.M., and Olson, C. 1977. Bovine leukemia virus–associated antigens in lymphocyte cultures. Am. J. Vet. Res. 38:1897–1898.

Evermann, J.F. 1983. Bovine leukemia virus infection. Mod. Vet. Pract. 64:103–105.

Ferrer, J.F. 1979. Bovine leukosis: Natural transmission and principles of control. J. Am. Vet. Med. Assoc. 175:1281–1286.

Ferrer, J.F. 1982. Eradication of bovine leukemia virus infection from a high-prevalence herd, using radioimmunoassay for identification of infected animals. J. Am. Vet. Med. Assoc. 180:890–893.

Ferrer, J.F., Marshak, R.R., Abt, D.A., and Kenyon, S.J. 1979. Relationship between lymphosarcoma and persistent lymphocytosis in cattle: A review. J. Am. Vet. Med. Assoc. 175:705–708.

Ghysdael, J., Bruck, C., Kettmann, R., and Burny, A. 1984. Bovine leukemia virus. Curr. Top. Microbiol. Immunol. 112:1–19.

Gupta, P., and Ferrer, J.F. 1978. A critical comparison of the virus neutralization, radioimmunoprecipitation and immunodiffusion tests for the serological diagnosis of BLV infection. Ann. Rech. Vét. 9:683–688.

Kahrs, R. 1981. Virus Diseases of Cattle. Iowa State University Press, Ames. Pp. 79–88.

Kawakami, T.G., Moore, A.L., Theilen, G.H., and Munn, R.J. 1970. Comparison of virus-like particles from leukotic cattle to feline leukosis virus. Bibl. Haematologica 36:471–475.

Kettmann, R., Cleuter, Y., Mammerickx, M., Meunier-Rotival, M., Bernardi, G., Burny, A., and Chantrenne, H. 1980. Genomic integration of bovine leukemia provirus: Comparison of persistent lymphocytosis with lymph node tumor form of enzootic bovine leukosis. Proc. Natl. Acad. Sci. USA 77:2577–2581.

Kettmann, R., Deschamps, J., Cleuter, Y., Couez, D., Burny, A., and Marbaix, G. 1982. Leukemogenesis of bovine leukemia virus: Proviral DNA integration and lack of RNA expression of viral long terminal repeat and 3' proximate cellular sequences. Proc. Natl. Acad. Sci. USA 79:2465–2469.

Levy, D., Deshayes, L., Parodi, A.L., Levy, J.P., Stephenson, J.R., Devare, S.G., and Gilden, R.V. 1977. Bovine leukemia virus specific antibodies among French cattle. II. Radioimmunoassay with the major structural protein (BLV p24). Int. J. Cancer 20:543–550.

Miller, J.M. 1986. Bovine leukemia virus. In J.L. Howard, ed., Current Veterinary Therapy: Food Animal Practice, 2d ed. W.B. Saunders, Philadelphia. Pp. 506–508.

Miller, J.M., and Van der Maaten, M.J. 1978. Evaluation of an inactivated bovine leukemia virus preparation as an immunogen in cattle. Ann. Rech. Vét. 9:871–877.

Miller, J.M., Miller, L.D., Olson, C., and Gillette, K.G. 1969. Virus-like particles in phytohemagglutinin-stimulated lymphocyte cultures with reference to bovine lymphosarcoma. J. Natl. Cancer Inst. 43:1297–1305.

Miller, J.M., Schmerr, M.J.F., and Van der Maaten, J.M. 1981. Comparison of four serologic tests for the detection of antibodies to bovine leukemia virus. Am. J. Vet. Res. 42:5–8.

Miller, J.M., Van der Maaten, J.M., and Schmerr, J.F. 1983. Vaccination of cattle with binary ethylenimine-treated bovine leukemia virus. Am. J. Vet. Res. 44:64–67.

Onuma, M., Hodatsu, T., Yamamoto, S., Higashihara, M., Masu, S., Mikami, T., and Izawa, H. 1984. Protection by vaccination against bovine leukemia virus infection in sheep. Am. J. Vet. Res. 45:1212–1215.

Rohde, W., Pauli, G., Paulsen, J., Harms, E., and Bauer, H. 1978. Bovine and ovine leukemia viruses. I. Characterization of viral antigens. J. Virol. 26:159–164.

Stock, N.D., and Ferrer, J.F. 1972. Replicating C-type virus in phytohemagglutinin-treated buffy-coat cultures of bovine origin. J. Natl. Cancer Inst. 48:985–996.

Straub, O.C. 1981. Enzootic bovine leukosis. In E.P.J. Gibbs, ed., Virus Diseases of Food Animals, vol. 2. Academic Press, New York. Pp. 683–718.

Theilen, G.H., Miller, J.M., Higgins, J., Ruppaner, R.N., and Garrett, W., 1982. Vaccination against bovine leukemia virus infection. Curr. Top. Vet. Med. Anim. Sci. 15:547–559.

Canine Oncoviruses

So far, retroviruses have not been shown to cause spontaneous neoplasia in the dog. Several reports in the literature, however, suggest that canine oncoviruses may exist. Retroviruslike particles have been described within neoplastic cells in several cases of canine lymphosarcoma (Chapman et al. 1967, Rudolph 1971, Seman et al. 1967) and in a case of a myeloproliferative disorder involving cells of the granulocytic series (Sykes et al. 1985). Borderline reverse transcriptase activity also has been reported in several lymphosarcoma cell cultures derived from clinical cases (Onions 1980). The role, if any, of retroviruses in canine neoplasms remains undetermined, however.

REFERENCES

Chapman, A.L., Bopp, W.J., Brightwell, A.S., Cohen, H., Nielsen, A.H., Gravelle, C.R., and Werder, A.A. 1967. Preliminary report on virus-like particles in canine leukemia and derived cell cultures. Cancer Res. 27:18–25.

Onions, D. 1980. RNA-dependent DNA polymerase activity in canine lymphosarcoma. Eur. J. Cancer Clin. Oncol. 16:345–350.

Rudolph, R. 1971. Virusähnliche Strukturen in Tumorzellen bei lymphatischer Leukose des Hundes. Berl. Münch. Tierärztl. Wochenschr. 84:68–70.

Seman, G., Proenca, G., Guillon, J.C., and Moraillon, R. 1967. Particles d'aspect viral dans les cellules du lymphosarcome du chien. Bull. Acad. Vét. 40:211–214.

Sykes, G.P., King, J.M., and Cooper, B.C. 1985. Retrovirus-like particles associated with myeloproliferative disease in the dog. J. Comp. Pathol. 95:559–564.

Porcine Oncoviruses

Retroviruses have been found in vitro in a number of stable porcine cell lines (Armstrong et al. 1971, Bouillant et al. 1975, Breese 1970, Frazier et al. 1979, Lieber et al. 1975, Suzuka et al. 1985, Todaro et al. 1974), and C-type oncovirus gene sequences are present in porcine genetic material (Todaro et al. 1974). Miniature swine with radiation-induced hematopoietic disorders express retroviral genes and produce virus particles that can be recovered from the blood (Frazier 1985). Leukemic swine that had not been exposed to radiation also were found to be retroviremic. To date, the exact role of oncoviruses in porcine neoplastic diseases remains obscure.

REFERENCES

Armstrong, J.S., Porterfield, J.S., and deMadrid, A.T. 1971. C-type virus particles in pig kidney cell lines. J. Gen. Virol. 10:195–198.

Bouillant, A.M.P., Greig, A.S., Lieber, M.M., and Todaro, G.J. 1975. Type C virus production by a continuous line of pig oviduct cells (PFT). J. Gen. Virol. 27:173–180.

Breese, S.S. 1970. Virus-like particles occurring in cultures of stable pig kidney cell lines. Arch. Gesam. Virusforsch. 30:401–404.

Frazier, M.E. 1973. Detection of virus-like particles from radiation-induced leukemia in swine. Ph.D. dissertation, University of Montana, Missoula.

Frazier, M.E. 1985. Evidence for retrovirus in miniature swine with radiation-induced leukemia or metaplasia. Arch. Virol. 83:83–97.

Frazier, M.E., Ushijima, R.N., Andrews, T.K., and Hooper, M.J. 1979. Comparative studies on cell lines established from normal and radiation-exposed miniature swine. In Vitro 15:1001–1012.

Lieber, M.M., Sherr, C.J., Benveniste, R.E., and Todaro, G.J. 1975. Biologic and immunologic properties of porcine type C viruses. Virology 66:616–619.

Suzuka, I., Sekiguchi, K., and Kodama, M. 1985. Some characteristics of a porcine retrovirus from a cell line derived from swine malignant lymphoma. FEBS Lett. 183:124–128.

Todaro, G.J., Benveniste, R.E., Lieber, M.M., and Sherr, C.J. 1974. Characterization of a type C virus released from the porcine cell line PK(15). Virology 58:65–74.

The Subfamily Lentivirinae

The lentiviruses are nononcogenic retroviruses that are structurally, antigenically, and biologically distinct from the oncoviruses. They produce persistent infections and diseases with slowly evolving pathology, such as maedi-visna of sheep, arthritis-encephalitis of goats, and the acquired immune deficiency syndrome of humans. The virus of equine infectious anemia is also provisionally placed in this subfamily.

Maedi-Visna

SYNONYMS: Ovine progressive pneumonia, *zwoegerziekte, la bouhite*

In 1954 Sigurdsson coined the term "slow virus infections" to describe the long incubation period and protracted course of several diseases that had appeared in epizootic form in Iceland between 1930 and 1950. Included among these diseases were *maedi* and *visna*. Maedi (Icelandic for "shortness of breath") and visna ("wasting") are chronic inflammatory conditions of the lungs and central nervous system, respectively, of adult sheep and less often of goats. The outcome of both diseases is inevitably fatal, despite the presence of an active immune response. The viruses that cause maedi and visna are so similar that they are generally regarded as variants of a single agent; visna is considered a secondary encephalitic form of maedi. In the United States maedi is known as ovine progressive peumonia and is prevalent in many of the major sheep-producing areas, particularly in the midwestern and northwestern states. The distribution of the maedi-visna agent is worldwide.

Several recent reviews of the virus are available (Brahic and Haase 1981, Cutlip 1986, Dawson 1980, Eklund and Hadlow 1981, Ellis and DeMartini 1983, McDaniel 1981, Nathanson et al. 1985).

Character of the Diseases. Three main types of disease are recognized:

Maedi (respiratory form). Sheep that are 2 years of age or older are affected by the disease. The incubation period can be months to years in length. Initial clinical signs include a relentlessly progressive loss of condition, emaciation, and dyspnea characterized by an increase in the respiratory rate. No fever is present. The signs eventually progress to severe respiratory distress, with double breathing and rhythmic jerks of the head. The disease is inevitably fatal, with death frequently attributable to complications arising from secondary bacterial pneumonia.

At necropsy the lungs are much enlarged and may weigh two or three times their normal weight. The interalveolar septa are thickened owing to a massive infiltration of mononuclear inflammatory cells, which may eventually obliterate the alveoli. Accumulations of lymphoid cells may be so extensive that the lesions come to resemble aberrant lymph nodes, with organized follicles and active germinal centers. In some cases the virus spreads to the central nervous system and produces clinical signs and/or lesions of visna.

Visna (neurological form). Like maedi, visna is a disease of adult animals, with a protracted incubation period and a chronic, inevitably fatal course. Early signs of illness include a slowly progressive ataxia, abnormal head posture, and trembling of the lips. As in maedi, there is no febrile response. The signs eventually progress to paresis or even total paralysis; unattended animals die of starvation. If they are assisted with eating and drinking, however, affected sheep may survive for 1 to 2 years.

Histopathologically, visna is characterized by a diffuse, demyelinating encephalomyelitis. Mononuclear inflammatory cell infiltrates are found in the brain parenchyma bordering the cerebral ventricles, in the meninges, and in the choroid plexus. The plexus infiltration may be so extensive that the lesions come to resemble aberrant lymph nodes, as in the pulmonary lesions of maedi. Demyelination occurs secondary to cell destruction within inflammatory foci (Georgsson et al. 1977, Sigurdsson et al. 1962). Histological examination of the lungs often reveals mononuclear inflammatory cell infiltrates characteristic of maedi.

Arthritic form. A polyarthritis resulting in severe lameness, especially of the carpal and tarsal joints, has been associated with ovine progressive pneumonia viral infections (Cutlip et al. 1985; Oliver, Gorham, Parish, et al. 1981a; Oliver, Gorham, Perryman, et al. 1981; Sheffield et al. 1980). Variable degrees of all three forms of the disease (respiratory, neurological, and arthritic) may be seen naturally in the same animals.

Properties of the Virus. The causative agent of maedi-visna is a typical member of the Lentivirinae subfamily of retroviruses. Like all retroviruses, it possesses a reverse transcriptase that produces DNA from the viral RNA. It is closely related to the virus of caprine arthritis-encephalitis (Gazit et al. 1983, Gogolewski et al. 1985, Roberson et al. 1982).

The virus particles are sensitive to ether and chloroform and are readily inactivated by heat. Most are stable between a pH of 7.2 and 9.2 and survive storage for months at $-70°C$. Phenol, formaldehyde, and ethanol readily inactivate the virus. It is relatively stable at refrigerator temperatures.

Cultivation. The virus replicates most efficiently in cells of ovine origin. It is commonly propagated in cell cultures of sheep choroid plexus, with the development of multinucleated giant cells. Fusion can be accomplished also by inactivated (irradiated) virus. Virions are released from infected cells by budding from the plasma membrane.

Epizootiology and Pathogenesis. Maedi-visna is a disease of adult sheep and to some extent of goats. The virus is spread by direct contact (probably in respiratory and salivary secretions) and by excretion in the milk. Vertical transmission across the placenta occurs but is thought to be of minor importance. The significance of fomite transmission is not known.

In general, infection and seroconversion are common, but clinical disease is infrequently seen. Rarely is there more than a 5 percent annual loss in a flock, although the prevalence of infection may be as high as 100 percent. Certain breeds of sheep (Icelandic, Finnish, border Leicester) seem to be more susceptible to clinical disease. Goats are the only other species known to be susceptible.

Maedi-visna virus apparently has a special affinity for monocytes and macrophages (Narayan et al. 1982). Normally proviral information appears to be repressed at the level of transcription (Brahic et al. 1981), with the virus residing in a covert state within the cell ("Trojan horse" effect) (Peluso et al. 1985). The core proteins of the virus are stable, but the envelope glycoproteins, important in neutralization by antibody, are subject to antigen drift (Clements and Narayan 1984). The evolution of antigenic mutants proceeds by a succession of minor mutations that accumulate under the selective pressure of neutralizing antibodies (Narayan et al. 1981). Both of these mechanisms promote viral persistence in the presence of a functional immune response, and this may contribute to the chronic nature of the disease, although this view has been seriously questioned (Lutley et al. 1983, Thormar et al. 1983). Fusion of infected macrophages with cells of the brain, lung, or synovium has been hypothesized to initiate the characteristic lesions (Narayan et al. 1982). The fusion factor that activates the disease process remains un-

identified but may be an enzyme involved in virion assembly.

Immunity. Sheep that show clinical signs of disease will eventually die. Most seropositive animals do not develop disease, but the mechanism of immunity remains unidentified. Viral persistence occurs in the presence of specific humoral and cell-mediated immune responses. Proviral DNA may be carried for the life of the animal in the absence of clinical disease, or it may induce fatal illness. At present, it is not known why some sheep succumb but most do not.

Diagnosis. Maedi and visna can be diagnosed by the clinical history, presenting signs, and characteristic histopathological lesions. Infection can be diagnosed by serologic testing (agar-gel immunodiffusion, neutralization, enzyme-linked immunosorbent assay) or by isolation of the virus from buffy coat cells of infected sheep.

Treatment. There is no treatment for either maedi or visna.

Prevention and Control. Maedi-visna virus was eradicated from Iceland by a test-and-slaughter program. The virus can be prevented from entering a flock by pretesting and quarantine of incoming animals. Once a flock is infected, however, the disease can be controlled only by removing seropositive animals, or by isolating lambs at birth, or by both. Annual serologic monitoring of virus-free flocks is considered essential to maintaining a virus-free status (Cutlip et al. 1986). No vaccines are available nor are any likely to be developed in the near future.

The Disease in Humans. Maedi-visna infections are not known to occur in humans.

REFERENCES

Brahic, M., and Haase, A.T. 1981. Lentivirinae: Maedi/visna virus group infections. In E. Kurstak and C. Kurstak, eds., Comparative Diagnosis of Viral Diseases, vol. 4, part B. Academic Press, New York. Pp. 619–643.

Brahic, M., Stowring, L., Ventura, P., and Haase, A.T. 1981. Gene expression in visna virus infection in sheep. Nature 292:240–242.

Clements, J.E., and Narayan, O. 1984. Immune selection of virus variants. In A.L. Notkins and M.B.A. Oldstone, eds., Concepts in Viral Pathogenesis. Springer-Verlag, New York. Pp. 152–157.

Cutlip, R.C. 1986. Maedi-visna (progressive pneumonia, zwoegerziekte). In J.L. Howard, ed., Current Veterinary Therapy: Food Animal Practice, 2d ed. W.B. Saunders, Philadelphia. Pp. 527–528.

Cutlip, R.C., and Lehmkuhl, H.D. 1986. Eradication of ovine progressive pneumonia from sheep flocks. J. Am. Vet. Med. Assoc. 188:1026–1027.

Cutlip, R.C., Lehmkuhl, H.D., Wood, R.L., and Brogden, K.A. 1985. Arthritis associated with ovine progressive pneumonia. Am. J. Vet. Res. 46:65–68.

Dawson, M. 1980. Maedi/visna: A review. Vet. Rec. 106:212–216.

Eklund, C.M., and Hadlow, W.J. 1981. Progressive interstitial pneumonia of sheep. In J.H. Steele, ed., CRC Handbook Series in Zoonoses, section B, vol. 2. CRC Press, Boca Raton, Fla. Pp. 355–360.

Ellis, J., and DeMartini, J.C. 1983. Retroviral diseases in small ruminants: Ovine progressive pneumonia and caprine arthritis-encephalitis. Compend. Cont. Ed. Pract. Vet. 5:S173–S183.

Gazit, A., Yaniv, A., Dvir, M., Perk, K., Irving, S.G., and Dahlberg, J.E. 1983. The caprine arthritis-encephalitis virus is a distinct virus within the Lentivirus group. Virology 124:192–195.

Georgsson, G., Pàlsson, P.A., Panitch, H., Nathanson, N., and Pètursson, G. 1977. The ultrastructure of early visna lesions. Acta Neuropathol. 37:127–135.

Gogolewski, R.P., Adams, D.S., McGuire, T.C., Banks, K.L., and Cheevers, W.P. 1985. Antigenic cross-reactivity between caprine arthritis-encephalitis, visna and progressive pneumonia viruses involves all virion-associated proteins and glycoproteins. J. Gen. Virol. 66:1233–1240.

Lutley, R., Petursson, G., Palsson, P.A., Georgsson, G., Klein, J., and Nathanson, N. 1983. Antigenic drift in visna: Virus variation during long-term infection of Icelandic sheep. J. Gen. Virol. 64:1433–1440.

McDaniel, H.A. 1981. Chronic viral pneumonias in sheep. In J.L. Howard, ed., Current Veterinary Therapy: Food Animal Practice. W.B. Saunders, Philadelphia. Pp. 557–558.

Narayan, O., Clements, J.E., Griffin, D.E., and Wolinsky, J.S. 1981. Neutralizing antibody spectrum determines the antigenic profiles of emerging mutants of visna virus. Infect. Immun. 32:1045–1050.

Narayan, O., Wolinsky, J.S., Clements, J.E., Strandberg, J.D., Griffin, D.E., and Cork, L.C. 1982. Slow virus replication: The role of macrophages in the persistence and expression of visna virus of sheep and goats. J. Gen. Virol. 59:345–356.

Nathanson, N., Georgsson, G., Palsson, P.A., Najjar, J.A., Lutley, R., and Petursson, G. 1985. Experimental visna in Icelandic sheep: The prototype lentiviral infection. Rev. Infect. Dis. 7:75–82.

Oliver, R.E., Gorham, J.R., Parish, S.F., Hadlow, W.J., and Narayan, O. 1981. Ovine progressive pneumonia: Pathologic and virologic studies on the naturally occurring disease. Am. J. Vet. Res. 42:1554–1559.

Oliver, R.E., Gorham, J.R., Perryman, L.E., and Spencer, G.R. 1981. Ovine progressive pneumonia: Experimental intrathoracic, intracerebral, and intra-articular infections. Am. J. Vet. Res. 42:1560–1564.

Peluso, R., Haase, A., Stowring, L., Edwards, M., and Ventura, P. 1985. A Trojan horse mechanism for the spread of visna virus in monocytes. Virology 147:231–236.

Roberson, S.M., McGuire, T.C., Klevjer-Anderson, P., Gorham, J.R., and Cheevers, W.P. 1982. Caprine arthritis-encephalitis virus is distinct from visna and progressive pneumonia viruses as measured by genome sequence homology. J. Virol. 44:755–758.

Sheffield, W.C., Narayan, O., Strandberg, J.D., and Adams, R.J. 1980. Visna-maedi-like disease associated with an ovine retrovirus infection in a Corriedale sheep. Vet. Pathol. 17:544–552.

Sigurdsson, B. 1954. Rida, a chronic encephalitis of sheep. Br. Vet. J. 110:341–354.

Sigurdsson, B., Pàlsson, P.A., and Van Bogaert, L. 1962. Pathology of visna: Transmissible demyelinating disease in sheep in Iceland. Acta Neuropathol. 1:343–362.

Thormar, H., Barshatsky, M.R., Arnesen, K., and Kozlowski, P.B. 1983. The emergence of antigenic variants is a rare event in long-term visna virus infection in vivo. J. Gen. Virol. 64:1427–1432.

Caprine Arthritis-Encephalitis

SYNONYMS: Viral leukoencephalomyelitis-arthritis of goats, infectious leukoencephalomyelitis of young goats, big knee; abbreviation, CAE

Caprine arthritis-encephalitis is a multisystemic disease of domestic goats, characterized by a primary demyelinating leukoencephalomyelitis, progressive hyperplastic villous synovitis, and interstitial pneumonia (Adams 1986, Crawford and Adams 1981, Crawford et al. 1980, Ellis and DeMartini 1983, Knight and Jokinen 1982, McGuire 1984). Encephalitis in young goats and an insidious arthritis in adult goats represent its most common clinical manifestations. The disease was first described in dairy kids in Washington in the early 1970s (Cork et al. 1974). The causative lentivirus is closely related to the maedi-visna agent. It is worldwide in distribution.

Character of the Disease. Clinical signs are first seen in young goats 1 to 4 months of age and can include ataxia and posterior paresis, body tremors, and an abnormal head posture. Affected animals frequently are stunted, have a rough, dry coat, and may have a subclinical or clinical interstitial pneumonia. Fever is absent, and the animals remain bright and alert. Signs frequently progress to tetraparesis and paralysis, with secondary complications, such as chronic bloating.

Adult goats (some of which may be survivors of the encephalitic form of the disease) are affected with an insidious, chronic arthritis, characterized by articular swelling ("big knee") of the carpal, hock, and stifle joints. The disease process affects all synovial membranes, including those of the joints, tendon sheaths, and bursae. Some animals develop swelling of the atlantal and supraspinous bursae. The disease may remain static or may progress rapidly to complete destruction of articular surfaces.

Lesions in the central nervous system occur in the white matter of the cerebrospinal leptomeninges of the brain and spinal cord and consist of extensive perivascular accumulations of mononuclear inflammatory cells, with primary demyelination of adjacent nerve fibers. Lesions are most numerous and severe from the mesencephalon caudally, with vessels near the aqueduct and ventricles affected most often. Articular lesions are composed of a proliferative synovitis characterized by villous hypertrophy, synovial cell hyperplasia, and infiltration by mononuclear inflammatory cells. Pulmonary lesions consist of a patchy interstitial pneumonia with hyperplasia of lymphoid tissues and an extensive mononuclear inflammatory cell infiltration into the alveolar septa. Severe lesions may progress to a bronchopneumonia.

Properties of the Virus. The virus has been placed in the Lentivirinae subfamily of retroviruses. Studies indicate a close antigenic relationship to the maedi–visna–progressive pneumonia agent (Gazit et al. 1983, Gogolewski et al. 1985, Roberson et al. 1982).

Cultivation. CAE virus (CAEV) is routinely grown in fetal caprine synovial membrane cells, with development of cellular vacuolation and formation of syncytia. Primary goat testicle cells also will support viral replication.

Epizootiology and Pathogenesis. All breeds of goats are susceptible to infection; experimentally, sheep have also been infected. Surveys for antibodies (agar-gel immunodiffusion) to the virus indicate that widespread subclinical infections occur. Of 1,160 serum samples tested from 24 states, 81 percent were positive for antibodies (Crawford and Adams 1981). Infections are more common among dairy goat breeds. Although the virus persists in infected goats and can be isolated long after initial infection, clinical disease does not develop in all animals. The percentage of infected goats with signs of arthritis varies by herd but is usually less than 25 percent. Goats that are seropositive are infected for life.

The natural route of infection is by ingestion of milk and colostrum from infected dams. Transmission across the placenta may occur but is not believed to be of major significance. Efficient horizontal transmission requires prolonged close contact (months). There is little environmental persistence of the agent.

The preponderance of lymphocytes in the mononuclear inflammatory cell response suggests an immunologically mediated reaction to chronic (viral) antigenic stimulation. Initially, the infection produces both local and systemic immune responses. Subsequent failure to remove provirus-infected, non-virus-producing cells allows for expression of viral antigens that can react with sensitized lymphocytes, resulting in chronic inflammation (McGuire 1984). The question of antigenic variation in CAE is under investigation. The importance of antigenic drift in the pathogenesis of CAE and the persistence of the agent was questioned by the failure, until relatively recently, to detect neutralizing antibody in infected goats (Klevjer-Anderson and McGuire 1982, Narayan et al. 1984). Recent evidence suggests that the lack of neutralizing antibody is due to a hyporesponsive state that can be overcome by simultaneous administration of virus and heat-inactivated *Mycobacterium tuberculosis* (Narayan et al. 1984). In the blood, the virus circulates in latent form in monocytes; activation apparently occurs during maturation to the macrophage stage (Anderson et al. 1983, Narayan et al. 1983).

Immunity. The factors regulating immunological responses to CAEV and controlling disease expression have not been identified. Animals infected with the virus are considered infected for life and a potential threat to susceptible animals with which they come into contact. Why only selected seropositive goats develop overt clinical signs is not yet known.

Diagnosis. CAE can be diagnosed by the clinical history, presenting signs, and characteristic histopathological lesions. Infection can be identified by serologic testing (agar-gel immunodiffusion, enzyme-linked immunosorbent assay) or by isolation of the virus in synovial membrane cell cultures.

Treatment. Treatment of the arthritic form of the disease is purely palliative. Good nutrition and nursing care are indicated. Severely affected goats may be made more comfortable by the administration of phenylbutazone. Treatment of the encephalitic form of the disease is not recommended.

Prevention and Control. Adams et al. (1983) have outlined measures for prevention of CAEV infection of newborn goats in infected heards. Kids should be separated from infected dams at birth and fed heat-inactivated colostrum (56°C for 1 hour) or colostrum from a doe known to be virus-free. Care should be taken to prevent any contact with secretions from the dam. Kids should be maintained in a well-ventilated isolation facility on virus-free goat milk, pasteurized cow milk, or milk replacer until weaning. The animals can then be tested by agar-gel immunodiffusion for evidence of antibody to CAEV at 6 months of age and at 6-month intervals thereafter. Any seropositive animals should be promptly removed. When no seropositive goats remain after two successive testing periods, the group can be considered free of CAEV (Adams 1986).

There is no available vaccine.

The Disease in Humans. CAE is not known to occur in humans.

REFERENCES

Adams, D.S. 1986. Caprine arthritis-encephalitis. In J.L. Howard, ed., Current Veterinary Therapy: Food Animal Practice, 2d ed. W.B. Saunders, Philadelphia. Pp. 528–529.

Adams, D.S., Klevjer-Anderson, P., Carlson, J.L., McGuire, T.C., and Gorham, J.R. 1983. Transmission and control of caprine arthritis-encephalitis virus. Am. J. Vet. Res. 44:1670–1675.

Anderson, L.W., Klevjer-Anderson, P., and Liggitt, H.D. 1983. Susceptibility of blood-derived monocytes and macrophages to caprine arthritis-encephalitis virus. Infect. Immun. 41:837–840.

Cork, L.C., Hadlow, W.J., Crawford, T.B., Gorham, J.R., and Piper, R.C. 1974. Infectious leukoencephalomyelitis of young goats. J. Infect. Dis. 129:134–141.

Crawford, T.B., and Adams, D.S. 1981. Caprine arthritis-encephalitis: Clinical features and presence of antibody in selected goat populations. J. Am. Vet. Med. Assoc. 178:713–719.

Crawford, T.B., Adams, D.S., Cheevers, W.P., and Cork, L.C. 1980. Chronic arthritis in goats caused by a retrovirus. Science 207:997–999.

Ellis, J., and DeMartini, J.C. 1983. Retroviral diseases in small ruminants: Ovine progressive pneumonia and caprine arthritis-encephalitis. Compend. Cont. Ed. Pract. Vet. 5:S173–S183.

Gazit, A., Yaniv, A., Dvir, M., Perk, K., Irving, S.G., and Dahlberg, J.E. 1983. The carpine arthritis-encephalitis virus is a distinct virus within the Lentivirus group. Virology 124:192–195.

Gogolewski, R.P., Adams, D.S., McGuire, T.C., Banks, K.L., and Cheevers, W.P. 1985. Antigenic cross-reactivity between caprine arthritis-encephalitis, visna and progressive pneumonia viruses involves all virion-associated proteins and glycoproteins. J. Gen. Virol. 66:1233–1240.

Klevjer-Anderson, P., and McGuire, T.C. 1982. Neutralizing antibody response of rabbits and goats to caprine arthritis-encephalitis virus. Infect. Immun. 38:455–461.

Knight, A.P., and Jokinen, M.P. 1982. Caprine arthritis-encephalitis. Compend. Cont. Ed. Pract. Vet. 4:S263–S270.

McGuire, T.C. 1984. Retrovirus-induced arthritis. In A.L. Notkins and M.B.A. Oldstone, eds., Concepts in Viral Pathogenesis. Springer-Verlag, New York. Pp. 254–259.

Narayan, O., Kennedy-Stoskopf, S., Sheffer, D., Griffin, D.E., and Clements, J.E. 1983. Activation of caprine arthritis-encephalitis virus expression during maturation of monocytes to macrophages. Infect. Immun. 41:67–73.

Narayan, O., Sheffer, D., Griffin, D.E., Clements, J., and Hess, J.H. 1984. Lack of neutralizing antibodies to caprine arthritis-encephalitis lentivirus in persistently infected goats can be overcome by immunization with inactivated *Mycobacterium tuberculosis*. J. Virol. 49:349–355.

Roberson, S.M., McGuire, T.C., Klevjer-Anderson, P., Gorham, J.R., and Cheevers, W.P. 1982. Caprine arthritis-encephalitis virus is distinct from visna and progressive pneumonia viruses as measured by genome sequence homology. J. Virol. 44:755–758.

Equine Infectious Anemia

SYNONYMS: Swamp fever, equine malarial fever; abbreviation, EIA

Equine infectious anemia is a disease of horses characterized by a diversity of signs and an exceedingly variable course (Cheevers and McGuire 1985; Coggins 1981a, 1981b, 1984; Knowles 1984; Tashjian 1984). It occurs in a variety of clinical forms ranging from acute to chronic, but it is essentially a chronic infection that results in a persistent carrier state and periodic exacerbations of clinical disease. It was first recognized and described in France in 1843, and since then it has been reported in nearly all parts of the world where horses are raised. It occurs frequently in rather small areas, from which it shows little tendency to spread. The name *swamp fever* is derived from the observation that flat, swampy lands tend to favor perpetuation of the disease. The disease has been seen in the United States for more than 75 years. In 1970 Coggins and Norcross developed an agar-gel immunodiffusion (AGID) test capable of detecting inapparent virus carriers. Through use of this test as a diagnostic screen, it has become apparent that EIA virus (EIAV) infection is much more common and widespread than clinical reports would indcate. This test, along with improved knowledge about EIAV transmission, has made effective control of the infection among horses a reality.

Character of the Disease. Infectious anemia may appear in an acute, subacute, or chronic form. The acute form occurs most often when EIAV is first introduced into a susceptible group of horses. The prominent clinical signs are pyrexia, anorexia, depression, rapid weight loss, severe hemolytic anemia, and dependent edema.

Affected horses often sweat profusely in warm weather and frequently develop a serous nasal discharge. Acute attacks generally last for 3 to 5 days. The majority of affected horses recover and become chronic, inapparent virus carriers after a few repeated episodes of clinical disease. The period between attacks may be months or years. During the first few months of infection, recurrent episodes may be surprisingly regular; after this period, attacks become much less frequent and severe and may be absent for long periods (Kono 1973). Any attack can be fatal; horses with severe, acute disease may die as early as 2 to 3 weeks after infection.

The chronic form of the disease consists, essentially, of a series of short acute attacks, between which the intervals of health may be quite long. Such animals may show no clinical signs whatsoever, but many of them develop anemia and hypergammaglobulinemia. The heart action becomes irregular, edematous swellings appear and disappear, and muscular weakness varies from slight to an inability to stand or walk. The gait may be very uncertain and wobbly. Chronically afflicted animals gradually become emaciated even though anorexia may not be present. Such animals have been kept under careful observation for many years, during which time their blood has been found to be continuously infective for susceptible horses.

The incubation period following inoculation is usually between 5 and 30 days but can be as long as several months. The morbidity rate is extremely variable but can approach 100 percent; mortality can be as high as 30 percent of infected horses. The number of fatal cases often increases during severely hot weather.

Horses dying of an acute episode of EIA show widespread hemorrhages in parenchymatous organs and on serous and mucous membranes. The spleen is usually enlarged and softened. The abdominal lymph nodes are swollen; the kidneys and liver show signs of parenchymatous degeneration. Subcutaneous edema, emaciation, and evidence of anemia usually are present.

Animals that die of the chronic form of the disease show lesions similar to those just described, but in addition there usually are characteristic changes in the bone marrow and liver. If the long bones are split lengthwise, the yellow marrow is frequently found to have been replaced, more or less completely, by red marrow—a reflection of massive hematopoiesis. The liver usually is reddish brown and enlarged because of a great proliferation of sinusoidal endothelial cells. These cells frequently are loaded with hemosiderin derived from damaged erythrocytes. Other abnormalities include generalized lymphoproliferative changes with perivascular and hepatic lymphoid infiltrations and hepatocyte necrosis. A proliferative glomerulonephritis with increased cellularity and thickening of glomerular tufts is prominent. The kidney lesion appears to be the result of immune complex deposition.

Properties of the Virus. EIAV has all the physicochemical and morphologic characteristics of a retrovirus and has tentatively been placed in the subfamily Lentivirinae. It is inactivated by heating (56°C for 1 hour) and by ether, phenol, formalin, and other chemicals. It survives lyophilization and freezing for long periods.

Neutralization tests have demonstrated a number of different strains of EIAV (Kono 1973). The virus possesses a hemagglutinin whose activity is resistant to the action of neuraminidase (Sentsui and Kono 1976).

Like other retroviruses, EIAV has a DNA-dependent stage in its replicative cycle and possesses reverse transcriptase. Specific proviral DNA has been identified in equine cells infected in vitro with the virus (Rice et al. 1978). Studies indicate that infected leukocytes from certain inapparent carrier horses do not produce mature virus particles until they have been activated by washing and inoculation into another host. Once again, there is persistence of virus in vivo in the presence of a specific immune response, a common finding in many retrovirus infections.

Cultivation. Equine leukocyte cultures derived from blood, spleen, or bone marrow have been used for the propagation of field virus (Kobayashi 1961). Several cell lines of equine, canine, or feline origin will support replication of stock virus (Benton et al. 1981, Malmquist et al. 1973). Ordinary laboratory animals are not susceptible to infection.

Epizootiology and Pathogenesis. EIAV is shed in all secretions and excretions of the body and is present in the blood. The potential for transmission appears to be greatest during episodes of clinical disease, at which time much higher levels of virus can be found in the blood and tissues (Kono 1973). Horses have been reported to carry EIAV in their blood for as long as 18 years (Stein et al. 1955). Currently available information continues to support the concept that infected horses carry the virus for life (Coggins (1984). Inapparent carriers generally are less infectious than clinically affected animals but under certain conditions are still able to effectively transmit the virus. At present, no test procedure is available that can assess the risk of virus transmission by individual carrier horses. The infected carrier is the only recognized reservoir of EIAV in nature.

Once it has entered the body, the virus travels through the bloodstream and is readily taken up by monocytes and macrophages, in which it is able to replicate. The highest titers of virus are found in the blood and tissues at the time of the initial febrile reaction. These titers then decline but rise again during each subsequent febrile episode (Kono et al. 1971). The likelihood of virus transmission to susceptible horses is greatest during febrile periods; nevertheless whole blood and washed leukocytes remain infective regardless of the animal's clinical state.

Anemia develops following the initial pyrexia and is a reflection both of decreased hematopoiesis and of complement-mediated hemolysis (Henson and McGuire 1974; McGuire et al. 1969a, 1969b). The anemia is Coombs-positive and thought to result from coating of red cells by antibody and complement, increasing their fragility and susceptibility to phagocytosis. A thrombocytopenia also occurs in concert with each febrile episode and may reflect clumping or aggregation of platelets in vessels and tissues. Thrombi secondary to disseminated intravascular coagulation may obstruct small vessels throughout the body, resulting in dependent edema and sometimes colic.

Infectious virus-antibody complexes circulate in the blood during and for a short period after acute disease (McGuire et al. 1972). It is thought that these complexes may be responsible for the subclinical glomerulonephritis often observed histologically in horses that have died of EIA.

The inability of EIAV-infected horses to eliminate the virus from the body has been well documented and most likely is attributable to a combination of mechanisms. These include a delayed and suboptimal neutralizing antibody response; a depression of cell-mediated immune responses during periods of rapid viral replication (clinical disease) (Banks and Henson 1973, Kono et al. 1978); and, most important, antigenic drift (Kono et al. 1970, Payne et al. 1984, Salinovich et al. 1986).

The virus is believed to be spread principally by insects, particularly bloodsucking flies (Issel and Foil 1984). Transmission is purely mechanical, and the pattern of spread is determined by the seasonal distribution of the vectors and by their flight habits. Tabanid horseflies are particularly important vectors because of the volume of blood carried on their mouthparts and because they are frequently interrupted during feeding. Stable flies, deerflies, and mosquitoes also may transmit the virus. The regional occurrence of EIA that has been recognized for many years is most probably a reflection of the geographic distribution of these insect vectors.

Rather conclusive evidence has been obtained that EIAV can be transmitted to susceptible horses by the careless use of hypodermic syringes, tattooing needles, and surgical instruments. Biologicals may become contaminated in this way, and the virus may survive in these products at refrigerator temperatures for many months.

Transfusion of blood products from infected horses is another means by which EIAV can be disseminated.

Natural transmission also occurs across the placenta to the developing fetus. Dams showing clinical signs of disease during gestation are much more likely to transmit the virus in utero than are healthy carrier mares (Kemen and Coggins 1972). Infected fetuses may be aborted or may be born as persistent carriers. Ingestion of colostrum containing virus-infected leukocytes by foals is yet another means by which the agent may be transmitted and infection perpetuated.

Immunity. Mechanisms of immunity in EIA remain poorly defined. It is clear, however, that in natural infections the virus persists in horses for prolonged periods (probably for a lifetime) despite the presence of precipitating, complement-fixing, and neutralizing antibodies. Horses that have recovered from EIAV infection usually are refractory to challenge with homologous virus but are hypersensitive to challenge with heterologous strains.

Diagnosis. History, presenting signs, and clinicopathological alterations are all important in making the diagnosis of EIA. Typically, affected horses show intermittent pyrexia, weakness, weight loss, anemia, and dependent edema. Sometimes clinical disease develops following a period of hard work or other forms of stress. Histopathological examination is indicated in horses that die of apparent EIAV infection. Piroplasmosis and equine viral arteritis (EVA) are important differential diagnoses.

Diagnosis of EIAV infection is usually made by serologic means. The AGID (Coggins) test (Figure 54.5) remains the most useful serodiagnostic aid for EIA (Coggins 1984, Coggins and Auchnie 1977, Coggins and Norcross 1970, Coggins et al. 1972, Evans et al. 1984, Issel and Coggins 1979, Knowles 1984, Pearson and Knowles 1984). It accurately and reliably (95 percent) identifies persistently infected horses by detecting precipitating antibody to the EIAV group-specific core protein, p28. Detection of this antibody has been shown to correlate well with viremia, except in young animals with maternally acquired antibody (which usually wanes after 6 months of age). Occasionally IgG(T) may interfere with the precipitin reaction, in which case confirmation of infection may require experimental horse inoculation.

Isolation of EIAV from field cases is currently impractical on a routine basis. Instead, the presence of virus is usually demonstrated by inoculation of susceptible horses with blood from suspect animals. Absence of fever and clinical illness for 45 days following inoculation is indicative of a negative test.

Treatment. There is no specific therapy for EIA.

Prevention and Control. EIA has been contained through use of the AGID test to identify and control the

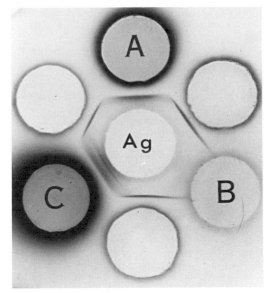

Figure 54.5. Agar-gel immunodiffusion (Coggins) test for the diagnosis of equine infectious anemia virus infection. Viral antigen is placed in the center well and a known antibody-positive control serum in the three outer, unmarked wells. Serums from horses A and C show a positive test. (Courtesy L. Coggins, North Carolina State University.)

movement of infected horses. The virus can be eradicated from a population of animals by detection and subsequent isolation or removal of all reactors (Coggins and Auchnie 1977, Cornell 1981). Freedom from EIA can be maintained by subsequent testing of all incoming horses. Annual testing of horses for carriers is the principal feature of the control program. A 90- to 120-day retest on the premises is also recommended, especially on breeding farms, until a completely negative EIA status is achieved.

In areas where the disease occurs, the use of common equipment—bridles, currycombs, and brushes—should be avoided. Surgical instruments, needles, and glass syringes should be thoroughly sterilized before use on each animal. Disposable instruments should be used only once. Flies and other insects should be controlled through use of insecticides and protective screens, if possible.

A vaccine to protect horses against EIA is desirable, but thus far progress in this area has been disappointing. Development of a protective vaccine is not expected soon.

The Disease in Humans. EIA is not known to occur in humans.

REFERENCES

Banks, K.L., and Hensen, J.B. 1973. Quantitation of immunoglobulin-bearing lymphocytes and lymphocyte response to mitogens in horses persistently infected by equine infectious anemia virus. Infect. Immun. 8:679–682.

Benton, C.V., Brown, B.L., Harshman, J.S., and Gilden, R.V. 1981. In vitro host range of equine infectious anemia virus. Intervirology 16:225–232.

Cheevers, W.P., and McGuire, T.C. 1985. Equine infectious anemia virus: Immunopathogenesis and persistence. Rev. Infect. Dis. 7:83–88.

Coggins, L. 1981a. Equine infectious anemia. In E. Kurstak and C. Kurstak, eds., Comparative Diagnosis of Viral Diseases, vol. 4, part B. Academic Press, New York. Pp. 647–658.

Coggins, L. 1981b. Equine infectious anemia. In E.P.J. Gibbs, ed., Virus Diseases of Food Animals, vol. 2. Academic Press, New York. Pp. 719–730.

Coggins, L. 1984. Carriers of equine infectious anemia virus. J. Am. Vet. Med. Assoc. 184:279–281.

Coggins, L., and Auchnie, J.A. 1977. Control of equine infectious anemia in horses in Hong Kong. J. Am. Vet. Med. Assoc. 170:1299–1301.

Coggins, L., and Norcross, N.L. 1970. Immunodiffusion reaction in equine infectious anemia. Cornell Vet. 60:330–335.

Coggins, L., Norcross, N.L., and Nusbaum, S.R. 1972. Diagnosis of equine infectious anemia by immunodiffusion test. Am. J. Vet. Res. 33:11–18.

Cornell, W.D. 1981. An effective program to control equine infectious anemia in Kentucky. Vet. Med./Small Anim. Clin. 76:485–488.

Evans, K.S., Carpenter, S.L., and Sevoian, M. 1984. Detection of equine infectious anemia virus in horse leukocyte cultures derived from horses in various stages of equine infectious anemia viral infection. Am. J. Vet. Res. 45:20–25.

Henson, J.B., and McGuire, T.C. 1974. Equine infectious anemia. Prog. Med. Virol. 18:143–159.

Issel, C.J., and Coggins, L. 1979. Equine infectious anemia: Current knowledge. J. Am. Vet. Med. Assoc. 174:727–733.

Issel, C.J., and Foil, L.D. 1984. Studies on equine infectious anemia virus transmission by insects. J. Am. Vet. Med. Assoc. 184:293–297.

Kemen, M.J., and Coggins, L. 1972. Equine infectious anemia: Transmission from infected mares to foals. J. Am. Vet. Med. Assoc. 161:496–499.

Knowles, R.C. 1984. An overview of equine infectious anemia control and regulation in the United States. J. Am. Vet. Med. Assoc. 184:289–292.

Kobayashi, K. 1961. Studies on the cultivation of equine infectious anemia virus in vitro. Propagation of the virus in leukocyte culture. Virus 11:249–256.

Kono, Y. 1973. Recurrences of equine infectious anemia. In J.T. Bryans and H. Gerber, eds., Proceedings of the 3d International Conference on Equine Infectious Diseases. S. Karger, Basel. Pp. 175–186.

Kono, Y., Kobayashi, K., and Fukunaga, Y. 1970. Immunization of horses against equine infectious anemia (EIA) with an attenuated EIA virus. Natl. Inst. Anim. Health Q. 10:113–122.

Kono, Y., Kobayashi, K., and Fukunaga, Y. 1971. Distribution of equine infectious anemia virus in horses infected with the virus. Natl. Inst. Anim. Health Q. 11:11–20.

Kono, Y., Sentsui, H., and Murakami, Y. 1978. Lymphocyte responses to specific viral antigen and nonspecific mitogens in horses infected with equine infectious anemia virus. In J.T. Bryans and H. Gerber, eds., Equine Infectious Diseases, vol. 4. Veterinary Publications, Princeton, N.J. Pp. 363–374.

McGuire, T.C., Crawford, T.B., and Henson, J.B. 1972. Equine infectious anemia. Detection of infectious virus-antibody complexes in the serum. Immunol. Commun. 1:545–551.

McGuire, T.C., Henson, J.B., and Quist, S.E. 1969a. Viral-induced hemolysis in equine infectious anemia. Am. J. Vet. Res. 30:2091–2097.

McGuire, T.C., Henson, J.B., and Quist, S.E. 1969b. Impaired bone marrow response in equine infectious anemia. Am. J. Vet. Res. 30:2099–2104.

Malmquist, W.A., Barnett, D., and Becvar, C.S. 1973. Production of equine infectious anemia antigen in a persistently infected cell line. Arch. Gesam. Virusforsch. 42:361–370.

Payne, S., Parekh, B., Montelaro, R.C., and Issel, C.J. 1984. Genomic alterations associated with persistent infections by equine infectious anaemia virus, a retrovirus. J. Gen. Virol. 65:1395–1399.

Pearson, J.E., and Knowles, R.C. 1984. Standardization of the equine infectious anemia immunodiffusion test and its application to the control of the disease in the United States. J. Am. Vet. Med. Assoc. 184:298–301.

Rice, N.R., Simek, S., Ryder, O.A., and Coggins, L. 1978. Detection of proviral DNA in horse cells infected with equine infectious anemia virus. J. Virol. 26:577–583.

Salinovich, O., Payne, S.L., Montelaro, R.C., Hussain, K.A., Issel, C.J., and Schnorr, K.L. 1986. Rapid emergence of novel antigenic and genetic variants of equine infectious anemia virus during persistent infection. J. Virol. 57:71–80.

Sentsui, H., and Kono, Y. 1976. Hemagglutination by equine infectious anemia virus. Infect. Immun. 14:325–331.

Stein, C.D., Mott, L.O., and Gates, D.W. 1955. Some observations on carriers of equine infectious anemia. J. Am. Vet. Med. Assoc. 126:277–287.

Tashjian, R.J. 1984. Transmission and clinical evaluation of an equine infectious anemia herd and their offspring over a 13-year period. J. Am. Vet. Med. Assoc. 184:282–288.

The Subfamily Spumavirinae

The spumaviruses have been isolated primarily as contaminants of primary cell cultures (Hooks and Detrick-Hooks 1981). The subfamily name is derived from the characteristically foamy degeneration the viruses produce in cultured cells. Like other retroviruses, these foamy viruses contain reverse transcriptase, mature by budding from the plasma membrane, and persist in the infected host for long periods in the presence of antiviral antibody. Unlike oncoviruses and lentiviruses, however, spumaviruses have not yet been shown to cause a specific disease in any species of animal.

Species in which foamy viruses have been found include cats, cattle, goats, hamsters, monkeys, and humans. Recently a spumavirus was recovered from a California sea lion (Kennedy-Stoskopf et al. 1986).

REFERENCES

Hooks, J.J., and Detrick-Hooks, B. 1981. Spumavirinae. Foamy virus group infections: Comparative aspects and diagnosis. In E. Kurstak and C. Kurstak, eds., Comparative Diagnosis of Viral Diseases, vol. 4, part B. Academic Press, New York. Pp. 599–618.

Kennedy-Stoskopf, S., Stoskopf, M.K., Eckhaus, M.A., and Strandberg, J.D. 1986. Isolation of a retrovirus and a herpesvirus from a captive California sea lion. J. Wildl. Dis. 22:156–164.

Bunyavirus. Rift Valley fever virus is a member of the genus *Phlebovirus*, whereas Nairobi disease of sheep virus is assigned to the genus *Nairovirus*.

REFERENCES

Bishop, D. 1985. Replication of Arenaviruses and Bunyaviruses. In B.N. Fields, D.M. Knipe, R.M. Chanock, J.L. Melnick, B. Roizman, and R.E. Shope, eds., Fields Virology. Raven Press, New York. Pp. 1083–1110.

Murphy, F.A., Harrison, A.K., and Whitfield, S.G. 1973. Bunyaviridae: Morphologic and morphogenetic similarities of Buyamwera serologic supergroup viruses and several other arthropod-borne viruses. Intervirology 1:297–316.

55 The Bunyaviridae

The family Bunyaviridae has four genera, *Bunyavirus*, *Phlebovirus*, *Nairovirus*, and *Uukuvirus*. Members of this family formerly were included under the general heading of arboviruses and comprise about 227 viruses in addition to some still unclassified viruses. Bishop (1985) believes the genus *Phlebovirus* belongs in separate family because the characteristics of the member viruses are significantly different from those of the viruses in the other three genera.

Viruses in this family contain single-stranded RNA in three or four linear segments. The molecular mass of the segments is 3.4 to 4.1, 2.1, and 0.5×10^6 daltons; and the total genome is 6×10^6 daltons and consists of three molecules of circular, negative-sense single-stranded RNA. The viruses have four major polypeptides, including a transcriptase. The particles are spherical, enveloped, and approximately 100 nm in diameter. Virions consist of a unit-membrane envelope with surface projections that may be randomly placed or clustered in arrays with icosahedral symmetry, and helically symmetric ribonucleocapsids with circular configuration. The particles, formed by budding from intracytoplasmic (primarily Golgi) members (Figure 55.1), have a buoyant density in potassium tartrate of 1.20 g/ml and are sensitive to ether, acid, and heat. The viruses hemagglutinate red blood cells by means of one or two surface glycoproteins.

Bunyaviridae includes three important diseases of domestic animals—akabane, Rift Valley fever, and Nairobi disease of sheep—which presently are limited to tropical climates. Akabane virus occurs in Australia, Japan, Kenya, and other tropical areas; it is a member of the genus

The Genus *Bunyavirus*

Akabane

Akabane virus, an arbovirus, causes infection in ruminants and is a disease of the bovine fetus. A member of the genus *Bunyavirus*, it falls into the Simbu group, which now includes four other distinct viruses—Douglas, Tinaroo, Aino, and Peaton—that also infect the biting midge *Culicoides brevitarsis* and livestock. The infection in cattle occurs in Australia, Japan, Kenya, Cyprus, Israel, and possibly Turkey and Syria. There is evidence that the virus infects sheep and goats but does not cause disease (Sellers and Herniman 1981). In Kenya neutralizing antibodies also have been detected in camels, horses, zebras, and wild ruminants that had no evidence of disease (Davies and Jessett 1985).

This virus causes abortions in cattle and congenital abnormalities in calves. In infected herds, stillborn or premature fetuses, as well as deformed or infirm neonatal calves that die within a few days after birth, are observed (Konno et al. 1982). A 3-month-old fetus had nonpurulent encephalomyelitis, characterized by necrosis of nerve tissue and endothelial proliferation, in the undifferentiated central nervous system. Polymyositis characterized by parenchymal degeneration and cellular infiltrates was observed in the skeletal muscles. During the early stage of the 1972–1974 Japanese epizootic the full-term fetuses and newborn calves had nonpurulent encephalomyelitis. In the middle or later stages of the epizootic a dysplastic muscular condition called runt-muscle disease, with a decrease in the number of ventral horn neurons in the spinal cord and arthrogryposis in the legs, was seen. Cystic cavities and thick vascular walls as well as hydranencephaly sometimes were seen in the central nervous systems of these calves.

The disease can be reproduced experimentally in cattle and goat fetuses by placental infection and also by intra-

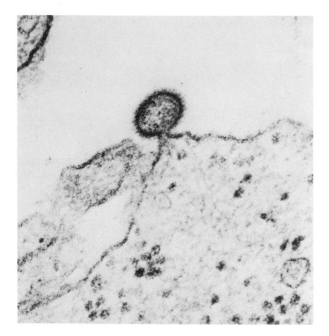

Figure 55.1. A clearly defined budding virus particle. Chagres, a member of the phlebotomus fever group. × 122,500. (From Murphy et al., 1973, courtesy of *Intervirology*.)

cerebral inoculation of calves (Konno and Nakagawa 1982). The encephalitogenic effect of Akabane virus on mice, hamsters, and guinea pigs has been described by Japanese investigators (Nakajima et al. 1980, Saito et al. 1981). Experimental infection of bulls caused a viremia that persisted for 2 to 9 days, and neutralizing antibodies were detected within 7 to 10 days. Virus was not isolated in the semen of the infected bulls, nor did the infection reduce the quality of the semen (Parsonson et al. 1981).

The virus replicates in cell-culture systems such as baby hamster kidney cell line, producing a cytopathic alteration (BHK-21). Two Australian strains of virus replicate in mosquito (*Aedes albopictus*) cells at 15°C after 1 to 2 days without producing a cytopathic effect (Hoffmann and St. George 1985). The virus replicates in hen's eggs and produces death and deformities in chick embryos (McPhee et al. 1984).

In Australia infection in livestock occurs principally in areas infested with the biting midge *Culicoides brevitarsis*, an insect from which the virus has been isolated (Cybinski 1984). The evidence at hand suggests that the infection is largely transmitted to livestock by a biting midge.

The bovine fetal disease can be prevented by the use of vaccine.

REFERENCES

Cybinski, D.H. 1984. Douglas and Tinaroo viruses: Two Simbu group arboviruses infecting *Culicoides brevitarsis* and livestock in Australia. Aust. J. Biol. Sci. 37:91–97.

Davies, F.G., and Jessett, D.M. 1985. A study of the host range and distribution of antibody to Akabane virus (genus *Bunyavirus*, family Bunyaviridae) in Kenya. J. Hyg. 95:191–196.

Hoffmann, D., and St. George, T.D. 1985. Growth of epizootic hemorrhagic disease, akabane, and ephemeral fever viruses in *Aedes albopictus* cells maintained at various temperatures. Aust. J. Biol. Sci. 38:183–188.

Konno, S., and Nakagawa, M. 1982. Akabane disease in cattle: Congenital abnormalities caused by viral infection. Experimental disease. Vet. Pathol. 19:267–279.

Konno, S., Moriwaki, M., and Nakagawa, M. 1982. Akabane disease in cattle: Congenital abnormalities caused by viral infection. Spontaneous disease. Vet. Pathol. 19:246–266.

McPhee, D.A., Parsonson, I.M., Della-Porta, A.J., and Jarrett, R.G. 1984. Teratogenicity of Australian Simbu serogroup and some other Bunyaviridae viruses: The embryonated chicken egg as a model. Infect. Immun. 43:413–420.

Nakajima, Y., Takahashi, E., and Konno, S. 1980. Encephalitogenic effect of Akabane virus on mice, hamsters, and guinea pigs. Natl. Inst. Anim. Health Q. (Tokyo) 20:81–82.

Parsonson, I.M., Della-Porto, A.J., Snowdon, W.A., and O'Halloran, M.L. 1981. Experimental infection of bulls with Akabane virus. Res. Vet. Sci. 31:157–160.

Saito, K., Fukuyama, Y., Ogata, T., and Oya, A. 1981. Experimental uterine infection of Akabane virus. Pathological studies of skeletal muscles and central nervous system of newborn hamsters with relevances to the Fukuyama type congenital muscular dystrophy. Brain Dev. 3:65–80.

Sellers, R.F., and Herniman, K.A. 1981. Neutralizing antibodies to Akabane virus in ruminants in Cyprus. Trop. Anim. Health Prod. 13:57–60.

The Genus *Phlebovirus*

Rift Valley Fever

SYNONYM: Infectious enzootic hepatitis of sheep and cattle

Rift Valley fever takes its name from a geographic area in Kenya, where the disease was first described. The causative virus is one of eight groups of viruses assigned to the genus *Phlebovirus*.

The disease occurs primarily in sheep and cattle, but outbreaks in goats have been described. It is highly contagious to humans, and cases invariably occur where the disease exists in animals. Antibodies have been found in camels and donkeys.

So far as is known, Rift Valley fever occurs only in Africa and the Middle East, where it is an important disease, although laboratory personnel in Europe, the United States, and Japan have also been infected with the virus. The disease was first described by Daubney et al. (1931) in Kenya, but there is much evidence that it had occurred for many years in parts of equatorial Africa. In 1950 it suddenly appeared in South Africa (Alexander 1951), and in 1978 it caused considerable mortality in humans and animals in Egypt. Outbreaks occur during warm, humid periods because mosquitoes are the principal transmitting agents.

Character of the Disease. The disease is most acute

and causes the heaviest losses in sheep. Very young lambs often die in large numbers. Mortality in ewes is lower, but still serious. In the original outbreak described by Daubney et al., 3,500 lambs and 1,200 ewes died in 2 weeks.

The incubation period of Rift Valley fever is very short. It may be no more than 24 hours in some cases and generally is not longer than 3 days.

In lambs the disease is characterized by high fever, prostration, and death generally within 24 hours; mortality is often 95 to 100 percent.

In ewes abortions frequently are seen before lamb losses occur. Some ewes appear sick only a few hours before they die, or they are simply found dead in the corrals. Some vomit. Many have thick, purulent nasal discharges. Some pass stools that consist of almost pure blood. Others show no signs other than abortion. Mortality does not exceed 20 percent, as a rule.

In cattle the disease resembles that in sheep in every way, but losses are not as high, averaging about 10 percent. Many pregnant cows abort.

The most characteristic lesion in ruminants is focal necrosis of the liver. In many lambs the necrosis is so complete that liver cells are hardly recognizable in histological section. Findlay (1933) and others have described inclusion bodies of an intensely acidophilic character in the nuclei of the liver cells. Other lesions consist principally of hemorrhages—in the lymph nodes, subendocardial and subepicardial, and in the gastric and intestinal mucosa. Blood examinations show severe leukopenia. In lambs especially it is sometimes difficult to find any mature leukocytes in blood films. Aborted fetuses show general hemorrhages and edema.

The disease is readily produced in cattle and sheep by inoculation. White mice of the Swiss type are very easily infected and die within 2 to 3 days after parenteral inoculation. Infections can be produced by inoculation in monkeys, ferrets, hamsters, white rats, and, possibly, rabbits. Horses, swine, guinea pigs, and domestic and wild birds are not susceptible.

Properties of the Virus. The Rift Valley Fever virus about 100 nm in diameter (Figure 55.2) (Murphy et al. 1973). Infective virus lives for 3 months at room temperature and almost 3 years in serum kept at −4°C. It withstands lyophilization, but is inactivated by a 1:1,000 dilution of formalin and by pasteurization.

The virus hemagglutinates red blood cells of day-old chicks at pH 6.5 and 25°C. Interference between yellow fever and Rift Valley fever viruses was the first reported for serologically unrelated viruses. The Zinga virus has been shown to be a strain of Rift Valley fever virus (Meegan et al. 1983).

Cultivation. Binn et al. (1963) described the virus propagation and plaque formation in primary cell cultures of lamb kidney and of hamster kidney. The virus also grows in primary cell cultures of the chick, rat, mouse, and human. Cell lines such as Vero, CER, and BHK-21 readily support replication. Most laboratories use the Vero cell line for plaque assay.

The virus produces a thickening of the chorioallantoic

Figure 55.2. Rift Valley virus particles. × 49,600. (From Murphy et al., 1973, courtesy of *Intervirology*.)

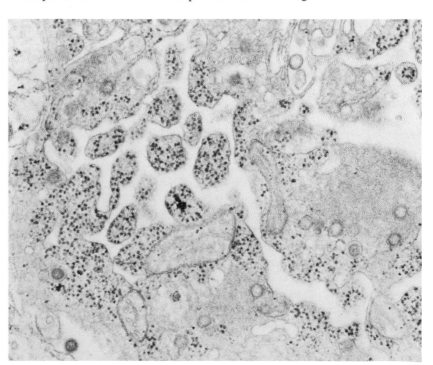

membrane of embryonated hens' eggs. Viral replication by the yolk-sac route is also successful.

Epizootiology. Daubney and Hudson, in their original investigations, found that Rift Valley fever could be easily transmitted by inoculating blood or tissue extracts with the blood of acutely infected sheep or cattle approaching 8 to 10 log mouse LD_{50} of virus (Shope 1985). All investigators who have worked with this disease in the field or the laboratory discovered that all persons who had intimate contact with infected animals developed the disease within 5 days after exposure. On the other hand, infected and susceptible sheep might be kept together and, in the absence of certain transmitting agents, the disease would not be transmitted. It was even shown that infected ewes did not infect their suckling lambs and that infected lambs did not infect their mothers. Other researchers (Callis 1979, Yedloutschnig and Walker 1979) suggested that direct contact and air-borne virus may also play a role in animal infection under certain conditions.

Smithburn et al. (1948) succeeded in isolating the virus from six different lots of mosquitoes in the Semliki Forest in an uninhabited part of Uganda. These mosquitoes included several species of the genus *Eretmapodites*, and it was later shown that some of these could transmit the disease. The present evidence points strongly to these and perhaps other species of mosquitoes as the principal transmitting agents. Because there were no cattle or sheep in the Semliki Forest, the presence of infected mosquitoes strongly suggests the existence of a reservoir of virus in wild animals.

Immunity. Animals and humans that recover from natural infection are solidly resistant thereafter. Sabin and Blumberg (1947) showed that neutralizing antibodies appeared in the blood of humans within a few days and persisted, in one patient, for as long as 12 years.

Smithburn (1949) passed strains of Rift Valley fever virus serially in white mice by intracerebral inoculation and found that as the strains acquired neurotropic properties, they lost viscerotropism. Finding that subcutaneously injected virus did not appear in the blood, he used these strains for immunizing ewes, and the animals suffered no damage. By this means the newborn lambs were protected during the period of greatest susceptibility.

Both neurotropic and field strains of Rift Valley fever virus have been adapted to embryonated eggs by Kaschula (1957). The neurotropic strains are used successfully for field immunization, but the immunity conferred is not as lasting or as solid as that conferred by natural disease.

Vaccines cannot be used on very young lambs or on pregnant ewes or cows. Only convalescent serum can confer protection to these animals.

Weiss (1962) suggested that the 102d intracerebral mouse passage level virus is a safe vaccine for 1-day-old lambs. Formalin-inactivated virus vaccines are also available for animals (Binn et al. 1963).

Abortions have occurred in both vaccinated ewes and cows after challenge with virulent Rift Valley fever virus (Yedloutschnig et al. 1981).

Diagnosis. The clinical course of the disease in sheep and cattle is at least highly suggestive. Extensive liver necrosis should confirm the suspicion. Inoculation of white mice results in prompt, fatal infections. Cell-culture systems also can be used to isolate the virus. Final confirmation must come from serologic tests with known antisera. These may be neutralization, complement-fixation, gel diffusion, or hemagglutination-inhibition tests, or enzyme-linked immunosorbent assay.

Prevention and Control. The original outbreak described by Daubney et al. (1931) was controlled promptly when the flocks were driven into pastures at a higher altitude. Presumably this put the animals above the mosquito range. Immunization with neurotropic vaccines is well tolerated by adult animals and protects flocks and herds that must remain in regions inhabited by vectors. Two injections of inactivated virus vaccine are recommended. A live attenuated virus vaccine (Smithburn 1949) is inexpensive and effective but may cause abortions.

The Disease in Humans. It has already been pointed out that veterinarians, laboratory workers, and herd and flock attendants almost invariably become infected when the disease appears. Butchers and housewives have also suffered from handling fresh meat from infected animals. The infections in these cases are obviously the result of direct contact with infected tissues. Humans can also be infected by air-borne contamination during contact with infected animal blood or aborted fetuses (Hoogstraal et al. 1979). It is not clear whether human infections can occur as a result of mosquito transmission, although there is epidemiologic and laboratory evidence to implicate *Culex pipiens* in Egypt (Meegan et al. 1980).

The disease can be fatal. Attacks occur within a few days after exposure, and symptoms resemble those of influenza or dengue fever. The onset is sudden, with malaise, headache, and chills. Fever develops quickly, and joint pains, often rather extreme, soon appear. Nausea and vomiting sometimes occur, and often there is some abdominal distress. The disease lasts only a few days, and recovery is complete. A formalin-inactivated virus vaccine is available for immunization of humans.

REFERENCES

Alexander, R.A. 1951. Rift Valley fever in the union. J. S. Afr. Vet. Med. Assoc. 22:105–111.

Binn, L.N., Randall, R., Harrison, V.R., Gibbs, C.J., Jr., and Aulisis, C.G. 1963. Immunization against Rift Valley fever: The development of vaccines from nonprimate cell cultures and chick embryos. Am. J. Hyg. 77:160–168.

Callis, J.A. 1979. Personal communication.

Daubney, R., Hudson, J.R., and Garnham, P.C. 1931. Enzootic hepatitis of Rift Valley fever. J. Pathol. Bact. 34:545–579.

Hoogstraal, H., Meegan, J.M., Khalil, G.M., and Adham, F. 1979. The Rift Valley fever epizootic in Egypt 1977–78. 2. Ecological and entomological studies. Trans. R. Soc. Trop. Med. Hyg. 73:624–629.

Findlay, G.M. 1933. Cytological changes in the liver in Rift Valley fever, with special reference to the nuclear inclusions. Br. J. Exp. Pathol. 14:207–219.

Kaschula, J. 1957. Personal communication.

Meegan, J.M., Digoutte, J.P., Peters, C.J., and Shope, R.E. 1983. Monoclonal antibodies to identify Zinga virus Rift Valley Fever virus (letter). Lancet 1:641.

Meegan, J.M., Khalil, G.M., Hoostrall, H., and Adham, F. 1980. Experimental transmission and field isolation studies implicating *Culex pipiens* as a vector of Rift Valley fever virus in Egypt. Am. J. Trop. Med. Hyg. 29:1405–1410.

Murphy, F.A., Harrison, A.K., and Whitfield, S.G. 1973. Bunyaviridae: Morphologic and morphogenetic similarities of Bunyamwera serologic supergroup viruses and several other arthropod-borne viruses. Intervirology 1:297–316.

Sabin, A.B., and Blumberg, R.W. 1947. Human infection with Rift Valley fever virus and immunity twelve years after single attack. Proc. Soc. Exp. Biol. Med. 64:385–389.

Shope, R.E. 1985. Bunyaviruses. In B.N. Fields, D.M. Knipe, R.M. Chanock, J.L. Melnick, B. Roizman, and R.E. Shope, eds., Fields Virology. Raven Press, New York. Pp. 1055–1082.

Smithburn, K.C. 1949. Rift Valley fever: The neurotropic adaptation of the virus and the experimental use of this modified virus as a vaccine. Br. J. Exp. Pathol. 30:1–16.

Smithburn, K.C., Haddow, A.J., and Gillett, J.D. 1948. Rift Valley fever. Isolation of the virus from wild mosquitoes. Br. J. Exp. Pathol. 29:107–121.

Weiss, K.E. 1962. Studies on Rift Valley fever. Passive and active immunity in lambs. Onderstepoort J. Vet. Res. 29:3–9.

Yedloutschnig, R.J., and Walker, J.S. 1979. Personal communication.

Yedloutschnig, R.J., Dardiri, A.H., Mevus, C.A., and Walker, J.B. 1981. Abortion in vaccinated sheep and cattle after challenge with Rift Valley fever virus. Vet. Rec. 109:383–384.

The Genus *Nairovirus*

Nairobi Disease of Sheep

Nairobi disease of sheep, an arbovirus disease, occurs in Kenya. Described by Montgomery (1917), the disease affects sheep that are annually brought down from the northern districts into Nairobi to be offered for sale. It may also cause disease in goats and, on occasion, mortality up to 10 percent. In sheep mortality varies from 30 to 70 percent. The disease is characterized by acute hemorrhagic gastroenteritis and respiratory signs. Abortions may occur. The blood and tissues are always infective during fever. The urine is said to be infective at this stage, but the feces ordinarily contain no virus.

The disease is transmitted by the adult forms of a tick, *Rhipicephalus appendiculatus*, which have fed as nymphs on infected sheep. Other species of *Rhipicephalus* and *Amblyomma* ticks may also act as vectors. Virus can be retained in the salivary glands of unfed nymphs and larvae for 1 year and may pass from one stage to another in the life cycle. Small rodents may act as a reservoir of the infection.

The virus was propagated in tissue-cultured cells of goat testes, goat kidney, and hamster kidney (Howarth and Terptra 1965). A consistent and uniform cytopathic effect occurred only with hamster kidney cells.

Cell-associated virus of a cell-culture–adapted virus strain in BHK21-13 cells was detected at 6 hours after exposure to a low multiplicity of virus. The virus titer increased until a cytopathic effect appeared at 48 hours and declined 72 hours after inoculation. Cell free virus was detected 10 hours after inoculation, but on the average its titer was two log units less than titer of cell-associated virus (Terptra 1983).

Intracerebral inoculation of suckling and adult mice with infective virus produces central nervous system signs and death within 10 days. Either mice or baby hamster kidney cells (BHK-21 cell line) support replication of virus and provide systems for research and diagnosis.

Recovered animals have lasting immunity. Antibodies can be detected by neutralization, hemagglutination inhibition, indirect immunofluorescent, and enzyme linked immunosorbent assay (Munz et al. 1983). Artificial immunization has been attempted only on a small scale. Control depends on eradication of the transmitting agent. *R. appendiculatus* also transmits East Coast fever of cattle; hence both sheep and cattle should be dipped, with benefit to both species.

REFERENCES

Howarth, J.A., and Terptra, C. 1965. The propagation of Nairobi sheep disease virus in tissue culture. J. Comp. Pathol. 75:347–441.

Montgomery, E. 1917. On a tick-borne gastro-enteritis of sheep and goats occurring in British East Africa. J. Comp. Pathol. Therap. 30:28–57.

Munz, E., Reimann, M., and Meier, K. 1983. An enzyme-linked immunosorbent assay (ELISA) for the detection of antibodies to Nairobi sheep disease in comparison with indirect immunofluorescent and hemagglutination test. I. Development and testing of the ELISA with sera of experimentally infected rabbits and sheep. Zentralbl. Veterinärmed. [B] 30:473–479.

Terptra, C. 1983. Physical and biological properties of Nairobi sheep disease. Vet. Microbiol. 8:531–541.

56 The Arenaviridae

Members of the family Arenaviridae belong to a single genus, *Arenavirus*, and contain single-stranded RNA in linear segments. The molecular mass of four large RNA segments is 2.1, 1.7, 1.1, and 0.7×10^6 daltons, respectively; one to three small RNA segments have a molecular mass of about 0.03×10^6 daltons. Virions are spherical or pleomorphic and 50 to 300 nm in diameter. They consist of a unit-membrane envelope with surface projections containing varying numbers of ribosome particles (20 to 25 nm) either free in the interior or, less commonly, connected by a linear structure. Virions are formed by budding from plasma membrane (Figure 56.1). Their buoyant density in cesium chloride is 1.19 to 1.20 g/ml, and their infectivity is sensitive to ether, acid, and heat. Most arenaviruses have a limited rodent host range in nature, and the host-pathogen relationship is maintained by persistent infection viruria. Some arenaviruses, such as Lassa fever virus and Junin and Machupo viruses, cause important diseases in humans, but there is no evidence that any of these viruses causes disease in domestic animals (Johnson 1985).

Lymphocytic Choriomeningitis

Lymphocytic choriomenigitis (LCM) of mice has great historical importance because it was the first viral disease in which immunological tolerance was suggested. Traub (1935) showed that mice infected in utero or at birth with LCM continue to harbor the virus in high titers in the blood and organs, but no antibody is produced. Such tolerant mice show no signs of illness, but develop a runtish condition later in life (Hotchin 1962). Mouse colonies infected by this virus have reduced birth and growth rates and elevated mortality rates (Seamer 1965). This chronic

Figure 56.1 Thin section of Lassa fever virus, an arenavirus. The virus is budding from plasma membrane and accumulating in extracellular spaces. × 55,500. (Courtesy F. A. Murphy, S. G. Whitfield, P. A. Webb, and K. M. Johnson, Centers for Disease Control.)

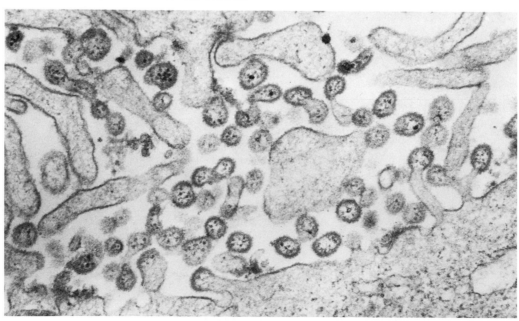

infection apparently leads to the development of an auto-immune disease (Seamer 1965).

Depending on the disease form that the infection assumes in mice, the pathological picture is one of a meningoplexal and perivascular infiltration by lymphoid cells, plasmacytes, macrophages, and other cells. Areas of focal gliosis are occasionally seen. There is often serous pleurisy, peritonitis, and hepatitis, as well as necrosis, hemorrhage, and serofibrinous exudate in the lymphatic organs. Lymphoid cell infiltrations are present in the kidneys, the salivary glands, and the pancreas. The renal lesions in this disease are comparable to those seen in Aleutian disease in mink, lupus glomerulitis in humans, and a spontaneous glomerulonephritis found in sheep in the United States and England (Abinanti 1967). A proliferation of the mesangial and endothelial cells occurs with occasional thickening of the basement membrane.

REFERENCES

Abinanti, F.R. 1967. The possible role of microorganisms and viruses in the etiology of chronic degerative diseases of man. Annu. Rev. Microbiol. 21:467–494.

Hotchin, J. 1962. The biology of lymphocytic choriomeningitis infection: Virus-induced immune disease. Cold Spring Harbor Symp. Quant. Biol. 27:479–499.

Johnson, K. 1985. Arenaviruses. In B.N. Fields, D.M. Knipe, R.M. Chanock, J.L. Melnick, B. Roizman, and R.E. Shope, eds., Fields Virology. Raven Press, New York. Pp. 1033–1053.

Seamer, J. 1965. The growth, reproduction and mortality of mice made immunologically tolerant to lymphocytic choriomeningitis virus by congenital infection. Arch. Gesam. Virusforsch. 15:169–177.

Traub, E. 1935. A filtrable virus recovered from white mice. Science 81:298–299.

The coronaviruses are a monogeneric family of single-stranded RNA viruses (Pensaert and Callebaut 1978; Robb and Bond 1979; Siddell, Anderson, et al. 1983; Siddell, Wege, et al. 1983; Tyrrell et al. 1978; Wege et al. 1983). The enveloped particles are pleomorphic but roughly spherical, with diameters ranging from 60 to 220 nm (average 100 nm). The nucleocapsid protein is complexed with the genome as a helical ribonucleoprotein. The surface has a characteristic fringe of radiating, club-shaped projections (peplomers) about 20 nm long (Figure 57.1), which resemble the rays, or corona, of the sun (Latin *corona,* "crown"). The buoyant density averages 1.18 g/ml in sucrose and 1.23–1.24 g/ml in cesium chloride. The particles are ether- and chloroform-labile but variably sensitive to pH. They are rapidly inactivated by heating (56°C) and by many common lipid solvents, detergents, and disinfectants.

The genomic RNA of coronaviruses is a linear, single-stranded molecule that is capped, polyadenylated, and infectious. The molecular weight is between 5 and 7×10^6, corresponding to about 15,000 to 20,000 nucleotides. Replication proceeds by production of multiple 3′ coterminal subgenomic RNAs that form a nested set extending for varying lengths in the 5′ direction. Structurally virions are composed of three major proteins: a phosphorylated nucleocapsid protein of 50 to 60×10^3 daltons; a glycosylated peplomer protein associated with glycopolypeptides of 90 to 180×10^3 daltons; and a transmembrane matrix protein associated with polypeptides of 20 to 35×10^3 daltons, with varying degrees of glycosylation.

Viral replication occurs in the cytoplasm of infected cells and is often accompanied by cytopathic changes. Reports conflict as to whether a nuclear function is required for coronavirus replication. Virion maturation occurs by budding from membranes of the endoplasmic reticulum and cytoplasmic vesicles (Figure 57.2). No budding occurs at the plasma membrane.

The type species for the single genus *Coronavirus* is avian infectious bronchitis virus. Antigenic relationships suggest two avian groups, each with one species (infectious bronchitis virus and turkey enteritis coronavirus), and two mammalian groups, one composed of transmissible gastroenteritis virus, canine coronavirus, feline infectious peritonitis virus, and human coronavirus 229E, and another composed of murine hepatitis virus, bovine coronavirus, hemagglutinating encephalomyelitis virus, rat (sialodacryoadenitis) coronavirus, and human coronavirus OC43.

Coronavirus infections are restricted predominantly to vertebrate hosts. They are characterized in general by respiratory and gastrointestinal tract disease signs (Table 57.1).

REFERENCES

Pensaert, M., and Callebaut, P. 1978. The coronaviruses: Clinical and structural aspects with some practical implications. Ann. Méd. Vét. 122:301–322.

Robb, J.A., and Bond, C.W. 1979. Coronaviridae. In H. Fraenkel-Conrat and R.R. Wagner, eds., Comprehensive Virology, vol. 14: Newly Characterized Vertebrate Viruses. Plenum Press, New York. Pp. 193–247.

Siddell, S.G., Anderson, R., Cavanagh, D., Fujiwara, K., Klenk, H.D., Macnaughton, M.R., Pensaert, M., Stohlman, S.A., Sturman, L., and van der Zeijst, B.A.M. 1983. Coronaviridae. Intervirology 20:181–189.

Siddell, S.G., Wege, H., and ter Meulen, V. 1983. The biology of coronaviruses. J. Gen. Virol. 64:761–776.

Tyrrell, D.A.J., Alexander, D.J., Almeida, J.D., Cunningham, C.H., Easterday, B.C., Garwes, D.J., Hierholzer, J.C., Kapikian, A., Macnaughton, M.R., and McIntosh, K. 1978. Coronaviridae: Second report. Intervirology 10:321–328.

Wege, H., Siddell, S., and ter Meulen, V. 1982. The biology and pathogenesis of coronaviruses. Curr. Top. Microbiol. Immunol. 99:165–200.

Feline Infectious Peritonitis
SYNONYM: Feline fibrinous peritonitis; abbreviation, FIP

Feline infectious peritonitis is an important immunologically mediated disease of domestic and exotic cats and is pathogenetically the most complex coronaviral disease of domestic species. It was first described by Holzworth in 1963, and its infectious nature was established experimentally by Wolfe and Griesemer in 1966. Reports indicate, however, that FIP has apparently been observed

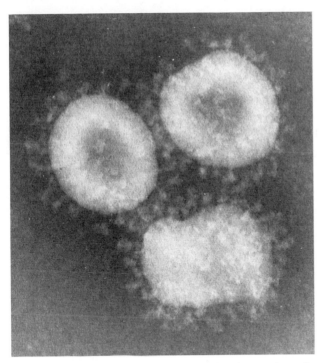

Figure 57.1. Avian infectious bronchitis virus in negative stain preparation showing surface projections. × 298,900. (Courtesy J. C. Hierholzer, E. L. Palmer, S. G. Whitfield, H. S. Kaye, and W. R. Dowdle, Centers for Disease Control.)

since the early 1950s but was not recognized as a specific disease entity. The disease is widespread in feline populations throughout the world.

Character of the Disease. Three forms of FIP are recognized: (1) effusive ("wet") FIP, characterized by peritoneal or pleural effusion or both; (2) noneffusive

Figure 57.2. Maturation by budding of avian infectious bronchitis virus into cytoplasmic vesicles of an embryonated hen's egg cell. (Courtesy B. Cowen.)

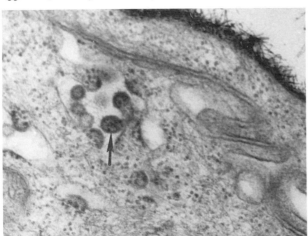

("dry") FIP, with minimal effusion but marked pyogranulomatous lesions involving especially the kidneys, liver, central nervous system, and eyes; and (3) combinations of the two (Barlough and Weiss 1983; Barlough and Stoddart 1986; Horzinek and Osterhaus 1979; Pedersen 1976a, 1987).

Effusive FIP is characterized by chronic weight loss, depression, variable anorexia, refractory fever, and progressive abdominal enlargement caused by ascites (Figure 57.3). Icterus may be present in animals in which there is severe liver involvement. Pleural effusion with clinical signs of respiratory insufficiency occurs in less than 25 to 30 percent of affected cats. The volume of fluid present in the abdomen or thorax varies and is generally a reflection of disease chronicity. In animals with more chronic disease a liter or more of fluid may accumulate within the abdomen. Typical FIP fluid is clear to slightly opaque, straw-colored to vivid yellow, and very viscous. It contains fibrin strands or flecks and often clots upon exposure to air. The fluid is an exudate of high specific gravity (1.017 to 1.047) and protein content (5–10 g/dl) and variable cell numbers (1,600 to 25,000 cells or more per microliter). In the early stages of the disease, the cells are primarily neutrophils. Later on, mononuclear and mesothelial cells predominate. In contrast with septic peritonitis, the majority of the leukocytes are intact. Fungal and bacterial (including mycoplasmal and chlamydial) isolation studies are usually negative.

Figure 57.3. Elevated fibrinous plaques on the visceral and parietal peritoneum observed in a typical case of feline infectious peritonitis. (Courtesy J. Gaskin.)

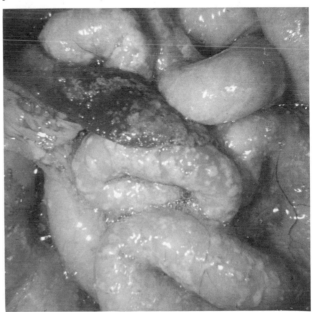

Table 57.1. Coronaviruses that cause diseases of importance in domestic animals

Virus	Natural host	Type of disease produced
Feline infectious per-itonitis virus, several serotypes?	Cats	Fibrinous serositis with fever, anorexia, depression, thoracic and/or abdominal effusion. High mortality rate. World-wide distribution
Transmissible gastroen-teritis virus, one serotype	Pigs	Acute, highly contagious diar-rheal disease in pigs of all ages. Epizootic and enzootic forms. Vomiting, diarrhea, dehydration, and high mor-tality rate in pigs less than 2 weeks of age. Adult pigs de-velop a milder or inapparent disease. Worldwide
Porcine epidemic diarrhea virus, one serotype?	Pigs	Acute, highly contagious diar-rheal disease closely resem-bling transmissible gastroenteritis. Worldwide
Hemagglutinating enceph-alomyelitis virus, one serotype	Pigs	Encephalomyelitis and vomiting and wasting disease in piglets. High morbidity and mortality in pigs under 2 weeks of age. Worldwide
Canine coronavirus, one serotype	Dogs	Enteritis in dogs of all ages, with some mortality in pups. Worldwide
Bovine coronavirus, one serotype	Cattle	Enteritis in neonatal calves, with some mortality. Probably worldwide
Avian infectious bron-chitis virus, multiple serotypes	Chickens	Acute, highly contagious respi-ratory disease with high mor-tality rate in young chicks. Kidney and oviduct damage may occur. Marked reduction in egg production and quality. Worldwide
Coronaviral enteritis virus, one serotype?	Turkeys	Acute, highly contagious enter-itis in turkeys of all ages. Mortality rate in young poults can be high. Probably worldwide

The onset of noneffusive FIP is often insidious; disseminated pyogranulomatous lesions frequently are present in one or more major organs. Clinical signs of renal and/or hepatic insufficiency, pancreatic disease, or central nervous system dysfunction may be seen in cats with severe organ impairment. Neurological signs can include posterior paresis, ataxia, nystagmus, behavioral changes, muscle rigidity, paralysis, and seizures. Ocular lesions, which occur in 25 percent or more of animals with noneffusive FIP, include iritis, hyphema, keratic precipi-

tates, retinal hemorrhage, retinal detachment, chorioreti-nitis, and panophthalmitis. Ophthalmoscopic examina-tion of cats showing signs of systemic disease is therefore an important diagnostic procedure.

Changes in the hemogram are variable and not specific for FIP. Commonly observed abnormalities are leuk-ocytosis due to an absolute neutrophilia (which may be accompanied by either a regenerative or a degenerative left shift), moderate monocytosis, and eosinopenia. Usu-ally an absolute lymphopenia, which may be profound, is present. Occasionally leukopenia may develop, especially in animals with more fulminating disease. Nearly half of all cats with FIP develop a mild to moderate normocytic, normochromic anemia. Total plasma protein levels are usually elevated, the result of a polyclonal hypergammaglobulinemia, with variable elevations of α_2 and β globulins.

In general, abnormalities in clinical chemistry profiles reflect the extent of involvement of different organ systems in the disease process. Extensive liver involvement may produce hyperbilirubinemia and mild to moderate elevations in serum enzyme levels. A proteinuria with or without increased urea nitrogen and creatinine concentrations may be seen in cases of renal involvement. Generalized peritoneal lesions involving the pancreas may result in clinical pancreatitis with elevations in serum lipase or amylase levels or both; in severe cases, this may lead to diabetes mellitus. Analysis of cerebrospinal fluid from cats with extensive meningeal lesions may reveal a nonseptic fluid high in protein (90–2,000 cells/μl), the latter predominantly neutrophils. Similar changes may occur in aqueous humor from cats with anterior chamber involvement.

At necropsy, effusive FIP is characterized by the presence of small necrotic lesions on the visceral and parietal surfaces of the peritoneum or pleura or both. Moderate to extensive accumulations of the yellowish viscous exudate containing fibrin are found in the body cavities. Focal necrotic lesions sometimes are observed in parenchymatous organs, usually the liver or kidneys or both. In noneffusive FIP there are disseminated gray lesions, up to 2 mm in diameter, that are most abundant in the kidneys, central nervous system, liver, and mesenteric lymph nodes. Lesions in the central nervous system are localized to the meninges, ependyma, choroid plexus, and along blood vessels in the parenchyma.

Fibrinous peritonitis or pleuritis or both, with areas of focal necrosis in the omentum, liver, spleen, kidneys, and other organs, is the principal histopathological feature of FIP. Necrotic foci are often subcapsular in location but also may be distributed throughout the organ parenchyma. Lesions contain necrotic neutrophils and debris surrounded by mononuclear cells (primarily macrophages). The necrotic foci have a perivascular orientation; a proliferative and necrotizing vasculitis is associated with the development of these necrotic lesions.

Properties of the Virus. FIP virus (FIPV) is a typical member of the coronavirus group. It is heat-labile, ether-sensitive, and inactivated by most common detergents and disinfectants. Maintenance of the virus at room temperature results in complete loss of infectivity within 24 to 48 hours. Virus particles are destroyed by formaldehyde,

sodium hypochlorite (bleach), and quaternary ammonium compounds, but they are resistant to phenol. FIPV is antigenically related to transmissible gastroenteritis virus, canine coronavirus, and human coronavirus 229E (Pedersen et al. 1978). There is some evidence that more than one serotype of FIPV may exist.

Cultivation. Studies of FIPV were hampered for many years by an inability to propagate the virus in cell culture. Early studies involved short-term growth in autochthonous peritoneal cell (macrophage) cultures from infected cats (Pedersen 1976b). The first successful in vitro isolation and propagation of FIPV in intestinal ring organ cultures (Hoshino and Scott 1978) was followed by isolations in several monolayer cell-culture systems, including feline embryonic lung cells, feline fetal fibroblasts and whole fetus cells, Crandell feline kidney cells, and canine A-72 cells. In vivo propagation of FIPV in suckling mouse brain has also been reported (Osterhaus, Horzinek, and Wirahadiredja 1978; Osterhaus, Horzinek, Wirahadiredja, and deKreek 1978). The isolates identified in these reports are apparently pathogenic field strains that have undergone adaptation for growth and continued passage outside the host. In this respect they are quite different from the majority of FIPV field strains, most of which are still not amenable to routine cell culture isolation. However, those strains that can be grown artificially have provided and will continue to provide valuable information about FIPV and its workings in nature.

Epizootiology and Pathogenesis. All breeds and ages of cats are susceptible to FIPV infection. In addition, FIP occurs in a number of exotic breeds, including cheetahs, lions, leopards, jaguars, lynxes, caracals, and sand cats. The effect of FIPV infection and disease on exotic cat populations can be devastating (Briggs et al. 1986, O'Brien et al. 1985, Pfeifer et al. 1983).

On the basis of serosurvey data, investigators have proposed that the majority of FIPV infections in nature result only in seroconversion without progression to lethal, disseminated disease (Barlough et al. 1983, Loeffler et al. 1978, Osterhaus et al. 1977, Pedersen 1976c). This conclusion was reached because serum coronavirus antibodies can be found not only in cats with FIP but also in many healthy cats and in many cats with other diseases. In general, in the healthy feline population—excluding cats in catteries and multiple cat households—approximately 10 to 40 percent of cats have coronavirus antibodies. A special situation is encountered when cats are artificially clustered together, as in catteries, in which case positive titers are either completely absent (i.e., there has been no coronavirus exposure) or are present in 80 to 90 percent of the cats within a household (indicating efficient spread of virus once it has been introduced). As discussed later in this section, these antibodies do not necessarily represent exposure to the FIP coronavirus, because cats are susceptible to infection with a number of cross-reacting coronaviruses in the FIPV group. In addition, the virulence of FIPV isolates can vary dramatically.

The route by which FIPV is spread in nature is still unknown, but it is most likely that initial infection results from ingestion or inhalation of the virus. FIPV is probably excreted into the environment by a number of routes: in oral and respiratory secretions, feces, and possibly urine. Close contact between cats is probably required for effective transmission of FIPV, although the possibility of virus being spread in excreta and by other indirect methods (fomites) also exists. The potential for transmission by bloodsucking arthropods is unknown. Transmission across the placenta to the developing fetus occurs occasionally (Pedersen 1987).

Experimental studies have demonstrated that initial exposure to FIPV can result in a localized upper respiratory disease manifested clinically as a mild to severe conjunctivitis or rhinitis or both, which may persist for as long as a month (Pedersen 1978). Although the vast majority of cats undergoing this primary form of the disease recover, many cats probably remain chronically infected (i.e., are chronic virus carriers). A very small number of exposed cats develop the lethal, disseminated (secondary) form of the disease weeks, months, or years after their primary infection.

Studies performed over the past decade have succeeded in identifying some of the major host-virus interactions in FIP (Jacobse-Geels et al. 1980, 1982; Pedersen and Boyle 1980; Weiss and Scott 1981a, 1981b, 1981c; Weiss et al. 1980). Following infection of large mononuclear cells in regional lymphoreticular tissue at or near the site of viral entry, a primary viremia involving virus or virus-infected cells or both occurs within 1 week after exposure. In this way virus is transported to other regions of the body, especially to such organs as the liver, spleen, and lymph nodes. These structures contain sizable populations of macrophages, which are believed to be the primary target cells of FIPV (Hayashi et al. 1980, Jacobse-Geels et al. 1983, Pedersen 1976b, Pedersen and Floyd 1985, Weiss and Scott 1981a). Hematogenous dissemination of virus also results in infection of circulating mononuclear cells (primarily monocytes) and, importantly, in localization of virus and virus-infected cells within the walls of small blood vessels (especially venules and small veins). A secondary cell-associated viremia may occur after initial infection of target tissues and result in further spread of virus throughout the body. Deposition of virus, virus-infected mononuclear cells, and immune complexes within blood vessel walls produces an intense perivascular

inflammatory response that damages vessels and allows for escape of fibrin-rich serum constituents into intercellular spaces, eventually accumulating as characteristic FIP fluid within body cavities.

Some studies have shown that certain cats with serum coronavirus antibodies may experience a more rapid, fulminating disease course following FIPV exposure than do cats without coronavirus antibodies who are similarly challenged. Moreover, intravenous administration of immune serum containing coronavirus antibodies to cats without antibodies results in the more fulminating form of the disease following FIPV challenge. A potential state of antibody-mediated hypersensitivity thus exists in FIP, with coronavirus antibody possibly accelerating uptake of FIPV (in the form of immune complexes) into mononuclear target cells, where production of additional infectious virus is enhanced, and promoting widespread destructive inflammatory reactions in blood vessel walls and tissues through immune complex deposition and complement activation (Weiss et al. 1980). This sensitization is FIPV strain–specific. Uptake of FIPV into macrophages appears to be enhanced by impaired T-lymphocyte function (Hayashi et al. 1983).

In addition to FIPV, cats are susceptible to natural infection with certain enteric coronaviruses that appear to be pathogenetic variants of FIPV, or vice versa (Boyle et al. 1984; Dea et al. 1983; McKeirnan et al. 1981; Pedersen et al. 1981; Pedersen, Black, et al. 1984; Pedersen, Evermann, et al. 1984). These feline enteric coronaviruses (FECVs) can produce a range of effects from asymptomatic infection of the gastrointestinal tract to severe enteritis in kittens and adult cats. Reports also indicate that at least two other coronaviruses in the FIPV antigenic cluster can infect cats under experimental conditions: transmissible gastroenteritis virus, which produces an asymptomatic infection and is excreted in feces for as long as 3 weeks (Reynolds and Garwes 1979), and canine coronavirus, which also produces an asymptomatic infection and is excreted from the oropharynx for at least 1 week (Barlough et al. 1984, Stoddart et al. 1985). At present, the frequency of infection of cats in nature with these latter two coronaviruses is unknown. Human coronavirus 229E does not appear to replicate to any extent in experimentally inoculated cats (Barlough et al. 1985).

In FIP hypersensitization by coronavirus antibody depends on the identity of the coronavirus(es) responsible for the antibody response. Thus antibodies resulting from exposure to FIPV or FECVs often hypersensitize, whereas antibodies resulting from exposure to canine coronavirus, transmissible gastroenteritis virus, or human coronavirus 229E usually do not. This phenomenon of virus-specific hypersensitization is of importance for the development of an effective FIP vaccine and is basic to a further understanding of pathogenetic mechanisms in FIP. It should be emphasized, however, that the mere presence of coronavirus antibodies in a cat's serum does not necessarily mean that FIP will ever develop in that animal. FIP is a relatively uncommon disease in nature, even in crowded catteries; the vast majority of cats with coronavirus antibodies never develop FIP. The factors that determine whether FIP *does* develop after exposure to the virus are multiple and probably include dose and virulence of the infecting viral strain and its ability to replicate within macrophages, route of exposure, age and immune status of the animal at the time of exposure, possibly genetic predisposition, concurrent viral infections (e.g., feline leukemia virus), and adverse environmental influences such as stress, overcrowding, or movement to unfamiliar surroundings.

Immunity. The presence of coronavirus antibodies in a cat is indicative only of prior exposure to a coronavirus in the FIPV group. A positive titer therefore is not diagnostic of clinical FIP, latent FIP, or viremia. Because the underlying basis of FIP is an immunopathological mechanism, however, a positive titer does not necessarily indicate protection either. Given that FIP occurs sporadically in the general population and that most cats in catteries with FIP problems are seropositive and yet will not contract the disease, it seems that many (if not most) cats are protected naturally against FIP. It appears unlikely, in light of current research, that this protection is conferred by humoral immunity. Rather, most researchers believe that cell mediated immunity is probably the critical determining factor in resistance (Hayashi et al. 1983, Pedersen and Black 1983, Pedersen and Floyd 1985, Takenouchi et al. 1985). Thus cats that recover from FIPV infection may produce a swift and highly efficient cell-mediated immune response; those that develop chronic, noneffusive FIP may have an immune response that is only partially successful; those that develop acute effusive FIP may have the least successful response (Pedersen and Floyd 1985). The virulence of the FIPV strain is also undoubtedly important in determining the outcome of infection. Immunity in FIP seems largely specific to the viral strain, with variable degrees of cross-protection. Such specificity of immunity is yet another potential impediment to development of an effective vaccine.

Diagnosis. The clinical diagnosis of FIP is made by evaluation of history and presenting signs and the results of supportive laboratory procedures (Barlough 1985, Barlough and Stoddart 1986, Pedersen 1987, Weiss and Scott 1980). Clinicopathological and serologic procedures useful in diagnosis include analysis of thoracic and abdominal effusions, hemogram, clinical chemistry profile, serum protein electrophoresis, serum coronavirus antibody titer (indirect immunofluorescence, enzyme-linked immunosorbent assay, virus neutralization), and biopsy (when possible). It is important to remember that biopsy is the only test procedure that can yield a definitive diagnosis of FIP in the living animal; hence any diagnosis of FIP made in the absence of histopathological examination (of either biopsy or necropsy specimens) must be considered presumptive. An antibody titer determination should be given no more weight than any of the other diagnostic procedures already listed (Barlough 1985). A combination of findings may point to a presumptive diagnosis of FIP; these findings should be heeded, regardless of the antibody titer. Most cats with FIP have serum coronavirus antibodies, often of high titer, but so do many cats that do not have FIP. Some cats with FIP have low or even negative titers, whereas some animals with long-standing chronic noneffusive FIP (e.g., ocular FIP) may have very elevated titers. In any cat with an elevated antibody titer, the titer must be considered supportive, not diagnostic. Exploratory laparotomy with organ punch biopsy of affected tissues—especially from liver, spleen, omentum, and mesenteric lymph nodes—is the preferred method of obtaining FIP biopsy samples. Percutaneous needle biopsy cannot be recommended because of the friability of diseased organs and the potential for occurrence of serious hemorrhage (Weiss and Scott 1980).

Treatment. Although it is possible that mild cases of FIP may occasionally occur in which clinical signs are minimal and spontaneously resolve, the vast majority of cats that develop disseminated FIP die, usually within a few weeks or months of onset.

Present-day treatment of cats with FIP is purely palliative, since no curative therapy exists. The aim of therapy is to alleviate the self-destroying, disseminated FIP inflammatory response, which represents the immune system's unsuccessful attempt to eliminate the virus. The most effective treatment protocols combine high levels of corticosteroids, cytotoxic drugs, and broad-spectrum antibiotics, with maintenance of nutrient intake and fluid and electrolyte balance (Barlough and Stoddart 1986). The best candidates for treatment are cats that are still in good physical condition and are still eating; that do not show severe anemia, neurological signs, or significant organ dysfunction; and that are not also infected with feline leukemia virus. Remissions are only occasionally achieved; progressive physical deterioration of the patient in the face of treatment is a poor prognostic sign.

Currently, there is no documented scientific evidence that supplemental multivitamin therapy is of any benefit in the treatment of FIP.

Prevention and Control. A safe and effective FIP vaccine is still unavailable. Experiments thus far with various preparations of FIPV and antigenically related coronaviruses have been unsuccessful in conferring consistently protective immunity. Because of the immunological nature of the disease, parenteral immunization with sensitizing coronavirus strains only predisposes cats to lethal, disseminated FIP. Until an effective vaccine is developed, control of FIPV infections must be based on identification and isolation of diseased animals and suspected chronic carriers. Current scientific information does not support a test-and-removal program for cats with coronavirus antibodies similar to the program used for cats with feline leukemia virus infection.

The Disease in Humans. There is no evidence that FIPV is a health hazard for humans.

REFERENCES

Barlough, J.E. 1985. Cats, coronaviruses and coronavirus antibody tests. J. Small Anim. Pract. 26:353–362.

Barlough, J.E., and Stoddart, C.A. 1986. Feline infectious peritonitis. In F.W. Scott, ed., Contemporary Issues in Small Animal Practice, vol. 3: Infectious Diseases. Churchill Livingstone, New York. Pp. 93–108.

Barlough, J.E., and Weiss, R.C. 1983. Feline infectious peritonitis. In R.W. Kirk, ed., Current Veterinary Therapy, vol. 8. W.B. Saunders, Philadelphia. Pp. 1186–1193.

Barlough, J.E., Jacobson, R.H., and Scott, F.W. 1983. Feline coronaviral serology. Feline Pract. 13(3):25–35.

Barlough, J.E., Johnson-Lussenburg, C.M., Stoddart, C.A., Jacobson, R.H., and Scott, F.W. 1985. Experimental inoculation of cats with human coronavirus 229E and subsequent challenge with feline infectious peritonitis virus. Can. J. Comp. Med. 49:303–307.

Barlough, J.E., Stoddart, C.A., Sorresso, G.P., Jacobson, R.H., and Scott, F.W. 1984. Experimental inoculation of cats with canine coronavirus and subsequent challenge with feline infectious peritonitis virus. Lab. Anim. Sci. 34:592–597.

Boyle, J.F., Pedersen, N.C., Evermann, J.F., McKeirnan, A.J., Ott, R.L., and Black, J.W. 1984. Plaque assay, polypeptide composition and immunochemistry of feline infectious peritonitis virus and feline enteric coronavirus isolates. Adv. Exp. Med. Biol. 173:133–147.

Briggs, M.B., Evermann, J.F., and McKeirnan, A.J. 1986. Feline infectious peritonitis. Feline Pract. 16(2):13–16.

Dea, S., Roy, R.S., and Elazhary, M.A.S.Y. 1982. Coronavirus-like particles in the feces of a cat with diarrhea. Can. Vet. J. 23:153–155.

Hayashi, T., Sasaki, N., Ami, Y., and Fujiwara, K. 1983. Role of thymus-dependent lymphocytes and antibodies in feline infectious peritonitis after oral infection. Jpn. J. Vet. Sci. 45:759–766.

Hayashi, T., Utsumi, F., Takahashi, R., and Fujiwara, K. 1980. Pathology of non-effusive type feline infectious peritonitis and experimental transmission. Jpn. J. Vet. Sci. 42:197–210.

Holzworth, J. 1963. Some important disorders of cats. Cornell Vet. 53:157–160.

Horzinek, M.C., and Osterhaus, A.D.M.E. 1979. The virology and pathogenesis of feline infectious peritonitis. Arch. Virol. 59:1–15.

Hoshino, Y., and Scott, F.W. 1978. Brief communication: Replication of feline infectious peritonitis virus in organ cultures of feline tissue. Cornell Vet. 68:411–417.

Jacobse-Geels, H.E.L., and Horzinek, M.C. 1983. Expression of feline infectious peritonitis coronavirus antigens on the surface of feline macrophage-like cells. J. Gen. Virol. 64:1859–1866.

Jacobse-Geels, H.E.L., Daha, M.R., and Horzinek, M.C. 1980. Isola-tion and characterization of feline C3 and evidence for the immune complex pathogenesis of feline infectious peritonitis. J. Immunol. 125:1606–1610.

Jacobse-Geels, H.E.L., Daha, M.R., and Horzinek, M.C. 1982. Antibody, immune complexes, and complement activity fluctuations in kittens with experimentally induced feline infectious peritonitis. Am. J. Vet. Res. 43:666–670.

Loeffler, D.G., Ott, R.L., Evermann, J.F., and Alexander, J.E. 1978. The incidence of naturally occurring antibodies against feline infectious peritonitis in selected cat populations. Feline Pract. 8(1):43–47.

McKeirnan, A.J., Evermann, J.F., Hargis, A., Miller, L.M., and Ott, R.L., 1981. Isolation of feline coronaviruses from two cats with diverse disease manifestations. Feline Pract. 11(3):16–20.

O'Brien, S.J., Roelke, M.E., Marker, L., Newman, A., Winkler, C.A., Meltzer, D., Colly, L., Evermann, J.F., Bush, M., and Wildt, D.E. 1985. Genetic basis for species vulnerability in the cheetah. Science 227:1428–1434.

Osterhaus, A.D.M.E., Horzinek, M.C., and Reynolds, D.J. 1977. Seroepidemiology of feline infectious peritonitis virus infections using transmissible gastroenteritis virus as antigen. Zentralbl. Veterinärmed. [B] 24:835–841.

Osterhaus, A.D.M.E., Horzinek, M.C., and Wirahadiredja, R.M.S. 1978. Feline infectious peritonitis virus. II. Propagation in suckling mouse brain. Zentralbl. Veterinärmed. [B] 25:301–307.

Osterhaus, A.D.M.E., Horzinek, M.C., Wirahadiredja, R.M.S., and deKreek, P. 1978. Feline infectious peritonitis (FIP) virus. III. Studies on the multiplication of FIP virus in the suckling mouse. Zentralbl. Veterinärmed. [B] 25:806–815.

Pedersen, N.C. 1976a. Feline infectious peritonitis: Something old, something new. Feline Pract. 6(3):42–51.

Pedersen, N.C. 1976b. Morphologic and physical characteristics of feline infectious peritonitis virus and its growth in autochthonous peritoneal cell cultures. Am. J. Vet. Res. 37:567–572.

Pedersen, N.C. 1976c. Serologic studies of naturally occurring feline infectious peritonitis. Am. J. Vet. Res. 37:1449–1453.

Pedersen, N.C. 1978. Feline infectious diseases. Proceedings of the Annual Meeting of the American Animal Hospital Association 45:125–146.

Pedersen, N.C. 1987. Coronavirus diseases (coronavirus enteritis, feline infectious peritonitis). In J. Holzworth, ed., Diseases of the Cat, vol. 1. W.B. Saunders, Philadelphia. Pp. 193–214.

Pedersen, N.C., and Black, J.W. 1983. Attempted immunization of cats against feline infectious peritonitis, using avirulent live virus or sublethal amounts of virulent virus. Am. J. Vet. Res. 44:229–234.

Pedersen, N.C., and Boyle, J.F. 1980. Immunologic phenomena in the effusive form of feline infectious peritonitis. Am. J. Vet. Res. 41:868–876.

Pedersen, N.C., and Floyd, K. 1985. Experimental studies with three new strains of feline infectious peritonitis virus: FIPV-UCD2, FIPV-UCD3, and FIPV-UCD4. Compend. Cont. Ed. Pract. Vet. 7:1001–1011.

Pedersen, N.C., Black, J.W., Boyle, J.F., Evermann, J.F., McKeirnan, A.J., and Ott, R.L. 1984. Pathogenic differences between various feline coronavirus isolates. Adv. Exp. Med. Biol. 173:365–380.

Pedersen, N.C., Boyle, J.F., Floyd, K., Fudge, A., and Barker, J. 1981. An enteric coronavirus infection of cats and its relationship to feline infectious peritonitis. Am. J. Vet. Res. 42:368–377.

Pedersen, N.C., Evermann, J.F., McKeirnan, A.J., and Ott, R.L. 1984. Pathogenicity studies of feline coronavirus isolates 79-1146 and 79-1683. Am. J. Vet. Res. 45:2580–2585.

Pedersen, N.C., Ward, J., and Mengeling, W.L. 1978. Antigenic relationship of the feline infectious peritonitis virus to coronaviruses of other species. Arch. Virol. 58:45–53.

Pfeifer, M.L., Evermann, J.F., Roelke, M.E., Gallina, A.M., Ott, R.L., and McKeirnan, A.J. 1983. Feline infectious peritonitis in a captive cheetah. J. Am. Vet. Med. Assoc. 183:1317–1319.

Reynolds, D.J., and Garwes, D.J. 1979. Virus isolation and serum antibody responses after infection of cats with transmissible gastroenteritis virus. Arch. Virol. 60:161–166.

Stoddart, C.A., Baldwin, C.A., and Scott, F.W. 1985. Unpublished data. Cornell Feline Health Center, Ithaca, N.Y.

Takenouchi, T., Ami, Y., Hayashi, T., and Fujiwara, K. 1985. Role of T cells in feline infectious peritonitis virus infection of suckling mice. Jpn. J. Vet. Sci. 47:465–468.

Weiss, R.C., and Scott, F.W. 1980. Laboratory diagnosis of feline infectious peritonitis. Feline Pract. 10(2):16–22.

Weiss, R.C., and Scott, F.W. 1981a. Pathogenesis of feline infectious peritonitis: Nature and development of viremia. Am. J. Vet. Res. 42:382–390.

Weiss, R.C., and Scott, F.W. 1981b. Pathogenesis of feline infectious peritonitis: Pathologic changes and immunofluorescence. Am. J. Vet. Res. 42:2036–2048.

Weiss, R.C., and Scott, F.W. 1981c. Antibody-mediated enhancement of disease in feline infectious peritonitis: Comparisons with dengue hemorrhagic fever. Comp. Immunol. Microbiol. Infect. Dis. 4:175–189.

Weiss, R.C., Dodds, W.J., and Scott, F.W. 1980. Disseminated intravascular coagulation in experimentally induced feline infectious peritonitis. Am. J. Vet. Res. 41:663–671.

Wolfe, L.G., and Griesemer, R.A. 1966. Feline infectious peritonitis. Pathol. Vet. 3:255–270.

Transmissible Gastroenteritis

Transmissible gastroenteritis (TGE) is a highly contagious gastroenteritis of swine (Bohl 1981, 1986; Hogg 1982; Underdahl and Torres-Medina 1981). The disease is frequently fatal in pigs less than 1 or 2 weeks old. Although swine of all ages are susceptible, most animals older than 5 weeks recover. In adult swine the disease is often inapparent or mild. Outbreaks of TGE are often explosive and occur in cycles over a period of years.

The disease was first reported in Indiana by Doyle and Hutchings in 1946, although it is clear that it had existed much earlier. It occurs throughout the densely populated swine belt of the United States (north central states) and sporadically in other areas where pigs are raised. Subsequent to its recognition in the United States, TGE was reported in England and other European countries, Japan, Taiwan, Central and South America, and Canada.

Character of the Disease. On a herd basis, there are two distinct forms of TGE: epizootic and enzootic.

Epizootic TGE occurs following entrance of the virus into a highly susceptible (i.e., nonimmune) herd. The disease spreads rapidly, involving animals of all ages. The older breeding animals show relatively mild signs, which can include anorexia, lethargy, diarrhea, weight loss, and some vomiting. These animals generally recover within a week, although the decrease in weight in feeder pigs may be a serious loss to the producer. The mortality in pigs less than 2 weeks old may approach 100 percent. The diarrhea in these young animals is profuse, the bowel discharge being watery and yellowish. Feces frequently contain small curds of undigested milk and are very fetid. The animals suffer from severe thirst and frequently collect around the watering troughs, from which they drink excessively. Most pigs less than 1 week old die within 2 to

7 days of the onset of clinical signs. Most sucklings more than 3 weeks old survive but often remain unthrifty afterward for a while.

Some infected lactating sows become very ill, showing fever, anorexia, agalactia, vomiting, and diarrhea. These severe signs may be due to a high degree of exposure to the virus from their infected offspring or possibly to endocrine effects that may influence disease susceptibility. Nonlactating sows without contact with infected piglets usually are only mildly affected, if at all.

The disease course of epizootic TGE in a herd usually lasts from 2 to 4 weeks, unless there is a continuing source of infection. The disease spreads more rapidly in winter.

Enzootic TGE is seen when the virus persists within a herd, usually as a result of continuous or frequent introduction of susceptible pigs; these animals, once infected, perpetuate the disease. This form of TGE is found in herds with a continuous farrowing program or with frequent additions of feeder pigs. Immune sows in such herds provide a variable degree of passive immunity to sucklings until weaning. Diarrhea usually is seen from 1 week of age to 2 weeks after weaning and results from an exposure to the virus that exceeds the protective capacity of maternally derived antibody. Clinical signs are similar to but less severe than those seen in fully susceptible pigs of comparable age. The mortality rate is low (10 to 20 percent), and sows usually are unaffected. In some herds, depending on management practice, enzootic TGE is seen primarily in the postweaning period.

Gross lesions in TGE usually are confined to the gastrointestinal tract. The stomach and intestines are often distended with liquid ingesta containing curdled milk, and the wall of the tract is thin and almost transparent. This thinning is caused by severe atrophy of the villi of the jejunum and ileum, a common feature of coronavirus-induced enteritides in many animal species. TGE virus infects the villus epithelial cells of the small intestine, producing necrosis, villus atrophy and focal fusion, shedding of epithelial cells and infectious virus into the gut lumen, and accumulation of unabsorbed, undigested fluid, resulting in diarrhea.

Properties of the Virus. TGE virus (TGEV) has the morphologic, physicochemical, and polypeptide characteristics of a typical member of the coronavirus group. The virus is ether- and chloroform-labile, trypsin-resistant, and relatively stable in bile. Virulent strains are more resistant to the activity of digestive enzymes and to pH than are attenuated strains (Chen 1985, Hess and Bachmann 1976, Laude et al. 1981). TGEV is relatively heat-labile and is highly photosensitive (Cartwright et al. 1965, Haelterman 1963, Laude 1981). The virus is quite stable when stored frozen, particularly in the tissue state.

Only a single serotype of TGEV is recognized at present (Kemeny 1976). The virus is antigenically related to feline infectious peritonitis virus, canine coronavirus, and human coronavirus 229E (Pedersen et al. 1978).

Cultivation. The cytopathic effects produced by field strains of TGEV usually are transient or slight in early passages; consequently, the piglet has been used as a sensitive experimental system for detecting field virus (Hooper and Haelterman 1966). Cell-culture systems useful for isolating and propagating TGEV include continuous swine testis (ST), primary pig kidney, secondary pig thyroid, and primary pig salivary gland cells. Of these, the ST cell line is probably the most sensitive and reliable (Kemeny 1978, McClurkin and Norman 1966). The interference phenomenon with bovine virus diarrhea virus or pseudorabies virus has been used to demonstrate noncytopathogenic strains of TGEV in cell cultures (McClurkin 1965, Pehl 1966).

Epizootiology and Pathogenesis. It seems certain that normal transmission of the virus occurs by the fecal-oral route, although the respiratory route and air-borne transmission may also be of importance (Kemeny et al. 1975; Laude et al. 1984; Reber 1956; Underdahl et al. 1974, 1975; Young et al. 1955). Virus has been recovered from intestinal material and lung homogenates for as long as 104 days after exposure and from nasal swabs for as long as 11 days. Fecal shedding under natural conditions may persist for up to 10 weeks in certain instances (Lee et al. 1954), although the duration is usually shorter. It has been suggested that chronic carrier pigs may harbor infections in the respiratory tract, possibly in alveolar or bronchiolar epithelial cells or in alveolar macrophages (Kemeny 1981, Laude et al. 1984, Underdahl et al. 1974, 1975).

Epizootic TGE usually occurs during the colder months of the year (November to April), possibly because the virus is more stable in the frozen state and less subject to direct sunlight in the winter. Birds may also be involved in its spread. Pilchard (1965) reported detection of TGEV in droppings of starlings for as long as 32 hours after ingestion of virus. Massive concentrations of these birds are commonly observed among swine in the midwestern region of the United States. Foxes, dogs, and cats also have been implicated as possible carriers of TGEV from farm to farm (Haelterman 1962, Larsen et al. 1979, McClurkin et al. 1970, Reynolds and Garwes 1979). Footware, clothing, and transport vehicles are potential mechanical vectors of the virus. Maintenance of TGEV in enzootic form in feeder pig operations may represent an important reservoir of infection between seasonal epizootics (Morin et al. 1978). Certain insect species, such as the housefly, may contribute to perpetuation of transmission during summer (Gough and Jorgenson 1983).

The pathogenesis of TGE is quite typical of coronavirus-induced diarrheas in a number of species. The virus replicates in the cytoplasm of the absorptive epithelial cells of the small intestine. These cells become susceptible to infection once they have migrated up from the crypts and onto the villi. Infection and rapid destruction or functional alteration of these cells produces a marked reduction in enzymatic activity in the small intestine, disrupting normal digestive processes and resulting in an acute malabsorption syndrome (Cross and Bohl 1969, Masek and Stepanek 1975, Thake 1968). Altered sodium transport in the jejunum (Butler et al. 1974) and loss of extravascular protein (Procházka et al. 1975) also occur. Morphologically, marked blunting and contraction of the villi occur, particularly in the jejunum and to a lesser extent in the ileum and duodenum, the result of epithelial cell desquamation. The higher survival rate of older piglets may be attributable in part to their ability to replace these cells at a faster rate than newborn pigs (Moon 1971). Attenuated strains of TGEV do not infect cells in the cranial portion of the small intestine, and this may explain their reduced virulence in vivo (Frederick et al. 1976, Furuuchi et al. 1979, Hess et al. 1977, Pensaert et al. 1970).

Immunity. It is generally agreed that pigs that have recovered from TGE usually are clinically protected when challenged with virulent test virus. Immunity to reinfection and disease is probably not complete, however, especially if the primary exposure occurred at a very young age and if the reexposure dose is severe and given some months later.

It has been observed that pigs born several weeks after the occurrence of an outbreak frequently escape the disease. When sows that have lost a litter are bred back immediately, the second litter is unaffected. It appears that the immunity of such animals is passive, but the protection transmitted to piglets by such immunized sows is not conferred by the absorption of antibodies from colostrum; rather, it depends on a continuous supply of IgA secreted in the sow's milk (lactogenic immunity) (Haelterman 1963). This IgA is produced only after the sow's intestine has been exposed to virulent TGEV (Bohl and Saif 1975, Bohl et al. 1972).

Some large swine farms that have suffered heavily from the disease follow the practice of feeding stored, frozen intestines from infected animals to their bred sows about a month before farrowing. The sows may experience a mild diarrhea but they recover, and their litters acquire enough immunity from their dams to protect them from the disease.

Diagnosis. A presumptive diagnosis of epizootic TGE can usually be made on the basis of clinical signs and a history of outbreaks on other premises in the area. The main features differentiating TGE from other enteric disorders of pigs are as follows: (1) rapidity of spread through all age groups, (2) lack of response to antibiotics, and (3) high mortality only in very young piglets and rapid recovery of older stock. Additional differences that separate TGE from other diseases include the absence of skin lesions, nervous signs, abortions, or stillbirths. Clinical signs may not differentiate TGE from porcine epidemic diarrhea (PED), which is caused by a coronavirus unrelated antigenically to TGEV (Pensaert 1981).

A presumptive diagnosis of enzootic TGE can be difficult, as it may not always be recognized by individuals familiar with only the more explosive epizootic form of TGE. It must be differentiated from other diseases such as coccidiosis, colibacillosis, and rotavirus diarrhea. A definitive diagnosis of TGE, in either its epizootic or enzootic form, is made by detection of viral antigen, with immunofluorescence microscopy, in frozen sections or mucosal scrapings of jejunum and ileum from piglets just beginning to have diarrhea (Black 1971, Konishi and Bankowski 1967, Pensaert et al. 1968). Subsequent isolation and identification of the virus in cell culture are confirmatory. The cell-culture immunofluorescence test is quite useful for detecting viral antigen at early passage levels (Bohl 1981). Negative-contrast electron microscopy does not differentiate TGEV from PED virus unless an immunoelectron microscopic approach is utilized (Saif et al. 1977). A serologic diagnosis may be made by demonstration of a rising antibody titer in paired acute and convalescent samples. If paired serums are unavailable, then simultaneous collection of samples from animals in different stages (acute, convalescent) of TGE can be used as an alternative method. If enzootic TGE is suspected, then serums from 2- to 6-month-old pigs should be tested. At this age, passively acquired antibody should be absent (Derbyshire et al. 1969), so that positive titers suggest enzootic TGEV infection. The most commonly utilized serologic procedure is the serum neutralization test, but many other techniques have been employed over the years. Other procedures described include an indirect immunofluorescence test (Benfield et al. 1978), indirect immunoperoxidase test (Kodama et al. 1980b, 1981), radioimmunoprecipitation (Kodama et al. 1980a), and enzyme-linked immunosorbent assay (Nelson and Kelling 1984).

Treatment. There is no specific treatment for TGE. Animal losses may be reduced by providing a warm, dry, draft-free environment and access to water, a glucose-electrolyte solution, or a milk replacer. However, most affected pigs less than 3 days of age will die regardless of treatment. Antibiotic therapy may be of some help in older animals if a concurrent bacterial infection (e.g., colibacillosis) is present.

Prevention and Control. Preventing entry of TGEV into a herd is frequently difficult. The virus is widespread in the swine population, and carrier pigs and pigs incubating the disease are ready sources of infection for susceptible animals (Bohl 1981, 1986; Hogg 1982; Underdahl and Torres-Medina 1981). Starlings, foxes, dogs, and cats may play a role in spreading the virus from one farm to another. In addition to these sources, muddy or feces-contaminated clothing and vehicles have accounted for many epizootics of TGE. Efforts at controlling entry of the virus should concentrate on several areas: (1) new stock should originate from TGEV-free herds, should be serologically negative, or should be placed in isolation for 2 to 4 weeks before they mix with the herd proper; (2) visitors should not be allowed onto the premises without clean boots and outer clothing; (3) trucks and their drivers should not be allowed near the main breeding herd; and (4) measures should be taken to control access of birds, dogs, and feral mammals to the herd.

If TGE has been diagnosed in a herd and piglets have died, the sows should be rebred, because the subsequent litters from these immune animals will be protected by lactogenic immunity. Among pregnant animals, those that are at least 2 or 3 weeks from farrowing can be fed minced intestines from pigs from the same herd that have died of TGE (material from another infected herd should not be used in order to prevent entry of other infectious agents). Sows that are 2 weeks or less from farrowing should be placed in individual isolation facilities or sold to market.

Several licensed vaccines are available for use in pregnant swine to provide passive immunity for sucklings. These vaccines are composed of modified live-virus and are given by the oral, intramuscular, or intramammary routes during the final 6 weeks of pregnancy. Most information suggests that these vaccines are of limited effectiveness when given to serologically negative pigs, that is, mortality is usually reduced but morbidity is unaffected (Bohl 1981, 1986; Crouch 1985). These vaccines may be useful for boosting existing immunity in previously infected swine, however, and thus are especially helpful for dealing with enzootic TGE.

A modified live small-plaque variant TGEV has received attention as a possible immunogen (Woods 1978, 1984). A viral subunit vaccine has been described that protected young, weaned swine against challenge with virulent virus (Gough et al. 1983).

The Disease in Humans. There is no conclusive evidence that TGEV causes disease in humans.

REFERENCES

Benfield, D.A., Haelterman, E.O., and Burnstein, T. 1978. An indirect fluorescent antibody test for antibodies to transmissible gastroenteritis of swine. Can. J. Comp. Med. 42:478–482.

Black, J.W. 1971. Diagnosis of TGE by FA: Evaluation of accuracy on field specimens. Proc. U.S. Anim. Health Assoc. 75:492–498.

Bohl, E.H. 1981. Transmissible gastroenteritis. In A.D. Leman, R.D. Glock, W.L. Mengeling, R.H.C. Penny, E. Scholl, and B. Straw, eds., Diseases of Swine, 5th ed. Iowa State University Press, Ames. Pp. 195–208.

Bohl, E.H. 1986. Transmissible gastro-enteritis virus. In J.L. Howard, ed., Current Veterinary Therapy: Food Animal Practice, 2d ed. W.B. Saunders, Philadelphia. Pp. 551–552.

Bohl, E.H., and Saif, L.J. 1975. Passive immunity in transmissible gastroenteritis of swine: Immunoglobulin characteristics of antibodies in milk after inoculating virus by different routes. Infect. Immun. 11:23–32.

Bohl, E.H., Gupta, R.K.P., McCloskey, L.W., and Saif, L. 1972. Immunology of transmissible gastroenteritis. J. Am. Vet. Med. Assoc. 160:543–549.

Butler, D.G., Gall, D.G., Kelly, M.H., and Hamilton, J.R. 1974. Transmissible gastroenteritis: Mechanisms responsible for diarrhea in an acute viral enteritis in piglets. J. Clin. Invest. 53:1335–1342.

Cartwright, S.F., Harris, H.M., Blandford, T.B., Fincham, I., and Gitter, M. 1965. A cytopathic virus causing a transmissible gastroenteritis in swine. I. Isolation and properties. J. Comp. Pathol. 75:387–396.

Chen, K.S. 1985. Enzymatic and acidic sensitivity profiles of selected virulent and attenuated transmissible gastroenteritis viruses of swine. Am. J. Vet. Res. 46:632–636.

Cross, R.F., and Bohl, E.H. 1969. Some criteria for the field diagnosis of porcine transmissible gastroenteritis. J. Am. Vet. Med. Assoc. 154:266–272.

Crouch, C.F. 1985. Vaccination against enteric rota and coronaviruses in cattle and pigs: Enhancement of lactogenic immunity. Vaccine 3:284–291.

Derbyshire, J.B., Jessett, D.M., and Newman, G. 1969. An experimental epidemiological study of porcine transmissible gastroenteritis. J. Comp. Pathol. 79:445–452.

Doyle, L.P., and Hutchings, L.M. 1946. A transmissible gastroenteritis in pigs. J. Am. Vet. Med. Assoc. 108:257–259.

Frederick, G.T., Bohl, E.H., and Cross, R.F. 1976. Pathogenicity of an attenuated strain of transmissible gastroenteritis virus for newborn pigs. Am. J. Vet. Res. 37:165–169.

Furuuchi, S., Shimizu, Y., and Kumagai, T. 1979. Multiplication of low and high cell culture passaged strains of transmissible gastroenteritis virus in organs of newborn piglets. Vet. Microbiol. 3:169–178.

Gough, P.M., and Jorgenson, R.D. 1983. Identification of porcine transmissible gastroenteritis virus in house flies (Musca domestica Linnaeus). Am. J. Vet. Res. 44:2078–2082.

Gough, P.M., Ellis, C.H., Frank, C.J., and Johnson, C.J. 1983. A viral subunit immunogen for porcine transmissible gastroenteritis. Antiviral Res. 3:211–221.

Haelterman, E.O. 1962. Epidemiological studies of transmissible gastroenteritis of swine. Proc. U.S. Livestock Sanit. Assoc. 66:305–315.

Haelterman, E.O. 1963. Transmissible gastroenteritis of swine. Proceedings of the World Veterinary Congress 17:615–618.

Hess, R.G., and Bachmann, P.A. 1976. In vitro differentiation and pH sensitivity of field and cell culture-attenuated strains of transmissible gastroenteritis virus. Infect. Immun. 13:1642–1646.

Hess, R.G., Bachmann, P.A., and Hänichen, T. 1977. Versuche zur Entwicklung einer Immunprophylaxe gegen die Übertragbare Gastroenteritis (TGE) der Schweine. I. Pathogenität des Stammes B1 im Verlaufe von Serienpassagen. Zentralbl. Veterinärmed. [B] 24:753–763.

Hogg, A. 1982. TGE: Epizootic and enzootic. Mod. Vet. Pract. 63:489–492.

Hooper, B.E., and Haelterman, E.O. 1966. Growth of transmissible gastroenteritis virus in young pigs. Am. J. Vet. Res. 27:286–291.

Kemeny, L.J. 1976. Antibody response in pigs inoculated with transmissible gastroenteritis virus and cross reactions among ten isolates. Can. J. Comp. Med. 40:209–214.

Kemeny, L.J. 1978. Isolation of transmissible gastroenteritis virus from pharyngeal swabs obtained from sows at slaughter. Am. J. Vet. Res. 39:703–705.

Kemeny, L.J. 1981. Isolation of transmissible gastroenteritis virus, pseudorabies virus, and porcine enterovirus from pharyngeal swabs taken from market-weight swine. Am. J. Vet. Res. 42:1987–1989.

Kemeny, L.J., Wiltsey, V.L., and Riley, J.L. 1975. Upper respiratory infection of lactating sows with transmissible gastroenteritis virus following contact exposure to infected piglets. Cornell Vet. 65:352–362.

Kodama, Y., Ogata, M., and Shimizu, Y. 1980a. Detection of antibody against transmissible gastroenteritis virus of pigs by indirect immunoperoxidase antibody test. Am. J. Vet. Res. 41:133–135.

Kodama, Y., Ogata, M., and Shimizu, Y. 1980b. Characterization of immunoglobulin A antibody in serum of swine inoculated with transmissible gastroenteritis virus. Am. J. Vet. Res. 41:740–745.

Kodama, Y., Ogata, M., and Shimizu, Y. 1981. Serum immunoglobulin A antibody response in swine infected with transmissible gastroenteritis virus, as determined by indirect immunoperoxidase antibody test. Am. J. Vet. Res. 42:437–442.

Konishi, S., and Bankowski, R.A. 1967. Use of fluorescein-labeled antibody for rapid diagnosis of transmissible gastroenteritis in experimentally infected pigs. Am. J. Vet. Res. 28:937–942.

Larson, D.J., Morehouse, L.G., Solorzano, R.F., and Kinden, D.A. 1979. Transmissible gastroenteritis in neonatal dogs: Experimental intestinal infection with transmissible gastroenteritis virus. Am. J. Vet. Res. 40:479–486.

Laude, H. 1981. Thermal inactivation studies of a coronavirus, transmissible gastroenteritis virus. J. Gen. Virol. 56:235–240.

Laude, H., Charley, B., and Gelfi, J. 1984. Replication of transmissible gastroenteritis coronavirus (TGEV) in swine alveolar macrophages. J. Gen. Virol. 65:327–332.

Laude, H., Gelfi, J., and Aynaud, J.M. 1981. In vitro properties of low- and high-passaged strains of transmissible gastroenteritis coronavirus of swine. Am. J. Vet. Res. 42:447–449.

Lee, K.M., Moro, M., and Baker, J.A. 1954. Transmissible gastroenteritis in pigs. Am. J. Vet. Res. 15:364–372.

McClurkin, A.W. 1965. Studies on transmissible gastroenteritis of swine. I. The isolation and identification of a cytopathogenic virus of transmissible gastroenteritis in primary swine kidney cell cultures. Can. J. Comp. Med. 29:46–53.

McClurkin, A.W., and Norman, J.O. 1966. Studies on transmissible gastroenteritis of swine. II. Selected characteristics of a cytopathogenic virus common to five isolates from transmissible gastroenteritis. Can. J. Comp. Med. 30:190–198.

McClurkin, A.W., Stark, S.L., and Norman, J.O. 1970. Transmissible gastroenteritis (TGE) of swine: The possible role of dogs in the epizootiology of TGE. Can. J. Comp. Med. 34:347–349.

Masek, J.J., and Stepanek, J. 1975. Biochemical changes in piglets infected with transmissible gastroenteritis virus. Acta Vet. Brno 44:79–85.

Moon, H.W. 1971. Epithelial cell migration in the alimentary mucosa of the suckling pig. Proc. Soc. Exp. Biol. Med. 137:151–154.

Morin, M., Solorzano, R.F., Morehouse, L.G., and Olson, L.D. 1978. The postulated role of feeder swine in the perpetuation of the transmissible gastroenteritis virus. Can. J. Comp. Med. 42:379–384.

Nelson, L.D., and Kelling, C.L. 1984. Enzyme-linked immunosorbent assay for detection of transmissible gastroenteritis virus antibody in swine sera. Am. J. Vet. Res. 45:1654–1657.

Pedersen, N.C., Ward, J., and Mengeling, W.L. 1978. Antigenic relationship of the feline infectious peritonitis virus to coronaviruses of other species. Arch. Virol. 58:45–53.

Pehl, K.H. 1966. Der Nachweis eines nichtzytopathogenen Stammes der Virus-Gastroenteritis der Ferkel (TGE-Typ) mit Hilfe von Interferenzerscheinungen zwischen diesem Stamm und dem Aujeszkyvirus in Ferkelnieren-Einschichtzellkulturen. Arch. Exp. Veterinärmed. 20:909–920.

Pensaert, M.B. 1981. Porcine epidemic diarrhea. In A.D. Leman, R.D. Glock, W.L. Mengeling, R.H.C. Penny, E. Scholl, and B. Straw, eds., Diseases of Swine, 5th ed. Iowa State University Press, Ames. Pp. 344–346.

Pensaert, M.B., Haelterman, E.O., and Burnstein, T. 1968. Diagnosis of transmissible gastroenteritis in pigs by means of immunofluorescence. Can. J. Comp. Med. 32:555–561.

Pensaert, M., Haelterman, E.O., and Burnstein, T. 1970. Transmissible gastroenteritis of swine: Virus-intestinal cell interactions. I. Immunofluorescence, histopathology and virus production in the small intestine through the course of infection. Arch. Gesam. Virusforsch. 31:321–334.

Pilchard, E.I. 1965. Experimental transmission of transmissible gastroenteritis virus by starlings. Am. J. Vet. Res. 26:1177–1179.

Prochàzka, Z., Hampl, J., Sedlàcek, M., Masek, J., and Stepànek, J. 1975. Protein loss in piglets infected with transmissible gastroenteritis virus. Zentralbl. Veterinärmed. [B] 22:138–146.

Reber, E.F. 1956. Airborne transmissible gastroenteritis. Am. J. Vet. Res. 17:194–195.

Reynolds, D.J., and Garwes, D.J. 1979. Virus isolation and serum antibody responses after infection of cats with transmissible gastroenteritis virus. Arch. Virol. 60:161–166.

Saif, L.J., Bohl, E.H., Kohler, E.M., and Hughes, J.H. 1977. Immune electron microscopy of transmissible gastroenteritis virus and rotavirus (reovirus-like agent) of swine. Am. J. Vet. Res. 38:13–20.

Thake, D.C. 1968. Jejunal epithelium in transmissible gastroenteritis of swine. An electron microscopic and histochemical study. Am. J. Pathol. 53:149–168.

Underdahl, N.R., and Torres-Medina, A. 1981. Transmissible gastroenteritis (TGE) of pigs. In J. L. Howard, ed., Current Veterinary Therapy: Food Animal Practice. W.B. Saunders, Philadelphia. Pp. 592–595.

Underdahl, N.R., Mebus, C.A., Stair, E.I., Rhodes, M.B., McGill, L.D., and Twiehaus, M.J. 1974. Isolation of transmissible gastroenteritis virus from lungs of market-weight swine. Am. J. Vet. Res. 35:1209–1216.

Underdahl, N.R., Mebus, C.A., and Torres-Medina, A. 1975. Recovery of transmissible gastroenteritis virus from chronically infected experimental pigs. Am. J. Vet. Res. 36:1473–1476.

Woods, R.D. 1978. Small plaque variant transmissible gastroenteritis virus. J. Am. Vet. Med. Assoc. 173:643–647.

Woods, R.D. 1984. Efficacy of vaccination of sows with serologically related coronaviruses for control of transmissible gastroenteritis in nursing pigs. Am. J. Vet. Res. 45:1726–1729.

Young, G.A., Hinz, R.W., and Underdahl, N.R. 1955. Some characteristics of transmissible gastroenteritis (TGE) in disease-free antibody-devoid pigs. Am. J. Vet. Res. 16:529–535.

Porcine Epidemic Diarrhea

In recent years coronaviruses antigenically distinct from transmissible gastroenteritis (TGE) virus and hemagglutinating encephalomyelitis virus have been incriminated in epizootics of porcine diarrhea in Europe, Canada, and Japan (Chasey and Cartwright 1978, Dea et al. 1985, Horvàth and Mocsàri 1981, Pensaert 1981, Pensaert and DeBouck 1978, Takahashi et al. 1983, Turgeon et al. 1980, Wood 1977). The most thoroughly studied of these agents associated with porcine epidemic diarrhea (PED) is coronavirus (CV) 777, first identified by Pensaert and DeBouck (1978) in Belgium.

Character of the Disease. Clinically, PED associated with CV 777 resembles an outbreak of TGE, characterized by acute diarrheal disease affecting pigs of all age groups. Morbidity is variable in sows but high (approaching 100 percent) in suckling pigs, which are most severely affected and exhibit vomiting, watery diarrhea, and dehydration. Mortality in piglets may be 50 percent or higher. Most fattening pigs and weaners recover from the disease, but some may remain unthrifty. In adults, anorexia, lethargy, and diarrhea are seen, but mortality is very low.

Pathological changes are limited primarily to the gastrointestinal tract. Histologically, lesions include blunting and fusion of small intestinal villi, with desquamation of infected epithelial cells into the gut lumen. The picture is generally typical of coronaviral enteritis.

Properties of the Virus. Morphologically, CV 777 and other agents associated with PED are typical of the coronavirus group. There is no apparent antigenic relationship between CV 777 and TGE virus, hemagglutinating encephalomyelitis virus, bovine coronavirus, canine coronavirus, feline infectious peritonitis virus, or avian infectious bronchitis virus (Pensaert et al. 1981); at least one PED-associated coronavirus appears to be unrelated to either TGE virus or CV 777 (Dea et al. 1985). There is no hemagglutinating activity associated with CV 777.

Cultivation. To date, no PED-associated coronavirus has been propagated in cell or explant culture. CV 777 has been successfully passaged in vivo in piglets (DeBouck and Pensaert 1980).

Epizootiology and Pathogenesis. PED-associated coronaviruses are spread primarily by the fecal oral route and by contaminated objects (fomites). There is no evidence that CV 777 persists on the premises after an epizootic. Outbreaks occur both in the winter and summer months. Little information is available on the prevalence and distribution of these coronaviruses in the swine population, but it is assumed that they are widespread (Pensaert 1981).

Replication of CV 777 occurs in the cytoplasm of villus epithelial cells of the small intestine and colon. The pathogenesis of the diarrhea is similar to that seen with TGE virus, bovine coronavirus, and canine coronavirus.

Immunity. Little is known about immunity in PED. One would expect colostral antibody and intestinal secretory antibody to be of primary importance in protection.

Diagnosis. Clinically, PED cannot be differentiated from TGE. A definitive diagnosis may be made by immunofluorescence microscopy of small intestinal tissue, using hyperimmune anti-TGEV, anti-CV 777 and anti-rotavirus reference serums for differentiation (Pensaert 1981).

Treatment. Treatment is entirely supportive and is aimed at fluid and electrolyte replacement and protection against secondary bacterial infection.

Prevention and Control. Pregnant sows that are more

than 2 weeks from farrowing should be fed minced fecal or intestinal material from affected pigs on the same premises in order to provide maternal immunity to neonates, in a manner similar to that employed for control of TGE (Pensaert 1981, Turgeon et al. 1980). No vaccine is available.

The Disease in Humans. PED is not known to occur in humans.

REFERENCES

Chasey, D., and Cartwright, S.F. 1978. Virus-like particles associated with porcine epidemic diarrhoea. Res. Vet. Sci. 25:255–256.

Dea, S., Vaillancourt, J., Elazhary, Y., and Martineau, G.P. 1985. An outbreak of diarrhea in piglets caused by a coronavirus antigenically distinct from transmissible gastroenteritis virus. Can. Vet. J. 26:108–111.

DeBouck, P., and Pensaert, M. 1980. Experimental infection of pigs with a new porcine enteric coronavirus, CV 777. Am. J. Vet. Res. 41:219–223.

Horvàth, I., and Mocsàri, E. 1981. Ultrastructural changes in the small intestinal epithelium of suckling pigs affected with a transmissible gastroenteritis (TGE)-like disease. Arch. Virol. 68:103–113.

Pensaert, M.B. 1981. Porcine epidemic diarrhea. In A.D. Leman, R.D. Glock, W.L. Mengeling, R.H.C. Penny, E. Scholl, and B. Straw, eds., Diseases of Swine, 5th ed. Iowa State University Press, Ames. Pp. 344–346.

Pensaert, M.B., and DeBouck, P. 1978. A new coronavirus-like particle associated with diarrhea in swine. Arch. Virol. 58:243–247.

Pensaert, M.B., DeBouck, P., and Reynolds, D.J. 1981. An immunoelectron microscopic and immunofluorescent study on the antigenic relationship between the coronavirus-like agent, CV 777, and several coronaviruses. Arch. Virol. 68:45–52.

Takahashi, K., Okada, K., and Ohshima, K. 1983. An outbreak of swine diarrhea of a new type associated with coronavirus-like particles in Japan. Jpn. J. Vet. Sci. 45:829–832.

Turgeon, D.C., Morin, M. Jolette, J., Higgins, R., Marsolais, G., and DiFranco, E. 1980. Coronavirus-like particles associated with diarrhea in baby pigs in Quebec. Can. Vet. J. 21:100–101.

Wood, E.N. 1977. An apparently new syndrome of porcine epidemic diarrhoea. Vet. Rec. 100:243–244.

Hemagglutinating Encephalomyelitis

SYNONYMS: Vomiting and wasting disease, Ontario encephalomyelitis, viral encephalomyelitis of piglets, suckling pig encephalomyelitis

In 1962 Greig et al. reported that they had isolated a hemagglutinating virus from baby pigs in Canada with encephalomyelitis. The signs and lesions of the disease were reproduced experimentally, and the virus was subsequently named hemagglutinating encephalomyelitis virus (HEV). In 1969 Cartwright et al. in England recovered a strain of HEV from suckling pigs affected with vomiting and wasting disease (VWD), a condition of previously unknown cause that, significantly, had first been recognized in Canada. This strain was subsequently shown to produce VWD in pigs (Cartwright and Lucas 1970). Al-

though clinical signs of neurological disease were not evident, histopathological examination revealed lesions of encephalomyelitis similar to those seen in Canada in about 25 percent of the diseased animals (Cartwright and Lucas 1970). Neurotropic differences in viral strains, differential susceptibilities of pigs, and immune status at the time of infection probably account for the variation in clinical signs seen in the two syndromes, encephalomyelitis and VWD, associated with HEV. In addition to Canada and England, the virus has been detected in the United States, Belgium, France, Germany, Switzerland, and Australia. The disease has been reviewed by Greig (1981).

Character of the Disease. The two clinical syndromes associated with HEV infection in piglets are peracute to acute nonsuppurative encephalomyelitis and subacute to chronic VWD.

Encephalomyelitis. In the original Canadian outbreaks, the affected animals were 4 to 7 days old when clinical signs first appeared, and morbidity and mortality in infected litters approached 100 percent (Mitchell 1963). The disease is characterized by anorexia, lethargy, loss of condition, vomiting, constipation, hyperesthesia, muscle tremors, and progressive posterior paresis. In advanced stages affected pigs exhibit prostration, paddling movements, progressive dyspnea, nystagmus, blindness, coma, and death. The disease course is usually 10 days or less and can be as short as 24 hours. In herds, only litters born within a few weeks of each other are affected; later litters are immune. Pigs that survive apparently recover completely (Alexander et al. 1959).

VWD. As in the encephalomyelitis syndrome, clinical signs are usually limited to animals less than a few weeks old. Clinical signs of VWD include anorexia, lethargy, progressive weight loss, vomiting, and constipation. Affected pigs appear thirsty but apparently cannot drink, possibly because of pharyngeal paralysis. Some animals die within 1 to 2 weeks, but in most the disease assumes a more chronic course, with death resulting from either starvation or concurrent disease. Those few that survive remain unthrifty.

Pathological changes are seen primarily in the central nervous system and the respiratory tract. Gross lesions generally are unremarkable, consisting of a mild catarrhal rhinitis in some animals with encephalomyelitis and gastroenteritis in those with VWD. Histological lesions frequently include a nonsuppurative encephalomyelitis characterized by perivascular mononuclear cell cuffing, gliosis, neuronal degeneration, and meningitis. The most severe lesions are almost always confined to the gray matter of the mesencephalon, pons, medulla, and upper spinal cord. Demyelination has not been reported (Werdin et al. 1976). Similar but less extensive lesions can be found during the early stages of VWD.

Experimentally, histological changes in the respiratory tract, consisting of focal or diffuse interstitial peribronchiolar pneumonia, hypertrophy of alveolar epithelium, alveolar emphysema, and mononuclear cell infiltration of turbinate and tracheal submucosal tissues, have been reported (Cutlip and Mengeling 1972). Lesions of such intensity have not been reported in field animals, however.

Properties of the Virus. Morphologically, HEV particles are typical of the coronavirus group (Greig et al. 1971, Phillip et al. 1971). There is no apparent antigenic relationship to porcine transmissible gastroenteritis virus or porcine epidemic diarrhea virus. Hemagglutination and hemadsorption of erythrocytes from several species (chicken, turkey, mouse, rat, hamster) have been demonstrated (Girard et al. 1964, Mengeling et al. 1972). There is no evidence of neuraminidase and thus no spontaneous elution. Red cells treated with receptor-destroying enzyme are still agglutinated by HEV, but hemagglutination is inhibited by mucins and animal serums.

The HEV is quite labile in the presence of heat but reasonably stable at refrigerator and freezer temperatures and in the lyophilized state (Greig and Girard 1963). Ether and chloroform destroy its infectivity and hemagglutinating activity.

Cultivation. HEV replicates in primary cultures of pig kidney and pig thyroid cells, with the formation of syncytia only in kidney cells (Greig et al. 1962). Most established porcine cell lines do not support HEV growth and replication. The virus has been adapted to the suckling mouse brain (Kaye et al. 1977).

Epizootiology and Pathogenesis. The virus is spread by aerosolization and direct physical contact with infected animals; it apparently enters the body through the upper respiratory tract (Appel et al. 1965, Mengeling and Cutlip 1972). Peripheral nerve tracts in the nasal and turbinate mucosa are invaded, with subsequent extension of infection to the brain, resulting in encephalomyelitis. Ultrastructural studies have demonstrated virus particles in neurons but not in glial (or other neural) cells, indicating a possible neuron-to-neuron transmission (Meyvisch and Hoorens 1978). The extent of central nervous system damage determines the character and severity of clinical signs. In VWD, spread of HEV occurs from the nasal mucosa to the tonsils, respiratory tract, brain, and stomach wall. Infection of the stomach wall apparently results in the characteristic vomiting syndrome of VWD (Andries and Pensaert 1980, Andries et al. 1978).

Immunity. The first appearance of disease in a herd frequently follows the introduction of new stock (Mitchell

1963). The virus spreads rapidly by direct contact and aerosolization and confers a strong herd immunity (Appel et al. 1965). Hence the disease can be considered essentially self-limiting. Infection is widespread, especially in areas of concentrated swine production, but it is usually subclinical, held in check by herd immunity. If, however, a susceptible nonimmune herd is infected during farrowing, then litters may be affected over several weeks, with high rates of morbidity and mortality.

Diagnosis. A tentative diagnosis of piglet encephalomyelitis or VWD is based on history, the occurrence of the characteristic clinical signs almost exclusively among pigs less than a few weeks of age, and postmortem histopathological findings. A definitive diagnosis requires isolation of HEV from brain or spinal cord or demonstration of HEV-infected neurons by immunofluorescence microscopy. Brain stem tissue from piglets that have shown clinical signs for no more than 48 hours, and preferably for less than 24 hours, is the material of choice for HEV isolation. Identification of the virus can be made by hemagglutination and hemadsorption tests, immunofluorescence or electron microscopy, and virus neutralization. Serologic tests used to demonstrate rising antibody titers (paired acute and convalescent serums) in infected piglets or dams are limited primarily to neutralization in pig kidney cell cultures and hemagglutination inhibition. A positive antibody titer in a single (unpaired) serum sample should be interpreted with extreme caution because subclinical HEV infections are widespread.

The differential diagnosis for piglet encephalomyelitis and VWD should include pseudorabies and Teschen disease (both often affect older pigs as well) and transmissible gastroenteritis (produces vomiting but also diarrhea, and central nervous system signs are absent).

Treatment. There is no specific treatment for HEV infection.

Prevention and Control. The outbreak generally is self-limiting. Neonates are well protected by colostral antibody, and this undoubtedly contributes to the relative rarity of clinical disease. Hence knowledge of the immune status of a herd, particularly the sows, would provide a basis on which the practitioner could devise means of control by appropriate management procedures. The sporadic nature of the disease makes vaccination economically unrealistic, and no commercial vaccine is available.

The Disease in Humans. There is no evidence that HEV causes disease in humans.

REFERENCES

Alexander, T.J.L., Richards, W.P.C., and Roe, C.K. 1959. An encephalomyelitis of suckling pigs in Ontario. Can. J. Comp. Med. 23:316–319.

Andries, K., and Pensaert, M.B. 1980. Virus isolation and immunofluorescence in different organs of pigs infected with hemagglutinating encephalomyelitis virus. Am. J. Vet. Res. 41:215–218.

Andries, K., Pensaert, M., and Callebaut, P. 1978. Pathogenicity of hemagglutinating encephalomyelitis (vomiting and wasting disease) virus of pigs, using different routes of inoculation. Zentralbl. Veterinärmed. [B] 25:461–468.

Appel, M., Greig, A.S., and Corner, A.H. 1965. Encephalomyelitis of swine caused by a hemagglutinating virus. IV. Transmission studies. Res. Vet. Sci. 6:482–489.

Cartwright, S.F., and Lucas, M. 1970. Vomiting and wasting disease in piglets. Virological and epidemiological studies. Vet. Rec. 86:278–280.

Cartwright, S.F., Lucas, M., Cavill, J.P., Gush, A.F., and Blandford, T.B. 1969. Vomiting and wasting disease of piglets. Vet Rec. 84:175–176.

Cutlip, R.C., and Mengeling, W.L. 1972. Lesions induced by hemagglutinating encephalomyelitis virus strain 67N in pigs. Am. J. Vet. Res. 33:2003–2009.

Girard, A., Greig, A.S., and Mitchell, D. 1964. Encephalomyelitis of swine caused by a hemagglutinating virus. III. Serological studies. Res. Vet. Sci. 5:294–302.

Greig, A.S. 1981. Hemagglutinating encephalomyelitis. In A.D. Leman, R.D. Glock, W.L. Mengeling, R.H.C. Penny, E. Scholl, and B. Straw, eds., Diseases of Swine, 5th ed. Iowa State University Press, Ames. Pp. 246–253.

Greig, A.S., and Girard, A. 1963. Encephalomyelitis of swine caused by a hemagglutinating virus. II. Virological studies. Res. Vet. Sci. 4:511–517.

Greig, A.S., Johnson, C.M., and Bouillant, A.M.P. 1971. Encephalomyelitis of swine caused by a hemagglutinating virus. VI. Morphology of the virus. Res. Vet. Sci. 12:305–307.

Greig, A.S., Mitchell, D., Corner, A.H., Bannister, G.L., Meads, E.B., and Julian, R.J. 1962. A hemagglutinating virus producing encephalomyelitis in baby pigs. Can. J. Comp. Med. 26:49–56.

Kaye, H.S., Yarbrough, W.B., Reed, C.J., and Harrison, A.K. 1977. Antigenic relationship between human coronavirus strain OC43 and hemagglutinating encephalomyelitis virus strain 67N of swine: Antibody responses in human and animal sera. J. Infect. Dis. 135:201–209.

Mengeling, W.L., and Cutlip, R.C. 1972. Experimentally induced infection of newborn pigs with hemagglutinating encephalomyelitis virus strain 67N. Am. J. Vet. Res. 33:953–956.

Mengeling, W.L., Boothe, A.D., and Ritchie, A.E. 1972. Characteristics of a coronavirus (strain 67N) of pigs. Am. J. Vet. Res. 33:297–308.

Meyvisch, C., and Hoorens, J. 1978. An electron microscopic study of experimentally-induced HEV encephalitis. Vet. Pathol. 15:102–113.

Mitchell, D. 1963. Encephalomyelitis of swine caused by a hemagglutinating virus. I. Case histories. Res. Vet. Sci. 4:506–510.

Phillip, J.I.H., Cartwright, S.F., and Scott, A.C. 1971. The size and morphology of TGE and vomiting and wasting disease viruses of pigs. Vet. Rec. 88:311–312.

Werdin, R.E., Sorensen, D.K., and Stewart, W.C. 1976. Porcine encephalomyelitis caused by hemagglutinating encephalomyelitis virus. J. Am. Vet. Med. Assoc. 168:240–246.

Canine Coronavirus Infection

Canine coronavirus (CCV) was first isolated in 1971 from military dogs in Germany during an epizootic of diarrheal disease (Binn et al. 1974). Pups experimentally infected with the virus developed a diarrheal syndrome similar to that seen in intestinal coronavirus infections of other species (Keenan et al. 1976, Takeuchi et al. 1976). The significance of CCV infections, however, was not widely appreciated until 1978, when outbreaks of CCV-associated diarrhea were reported in dogs throughout the United States (Appel et al. 1978, Carmichael 1978). Serologic and electron microscopic studies indicate that CCV infections are common in many parts of the world.

Character of the Disease. Infections range in severity from inapparent to fatal, with younger animals more severely affected (Carmichael and Binn 1981). Clinical signs include anorexia, lethargy, vomiting, dehydration, and diarrhea. There may be mucus or blood or both in the feces. Stools are loose, often yellow-orange, and characteristically fetid. Watery or bloody projectile diarrhea has been observed. Some pups may be extremely dehydrated. Many animals remain afebrile. Recovery without treatment usually occurs in 7 to 10 days. Relapses after 1 to 3 weeks have been reported, with deaths in a few instances (Carmichael 1978). Occasionally diarrhea persists for 3 to 4 weeks even with treatment. Young pups with severe diarrhea may die suddenly, especially if they are stressed by fatigue, concurrent disease (canine parvovirus infection, intestinal parasitism), or sudden changes in temperature. Morbidity is variable, but mortality is usually low.

In experimental studies in neonates, CCV caused diarrhea that persisted for about a week (Keenan et al. 1976). Virus could be recovered from rectal swabs for 6 to 9 days after infection and was present in all sections of the small intestine, colon, and mesenteric lymph nodes. No mortality or complications were reported.

Pathological changes are seen primarily in the gastrointestinal tract (Keenan et al. 1976, Takeuchi et al. 1976). Histologically, the intestinal villi are shortened and show blunting and focal fusion. The crypts are lengthened, and there is an initial increase in cellularity in the lamina propria. The virus infects apical epithelial cells along the entire length of the small intestine, with diarrhea accompanying morphologic and functional alteration of the villi. Virus particles are released in high titers into the gut lumen within exfoliated cells and from ruptured cell membranes. With the return of structural integrity of the small intestinal cells, usually by postinfection day 10, clinical signs disappear and the amount of virus excreted drops to a low level. Experimentally, infected dogs may excrete virus in feces for as long as 2 weeks. Recovery is accompanied by the development of neutralizing antibodies.

Infection of the colonic mucosa of diarrheic dogs with an unidentified coronavirus has been reported (Vandenberghe 1980), but this is atypical for CCV.

Properties of the Virus. Morphologic and physicochemical studies indicate that CCV particles are typical of the coronavirus group (Binn et al. 1974, Carmichael 1978). Virions are acid-stable, enveloped, and contain RNA and three major structural polypeptides. Antigenic cross-reactivity with both transmissible gastroenteritis virus and feline infectious peritonitis virus has been reported (Pedersen et al. 1978, Reynolds et al. 1980). Antigenic variation among CCV isolates has been observed (Appel et al. 1979, Carmichael and Binn 1981), but variants appear to belong to a single viral serotype.

Cultivation. CCV replicates in a variety of primary and continuous canine cell cultures, and in Crandell feline kidney cells and feline embryonic fibroblasts. The canine A-72 cell line (Binn et al. 1980) is especially useful for propagation of CCV strains. Syncytium formation in infected cultures is a characteristic but not universal finding (Yasoshima et al. 1983).

Epizootiology and Pathogenesis. Dogs of all breeds and ages are susceptible to CCV infection, as are coyotes (Evermann et al. 1980). The disease is acquired by contact with infected animals or their feces; infection occurs primarily by the oral route. Contaminated fomites may remain infectious for extended periods during the winter months (Carmichael and Binn 1981). The virus is highly contagious. Serologic evidence exists of widespread (probably subclinical) infection in the canine population.

In general, the pathology and pathogenesis of CCV infection are remarkably similar to those of porcine transmissible gastroenteritis virus and bovine coronavirus.

In addition to canids, CCV also infects cats, producing an asymptomatic infection with excretion of the virus from the oropharynx for as long as a week (Barlough et al. 1984, Stoddart et al. 1985).

Immunity. As in other intestinal coronavirus infections, local secretory antibody (IgA) in the gut is probably of primary importance in protection. It is likely that maternal immunity protects most neonates.

Diagnosis. A tentative diagnosis is based on history, the appearance of characteristic clinical signs, identification of coronavirus particles in feces by negative-contrast electron microscopy, and, in animals that have died, on postmortem histopathological findings. Mixed infections with other etiological agents must also be considered. A definitive diagnosis requires isolation of CCV from feces, gut scrapings, or intestinal tissue and immunofluorescence microscopy of infected intestinal cells. Fresh tissues obtained at necropsy are the material of choice for CCV isolation. Immunoelectron microscopy with hyperimmune anti-CCV reference serum and paired (acute and convalescent) serum neutralization tests are also useful in making a diagnosis.

Treatment. Treatment is primarily supportive and should be directed at the control of vomiting and fluid and electrolyte losses in severely affected pups. Warmth and reduction of stress also promote recovery.

Prevention and Control. Recently a modified live-

CCV vaccine was developed and marketed, but it was voluntarily withdrawn following widespread reports of adverse reactions (Martin 1985, Payton et al. 1984). Because subclinical CCV infections are common, vaccines may have limited efficacy, and the cost and risk of vaccination may outweigh any potential benefits (Pollock and Zimmer 1986).

The Disease in Humans. There is no evidence that CCV causes disease in humans.

REFERENCES

Appel, M.J.G., Cooper, B.J., Greisen, H., and Carmichael, L.E. 1978. Status report: Canine viral enteritis. J. Am. Vet. Med. Assoc. 173:1516–1518.

Appel, M.J.G., Meunier, P., Greisen, H., Carmichael, L.E., and Glickman, L. 1979. Enteric viral infections of dogs. Gaines Vet. Symp. 29:3–8.

Barlough, J.E., Stoddart, C.A., Sorresso, G.P., Jacobson, R.H., and Scott, F.W. 1984. Experimental inoculation of cats with canine coronavirus and subsequent challenge with feline infectious peritonitis virus. Lab. Anim. Sci. 34:592–597.

Binn, L.N., Lazar, E.C., Keenan, K.P., Huxsoll, D.L., Marchwicki, R.H., and Strano, A.J. 1974. Recovery and characterization of a coronavirus from military dogs with diarrhea. Proc. U.S. Anim. Health Assoc. 78:359–366.

Binn, L.N., Marchwicki, R.H., and Stephenson, E.H. 1980. Establishment of a canine cell line: Derivation, characterization, and viral spectrum. Am. J. Vet. Res. 41:855–860.

Carmichael, L.E. 1978. Infectious canine enteritis caused by a corona-like virus. Canine Pract. 5(4):25–27.

Carmichael, L.E., and Binn, L.N. 1981. New enteric viruses in the dog. Adv. Vet. Sci. Comp. Med. 25:1–37.

Evermann, J.F., Foreyt, W., Maag-Miller, L., Leathers, C.W., McKeirnan, A.J., and LeaMaster, B. 1980. Acute hemorrhagic enteritis associated with canine coronavirus and parvovirus infections in a captive coyote population. J. Am. Vet. Med. Assoc. 177:784–786.

Keenan, K.P., Jervis, H.R., Marchwicki, R.H., and Binn, L.N. 1976. Intestinal infection of neonatal dogs with canine coronavirus 1-71: Studies by virologic, histologic, histochemical, and immunofluorescent techniques. Am. J. Vet. Res. 37:247–256.

Martin, M.L. 1985. Canine coronavirus enteritis and a recent outbreak following modified live virus vaccination. Compend. Cont. Ed. Pract. Vet. 7:1012–1017.

Payton, A.J., Martin, M.L., Glickman, L.T., and Morris, C.F. 1984. Adverse reactions to a new canine coronavirus vaccine. Lab. Anim. Sci. 34:508.

Pedersen, N.C., Ward, J., and Mengeling, W.L. 1978. Antigenic relationship of the feline infectious peritonitis virus to coronaviruses of other species. Arch. Virol. 58:45–53.

Pollock, R.V.H., and Zimmer, J.F. 1986. Canine enteric infections. In F.W. Scott, ed., Contemporary Issues in Small Animal Practice, vol. 3: Infectious Diseases. Churchill Livingstone, New York. Pp. 55–80.

Reynolds, D.J., Garwes, D.J., and Lucey, S. 1980. Differentiation of canine coronavirus and porcine transmissible gastroenteritis virus by neutralization with canine, porcine and feline sera. Vet. Microbiol. 5:283–290.

Stoddart, C.A., Baldwin, C.A., and Scott, F.W. 1985. Unpublished data. Cornell Feline Health Center, Ithaca, N.Y.

Takeuchi, A., Binn, L.N., Jervis, H.R., Keenan, K.P., Hildebrandt, P.K., Valas, R.B., and Bland, F.F. 1976. Electron microscope study of experimental enteric infection in neonatal dogs with a canine coronavirus. Lab. Invest. 34:539–549.

Vandenberghe, J., Ducatelle, R., DeBouck, P., and Hoorens, J. 1980. Coronavirus infection in a litter of pups. Vet. Q. 2:136–141.

Yasoshima, A., Fujinami, F., Doi, K., Kojima, A., Takada, H., and Okaniwa, A. 1983. Case report on mixed infection of canine parvovirus and canine coronavirus—Electron microscopy and recovery of canine coronavirus. Jpn. J. Vet. Sci. 45:217–225.

Bovine Coronavirus Infection

SYNONYMS: Neonatal calf diarrhea coronavirus infection; Nebraska calf diarrhea coronavirus infection

Bovine coronavirus (BCV) infection was first described by Mebus and colleagues during a field trial of an oral rotavirus vaccine (Mebus et al. 1972, 1973a, 1973b, 1975; Sharpee et al. 1976; Stair et al. 1972). Coronavirus particles were identified by electron microscopy in feces of diarrheic calves from several herds. Feces collected from one affected herd produced enteric disease in experimentally inoculated calves.

BCV infection is a component of the acute diarrheal disease complex of neonatal calves—a very common and serious economic problem in dairy and beef operations.

Character of the Disease. The disease occurs in farm and ranch calves 1 day to 3 or more weeks old. The principal clinical sign is acute diarrhea. The appearance of the initial diarrhea is similar to that seen in rotavirus diarrhea: feces are liquid and yellow and may contain curd or mucus. The volume depends on the quantity of milk consumed before onset. The diarrhea can persist for 5 to 6 days, during which time calves may continue to eat and accept milk; however, weakness, lethargy, severe dehydration, and hypovolemic shock may develop in some severely affected animals. Factors contributing to the severity of the disease are multiple and probably include immune status of the dam and calf, dose of virus received, failure to ingest colostrum, secondary bacterial infection, and coinfection with other viral agents.

Gross pathological findings in uncomplicated cases are generally unremarkable. There may be a reddening of the intestinal mucosa resulting from secondary bacterial infection and fluid contents or a greenish mucoid fecal cast in the colon. Histopathological lesions consist of blunting and fusion of small intestinal villi (Figure 57.4), desquamation of villus epithelial cells, and replacement by immature cells that have a squamous or cuboidal morphology and are deficient in enzymatic activity. Viral rep-

Figure 57.4. Scanning electron micrograph of lower ileum from a gnotobiotic calf infected with bovine coronavirus. Villi are of irregular length, and numerous adjacent villi are fused. × 100. (From C. A. Mebus, 36 [1975]:1723, courtesy of *American Journal of Veterinary Research.*)

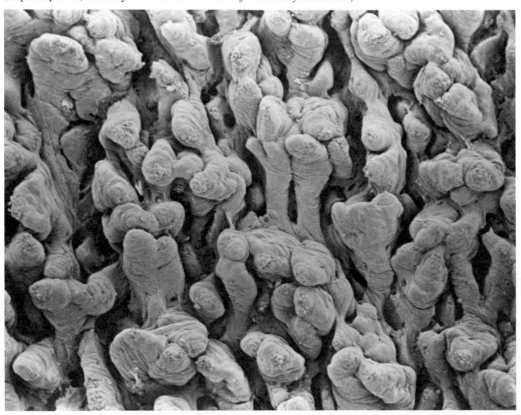

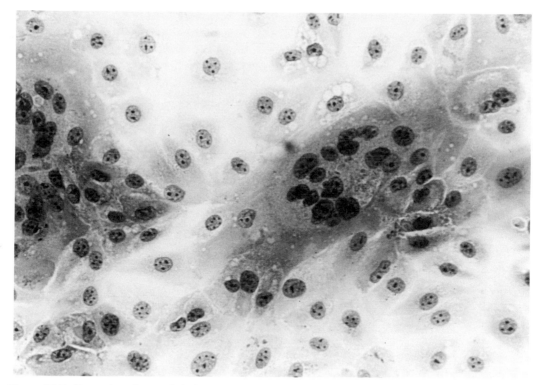

Figure 57.5. Formation of syncytia in fetal bovine kidney cells infected with bovine coronavirus. (Courtesy C. A. Mebus, Plum Island Animal Disease Center, U.S. Dept. of Agriculture.)

lication occurs in the cytoplasm of intestinal epithelial cells and in some cells in the lamina propria (Storz et al. 1978).

Certain strains of BCV are capable of infecting the respiratory tract and producing disease (McNulty et al. 1984, Reynolds et al. 1985, Thomas et al. 1982). The significance of such infections in the general bovine population, however, is not yet well understood.

Properties of the Virus. BCV is a typical member of the coronavirus group. It is antigenically related to murine hepatitis virus, hemagglutinating encephalomyelitis virus, rat (sialodacryoadenitis) virus, and human coronavirus OC43 (Gerna et al. 1981, 1982; Hogue et al 1984; Pedersen et al. 1978). Hemagglutinating and hemadsorptive activities have been reported for BCV (Sharpee et al. 1976).

Cultivation. The virus replicates in a number of cell-culture systems, including primary and secondary bovine fetal kidney, bovine embryonic kidney, Madin-Darby bovine kidney, Vero, and pig kidney-15 (PK-15) cells (Figure 57.5). Its cytopathic effects are often inconsistent, however, and not evident on primary isolation; the virus frequently requires adaptation to a given cell line before cytopathology becomes a useful tool in identification. Degree of cytopathogenicity and production of the

virus can be enhanced by treatment of the cell sheets with dactinomycin, trypsin, DEAE dextran, or hypertonic medium (Dea et al. 1980, Storz et al. 1981). The virus has also been adapted to the suckling mouse brain (Figure 57.6).

Epizootiology and Pathogenesis. The most likely sources of infection are carrier cows and their infected calves, with transmission accomplished primarily by the fecal-oral route (Crouch et al. 1985). Seroepizootiological and other studies indicate a wide geographic distribution for BCV in North America and Europe.

Following ingestion, the virus replicates in villus epithelial cells of the small intestine, resulting in loss of mature absorptive cells and their replacement by immature squamous to cuboidal epithelium (Mebus 1978). Continued ingestion of milk and prolonged presence of immature intestinal epithelium combine to accentuate the degree and duration of diarrhea, which is believed to be initiated by the initial viral infection with redirection of cell function from absorption to virion production. The amount of virus excreted in feces during the initial stages of diarrhea can be as high as 10^{10} particles per milliliter. Severely affected calves may become quite dehydrated and require extensive care to prevent development of hypovolemic shock and its consequences. In essence, BCV

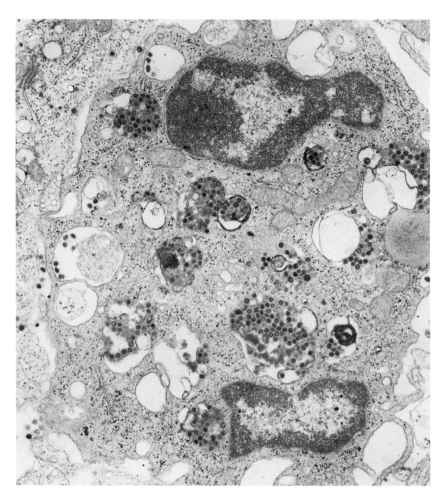

Figure 57.6. Bovine coronavirus in suckling mouse brain. Virions have accumulated in vacuoles within a macrophage. × 25,000. (Courtesy A. K. Harrison, Centers for Disease Control.)

infection presents a clinicopathological picture that is quite typical of coronavirus-induced diarrheas.

In addition to domestic cattle, certain wild ruminants—caribou, sitatunga, and waterbuck—appear to have been infected with BCV or a closely related coronavirus (Chasey et al. 1984, Elazhary et al. 1981).

Immunity. As with other intestinal coronavirus infections, local secretory antibody in the intestinal lumen is of primary importance in protection (Saif and Smith 1985). Maternal IgA will protect neonates for a limited time. In ideal situations, calves should become infected when some antibody is present, develop a subclinical infection, and thus become immunized.

Diagnosis. A definitive diagnosis of BCV-induced diarrhea can be made by identification by immunofluorescence microscopy of BCV antigen in frozen sections of spiral colon collected from a calf killed 1 to 4 days after the onset of diarrhea (Mebus 1978, 1986). Use of the serum neutralization test to demonstrate a rising antibody titer with acute and convalescent serums is another approach. Isolation of BCV in cell culture may also be attempted.

Treatment. No specific therapy exists for BCV infections; treatment is entirely supportive (fluid and electrolyte replacement, protection against secondary bacterial infection).

Prevention and Control. Programs for hygienic parturition and assurance of colostral acquisition should be initiated in a herd once BCV infection has been detected (Kahrs 1981). Extreme sanitary measures for rearing calves should be instituted, and immunization of all neonates and pregnant cattle should be considered. Halting an outbreak depends largely on correcting conditions that permit BCV transmission to stressed or colostrum-deprived calves and on initiating prompt therapeutic and preventive measures, including vaccination.

A modified live-virus vaccine, combined with proper hygienic measures, can reduce morbidity and mortality due to BCV infection. The vaccine, generally combined with a rotavirus component, should be administered orally to calves as soon as possible after birth and may also be used in pregnant cattle to stimulate production of colostral antibodies. Because of the multifactorial nature of the diarrhea complex in the neonatal calf, however, the vaccine may at times be only partially effective in preventing diarrhea. Assurance of colostral intake from immunized cows remains the most reliable means of protecting neonates against BCV disease.

The Disease in Humans. BCV infection is not known to occur in humans.

REFERENCES

Chasey, D., Reynolds, D.J., Bridger, J.C., Debney, T.G., and Scott, A.C. 1984. Identification of coronaviruses in exotic species of Bovidae. Vet. Rec. 115:602–603.

Crouch, C.F., Bielefeldt Ohmann, H., Watts, T.C., and Babiuk, L.A. 1985. Chronic shedding of bovine enteric coronavirus antigen-antibody complexes by clinically normal cows. J. Gen. Virol. 66:1489–1500.

Dea, S., Roy, R.S., and Begin, M.E. 1980. Bovine coronavirus isolation and cultivation in continuous cell lines. Am. J. Vet. Res. 41:30–38.

Elazhary, M.A.S.Y., Frechette, J.L., Silim, A., and Roy, R.S. 1981. Serological evidence of some bovine viruses in the caribou (*Rangifer tarandus caribou*) in Quebec. J. Wildl. Dis. 17:609–612.

Gerna, G., Battaglia, M., Cereda, P.M., and Passarani, N. 1982. Reactivity of human coronavirus OC43 and neonatal calf diarrhoea coronavirus membrane-associated antigens. J. Gen. Virol. 60:385 390.

Gerna, G., Cereda, P.M., Revello, M.G., Cattaneo, E., Battaglia, M., and Gerna, M.T. 1981. Antigenic and biological relationships between human coronavirus OC43 and neonatal calf diarrhoea coronavirus. J. Gen. Virol. 54:91–102.

Hogue, B.G., King, B., and Brian, D.A. 1984. Antigenic relationships among proteins of bovine coronavirus, human respiratory coronavirus OC43, and mouse hepatitis coronavirus A59. J. Virol. 51:384–388.

Kahrs, R.F. 1981. Virus Diseases of Cattle. Iowa State University Press, Ames. Pp. 107 113.

McNulty, M.S., Bryson, D.G., Allan, G.M., and Logan, E.F. 1984. Coronavirus infection of the bovine respiratory tract. Vet. Microbiol. 9:425–434.

Mebus, C.A. 1978. Pathogenesis of coronaviral infection in calves. J. Am. Vet. Med. Assoc. 173:631–632.

Mebus, C.A. 1986. Calf coronavirus diarrhea. In J.L. Howard, ed., Current Veterinary Therapy: Food Animal Practice, 2d ed. W.B. Saunders, Philadelphia. P. 493.

Mebus, C.A., Newman, L.E., and Stair, E.L. 1975. Scanning electron, light, and immunofluorescent microscopy of intestine of gnotobiotic calf infected with calf diarrheal coronavirus. Am. J. Vet. Res. 36:1719–1725.

Mebus, C.A., Stair, E.L., Rhodes, M.B., and Twiehaus, M.J. 1973a. Neonatal calf diarrhea: Propagation, attenuation, and characteristics of a coronavirus-like agent. Am. J. Vet. Res. 34:145–150.

Mebus, C.A., Stair, E.L., Rhodes, M.B., and Twiehaus, M.J. 1973b. Pathology of neonatal calf diarrhea induced by a coronavirus-like agent. Vet. Pathol. 10:45–64.

Mebus, C.A., White, R.G., Stair, E.L., Rhodes, M.B., and Twiehaus, M.J. 1972. Neonatal calf diarrhea: Results of a field trial using a reo-like virus vaccine. Vet. Med./Small Anim. Clin. 67:173–178.

Pedersen, N.C., Ward, J., and Mengeling, W.L. 1978. Antigenic relationship of the feline infectious peritonitis virus to coronaviruses of other species. Arch. Virol. 58:45–53.

Reynolds, D.J., Debney, T.G., Hall, G.A., Thomas, L.H., and Parsons, K.R. 1985. Studies on the relationship between coronaviruses from the intestinal and respiratory tracts of calves. Arch. Virol. 85:71–83.

Saif, L.J., and Smith, K.L. 1985. Enteric viral infections of calves and passive immunity. J. Dairy Sci. 68:206–228.

Sharpee, R.L., Mebus, C.A., and Bass, E.P. 1976. Characterization of a calf diarrheal coronavirus. Am. J. Vet. Res. 37:1031–1041.

Stair, E.L., Rhodes, M.B., White, R.G., and Mebus, C.A. 1972. Neonatal calf diarrhea: Purification and electron microscopy of a coronavirus-like agent. Am. J. Vet. Res. 33:1147–1156.

Storz, J., Doughri, A.M., and Hajer, I. 1978. Coronaviral morphogenesis and ultrastructural changes in intestinal infections of calves. J. Am. Vet. Med. Assoc. 173:633–635.

Storz, J., Rott, R., and Kaluza, G. 1981. Enhancement of plaque formation and cell fusion of an enteropathogenic coronavirus by trypsin treatment. Infect. Immun. 31:1214–1222.

Thomas, L.H., Gourlay, R.N., Stott, E.J., Howard, C.J., and Bridger, J.C. 1982. A search for new microorganisms in calf pneumonia by the inoculation of gnotobiotic calves. Res. Vet. Sci. 33:170–182.

Avian Infectious Bronchitis

SYNONYMS: Chick bronchitis, gasping disease; abbreviation, IB

Avian infectious bronchitis is an acute, highly contagious respiratory disease of chickens, with a high mortality rate in young chicks. It was first described by Schalk and Hawn in North Dakota in 1931. In 1936 Beach and Schalm showed that the causative agent was a virus and that it differed in several respects from the agent of infectious laryngotracheitis (a herpesvirus). The disease is characterized by a lightning-fast spread, such that nearly all exposed birds develop clinical signs at almost the same time. It occurs worldwide. The disease has been reviewed by Hofstad (1984).

Character of the Disease. The chicken is the primary natural host for IB virus (IBV). Birds of all ages are susceptible, but clinical signs are most severe in baby chicks. The incubation period is 2 to 4 days. The disease is characterized by sudden onset of listlessness, depression, gasping, coughing, tracheal rales, and nasal discharge. The outbreak usually runs a rapid course. Morbidity is practically 100 percent, although the severity of signs may vary. The mortality rate may be as high as 25 percent in young chicks but is usually negligible in chickens more than 5 to 6 weeks old. The effect on birds from 6 weeks to shortly before the first egg is laid is usually little more than slight retardation in development. In adult laying flocks, the damage results from depression of egg yield rather than death. Generally, the egg yield drops to half the preoutbreak level, but the decrease varies with the period of lay. Flocks infected in the latter portion of the laying year usually show a marked drop in egg yield. Such flocks may require long periods to recover production and usually become unprofitable. In addition to depressed yield, those eggs that are produced may be misshapen, soft- or rough-shelled, and have poor internal quality. Frequently, egg quality is permanently impaired.

An exudate, which may be serous, catarrhal, or caseous, is regularly found in the trachea, nasal passages, and sinuses of these chickens. In chicks that die, caseous plugs often are found in the lower portion of the trachea or in the larger bronchi. Ova in laying fowl are flaccid; often yolks and eggs with shells are found in the abdominal cavity. This latter condition is nonspecific, however, and not uncommon in other diseases that produce a marked drop in egg yield. Certain strains of IBV cause a nephrosis in addition to respiratory tract lesions (Chong and Apostolov 1982, Cumming 1963, Winterfield and Albassam 1984). Kidneys of affected birds are pale and swollen, with tubules and ureters often distended by uric acid crystals.

Histopathological lesions in the respiratory tract include cellular infiltration and edema of the mucosa and submucosa, vascular congestion, hyperplasia and vacuolation of the epithelium, and submucosal hemorrhage. The principal oviduct lesion is a localized hypoplasia. Kidney lesions in birds with nephrosis originate in the tubules. Initially necrosis occurs, followed by formation of cystic tubules containing epithelial cell debris and polymorphonuclear leukocytes in both the cortex and medulla.

Mixed infections sometimes occur when chicks harbor *Mycoplasma gallisepticum* or infectious bursal disease virus and become infected with IBV. The resulting disease may be more severe than usual (Chu and Uppal 1975, Rosenberger and Gelb 1978).

Properties of the Virus. Avian IBV is considered the type species of the genus *Coronavirus* of the family Coronaviridae (Siddell et al. 1983) (see Figure 57.1). At least eight serotypes have been described (Dawson and Gough 1971, Hopkins 1974). These serotypes can be separated into two main groups, the Massachusetts and Connecticut types (Hofstad 1958), which differ in their antigenic relatedness. The virulence of many different isolates of IBV varies markedly. The virus is unrelated antigenically to other avian or mammalian coronaviruses. Treatment with phospholipase C enables the virus to hemagglutinate erythrocytes (Alexander and Chettle 1977).

Heat stability at 56°C varies with viral strain, but none consistently survives for longer than 45 minutes at that temperature. Virus has been successfully stored at −30°C for as long as 24 years. Artificially contaminated surfaces remain infective for up to 12 days in spring weather and for at least 56 days in winter. The virus is ether-labile, variably resistant to pH 3, and sensitive to most common disinfectants. It is resistant, however, to the action of phenol.

Cultivation. Initial isolation is usually performed in the developing chick embryo (Beaudette and Hudson 1937) (see Figure 57.2). Dwarfing of a few embryos with survival of 90 percent through the 19th day of incubation is characteristic of initial passage material. Mortality and dwarfing then increase with subsequent passaging; by the 10th passage level most embryos are stunted, and survival may be as low as 20 percent. Subsequent adaptation to cell-culture systems has often been successful only after several egg passages.

Titration of the virus may be performed in chick embryonic kidney cells with egg-adapted strains by using cytopathic effects, as revealed by the formation of large syncytia followed by necrosis (Figure 57.7) and by the plaque technique (Figure 57.8). Plaque formation is enhanced in chick embryonic fibroblasts by the addition of trypsin (Otsuki and Tsubokura 1981). The virus will also grow in organ cultures derived from trachea or oviduct (Pradhan et al. 1983, Sawaguchi et al. 1985).

Epizootiology and Pathogenesis. Avian IBV infection

Figure 57.7 (*left*). Syncytia with necrosis induced by replication of avian infectious bronchitis virus in chicken kidney cell culture. Giemsa stain. × 60. (Courtesy B. Cowen.)

Figure 57.8 (*right*). Necrosis of syncytia in Figure 57.7 manifested as plaques by the agar overlay method. (Courtesy B. Cowen.)

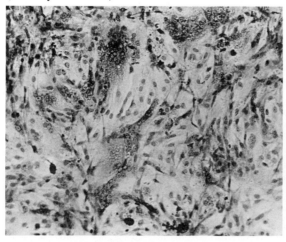
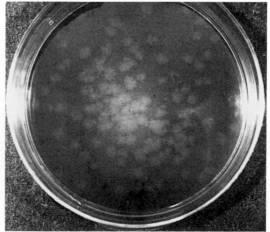

can be readily induced by inoculating minute amounts of virus into the respiratory tract. Natural infections are contracted through inhalation of infective droplets or fecal-oral contamination. Levine and Hofstad (1947) demonstrated experimentally that the virus can be air-borne for a distance of at least 5 feet, but the potential distance of transmission in the outside atmosphere (i.e., in the direction of the prevailing wind) is unknown. Frequently a prolonged infection occurs following recovery, which results in shedding of virus in the feces for several months (Alexander and Gough 1977, Alexander et al. 1978). The virus can also be spread by contamination of feed sacks, equipment, and outer garments and boots of caretakers.

The primary target tissue for infection is the trachea (Darbyshire et al. 1975, Purcell and McFerran 1972). Replication occurs also in bronchial tissue, lungs, kidneys, ovaries, and oviducts. Respiratory lesions are characterized by desquamation of the ciliated and glandular epithelium of the trachea, followed by a rapid proliferation of basal cells with formation of a stratified, undifferentiated epithelial covering. Lymphocyte infiltration occurs in small areas of the tracheal submucosa. Regeneration usually is complete on or about the 12th day after infection. Small patches of fluorescent cells are still present on immunofluorscence microscopy 6 weeks after infection, but the regenerated tracheal epithelium is resistant to viral injury.

Immunity. Chickens that recover from natural infection are solidly immune to reinfection with the homologous viral strain for at least 6 to 8 months. Resistance is probably mediated by the local immune response in the trachea, nasal mucosa, and harderian gland, although the details are not yet fully understood (Gillette 1981). The level of humoral neutralizing antibody does not necessarily correlate with immunity. Maternal immunity seems to be effective in providing passive protection for 2 to 4 weeks after the chick is hatched (Cunningham 1975, Darbyshire and Peters 1985). Passive antibody reduces the severity of the disease but does not prevent infection of the respiratory tract. Matters are complicated, however, by strain and serotype variation and by the presence of chronic virus carriers.

Diagnosis. In the absence of nervous signs, coughing and gasping in young chicks suggest IB. The primary differential diagnoses are Newcastle disease and infectious laryngotracheitis. A presumptive clinical diagnosis early in the course of the disease may be difficult, but as the outbreak progresses, the clinicopathological picture comes to resemble IB. A definitive diagnosis rests on isolation of the virus or detection of rising antibody titers in paired (acute and convalescent) serum samples.

Respiratory tract tissues are the most useful for virus isolation. This is usually done by inoculating 10- or 11-day-old embryonating chicken eggs with tracheal swab material from several birds in the acute stages of the disease. In initial passages dwarfing will not be prominent, but on continued passage most embryos will be dwarfed and will die after 5 or 6 days' incubation. IBV can be identified also in tracheal organ culture or by intratracheal inoculation of susceptible chicks with allantoic fluid from egg passage material. If IBV is present, chicks develop tracheal rales within 24 to 36 hours. Hemagglutinating activity is absent from allantoic fluid (in contrast to that observed with Newcastle disease virus).

Antibodies may be detected by a number of methods, including neutralization and plaque reduction, hemagglutination-inhibition, agar-gel immunodiffusion, and enzyme-linked immunosorbent assay (Hofstad 1984). Immunofluorescence microscopy has been used to detect IBV in tracheal smears of acutely affected chickens (Braune and Gentry 1965).

Treatment. There is no specific therapy for IB. Affected birds should be maintained in a warm, draft-free environment and allowed to recover as the flock acquires immunity to the infecting strain. The use of broad-spectrum antibiotics in the drinking water may be indicated if the outbreak is complicated by air sac infection or chronic respiratory disease.

Prevention and Control. The disease is best controlled by strict isolation of the infected flock and by rearing replacement chicks in separate quarters. Even under the best of management circumstances, however, outbreaks of IB can occur, and immunization may be the only practical means of control.

For some years in the northeastern United States, a method of immunization recommended by Van Roekel et al. (1950) was used with excellent success. This involved inoculating a small number of birds in a flock with virulent field virus when the birds were from 7 to 15 weeks of age. At this stage of their development, the birds were not seriously damaged by the disease. Following recovery, the flock would then be immune for the laying year. This technique worked quite well, but because the pathogenic field strains perpetuated the disease in the flock and in the community, the procedure was given up in favor of modified live-virus vaccines (Hofstad 1975). These vaccines are not necessarily avirulent, and problems sometimes result from their use. In general, however, they are safer than and just as efficacious as virulent field virus. Vaccines are usually given to flocks in their drinking water or by spraying or dusting. At least six serotypes are now being used in commercial vaccine preparations (Hofstad 1984). The plurality of serotypes is a complication. No single strain has been identified that is capable of producing reliable immunity against many heterologous serotypes. There is some degree of cross-protection, however, which may help protect vaccinated flocks that are exposed to heterologous strains (Hofstad 1981).

Chicks usually are vaccinated at 4 to 5 days of age and given a booster dose at 4 weeks. The best immune response is obtained in birds 6 weeks of age or older, however. Replacement flocks should be vaccinated at 2 to 4 months.

The Disease in Humans. There is no evidence that IBV is hazardous to human health.

REFERENCES

Alexander, D.J., and Chettle, N.J. 1977. Procedures for the haemagglutination and the haemagglutination inhibition tests for avian infectious bronchitis virus. Avian Pathol. 6:9–17.

Alexander, D.J., and Gough, R.E. 1977. Isolation of infectious bronchitis virus from experimentally infected chickens. Res. Vet. Sci. 23:344–347.

Alexander, D.J., Gough, R.E., and Pattison, M. 1978. A long-term study of the pathogenesis of infection of fowls with three strains of avian infectious bronchitis virus. Res. Vet. Sci. 24:228–233.

Beach, J.R., and Schalm, O.W. 1936. A filterable virus, distinct from that of laryngotracheitis, the cause of a respiratory disease of chicks. Poultry Sci. 15:199–206.

Beaudette, F.R., and Hudson, C.B. 1937. Cultivation of the virus of infectious bronchitis. J. Am. Vet. Med. Asoc. 90:51–60.

Braune, M.O., and Gentry, R.F. 1965. Standardization of the fluorescent antibody technique for the detection of avian respiratory viruses. Avian Dis. 9:535–545.

Chong, K.T., and Apostolov, K. 1982. The pathogenesis of nephritis in chickens induced by infectious bronchitis virus. J. Comp. Pathol. 92:199–211.

Chu, H.P., and Uppal, P.K. 1975. Single and mixed infections of avian infectious bronchitis virus and *Mycoplasma gallisepticum*. Dev. Biol. Stand. 28:101–114.

Cumming, R.B. 1963. Infectious avian nephrosis (uraemia) in Australia. Aust. Vet. J. 39:145–147.

Cunningham, C.H. 1975. Immunity to avian infectious bronchitis. Dev. Biol. Stand. 28:546–562.

Darbyshire, J.H., and Peters, R.W. 1985. Humoral antibody response and assessment of protection following primary vaccination of chicks with maternally derived antibody against avian infectious bronchitis virus. Res. Vet. Sci. 38:14–21.

Darbyshire, J.H., Cook, J.K.A., and Peters, R.W. 1975. Comparative growth kinetic studies on avian infectious bronchitis virus in different systems. J. Comp. Pathol. 85:623–630.

Dawson, P.S., and Gough, R.E. 1971. Antigenic variation in strains of avian infectious bronchitis virus. Arch. Gesam. Virusforsch. 34:32–39.

Gillette, K.G. 1981. Local antibody response in avian infectious bronchitis: Virus-neutralizing antibody in tracheobronchial secretions. Avian Dis. 25:431–443.

Hofstad, M.S. 1958. Antigenic differences among isolates of avian infectious bronchitis virus. Am. J. Vet. Res. 19:740–743.

Hofstad, M.S. 1975. Immune response to infectious bronchitis virus. Am. J. Vet. Res. 36:520–521.

Hofstad, M.S. 1981. Cross-immunity in chickens using seven isolates of avian infectious bronchitis virus. Avian Dis. 25:650–654.

Hofstad, M.S. 1984. Avian infectious bronchitis. In M.S. Hofstad, H.J. Barnes, B.W. Calnek, W.M. Reid, and H.W. Yoder, eds., Diseases of Poultry, 8th ed. Iowa State University Press, Ames. Pp. 429–443.

Hopkins, S.R. 1974. Serological comparisons of strains of infectious bronchitis virus using plaque-purified isolants. Avian Dis. 18:231–239.

Levine, P.P., and Hofstad, M.S. 1947. Attempts to control air-borne infectious bronchitis and Newcastle disease of fowls with sterilamps. Cornell Vet. 37:204–211.

Otsuki, K., and Tsubokura, M. 1981. Plaque formation by avian infectious bronchitis virus in primary chick embryo fibroblast cells in the presence of trypsin. Arch. Virol. 70:315–320.

Pradhan, H.K., Mohanty, G.C., and Rajya, B.S. 1983. Comparative sensitivities of oviduct and tracheal organ cultures and chicken embryo kidney cell cultures to infectious bronchitis virus. Avian Dis. 27:594–601.

Purcell, D.A., and McFerran, J.B. 1972. The histopathology of infectious bronchitis in the domestic fowl. Res. Vet. Sci. 13:116–122.

Rosenberger, J.K., and Gelb, J. 1978. Response to several avian respiratory viruses as affected by infectious bursal disease virus. Avian Dis. 22:95–105.

Sawaguchi, K., Yachida, S., Aoyama, S., Takahashi, N., Iritani, Y., and Hayashi, Y. 1985. Comparative use of direct organ cultures of infected chicken tracheas in isolating avian infectious bronchitis virus. Avian Dis. 29:546–551.

Schalk, A.F., and Hawn, M.C. 1931. An apparently new respiratory disease of baby chicks. J. Am. Vet. Med. Assoc. 78:413–422.

Siddell, S.G., Anderson, R., Cavanagh, D., Fujiwara, K., Klenk, H.D., Macnaughton, M.R., Pensaert, M., Stohlman, S.A., Sturman, L., and van der Zeijst, B.A.M. 1983. Coronaviridae. Intervirology 20:181–189.

Van Roekel, H., Bullis, K.L., Clarke, M.K., Olesiuk, O.M., and Sperling, F.G. 1950. Infectious bronchitis. Mass. Agric. Exp. Stn. Bull. 460:1–47.

Winterfield, R.W., and Albassam, M.A. 1984. Nephropathogenicity of infectious bronchitis virus. Poultry Sci. 63:2358–2363.

Coronaviral Enteritis of Turkeys

SYNONYMS: Bluecomb disease, transmissible enteritis, infectious enteritis, mud fever; abbreviation, CE

Coronaviral enteritis is an acute, highly infectious disease affecting turkeys of all ages. It was first described by Peterson and Hymas in Washington state in 1951, although it is clear that it had existed much earlier. In addition to the United States, CE has been reported in Canada and Australia. The disease was reviewed in 1984 by Pomeroy.

Character of the Disease. CE affects turkeys of all ages, and outbreaks are frequently severe. The onset of the disease is sudden. The birds become depressed, anorectic, and hypothermic, losing weight and producing watery droppings. Darkening of the head and skin, with development of discolored, purple combs (associated with cyanotic changes) is also seen. Droppings are green to brown and frequently contain mucus threads or casts. In breeder hens a rapid drop in egg production occurs. Morbidity may approach 100 percent, with mortality as high as 50 percent; the disease is more severe in younger birds. In range turkeys losses may depend on the prevailing weather. The course of the disease is usually 10 to 14 days. Many affected older birds never regain a satisfactory weight.

The lesions of CE are confined chiefly to the intestinal tract and consist of inflammatory cellular reactions in the lamina propria, with infiltration of heterophils, lymphocytes, and reticuloendothelial cells. As with other coronaviral enteritides, infection and disruption of villus cells of the intestine occur. Lesions appear to be most distinct in the jejunum but are also present in the duodenum, ileum, and cecum (Adams et al. 1970).

Properties of the Virus. Physicochemical and morphologic parameters of the CE virus place it within the coronavirus group, but it is antigenically unrelated to other coronaviruses.

Cultivation. The agent has been cultivated successfully in embryonating turkey eggs and in chicken eggs but not in monolayer cell cultures. In vitro interference against Newcastle disease virus has been demonstrated (Deshmukh and Pomeroy 1974).

Epizootiology and Pathogenesis. CE virus infects only turkeys. The primary route of transmission is fecal-oral. The disease spreads rapidly through a flock and from flock to flock on the same premises. Wild birds and fomites (boots, outer garments, equipment, or vehicles) are probably of importance in spreading the virus to other farms. The virus can also overwinter in frozen feces, even after a farm has been depopulated of birds, unless appropriate decontamination procedures are followed (Pomeroy and Sieburth 1953). To date, there is no evidence that the infection is transmitted through the egg.

The pathogenesis of the disease is similar to that of other coronaviral enteritides (Adams et al. 1970, Pomeroy et al. 1978).

Immunity. Turkeys that recover from CE remain immune carriers for life and hence will always be a potential hazard to new flocks on the premises or nearby (Pomeroy and Sieburth 1953, Pomeroy et al. 1975). Protection is probably mediated by local synthesis of secretory IgA in the intestine (Nagaraja and Pomeroy 1978, 1980a, 1980b). Poults exposed less than 1 week after hatching have the same immunological response to natural infection as older birds.

Diagnosis. A definitive diagnosis of CE is made by detection of viral antigen in intestinal epithelial cells of affected birds by immunofluorescence microscopy. Serum neutralization tests are also helpful in diagnosing the disease (Pomeroy et al. 1975).

Treatment. There is no specific therapy for CE. Supportive measures that may help to reduce losses include provision of warmth and addition of antibiotics, potassium chloride, and calf milk replacer to the drinking water (Pomeroy 1984).

Prevention and Control. Once the virus has infected a flock, the only solution is controlled depopulation and decontamination; restocking should be delayed for at least a few weeks (Pomeroy 1984). The entire process should preferably be carried out during the summer, in order to facilitate inactivation of virus in feces, litter, and soil. There is no available vaccine.

The Disease in Humans. CE is not known to occur in humans.

REFERENCES

Adams, N.R., Ball, R.A., and Hofstad, M.S. 1970. Intestinal lesions in transmissible enteritis of turkeys. Avian Dis. 14:392–399.

Deshmukh, D.R., and Pomeroy, B.S. 1974. In vitro test for the detection of turkey bluecomb coronavirus—Interference against Newcastle disease virus. Am. J. Vet. Res. 35:1553–1556.

Nagaraja, K.V., and Pomeroy, B.S. 1978. Secretory antibodies against turkey coronaviral enteritis. Am. J. Vet. Res. 39:1463–1465.

Nagaraja, K.V., and Pomeroy, B.S. 1980a. Cell-mediated immunity against turkey coronaviral enteritis (bluecomb). Am. J. Vet. Res. 41:915–917.

Nagaraja, K.V., and Pomeroy, B.S. 1980b. Immunofluorescent studies on localization of secretory immunoglobulins in the intestines of turkeys recovered from turkey coronaviral enteritis. Am. J. Vet. Res. 41:1283–1284.

Peterson, E.H., and Hymas, T.A. 1951. Antibiotics in the treatment of an unfamiliar turkey disease. Poultry Sci. 30:466–468.

Pomeroy, B.S. 1984. Coronaviral enteritis of turkeys (bluecomb disease). In M.A. Hofstad, H.J. Barnes, B.K. Calnek, W.M. Reid, and H.W. Yoder, eds., Diseases of Poultry, 8th ed. Iowa State University Press, Ames. Pp. 553–559.

Pomeroy, B.S., and Sieburth, J.M. 1953. Bluecomb disease of turkeys. Proceedings of the Annual Meeting of the American Veterinary Medical Association 90:321–328.

Pomeroy, B.S., Larsen, C.T., Deshmukh, D.R., and Patel, B.L. 1975. Immunity to transmissible (coronaviral) enteritis of turkeys (bluecomb). Am. J. Vet. Res. 36:553–555.

Pomeroy, K.A., Patel, B.L., Larsen, C.T., and Pomeroy, B.S. 1978. Combined immunofluorescence and transmission electron microscopic studies of sequential intestinal samples from turkey embryos and poults infected with turkey enteritis coronavirus. Am. J. Vet. Res. 39:1348–1354.

Equine Coronavirus Infection

In 1975 Bass and Sharpee reported electron microscopic identification of coronavirus particles in feces from foals with diarrhea. The disease syndrome was characterized by fever, profuse watery diarrhea, extensive lymphatic involvement, and a high mortality rate. Similar cases, with histological evidence of denuded small intestinal villus epithelium, were reported in 1983 (Ward et al.). Others have reported coronaviruslike particles in feces of adult horses with diarrhea (Eugster and Jones 1980, Huang et al. 1983). One of these latter agents has been propagated in cell culture and shown to be antigenically unrelated to bovine coronavirus, transmissible gastroenteritis virus, or avian infectious bronchitis virus (Huang et al. 1983). A single report has also been published of coronavirus particles in lung tissue from an aborted equine fetus (Eugster and Jones 1980).

REFERENCES

Bass, E.P., and Sharpee, R.L. 1975. Coronavirus and gastroenteritis in foals. Lancet 2:822.

Eugster, A.K., and Jones, L.P. 1980. Coronaviruses in an aborted equine fetus. Southwest Vet. 33:12.

Huang, J.C.M., Wright, S.L., and Shipley, W.D. 1983. Isolation of coronavirus-like agent from horses suffering from acute equine diarrhoea syndrome. Vet. Rec. 113:262–263.

Ward, A.C.S., Evermann, J.F., and Reed, S.M. 1983. Presence of coronavirus in diarrheic foals. Vet. Med./Small Anim. Clin. 78:563–565.

Lapine Coronavirus Infections

Pleural effusion disease (PED) is an acute illness of rabbits characterized by fever, anorexia, weakness, pleural and peritoneal effusions, myocardial degeneration and necrosis, and depletion of thymic lymphocytes (Fennestad et al. 1975, 1981; Small et al. 1979). The condition has been associated with a coronavirus antigenically related to human coronaviruses 229E and OC43 (Small et al. 1979). Viral antigen was demonstrated in myocardial tissue by immunofluorescence microscopy with hyperimmune anti-229E reference serum. To date, the agent has not been successfully propagated in cell or explant cultures but can be passaged in vivo in rabbits. Baby rabbits surviving initial challenge develop a persistent viremia lasting for at least 6 months, despite the presence of antiviral antibody (Fennestad et al. 1981).

Coronaviruses have also been implicated in diarrheal disease in rabbits (Descôteaux et al. 1985, Eaton 1984, Lapierre et al. 1980, Osterhaus et al. 1982). Descôteaux et al. (1985) examined one of these agents closely and showed that its structural polypeptide pattern is similar to that of other coronaviruses. The agent cross-reacts antigenically with avian infectious bronchitis and transmissible gastroenteritis viruses. Chronic carriers of the virus appear to be common and are probably responsible for persistence of the agent in certain colonies where deaths due to enteritis are frequent.

REFERENCES

Descôteaux, J.P., Lussier, G., Berthiaume, L., Alain, R., Seguin, C., and Trudel, M. 1985. An enteric coronavirus of the rabbit: Detection by immunoelectron microscopy and identification of structural polypeptides. Arch. Virol. 84:241–250.

Eaton, P. 1984. Preliminary observations on enteritis associated with a coronavirus-like agent in rabbits. Lab. Anim. 18:71–74.

Fennestad, K.L., Mansa, B., and Larsen, S. 1981. Pleural effusion disease in rabbits. Observations on viraemia, immunity and transmissibility. Arch. Virol. 70:11–19.

Fennestad, K.L., Skovgaard Jensen, H.J., Moller, S., and Weis Bentzon, M. 1975. Pleural effusion disease in rabbits. Clinical and post mortem observations. Acta Pathol. Microbiol. Scand. B83:541–548.

Lapierre, J., Marsolais, G., Pilon, P., and Descôteaux, J.P. 1980. Preliminary report on the observation of a coronavirus in the intestine of the laboratory rabbit. Can J. Microbiol. 26:1204–1208.

Osterhaus, A.D.M.E., Teppena, J.S., and van Steenes, G. 1982. Coronavirus-like particles in laboratory rabbits with different syndromes in the Netherlands. Lab. Anim. Sci. 32:663–665.

Small, J.D., Aurelian, L., Squire, R.A., Strandberg, J.D., Melby, E.C., Turner, T.B., and Newman, B. 1979. Rabbit cardiomyopathy associated with a virus antigenically related to human coronavirus strain 229E. Am. J. Pathol. 95:709–724.

Enteric Coronaviruslike Particles

Enteric coronaviruslike particles (CVLPs) are an enigmatic group of morphologically distinctive entities that have been identified by electron microscopy in feces of humans and a number of animal species (Macnaughton and Davies 1981). Particles are moderately to markedly pleomorphic, ranging in diameter from 60 to 1200 nm, and possess regularly spaced radiating surface projections somewhat similar to coronavirus peplomers (Figure 57.9). Closer examination, however, reveals that CVLP projections consist of delicate, round to oval, knoblike structures anchored to the particle by slender stalks, and thus they are distinguishable from the larger, more massive petal-shaped peplomers of coronaviruses (see Figure 57.1). CVLP surface projections are approximately 18 to

Figure 57.9. Negative-contrast electron micrograph of three enteric coronaviruslike particles in feline feces, demonstrating the characteristic knob-shaped peplomers attached by slender stalks. × 174,000. (Courtesy C. Stoddart.)

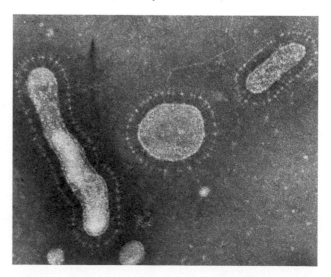

28 nm long; some particles have an additional T-shaped structure at the distal end, yielding an overall projection length of 44 nm. Although enteric CVLPs have been identified most commonly in diarrheic feces, they have not been proved to cause disease.

Enteric CVLPs were detected in 1979 in the feces of cats raised in a barrier-maintained breeding colony (Hoshino and Scott 1980), and since then the particles have been detected in fecal samples from hospitalized pet cats (Hoshino et al. 1981). Cats that have been experimentally infected with feline enteric CVLPs have not shown signs of disease (Stoddart et al. 1984). Soon after birth kittens become infected with CVLPs excreted by their dams and remain healthy. Particles morphologically indistinguishable from feline enteric CVLPs have been identified in humans (Macnaughton and Davies 1981), dogs (Schnagl and Holmes 1978), sheep (Pass et al. 1982, Tzipori et al. 1978), and nonhuman primates (Caul and Egglestone 1979, Smith et al. 1982).

Further understanding of the relationship of these particles, if any, to the family Coronaviridae must await their successful isolation and propagation in the laboratory, and subsequent physicochemical, virological, and immunological investigations.

REFERENCES

Caul, E.O., and Egglestone, S.I. 1979. Coronavirus-like particles present in simian faeces. Vet. Rec. 14:168–169.

Hoshino, Y., and Scott, F.W. 1980. Coronavirus-like particles in the feces of normal cats. Arch. Virol. 63:147–152.

Hoshino, Y., Baldwin, C.A., and Scott, F.W. 1981. New insights in gastrointestinal viruses. Cornell Feline Health Center News 2:2–4.

Macnaughton, M.R., and Davies, H.A. 1981. Human enteric coronaviruses. Arch. Virol. 70:301–313.

Pass, D.A., Penhale, W.J., Wilcox, G.E., and Batey, R.G. 1982. Intestinal coronavirus-like particles in sheep with diarrhoea. Vet. Rec. 111:106–107.

Schnagl, R.D., and Holmes, I.H. 1978. Coronavirus-like particles in stools from dogs from some country areas of Australia. Vet. Rec. 102:528–529.

Smith, G.C., Lester, T.L., Heberling, R.L., and Kalter, S.S. 1982. Coronavirus-like particles in nonhuman primate feces. Arch. Virol. 72:105–111.

Stoddart, C.A., Barlough, J.E., and Scott, F.W. 1984. Experimental studies of a coronavirus and coronavirus-like agent in a barrier-maintained feline breeding colony. Arch. Virol. 79:85–94.

Tzipori, S., Smith, M., Makin, T., and McCaughan, C. 1978. Enteric coronavirus-like particles in sheep. Aust. Vet. J. 54:320–321.

58 Diseases Caused by Unclassified Viruses and Diseases of Uncertain Viral Etiology

Astrovirus Infection

The term *astrovirus* was introduced by Madeley and Cosgrove (1975a, 1975b) to describe certain small round virus particles, 28 to 30 nm in diameter, that had been observed by electron microscopy in diarrheic stools of human infants. Since then, astroviruses and astroviruslike particles have been identified in fecal specimens, gut contents, or tissues from a variety of animal species, including cattle, sheep, pigs, dogs, cats, deer, mice, turkeys, and ducks (Bridger 1980; Bridger et al. 1984; Gough et al. 1984, 1985; Harbour et al. 1987; Hoshino et al. 1981; Kjeldsberg and Hem 1985; McNulty et al. 1980; Reynolds and Saif 1985; Shirai et al. 1985; Snodgrass and Gray 1977; Tzipori et al. 1981; Williams 1980; Woode and Bridger 1978). They are found most frequently in the young of most of these species. In humans, several outbreaks of gastroenteritis among young children have been associated with astrovirus, but older children and some adults also have been affected (Ashley et al. 1978, Konno et al. 1982, Kurtz et al. 1977).

Astrovirus particles are nonenveloped and possess a characteristic surface configuration that resembles a five- or six-pointed star rimmed by an unbroken circular border (Figure 58.1). They frequently occur in large clusters or aggregates, with occasional "bridging" structures visible between individual particles. It has been proposed that these structures might represent surface fibers similar to those of adenoviruses (Madeley 1979). To date, human, bovine, feline, and porcine astroviruses can be propagated serially with the aid of trypsin in cell culture (Har-

bour et al. 1987, Lee and Kurtz 1981, Shirai et al. 1985, Woode et al. 1984). Erratic growth in embryonating chicken eggs has been reported for the duck agent (Gough et al. 1985). Limited studies of purified ovine astrovirus indicate that the capsid consists of two major polypeptides and that the genome is a single molecule of single-stranded RNA with a poly(A) tract (Herring et al. 1981). The genome thus resembles that of caliciviruses and picornaviruses, but the polypeptide composition is unlike that of either family (one capsid polypeptide for caliciviruses, four capsid polypeptides for picornaviruses). The name *astrovirus* has not been officially approved for use by the International Committee on Taxonomy of Viruses, but it has found considerable favor with those actively working in the field of viral gastroenteritis.

In experimental studies, astroviruses have produced mild gastroenteritis in adult human volunteers and in lambs, cats, and turkeys (Harbour et al. 1987, Kurtz et al. 1979, Reynolds and Saif 1985, Snodgrass et al. 1979). The ovine agent has been shown to infect mature villus epithelial cells and subepithelial macrophages in the small intestine, producing partial villus atrophy (Snodgrass et al. 1979). Astrovirus-infected cells were found scattered throughout the apical half of the villi. Histological alterations and the presence of viral antigen were confined to the middle and distal segments of the small intestine. Examination of thin sections of lamb intestine showed that the virus is present in viroplasm or in quasicrystalline arrays in the cytoplasm of infected cells and occasionally within membranous structures or vacuoles (Gray et al. 1980). Bovine astroviruses appear to be relatively in-

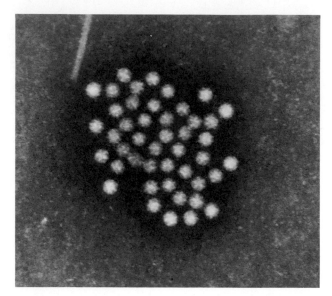

Figure 58.1. Electron micrograph of negatively stained feline astrovirus particles, from a 4-month-old kitten with diarrhea. Both five- and six-pointed star-shaped surface configurations are seen. × 93,000. (From Hoshino et al., 1981, courtesy of *Archives of Virology.*)

nocuous according to experiments conducted thus far (Bridger et al. 1984, Woode and Bridger 1978). One of these agents has been shown to infect the dome epithelial cells of the ileum, but the infected calves did not develop diarrhea unless coinfected with rotavirus or Breda virus 2, in which case more extensive astrovirus infection of the dome epithelium occurred (Woode et al. 1984). The duck astrovirus appears to be unique in that it produces outbreaks of severe hepatitis (duck hepatitis type 2) in ducklings, often with significant mortality (Gough et al. 1984, 1985).

Astroviruses of the different species appear to be antigenically distinct. Limited serologic studies indicate that infections are common in at least two susceptible hosts, humans and cattle (Kurtz and Lee 1978, Woode and Bridger 1978), and there is evidence for a multiplicity of astrovirus serotypes in both of these species (Kurtz and Lee 1984, Woode et al. 1985).

REFERENCES

Ashley, C.R., Caul, E.O., and Paver, W.K. 1978. Astrovirus-associated gastroenteritis in children. J. Clin. Pathol. 31:939–943.

Bridger, J.C. 1980. Detection by electron microscopy of caliciviruses, astroviruses and rotavirus-like particles in the faeces of piglets with diarrhoea. Vet. Rec. 107:532–533.

Bridger, J.C., Hall, G.A., and Brown, J.F. 1984. Characterization of a calici-like virus (Newbury agent) found in association with astrovirus in bovine diarrhea. Infect. Immun. 43:133–138.

Gough, R.E., Borland, E.D., Keymer, I.F., and Stuart, J.C. 1985. An outbreak of duck hepatitis type II in commercial ducks. Avian Pathol. 14:227–236.

Gough, R.E., Collins, M.S., Borland, E., and Keymer, L.F. 1984. Astrovirus-like particles associated with hepatitis in ducklings. Vet. Rec. 114:279.

Gray, E.W., Angus, K.W., and Snodgrass, D.R. 1980. Ultrastructure of the small intestine in astrovirus-infected lambs. J. Gen. Virol. 49:71–82.

Harbour, D.A., Ashley, C.R., Williams, P.D., and Gruffydd-Jones, T.J. 1987. Natural and experimental astrovirus infection of cats. Vet. Rec. 120:555–557.

Herring, A.J., Gray, E.W., and Snodgrass, D.R. 1981. Purification and characterization of ovine astrovirus. J. Gen. Virol. 53:47–55.

Hoshino, Y., Zimmer, J.F., Moise, N.S., and Scott, F.W. 1981. Detection of astroviruses in feces of a cat with diarrhea. Arch. Virol. 70:373–376.

Kjeldsberg, E., and Hem, A. 1985. Detection of astroviruses in gut contents of nude and normal mice. Arch. Virol. 84:135–140.

Konno, T., Suzuki, H., Ishida, N., Chiba, R., Mochizuki, K., and Tsunoda, A. 1982. Astrovirus-associated epidemic gastroenteritis in Japan. J. Med. Virol. 9:11–17.

Kurtz, J., and Lee, T. 1978. Astrovirus gastroenteritis age distribution of antibody. Med. Microbiol. Immunol. (Berlin) 166:227–230.

Kurtz, J.B., and Lee, T.W. 1984. Human astrovirus serotypes. Lancet 2:1405.

Kurtz, J.B., Lee, T.W., Craig, J.W., and Reed, S.E. 1979. Astrovirus infection in volunteers. J. Med. Virol. 3:221–230.

Kurtz, J.B., Lee, T.W., and Pickering, D. 1977. Astrovirus associated gastroenteritis in a children's ward. J. Clin. Pathol. 30:948–952.

Lee, T.W., and Kurtz, J.B. 1981. Serial propagation of astrovirus in tissue culture with the aid of trypsin. J. Gen. Virol. 57:421–424.

Madeley, C.R. 1979. Comparison of the features of astroviruses and caliciviruses seen in samples of feces by electron microscopy. J. Infect. Dis. 139:519–523.

Madeley, C.R., and Cosgrove, B.P. 1975a. Viruses in infantile gastroenteritis. Lancet 2:124.

Madeley, C.R., and Cosgrove, B.P. 1975b. 28 nm particles in faeces in infantile gastroenteritis. Lancet 2:451–452.

McNulty, M.S., Curran, W.L., and McFerran, J.B. 1980. Detection of astroviruses in turkey faeces by direct electron microscopy. Vet. Rec. 106:561.

Reynolds, D.L., and Saif, Y.M. 1985. Experimental infections of turkeys with an astro-like virus. Proceedings of the Conference of Research Workers in Animal Disease 66:55.

Shirai, J., Shimizu, M., and Fukusho, A. 1985. Coronavirus-, calicivirus-, and astrovirus-like particles associated with acute porcine gastroenteritis. Jpn. J. Vet. Sci. 47:1023–1026.

Snodgrass, D.R., and Gray, E.W. 1977. Detection and transmission of 30-nm virus particles (astroviruses) in faeces of lambs with diarrhoea. Arch. Virol. 55:287–291.

Snodgrass, D.R., Angus, K.W., Gray, E.W., Menzies, J.D., and Paul, G. 1979. Pathogenesis of diarrhoea caused by astrovirus infections in lambs. Arch. Virol. 60:217–226.

Tzipori, S., Menzies, J.D., and Gray, E.W. 1981. Detection of astrovirus in the faeces of red deer. Vet. Rec. 108:286.

Williams, F.P. 1980. Astrovirus-like, coronavirus-like, and parvovirus-like particles detected in the diarrheal stools of beagle pups. Arch. Virol. 66:215–226.

Woode, G.N., and Bridger, J.C. 1978. Isolation of small viruses resembling astroviruses and caliciviruses from acute enteritis of calves. J. Med. Microbiol. 11:441–452.

Woode, G.N., Gourley, N.E.K., Pohlenz, J.F., Liebler, E.M., Mathews, S.L., and Hutchinson, M.P. 1985. Serotypes of bovine astrovirus. J. Clin. Microbiol. 22:668–670.

Woode, G.N., Pohlenz, J.F., Gourley, N.E.K., and Fagerland, J.A. 1984. Astrovirus and Breda virus infections of dome cell epithelium of bovine ileum. J. Clin. Microbiol. 19:623–630.

Hepadnavirus Infection

The family name Hepadnaviridae has recently been proposed for a small and unique group of DNA viruses (the hepatitis B viruses, or HBVs) found in humans, woodchucks, ground squirrels, and Pekin ducks (Gust et al. 1986; Marion and Robinson 1983; Marion et al. 1980, 1984; Mason et al. 1980; Summers et al. 1978; Tiollais et al. 1985). Because these viruses have been identified only recently and as yet have not been serially propagated in cell culture, many details of their structure and replication cycle remain obscure. Nevertheless, a number of distinctive features have been delineated:

1. The viral genome is composed of a single molecule of circular DNA that is partially double-stranded and partially single-stranded. One strand (*minus* strand, complementary to mRNA) is full length, whereas the other strand (*plus* strand) varies in length in different molecules. Neither strand is a covalently closed circle; rather, the 5' ends overlap by approximately 200 base pairs, so that the overall circular conformation is maintained by base pairing of the cohesive ends. A virion-associated DNA polymerase activity can repair the single-stranded region to make fully double-stranded DNA molecules.

2. Replication proceeds by way of an RNA intermediate that serves as a template for synthesis of the full-length DNA strand (reverse transcription). The full-length strand itself subsequently serves as a template for synthesis of the plus strand, which is left incomplete in most particles at the time of assembly and release.

3. The virion is a 28-nm icosahedral nucleocapsid core composed of a single major polypeptide and surrounded by a detergent-sensitive envelope. The overall diameter of complete, enveloped virions (Dane particles) (Figure 58.2) is approximately 42 nm. The nucleocapsid carries the hepatitis B core antigen (HBcAg) on its surface, whereas the envelope protein appears to contain the serologically important hepatitis B surface antigen (HBsAg) (Australia antigen). Particulate forms (22-nm spherical and filamentous particles) found in high concentrations in the blood of infected individuals also bear HBsAg and are believed to represent empty viral envelopes (Figure 58.2). The presence in serum of HBsAg, in either complete or incomplete viral form, is the most useful marker for the detection of active HBV infection. A third antigen, HBeAg, is also found in the blood and is thought to be associated with the virion core.

Hepadnaviruses display a striking tropism for hepatocytes and have been associated with acute and chronic hepatitis, cirrhosis, and hepatocellular carcinoma (Beasley et al. 1981, Gust et al. 1986, Peters 1975, Popper et al. 1981, Redeker 1975, Summers et al. 1978, Szmuness

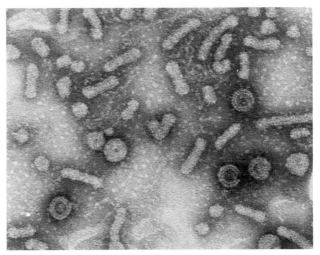

Figure 58.2. Electron micrograph of negatively stained woodchuck hepatitis B virus particles, obtained from woodchuck serum. The larger circular forms are complete, enveloped virions (Dane particles), whereas the smaller circular and rod-shaped forms are believed to represent empty viral envelopes. × 145,350. (Courtesy E. C. Ford and J. L. Gerin, Georgetown University.)

1978). The precise mechanism of liver cell injury is unknown, but the host immune response to viral antigens on hepatocyte membranes apparently plays a major role in the pathogenesis (Thomas et al. 1984, Tiollais et al. 1985). Immunological phenomena may also be involved in some of the extrahepatic manifestations of hepadnavirus infection (arthritis, polyarteritis, glomerulonephritis, and a syndrome resembling serum sickness) (Fye et al. 1977, Gocke 1975, Kohler et al. 1974, Wands et al. 1975).

Another characteristic biological feature of hepadnaviruses is the relatively common occurrence of persistent infections (for human HBV, 5 to 10 percent of infected adults, more frequently in neonates), with viral antigens and infectious virus remaining in the blood circulation in high concentrations for years (Marion and Robinson 1983). Production and release of HBsAg, however, may also occur in the absence of viral DNA replication and infectious virion production. The primary modes of spread of these viruses are by transfer of infected blood or blood products, by sexual encounter or other close physical contact, and by vertical transmission from mother to offspring.

Variations on the common hepadnavirus theme are observed for the animal agents. Woodchuck HBV produces a severe, progressive hepatitis that does not lead to cirrhosis but that is associated with the development of hepatocellular carcinomas in a significant percentage of persistently infected animals (Popper et al. 1981, Summers et al. 1978). By contrast, ground squirrel HBV infections have been associated with only the mildest forms of hepatitis in carrier animals (Marion and Robinson 1983, Marion et al. 1980). Duck HBV apparently causes mild to severe hepatitis, but to date no association with hepatocellular carcinoma has been made (Marion et al. 1984, Omata et al. 1983).

Preliminary observations suggest that a pathogenic HBV may be present in certain species of exotic felids (Gupta 1978, Raphael 1982, Worley 1983). More recently, a transmissible hepatitis has been reported in the dog, but evidence of hepadnavirus involvement was not presented (Jarrett and O'Neil 1985).

REFERENCES

Beasley, R.P., Lin, C.C., Hwang, L.Y., and Chien, C.S. 1981. Hepatocellular carcinoma and hepatitis B virus. A prospective study of 22,707 men in Taiwan. Lancet 2:1129–1133.

Fye, K.H., Becker, M.J., Theofilopoulos, A.N. Moutsopoulos, H., Feldman, J.L., and Talal, N. 1977. Immune complexes in hepatitis B antigen-associated periarteritis nodosa. Detection by antibody-dependent cell-mediated cytotoxicity and the Raji cell assay. Am. J. Med. 62:783–791.

Gocke, D.J. 1975. Extrahepatic manifestations of viral hepatitis. Am. J. Med. Sci. 270:49–52.

Gupta, P.P. 1978. Inclusion body hepatitis in a black panther (*Panthera pardus pardus*). Zentralbl. Veterinärmed. [B] 25:858–860.

Gust, I.D., Burrell, C.J., Coulepis, A.G., Robinson, W.S., and Zuckerman, A.J. 1986. Taxonomic classification of human hepatitis B virus. Intervirology 25:14–29.

Jarrett, W.F.H., and O'Neil, B.W. 1985. A new transmissible agent causing acute hepatitis, chronic hepatitis and cirrhosis in dogs. Vet. Rec. 116:629–635.

Kohler, P.F., Cronin, R.E., Hammond, W.S., Olin, D., and Carr, R.I. 1974. Chronic membranous glomerulonephritis caused by hepatitis B antigen-antibody immune complexes. Ann. Int. Med. 81:448–451.

Marion, P.L., and Robinson, W.S. 1983. Hepadna viruses: Hepatitis B and related viruses. Curr. Top. Microbiol. Immunol. 105:99–121.

Marion, P.L., Knight, S.S., Ho, B.K., Guo, Y.Y., Robinson, W.S., and Popper, H. 1984. Liver disease associated with duck hepatitis B virus infection of domestic ducks. Proc. Natl. Acad. Sci. USA 81:898–902.

Marion, P.L., Oshiro, L.S., Regnery, D.C., Scullard, G.H., and Robinson, W.S. 1980. A virus in Beechey ground squirrels that is related to hepatitis B virus of humans. Proc. Natl. Acad. Sci. USA 77:2941–2945.

Mason, W.S., Seal, G., and Summers, J. 1980. Virus of Pekin ducks with structural and biological relatedness to human hepatitis B virus. J. Virol. 36:829–836.

Omata, M., Uchiumi, K., Ito, Y., Yokosuka, O., Mori, J., Terao, K., Wei-Fa, Y., O'Connell, A.P., London, W.T., and Okuda, K. 1983. Duck hepatitis B virus and liver diseases. Gastroenterology 85:260–267.

Peters, R.L. 1975. Viral hepatitis: A pathologic spectrum. Am. J. Med. Sci. 270:17–31.

Popper, H., Shih, J.W.K., Gerin, J.L., Wong, D.C., Hoyer, B.H., London, W.T., Sly, D.L., and Purcell, R.H. 1981. Woodchuck hepatitis and hepatocellular carcinoma: Correlation of histologic with virologic observations. Hepatology 1:91–98.

Raphael, B.L. 1982. Hepatitis in a spotted leopard (*Panthera pardus*). Proceedings of the American Association of Zoo Veterinarians. Pp. 61–63.

Redeker, A.G. 1975. Viral hepatitis: Clinical aspects. Am. J. Med. Sci. 270:9–16.

Summers, J., Smolec, J.M., and Snyder, R. 1978. A virus similar to human hepatitis B virus associated with hepatitis and hepatoma in woodchucks. Proc. Natl. Acad. Sci. USA 75:4533–4537.

Szmuness, W. 1978. Hepatocellular carcinoma and the hepatitis B virus: Evidence for a causal association. Prog. Med. Virol. 24:40–69.

Thomas, H.C., Pignatelli, M., Goodall, A., Waters, J., Karayiannis, P., and Brown, D. 1984. Immunologic mechanisms of cell lysis in hepatitis B virus infection. In G.N. Vyas, J.L. Dienstag, and J.H. Hoofnagle, eds., Viral Hepatitis and Liver Disease. Grune & Stratton, New York. Pp. 167–177.

Tiollais, P., Pourcel, C., and Dejean, A. 1985. The hepatitis B virus. Nature 317:489–495.

Wands, J.R., Mann, E., Alpert, E., and Isselbacher, K.J. 1975. The pathogenesis of arthritis associated with acute hepatitis-B surface antigen-positive hepatitis. Complement activation and characterization of circulating immune complexes. J. Clin. Invest. 55:930–936.

Worley, M.B. 1983. The continuing role of a feline hepatitis B-like virus in the pathogenesis of liver disease in exotic felids. Proceedings of the American Association of Zoo Veterinarians. Pp. 17–20.

Torovirus Infection

The family name Toroviridae has been proposed for a small and intriguing group of RNA viruses found in animals and humans (Beards et al. 1984; Horzinek and Weiss 1984; Horzinek et al. 1984; Moussa et al. 1983; Weiss and Horzinek 1987; Weiss et al. 1983; Woode et al. 1982, 1985). At present, the members of this group that are associated with animals consist of (1) Berne virus, isolated in Switzerland from a horse that died with pseudomembranous enteritis and miliary granulomas and necrosis in the liver (Weiss et al. 1983); (2) Breda virus serotypes 1 and 2, from scouring calves in the United States (Woode et al. 1982, 1985); and (3) Lyon 4 virus, from cattle in France (Moussa et al. 1983, Weiss et al. 1983). Similar agents that are cross-reactive with Breda virus have been observed in France and England in feces of humans with diarrhea (Beards et al. 1984). To date, the equine Berne agent remains the only torovirus isolated in cell culture. On the basis of available scientific data (and extrapolating largely from studies of Berne virus), the following features appear to be characteristic of this newly recognized group of viruses:

1. The genome is composed of single-stranded RNA. Nevertheless, replication depends on some nuclear function of the host cell (Horzinek et al. 1984, Pohlenz et al. 1984).

2. The nucleocapsid is an elongated, tubular structure of presumably helical symmetry. It may be bent into the shape of an open torus, conferring a disk- or kidney-shaped morphology to the virion (diameter 120 to 140 nm) (Figure 58.3), or it may appear as a straight tube, producing a rod-shaped particle (dimensions: 35 by 170 nm) (Horzinek and Weiss 1984, Horzinek et al. 1985). The curved or toroid shape apparently is maintained by the

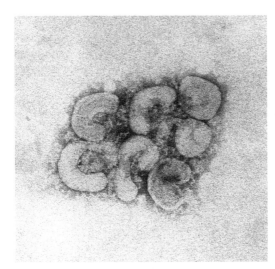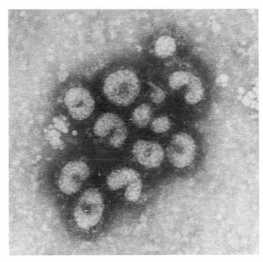

Figure 58.3. Toroviruses, illustrating the characteristic toroid or kidney-shaped morphology of the virions. (*Left*) Berne virus, semipurified preparation from a cell-culture supernatant. Phosphotungstic acid. × 130,380. (Courtesy M. Weiss, University of Berne.) (*Right*) Breda virus 2, immune electron microscopic preparation. Phosphotungstic acid. × 109,620. (From Woode et al., 1985, by permission of *American Journal of Veterinary Research*. Photo courtesy of L. J. Saif, OARDC, Ohio State University.)

tight-fitting viral envelope, which is studded with drumstick-shaped peplomers and contains a hemagglutinin (Weiss et al. 1983, Woode et al. 1982, Zanoni et al. 1986). The overall morphology superficially resembles that of the Coronaviridae, but data on protein composition (only two major structural polypeptides), replication strategy, physicochemical properties, and antigenic structure indicate that toroviruses are distinct from coronaviruses.

3. Experimental studies suggest a relatively narrow in vivo host cell spectrum, consisting primarily of epithelial cells in the jejunum, ileum, cecum, and colon (Pohlenz et al. 1984, Woode et al. 1982). Enteropathogenicity has been definitively demonstrated for the Breda agent in calves, but experimental inoculation of horses with Berne virus has not resulted in clinical disease (Pohlenz et al. 1984, Weiss et al. 1984, Woode et al. 1982, 1985).

Seroepizootiological studies indicate that Berne virus infections are widespread in horses in Switzerland and have been so for at least a decade (Weiss et al. 1984). A number of seropositive horses have also been identified in France, Germany, and the United States. Antibody titers have also been demonstrated in cattle, goats, sheep, pigs, rabbits, and mice. In limited studies in the United States, a high percentage of cattle have been found to have antibodies to Breda virus (Woode et al. 1985).

At the time of this writing, (1987), it is clear that at least one torovirus—the Breda agent—is probably involved in the pathogenesis of the neonatal calf diarrhea complex, a multifactorial disease entity of great economic impor-

tance to the livestock industry. Further studies are required, however, to elucidate the relative importance of this agent (and other toroviruses) in livestock disease outbreaks. In addition, the significance of Berne virus in diseases of horses and ruminants remains to be determined.

REFERENCES

Beards, G.M., Green, J., Hall, C., Flewett, T.H., Lamouliatte, F., and du Pasquier, P. 1984. An enveloped virus in stools of children and adults with gastroenteritis that resembles the Breda virus of calves. Lancet 1:1050–1052.

Horzinek, M.C., and Weiss, M. 1984. Toroviridae: A taxonomic proposal. Zentralbl. Veterinärmed. [B] 31:649–659.

Horzinek, M.C., Ederveen, J., and Weiss, M. 1985. The nucleocapsid of Berne virus. J. Gen. Virol. 66:1287–1296.

Horzinek, M.C., Weiss, M., and Ederveen, J. 1984. Berne virus is not "coronavirus-like." J. Gen. Virol. 65:645–649.

Moussa, A., Dannacher, G., and Fedida, M. 1983. Nouveaux virus intervenant dans l'étiologie des entérites néonatales des bovins. Rec. Méd. Vét. 159:185–190.

Pohlenz, J.F.L., Cheville, N.F., Woode, G.N., and Mokresh, A.H. 1984. Cellular lesions in intestinal mucosa of gnotobiotic calves experimentally infected with a new unclassified bovine virus (Breda virus). Vet. Pathol. 21:407–417.

Weiss, M., and Horzinek, M.C. 1987. The proposed family Toroviridae: Agents of enteric infections. Arch. Virol. 92:1–15.

Weiss, M., Steck, F., and Horzinek, M.C. 1983. Purification and partial characterization of a new enveloped RNA virus (Berne virus). J. Gen. Virol. 64:1849–1858.

Weiss, M., Steck, F., Kaderli, R., and Horzinek, M.C. 1984. Antibodies to Berne virus in horses and other animals. Vet. Microbiol. 9:523–531.

Woode, G.N., Reed, D.E., Runnels, P.L., Herrig, M.A., and Hill, H.T. 1982. Studies with an unclassified virus isolated from diarrheic calves. Vet. Microbiol. 7:221–240.

Woode, G.N., Saif, L.J., Quesada, M., Winand, N.J., Pohlenz, J.F., and Gourley, N.K. 1985. Comparative studies on three isolates of Breda virus of calves. Am. J. Vet. Res. 46:1003–1010.

Zanoni, R., Weiss, M., and Peterhans, E. 1986. The haemagglutinating activity of Berne virus. J. Gen. Virol. 67:2485–2488.

Borna Disease

SYNONYMS: Meningoencephalomyelitis enzootica equorum, enzootic encephalomyelitis, hot head, nerve fever

Borna disease is a rare viral meningoencephalomyelitis of horses and sheep that has been enzootic in certain areas of Germany and Switzerland for over 150 years (Blood et al. 1983; Buxton and Fraser 1977; Dietz and Wiesner 1984; Gosztonyi and Ludwig 1984; Ludwig and Becht 1977; Metzler et al. 1976; Metzler, Ehrensperger, et al. 1979; Metzler, Minder, et al. 1979; Waelchli et al. 1985; Zwick 1939). The name derives from a town near Leipzig in which a particularly severe epizootic occurred in the 1890s. Confirmed cases appear to be limited to middle and eastern Europe, with a pattern of sporadic spread within circumscribed geographic areas. Persistence of the virus in infected animals is an important pathogenetic feature of the disease (Ludwig and Becht 1977; Metzler, Ehrensperger, et al. 1979; Metzler, Minder, et al. 1979).

Character of the Disease. *In horses* the incubation period is characteristically prolonged (at least 4 to 6 weeks and possibly as long as 6 months). Initial clinical signs are generally nonspecific and can include anorexia, fever, excessive salivation, chewing movements, frequent yawning, and lassitude. Diarrhea, mild colic, and coughing also may be present. As the disease progresses, neurological signs—ataxia, nystagmus, head-pressing, saw-horse stance, somnolence, paresis, and disturbances of equilibrium—gain increasing prominence. The disequilibrium is especially pronounced if a blindfold is placed over the animal's eyes. A transient stage of restlessness may be seen, which is characterized by hyperesthesia, reflex irritability, and biting, kicking, or other compulsive movements. The animal is easily startled and may fall into convulsions. Usually the disease course is progressive, with recumbency occurring after 1 to 2 weeks. Sometimes, however, the course is more gradual, with days or even weeks of temporary improvement. These periods are usually interrupted by recurrent fevers and neurological signs. Low morbidity and high mortality are characteristic of the disease; the mortality rate in animals showing signs of encephalomyelitis averages 90 to 95 percent or more. Residual neurological deficits are common in those animals that survive.

In sheep the clinical signs and disease course are comparable to those in horses (Metzler et al. 1976; Metzler, Ehrensperger, et al. 1979; Waelchli et al. 1985).

No characteristic gross lesions have been identified. Histologically, lesions of meningoencephalomyelitis—perivascular cuffing, ganglion cell degeneration, neuronophagia, gliosis—are evident, being most conspicuous in the midbrain. Characteristic eosinophilic intranuclear inclusions (Joest-Degen bodies), when present, can be found in ganglion cells of the hippocampus and olfactory lobes of the cerebral cortex and are considered pathognomonic for the disease (Figure 58.4). Typically, they are located near the nucleolus and are surrounded by a colorless halo. In general, lesions in the spinal cord are much less severe than those in the brain.

Properties of the Virus. Borna disease is caused by an

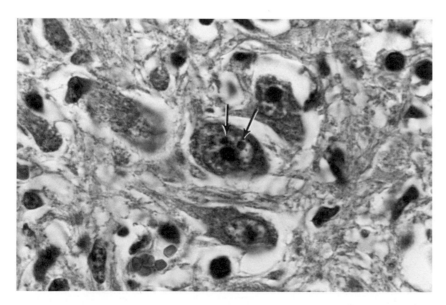

Figure 58.4. Borna disease. Intranuclear (Joest-Degen) inclusion bodies (*arrows*) in a neuron of the hippocampus, from the brain of a sheep with Borna disease. Hematoxylin and eosin stain. × 1,023. (Courtesy F. Ehrensperger, University of Zurich.)

unclassified RNA virus that appears to be enveloped and closely associated with host cell membranes (Danner and Mayr 1979, Danner et al. 1978, Herzog and Rott 1980, Hirano et al. 1983, Ludwig and Becht 1977, Ludwig et al. 1973, Mayr and Danner 1972). It replicates only very slowly in cell culture, producing a persistent non-cytopathic infection, and spreads mainly by direct cell-to-cell contact without the release of infectious virions into the culture medium (although a particulate, complement-fixing antigen is produced). As might be expected, for decades these properties have hampered attempts to further characterize the virus. Data accumulated thus far indicate that the agent is heat- and acid-labile but relatively resistant to drying and can survive in the environment for lengthy periods if protected from direct light. Discrete virus particles have only rarely been demonstrated by electron microscopy (Ludwig and Becht 1977); filtration studies suggest a diameter of between 80 and 100 nm. Experiments have shown that DNA synthesis is not required for Borna virus replication; yet viral antigen is consistently found in the nucleus of infected cells examined by immunofluorescence microscopy and, probably, is recognized histologically as Joest-Degen inclusions. There appears to be only a single virus serotype, although individual strains can show differences in virulence and the range of hosts they infect. Consideration must be given to placement of the virus in a new and distinct group, since its known properties are not shared by any recognized virus family.

Cultivation. Ironically, Borna disease virus produces persistent, noncytolytic infections in a variety of primary cell cultures and established cell lines. Presence of the virus can be readily demonstrated by immunofluorescence microscopy. Titer yields from disrupted monolayers are very low, however, but can be boosted somewhat by *n*-butyrate or hypertonic media (Pauli and Ludwig 1985). The virus can also be propagated in embryonating chicken eggs and in a number of laboratory animal species, especially rabbits. Guinea pigs, rats, monkeys, and tree shrews are also susceptible. Dogs and cats appear to be resistant.

Epizootiology and Pathogenesis. Borna disease occurs naturally in horses and sheep and occasionally in rabbits (Buxton and Fraser 1977; Dietz and Wiesner 1984; Ludwig and Becht 1977; Metzler et al. 1976, 1978; Metzler, Ehrensperger, et al. 1979; Metzler, Minder, et al. 1979; Waelchli et al. 1985). Antibodies have been found in cattle and goats, but spontaneous cases of the disease have not been reported in these species. Wildlife reservoirs have not been identified; the natural reservoir is assumed to be infected domestic animals, with shedding by convalescent and immune carriers considered likely. Al-

though most cases are seen during late spring and early summer, the disease may occur at any time. The decline in the number of new cases seen late in the year suggests that arthropod vectors may play a role in transmission of the virus. Despite decades of study, however, the generally sporadic nature of the disease and its striking geographic isolation have never been adequately explained.

The principal means of natural infection is apparently by way of the nasal mucosa and olfactory nerve following droplet inhalation (Dietz and Wiesner 1984, Krey et al. 1979). The virus has an affinity for ganglionic neurons, especially those of the limbic system. Evidence suggests that it invades the central nervous system along neural (axonal) pathways and then spreads centrifugally to the mucous membranes, salivary glands, kidneys, and mammary glands, thus disseminating in a manner reminiscent of its behavior in cell culture (Dietz and Wiesner 1984, Gosztonyi and Ludwig 1984, Krey et al. 1979, Narayan et al. 1983). The largest amount of viral antigen is always found in the nuclei of infected neurons; the presence of this antigen appears to trigger self-destructive inflammatory reactions, producing an encephalomyelitis (Gosztonyi and Ludwig 1984). Spread of infection probably results from contamination of food and water by virus shed in nasal and salivary secretions during the period of acute illness. The virus is also excreted in urine and milk.

Immunity. Seroconversion in the absence of clinical disease is recognized, but most animals that develop clinical signs of encephalomyelitis die. Animals that recover are immune, but the duration of immunity is not known. Convalescent and immune carriers are believed to be important in the maintenance of infections in nature.

Diagnosis. A presumptive diagnosis may be made in enzootic areas on the basis of clinical signs, but a definitive diagnosis requires laboratory confirmation. Several techniques are available, including rabbit inoculation, virus isolation, and immunofluorescence microscopy or complement fixation for detection of viral antigen in tissues or in cell culture. Histological identification of Joest-Degen inclusion bodies in ganglion cell nuclei is considered diagnostic. In animals that survive, paired (acute and convalescent) serum or cerebrospinal fluid samples may be collected for detection of an antibody titer rise by indirect immunofluorescence.

Treatment. There is no specific therapy for Borna disease. Cerebral edema can be relieved temporarily by intravenous administration of mannitol, and antiinflammatory drugs may make affected animals more comfortable. The prognosis is exceedingly poor; more than 90 percent of animals showing signs of encephalomyelitis die.

Prevention and Control. Both inactivated and modified live virus vaccines have been investigated for preven-

Sporadic Bovine Encephalomyelitis

SYNONYM: Sporadic bovine
meningoencephalomyelitis; abbreviation,
SBE

Sporadic bovine encephalomyelitis is an extremely rare acute to subacute disease of young cattle primarily between 1 and 3 years of age (Bachmann 1986, Bachmann et al. 1975, Billing 1974, Fankhauser 1961, Fatzer 1971). It was first described in 1961 in Switzerland and has since been recognized also in Germany. Despite the name, it is etiologically and pathogenetically distinct from chlamydial SBE.

The onset of the disease is often sudden. Nonspecific clinical signs include anorexia, weight loss, lethargy, and fever. Hyporeactivity, somnolence, incoordination, abnormal carriage of the head and ears, and changes in behavior result from pathological changes in the central nervous system. Other neurological signs include pharyngeal paralysis and hypersalivation, abnormal stance and gait, muscular spasms, restlessness, excitation, frequent falling, timidity, aggression, grinding of the teeth, running against fixed objects, and bellowing. With progressive paralysis of the limbs the animal goes down, showing opisthotonus, tympany of the rumen, occasional diarrhea, and tenesmus. The expression of the eyes is altered, and slight miosis and ptosis are seen. Extreme weakness and dyspnea follow, terminating in death. The duration of the clinical course in most animals is between 2 and 5 days, but some animals may linger on for weeks. There is no recognized seasonality in the occurrence of the disease, and generally only a single animal in a herd is affected at any one time.

No characteristic gross lesions are seen. Histopathological changes in the brain include perivascular cuffing, diffuse infiltration of lymphocytes into the parenchyma, proliferation of microglial cells and astrocytes, neuronal loss, massive neuronophagia, and eosinophilic intranuclear and intracytoplasmic inclusion bodies within affected neurons. Demyelination and sclerosis do not occur. The histological alterations generally are distributed over all portions of the brain and brain stem, although the cerebellum may be spared.

The causative agent of SBE has not been identified, but a cell-associated paramyxovirus (probably morbillivirus) has been isolated from one diseased animal in southern Germany (Bachmann et al. 1975). Antibodies to this virus have been found in cattle in several countries, including Germany, Australia, and the United States, but inoculation experiments thus far have failed to reproduce the disease (Bachmann 1986). The agent appears to be very distantly related antigenically to rinderpest virus and to the virus of subacute sclerosing panencephalitis (SSPE) (Bachmann et al. 1975). This latter agent is now recognized as a persistent variant of measles virus that causes a late, progressive, noncontagious encephalitis in children and young adults (Fujinami and Oldstone 1984, Norrby 1985). The clinical signs and neuropathological lesions of SBE somewhat resemble those seen in calves experimentally inoculated with SSPE virus (Thein et al. 1972), and some investigators have suggested that animals may be involved in the epizootiology of SSPE because of this disease's predominance in rural areas (Brody and Detels 1970).

Definitive diagnosis of SBE can be made only by histopathological examination of brain tissue. The disease is inevitably fatal, and no specific therapy or immunoprophylaxis is available.

REFERENCES

Bachmann, P.A. 1986. Sporadic bovine encephalomyelitis (SBE). In J.L. Howard, ed., Current Veterinary Therapy: Food Animal Practice, 2d ed. W.B. Saunders, Philadelphia. Pp. 499–501.
Bachmann, P.A., ter Meulen, V., Jentsch, G., Appel, M., Iwasaki, Y., Meyermann, R., Koprowski, H., and Mayr, A. 1975. Sporadic bovine meningo-encephalitis—Isolation of a paramyxovirus. Arch. Virol. 48:107–120.
Billing, J. 1974. Epizootologische Untersuchungen über sporadisch auftretende, nichteitrige Encephalomyelitiden beim Rind. Inaugural dissertation, Tierärztliche Fakultät, Munich. 102 pp.
Brody, J.A., and Detels, R. 1970. Subacute sclerosing panencephalitis: A zoonosis following aberrant measles. Lancet 2:500–501.
Fankhauser, R. 1961. Sporadische Meningo-Encephalomyelitis beim Rind. Schweiz. Arch. Tierheilkd. 103:225–235.
Fatzer, R. 1971. Untersuchungen an Gehirnen tollwutnegativer Haustiere. Schweiz. Arch. Tierheilkd. 112:59–65.
Fujinami, R.S., and Oldstone, M.B.A. 1984. Antibody initiates virus persistence: Immune modulation and measles virus infection. In A.L. Notkins and M.B.A. Oldstone, eds., Concepts in Viral Pathogenesis. Springer-Verlag, New York. Pp. 187–193.
Norrby, E. 1985. Measles. In B.N. Fields, ed., Virology. Raven Press, New York. Pp. 1305–1321.
Thein, P., Mayr, A., ter Meulen, V., Koprowski, H., Käckell, M.Y., Müller, D., and Meyermann, R. 1972. Subacute sclerosing panencephalitis. Transmission of the virus to calves and lambs. Arch. Neurol. 27:540–548.

Scrapie

SYNONYMS: *Rida, la tremblante, die
Traberkrankheit,* brushing disease,
trotting disease, trembling disease,
nibbling disease, the rubs, cuddy trot,
yeuky pine

Several diseases of animals and humans are characterized by a prolonged incubation period, insidious onset, protracted course, and inevitable fatality, and produce histopathological alterations atypical of acute viral infections. The term *slow infection* was introduced by

Sigurdsson in 1954, based on his studies of several such diseases that had appeared in Iceland following importation of sheep from Germany and on his studies of scrapie, which had been known in Iceland for many years as *rida* (Eklund and Hadlow 1981, Kimberlin 1981, Sigurdsson 1954). One of the central tenets of Sigurdsson's work was that an initially mild clinical disease that over several months progressed to a fatal conclusion could be the result of an infection that had occurred years earlier. Today there is great interest in the study of such slow diseases of animals because of the unconventional properties of certain of their causative agents and because some of them show similarities to comparable intractable conditions of humans. One of the most unusual and intriguing of these agents is the cause of scrapie, a disease of sheep and goats. Scrapie, transmissible mink encephalopathy, chronic wasting disease of captive mule deer and elk, and the human maladies kuru and Creutzfeldt-Jakob disease constitute a cluster of so-called slow virus diseases of the central nervous system known as the subacute spongiform viral encephalopathies (Gajdusek 1985).

Character of the Disease. Scrapie is an afebrile, chronic, progressive degenerative disorder of the central nervous system of sheep and occasionally of goats (Eklund and Hadlow 1981, Kimberlin 1981, Mitchell and Stamp 1983, Parry and Oppenheimer 1983). It has been known in many parts of Europe for more than 200 years and has also been recorded in Asia, Africa, and the Americas (Gajdusek 1985, Stockman 1913). It has been a particular problem in England, Scotland, Iceland, France, and Germany. On occasion it has been imported into Australia, New Zealand, South Africa, and Kenya, but its prompt recognition and the subsequent slaughter of all affected animals have led to its eradication from those areas. It was first recognized in Canada in 1938 and in the United States in 1947 and still exists in both of these countries.

Scrapie is clearly an age-related disorder, first appearing in animals between the ages of 2 and 5 years and progressing slowly, over 3 to 6 months or longer, to death. The most commonly affected sheep breeds are Suffolk, Cheviot, and Swaledale. There is no recognized sex predilection, although rams appear to manifest the disease at a slightly younger age. The incubation period is extraordinarily long, ranging on the average from 1 to 4 years.

In sheep the onset of the disease is insidious; several months may elapse before specific signs of illness are recognized. During this initial stage, however, subtle changes of behavior may be noted by the experienced observer: a slight apprehensiveness or general nervousness, a staring or fixed gaze, distrust of humans and failure to respond to herding dogs, and a certain jitteriness while being shorn. As the disease progresses, intolerance to exercise and a clumsy, unsteady gait begin to be noticed. Often the ears flop unduly while the animal is walking, and the fleece may show a whitish tip to the staple over the back. Affected sheep make frequent trips to the watering trough but drink very little each time. Later the animals begin to rub themselves against firm, immobile objects, wearing away the fleece and hair, hence the name *scrapie*. The rubbing usually is confined to localized areas around the base of the tail, the sides of the body just above and below the elbow, and the lower lateral neck (Figure 58.5). Sometimes there is a general brushing of the entire side of the body ("shrugginess"). A compulsive nibbling

Figure 58.5. Scrapie in a Herwick sheep, showing severe wool loss caused by compulsive nibbling and rubbing. (From Kimberlin, 1981, courtesy of Academic Press.)

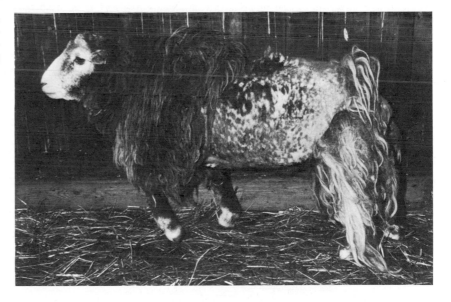

at the haired skin below the knee and hock is seen. This response can be elicited manually by sharply stroking the lumbar spine and the hips; nibbling motions, a raising of the head, extrusion of the tongue and smacking of the lips, and a general ovine "air of satisfaction" with the process are the result. At this stage of the disease, usually some 2 months after the onset of recognizable clinical signs, loss of weight and a general unthriftiness first become apparent, although the appetite usually is unaffected. The fleece and hair are lusterless. A rash may appear over the haired portions of the body, with papular eruptions and production of a serous exudate. The gait is noticeably ataxic and is accentuated when the animals are driven. The stance is wide-based, with the head held up and the nose in the air. A fine trembling of the body and head and coarsely adjusted posturing movements that attempt to maintain the animal on an "even keel" are seen.

Within 3 or 4 months of onset, the late and final stages of the disease develop. Most animals now lose weight to an alarming degree, wasting away despite all attempts at medical intervention. They become extremely difficult to handle because they can no longer be driven and may become quite agitated and confused if separated from familiar companions. The gait becomes extremely unsteady, and frequently they attempt to move forward in a sort of clumsy gallop, using both hind limbs simultaneously, in antelope fashion, in order to maintain balance. Animals that are frightened or alarmed may fall down repeatedly owing to their incoordination of locomotion. Partial paralysis, particularly of the hind quarters, then develops in many animals. In the terminal stage the sheep cannot rise to their feet, and display hypertonicity of the limbs, particularly of the side on which they are lying. Blindness and seizures are occasionally seen. The ability to swallow food without assistance is lost, and death follows soon after. Often the animal is found dead in the morning by the shepherd or flockmaster. Not all signs of scrapie are manifested in every affected animal; however, most do exhibit the classic clinical triad of rubbing, ataxia, and wasting. The mortality rate is essentially 100 percent.

In goats the clinical signs of scrapie are generally comparable to those in sheep. *In mink* a rare transmissible encephalopathy with signs similar to those of scrapie has been observed and may in fact be caused by the scrapie agent or a variant of it (Burger and Hartsough 1965, Hartsough and Burger 1965, Kimberlin and Marsh 1975, Marsh and Kimberlin 1975).

No characteristic gross lesions are found in scrapie. Histologically, the only consistent lesions occur in the central nervous system and are degenerative rather than inflammatory (Bignami and Parry 1972a, 1972b; Brown-lee 1940; Holman and Pattison 1943; Jubb et al. 1985; Kimberlin 1981; Zlotnick 1958). Of these, the most striking is a bilaterally symmetrical vacuolation of neurons in the brain stem and spinal cord (Figure 58.6). The vacuoles can be either single or multiple and are located in the cytoplasm, often producing a bulging or distention of the affected cells. Some vacuoles contain eosinophilic globules, but most appear to be empty. Accompanying interstitial spongy degeneration is usually found in the same areas as neuronal vacuolation, and occasionally neuronal loss occurs. Astrogliosis is a common finding, but amyloid plaques are rare. There is no gross tract demyelination and little perivascular cuffing or meningitis. In general the cerebral cortex is spared.

Although it is consistently associated with scrapie, neuronal vacuolation is not considered to be pathognomonic, since it can be found in varying degrees in other diseases and, to a much lesser extent, in apparently healthy sheep. However, the lesions are considered specific and dramatic enough for diagnostic purposes, especially when combined with the history, clinical picture, and concomitant presence of other signs of degeneration, which are not found in normal sheep (Jubb et al. 1985, Kimberlin 1981, Zlotnick 1958, Zlotnick and Rennie 1958).

Properties of the Agent. Identification and characterization of the causative agent of scrapie (and agents of the other spongiform encephalopathies) is an area of fertile research interest today (Carp et al. 1985; Gajdusek 1985; Kimberlin 1981; Prusiner 1982, 1984a, 1984b). The scrapie agent, whatever its nature, certainly behaves unconventionally. It is extremely resistant to heat, formalin, pH variation, and a number of enzymes, including nucleases. It is sensitive, however, to phenol, 2-chloroethanol, proteases, urea, and sodium dodecylsulfate. Scrapie infectivity is intimately associated with cellular membranes, and thus the agent has proved extremely difficult to purify. Studies indicate that the infectious unit is probably larger than about 30 nm, but conventional virionlike particles have never been visualized by electron microscopy. Instead, filamentous structures known as *scrapie-associated fibrils* (SAFs) are found in negatively stained, detergent-treated membrane fractions from scrapie-infected brain tissue (Figure 58.7) (Diringer et al. 1983, Merz et al. 1981, Prusiner 1982, Prusiner et al. 1983). Structurally they do not resemble any known animal virus or virus product, but they do bear a superficial resemblance to amyloid (DeArmond et al. 1985; Merz et al. 1981,1982; Prusiner 1984b; Prusiner et al. 1983). They appear to be quite heterogeneous in character and are specific for different strains of the scrapie agent (Kascsak et al. 1985). It remains undetermined whether these fibrils are the result of a unique pathological

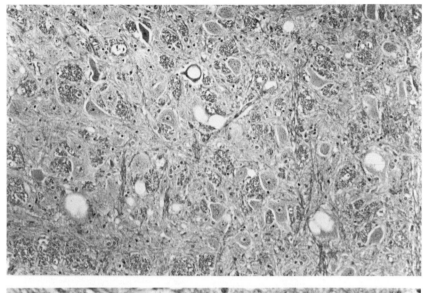

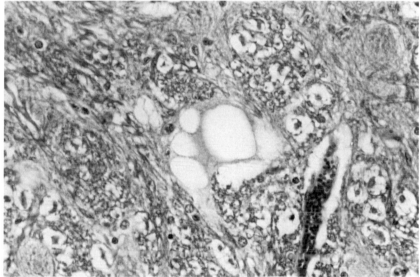

Figure 58.6. Vacuolation of several neurons and of the neuropil in the medulla oblongata of a sheep with scrapie (*top*). Hematoxylin and eosin. × 40. Higher magnification of a neuron containing several intracytoplasmic vacuoles (*bottom*). Hematoxylin and eosin. × 98. (Courtesy B. A. Summers, Cornell University.)

response to the scrapie agent or represent the actual agent itself (Carp et al. 1985, Chesebro et al. 1985, Cho 1986, Gajdusek 1985, Liao et al. 1986, Merz et al. 1984, Somerville et al. 1986). Related structures can also be found in certain other unconventional slow virus diseases that have similarities to scrapie (kuru, Creutzfeldt-Jakob disease) (Bendheim et al. 1985, Gajdusek 1985, Manuelidis et al. 1985, Merz et al. 1983).

These and other unusual physicochemical and biological properties of the scrapie agent have led, not unexpectedly, to an abundance of hypotheses concerning its exact nature and mode of replication. The following are among the current hypotheses (Carp et al. 1985):

The filamentous virus hypothesis. In this hypothesis the SAFs are interpreted as representing a visible form of the scrapie agent, that is, the agent is a filamentous virus, analogous to the filamentous bacteriophages and plant viruses (Carp et al. 1985, Merz et al. 1983).

The prion hypothesis. The term *prion* is derived from the words *proteinaceous infectious particle;* in its strictest sense, it describes a small infectious protein, either completely devoid of nucleic acid or containing a polynucleotide too small to code for its own biosynthesis, which nevertheless is capable of being replicated (Bolton et al. 1984; Diener et al. 1982; Prusiner 1982, 1984a, 1984b). The SAFs are thus interpreted as polymeric forms of the prion protein (prion rods).

The virino hypothesis. According to this theory, the agent is composed of an extremely low molecular weight regulatory nucleic acid that acquires a protective protein

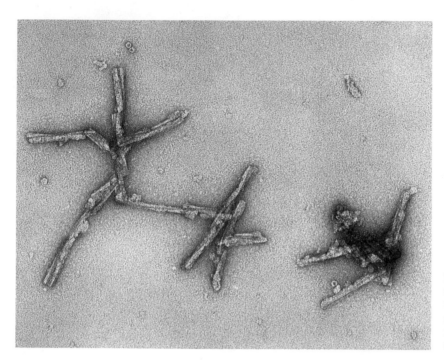

Figure 58.7. Scrapie-associated fibrils from scrapie strain ME7 in affected mouse brain. Uranyl acetate. × 132,828. (Courtesy P. M. Merz, New York State Institute for Basic Research in Developmental Disabilities.)

coat encoded by the host cell DNA; the nucleic acid is replicated by host cell enzymes (Dickinson and Outram 1979, Kimberlin 1982).

The requirement of the scrapie agent for protein (i.e., its sensitivity to proteases) clearly rules out the possibility that it is a *viroid* (Carp et al. 1985, Diener et al. 1982). Viroids are higher plant pathogens, composed exclusively of RNA, which probably induce pathological changes by disrupting host cellular regulatory functions. Other hypotheses suggest that the scrapie agent is composed exclusively of polysaccharide or oligosaccharide, is a replicating membrane component or macromolecular membrane complex, or perhaps is a more conventional virus whose close association with membrane material in crude tissue preparations affords it a degree of protection against harsh treatments and dissociative purification procedures (Dees et al. 1985a, 1985b; Dees, Wade, et al. 1985; Gajdusek 1985; Gibbons and Hunter 1967; Marsh et al. 1974, 1984; Rohwer 1984a, 1984b). A most interesting hypothesis is that the scrapie agent and others like it act by derepressing host genetic information that codes for their own biosynthesis (Gajdusek and Gibbs 1973).

Cultivation. The scrapie agent can be replicated in a small number of murine cell-culture systems, but the efficiency of infection is extremely low, and cytopathic effects are not observed (Clarke and Haig 1970a, 1970b; Clarke and Millson 1976; Elleman 1984). Thus the only quantitative method available for assay of the agent is titration in experimental animals. Successful transmission of scrapie has been accomplished by inoculation of sheep,

goats, mink, rats, hamsters, gerbils, and mice. Of these, the mouse represents the most important and useful animal model of the disease, and much of our knowledge about the agent and the genetics and pathogenesis of scrapie has been gleaned from experimental infections in this species (Kimberlin 1981, Mitchell and Stamp 1983). It has thus been possible to differentiate strains of the scrapie agent on the basis of genetically controlled parameters of incubation period and lesion distribution in inbred mice of defined phenotypes (Dickinson and Fraser 1977).

Epizootiology and Pathogenesis. Sheep are considered the natural hosts for the scrapie agent. A considerable body of evidence indicates that most sheep with scrapie were infected early in life and that the agent has persisted within them in a quiescent state during the intervening period (Mitchell and Stamp 1983). It is well established that maternal transmission accounts for much of the familial pattern commonly seen in outbreaks of scrapie (Dickinson et al. 1965, 1974). The route by which maternal transmission occurs is not known; there is evidence both for prenatal and postnatal infections, and the agent is known to be present in the fetal membranes (Pattison et al. 1972). Horizontal transmission also occurs and can be accomplished experimentally by oral dosing, scarification, and instillation within the conjunctiva (Kimberlin 1981). Relatively little is known about the persistence of the scrapie agent in the environment, but its general stability, together with certain clinical observations, suggests that persistence in the pasture or in buildings is a real possibility. Dissemination at parturition through contaminated fetal membranes may be an extremely important means by which the agent is liberated into the environment (Pattison et al. 1972).

In the mouse model, initial replication of the scrapie agent appears to take place in the lymphoid organs and in the lower intestine, possibly within mucosal-associated lymphoid tissue (Eklund et al. 1967, Kimberlin 1981). Viremia (or, perhaps, "agentemia") is either absent or of extremely low titer, and the route of invasion of the central nervous system is still not clearly defined. Possibly the agent enters at the level of the spinal cord and then travels along neural pathways to the brain (Kimberlin 1981, Kimberlin and Walker 1986). Infective titers in the brain are higher than those in extraneural tissues and are highest in those areas in which the most severe histopathological changes are observed. The mechanism by which the agent induces these changes has not been elucidated (Kretzschmar et al. 1986).

Immunity. Scrapie occurs naturally in the absence of any detectable host humoral or cellular immune response and is inevitably fatal once clinical signs are manifest. Artificially, antibodies can be raised to SAF-prion rods in rabbits by hyperimmunization procedures (Barry et al. 1985, Bendheim et al. 1984). Neither lymphocytes nor interferon appears to be effective in controlling scrapie (Fraser and Dickinson 1978, Gresser and Pattison 1968, Kasper et al. 1982, Katz and Koprowski 1968, Kingsbury et al. 1981, McFarlin et al. 1971, Worthington 1972, Worthington and Clark 1971). There is considerable evidence, however, both in sheep and in mice, that host genetic factors and strain variation in the agent are of great importance in susceptibility to and development of natural scrapie infections (Dickinson and Fraser 1977; Dickinson et al. 1974; Gordon 1959; Kimberlin 1979, 1981; Mitchell and Stamp 1983; Nussbaum et al. 1975; Parry 1962; Parry and Oppenheimer 1983).

Diagnosis. At present the diagnosis of scrapie rests largely on the history and clinical signs and on postmortem demonstration of neuronal vacuolation and associated degenerative changes in the brain (Kimberlin 1981, Mitchell and Stamp 1983, Parry and Oppenheimer 1983). Transmission of the disease to mice by inoculation with suspect brain material aids in confirmation of the diagnosis. In general, the clinical diagnosis of scrapie is complicated by variability in the clinical signs manifested by different animals and by breed predisposition and agent strain variation. The clinical features in a given flock, however, tend to be similar and thus become more readily identifiable as time passes.

Treatment. There is no treatment for scrapie, and none should be attempted.

Prevention and Control. The complete eradication of

scrapie from enzootic areas seems impossible in light of the current absence of a sensitive diagnostic test to identify all infected animals (Kimberlin 1981). In several countries, including the United States, Canada, and Iceland, attempts to control the disease through quarantine and depopulation have failed. In Iceland, slaughter of all sheep in areas where maedi-visna and scrapie occurred eliminated maedi-visna but not scrapie (Pálsson 1979). Vigorous attempts at eradication have been made in the United States by slaughtering sheep in affected flocks as well as those in source flocks (Klingsporn et al. 1969). In 1983 the bloodline scrapie program was established to protect certain valuable breeding stock and reduce indemnity expenditures, and it has apparently fostered better reporting of the disease by flock owners (Howard and Pitcher 1985). In certain countries (e.g., Australia and New Zealand) scrapie was successfully eradicated before an enzootic foothold became established after animal health officials quickly recognized the disease and ordered the slaughter of all affected animals (Eklund and Hadlow 1981, Kimberlin 1981).

Despite the general lack of success in eradication, the only practical method of at least controlling the disease in enzootic areas is by instituting some type of slaughter policy (Kimberlin 1981). Slaughter of infected flocks and source flocks is the most effective procedure but is frequently overruled by economic and genetic considerations. Selective culling involving slaughter of bloodline relatives of scrapie cases limits the effects of maternal transmission and reduces the number of genetically susceptible sheep. Less drastic control measures involve culling of the female line and careful husbandry when sheep are kept closely confined (Kimberlin 1981). Because the fetal membranes are very likely an important source of infection (Pattison et al. 1972), the risk of contagion can be reduced by prompt removal of the afterbirth, avoidance of lambing pens, and yearly rotation of lambing areas.

Attempting to eradicate scrapie by identifying sires whose genotype should produce exclusively resistant progeny is both expensive and labor-intensive (Kimberlin 1979, Mitchell and Stamp 1983). Progeny testing is required, and the interval necessary for determination of scrapie status of the progeny is usually from 3 to 5 years. A supply of ewes with predictable susceptibility to scrapie is also required so that test matings of suspected negative rams can be conducted. Sometimes the environmental contamination with the scrapie agent that occurs over the course of the testing program may outweigh any potential benefits accruing from the program itself. If, however, during the course of normal breeding, rams are identified that produce apparently resistant progeny, then their use in future breeding programs should of course be encouraged.

The Disease in Humans. Although many features of kuru and Creutzfeldt-Jakob disease are similar to those of scrapie, these diseases are not believed to be caused by the scrapie agent (Gajdusek 1985). There is no evidence at this time that scrapie is transmissible to human beings; however, certain nonhuman primate species develop a condition resembling Creutzfeldt-Jakob disease following experimental inoculation with the scrapie agent (Gajdusek 1985, Gibbs and Gajdusek 1972).

REFERENCES

Barry, R. A., McKinley, M. P., Bendheim, P. E., Lewis, G. K., DeArmond, S. J., and Prusiner, S. B. 1985. Antibodies to the scrapie protein decorate prion rods. J. Immunol. 135:603–613.

Bendheim, P. E., Barry, R. A., DeArmond, S. J., Stites, D. P., and Prusiner, S. B. 1984. Antibodies to a scrapie prion protein. Nature 310:418–421.

Bendheim, P. E., Bockman, J. M., McKinley, M. P., Kingsbury, D. T., and Prusiner, S. B. 1985. Scrapie and Creutzfeldt-Jakob disease prion proteins share physical properties and antigenic determinants. Proc. Natl. Acad. Sci. USA 82:997–1001.

Bignami, A., and Parry, H. B. 1972a. Electron microscopic studies of the brain of sheep with natural scrapie. I. The fine structure of neuronal vacuolation. Brain 95:319–326.

Bignami, A., and Parry, H. B. 1972b. Electron microscopic studies of the brain of sheep with natural scrapie. II. The small nerve processes in neuronal degeneration. Brain 95:487–494.

Bolton, D. C., McKinley, M. P., and Prusiner, S. B. 1984. Molecular characteristics of the major scrapie prion protein. Biochemistry 23:5898–5906.

Brownlee, A. 1940. Histo-pathological studies of scrapie, an obscure disease of sheep. Vet. J. 96:254–264.

Burger, D., and Hartsough, G. R. 1965. Encephalopathy of mink. II. Experimental and natural transmission. J. Infect. Dis. 115:393–399.

Carp, R. I., Merz, P. A., Kascsak, R. J., Merz, G. S., and Wisniewski, H. M. 1985. Nature of the scrapie agent: Current status of facts and hypotheses. J. Gen. Virol. 66:1357–1368.

Chesebro, B., Race, R., Wehrly, K., Nishio, J., Bloom, M., Lechner, D., Bergstrom, S., Robbins, K., Mayer, L., Keith, J. M., Garon, C., and Haase, A. 1985. Identification of scrapie prion protein-specific mRNA in scrapie-infected and uninfected brain. Nature 315:331–333.

Cho, H. J. 1986. Antibody to scrapie-associated fibril protein identifies a cellular antigen. J. Gen. Virol. 67:243–253.

Clarke, M. C., and Haig, D. A. 1970a. Evidence for the multiplication of scrapie agent in cell culture. Nature 225:100–101.

Clarke, M. C., and Haig, D. A. 1970b. Multiplication of scrapie agent in cell culture. Res. Vet. Sci. 11:500–501.

Clarke, M. C., and Millson, G. C. 1976. Infection of a cell line of mouse L fibroblasts with scrapie agent. Nature 261:144–145.

DeArmond, S. J., McKinley, M. P., Barry, R. A., Braunfeld, M. B., McColloch, J. R., and Prusiner, S. B. 1985. Identification of prion amyloid filaments in scrapie-infected brain. Cell 41:225–235.

Dees, C., German, T.L., Wade, W.F., and Marsh, R.F. 1985a. Characterization of proteins in membrane vesicles from scrapie-infected hamster brain. J. Gen. Virol. 66:851–859.

Dees, C., German, T.L., Wade, W.F., and Marsh, R.F. 1985b. Characterization of lipids in membrane vesicles from scrapie-infected hamster brain. J. Gen. Virol. 66:861–870.

Dees, C., Wade, W.F., German, T.L., and Marsh, R.F. 1985. Inactivation of the scrapie agent by ultraviolet irradiation in the presence of chlorpromazine. J. Gen. Virol. 66:845–849.

Dickinson, A.G., and Fraser, H. 1977. The pathogenesis of scrapie in inbred mice: An assessment of host control and response involving many strains of agent. In V. ter Meulen and M. Katz, eds., Slow Virus Infections of the Central Nervous System. Springer-Verlag, New York. Pp. 3–14.

Dickinson, A.G., and Outram, G. 1979. The scrapie replication-site hypothesis and its implications for pathogenesis. In S.B. Prusiner and W.J. Hadlow, eds., Slow Transmissible Diseases of the Nervous System, vol. 2. Academic Press, New York. Pp. 13–31.

Dickinson, A.G., Stamp, J.T., and Renwick, C.C. 1974. Maternal and lateral transmission of scrapie in sheep. J. Comp. Pathol. 84:19–25.

Dickinson, A.G., Young, G.B., Stamp, J.T., and Renwick, C.C. 1965. An analysis of natural scrapie in Suffolk sheep. Heredity 20:485–503.

Diener, T.O., McKinley, M.P., and Prusiner, S.B. 1982. Viroids and prions. Proc. Natl. Acad. Sci. USA 79:5220–5224.

Diringer, H., Gelderbloom, H., Hilmert, H., Özel, M., Edelbluth, C., and Kimberlin, R.H. 1983. Scrapie infectivity, fibrils and low molecular weight protein. Nature 306:476–478.

Eklund, C.M., and Hadlow, W.J. 1981. Scrapie. In J.H. Steele, ed., CRC Handbook Series in Zoonoses, vol. 2, section B. CRC Press, Boca Raton, Fla. Pp. 344–346.

Eklund, C.M., Kennedy, R.C., and Hadlow, W.J. 1967. Pathogenesis of scrapie virus infection in the mouse. J. Infect. Dis. 117:15–22.

Elleman, C.J. 1984. Attempts to establish the scrapie agent in cell lines. Vet. Res. Comm. 8:309–316.

Fraser, H., and Dickinson, A.G. 1978. Studies of the lymphoreticular system in the pathogenesis of scrapie: The role of spleen and thymus. J. Comp. Pathol. 88:563–573.

Gajdusek, D.C. 1985. Unconventional viruses causing subacute spongiform encephalopathies. In B.N. Fields, ed., Virology. Raven Press, New York. Pp. 1519–1557.

Gajdusek, D.C., and Gibbs, C.J. 1973. Subacute and chronic diseases caused by atypical infections with unconventional viruses in aberrant hosts. Perspect. Virol. 8:279–311.

Gibbons, R.A., and Hunter, G.D. 1967. Nature of the scrapie agent. Nature 215:1041–1043.

Gibbs, C.J., and Gajdusek, D.C. 1972. Transmission of scrapie to the cynomolgus monkey (*Macaca fascicularis*). Nature 236:73–74.

Gordon, W.S. 1959. Scrapie panel. Proc. U.S. Livestock Sanit. Assoc. 63:286–294.

Gresser, I., and Pattison, I.H. 1968. An attempt to modify scrapie in mice by the administration of interferon. J. Gen. Virol. 3:295–297.

Hartsough, G.R., and Burger, D. 1965. Encephalopathy of mink. I. Epizootiologic and clinical observations. J. Infect. Dis. 115:387–392.

Holman, H.H., and Pattison, I.H. 1943. Further evidence on the significance of vacuolated nerve cells in the medulla oblongata of sheep affected with scrapie. J. Comp. Pathol. 53:231–236.

Howard, M.C., and Pitcher, J.R. 1985. Report of the committee on sheep and goats. Proceedings of the U.S. Animal Health Association 89:439–442.

Jubb, K.V.F., Kennedy, P.C., and Palmer, N. 1985. Pathology of Domestic Animals, 3d ed., vol. 1. Academic Press, New York. Pp. 305–307.

Kascsak, R.J., Rubenstein, R., Merz, P.A., Carp, R.I., Wisniewski, H.M., and Diringer, H. 1985. Biochemical differences among scrapie-associated fibrils support the biological diversity of scrapie agents. J. Gen. Virol. 66:1715–1722.

Kasper, K.C., Stites, D.P., Bowman, K.A., Panitch, H., and Prusiner, S.B. 1982. Immunological studies of scrapie infection. J. Neuroimmunol. 3:187–201.

Katz, M., and Koprowski, H. 1968. Failure to demonstrate a relationship between scrapie and production of interferon in mice. Nature 219:639–640.

Kimberlin, R.H. 1979. An assessment of genetical methods in the control of scrapie. Livestock Prod. Sci. 6:233–242.

Kimberlin, R.H. 1981. Scrapie as a model slow virus disease: Problems, progress, and diagnosis. In E. Kurstak and C. Kurstak, eds., Comparative Diagnosis of Viral Diseases, vol 3, part A. Academic Press, New York. Pp. 349–390.

Kimberlin, R.H. 1982. Scrapie agent: Prions or virions? Nature 297:107–108.

Kimberlin, R.H., and Marsh, R.F. 1975. Comparison of scrapie and transmissible mink encephalopathy in hamsters. I. Biochemical studies of brain during development of disease. J. Infect. Dis. 131:97–103.

Kimberlin, R.H., and Walker, C.A. 1986. Pathogenesis of scrapie (strain 263K) in hamsters infected intracerebrally, intraperitoneally or intraocularly. J. Gen. Virol. 67:255 263.

Kingsbury, D.T., Smeltzer, D.A., Gibbs, C.J., and Gajdusek, D.C. 1981. Evidence for normal cell-mediated immunity in scrapie-infected mice. Infect. Immun. 32:1176–1180.

Klingsporn, A.L., Hourrigan, J.L., and McDaniel, H.A. 1969. Scrapie—Eradication and field trial study of the natural disease. J. Am. Vet. Med. Assoc. 155:2172–2177.

Kretzschmar, H.A., Prusiner, S.B., Stowring, L.E., and DeArmond, S.J. 1986. Scrapie prion proteins are synthesized in neurons. Am. J. Pathol. 122:1–5.

Liao, Y.C.J., Lebo, R.V., Clawson, G.A., and Smuckler, E.A. 1986. Human prion protein cDNA: Molecular cloning, chromosomal mapping, and biological implications. Science 233:364–367.

Manuelidis, L., Valley, S., and Manuelidis, E.E. 1985. Specific proteins associated with Creutzfeldt-Jakob disease and scrapie share antigenic and carbohydrate determinants. Proc. Natl. Acad. Sci. USA 82:4263–4267.

Marsh, R.F., and Kimberlin, R.H. 1975. Comparison of scrapie and transmissible mink encephalopathy in hamsters. II. Clinical signs, pathology, and pathogenesis. J. Infect. Dis. 131:104–110.

Marsh, R.F., Castle, B.E., Dees, C., and Wade, W.F. 1984. Equilibrium density gradient centrifugation of the scrapie agent in Nycodenz. J. Gen. Virol. 65:1963–1968.

Marsh, R.F., Semancik, J.S., Medappa, K.C., Hanson, R.P., and Rueckert, R.R. 1974. Scrapie and transmissible mink encephalopathy: Search for infectious nucleic acid. J. Virol. 13:993–996.

McFarlin, D.E., Raff, M.C., Simpson, E., and Nehlsen, S.H. 1971. Scrapie in immunologically deficient mice. Nature 233:336.

Merz, P.A., Rohwer, R.G., Kascsak, R., Wisniewski, H.M., Somerville, R.A., Gibbs, C.J., and Gajdusek, D.C. 1984. Infection-specific particle from the unconventional slow virus diseases. Science 225:437 440.

Merz, P.A., Somerville, R.A., and Wisniewski, H.M. 1982. Comparative ultrastructure of scrapie associated fibrils and CNS amyloid fibrils. J. Neuropathol. Exp. Neurol. 41:359.

Merz, P.A., Somerville, R.A., Wisniewski, H.M., and Iqbal, K. 1981. Abnormal fibrils from scrapie-infected brain. Acta Neuropathol. (Berlin) 54:63–74.

Merz, P.A., Somerville, R.A., Wisniewski, H.M., Manuelidis, L., and Manuelidis, E.E. 1983. Scrapie-associated fibrils in Creutzfeldt-Jakob disease. Nature 306:474–476.

Mitchell, B., and Stamp, J.T. 1983. Scrapie. In W.B. Martin, ed., Diseases of Sheep. Blackwell Scientific Publications, Oxford. Pp. 71–75.

Nussbaum, R.E., Henderson, W.M., Pattison, I.H., Elcock, N.V., and Davies, D.C. 1975. The establishment of sheep flocks of predictable susceptibility to experimental scrapie. Res. Vet. Sci. 18:49–58.

Pálsson, P.A. 1979. Rida (scrapie) in Iceland and its epidemiology. In S.B. Prusiner and W.J. Hadlow, eds., Slow Transmissible Diseases of the Nervous System, vol. 1. Academic Press, New York. Pp. 357–366.

Parry, H.B. 1962. Scrapie: A transmissible and hereditary disease of sheep. Heredity 17:75–105.

Parry, H.B., and Oppenheimer, D.R. 1983. Scrapie Disease in Sheep. Academic Press, New York. 192 pp.

Pattison, I.H., Hoare, M.N., Jebbett, J.N., and Watson, W.A. 1972. Spread of scrapie to sheep and goats by oral dosing with foetal membranes from scrapie-affected sheep. Vet. Rec. 90:465–467.

Prusiner, S.B. 1982. Novel proteinaceous infectious particles cause scrapie. Science 216:136–144.

Prusiner, S.B. 1984a. Prions: Novel infectious pathogens. Adv. Virus Res. 29:1–56.

Prusiner, S.B. 1984b. Some speculations about prions, amyloid, and Alzheimer's disease. N. Engl. J. Med. 310:661–663.

Prusiner, S.B., McKinley, M.P., Bowman, K.A., Bolton, D.C., Bendheim, P.E., Groth, D.F., and Glenner, G.G. 1983. Scrapie prions aggregate to form amyloid-like birefringent rods. Cell 35:349–358.

Rohwer, R.G. 1984a. Virus-like sensitivity of the scrapie agent to heat inactivation. Science 223:600–602.

Rohwer, R.G. 1984b. Scrapie infectious agent is virus-like in size and susceptibility to inactivation. Nature 308:658–662.

Sigurdsson, B. 1954. Rida, a chronic encephalitis of sheep. Br. Vet. J. 110:341–354.

Somerville, R.A., Merz, P.A., and Carp, R.I. 1986. Partial copurification of scrapie-associated fibrils and scrapie infectivity. Intervirology 25:48–55.

Stockman, S. 1913. Scrapie: An obscure disease of sheep. J. Comp. Pathol. 26:317–327.

Worthington, M. 1972. Interferon system in mice infected with the scrapie agent. Infect. Immun. 6:643–645.

Worthington, M., and Clark, R. 1971. Lack of effect of immunosuppression on scrapie infection in mice. J. Gen. Virol. 13:349–351.

Zlotnick, I. 1958. The histopathology of the brain stem of sheep affected with natural scrapie. J. Comp. Pathol. 68:148–166.

Zlotnick, I., and Rennie, J.C. 1958. A comparative study of the incidence of vacuolated neurones in the medulla from apparently healthy sheep of various breeds. J. Comp. Pathol. 68:411–415.

Winter Dysentery

SYNONYMS: Bovine epizootic diarrhea, epizootic enteritis, winter scours, black scours, barn scours; abbreviation, WD

Winter dysentery is an acute, highly contagious gastrointestinal disease of adult stabled cattle that is characterized by a brief, explosive attack of diarrhea or dysentery or both (Blood et al. 1983, Campbell and Cookingham 1978, Hillman 1986, Van Kruiningen et al. 1985). It is epizootic most commonly from November to March in the northern United States and Canada and has also been reported in Europe, Israel, and Australia. In affected herds almost all animals may become ill, but mortality usually is quite low.

Character of the Disease. Following an incubation period of 3 to 7 days, affected animals exhibit a profuse, explosive, projectile diarrhea that is homogeneous, watery, deep brown to greenish black, and sometimes flecked with blood or mucus. A transient febrile response may precede the onset of diarrhea, but in most cases fever and hematological abnormalities are absent once clinical signs of the disease are manifest, and the appetite remains normal. Black or blood-tinged feces frequently have a characteristic offensive odor; some investigators claim to be able to diagnose WD on the basis of the aroma encountered in barns where affected herds are housed (Campbell and Cookingham 1978). The disease spreads rapidly, and within 4 or 5 days nearly all susceptible individuals in the herd are ill. Approximately 5 to 10 percent may develop severe intestinal hemorrhage (dysentery). A mild cough, with or without nasolacrimal discharge, occurs in some animals and may be accompanied by the explosive expulsion of feces. In most individuals a marked reduction in milk yield and a mild loss of body condition are the only consistent additional clinical signs. Animals exhibiting severe dysentery, however, may also develop anorexia, depression, anemia, weakness, and extreme dehydration. The mortality rate in uncomplicated outbreaks usually is less than 1 percent, but milk loss may be severe. Animals that have recently calved seem to be more seriously affected, and their milk production may drop 25 to 95 percent for a few days to a week (Campbell and Cookingham 1978). Although the diarrhea typically lasts from 1 to 4 days, milk production, while tending to increase following recovery, may not return to normal during that lactational year (Fox 1970). Postparturient, young adult cattle are the most severely affected in most WD outbreaks; heifers usually experience a milder disease, and calves less than 4 to 6 months of age are unaffected.

Properties and Cultivation of the Agent. The cause of WD has not been definitively determined. The disease was originally believed to be caused by *Vibrio (Campylobacter) jejuni* (Jones and Little 1931a, 1931b; Jones et al. 1931, 1932), but this has not been proved (see p. 159). Several candidate viruses have been identified in a number of countries, but extensive work in the United States has failed to confirm these findings (Andersen and Scott 1976, Charton et al. 1963, Komarov et al. 1959, Scott et al. 1973, Takahashi et al. 1983). Despite these results, a virus is still considered the most likely cause (Scott et al. 1973, Van Kruiningen et al. 1985).

Epizootiology and Pathogenesis. WD commonly occurs as a localized epizootic, spreading rapidly from farm to farm within a given area, affecting primarily adult stabled dairy cattle (Blood et al. 1983, Campbell and Cookingham 1978, Hillman 1986). In the northern hemisphere, WD is seen almost exclusively during winter. The disease is highly contagious and is apparently transmitted by the fecal-oral route. Abrupt changes in feeding or in the weather have been cited as possible predisposing stress factors (Campbell and Cookingham 1978). Generally, it is unusual for herds to experience another outbreak of WD sooner than 2 or 3 years after the last one (Hillman 1986, Roberts 1957). When they are affected, herds that have encountered WD in the previous year or two have a lower attack rate, with primarily the new young adult cattle involved; herds without a recent history of the disease may have attack rates of between 80 and 100 percent.

The pathogenesis of WD appears to involve a relatively straightforward gastroenteritis that affects the small intestine primarily but also the colon (Campbell and Cookingham 1978, Van Kruiningen et al. 1985). Histopathological changes in the colon include focal degeneration and necrosis of crypt epithelium, which are consistent with the proposed viral etiology (Van Kruiningen et al. 1985). Hemorrhage apparently occurs by petechiation of colonic ridges. It has been suggested that the causative agent is present only before the onset of diarrhea and that this may account for difficulties in recovering it (Van Kruiningen et al. 1985).

Immunity. A moderate immunity of short duration (at least 6 months) is believed to follow natural WD outbreaks (Blood et al. 1983, Hillman 1986). Yearly recurrences of the disease in the same animal are uncommon.

Diagnosis. Occurrence during the winter, explosive onset of the diarrhea, localized distribution of the outbreak, high attack rate, and short duration of disease make a diagnosis of WD quite likely (Hillman 1986).

Treatment. There is no specific therapy for WD. Supportive care is required to replenish lost fluid and electrolytes in severely dehydrated animals, and antibiotics or intestinal sulfonamides may be administered to prevent secondary bacterial infection. In most animals, however, the disease is self-limiting.

Prevention and Control. Owing to the explosive nature of the disease and the current paucity of information regarding its cause, control of WD must rely on strict measures aimed at minimizing the spread of infection on fomites (boots, clothing, feeding utensils, bedding, motor vehicles, farm equipment). Careful disinfection of footware and equipment is an absolute requirement. In outbreaks involving only a small number of animals, isolation of the affected individuals for the duration of illness may help limit the spread of the disease.

There is no effective prophylactic vaccine.

The Disease in Humans. WD is not known to occur in humans.

REFERENCES

Andersen, A.A., and Scott, F.W. 1976. Serological comparison of French WD-42 enterovirus isolate with bovine winter dysentery in New York state. Cornell Vet. 66:232–239.

Blood, D.C., Radostits, O.M., and Hendersen, J.A. 1983. Veterinary Medicine, 6th ed. Baillère Tindall, London. Pp. 674–675.

Campbell, S.G., and Cookingham, C.A. 1978. The enigma of winter dysentery. Cornell Vet. 68:423–441.

Charton, A., Faye, P., Lecoanet, J., Desbrosse, H., and LeLayec, C. 1963. Etude clinique et expérimentale d'une entérite hémorragique hivernale des bovins, associée à la présence, dans le tube digestif, d'un ultra-virus pathogène. Rec. Méd. Vét. 139:897–908.

Fox, F.H. 1970. The esophagus, stomach, intestines, and peritoneum. In W.J. Gibbons, E.J. Catcott, and J.F. Smithcors, eds., Bovine Medicine and Surgery. American Veterinary Publications, Wheaton, Ill. Pp. 417–442.

Hillman, R.B. 1986. Winter dysentery. In J.L. Howard, ed., Current Veterinary Therapy: Food Animal Practice, 2d ed. W.B. Saunders, Philadelphia. Pp. 956–957.

Jones, F.S., and Little, R.B. 1931a. The etiology of infectious diarrhea (winter scours) in cattle. J. Exp. Med. 53:835–843.

Jones, F.S., and Little, R.B. 1931b. Vibrionic enteritis in calves. J. Exp. Med. 53:845–851.

Jones, F.S., Little, R.B., and Orcutt, M. 1932. A continuation of the study of the etiology of infectious diarrhea (winter scours) in cattle. J. Am. Vet. Med. Assoc. 81:610–619.

Jones, F.S., Orcutt, M., and Little, R.B. 1931. Vibrios (*Vibrio jejuni*, n. sp.) associated with intestinal disorders of cows and calves. J. Exp. Med. 53:853–863.

Komarov, A., Goldsmit, L., Kalmar, E., Adler, J.H., and Egyed, M. 1959. Isolation of a viral agent from winter dysentery of cattle. Refuah Vet. (Israel) 16:149–152.

Roberts, S.J. 1957. Winter dysentery in dairy cattle. Cornell Vet. 47:372–388.

Scott, F.W., Kahrs, R.F., Campbell, S.G., and Hillman, R.B. 1973. Etiologic studies on bovine winter dysentery. Bovine Practit. 8:40–43.

Takahashi, E., Akashi, H., and Inaba, Y. 1983. Bovine epizootic diarrhea resembling winter dysentery caused by bovine coronavirus. Jpn. Agric. Res. Q. 17:185–190.

Van Kruiningen, H.J., Hiestand, L., Hill, D.L., Tilton, R.C., and Ryan, R.W. 1985. Winter dysentery in dairy cattle: Recent findings. Compend. Cont. Ed. Pract. Vet. 7:S591–S601.

Kitten Mortality Complex

Kitten mortality complex (KMC) is a general term used to describe a specific cluster of diseases that may or may not be etiologically related. It was first described in the late 1970s, at which time it appeared as a new and apparently discrete disease affecting many catteries and feline breeding colonies throughout the United States (Norsworthy 1979, Scott 1980, Scott et al. 1979). The complex has been divided into two major syndromes: reproductive failure in queens (repeat breeding, fetal resorption, abortion, stillbirths, congenital birth defects) and kitten mortality from acute congestive cardiomyopathy (Figure 58.8), feline infectious peritonitis (FIP), or nonspecific illness (fading kitten syndrome). In addition to these disorders, respiratory disease, recurrent fever spikes, endometritis, and cardiovascular disease have been reported in adults living in affected catteries.

The cause of KMC has not been determined, although a virus is suspected. Early reports and serologic studies suggested the possible involvement of the FIP virus (Norsworthy 1979, Scott 1980, Scott et al. 1979), but the experimental data remain equivocal. Thus although a strain of FIP virus has been isolated from a fading kitten (McKeirnan et al. 1981), subsequent inoculation experiments have failed to reproduce any component of KMC except FIP itself (Pedersen et al. 1984). Animals in most affected catteries have been negative for the presence of feline leukemia virus, and most breeders routinely vaccinate against panleukopenia and the feline respiratory viruses (herpesvirus and calicivirus). The role of stud cats in KMC is unknown.

It is important to remember that reproductive disturbances in domestic species are frequently the result of a combination of factors (Johnston 1983, Noden 1986). Viruses, bacteria, fungi, nutrition, heredity, husbandry, stress, and environmental conditions can all contribute to reproductive disorders. Although it is true that the FIP virus is indeed the cause of some mortality in kittens, it may be that a number of factors, acting either independently or synergistically, are capable of producing the syndrome currently recognized as KMC.

REFERENCES

Johnston, S.D. 1983. Management of pregnancy disorders in the bitch and queen. In R.W. Kirk, ed., Current Veterinary Therapy, vol. 8. W.B. Saunders, Philadelphia. Pp. 952–955.

McKeirnan, A.J., Evermann, J.F., Hargis, A., Miller, L.M., and Ott, R.L. 1981. Isolation of feline coronaviruses from two cats with diverse disease manifestations. Feline Pract. 11(3):16–20.

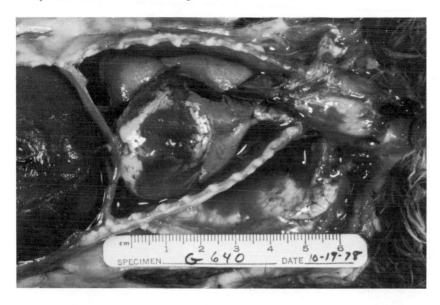

Figure 58.8. Acute congestive cardiomyopathy in a specific pathogen-free kitten. (Courtesy J. E. Post, Cornell University.)

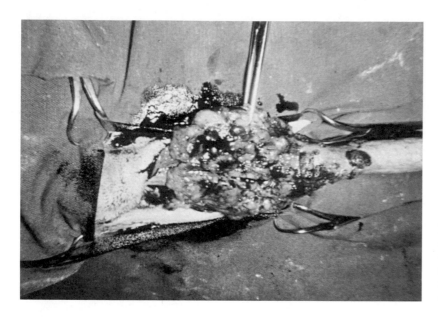

Figure 58.9. Typical fungating appearance of a transmissible venereal tumor at the base of the penis in an adult dog. The development of phimosis necessitated surgical removal. (Courtesy G. H. Theilen, University of California, Davis.)

Noden, D.M. 1986. Normal development and congenital birth defects in the cat. In R.W. Kirk, ed., Current Veterinary Therapy, vol. 9. W.B. Saunders, Philadelphia. Pp. 1248–1257.

Norsworthy, G.D. 1979. Kitten mortality complex. Feline Pract. 9(2):57–60.

Pedersen, N.C., Evermann, J.F., McKeirnan, A.J., and Ott, R.L. 1984. Pathogenicity studies of feline coronavirus isolates 79-1146 and 79-1683. Am. J. Vet. Res. 45:2580–2585.

Scott, F.W. 1980. Kitten mortality complex. In R.W. Kirk, ed., Current Veterinary Therapy, vol. 7. W.B. Saunders, Philadelphia. Pp. 1313–1316.

Scott, F.W., Weiss, R.C., Post, J.E., Gilmartin, J.E., and Hoshino, Y. 1979. Kitten mortality complex (neonatal FIP?). Feline Pract. 9(2):44–56.

Canine Transmissible Venereal Tumor

SYNONYMS: Contagious venereal tumor, venereal granuloma, infectious sarcoma, Sticker venereal sarcoma; abbreviation, TVT

Canine transmissible venereal tumor was the first neoplasm to be transmitted experimentally (Novinsky 1876). Although a viral cause has been suspected, the bulk of the experimental evidence now argues against this; the disease is apparently spread by transfer of neoplastic cells (Barski and Cornefert-Jensen 1966; Calvert 1984; Cohen 1974, 1978; Epstein and Bennett 1974; Makino 1963). Canine TVT has been reported from many areas of the world and is enzootic wherever there are large populations of free-roaming dogs (Calvert 1984, Cohen 1978, Theilen and Madewell 1979). There is no recognized breed or sex predilection. Most cases apparently occur in animals from 1 to 6 years old, the ages of greatest sexual activity.

In male dogs the tumor may be located anywhere on the penis or the mucosa of the prepuce. In females it is frequently found in the vestibule of the vagina and often surrounds the urethral orifice. The tumor appears initially as a group of small hyperemic papules that progress to form lobulated, fungating, sessile masses (Figure 58.9). During the period of rapid growth, the tumor tissue is bright red owing to its extensive vascular supply; later it ulcerates and becomes necrotic. The tumor masses are very friable and frequently ooze a serosanguineous or overtly bloody fluid in which neoplastic cells may be found. Cytologically these cells are histiocytic, with large rounded nuclei and a vacuolated cytoplasm, and they are readily transmitted from dog to dog during coitus. Extragenital tumors in the mouth or nostrils, on the skin, or in the subcutis may arise following direct cell transplantation by licking or biting; true metastases are uncommon. Although spontaneous regression of experimentally induced canine TVT is frequently observed, most natural cases appear to persist (Bennett et al. 1975, Brown et al. 1980, Calvert et al. 1982, Karlson and Mann 1952).

Recurrence of canine TVT following surgical excision is common; therefore, this treatment is best reserved for small, solitary tumors (Brown et al. 1980, Calvert 1984, Calvert et al. 1982). Cures have been reported with orthovoltage radiotherapy, often following a single dose of radiation (Thrall 1982). Cytotoxic chemotherapy has been used with varying degrees of success, although vincristine, either alone or in combination with cyclophosphamide and methotrexate, has been reported to be effective (Brown et al. 1980, Calvert et al. 1982). Doxorubicin has also been successful. Immunotherapy has produced good results (Hess et al. 1977), but autogenous vaccines and extracts of irradiated tumor cells have not been consistently effective (Pandey et al. 1977, Prier and Johnson 1964).

REFERENCES

Barski, G., and Cornefert-Jensen, F. 1966. Cytogenetic study of Sticker venereal sarcoma in European dogs. J. Nat. Cancer Inst. 37:787–797.

Bennett, B.T., Taylor, Y., and Epstein, R. 1975. Segregation of the clinical course of transmissible venereal tumor with DL-A haplotypes in canine families. Transplant. Proc. 7:503–505.

Brown, N.O., Calvert, C., and MacEwen, E.G. 1980. Chemotherapeutic management of transmissible venereal tumors in 30 dogs. J. Am. Vet. Med. Assoc. 176:983–986.

Calvert, C.A. 1984. Canine viral and transmissible neoplasias. In C.E. Greene, ed., Clinical Microbiology and Infectious Diseases of the Dog and Cat. W.B. Saunders, Philadelphia. Pp. 461–478.

Calvert, C.A., Leifer, C.E., and MacEwen, E.G. 1982. Vincristine for treatment of transmissible venereal tumor in the dog. J. Am. Vet. Med. Assoc. 181:163–164.

Cohen, D. 1974. The mechanism of transmission of the transmissible venereal tumour of the dog. Transplantation 17:8–11.

Cohen, D. 1978. The transmissible venereal tumor of the dog—A naturally occurring allograft? Isr. J. Med. Sci. 14:14–19.

Epstein, R.B., and Bennett, B.T. 1974. Histocompatibility typing and course of canine venereal tumors transplanted into unmodified random dogs. Cancer Res. 34:788–793.

Hess, A.D., Catchatourian, R., Zander, A.R., and Epstein, R.B. 1977. Intralesional *Bacillus Calmette-Guerin* immunotherapy of canine venereal tumors. Cancer Res. 37:3990–3994.

Karlson, A.G., and Mann, F.C. 1952. The transmissible venereal tumor of dogs: Observations on forty generations of experimental transfers. Ann. N.Y. Acad. Sci. 54:1197–1213.

Makino, S. 1963. Some epidemiologic aspects of venereal tumors of dogs as revealed by chromosome and DNA studies. Ann. N.Y. Acad. Sci. 108:1106–1122.

Novinsky, M.A. 1876. Zur Frage über die Impfung der krebsigen Geschwulste. Zentralbl. Med. Wissenschr. 14:790–791.

Pandey, S.K., Dhawedkar, R.G., and Patel, M.R. 1977. Canine transmissible venereal sarcoma: Clinical trial with autogenous formolized vaccine. Ind. Vet. J. 54:852–853.

Prier, J.E., and Johnson, J.H. 1964. Malignancy in a canine transmissible venereal tumor. J. Am. Vet. Med. Assoc. 145:1092–1094.

Theilen, G.H., and Madewell, B.R. 1979. Tumors of the skin and subcutaneous tissues. In G.H. Theilen and B.R. Madewell, eds., Veterinary Cancer Medicine. Lea & Febiger, Philadelphia. Pp. 123–191.

Thrall, D.E. 1982. Orthovoltage radiotherapy of canine transmissible venereal tumors. Vet. Radiol. 23:217–219.

Index